Atlas of Neurosurgical Techniques

Brain

Thieme

Atlas of Neurosurgical Techniques

Brain

Laligam N. Sekhar, M.D., F.A.C.S.
Professor and Vice Chairman
Department of Neurological Surgery
University of Washington
Director, Cerebrovascular Surgery
Co-Director, Skull Base Surgery
Harborview Medical Center
Seattle, Washington

Richard G. Fessler, M.D., Ph.D.
John Harper Seeley Professor and Chief
Section of Neurosurgery
Department of Surgery
The University of Chicago Hospitals
Chicago, Illinois

Thieme
New York • Stuttgart

Thieme Medical Publishers, Inc.
333 Seventh Ave.
New York, NY 10001

Editor: Timothy Hiscock
Associate Editor: Birgitta Brandenburg
Assistant Editor: Ivy Ip
Vice President, Production and Electronic Publishing: Anne T. Vinnicombe
Production Editor: Print Matters, Inc.
Sales Director: Ross Lumpkin
Associate Marketing Director: Verena Diem
Chief Financial Officer: Peter van Woerden
President: Brian D. Scanlan
Compositor: Thomson Digital
Printer: Everbest

Library of Congress Cataloging-in-Publication Data

Atlas of neurosurgical techniques. Brain/[edited by] Laligam N. Sekhar, Richard G. Fessler.
p. ; cm.
Includes bibliographical references and index.
ISBN 0-86577-920-1 (US-HC) – ISBN 3-13-127541-3 (GTV-HC)
1. Brain – Surgery – Atlases. 2. Nervous system – Surgery – Atlases. I. Title: Brain.
II. Sekhar. Laligam N. III. Fessler, Richard G.
[DNLM: 1. Brain – surgery – Atlases. 2. Neurosurgical Procedures – methods – Atlases.
WL 17 A8838 2006]
RD594. A75 2006
617.4′8100223 – dc22

2005046723

Important note: Medical knowledge is ever-changing. As new research and clinical experience broaden our knowledge, changes in treatment and drug therapy may be required. The authors and editors of the material herein have consulted sources believed to be reliable in their efforts to provide information that is complete and in accord with the standards accepted at the time of publication. However, in view of the possibility of human error by the authors, editors, or publisher of the work herein or changes in medical knowledge, neither the authors, editors, or publisher, nor any other party who has been involved in the preparation of this work, warrants that the information contained herein is in every respect accurate or complete, and they are not responsible for any errors or omissions or for the results obtained from use of such information. Readers are encouraged to confirm the information contained herein with other sources. For example, readers are advised to check the product information sheet included in the package of each drug they plan to administer to be certain that the information contained in this publication is accurate and that changes have not been made in the recommended dose or in the contraindications for administration. This recommendation is of particular importance in connection with new or infrequently used drugs.

Printed in China

5 4 3 2 1

TMP ISBN 0-86577-920-1
GTV ISBN 3 13 127541 3

Dedication

This book is dedicated to my residents, fellows, and students. Their curiosity and eagerness to learn continues to inspire me. It is also dedicated to my children, Raja, Daniela, and Krishna. They have taught me that the world is constantly changing and it is our responsibility to create happiness and a good future for children all over the world. I dedicate this book to the Universal Force, who continues to guide me, and has rescued me and my patients from some very difficult situations in neurosurgery.

—L. N. S.

Contents

Foreword

Those of us who practice neurological surgery are forever grateful to the surgical educators who are dedicated to publishing descriptions of operative techniques and anatomy that elevate our art and advance our ability to operate upon challenging neurological conditions. The field of neurological surgery is evolving rapidly and requires constant attention to the operative nuances within the craft. Techniques that were once standard are either discarded or metamorphosed to a more sophisticated level. For that reason, many surgeons, like myself, cherish and guard each surgical atlas we purchase because of how much we learn from them. And, years later these editions astoundingly continue to inspire us to do better for our patients.

Professors Sekhar and Fessler have, to no one's surprise, produced an atlas of unparalleled breadth and practical importance. It promises to be a cherished edition for both those just entering our beloved field and those who are at the "top of their game." The publisher has chosen unique and highly respected editors to produce this impressive compilation. Professors Sekhar and Fessler are two of the most splendid examples of creativity and innovation in neurological surgery. Each has advanced his subspecialty by novel and ingenious technical contributions. Their superior psychomotor skills, technical mastery, original perspective, and effective educational style permit them to practice precisely in the manner they educate, write, and illustrate.

The editors carefully and thoughtfully chose other surgical masters and surgical educators in their respective field of expertise to verbally and visually illustrate accepted approaches to these neurological conditions and diseases. These are done in a beautifully written and simply illustrated fashion so that both the novice resident who may assist and the experienced surgeon who will perform the operation can interpret, absorb, and assimilate the material for the next morning's surgical procedure.

This atlas is thoroughly modern, presenting the endovascular, endoscopic, minimally invasive, and stereotactic approaches to neurological disease. The architectural plan of the chapters is in precisely the manner a thorough and diligent neurosurgeon thinks. Each author starts with a bit of history and then progresses to the indications, approaches, alternative approaches, anesthesia, positioning, incision, dissection, closure, and postoperative care. Complication avoidance is dealt with in a real-world, practical, and honest manner. There is barely a wasted word in the text. The sentences and paragraphs are concise yet supported by the latest literature. Each chapter is meticulously devised so that the surgical thought process is crisp, sequential, and transferable to any reader's practice, regardless of his or her sophistication. The tables contain bulletlike information suitable for quickly organizing the reader's perspective on the subject. The figures are accurately drawn and meticulously labeled without the clutter of nonessential detail.

Atlas of Neurosurgical Techniques is an absolutely up-to-date gem, written and edited by a team of neurosurgical masters who present a virtual colloquia of the most common, the most cutting edge, and the complex surgical conditions that face us today. This book will no doubt inspire the next generation of neurological surgeons toward future surgical innovation and advancement, while keeping the current generation well educated.

Richard G. Ellenbogen, M.D., F.A.C.S.
Professor and Chairman
Theodore S. Roberts Endowed Chair
Department of Neurological Surgery
University of Washington
Seattle, Washington

Preface

When I was a resident in neurosurgery at the University of Pittsburgh, I frequently studied Ludwig Kempe's *Operative Neurosurgery*, which was my constant companion and allowed me to learn many operative techniques. Later, I edited two books of my own: *Surgery of Cranial Base Tumors* and *Cranial Microsurgical Techniques and Approaches*. These proved to be extremely popular with residents, fellows, and many neurosurgeons around the world. The success of these books stimulated me and Richard Fessler to collaborate on two multiauthored volumes on cranial and spinal neurosurgery, focusing on neurosurgical operations, indications, techniques, complications, and results. The strength of this volume lies in the fact that almost all current areas of cranial neurosurgery are covered by internationally renowned experts in the field, and they have used the same format to convey the information in a succinct and simple manner. The advantage of a multiauthored text such as this is that readers have access to different viewpoints and styles, although most of the techniques discussed are used by a large number of neurosurgeons and are considered a "treatment standard."

Neurosurgery is a constantly evolving and changing discipline; advances are made every 5 years, and the field changes significantly every 10 years. Yet many basic operative techniques remain the same, and new operative techniques are built on a foundation of existing techniques. Young neurosurgeons, who themselves want to become experts some day, should use this book in conjunction with other modalities of learning, such as preceptorships (residency or fellowship), operative videotapes, practical courses, and educational seminars.

I advise all young neurosurgeons to keep personal records of all operations they perform, including indications, results, and anatomical drawings of the procedure. The surgeon must analyze his personal results every year and try continuously to improve his performance for as long as he remains a neurosurgeon. The acquisition of new knowledge and skills keeps the surgeon constantly challenged and young. Neurosurgery is an art as well as a science, and while there will be differences in the skill level between individual surgeons, every surgeon can improve with constant practice and learning. *Experience* is simply the number of patients one takes care of, whereas *expertise* is achieved by actively learning from each patient. The goal of every neurosurgeon should be to acquire both, but especially the latter.

I believe firmly in the concept of a superior force that can help us in our daily life, through prayer and meditation. Neurosurgeons will be very familiar with the exhilaration they feel when a patient makes a great recovery after a life-threatening illness, but they also will feel the acute depression that follows a major complication in one of their patients, even after a perfectly executed operation. It is advisable to preserve humility and self-critical thinking throughout one's life.

As neurosurgeons, we are blessed to be able to take care of our patients with serious brain or spinal problems. In our practices, we are influenced every day by many external forces: the need to perform more operations in order to keep the practice profitable, the practice of defensive medicine due to the fear of malpractice suits, and other types of pressures from hospital administrators and insurance companies. Every neurosurgeon must develop a personal set of principles and ethics and adhere to them strictly in order to do the right thing for each patient.

—L. N. S.

Acknowledgments

A multiauthored book of this kind is truly a labor of love. For the amount of time spent on creating the chapters, editing them, working on illustrations, and all the other tasks involved in creating the book, the financial rewards are minimal or not existent. The real reward is the feeling of happiness in being able to educate a new generation of neurosurgeons. The many authors who have contributed chapters to this book and have waited patiently for the book to be published truly deserve medals of honor. Some authors accepted assignments to contribute chapters but did not send them for various reasons. Because of this, the editors had to write the chapters themselves or find substitute authors, who completed them on short notice. For this, I am even more grateful. A number of my past fellows and residents have either assisted in the preparation of the chapters, or in other stages, such as checking references and reading proofs. In addition to those who have coauthored chapters with me, I would like to mention Dr. Sabareesh Kumar Natarajan, who has worked for many hours on this book.

A major feature of this book is the illustrations. In addition to the artists used by the authors themselves, Jennifer Pryll and Tony Pazos have worked on a number of illustrations for many chapters and produced drawings of outstanding quality.

Finally, the many people at Thieme who have worked with me, Richard Fessler, and the various authors during the production of this book deserve appreciation. I would like to particularly mention Brian Scanlon, Richard Rothschild, Anne Vinnicombe, Timothy Hiscock, Birgitta Brandenburg, and Ave McCracken, who have produced an outstanding volume which is pleasing to the eye, and have maintained the high standard for which Thieme is known.

—L. N. S.

Contributors

Bizhan Aarabi, M.D.
Associate Professor
Director of Neurotrauma
University of Maryland Medical Center
Baltimore, Maryland

Amal Abou-Hamden, M.B.B.S., B.Med.Sc.(Hons)
Neurosurgery Registrar
Department of Neurosurgery
Royal Adelaide Hospital
South Australia, Australia

Saleem I. Abdulrauf, M.D., F.A.C.S.
Director
Cerebrovascular and Skull Base Surgery Program
Division of Neurological Surgery
Saint Louis University School of Medicine
St. Louis, Missouri

Carlos Acevedo, M.D.
Professor and Chairman
Centro Medico Clinica de Occidente
Cali, Columbia

Ossama Al-Mefty, M.D.
Department of Neurosurgery
University of Arkansas for Medical Sciences
Little Rock, Arkansas

Cargill H. Alleyne Jr, M.D.
Associate Professor
Department of Neurological Surgery
Medical College of Georgia
Augusta, Georgia

James I. Ausman, M.D., Ph.D.
Professor
Department of Neurosurgery
University of California, Los Angeles, Medical Center
Los Angeles, California

Tipu Z. Aziz, M.D., F.R.C.S.
Professor
Nuffield Department of Surgery
University of Oxford
Consultant Neurosurgeon
Department of Neurosurgery
Radcliffe Infirmary
Oxford Radcliffe Hospitals NHS Trust
Oxford, United Kingdom

Roy A. E. Bakay, M.D.
Professor and Vice Chairman
Department of Neurological Surgery
Rush Presbyterian-St. Luke's Medical Research Center
Chicago, Illinois

Jeffrey R. Balzer, M.D.
Associate Professor
Department of Neurological Surgery
University of Pittsburgh Medical Center
Pittsburgh, Pennsylvania

Daniel L. Barrow, M.D.
Professor and Chairman
Department of Neurological Surgery
Emory University School of Medicine
Atlanta, Georgia

H. Hunt Batjer, M.D.
Professor and Chairman
Department of Neurosurgery
Northwestern University Feinberg School of Medicine
Chicago, Illinois

Ghassan K. Bejjani, M.D.
Clinical Assistant Professor
Department of Neurosurgery
University of Pittsburgh Medical Center
Pittsburgh, Pennsylvania

Mitchel S. Berger, M.D.
Professor and Chairman
Department of Neurosurgery
University of California at San Francisco
San Francisco, California

Sumon Bhattacharjee, M.D.
Fellow
Department of Neurosurgery
University of Virginia Medical Center
Charlottesville, Virginia

Karin S. Bierbrauer, M.D.
Associate Professor of Neurosurgery
Cincinnati Children's Hospital Medical Center
Division of Pediatric Neurosurgery
Cincinnati, Ohio

Christopher A. Bogaev, M.D.
Assistant Professor
Division of Neurosurgery
University of Texas Health Science Center at San Antonio
San Antonio, Texas

Francis J. Bova, Ph.D.
University of Florida
Gainesville, Florida

Derald E. Brackmann, M.D.
House Ear Institute
Los Angeles, California

Albino Bricolo, M.D.
Professor and Chairman
Department of Neurosurgery
University Hospital
Verona, Italy

Jacques Brotchi, M.D., Ph.D.
Professor and Chairman
Department of Neurosurgery
Erasme Hospital-Free University of Brussels
Brussels, Belgium

Jeffrey A. Brown, M.D.
Long Island, New York

Jeffrey N. Bruce, M.D.
Professor of Neurological Surgery
Director
Bartoli Brain Tumor Laboratory
Department of Neurological Surgery
Columbia-Presbyterian Medical Center
New York, New York

John M. Buatti, M.D.
Laboratory Profesor and Head
Department of Radiation Oncology
University of Iowa
Iowa City, Iowa

Ketan Bulsara, M.D.
Department of Surgery
Division of Neurosurgery
Duke University
Durham, North Carollina

Dawn Carroll
Pain Research Unit
University of Oxford and Oxford Radcliffe Hospitals NHS Trust
Oxford, United Kingdom

Michael Cawley, M.D.
Assistant Professor
Department of Neurological Surgery
Emory University School of Medicine
Atlanta, Georgia

Feres E. A. Chaddad, M.D.
Neurosurgeon
Instituto de Ciências Neurológicas
São Paulo, Brazil

Amitabha Chanda, M.D.
Calcutta, India

James P. Chandler, M.D.
Associate Professor
Department of Neurological Surgery
Northwestern Memorial Hospital
Chicago, Illinois

Fady T. Charbel, M.D.
Professor and Chairman
Department of Neurosurgery
University of Illinois at Chicago
Chicago, Illinois

Chun Siang Chen, M.D.
Department of Neurosurgery
St. Luke's Roosevelt Hospital Center
New York, New York

Michael R. Chicoine, M.D.
Assistant Professor
Department of Neurological Surgery
Washington University School of Medicine
St. Louis, Missouri

Greg Christoforidis, M.D.
Institute of Neuroradiology
University Hospital of Zurich
Zürich, Switzerland

Harry J. Cloft, M.D., Ph.D.
Professor
Department of Radiological Neurosurgery
Mayo Clinic College of Medicine
Rochester, Minnesota

Fabrizio Cohn, M.D.
Department of Neurosurgery
Hospital de Especialidades
University of Mexico
Mexico City, Mexico

Ernesto Coscarella, M.D.
Research Assistant Professor
Department of Neurosurgery
University of Miami
Miami, Florida

Donald Crammond, M.D.
Assistand Professor
Department of Neurological Surgery
University of Pittsburgh Medical Center
Pittsburgh, Pennsylvania

Kerry Crone, M.D.
Professor of Neurosurgery and Pediatrics
Department of Pediatric Neurosurgery
University of Cincinnati Medical Center
Cincinnati, Ohio

Ralph G. Dacey Jr., M.D.
Professor and Chairman
Department of Neurosurgery
Washington University School of Medicine
St. Louis, Missouri

Chris Danner, M.D.
Department of Head and Neck Surgery
University of California at San Diego
San Diego, California

Carlos A. David, M.D.
Director
Cerebrovascular and Skull Base Surgery
Lahey Clinic Medical Center
Burlington, Massachusetts
Clinical Assistant Professor
Tufts University School of Medicine
Boston, Massachusetts

Arthur L. Day, M.D.
Professor, Associate Chair, and Program Director
Department of Neurovascular Surgery
Harvard Medical School
Brigham and Woman's Hospital
Boston, Massachusetts

Evandro de Oliveira, M.D., Ph.D.
Director
Instituto de Ciências Neurológicas
Professor
Department of Neurological Surgery
University of Campinas
São Paulo, Brazil

Gerard M. Debrun, M.D.
Professor Emeritus
Department of Neurosurgery
University of Illinois at Chicago
Chicago, Illinois

Jacques E. Dion, M.D., F.R.C.P. (C)
Professor
Departments of Radiology and Neurosurgery
Emory University School of Medicine
Atlanta, Georgia

John Dornhoffer, M.D.
Assistant Professor, Director of Residency Program
Department of Otolaryngology
University of Arkansas for Medical Sciences
Little Rock, Arkansas

Colleen B. Duffy, R.N., B.S.N., C.N.R.N.
Department of Neurosurgery
Wayne State University
Detroit, Michigan

Felix Durity, M.D.
Professor Emeritus
Division of Neurosurgery
University of British Columbia
Vancouver, Canada

Kevin M. Dwyer, M.D.
Trauma Services
INOVA Fairfax Hospital
Falls Church, Virginia

Howard M. Eisenberg, M.D.
Chairman
Department of Neurosurgery
University of Maryland Medical Center
Baltimore, Maryland

Foad Elahi, M.D.
Neurosurgery Research Fellow
Department of Neurological Surgery
University of Washington
Seattle, Washington

Fred Epstein, M.D.
Director, INN Foundation
Institute for Neurology and Neurosurgery
Beth Israel Institute for Neurology and Neurosurgery
New YorK, New York

Samir M. Fakhry, M.D.
Trauma Services
INOVA Fairfax Hospital
Falls Church, Virginia

Jose N. Fayad, M.D.
Clinical Studies Department
House Ear Institute
Los Angeles, California

Kelly D. Foote, M.D.
University of Florida
Gainesville, Florida

Allan Friedman, M.D.
Professor
Chief of Neurosurgery
Department of Surgery
Division Of Neurosurgery
Duke Medical Center
Durham, North Carolina

William A. Friedman, M.D.
Professor and Chairman
Department of Neurosurgery
University of Florida
Gainesville, Florida

Mauricio Gallardo, M.D.
Department of Neurosurgery
Hospital de Especialidades
University of Mexico
Mexico City, Mexico

Hani El Garem, M.D.
Assistant Professor
Department of Otorhinolaryngology
University of Alexandria
Alexandria, Egypt

Bernard George, M.D.
Professor
Department of Neurosurgery
Hospital Lariboisiere
Paris, France

Christopher C. Getch, M.D.
Associate Professor
Department of Neurological Surgery
Northwestern University Feinberg School of Medicine
Chicago, Illinois

Fábio L. F. Godinho, M.D.
Neurosurgeon
Instituto de Ciências Neurológicas
São Paulo, Brazil

Keith Y. C. Goh, M.D.
Department of Neurosurgery
Singapore General Hospital
Singapore, Singapore

Gabriel A. Gonzales-Portillo, M.D., F.A.C.S.
Neurological Surgeon
Tampa, Florida

Yannick Grenier, M.D.
Department of Neurological Surgery
Northwestern University Feinberg School of Medicine
Chicago, Illinois

Gerardo Guinto, M.D.
Professor and Chairman
Department of Neurosurgery
Hospital de Especialidades
University of Mexico
Mexico City, Mexico

Kern H. Guppy, M.D., Ph.D.
Department of Neurosurgery
University of Illinois at Chicago
Chicago, Illinois

Murali Guthikonda, M.D.
Professor and Chairman
Department of Neurosurgery
Wayne State University
Detroit, Michigan

Philip H. Gutin, M.D.
Director
Department of Neurosurgery Service
Memorial Sloan Kettering Cancer Center
New York, New York

Lisa L. Guyot, M.D., Ph.D., M.B.A.
Genesys Regional Medical Center
Grand Blanc, Michigan

Miguel E. Habeych, M.D., M.P.H.
Assistant Professor
University of Pittsburgh Medical Center
Pittsburgh, Pennsylvania

Ehab Hanna, M.D.
Professor and Director of Skull Base Surgery
Department of Head and Neck Surgery
University of Texas M. D. Anderson Cancer Center
Houston, Texas

Roberto C. Heros, M.D.
Professor and Co-Chairman
Department of Neurosurgery
University of Miami
Miami, Florida

Brian Holmes, M.D., F.A.C.S.
Neurological Specialists LLC
Hagerstown, Maryland

Kazuhiro Hongo, M.D.
Professor and Chairman
Department of Neurosurgery
Shinshu University School of Medicine
Matsumoto, Japan

Michael Horowitz, M.D.
Associate Professor
Department of Neurological Surgery
University of Pittsburgh Medical Center
Pittsburgh, Pennsylvania

George I. Jallo, M.D.
Assistant Professor
Department of Neurosurgery
Johns Hopkins University
Baltimore, Maryland

Jack Jallo, M.D.
Assistant Professor
Department of Neurosurgery
Temple University
Philadelphia, Pennsylvania

Rashid M. Janjua M.D.
Department of Neurosurgery
University of Louisville
Louisville, Kentucky

Hae-Dong Jho, M.D., Ph.D.
Department of Neurosurgery
Allegheny General Hospital
Pittsburgh, Pennsylvania

Chandrasekar Kalavakonda, M.D.
Neurosurgeon
Appollo Hospital
Chennai, India

Yoko Kato
Professor
Department of Neurosurgery
Fujita Health University
Toyoake, Japan

G. Evren Keles, M.D.
Department of Neurosurgery
University of California at San Francisco
San Francisco, California

Shigeaki Kobayashi, M.D., Ph.D.
Professor Emeritus
Department of Neurosurgery
Komoro Kosei General Hospital
Matsumoto, Japan

Douglas Kondziolka, M.D., M.Sc., F.R.S.C., F.A.C.S.
Peter J. Jannetta Professor and Vice-Chairman
Department of Neurological Surgery
University of Pittsburgh Medical Center
Pittsburgh, Pennsylvania

Thomas Kopitnik, M.D.
Casper, Wyoming

Donald N. Krieger
Associate Research Professor
Department of Neurosurgery
Presbyterian University Hospital
Pitsburg, Pennsylvania

Satish Krishnamurthy, M.D., M.Ch.
Assistant Professor
Department of Neurosurgery
SUNY Upstate Medical University
Syracuse, New York

Ali F. Krisht, M.D.
Professor
Department of Neurosurgery
University of Arkansas for Medical Sciences
Little Rock, Arkansas

Sun-Ho Lee, M.D.
Department of Neurological Surgery
College of Medicine
Seoul National University
Seoul, Korea

Mark Linskey, M.D.
Professor and Chairman
Department of Neurosurgery
University of California, Irvine
Irvine, California

Christopher Loftus, M.D.
Professor and Chairman
Department of Neurosurgery
Temple University Medical Center
Philadelphia, Pennsylvania

L. Dade Lunsford, M.D., F.A.C.S.
Lars Leksell Professor and Chairman
Department of Neurological Surgery
University of Pittsburgh Medical Center
Pittsburgh, Pennsylvania

Nikki Maartens
Department of Neurosurgery
Radcliffe Infirmary
Oxford Radcliffe Hospitals NHS Trust
Oxford, United Kingdom

Jacques Magnan, M.D.
Professor
University Aix Marseille II
Department of Otorhinolaryngology
Hospital Nord
Marseille, France

Gary Magram, M.D.
Clinical Associate Professor
Department of Neurosurgery
George Washington University
INOVA Fairfax Hospital
Falls Church, Virginia

Jonathan E. Martin, M.D.
Resident
Department of Neurosurgery
Walter Reed Army Medical Center (previously)
Washington, D.C.

J. Parker Mickle, M.D.
Professor
Department of Neurosurgery
University of Florida
Gainesville, Florida

Jacques J. Morcos, M.D., F.R.C.S. Eng., F.R.C.S. Ed.
Associate Professor
Department of Neurology and Otolaryngology
University of Miami
Miami, Florida

Akio Morita, M.D.
Associate
Department of Neurosurgery
University of Tokyo
Tokyo, Japan

Dipankar Mukherjee, M.D., P.C., F.A.C.S., V.CERT., R.V.T.
Clinical Associate Professor
Georgetown University School of Medicine
INOVA Fairfax Hospital
Falls Church, Virginia

Antônio C. M. Mussi, M.D.
Department of Neurological Surgery
University of Florida
Gainesville, Florida

Dipankar Nandi, M.D.
Department of Neurosurgery
Radcliffe Infirmary
Oxford Radcliffe Hospitals NHS Trust
Oxford, United Kingdom

Prithvi Narayan, M.D.
Assistant Professor
Department of Neurosurgery
Mount Sinai School of Medicine
New York, New York

Raj K. Narayan, M.D.
Mayfield Professor and Chairman
Department of Neurosurgery
University of Cincinnati College of Medicine
Mayfield Clinic
Cincinnati, Ohio

Sabareesh Kumar Natarajan, M.D., M.S.
Senior Fellow, Cerebrovascular Surgery
Department of Neurological Surgery
University of Washington
Seattle, Washington

Rodrigo F. F. Naufal, M.D.
Neurosurgeon
Instituto de Ciências Neurológicas
São Paulo, Brazil

Michael Olding, M.D., F.A.C.S.
Associate Professor of Surgery
Division of Plastic and Reconstructive Surgery
George Washington University Medical Center
Washington, D.C.

Bert W. O'Malley, M.D.
Chairman
Department of Otorhinolaryngology
Director
PENN Otolyrngology Residency Program
Co-Director
Head and Neck Cancer Center
Hospital of the University of Pennsylvania Health System
Philadelphia, Pennsylvania

Sarah L. F. Owen, B.A.
Department of Neurosurgery
Radcliffe Infirmary
Oxford Radcliffe Hospitals NHS Trust
Oxford, United Kingdom

Robert M. Owens, M.D.
Owens Ear Clinic
Dallas, Texas

Ioannis Panourias
Department of Neurosurgery
Radcliffe Infirmary
Oxford Radcliffe Hospitals NHS Trust
Oxford, United Kingdom

Sunil J. Patel, M.D.
Professor and Chairman
Department of Neurological Surgery
Medical University of South Carolina
Charleston, South Carolina

Ramiro Perez-de la Torre, M.D.
Department of Neurosurgery
Hospital de Especialidades
University of Mexico
Mexico City, Mexico

Richard Peterson, M.D.
Department of Neurology
University of Washington
Seattle, Washington

Daniel Pieper, M.D.
Michigan Head and Spine Institute, PLLC
Southfield, Montana

Fernando C. G. Pinto, M.D.
Neurosurgeon
Instituto de Ciências Neurológicas
São Paulo, Brazil

Benoit Pirotte, M.D.
Associate Professor
Department of Neurosurgery
Erasme Hospital-Free University of Brussels
Brussels, Belgium

Ian F. Pollack, M.D.
Professor
Department of Neurosurgery
University of Pittsburgh
Children's Hospital of Pittsburgh
Pittsburgh, Pennsylvania

Fabrizio R. F. Porro, M.D.
Neurosurgeon
Instituto de Ciências Neurológicas
São Paulo, Brazil

Ramin Rak, M.D.
Resident
University of New Mexico
Albuquerque, New Mexico

H. David Reines, M.D.
Vice Chair
Department of Surgery
INOVA Fairfax Hospital
Falls Church, Virginia

Albert L. Rhoton, M.D.
Professor
Department of Neurological Surgery
University of Florida–Shands Hospital
Gainesville, Florida

Fabio Roberti, M.D.
Chief Resident in Neurosurgery
Department of Neurological Surgery
George Washington University Medical Center
Washington, D.C.

Jack P. Rock, M.D.
Associate Professor
Department of Neurosurgery
Henry Ford Medical Center
Detroit, Michigan

Jack Rootman, M.D.
Professor
Ophthalmology and Pathology
Department of Ophthalmology
University of British Columbia
Eye Care Centre
Vancouver, Canada

Mark L. Rosenblum, M.D.
Professor and Chairman
Department of Neurosurgery
Henry Ford Medical Center
Detroit, Michigan

Robert C. Rostomily, M.D.
Associate Professor
Department of Neurological Surgery
University of Washington School of Medicine
Seattle, Washington

Eric J. Russell, M.D.
Department of Radiology
Northwestern Memorial Hospital
Chicago, Illinois

Duke Samson, M.D.
Professor and Chairman
Department of Neurological Surgery
University of Texas Southwestern Medical Center
Dallas, Texas

Hirotoshi Sano, M.D.
Professor and Chairman
Department of Neurosurgery
Fujita Health University
Toyoake, Japan

Sajjan Sarma, M.D.
Ruby General Hospital
Kolkata, India

Raymond Sawaya, M.D.
Professor and Chairman
Department of Neurosurgery
Baylor Medical College
Houston, Texas

David A. Schessel, M.D., Ph.D.
Associate Professor of Otolaryngology/Neurosurgery
George Washington University Medical Center
Washington, D.C.

Theodore H. Schwartz, M.D.
Assistant Professor
Department of Neurological Surgery
Weill Medical College of Cornell University
New York Presbyterian Hospital
New York, New York

Robert J. Sclabassi, M.D., Ph.D.
Professor
Department of Neurosurgery
Presbyterian University Hospital
Pittsburgh, Pennsylvania

Laligam N. Sekhar, M.D., F.A.C.S.
Professor and Vice Chairman
Department of Neurological Surgery
University of Washington
Director, Cerebrovascular Surgery
Co-Director, Skull Base Surgery
Harborview Medical Center
Seattle, Washington

Chandranath Sen, M.D.
Chairman
Department of Neurosurgery
Co-Director
The Center for Cranial Base Surgery
Department of Neurosurgery
St. Luke's Roosvelt Hospital
New York, New York

Ram Prasad (Robin) Sengupta, M.D.
Regional Neurosciences Center
Newcastle General Hospital
Newcastle upon Tyne, United Kingdom

Scott R. Shepard, M,D.
Clinical Instructor
Division of Neurosurgery
University of Medicine and Dentistry of New Jersey
Robert Wood Johnson Medical School
New Brunswick, New Jersey

Marc Sindou, M.D., D.Sc.
Professor and Chairman
Department of Neurosurgery
Hospital Neurologique P. Wertheimer
University of Lyon
Lyon, France

Michael B. Sisti, M.D.
Department of Neurosurgery
Columbia University College of Physicians and Surgeons
New York, New York

Robert F. Spetzler, M.D.
Director
Barrow Neurological Institute
J.N. Harber Chairman of Neurological Surgery
Phoenix, Arizona
Professor
Section of Neurosurgery
University of Arizona
Tucson, Arizona

Dinko Stimac, M.D., Ph.D.
Assisant Professor
Osijek University
Clinical Hospital Osijek
Osijek, Croatia

Jamal M. Taha, M.D.
Department of Neurosurgery
Wallace-Kettering Neuroscience Institute
Kettering Medical Network
Advanced Neurosurgery, Inc.
Kettering, Ohio

Yuichiro Tanaka, M.D.
Associate Professor
Department of Neurosurgery
Shinshu University School of Medicine
Matsumoto, Japan

Ronald R. Tasker, M,D., F.R.C.S (C.)
Professor Emeritus
University of Toronto
Division of Neurosurgery
Toronto Western Hospital
Toronto, Canada

Helder Tedeschi, M.D.
Neurosurgeon
Instituto de Ciências Neurológicas
São Paulo, Brazil

Anton Valavanis, M.D.
Professor
Department of Neuroradiology
Universitat Hospital Zurich
Zurich, Switzerland

J. J. van Overbeeke, M.D., Ph.D.
Professor of Neurosurgery
St. Elizabeth Hospital Medical Center
Tilburg, The Netherlands

A. Giancarlo Vishteh, M,D.
Director of Neurosurgery
J. C. Lincoln Health Network
Phoenix, Arizona

Hung Tzu Wen, M.D.
Attending Neurologist
Hospital das Clínicas
University of São Paulo
São Paulo, Brazil

Akira Yamamura, M.D.
Professor and Chairman
Department of Neurosurgery
Chiba University School of Medicine
Chiba-shi, Japan

Gregory J. Zipfel, M.D.
Assistant Professor
Department of Neurological Surgery and Neurology
Washington University School of Medicine
St. Louis, Missouri

Ibrahim M. Ziyal, M.D.
Associate Professor
Department of Neurosurgery
University of Ankara
Ankara, Turkey

Section I

Introduction

1

General Principles of and Instrumentation for Cranial Surgery

Albert L. Rhoton Jr.

The introduction of the operating microscope in neurosurgery brought about the greatest improvement in operative techniques that has occurred in the history of the specialty. The microscope has resulted in profound changes in the selection and use of instruments and in the way neurosurgical operations are completed. The advantages provided by the operating microscope in neurosurgery were first demonstrated during the removal of acoustic neuromas.[1] The benefits of magnified stereoscopic vision and intense illumination provided by the microscope were quickly realized in other neurosurgical procedures. The operating microscope is now used for the intradural portion of nearly all operations on the head and spine and for most extradural operations along the spine and skull base, converting almost all of neurosurgery into micro-operative specialty.[2]

Microsurgery has improved the technical performance of many standard neurosurgical procedures (e.g., brain tumor removal, aneurysm obliteration, neurorrhaphy, lumbar and cervical diskectomy) and has opened new dimensions previously unattainable to the neurosurgeon. It has improved operative results by permitting neural and vascular structures to be delineated with greater visual accuracy, deep areas to be reached with less brain retraction and smaller cortical incisions, bleeding points to be coagulated with less damage to adjacent neural structures, nerves distorted by tumor to be preserved with greater frequency, and anastomosis and suture of small vessels and nerves not previously possible. Its use has resulted in smaller wounds, less postoperative neural and vascular damage, better hemostasis, more accurate nerve and vascular repairs, and operations for some previously inoperable lesions. It has introduced a new era in surgical education by permitting the observation and recording, for later study and discussion, of minute operative detail not visible to the naked eye. Some general considerations are reviewed prior to the discussion of instrument selection and operative techniques.

◆ General Considerations

Achieving a satisfactory operative result depends not only on the surgeon's technical skill and dexterity but also on a host of details related to accurate diagnosis and careful operative planning. Essential to this plan is having a patient and family members who are well informed about the operation and understand the side effects and risks. The surgeon's most important ally is a well-informed patient.

Scheduling in the operating room should include information about the side and site of the pathology and the position of the patient so that the instruments and equipment can be positioned properly before the patient arrives (**Fig. 1–1**). Any unusual equipment needs should be listed at the time of scheduling. There are definite advantages to operating rooms dedicated to neurosurgery and to having a team of nursing personnel who know the equipment and procedures for neurosurgical cases.

Before induction, the surgeon and anesthesiologist should reach an understanding regarding the need for steroids, hyperosmotic agents, anticonvulsants, antibiotics, barbiturates, and lumbar and ventricular drainage, and intraoperative evoked potential, electroencephalogram, or other specialized monitoring. Elastic or pneumatic stockings are placed on the patient's lower extremities to prevent venous stagnation and postoperative phlebitis and emboli. A urinary catheter is inserted if the operation is expected to last more than 2 hours. If the patient is positioned so that the operative site is significantly higher than the right atrium, a Doppler monitor is attached to the chest or inserted in the esophagus, and a venous catheter is passed into the right atrium so that venous air emboli may be detected and treated. At least two intravenous lines are established if significant bleeding is likely to occur.

Most intracranial procedures are done with the patient in the supine, three-quarter prone (lateral oblique or park bench), or full prone position, with the surgeon sitting at the head of the table (**Figs. 1–1A–C**). The supine position, with appropriate turning of the patient's head and neck and possibly elevating one shoulder to rotate the upper torso, is

A

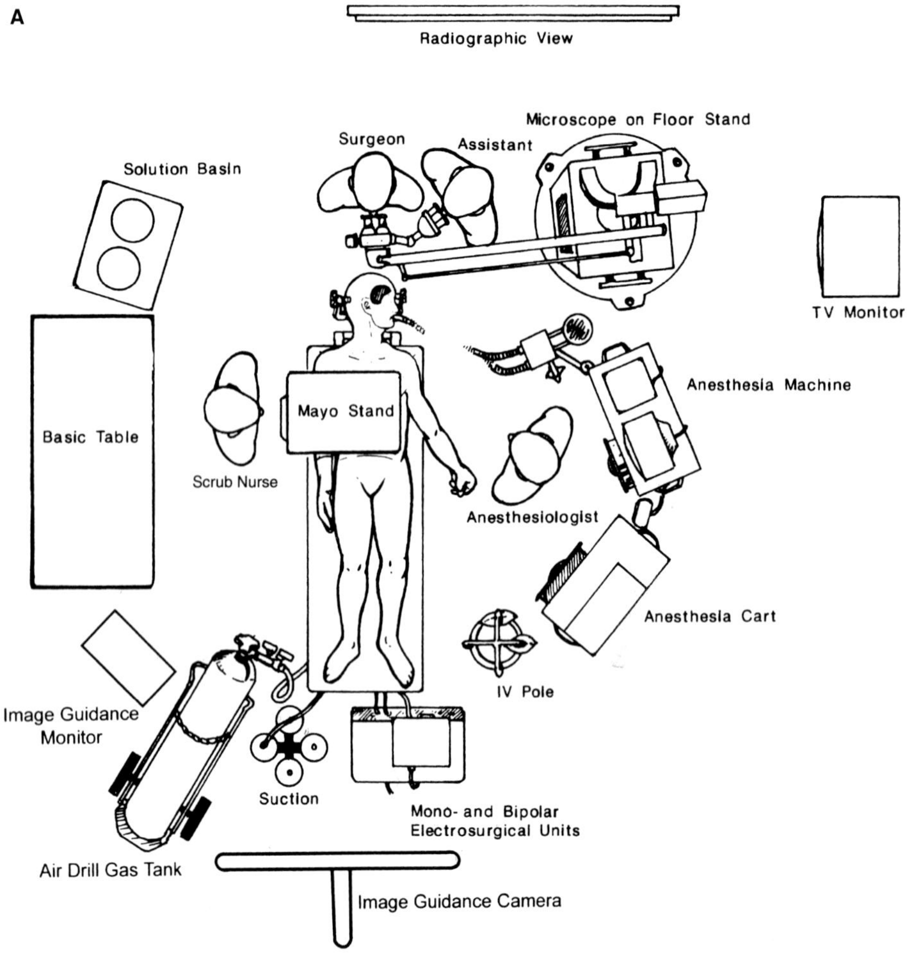

Figure 1–1 Positioning of staff and equipment in the operating room. **(A)** For performing a right frontotemporal craniotomy, the anesthesiologist is positioned on the patient's left side for easy access to the airway, monitors on the chest, and the intravenous and intra-arterial lines. The microscope stand is positioned to the right of the anesthesiologist. The scrub nurse, positioned on the right side of the patient, passes instruments to the surgeon's right hand. The position is reversed for a left frontotemporal craniotomy, placing the anesthesiologist and microscope on the patient's right side and the nurse on the left side. Mayo stands have replaced the large, heavy instrument tables that were positioned above the patient's trunk and restricted access to the patient. The suction, compressed air for the drill, and electrosurgery units are situated at the foot of the patient, and the lines from these units are led up near the Mayo stand so that the nurse can pass them to the surgeon as needed. A television monitor is positioned so that the nurse can anticipate the instrument needs of the surgeon. The infrared image guidance camera is positioned so that the surgeon, assistants, and equipment do not block the camera's view of the markers at the operative site. **(B)** Positioning for a right suboccipital craniotomy directed to the upper part of the posterior fossa, such as a decompression operation for trigeminal neuralgia. The surgeon is seated at the head of the patient. The anesthesiologist and microscope are positioned on the side the patient faces. The anesthesiologist and nurse shift sides for an operation on the left side. **(C)** Positioning for a left suboccipital craniotomy for removal of an acoustic neuroma. The surgeon is seated behind the head of the patient. For removal of a left acoustic tumor, the scrub nurse and Mayo stand may move up to the shaded area, where instruments can be passed to the surgeon's right hand. For right suboccipital operations or for a midline exposure, the position is reversed, with the scrub nurse and Mayo stand positioned above the body of the patient, allowing the nurse to pass instruments to the surgeon's right hand. In each case, the anesthesiologist is positioned on the side toward which the patient faces.

(*Continued on pages 5 and 6*)

B

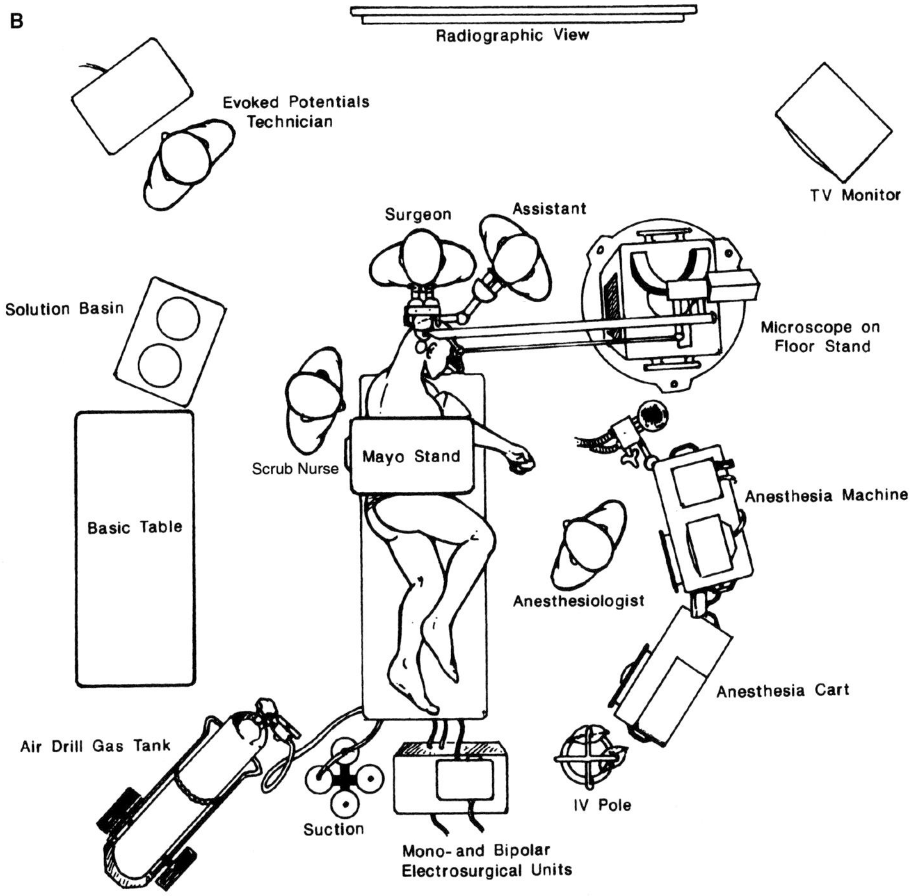

Radiographic View
Evoked Potentials
Technician
TV Monitor
Surgeon
Assistant
Solution Basin
Microscope on
Floor Stand
Mayo Stand
Scrub Nurse
Basic Table
Anesthesia Machine
Anesthesiologist
Anesthesia Cart
Air Drill Gas Tank
IV Pole
Suction
Mono- and Bipolar
Electrosurgical Units

C

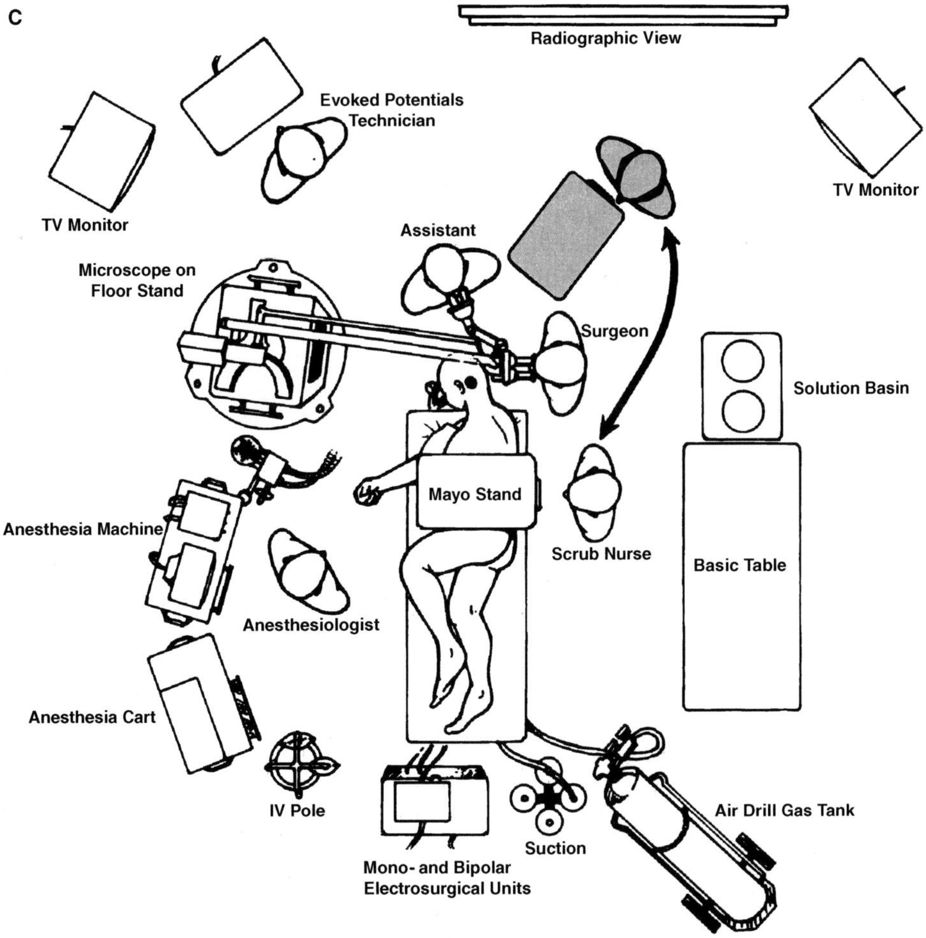

Radiographic View
Evoked Potentials
Technician
TV Monitor
TV Monitor
Assistant
Microscope on
Floor Stand
Surgeon
Solution Basin
Mayo Stand
Anesthesia Machine
Scrub Nurse
Basic Table
Anesthesiologist
Anesthesia Cart
IV Pole
Air Drill Gas Tank
Suction
Mono- and Bipolar
Electrosurgical Units

D

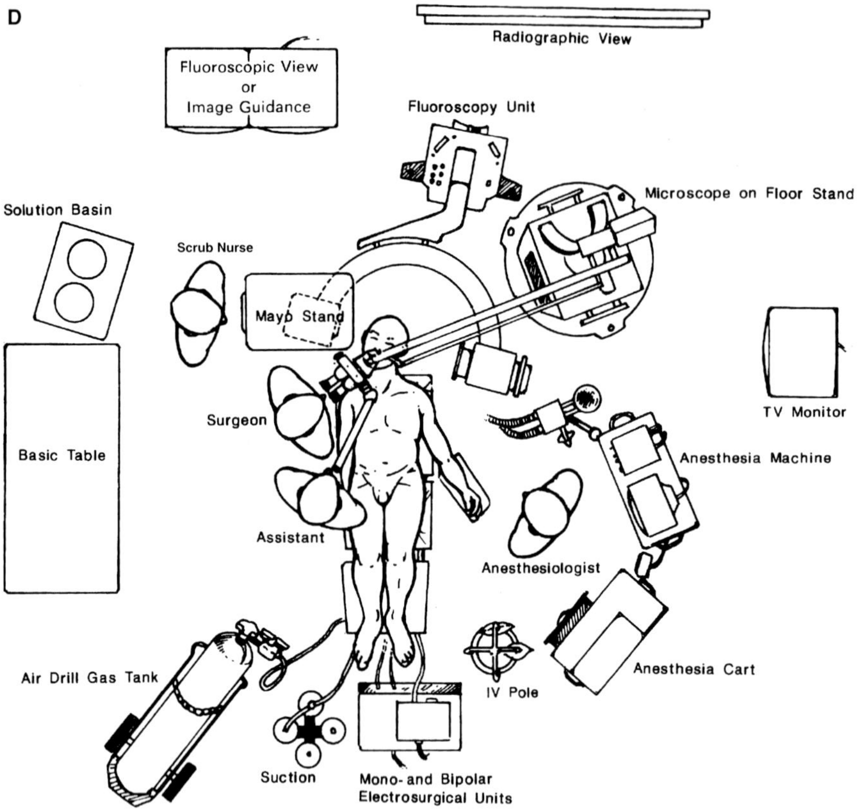

(*Continued*) **Figure 1–1** **(D)** Positioning for transsphenoidal surgery. The surgeon is positioned on the right side of the patient and the anesthesiologist on the left side. The patient's head is rotated slightly to the right and tilted to the left to provide the surgeon with a view directly up the patient's nose. The microscope stand is located just outside the C-arm on the fluoroscopy unit. The scrub nurse and Mayo stand are positioned near the patient's head above one arm of the fluoroscopy unit. The image-guiding camera is positioned so the surgeon does not block its view of the operative site.

selected for procedures in the frontal, temporal, and anterior parietal areas and for many skull base approaches. The three-quarter prone position with the table tilted to elevate the head is used for exposure of the posterior parietal, occipital, and suboccipital areas (**Figs. 1–1B,C** and **1–3A**). Some surgeons still prefer to have the patient in the semisitting position for operations in the posterior fossa and cervical region because the improved venous drainage may reduce bleeding and because cerebrospinal fluid and blood do not collect in the depth of the exposure. Tilting the whole table to elevate the head of the patient in the lateral oblique position also reduces venous engorgement at the operative site. Extreme turning of the head and neck, which may lead to obstruction of venous drainage from the head, should be avoided. Points of pressure or traction on the patient's body should be examined and protected.

Careful positioning of operating room personnel and equipment ensures greater efficiency and effectiveness. The anesthesiologist is positioned near the head and chest on the side toward which the head is turned to provide easy access to the endotracheal tube and the intravenous and intra-arterial lines, rather than at the foot of the patient, where access to support systems is limited (**Fig. 1–1**). If the patient is in the supine or three-quarter prone position, the anesthesiologist is positioned on the side toward which the face is turned, and the surgical technologist is positioned at the other side, with the surgeon seated at the head of the patient (i.e., for a left frontal or frontotemporal approach, the anesthesiologist is positioned on the patient's right side, and the scrub nurse is on the left side).

It is easiest to position the operating team when instruments are placed on Mayo stands that can be moved around the patient. In the past, large, heavy overhead stands with many instruments were positioned above the body of the patient. Mayo stands, which are lighter and more easily moved, allow the scrub nurse and the instruments to be positioned and repositioned at the optimal site to assist the surgeon. They also allow the flexibility required by the more frequent use of intraoperative fluoroscopy, image guidance, and angiography. The control console for drills, suction, and coagulation is usually positioned at the foot of the operating table, and the tubes and lines are led upward to the operative site.

In the past, it was common to shave the whole head for most intracranial operations, but hair removal now commonly extends only 1.5 to 2.0 cm beyond the margin of the incision. Care must be taken to shave and drape a wide enough area to allow extension of the incision if a larger operative field is needed and to allow drains to be led out through stab wounds. Some surgeons currently do not remove hair in preparation for a scalp incision and craniotomy. It may be helpful in supratentorial operations to outline several important landmarks on the scalp prior to applying the drapes. Sites commonly marked include the coronal, sagittal, and lambdoid sutures; the rolandic and sylvian fissures; and the pterion, inion, asterion, and keyhole (**Fig. 1–4**).

Scalp flaps should have a broad base and adequate blood supply (**Fig. 1–2**). A pedicle that is narrower than the width of the flap may result in the flap edges becoming

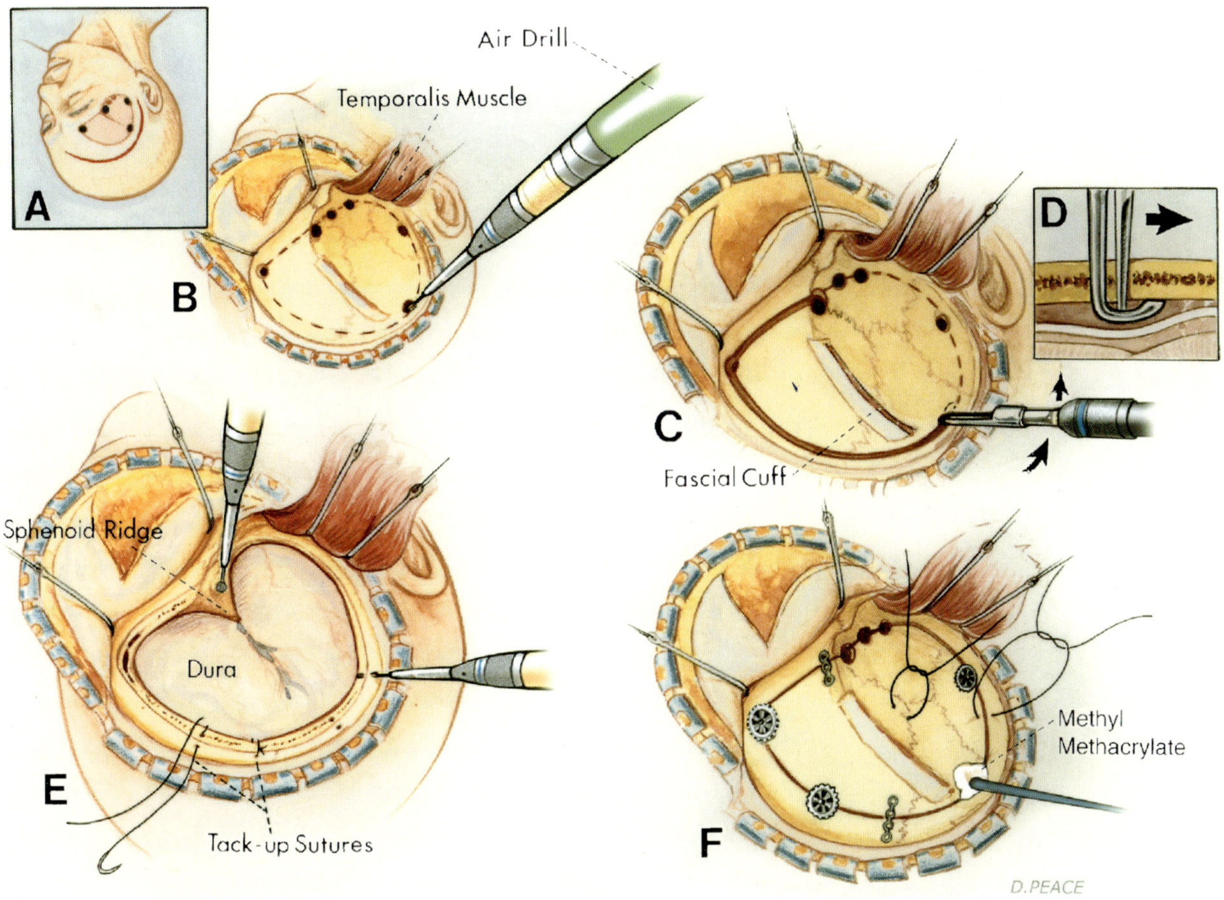

Figure 1–2 Technique of craniotomy using a high-speed air or electric drill. **(A)** Right frontotemporal scalp and free bone flaps are outlined. **(B)** The scalp flap has been reflected forward and the temporalis muscle downward. Elevating the temporalis muscle with careful subperiosteal dissection using a periosteal elevator, rather than the cutting Bovie, aids in preserving the muscle's nerve and vascular supply, which course in the periosteal attachments of the muscle to the bone. The high-speed drill prepares bur holes along the margin of the bone flap (dashed line). **(C)** A narrow tool with a foot plate to protect the dura connects the holes. **(D)** Cross-sectional view of the cutting tool to show how the foot plate strips the dura away from the bone. **(E)** The high-speed drill removes the lateral part of the sphenoid ridge. A drill bit makes holes in the bone edge for tack-up sutures to hold the dura against the bony margin. **(F)** After completion of the intradural part of the operation, the bone flap is held in place with plates and screws, or bur hole covers that align the inner and outer tables of the bone flap and adjacent skull. Silk sutures brought through drill holes in the margin of the bone flap may be used but do not prevent the degree of inward settling of the bone flap that is achieved with plating. Some methylmethacrylate may be molded into some bur holes or other openings in the bone to give a firm cosmetic closure. (With permission from Rhoton AL Jr. Operative techniques and instrumentation for neurosurgery. Neurosurgery 2003;53:907–934.[2])

gangrenous. An effort is made to make scalp incisions behind the hair line and not on the exposed part of the forehead. A bicoronal incision situated behind the hair line is preferred to extending an incision low on the forehead for a unilateral frontal craniotomy. An attempt is made to avoid the branch of the facial nerve that passes across the zygoma to reach the frontalis muscle. Incisions reaching the zygoma more than 1.5 cm anterior to the ear commonly interrupt this nerve unless the layers of the scalp in which it courses are protected.[3] The superficial temporal and occipital arteries should be preserved if there is the possibility that they will be needed for an extracranial to intracranial arterial anastomosis.

In elevating a scalp flap, the pressure of the surgeon's and assistant's fingers against the skin on each side of the incision is usually sufficient to control bleeding until hemostatic clips or clamps are applied. The skin is usually incised with a sharp blade, but the deeper fascial and muscle layers may be incised with cutting Bovie electrocautery. The ground plate on the electrocutting unit should have a broad base of contact to prevent the skin at the ground plate from being burned. Achieving a satisfactory cosmetic result with a supratentorial craniotomy often depends on preservation of the bulk and viability of the temporalis muscle. This is best achieved by avoiding use of the cutting Bovie in elevating the muscle from the bone. Both the vascular and nerve supply of the temporalis muscle course tightly along the fascial attachments of the muscle to the bone where they could easily be damaged by a hot cutting instrument.[3] Optimal preservation of the muscle's bulk is best achieved by separation of the muscle from the bone using accurate dissection with a sharp periosteal elevator.

Bipolar coagulation is routinely used to control bleeding from the scalp margins, on the dura, and at intracranial sites.

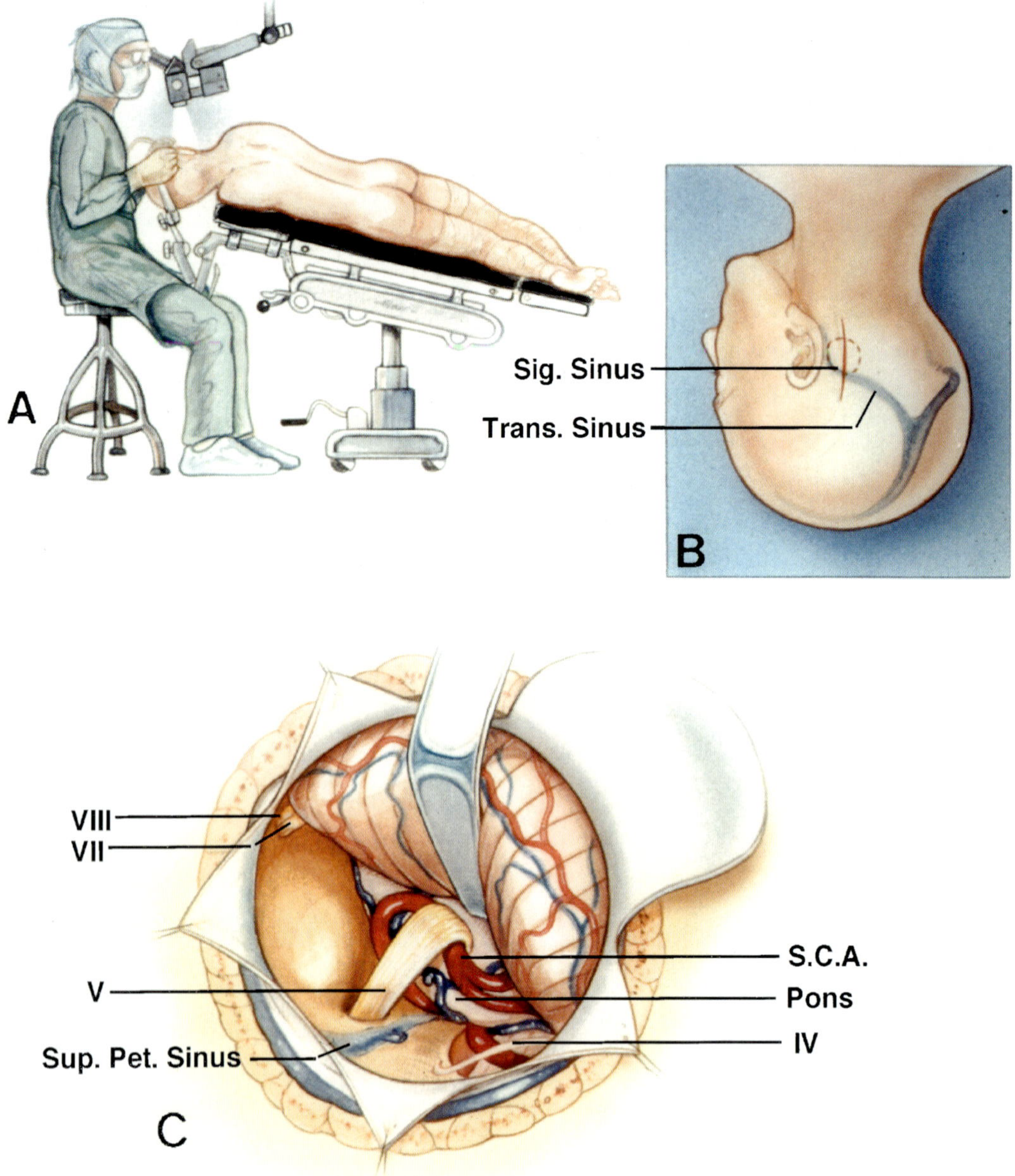

Figure 1–3 Retrosigmoid approach to the trigeminal nerve for a decompression operation. **(A)** The patient is positioned in the three-quarter prone position. The surgeon is at the head of the table. The patient's head is fixed in a pinion head holder. The table is tilted to elevate the head. **(B)** The vertical paramedian suboccipital incision crosses the asterion. A small craniotomy flap, rather than a craniectomy, is utilized for approaches to the cerebellopontine angle. The superolateral margin of the craniotomy is positioned at the lower edge junction of the transverse and sigmoid sinuses. **(C)** The superolateral margin of the cerebellum is gently elevated using a tapered brain spatula to expose the site at which the superior cerebellar artery loops down into the axilla of the trigeminal nerve. The brain spatula is advanced parallel to the superior petrosal sinus. The trochlear, facial, and vestibulocochlear nerves are in the exposure. The dura along the lateral margin of the exposure is tacked up to the adjacent muscles to maximize the exposure. The bone flap is held in place with magnetic resonance imaging–compatible plates at the end of the procedure. (With permission from Rhoton AL Jr. Microsurgical anatomy of decompression operations on the trigeminal nerve. In: Rovit RL, ed. Trigeminal Neuralgia. Baltimore: Williams & Wilkins; 1990:165–200.)

At sites where even gentle bipolar coagulation could result in neural damage, such as around the facial or optic nerves, an attempt is made to control bleeding with a gently applied hemostatic gelatinous sponge (Surgifoam, Ethicon, Inc., New Brunswick, NJ). Alternatives to gelatinous sponge include oxidized regenerated cellulose (Surgicel, Ethicon, Inc., New Brunswick, NJ), oxidized cellulose or a microfibrillar collagen hemostat (Avitene, Bard, Inc., Murray Hill, NJ). Venous bleeding can often be controlled with the light application of gelatinous sponge. Metallic clips, often used on the dura and vessels in the past, are now applied infrequently except on the neck of an aneurysm because they interfere with the quality of the computed tomography scan. If used, they should be composed of nonmagnetic alloys or titanium.

Elevation of bone flaps, using a series of bur holes made with a manual or motor-driven trephine, that are connected

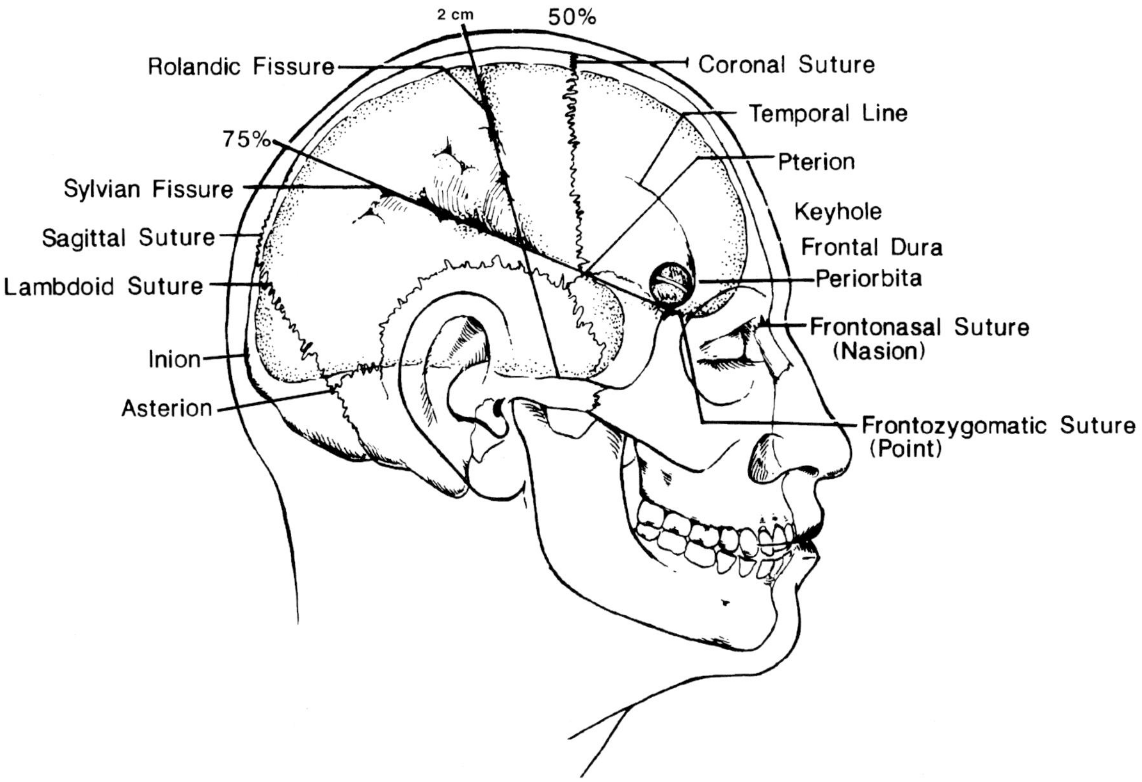

Figure 1–4 Sites commonly marked on the scalp before applying the drapes include the coronal, sagittal, and lambdoid sutures; the rolandic and sylvian fissures; and the pterion, inion, asterion, and keyhole. Approximating the site of the sylvian and rolandic fissures on the scalp begins by noting the position of the nasion, inion, and frontozygomatic point. The nasion is located in the midline at the junction of the nasal and frontal bones. The inion is the site of a bony prominence that overlies the torcula. The frontozygomatic point is located on the orbital rim 2.5 cm above the level where the upper edge of the zygomatic arch joins the orbital rim and just below the junction of the lateral and superior margins of the orbital rim. The next steps are to construct a line along the sagittal suture and, using a flexible measuring tape, to determine the distance along this line from the nasion to the inion and mark the midpoint and three-quarter points (50 and 75% points). The sylvian fissure is located along a line that extends backward from the frontozygomatic point across the lateral surface of the head to the three-quarter point. The pterion, the site on the temple approximating the lateral end of the sphenoid ridge, is located 3 cm behind the frontozygomatic point on the sylvian fissure line. The rolandic fissure is located by identifying the upper and lower rolandic points. The upper rolandic point is located 2 cm behind the midpoint (50% plus 2 cm point) on the nasion to inion midsagittal line. The lower rolandic point is located where a line extending from the midpoint of the upper margin of the zygomatic arch to the upper rolandic point crosses the line defining the sylvian fissure. A line connecting the upper and lower rolandic points approximates the rolandic fissure. The lower rolandic point is located ~2.5 cm behind the pterion on the sylvian fissure line. Another important point is the keyhole, the site of a bur hole, which if properly placed, has the frontal dura in the depths of its upper half and the periorbita in its lower half. It is ~3 cm anterior to the pterion, just above the lateral end of the superior orbital rim and under the most anterior point of attachment of the temporalis muscle and fascia to the temporal line. (With permission from Rhoton AL Jr. The cerebrum. Neurosurgery 2002;51(Suppl 4): S11–S51.)

with a Gigli's wire saw, has given way to the use of high-speed drills for making bur holes and cutting the margin of a bone flap (**Fig. 1–2**). Commonly, a hole is prepared using a cutting bur on a high-speed drill, and a tool with a foot plate to protect the dura cuts around the margins of the flap. Extremely long bone cuts should be avoided, especially if they extend across an internal bony prominence such as the pterion or across a major venous sinus. The risk of tearing the dura or injuring the brain is reduced by drilling several holes and making shorter cuts. A hole is placed on each side of a venous sinus, and the dura is carefully stripped from the bone, after which the bone cut is completed rather than cutting the bone above the sinus as a part of a long cut around the whole margin of the flap. Bleeding from bone edges is stopped by the application of bone wax. Bone wax is also used to close small openings into the mastoid air cells and other sinuses, but larger openings in the sinuses are closed with other materials, such as fat, muscle, or a pericranial graft, sometimes used in conjunction with a thin plate of methylmethacrylate or other bone substitute.

After elevating the bone flap, it is common practice to tack the dura up to the bony margin with a few 3–0 black silk sutures brought through the dura and then through small drill holes in the margin of the cranial opening (**Fig. 1–2**). If the bone flap is large, the dura is also "snugged up" to the intracranial side of the bone flap with the use of a suture brought through drill holes in the central part of the flap. Care is taken to avoid placing drill holes for tack-up sutures that might extend into the frontal sinus or mastoid air cells. Tack-up sutures are more commonly used for dura over the cerebral hemispheres than over the cerebellum. If the brain is pressed tightly against the dura, the tack-up sutures are placed after dealing with the intradural pathology when the brain is relaxed and the sutures can be placed with direct vision of the deep surface of the dura. Tack-up sutures can also be led through adjacent muscles or pericranium rather than a hole in the margin of the bone flap.

In the past, there was a tendency for bone flaps to be elevated and replaced over the cerebral hemispheres and for exposures in the suboccipital region to be done as craniectomies without replacement of the bone. Laterally placed suboccipital exposures are now commonly done as craniotomies with replacement of the bone flaps. Midline suboccipital operations are more commonly done as craniectomies, especially if decompression at the foramen magnum is needed, because this area is protected by a greater thickness of overlying muscles.

Bone flaps are usually held in place with nonmagnetic plates and screws or small metal disks or bur hole covers that compress and align the inner and outer table of the bone flap and the adjacent skull (**Fig. 1–2F**). Remaining defects in the bone are commonly covered with metal disks or filled with methylmethacrylate that is allowed to harden in place before the scalp is closed.

The dura is closed with 3–0 silk interrupted or running sutures. Small bits of fat or muscle may be sutured over small openings caused by shrinkage of the dura. Larger dural defects are closed with pericranium or temporalis fascia taken from the operative site or with sterilized cadaveric dura or fascia lata, or other approved dural substitutes. The deep muscles and fascia are commonly closed with 1–0, the temporalis muscle and fascia with 2–0, and the galea with 3–0 synthetic absorbable suture. The scalp is usually closed with metallic staples, except at sites where some 3–0 or 5–0 nylon reinforcing sutures may be needed. Skin staples are associated with less tissue reaction than other forms of closure with sutures.

Head Fixation Devices

Precise maintenance of the firmly fixed cranium in the optimal position greatly facilitates the operative exposure (**Figs. 1–5, 1–6**). Fixation is best achieved by a pinion head

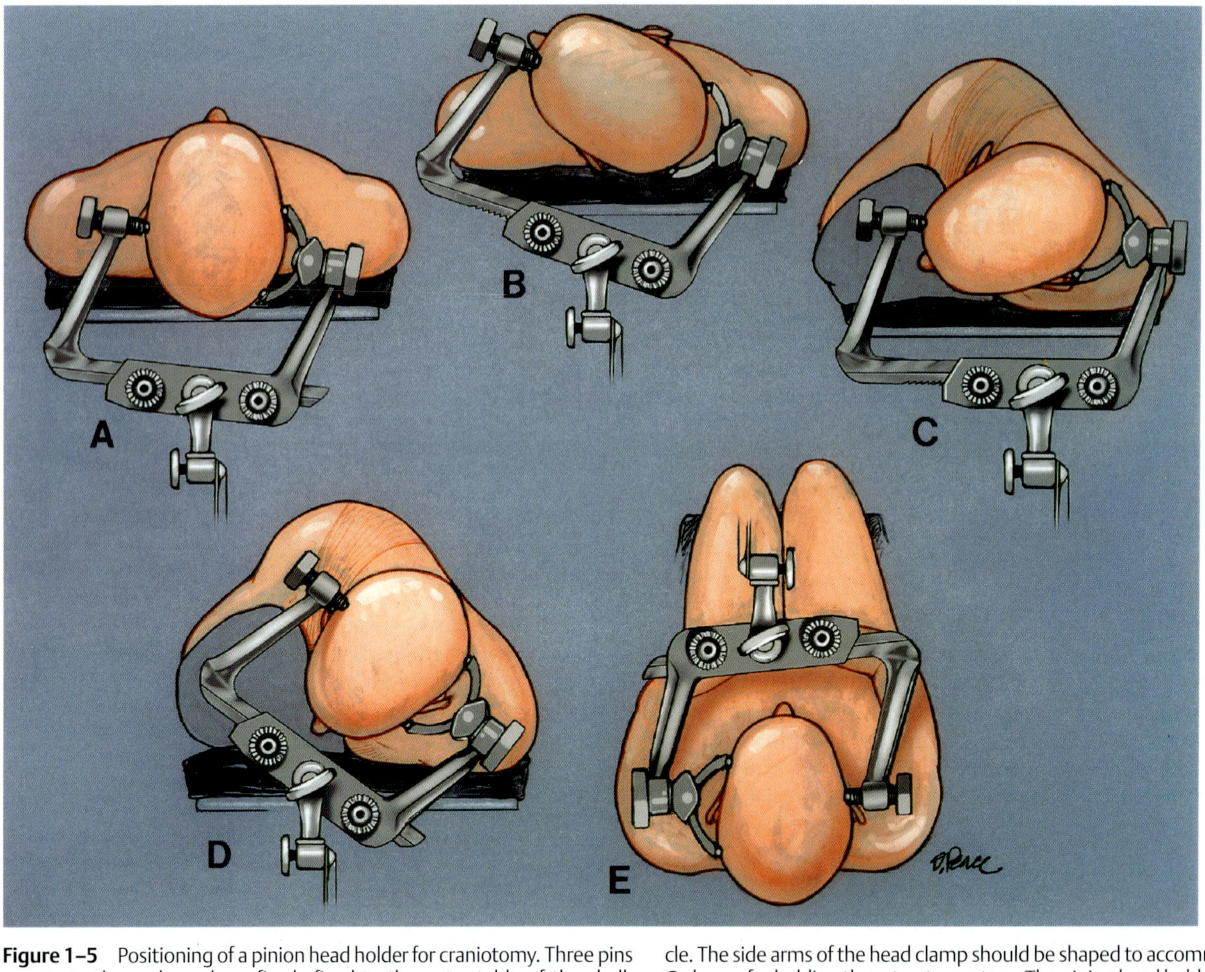

Figure 1–5 Positioning of a pinion head holder for craniotomy. Three pins penetrate the scalp and are firmly fixed to the outer table of the skull. **(A)** Position of the head holder for a unilateral or bilateral frontal approach. **(B)** Position for a pterional or frontotemporal craniotomy. **(C)** Position for retrosigmoid approach to the cerebellopontine angle. **(D)** Position for a midline suboccipital approach. **(E)** Position for a midline suboccipital approach with the patient in the semisitting position. The pins are positioned to avoid the thin bone over the frontal sinus or mastoid air cells and the temporalis muscle. The side arms of the head clamp should be shaped to accommodate the C-clamps for holding the retractor system. The pinion head holder has a bolt that resembles a sunburst for attaching it to the surgical table. Placing three sunburst sites on the head clamp, rather than only one, allows greater flexibility in attaching the head clamp to the surgical table and provides extra sites for the attachment of retractor systems and instruments for instrument guidance. (With permission from Rhoton AL Jr. Operative techniques and instrumentation for neurosurgery. Neurosurgery 2003;53:907–934.)

holder in which the essential element is a clamp made to accommodate three relatively sharp pins. When the pins are placed, care should be taken to avoid a spinal fluid shunt, thin bones such as overlie the frontal and mastoid sinuses, and the thick temporalis muscle, where the clamp, however tightly applied, tends to remain unstable. The pins should be applied well away from the eye or where they would be a hindrance to making the incision. Special shorter pediatric pins are available for thin skulls. The pins should not be placed over the thin skulls of some patients with a history of hydrocephalus. After the clamp is secured on the head, the final positioning is done, and the head holder is fixed to the operating table.

This type of immobilization allows intraoperative repositioning of the head. The clamp avoids the skin damage that may occur if the face rests against a padded head support for several hours. The skull clamps do not obscure the face during the operation as do padded headrests, facilitating intraoperative electromyographic monitoring of the facial muscles and monitoring of auditory or somatosensory evoked potentials. Until recently, all the head clamps were constructed of radiopaque metals, but the increasing use of intraoperative fluoroscopy and angiography has prompted the development of head holders constructed of radiolucent materials. The pinion head clamp commonly serves as the site of attachment of the brain retractor system. The side

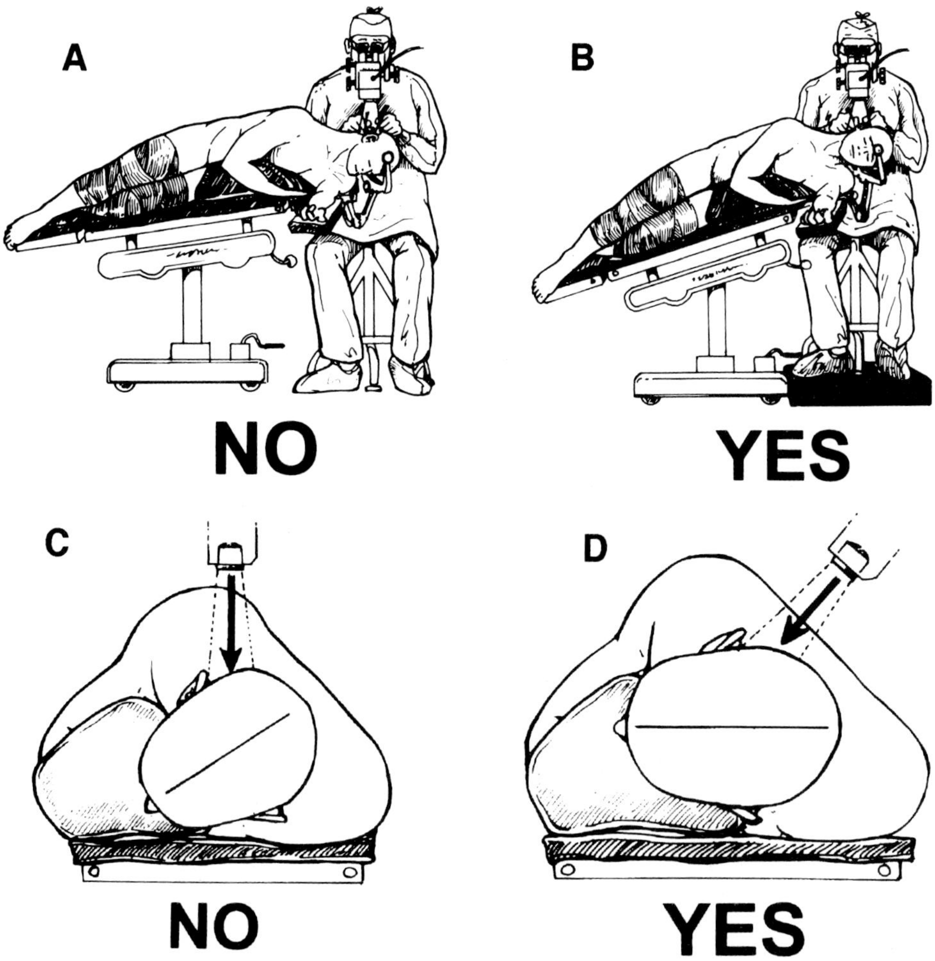

Figure 1–6 Positioning patients for acoustic neuroma removal and decompression for hemifacial spasm. **(A)** and **(B)** Elevation of the head of the table. **(A)** In our initial use of the three-quarter prone position, the head of the operating table was tilted to elevate the head only slightly, but it was later found that **(B)** more marked tilting of the table significantly elevated the head and reduced the venous distension and intracranial pressure. The author usually does operations for acoustic neuromas and hemifacial spasm sitting on a stool positioned behind the head of the patient. In recent years, we have tilted the table to elevate the head to a degree that the surgeon's stool must be placed on a platform. The patient should be positioned on the side of the table nearest the surgeon. **(C)** and **(D)** Rotation of the head. **(C)** There is a tendency to rotate the face toward the floor for acoustic neuroma removal. **(D)** However, better operative access is obtained if the sagittal suture is placed parallel to the floor. Rotating the face toward the floor as in **(C)** places the direction of view through the operating microscope forward toward the shoulder, thus blocking or reducing the operative angle. Positioning the head so that the sagittal suture is parallel to the floor as in **(D)** allows the direction of view of the operating microscope to be rotated away from the shoulder and provides easier and wider access to the operative field. The position shown in **(D)** is also used for decompression operations for hemifacial spasm. The position shown in **(C)** is used for decompression operations for trigeminal neuralgia, in which the surgeon is seated at the top of the patient's head as shown in **Fig. 1–3A** rather than behind the patient's head as shown in **(B).**

(Continued on page 12)

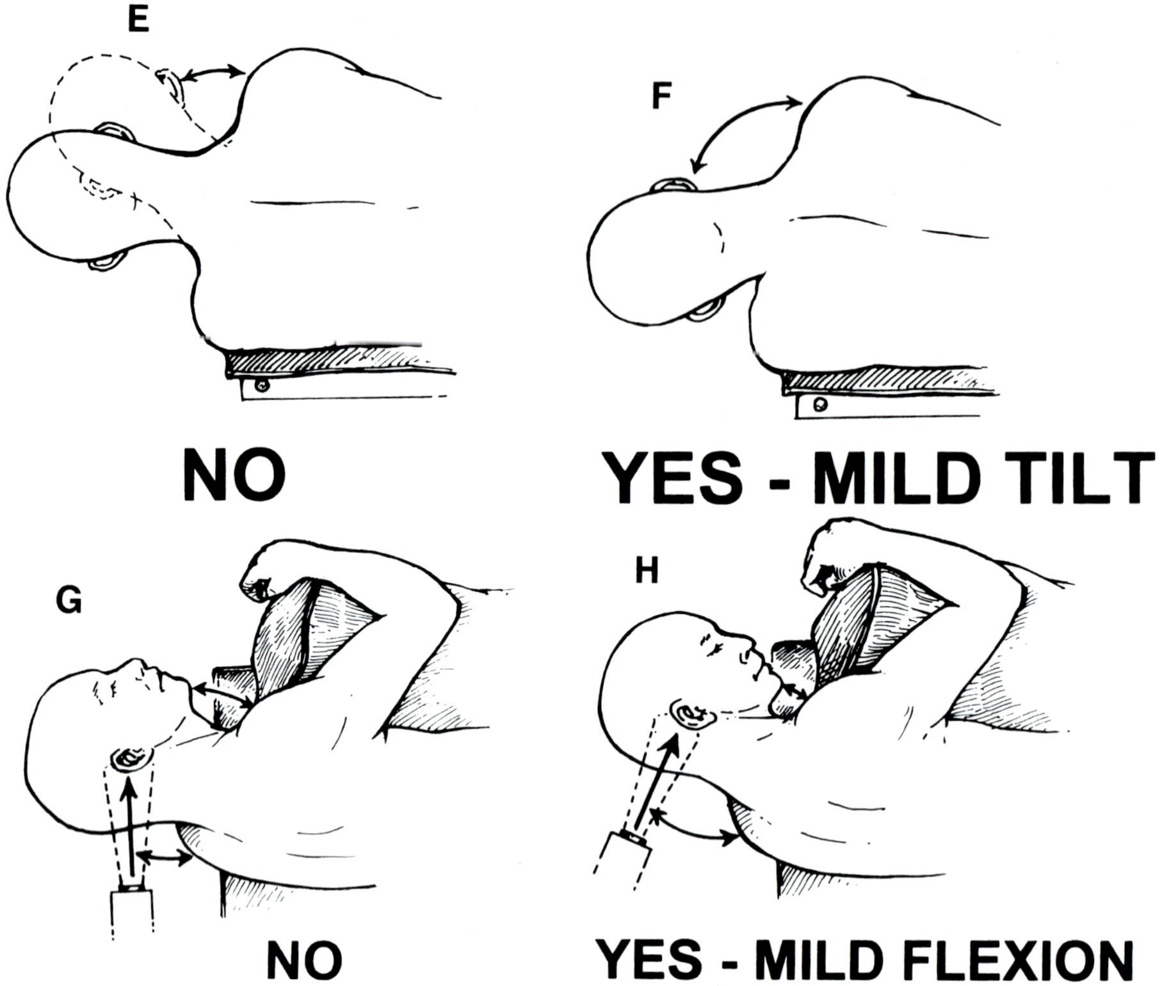

(*Continued*) **Figure 1–6** **(E)** Rather than tilting the head toward the ipsilateral shoulder, it is better to **(F)** tilt the head gently toward the contralateral shoulder. Tilting the vertex toward the floor with the sagittal suture parallel to the floor aids in opening the angle between the shoulder and head and increases operative access. **(G)** Extending the neck tends to shift the operative site toward the prominence of the shoulder and upper chest, whereas **(H)** gentle flexion opens the angle between the upper chest and operative site and broadens the range of access to the operative site. (With permission from Rhoton AL Jr. Operative techniques and instrumentation for neurosurgery. Neurosurgery 2003;53: 907–934.[2])

arms of the head clamp should be shaped to accommodate the C-clamps for holding the retractor system. The pinion head holder has a bolt that resembles a sunburst for attaching it to the surgical table. Placing three sunburst sites on the head clamp, rather than only one, allows greater flexibility in attaching the head clamp to the surgical table and provides extra sites for the attachment of retractor systems and components of the image guidance system.

◆ Instrument Selection

Optimizing operative results requires the careful selection of instruments for the macrosurgical portion of the operation done with the naked eye and the microsurgical part done with the eye aided by the operating microscope.[4,5] In the past, surgeons commonly used one set of instruments for performing conventional macrosurgery with the naked eye and another set with different handles and smaller tips for microsurgery done with the eye aided by the microscope. A trend is to select instruments having uniform handles and tactile characteristics for macrosurgery and microsurgery and to change only the size of the tip of the instrument, depending on whether the use is to be macro- or microsurgical. For example, forceps for macrosurgery have grasping tips as large as 2 to 3 mm, and those for microsurgery commonly have tips measuring 0.3 to 1.0 mm.

If possible, the instruments should be held in a pencil grip between the thumb and the index finger rather than in a pistol grip with the whole hand (**Fig. 1–7**). The pencil grip permits the instruments to be positioned by delicate movements of the fingers, but the pistol grip requires that the instruments be manipulated with the coarser movements of the wrist, elbow, and shoulder.

The author prefers round-handled forceps, scissors, and needle holders because they allow finer movement. It is possible to rotate these instruments between the thumb and forefinger rather than having to rotate the entire wrist (**Fig. 1–8**). The author first used round-handled needle holders and scissors in performing superficial temporal to middle cerebral artery anastomosis and later found that the advantage of being able to rotate the instrument between

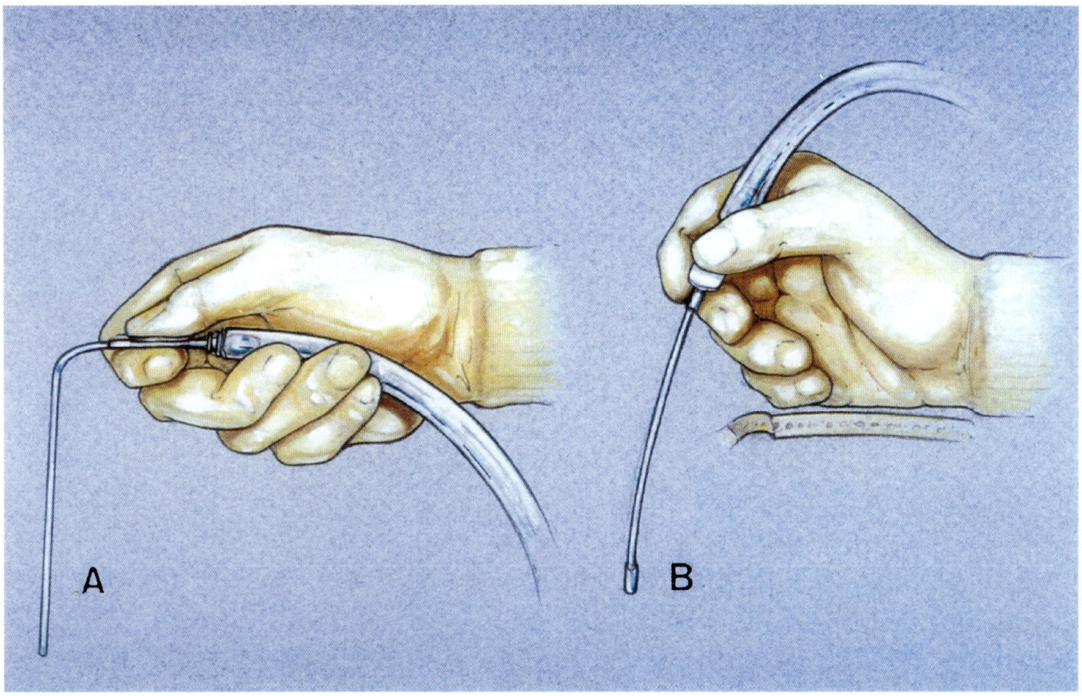

Figure 1–7 Common hand grips for holding a surgical instrument. The grip is determined largely by the design of the instrument. **(A)** A suction tube is held in a pistol grip. The disadvantage of this type of grip is that it uses movements at the wrist and elbow rather than fine finger movements to position the tip of the instrument, and the hand cannot be rested and stabilized on the wound margin. **(B)** A suction tube is held in a pencil grip, permitting manipulation of the tip with delicate finger movements while the hand rests comfortably on the wound margin.

the thumb and the fingers also improved the accuracy of other straight and bayonet instruments used for dissection, grasping, cutting, and coagulation (**Figs. 1–9, 1–10**). Round-handled straight and bayonet forceps may be used for both macrosurgery and microsurgery.

The addition of straight round-handled forceps with teeth, called tissue forceps, increases the use of the set of round-handled instruments to include grasping muscle, skin, and dura (**Fig. 1–11**). A tissue forceps with large teeth is used on the scalp and muscle, and ones with small teeth are used on dura. The addition of round-handled dressing forceps, which have fine serrations inside the tips, makes the set suitable for grasping arterial walls for endarterectomy and arterial suturing.

The instruments should have a dull finish because the brilliant light from highly polished instruments reflected back through the microscope can interfere with the surgeon's vision and detract from the quality of photographs taken through the microscope. Sharpness and sterilization are not affected by the dull finish. The separation between the instrument tips should be wide enough to allow them to straddle the tissue, the needle, or the thread to cut or grasp it accurately. The excessive opening and closing movements required for widely separated tips reduce the functional accuracy of the instrument during delicate manipulation under the operating microscope. The finger pressure required to bring widely separated tips together against firm spring tension often initiates a fine tremor and inaccurate movement. Microsurgical tissue forceps should have a tip separation of no more than 8 mm; microneedle holder tips should open no more than 3 mm; and microscissors tips should open no less than 2 mm and no more than 5 mm, depending on the length of the blade and the use of the scissors.

The length of the instruments should be adequate for the particular task that is being contemplated (**Figs. 1–9, 1–10**). Bayonet instruments (e.g., forceps, needle holders, and scissors) should be available in at least the three lengths needed for the hand to be rested while the surgeon operates at superficial, deep, and extra deep sites.

Bayonet Forceps

Bayonet forceps are standard neurosurgical instruments (**Figs. 1–9, 1–10**). The bayonet forceps should be properly balanced so that when its handle rests on the web between the thumb and index finger and across the radial side of the middle finger it remains there without falling forward when the grasp of the index finger and thumb is released. Poor balance prevents the delicate grasp needed for microsurgical procedures.

It is preferable to test forceps for tension and tactile qualities by holding them in the gloved rather than the naked hand. Forceps resistance to closure that is perceived as adequate in the naked hand may become almost imperceptible in the gloved hand. The forceps may be used to develop tissue planes by inserting the closed forceps between the structures to be separated and releasing the tension so that the blades open and separate the structures. This form of dissection requires greater tension in the handles than is found in some delicate forceps.

In selecting bayonet forceps, the surgeon should consider the length of the blades needed to reach the operative site

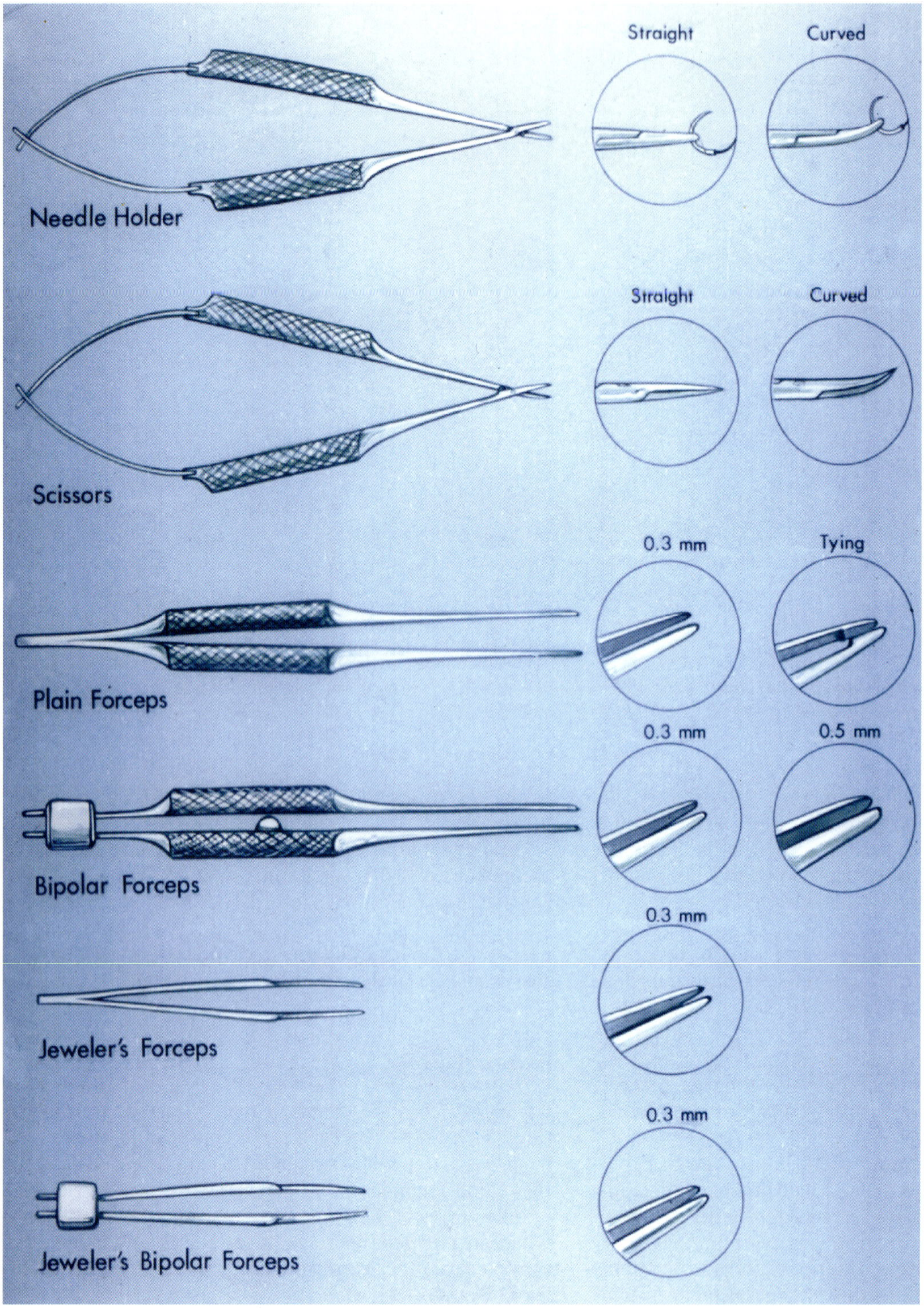

Figure 1–8 Straight Rhoton instruments with round handles and fine tips for use at the surface of the brain. These instruments are suitable for microsurgical procedures, such as an extracranial to intracranial arterial anastomosis. The instruments include needle holders with straight and curved tips, scissors with straight and curved tips, forceps with platforms for tying fine suture, bipolar forceps with 0.3 and 0.5 mm tips, and plain and bipolar jeweler's forceps. The jeweler's forceps can be used as a needle holder for placing sutures in a fine microvascular anastomosis on the surface of the brain, but the author prefers a straight, round-handled needle holder for that use.

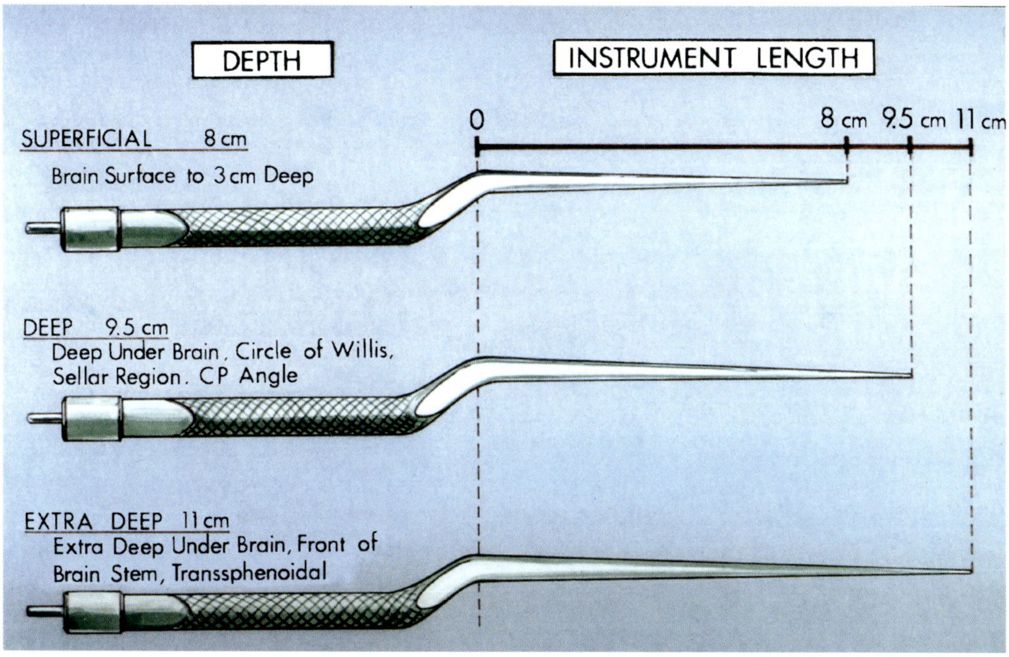

Figure 1–9 Rhoton bayonet bipolar coagulation forceps for use at different depths. Bayonet forceps with 8 cm blades are suitable for coagulation on the surface of the brain and down to a depth of 3 cm. Bayonet forceps with 9.5 cm blades are needed for coagulation deep under the brain in the region of the circle of Willis, suprasellar area, or cerebellopontine (CP) angle. Bayonet forceps with 11 cm blades are suitable for coagulation in extra deep sites, such as in front of the brain stem or in a transsphenoidal exposure. Some surgeons prefer that the forceps be coated to ensure that the current is delivered to the tips, but the coating may obstruct the view at the tips when operating under the microscope.

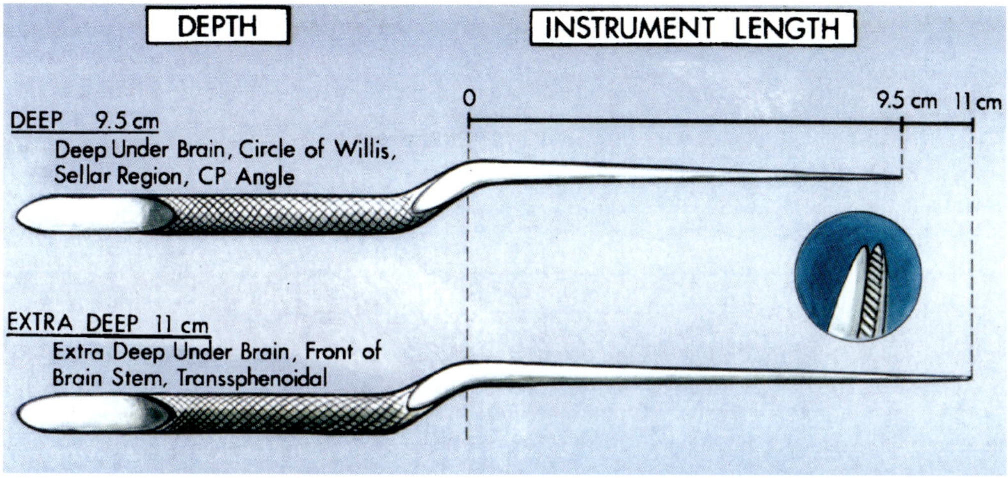

Figure 1–10 Rhoton dissecting bayonets with fine (0.5 cm) tips for use at deep and extra deep sites. Fine cross-serrations (inset) inside the tips aid in grasping and manipulating tissue. CP, cerebellopontine.

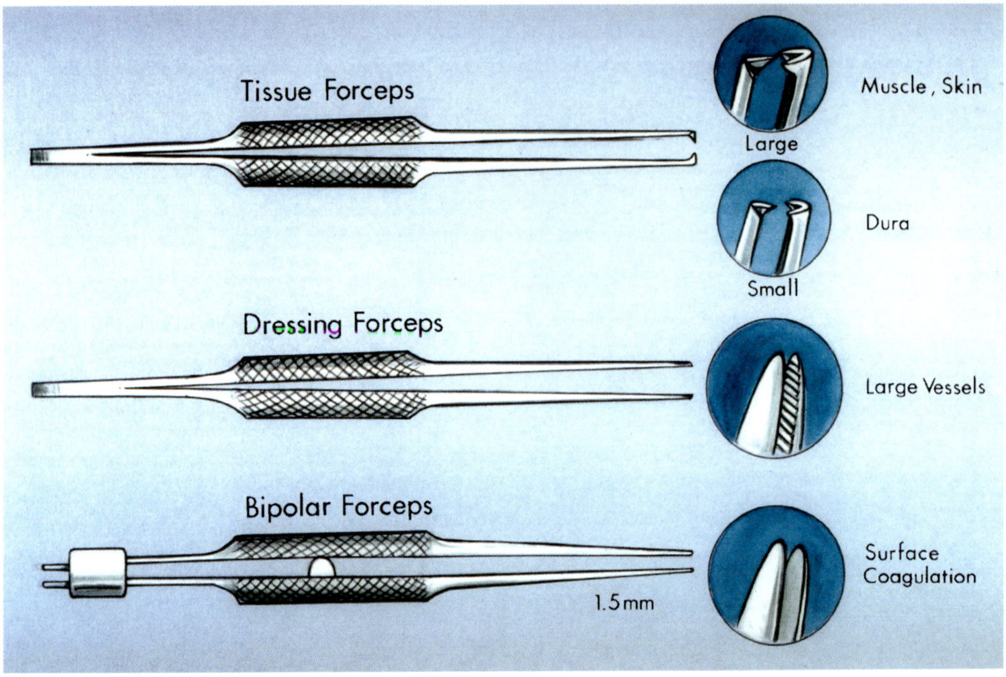

Figure 1–11 Rhoton straight instruments with round handles are needed to complete the set so that the same type of handles can be used for macrosurgery done with the naked eye and microsurgery done with the eye aided by the microscope. Forceps with teeth, called tissue forceps, are needed for grasping dura, muscle, and skin. Small teeth are used on dura, and large teeth are used for skin and muscle. Forceps with cross-serrations, called dressing forceps, may be used during an endarterectomy on larger arteries. Smooth-tip bipolar coagulation forceps with 1.5 mm tips are used for macrocoagulation of large vessels in the scalp, muscle, or dura.

and the size of the tip needed for the specific task to be completed. Bayonet forceps with 8.0, 9.5, and 11.0 cm blades in a variety of tip sizes ranging from 0.5 to 2.0 mm are needed (**Figs. 1–9** and **1–10**). Bayonet forceps with an 8.0 cm shaft are suitable for use on the brain surface and down to a depth of 2.0 cm below the surface. Bayonet forceps with blades of 9.5 cm are suitable for manipulating tissues deep under the brain at the level of the circle of Willis (e.g., in an aneurysm operation), in the sellar region (e.g., in a transcranial approach to a pituitary tumor), and in the cerebellopontine angle (e.g., for removal of an acoustic neuroma or decompression of a cranial nerve). For dissection and coagulation in extra deep sites, such as in front of the brain stem or in the depths of a transsphenoidal exposure, forceps having blades of 11 cm are used. Some surgeons prefer that the forceps be coated with an insulating material except at the tips to ensure that the current is delivered to the tips, but the coating, if thick, may obstruct the view of the tissue being grasped when operating under the microscope.

A series of bipolar bayonet forceps having tips of 0.3 to 2.0 mm will allow coagulation of a vessel of almost any size encountered in neurosurgery (**Fig. 1–12**). For coagulating larger structures, tips with widths of 1.5 and 2.0 mm are needed. For microcoagulation, forceps with 1.0, 0.7, or 0.5 mm tips are selected. The fine 0.3 mm tips, like those found on jeweler's forceps, when placed on bayonet forceps may scissor rather than firmly opposing unless carefully aligned. A 0.5 mm tip is the smallest that is practical for use on many bayonet forceps. The forceps should have smooth tips if they are to be used for bipolar coagulation. If they are used for dissecting and grasping tissue and not for coagulation, the inside tips should have fine cross-serrations like dressing forceps (**Fig. 1–10** and **11**). For grasping large pieces of tumor capsule, forceps with small rings with fine serrations at the tips may be used.

Bipolar Coagulation

The bipolar electrocoagulator has become fundamental to neurosurgery because it allows accurate, fine coagulation of small vessels, minimizing dangerous spread of current to adjacent neural and vascular structures (**Figs. 1–9, 1–12, 1–13**).[6,7] It allows coagulation in areas where unipolar coagulation would be hazardous, such as near the cranial nerves, brain stem, cerebellar arteries, and fourth ventricle.

When the electrode tips touch each other, the current is short-circuited, and no coagulation occurs. There should be enough tension in the handle of the forceps to allow the surgeon to control the distance between the tips because no coagulation occurs if the tips touch or are too far apart. Some types of forceps, attractive for their delicacy, compress with so little pressure that a surgeon cannot avoid closing them during coagulation, even with a delicate grasp. The cable connecting the bipolar unit and the coagulation forceps should not be excessively long because longer cables can cause an irregular supply of current.

Surgeons with experience in conventional coagulation are conditioned to require maximal dryness at the surface of application, but with bipolar coagulation, some moistness is preferable. Coagulation occurs even if the tips are immersed

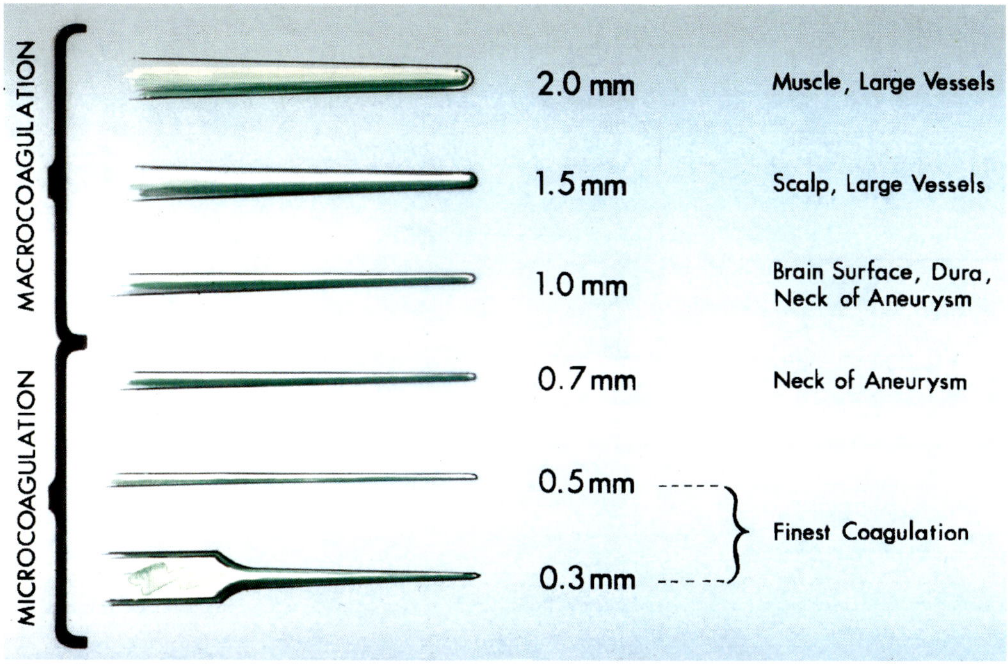

Figure 1–12 Forceps tips needed for macro- and microcoagulation. Bipolar forceps with 1.5 and 2.0 mm tips are suitable for coagulating large vessels and bleeding points in the scalp, muscle, and fascia. The 0.7 and 1.0 mm tips are suitable for coagulation on the dura and brain surface and for coagulation on the surface of a tumor capsule. Fine coagulation at deep sites in the posterior fossa is done with bayonet forceps with 0.5 mm tips. The 0.3 mm tip is suitable for use on a short instrument like a jeweler's forceps. When tips as small as 0.3 mm are placed on a bayonet forceps, the tips may scissor rather than oppose.

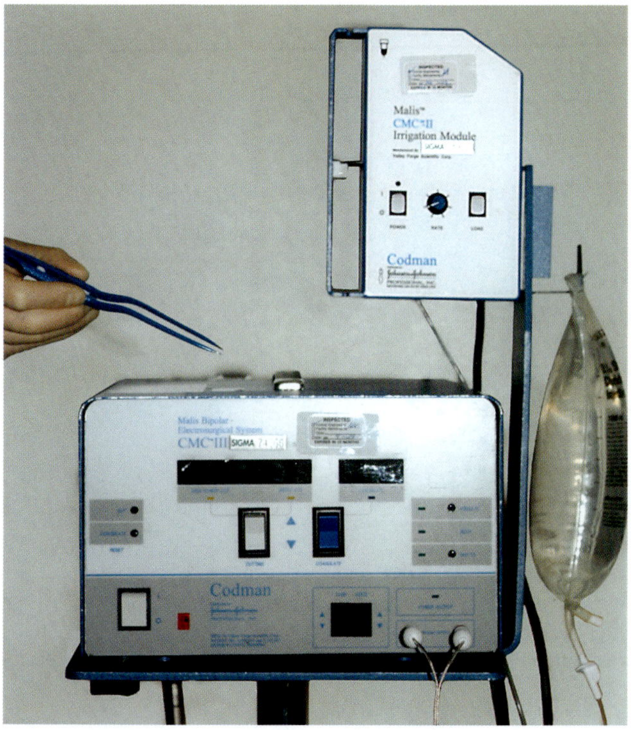

Figure 1–13 A. Malis Bipolar Electrosurgical System and Irrigation Module (Codman & Shurtleff, Inc., Raynham, MA) with coated Rhoton bayonet coagulation forceps. A small amount of fluid is dispensed at the tip of the forceps during each coagulation.

in saline, and keeping the tissue moist with local cerebrospinal fluid or saline irrigation during coagulation reduces heating and minimizes drying and sticking of tissue to the forceps. Fine irrigation units and forceps have been developed that dispense a small amount of fluid through a long tube in the shaft of the forceps to the tip with each coagulation (**Fig. 1–14**). To avoid sticking after coagulation, the points of the forceps should be cleaned after each application to the tissue. If charred blood coats the tips, it should be removed with a damp cloth rather than by scraping with a scalpel blade because the blade may scratch the tips and make them more adherent to tissue during coagulation. The tips of the forceps should be polished if they become pitted and rough.

Scissors

Scissors with fine blades on straight and bayonet handles are frequently used in microsurgical procedures (**Figs. 1–8, 1–15**). Cutting should be done by the distal half of the blade. If the scissors open too widely, cutting ability and accuracy suffer. Delicate cutting near the surface, such as opening the middle cerebral artery for anastomosis or embolectomy, should be done with straight, not bayonet, scissors with fine blades ~5 mm long that open ~3 mm. Only delicate suture material and tissue should be cut with such small blades. Bayonet scissors with an 8 cm shaft and curved or straight blades are selected for areas 3 to 4 cm below the cranial surface. Bayonet

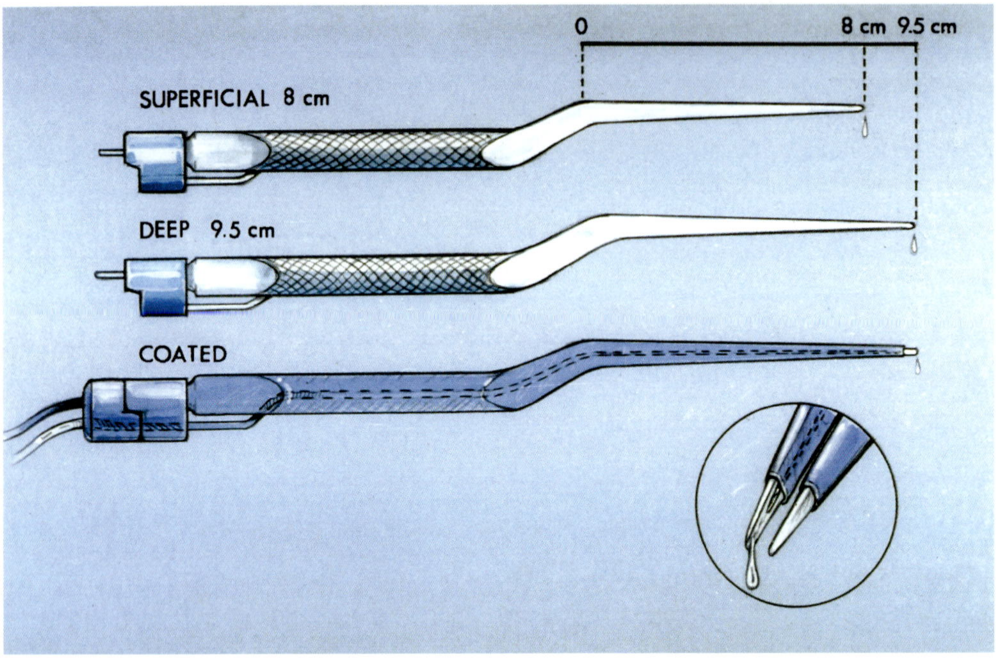

Figure 1–14 Rhoton irrigating bipolar forceps. A small amount of fluid is dispensed at the tip of the forceps during each coagulation. The small metal tube that carries the irrigating fluid is inlaid into the shaft of the instrument so that it does not obstruct the view when the surgeon is looking down the forceps into a deep, narrow operative site. The irrigating forceps with 8 cm blades are suitable for coagulation at or near the surface of the brain. Bayonet forceps with 9.5 cm blades are used for coagulation deep under the brain. Some surgeons prefer that the forceps be coated to ensure that the current is delivered to the tips, but the coating may obstruct the view at the tips when operating under the microscope.

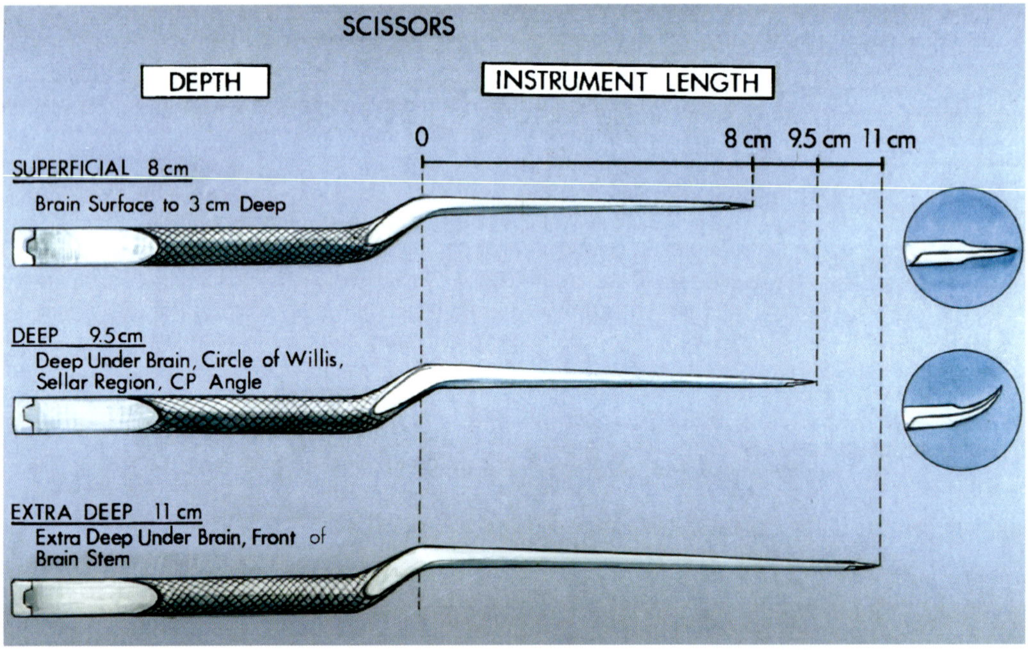

Figure 1–15 Rhoton bayonet scissors with straight and curved blades. The bayonet scissors with 8 cm shafts are used at the surface of the brain and down to a depth of 3 cm. The scissors with 9.5 cm shafts are used deep under the brain, at the level of the circle of Willis, suprasellar area, and in the cerebellopontine (CP) angle. The scissors with 11 cm shafts are used at extra deep sites such as in front of the brain stem. The straight, nonbayonet scissors shown in **Fig. 1–8** may also be used at the brain's surface.

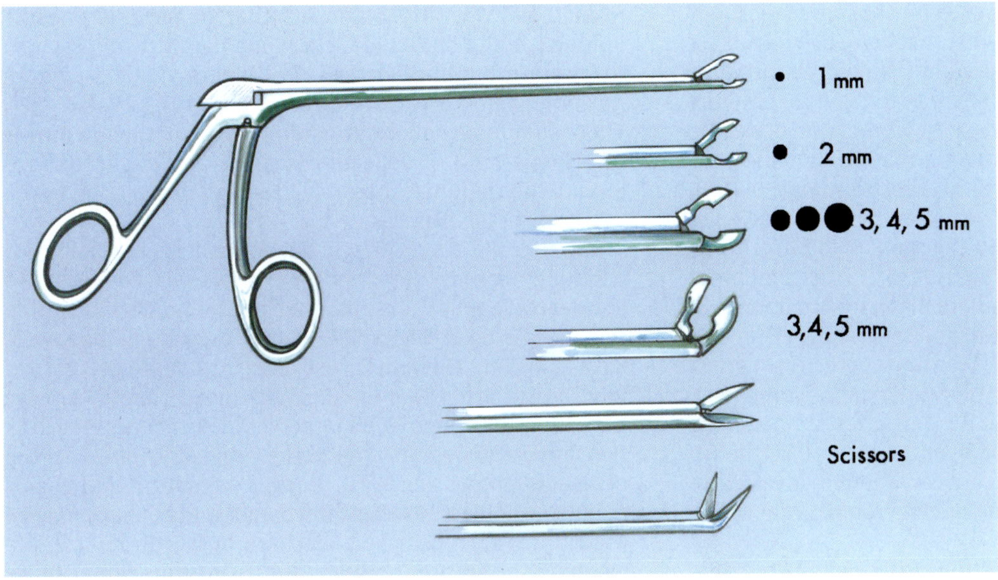

Figure 1–16 Straight and angled alligator cup forceps and scissors. These fine cup forceps are used for grasping and removing tumor in deep, narrow exposures. A 2, 3, or 4 mm cup is required for most microsurgical applications, but cup forceps as small as 1 mm or as large as 5 mm are occasionally needed. Straight and angled alligator scissors with the same mechanism of action as the cup forceps are needed in deep, narrow exposures, as in the depths of a transsphenoidal operation.

scissors with a 9.5 cm shaft are selected for deep areas, such as the cerebellopontine angle or suprasellar region. The blade should measure 14 mm long and should open ~4 mm. For extra deep sites, such as in front of the brain stem, the scissors should have an 11 cm shaft. Scissors on an alligator-type shank with a long shaft are selected for deep, narrow openings, as in transsphenoidal operations (**Fig. 1–16**).

Dissectors

The most widely used neurosurgical macrodissectors are of the Penfield or Freer types; however, the size and weight of these instruments make them unsuitable for microdissection around the cranial nerves, brain stem, and intracranial vessels. The smallest Penfield dissector, the no. 4, has a width of 3 mm. For microsurgery, dissectors with 1 and 2 mm tips are needed (**Fig. 1–17**). Straight, rather than bayonet, dissectors are preferred for most intracranial operations because rotating the handles of the straight dissector does not alter the position of the tip, but rotating the handle of a bayonet dissector causes the tip to move through a wide arc.

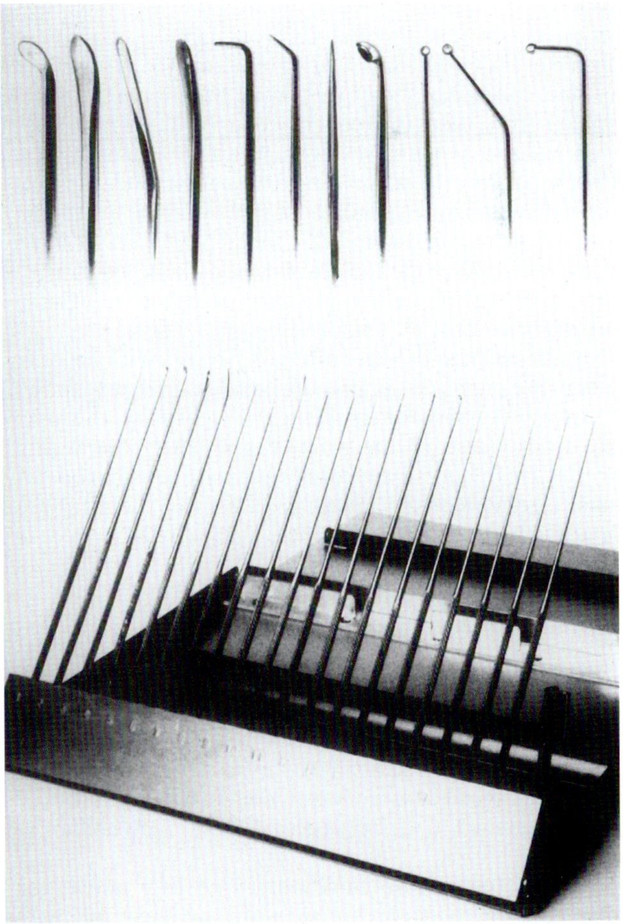

Figure 1–17 Rhoton microdissectors for neurosurgery. Beginning on the left of the top row are four types of dissectors: round, spatula, flat, and micro-Penfield. The next instruments, in order, along the top row are a right-angled nerve hook, angled and straight needle dissectors, and a microcurette. The last three instruments in the top row are straight, and 40 degree, and right-angled teardrop dissectors. A storage case of the type shown below the instruments permits easy access to instruments and protects the delicate tips when not in use. The full set includes round and spatula dissectors in 1, 2, and 3 mm widths, straight and angled microcurettes, long and short teardrop dissectors in 40 degree and right-angled configurations, and one straight teardrop dissector.

Round-tipped dissectors are used for separation of tumor from nerve (**Figs. 1–17, 1–18, 1–19**). An alternative method of fine dissection is to use the straight, pointed instruments that the author calls needles.[8] It may be difficult to grasp the margin of the tumor with forceps; however, a small needle dissector introduced into its margin may be helpful in retracting the tumor in the desired direction (**Figs. 1–18B, 1–19A**). This type of pointed instrument can also be used to develop a cleavage plane between tumor and arachnoid membrane, nerves, and brain. Spatula dissectors similar to, but smaller than, the no. 4 Penfield dissector are helpful in defining the neck of an aneurysm and separating it from the adjacent perforating arteries. Teardrop dissectors with a 40 degree angle are especially helpful in defining the neck of an aneurysm and in separating arteries from nerves during vascular decompression operations because the tip slides easily in and out of tight areas without inadvertently avulsing perforating arteries or catching on delicate tissue (**Figs. 1–20, 1–21**).[9,10]

Any vessel that stands above the surface of an encapsulated tumor, such as an acoustic neuroma or a meningioma, should be dealt with initially as if it were a brain vessel that runs over the tumor surface and can be preserved with accurate dissection. The surgeon should try to displace the vessel and adjacent tissue off the tumor capsule toward the adjacent neural tissues by using a small dissector after the tumor has been removed from within the capsule. Vessels that initially appear to be adherent to the capsule often prove to be neural vessels on the pial surface when dissected free of the capsule.

If the pia-arachnoid membrane is adherent to the tumor capsule or if a tumor mass is present within the capsule and prevents collapse of the capsule away from brain stem and cranial nerves, there is a tendency to apply traction to both layers and to tear neural vessels running on the pial surface. Before separating the pia-arachnoid from the capsule, it is important to remove enough tumor so that the capsule is so thin that it is almost transparent. If the surgeon is uncertain about the margin between the capsule and the pia-arachnoid membrane, several gentle sweeps of a small dissector through the area will help clarify the appropriate plane for dissection.

For transsphenoidal operations, dissectors with bayonet handles are preferred because the handles aid in preventing the surgeon's hand from blocking the view down the long, narrow exposure of the sella (**Fig. 1–22**).[11] Blunt ring curettes are frequently used during transsphenoidal operations to remove small and large tumors of the pituitary gland and to explore the sella (**Figs. 1–23** to **1–26**).

Needles, Sutures, and Needle Holders

The operating room should have readily available microsuture, ranging from 6–0 to 10–0, on a variety of needles ranging in diameters from 50 to 130 µm (**Table 1–1**).[12,13] For the most delicate of suturing, as in an extracranial to intracranial arterial anastomosis, nylon or Prolene suture of 22 µm diameter (10–0) on needles ~50 to 75 µm in diameter is used.

Jeweler's forceps are commonly used as a holder for grasping a microneedle, but they are too short for most intracranial operations. The handles of the microneedle holders should be round rather than flat or rectangular so that rotating them between the fingers yields a smooth movement that drives the needle easily (**Figs. 1–8, 1–27**). There should be no lock or holding catch on the microneedle. No matter how delicately such a lock is engaged or released, the tip jumps, possibly causing misdirection of the needle or tissue damage.

Jeweler's forceps or straight needle holders are suitable for handling microneedles near the cortical surface (**Fig. 1–8**). For deeper applications, bayonet needle holders with fine tips may be used (**Fig. 1–27**). Bayonet needle holders with 8 cm shafts are suitable for use down to a depth of 3 cm below the surface of the brain. Shafts measuring 9.5 cm are needed for suturing vessels or nerves in deeper areas such as the suprasellar region, around the circle of Willis, or in the cerebellopontine angle. For tying microsuture, either microneedle holders, jeweler's forceps, or tying forceps may be used. Tying forceps have a platform in the tip to facilitate grasping the suture; however, most surgeons prefer to tie suture with jeweler's forceps or fine needle holders.

Suction Tubes

Suction tubes with blunt, rounded tips are preferred. Dandy designed and used blunt suction tubes, and his trainees have continued to use the Dandy type of tube (**Fig. 1–28**).[14] Yaşargil and colleagues and Rhoton and Merz reported using suction tubes having blunt, rounded tips that allowed them to be used for the manipulation of tissue as well as for suction.[14,15] The thickening and rounding of the tips reduce the problem of the small 3 and 5 French tubes becoming sharp when cut smoothly at right angles to the shaft. Some suction tubes, such as those of the curved Adson type, become somewhat pointed when prepared in sizes as small as 3 or 5 French because the distal end of the tube is cut obliquely to the long axis of the shaft, making them less suitable for use around the thin walls of aneurysms.

The suction tube should be designed to be held like a pencil rather than like a pistol (**Fig. 1–7**). Frazier suction tubes are designed to be held like a pistol. The pencil grip design frees the ulnar side of the hand so that it can be rested comfortably on the wound margin, affording sturdier and more precise, delicate manipulation of the tip of the suction tube than is allowed by the unsupported pistol grip.

Selecting a tube of appropriate length is important because the arm tires during extended operations if the suction tube is too long to allow the hand to be rested (**Figs. 1–29, 1–30**). Tubes with 8 cm shafts (i.e., the length between the angle distal to the thumb piece and the tip) are used for suction at the level of the skull or near the surface of the brain (**Fig. 1–31**). Tubes with 10 cm shafts allow the hand to rest along the wound margin during procedures performed in deep operative sites, such as the regions of the cerebellopontine angle, suprasellar region, and basilar apex or around the circle of Willis (**Fig. 1–32**). Suction tubes with 13 cm shafts may be used at extra deep sites such as in front of the brain stem and also for transsphenoidal operations. The suction tubes with 13 cm shafts, as used for transsphenoidal operations, in addition to having straight tips have

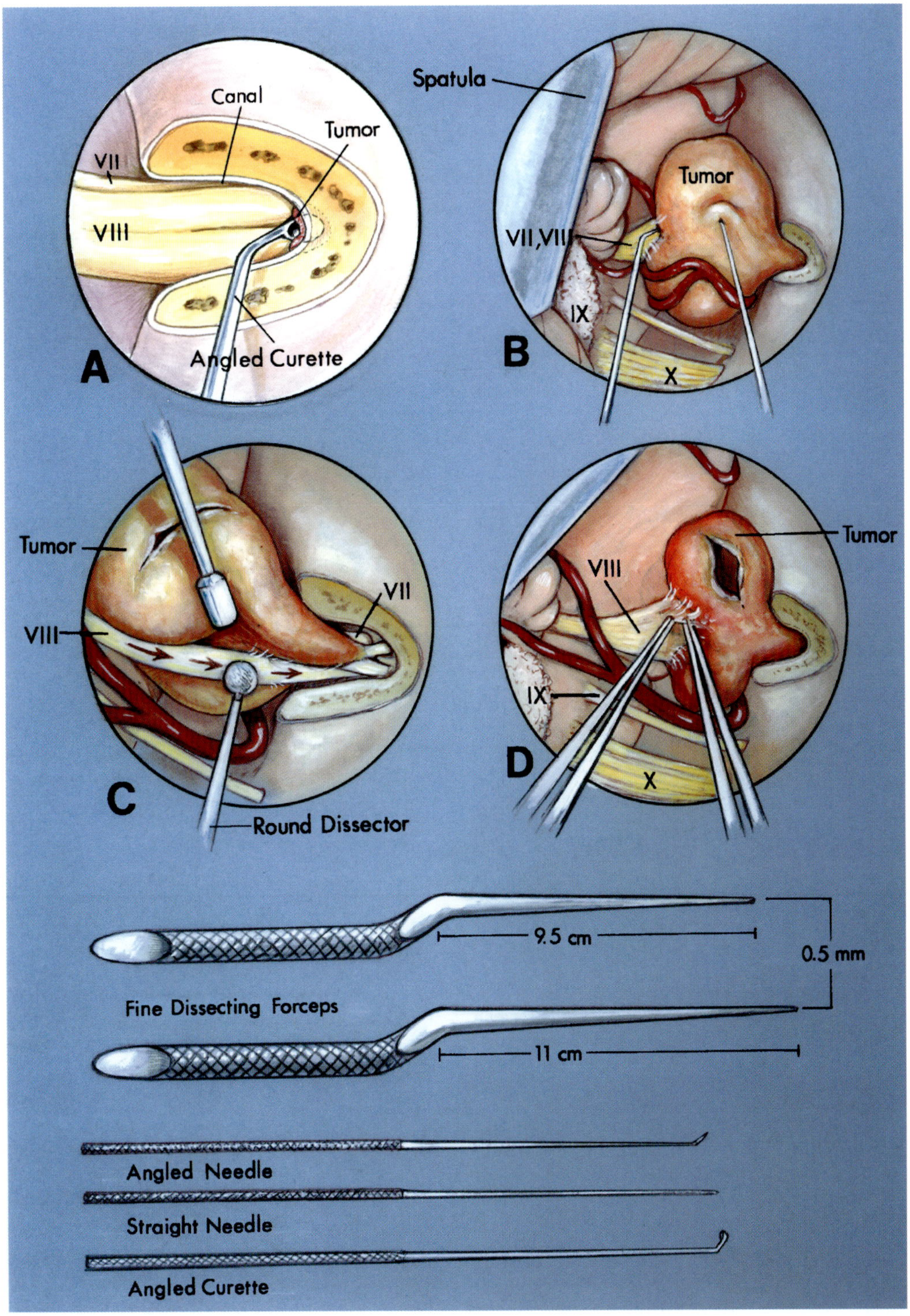

Figure 1–18 Four methods of fine dissection for separating the capsule of an acoustic neuroma from the nerves in the cerebellopontine angle. **(A)** The posterior wall of the internal auditory canal has been removed, and the entire tumor has been removed except for a small fragment of the capsule in the lateral end of the canal behind the vestibulocochlear and facial nerves. The angled curette is inserted in the meatal fundus behind the nerves and lifts the last fragment of capsule out of the lateral end of the meatus after the tumor has been separated from the posterior surface of the nerves. **(B)** A small acoustic neuroma is removed from the posterior surface of the vestibulocochlear nerve using angled and straight needles. The straight needle is used to retract the tumor capsule, and the angled needle separates the tumor capsule and nerve. **(C)** The nerve and tumor capsule are separated with a round dissector. The strokes of the dissectors should be directed from medial to lateral if there is a chance of preserving hearing. The facial nerve is exposed at the lateral end of the meatus. **(D)** Removal of the capsule of a large tumor from the posterior surface of the vestibulocochlear nerve using fine dissecting bayonet forceps having 0.5 mm tips with small serrations on the inside of the tip to aid in grasping tissue. Bayonet dissecting forceps with 9.5 cm shafts are used in deep sites such as the cerebellopontine angle, and bayonet forceps with an 11 cm shaft are used at extra deep sites, as in front of the brain stem. The glossopharyngeal and vagus nerves are below the tumor. (With permission from Rhoton AL Jr. Operative techniques and instrumentation for neurosurgery. Neurosurgery 2003;53:907–934.[2])

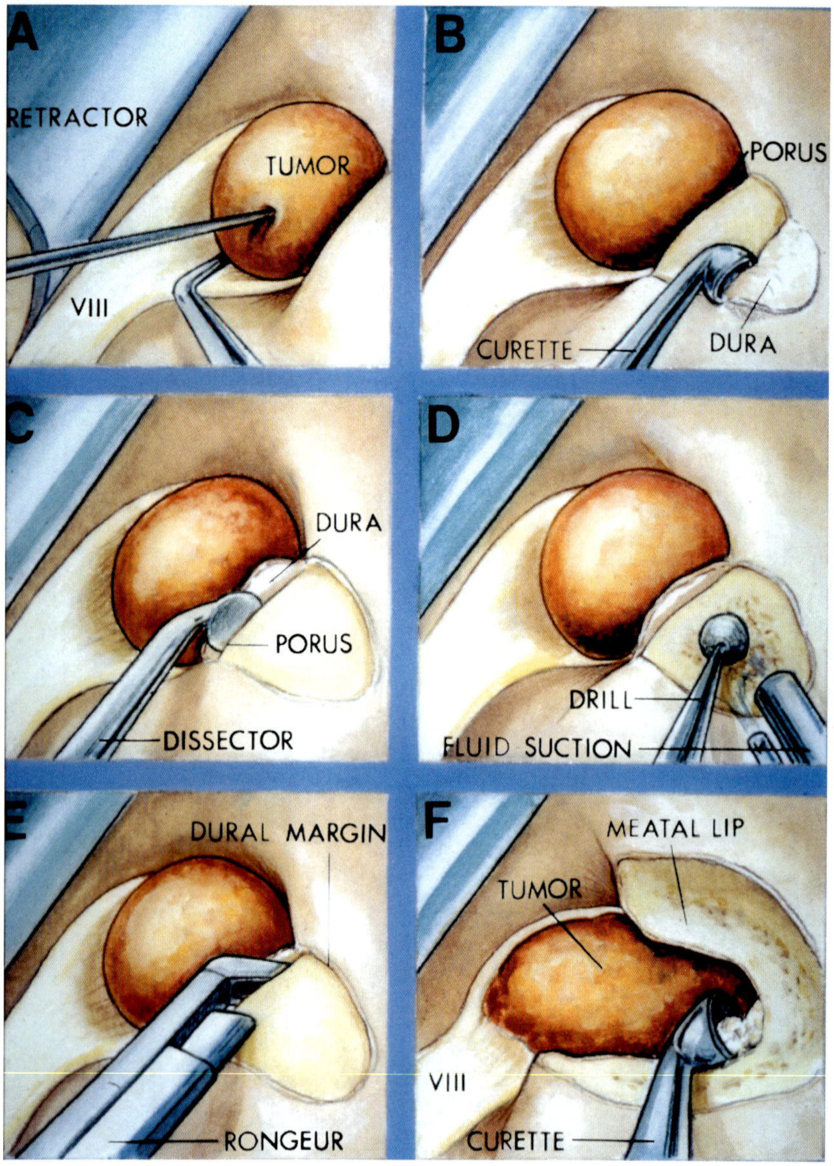

Figure 1–19 Microinstruments used in the cerebellopontine angle. This illustration was prepared from 16 mm movie frames taken at the time of removal of an acoustic neuroma in the right cerebellopontine angle. This operation resulted in preservation of the facial, acoustic, and vestibular nerves. **(A)** A brain spatula gently elevates the right cerebellum to expose the tumor. Small, pointed instruments called needles separate the tumor from the eighth nerve. The straight needle retracts the tumor, and the 45 degree needle develops a cleavage plane between the tumor and the nerve. The facial nerve is hidden in front of the vestibulocochlear nerve. **(B)** The microcurette with a 1.5 mm cup strips dura mater from the posterior wall of the meatus. **(C)** The 1 mm round dissector separates dura from the bone at the porus and within the meatus. **(D)** A drill is used to remove the posterior wall of the meatus. Suction irrigation cools and removes bone dust. **(E)** Alternative method of removal of the posterior wall after it has been thinned by a drill using a Kerrison rongeur with a 1 mm wide bite. **(F)** The microcurette with a 1.5 mm cup removes the last bit of bone from the posterior meatal wall.

tips angled up and down for suction around the curves within the capsule of a tumor or for following asymmetrical extensions of tumor (**Figs. 1–24, 1–33**).

The suction tubes should encompass a range of diameters from 3 to 12 French, which allows them to be used for macroneurosurgery and microneurosurgery (**Table 1–2**) (**Fig. 1–30**). Conventional surgery done with the naked eye uses 9, 10, or 12 French tubes. The French designation applies to the outer diameter. Three French units equal 1 mm; thus a 9 French tube has an outer diameter of 3 mm. The 10 and 12 French tubes are used during the opening of the scalp, muscle, and bone and for heavy bleeding. The most commonly used macrosuction tubes, the 9 and 10 French sizes, are too large for use after the dura is open. Stretched nerve fascicles or small vessels can easily become entrapped in such large tubes. Most microsurgical procedures require tube diameters of 5 and 7 French. The 3 or 5 French sizes are suitable for delicate applications such as suction around the facial nerve during the removal of an acoustic neuroma. The 5 French suction tube with a 10 cm shaft may be used as a suction-dissector in defining the neck of an aneurysm or as a suction-dissector in the cerebellopontine angle and near the cerebellar arteries and cranial nerves (**Fig. 1–32**). The 7 French tube is commonly used in completing the intracapsular removal of an acoustic neuroma or meningioma of medium or large size. The 3 French tube is too small for most microsurgical procedures, but it is suitable for applications such as suction along the suture line of an extracranial to intracranial arterial bypass (**Fig. 1–31**).

The power of the suction is regulated by adjusting the degree to which the thumb occludes an air hole. The air holes should be large enough that the suction at the tip is markedly reduced when the thumb is off the hole; however, the suction pressure may need to be adjusted at its source to avoid the danger of entrapping and damaging fine neural and vascular structures.

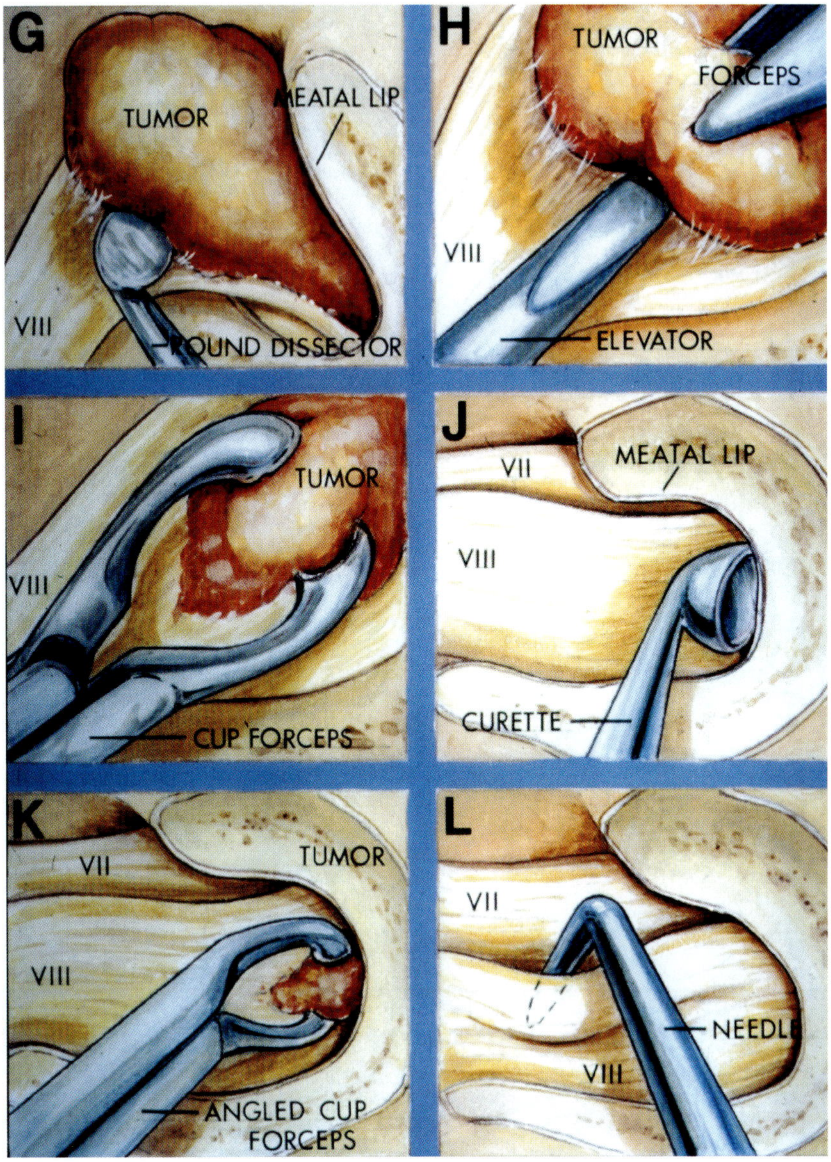

(*Continued*) **Figure 1–19** **(G)** The 1 mm round dissector separates tumor from the eighth nerve. **(H)** The flat dissector with a 1 mm tip separates tumor from the eighth nerve. **(I)** The microcup forceps with a 1 mm cup removes a nodule of tumor from the nerve. **(J)** The microcurette reaches into the meatus behind the eighth nerve to bring a nodule of tumor into view. The facial nerve is anterior and superior to the vestibulocochlear nerve. **(K)** The microcup forceps angled to the right removes the last remaining fragment of tumor from the lateral part of the meatus. **(L)** The angled needle examines the area between the facial and vestibulocochlear nerves for residual tumor. (With permission from Rhoton AL Jr. Operative techniques and instrumentation for neurosurgery. Neurosurgery 2003;53:907–934.[2])

A continuous stream of irrigating fluid, which is often delivered through another tube that is fused to the suction tube, can be helpful during part of the operation (**Fig. 1–19D**). Irrigation discourages the formation of small blood clots and their adherence to the dissected surfaces; it also increases the effectiveness of the bipolar coagulation forceps and reduces the adhesiveness of the tips to tissue. Constant bathing by cerebrospinal fluid has the same effect.

Irrigation with physiological saline is also helpful in cooling the drill, which may transmit heat to nearby neural structures, and in washing bone dust from the incision (**Fig. 1–19D**). The irrigation should be regulated so that the solution does not enter the operative field unless the surgeon's finger is removed from the suction release hole.

Brain Retractors

Self-retaining retraction systems are routinely used for most intracranial operations.[4,15,16] They allow the surgeon to work in a relatively confined space unhindered by an assistant's hand. They are more dependable than the surgeon's or assistant's hand in maintaining constant, gentle elevation of the brain. The retraction system should include tapered and rectangular brain spatulas that are applied to the protected surface of the brain; flexible arms that can support the brain spatulas in any position within the operating field; and a series of clamps and bars for attaching the system to the pinion head holder or the operating table (**Fig. 1–34**). The most frequently used self-retaining retractor systems have flexible arms that consist of a series of ball-and-socket units, resembling a string of

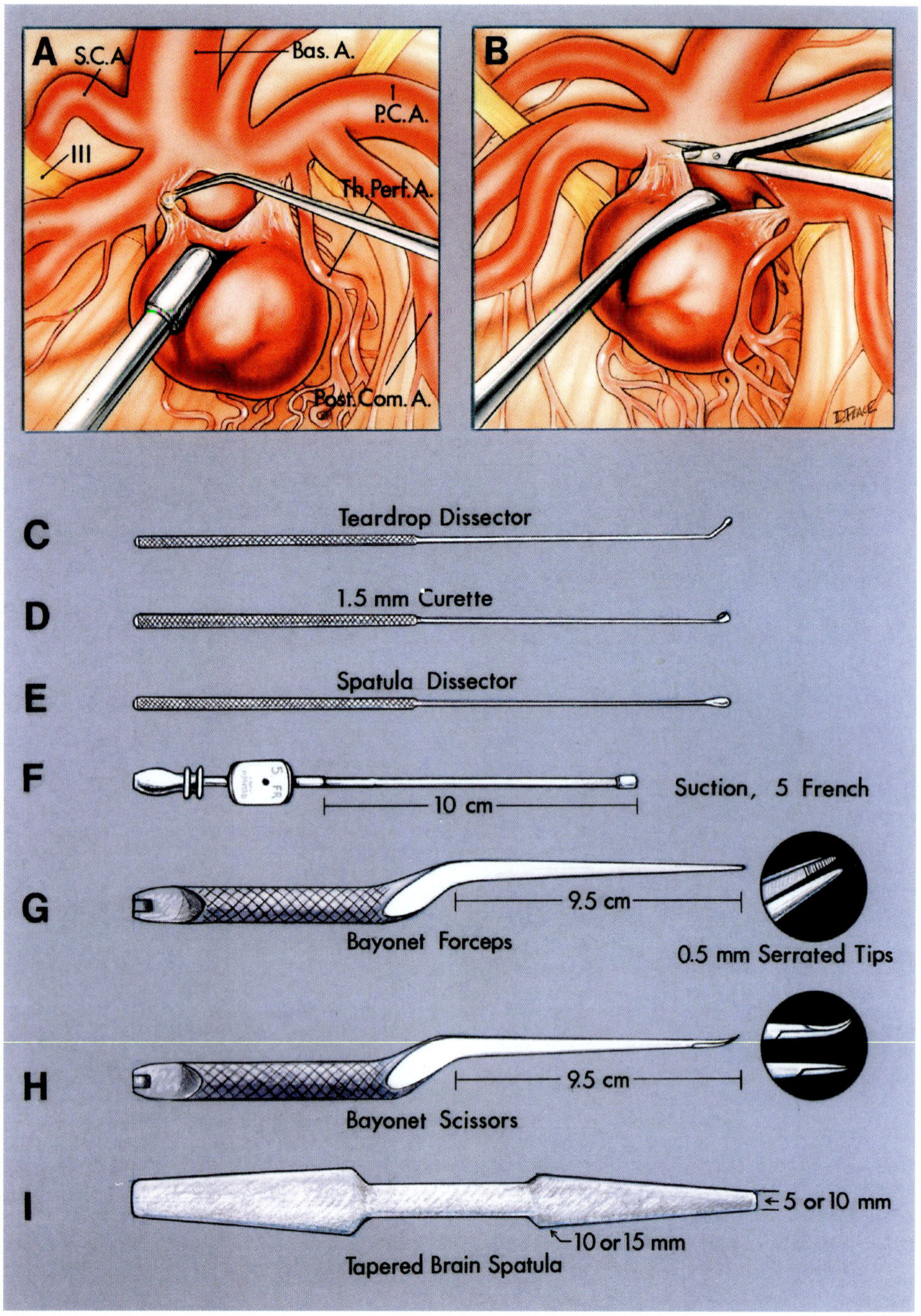

Figure 1–20 Instruments for aneurysm dissection. **(A)** The 40 degree teardrop dissector separates perforating branches and arachnoidal bands from the neck of an aneurysm of the basilar artery (Bas. A.). The blunt-tip suction of a 5 French tube provides suction and aids in the retraction of the aneurysm neck for dissection. Structures in the exposure include the basilar artery (Bas. A.), Superior Cerebellar artery (SCA), posterior communicating artery (Post. com. A.), Posterior cerebral and posterior thalamoperforating arteries (PCA and Th. Perf. A.), and the occulomotor nerve(III). **(B)** The wall of the aneurysm is being retracted with a spatula dissector, and tough arachnoidal bands around the neck are divided with a microscissors. **(C)** A 40 degree teardrop dissector for defining the neck and separating perforating vessels from the neck of an aneurysm. **(D)** The angled microcurette with 1.5 mm cup is useful in removing the dura from the anterior clinoid process. **(E)** Spatula dissector for defining the neck and separating perforating vessels from the wall of an aneurysm. **(F)** Blunt-tip suction with a 10 cm shaft and a 5 French tip for suction and dissection of an aneurysm. A 7 or 9 French blunt-tip suction may be needed if heavy bleeding should occur. **(G)** Bayonet forceps with 0.5 mm serrated tips. **(H)** Bayonet scissors. **(I)** Tapered brain spatula with the tip tapered to 5 or 10 mm. (With permission from Rhoton AL Jr. Aneurysms. Neurosurgery 2002;51 (Suppl 4):S121–S158.)

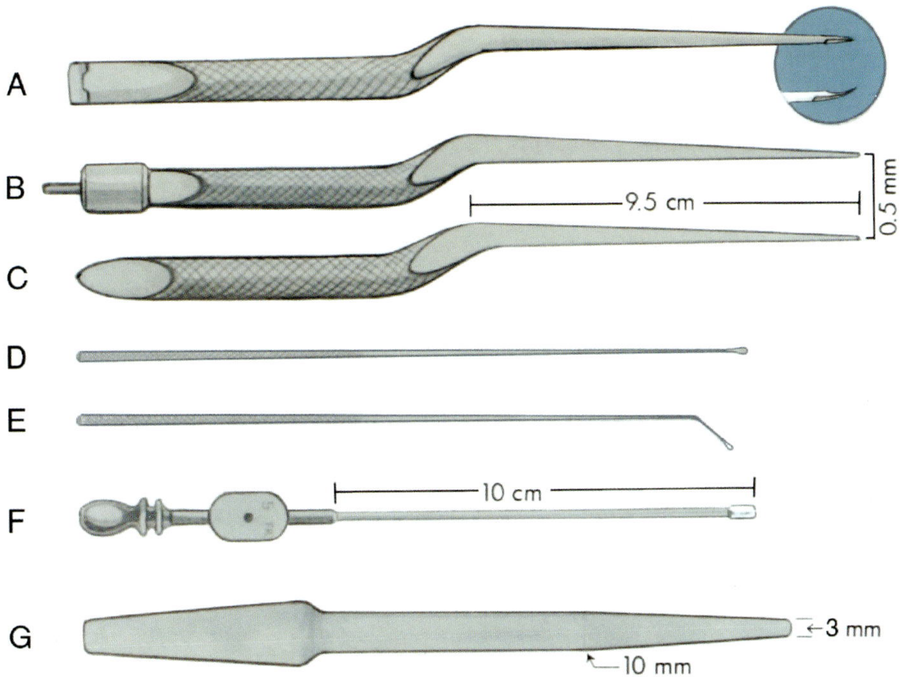

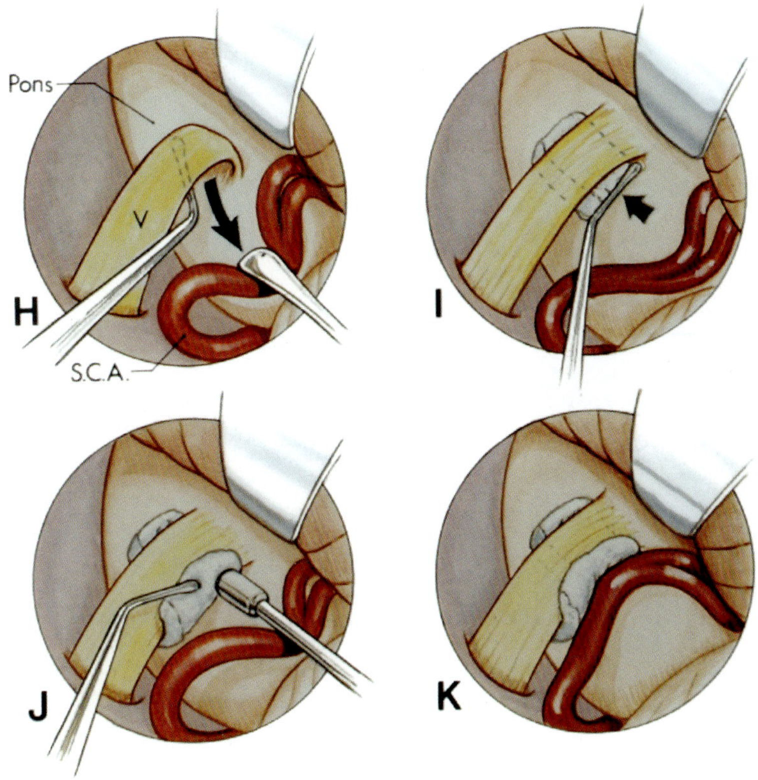

Figure 1–21 Commonly used instruments for the microsurgical portion of a decompression operation for trigeminal neuralgia. **(A)** Bayonet scissors with 9.5 cm shafts and straight and curved blades are used for opening the arachnoid membrane and cutting in the depths of the exposure. **(B)** A bipolar bayonet forceps with 9.5 cm shaft and 0.5 cm tip is used for coagulation near the nerves or brain stem. A bipolar bayonet forceps with a 0.7 mm tip is used for coagulating large vessels in the superficial part of the exposure and a forceps with a 0.5 mm tip is used for deep coagulation. **(C)** Fine dissection around the arteries and nerves is done with a plain bayonet forceps with 9.5 cm shaft and 0.5 mm tip. **(D)** The two dissectors most commonly used around the trigeminal nerve are the small spatula microdissector and **(E)** a 40 degree teardrop dissector. **(F)** Suction around the nerve is done with a blunt-tip suction tube having a 10 cm shaft and a 5 French tip. **(G)** Retraction is done with a tapered brain spatula having a 10 or 15 mm width at the base and a 3 or 5 mm width at the tip. A self-retaining brain retractor system is used to hold the brain spatula in place. **(H)** The orientation is the same as in **Fig. 1–3**. The right superior cerebellar artery (SCA) is gently elevated away from the trigeminal nerve with the spatula dissector, and the area medial to the nerve is explored with a 40 degree teardrop dissector. **(I)** A small foam pad is fitted into the axilla of the nerve using the teardrop dissector. **(J)** The separation between the superior surface of the nerve and the artery is maintained with a small foam prosthesis. A blunt-tip suction of 5 French size aids in positioning the small foam pad above the nerve. **(K)** The small foam pad protects the medial and superior surfaces of the nerve. (With permission from Rhoton AL Jr. Microsurgical anatomy of decompression operations on the trigeminal nerve. In Rovit RL, ed. Trigeminal Neuralgia. Baltimore: Williams & Wilkins; 1990:165–200.)

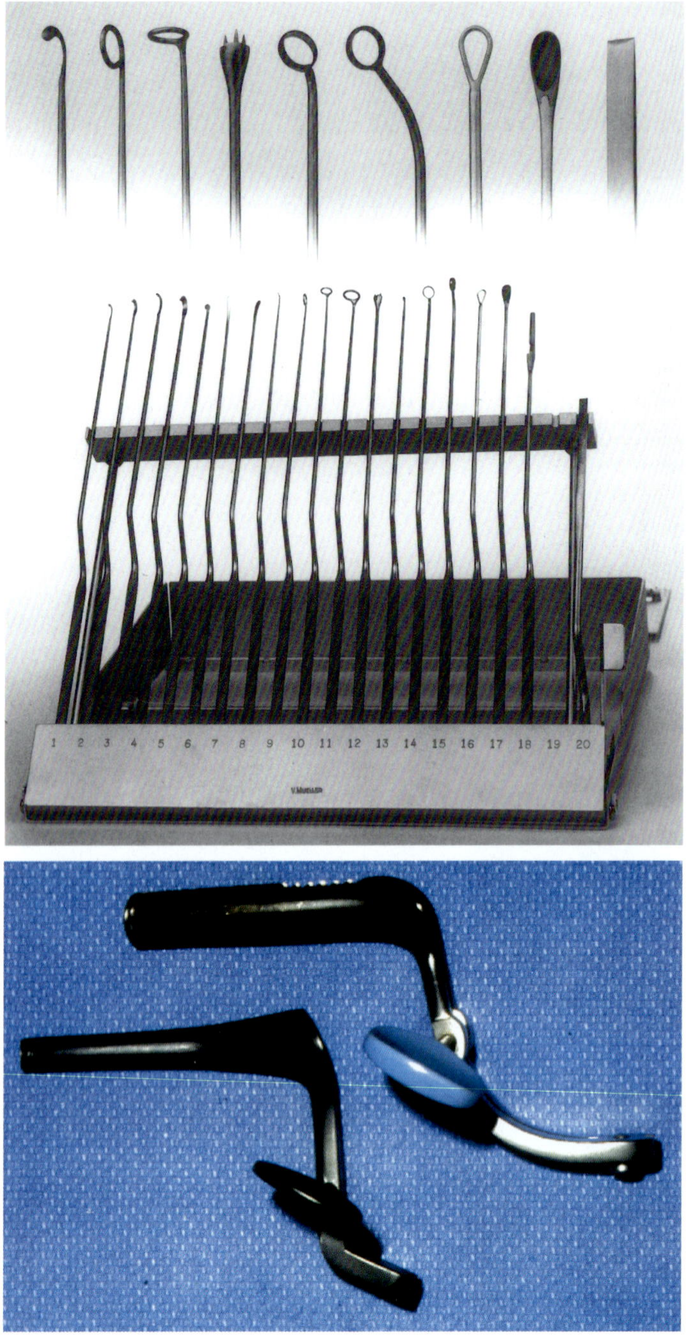

A

B

Figure 1–22 **(A)** Rhoton microinstruments from transsphenoidal operations. The set includes, from left to right (top), Hardy-type curettes, Rhoton-type blunt ring curettes, and a three-pronged fork for manipulating cartilage into the sellar opening, Ray-type curettes, malleable loop and spoon, and an osteotome for opening the sellar wall. **(B)** Speculums for transsphenoidal surgery. (Upper right) Traditional transsphenoidal speculum with thick, wide blades. (Lower left) Rhoton endonasal speculum with smaller, thinner blades used for endonasal transsphenoidal tumor removal.

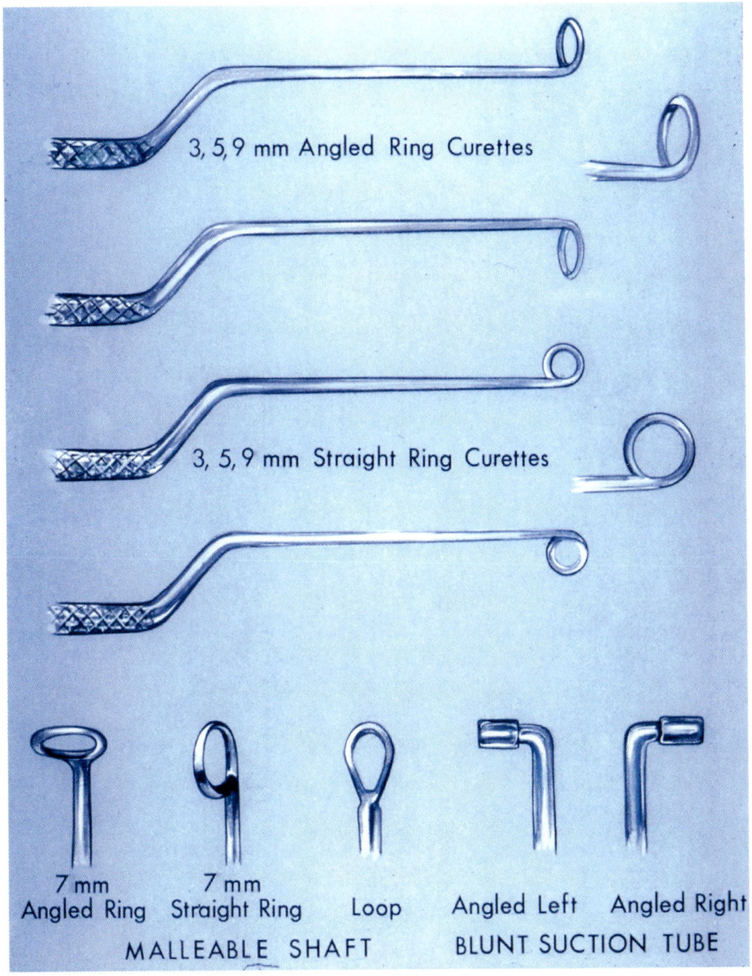

Figure 1–23 Rhoton blunt ring curettes for transsphenoidal operations. These blunt ring curettes have small circular loops on the dissecting tip and are of two types. One type, called angled rings, has a loop, the circumference of which is in a plane at right angles to the long axis of the shaft (upper set); the other type, called straight rings, has a circular loop, the circumference of which is in the same plane as the long axis of the shaft (lower set). The rings on the angled and straight curettes have 3, 5, and 9 mm diameters. The instruments have 12 cm shafts, needed for reaching the intracapsular-suprasellar area through the transsphenoidal exposure, and bayoneted handles that facilitate visualization of the tips of the instruments in the deep, narrow transsphenoidal exposure. The set includes curettes with tips directed upward and downward. The instruments shown below on the left have a malleable shaft that allows them to be bent for removal of unusual extensions of the tumor. The angled blunt-tip suction tubes are helpful in removing soft parasellar and suprasellar extensions of tumor.

pearls, with an internal cable that holds in the desired position when tightened.

The stability of the system is increased if the flexible arms that hold the brain spatulas are constructed so that they are tapered, having the largest pearls near the bar to which the arm attaches and the smallest pearls on the end that holds the brain spatulas (**Fig. 1–34A**). Three lengths of flexible arms (20, 30, and 48 cm) will allow the system to be used at diverse operative sites. Greater flexibility in positioning the flexible arms can be achieved if the arms are attached to the rigid bars with the use of a coupling that allows them to be rotated through a 360 degree arc (**Fig. 1–34B**). The flexible arms may be affixed to a short bar that is fixed to the pinion head holder, or they may be attached to longer bars that are attached to the operating table or head holder. The short handles used to tighten the flexible arms and joints in the system should be broad and flat rather than narrow and round, as found in some systems (**Fig. 1–34C**). The broad, flat handles increase the ease of adjustment of the arms and joints.

The clamps that attach the retractor system to the head holder or operating table should be firmly fixed in place prior to affixing the flexible arm to them. The clamps should be affixed to the head holder as close to the operative field as possible and yet should not block the ease and freedom with which the surgeon moves other instruments into the operative site. The retractor system should include straight and curved bars, a jointed bar, and clamps for attaching the bars to the head holder or the operating table (**Fig. 1–34D**). The retractor set may also include two semicircular rings that can be positioned to create a circular halo around the operative site (**Fig. 1–34E**). It is helpful if the arms on the pinion head holder are shaped to accommodate the C-clamp that holds the bars to which the flexible arms are attached.

The flexible arms should be led into the operative site in such a way that they rest closely against the drapes around the margin of the operative site. If the flexible arms are not positioned close to the drapes, the suctioned tubing or cable on the bipolar coagulator may become entangled with the arms and brain spatulas. Positioning near the drapes also reduces the chance that the nurse who is passing instruments will bump the flexible arms. If the bar for holding the flexible arms is positioned between the head of the patient and the surgeon, the bar should be sufficiently close to the patient's head that the surgeon does not bump against it when moving from one position to another around the head of the patient.

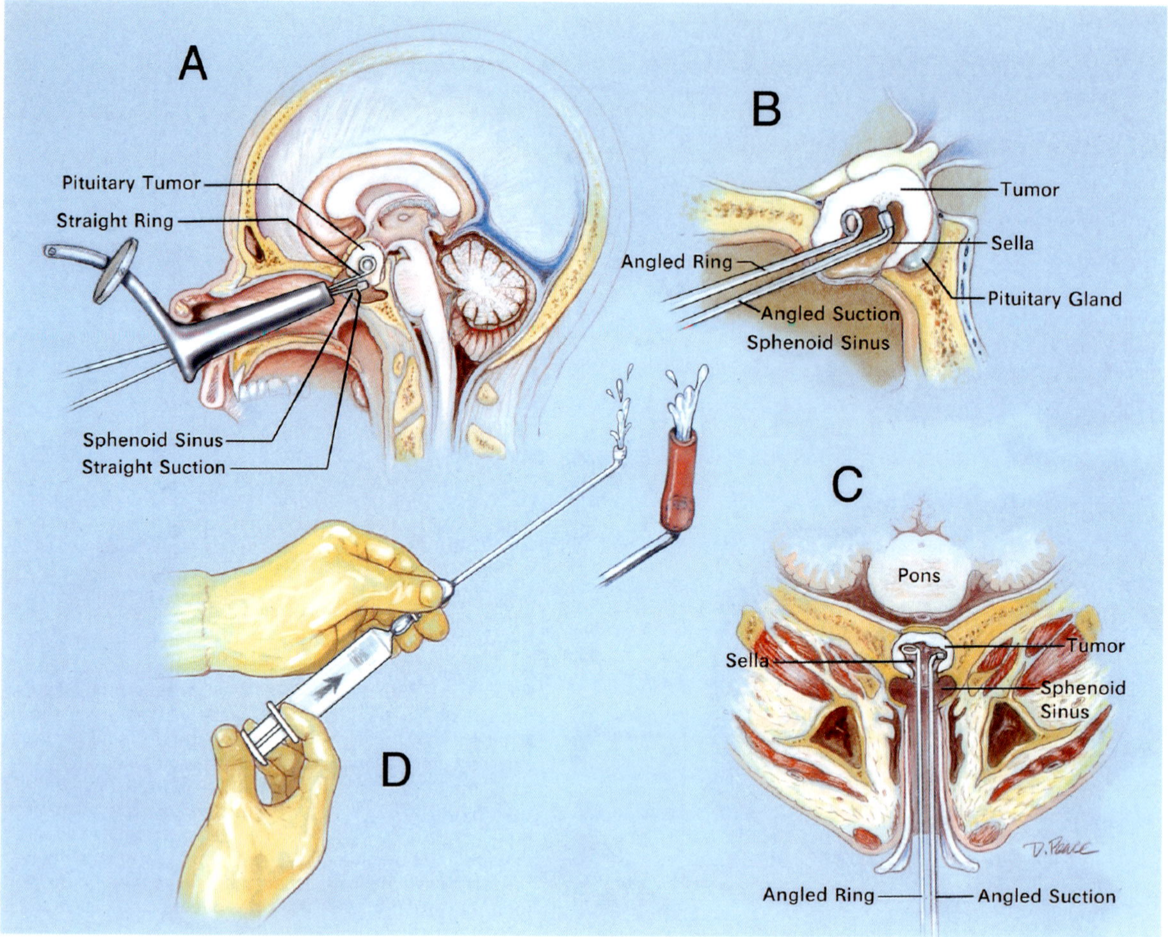

Figure 1–24 Endonasal transsphenoidal removal of a large pituitary tumor with suprasellar extension. **(A)** and **(B)** are midsagittal sections and **(C)** is an oblique horizontal section through the plane along the transnasal route to the sphenoid sinus and sella turcica. **(A)** The endonasal speculum has been advanced through the left nostril and along the side of the nasal septum to the sphenoid. The straight ring breaks up the intracapsular contents of a suprasellar tumor, and the straight transsphenoidal suction tube aspirates tumor tissue from within the capsule. **(B)** The angled ring and angled suction tube are directed upward to remove the intracapsular contents of the suprasellar extension. **(C)** The angled ring and suction tube remove tumor tissue that extends into the parasellar region. **(D)** Placing a syringe on the curved and straight tubes, with the thumb covering the thumb hole, allows the tube to be used for irrigation inside the tumor capsule to soften, fragment, and remove tumor. A piece of red rubber catheter may be placed on the angled tubes for suction and irrigation inside the capsule of large tumors. (With permission from Rhoton AL Jr. Operative techniques and instrumentation for neurosurgery. Neurosurgery 2003;53:907–934.[2])

A series of tapered and rectangular brain spatulas should be available at the various operative sites (**Figs. 1–35, 1–36, 1–37**). Paired brain spatulas of the same size are frequently used for separating the edges of the sylvian fissure or a cortical incision, and a single spatula is commonly used for elevating the surface of the brain away from the cranial base, tentorium, or falx. A single spatula tapered from 15 to 25 mm at the base to 10 to 20 mm at the tip is commonly used for elevating the frontal or temporal lobes or the cerebellum for tumor removal. A spatula with a 10 mm base that tapers to a 3 mm tip is commonly used during operations for trigeminal neuralgia or hemifacial spasm.

The surgeon should learn to manipulate the retractor while looking through the microscope. The retractor should not be applied so firmly that it blanches the vessels on the surface of the brain and causes infarction of the underlying brain. Infarction occurs infrequently if blood pressure is normal; however, if induced hypotension is used intraoperatively, inadequate perfusion under the retractor may cause infarction and subsequent hemorrhage after the retractor is removed.

Drills

High-speed drills have replaced the trephine and Gigli's wire saw for removal of thick plates of bone. In the past, removal of thick plates of bone with rongeurs required great strength, but today, drills are commonly used to reduce the thickness of bone so that it can be removed gently without the use of great force (**Fig. 1–2**). A drill and its cutting attachments are commonly used during most operations for placing bur holes and evaluating bone flaps. Fine burs are also available for delicate tasks such as removing the wall of the internal acoustic meatus, the anterior clinoid process, part of the temporal bone, or protrusions of the cranial base (**Fig. 1–19D**). After a drill has reduced

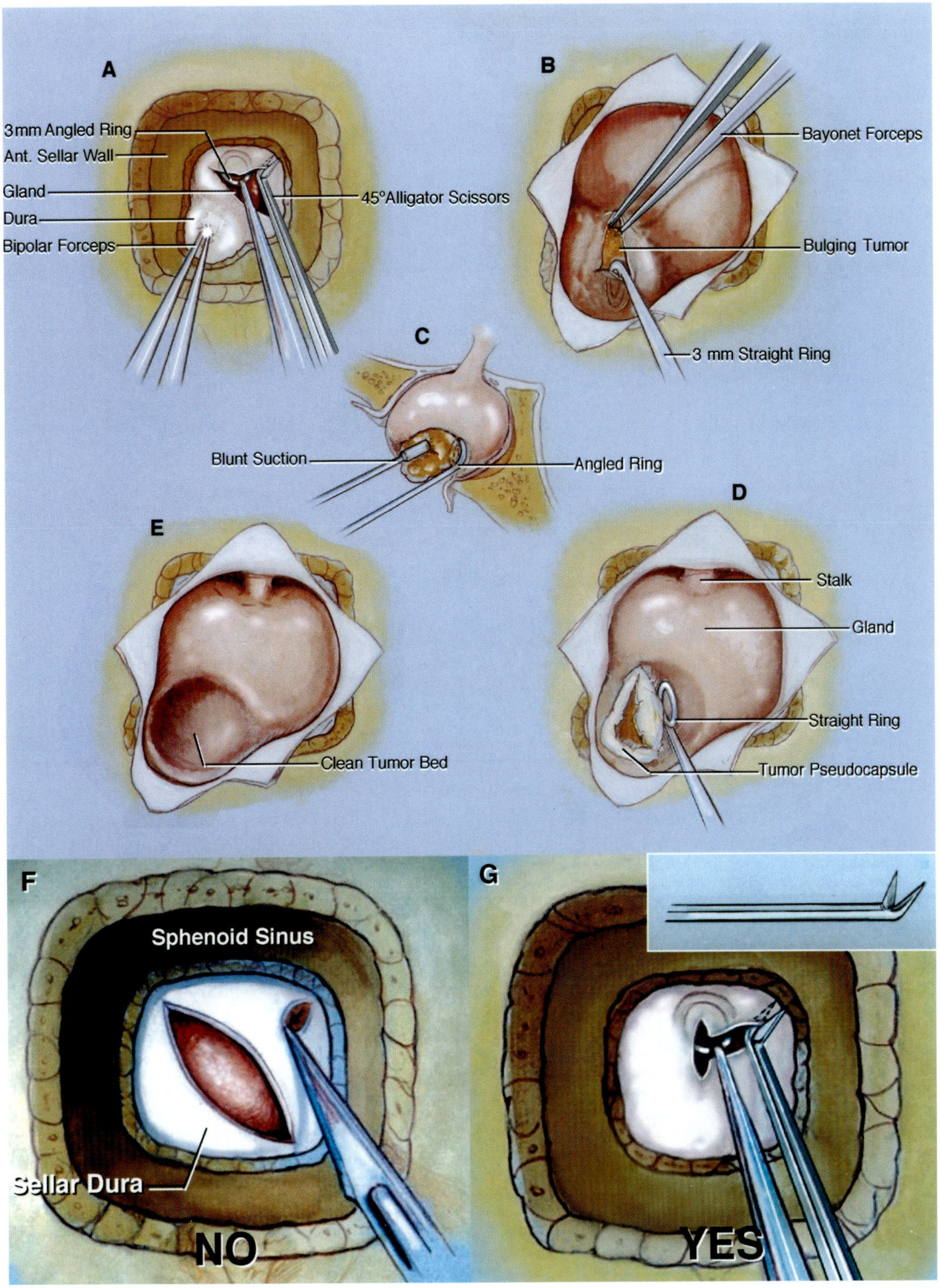

Figure 1–25 Steps in the removal of a microadenoma. **(A)** The sphenoid sinus and the anterior sellar wall have been opened. The thin bone and dura anterior to the tumor bulges in the inferior part of the right half of the sphenoid sinus. The bipolar forceps coagulate a vascular channel in the dura mater before the dura mater is opened. The dura is opened with a small vertical incision in the midline. A 3 mm angled ring, inserted through the vertical incision, separates the dura from the anterior surface of the gland. A 40 degree angled alligator scissors, inserted through the vertical dural incision, opens the dura from corner to corner. Incising the dura in the corners and lateral margins of the sellar opening with a sharp, pointed knife risks injury to the internal carotid arteries. **(B)** The bulge at the site of the tumor is opened with the tips of a bayonet forceps or a small straight ring. The initial opening into the gland and the tumor is enlarged with the small, straight ring curette. **(C)** Tumor tissue is removed from within the gland using the blunt-tip suction tube and the small-angled ring curettes. The center of the tumor is often soft and gelatinous. **(D)** The straight ring curette develops a cleavage plane between the firmer margin of tumor, which forms a pseudocapsule, and the gland. **(E)** The cavity within the gland, after removal of the tumor, is cleaned with irrigation. If the subarachnoid space was not opened during the procedure, a small tumor bed may be cleaned of tumor cells by placing small pledgets of cottonoid immersed in absolute alcohol in the tumor bed. **(F)**, **(G)**. Show that only an angled microscissors should be used for incision of the sellar dura.

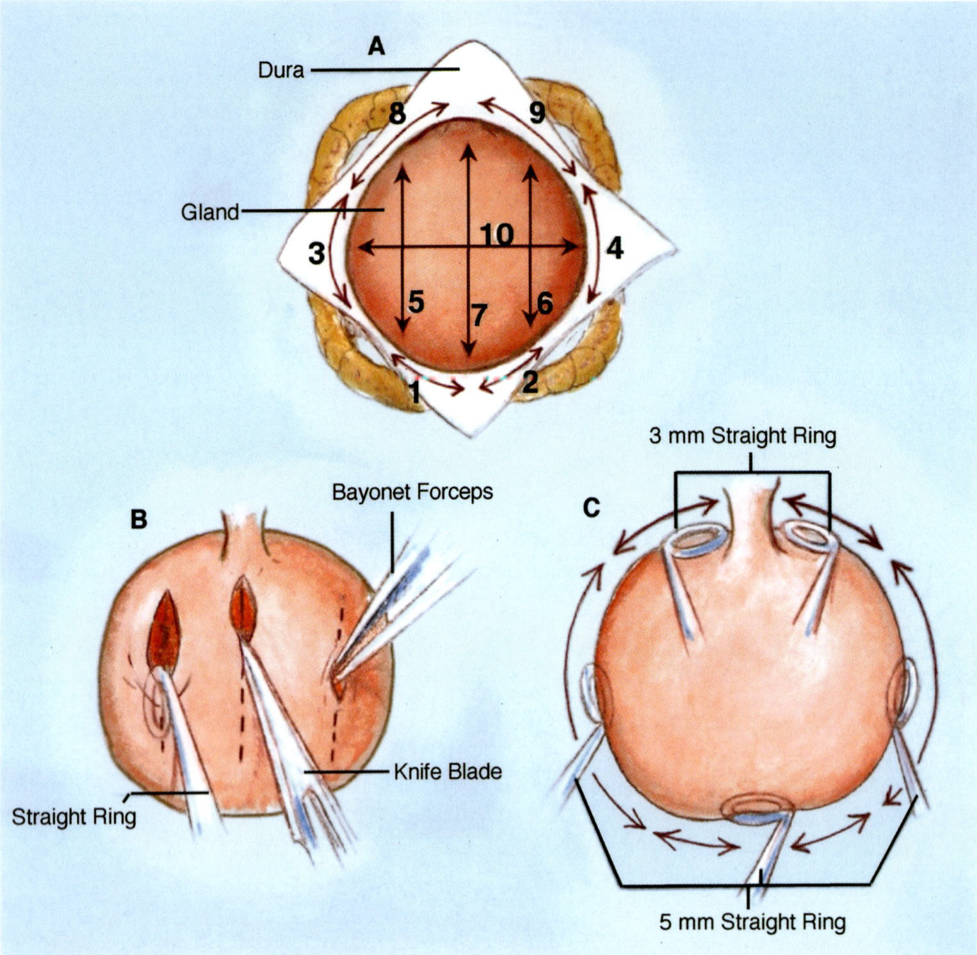

Figure 1–26 Steps in the exploration of the pituitary gland when a hypersecreting adenoma is known to be present but is not obvious upon initial exposure of the gland. The order in which these steps is performed should be selected so that the fewest steps are needed to find the tumor. If there are equivocal or clear-cut radiological findings or results from petrosal sinus sampling that suggest the tumor is confined to a specific part of the sella, the exploration should begin in that area. Knowledge of the most common locations of each type of microadenoma is helpful in selecting the area in which to begin the exploration. Tumors secreting growth hormone and prolactin commonly occur in the lateral aspect, and corticotropin-secreting tumors in the central part of the gland. **(A)** Anterior view of the gland with the dura mater opened. Steps in the exploration of the gland: (1) Separation of the inferior surface of the right half of the gland from the sellar floor. (2) Separation of the left half of the inferior surface of the gland from the sellar floor. (3) Separation of the right lateral surface of the gland from the medial wall of the cavernous sinus. (4) Separation of the left lateral surface of the gland from the medial wall of the cavernous sinus. (5) Vertical incision into the right half of the gland. The exploratory incisions into the gland are not carried through the superior, inferior, or lateral surfaces of the gland but are performed so as to preserve a margin of the gland at both ends of the incision. (6) Vertical incision into the left half of the gland. (7) Vertical incision into the midportion of the gland. (8) Separation of the superior surface of the right half of the gland from the diaphragm. (9) Separation of the superior surface of the left half of the gland from the diaphragm. (10) Transverse incision into the gland. **(B)** Methods of incising the gland. The openings in the gland can be started with a no. 11 knife blade or by introducing the closed tips of a pointed bayonet forceps into the surface of the gland and allowing the tips to open, splitting the gland. These incisions are enlarged with the 3 mm straight ring. **(C)** The arrows show the direction in which the straight ring curettes are slipped around the outer circumference of the gland to separate its surfaces from the sellar floor, the medial walls of the cavernous sinus, and the diaphragm. The 5 mm straight ring is used to separate the gland from the floor and medial walls of the cavernous sinus. The 3 mm straight ring is used to separate the superior surface of the gland from the diaphragm. Exploration of the superior surface of the gland is done as a late step to avoid entering the subarachnoid space and reduce the risk of cerebrospinal fluid leakage and injury to the pituitary stalk. Most microadenomas can be removed without disturbing the superior surface of the gland and without making an opening into the subarachnoid space. (With permission from Rhoton AL Jr. Operative techniques and instrumentation for neurosurgery. Neurosurgery 2003;53:907–934.[2])

Table 1–1 Recommended Suture Size in Relation to Vessel Size

Suture Size	Diameter Vessel (mm)	Example of Blood Vessel Size
6–0	5.0–6.0	Common carotid artery
7–0	4.0–5.0	Internal carotid or vertebral artery
8–0	3.0–4.0	Basilar and middle cerebral arteries
9–0	2.0–3.0	Anterior and posterior cerebral arteries
10–0	0.8–1.5	Sylvian and cortical arteries

Microsurgery Suture Diameters

Size	Microns
11–0	18
10–0	22
9–0	35
8–0	45

Source: By permission from Yaşargil MG. Suturing techniques. In: Yaşargil MG, ed. Microsurgery Applied to Neurosurgery. New York: Academic; 1969:51–58.

the thickness of an area such as the posterior lip of the internal acoustic meatus or anterior clinoid process, a microcurette or a Kerrison microrongeur with a 1 mm lip may be used to remove the remaining thin layer of bone (**Fig. 1–19E**).

For delicate bone work, a drill that can reverse its direction may be preferred to one that cuts in only one direction. Most electric drills, but only a few air drills, are reversible. When reversible drills are used, the operation should be planned so that the bur rotates away from critical structures; if skidding occurs, it will be away from these areas. Diamond burs are used near important structures. It is better for the surgeon to become acquainted with and skilled in the application of the drill in the laboratory before using it in a neurosurgical operation. Use of the drill can also be learned by assisting a surgeon experienced in its use before beginning its use under supervision of a skilled operator.

Drills are available that function at speeds from 10,000 to almost 100,000 rpm. At speeds greater than 25,000 rpm, the bone melts away so easily that the drill poorly transmits the tactile details of bony structure to the surgeon's hand. Slower speeds may be used for delicate procedures in which tactical control of the drill is important. A diamond bit is preferable for the most delicate bone removal.

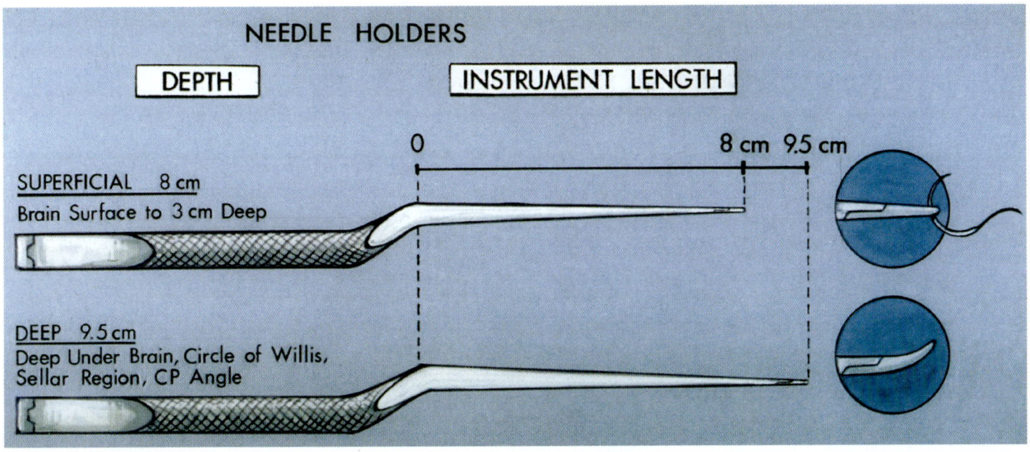

Figure 1–27 Rhoton bayonet needle holders with round handles. The bayonet needle holders with 8 cm shafts are used at the surface of the brain and down to a depth of 3 cm. The needle holders with 9.5 cm shafts are used deep under the brain at the level of the circle of Willis, the suprasellar region, and the cerebellopontine (CP) angle. Needle holders with straight and curved tips (round insets) may be needed. The straight needle holders shown in **Fig. 1–8** may also be used at the surface of the brain.

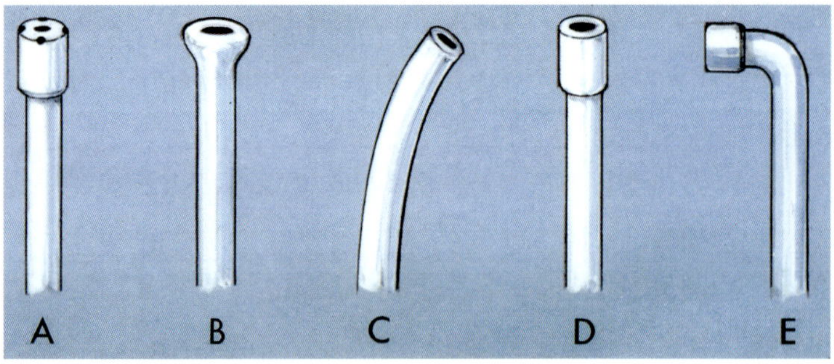

Figure 1–28 Different types of suction tubes. **(A)** Yankauer type suction tube with a blunt tip. This tip is commonly used in general surgery. **(B)** Dandy suction tube with a blunt tip. **(C)** Curved tip on Adson suction tube. The distal tip of the Adson suction tube is oriented obliquely to the long axis of the shaft. **(D)** Straight blunt tip for neurosurgery. **(E)** Angled blunt suction tubes for transsphenoidal surgery.

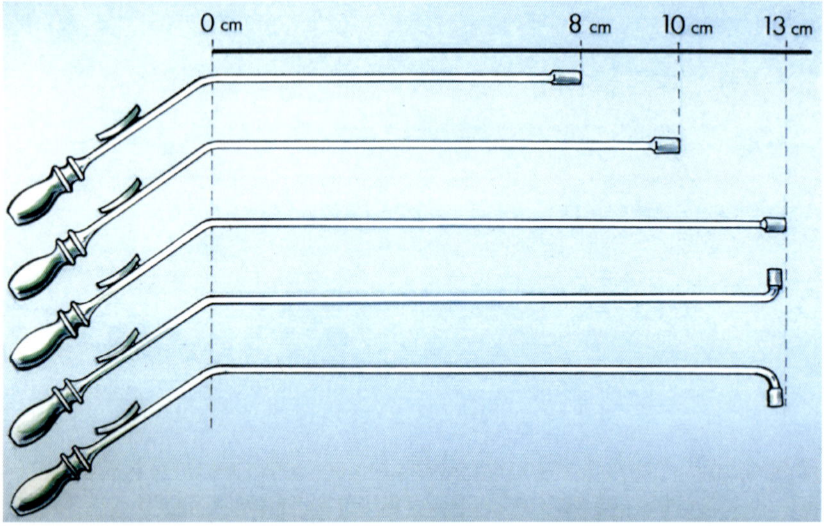

Figure 1–29 Rhoton-Merz suction tubes of the three lengths needed for superficial, deep, and transsphenoidal or extra deep neurosurgery. The 8 cm tube is used during the opening of the cranium and at superficial intracranial sites. The 10 cm tube is used for deep intracranial sites, as around the circle of Willis, the suprasellar area, and the cerebellopontine angle. The 13 cm tube is used at extra deep sites, as in front of the brain stem and for transsphenoidal operations. The transsphenoidal suction tubes have straight, angled up, and angled down tips in each of the 5, 7, and 10 French sizes.

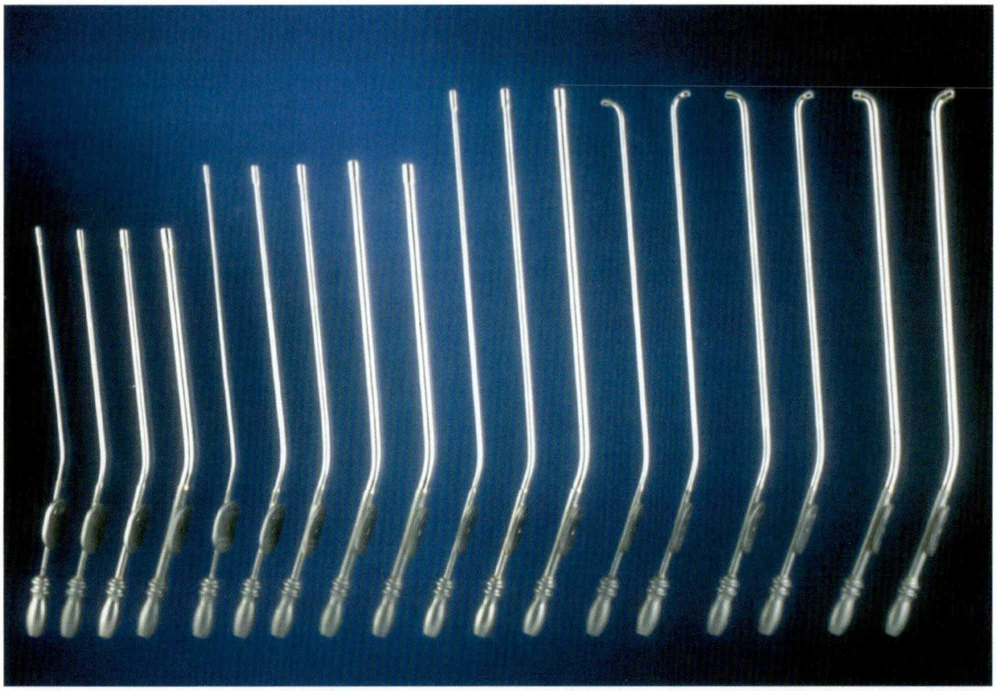

Figure 1–30 Complete set of suction tubes for macroneurosurgery and microneurosurgery. The four short tubes (8 cm shaft) on the left have diameters of 3, 5, 7, and 10 French and are used at superficial sites. The five longer tubes (10 cm shaft) in the center have diameters of 3, 5, 7, 10, and 12 French and are used at deep sites. The set of nine longest tubes (13 cm shaft) on the right have three diameters (5, 7, and 10 French) and three tip configurations: straight, angled up, and angled down tips. They are used at extra deep sites and for transsphenoidal operations. The angled tubes are used for transsphenoidal operations.

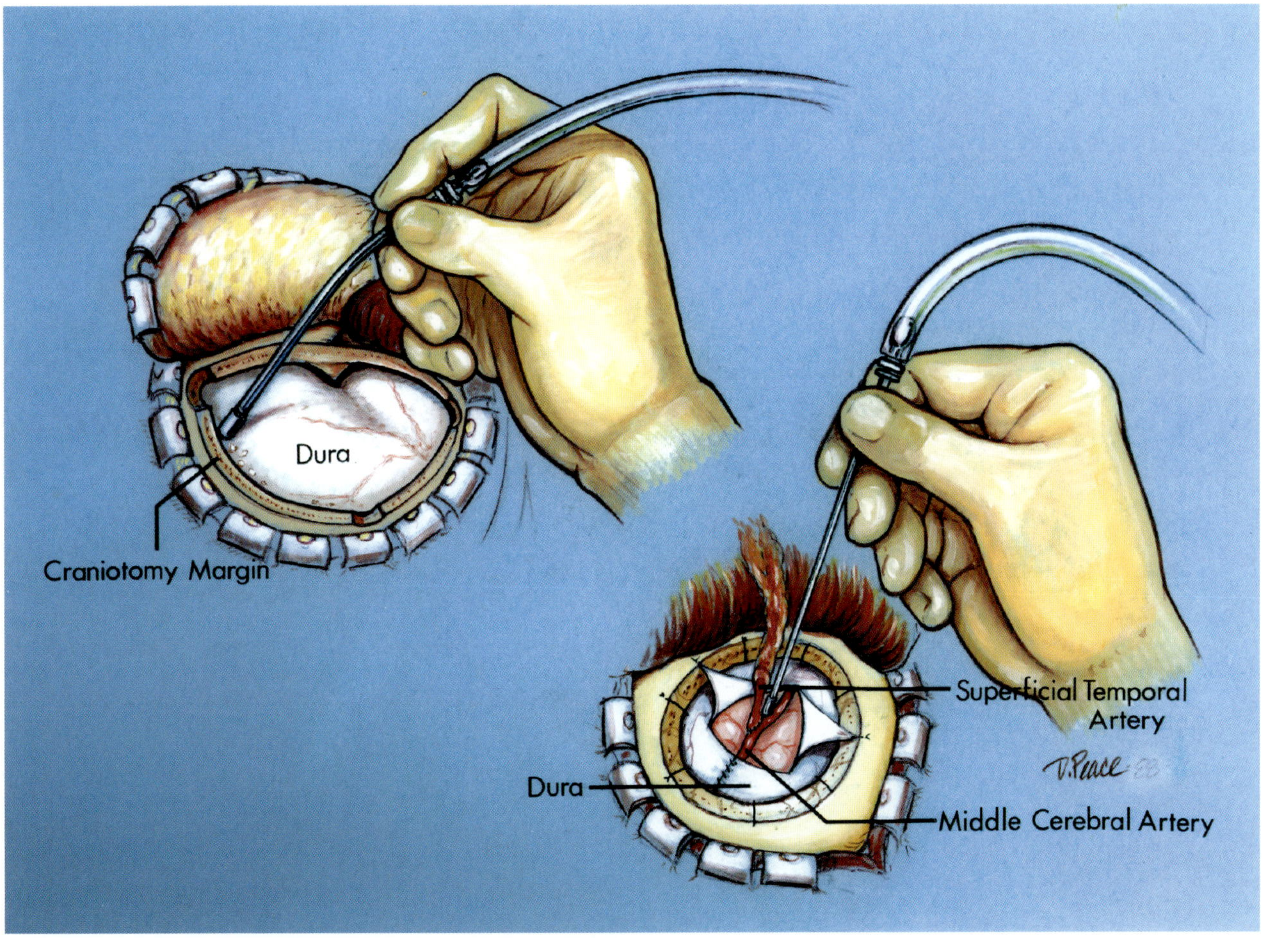

Figure 1–31 The short tubes (8 cm shafts) are used for suction when turning a bone flap or during other operations near the surface of the brain. When held in a pencil grip for suction near the surface of the brain, the short tubes permit the hand to be rested on the wound margin and the tip to be manipulated by delicate finger movements. Use of a longer tube or a tube held in a pistol grip would not allow the hand to be rested on the wound margin. The short tube (upper left) with a large diameter (10 French) is used for aspirating bone dust and heavy bleeding while elevating a craniotomy flap. The short tube (lower right) with the narrowest diameter (3 French) is used for suction in the area of a superficial temporal to middle cerebral artery bypass; a larger suction tube could injure the vessels or disrupt the suture line. (With permission from Rhoton AL Jr. Operative techniques and instrumentation for neurosurgery. Neurosurgery 2003;53:907–934.)

The drill is held like a pen. Cutting is done with the side rather than with the end of the bur except when making small calibrated holes for placement of sutures or screws at the margin of a bone flap. A large bur is used when possible. The greatest accuracy and control of the drill are obtained at higher speeds if a light brush action is used to remove the bone. Dangerous skidding may ensue at lower speeds because greater pressure is needed to cut the bone. The surgeon avoids running the bur across bone by using light, intermittent pressure rather than constant pressure of the bur on one spot. Overheating near nerves may damage them. Constant irrigation with physiological saline reduces heat transmission to the bone and nearby neural structures and prevents heat necrosis of bone. Directing irrigating fluid toward the bur ensures optimal cleaning of the bur while it irrigates the operating field. The field may also be irrigated by the use of a suction-irrigation system. The teeth of the bur should be kept clean of bone dust. A coarse bur that clogs less easily is harder to control and skids across bone more easily, but this is reduced with irrigation. A bur should not be used to make a long, deep hole, but rather the hole should be beveled and as wide open as possible to ensure visibility. The surgeon should use a small curette to follow a small track rather than pursuing it with a drill. Bone dust should be meticulously removed because of its potent osteogenic properties.

Bone Curettes

Small curettes are frequently used for removing the last shell of bone between a drill surface and neural or vascular structures. Straight and angled curettes are needed (**Figs. 1–17, 1–18A, 1–19B,F,J**). Curettes angled at 45 degrees are frequently used for special purposes, such as removing the last thin shell of bone over the internal acoustic meatus or curetting a fragment of tumor from the lateral margin of the

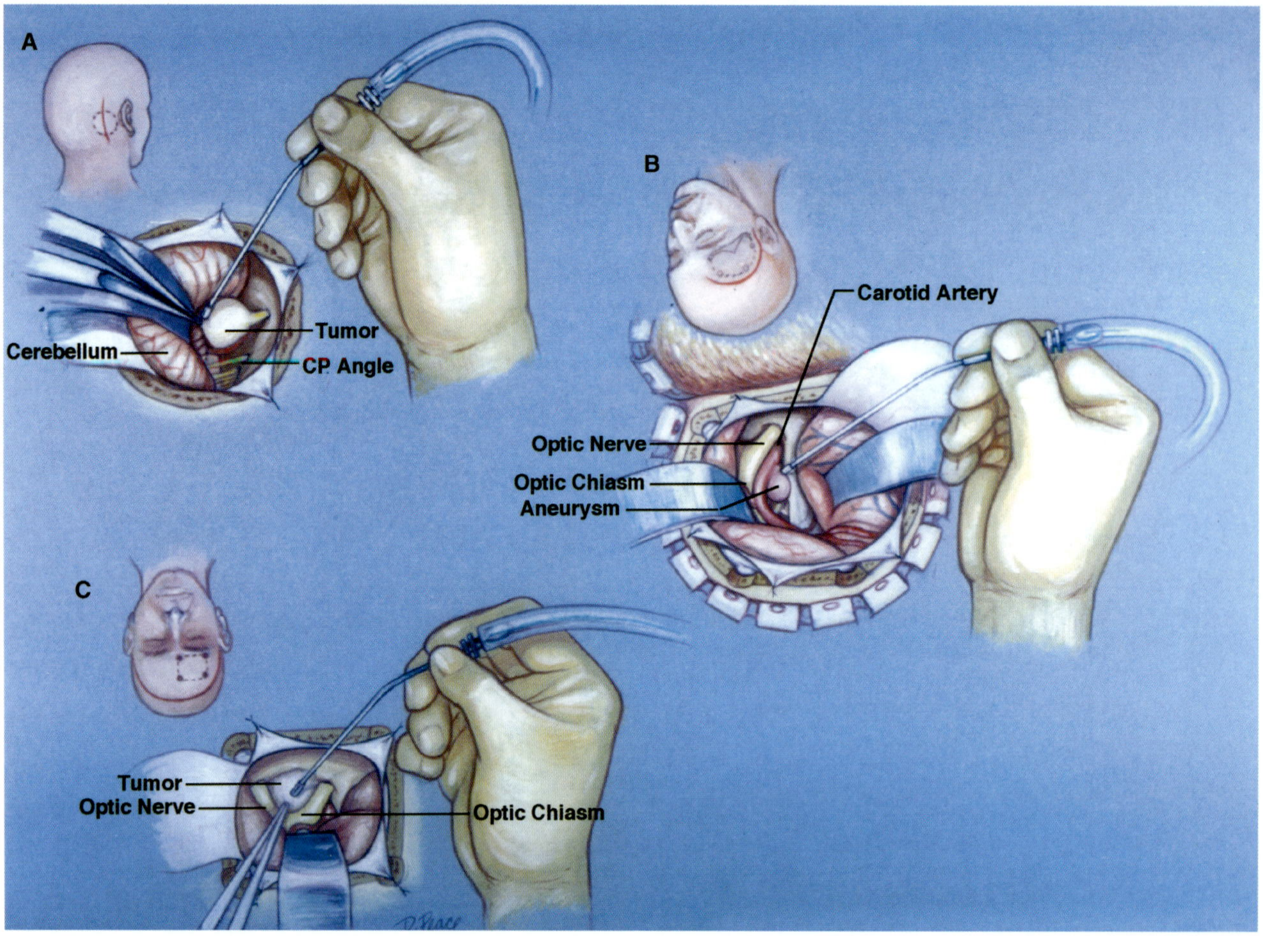

Figure 1–32 Suction tubes with a 10 cm shaft are used in deep intracranial operations in the cerebellopontine angle (CP), suprasellar region, and around the circle of Willis. The smaller drawings, show the scalp incisions (solid line) and the craniectomy or craniectomy sites (dotted line), and the larger drawings show the operative sites. **(A)** The 10 cm suction tube aids in exposing a tumor in the right cerebellopontine angle. **(B)** The 10 cm suction tube aspirates tumor from within the capsule of a suprasellar tumor. **(C)** The 10 cm suction tube aspirates clot and aids in dissection of the neck for an aneurysm arising on the internal carotid artery.

acoustic meatus, or other areas on the cranial base. Curettes with tips as small as 1.5 mm are frequently needed. The curette is held so that the cutting edge is in full view. Cutting is done, when possible, with the side rather than the tip. Pressure should be directed parallel to or away from important structures rather than perpendicularly toward them. Properly sharpened curettes cut with less pressure and are safer than dull ones. The surgeon should try to use the largest curette that can do the job.

Cup Forceps

A cup forceps such as that used for intravertebral disk removal is commonly used for removal of tumors (**Figs. 1–16, 1–19I,K**). The most frequently used cup forceps have a tip 3, 4, or 5 mm wide, which is suitable for the intracapsular removal of large tumors. For removal of small tumors or small fragments of tumor in critical locations, such as on the cranial nerves, in the acoustic meatus, or within the fourth ventricles, cup forceps with a diameter

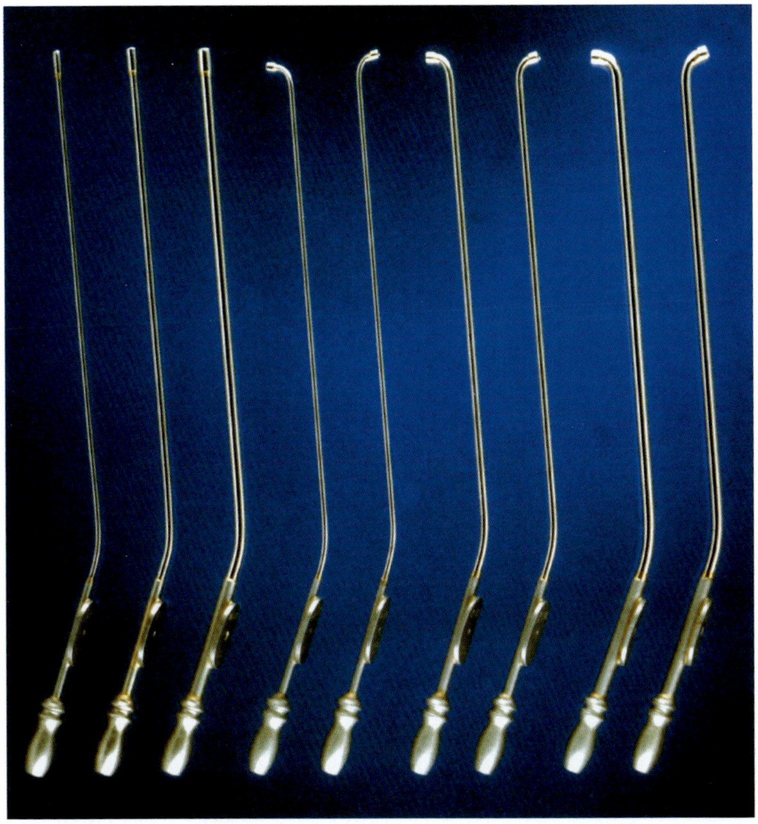

Figure 1–33 Rhoton-Merz suction tubes for transsphenoidal operations. The transsphenoidal tubes have a 13 cm shaft and are of three sizes: 5, 7, and 10 French. They have straight, angled up, and angled down tips in each of the three sizes. (With permission from Rhoton AL Jr. Operative techniques and instrumentation for neurosurgery. Neurosurgery 2003;53:907–934.)

of 1 to 2 mm are used. For grasping small bits of tumor directly on or within the cranial nerves, the 1 mm cup forceps is used. The 2, 3, and 4 mm cups are suitable for the intracapsular removal of small tumors. Angled microcup forceps enable the surgeon to reach around a corner to grasp tissue or remove tumor. A cup forceps angled to the right is used to reach laterally to the right (e.g., to reach a right parasellar extension of a pituitary adenoma or behind the facial and acoustic nerves in the right acoustic meatus), and the cup forceps angled to the left is used on the left side (**Fig. 1–19K**). The angled cup forceps can also be used to reach to either side of a small capsular opening for intracapsular removal or for reaching laterally into an intervertebral foramen for disk removal.

Table 1–2 Uses for Suction Tubes

Diameter[a]	Use
3 French	Smallest nerves, vessel anastomosis
5 French	Aneurysm neck, pituitary gland, medium nerves
7 French	Microsurgical resection of larger tumors
10–12 French	Heavy bleeding, bone dust, flap elevation

[a]3 French = 1 mm outer diameter.

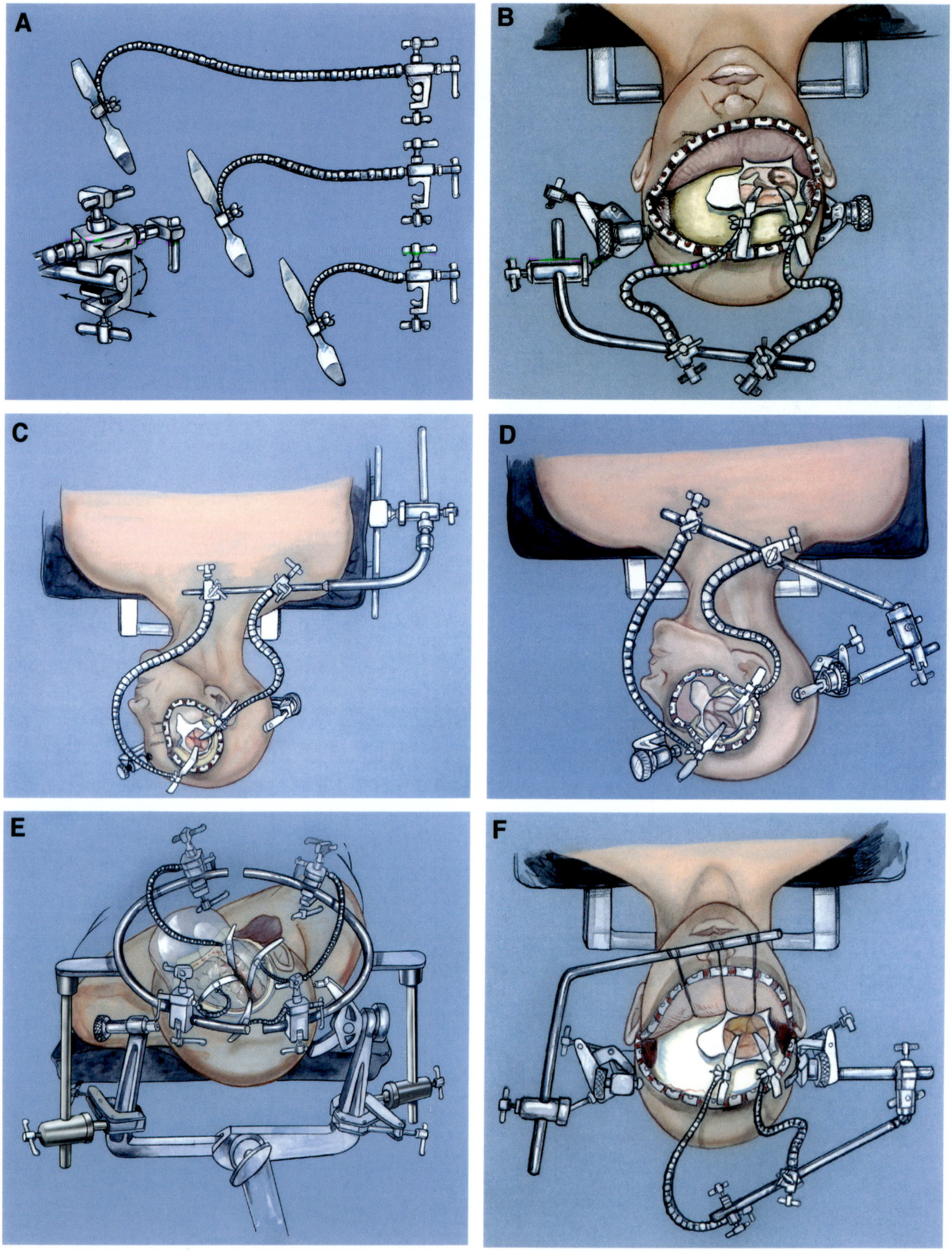

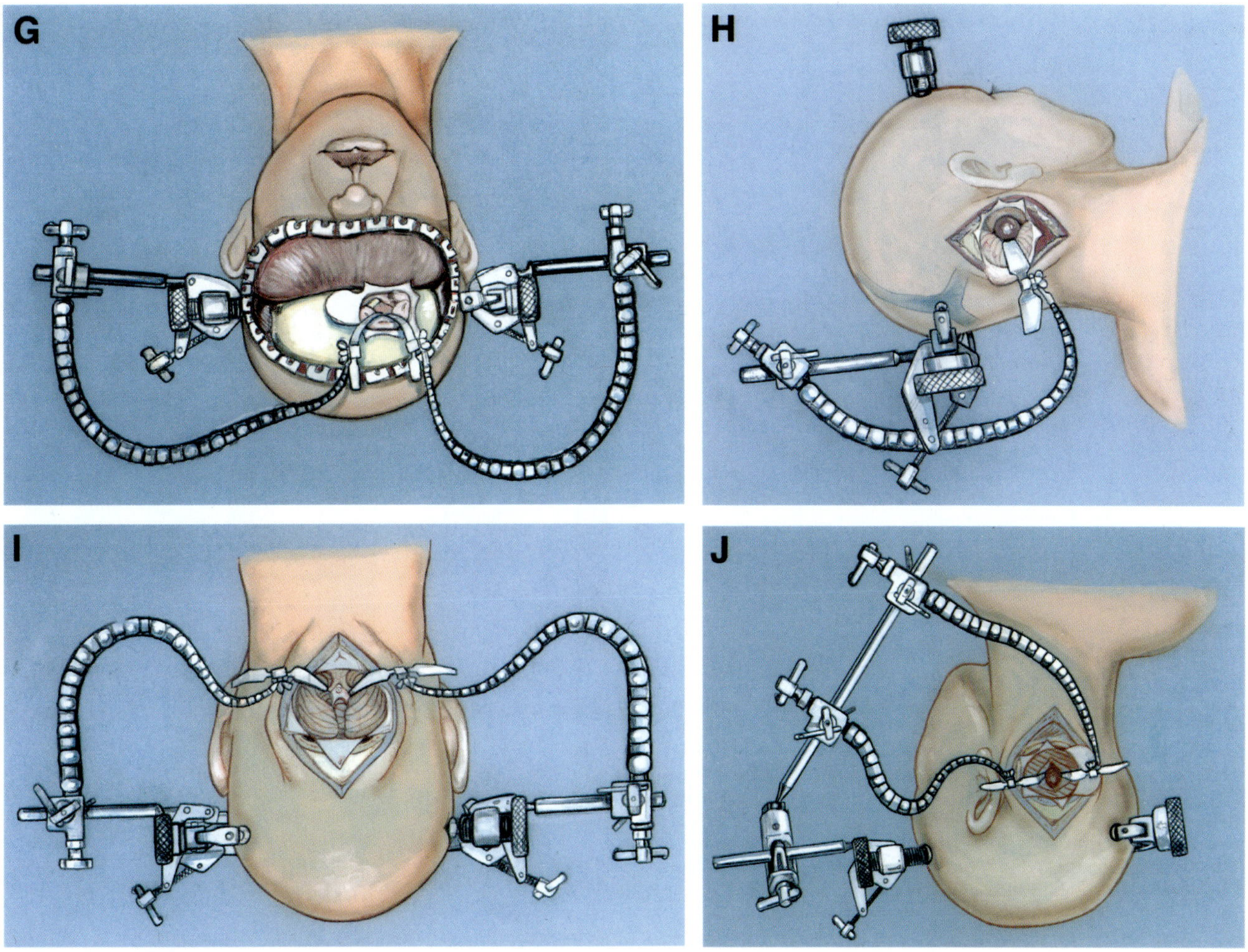

Figure 1–34 Self-retaining retractor system developed by Rhoton and Merz (V. Mueller, Chicago, IL). **(A)** The flexible arms that hold the brain spatulas are composed of a series of ball and sockets that resemble a string of pearls. The arms are tapered by having the largest "pearls" near the site where the arms attach to a stabilizing bar and the smallest "pearls" near the tip that holds the brain spatula. The system includes short (20 cm), medium (30 cm), and long (48 cm) flexible arms. The flexible arms are attached to the stabilizing bar by a coupling that allows the arms to slide and rotate on the bar (lower left). The site of attachment of the flexible arm to the coupling can also be rotated through 360 degrees for greater flexibility in positioning the flexible arms. The handles used to tighten the flexible arms and joints are broad and flat rather than being small and round as found on some systems. The broad, flat handles aid in adjustment of the arms and joints. **(B)** The system may be attached to the pinion head holder or to the rail on the side of the operating table. In this illustration, a curved bar attached to the pinion headrest holds the flexible arms for elevation of the frontal lobe. **(C)** A long bar attached to the operating table holds the flexible arms for opening the sylvian fissure. **(D)** A joined bar attached to the pinion headrest holds the flexible arms for separating the margins of the sylvian fissure. **(E)** Two semicircular bars, attached by C-clamps to the pinion headrest, form a halo or ring around the craniotomy site that holds the flexible arms for splitting the sylvian fissure. **(F)** The jointed bar, attached to the right side of the pinion head holder, serves as the site of attachment of the flexible arms for elevating the frontal lobe. A bar attached to the left side of the head holder serves as the site of attachment for the scalp retractors. **(G)** The flexible arms are attached directly to the clamps on the pinion head holder for elevation of the frontal lobe. **(H)** A flexible arm is attached to the clamp on the pinion head holder for removal of an acoustic neuroma. **(I)** The flexible arms are attached to the clamp on the pinion head holder for separation of the cerebellar tonsils. **(J)** The jointed bar holds the flexible arms for separation of the edges of an incision in the cerebellar hemisphere. (With permission from Rhoton AL Jr. Operative techniques and instrumentation for neurosurgery. Neurosurgery 2003;53:907–934.)

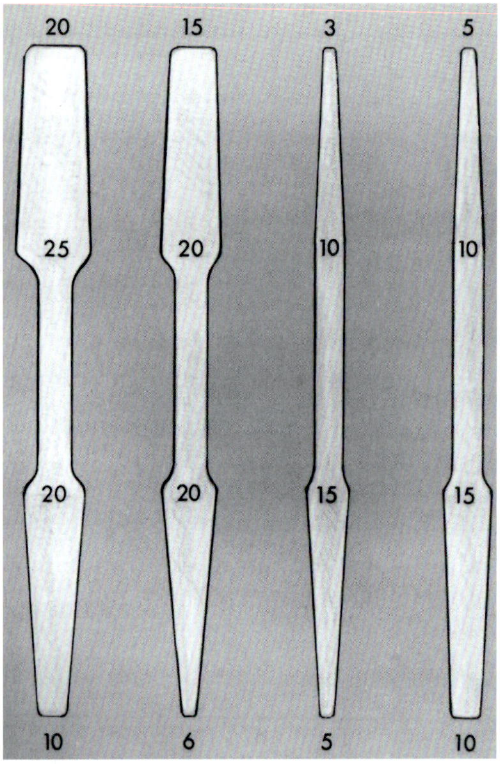

Figure 1–35 Rhoton tapered brain spatulas of various widths. Spatulas of different widths may be needed depending on the site and size of the lesion. A spatula tapered from 10 or 20 mm at the base to 5 to 15 mm at the tip is commonly selected for separating the margins of the sylvian fissure, elevating the frontal or temporal lobe, or exposing lesions in the posterior fossa. A brain spatula tapered from 10 mm at the base to 3 or 5 mm at the tip is commonly selected for operations for trigeminal neuralgia or hemifacial spasm. A brain spatula with a 20 or 25 mm base and a 15 or 20 mm tip commonly serves for acoustic neuroma removal.

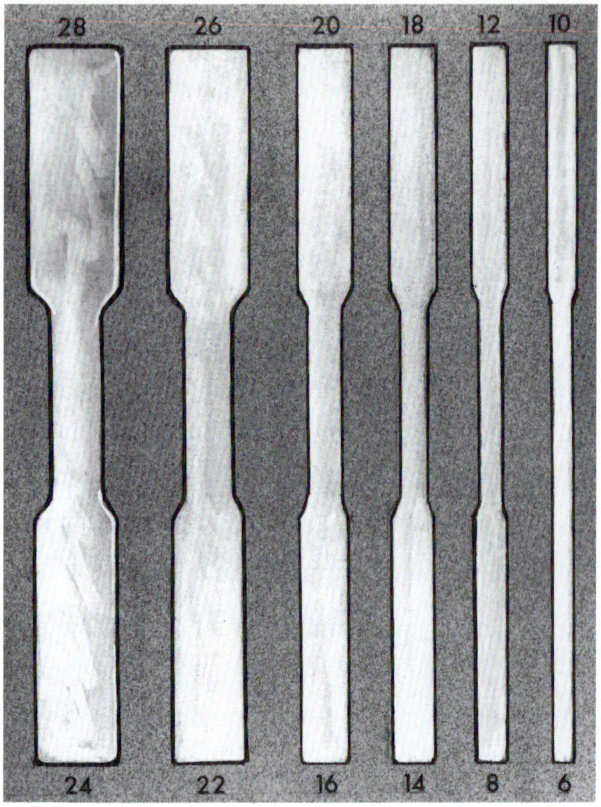

Figure 1–36 Rhoton rectangular brain spatulas in a range of widths from 6 to 28 mm. Opposing brain spatulas of almost the same size are commonly used when opening the sylvian fissure or fourth ventricle or when exposing lesions in the cerebral or cerebellar hemispheres. Each end of the brain spatulas has a different width. The widths of the two ends of the spatulas are arranged so that the next smaller and larger sizes, which could serve as an opposing retractor, are not on the opposite end of the same spatula but are instead on a different spatula.

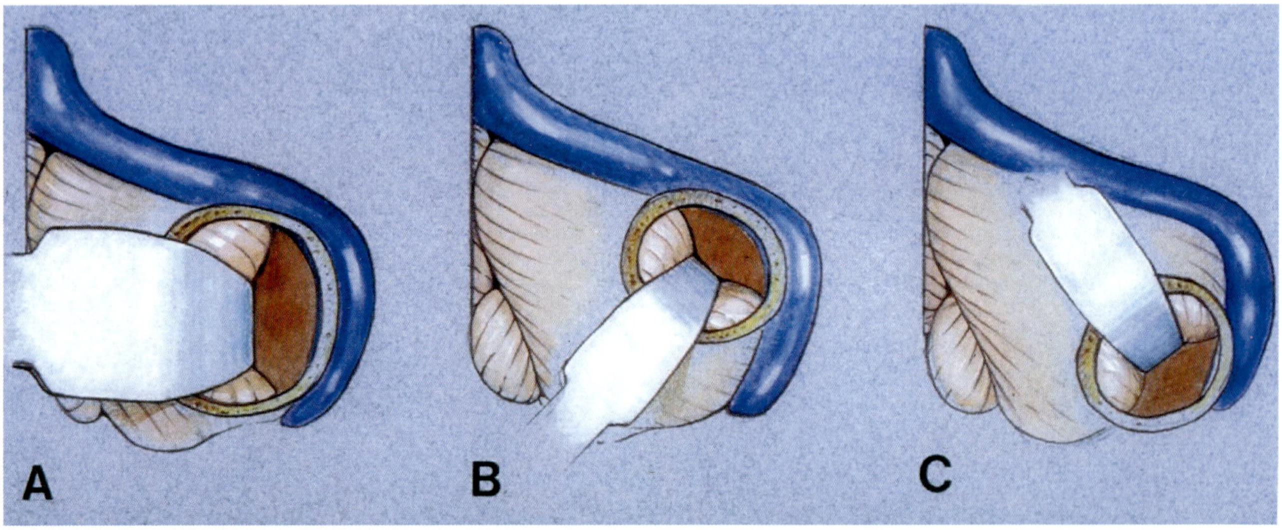

Figure 1–37 Direction of application of brain spatulas for surgery in the various compartments of the cerebellopontine angle. **(A)** Retractor application for exposing a lesion in the midportion of the cerebellopontine angle. The craniotomy is situated below the transverse sinus and medial to the sigmoid sinus. A brain spatula tapered from 20 or 25 mm at the base to 15 mm or 20 mm at the tip, depending on the size of the tumor, is commonly selected for elevation of the lateral surface of the cerebellum for acoustic neuroma removal. **(B)** Retractor application for exposing the superolateral compartment of the posterior fossa for a vascular decompression operation for treating trigeminal neuralgia. A spatula tapered from 10 mm at the base to 3 mm at the tip is commonly selected. **(C)** Retractor application for exposure of the inferolateral compartment of the posterior fossa as for an operation for hemifacial spasm or glossopharyngeal neuralgia. A brain spatula tapered from 10 mm at the base to 3 mm at the tip is commonly used for operations for hemifacial spasm. (With permission from Rhoton AL Jr. The cerebellopontine angle and posterior fossa cranial nerves by the retrosigmoid approach. Neurosurgery 2000;47(Suppl 1):S93–S129.)

◆ Operating Microscope

The use of the operating microscope and microsurgical techniques has disadvantages. Use of the microscope requires training and a shift away from a tactile-manual technique using fingers to one that relies on vision-oriented instruments (**Fig. 1–38**). The equipment is moderately expensive and requires added space in the operating room, and its care places an added burden on the nursing staff. It has been speculated that by prolonging some procedures, microsurgical techniques may increase the risks of anesthesia and infection. However, by allowing operations to be done through smaller openings and by permitting increasing accuracy of dissection, microsurgical techniques may reduce the duration of the procedure.

Performing operations with loupes (i.e., magnifying lenses attached to eyeglasses) is a form of microsurgery. Loupes are an improvement over the naked eye, but even

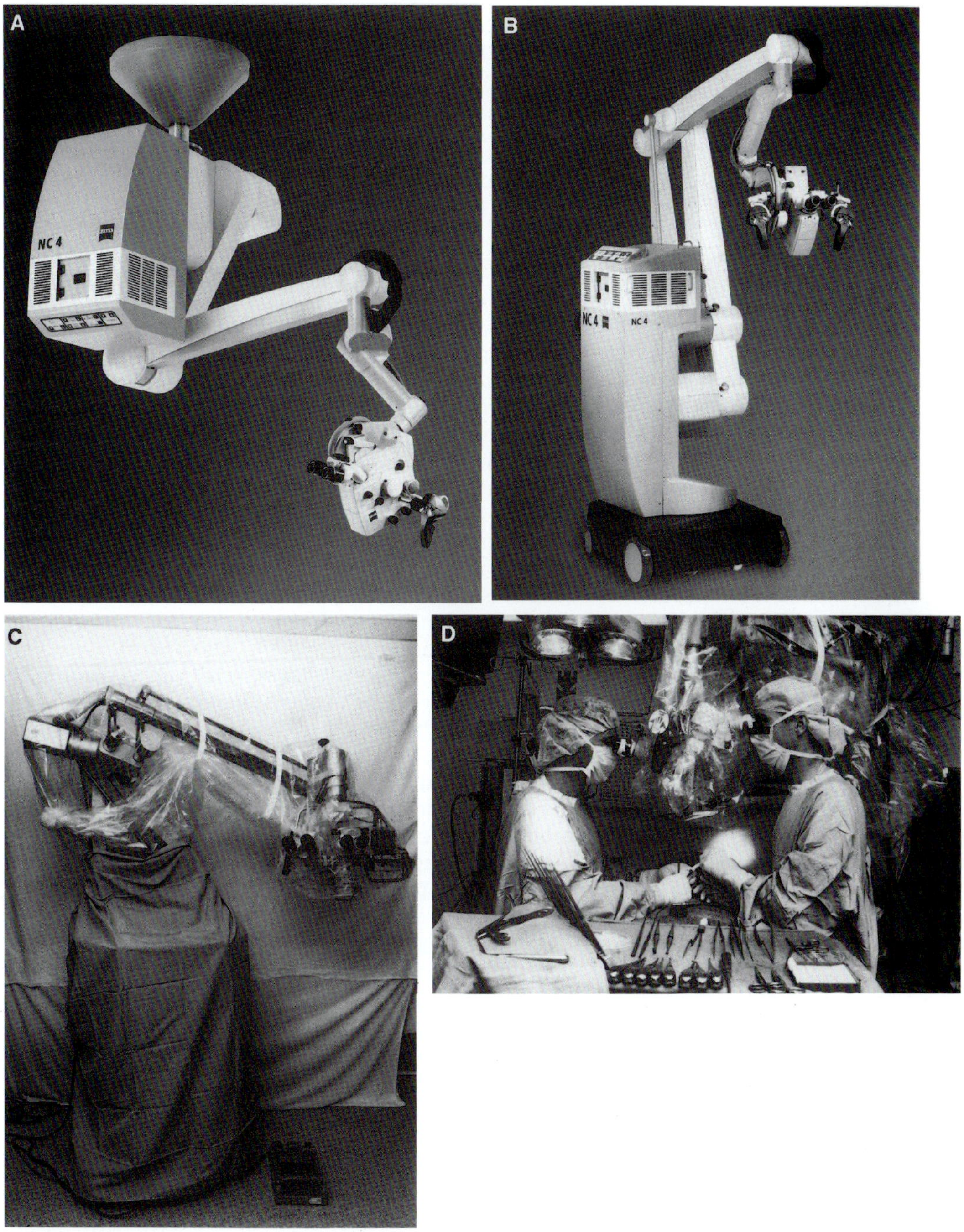

Figure 1–38 Microscope mounts. **(A)** Zeiss NC4 microscope mounted on the ceiling. **(B)** Zeiss motorized microscope on a floor stand. **(C)** Motorized zoom microscope draped for surgery. The motorized functions are controlled by foot switches on the floor or by switches on the handles beside the microscope body. **(D)** Microscope being used for a spinal operation. The surgeon is on the left. The assistant, on the right, has a binocular viewing tube.

(*Continued on page 40*)

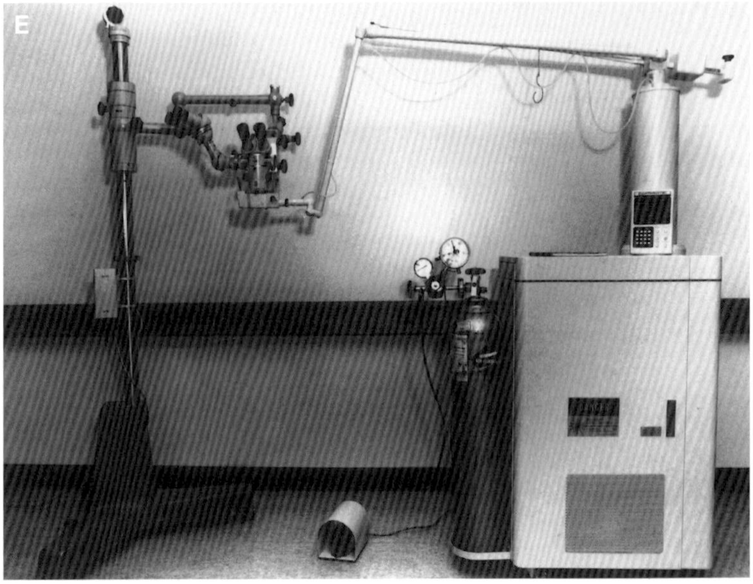

(*Continued*) **Figure 1–38** Microscope mounts. **(E)** Carbon dioxide laser coupled to the operating microscope. The laser is activated by a foot switch. The power output and length of exposure are determined by settings on the control console. The site of impact of the beam is moved about using the straight lever to the left of the objective lens. The beam is delivered to the target using a series of deflecting mirrors that are located inside articulating tubular arms, which are coupled mechanically to the microscope.

when combined with a headlight, they lack many of the advantages of the microscope. Most surgeons are unable to use loupes that provide more than two to three times magnification, the lower limit of resolution provided by the operating microscope. For craniotomy, many surgeons use loupes during the initial part of the operation and bring the microscope into the operative field just before or after opening the dura mater.

Only when the surgeon has acquired proficiency in the use of the microscope should operations be undertaken. Clinical microtechnique should be applied first to procedures with which the surgeon is entirely familiar, such as excision of ruptured disks, before its use is expanded to new and technically more difficult procedures. Early in their experience with the microscope, surgeons tend to use it in less demanding situations and to discontinue its use when they encounter hemorrhage or problems of unusual complexity. Increasing experience, however, makes it apparent that bleeding is more accurately and quickly stopped and usually of lesser magnitude in operations using magnification.

The surgeon should be knowledgeable about the basic optical and mechanical principles of the operating microscope; the common types of mechanical illumination and electrical failure that affect it and how to correct them; and the selection of lenses, eyepieces, binocular tubes, light sources, stands, and accessories for different operations (**Fig. 1–38**). The laboratory provides a setting in which the mental and physical adjustments required for doing microsurgery can be mastered. Training in the laboratory is essential before the surgeon undertakes microanastomotic procedures on patients (e.g., superficial temporal to middle cerebral artery anastomosis). These techniques cannot be learned by watching others do them; they must be perfected on specimens of cerebral vessels taken at autopsy and on animals.

Using the microscope for dissection of tissues taken from cadavers or at autopsy may increase the surgeon's skill (**Fig. 1–39**). The performance of temporal bone dissection in the laboratory is an accepted component of the microsurgical training for otological operations, and such exercises are of value to the neurosurgeon. The surgeon may gain skill in procedures in the cerebellopontine angle by dissecting temporal bone specimens and in transsphenoidal operations by dissecting sphenoid and sellar blocks.[17,18] A detailed microscopic exploration of the perforating branches of the circle of Willis and other common sites of aneurysm occurrence may improve the surgeon's technique with aneurysms. As the need arises, other selected specimens may also be used to increase the surgeon's acquaintance with other operative sites, such as the jugular foramen, cavernous sinus, pineal region, or ventricles.

The surgical nurse plays an especially important role in microneurosurgery.[19] The nurse should make a constant effort to reduce the number of times the surgeon looks away from the microscope and to limit any distraction. The scrub nurse may need to guide the surgeon's hands to the operative field. Communication between the nurse and the surgeon can be facilitated by a television system that allows the nurse to view the operative field displayed on a nearby monitor and to place the proper instrument in the surgeon's hands without obliging the surgeon to look away from the microscope (**Fig. 1–1**). The nurse should be skilled in the operation and maintenance of the microscope; be able to balance and prepare it for the particular operation, including selecting the appropriate lenses; and be able to prepare it for use with the patient in the supine, prone, or sitting position. The nursing staff should also be able to drape the microscope quickly and deal with commonly encountered mechanical and electronic malfunctions. The circulating nurse must be immediately available to adjust the bipolar coagulator and suction, rapidly change the microscope bulb or other light source, replace clouded or dirty objective lenses or eyepieces, and adjust all foot pedals and controls for the microscope. The nurse should record the surgeon's eyepiece settings so that all replacement eyepieces are properly adjusted for use.

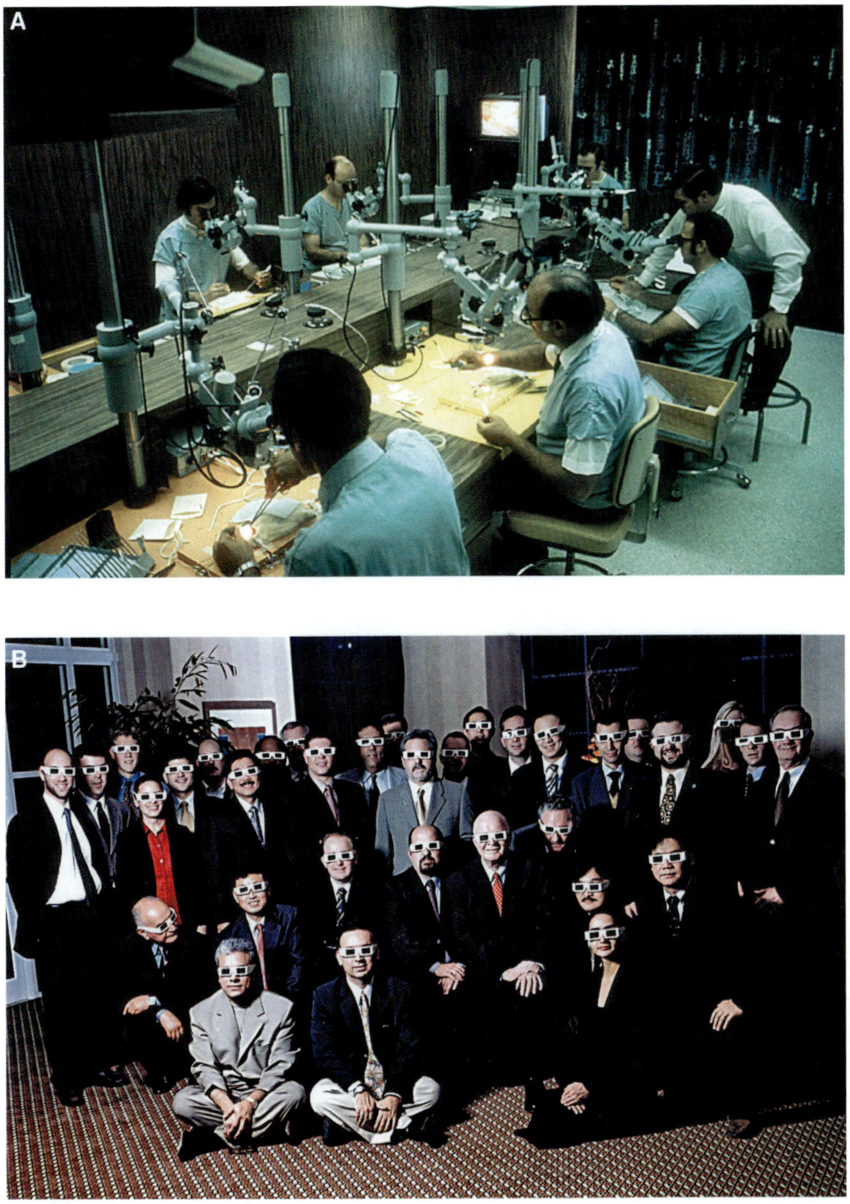

Figure 1–39 **(A)** Participants working at the first microneurosurgery course held at the University of Florida in 1975. **(B)** Participants from a recent course held at the McKnight Brain Institute at the University of Florida in 3-D stereo glasses; 3-D presentations have become an increasingly important part of the courses.

Developments in frameless stereotaxic surgery permit the microscope to function as part of a stereotactic surgical system. An infrared localizing system for the microscope, when combined with digitization of the angle of view and the focal length, enables the surgeon to simultaneously view a reconstructed magnetic resonance or computed tomography scan that can match the focal point of the image seen through the microscope. The surgeon knows exactly where the focal point of the image being viewed in the microscope is located in relation to the normal and pathological structures seen on computed tomography and magnetic resonance imaging.

◆ Ultrasonic and Laser Dissection

Alternatives to the use of cup forceps and suction for tumor removal are the ultrasonic and laser dissection units. The latter instruments are applied with the greatest degree of accuracy when guided by the magnified vision provided by the operating microscope. They are most commonly used to debulk tumors. The ultrasonic aspirator is preferred over the laser because it can remove tumor tissue more rapidly. Tumor removal with the laser proceeds much more slowly. Neither instrument should be used to remove small fragments of tumor on the surface of vessels or nerves. A special application of the laser is to coagulate the attachment of a tumor to the skull base, but the author feels this has no significant advantage over carefully applied bipolar coagulation.

Ultrasonic Aspirators

Ultrasonic aspirators enjoy wider usage than the laser because of their ability to rapidly debulk large tumors, but they must be used with extreme care because they can quickly open through the surface of a tumor capsule and damage vessels and nerves that are adherent to the surface of the tumor. The aspirators are commonly used for the removal of large tumors. These vibrating suction devices fragment and aspirate tumor tissue. These units have a control console that regulates the amount of irrigation and suction to the hand piece and the vibration of the cutting tip. They are suitable for fragmenting firm tumors such as meningiomas, acoustic neuromas, and some gliomas. They rapidly debulk the center of all but the most calcified tumors. They are commonly used to debulk a neoplasm rapidly, after which the capsule is removed from nerves and vessels using fine dissecting instruments. These devices do not control bleeding, although some are designed to allow coagulation to be applied through the tip.

Laser Microsurgery

The fact that a laser beam can be focused to a fine point makes it an ideal tool to be directed by a magnified vision of the operating microscope (**Fig. 1–38**). The carbon dioxide laser, the one most commonly utilized in neurosurgery, can be used freehand, but it is more commonly linked to the operating microscope by means of a direct mechanical or electromechanical manipulator. The beam from the carbon dioxide laser is invisible and must be identified by a coincident pilot helium-neon laser. The carbon dioxide and helium-neon beams must be absolutely coaxial; if not, error will result in the direction of the destructive carbon dioxide beam. The carbon dioxide laser energy is immediately absorbed by and vaporizes tissues containing fluid. Because the beam cannot pass through fluid, its maximal effect is on the surface. The vaporized tissue is removed by a routine suction system.

The carbon dioxide laser is most commonly used for the removal of extra-axial tumors. The basic actions of incision, coagulation, and vaporization of tissue are a function of the amount of energy measured in terms of watts applied to tissue. Lower wattages are used for coagulation, and higher wattages are used for incision and removal of tissue. The radiant energy is manipulated by altering the variables of power input, length of exposure, and surface area of the impact site. The beam is turned on by depressing a foot switch, and the power and length of exposure are determined by settings on the control console. The micromanipulator for directing the site of impact of the beam is a straight lever situated near the objective lens of the microscope.

It is best to begin with low power and increase the power as the situation dictates. The cross-sectional area of the impact zone is increased by defocusing the beam. Shortening the times of exposure tends to reduce buildup of heat and thermal effects on the tissues adjacent to the target. Adjacent tissue is protected by cottonoids soaked in saline. The laser is used predominantly for debulking tumor. It decreases bleeding by coagulating the adjacent tissue; however, the author prefers accurately applied bipolar coagulation for hemostasis near critical neural structures. Accurate microdissection with fine instruments is the preferred method for removing the final fragments of tumor from neural and vascular structures.

Argon and neodymium:yttrium-aluminum-garnet (Nd:YAG) lasers, although used less frequently than carbon dioxide lasers in neurosurgery, have some promise in the treatment of vascular tumors of the nervous system. The argon laser has found use in ophthalmology because of the affinity of its wavelength for the melanin pigment in the retinal epithelium of the eye. The affinity of the Nd:YAG laser for the red color of hemoglobin has led to its use in managing lesions with a high blood content. Argon and Nd:YAG lasers can be delivered through an optic fiber, but this fiber, when used with a carbon dioxide laser, leads to an unacceptable loss of energy. The carbon dioxide beam is delivered to the target using a series of deflecting mirrors that are located inside articulating tubular arms coupled mechanically to the microscope. Individuals working around laser systems should wear protective lenses that are color-specific for the wavelength involved.

References

1. Kurze T. Microtechniques in neurological surgery. Clin Neurosurg 1964;11:128–137
2. Rhoton AL Jr. Operative techniques and instrumentation for neurosurgery. Neurosurgery 2003;53:907–934
3. Rhoton AL Jr. The anterior and middle cranial base. Neurosurgery 2002;51(Suppl 4):S273–S302
4. Rhoton AL Jr. Instrumentation. In: Apuzzo MJL, ed. Brain Surgery: Complication, Avoidance and Management. Vol 2. New York: Churchill-Livingstone; 1993:1647–1670
5. Rhoton AL Jr. General and micro-operative techniques. In: Youmans JR, ed. Neurological Surgery. Vol 1. Philadelphia, WB Saunders; 1996:724–766
6. Greenwood J. Two point coagulation: a new principle and instrument for applying coagulation current in neurosurgery. Am J Surg 1940;50:267–270
7. Malis LL. Bipolar coagulation in microsurgery. In: Yaşargil MG, ed. Microsurgery Applied to Neurosurgery. New York: Academic; 1969:41–45
8. Rhoton AL Jr. Microsurgery of the internal acoustic meatus. Surg Neurol 1974;2:311–318
9. Rhoton AL Jr. Microsurgical anatomy of decompression operations on the trigeminal nerve. In: Rovit RL, ed. Trigeminal Neuralgia. Baltimore: Williams & Wilkins; 1990:165–200
10. Rhoton AL Jr. Aneurysms. Neurosurgery 2002;51(Suppl 4):S121–S158
11. Rhoton AL Jr. Ring curettetes for transsphenoidal pituitary operations. Surg Neurol 1982;18:28–33
12. Yaşargil MG. Suture material. In: Yaşargil MG, ed. Microsurgery Applied to Neurosurgery. New York: Academic; 1969:55
13. Yaşargil MG. Suturing techniques. In: Yaşargil MG, ed. Microsurgery Applied to Neurosurgery. New York: Academic; 1969:51–58
14. Rhoton AL Jr, Merz W. Suction tubes for conventional or microscopic neurosurgery. Surg Neurol 1981;15:120–124
15. Yaşargil MG, Vise WM, Bader DC. Technical adjuncts in neurosurgery. Surg Neurol 1977;8:331–336
16. Greenberg IM. Self-retaining retractor and handrest system for neurosurgery. Neurosurgery 1981;8:205–208
17. Pait TG, Harris FS, Paullus WS, et al. Microsurgical anatomy and dissection of the temporal bone. Surg Neurol 1977;8:363–391
18. Rhoton AL Jr, Hardy DG, Chambers SM. Microsurgical anatomy and dissection of the sphenoid bone, cavernous sinus and sellar region. Surg Neurol 1979;12:63–104
19. Bader DC. Microtechnical nursing in neurosurgery. J Neurosurg Nurs 1975;7:22–24

2

Anesthesia Techniques for Cranial Base Surgery

Richard Peterson

Neuroanesthesia has evolved rapidly over the last few years. Neurosurgical techniques and supportive management have improved, making it possible to treat the most complex tumor and vascular disorders of the central nervous system. These neurosurgical procedures present the risk of ischemia or injury to the brain. The anesthesiologist seeks to understand the mechanism of these injuries and to devise therapies to protect against insults such as vascular occlusion, increased intracranial pressure (ICP), unrelieved retraction pressure, or embolic phenomenon.

Intraoperative cerebral protection is aimed at the prevention of focal ischemic events by pharmacological and physiological interventions before and after the detected insults, as well as beginning resuscitative measures before neuronal damage becomes irreversible. Cerebral protection includes the management of all patient interventions, including the smooth insertion of the intravenous and arterial lines, preparedness for head pin placement, avoidance of wide blood pressure swings on incision and craniectomy, provision of optimal surgical conditions, and ability to utilize neurophysiological monitoring to optimize both central nervous system (CNS) and cardiovascular parameters. Paying close attention to all the details will enable the anesthesia team to provide a smooth intraoperative course and emergence.

Unfortunately, there is no single magic bullet or pharmacological or procedural intervention that can protect the CNS from ischemic injury. The material that follows utilizes modalities blended into procedural guidelines that take advantage of current information to provide a logical clinical management plan. Standardization of anesthetic regimens helps familiarize all practitioners with the temporal sequence of surgical events and enables them to be proactive in preventing unfavorable intracranial conditions.

◆ Pathophysiology of Ischemia

To more thoroughly appreciate the therapy modalities, one must understand the pathways that lead to ischemic damage. The ischemic insult initiates a cascade of pathophysiological events that lead to neural cell death. First is the accumulation of lactic acid due to anaerobic metabolism. This condition leads to increased membrane permeability and resultant cellular edema. Anaerobic metabolism cannot maintain the intracellular energy state, resulting in adenosine triphosphate (ATP) store depletion and failure of energy-dependent ion pumps. As ionic pumps fail, the neuron partially or fully depolarizes as well as releases excitatory amino acids (glutamate, aspartate). Activation of NMDA, AMPA, and voltage-dependent calcium and sodium channels allow Ca^{2+} and Na^{+} influx leading to increased energy-requiring processes. Calcium activates proteases and phospholipases, which release intracellular free fatty acids

Table 2–1 Concepts of Anesthetic Brain Protection

1. Increase CBF to potential ischemic areas
2. Pharmacological and physiological reduction of $CMRO_2$ and ICP
3. Hypothermia
4. Suppression of seizure activity
5. Depress excitatory neurotransmitter activity
6. Prevention of calcium and sodium influx
7. Inhibit lipid breakdown
8. Free radical scavenging
9. Neurophysiological monitoring of specific pathways at risk of injury

CBF, cerebral blood flow; $CMRO_2$, cerebral metabolic rate for oxygen; ICP, intracranial pressure.

(FFAs) and free radicals, which interfere with membrane function. Other proteases break down deoxyribonucleic acid (DNA) and mitochondrial membranes and promote necrosis or apoptosis [programmed cell death (PCD)]. Phospholipase activation results in elevated arachidonic acid, which on reperfusion leads to production of eicosanoids (i.e., thromboxane, prostaglandin, and leukotrienes), which are potent vasoconstrictors. Reperfusion, which is undoubtedly necessary, may be a very destructive process. Literature on cerebral protection supports measures taken early in the ischemic cascade to prevent or modulate further neuronal deterioration. Techniques instituted in the management of neurosurgical cases to prevent the ischemic insult are perhaps the most effective way to protect the CNS from injury (**Table 2–1**.)

◆ Anesthetic Pharmacological Cerebral Protection

Reducing cerebral metabolic rate is the cornerstone of pharmacological cerebral protection. Anesthetic drugs routinely used for all types of anesthesia and surgical cases make up the majority of agents studied in brain protection. These agents are also the ones that have shown the most promise in providing a cerebral protectant effect during neurosurgical cases. The goal is to maximize oxygen delivery and decrease oxygen demand. Candidates for cerebral protection include patients with space-occupying lesions, those for intracranial vascular procedures, and cardiac patients at risk for low flow state or embolic phenomenon.

Barbiturates

Barbiturates have been the most studied and most utilized agents for pharmacological cerebral protection and have the most literature support showing usefulness in humans.[1–3] Studies in laboratory animals have shown that barbiturates and propofol reduce infarct size and improve neurological outcome following total or incomplete global ischemia provided physiological variables were controlled during the experiment.[4–9] Mechanisms of protection are attributed to decreased CMR, decreased transient ischemic depolarizations,[10–12] inhibition of membrane depolarization,[13] decreased NMDA receptor stimulus,[14,15] and decreased lipid membrane breakdown.[16]

The advantages of barbiturates include a predictable decrease in CMR and cerebral blood flow (CBF) with a resultant decrease in intracranial pressure. Barbiturates have been shown to decrease calcium ion influx, inhibit free radical formation, increase inhibitory transmission or secretion of γ-aminobutyric acid (GABAergic activity), decrease cerebral edema, inhibit glucose transfer across the blood–brain barrier and decrease glucose transport into cells, and block sodium channels. These properties cover many of the steps in the ischemic cascade to inhibit progression of the cascade.

Propofol

Propofol has recently gained popularity as a neuroanesthetic agent due to its favorable clinical attributes such as ease of titration, rapid metabolism and elimination, and predictability. Propofol, like the barbiturates, decreases CMR but may aggravate glutamate excitotoxicity and increase neuronal damage.[15] More studies are needed for propofol to supplant barbiturates, but it does have a favorable clinical profile. Propofol also has potent antiemetic effects. In a prospective, randomized clinical trial comparing three anesthetic techniques (propofol/fentanyl, isoflurane-/N_2O, and fentanyl/N_2O) in 100 patients with supratentorial mass lesions, there was no difference in the anesthetic regimens comparing hemodynamic stability, brain swelling, and awakening.[17]

Etomidate

The effects of etomidate on neurological outcome are not well defined, although it remains the standard regimen for cerebral protection at several institutions.[18] There is evidence to show that the neuroprotective potential of etomidate is minor when compared with barbiturates or propofol. There is now clinical evidence that the standard propylene glycol formulation of etomidate[19] induces more tissue hypoxia, acidosis, and neurological defects than an electroencephalographic (EEG) equivalent of desflurane.[20] In addition, there was no electrophysiological recovery following anoxia of rat hippocampal slices.[21,22] Etomidate may cause myoclonic activity and possibly seizures in some patients. Etomidate also causes adrenocortical suppression and postoperative nausea and vomiting. Etomidate is avoided in the management of neurosurgical cases at our institution.

Volatile Agents

All potent inhalational agents decrease CMR. They increase CBF and ICP, but the effects are attenuated by hyperventilation (i.e., CO_2 responsiveness is maintained). Animal studies with focal ischemia and tight physiological control including temperature show that isoflurane and sevoflurane may decrease infarct size and improve neurological outcome when administered prior to ischemic insult.[23,24] Patients undergoing carotid endarterectomy anesthetized with isoflurane and sevoflurane show increased tolerance to lower levels of CBF with preserved neuronal function during carotid cross-clamp[25] (i.e., critical CBF is lowered to 8 mL/100 g tissue/min). Inhalational agents are easily titrated and are a standard part of our anesthetic regimen.

N_2O, on the other hand, may reverse the protective effects of barbiturates and volatile agents.[26] As well, N_2O may worsen pneumocephalus if not discontinued prior to dural closure. The effect of N_2O on air bubbles is also well known and can increase the size of an air embolism quickly or conversely enhance its detection by the precordial Doppler. Treatment can begin by discontinuing N_2O immediately, allowing the air bubble to shrink. By eliminating N_2O, deleterious effects can be avoided and oxygen content can be increased to provide optimal O_2 delivery at critical junctures in the operation.

Hypothermia

For decades the mechanism of cerebral protection for mild hypothermia was thought to be its attenuation of CMR. However, because the decrease in CMR is minimal to moderate with the degree of mild hypothermia (30%), other factors must have a role. The protection by mild intraoperative hypothermia is attributable to retardation of the destructive consequences of ischemia by diminishing the synergists of the ischemic cascade.[27] One degree of hypothermia (36°C) maintains ATP levels during a hypoxic episode that depletes ATP in half at 37°C. At 34°C phosphocreatine preservation more than doubled. Ischemic depolarizations in the penumbra zone of an ischemic insult are greatly diminished also.[28] Disadvantages of hypothermia include coagulopathy, cardiac dysrhythmias, increased duration of muscle relaxants, and decreased minimum alveolar concentration (MAC) for volatile anesthetics. The potential benefit of mild hypothermia far outweighs the detrimental effects because these effects occur at temperatures lower than 34°C in most instances. In a recent poll of the Society of Neuroanesthesia and Critical Care 40% of clinicians practice induced hypothermia in patients undergoing cerebral aneurysm surgery.[29] In a randomized prospective clinical pilot study of mild (33.5°C) hypothermia as a protective therapy during intracranial aneurysm clipping, patients with subarachnoid hemorrhage (SAH) in the hypothermia group had less neurological deterioration at 24 and 72 hours, greater frequency of discharge to home, and better long-term outcome.[30] A large prospective study is in progress.

◆ Anesthesia Guidelines for Intracranial Vascular Surgery

Approximately 1:20/1:100 adults have an intracranial aneurysm. However, only ~1:10,000 experience SAH. Unruptured aneurysms are usually found incidentally during a medical workup for headaches. However, a few will present with seizures or cranial nerve difficulties (i.e., visual disturbances). Surgery is recommended for unruptured aneurysms even though 20 to 25% will still have less than an optimal outcome.

Sudden onset of a severe headache is a universal symptom of SAH. The patient may experience warning signs for weeks preceding the event. The headache is caused by blood gushing into the subarachnoid space. Intracranial pressure may increase tremendously after the initial rupture.

Blood flow to the aneurysmal area is decreased due to vasoconstriction (not vasospasm). If ICP remains elevated and the vasoconstriction and clot formation do not control the bleeding, the patient will die or suffer a severe neurological disaster. SAH will also initiate autonomic imbalance, resulting in severe hypertension and dysrhythmias. Most patients presenting to the operating room have had aneurysmal rupture (SAH). The incidence of SAH is ~1/10,000 adults. Nearly 50% die immediately. Of the survivors, another 50% will die or be permanently impaired. Even after a successful operation, 25% will still have a less than normal neurological outcome.

Complications of SAH are rebleeding, vasospasm, hydrocephalus, and metabolic disturbances. Hydrocephalus and metabolic disturbances are anticipated and easily treated. However, rebleeding and vasospasm can be devastating. Early surgery in the first 24 to 48 hours after rupture is recommended to prevent rebleeding in at least the nonmoribund patient. Early surgery allows aggressive therapy to prevent or lessen vasospasm that develops 3 to 7 days postrupture.

Clinical vasospasm is essentially a postoperative management problem. The mechanism of vasospasm is thought to be an imbalance of nitric oxide–mediated vasodilation and increase of concentration of endothelin. Vasospasm treatment relies on administration of nimodipine, a calcium channel blocker that reduces angiographic vasospasm and increases CBF, and the institution of triple-H therapy (hypervolemia, hypertension, hemodilution).

Triple-H therapy is used to treat and help prevent vasospasm. The goals of therapy are to maintain cerebral perfusion by augmenting blood pressure and cardiac output via inotropic support. Spasm is treated with nimodipine. Intravascular volume expansion with appropriate crystalloids and colloids will result in a relative hemodilution. Generous fluids are administered to maintain central venous pressure (CVP) at 10 to 15 mm Hg. Correcting hypernatremia is important to prevent further neural injury. Interventional radiology may be able to perform intracerebral transluminal angioplasty on vasospastic vessels. Transcranial Doppler monitoring is done daily to assess cerebral blood velocity and detect vasospasm.

Guidelines

In an effort to provide an anesthetic that offers a degree of cerebral protection as well as a chance at rapid emergence and recovery, the following guidelines have been established for intracranial vascular surgery management.

In preoperative holding, chart review and discussion of anesthetic events with the patient and family are important first to compare the previous day's visit for any neural changes and to take note of any existing deficits to distinguish between baseline deficits and residual anesthetic effects. In an area free from bright lights and noise (e.g., a post-anesthesia care unit in early morning), sedate the patient as needed to prevent agitation and possible hypertension. Arterial and CVP monitoring are a requirement.

A Berman pulmonary angiography catheter via an antecubital (basilic) vein is utilized on most occasions. These catheters are flow directed, multiorificed, and able to siphon blood back adequately. If the antecubital site has been used or is nonexistent, the internal jugular or subclavian vein opposite the side of surgery is used to avoid obstructing the ipsilateral neck. The carotid artery is frequently exposed for clamping prior to aneurysm clipping. Ensure blood is available, administer the requested antibiotics, and avoid glucose-containing solutions. Additional monitoring will include precordial Doppler placed over the right fourth interspace near the sternum. The Doppler position is tested with the injection of 10 mL saline with microbubbles. Neurophysiological monitoring (NPM) is used routinely. Somatosensory evoked potentials (SSEPs) and EEG will give a general idea of the well-being of cerebral tissue beyond an area of clipping either temporary or permanent. EEG is used to monitor and guide barbiturate therapy. NPM can be effective if communication exists with experienced teams of anesthesia, surgery, and monitoring. The majority of intracranial vascular surgical procedures at our institution incorporate an intraoperative angiogram. The groin is prepped and a 5F sheath is placed after induction of anesthesia and preserved for the radiology team later in the case. Induction is designed to prevent wide swings in blood pressure. There is a risk of rebleeding in the peri-induction period on the order of 1 to 2%, presumably due to uncontrolled blood pressure. The most stimulating events in the initial operation phase are laryngoscopy and intubation, pin placement, and incision/craniectomy. After providing head up position, induction proceeds with propofol or thiopental, fentanyl 8 to 10 µg/kg (fentanyl dosing is described here; however, any synthetic opioid may be used), lidocaine, and a muscle relaxant. Waiting a full 90 seconds or more ensures that the muscle relaxant has taken effect; thus coughing and bucking cannot occur. The dose of narcotics will blunt the hemodynamic responses to all the initial stimulating events in the first phase of the pro-cedure. Administration of an additional dose of propofol (0.5–1.0 mg/kg) prior to head pin placement is sometimes necessary to prevent a dramatic increase in blood pressure. Adding an inhalational agent during induction while moderately hyperventilating the patient will also help prevent increases in blood pressure (BP). After induction, maintenance anesthesia is provided by isoflurane at less than 1% end tidal concentrations. N_2O is avoided, and optimal oxygenation during potentially ischemic periods is maintained. Little stimulation occurs during brain dissection. Adequate surgical conditions are maintained by ensuring adequate cerebral perfusion pressure (CPP), moderate hyperventilation (28–32 mm Hg). Lower arterial CO_2 tensions are not recommended due to severe vasoconstriction and metabolic changes. Mannitol (0.5–1.0 g/kg) is standard, and cerebrospinal fluid (CSF) drainage either through the incision or via a lumbar CSF drain is performed. Craniotomy with orbitectomy provides a much better exposure to cranial-based aneurysms. Less retraction is needed, and theoretically less neuronal damage is encountered.

As the surgeon dissects near the aneurysm, thiopental (2–3 mg/kg) is administered to achieve EEG burst suppression. After the bolus an infusion at 1 mg/kg/hr is begun to maintain burst suppression. The infusion is titrated upward to maintain EEG burst suppression. The infusion is discontinued after the aneurysm is clipped. Much smaller doses of thiopental are needed when used in conjunction with hypothermia, inhalational agents, and intravenous anesthetics. The result is patients who are awake and responsive at the end of surgery. Passive hypothermia to 34°C is allowed to aid in depressing cerebral metabolic rate. A decrease of 1 to 2°C per mg depresses $CMRO_2$ up to 14 to 20%. A warming blanket is placed over the patient, and warming begins to prevent the temperatures from falling to levels lower than 34°C. More severe levels of hypothermia may cause coagulopathy, prevent reversal of muscle relaxation, and exaggerate effects of anesthetics. Conversely, patients are not rewarmed to greater than 36°C.

During dissection near the aneurysm maintain the BP at levels lower than baseline and then elevate the BP to 10 to 20% above baseline when temporary clipping begins. BP manipulation is easily achieved using anesthetic or vasoactive agents. After the permanent clip is placed, maintain the BP at or slightly above baseline. Continuation of triple-H therapy is suggested. Except for patients grade III or worse or for longer, more complicated surgery, the aim is to have patients awake and responsive and extubated at the end of the case.

Special Circumstances

Some more complex aneurysms may require saphenous vein or radial artery grafting to bypass the aneurysmal vessel. The anatomy of these vessels may preclude adequate clipping because of a wide irregular base or the inclusion of feeding vessels in the aneurysm wall. Long periods of temporary clipping, heparin administration, and preoperative planning for potential harvest site (vein or artery) make management of these cases very difficult. Communication between the surgeon and anesthesiologist relieves any uncertainty concerning the intraoperative management of these patients.

◆ Anesthesia Guidelines for Arteriovenous Malformation

The anesthetic management of arteriovenous malformations (AVMs) is similar to that of aneurysm clipping. Many times the patient will have an interventional radiological procedure for embolization a day or two prior to the procedure. Bleeding might be more vigorous postresection. Blood pressure must be kept at levels below baseline to prevent normotensive breakthrough. Areas around the resected AVM are fragile and may easily bleed and rebleed if not managed carefully.

◆ Anesthesia Guidelines for Skull-based Tumors

Brain tumors that arise near the floor of the cranium are difficult to approach from a routine craniotomy. The tumors may be benign or malignant but are largely malignant by location. Common types of tumors are meningioma, acoustic neuroma, pituitary adenoma, chordoma, and chondrosarcoma. The tumors frequently involve major arteries, veins, and cranial nerves; thus surgical treatment is difficult. Cranial nerves may need to be sacrificed and major vessels ligated or bypassed. Proximity to brain stem structures makes loss of brain stem reflexes a major concern after surgery. Exposure may involve extensive craniectomy, including bilateral orbital unroofing and extensive drilling of the cranial floor. The operation may be long and arduous (> 10 hours) and involves not only neurosurgery but also ear, nose, and throat (ENT) and plastic surgery. These patients are at risk for extensive blood loss, and cerebral protection measures for internal carotid artery bypass may occasionally be required. Some tumors are extensive and may be staged into more than one operation. Chart review and familiarity with the radiographic studies help the anesthesiologist plan and prepare for the operative procedure along with a detailed discussion with the surgeon. For example, if magnetic resonance imaging studies reveal encasement of the internal carotid artery, certainly cerebral protection measures should be taken and intraoperative angiogram may be indicated.

After evaluation and discussion of the anesthesia and monitoring required, intravenous access is obtained with large-bore IVs, avoiding glucose-containing solutions. Sedation is titrated as necessary after the surgeon visits the patient in the holding area. An arterial line is placed, and if accessible the right antecubital basilic vein is cannulated with an introducer for the placement of a central venous line. At our institution a Berman pulmonary angiography catheter is inserted to 20 cm, then floated to position in the operating room. Advantages of the pulmonary angiography catheter are that it is flow directed, multiorificed, and easy to place nearly 90% of the time via the basilic vein. Antibiotics are administered per surgeon's request in the holding area, and blood availability is checked.

Monitoring

The usual American Society of Anesthesiologists standard monitoring is utilized as well as the arterial line and central venous line as already described. A precordial Doppler is placed over the right fourth intercostal space near the sternum and tested for detection of characteristic Doppler sounds indicating air entrainment. These patients are positioned head up so that the incision is at least 10 to 15 cm above the right atrium. Air entrainment is much more likely than that in the supine or lateral position and possibly as great as that in the sitting position.

NPM is used to monitor neural pathways at risk and to aid in the titration of cerebral protective agents. Most cranial-based procedures require brain stem auditory evoked responses (BAERs), which monitor adequacy of brain stem function, and EEG to monitor cortical function and to aid in titration of cerebral protectant drugs to burst suppression. SSEPs are sometimes utilized to monitor pathways in the brain stem to the cortex. Electromyography (EMG) is utilized if the facial nerve is at risk.

Induction

Induction of the anesthetic occurs with the head 180 degrees from the anesthesia machine to aid in preventing the confusion and tangling that occur with turning. Induction in this manner requires the anesthesia team to work together in airway management. The head is elevated for all inductions for cranial-based surgery to alleviate cerebral volume problems (CSF drainage and cerebral venous drainage). All patients will have some decrease in intracranial compliance or elastance. Preoxygenation with the patient voluntarily slightly hyperventilating aids in improving intracranial conditions. Propofol (2 mg/kg) is administered along with lidocaine (0.15 mg/kg) and fentanyl (8–10 µg/kg). When unconsciousness is attained and the airway assured, rocuronium (0.75 mg/kg) is administered and the patient's mask ventilated until full muscle relaxation is obtained. Coughing and bucking are avoided with this technique. The patient is then intubated and moderately hyperventilated to an end total CO_2 of 28 to 30 mm Hg or a corresponding $PaCO_2$ of 28 to 30 mm Hg. Decadron (0.15 m/kg) is given peri-induction for cerebral swelling, and phenytoin (15 mg/kg) to a maximum of 1 g is given slowly over 30 minutes. Vasoactive drugs are immediately available to counteract wide swings in BP. Additional propofol (1–2 mg/kg) may be needed prior to head pin placement. A lumbar CSF drain is frequently requested to aid in surgical exposure.

Maintenance

Anesthesia for cranial-based surgery is maintained with isoflurane in an oxygen/air mixture. N_2O is avoided as discussed earlier. End tidal concentrations of 1% or less are more than sufficient for maintenance for the nonstimulating portions of the procedure. The initial dose of fentanyl at induction is sufficient to cover the most stimulating periods of the procedure such as laryngoscopy and intubation, head pin placement, incision and craniectomy, and lengthy drilling.

If EMG is used to monitor cranial nerve (CN) VII function during long drilling and brain stem retraction, a muscle relaxant infusion is started to maintain two or more twitches on the nerve stimulator. BP must be carefully controlled and may be elevated with vasoactive drugs (phenylephrine/dopamine) to 20% above baseline during vascular bypass. If vascular bypass is indicated, then cerebral protection is utilized. Pentothal is the drug of choice (see Anesthetic Pharmacological Cerebral Protection). A bolus of pentothal (2–3 mg/kg) is administered just prior to vascular clamping and titrated to EEG burst suppression (usually 5:1). After the bolus, a pentothal infusion is begun at 1 mg/kg/hr to maintain burst suppression.

Emergence

Procedures for cranial-based surgery may be long, and blood loss may be extensive, so postoperative ventilation may be likely. However, if anesthetics are managed sensibly and the surgery proceeds without incident, then extubation is predominantly accomplished in the operating room. Frequent postoperative assessments of the patient are made, screening for developing neural deficits.

◆ Anesthesia Guidelines for Cranial Nerve V (Trigeminal Nerve)

Trigeminal neuralgia or tic douloureux is the most common syndrome of cranial nerve dysfunction. Patients experience paroxysms of excruciating lancinating pain, usually to the teeth or gums. The pain can be elicited easily by trigger point stimulation (e.g., eating or drinking). In severe cases patients may present to the operating room malnourished and dehydrated. The mechanism of trigeminal neuralgia is thought to be in small vessels (usually arteries but occasionally veins, AVMs, or tumors) impinging on CN V as it enters the brain stem. Through a microscope the surgeon either lifts the vessel off the nerve and tethers it away with suture or places a Teflon graft between the vessel and the nerve.

Although specific monitoring is not available for CN V, monitoring of CN VII, BAER, and SSEP in some cases will aid in detecting stretch or injury to the facial nerves or brain stem.

Intraoperative problems may include any combination of hypo/hypertension, brady/tachycardia due to retraction or cautery on the brain stem. Venous air embolism (VAE) is rare due to the surgical approach and easily prevented by adequate fluid management and control of the patient's head position. Central venous monitoring is not routinely used. However, the sigmoid sinus may be entered during the approach, causing brisk bleeding and the possibility of entraining large amounts of air.

Pain relief is usually immediate but may take weeks. The syndrome may recur at a rate of 15 to 20% in 5 years. Older, more fragile patients may be offered percutaneous trigeminal rhizolysis (PTR). These patients may be on a variety of medications (narcotics, antidepressants, and antiseizure) for their painful syndrome. The anesthesiologist should be aware of the potential side effects and drug interactions.

◆ Anesthesia Guidelines for Cranial Nerve VII

Dysfunction of the seventh cranial nerve is also known as hemifacial spasm. It is caused by the pulsatile vascular irritation at the root entry zone of CN VII into the brain stem. The syndrome presents as painful paroxysms of facial contraction. Monitoring of BAERs and CN VII EMG responses during surgery may demonstrate the success of the vascular decompression as well to avoid facial paralysis and deafness.

The surgical approach is from a small retromastoid craniectomy with the patient in the lateral position. Intraoperative problems are those associated with brain stem retraction and cautery, as discussed previously with CN V surgery.

◆ Anesthesia Guidelines for Acoustic Neuroma

Acoustic neuromas or vestibular schwannomas arise from the neural covering of CN VIII. They are usually unilateral;

Table 2–2 Guidelines for Microvascular Decompression

I. Holding area preparation

- A. Chart review and patient interview
  1. Laboratories and electrocardiogram
  2. Angiograms and magnetic resonance imaging
- B. Patient preparation
  1. Large-bore IV
  2. Arterial line
  3. Central venous line (periphera)
  4. Antibiotics and sedatives as needed
  5. Lumbar cerebrospinal fluid drain if requested (in holding area if possible)
- C. Monitors
  1. ASA standard
  2. Invasive
     - a. Arterial line
     - b. Central venous line (optional)
  3. Noninvasive
     - a. Precordial Doppler
     - b. Neurophysiological monitoring (BAER, EMG, SSEP, EEG as indicated)

II. Operating room preparation

- A. Induction
  1. Head elevated
  2. Lidocaine 0.5–1.5 mg/kg IV
  3. Propofol 2 mg/kg IV
  4. Fentanyl 8–10 μg/kg IV
  5. Rocuronium 0.75 mg/kg IV (wait 90 seconds prior to intubation)
- B. Maintenance
  1. Isoflurane/sevoflurane; air/O_2
  2. Titrate muscle relaxant infusion to maintain TOF > 2 twitches
  3. $PaCO_2$ 28–30 mm Hg
  4. CVP > 10 mm Hg
- C. Special considerations
  1. Cardiovascular lability (any combination of brady/tachycardia and hypo/hypertension): notify surgeon immediately; treat as necessary
  2. Mannitol as needed
  3. VAE (rare but may be severe if sigmoid sinus entered, blood loss)

BAER, brain stem auditory evoked response; CVP, central venous pressure; EEG, electroencephalography; EMG, electromyography; $PaCO_2$, partial pressure of CO_2; SSEP, somato sensory evoked potential; VAE, venous air embolism.

however, bilateral tumors are common in neurofibromatosis. The tumor arises in the internal auditory canal and expands posteriorly and medially into the posterior fossa. Here the tumor may press on the cerebellum, cranial nerves, and brain stem. Tinnitus is an early sign, followed by a gradual, usually unnoticeable hearing loss. Ataxia is a common correlating symptom. Small tumors are usually approached via a retrosigmoid craniectomy in the lateral position. Monitoring will include BAER and facial nerve EMG to preserve as much function as possible. Larger acoustic neuromas are approached transcranially. Anesthetic guidelines utilized at our institution are referenced in **Table 2–2.**

References

1. Bendo et al. In: Barash, Cullen, Stoelting, eds. Clinical Anesthesia. Philadelphia: JB Lippincott; 1992:880
2. Zaidan JR, et al. Effect of thiopental on neurologic outcome following coronary bypass surgery. Anesthesiology 1991;74:406–411
3. Todd MM, et al. Barbiturate protection and cardiac surgery: a different result. Anesthesiology 1991;74:402–405
4. Warner DS, et al. Electroencephalographic burst suppression is not required to elicit maximal neuroprotection from pentobarbital in a rat model of focal cerebral ischemia. Anesthesiology 1996;84:1475–1484
5. Kochs E, et al. The effects of propofol on brain electrical activity, neurologic outcome, and neuronal damage following incomplete ischemia in rats. Anesthesiology 1992;76:245–252
6. Yamaguchi S, et al. Propofol prevents delayed neuroma: death following transient forebrain ischemia in gerbils. Can J Anaesth 1999;46: 593–598
7. Young Y, et al. Propofol neuroprotection in a rat model of ischaemia reperfusion injury. Eur J Anaesthesiol 1997;14:320–326
8. Ridenour TR, et al. Comparative effects of propofol and halothane on outcome from temporary middle artery occlusion in the rat. Anesthesiology 1992;76:807–812
9. Pittman JE, et al. Comparison of the effects of propofol and pentobarbital on neurologic outcome and cerebral infarct size after temporary focal ischemia in the rat. Anesthesiology 1997;87:1139–1144
10. Patel PM, et al. Isoflurane and pentobarbital reduce the frequency of transient ischemic depolarizations during focal ischemia in rats. Anesth Analg 1998;86:773–780
11. Nakashima K, et al. The relation between cerebral metabolic rate and ischemic depolarization. Anesthesiology 1995;82:1199–1208
12. Wang T, et al. Thiopental attenuates hypoxic changes of electrophysiology, biochemistry, and morphology in rat hippocampal slice CA1 pyramidal cells. Stroke 1999;30:2400–2407
13. Zhan RZ, et al. Thiopental inhibits increases in Ca++ induced membrane depolarization, NMDA receptor activation, and ischemia in rat hippocampal and cortical slices. Anesthesiology 1998;89:456–466
14. Beirne JP, et al. Effect of halothane in cortical cell cultures exposed to NMDA. Neurochem Res 1998;23:17–23
15. Zhu H, et al. The effect of thiopental and propofol on NMDA and AMPA mediated glutamate excitotoxicity. Anesthesiology 1997;87:944–950
16. Almaas R, et al. Effects of barbiturates on hydroxyl radicals, lipid peroxidation, and hypoxic cell death in human NT2-N neurons. Anesthesiology 2000;92:764–774
17. Sato K, Karibe H, Yoshimoto T. Advantage of intravenous anaesthesia for acute stage surgery of aneurysmal subarachnoid hemorrhage. Acta Neurochir (Wien) 1999;141:161–164
18. Samson D, et al. A clinical study of the parameters and effects of temporary arterial occlusion in the management of intracranial aneurysms. Neurosurgery 1994;34:22–28
19. Doenicke A, et al. Haemolysis after etomidate: comparison of propylene glycol and lipid formulation. Br J Anaesth 1997;79:386–388
20. Hoffman WE, et al. Comparison of the effect of etomidate and desflurane on brain tissue gases and pH during prolonged middle cerebral artery occlusion. Anesthesiology 1998;88:1188–1194
21. Guo J, et al. Limited protective effects of etomidate during brainstem ischemia in dogs. J Neurosurg 1995;82:278–283
22. Amadeu ME, et al. Etomidate does not alter recovery after anoxia of evoked population spikes recorded from the CA1 region of rat hippocampal slices. Anesthesiology 1998;88:1274–1280
23. Werner C, et al. Sevoflurane improves neurological outcome following incomplete cerebral ischemia in rats. Br J Anaesth 1995;75: 756–760
24. Engelhard K, et al. Desflurane and isoflurane improve neurologic outcome after incomplete cerebral ischemia in rats. Br J Anaesth 1999;83:415–421
25. Grady RE, et al. Correlation of regional cerebral blood flow with ischemic electroencephalographic changes during sevoflurane-nitrous oxide anesthesia for carotid endarterectomy. Anesthesiology 1998;88:892–897
26. Hartung J, Cottrell JE. Nitrous oxide reduces thiopental-induced prolongation of survival in hypoxic and anoxic mice. Anesth Analg 1987;66:47–52
27. Hartung J, et al. Mild hypothermia and cerebral metabolism. J Neurosurg Anesthesiol 1994;6:1–3
28. Chen Q, et al. Temperature modulation of cerebral depolarization during focal cerebral ischemia in rats: correlation with ischemic injury. J Cereb Blood Flow Metab 1993;13:389–394
29. Craen R, et al. Current anesthetic practices and use of brain protective therapies for cerebral aneurysm surgery at 41 North American centers [abstract]. J Neurosurg Anesth 1994;6:303
30. Hindman BJ, et al. Mild hypothermia as a protective therapy during intracranial aneurysm surgery: a randomized prospective pilot trial. Neurosurgery 1999;44:23–32

3

Neurophysiological Monitoring: A Tool for Neurosurgery

Robert J. Sclabassi, Jeffrey R. Balzer, Donald Crammond, and Miguel E. Habeych

Limitations in the ability to clinically assess nervous system function during surgery have led to the development of neurophysiological intraoperative monitoring (IOM). IOM provides a real-time control loop around the surgeon and the patient. This control loop provides a dynamic assessment of the effects of surgical manipulations on the structure–function relationships of the patient's nervous system to facilitate the surgeon's decision making. Specific and sensitive measurements reflect the interactions between the surgeon's intraoperative manipulations and the functioning of the patient's nervous system.

This requires both rapid (as close as possible to real time) and multiple, simultaneous measurements of central nervous system (CNS) function. This combination allows a close and dynamic correlation with operative manipulations.

This chapter reviews our approach to IOM and summarizes pertinent literature with respect to this developing field. The emphasis is on the simultaneous acquisition of multiple neurophysiological measures. Depending on the surgical procedure, measures may be directly dependent on the functioning of the cortex [the electroencephalogram (EEG), somatosensory evoked potentials (SEPs) and visual evoked potentials (VEPs), direct cortical stimulation], the brain stem [brain stem auditory evoked potentials (BAEPs) and brain stem somatosensory evoked potentials (BSEPs)], and cranial nerves (CN) II, III, IV, V, VI, VII, VIII, IX, X, XI, and XII spontaneous and evoked electromyography (EMG), the spinal cord (sensory and motor potentials), and peripheral nerves (evoked EMG and compound action potentials).

◆ Neuroanesthetic Considerations

It is well known that the type of anesthesia, the patient's blood pressure, cerebral blood flow, body temperature, hematocrit, and blood gas tensions all affect the patient's CNS function and thus the observed intraoperative neurophysiological measures.[39] Many of the monitoring techniques place competing and complex demands on anesthetic management, with a variety of techniques being used at different times during a single operative procedure to enable the appropriate neurophysiological measures.[96]

Halogenated inhalational agents are favored by anesthesiologists for many procedures; however, they tend to significantly reduce the amplitude and shift the frequency components of the EEG, reduce the amplitude and increase the latencies of somatosensory and motor evoked potentials,[91] eliminate visual responses, and confound evoked EMGs.[104] We have found the optimal anesthetic technique to be a balanced narcotic technique, usually fentanyl, nitrous oxide ($< 50\%$), a low level of isoflurane ($< 0.5\%$), and a short-acting muscle relaxant that can be rapidly reversed when it is necessary to observe evoked EMGs. This technique may need to be modified if motor potentials are recorded to predominantly total intravenous anesthesia.

In many situations, halogenated hydrocarbon inhalation agents are desired to help control blood pressure. In our experience this problem is best approached by beginning the operative procedure under balanced narcotic technique, and then once baseline responses have been obtained and compared with the preoperative responses, introducing inhalation agents in a controlled fashion. It has also been our experience, particularly in children, that responses can be maintained at an isoflurane level of ~0.3 minimum alveolar concentration (MAC), whereas many adults can maintain their responses at 0.5 MAC.

Of the inhalation agents, isoflurane produces the weakest effects on cortical activity. Thus, in those cases where a balanced narcotic technique can not be used, isoflurane is recommended as the anesthetic from a monitoring perspective. These effects are very individualized, and even low levels of inhalation agents may reduce the amplitudes of cortically generated activity in some patients (**Fig. 3–1**).[92] The somatosensory short latency potentials (BSEPs) behave similarly to those from the auditory system (BAEPs) and are unaffected by most anesthetic manipulation.[29,40,65]

◆ Monitoring Systems

The presently available systems supporting IOM allow the simultaneous acquisition of evoked potentials, EEGs, and EMGs along with data from the anesthesiology monitoring unit,[95] and have significantly increased the utility and sensitivity of IOM (**Fig. 3–2**).

Neurophysiological signals are amplified using differential amplifiers[36] in which two input channels to the amplifier are differenced. This differencing has the effect of eliminating identical (in-phase) signal components that might be present at each recording electrode (presumably noise), and retaining the signals that are different (out-of-phase) and presumably produced by physiological generators. The effectiveness with which a differential amplifier rejects in-phase signals compared with its ability to amplify out-of-phase signals is called the common mode rejection ratio (CMRR). Differential amplifiers typically have CMRRs of greater that 10,000:1 (80 dB). For efficient rejection of in-phase signals, it is extremely important that the electrode impedances of each electrode of a pair not only be as low as possible but as similar as possible because any inequality in electrode impedance will produce amplitude differences in the in-phase activity that will be amplified along with the desired signal.

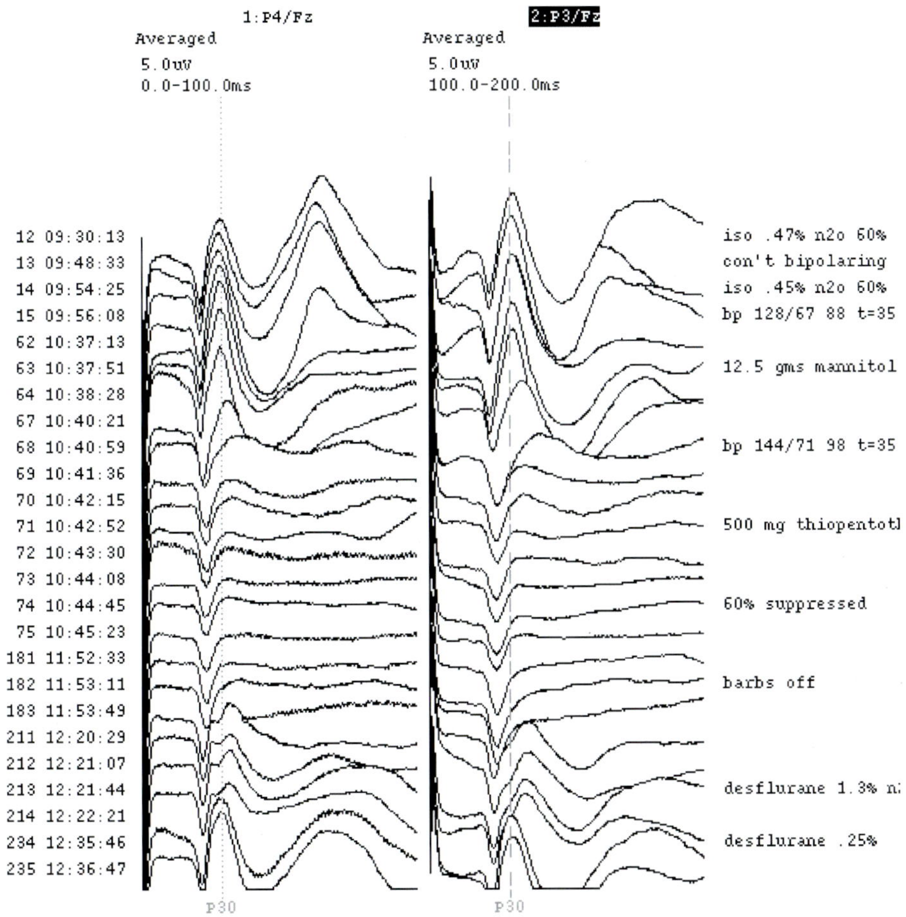

Figure 3–1 Bilateral median nerve evoked potentials demonstrating effects of multiple anesthetic agents during carotid endarterectomy. Sequential recordings start at the top of the figure. Initial responses are within normal limits. Recordings start to deteriorate, and thiopental is given, reducing P30. When thiopental is turned off, recordings return rapidly, but the effect of desflurane can be seen. As desflurane levels are decreased, recordings return to baseline at the bottom of the figure.

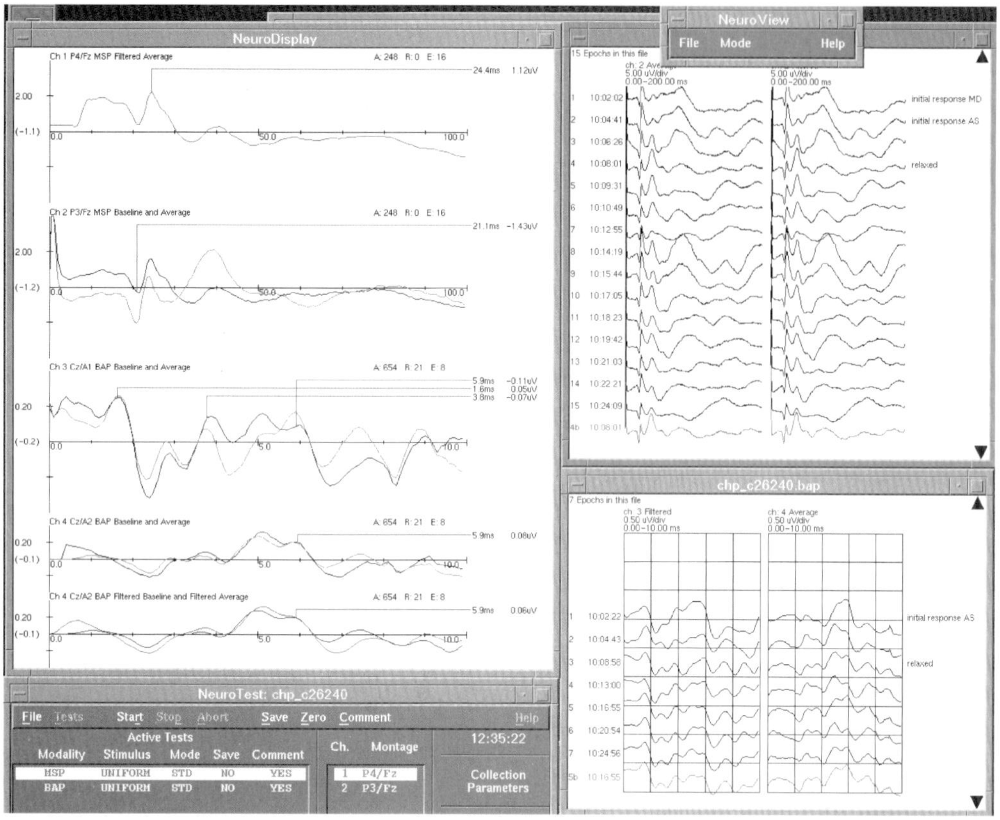

Figure 3–2 Example of median nerve evoked potentials (MSPs) and BAEPs being acquired simultaneously with the second channel (ch 4) of BAEPs being digitally filtered. Channels 2, 3, and 4 are also being compared against baseline data. Waterfall displays of both modalities are also shown with baseline responses at the bottom of each waterfall, and annotating comments are attached to the appropriate recording.

In evoked potential recording, the observed neuroelectric activity, either from the scalp or propagating activity from the cord, is assumed to consist of a signal component representative of underlying activity evoked by the stimulus and random noise consisting of both physiological signals not relevant to the study and environmental noise generated by ubiquitous sources of electrical signals. Evoked potentials are typically a fraction of the size of the spontaneous brain activity appearing in the background EEG, and about one thousandth the size of the other physiological and extraneous potentials with which they are intermixed. The aim of evoked potential recording is to acquire a large, clear response with the least possible noise contamination (i.e., the best signal to noise ratio possible); thus the elimination of unwanted signal components is essential. This elimination is accomplished through the use of both analog and digital filtering techniques and signal averaging.

After signal amplification, the most effective method for extracting a signal of interest from background noise is signal averaging. Signal averaging is in effect a cross-correlation between a point-process defined by the occurrence of the stimuli and the recorded evoked activity (i.e., an optimal filter).[58] In averaging, the signal component at each point is coherent and adds directly, whereas the background and noise components tend to be statistically independent and summate in a more or less root-mean-square (RMS) fashion.

Neurophysiological Measures

Neurophysiological measures are available that provide a functional map of nearly the entire neuroaxis. These measures include the EEG, an unstimulated measure of cortical function suitable for providing information concerning the degree of cortical activation related to either metabolic processes (e.g., hypoxia) or pharmacological manipulation (e.g., pentobarbital-induced burst suppression to protect the patient's cortical function)[75]; the somatosensory and visual cortical potentials (SEPs and VEPs), which provide additional measures of cortical function specific to certain pathways and vasculature; the auditory and somatosensory brain stem potentials (BAEPs and BSEPs), which provide information about the brain stem function specific to certain pathways[86]; compound nerve action potentials (CNAPs) providing information from both the spinal cord (SCAPs) and the peripheral nerves; and, finally, both continuous and evoked EMGs recorded from muscles [compound muscle action potentials (CMAPs)] innervated by the various cranial and peripheral nerves, which provide direct information about the integrity of the cranial nerves, their underlying brain stem nuclei,[51] the spinal cord, and peripheral nerves.

All measured potentials may be characterized as either near-field or far-field potentials (NFPs or FFPs). These concepts express observed differences between types of potentials and are meant to distinguish between two different manifestations of volume-conducted fields.[54]

FFPs are recorded at some distance from the presumed generator, however, and the point at which a "near field" becomes a "far field" has never been clearly defined. A useful definition for the FFP is one that fails to decay in proportion to the square of the distance from the generator.

Electroencephalogram

The EEG is a valuable monitoring tool in almost all cerebrovascular procedures or tumor resections where significant risk for interruption of blood flow to the brain occurs.

Cerebral blood flow alterations may occur during carotid endarterectomy, clipping or coiling of cerebral aneurysms, or repair of the internal carotid artery associated with tumor removal from the cavernous sinus. In most open cases, proximal and distal control of the feeding artery is required, potentially reducing blood flow to the brain. Associated with this decreased availability of blood may be hypoxia caused by an inability of the collateral circulation to adequately supply blood to the brain (**Fig. 3–3**).

The second most useful application of EEG monitoring has been to help define the occurrence of embolic phenomena during these same procedures, which results in decreased blood flow and a potentially ischemic event, but which may be treated intraoperatively if recognized.[12]

In all of these situations EEG monitoring can help identify the presence of an insult, define the possibility for immediate therapy, and define the degree of burst suppression if barbiturate brain protection is instituted.

The typical pattern seen in the EEG during cerebral hypoperfusion is a reduction or loss in high-frequency activity and the appearance of large-amplitude slow waves in the range of 1 to 4 Hz. There are situations where the EEG may be acutely depressed upon injection of an anesthetic that rapidly passes the blood–brain barrier. Such situations may be found in high-dose opioid anesthesia, where fentanyl induces an immediate and marked reduction of fast frequency activity in the EEG, with an increase in low-frequency, high-amplitude activity.[33]

A simple but useful summary of possible changes is that decreased frequency with increased amplitude implies an ischemic event to the cortex,[106] widespread frequency slowing and decreased amplitude usually imply brain stem ischemia,[87] whereas ischemic events affecting the thalamus and the internal capsule produce unremarkable changes in the EEG[106] but possibly significant changes in the SEPs.

Somatosensory Evoked Potentials (Ascending Spinal Cord Activity)

SEPs are used during spinal surgery, vascular procedures, and cranial base procedures. For most cases we simultaneously stimulate the median or ulnar nerve at the wrist, and the common peroneal nerve as it passes under the head of the fibula, or the posterior tibial nerve at the medial malleolus.

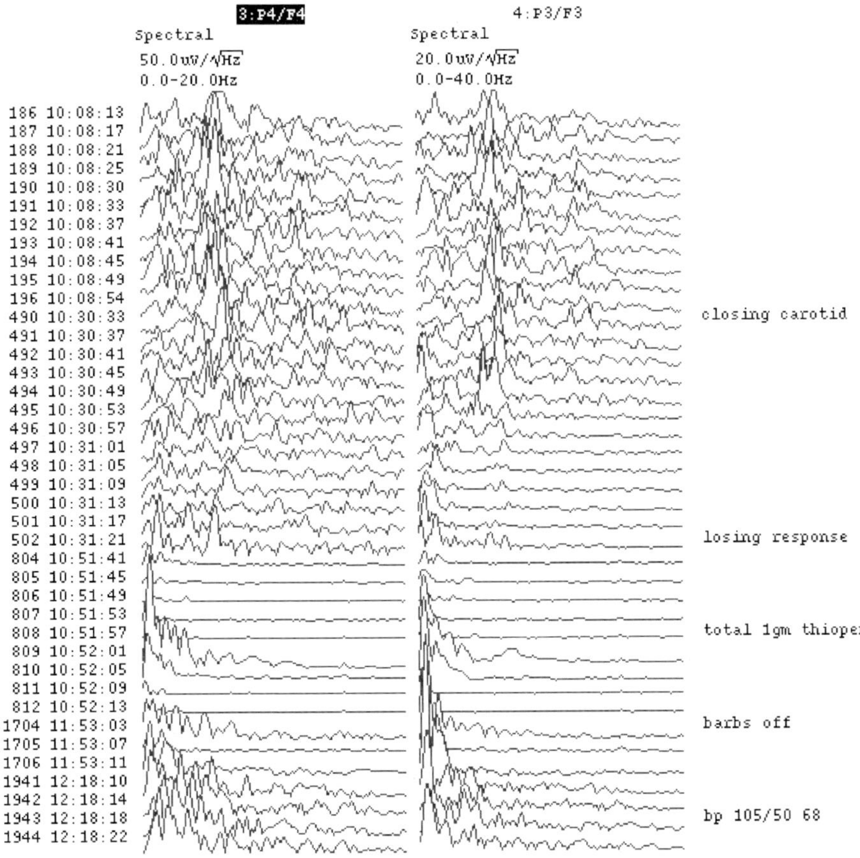

Figure 3–3 Power spectrum of two channels of electroencephalography recorded during temporary clipping of the left middle cerebral artery. Data are sequentially presented starting at the top of the figure. The spectra in column 2 demonstrate changes associated with cross-clamping and recovery after removal of the clip. Both channels of data reflect the generalized effect of thiopental on cortical activity and its underlying metabolic demand.

In addition, dermatomal SEPs are of use in selected cases where concern exists about protecting particular nerve roots, such as during tethered cord release.

SEPs are dependent on the stimulation of large afferent fibers of peripheral nerves. Following stimulation of peripheral nerves in the arms or the legs, SEPs can be reproducibly recorded over the spine and scalp. In the spinal cord, the SEPs are conducted primarily through the dorsal columns; however, extensive work has been done to clarify the generators for the various components of the SEPs.[24,25] In humans, loss of posterior column function is associated with abnormality of the SEPs; however, extralemniscal pathways may also mediate some mid- and long-latency scalp SEP components.

In our experience, SEPs are extremely sensitive and specific to spinal cord injury whether it occurs in the dorsal or in the ventral pathways. This is confirmed in the literature,[76] where a false-negative rate of 0.063% was found for 51,263 spinal cases in which SEPs were the only modality monitored. Furthermore, the negative predictive value (i.e., the likelihood of normal spinal cord function in the presence of stable SEPs) was 99.93%. This is a significant improvement over the 0.72 to 1.4% incidence of spinal cord injury reported for unmonitored cases.[62]

Temperature changes significantly influence the SEP latency. For each degree Celsius of local cooling, the nerve conduction velocity decreases by ~2.5 msec. During long operations, a drop in temperature around the nerve being stimulated can result in a progressive increase in latencies unrelated to surgical manipulation. Also, latencies may be transiently affected when the surgeon irrigates with physiological solution at cooler temperatures. Significant changes are also seen related to hypotension. Attention must be paid to these changes because spinal cord hypotension in patients with myelopathy may lead to an extension of the myelopathic lesion.

Upper Extremity (Median and Ulnar Nerve) Evoked Potentials

Median and ulnar nerve evoked potentials (MSPs and USPs) are both useful in assessing the brachial plexus, cervical spinal cord, brain stem, and telencephalon. These potentials are useful in preventing and reducing surgical morbidity during procedures that pose potential harm to the cervical cord and in assessing the level of hypoxia in cortical and spinal tissue.[35] Only the MSPs are described in detail here because the USPs are usually identical except for their level of entry into the spinal cord.

Stereotypical MSPs are simultaneously recorded from the ipsilateral Erb's point referenced to the contralateral Erb's point, the neck (cervical CV_7) and parietal (P_3 or P_4) (electrode locations are given in the International 10/20 system[49]) scalp with a reference to a frontal electrode (**Fig. 3–4**).

At Erb's point, the response is an NFP consisting of an apparently triphasic (positive-negative-positive) nerve action potential, reflecting the passage of a mixed nerve volley passing the brachial plexus. This component is usually labeled N_{11} for the large negative-going component generated at 11 msec (all waves will be identified as N or P for their polarity subscripted by the latency of the wave). At the cervical C_7 recording site, the NFP consists of an N14 wave with an associated complex waveform. It has been postulated that these waves are generated in the dorsal roots, dorsal horn, posterior columns, and structures of the lower brain stem.[27,28] The response recorded from scalp electrodes placed (roughly over the hand area of the sensory cortex) contralateral to the stimulated arm consists of a P_{15}, N_{20}, P_{30} complex. Some data suggest that P_{15} is thalamic in origin,[93] whereas N_{20} is generated in thalamocortical pathways, and P_{30} is generated in parietal cortex.[2,37] After this wave, there is considerable disagreement as to the identity of the cortical underlying generators; however, it is clear that the parietal cortex is involved in the generation of the N_{20}/P_{30} complex and that the parietal association areas are involved in the generation of the later waves.

Lower Extremity (Common Peroneal and Tibial Nerve) Evoked Potentials

In the lower limbs, nerves used to elicit SEPs include the tibial and peroneal nerves. Occasionally the femoral nerve is also used. Spinal potentials are most consistently obtained by stimulation of the tibial nerve at the medial malleolus or peroneal nerve in the popliteal fossa.

Recordings are made routinely at the lumbar spine and the cerebral cortex (Pz/Fz). SEPs also can be recorded along the thoracic or cervical spine as clinically indicated. Stimulation of the posterior tibial nerve at the ankle evokes P_{32} and N_{42} potentials in the younger population,[24] which gradually increases in latency until adult values of 40 and 48 msec, respectively, are obtained.[108] Stimulation of the common peroneal nerve at the popliteal fossa produces waves that are slightly shorter in latency.[25] The first useful component is an N_{20} wave, which is usually maximal over the T12 or L1 vertebra. At more rostral and caudal levels it may be possible to record small "traveling" waves, representing the envelope of action potentials in the dorsal roots and sensory tracts of the spinal cord.

Spinal SEPs are relatively easy to obtain in children, with the amplitude and definition of the waves decreasing with increasing age such that by the midteenage years these responses are more difficult to obtain. The response over the mid and lower lumbar spine consists of an initially positive triphasic potential. This reflects the NFP produced by a volley of action potentials ascending through the cauda equina (**Fig. 3–5**).

Dermatomal Responses

A disadvantage of SEPs produced by stimulation of large nerve trunks is that input to the spinal cord usually occurs over more than one level. This problem can be addressed by delivering the stimulus to small cutaneous nerves that are derived from a single dorsal root and which innervate the "signature area" of a particular dermatome.

Pudendal nerve responses are a special case of dermatomal responses, particularly useful in patients with spina bifida or tethered cords. The pudendal nerve carries sensory fibers from the penis, urethra, anus, and pelvic floor muscles, and supplies motor innervation to the bulbocavernosus and pelvic floor muscles, the external urethral sphincter, and the external anal sphincter. Cortical responses to

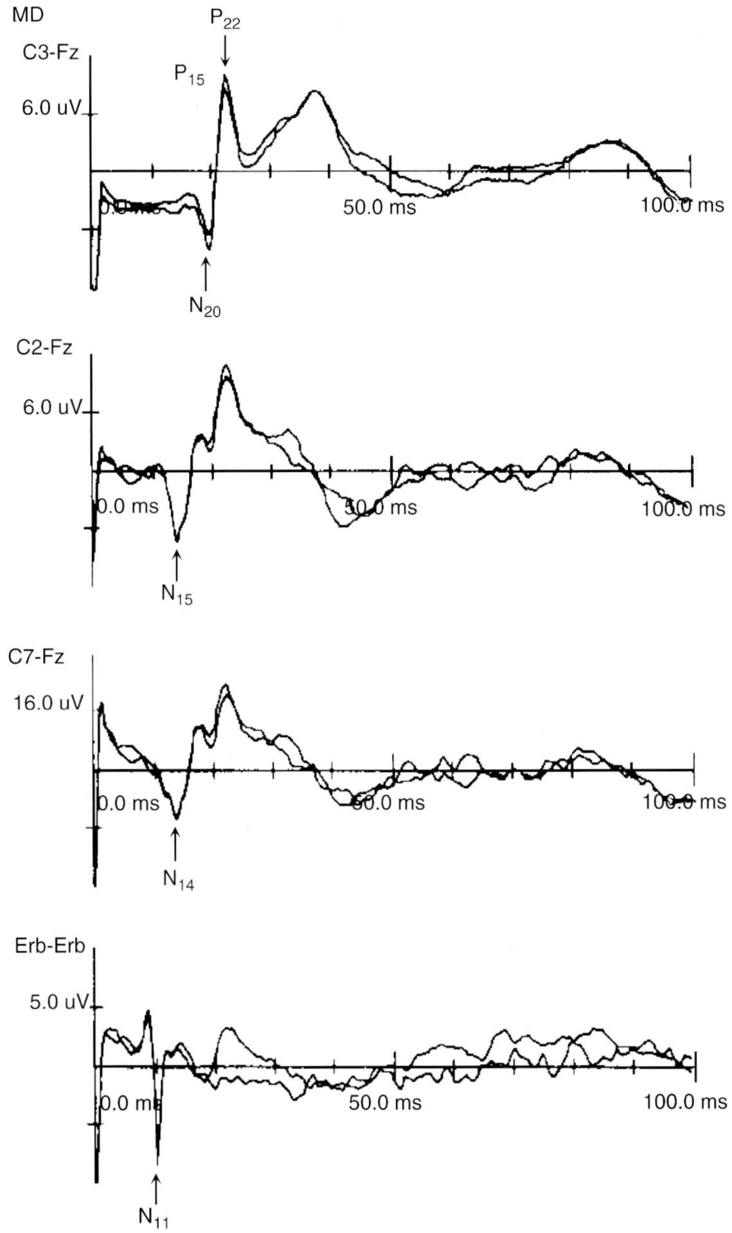

Figure 3–4 Median nerve evoked potentials (MSPs) demonstrating the significant waves at different levels along the neuraxis from Erb's point (ch 4) to the contralateral scalp (ch 1).

electrical stimulation of the dorsal nerve of the penis, the urethra,[41] and the urinary bladder[4] have all been described. Pudendal nerve responses are similar in morphology to the tibial nerve SEP and are best recorded from the same area of the scalp.[42]

Brain Stem Evoked Responses

BSEPs are monitored routinely during all procedures in which SEPs are recorded. We routinely record between electrode locations M_1 (left mastoid) and Fz, similar to the recording locations for BAEPs. The waves and their generators[27] are (1) P_{10}, the brachial plexus; (2) P_{12}, dorsal column nuclei; (3) P_{15} medial lemniscus; (4) N_{16}, thalamus; and (5) later peaks representing the thalamocortical projections. It is believed that multiple parallel spinal cord pathways are activated by suprathreshold stimulus intensities and that they contribute differentially to the various BSEP peaks.[85]

Ventral Cord Monitoring

Even though the results of SEP monitoring in preventing both motor and sensory iatrogenic injury during spinal surgery have been excellent, they cannot provide complete coverage of the spinal cord, and several cases have been reported of spinal injury going undetected using only SEP monitoring.[19,59]

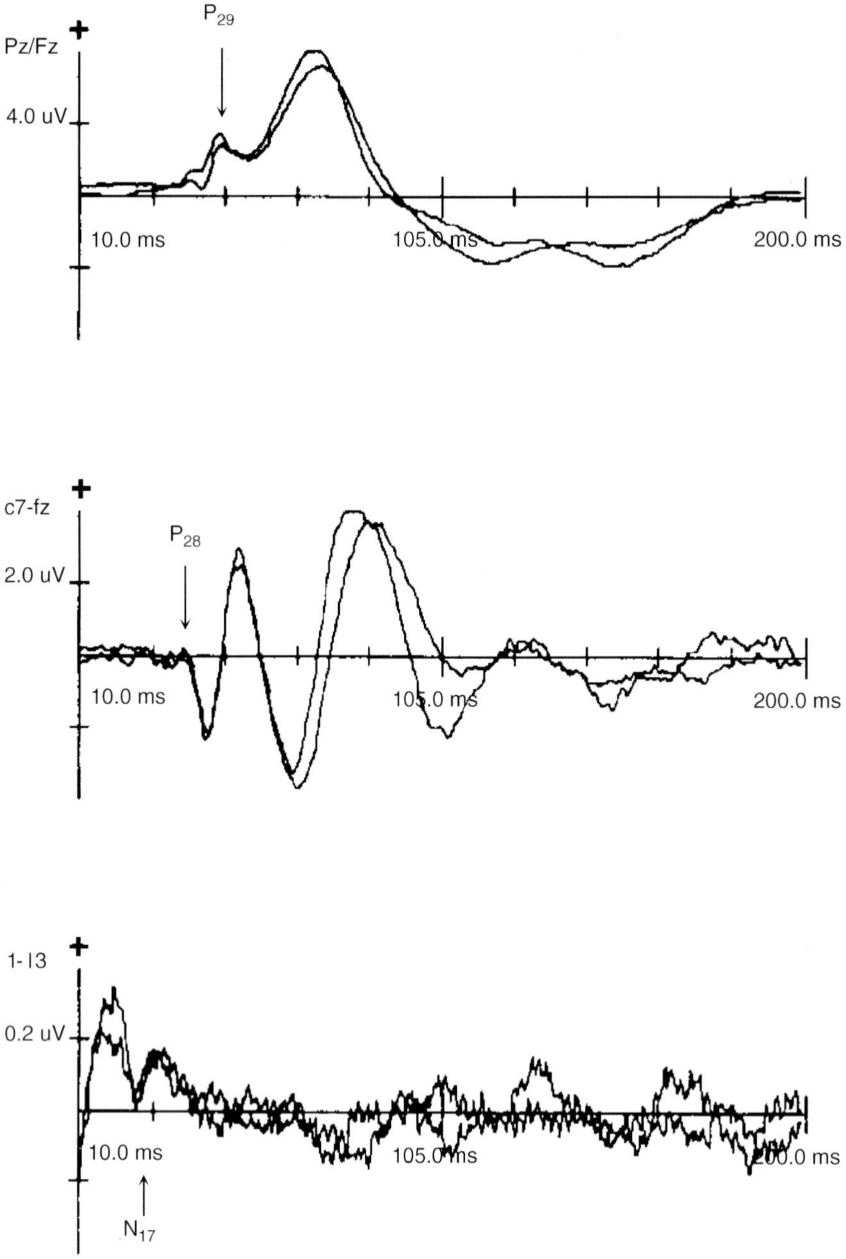

Figure 3–5 Posterior tibial nerve evoked potentials demonstrating components at different levels of the neuroaxis from the lumbar region bottom to the scalp top.

Thus considerable attention has been paid to developing robust and reliable methods for monitoring the more ventral corticospinal tracts.[47] Two methods briefly reviewed here are cerebellar and motor potentials (evoked EMGs).

Cerebellar Potentials (Ascending Activity)

In addition to the ascending dorsal columns and spinothalamic tracts and descending ventral motor tracts, several other ascending long tracts exist and are useful for IOM purposes. These pathways include the ventral and lateral spinocerebellar and cuneocerebellar tracts, which provide dense input to the cerebellum. Several studies have demonstrated that stimulation of the peripheral nerves commonly utilized to generate SEPs also generates a cerebellar evoked potential (CEP).[45] Moreover, animal models have demonstrated that the evoked potential recorded from the cerebellum is generated via ascending ventral spinal cord tracts.[44] Thus this stimulation and recording technique provides an assay of the ventral spinal cord utilizing conventional techniques developed for SEP monitoring. These responses may be obtained reliably and are reproducible from an additional electrode placed over the occiput and require the same anesthetic technique used to record SEPs.

Motor Evoked Potentials (Descending Activity)

Motor evoked potentials (MEP) have been under serious investigation in the IOM field for ~20 years.[47,66] In general, stimulation has involved either cortical or spinal cord sites. Noninvasive stimulation has been investigated using either electrical[63] or magnetic[9] stimulation of the motor cortex,[89] indirect stimulation of the spinal cord via spinous processes,[79] or direct stimulation of the spinal cord[100] by placing subdural or epidural stimulation electrodes. Various responses are recorded distal to the operative site for these assorted stimulation techniques. **Fig. 3–6** summarizes both the stimulating and the recording techniques currently available.[105] Recording sites include (1) spinal cord evoked potentials (SCEPs) using transcutaneous or direct (epidural or subdural) recording electrodes; (2) direct (D) and indirect (I) waves from the spinal cord using epidural recording sites; (3) CNAPs, referred to as NMEPs in **Fig. 3–6** recorded from peripheral nerves using transcutaneous or subdermal needle electrodes; and (4) CMAPs from muscle groups of the upper and lower extremities using transcutaneous or subdermal needle electrodes. CMAPs are referred to as myogenic potentials, whereas CNAPS have been termed neurogenic responses (**Fig. 3–6**).

Transcranial Stimulation

The motor cerebral cortex or brain stem can be activated by either electrical or magnetic stimulation; however, only electrical stimulators are currently approved by the Food and Drug Administration (FDA) for transcranial stimulation. Scalp electrodes or electrode plates placed adjacent to the scalp or hard palate can be used to stimulate the cortex and underlying tissues. Stimulation voltages are typically in the range of 100 to 250 V. SCEPs have been observed with between 100 and 4000 stimuli being averaged. CMAPs obtained following transcranial stimulation do not require averaging and provide a rapid assessment of motor pathway function; however, these responses are very susceptible to anesthetic influence and have considerable intrinsic variability, making their interpretation difficult. CNAPs have been extremely unreliable, again due to anesthetic effects.

Transcranial electrical stimulation through the intact scalp has been shown to result in a charge density that might result in neuronal damage if applied directly to the cortex.[78] However, electrical stimuli are attenuated by a factor of 30 due to the high resistance of the intervening muscle, skull, and meninges. Thus the charge density at the surface of the brain with electrical stimulation is estimated to fall well within acceptable safe limits.[3] One of the most important stimulation parameters for eliciting reliable transcranial Motor evoked potentials (MEPs) is the interstimulus interval (ISI) of a burst of stimuli, applied at the above-referenced rate.[101] It has been found that bursts of stimuli with an ISI between 2 and 5 msec produce a maximal response by overcoming the depressant effects of general anesthesia.[50,52] The significant parameters and morphological fea- tures of CMAPs generated via transcranial stimulation are response threshold, onset latency, central conduction time, and response size[48] (**Fig. 3–7**).

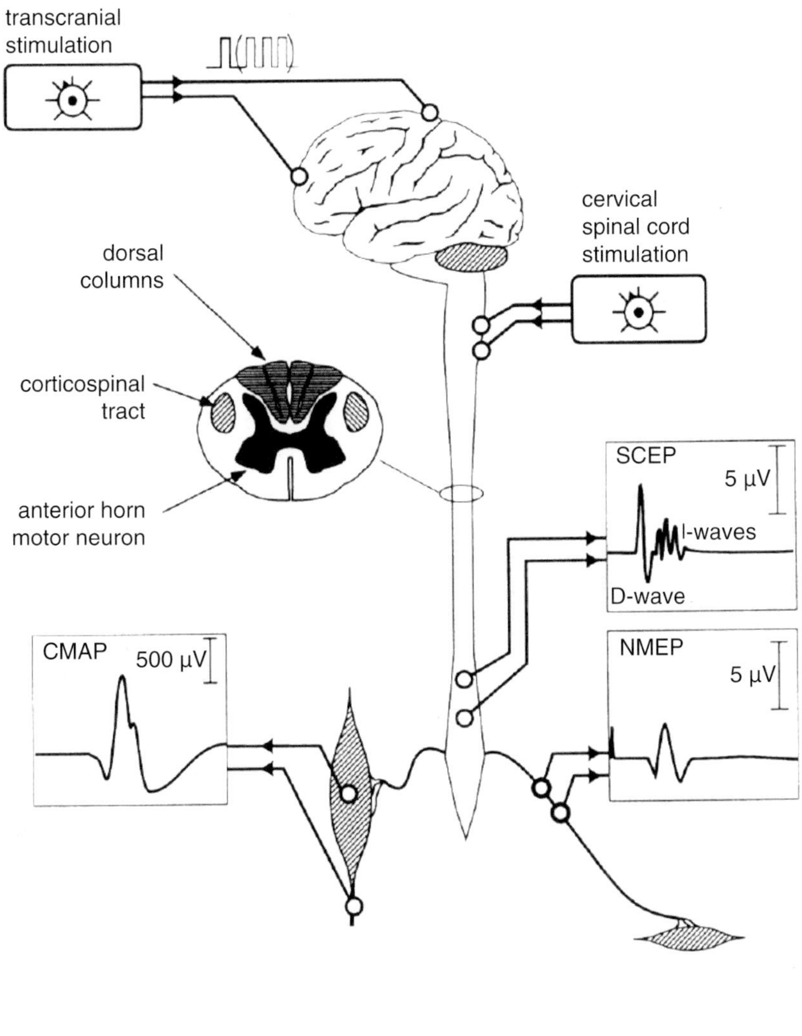

Figure 3–6 Various stimulating and recording sites for intraoperative motor evoked potential (MEP) monitoring. SCEPs are spinal cord evoked potentials. NMEPs are neurogenic motor evoked potentials, which are also referred to as compound nerve action potentials (CNAPs). CMAPs are compound muscle action potentials. (Printed with permission from Kalkman CJ, Ubags LH. Motor evoked potential monitoring. Current Opinion in Anaesthesiology 1997; 10:327–332.)

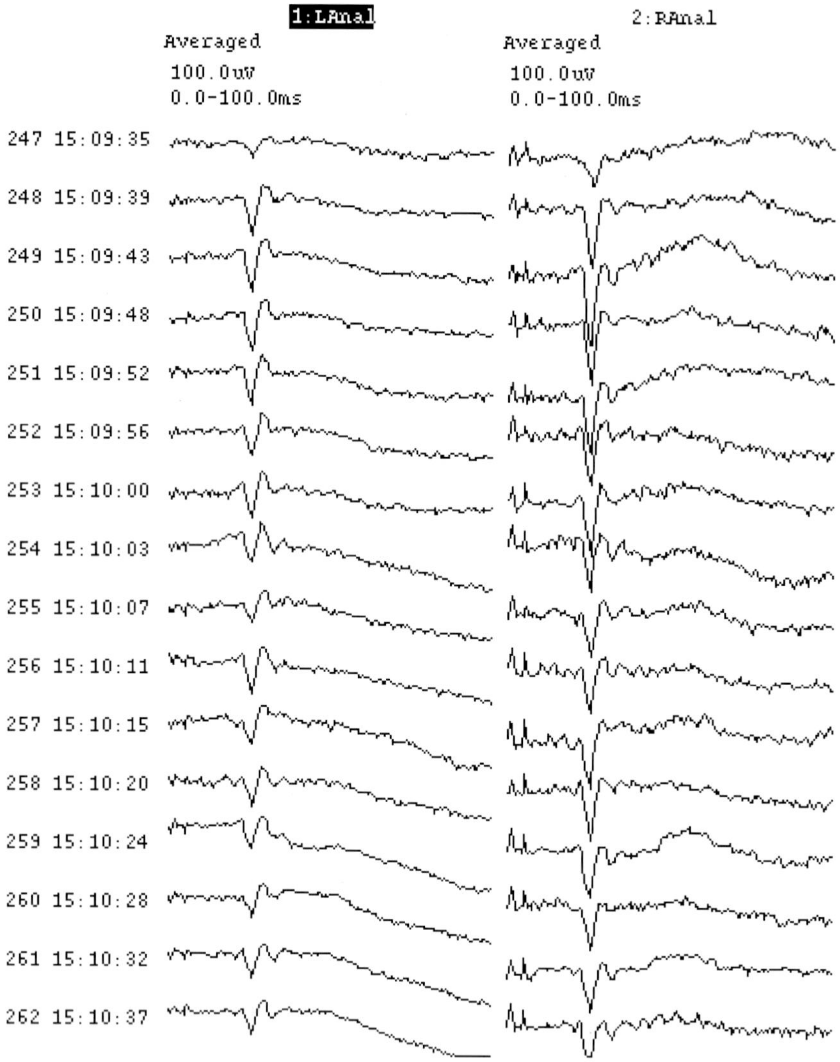

Figure 3–7 Compound muscle action potentials obtained by transcranial electrical stimulation during lumbosacral instrumentation from the external anal sphincter muscle.

Epidural spinal recordings of corticospinal tract activity following transcranial stimulation produce a complex of positive and negative components composed of I and D waves[48,84] **(Fig. 3–8).**

Indirect Spinal Cord Stimulation

Indirect stimulation of the spinal cord through vertebral bone has been used to produce descending neural activity recorded peripherally from mixed nerves (CNAP).[80] The CNAPs are typically recorded at the popliteal fossa, with stimulation provided through a pair of electrodes positioned at adjacent spinal processes in the cervical region. Considerable controversy exists over the relative contribution of the sensory and motor pathways to these neurogenic spinal evoked potentials. Thus the term *descending neurogenic evoked potential (DNEP),* which describes the stimulation method and the direction of the neural volley along the spinal cord, but not necessarily its composition, has been adopted. Collision studies[56] have raised serious doubts about the independent utility of this method because both modalities (SEPs and DNEPs) appear to be primarily mediated by the same neural pathways, namely, the dorsal columns.[103] The consensus, based on these experiments, is that these responses are not a pure motor response but are largely composed of antidromic sensory activity and minimal orthodromic motor activity.[82]

Direct Cord Stimulation

Considerable work has been done with direct stimulation over the midline of the posterior, rostral spinal cord and recordings made either with epidural or subdural[30] strip electrodes or peripheral CMAPs.[74] Epidural SCEPs recorded from the midline of the posterior spinal cord produced by a descending spinal cord volley of action potentials can vary in morphology depending on both the stimulating and the recording sites. The dominant waves seem to be an initial negative spike (N_1) followed by a slow negative component (N_2). The conduction velocity of the N_1 component has varied greatly, ranging from 47 to 90 m/s, whereas the average conduction velocity of the N_2 component has ranged from 46 to 53 m/s.[56,63]

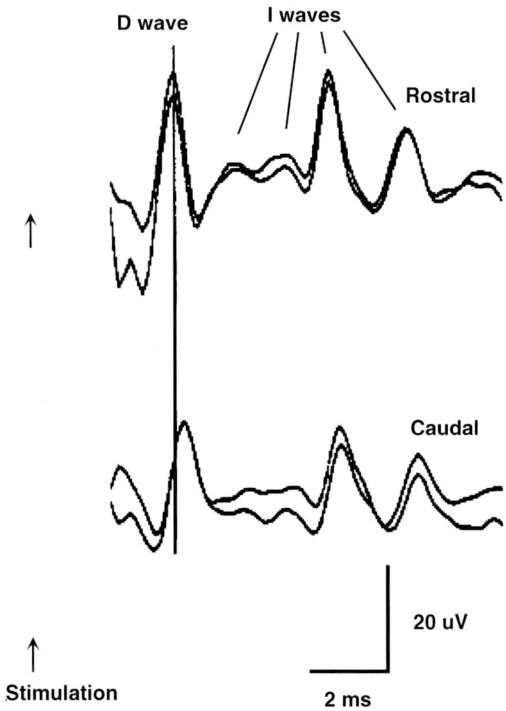

Figure 3–8 Typical direct (D) and indirect (I) waves recorded from the epidural space.

Spinal Cord and Peripheral Nerve Electromyography

The EMG, a useful indicator of the integrity of descending activity in the spinal cord, is electrical activity produced in muscle fibers below the skin and has a frequency content ranging from 15 to 150 Hz.[26] The EMG is either spontaneous (e.g., anal sphincter activity produced by irritation of the S_3 to S_5 roots during an untethering procedure involving the lower portion of the cauda equina) or evoked, of the type produced in selective rhyzotomy for the treatment of spasticity, for pedicle screw placement, or as already discussed for spinal cord evaluation. Evoked EMGs have a considerably larger amplitude ($\geq 100\ \mu V$) than sensory evoked potential data ($\geq 0.2\ \mu V$), and therefore these signals do not require averaging to extract them from the background noise.

Cranial Nerve Electromyography

Cranial nerve function is monitored continuously during many cases for two reasons: first, to identify the location and orientation of the cranial nerves in the operative field; and second, to preserve functioning in the cranial nerves and their related brain stem nuclei.[70]

The major observed variables are the EMGs recorded from the appropriate muscle group innervated by the cranial nerves of interest. The cranial nerves, along with the associated muscle groups, which are usually monitored using EMG techniques, are the facial nerve (VII) through the orbicularis oculi, orbicularis oris, and the mentalis muscles innervated by the zygomatic branch, the buccal branch, and the mandibular branch, respectively; the abducens nerve (VI) through the lateral rectus muscle; the trigeminal nerve (V) through the masseter muscle; the trochlear nerve (IV) from the superior oblique muscle; and the oculomotor nerve (III) through the medial and inferior rectus and the inferior oblique muscles of the eye. When appropriate, the functioning of the glossopharyngeal (IX), vagus (X), spinal accessory (XI), and hypoglossal (XII) cranial nerves is monitored by placing electrodes in the stylopharyngeus, cricothyroid, trapezius, and intrinsic muscles of the tongue, respectively. In general, the cranial nerves ipsilateral to the operative side are monitored; however, bilateral activity is monitored as necessary.

The amplifier band pass is set from 10 to 1000 Hz. The unstimulated EMG activity from multiple channels is monitored continuously throughout the case. Most importantly, the activity from all recorded muscle groups is made continuously audible. The audio system is of paramount importance in identifying the level of activity in the muscle groups. These signals are listened to continuously for evaluation of nerve function by both the neurophysiologists and the surgeons.

Four categories of EMG activity are observed: (1) no activity, which in an intact nerve is the best situation, but which also may be the case in a sharply dissected nerve; (2) irritation activity, which sounds like soft intermittent flutter and is consistent with working near the nerve; (3) injury activity, which sounds like a continuous, nonaccelerating tapping and can indicate permanent injury to the cranial nerve; and (4) a "killed-end" response, which sounds like an accelerating firing pattern and is an unequivocal indicator of nerve injury.[83] It is important to note that a sharply cut nerve may produce only a brief burst of activity; thus monitoring cannot be expected to replace extreme caution when working near the cranial nerves (**Fig. 3–9**).

In addition to monitoring the ongoing EMG activity, the various cranial nerves may be electrically stimulated. This is usually done to determine the location of the nerve in the operative field because many times the nerve is encased by tumor and may not be directly observable, or to determine the functional integrity of the nerve.[83] The most common example of this procedure is the direct stimulation of the seventh nerve. The stimulus utilized is a constant voltage, with a pulse frequency of 10 Hz and a pulse width of 100 µsecs. The voltage amplitude is typically varied between 0.1 and 1 V. In some situations, where very precise localization of the nerve is required, bipolar stimulating electrodes are utilized.[43]

Auditory Evoked Potentials (Brain Stem) and Direct Recording

Monitoring the function of the eighth cranial nerve is used to preserve hearing, locate the eighth nerve, and determine if the overall function of the brain stem is altered.

Brain Stem Auditory Evoked Potentials (BAEPs)

The classic BAEP consists of a minimum of five and a maximum of seven peaks. The first five peaks, Jewett waves I through V, are the principal peaks used in clinical practice. All occur within 10 msec of a brief click or tone presentation.

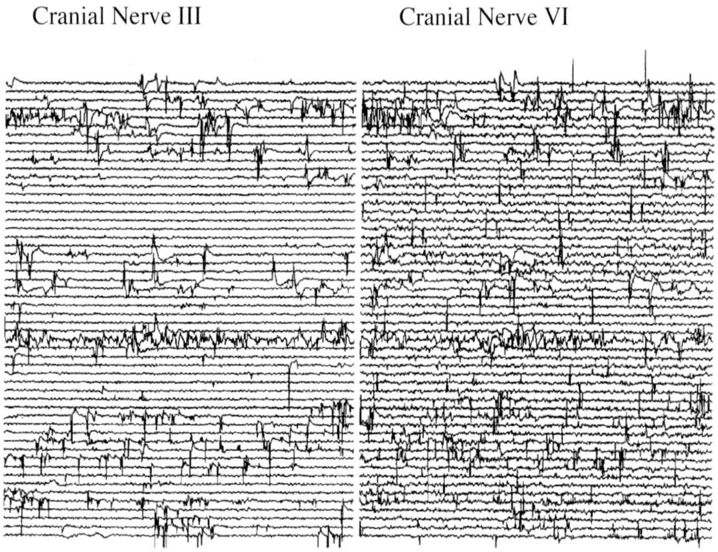

Figure 3–9 Spontaneous electromyographic recorded from the medial rectus and lateral rectus muscles of the eye, innervated by cranial nerves III and VI during resection of a cranial base tumor.

Wave I is generated in the cochlear portion of the eighth nerve. Its latency is ~1.5 to 2.1 msec in a normal adult. Wave I is present in recordings made on the ipsilateral side to the stimulus but is not usually seen on contralateral-side recordings. Wave II is generated bilaterally at or in the proximity of the cochlear nucleus. The latency between waves I and II is ~0.8 to 1.0 msec. The amplitude of wave II on the contralateral side may be greater than on the ipsilateral side. Wave III is generated bilaterally from the lower pons near the superior olive and trapezoid body. The latency between waves I and III is ~2.0 to 2.3 msec in a normal adult. Wave III may be smaller on the contralateral side than on the ipsilateral side. Waves IV and V are probably generated in the upper pons or lower midbrain, near the lateral lemniscus or possibly near the inferior colliculus.[17] In ipsilateral recordings waves IV and V may fuse into a complex that can vary between two identifiable components with a common base to a single wave with a tall, wide peak. On the contralateral side the peaks tend to be more easily identified. Wave V tends to be the most robust peak and is typically the last to disappear when stimulus intensity is reduced. In addition, there tends to be a large negative-going wave following wave V, which aids in its identification. Wave V, being the most robust is most closely followed during intraoperative procedures (**Fig. 3–10**).

The intensity level of the click is set to ~90 dB sound pressure level SPL. However, when the patient is known to have a hearing loss or a given patient's responses are not well

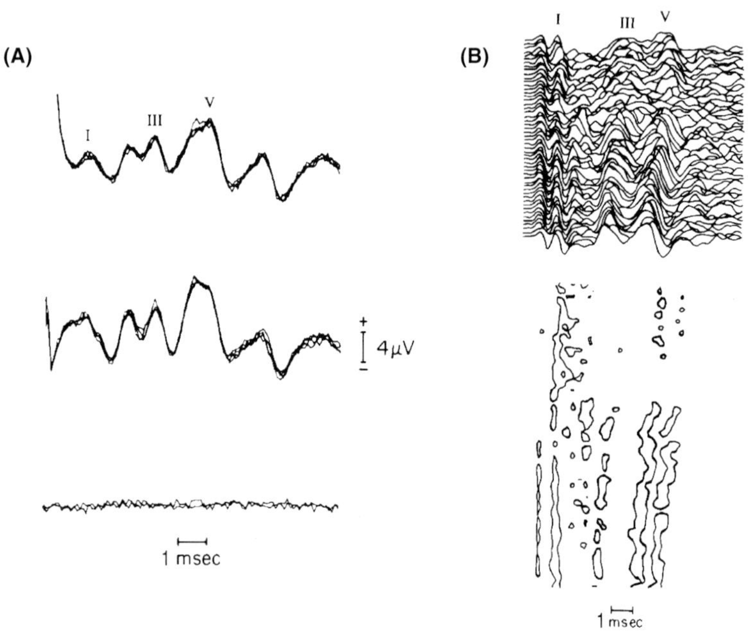

Figure 3–10 **(A)** Normal BAEPs and **(B)** BAEPs recorded during microvascular decompression for trigeminal neuralgia showing increase in latency as a function of retraction.

defined, higher intensity levels may be required. In such cases an intensity level of 95 dB SPL is typical. Rarefaction and compression clicks are applied in an alternating fashion to minimize apparent stimulus artifact. The stimulus rate is usually set between 9.3 and 19.3 Hz because of the well-known effects of higher stimulus rates on response latencies.[107]

Baseline responses for each ear are acquired prior to the beginning of surgery. These data are compared with the preoperative evaluation and used as baselines throughout the case.

Waves I to V are relatively resistant to sedative medication and general anesthetics. Thus BAEP recording places no constraints on the anesthesiologist. However, they are sensitive to temperature changes, with absolute and interpeak latencies increasing by ~0.20 msec/°C.

The latency of wave V is the primary concern in IOM of the BAPs because this is the most robust and easily identifiable of the waves. Latency shifts of greater than 0.3 msec are reported to the surgeon. However, clear changes in the wave morphology, even with latency shifts less than 0.3 msec, are reported. The next average is recorded as soon as possible to confirm the presence of a significant change. In cases where potentials are completely lost, the neurophysiologist reports the loss and then immediately checks to ensure that both the stimulating system and the recording electrodes are functioning properly.

Auditory Nerve Compound Action Potentials (Direct Recording)

CNAPs may be recorded directly from the cochlear portion of the eighth cranial nerve ($CNAP_a$).[72] To accomplish this recording, the intracranial portion of the eighth nerve must be exposed during the operation. The eighth nerve is composed of the vestibular and cochlear divisions. Near the brain stem the cochlear division is located on the caudal side of the eighth nerve and is anterioventral to the eighth nerve near the porus acusticus. Moller and Jannetta[68] reported a technique for recording the $CNAP_a$ by placing a recording electrode on the exposed eighth nerve. They recommended that the electrode be made of fine, malleable, multistrand, Teflon-insulated silver wire with a cotton wick sutured to the wire.

The recording electrode need not be placed directly on the cochlear portion of the nerve to record $CNAP_a$. The amplitude of the recorded potentials is largest, however, when the recording electrode is placed on the cochlear division. Even when placed on the vestibular portion of the eighth nerve the amplitude of the potentials is normally several microvolts. The $CNAP_a$ recorded in a patient with normal hearing appears as the triphasic waveform previously described. This recording technique provides the capability to detect changes in neural conduction almost instantaneously on the basis of recording click-evoked CNAP and can be valuable in patients with preexisting hearing loss and, as a consequence, poor BAP recordings.

Visual Evoked Potentials

VEPs are used to aid in determining the functional integrity of the visual system, primarily in the region of the optic nerves, chiasm, and optic radiations.[1] The recorded activity is generated either at the retina (electroretinogram) or at the occipital cortex.

Except in selected situations, stimulation of the visual system using a bright flash is not recommended for diagnostic purposes due to intersubject variability;[22] however, in the operating room this is a very helpful and effective technique. Four waves are typically seen in the VEP: P_{60}, which is thought to be generated in subcortical structures; and N_{70}, P_{100}, and N_{120}, which are all thought to be generated in the primary visual cortex.[55]

Peripheral Nerve Compound Action Potentials

The recording of CNAPs from the peripheral nerve, evoked by supramaximal stimulation, provides a measure of the functional integrity of the nerve and may be thought of as a physiological biopsy of the nerve. Pathophysiological mechanisms produce reductions in conduction velocities, desynchronization of CNAPs and CMAPs, and complete conduction block.

Measurements of this type are used to protect a particular peripheral nerve from damage during surgical repair of some other structure and to aid the surgeon in determining the correct approach to repairing a damaged peripheral nerve[34] (e.g., repair of a neuroma-in-continuity by neurolysis or anastomosis). CNAP recording is useful because the amplitude of the CNAP is approximately correlated with the number of moderately sized early myelinating fibers present in the recovering nerve. The presence of these fibers in a recovering nerve indicates that neurolysis alone will be effective, as opposed to resection and repair, in reestablishing useful distal function.[102] The appearance of a CNAP in a damaged nerve precedes the reinnervation of the muscle and is therefore detectable considerably earlier than EMG evidence of reinnervation and even longer before clinical recovery. The absence of a CNAP 3 to 4 months after injury demonstrates failed regeneration and allows for repair to be undertaken at a time when denervated muscle is still receptive to returning axons.

The major focus of CNAP recording is the presence or absence of a CNAP across a segment of the damaged nerve. When a CNAP is present, the surgeon may stop with neurolysis and be assured that the damaged nerve will likely recover to a reasonable degree. When the CNAP is absent, the surgeon must be prepared to resect and repair the damaged section of peripheral nerve (**Fig. 3–11**).

Other Monitoring Modalities

Oximetry

The use of near infrared spectroscopy (NIRS) to measure cerebral oxygenation is a developing field.[18] The systems that are currently available are based on reflectance spectrophotometry.[6] These devices provide a very localized regional oxygen saturation index (rSO_2) or relative hemoglobin oxygen, deoxyhemoglobin, total hemoglobin, and cytochrome oxidase, and a total oxygen index. The difficulties with this technique pertain to the fact that the distance between where the light enters the tissue and the point of detection is unknown and variable depending on the degree

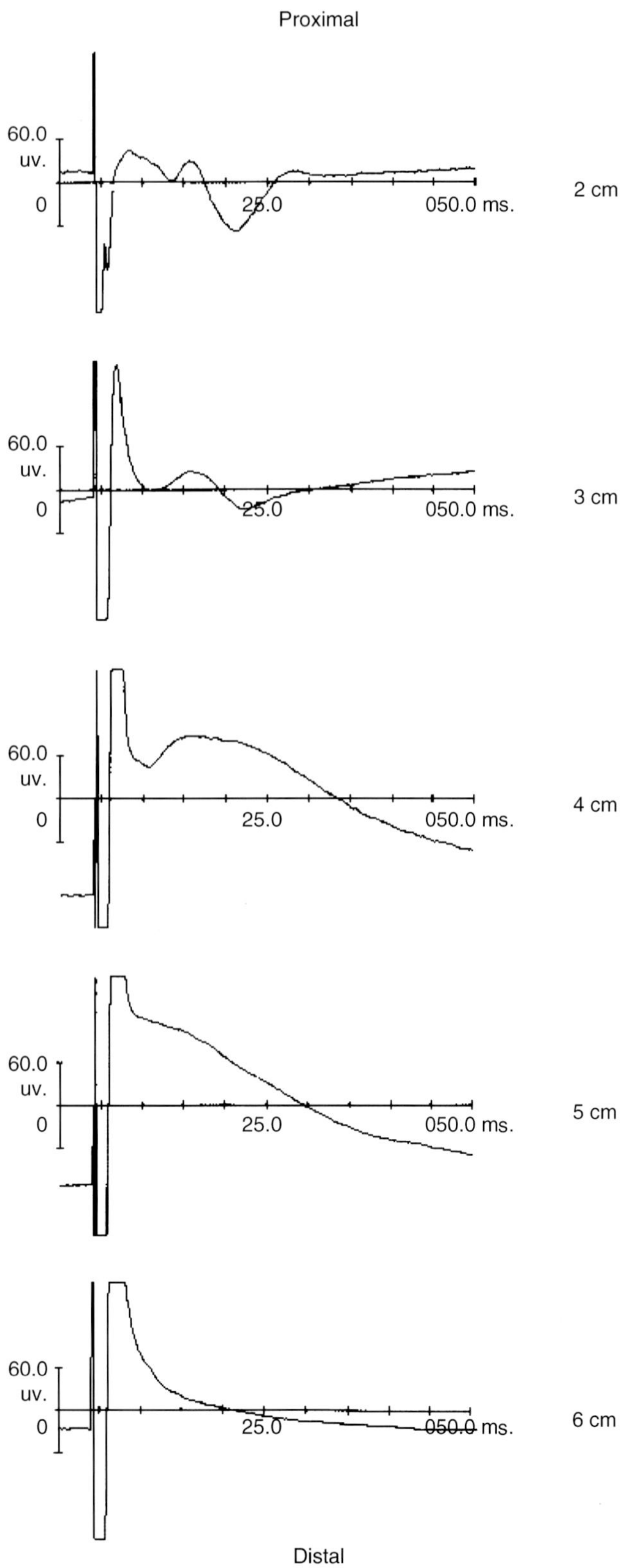

Figure 3–11 Compound nerve action potentials recorded above and below a neuroma-in-continuity, suggesting that an anastomosis was the appropriate treatment.

of light scattering and on the amount of absorbing material in the tissue.

All calibrations must be tested on the basis of jugular venous and arterial blood oxygen saturation. Studies have examined the relationship between regional oxygen saturation of hemoglobin and jugular venous saturation.[16] The cerebral oximeter was less accurate and precise and also demonstrated a systematic error in bias unrelated to cerebral perfusion pressure. Comparisons have been made between MSPs and cerebral oximetry during carotid endartectomy.[21] This technology will play an important role in IOM as it develops further.

Transcranial Doppler

Transcranial Doppler (TCD) sonography has proven to be a safe and reliable intraoperative tool for measuring blood flow velocities within the major vessels of the cerebrovasculature. Pulses of ultrasound, delivered at frequencies of 2 MHz, are directed using a probe that can either be handheld or fastened securely with a head holder. The pulses are directed toward the major vessels at the base of the skull through various bony windows located on the skull.

The frequency shift, or Doppler effect, in the reflected sound indicates the velocity of the reflecting substance within the artery. Images can then be rendered from the time-dependent intensity of the reflected sound.

TCD sonography has been used extensively during carotid endarterectomy for both the detection of changes in blood flow velocity during cross-clamping of the internal carotid artery and detection of embolus during dissection, shunt placement, and reopening of the carotid artery. Blood flow velocities can also be useful as a measure of a lack of autoregulation after the artery has been cleared of debris. The lack of autoregulation is revealed as a sustained increase in velocity, which presumably is an indication of a hyperemic blood flow state.

Microvasculature Doppler

Microvasculature Doppler sonography has also proven to be an invaluable tool during various neurosurgical procedures. A sterile handheld 20 mHz, 1 mm pulsed Doppler may be employed to insonate arterial vasculature directly within the surgical site. The Doppler is placed either directly on the vessel or on a vessel that may be encased in either bone or tumor. The Doppler probe is able to insonate at various depths beginning at 1 mm. The depth of insonation can be advanced in 1 mm steps up to 10 mm.

Microvasculature Doppler sonography has been used extensively during aneurysm surgery, providing real-time assessment of vasculature patency after aneurysm clipping[5,57,97] and thus preventing permanent ischemic damage. Microvasculature Doppler sonography during aneurysm surgery utilizes direct insonation of exposed vasculature and feedback concerning patency of parent and daughter vessels as well as information regarding the successful obliteration of the aneurysm itself. Several reports have demonstrated either or both the readjustment and the replacement of aneurysm clips based on feedback provided by the handheld Doppler.[5]

Microvasculature Doppler sonography can also be utilized during skull base procedures for the identification of critical vasculature in either tumor or bony dissection. In contrast to aneurysm surgery, microvascular Doppler sonography during skull base procedures utilizes insonation of vasculature through bony structures or intracerebral masses, that is, when the vessels are not visible to the surgeon. It has been reported that intraoperative Doppler sonography is an effective means by which to locate and identify critical vascular structures during skull base tumor resection.[7] The identification of this vasculature allows for the successful approach and resection of intracerebral masses in a situation where simple visual identification is not possible. Doppler sonography also allows for confirmation of vascular patency after exposure of the vasculature in question and serves as a valuable adjuvant to other forms of IOM known to improve outcome during skull base procedures.

◆ Neurosurgical Procedures

Cortical Localization

The surgical resection of cerebral cortex is often limited by neighboring regions of essential functional cortex. There is a high degree of individual variability with respect to cortical topography and functional localization.[77] Intraoperative brain-mapping techniques have been used to localize language cortex, sensorimotor pathways, and seizure foci. Methods of direct cortical recording and stimulation as well as subcortical stimulation enable maximum tumor resection and minimal morbidity.

Phase Reversal

MSPs recorded from the cortex are similar in appearance to the data previously presented. P_{15} is approximately equally distributed over the entire scalp because it is generated in the subcortical structure. N_{20} and P_{30} have extensive distribution over the scalp with a maximum over the parietal area contralateral to the stimulus and phase reversal across the central sulcus. MSPs are easily recorded directly from the human cortex, using surface point contact electrodes due to their large amplitude, and in contrast to their widespread scalp distribution, N_{20} and P_{30} are highly localized to the immediate rolandic-perirolandic area in direct recordings. Thus three characteristics make MSPs ideally suitable for functional localization studies: (1) localization close to the rolandic fissure, (2) their large amplitude in this location, and (3) the amplitude reversal of N_{20} and P_{30} across the rolandic fissure (**Fig. 3–12**).

Evoked potentials from the scalp either from a parietal electrode or from an electrode placed between the contralateral parietal and central position and are used to compare the polarity of corresponding peaks recorded from scalp and subdural electrodes. The cortical electrodes are positoned prerolandic when the peaks recorded from the cortex are phase reversed with respect to the parietal scalp electrodes. If the peaks are in phase, the electrodes are postrolandic.[61] All somatosensory evoked responses produce results; however, the best results are obtained with the MSPs.

Cortical Stimulation

We have found the techniques described by Berger at al,[15] with slight modification, to be very effective. Simultaneous electrocorticography (ECoG) is performed to monitor for after-potential discharge indicating that the direct stimulation is too intense and should be reduced to avoid the induction of seizure activity. Patients under general anesthesia remain unparalyzed until the motor mapping is completed.

Direct application of current to the sensory cortex may elicit paresthesias in the appropriate somatic area in awake patients, especially when the face and hand areas are

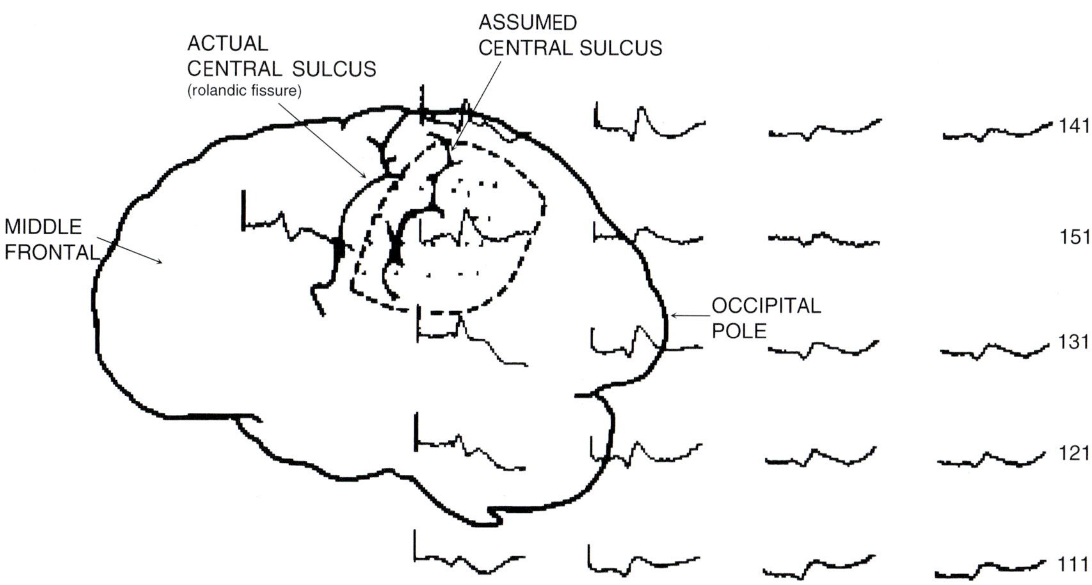

Figure 3–12 Median nerve evoked potentials phase reversal across the central sulcus allowing localization of motor and sensory strips.

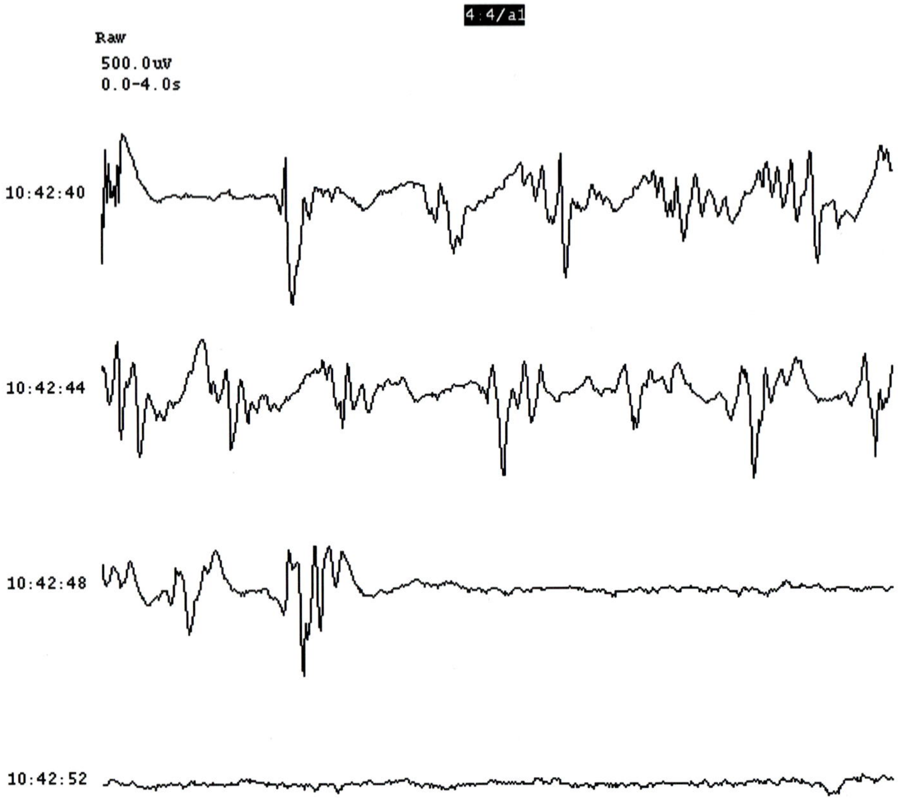

Figure 3–13 Seizure activity induced by prior direct cortical stimulation, which is turned off at the beginning of the top trace. In this situation the afterdischarge lasted for ~10 seconds.

stimulated. Language mapping is performed using the maximal current that does not evoke afterdischarges yet is effective in altering language function. Patients are asked to repeat standard phrases and name standard objects during the stimulation. Repeated instances of speech arrest or anomia accompanying stimulation are the end points used to determine language localization.

Focal seizure activity may occur with increasing current intensity during any of these testing procedures and is detected by the simultaneous ECoG. If this activity does not cease spontaneously within 10 to 30 seconds, intravenous Valium or a short-acting barbiturate should be given. Cold saline applied to the cortex will also suppress seizure activity and has the advantage of not interfering with further recording (**Fig. 3–13**).

◆ Vascular Procedures

The functioning of the cerebral cortex is extremely sensitive to changes in arterial oxygenation, cerebral blood flow, or partial pressure of oxygen. This sensitivity is rapidly reflected by changes in EEG,[67] SEPs, and cerebral oximetry. Some factors that may contribute to ischemic events are decreased oxygen-carrying capacity due to hypovolemia or decreased cerebral perfusion pressure due to factors associated with decreased systemic arterial pressure, increased intracranial pressure, or mechanical obstruction of cerebral vessels.[33]

Critical information is gained from monitoring the EEG and SEPs (both median nerve and tibial or peroneal nerve). Changes in observed activity may be due to retraction, brain stem compression, or impairment of blood flow to cortical and subcortical structures. Cortical activity also guides the surgeon regarding the adequacy of collateral flow when hypotension, intentional temporary occlusion, or cerebrovascular bypass is necessary for treatment of vascular anomalies. In addition, functional information may be obtained prior to the removal of cortical tumors.

For cortical responses, the amplitude and latency of the N_{20}/P_{30} complex are of primary concern. In general, a decrease of more than 50% in amplitude or an increase of more than 10% in latency is communicated to the surgeon. Another average is obtained as soon as possible to confirm the stability or persistence of the response change. The neurophysiologist consults with the anesthesiologist to determine if a change in blood pressure, level of anesthesia, or type of anesthesia could have contributed to the observed variations in either or both the amplitude and the latency of the evoked potential.

Intracranial Aneurysms

Cerebral aneurysm obliteration carries risks associated with cerebral ischemia secondary to occlusion of parent and perforating arteries, cerebral vasospasm, as well as embolic events associated with vessel manipulation and clip application.

To reduce ischemic insult, multimodality IOM has been successfully implemented and shown to be a useful adjunct during these procedures.[60] The evoked potential modalities recorded during aneurysm clipping will be dictated by the location of the lesion. For posterior circulation aneurysms, both BAPs and SEPs should be recorded simultaneously. These modalities will provide physiological feedback concerning the integrity of several different brain stem pathways as well as provide information concerning the integrity of the somatosensory cerebral cortices. For anterior circulation aneurysms, SEP recording in response to median nerve and tibial nerve stimulation is essential. These modalities provide information about the normal functioning of both midline and lateral somatosensory cortical function secondary to potential disruptions in blood flow during the procedure. In addition to evoked potential monitoring, bihemispheric EEG should be recorded during these procedures.[81]

Endovascular Treatment of Intracranial Aneurysms

IOM has been useful in the surgical treatment of intracranial aneurysms, and this usefulness has carried over to the endovascular treatment of intracranial aneurysms.[8] MSPs, tibial nerve evoked potentials (TSPs), BAPs, and EEGs have been recorded in 43 consecutive patients undergoing Guglielmi detachable coiling (GDC) of anterior and posterior circulation cerebral aneurysms using methods already described. Thirty-one procedures (72.1%) had no neurophysiological changes during the procedure. Twelve procedures (27.9%) were observed to have significant alterations in monitored parameters. All 12 of these procedures involved coiling of the anterior circulation aneurysms. No posterior circulation aneurysm embolizations ($N = 14$) have been associated with BAP changes. Of those with significant changes, nine (20.9%) were transient, whereas three (7.0%) persisted throughout the procedure. No significant change in baseline neurological status was observed in 39 (90.6%) patients. Transient neurological change, as defined by a return to baseline within 2 months of the procedure, was observed in three (6.9%), and one (2.3%) patient experienced a persistent neurological deficit (**Fig. 3–14**).

Carotid Endarterectomies

The majority of patients with either asymptomatic or symptomatic carotid artery stenosis undergo carotid endarterectomy (CEA) under general anesthesia with and without mandatory intraluminal bypass shunting of carotid artery blood flow and using IOM to determine the need for selective use of intraluminal carotid shunts. The latter option makes no assumption of the patient's ability to tolerate cerebral hypoperfusion. Instead, IOM can be used to evaluate the patient for cerebral ischemia and to identify those patients that do not have adequate collateral cerebral perfusion and require supplemental perfusion through use of a carotid artery shunt. Using IOM in carotid endarterectomy

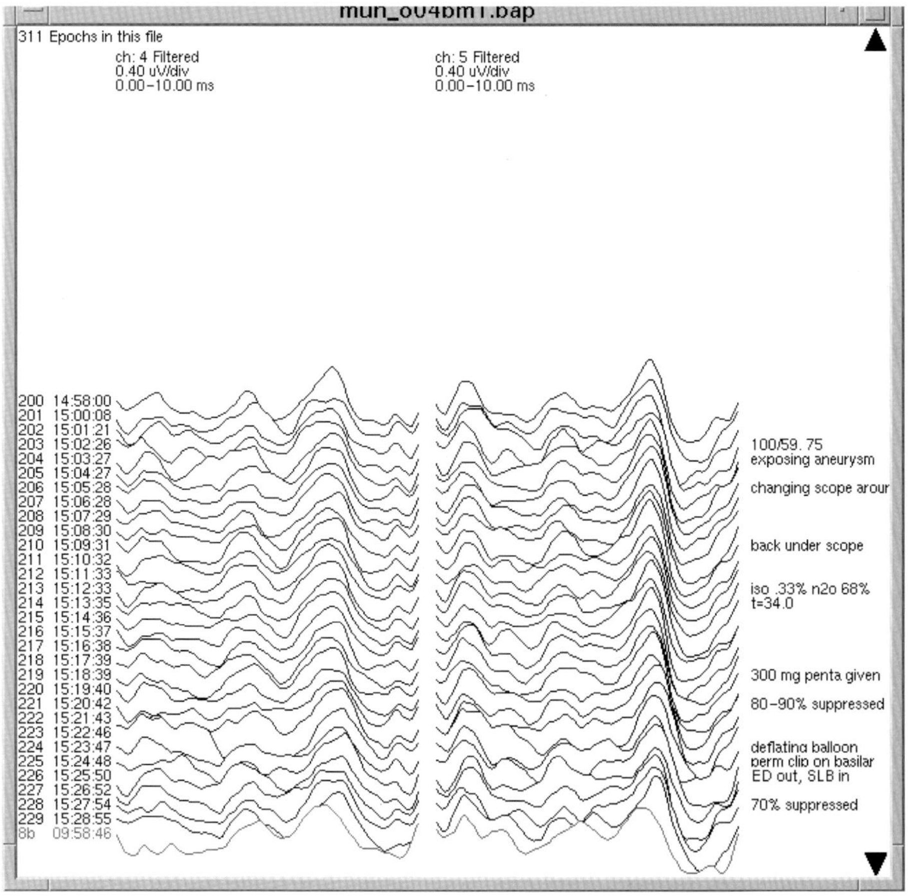

Figure 3–14 Bilateral BAEPs during clipping of basilar tip aneurysm.

reduces the frequency of shunt placement, which has been associated with iatrogenic injury.[46,99] In addition, IOM allows the blood flow through carotid shunts to be evaluated for adequacy during carotid endarterectomy and is also sensitive to intraoperative thromboembolic events.[12]

Pallidotomy and Deep Brain Stimulation

In pallidotomy, the goal is to place large, destructive radiofrequency, thermal lesions within as much of the internal segment of the globus pallidus as possible without causing iatrogenic injury to adjacent structures, specifically the internal capsule and the optic tract. Although the lesion-making electrode is placed under stereotactic guidance, even small deviations in the final electrode tip position can result in misplaced lesions with devastating consequences to the patient. Because of this, small, reversible test lesions are made that are evaluated in two ways. Because the patient is awake, the integrity of the internal capsule can be continuously examined by having the patient follow commands to make arm, leg, or facial movements. Having the patient repeat complex sentences can assess dysarthric speech. The optic tract can be continuously evaluated electrophysiologically with use of flash visual evoked potentials (FEP). Typically the large P100 cortical response is monitored before, during, and after test lesions, and changes in either or both the FVP and voluntary motor commands are used to change the electrode tip location until there is a return to baseline behavioral and electrophysiological values. A permanent lesion is then placed.

IOM would be an important adjunct to the procedure to confirm the electrode tip has not strayed off target. To ensure proper electrode placement and to minimize morbidity, MSP, MEP, and FVP tests may be utilized. In addition, more advanced IOM methods such as recording from single neurons to identify gross firing patterns of cell groups may be necessary to determine where the electrode tip is, given the small cell volume of structures such as the subthalamic nucleus.

◆ Microvascular Decompression Procedures

IOM has been a significant factor in reducing the incidence of hearing loss in microvascular decompression (MVD) operations.[69] In neurovascular compression syndromes (of cranial nerves V, VII, VIII, IX, X, and XI and the lateral medulla), we routinely monitor BAEPs and appropriate cranial nerve EMGs. The eighth cranial nerve is more sensitive to mechanical manipulation than other cranial nerves of the cerebellopontine angle, and monitoring BAPs has proven to be important in reducing risks of hearing loss by detecting changes in neural conduction in the auditory nerve. It has been shown that changes in the BAP caused by retraction could be reversed by releasing the retraction, resulting in preservation of hearing. It has been our experience in MVD procedures that an increase in the wave V latency of greater than 1.5 msec and a decrease in wave V amplitude of greater than 50% at least three times in a single operation significantly increases the risk of ipsilateral hearing loss to greater than 10%.[53]

Trigeminal Neuralgia

Trigeminal neuralgia (TN) is thought to be due to ephaptic transmission in the trigeminal nerve between large-diameter myelinated A-fibers and poorly myelinated A-delta and C (nociceptive) fibers. Vascular compression of the trigeminal nerve occurs most commonly at the root entry zone by the superior cerebellar artery. Monitoring a CN V MVD procedure requires only the use of BAPs, although monitoring fifth nerve EMG during reexploration procedures is worthwhile using subdermal electrodes over the masseter muscle. Via the retromastoid approach, cerebellar retraction is adjusted or eliminated if the latency of wave V changes more than 1.0 msec[32]; however, latency shifts greater than 0.3 msec are noted. Failure to respond to such changes could result in iatrogenic injury, causing, for example, loss of hearing. In one series of over 3000 patients, 75% were pain free at 15 years with an incidence of hearing loss of just over 0.5%[11] (**Fig. 3–10**).

Two patients of 300 having an MVD for TN over a recent 12-month period have had their BAPs disappear completely during dural closure. The CP angle was immediately reexplored, and a prominent vascular compression of the cochlear nerve was observed. MVD of this nerve was then performed with an immediate restoration of the BAPs.[109]

Hemifacial Spasm

Hemifacial spasm (HFS) is thought to be due to either ephaptic transmission[90] or hypersensitization of the facial nucleus.[31] The pathogenesis is from vascular compression of the facial nerve at the root entry zone most commonly by the posterior inferior cerebellar artery. Facial nerve EMGs in patients with HFS are notable for "lateral spread," or the abnormal dispersion of action potentials through branches of CN VII. Successful treatment of HFS may depend on the elimination of lateral spread with removal of an offending vessel from the root entry zone of CN VII.[10] This is confirmed intraoperatively with facial nerve EMG produced by stimulating the zygomatic branch of CN VII and recording a direct evoked EMG from the orbicularis oculi and an abnormal indirect evoked EMG from the mentalis muscle.[71] In this operation the disappearance of the abnormal indirect evoked EMG is used to determine the end point of the decompression, as opposed to its use in other operative procedures where the EMG activity serves either a warning or identifying function. In a series of 684 patients, 84% were spasm free after 10 years.[10] In this series 2.6% had an ipsilateral deaf ear, and 0.9% had severe facial weakness (**Fig. 3–15**).

We have also noticed in a series of 67 patients having MVD for HFS that, of 46 (69%) who had multiple previous Botox injections, six (13%) were surgical failures, whereas all 21 Botox-naive patients had complete or dramatic improvement. All the failed Botox patients had a nonclassical lateral spread (indirect response).[53]

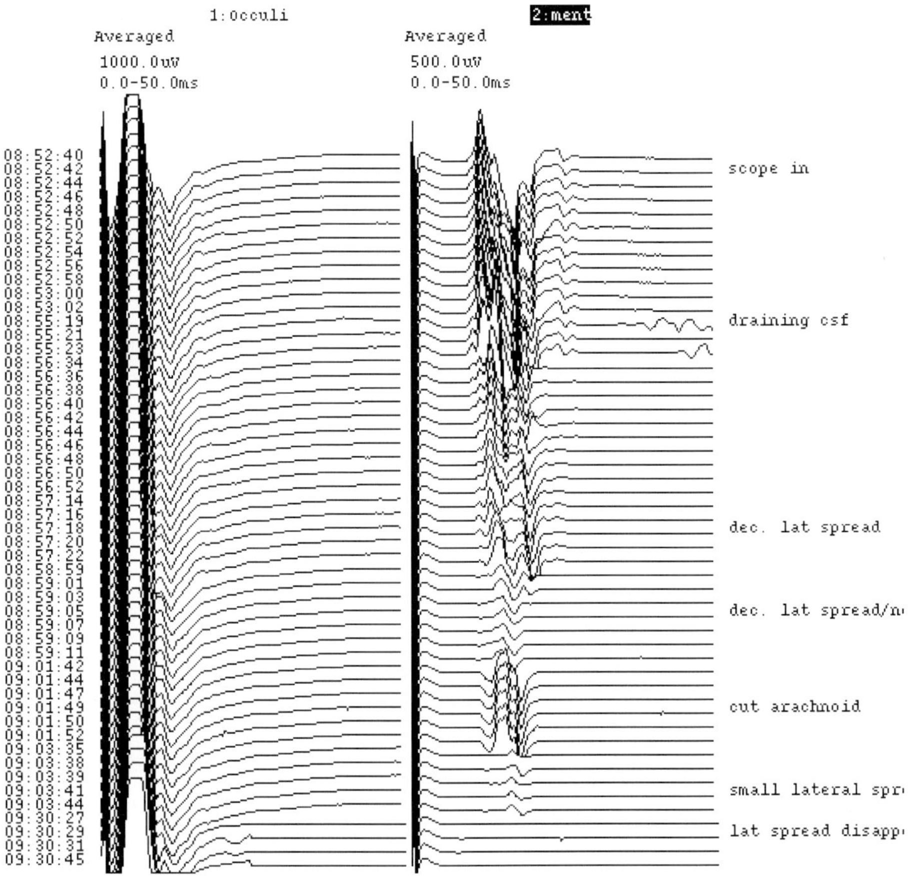

Figure 3–15 Lateral spread serving as an end point for surgical decompression. These data were recorded from a 59-year-old female with left hemifacial spasm. The direct responses are shown in the left column, and the indirect responses are shown in the right column.

Cranial Base Procedures

Neurophysiological monitoring during cranial base procedures can rapidly become quite complex. It is not unusual to monitor as many as nine different neurophysiological variables simultaneously; for example, EEG, BAPs and BSEP, SEPs, and EMGs relating to five cranial nerves (III, IV, V, VI, and VII). The major risks in these procedures are due to problems associated with maintaining adequate blood supply to the brain stem and cerebral hemispheres and to the effect of various operative manipulations aimed at adequately exposing the tumor and removing it.

In removing tumors from the cavernous sinus, clival region, fourth ventricle, or posterior fossa or within the cerebellopontine angle, appropriate cranial nerve EMG recording is critical.[94]

Acoustic Neuromas

From an IOM perspective, one must first determine whether the patient has useful hearing prior to surgery. This is best accomplished via an audiogram and baseline BAEP testing. If the patient does have useful hearing and a reasonable BAEP tracing is obtained, then a hearing preservation approach to the tumor may be chosen (middle fossa, retrosigmoid).[13] As with other IOM strategies employed with procedures involving masses of the posterior fossa, a multimodality approach is utilized. BAEPs should be recorded in response to auditory stimulation delivered to the ipsilateral ear. It has also been shown that compound nerve action potentials recorded directly from the eighth nerve can assist in hearing preservation during these procedures.[23] Additionally, facial nerve free-running EMG should be continuously recorded from the orbicularis oculi, orbicularis oris, and mentalis muscle groups and made audible to the surgeon.[88]

Evoked facial nerve EMG activity should also be elicited via monopolar stimulation to map the course of the seventh nerve through the cerebellopontine angle. This is vital in attaining a favorable outcome with regard to facial nerve function.[38] In larger tumors (and in those patients without useful hearing), it is useful to record BAPs in response to stimulation of the contralateral ear as a measure of brain stem function. It is also essential to measure brain stem function via MSP recordings in response to median nerve stimulation in cases where large tumors cause significant brain stem displacement. Additional cranial nerves should also be monitored in larger lesions. The fifth cranial nerve, which is usually adjacent to the rostral border of the tumor, can be monitored via EMG recording from the messeter muscle and the ninth and tenth cranial nerves, which are usually adjacent to the caudal tumor edge and can be monitored via recording from the soft palate and vocal cords. Overall, IOM techniques for acoustic neuroma surgery can be very challenging and complicated; constant vigilance on the part of the neurophysiologist and interaction with the surgeon are necessary (**Fig. 3–16**).

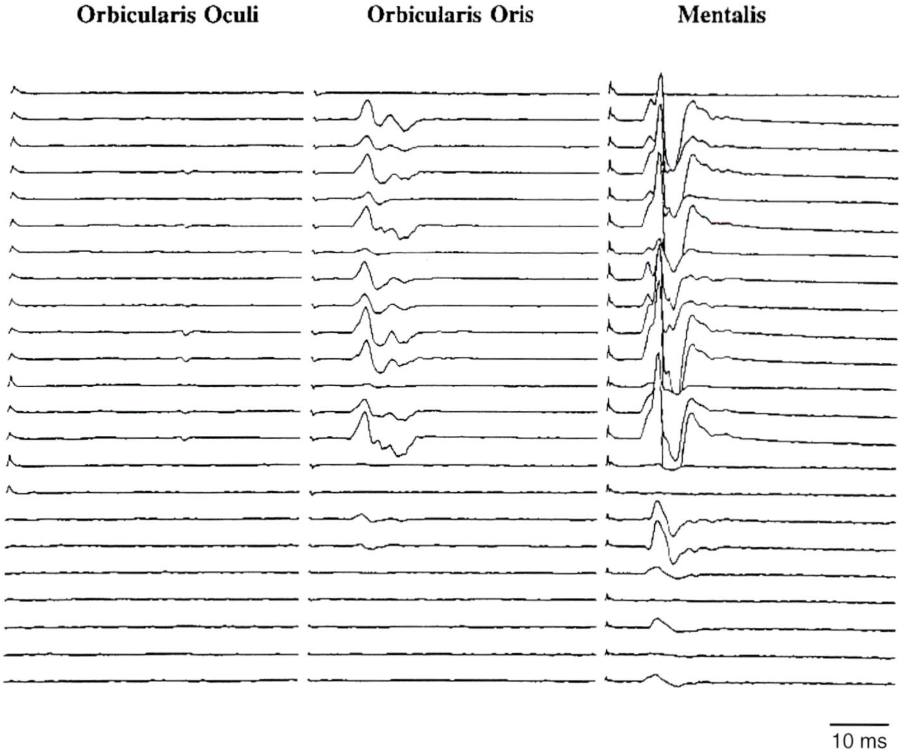

Figure 3–16 Compound muscle action potentials obtained from stimulation of CN VII during removal of an acoustic neuroma.

Mapping the Floor of the IV Ventricles

In the normal posterior fossa, the motor nuclei of the cranial nerves are located on the floor of the fourth ventricle relative to various anatomical landmarks. In cases where pathology is present, these normal landmarks can be distorted and, as a consequence, may not be identified. In persons with fourth ventricular brain stem masses that are adherent to or growing from the floor of the fourth ventricle or in pathologies that are intrinsic to the brain stem (e.g., cavernoma), techniques have been developed that allow identification of motor nuclei using direct electrical stimulation. The facial colliculus and the motor nuclei of CN IX/X and XII can be located,[73,98] and decisions concerning further tumor dissection or brain stem myelotomy can be made. Procedurally, different points along the floor of the fourth ventricle are stimulated with a monopolar or bipolar probe, and EMG responses are recorded from various muscle groups, including the orbicularis oculi, orbicularis oris, mentalis, soft palate, and intrinsic muscles of the tongue. Once the extent and borders of the nuclei have been identified, the surgeon can proceed.

Posterior Fossa Procedures

Intra-axial posterior fossa tumors can be of a wide variety, occurring in both adults and children. Whatever the age or tumor type, a multimodality approach to IOM is preferred when the surgical procedure involves the posterior fossa.[20] Specifically, with tumors filling the fourth ventricle, BAEP and SEP recordings are essential. SEP recordings should be made in response to at least median nerve stimulation, and care should be taken to record a subcortical brain stem potential in addition to cortical recordings during these procedures. The BAEP should be recorded in response to either right or left ear stimulation, although if the tumor is eccentric to one side, the ipsilateral ear should be stimulated. In addition to evoked potential monitoring, multiple bilateral cranial nerve EMG recordings should be obtained during these procedures.[64]

◆ Discussion

The commonly accepted goal of IOM is to prevent morbidity; however, the more fundamental goal is to provide information that allows the surgeon to accomplish the desired operative objective with as little morbidity as possible. This requires rapid and reliable interpretation of the data under sometimes suboptimal circumstances, and excellent communication between the surgeon and the neurophysiologist.

Several general rules have been found to be useful in our experience. We consider all increases in latency from baseline, for early and middle latency components (< 50 msec), of 10% to be significant. We also consider all amplitude reductions greater than 50% from baseline to be significant, requiring the immediate attention of the surgical team. Finally, we consider the degree of variability in the responses to be highly correlated with the degree of pathology. For example, a normal spinal cord will produce very consistent and nonvariable responses, but a spinal cord with a significant lesion will produce highly variable responses. And most importantly, responses that are highly stable at the beginning of a case but start to demonstrate increasing variability in either amplitude or latency are indicative of a potentially developing lesion.

The issue of cost benefits of monitoring has only been addressed partially and incompletely in the literature. In one paper[14] the financial records of 193 patients were evaluated for monitoring during cranial base surgery. In this series, the average cost of monitoring was $555 per case, whereas the estimated cost of the additional hospital stay for a patient with a major preventable deficit was $52,500. In this series there were 47 patients with significant monitoring changes that were acted on and who demonstrated no postoperative deficits. If deficits were prevented in only three of these patients because of monitoring, then IOM is cost-effective.

References

1. Albright AL, Sclabassi RJ. Cavitron ultrasonic surgical aspirator and visual evoked potential monitoring for chiasmal gliomas in children. J Neurosurg 1985;63:138–140
2. Allison T. Developmental and aging changes in human evoked potentials. In: Barber C, Blum T, Nodar R, eds. Evoked Potentials III. Boston: Butterworth; 1987:72–90
3. Amassian VE, Cracco RQ, Maccabee PJ. Focal stimulation of human cerebral cortex with the magnetic coil: a comparison with electrical stimulation. Electroencephalogr Clin Neurophysiol 1989;74:401–416
4. Badr G, Carlsson CA, Fall M, et al. Cortical evoked potentials following stimulation of the urinary bladder in man. Electroencephalogr Clin Neurophysiol 1982;54:494–498
5. Bailes JE, Tantuwaya LS, Fukushima T, Schurman GW, Davis D. Intraoperative microvascular Doppler sonography in aneurysm surgery. Neurosurgery 1997;40:965–972
6. Balzer JR, Nemoto EM. Cerebral oximetry during carotid endarterectomy. ASNM Monitor 1999;7:35–42
7. Balzer JR, Kassam AB, Crammond D, et al. Intraoperative microvascular Doppler sonography for arterial localization during skull base surgery. In press.
8. Balzer JR, Horowitz M, Krieger D, et al. Neuphysiological monitoring during Guglielmi detachable coiling for cerebral aneurysms. In press.
9. Barker AT, Jalinous R, Freeston IL. Non-invasive magnetic stimulation of the human motor cortex. Lancet 1985;1:1106–1107
10. Barker FG, Jannetta PJ, Bissonette DJ, Shields PT, Larkins MV, Jho HD. Microvascular decompression for hemifacial spasm. J Neurosurg 1995;82:201–210
11. Barker FG, Jannetta PJ, Bissonette DJ, Larkins MV, Jho HD. The long-term outcome of microvascular decompression for trigeminal neuralgia. N Engl J Med 1996;334:1077–1083
12. Barr JD, Horowitz MB, Mathis JM, Sclabassi RJ, Yonas H. Intraoperative urokinase infusion for embolic stroke during carotid endarterectomy. Neurosurgery 1995;36:606–611
13. Battista RA, Wiet RJ, Paauwe L. Evaluation of three intraoperative auditory monitoring techniques in acoustic neuroma surgery. Am J Otol 2000;21:244–248
14. Bejjani GK, Nora PC, Vera PL, Broemling L, Sekhar LN. The predictive value of intraoperative somatosensory evoked potential monitoring: review of 244 procedures. Neurosurgery 1998;43:491–500
15. Berger MS, Kincaid J, Ojemann GA, Lettich A. Brain mapping techniques to maximize resection, safety, and seizure control in children with brain tumors. Neurosurgery 1989;25:786–792
16. Brown R, Wright G, Royston D. A comparison of two systems for assessing cerebral venous oxyhaemoglobin saturation during cardiopulmonary bypass in humans. Anaesthesia 1993;48:697–700
17. Buchwald JS, Huang CM. Far-field acoustic responses: origins in the cat. Science 1975;189:382–384
18. Chance B, Cope M, Gratton E, Ramanujam N, Tromberg B. Phase measurement of light absorption and scatter in human tissue. Rev Sci Instru 1998;689:3457–3481
19. Chatrian GE, Berger MS, Wirch AL. Discrepancy between intraoperative SSEPs and postoperative function: case report. J Neurosurg 1988;69:450–454
20. Cheek JC. Posterior fossa intraoperative monitoring. J Clin Neurophysiol 1993;10:412–424
21. Cho H, Nemoto EM, Yonas H, Balzer J, Sclabassi RJ. Cerebral monitoring by means of oximetry and somatosensory evoked potentials during carotid endarterectomy. J Neurosurg 1998;89:533–538
22. Ciganek L. The EEG response (evoked potential) to light stimulus in man. Electroencephalogr Clin Neurophysiol 1961;13:165–172
23. Colletti V, Bricolo A, Fiorino FG, Bruni LC. Changes in directly recorded cochlear nerve compound nerve action potentials during acoustic tumor surgery. Skull Base Surg 1994;4:1–9
24. Cracco JB, Cracco RQ, Stolove R. Spinal evoked potentials in man: a maturational study. Electroencephalogr Clin Neurophysiol 1979;46:58–64
25. Cracco JB, Cracco RQ. Spinal, brainstem, and cerebral SEP in the pediatric age group. In: Cracco RQ, Bodis-Wollner I, eds. Evoked Potentials. New York: Alan R. Liss; 1986;471–482
26. Daube JR, Harper CM. Surgical monitoring of cranial and peripheral nerves. In: Desmedt JE, ed. Neuromonitoring in Surgery. Amsterdam: Elsevier; 1989;115–138
27. Desmedt JE, Cheon G. Central somatosensory conduction in man: neural generators and interpeak latencies in the far-field components recorded from neck and right or left scalp and earlobes. Electroencephalogr Clin Neurophysiol 1980;50:382–403
28. Desmedt JE. Generator sources of SEPs in man. In: Cracco RQ, Bodis-Wollner I, eds. Evoked Potentials. New York: Alan R. Liss; 1986:235–245
29. Domino KB. Anesthesia for cranial base tumor operations. In: Sekhar LN, Schramm VL, eds. Tumors of the Cranial Base: Diagnosis and Treatment. Mount Kisco, NY: Futura; 1987;107–122
30. Ertekin C. Intradural spinal recordings (particular reference to invasive methods). In: Ducker TB, Brown RH, eds. Neurophysiology and Standards of Spinal Cord Monitoring. New York: Springer-Verlag; 1988:82–99
31. Ferguson JH. Hemifacial spasm and the facial nucleus. Ann Neurol 1978;4:97–103
32. Fischer C. Brainstem auditory evoked potential (BAEP) monitoring in posterior fossa surgery. In: Desmedt JE, ed. Neuromonitoring in Surgery. New York: Elsevier; 1989;191–207
33. Freye E. Cerebral Monitoring in the Operating Room and the Intensive Care Unit. Boston: Kluwer Academic; 1990
34. Friedman W. The electrophysiology of peripheral nerve injuries. Neurosurg Clin N Am 1991;2:43–56
35. Gentili F, Lougheed WM, Yamashiro K, Corrado C. Monitoring of sensory evoked potentials during surgery of skull base tumors. Can J Neurol Sci 1985;12:336–340
36. Goff WR. Human average evoked potentials: procedures for stimulating and recording. In: R. Thompson F, Patterson MM, eds. Bioelectric Recording Techniques. Part B: Electroencephalography and Human Brain Potentials. New York: Academic; 1974:101–156
37. Goff WR, Williamson PD, Vangilder JC, Allison T, Fisher TC. Neural origins of long latency evoked potentials recorded from the depths and from the cortical surface of the brain in man. In: Desmedt JE, ed. Progress in Clinical Neurophysiology. Vol 2. Basel: Karger; 1980: 126–145
38. Goldbrunner RH, Schlake HP, Milewski C, Tonn JC, Helms J, Roosen K. Quantitative parameters of intraoperative electromyography predict facial nerve outcomes for vestibular schwannoma surgery. Neurosurgery 2000;46:1140–1148
39. Grundy BL. Intraoperative monitoring of sensory-evoked potentials. Anesthesiology 1983;58:72–87
40. Grundy BL. Anesthetic considerations in spinal surgery. In: Salzman SK, ed. Neural Monitoring: The Prevention of Intraoperative Injury. Clifton, NJ: Humana Press; 1990:253–270
41. Haldeman S, Bradley WE, Bhatia N. Evoked responses from the pudendal nerve. J Urol 1982;128:974–980
42. Haldeman S, Bradley WE, Bhatia NN, Johnson BK. Cortical evoked potentials on stimulation of the pudendal nerve in women. Urology 1983;21:590–593

43. Harner SG, Daube JR, Beatty CW, Ebersold MJ. Intraoperative monitoring of the facial nerve. Laryngoscope 1988;98:209–212
44. Hurlbert RJ, Koyanagi I, Tator CH. Sensory evoked potentials for selective monitoring of ventral rat spinal cord: a cerebellar evoked potential for assessing ventral cord integrity. J Neurotrauma 1993;10:181–200
45. Hurlbert RJ, Fehlings MG, Moncada MS. Use of sensory-evoked potentials recorded from the human occiput for intraoperative physiological monitoring of the spinal cord. Spine 1995;20:2318–2327
46. Isley MR, Cohen MJ, Wadsworth JS, Martin SP Jr, O'Callaghan MA. Multimodality neurophysiological/electroencephalographic monitoring for carotid endarterectomy surgery determination of critical cerebral ischemic thresholds. Am J END Technol 1998;38: 65–122
47. Isley MR, Balzer JR, Pearlman RC, Zhang X-F. Intraoperative motor evoked potentials. Am J END Technol 2001;41:266–338
48. Inghilleri M, Berardarelli A, Cruccu G, et al. Corticospinal potentials after transcranial stimulation in humans. J Neurol Neurosurg Psychiatry 1989;52:970–974
49. Jasper HH. Report of Committee on Methods of Clinical Examination in EEG: Appendix: The ten twenty system of the International Federation. EEG Clin Neurophysiol 1958;10:370–375
50. Jones SJ, Harrison R, Koh KF, Mendoza N, Crockard HA. Motor evoked potential monitoring during spinal surgery: responses of distal limb muscles to transcranial cortical stimulation with pulse trains. Electroencephalogr Clin Neurophysiol 1996;100:375–383
51. Kamura J. Electrodiagnosis in Diseases of Nerve and Muscle. Philadelphia: FA Davis; 1983
52. Kalkman CJ, Ubags LH, Been JD, Swaan A, Drummond JC. Improved amplitude of intraoperative myogenic evoked response after paired transcranial electrical stimulation during sufentanil/nitrous oxide. Anesthesiology 1995;83:270–276
53. Kassam A, Horowitz M, Scarrow A, et al. Outcomes following microvascular decompression for hemifacial spasm in 121 patients. J Neurosurg Submitted
54. Kimura J. Field theory as it pertains to SEP analysis. In: Salzman SK, ed. Neural Monitoring. Clifton, NJ: Humana Press; 1990:5–21
55. Kraut MA, Arezzo JC, Vaughan HG Jr. Intracortical generators of the flash VEP in monkeys. Electroencephalogr Clin Neurophysiol 1985;62:300–312
56. Leppanen R, Madigan R, Sears C, MaGuire J, Wallace S, Captain J. Intraoperative collision studies demonstrate descending spinal cord stimulated evoked potentials and ascending somatosensory evoked potentials are mediated through common pathways [abstract]. J Clin Neurophysiol 1999;16:170.
57. Laborde G, Gilsbach J, Harders A. The microvascular Doppler: an intraoperative tool for the treatment of large and giant aneurysms. Acta Neurochir Suppl (Wien) 1988;42:75–80
58. Lee YW. Statistical Theory of Communication. New York: Wiley; 1960
59. Lesser RP, Raudzens P, Leuders H, et al. Postoperative neurological deficits may occur despite unchanged intraoperative somatosensory evoked potentials. Ann Neurol 1986;19:22–25
60. Lopez JR, Chang SD, Steinberg GK. The use of electrophysiological monitoring in the intraoperative management of intracranial aneurysms. J Neurol Neurosurg Psychiatry 1999;66:189–196
61. Luders H, Dinner DS, Lesser RP, Morris HH. Evoked potentials in cortical localization. J Clin Neurophysiol 1986;3:75–84
62. MacEwen GD, Bunnell WP, Sriram K. Acute neurological complications in the treatment of scoliosis. J Bone Joint Surg Am 1975;57:404–408
63. Machida M, Weinstein SL, Yamada T, Kimura J. Spinal cord monitoring: electrophysiological measures of sensory and motor function during spinal surgery. Spine 1985;10:407–413
64. Manninen PH, Patterson S, Lam AM, Gelb AW, Nantau WE. Evoked potential monitoring during posterior fossa surgery: a comparison of two modalities. Can J Anaesth 1994;41:92–97
65. McPherson RW. General anesthetic considerations in intraoperative monitoring: effects of anesthetic agents and neuromuscular blockade on evoked potentials, EEG, and cerebral blood flow. In: Loftus CM, Traynelis VC, eds. Intraoperative Monitoring Techniques in Neurosurgery. New York: McGraw-Hill; 1994:97–106
66. Merton PA, Morton HB. Stimulation of the cerebral cortex in the intact human subject. Nature 1980;285:227
67. Meyer JS, Marx PW. The pathogenesis of EEG changes during cerebral anoxia. In: Van der Drift JHA, ed. Cardiac and Vascular Diseases/Handbook of Electroencephalography and Clinical Neurophysiology. Vol 14A. Amsterdam: Elsevier; 1972:5–11
68. Moller AR, Jannetta PJ. Monitoring auditory function during cranial microvascular decompression operations by direct recording from the eighth nerve. J Neurosurg 1983;59:493–499
69. Moller MB, Moller AR. Loss of auditory function in microvascular decompression for hemifacial spasm: results in 143 consecutive cases. J Neurosurg 1985;63:17–20
70. Moller AR. Electrophysiological monitoring of cranial nerves in operations in the skull base. In: Sekhar LN, Schramm VL, eds. Tumors of the Cranial Base: Diagnosis and Treatment. Mount Kisco, NY: Futura; 1987: 120–132
71. Moller AR, Jannetta PJ. Monitoring facial EMG during microvascular decompression operations for hemifacial spasm. J Neurosurg 1987; 66:681–685
72. Moller AR. Intraoperative Neurophysiological Monitoring. Luxemburg: Harwood Academic; 1995
73. Morota N, Deletis V, Epstein FJ, et al. Brain stem mapping: neurophysiological localization of motor nuclei on the floor of the fourth ventricle. Neurosurgery 1995;37:922–929
74. Nagle KJ, Emerson RG, Adams DC, et al. Intraoperative monitoring of motor evoked potentials: a review of 116 cases. Neurology 1996;47:999–1004
75. Niedermeyer E, Lopes da Silva F. Electroencephalography, Urban and. Baltimore: Schwarzenberg; 1987
76. Nuwer MR. Evoked Potential Monitoring in the Operating Room. New York: Raven; 1986
76. Nuwer MR, Dawson EG, Carlson LG, Kanim LEA, Sherman JE. Somatosensory evoked potential spinal cord monitoring reduces neurological deficits after scoliosis surgery: results of a large multicenter survey. Electroencephalogr Clin Neurophysiol 1995;9 6:6–11
77. Ojemann G, Ojemann J, Lettich E, Berger M. Cortical language localization in left, dominant hemisphere: an electrical stimulation mapping investigation in 117 patients. J Neurosurg 1989;71:316–326
78. Osenbach RK, Yamada T, Traynelis VC. Transcranial magnetic stimulation of the motor cortex. In: Loftus CM, Traynelis VC, eds. Intraoperative Monitoring Techniques in Neurosurgery. New York: McGraw-Hill; 1994:239–250
79. Owen JH, Laschinger J, Bridwell KH. Sensitivity and specificity of somatosensory and neurogenic motor potentials in animals and humans. Spine 1988;13:1111–1118
80. Owen JH, Bridwell KH, Grubb R, et al. The clinical application of neurogenic motor evoked potentials to monitor spinal cord function during surgery. Spine 1991;16;8:S385–S390
81. Parenti G, Marconi F, Fiori L. Electrophysiological (EEG-SSEP) monitoring during middle cerebral aneurysm surgery. J Neurosurg Sci 1996;40:195–205
82. Pereon Y, Tich SNT, Delacroix I A, Passuti N. Letters to the editor. Spine 1999;11:1169–1170
83. Prass RL, Kinney SE, Hardy RW Jr, Hahn JF, Luders H. Acoustic (loudspeaker) facial EMG monitoring, II: Use of evoked EMG activity during acoustic neuroma resection. Otolaryngol Head Neck Surg 1987;97:541–551
84. Patton HD, Amassian VE. Single and multiple unit analysis of cortical state of pyramidal tract activation. J Neurophysiol 1954;17:345–363
85. Powers SK, Bolger CA, Edwards MSB. Spinal cord pathways mediating somatosensory evoked potentials. J Neurosurg 1982;57:472–482
86. Regan D. Human Brain Electrophysiology: Evoked Potentials and Evoked Magnetic Fields in Science and Medicine. New York: Elsevier; 1989
87. Roger J, Roger A, Gastaut H. Electro-clinical correlation in 36 cases of vascular syndromes of brainstem [abstract]. Electroencephalogr Clin Neurophysiol 1954;6:164
88. Romstock J, Strauss C, Fahlbusch R. Continuous electromyography monitoring of motor cranial nerves during cerebellopontine angle surgery. J Neurosurg 2000;93:586–593
89. Rothwell JC, Day BL, Thompson PD, Dick JPR, Marsden CD. Some experiences of techniques for stimulation of the human cerebral motor cortex through the scalp. Neurosurgery 1987;20:156–163
90. Sadjadpour K. Postfacial palsy phenomena: faulty nerve regeneration or ephaptic transmission? Brain Res 1975;95:403–406
91. Salzman SK, Beckman AL, Marks HG, Naidu R, Bunnell WP, MacEwen GD. Effects of halothane on intraoperative scalp-recorded somatosensory-evoked potentials to posterior tibial nerve stimulation in man. Electroencephalogr Clin Neurophysiol 1986;65:36–45
92. Samra SK. Effect of isofluvase on human median nerve evoked potentials. In: Ducker TB, Brown RH, eds. Neurophysiology and Standards of Spinal Cord Monitoring. New York: Springer-Verlag; 1988:147–156
93. Sclabassi RJ, Kroin JS, Hinman CL, Risch HA. The effect of cortical ablation on afferent activity in the cat somatosensory system. Electroencephalogr Clin Neurophysiol 1986;64:31–40
94. Sclabassi RJ, Krieger DN, Weisz D, Durrant J. Electrophysiological monitoring. In: Sekhar LN, Janecka I, eds. Surgery of Cranial Base Tumors: A Color Atlas. New York: Raven; 1993:83–98
95. Sclabassi RJ, Krieger DN, Simon R, Lofink R, Gross G, DeLauder D. NeuroNet: collaborative intraoperative guidance and control. IEEE Comput Graph Appl 1996;16:39–45
96. Sloan TB. Anesthetic effects on electrophysiologic recordings. J Clin Neurophysiol 1998;15:217–226

97. Stendel R, Pietila T, Al Hassan AA, Schilling A, Brock M. Intraoperative microvascular Doppler ultrasonography in cerebral aneurysm surgery. J Neurol Neurosurg Psychiatry 2000;68:29–35

98. Strauss C, Romstock J, Nimsky C, Fahlbusch R. Intraoperative identification of motor areas of the rhomboid fossa using direct stimulation. J Neurosurg 1993;79:393–399

99. Sundt TM Jr, Ebersold MJ, Sharbrough FW, Piepgras DG, Marsh WR, Messick JM. The risk-benefit ratio of intraoperative shunting during carotid endarterectomy. relevancy of operative and post-operative results and complications. Ann Surg 1986;203:196–204

100. Tamaki T. Spinal cord monitoring with spinal evoked potentials evoked by direct stimulation of the spinal cord. In: Desmedt JE, ed. Neuromonitoring in Surgery. Amsterdam: Elsevier; 1989:139–149

101. Taylor BA, Fennelly ME, Taylor A, Farrell J. Temporal summation: the key to motor evoked potential spinal cord monitoring in the humans. J Neurol Neurosurg Psychiatry 1993;56:104–106

102. Tiel RL, Happel L, Kline DG. Nerve action potential recording. Neurosurgery 1996;39:103–109

103. Toleikis JR, Skelly JP, Carlvin AO, Burkus JK. Spinally elicited peripheral nerve responses are sensory rather than motor. Clin Neurophysiol 2000;111:736–742

104. Ubags LH, Kalkman CJ, Been HD. Influence of isoflurane on myogenic motor evoked potentials to single and multiple transcranial stimuli during nitrous oxide/opioid anesthesia. Neurosurgery 1998;43:90–95

105. Kalkman CJ, Ubags LH. Motor evoked potential monitoring. Current Opinion in Anaesthesiol 1997;10:327–332

106. Van der Drift JHA. The EEG in cerebro-vascular disease. In: Vinken PJ, Bruyn GW, eds. Handbook of Clinical Neurology. Vol 11. Amsterdam; Noft-Holland; 1972:267–291

107. Van Olphen AF, Rodenberg M, Verwey C. Influence of stimulus repetition rate on brainstem evoked responses in man. Audiology 1979;18:388–394

108. Verroust J, Blinowska A, Vilfrit R, Couperie D, Malapert D, Perrier M. Somatosensory evoked potentials from posterior tibial nerve; normative data. Electromyogr Clin Neurophysiol 1989;29:299–303

109. Wahlig JB, Kaufmann AM, Balzer JR, Lovely TL, Jannetta PJ. Intraoperative loss of auditory function relieved by microvascular decompression of the cochlear nerve. Can J Neurol Sci 1999;26:44–47

4

Postoperative Critical Care for Neurosurgery

Kevin M. Dwyer, H. David Reines, and Samir M. Fakhry

The management of the postoperative neurosurgical patient depends on the patient's underlying physiology, the procedure performed, and the expectation of postoperative complications. A significant number of patients undergoing intracranial surgery or those afflicted with severe spinal or head trauma or acute intracranial hemorrhage need to be managed in an intensive care unit (ICU). The ICU has specially trained nurses providing one-to-one or one-to-two patient care. The ICU is equipped with the latest technology to monitor and treat the critically ill patient. The nursing staff that manages the neurosurgical patient should have expertise in recognizing neurological deterioration and in working with intracranial pressure (ICP) monitors. Ideally, the ICU will have intensivists to manage the multiple needs of the critically ill patient.[1]

Patients who meet the following criteria should be considered for ICU admission:

1. Major intracranial procedures
2. Acute intracerebral or subarachnoid hemorrhage (SAH)
3. Moderate to severe head or spinal cord trauma
4. Neurosurgical procedure combined with history of recent myocardial infarction, severe congestive heart failure, or significant pulmonary disease
5. Significant intraoperative blood loss, ongoing coagulopathy, hemodynamic instability, hypo- or hypertension, or continued ventilatory support
6. Continuous monitoring and treatment of ICP
7. Acute stroke

Medical centers that manage a large volume of neurosurgical patients frequently have a separate neuroscience ICU. Many of these centers have intensivists participate in the care of these patients. The intensivist should be board certified in critical care and be familiar with the unique aspects of care required by neurosurgical patients. The neurosurgeon, who directs the overall plan of care, relies on the intensivist to manage all aspects of the patient's care in the ICU. The availability of an experienced intensivist at the bedside who can coordinate the care of the patient and respond rapidly to changes in the patient's condition has resulted in better outcomes for intensive care patients as well as a decrease in the cost of ICU care.[2]

This chapter outlines the management of neurosurgical patients in the ICU, including cardiac and pulmonary physiology, invasive monitoring, ventilator management, intracranial hypertension, fluid and electrolyte dynamics, hemodynamic manipulation, sedation, analgesia, and nutrition.

Cardiovascular Physiology

Oxygen delivery to the cells is dependent upon cardiovascular function. Though many neurointensive care patients have normal cardiac function, a few will have cardiovascular disease. Some neurological insults, such as SAH, will depress cardiac function. These patients will require invasive monitoring for optimal treatment.

Formulas that define cardiac function are listed in **Table 4–1**. The quantity of blood that leaves the ventricle with each systolic heartbeat is the stroke volume (SV). The amount of blood that is ejected from the heart in 1 minute is the cardiac output (CO), which is the SV × the heart rate (HR). The CO is the measurable result of the function of the left ventricle and is directly related to delivery of oxygen to the cells. This equation for oxygen delivery (DO_2) is (**Table 4–1**):

$$\begin{aligned} DO_2 &= CO \times CaO_2 \\ &= CO \times (O_2 \text{ bound to Hgb}) \\ &\quad + (O_2 \text{ dissolved in blood}) \\ &= CO \times [(1.34 \times Hgb \times SaO_2) \\ &\quad + (0.0034 \times PaO_2)] \end{aligned}$$

In the foregoing equation, arterial oxygen content ($CaCO_2$) is mainly the oxygen carried on saturated (SaO_2) hemoglobin. The dissolved arterial oxygen (PaO_2) adds little to the amount of oxygen delivered to the cells and is frequently ignored in the equation. Oxygen content will be discussed in more detail in the section on pulmonary physiology. The maintenance of an acceptable CO is crucial to tissue oxygenation.[3]

The amount of oxygen consumed at a cellular level is related to the delivery of oxygen as well as cellular utilization. Therefore, the equation for oxygen consumption is similar:

$$\begin{aligned} VO_2 &= CO \times CaO_2 - CvO_2 \\ &= CO\,[(1.34 \times Hgb \times (SaO_2 - SvO_2)] \end{aligned}$$

CvO_2 is venous oxygen content, and SvO_2 is the mixed venous oxygen saturation. A low VO_2 is reflective of either a low oxygen delivery or decreased oxygen utilization by the cells. Normally, oxygen consumption is ~25% of oxygen delivery, also known as the oxygen extraction rate (O_2ext). If O_2ext is higher than 25%, then delivery is inadequate for the amount of oxygen required by the cells. This is an oxygen debt that needs to be relieved by increasing oxygen delivery. This could also be due to an increase in oxygen consumption, as seen, for example, with seizure activity. Under normal conditions, the SvO_2 is 70 to 75%. The O_2ext can be simply derived as $SaO_2 - SvO_2$. If SvO_2 is low, there is either a low SaO_2 or an increase in oxygen consumption and an increase in oxygen debt. Oxygen delivery can be increased by increasing the CO or the level of saturated hemoglobin. If the hemoglobin level is adequate, then the CO must be increased. A high SvO_2 may reflect poor utilization of oxygen at the cellular level, such as in sepsis. Therefore, a low O_2ext may be a sign of cellular dysfunction and shock.

Though the oxygen delivery and consumption equations are important guides to resuscitation, they frequently do not correlate with oxygen metabolism at the cellular level. If there is not enough oxygen available to the cells, or if it is not utilized, anaerobic metabolism will occur. This will lead to an increase in lactic acid and an increase in the base deficit on an arterial blood gas. In shock, an increase in serum lactic acid is caused by systemic hypoperfusion, but it may be normal with isolated organ hypoperfusion. In shock, an increasing level of lactic acid is a sign of an ongoing deficit in cellular perfusion.

The stroke volume, and therefore CO, is determined by four factors[1]: ventricular preload,[2] afterload,[3] contractility, and HR.[4]

The preload for the left ventricle is the left ventricular end diastolic volume (LVEDV). The force of contraction of the left ventricle is related to the volume of the ventricle. As the volume increases, the muscle cells stretch and the force of contraction is greater. This is Starling's law. Therefore, preload and contractility are directly related. The LVEDV is difficult to measure. LVEDV can be estimated by echocardiogram or a nuclear scan. When the chambers of the heart fill, the pressures generated can be measured directly on the right side and indirectly on the left with a pulmonary artery catheter (PAC). Because pressure and volume are closely related, measuring the pressure (LVEDP) will reflect the LVEDV in a compliant system. In a noncompliant left ventricle, the LVEDP may not accurately reflect the LVEDV. However, changes in LVEDP will reflect the changes of LVEDV, even in a noncompliant left ventricle. The LVEDP is not measured directly. Rather, the LVEDP is measured indirectly by the pulmonary artery wedge pressure (PAWP), obtainable from the PAC. In the absence of significant mitral valve disease, the PAWP reflects the pressure of the left ventricle in diastole. Central venous pressure (CVP) measures the filling pressure of the right ventricle. In many patients, CVP alone is adequate to measure filling pressures and preload. For patients with heart failure or pulmonary hypertension, PAC monitoring is recommended.

Decreased CO secondary to decreased preload is common. Hypovolemia, hemorrhage, and systemic vasodilation such as with septic shock will result in a decrease in preload. When preload is decreased, the fastest way to increase CO is to infuse fluids. If the clinical situation suggests that intravascular hypovolemia is the cause of poor perfusion, confirmation with a central monitor (CVP or PAC) is not necessary. However, in situations in which the cause of poor perfusion may be mixed, such as a patient with a myocardial infarction or decreased contractility secondary to SAH, central monitoring with a CVP or PAC will aid in the choice of intervention. Regardless of whether the reason for poor perfusion is a decrease in preload, cardiac dysfunction, or an increase in afterload, a fluid bolus will usually increase CO. This is the initial intervention to increase perfusion until more patient-specific data can be obtained.

The afterload is the resistance to CO. Cardiac factors that determine afterload include ventricular wall compliance, ventricular geometry, and the pericardium. For example, the afterload will be increased if the ventricle muscle is less compliant because of an infarction or hypertrophy, such as with long-standing hypertension. Left ventricular filling space will decrease with a dilated right ventricle that displaces the septum. Cardiac tamponade or pericarditis will increase afterload as well as limit cardiac filling (preload), severely decreasing CO.

Table 4–1 Cardiovascular and Pulmonary Variables

Variable	Definition	Derivation	Unit	Normal Value	Acceptable Value
PaO_2	Partial pressure of oxygen in arterial blood	Direct measurement	mm HG	85–95	> 65
SaO_2	% arterial hemoglobin saturated with oxygen	Direct measurement	%	95–100	> 90
Hgb	Hemoglobin	Direct measurement	g/dL	13–16	> 7–8
$PaCO_2$	Partial pressure of carbon dioxide in artery	Direct measurement	mm HG	35–45	32–47
R	Respiratory quotient	Ratio of carbon dioxide produced over the oxygen consumed		0.8	0.7–0.8
FiO_2	Percentage of oxygen delivered to patient	Direct measurement	%	21 (room air)	21–60
Pb	Barometric pressure	Direct measurement	mm Hg	760 (sea level)	same
PH_2O	Partial pressure of water vapor at 37°C	Direct measurement	mm HG	47	same
PAO_2	Partial pressure of oxygen in alveolus	$PAO_2 = (Pb - PH_2O)FiO_2 - PaCO_2/R$ (alveolar gas equation)	mm HG	100 (room air and sea level)	same
SvO_2	% venous hemoglobin saturated with oxygen	Direct measurement	%	70–75	67–77
CaO_2	Arterial oxygen content	$CaO_2 = 1.36\ Hgb \times SaO_2 + (0.0031 \times PaO_2)$	mL/dL	18–20 (Hgb 14–16)	13–20
CvO_2	Venous oxygen content	CvO2 = 1.36 Hgb×SvO2 + (0.0031 × PvO2)	mL/dL	13–15 (Hgb 14–16)	15-Aug
CO	Cardiac output	Direct measurement	L/min	5	3.5–7.0
CI	Cardiac index	CI = CO/body surface area	L/min × m^2	3	2.3–6.0
DO_2	Oxygen delivery	$DO_2 = CI \times CaO_2 \times 10$	mL/min × m^2	520–560	500–700
VO_2	Oxygen consumption	$VO_2 = CI \times C(a\text{-}v)O_2 \times 10$	mL/min × m^2	130–140	120–180
O_2ext	Oxygen extraction	$O_2\ ext = VO_2/DO_2$	%	25	20–30
PAWP	Pulmonary artery wedge pressure	Direct measurement	mm HG	2.5–10	0–18
PAP	Pulmonary artery pressure	Direct measurement	mm HG	15–28/5–12	10–35/4–17
RVP	Right ventricular pressure	Direct measurement	mm HG	20–30/0–6	20–35/0–10
CVP	Central venous pressure	Direct measurement	mm HG	0–5	0–10
SV	Stroke volume	CO/Heart rate (HR)	mL	70–130	Stroke volume index 40–50
SI	Stroke index	SV/body surface area	mL/m^2	40–50	40–50
MAP	Mean arterial pressure	Direct measurement $^1/_3$ systolic BP + $^2/_3$ diastolic BP	mm HG	80–95	70–105
SVR	Systemic vascular resistance	SVR = MAP − CVP/CO × 80	dyne/sec/cm-5	1100–1500	800–1500
PVR	Pulmonary vascular resistance	PVR = mean PAP/CO × 80	dyne/sec/cm-5	120–250	100–250
LVEDVI	Left ventricular end diastolic volume index	Direct measurement	mL/m^2	50–80	50–100
LVEDP	Left ventricular end diastolic pressure	Direct measurement	mm HG	2.5–10	2.5–20

(*Continued*) **Table 4–1**

Variable	Definition	Derivation	Unit	Normal Value	Acceptable Value
LVSW	Left ventricular stroke work	LVSW = SI × MAP × 0.144	gm × mL/m^2	50–60	45–60
RVSW	Right ventricular stroke work	RVSW = SI × MPAP × 0.144	gm × mL/m^2	8.1–9.8	7–9.8
EF	Ejection fraction	EF = SV/LVEDV	%	55–75	40–80
Vt	Tidal volume	Direct measurement	mL	500–800	400–1000
C	Compliance	C = change V/change P	mL/cm H_2O	Static: 60–100	40–100
PEEP	Positive end-expiratory pressure	Direct measurement	cm H_2O	0–5	0–15

The principle resistance to CO is the systemic vascular resistance (SVR). Baseline SVR is high, and the muscular left ventricle adapts well to acute changes in SVR. Diffuse vascular vasoconstriction may decrease CO, but the normal left ventricle will adjust with an increase in HR and contractility. The pulmonary vasculature resistance (PVR), however, is normally quite low, and acute changes causing significant pulmonary hypertension such as with a pulmonary embolism (PE) or acute respiratory distress syndrome (ARDS) can cause acute right heart failure. A PAC can directly measure right heart filling pressure and pulmonary vascular pressure and is indicated in these patients. The normal PAC values are shown in **Table 4–1.**

The force of contractility is related to preload. The ejection fraction (EF) is useful to measure contractility. EF is the percent of blood ejected from the left ventricle with each heartbeat. This is estimated with echocardiography or nuclear scan. This corresponds to the end systolic volume over the end diastolic volume. EF measures contractility if the preload, afterload, and HR remain the same from beat to beat. Because these variables constantly change, the contractility can only be inferred by EF. Specialized PACs can measure the EF in the right heart as well as right ventricular stroke work. These data may be a better reflection of volume status and cardiac function than PAWP, with questionable clinical significance. Contractility will decrease with previous myocardial infarction, ischemia, and myopathy. Neurohumeral factors may also decrease contractility such as seen with poor-grade SAH. If CO is low with adequate preload, treatment with inotropic agents may be indicated.[4]

Because CO equals SV × HR, increasing the HR will increase the CO. Tachycardia is the normal heart's response to stress and conditions of poor perfusion. The CO will increase with sinus tachycardia in the healthy heart. The infarcted or ischemic heart may not respond well to tachycardia. Coronary insufficiency increases with tachycardia. Very high HRs will not allow time for ventricular filling and may lead to a decrease of CO. Tachycardia in most patients will increase perfusion, and overly aggressive treatment of tachycardia may lead to hypotension. Before tachycardia is treated, the primary cause of the poor perfusion should first be sought and treated.

◆ Hemodynamic Monitoring

Noninvasive Monitoring

An essential component of quality ICU care is a well-trained ICU nurse who understands the neurological assessment as well as overall patient management. This includes frequent assessment of mental status, pupillary size and reaction, cranial nerve function, and sensory and motor exam. Hemodynamic status, urinary and drain output, as well as patient well-being and comfort are also monitored by the bedside nurse.

All ICU patients should have at minimum noninvasive monitoring. This includes continuous electrocardiography (ECG), electronic Doppler sphygmomanometers, and oxygen saturation probes. The cardiac monitors will detect episodes of tachycardia, bradycardia, arrythmias, and ECG changes. The sphygmomanometer will automatically cycle blood pressures (BPs) at a set interval, usually every 5 minutes. These measurements are not continuous and may not be as accurate as an arterial line if the cuff does not fit well. The O_2 saturation monitor, which works by photoelectric diodes that measure the saturation of hemoglobin in pulsating flow, is placed on a finger, toe, or earlobe. It is essential for picking up acute drops in O_2 saturation requiring immediate intervention. The probe can be inaccurate in patients who are vasoconstricted either from poor perfusion or from hypothermia. The probe also measures the pulse rate, which, if it equals the HR, tests the reliability of the O_2 saturation readings.

The indwelling urinary catheter (an invasive monitor in the bladder) measures urine output, which is a most basic assessment of adequate circulating volume to an end organ, the kidney. Hyperglycemia, diabetes insipidus, and diuretics will elevate urine output, and its sensitivity as a monitor of perfusion is lost. However, urine output is essential as a measurement of output and fluid balance in critically ill patients. A temperature probe is an added feature available on some catheters.

Invasive Monitoring

Arterial Lines

Many critically ill neurosurgical patients will require invasive monitoring. Patients who need continuous monitoring and control of their BP are best managed with an indwelling arterial catheter (A-line). Typically, the A-line is placed in the radial artery, but it can be inserted in the femoral artery in the absence of overt atherosclerotic changes, or into the dorsalis pedis artery. The smaller and more distal the artery that an A-line is placed into, the higher and sharper is the slope of the tracing, and the pulse pressure (difference of systolic and diastolic readings) is wider. In normal arteries, the mean arterial pressure should be the same no matter where the A-line is placed. The A-line values can be misleading if the catheter is kinked or clotted, with a dampened, falsely low BP; or if the catheter has excessive stiffness and whip, resulting in a falsely elevated BP reading. The A-line also provides easy access for blood withdrawal for frequent laboratory tests such as arterial blood gases and electrolytes. Infrequent complications of A-lines are infection and arterial thrombosis.

Central Venous Catheters

The use of a CVP catheter contributes information on the patient's volume status and the right heart preload. CVP monitoring is beneficial for patients who are to receive large amounts of intravenous fluid or blood products, for patients who are in shock and require resuscitation, or for patients who may have some degree of heart failure. Patients with increased ICP and patients with vasospasm will require aggressive fluid infusion and the use of vasopressors. CVP monitoring provides an important measure of central volume status in these patients.

CVP catheters are typically placed in the subclavian or internal jugular vein (**Fig. 4–1**). A longer catheter may also be placed in the brachial vein and advanced to the superior vena cava (SVC). The CVP catheter has the additional advantage of central delivery of pressors and hyperalimentation, which are not well tolerated in peripheral veins. The complications of central lines are infrequent but many. Insertion of a subclavian catheter may lead to subclavian artery injury, air embolism, or a pneumothorax. Insertion of the internal jugular catheter may lead to carotid artery injury, air embolism, pneumothorax, thoracic duct injury, or tracheal injury. A chest x-ray (CXR) postinsertion is essential to check for catheter position in the SVC and to confirm the absence of a pneumothorax. Ventricular ectopy may occur during insertion with irritation of the myocardium. The infection rate is low but does increase with the length of time the catheter is in place. Infection rates have been reported to rise significantly after 7 days. Line sepsis can add significant morbidity and cost to the patient's care. If a central catheter is to be in place for more than 4 to 7 days, an antibiotic-impregnated line should be considered to decrease the risk of catheter-related infections. Thrombosis of central veins is also a complication of CVP catheters.

Pulmonary Artery Catheters

The PAC developed by Swan and Ganz in 1970 provides additional information on cardiac function that may be useful in the management of the most critically ill patients. The PAC is an elongated catheter with a balloon at the tip. It is placed through a large central vein catheter (the introducer). The balloon is inflated to carry the catheter through the right heart to the pulmonary artery and beyond to a pulmonary arteriole (**Fig. 4–2**). In the pulmonary artery it continuously records pulmonary artery pressures (PAPs). With the balloon inflated, the catheter lodges in an end arteriole where it can measure the PAWP. The PAWP reflects the left end diastolic pressure in a patient without mitral valvular disease. This provides the intensivist with an estimate of the left heart filling pressures. The PAC also measures CO with a thermistor at the tip that can detect the change of temperature over time and distance. This allows the estimation of CO. Some PACs have added features that provide right heart function data, continuous CO, or continuous mixed venous oxygen saturation values.

The information obtained from the PAC is of value for treating patients who have heart disease or a potential for cardiac failure. Patients suffering from septic shock, ARDS, or multiple organ failure may also benefit from monitoring with the PAC. These catheters are frequently used in the management of severe head trauma, SAH with vasospasm, and patients with increased ICP.

The complications of PACs are the same as for central venous catheters. Additional rare complications include pulmonary hemorrhage, significant cardiac ectopy, cardiac perforation, or the development of a knot in the catheter within the heart. Because the PAC has significant associated complications, only physicians knowledgeable in the use of the catheter should place it, and it should be removed from the patient as soon as the information gained is no longer needed for patient management.

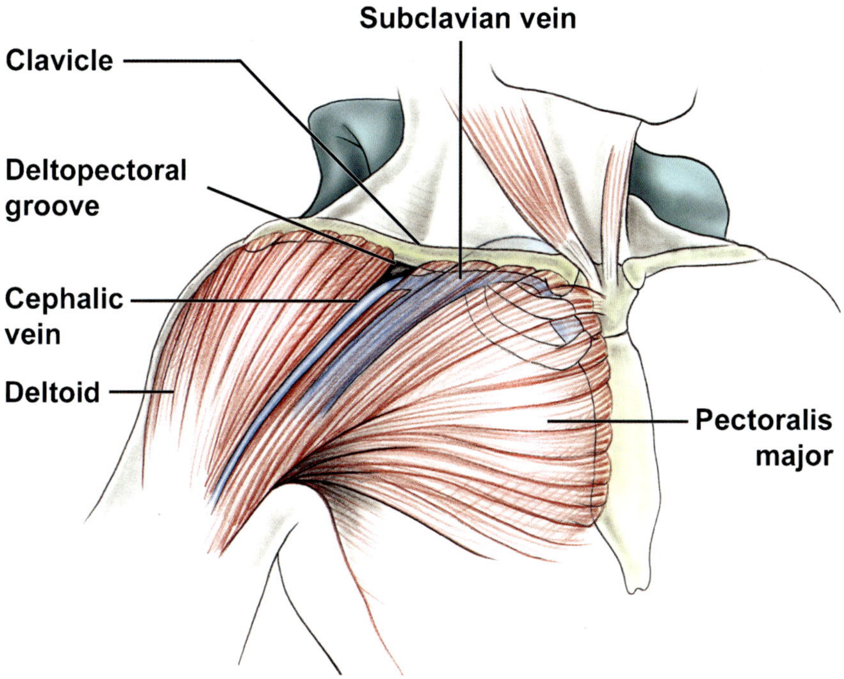

A

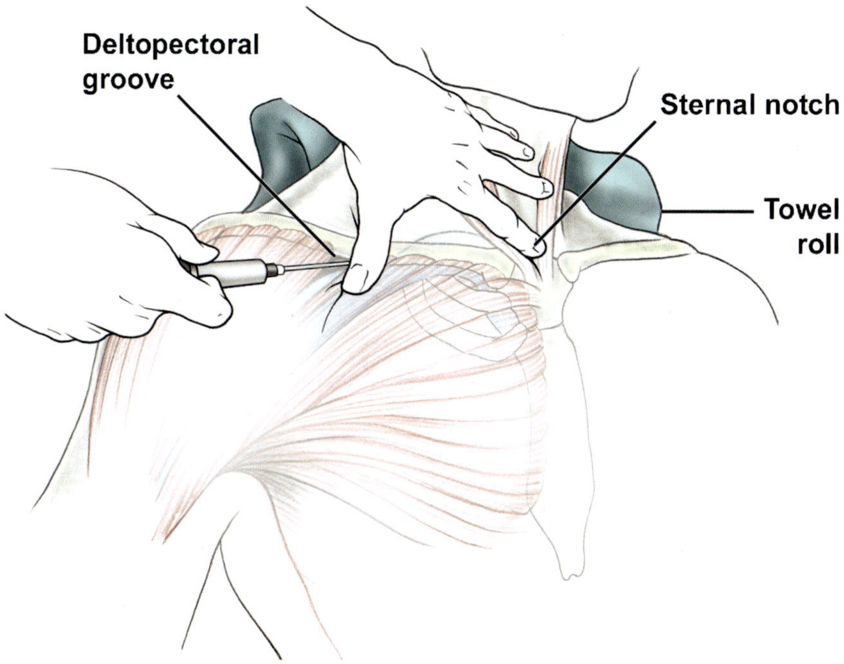

B

Figure 4–1 **(A)** The approach to the subclavian vein is at the deltopectoral groove, where the clavicle bends toward the chest. The patient should have a towel roll placed between the shoulder blades to let the shoulders fall laterally. This may not be possible for patients with potential C-spine injuries. The patient should be placed in the Trendelenburg position to distend the vein with blood. The area should be prepped and anesthetized prior to head-down positioning for patients with increased intracranial pressure. The operator should wear a cap, mask, gown, and gloves, and the area should be cleaned with antiseptic. The skin and area underneath the clavicle at the insertion site needs local anesthesia with 1% lidocaine, plain. **(B)** The skin is punctured 2 to 3 cm lateral to the point where the insertion of the pectoralis major muscle to the clavicle is palpated. The needle is directed at this groove, at the clavicle, ~20 degrees toward the head off the transverse plane. The needle makes contact with the clavicle and is marched carefully underneath the clavicle to avoid an acute angle into the chest and an increased chance of lung injury. The thumb of the other hand should be placed on the needle at the insertion site to gently push the needle down at the chest to keep the needle in a horizontal position with the chest. The index finger of that hand should be placed in the sternal notch. Once the needle moves beneath the clavicle, the needle is aimed at the sternal notch, which should be at 0 degrees in a transverse plane. Once the vein is entered, the syringe is removed, and a guidewire is threaded through the needle, with care not to introduce air into the vein. The needle is removed, and a stab incision is made at the skin so the catheter will slide over the wire easily. The catheter is slid over the wire (Seldinger technique), and the wire is removed. All ports of the catheter should be closed to avoid air embolism. Blood is withdrawn through the ports, and the ports are flushed with saline. The catheter is then sutured to the skin. Chest X-ray is obtained to check catheter position and to check for a pneumothorax.

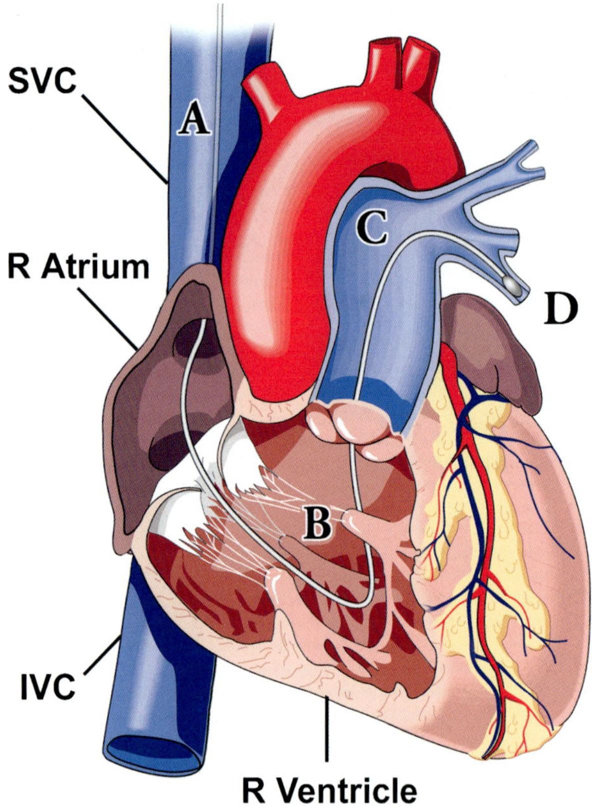

Figure 4–2 The Swan-Ganz pulmonary artery catheter (Baxter International; Deerfield, Illinois) is floated through the chambers of the heart from the superior vena cava (SVC) **(A)** with the aid of an inflated balloon at the tip of the catheter. The progress of the catheter through the heart can be identified by the difference in the pressure tracings that are generated as the catheter courses to the pulmonary artery. The pressure tracing of the SVC **(A)** dramatically increases as the catheter enters the right ventricle **(B)**. The diastolic inflection of the pressure tracing further decreases as the catheter enters the pulmonary artery **(C)**, and the tracing noticeably decreases as it progresses to the pulmonary arterial tracing **(D)**. When the balloon is "wedged" in the artery, the tracing is typically flatter. When the balloon is deflated, it should return to the arterial tracing **(D)**. This is the correct position. If the wedge remains despite balloon deflation, the catheter is "overwedged" and should be withdrawn a few centimeters until the arterial tracing **(D)** returns. IVC, inferior vena cava.

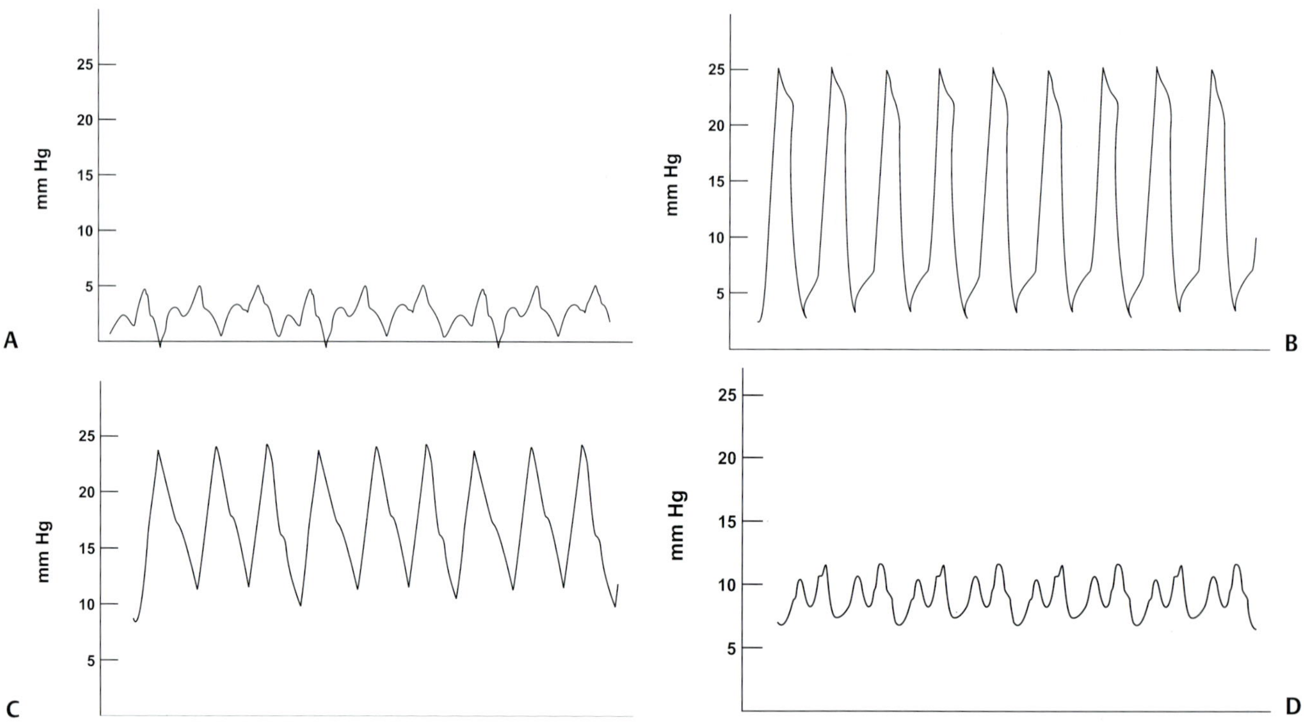

◆ Ventilator Management

Mechanical ventilation is required whenever a patient cannot maintain ventilation without assistance. Postanesthetic patients, after lengthy operations, may require short-term mechanical ventilation. Patients with preexisting pulmonary or cardiac disease, severe brain injury, or cerebral edema may require prolonged ventilator management to prevent hypoxia, hypercarbia, and secondary brain injury. It is essential to have an understanding of pulmonary physiology to manage mechanical ventilation.

Pulmonary Physiology

Oxygenation

The goal of ventilator management is to maintain oxygenation and to eliminate carbon dioxide. The partial pressure of oxygen available in the alveolus can be determined by the alveolar gas equation:

$$PAO_2 = Pb - 47(FiO_2) - PaCO_2/R$$

The FiO_2 (concentration of oxygen) of air is 21%, the $PaCO_2$ (partial pressure of carbon dioxide) is normally 40 mm Hg, Pb is barometric pressure (760 mm Hg at sea level), 47 is the partial pressure of water vapor, and R is the respiratory quotient, normally 0.8. At sea level, the PAO_2 is 100. The PaO_2, which is the partial pressure of oxygen in arterial blood, is 90 to 95 in healthy people at sea level. This difference between the PAO_2 and the PaO_2 is the percent of CO not oxygenated. This is a physiological shunt and is also called the A–a gradient. The A–a gradient is 8 to 12 mm Hg and increases with age. An easier way to quantify an abnormality with oxygenation is to determine the ratio of PaO_2:FiO_2 (the P:F ratio). Normally the P:F ratio will be above 300. If the P:F ratio is between 200 and 300, the patient is considered to have acute lung injury. In ARDS, the degree of shunt (venous blood that is not exposed to aerated alveoli) will increase with the severity of pulmonary injury, and progressive hypoxemia will occur. The P:F ratio in ARDS is < 200.

The first intervention in hypoxemia is to increase the FiO_2. This may be the only maneuver necessary in mild lung failure, but other strategies will be necessary to keep the FiO_2 at nontoxic levels. Oxygen at high concentrations for a prolonged period of time has been shown to be toxic to the alveolar cells in experimental models. The goal of therapy is to keep the $FiO_2 < 60\%$. When the pulmonary shunt approaches 50%, as in severe ARDS, increasing ventilation will decrease the $PaCO_2$ and may increase the PaO_2 through the relationship seen in the alveolar gas equation.[5]

The oxygen delivery equation, as previously discussed, relies on the arterial oxygen content (CaO_2) and the CO. The CaO_2 is mainly determined by the concentration of saturated hemoglobin.

$$DO_2 = CO \times CaO_2 = CO \times [(1.34 \times Hgb \times SaO_2) - (0.0034 \times PaO_2)]$$

There is a relationship between the PaO_2 and the saturation of hemoglobin, as shown by the oxygen hemoglobin saturation curve (**Fig. 4–3**). As long as the PaO_2 is kept above 60, the saturation of hemoglobin is above 90%. Increasing the oxygen to PaO_2 above 60 does not increase oxygen content significantly because most of the hemoglobin is already saturated, as shown by the curve. As soon as the PaO_2 drops below 60, the saturation drops quickly, decreasing the concentration of oxygen being delivered to the cells. Maintaining the SaO_2 above 89% is essential to avoid hypoxemia.

For many years, the optimal Hgb level was felt to be between 10 and 12 g/dL. There are little data to support this concept. Recent class 1 data suggest that Hgb levels of 10 g/dL

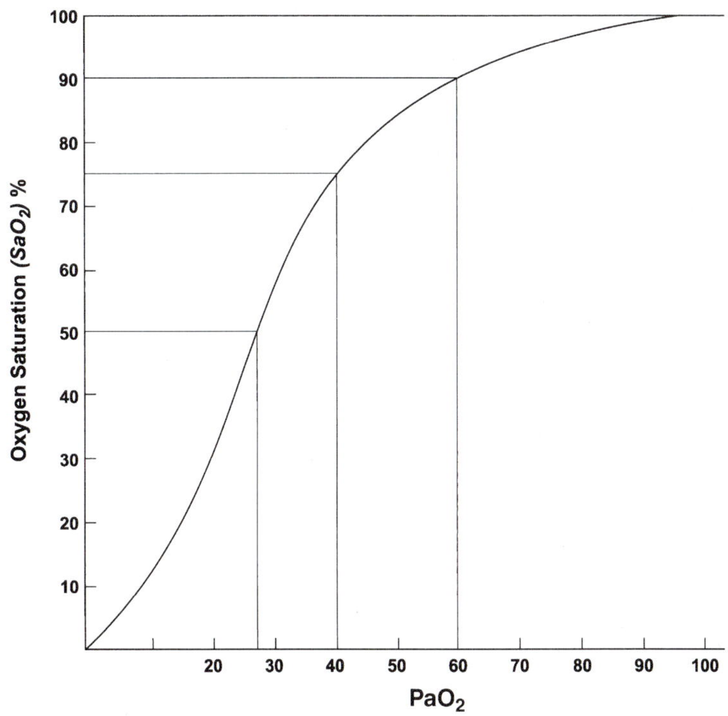

Figure 4–3 The oxyhemoglobin dissociation curve. This figure shows the nonlinear relationship of the saturation of the oxygen-binding site on hemoglobin (SaO_2) with the partial pressure of arterial oxygen (PaO_2). At a PaO_2 of 27, 50% of the hemoglobin is saturated; this is the P50. When the PaO_2 is 40, 75% of the hemoglobin is saturated with oxygen, and at a PaO_2 of 60, 90% is saturated. Raising the PaO_2 above 60 will not raise the content of arterial oxygen significantly. If this curve is shifted to the right, the hemoglobin will release the oxygen to the tissues more rapidly than if shifted to the left. This is a positive effect. Conditions of acidosis, increased $PaCO_2$, increased blood levels of 2,3-diphosphoglycerate (2,3-DPG), and increased temperature shift the curve to the right.

are not necessary to avoid cellular hypoxia and increased morbidity. Hgb levels above 7 g/dL were adequate in the ICU patient when compared with patients with Hgb levels of 10 g/dL.[6] Patients who receive many transfusions may fare worse than patients with a lower Hgb because of the immunomodulating effects of transfusion and the increased viscosity of a greater quantity of red blood cells (RBCs).

Ventilation

The $PaCO_2$ is affected directly by ventilation. When a patient is hyperventilated, the $PaCO_2$ will decrease. If the patient is hypoventilating, the $PaCO_2$ will increase. Tidal volume (Vt) and respiratory rate (RR) determine ventilation. The Vt is the volume of air inspired during a single breath. The RR is the number of breaths per minute. The $PaCO_2$ can be decreased by increasing the Vt or RR. The minute ventilation is the Vt $\times$ RR/min. Normal minute ventilation is 6 to 10 L/min. Patients who are under stress secondary to sepsis, injury, or shock will expend more energy, which may be reflected by a high minute ventilation. These patients are not ready to be removed from the ventilator. Patients with severe head injury frequently hyperventilate for a prolonged period. This may be due to central brain injury rather than a pulmonary or metabolic cause.

Mechanical Ventilation

There are several different ventilator modes. These are listed in **Table 4–2.** In the operating room, controlled mandatory

Table 4–2 Modes of Ventilation

Mode	Support Level	Pharmacological Support	Advantages	Disadvantages	Utilization
Controlled mandatory ventilation (CMV)	Full support; mandatory TV at a set rate	Heavy sedation or general anesthesia	Simple mode for a patient with little or no ventilatory effort	Patient will fight ventilator with own effort; not for patients with poor compliance	Operating room primarily; can be used for paralyzed patients
Assist control	Full support; mandatory TV at set rate, or rate driven by patient effort	Sedation requirement not as high	Resting mode; ideal for patients that fight or "buck" the ventilator	Not a weaning mode	For nonparalyzed patients that buck the ventilator
Pressure-regulated volume control(PRVC)	Full support; mandatory TV at a set rate; machine regulates delivery of pressure secondary to compliance to achieve set TV	Heavy sedation; machine will work with patient's respiratory effort in an assist control mode	Ideal mandatory ventilation for patients with low compliance and patients needing full support in ICU; lowers risk of barotrauma	Not a weaning mode	Desired mode for patients with prolonged ventilation therapy, ALI, and ARDS
Synchronized intermittent mandatory ventilation (SIMV)	Full or partial support if spontaneous rate > than set rate; machine attempts to match set TV with inspiratory effort	Sedation requirement not as high	Classic mode to decrease ventilatory support while allowing increased patient effort; patient bucks ventilator less	Partial weaning mode; patient may still buck ventilator; increased peak pressures in patients with ARDS	Initial waking postoperative mode in ICU, and mode used as transition to weaning
Pressure control (PC)	Full support; set pressure above PEEP at set rate	Heavy sedation, likely paralysis as patients sense air hunger	Severe ARDS where volume-limited ventilation triggers high pressure and barotrauma	Very heavy sedation or paralysis; promotes low tidal volume, mucous plugs, and hypercarbia	Severe ARDS; used frequently with inverse I:E ratio to oxygenate
Pressure support	Partial support of spontaneous breaths with decreasing pressure as needed	Light to moderate sedation	Weaning mode; as the patient awakens or strengthens, pressure support is decreased	If support inadequate, then mucous plugging may occur with low TV; beware of apnea	Popular weaning mode
Volume support	Partial support of spontaneous breaths with decreasing volume as needed	Light to moderate sedation	Weaning mode; inspiratory pressure decreases as patient's ventilation strengthens	End point of support not as easy to measure as pressure support; mucous plugging	Weaning mode; can set ventilator to switch to PRVC as needed
Continuous positive airway pressure (CPAP)	Low constant pressure during spontaneous breathing through ET tube or tracheotomy	Light to moderate sedation	If patient tolerates CPAP, may be ready for extubation or ventilator removal	Minimal support; may lead to tiring in patient who is not ready for ventilator removal	Weaning method T-piece trials are similar in leading to extubation

ALI, acute lung injury; ARDS, acute respiratory distress syndrome; CPAP, continuous positive airway pressure; ET, continuous positive airway pressure; ICU, intensive care unit; I:E, inspiratory:expiratory; TV, tidal value (also Vt).

ventilation (CMV) is used. Typical operating room parameters are TV of 8 to 10 cc/kg, 80 to 100% FiO_2, slight hyperventilation, and minimal positive end-expiratory pressure (PEEP). In the ICU, PEEP of 5 is added, the $PaCO_2$ is normalized, and the FiO_2 is dropped to keep O_2 saturation above 90%.

Respiratory Failure and Adult Respiratory Distress Syndrome

A group of patients that include those with severe head injury and multiple trauma, grade IV or V SAH, significant cerebral edema, and hemorrhagic or septic shock may develop respiratory failure, acute lung injury (ALI), and, possibly, ARDS. The ventilator management of these patients will require additional techniques to avoid hypoxia.

ARDS is a diffuse, patchy infiltrative process that leads to severe hypoxemia, noncardiogenic pulmonary edema, and poor lung compliance. It occurs secondarily to shock, sepsis, or any process that leads to the systemic inflammatory response syndrome (SIRS). The definitive treatment of ARDS is to cure the underlying disease process, but ventilator management is essential to avoid sustained hypoxemia. The first signs of ARDS are hypoxemia and increased work of breathing. Patients on mechanical ventilation may develop increased ventilatory pressures. Initially, increasing the FiO_2 will maintain oxygen saturation. As the disease progresses, other modes of therapy are necessary to maintain oxygenation and avoid further alveolar damage.

PEEP is applied at the end of a ventilator breath to prevent the airway pressure from falling to 0, thus promoting alveolar collapse. In a normal lung, this would not cause a significant problem. In noncompliant lungs, the collapsed alveoli become difficult to reopen, leading to persistent atelectasis and ventilation/perfusion mismatch. When alveoli in ARDS are filled with inflammatory fluid or collapsed, increased PEEP may "recruit" some of the alveoli back into effective ventilation. Increasing the PEEP has been shown to decrease hypoxemia from ARDS. High levels of PEEP can lead to a decrease in cardiac compliance and decreased venous return to the heart. In patients receiving high levels of PEEP, preload needs to be increased by fluid infusion to maintain CO. There is also concern that PEEP may increase ICP. This effect is minimal compared with the effect of hypoxia on ICP. High PEEP may contribute to barotrauma, but to a lesser extent than high peak and plateau airway pressures. It has been shown in large multicenter randomized trials that large-volume ventilation with resultant high peak and plateau pressures leads to increases in mortality from ARDS.[7] Vts of 4 to 6 mg/kg result in less alveolar barotrauma and may promote earlier resolution of ARDS. Newer ventilator modes, such as pressure-regulated volume control (PRVC), may lead to less barotrauma by varying flow and volume delivery to the patient depending on lung compliance. This is an ideal mode of ventilation for patients with ALI or ARDS.

Pressure control (PC) ventilation is another mode utilized in severe ARDS. In this mode, the ventilator delivers airflow to a target peak pressure, and the Vt varies depending on lung compliance. In some cases where the airway pressure is kept to a minimum to avoid barotrauma, ventilation may suffer with an increase in $PaCO_2$. This is permissive hypercapnea, and if attained gradually, it is well tolerated by most patients. Increased $PaCO_2$ may be a concern in patients with cerebral edema because ICP may rise. If the $PaCO_2$ is allowed to rise slowly, this may not occur. Another manipulation used to increase oxygenation is to increase the inspiratory:expiratory (I:E) ratio, normally at 1:3. Increasing the inspiratory time will increase mean airway pressure and may increase PaO_2. This will also lead to less ventilation in patients with stiff lungs. Patients on these advanced modes of therapy need to be heavily sedated, and many need to be chemically paralyzed. An intensivist experienced in the management of patients with ALI and ARDS is crucial to the successful, safe management of such patients.

Weaning

A patient who is receiving minimal ventilator support and whose condition originally requiring mechanical ventilation has abated is ready to be weaned from the ventilator. To be weaned successfully from mechanical ventilation, the patient must have a spontaneous breathing drive, be awake enough to maintain the airway and effectively clear secretions (cough), and be able to achieve an adequate Vt. Despite normal pulmonary physiology, many neurosurgical patients cannot be weaned due to a decreased mental status. A patient who can follow commands may successfully wean from the ventilator. Sedation should be kept to a minimum when weaning, and short-acting sedatives such as propofol may be ideal at the time of weaning from mechanical ventilation.

Synchronized intermittent mandatory ventilation (IMV), with pressure support, pressure or volume support alone, and CPAP or T-piece trials are modes used for weaning. A patient who is breathing comfortably on little or no support and is not comatose is ready for extubation. One objective measure of predicting success of extubation is the rapid breathing index or RR/vT. If this rate is < 100, there is an 85% success of extubation.[8] Other "weaning parameters" include $Vt > 5$ cc/kg, vital capacity > 10 cc/kg, maximum inspiratory force > 20, and a spontaneous minute ventilation < 11 L/min.

Patients who have no hope of weaning from the ventilator after 3 to 7 days of mechanical ventilation and patients who will be predictably in a prolonged coma should be considered for a tracheotomy.

◆ Intracranial Pressure and Cerebral Oxygen Delivery

Patients who have had major intracranial surgery, intracranial hemorrhage, ischemia, or trauma may develop cerebral edema. These patients are at risk for increased ICP and, thereby, inhibiting cerebral blood flow (CBF) leading to ischemia and herniation. These patients need monitoring of their ICP. The two most common types of monitors are ventriculostomies and intraparenchymal monitors.

Ventriculostomies are accurate monitors of ICP. They also allow for therapeutic intervention for increased ICP by drain-ing cerebrospinal fluid (CSF). The disadvantages include greater difficulty of placement in brains with compressed ventricles, a slightly higher incidence of bleeding, and a higher infection rate.[9] Ventriculostomies may occlude and malfunction when there is blood in the ventricles.

Intraparenchymal (IP) monitors are placed into the cerebral parenchyma and may not reflect global changes in ICP as well as ventriculostomies. CSF cannot be drained as a therapeutic maneuver from IP monitors.

The normal ICP is below 20 mm Hg. In general, ICP elevations above 20 mm Hg need to be treated. Patients who have more frequent instances of ICP elevations greater than 20 mm Hg have a progressively worse outcome. Acute unexpected elevations of ICP should be evaluated by head computed tomography (CT) to look for surgically treatable causes. One early intervention to decrease ICP is to increase sedation and to treat any seizure activity. Lidocaine instilled into the endotracheal tube may help prevent ICP increases with suctioning. If a ventriculostomy is in place, CSF can be drained off. Hypoxia and hypotension need to be corrected. Mannitol can be given as an osmotic diuretic and is effective in reducing ICP. Hyperventilation will also decrease ICP, but this effect will only last for a short period as the brain pH equalizes. Hyperventilation may also lead to cerebral ischemia via cerebral vasoconstriction.[10,11] ICP will also decrease if the brain metabolism is decreased. Medication such as barbiturates will have this effect.[12] Propofol will also decrease cerebral metabolism at high doses.[13] The drawback is that both medications will decrease CO and BP.

The current principle in managing increases in ICP is to maintain cerebral perfusion pressure (CPP).[14]

$$CPP = MAP - ICP$$

MAP is mean arterial pressure. Normally, CBF is maintained by autoregulation, for a MAP as low as 50 mm Hg. In a damaged brain, autoregulation is lost, and CBF will be severely decreased, with CPP $<$ 60 mm Hg. It is important to maintain a CPP of at least 60 to 70 mm Hg as the ICP rises. Maneuvers to increase CPP include fluid boluses or increasing doses of pressors (**Table 4–3**) if the patient is euvolemic or hypervolemic.

Jugular bulb venous saturation ($SjvO_2$) can be used as a monitor of cerebral oxygen consumption. This can be of assistance in identifying events that decrease oxygen delivery such as alterations in CBF. The cerebral oxygen equations are:

$$\text{Cerebral } DO_2 = CBF \times \text{arterial oxygen content } (CaO_2)$$

$$\text{Cerebral } VO_2 = CBF \times CaO_2 - \text{venous oxygen content } (CvO_2)$$

$$\text{Cerebral } VO_2 = CBF \times (1.34 \times Hgb \times SaO_2 - 1.34 \times Hgb \times SjvO_2)$$

$$\text{Cerebral } VO_2 = CBF \times (1.34 \times Hgb\,(SaO_2 - SjvO_2))$$

Table 4–3 Antihypertensives

Agent	Action	Utility	Onset	Duration	Dosage	Adverse Reactions
Sodium nitroprusside	Most effective and rapid intravenous controller of systemic hypertension; potent vasodilator of both veins and arteries	Used in intensive care units as a front-line control of acute, severe hypertension	Immediate	1–2 min	Should be started at a low dose, 0.3 mg/kg/min, and titrated up to 10 mg/kg/min to the desired effect	Can lead to cyanide poisoning if left at > 10 mg/kg/min for 30 min or > 2 mg/kg/min for 72 h; cerebral vasodilator and can acutely increase CBF and increase ICP
Nitroglycerin	Venodilator that can lower BP at high doses (these effects can be controlled via titration); vasodilator of coronary arteries	Protective for patients with possible myocardial ischemia	1–2 min	1–3 min	5–300 μg/min IV drip	Headache, mild hypotension
Lebetalol	Parenteral α-adrenergic and nonselective β-blocker that reduces BP within minutes without increasing heart rate; no effect on CBF or metabolism, and autoregulation remains intact	Easily titratable to response; can be used as a drip infusion	3–5 min	2–6 h	10 mg bolus IV; may redose q10min until desired BP; drip of 5 mg/hr and increase as necessary	Mild bradycardia

(*Continued*) **Table 4–3**

Agent	Action	Utility	Onset	Duration	Dosage	Adverse Reactions
Hydralazine	Arterial vasodilators; effectively lowers BP	Variable drop in BP	10–30 min	2–6 h	5–20 mg IV	Difficult to titrate; causes reflex tachycardia; contraindicated with coronary disease, MI
Diazoxide	Potent arterial vasodilator; better titration than hydralazine	Rapid drop in BP	1–5 min	6–8 h	25–100 mg IV q5min drip: 7.5–30 mg/min, total dose 300 mg	Reflex tachycardia as above; not for long-term use because of additional severe side effects
Nimodipine	Calcium channel blocker used to lower risk of adverse effects of vasospasm; will lower BP; half dose if hypotension not desired	Improves outcome after SAH by decreasing effects of vasospasm	1 h	2–4 h	30–60 mg PO	Hypotension
Nicardipine	Calcium channel blocker; vascular and coronary vasodilator	Effective in lowering BP rapidly; cardioprotective	1–3 minute	15–45 minute	5–15 mg/hr IV	Headache, hypotension, nausea, mild tachycardia
Diltiazem	Calcium channel blocker; decrease conduction of AV node	Treatment of atrial fibrillation with rapid response; also used for coronary disease	5–15 min	IV 2–4 h PO 4–8 h	5 –10 mg IV for atrial fibrillation; 30–60 mg PO for chronic treatment of hypertension	Hypotension
Metoprolol	β-blocker; lowers heart rate, cardioprotective, and effective antihypertensive	Excellent for patients with tachycardia, coronary vascular disease	IV 5–15 min	3–7 h	2.5–5.0 mg IV 50–100 mg PO for long-term treatment	Prolonged β-blocker effect
Esmolol	β-blocker; same effects as metoprolol but very short acting	Short-acting IV treatment of tachycardia	1–2 min	10–20 min	Bolus 250–500 μg/kg/min, then 50–250 μg/kg/min	Severe hypotension
Propranolol	β-blocker; same effects, longer acting	May decrease sympathetic effects of severe head injury	PO 30–60 min	6–8 h	1 mg IV 10– 20 mg PO	Hypotension at higher doses
Enalaprilat	ACE inhibitor; long-acting antihypertensive	IV form available to start on long-term treatment for hypertension in ICU	IV 10–15 min	IV 4–6 h PO 8–12 h	1.25 mg IV q6h 10–25 mg PO q8–12h	May increase creatinine in patients with renovascular diseases; slow acting
Pressors						
Agent	**Action**	**Utility**		**Duration**	**Dosage (IV Drip)**	**Adverse Reactions**
Dopamine	Dopaminergenic receptors; low doses—tachycardia, increases cardiac output, splanchnic arteriole vasodilator; higher doses—tachycardia, primary increase in BP	Most common pressor initially used for hypotension due to combined cardiac and pressor effect as well as believed increase in organ perfusion at lower doses	Immediate	min	Low doses 1–5 μg/kg/h; high doses: 5–30 μg/kg/h	Severe tachycardia, renal diuresis

(*Continued on page 84*)

(*Continued*) **Table 4–3**

Agent	Action	Utility	Onset	Duration	Dosage	Adverse Reactions
Neosynephrine	Pure α_1-agonist; vasoconstriction, increase in BP	Commonly used for neurosurgical patients, does not cross blood–brain barrier	Immediate	min	20–300 mg/min	Reflex bradycardia may be symptomatic; potential end organ malperfusion
Norepinephrine	Strong α_1-agonist, with some B1 effects; profound increase in BP and some increase in cardiac output	Excellent to increase BP	Immediate	min	1–20 µg/kg/min	May cause severe hypoperfusion and tissue necrosis in patients who are hypovolemic
Epinephrine	Profound B1 effects, α_1 effects increase with high doses	Primary	Immediate	min	1 mg bolus for cardiac arrest q3–5min; drip 0.1–10 mg/hr for sustained effect	Increase in cardiac ischemia; malperfusion with hypovolemia
Dobutamine	B1-agonist; increases cardiac output and heart rate; mild vasodilator	Cardiogenic shock, increase cardiac output	Immediate	min	2–20 µg/kg/min	Tachycardia, reflex hypotension
Amrinone Milrinone	Phosphodiesterase inhibitors; increase cardiac output, but may cause hypotension; pulmonary vasodilators	Cardiogenic shock, especially with pulmonary hypertension	5–10 min	2–3 h	Milrinone: loading 50 µg/kg; drip: 0.25–1 µg/kg/min	Vasodilatation with hypotension may negate its use; amiodarone causes thrombocytopenia
Vasopressin	Profound increases in BP	Recent data support its use in cardiac arrest and as a vasopressor; additional effect for diabetes insipidus	Immediate	longer effect	40 units IV for cardiac arrest; IV drip: 0.1–2 U/min	Malperfusion of organs with hypovolemia
Norepinephrine	Strong α_1-agonist, with some B1 effects; profound increase in BP and some increase in cardiac output	Excellent to increase BP	Immediate	min	1–20 µg/kg/min	May cause severe hypoperfusion and tissue necrosis in patients who are hypovolemic

ACE, angiotensin converting enzyme; BP, blood pressure; CBF, cerebral blood flow; ICU, intensive care unit; IV, intravenous; MI, myocardial infarction; SAH, subarachnoid hemorrhage.

The $SjvO_2$ will decrease if the oxygen delivery decreases either from decreased CBF or from hypoxemia.

The $SjvO_2$ is measured by placing a catheter with a co-oximeter tip into the jugular vein and advancing it up to the jugular bulb at the level of the first cervical vertebra. The $SjvO_2$ has been studied extensively and does correlate well with changes in CBF and cerebral oxygenation. Its drawbacks are frequent malfunction and its inability to measure oxygenation of specific parts of the brain.[15] It can only be a measure of global oxygenation of the brain and will not identify specific areas of or decreased blood flow. Placement is in the dominant jugular vein, usually the right. Placement in the jugular bulb must be accurate to assure no admixture from the facial veins.

$SjvO_2$ correlates well with decreased blood flow secondary to increases in ICP. $SjvO_2$ may guide the use of hyperventilation in the refractory increase in ICP.[16] $SjvO_2$ usually decreases with hyperventilation because of decreased CBF. This could lead to brain ischemia. If there is jugular bulb desaturation with hyperventilation, then it should be avoided as a treatment of elevated ICP.

There are now cerebral tissue oxygenation probes that can be used to directly measure brain tissue oxygen tension. The risks of placement are the same as those risks of ICP monitor placement. These probes correlate well with $SjvO_2$. They can be placed in an area of injury or ischemia, which may be useful in directing therapy for the most vulnerable part of the brain.[17]

◆ Fluid and Sodium Balance

Total body water (TBW) in a normal adult is ~60% of the body weight. Men, with more lean body mass, have a higher percentage of TBW than women, and infants and children have higher body water content than adults. Approximately two thirds of the body water is intracellular fluid (ICF), and one third is extracellular. Three fourths of the extracellular fluid (ECF) is in the interstitial space, and one fourth is in the intravascular compartment. The third space is where water is actively transported across an epithelial membrane such as the gastrointestinal tract or CSF. Under conditions of injury or inflammation the third space may accumulate large amounts of fluid by passive shifts. Increased tissue edema that is difficult to mobilize may also be referred to as a third space though it is in the interstitial space.

Total body sodium is ~40 mEq/kg, and over 95% is extracellular. The Na^+K^+-ATPase pump maintains this gradient and the resting membrane potential. The extracellular Na concentration ranges from 135 to 145 mEq/L, whereas the intracellular concentration is 5–15 mEq/L. Osmotic neutrality with cells is maintained primarily by the intracellular concentration of potassium, which ranges from 140 to 150 mEq/L with an extracellular concentration of 3.5 to 5.0 mEq/L.

Under normal physiological conditions, D5W will move intracellular, crystalloid will remain in the extracellular space, and colloid will remain mostly intravascular. When resuscitating hemorrhagic shock, the replacement for blood with crystalloid is 3 liters to 1. In shock, albumin leaks into the extravascular space, losing its oncotic effect.

Osmolality, Tonicity, and the Blood–Brain Barrier

Osmolality is the molal concentration of all solutes in water. Across a water-permeable membrane, water will move freely from a compartment of low osmolality to higher osmolality. The ECF osmolality is primarily determined by the concentration of Na^+ and its associated anions, primarily chlorine (Cl^-). The equation to determine the serum osmolality is:

$$\text{Osmolality (mOsm/kg)} = 2 \times (Na^+) + \text{glucose}/18 = \text{BUN}/2.8$$

ECF measured osmolality is ~10 mOsm/kg higher than the calculated osmolality. Any increase of the measured osmolality higher than 10 mOsm/kg over the calculated osmolality is known as the osmolar gap. The gap is caused by unmeasured solutes such as alcohol or mannitol, or with significant hyperlipidemia or hyperproteinemia.

In most compartments of the body, water will move across cell membrane in the direction of an osmotic gradient. However, the movement of water will be affected by the permeability of the membrane to water and to the particles providing the gradient. Therefore, the osmotic effectiveness or tonicity of solutes will be the major factor as to the movement of water. The osmotic effectiveness helps determine the movement of particles across the blood–brain barrier. What is permeable to transport in most tissues is much less permeable across the blood–brain barrier and its tight junctions. Tonicity can be expressed mathematically for a certain capillary membrane system as the osmotic reflection coefficient. A value of 1 is given to a particle that is impermeable to a membrane and has strong osmotic activity. Sodium and chloride have a reflection coefficient ~0.95. Urea and glucose contribute to serum osmolality but are more permeable across the blood–brain barrier. They have a short-term osmotic effect.[18]

Water is less permeable across the blood–brain barrier. This will effect its movement to a higher osmolar concentration. The movement of water through a membrane is the hydraulic conductivity of that membrane. The hydraulic conductivity of the blood–brain barrier is much lower than in extracerebral vessels. In most body regions, the capillaries are permeable to water, and the osmotic effectiveness of sodium and other small solutes is small. The impermeable serum proteins exert a large osmotic effect, and it is this oncotic pressure effect that helps to counterbalance the hydrostatic pressure movement of water out of the capillary. In the brain, because solutes such as sodium and chloride are impermeable, their effect is much greater than that of serum proteins. Therefore, colloid solutions have very little effect on fluid movement in the brain. There have been no definitive trials showing any advantage for using colloid solutions in neurosurgical patients. There is no evidence of any benefit for infusing albumin in postsurgical or trauma patients. There is some evidence that suggests a higher patient mortality with routine use of albumin, and therefore, it should not be used in the neurosurgical critical care unit.[19,20]

Sodium and chloride have the most profound effect on fluid movement across the blood–brain barrier. The low hydraulic conductivity of the blood–brain barrier helps avoid massive fluid shifts with quick changes of serum osmolality. However, due to the greater tonicity across the blood–brain barrier, fast changes in sodium concentration could shift the brain's extracellular and intracellular concentration of water too quickly, leading to decreased brain function, seizures, and permanent damage. Mannitol, like sodium, is much more effective in causing an osmotic gradient in the brain than in other organs. Mannitol, with its high reflection coefficient, will selectively move fluid from the ECF of the brain, and perhaps some from the ICF. This "brain shrinkage" is one theory of mannitol's effect in lowering ICP. However, mannitol's half-life as producing an osmotic gradient lasts just minutes after circulation because it will draw fluid in from the rest of the system and its gradient will be gone. Perhaps its greater effect is its hemodynamic effect on the flow of blood to the brain.[21]

Mannitol will acutely increase preload and will temporarily increase cerebral perfusion pressure. Mannitol may also increase flow to the brain by decreasing viscosity of the blood. It does this by decreasing the hematocrit, and also by moving fluid out of red blood cells, decreasing their volume and rigidity. This increased oxygen delivery to the brain increases perfusion to the brain and actually causes a reflex decrease in CBF and thereby a decrease in ICP. Perhaps mannitol also enhances flow and oxygen delivery to damaged brain by the rheologic effect. Mannitol also has a free radical scavenger effect that may help with clearance of these products away from damaged brain. Indomethacin may help damaged brain by a similar mechanism.[22]

Many studies have compared the use of various percents of hypertonic saline to mannitol as an osmotherapy substitute. These studies have shown favorable results in the reduction of ICP and the increase in CPP, with a tendency to sustained effect in the hypertonic saline groups.[23] This treatment has not been adopted because of the low number of patients in these studies. Osmotherapy may have its limitations, which include dehydration and hypovolemia resulting in decreased CPP. In some patients, osmotherapy may lead to an unusual rebound hyperemia and severe increase in ICP.

Sodium Balance

The effect of sodium on the osmotic gradient of the brain has been emphasized. It is important to regulate the extracellular sodium level closely to maintain ICP control and brain cell function. Hyponatremia is a frequent consequence of neurosurgical procedures and brain injury. The common causes of hyponatremia include iatrogenic fluid overloading the syndrome of inappropriate release of antidiuretic hormone (SIADH), and cerebral salt wasting. The infusion of hypotonic solutions or ingestion of free water may cause hyponatremia. Hyponatremia may increase brain edema. Normal saline is the intravenous fluid of choice for the neurosurgical patient. The serum sodium level, as well as other electrolytes, should be obtained regularly in the postoperative or postinjury period to avoid the complications of severe hyponatremia, which include obtundation, seizure, and coma.[24]

Historically, hyponatremia in the neurosurgical patient was attributed to SIADH. Antidiuretic hormone (ADH) conserves free water in the collecting ducts of the kidney in response to a slight elevation (7 mmol) of serum osmolality above normal. Hypo-osmolality will shut off ADH as a feedback mechanism. Patients with moderate to severe neurological insult may secrete ADH despite becoming hypo-osmolar. The hyponatremia is secondary to hypervolemia with the retention of free water. The treatment of SIADH is fluid restriction (which may be difficult and maintaining CPP).

Many neurosurgical patients with hyponatremia will not respond to fluid restriction and are not found to have high levels of ADH. They may have cerebral salt wasting (CSW). CSW may be caused by the secretion of a natriuretic peptide similar to atrial natriuretic peptide. This hormone promotes salt secretion in the kidney. As salt leaves, so does water, which leads to hypovolemia. Hypovolemia may distinguish these patients from those with SIADH. In practice, it may be very difficult to determine which is the cause of hyponatremia. Urine sodium is increased in both syndromes. Treatment would be to assess volume status and resuscitate with intravenous saline if the patient is hypovolemic. If the patient's volume status is normal or perhaps high, a trial of fluid restriction may correct the hyponatremia. If the patient remains hyponatremic, salt supplement should be started. Patients with hyponatremia are rarely symptomatic with serum sodium levels above 125. If a patient is symptomatic or if the sodium level dips below 125, infusion of 3%N hypertonic saline should be started. Infusion rate is low (30 – 40 mL/hr) because too aggressive correction of the hyponatremia may lead to central pontine myelinolysis (leading to "locked in state"). The correction of the serum sodium should not be faster than 1 mEq every 2 hours.

Hypernatremia is also frequent in the postoperative neurosurgical patient and may be the result of osmotherapy to decrease brain fluid volume and perhaps ICP. Hypernatremia may also be caused by the maintenance infusion of normal saline over time. This will also lead to hyperchloremic acidosis. Large volumes of fluid replacement to maintain hypervolemia or CPP may lead to large volumes of renal output. If this volume is not maintained, hypernatremia and dehydration may develop. Hypernatremia may be caused by central diabetes insipidus (DI), with a loss of ADH secondary to hypophyseal or hypothalamic surgery or injury. It can occur as a sign of severe cerebral edema and herniation. Central DI is diagnosed by the presence of a low urine osmolality (< 250 mmol), with a high serum osmolality (> 300 mmol), or serum Na > 150. In the setting of a very high urine output (> 600 mL/hr), a trial of intravenous DDAVP (2–4 mg) may be warranted. A dramatic reduction in urine output would suggest the diagnosis of DI and the need for continued therapy with DDAVP. Hypernatremia should be treated with fluid hydration, initially with normal saline until hypovolemia is corrected, and then with slow replacement of the free water deficit over a few days to avoid reflex intracerebral edema.

Electrolytes other than sodium need to be followed in the ICU. Critical care patients frequently develop hypokalemia with diuresis and large volume shifts. Potassium needs to be replaced. Hypomagnesemia is common, and magnesium needs to be replaced to replenish energy stores as well as avoid arrythmias. Patients will also appear to be hypocalcemic secondary to low albumin levels. Usually, the ionized calcium level is normal, and calcium rarely needs replacement. Hyperkalemia, hypermagnesemia, and hyperphosphatemia develop in the patient with renal dysfunction. Hyperkalemia that causes electrocardiographic (EKG) change (peaked T waves, broadened QRS) requires emergency treatment. This consists of intravenous calcium to counteract the cardiac effects, an ampule of glucose and IV insulin, β-agonists, sodium bicarbonate (these all increase cellular uptake of potassium), and a potassium-wasting diuretic, such as Lasix.

◆ Subarachnoid Hemorrhage

The management of the patient with acute SAH, usually secondary to a ruptured cerebral aneurysm, is complex and requires both pre- and postoperative-procedure critical care.[25] All patients with spontaneous SAH are placed in the ICU regardless of cause or grade because there is potential for deterioration, rebleeding, and acute hydrocephalus. Patients with poor clinical status after SAH have a worse prognosis, with a greater chance of complications. Clinical status is graded on a scale, such as the Hunt and Hess scale. In general, patients with grade I through III have a better prognosis and present without severe obtundation, requiring less critical care support. Patients who present in grades IV to V have severe neurological deficits, present in coma, and are near death. They require ventilatory support, intracerebral monitoring with ventriculostomy, and at times resuscitation.

Hypertension

Many patients with SAH present with hypertension. The cause of SAH is frequently a ruptured cerebral aneurysm. Prior to obliteration of the aneurysm, control of hypertension may prevent rebleeding. This section discusses management of hypertension for these patients.[26] These principles can be applied to any patient within the neurosurgical ICU in which control of BP is desired.

The most effective and rapid intravenous control of systemic hypertension is sodium nitroprusside (Nipride, F. Hoffmann-La Roche Ltd, Basel, Switzerland). Nipride may cause cerebral vasodilation resulting in increased ICP, and toxicity is a concern with use beyond 24 to 48 hours. At some point, it is advantageous to switch the patient to lebetalol, which is effective and does not interfere with intracerebral circulation. These and other agents for IV control of hypertension are listed in **Table 4–3.**

Patients with SAH are placed on nimodipine to decrease the clinical effects of vasospasm. Nimodipine is also an antihypertensive. Once the BP is controlled, the patient should be switched to oral therapy. Choices include angiotensin converting enzyme (ACE) inhibitors, β-blockers, nitrates, and calcium channel blockers. Clonidine may also be considered for subacute, long-term therapy. Some of these choices are listed in **Table 4–3**.

Vasospasm

Vasospasm occurs in 50% of patients with SAH and is symptomatic in over 30%.[27,28] It can lead to cerebral ischemia, infarction, and death. Vasospasm occurs after the first 3 days and lasts up to 14 days. The cause of cerebral vasospasm is unknown, but the exposure of the cerebral blood vessels to the breakdown products of blood and RBCs is considered to be the cause. Oxyhemoglobin and superoxide radicals may promote vasospasm by stimulation of endothelin and inflammatory mediators and inhibition of nitric oxide, resulting in vasoconstriction. The incidence of vasospasm is related to the volume of subarachnoid blood as well as the worst clinical grade of SAH.

Current treatment of vasospasm revolves around early diagnosis, prophylactic use of nimodipine, aggressive use of angioplasty to dilate vasoconstricted vessels, and hypervolemic, hypertensive, hemodilution (HHH) therapy to maintain CBF. As previously discussed, there have been large randomized studies to show that nimodipine improves the outcome of patients with vasospasm after SAH. The incidence of vasospasm remains the same despite nimodipine, so perhaps nimodipine outcome advantage is not related to its vasodilatory effects but to limitation of calcium influx in marginally ischemic neurons.[29]

Vasospasm does not usually occur until 3 days after SAH. Change in neurological status will be the first manifestation of vasospasm. In the anterior and middle circulation, lateralizing deficits may occur. In the posterior circulation, the patient may have a decreased level of consciousness. A new severe headache or seizure may be the presenting symptom. These patients should undergo CT scan to look for the cause of deterioration, followed by angiography to diagnose and possibly treat vasospasm with angioplasty.

Vasospasm is present 50% of the time in asymptomatic patients. To diagnose vasospasm prior to symptoms, serial transcranial Doppler (TCD) exams have been advocated.[30] Either high flow through a vessel (> 120 cm/s) or a great increase of vessel flow over a baseline TCD is suggestive of vasospasm. TCD velocity > 200 cm/s has been associated with severe vasospasm and infarction. Absolute velocities of TCD and its association with clinical and angiographic vasospasm have been questioned in other studies. TCD's role in predicting symptomatic vasospasm may be limited, but as a screening exam for vasospasm, it may function as a guide to initiate HHT, angiographic evaluation, or continued observation in an ICU.

Hypervolemic, hypertensive, hemodilution therapy (HHH, or currently HHT) was developed in the late 1970s and throughout the 1980s as a treatment for vasospasm.[31] Though there has not been any large multicenter randomized, prospective study to support the use of HHT for vasospasm, there are clinical data to support the theory that hypovolemia and hypotension potentiate the clinical severity of vasospasm. The theory behind HHT is to promote hypervolemia (causing hemodilution) and hypertension to maintain CBF through narrowing vessels. Increasing cerebral perfusion pressure in some patients with symptomatic vasospasm can lead to dramatic reversal of neurological deficits. In others, it will not change the course of vasospasm.

A CVP catheter is used to monitor volume status for HHT. Frequently, a pulmonary catheter is required for patients with cardiac malfunction (cardiac depression is common with severe SAH), pulmonary failure, or other organ dysfunction. The numeric end points of HHT [ideal MAP, CVP, or pulmanary wedge pressure (PWP)] are not established and are surgeon dependent. If HHT leads to complications of end organ failure, then the aggressive treatment should be adjusted to balance hypervolemia with maintenance of pulmonary and cardiac function. HHT can be maintained with crystalloid infusion, and there are no data to support that the transfusion of blood to hemoglobin of 10 matters. Previously healthy patients with SAH and HHT diurese with large volumes of urine. The use of an analogue of aldosterone, fludrocortisone, may help in reducing water and sodium urinary losses. Patients with SAH who become hyponatremic should have sodium replacement because fluid restriction may promote vasospasm.

◆ Perioperative Pharmocotherapy and Prophylaxis

Steroids

Steroids, primarily dexamethasone (1–10 mg q6h), are frequently used postoperatively in neurosurgical patients. For patients with brain tumors, steroids help decrease cerebral peritumor edema. The efficacy of steroids is controversial in patients with acute intracranial hemorrhage. There is no use for steroids in head trauma; however, a short course of high-dose steroids is used for patients with spinal cord injury. With the exception of patients with residual tumors, steroids will likely be tapered after surgery, and rapidly if the therapy has been short. Complications of delayed wound healing, gastric ulceration, and infection should be monitored.

Ulcer Prophylaxis

The patient with an acute intracerebral hemorrhage, head trauma, or a neurosurgical procedure with excessive blood loss is at risk for gastric or duodenal ulceration. Initial prophylaxis with histamine$_2$ receptor blockers [ranitadine (50 mg IV q8h, famotidine (20 mg IV q12h)] or proton-pump inhibitor is reasonable in the immediate postoperative period. Sucralfate (1 g PO q6h) has been found to be just as gastroprotective in the head-injured and multiple-trauma patient. Early enteral nutrition is desired in all postoperative patients, and, once instituted, there is no need for ulcer prophylaxis. Patients receiving prolonged steroid therapy could be considered for continued ulcer prophylaxis.

Seizure Prophylaxis

All patients with an insult to the brain have some increased risk of seizure activity. This risk may be relatively high, $>$ 50% in patients with certain brain tumors or penetrating head trauma, to relatively low, such as in patients with blunt trauma or uncomplicated SAH. The anticonvulsant used most often is phenytoin. Phenytoin is given as a 1 g loading dose to an adult patient and 300 to 400 mg in divided doses per day. Serum levels should be followed periodically. Phenobarbital can be used if there is a contraindication to phenytoin.

Deep Venous Thrombosis Prophylaxis

The rate of deep venous thrombosis (DVT) in postoperative or postinjury neurosurgical patients can be as high as 20 to 50%, and the rate of PE can be 0.4 to 5%, with a mortality rate up to 50%. Because of the fear of operative and postoperative intracranial hemorrhage, there is a reluctance to use heparin prophylaxis. Mechanical prevention of DVT may not alter the risk of DVT. Studies have demonstrated the safety of subcutaneous unfractionated heparin begun at the time of surgery without serious bleeding side effects in neurosurgical patients.[32] There is also a large, prospective, randomized study showing the decreased risk of DVT and PE using low molecular weight heparin versus compression stockings without increased risk of intracranial hemorrhage for elective neurosurgery.[33] More research is needed to determine the risk of DVT prophylaxis for patients with SAH and head trauma.

There is significant risk for patients with complete spinal cord injury to develop DVT and fatal PE. Many trauma surgeons recommend prophylactic inferior vena cava (IVC) filters for these patients. If a patient with increased risk for intracranial hemorrhage develops DVT or PE, then an IVC filter should be placed for prevention of fatal PE. The safety of early anticoagulation as treatment for DVT and PE in the neurosurgical patient has not been established.

◆ Sedation and Analgesics

The use of sedation and analgesics is essential in the critical care unit. Patients can experience significant postoperative pain and frequently remember the discomfort of intubation and other painful procedures in the ICU. Mechanically ventilated patients need adequate sedation to tolerate intubation and prevent self-injury.

The titration of sedation and analgesia is challenging in the neurosurgical critical care patient. Although adequate sedation and control of pain is desired, too much sedation or analgesics can severely limit the neurological exam, which is essential in these patients. Oversedation can lead to unnecessary CT scans and prolonged mechanical ventilation and ICU stay. Strategies need to be developed to choose the correct sedatives and analgesics and the most effective way to dose these medications. The management of pain and sedation in the ICU is most efficient if done by protocol.

Pain in the ICU can be assessed by asking the patient. The comatose patient will reveal pain physiologically with an increase in HR, BP, agitation, grimacing, and tearing. Other serious causes of tachycardia and agitation such as hypoxia, hypovolemia, and bleeding need to be assessed before assuming pain is the cause.

Intravenous morphine is the standard for analgesia in the ICU. It is effective and titratable, and its side effects can be avoided by careful dosing. Synthetic opioids such as fentanyl are also available. Ketorolac and other nonsteroidal anti-inflammatory agents would avoid the sedative effect of narcotics but have not been used often in the neurosurgical patient, probably for fear of their antiplatelet effects and increased risk of bleeding. The new α_2-agonist, dexmedetomidine has both sedative and analgesic properties, with less effect on neurological function. Currently, it has not been evaluated for this population and is used short term in the postoperative patient. A listing of analgesics can be found in **Table 4–4.**[34]

Sedation in the ICU should be monitored by a scoring system to help prevent under- and oversedation. Monitoring systems have demonstrated effectiveness in decreasing ICU length of stay and ventilator time, and the excess use of diagnostic tests. There is a multitude of subjective scales, including the commonly used Ramsay scale, or Riker Sedation-Agitation scale. The bispectral index provides a somewhat objective measure of sedation with gradation of continuous electroencephalographic monitoring. Although the bispectral index (BIS) utility is questionable in the awake, agitated, or lightly sleeping patient, there are data supporting its use to determine the depth of sedation in patients under general anesthesia, heavy sedation, barbiturate coma, and neuromuscular blockade.

Benzodiazepines are the most commonly used sedatives that bind to γ-aminobutyric acid (GABA) receptors.[35] They provide anxiolysis, hypnosis, antiseizure activity, muscle

Table 4–4 Analgesics, Sedatives, and Paralytics

Analgesic	Dosage	Duration	Advantages	Disadvantages
Morphine	1–10 mg IV q1–2h or 1–20 mg/hr	1–3 h	Effective and easily titratable	May cause hypoventilation, and decreased sensorium if dose is too high
Fentanyl synthetic opioid	25–100 μg IV q30–60min or 25–250 μg/h continuous IV	30–60 min	More potent and less of a hypotensive effect than morphine; shorter half-life (30 min) than morphine; excellent for short procedures	Same as morphine though much more potent
Alfentanil	10–25 μg/kg IV or 0.5–3 μg/kg/min	15–30 min	Potent, shorter acting than fentanyl; may be considered for short-term neuro exam	Expensive for the long term
Remifentanil	0.05 μg/kg IV or 0.01–0.025 μg/kg/min	3–5 min	Ultrashort half-life	Expensive
Ketorolac nonsteroidal anti-inflammatory agent	Loading dose: 60 mg IM or 30 mg IV; 15 mg IV q6h for 24–48 h	6 h	Does not cause sedative effect of narcotics and works well synergistically	Antiplatelet effect with possible increased risk of bleeding, renal tubular damage, ulcerogenic
Dexmedetomidine α_1-agonist	Loading dose: 1 μg/kg IV; 0.2–0.7 μg/kg/hr IV infusion	Onset 30 min to desired level; 6–30 min off	Has beneficial analgesic and sedative properties with an apparently lesser effect on neurological function	May cause hypotension, but this can be avoided with careful dosing and adequate hydration of the patient; expensive
Sedative	**Dosage**	**Duration**	**Advantages**	**Disadvantages**
Benzodiazepines—Midazolam	1–5 mg IV q1–2h; 1–10 mg/h IV continuous	1–3 h, increases with use	Provides anxiolysis, hypnosis, antiseizure activity, muscle relaxation, and antegrade and some retrograde amnesia; 1–3 min onset of action and short half-life (2 h)	Increased half-life, > 8 h with advanced age, hepatic and renal failure, and continuous infusion
Diazepam	5–10 mg IV or PO	12–48 h	Very fast onset of action; effective when used as an anticonvulsant and for benzodiazepine withdrawal	Very prolonged and variable half-life; not used as continuous infusion
Loraxepam	1–5 mg IV q2–6h; 1–10 mg/h continuous IV	8–20 h	Potent and inexpensive; ideal for patients who will receive prolonged mechanical ventilation (i.e., patients with increased ICP or grade III–V SAH being treated for vasospasm)	Delayed onset of action, and long half-life (10–20 h); prolonged infusions of very high doses may lead to lactic acidosis and renal failure secondary to accumulation of the polyethylene glycol 400 solvent in children
Etomidate	0.2–0.6 mg IV for intubation	30–60 min	Quick onset of action and short half-life; does not affect ICP	Continuous infusion may induce seizures or cause adrenocortical suppression with increased mortality

(*Continued on page 90*)

(*Continued*) **Table 4–4**

Analgesic	Dosage	Duration	Advantages	Disadvantages
Propofol	0.2 mg/kg/h IV and titrate to doses for level of sedation desired, usually 1–3 mg/kg/min IV continuous; higher doses may be necessary	Rapid onset; patients are conscious 5–30 min when discontinued depending on length of time of drip	Rapid onset and rapid offset of action is ideal for patients requiring periodic neuro exams; useful for patients who are weaning from mechanical ventilation with shorter times to extubation; high-dose therapy 8–10 mg/kg/min decreases brain metabolism and ICP	Expensive, useful in short-term sedation; increased serum triglycerides with theoretical thrombotic and inflammatory side effects; high continuous doses depress cardiovascular function and may rarely cause severe acidosis in some patients, primarily children and adolescents
Haldoperidol	2–10 mg q1h until desired effect	4–12 h	Complements benzodiazepines with less respiratory effect; good for ICU psychosis	May have acute psychosis rarely (neuroleptic syndrome); does not lower ICP and not indicated in heavily sedated patients
Barbiturates–thiopental	Thiopental 5–10 mg bolus and IV continuous of 2–6 mg/kg/h	Builds up in lipid stores with prolonged use; half-life lasts for days	Effective at treating sustained increases in ICP by decrease in cerebral metabolism and oxygen consumption	Patients must be closely monitored with continuous EEG to ensure the lowest possible dose is administered for the desired effect because of severe effect on cardiopulmonary function; monitoring with a pulmonary artery catheter is highly recommended to avoid organ failure
Paralytics	**Dosage**	**Duration**	**Advantages**	**Disadvantages**
Succinylcholine	1 mg/kg IV	5–10 min	Rapid onset, for intubation	Depolarizing agent, may cause hyperkalemia; contraindicated with malignant hyperthermia, large burn or crush injury; may increase ICP
Pancuronium	Loading: 0.04–0.1 mg/kg IV; then 0.1–0.2 mg/kg q1–3h	1–4 h	Inexpensive, good for long-term (> 24 h) paralysis	Delayed onset; histamine release, tachycardia, more difficult to titrate
Vecuronium	Loading: 0.1 mg/kg IV; continuous: IV 0.05–0.1 mg/kg/h	20 min–24 h after prolonged use	Onset within minutes without depolarizing effects; most popular, easy to titrate, short acting over short term	Paralytic most associated with prolonged paralysis after long-term use (> 48–72 h), may be increased with steroids and liver failure
Atricurium	Loading: 0.04–0.1 mg/kg IV; continuous: IV 0.06–0.1 mg/kg/h	15–30 min	Short acting, metabolized by Hoffman degradation, making it ideal choice for patients with significant hepatic and renal failure	Slow onset, high doses for prolonged use

EEG, electroencephalography; ICP, intracranial pressure; ICU, intensive care unit; IV, intravenous; SAH, subarachnoid hemorrhage.

relaxation, and antegrade with some retrograde amnesia. **Table 4–4** provides a listing of the benzodiazepines. We use midazolam for procedures and short-term sedation, and loraxepam for longer sedation.

Etomidate is used for induction of anesthesia because of its quick onset of action and its short half-life, and it does not increase ICP. It is not used for continuous infusion because it may induce seizures and causes adrenocortical suppression with increased mortality.[36,37]

Propofol is frequently used in neurosurgical critical care because of its rapid onset of action and, more important, its rapid recovery.[36,37] A patient can be given a neurological exam minutes after the drug is stopped. Propofol is also excellent when a patient is weaning from the ventilator. However, for prolonged use it is expensive and has increased toxicity. At high doses, it does decrease cerebral metabolism like barbiturates. However, its adverse reactions also increase, and it has been associated with mortality at these prolonged high doses.

Barbiturates are used in the neurosurgical ICU for deep sedation of a patient with sustained high ICP. As mentioned previously, barbiturates decrease cerebral metabolism and, thereby, ICP. They are often used as a last resort because of the side effects of significant cardiopulmonary depression. Patients in barbiturate coma need a PAC for monitoring.

◆ Nutrition

Early nutrition is considered essential to the recovery of the critically ill patient. Although early nutrition is not necessary in the routine postoperative patient, patients who have significant stress, such as head injury and multiple trauma, shock, or high-grade SAH, benefit from early feeding. These patients have increased metabolism and catabolism of lean body mass secondary to elevated cortisol, epinephrine, norepinephrine, and glucagon. The metabolic rate can increase from 30 to 100%, and there is a negative nitrogen balance. A 24-hour measurement of urinary urea nitrogen (UUN) is used as a measure of nitrogen loss per day. The normal UUN/day loss is 5 to 10 g. Patients with severe brain injury can lose up to 20 to 30 g of UUN/day.[38]

Although a negative nitrogen balance secondary to the stress of injury or sepsis cannot be reversed, early nutrition enhances patients' recovery. Patients with severe neurological injury should receive an increase in calories and protein to try to match their increase in metabolism. Patients may require 25 to 30 kcal/day and 1.5 to 2.0 g protein/day depending on the severity of injury. The protein or nitrogen intake can be adjusted to match the UUN/day. Every gram of nitrogen equals 6.25 g of protein. The nitrogen intake per day should match the UUN/day plus 2 to 4 g of additional loss.

One of the original studies that demonstrated a better outcome for patients who were given early nutrition was in head-injured patients.[39] These patients were given more calories and protein per day via total parenteral nutrition (TPN) than they were receiving via enteral feedings. The TPN patients had less mortality and sepsis. This study had a low number of patients, and the improvement was due to adequate nutrition, not TPN. It has been shown in much larger, well controlled, and randomized studies that adequate early nutrition leads to fewer episodes of infection when given via an enteral route, versus parenterally.[40] It has been shown more recently that patients with severe stress from multiple trauma also have fewer episodes of infection if they are given immune-enhancing enteral formulas.[41] It may be wise to use these formulas in patients suffering severe neurological injury as well.

◆ Conclusion

Critical care of postoperative and postinjury neurosurgical patients is complex and requires a highly trained staff of therapists, nurses, and physicians. This chapter outlines the detailed care that these patients require, not the least of which is frequent clinical assessment by experienced staff. As further scientific research and technological advances become available to improve upon the management of these patients, an experienced critical care service in concert with neurosurgeons can utilize these advances to enhance the quality of care in the neurosurgical ICU.

References

1. Hyman SA, Williams V, Maiunas RJ. Neurosurgical intensive care unit organization and function: an American experience. J Neurosurg Anesthesiol 1993;5:71–80
2. Hanson CW III, Deutschman CS, Anderson HL III, et al. Effects of an organized critical are service on outcomes and resource utilization: a cohort study. Crit Care Med 1999;27:270–274
3. Shoemaker WC. Diagnosis and treatment of shock and circulatory dysfunction. In: Shoemaker WC, Ayres SM, Grenvik A, Holbrook PR, eds. Textbook of Critical Care. Philadelphia: WB Saunders; 2000: 92–114
4. Hess ML, Sibbald WS. Applied cardiovascular physiology in the critically ill. In: Shoemaker WC, Ayres SM, Grenvik A, Holbrook PR, eds. Textbook of Critical Care. Philadelphia: WB Saunders; 2000: 1001–1015
5. Sheldon GF, Fakhry SM, Messick WJ, Rutherford EJ. Respiratory failure and ventilatory support. In: Baker RJ, Fischer JE, eds. Mastery of Surgery. Vol 1. 4th ed. Philadelphia: Lippincott Williams & Wilkins; 2001:107–127
6. Hebert PC, Wells G, Blajchman MA, et al. A multicenter, randomized, controlled clinical trial of transfusion requirements in critical care. N Engl J Med 1999;340:409–417
7. The Acute Respiratory Distress Syndrome Network. Ventilation with lower tidal volumes as compared with traditional tidal volumes for acute lung injury and the acute respiratory distress syndrome. N Engl J Med 2000;342:1301–1308
8. Yang KL, Tobin MJ. A prospective study of indexes predicting the outcome of trials of weaning form mechanical ventilation. N Engl J Med 1991;324:1445–1450
9. Rebuck JA, Murry KR, Rhoney DH, et al. Infection related to intracranial pressure monitors in adults: analysis of risk factors and antibiotic prophylaxis. J Neurol Neurosurg Psychiatry 2000;69:381–384
10. Muizelaar JP, Marmarou A, Ward JD, et al. Adverse effects of prolonged hyperventilation in patients with severe head injury: a randomized clinical trial. J Neurosurg 1991;75:731–739
11. Yundt KD, Diringer MN. The use of hyperventilation and its impact on cerebral ischemia in the treatment of traumatic brain injury. Crit Care Clin 1997;13:163–184
12. Cormio M, Gopinath SP, Valadka A, Robertson CS. Cerebral hemodynamic effects of pentobarbital coma in head-injured patients. J Neurotrauma 1999;16:927–936
13. Kelly DF, Goodale DB, Williams J, et al. Propofol in the treatment of moderate and severe head injury: a randomized, prospective double-blinded pilot trial. J Neurosurg 1999;90:1042–1052
14. Rosner MJ. Pathophysiology and management of increased intracranial pressure. In: Andrews BT, ed. Neurosurgical Intensive Care. San Francisco: McGraw-Hill; 1993:57–112
15. Feldman Z, Robertson CS. Monitoring of cerebral hemodynamics with jugular bulb catheters. Crit Care Clin 1997;13:51–77
16. Unterberg AW, Kiening KL, Hartl R, et al. Multimodal monitoring in patients with head injury: evaluation of the effects of treatment on cerebral oxygenation. J Trauma 1997;42:S32–S37
17. Gopinath SP, Valadka AB, Uzura M, et al. Comparison of jugular venous saturation and brain tissue PO_2 as monitors of cerebral ischemia after head injury. Crit Care Med 1999;27:2337–2345

18. Paczynski RP. Osmotherapy: basic concepts and controversies. Crit Care Clin 1997;13:105–129
19. Varney KL, Hatton-Kolpek J, Young B. Albumin use in neurosurgery patients [abstract #183]. Crit Care Med 1999;27(12S):447
20. Boldt J. The good, the bad and the ugly: should we completely banish human albumin from our intensive care units. Anesth Analg 2000;91:887–895
21. Mendelow AD, Teasdale GM, Russell T, et al. Effect of mannitol on cerebral blood flow and cerebral perfusion pressure in human head injury. J Neurosurg 1985;63:43–48
22. Bundgaard H, Jenson K, Cold GE, et al. Effects of perioperative indomethacin on intracerebral pressure, cerebral blood flow and cerebral metabolism in patients subjected to craniotomy for cerebral tumors. J Neurosurg Anesthesiol 1996;8:273–279
23. Qureshi AI, Suarez JI, Bhardwaj A, et al. Use of hypertonic (3%) saline/acetate infusion in the treatment of cerebral edema: effect on intracranial pressure and lateral displacement of the brain. Crit Care Med 1998;26:440–446
24. Sivakumar V, Rajshekhar V, Chandy MJ. Management of neurosurgical patients with hyponatremia and natriuresis. Neurosurgery 1994;34: 269–274
25. McKhann GM II, Le Roux PD. Perioperative and intensive care unit care of patients with aneurysmal subarachnoid hemorrhage. Neurosurg Clin N Am 1998;9:595–613
26. Adams RE, Powers WJ. Management of hypertension in acute intracerebral hemorrhage. Crit Care Clin 1997;13:131–161
27. Mayberg MR. Cerebral Vasospasm. Neurosurg Clin N Am 1998;9: 615–627
28. McGrath BJ, Guy J, Borel CO, et al. Perioperative management of aneurysmal subarachnoid hemorrhage, II: Postoperative management. Anesth Analg 1995;81:1295–1302
29. Petruk KC, West M, Mohr G, et al. Nimodipine treatment in poor-grade aneurysm patients: results of multicenter double-blind placebo-controlled trial. J Neurosurg 1988;68:505–517
30. Sekhar LN, Wechsler LR, Yonas H, et al. Value of transcranial Doppler examination in the diagnosis of cerebral vasospasm after subarachnoid hemorrhage. Neurosurgery 1988;22:813–821
31. Origitano TC, Wascher TM, Reichman H, et al. Sustained increased cerebral blood flow with prophylactic hypertensive hypervolemic hemodilution ("triple-H therapy") after subarachnoid hemorrhage. Neurosurgery 1990;27:729–740
32. Cerrato D, Ariano C, Fiacchino FF. Deep vein thrombosis and low-dose heparin prophylaxis in neurosurgical patients. J Neurosurg 1978;49: 378–381
33. Agnelli G, Piovella F, Buoncristiani P, et al. Enoxaparin plus compression stockings compared with compression stockings alone in the prevention of venous thromboembolism after elective neurosurgery. N Engl J Med 1998;339:80–85
34. Hall LG, Oyen LJ, Murray, MJ. Analgesic agents: pharmacology and application in critical care. Crit Care Clin 2001;17:899–923
35. Young CC, Prielipp RC. Benzodiazepines in the intensive care unit. Crit Care Clin 2001;17:843–862
36. Angelini G, Ketzler JT, Coursin DB. Use of propofol and other nonbenzodiazepine sedatives in the intensive care unit. Crit Care Clin 2001;17:863–880
37. Cheng MA, Theard MA, Tempelhoff R. Intravenous agents and intraoperative neuroprotection. Crit Care Clin 1997;13:185–199
38. Twyman D. Nutritional management of the critically ill neurologic patient. Crit Care Clin 1997;13:39–49
39. Haider W, Lackner F, Schlick W, et al. Metabolic changes in the course of severe acute brain damage. Eur J Intensive Care Med 1975;1: 19–25
40. Kudsk KA, Croce MA, Fabian TC, et al. Enteral vs. parental feeding effects on septic morbidity following blunt and penetrating abdominal trauma. Ann Surg 1992;215:503–513
41. Kudsk KA, Minard G, Croce MA, et al. A randomized trial of isonitrogenous enteral diets after severe trauma. Ann Surg 1996;224: 531–543

Section II

Aneurysms

5

General Principles of Aneurysm Surgery

Yuichiro Tanaka, Kazuhiro Hongo, and Shigeaki Kobayashi

Contemporary treatments of cerebral aneurysms include neck clipping, wrapping or coating, proximal ligation or trapping of the aneurysm with or without bypass, and coil embolization. The goal of aneurysm surgery is to occlude the aneurysm completely while preserving the patency of parent vessels and their perforating arteries. The majority of aneurysms are treated by aneurysmal neck occlusion with clips, but other methods are required when clipping surgery is inappropriate. This chapter describes general principles of clipping surgery and introduces useful technical points.

◆ Surgical Technique

Instrumentation

An operating microscope, operating chair, operating table, instrument table, and head frame are essential for microneurosurgery. The choice of microsurgical instruments varies according to the surgeon's preference and familiarity with the mechanism of these instruments. We use the microsurgical system developed by Sugita (Mizuho-Ika Co., Tokyo, Japan).[15] One of the characteristics of this system is hands-free control of the microscope. Foot pedals in the mobile operating chair are used to control changes in magnification, focus, and axis of the microscope. A tapered self-retaining retractor, tapered spatula, bipolar forceps, balanced suction with eight different suction tips, and silver dissector are also designed to facilitate accurate microsurgical manipulation. The retractor system, housed in the semicircular rail of the multipurpose frame, is very steady and accurate. Various kinds of clips should be prepared for possible use. The choice of clip applicator is another important issue to be considered in aneurysm surgery. All of these instruments must be checked prior to surgery.

Positioning

The patient's head is fixed in the head holder and is held higher than the heart by adjusting the operating table. The head is positioned depending on the location of the aneurysm. We often change the location and height of the operating chair, incline the operating table, rotate the head holder, and shift the microscope during the operation for the most comfortable access to the surgical field (**Fig. 5–1A,B**). Although tilting the microscope or the operating table is enough for temporary change of the operative view through the microscope (**Fig. 5–1C,D**), the head holder should be rotated for longer periods (**Fig. 5–1E**). The cervical carotid artery is occasionally prepared for proximal control in the case of juxtadural ring aneurysms.[10] Catheters for intraoperative angiography or balloon occlusion are placed proximal to the parent artery if technical difficulty is anticipated.

Approach

The appropriate craniotomy is selected, depending on the location of each aneurysm and required approach, which may include interhemispheric, subfrontal, pterional, subtemporal, and suboccipital approaches, among others. A contralateral approach is very effective in selected cases, especially for internal carotid artery aneurysms projecting medially in the prechiasmatic cistern. This approach is complicated when the proximal neck is close to the dural ring. Skull base techniques (i.e., frontobasal osteotomy, orbitotomy, zygomatic osteotomy, petrosectomy, resection of occipital condyle, and laminectomy) provide additional spaces to conventional craniotomies. These techniques provide a wider operative field with less brain retraction. A frontobasal interhemispheric approach is recommended

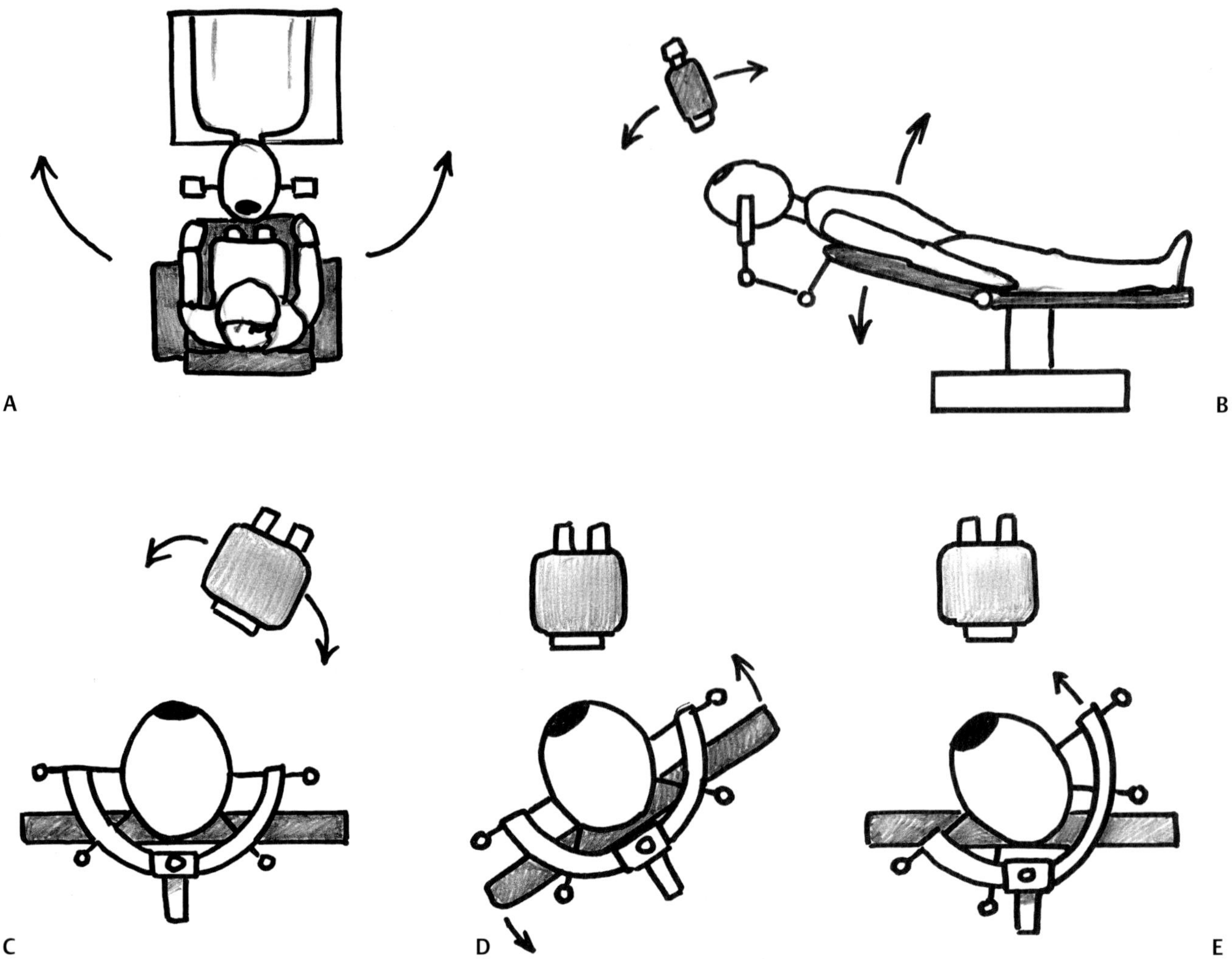

Figure 5–1 Schema showing spatial relations among microscope, patient's head, head frame, operating table, and operator. **(A)** Considerable space is necessary around the patient's head to allow the mobile chair to get the best operating view. **(B)** Sagittal theoretical view showing the relationship between the level of operating table and direction of the microscope. Axis of the operating view is adjusted by tilting the **(C)** microscope or **(D)** operating table for a short period, and **(E)** by rotating the head frame for a long period.

for unusual anterior communicating artery aneurysms. Removal of the anterior clinoid process is an important procedure for exposing juxtadural ring aneurysms.[10] Zygomatic, transcavernous, and extradural temporopolar approaches are methods for reaching unusual distal basilar aneurysms.[2,3,6] Anterior petrosectomy provides an approach route to mid-basilar artery aneurysms, and a transcondylar approach to large vertebral aneurysms.[8]

Intradural Procedure

The brain should be made as slack as possible by means of osmotic diuretics, cerebrospinal fluid drainage, or hyperventilation before opening the dura. The brain is retracted gently, and superficial veins are preserved as much as possible. The brain should be minimally retracted; brain spatulas are often unnecessary in elderly patients. Hemostasis of minor venous bleeding can easily be achieved with mild compression with oxycellulose cotton; electrocoagulation should be avoided as much as possible during brain dissection. Subarachnoid clots should be removed by suctioning with irrigation of saline in the ruptured case. Never approach an aneurysm directly, especially the dome. Parent arteries adjacent to the aneurysm should first be dissected. Sharp dissection with microscissors is recommended around the aneurysm to lessen the stress to the aneurysm. An appropriate clip and clip holder should be at hand at each stage of dissection in preparation for an inadvertent rupture of the aneurysm. The suction to be used around the aneurysm should be the smallest available, and a small piece of cotton should be used with it to avoid accidental injury to the aneurysmal body.

Direct retraction of parent arteries, aneurysms, and nerves is often necessary using a tapered spatula with a tip of 2 mm in width[16] (**Fig. 5–2**). A small, unruptured aneurysm can be exposed by rotating the parent artery with a tapered spatula (**Fig. 5–3A**). This technique is effectively coupled with a microsurgical mirror to observe the dead

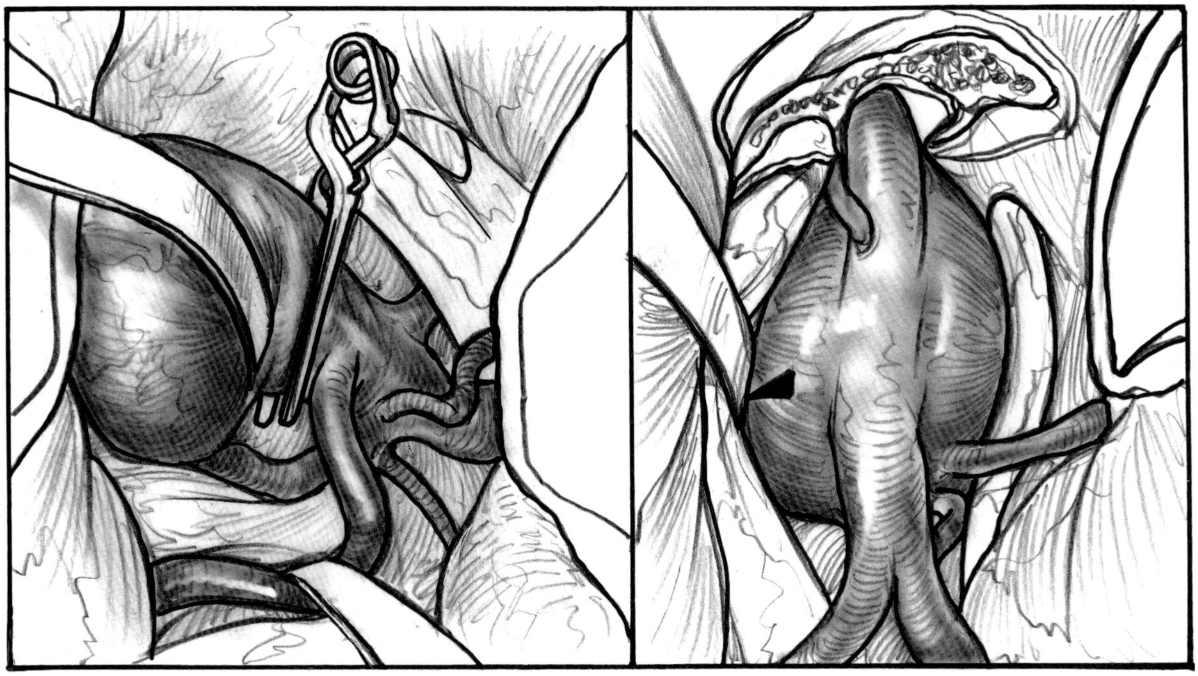

A B

Figure 5–2 **(A)** Schema showing direct retraction of the aneurysm and the A2 segment of the right anterior cerebral artery in the case of an anterior communicating artery aneurysm and **(B)** direct retraction of the optic nerve medially after being unroofed in the case of a large internal carotid artery aneurysm.

angles (**Fig. 5–3B**). A temporary clip applied on the parent artery can be gently retracted to gain efficient rotation of the parent artery (**Fig. 5–3C**). Lightweight titanium spatulas and self-retaining retractors allow the surgeon to "feel" the spatula tip when it is applied over the artery or aneurysm body.

Temporary Occlusion of the Parent Artery or Induced Hypotension

Temporary arterial occlusion is a useful tactic with some large or unusual aneurysms. We use temporary clipping for no more than 10 minutes at a time, releasing for 5 minutes to lessen the danger of ischemic complications. Temporary balloon occlusion of the parent artery is useful when the parent artery cannot be exposed in the operative field. Suction decompression of the aneurysm is useful for large aneurysms under temporary occlusion of the parent artery to obtain space for microdissection of the aneurysm neck (**Fig. 5–4**). Suction decompression can be performed by puncturing the aneurysm in the operative field or by suctioning blood through a balloon catheter placed in the proximal segment of the parent artery before craniotomy.[1,4,19] Temporary clipping of the aneurysm body before neck clipping (tentative clipping) is recommended to avoid premature rupture of the aneurysm before complete exposure of the neck.[19] Step clipping can be used to perform tentative clipping of the aneurysmal body before complete exposure of the neck; the primary clip is removed after placement of the final clip to the aneurysmal neck (**Fig. 5–5**). A bayonet clip is recommended for the initial tentative clipping because the final clip can be easily inserted without interfering with the primary clip. A similar method was described by Yasargil as stepwise "staging" elimination of an aneurysm.[22] Induced systemic hypotension provides a similar effect to temporary clipping of the parent artery. The operator should pay attention to an aneurysm when the blood pressure returns to normal range because the clip is occasionally shifted by arterial pulsation, especially in large aneurysms. Profound hypothermia and circulatory arrest are ultimate methods for highly complicated aneurysms if the patient's condition is good enough to tolerate the procedures.[14]

Clip Selection

The clip must have the most suitable shape and size to apply to the aneurysm neck. The surgeon should consider all the available shapes of aneurysm clip. The closing force of the clip blade is not consistent along the blades; the force close to the spring is stronger than that at the blade tips. Appropriate clipping is ordinarily possible with a regular clip from the standard clip set. If a clip with short blades is used for a wide-necked aneurysm, however, there is a risk of clip slippage because the closing force is dispersed over the total length of the blades. Miniclips are useful for small aneurysms and are combined with regular clips for multiple clipping. Long clips are preferred for aneurysms in a deep, narrow space (e.g., a basilar bifurcation aneurysm) because the longer blades can lessen the dead angle created by the clip head and the jaw portion of the applicator.[21] Specially designed clips are occasionally needed for unusual aneurysms[17]. A right-angled fenestrated clip with side-curved blades is required for the carotid

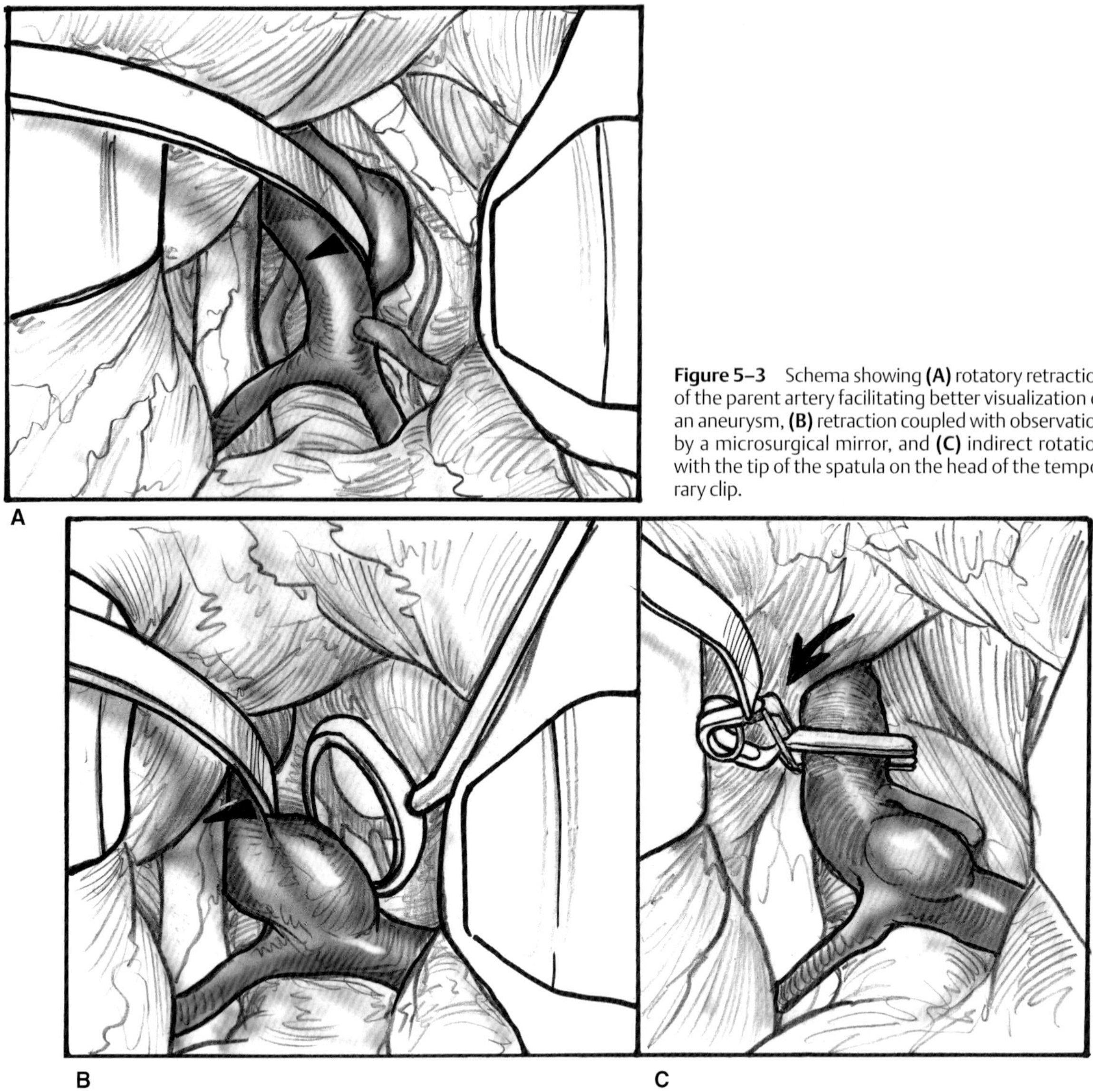

Figure 5–3 Schema showing **(A)** rotatory retraction of the parent artery facilitating better visualization of an aneurysm, **(B)** retraction coupled with observation by a microsurgical mirror, and **(C)** indirect rotation with the tip of the spatula on the head of the temporary clip.

cave aneurysm and a right-angled fenestrated clip with deviated blades for internal carotid artery aneurysms[5,10] (**Fig. 5–6A,B**). Multiple clipping using two or more clips is occasionally required for wide-based aneurysms, although it should be avoided if a single clip can replace the two or more clips. Shank clipping, which is a method that uses a genu portion of the bayonet clip, is one of the methods used to avoid multiple clipping.[13] A crankshaft-shaped clip, which is a modified bayonet clip, is designed to be more suitable for shank clipping (**Fig. 5–6C**). Clipping with wrapping materials is utilized for unclippable aneurysms.[9] Wrap clipping with a thinned surgical patty or silicone sheet or clipping with a Heifetz encircling clip is useful for a blisterlike aneurysm, such as a dorsal aneurysm of the internal carotid artery[12] (**Fig. 5–7**). However, one should be aware of possible occlusion of the parent artery or occurrence of a foreign body granuloma in the future.[7]

Multiple clipping serves several purposes: (1) reinforcement of the closing force of the clip blades (**Fig. 5–8**), (2) closure of an aneurysmal neck with uneven thickness (**Fig. 5–9**), (3) creation of a branch artery using an aneurysmal wall (**Fig. 5–10A**), (4) neck plasty before final neck closure (**Fig. 5–10B**), and (5) prolongation of the total span of clip blades (**Fig. 5–11**). Combinations of aneurysm clips to reinforce the closing pressure (booster clipping) include three different methods using a booster clip, using another clip parallel to the primary clip blades, or perpendicular to the primary clip[18] (**Fig. 5–8**). The second method can be modified using a straight fenestrated clip to occlude the neck with a lumen that is uneven due to the atheroma (**Fig. 5–9**). Endarterectomy of the aneurysmal neck is required if the atherosclerotic change is severe. In the last method, silicone tubing to the clip blades is recommended to avoid twisting the clip blades (**Fig. 5–8C**). These booster-clipping methods are often useful for wide-necked aneurysms to prevent clip slippage, although slippage may happen postoperatively even in a patient with "perfect clipping," due to an abrupt rise in systemic blood pressure. The important point before performing multiple clip.ping is to imagine the best arrangement and combination of clips.

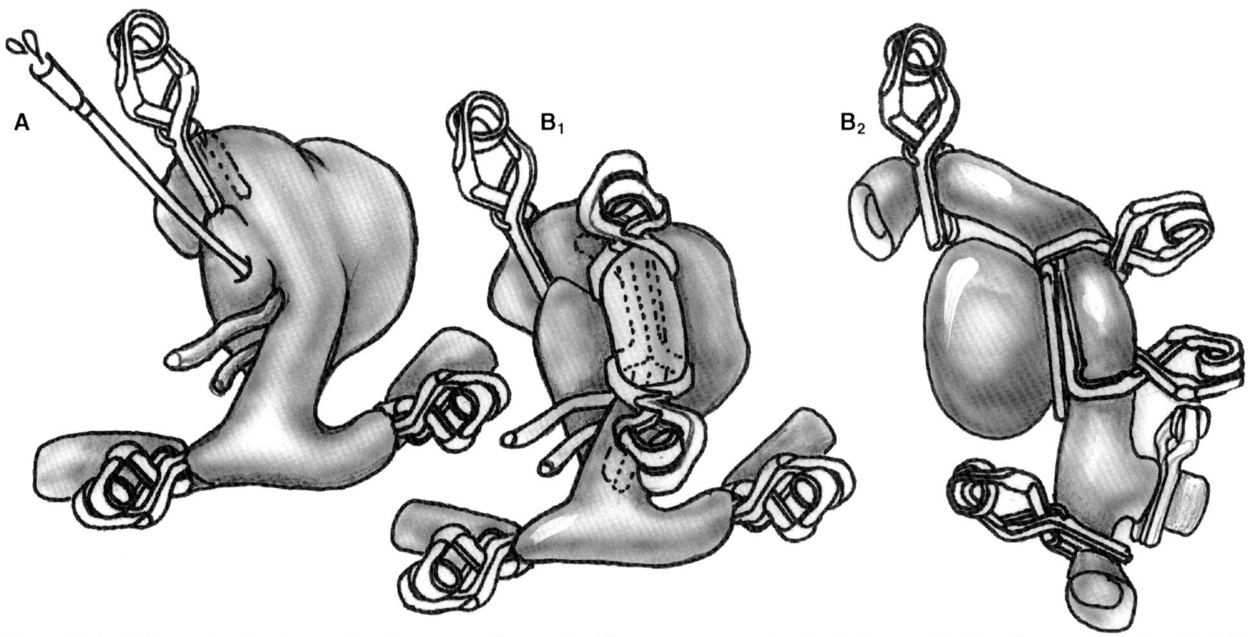

Figure 5–4 Schema showing the suction-decompression method for a giant aneurysm. **(A)** Temporary clipping of three parent arteries and continuous suctioning of blood from the aneurysm reduce the aneurysm tension before application of permanent clips. **(B_1,B_2)** Seen in two views, the neck was occluded with two right-angled fenestrated clips in crosswise fashion.

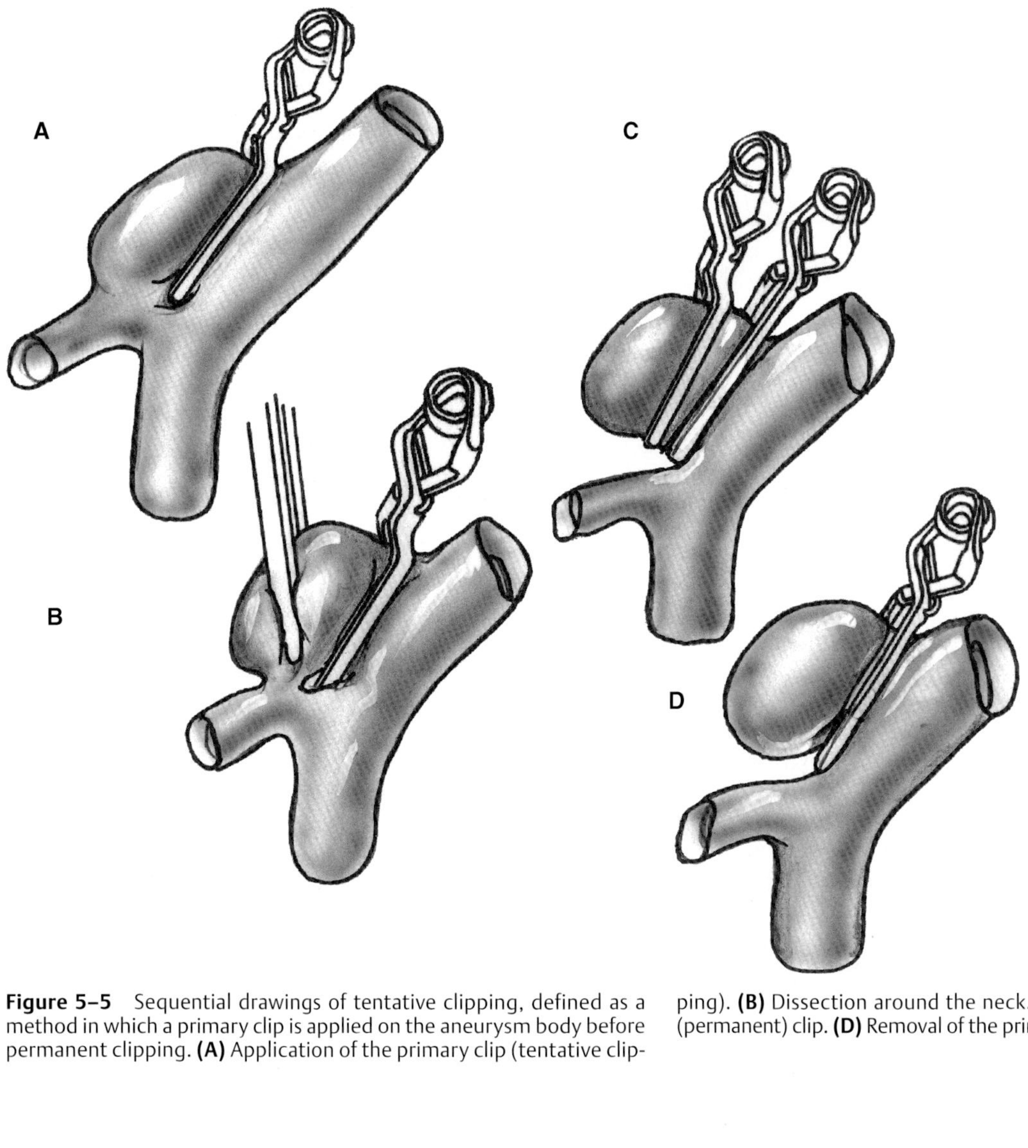

Figure 5–5 Sequential drawings of tentative clipping, defined as a method in which a primary clip is applied on the aneurysm body before permanent clipping. **(A)** Application of the primary clip (tentative clipping). **(B)** Dissection around the neck. **(C)** Application of the second (permanent) clip. **(D)** Removal of the primary clip.

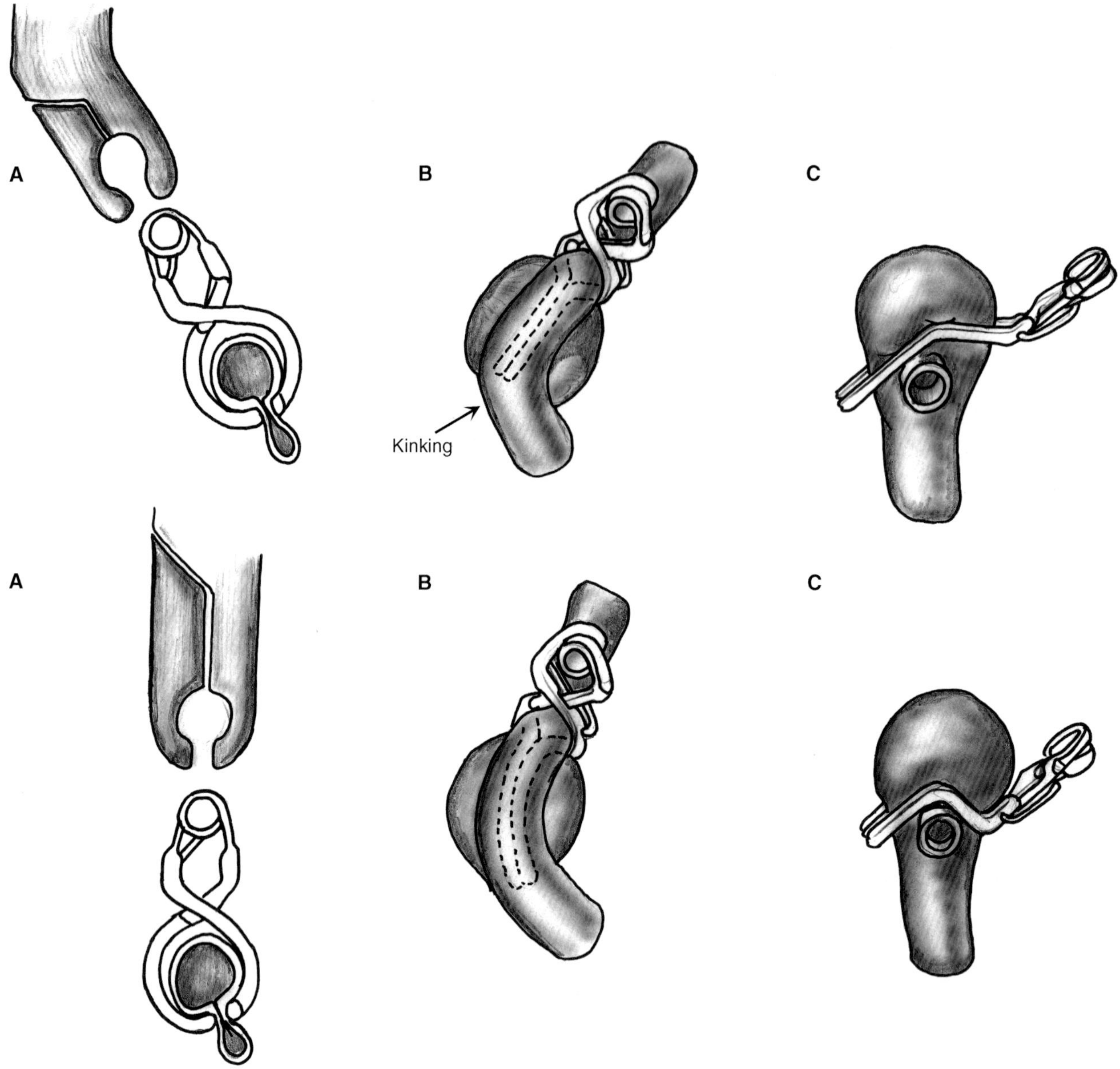

Figure 5–6 Schema showing examples of the modified Sugita's clips. **(A)** A wide operative field is necessary when a right-angled fenestrated clip is applied with a side-bent applicator (upper). If a fenestrated clip with deviated blades (Fujita's modification[5]) is used, a straight applicator can be used in a narrow space with minimal brain retraction (lower). **(B)** If a right-angled fenestrated clip with straight blades is applied to an aneurysm of the carotid siphon, straightening and kinking of the artery occur (upper). A fenestrated clip with curved blades (Kobayashi's modification[10]) should be selected to keep the original curvature of the artery. **(C)** Note that the residual neck formed by an original bayonet clip (shank clipping, upper) is completely occluded by a crankshaft clip (Osawa's modification,[13] lower).

Large aneurysms often involve the origins of branch arteries. These can be reconstructed using a part of the aneurysm wall with fenestrated clips (**Fig. 5–10A**). Neck plasty clipping that does not occlude the neck makes final neck clipping easier (**Fig. 5–10B**). When right-angled clips are needed in the deep operative field, clips with long blades cannot be inserted. Therefore, to prolong the total span of blades, two or more clips are required. The operator should search for the best combination of fenestrated clips if more than two clips are required because fenestrated clips have more combinations, such as a tandem, facing, or crosswise combinations, than nonfenestrated ones[20] (**Fig. 5–11**). Clipping by the crosswise fashion is useful in a deep, narrow space because the procedures can be performed in the narrower space than by the facing or tandem fashions[17]. Clip blades may slip in or out at the junction between a fenestrated portion of the primary clip and the tip of the second clip (**Fig. 5–12**). These clips should be arranged most suitably for each aneurysms. If slip-in is a concern, the blade tips of the second clip should be placed outside the fenestration of the primary clip. If slip-out is anticipated, the blade tips should be placed inside the fenestration.

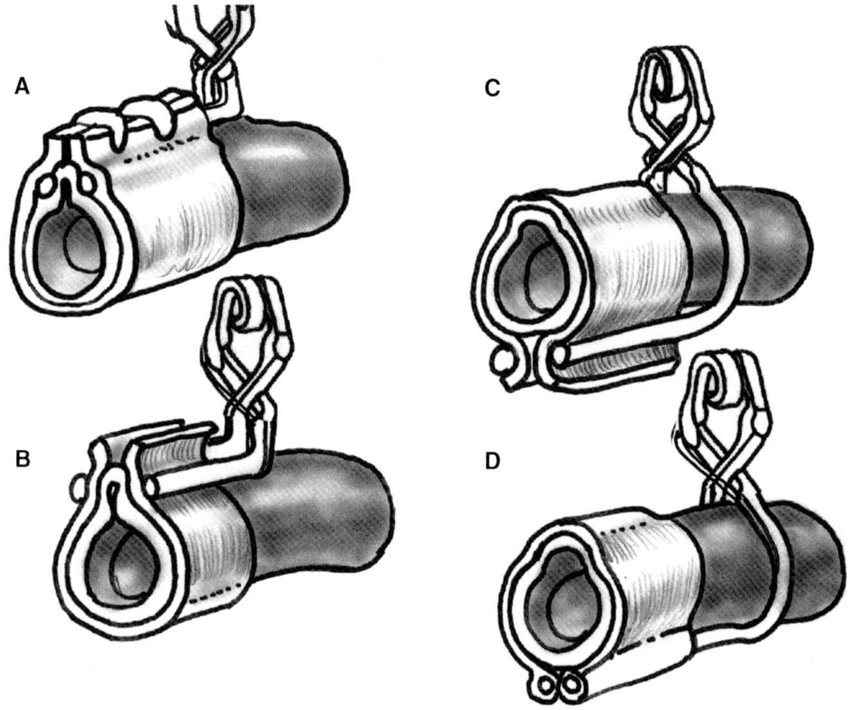

Figure 5–7 Schema showing clipping methods for a blisterlike aneurysm, such as a dorsal aneurysm of the internal carotid artery, with wrapping materials (wrap clipping). **(A)** Wrapping with a thinned surgical patty is added over the clip blades. **(B)** Clipping is performed with a right-angled clip or a **(C)** right-angled fenestrated clip after wrapping. **(D)** Wrap clipping is performed with a Vascwrap silicon sheet (Mizuhe-Ika, Tokyo, Japan[9]).

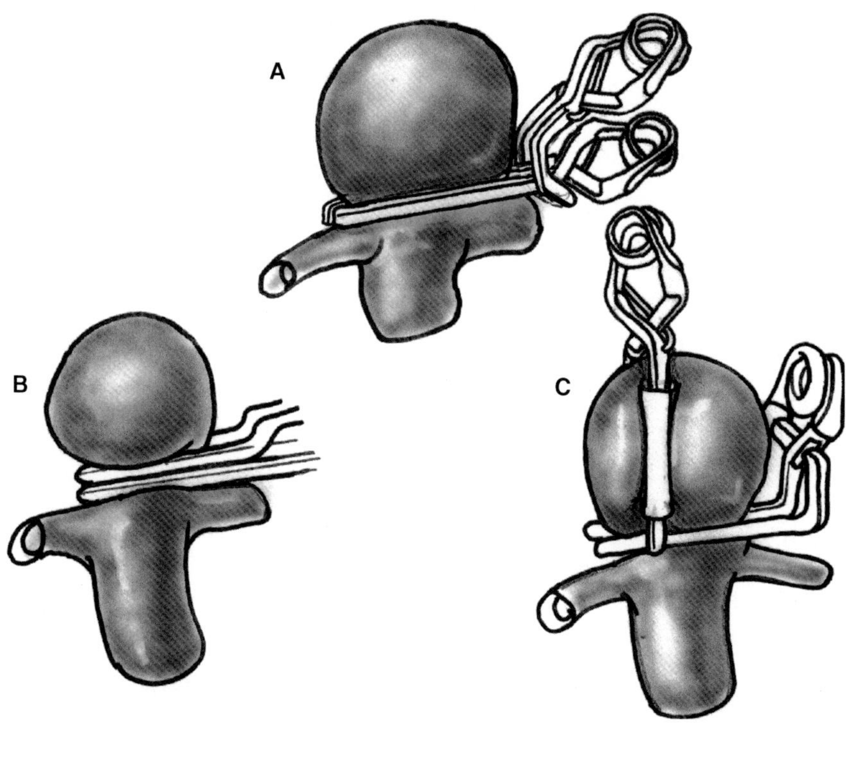

Figure 5–8 Schema of booster clipping. **(A)** A booster clip is applied on blades of the primary clip. **(B)** The second clip is applied parallel or **(C)** perpendicular to the primary clip.

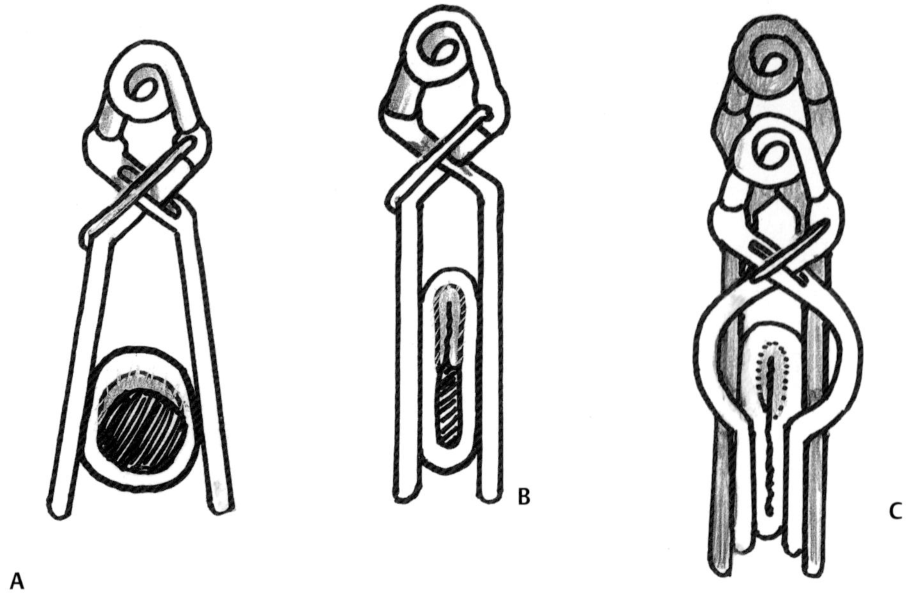

Figure 5–9 Sequential drawings showing a cross section of the aneurysmal neck and clips. **(A,B)** An atheromatous uneven neck is not closed by a primary clip. **(C)** A fenestrated straight clip is added to the primary one to jump the atheroma.

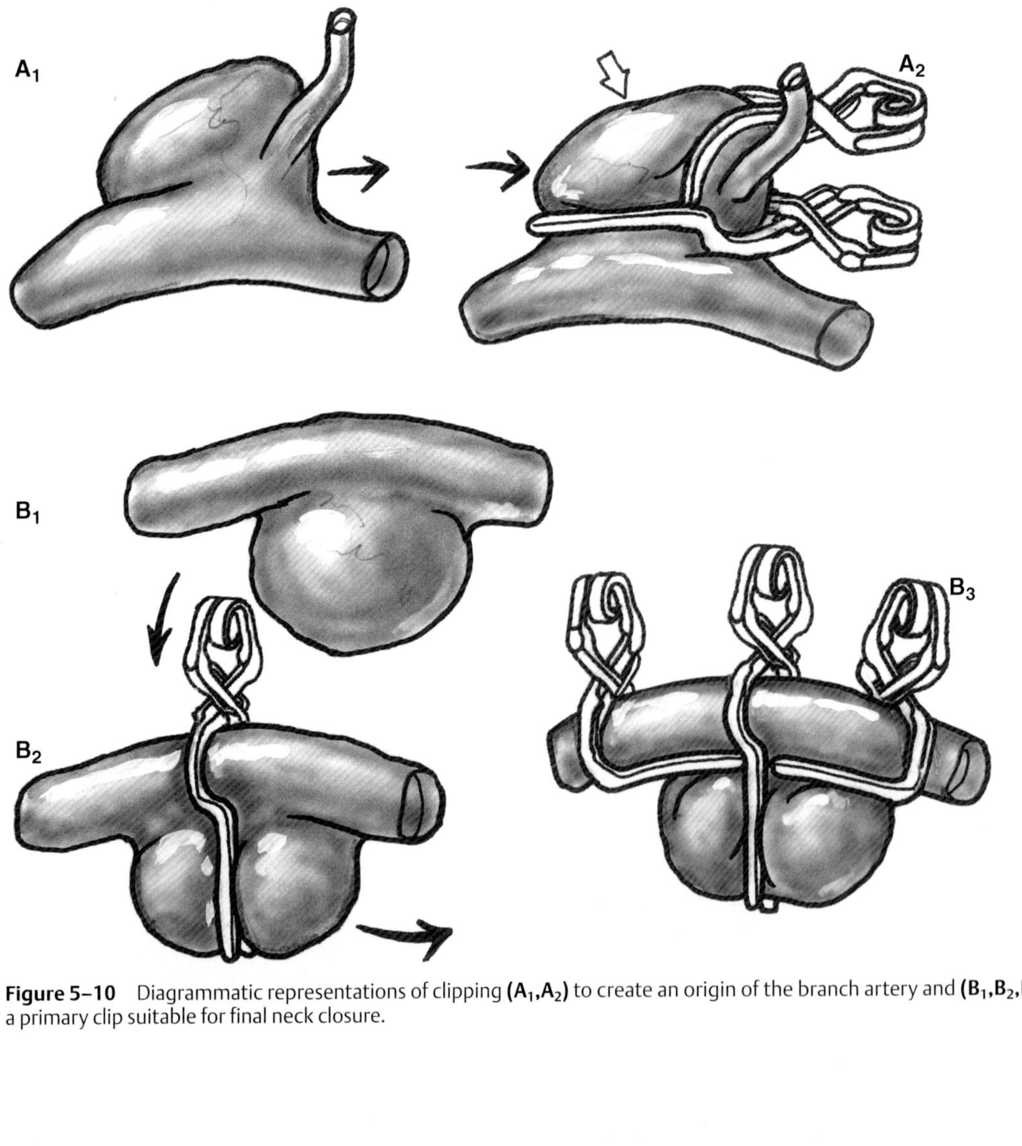

Figure 5–10 Diagrammatic representations of clipping **(A_1,A_2)** to create an origin of the branch artery and **(B_1,B_2,B_3)** to reconstruct the neck with a primary clip suitable for final neck closure.

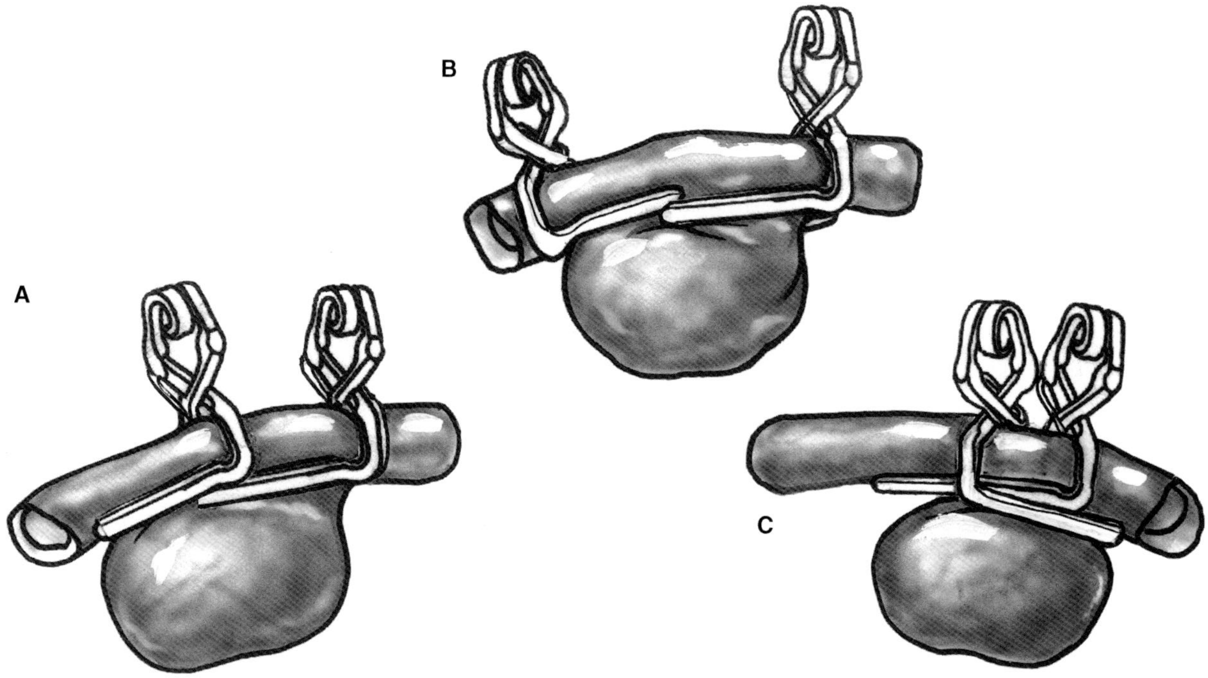

Figure 5–11 Schema showing three basic combinations of right-angled fenestrated clips: **(A)** tandem, **(B)** facing, and **(C)** crosswise.

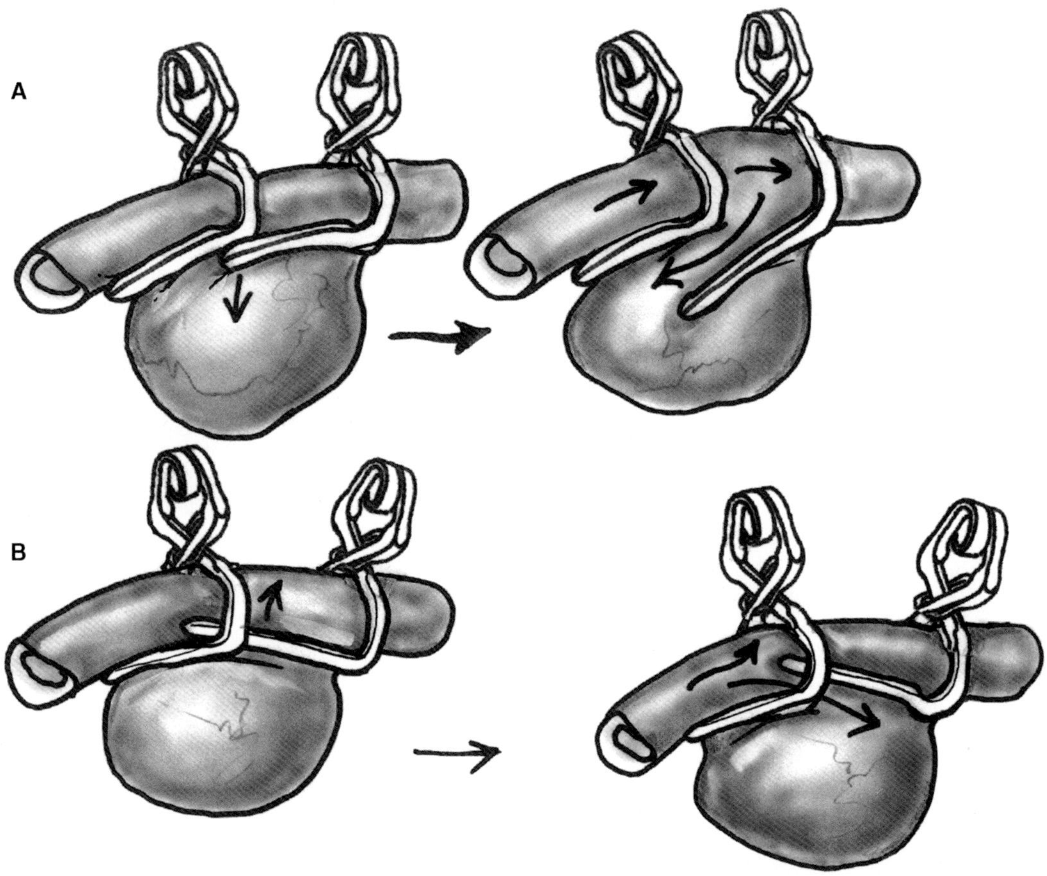

Figure 5–12 Schema showing multiple clipping with right-angled fenestrated clips in tandem fashion. The clip blades of the second clip are arranged **(A)** outside and **(B)** inside the fenestration of the primary clip. Be careful of slip-out motion of blades in **(A)** and slip-in motion in **(B)**. Arrows indicate the directions that the clip blades tend to move (left). Black arrows indicate direction of the bloodstream (right).

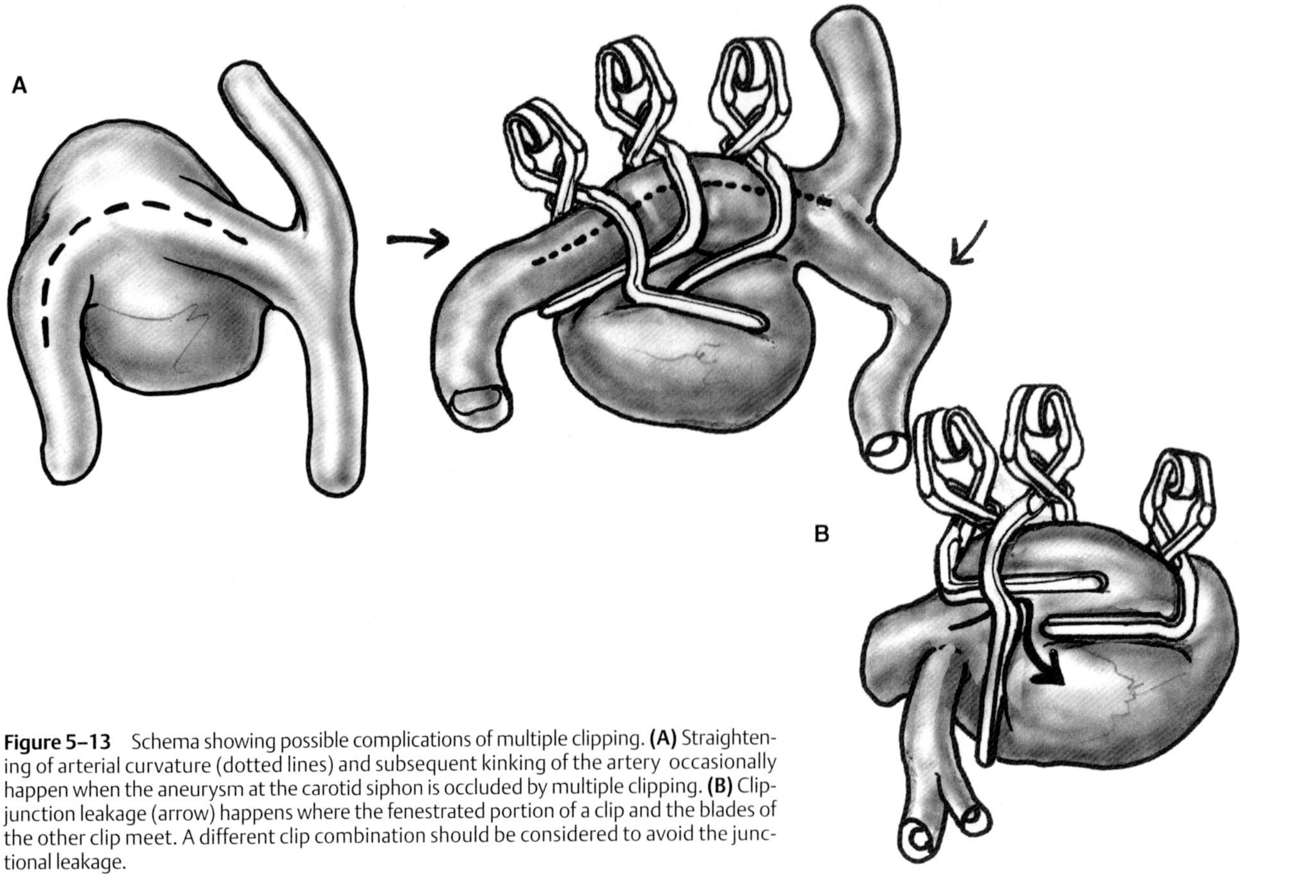

Figure 5–13 Schema showing possible complications of multiple clipping. **(A)** Straightening of arterial curvature (dotted lines) and subsequent kinking of the artery occasionally happen when the aneurysm at the carotid siphon is occluded by multiple clipping. **(B)** Clip-junction leakage (arrow) happens where the fenestrated portion of a clip and the blades of the other clip meet. A different clip combination should be considered to avoid the junctional leakage.

Slip-in tends to occur when a large aneurysmal dome is left unruptured. Slip-out happens when the aneurysm is sectioned. Arrangement of the two clips in tandem fashion should consider the fact that the jaw portion of an angled fenestrated clip has a stronger closing force than the tip portion of the blades.

One of the technical complications with using multiple clip application is straightening of the parent artery[20] (**Fig. 5–13A**). This kind of arterial deformity often occurs following the neck obstruction of broad-based aneurysms; the parent or branch arteries are indirectly kinked by a remote effect. To avoid straightening of the parent arteries, the anatomical structures around the aneurysm should be dissected widely, including separation of the dural ring if necessary. Clip junction leakage may happen through a narrow cleft that remains between the fenestrated portion and blade tips of the other clip (**Fig. 5–13B**). Such leakage should be avoided by rearranging or replacing clips.

Clip Placement

Selection and manipulation of clip applicators are also important issues for appropriate clipping. Angled or vari-angled applicators are useful in some situations for obtaining a desirable direction for clip application. A side-bent applicator is also useful, although more space is needed around the aneurysm than with regular applicators (**Fig. 5–6A** upper). Compressive application of the clip against the parent artery is effective for a broad-based and relatively small aneurysm (**Fig. 5–14A**). Twisting the applicator to advance the clip blades to fit the aneurysmal neck is necessary to avoid leaving residual neck in proximal aneurysms of the internal carotid artery (**Fig. 5–14B**). Relocation of the clip by changing to an applicator with a different angle is useful in the narrow, deep operative field(**Fig 5-14C_1,C_2**). To preserve perforating arteries behind the aneurysm neck, a closing and releasing maneuver is advisable as well as insertion of oxidized cellulose balls between the neck and perforators. Another method to protect perforating arteries uses silicone sheets[11] (**Fig. 5–15**). It may be important to keep in mind that a straight, regular applicator is in principle best suited for clip adjustment maneuvers.

Techniques after Clip Placement

Exploration of the operative field after clipping should be done meticulously to search for unexpected inclusion of the perforating arteries and residual neck. Therefore, aneurysms

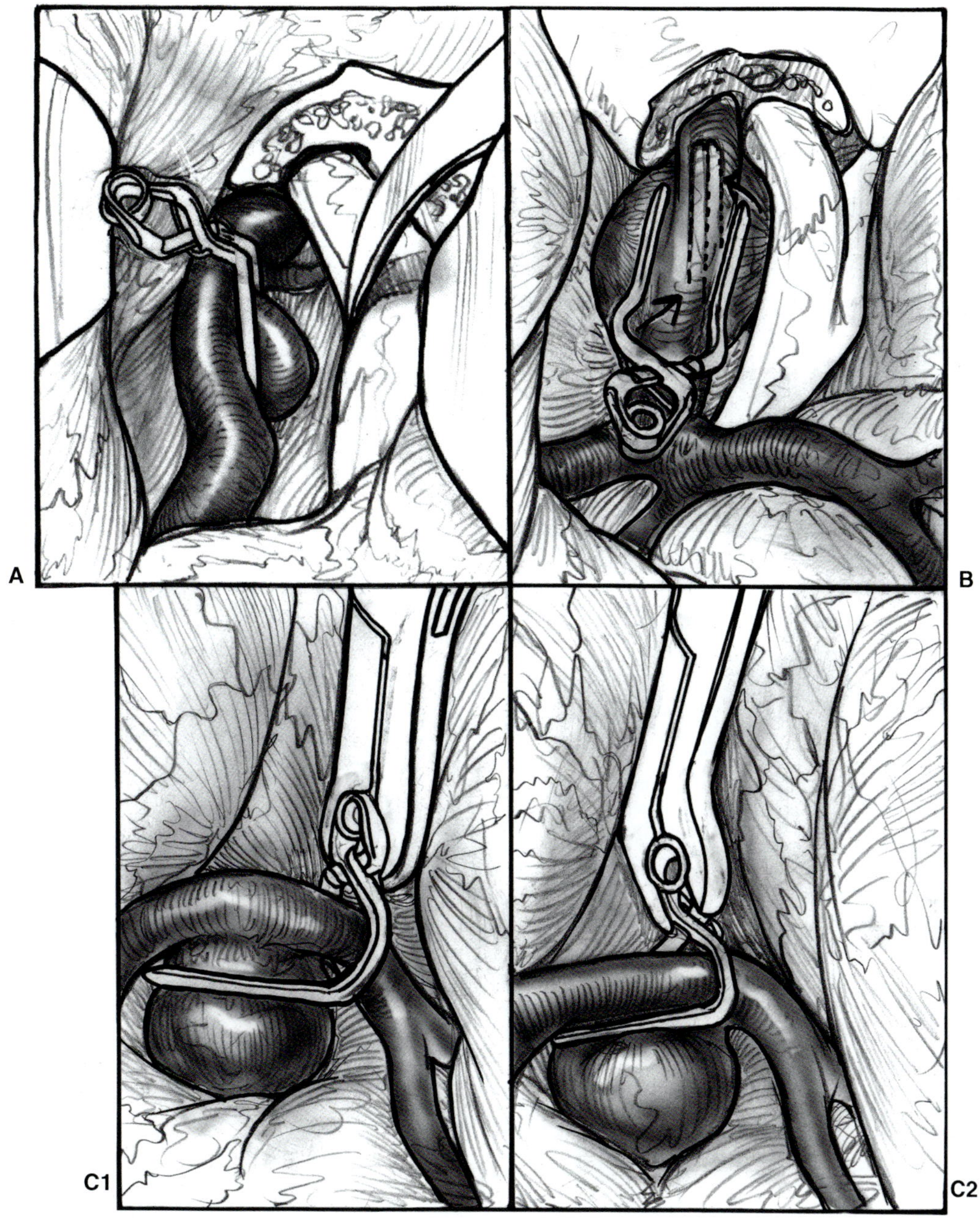

Figure 5–14 Schema showing various methods to manipulate with clip applicator: **(A)** compressive application, **(B)** rotational application, and **(C_1,C_2)** switching applicators for clip repositioning.

should be dissected sufficiently from the surrounding tissue, and aneurysmectomy or electrical shrinkage is performed if necessary. A small probe of a Doppler flowmeter is routinely used for confirmation of vascular patency. Intraoperative angiography is indispensable in a few unusual aneurysms to detect residual neck and deformity of parent arteries. A microsurgical mirror or rigid endoscope is useful for observing the dead angle behind the aneurysm and clip. Wrapping may be added to the residual neck if complete clipping is impossible. When a clip head is displaced by compression with brain when removing the spatula, a small amount of the brain should be removed to create a room for the clip head, or the clip should be changed to one with a shape that will not make contact with the brain (**Fig. 5–16**).

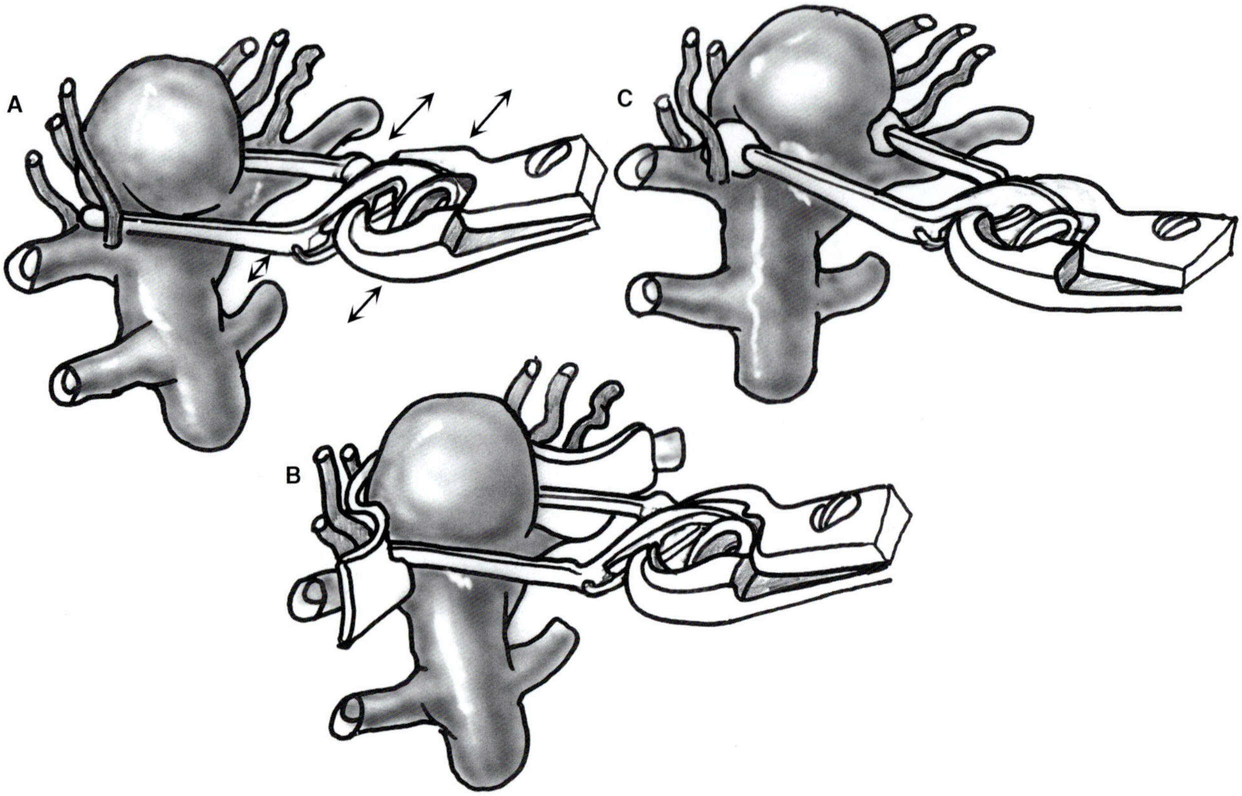

Figure 5–15 Schema showing methods for preserving perforators around the aneurysm neck. **(A)** Closing and releasing maneuver with the clip applicator is helpful to find perforating arteries behind the aneurysm before final closure. **(B)** Silastic sheets interposed between the aneurysmal neck and perforators avoid including the perforators. **(C)** Balls made of oxidized cellulose are inserted between the neck and perforators and clip blades are advanced to push out them (Kodama's method[11]).

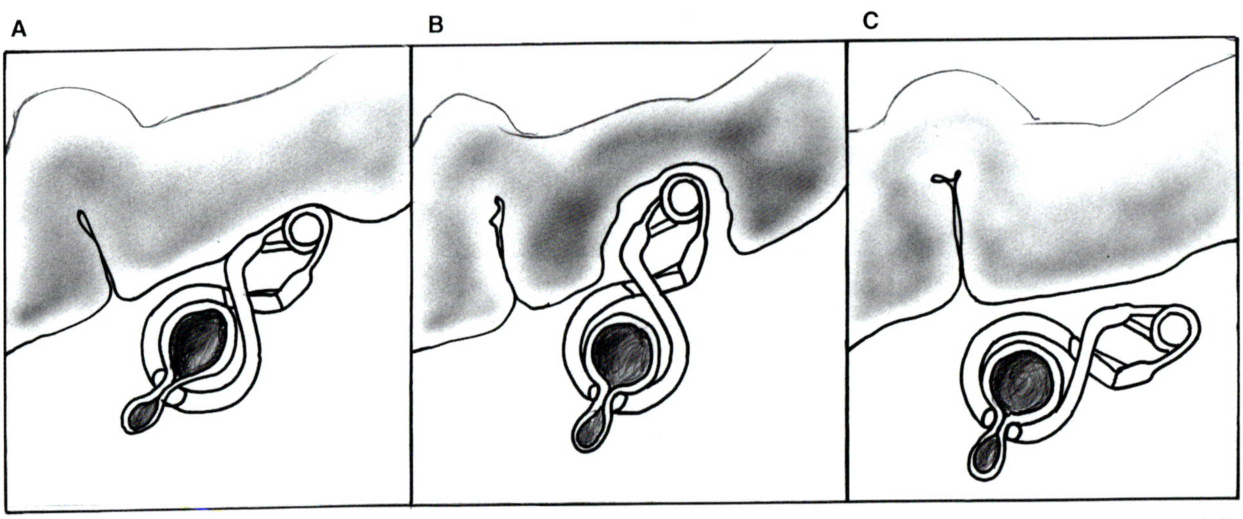

Figure 5–16 Drawings showing methods to avoid shearing the neck after releasing a brain retractor. **(A)** The restored brain pushes a clip downward and subjects the aneurysm to the danger of rupture. **(B)** A method of embedding the clip head into the brain tissue. **(C)** The primary clip is replaced with another design (by Fujita[5]) to prevent the clip from being displaced by the brain.

◆ Postoperative Care

The postoperative care of aneurysm patients varies according to whether the patient has had a subarachnoid hemorrhage and general medical condition of the patient. It is discussed under the special sections regarding various aneurysms.

◆ Conclusions

The general principles of aneurysm surgery are discussed in this chapter.

References

1. Batjer HH, Samson DS. Retrograde suction decompression of giant paraclinoidal aneurysms: technical note. J Neurosurg 1990;73:305–306
2. Day JD, Giannotta SL, Fukushima T. Extradural temporopolar approach to lesions of the upper basilar artery and infrachiasmatic region. J Neurosurg 1994;81:230–235
3. Dolenc VV, Skrap M, Sustersic J, et al. A transcavernous-transsellar approach to the basilar tip aneurysms. Br J Neurosurg 1987;1:251–259
4. Flamm ES. Suction decompression of aneurysms: technical note. J Neurosurg 1981;54:275–276
5. Fujita S. Fenestrated clips for internal carotid artery aneurysms: technical note. J Neurosurg 1986;65:122–123
6. Fujitsu K, Kuwabara T. Zygomatic approach for lesions in the interpeduncular cistern. J Neurosurg 1985;62:340–343
7. Heifetz MD. A new intracranial aneurysm clip. J Neurosurg 1969;30:753
8. Kawase T, Toya S, Shiobara R. Transpetrosal approach for aneurysms of the lower basilar artery. J Neurosurg 1985;63:857–861
9. Kawase T, Gotoh K, Toya S. A wrapping clip combined with Silastic sheet for emergent hemostasis: technical note. Neurosurgery 1994;35:769–770
10. Kobayashi S, Kyoshima K, Gibo H, et al. Carotid cave aneurysms of the internal carotid artery. J Neurosurg 1989;70:216–221
11. Kodama N, Matsumoto M, Sasaki T. Techniques to preserve arteries around the aneurysm. Surgery for Cerebral Stroke 1991;585–589
12. Nakagawa F, Kobayashi S, Takemae T, Sugita K. Aneurysms protruding from the dorsal wall of the internal carotid artery. J Neurosurg 1986;65:303–308
13. Osawa M, Obinata C, Kobayashi S, Tanaka Y. Newly designed bayonet clips for complicated aneurysms: technical note. Neurosurgery 1995;36:425–427
14. Spetzler RF, Hadley MN, Rigamonti D. Aneurysms of the basilar artery treated with circulatory arrest, hypothermia, and barbiturate cerebral protection. J Neurosurg 1988;68:868–879
15. Sugita K. Microneurosurgical Atlas. Berlin: Springer-Verlag; 1985:62–65
16. Sugita K, Kobayashi S, Takemae T, et al. Direct retraction method in aneurysm surgery. J Neurosurg 1980;53:417–419
17. Sugita K, Kobayashi S, Inoue T, Banno T. New angled fenestrated clips for fusiform vertebral artery aneurysms. J Neurosurg 1981;54:346–350
18. Sundt TM Jr, Piepgras DG, Marsch WR. Booster clips for giant and thick-based aneurysms. J Neurosurg 1984;60:751–762
19. Tamaki N, Kim S, Ehara K. Giant carotid-ophthalmic artery aneurysms utilizing the 'trapping-evacuation' technique. J Neurosurg 1991;74:567–572
20. Tanaka Y, Kobayashi S, Kyoshima K, Sugita K. Multiple clipping technique for large and giant internal carotid artery aneurysms and complications: angiographic analysis. J Neurosurg 1994;80:635–642
21. Tanaka Y, Kobayashi S, Sugita K, Gibo H, Kyoshima K, Nagasaki T. Characteristics of pterional routes to basilar bifurcation aneurysm. Neurosurgery 1995;36:533–540
22. Yasargil MG. Microneurosurgery. Vol 2. Clinical Considerations, Surgery of the Intracranial Aneurysms and Results. New York: Thieme Stratton, 1987

6

Internal Carotid Artery Supraclinoid Aneurysms

Cargill H. Alleyne Jr. and Daniel L. Barrow

Historical Background

Although Biumi of Milan described the clinical aspects and autopsy appearance of a ruptured aneurysm in 1765, it was not until the 1930s that Dandy and Dott treated carotid aneurysms by ligation of the cervical internal carotid artery (ICA).[1] Dandy subsequently treated intracranial aneurysms by clip ligation.[1] A precursor to the now commonly used standard pterional approach to ICA aneurysms was first performed around 1850. This was essentially an osteoplastic frontotemporal flap that was used in traumatic cases.[2] Yasargil repopularized the pterional approach with a description of his experience with ICA and other aneurysms.[3]

Classification

The classification of aneurysms that arise from the proximal portion of the intracranial ICA has recently undergone significant revision. Traditionally, these aneurysms have been classified on the basis of their anatomical relationship to the anterior clinoid process. Aneurysms that lay above the clinoid process were considered to be in the subarachnoid space and thus at risk for subarachnoid hemorrhage (SAH). Conversely, infraclinoid aneurysms were believed to be intracavernous, at low risk for SAH, and often inoperable. We now know that this arbitrary scheme insufficiently addresses the complex anatomy of this relatively small segment of the ICA.

The further characterization of the clinoidal segment of the ICA (i.e., the portion that lies between the proximal and distal dural rings) has led to the recognition of the "clinoidal aneurysm," of which there are the anterolateral and anteromedial varieties. The anteromedial variety may also be termed "carotid cave" aneurysms, as first emphasized by Kobayashi et al.[4] These arise from the ventral aspect of the ICA, project ventromedially, and may extend into the cavernous sinus. Day[5] has emphasized the distinction between ophthalmic and superior hypophyseal artery aneurysms. The former arises just distal to the ophthalmic artery origin and projects dorsally or dorsomedially. Superior hypophyseal artery aneurysms have been further subdivided by Day. The paraclinoid variant extends inferiorly or inferomedially toward and beneath the anterior clinoid, and the suprasellar variant extends medially or superomedially above the diaphragma sellae.

Posterior communicating artery (PComm) and anterior choroidal artery aneurysms are associated with their respective named vessels. Carotid terminus aneurysms arise from the bifurcation of the ICA into the A1 and M1 segments.

Giant Aneurysms

A specific subgroup of ICA aneurysms that warrants special mention is those that achieve giant proportions. An analysis of 1167 giant aneurysms reported in the literature until 1992 revealed that 53% originated from the ICA (including the cavernous carotid segment).[6] In addition to presenting with SAH and rarely intracerebral hemorrhage, giant supraclinoid aneurysms may also present with signs and symptoms of mass effect. These can include cranial neuropathy (e.g., optic neuropathy in carotid ophthalmic aneurysms) and hemiparesis.[6] Intrasaccular thrombus and calcification may result in spontaneous distal thromboembolism, or propagation of thrombus in the parent artery or perforating branches. These processes may lead to minor transient ischemic attacks (TIAs) or devastating infarctions. Rarely, giant supraclinoid ICA aneurysms may also present with focal seizures and intracranial hypertension. The prognosis of patients harboring giant aneurysms is somewhat worse than that of patients with smaller aneurysms. This is true for both ruptured and unruptured aneurysms.[7,8]

◆ Indications

Treatment is indicated for virtually all symptomatic supraclinoid aneurysms. Although the indications for treatment of incidental or asymptomatic aneurysms are controversial, intervention should be considered for all patients with a reasonable life expectancy. The therapeutic options must be individualized for each patient and include no therapy, antiplatelet or anticoagulant therapy, deconstructive procedures (i.e., proximal parent artery occlusion by surgical or endovascular means with or without bypass), or reconstructive procedures including open surgical clip ligation and endosaccular embolization. Factors influencing the choice of a particular modality include those pertaining to the patient (i.e., age, neurological status, symptoms, and potential collateral blood flow) and those pertaining to the aneurysm (i.e., size, location, configuration, and the presence of thrombus or calcification). Adjunctive measures that may be utilized with surgery include hypothermic circulatory arrest, revascularization, skull base approaches, and endovascular techniques.[9]

The most versatile surgical approach to aneurysms involving the supraclinoid carotid artery remains the frontotemporal or pterional approach. This provides direct access to clinoidal segment, ophthalmic, superior hypophyseal, posterior communicating, anterior choroidal, and carotid terminus aneurysms. For clinoidal or ophthalmic segment aneurysms, removal of bone from the anterior skull base is usually necessary. Modifications of the pterional approach may be made in certain instances. The orbitozygomatic approach may be used to achieve a flatter angle to the circle of Willis with more working room. The contralateral pterional approach, interhemispheric approach, or a combination thereof has been used successfully in carotid ophthalmic or superior hypophyseal aneurysms, as previously discussed.

◆ Preparation

Currently there is no substitute for a complete four-vessel cerebral angiogram to diagnose the presence of an aneurysm and to begin to formulate a treatment strategy. Items of interest on the angiogram are the size, configuration, and location of the dome, and the size and configuration of the neck of the aneurysm. Also important is its relationship to important perforating vessels, the presence of associated vascular anomalies, and the presence within the aneurysm of a flow void that might indicate a thrombus. If a large or giant aneurysm is present, a magnetic resonance image may give invaluable information concerning the presence of thrombus in the lumen of the aneurysm and the anatomy of the surrounding neural tissue. Large or giant aneurysms often develop calcification in the wall. The presence of calcium in the neck of the aneurysm may severely hinder optimal placement of a clip. A computed tomographic (CT) scan with thin cuts through the aneurysm would greatly facilitate the planning phase and may help predict whether aneurysmorraphy or cerebral revascularization will be necessary. Newer techniques that await their proper place in the preoperative assessment of aneurysm patients include spiral CT and CT angiography.[10,11]

All patients undergo a preoperative workup by the anesthesiology service. For almost all patients undergoing aneurysm surgery, a femoral sheath is placed preoperatively by the interventional neuroradiologist. If the ipsilateral carotid is to be exposed, this step is eliminated because a direct carotid puncture will easily facilitate intraoperative angiography. For those select cases of giant aneurysms that may be better treated by trapping, a preoperative balloon test occlusion is indicated to determine the patient's tolerance of carotid occlusion and the need for revascularization. Those patients undergoing hypothermic circulatory arrest undergo a preoperative evaluation by the cardiology service. This is very rarely indicated in patients with anterior circulation aneurysms.

◆ Surgical Technique

Alternative Approaches

This chapter addresses the frontotemporosphenoidal or pterional approach to aneurysms of the supraclinoid carotid artery. Advantages of this approach include easy access to cisternal compartments, the ICA, and circle of Willis. Various modifications of this standard approach have been described.

The orbitozygomatic technique permits a flatter angle of approach to the circle of Willis by removal of the lateral and superior orbital walls of the zygoma.[12] A contralateral pterional approach to carotid ophthalmic aneurysms has been described.[13,14] Also reported have been the interhemispheric approach[15,16] and the combined contralateral pterional and interhemispheric approach.[17]

The contralateral pterional approach may be considered for proximal ICA aneurysms that displace the optic nerve superolaterally because it makes use of the space-occupying effect of the aneurysm.[13] If a contralateral pterional approach is planned for a subchiasmal aneurysm, it has been recommended that this approach be combined with the interhemispheric approach when the chiasm is prefixed. The latter approach facilitates unroofing the optic canal.[17]

Anesthesia

If temporary vascular occlusion is planned, the administration of cerebral protective agents will increase the length of time the brain can tolerate ischemia. Barbiturates decrease cerebral metabolic requirement of oxygen, decrease the production of free radicals that contribute to cell death, and enhance the binding of γ-aminobutyric acid (GABA) to its receptors, thus decreasing central nervous system excitation.[18] Etomodiate and propofol also induce burst suppression of the electroencephalogram (EEG), but their protective effects comparative to barbiturates remain controversial and await further elucidation.[19,20] Moderate hypothermia to 32–33°C provides safe and inexpensive cerebral protection. This can usually be accomplished by avoiding warming blankets and the use of warm intravenous fluids.

Neurophysiological Monitoring

Intraoperative EEG monitoring or compressed spectral analysis is useful during surgery for aneurysms that require temporary occlusion of the ICA. This modality can help determine the need for administration of cerebral protectants by revealing significant slowing or asymmetry. EEG is also used to document burst suppression to optimize cerebral protection after the administration of cerebral protectants. Somatosensory evoked potentials (SEPs) are also of use in procedures that will potentially comprise cerebral blood flow. Motor evoked potentials, although promising, are still considered investigational at the time of this writing.[21]

Positioning

The vast majority of patients with aneurysms involving the supraclinoid carotid artery are positioned supine on the operating room table. The ipsilateral upper extremity is generally tucked and appropriately padded. A contralateral upper extremity may be left abducted for anesthesia access. A pillow or set of sheets is placed under the knees to reduce traction of the sciatic nerves. The head is then turned 10 to 30 degrees to the contralateral side and placed in a three-point fixation using the Ohio Medical Radiolucent head frame (Ohio Medical Instruments, Cincinnati, OH). Care should be taken to ensure that the head does not lie below the level of the heart because this can impair venous return.

Initial Steps

The frontotemporal scalp is shaved, prepped, and sterilely draped. The first author routinely performs a minimal scalp shave. For situations that call for proximal control, the ipsilateral neck can also be prepped and draped for eventual exposure. In most cases, a femoral sheath is placed in the ipsilateral groin in the holding area, or after induction of anesthesia. This area is now draped. The skin incision is made from the zygomatic arch inferiorly, and arched superiorly and anteriorly within the hairline to the midline. It is important not to violate the forehead for obvious cosmetic reasons. For patients with greatly receded hairlines, the incision can be carried across the midline to improve exposure. The temporalis muscle and fascia are incised and reflected anteriorly with the skin flap. The musculocutaneous flap is held in position by rubber-banded fishhooks attached to a Leyla bar. With the pterion exposed, one bur hole is placed in each of two locations: the inferior temporal bone just above the zygomatic arch, and at the keyhole. We use the Midas Rex drill (Midas Rex Pneumatic Tools, Inc., Fort Worth, TX) with a B-1 attachment and foot plate to elevate the craniotomy flap (**Fig. 6–1**).

Surgical Dissection

Once the craniotomy is raised, the M-35 drill bit is substituted and the lesser wing of the sphenoid bone drilled away until it is flush with the floor of the frontal fossa. For proximal ICA aneurysms, the posterior third of the orbit is unroofed back to the sphenoid ridge (**Fig. 6–2**). Bone wax and Avitene powder (MedChem, Woburn, MA) are used for hemostasis. Wire pass drill holes are created at the periphery of the craniotomy and of the bone flap to facilitate eventual replacement. Alternatively, peripheral wire pass holes may be omitted from the flap if titanium miniplates and screws are to be used for bone flap replacement. Dural tack-up sutures are placed.

The Budde Halo Retraction System (Ohio Medical Instruments Co., Cincinnati, OH) is attached to the headframe and a semicircular durotomy created based on the sphenoid wing. A separate linear durotomy is created posteriorly from the midpoint of the initial durotomy to facilitate exposure of the sylvian fissure. The dura is tacked up with 4-0 Nurolon sutures. At this point, the operating microscope is brought into the field, and the sylvian fissure is opened sharply with a no. 11 knife blade. The fissure is then progressively opened proximally, following the middle cerebral artery to the carotid bifurcation. This maneuver separates the frontal and temporal lobes and provides for the egress of cerebrospinal fluid (CSF), thus minimizing

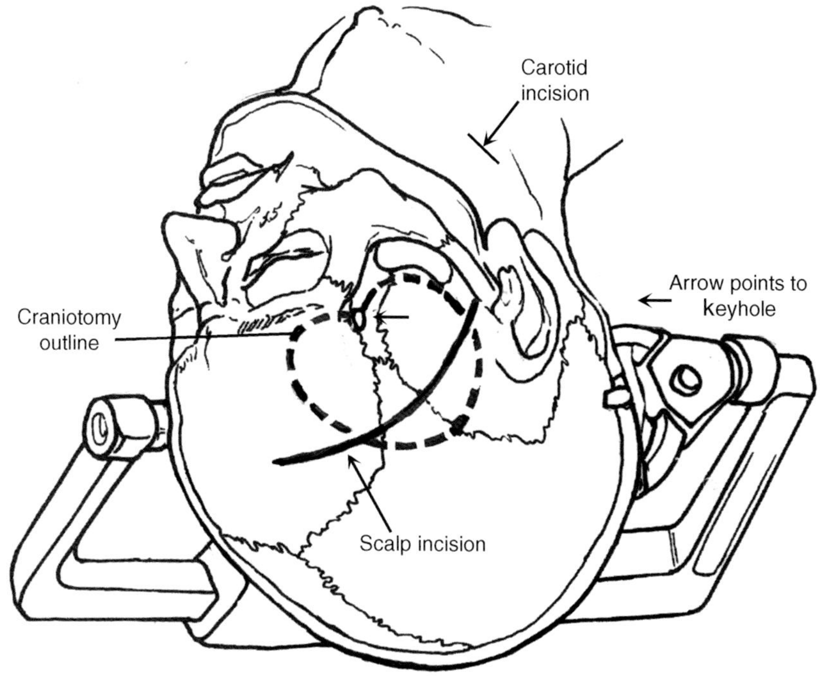

Figure 6–1 Artist's illustration of head position, scalp incision, and craniotomy for exposure of carotid aneurysms.

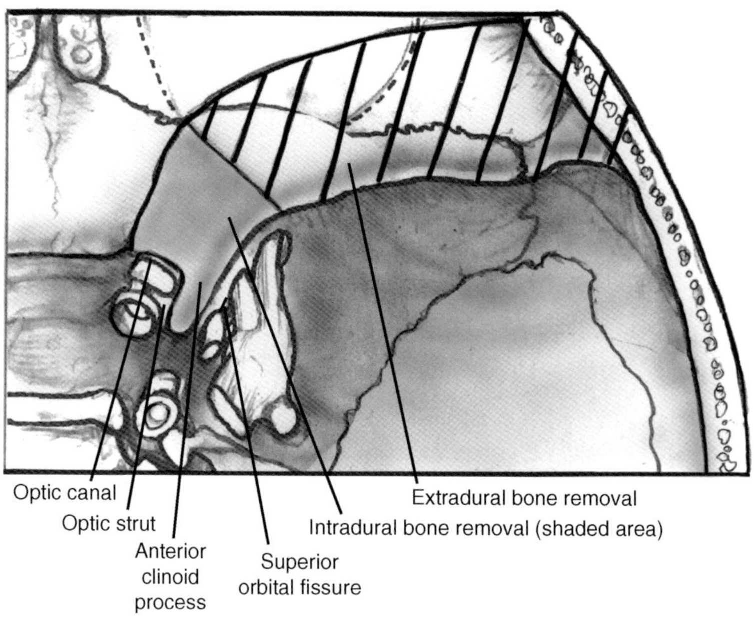

Figure 6–2 Illustration of anterior skull base demonstrating area of bone removal (shaded area) for exposure of internal carotid artery aneurysm. The lesser wing of the sphenoid is removed using rongeurs and a cutting LINAC on a high-speed drill. For an ophthalmic segment aneurysm, the posterior third of the orbit is unroofed as well.

the need for brain retraction (**Fig. 6–3**). Once the fissure is opened, self-retaining retractors may be placed to maintain exposure of the carotid artery and optic nerve. Under direct microscopic vision, the optic nerve is identified and the optic cistern sharply opened to allow further egress of CSF. On occasion, ventricular drainage may be necessary. The carotid cistern, sylvian cistern, lamina terminalis, and interpeduncular cisterns are all widely opened. This release of CSF greatly reduces the need for brain retraction. Bridging veins from the temporal lobe to the sphenoid parietal sinus are coagulated and divided only if necessary. The microanatomy of the aneurysm is clearly defined before application of any clips.

Proximal Internal Carotid Artery Aneurysms

Proximal carotid aneurysms (i.e., anterolateral or anteromedial variant of the clinoidal aneurysm and ophthalmic segment aneurysms) require special preparation before clip placement. The ipsilateral cervical ICA is frequently exposed to facilitate proximal control. Alternatively, intraoperative balloon occlusion of the cervical or petrous ICA may be performed using intraoperative angiography. To enhance visualization of the proximal neck of the aneurysm and proximal carotid, the anterior clinoid process is removed. The dura overlying the structure is first sharply incised in a semicircular fashion from the medial aspect of the optic

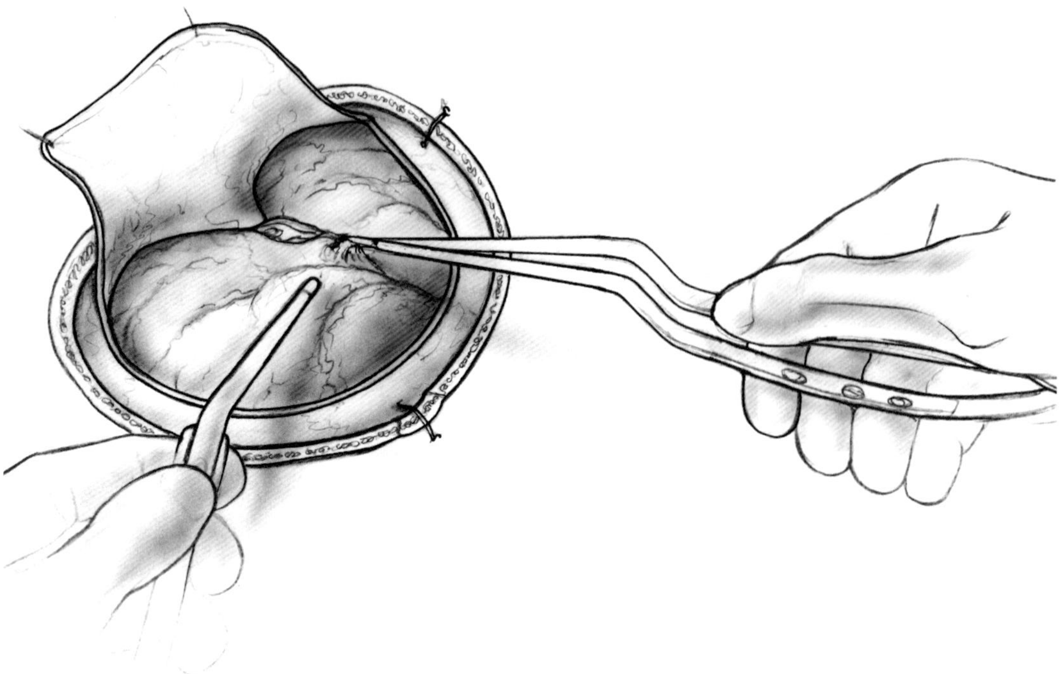

Figure 6–3 The sylvian fissure is opened distally with a no. 11 knife blade and split proximally using microscissors. The middle cerebral artery is followed proximally to the carotid bifurcation, the egress of cerebrospinal fluid from the sylvian and basilar cisterns. The brain is relaxed, and the frontal and temporal lobes are separated. Once the sylvian fissure is fully opened, self-retaining retractors are used only to maintain exposure.

nerve (falciform ligament) to the lateral aspect of the anterior clinoid. This broad-based dural flap is then reflected posteriorly to provide a protective covering for the underlying neurovascular structures (**Fig. 6–4**). The clinoid process is then drilled away with a high-speed drill using a small diamond bur. A House curet may be used to complete bony removal of the clinoid, lateral optic canal, and optic strut. The dural flap and distal dural ring are excised to expose the

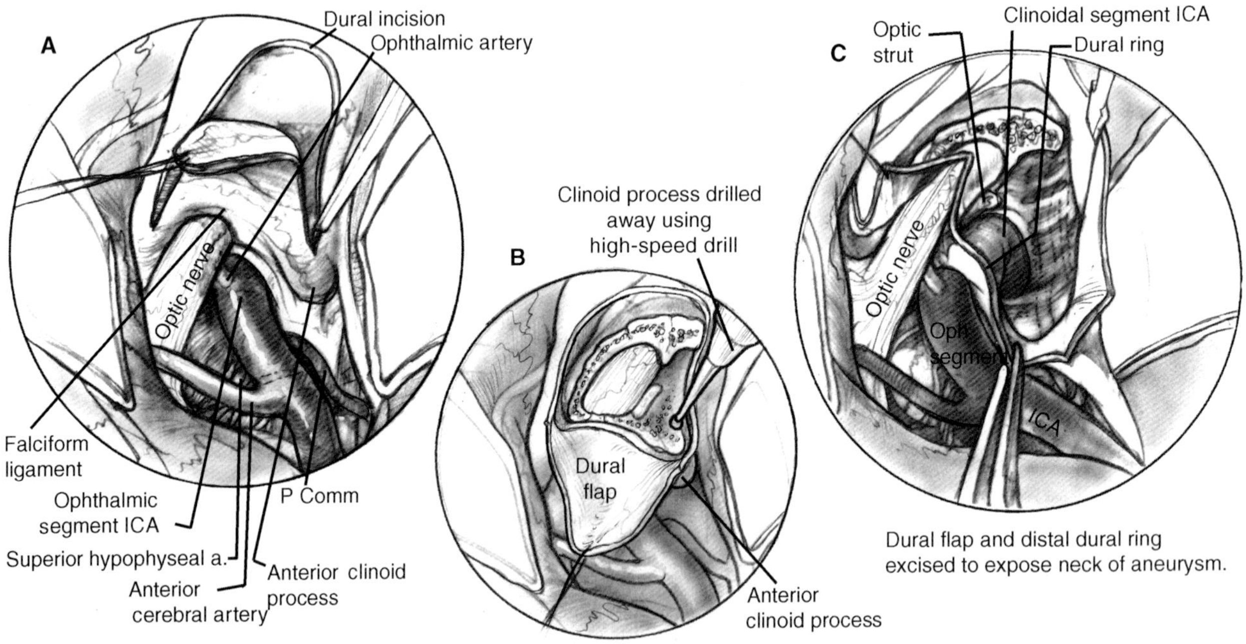

Figure 6–4 For proximal ICA aneurysms, the anterior clinoid process is usually removed intradurally. A no. 11 knife blade is used to open a curvilinear flap of dura over the optic canal and anterior clinoid process, which is elevated posteriorly. A high-speed drill with a diamond bur is used to drill away the roof of the optic canal and clinoid process, disconnecting the anterior clinoid from the optic stent. This exposes the clinoidal segment of the internal carotid artery (ICA). The dural flap previously covering the clinoid and optic canal is removed with microscissors, and the dural ring and falciform ligament are opened. This mobilizes the optic nerve, exposes the origin of the ophthalmic artery, and exposes the junction of the clinoidal and ophthalmic segments of the ICA. PComm, posterior communicating artery.

neck of the aneurysm and the clinoidal segment of the ICA. Bleeding from cavernous sinus tributaries may be controlled by judicious use of Surgicel (Johnson & Johnson, Arlington, TX) and Avitene. By opening the falciform ligament over the optic nerve, the nerve may now be gently manipulated to enhance exposure of the aneurysm. Batjer et al[23] have described a method of trapping large, unwieldy aneurysms by temporarily occluding the ICA just proximal to the PComm and in the cervical region. They then apply a retrograde suction of the cervical ICA to decompress the aneurysm.

Although clip application is dictated by the particular anatomy of each aneurysm, certain basic principles hold. Attempts should be made to align the blades of the clip so that they are parallel to the ICA. Carotid-ophthalmic artery aneurysms are usually best occluded by use of a side-angled clip so that the blades are parallel to the ICA and in a proximal to distal direction (**Fig. 6–5**). Superior hypophyseal aneurysms are best ligated using a fenestrated clip with the ICA passing through the fenestration and the blades parallel to the long axis of the ICA in a distal to proximal direction (**Fig. 6–6**). It may also be possible to use a conventional nonfenestrated clip from distal to proximal in this instance.

Distal Internal Carotid Artery Aneurysms

PComm and anterior choroidal aneurysms are usually ligated with a slightly curved clip to eliminate a potential "dog ear" (**Fig. 6–7**). With PComm aneurysms, manipulation of the temporal lobe should be avoided before securing proximal control of an ICA because the aneurysm dome may be adherent to the medial temporal lobe. This is more likely to be true if the aneurysm points laterally on the anteroposterior angiogram. It is of paramount importance that before clip ligation of the PComm and anterior choroidal aneurysms the anterior choroidal artery be identified at its origin and preserved. If the preoperative angiogram illustrates filling of the P1 segment of the posterior cerebral artery from the posterior circulation, then the PComm artery may be occluded proximally if necessary.

Aneurysms of the carotid terminus may be intimately associated with branches of the medial or lateral lenticulostriate arteries. These perforators must be carefully moved out of harm's way before clip application. Wide opening of the sylvian fissure provides an excellent view of the back of the aneurysm and facilitates application of a clip that is perpendicular to the axis of the ICA (**Fig. 6–8**).

Although distal ICA aneurysms usually require less preparation and are usually more straightforward than more proximal ICA aneurysms, one should be prepared for the unexpected. We have recently operated on a patient with a "standard" PComm aneurysm as diagnosed on preoperative angiogram. At surgery, the PComm was nowhere to be seen. It was only after removal of the anterior clinoid process and excision of the distal dural ring that a clinoidal origin of the PComm (and neck of the aneurysm) became apparent (unpublished data, Barrow DL). In most cases, once the aneurysm is ligated, an intraoperative angiogram

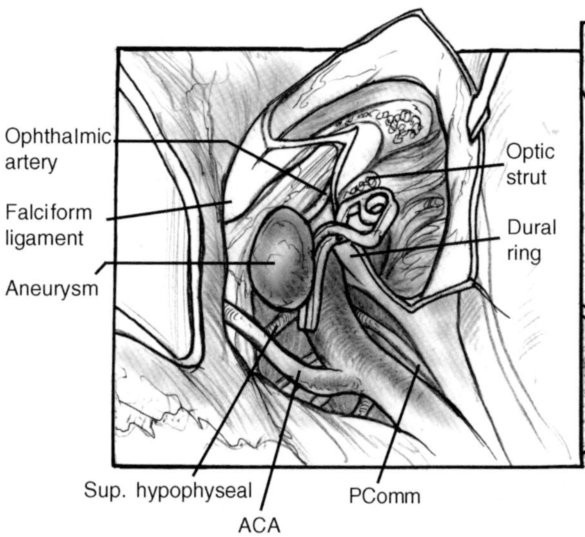

Figure 6–5 Clip ligation of a carotid-ophthalmic aneurysm. The ophthalmic artery aneurysm arises just distal to the origin of the ophthalmic artery and points superiorly. A side-angled clip is most commonly used to initially place the blades of the clip perpendicular to the axis of the internal carotid artery (ICA). The clip applier is then moved anteriorly to allow the blades to align parallel to the ICA. ACA, anterior cerebraling artery; PComm, posterior communicating artery.

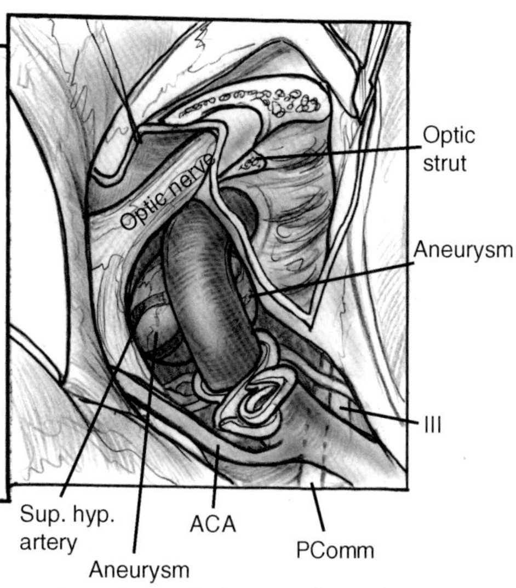

Figure 6–6 Clip ligation of carotid–superior hypophyseal aneurysm. The superior hypophyseal aneurysm arises at the origin of the superior hypophyseal branches on the ventro-medial side of the internal carotid artery (ICA). A fenestrated clip is usually used, allowing the fenestration to reconstruct the lumen of the ICA and the blades to neck occlude the rest of the aneurysm. For wide-necked aneurysms, multiple clips in tandem are frequently required.

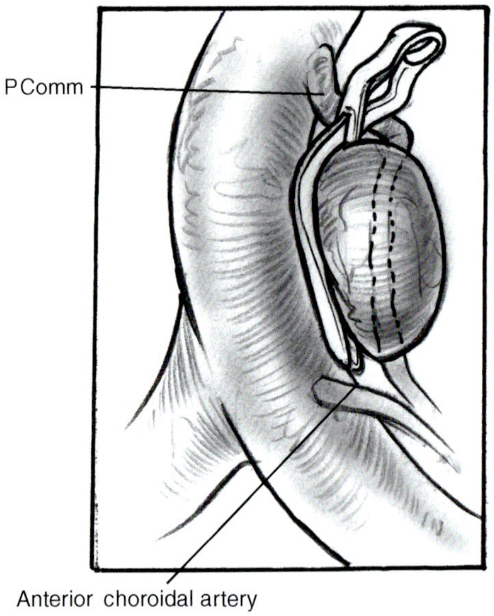

Figure 6–7 Clip ligation of carotid–posterior communicating artery aneurysm. Most commonly, a slightly curved clip is used to reconstruct the curve of the internal carotid artery (ICA) and to eliminate any residual "dog ear." PComm, posterior communicating artery.

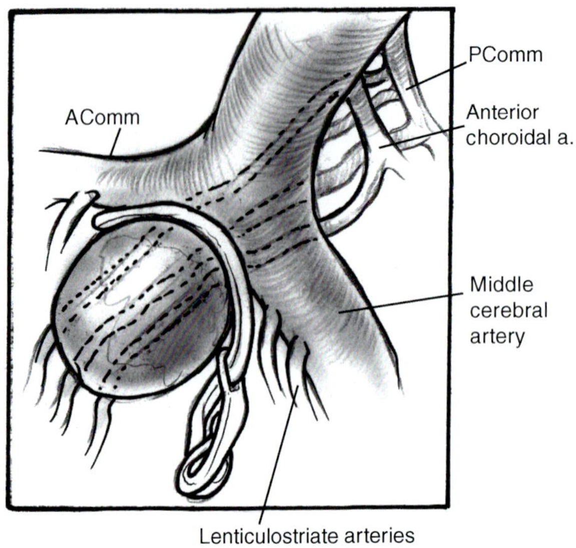

Figure 6–8 Clip ligation of internal carotid artery (ICA) bifurcation aneurysm. Wide opening of the sylvian fissure facilitates exposure of ICA bifurcation aneurysms and enhances the surgeon's ability to identify all perforators and dissect them out of harm's way. A slightly curved clip applied from lateral to medial will usually provide for optimal reconstruction of the ICA bifurcation.

is performed to verify complete obliteration of the aneurysm and to ensure patency of the surrounding normal vasculature.

Closure

The basal cisterns are irrigated with saline, and the dura is closed in a watertight fashion. The craniotomy flap is replaced and secured with titanium miniplates and screws. The temporalis muscle and fascia are reapproximated with 2–0 Vicryl sutures, a subgaleal drain is placed, and the galeal layer is closed with interrupted 2–0 Vicryl sutures. Staples are placed on the scalp, and a sterile dressing is applied.

◆ Postoperative Care

Patients with uncomplicated, unruptured aneurysms are observed postoperatively in the intensive care unit (ICU) for 24 to 48 hours. Longer ICU stays are often required for patients with complicated or ruptured aneurysms. Patients with clinical or angiographic vasospasm undergo standard ICU management, including central venous line placement or Swan-Ganz monitoring, hemodilution, hypertensive and hypervolemic therapy, serial transcranial Doppler studies, selected postoperative angiograms, and angioplasty as necessary. Intracranial pressure monitoring is performed with ventriculostomy if necessary.

Dressings and the subgaleal drain are removed on postoperative day 2, and antibiotics are continued for three doses after surgery unless an indwelling ventriculostomy is present. Along with standard medication regimens, nimodipine is continued for 21 days postbleed for all patients with ruptured aneurysms. Upon discharge from the hospital, the patient is instructed to return for suture removal 10 days to 2 weeks after surgery.

◆ Complications

Intraoperative Rupture

The premature rupture of a supraclinoid carotid aneurysm is the most dramatic and perhaps the most feared complication of aneurysm surgery. The risk of this complication can be significantly reduced by the use of sharp dissection in exposing the aneurysm.[23] The management of intraoperative rupture is determined to some extent by the stage at which the rupture occurs. The prior exposure of the ipsilateral carotid facilitates control of a ruptured aneurysm that has not been completely exposed. If the parent artery has been isolated, placement of a proximal and distal clip will permit continued dissection and isolation of the aneurysm neck. If all of the surrounding anatomy has been exposed, tamponade of the bleeding aneurysm with a piece of cotton and a suction tip may be all that is necessary to promote a clear field and application of the definitive clip.

Simultaneous with the temporary occlusion of the carotid artery, mild hypertension, the administration of cerebral protectants, and passive cooling of the core temperature is achieved. Barbiturates, etomidate, or propofol is typically used.

Parent or Branch Vessel Occlusion

Perhaps the most important factor in preventing inadvertent occlusion of the parent artery or branch is complete exposure of the pertinent anatomy. This is achieved by complete removal of the anterior clinoid processes and opening of the dural ring for more proximally placed ICA aneurysms, and meticulous sharp dissection of the arachnoid in the vicinity of the aneurysm and the adjacent cisternal compartments. We typically use intraoperative angiography to assess patency of parent and branch vessels.[24] Intraoperative microDoppler recordings may also be used for this purpose.

Incomplete Elimination of the Aneurysm from the Circulation

A failure to eliminate an aneurysm from the circulation may result from a variety of factors, including incomplete bony removal or calcification or atherosclerosis in the vessel wall. Use of some of the techniques described earlier will help reduce the incidence of this complication. Again, intraoperative angiography is used to diagnose this problem, and repositioning of the clip or clips is performed if necessary.

Postoperative Vasospasm

As advocated by various authors,[25] we generally irrigate the basal cistern with saline and widely open the lamina terminalis and membrane of Lillequist to decrease the concentration of blood products that might induce vasospasm. The intracisternal instillation of thrombolytic agents in certain patients may decrease the risk of vasospasm.[26–29] Patients at significant risk for vasospasm are treated prophylactically with "triple-H" therapy including hemodilution to a hematocrit of 30 to 32, relative hypertension using pressors, and hypervolemia (central venous pressure $\geq$ 6 mmHg) using colloid and crystalloid. Patients manifesting clinical or radiographic vasospasm refractory to medical therapy are treated with endovascular techniques. Currently, we use intra-arterial papaverine therapy and angioplasty as the need for them materializes. Nimodipine is used to decrease the risk of ischemic deficit posthemorrhage.[29] Serial transcranial Doppler studies or serial angiograms are used to document the efficacy of therapy.

Retractor Injury to Neural Tissue

Injury to the frontal or temporal lobes may occur from excessive or prolonged use of retractors. Widely opening the basal cisterns and evacuating CSF will greatly reduce the need for retraction and its concomitant risks. Treatment of lobar retraction injuries will depend on the size and extent of the lesion and symptomatology of the patient. A wide spectrum of treatment options exists, including conservative management and operative intervention.

Postoperative Hydrocephalus

Hydrocephalus may result after SAH regardless of whether surgery is performed. Widely incising arachnoid barriers to free CSF flow may decrease the risk of subsequent hydrocephalus. The need for a shunting procedure (e.g., ventriculostomy, serial lumbar punctures, or ventriculoperitoneal shunt) can be determined from serial CT scans and neurological examinations.

Postoperative Infection

The use of prophylactic antibiotic therapy in craniotomies was analyzed in a meta-analytical study by Barker.[30] An advantage of antibiotics over placebo was noted. We administer a dose of nafcillin preoperatively and continue for three doses postoperatively. Infections, including local skin infections, bone flap infections, meningitis, and abscess, may occur at any point after surgery. Treatment can include local wound care, antibiotic administration, or surgical debridement.

Postoperative Cerebrospinal Fluid Leaks

The risk of CSF rhinorrhea can be significantly reduced by the careful obliteration of any potential site of CSF egress. These sites include air cells in the temporal bone, the frontal sinus, and the anterior clinoid process. Bone wax or muscle with an overlying layer of pericranial tissue may all be used after exenteration of sinus mucosa. A concerted effort to achieve watertight dural closure will help prevent postoperative subgaleal fluid collections. A temporary period of ventricular or lumbar drainage may be instituted to treat this complication.

◆ Conclusion

Aneurysms of the supraclinoid ICA represent a heterogeneous group of lesions that require different treatment strategies depending on their location and presentation. A careful consideration of the preoperative neurological status and of the preoperative radiological studies that include a four-vessel angiogram will dictate the surgical strategy. The pterional approach remains the most versatile in exposing these aneurysms, but various modifications may be indicated. Meticulous surgical technique, the use of various adjuncts, and the prompt attention to postoperative complications will optimize outcome.

References

1. Walker AE. Manifestations of cerebral disorders: headache, epilepsy, sleep disorders, and cerebrovascular disease. In: Laws ER Jr, Udvarhelyn GB, eds. The Genesis of Neuroscience. Park Ridge, IL: AANS Publications; 1998:187–189
2. Ljunggren B, Fox JL. History of the pterional approach. In: Fox JL, ed. Atlas of Neurosurgical Anatomy: The Pterional Perspective. New York: Springer-Verlag; 1989:1–9
3. Yasargil MG. Microneurosurgery. Stuttgart: Georg Thieme Verlag; 1984:33–122
4. Kobayashi S, Kyoshima K, Gibo H, et al. Carotid cave aneurysms of the internal carotid artery. J Neurosurg 1989;70:216–221
5. Day AL. Aneurysms of the ophthalmic segment: a clinical and anatomical analysis. J Neurosurg 1990;72:677–691
6. Barrow DL, Alleyne C. Natural history of giant intracranial aneurysms and indications for intervention. Clin Neurosurg 1995;42:214–244
7. Ljunggren B, Brandt L, Sundbarg G, et al. Early management of aneurysmal subarachnoid hemorrhage. Neurosurgery 1982;11: 412–418
8. Pakarinen S. Incidence, aetiology, and prognosis of primary subarachnoid hemorrhage: a study based on 589 cases diagnosed in a defined urban population during a defined period. Acta Neurol Scand Suppl 1967;43:1–28
9. Lawton MT, Spetzler RF. Surgical management of giant intracranial aneurysms: experience with 171 patients. Clin Neurosurg 1995; 42:245–266
10. Schwartz RB. Neuroradiological applications of spiral CT. Semin Ultrasound CT MR 1994;15:139–147
11. Anderson GB, Findlay JM, Steinke DE, et al. Experience with computed tomographic angiography for the detection of intracranial aneurysms in the setting of acute subarachnoid hemorrhage. Neurosurgery 1997;41:522–527
12. Al-Mefty O. The cranio-orbital zygomatic approach for intracranial lesions. Contemp Neurosurg 1992;14:1–6
13. Fries G, Perneczky A, van Lindert E, et al. Contralateral and ipsilateral microsurgical approaches to carotid-ophthalmic aneurysms. Neurosurgery 1997;41:333–342
14. Milenkovic Z, Gopic H, Antovic P, et al. Contralateral pterional approach to a carotid-ophthalmic aneurysm ruptured at surgery: case report. J Neurosurg 1982;57:823–825
15. Aoki N. Interhemispheric approach to carotid-ophthalmic artery aneurysm clipping. Case report. J Neurosurg 1987;67:293–295
16. Suzuki J, Kinjo T, Mizoi K. Bifrontal interhemispheric approach to carotid-ophthalmic aneurysms. No Shinkei Geka 1986;14:1175–1181
17. Shiokawa Y, Aoki N, Saito I, et al. Combined contralateral pterional and interhemispheric approach to a subchiasmal carotid-ophthalmic aneurysm. Acta Neurochir (Wien) 1988;93:154–158
18. McQueen KAK, Shedd S. Neuroanesthesiology. Operative Techniques in Neurosurgery 1998;1:14–22
19. Ravussin P, de Tribolet N. Total intravenous anesthesia with propofol for burst suppression in cerebral aneurysm surgery: preliminary report of 42 patients. Neurosurgery 1993;32:236–240
20. Modica PA, Tempelhoff R. Intracranial pressure during induction of anaesthesia and tracheal intubation with etomidate-induced EEG burst suppression. Can J Anaesth 1992;39:236–241
21. Lopez JR. The use of evoked potentials in intraoperative neurophysiologic monitoring. Phys Med Rehabil Clin N Am 2004;15:63–84
22. Batjer HH, Kopitnik TA, Giller CA, et al. Surgery for paraclinoid carotid artery aneurysms. J Neurosurg 1994;80:650–658
23. Batjer H, Samson D. Intraoperative aneurysmal rupture: incidence, outcome, and suggestions for surgical management. Neurosurgery 1986;18:701–707
24. Barrow DL, Boyer KL, Joseph GJ. Intraoperative angiography in the management of neurovascular disorders. Neurosurgery 1992;30: 153–159
25. Sindou M. Favourable influence of opening the lamina terminalis and Lillequist's membrane on the outcome of ruptured intracranial aneurysms: a study of 197 consecutive cases. Acta Neurochir (Wien) 1994;127:15–16
26. Findlay JM, Kassell NF, Weir BK, et al. A randomized trial of intraoperative, intracisternal tissue plasminogen activator for the prevention of vasospasm. Neurosurgery 1995;37:168–176
27. Steinberg GK, Vanefsky MA, Marks MP, et al. Failure of intracisternal tissue plasminogen activator to prevent vasospasm in certain patients with aneurysmal subarachnoid hemorrhage. Neurosurgery 1994;34: 809–813
28. Usui M, Saito N, Hoya K, et al. Vasospasm prevention with postoperative intrathecal thrombolytic therapy: a retrospective comparison of urokinase, tissue plasminogen activator, and cisternal drainage alone. Neurosurgery 1994;34:235–244
29. Barker FG II, Ogilvy CS. Efficacy of prophylactic nimodipine for delayed ischemic deficit after subarachnoid hemorrhage: a meta-analysis. J Neurosurg 1996;84:405–414
30. Barker FG II. Efficacy of prophylactic antibiotics for craniotomy: a meta-analysis. Neurosurgery 1994;35:484–490

7

Internal Carotid Artery Infraclinoid/ Clinoid Aneurysms

Gregory J. Zipfel, C. Michael Cawley, and Arthur L. Day

Over the years, several classification systems addressing aneurysms of the paraclinoid area have been introduced, most of which reference the aneurysm's location to adjacent structures (proximal carotid, paraclinoid, supraclinoid, infraclinoid, paraophthalmic, supraophthalmic, infraophthalmic, parachiasmal, subchiasmal, and suprachiasmal). With improved anatomical clarification of the paraclinoid internal carotid artery (ICA), a more traditional classification system based on the exact point of origin from the carotid artery has been established.[1–4] Paraclinoid aneurysms are now typically categorized into ophthalmic, clinoid, and intracavernous segment aneurysms. Each subtype is associated with its own unique set of clinical features, risk of future hemorrhage, and indications and methods for safe and effective treatment.

Options for treatment of an individual harboring a paraclinoid aneurysm include observation only, direct or indirect surgical methods, and endovascular techniques. Direct surgical approaches include aneurysm clipping, aneurysm obliteration with sacrifice of the ICA, exploration and reinforcement, or aneurysm excision with primary repair of the parent artery. Indirect surgical approaches include proximal cervical ICA ligation or trapping, with or without a superficial temporal artery–middle cerebral artery (STA-MCA) anastomosis or an interposition saphenous vein graft to augment the distal circulation.[5,6] Endovascular methods utilize detachable balloons or coils to selectively obliterate the aneurysm or to occlude the ICA, sometimes in combination with a blood flow augmentation procedure.[7]

This chapter addresses clinoidal segment aneurysms; those arising from the ophthalmic and intracavernous segments are described elsewhere in this book. The pertinent paraclinoid anatomy, aneurysm classification, clinical features, and step-by-step description of direct aneurysm clipping are provided.

◆ Anatomy

The paraclinoid region is a complex anatomical arrangement of bony ridges, dural folds, vascular structures (ICA, ophthalmic artery, superior hypophyseal arteries, cavernous sinus, and superior orbital fissure veins), and nerves (optic, oculomotor, trochlear, abducens, trigeminal, sympathetic, and parasympathetic).

Osseous Relationships

The anterior clinoid process (ACP) is the anatomical landmark around which this region is defined (**Fig. 7–1**). The most medial extension of the lesser wing of the sphenoid, the ACP forms the roof of the superior orbital fissure (SOF) and the anterior cavernous sinus (CavSin), and borders the anterior and lateral walk of the ICA as the vessel leaves the CavSin to enter the subarachnoid space. The optic strut (OS) attaches to the inferomedial ACP surface and extends

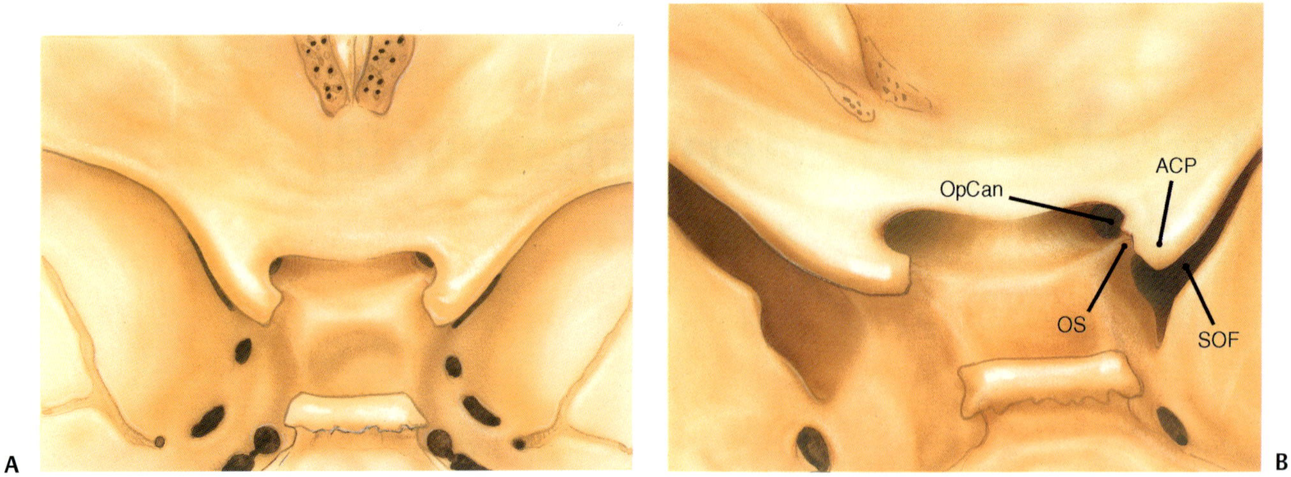

Figure 7–1 Paraclinoid osseous anatomy, **(A)** dorsal and **(B)** posterior oblique views. The anterior clinoid process (ACP) is the most medial extension of the lesser wing of the sphenoid. It forms the roof over the superior orbital fissure (SOF), an anterolateral margin to the cavernous sinus roof, and an anterior and lateral border to the clinoid segment of the internal carotid artery. The optic strut (OS) projects from the inferomedial ACP to the body of the sphenoid body. It separates the optic canal (OpCan) superomedially from the SOF inferolaterally.

to the body of the sphenoid bone, separating the optic canal superomedially from the SOF inferolaterally.

The CavSins are located lateral to the sella turcica and body of the sphenoid bone. Each CavSin extends from the SOF anteriorly to the apex of the petrous ridge posteriorly. The CavSin roof is defined anteriorly by the ACP and posteriorly by the posterior clinoid process. The remaining sinus boundaries are delineated by dural folds (see following section).[3]

Dural Relationships

Multiple dural folds (**Fig. 7–2**) attach at the ACP, including the anterior petroclinoid fold (extending from the petrous apex to the ACP), the interclinoid fold (extending from the posterior clinoid process to the ACP), and the falciform ligament. In conjunction with the medial tentorial edge, the diaphragma sella, and the dura overlying the middle fossa floor, these dural folds form the superior, medial, and lateral boundaries of the CavSin.

Two distinctly discernible dural membranes are formed from the superior and inferior periosteal reflections off the ACP—the dural ring (DR) and the carotid–oculomotor membrane (COM). The DR represents a portal through the superomedial dural continuation off the roof of the ACP that merges and blends with the diaphragma sella and optic canal floor. The ICA penetrates this plane of dura to enter the subarachnoid space. The periosteal attachments that extend to and encircle the ICA at this site (the DR) have an oblique orientation with a downward slope from anterior to posterior and lateral to medial. This downward slant of the thin, medial portion of the DR creates a small subarachnoid pocket medial to the ICA termed the carotid cave.

The COM is formed by the inferior and medial periosteal reflections off the ACP. The COM blankets and extends from the ICA medially to the oculomotor nerve laterally, beneath the plane of the ACP. This thin periosteal membrane fuses with the venous wall and marks the exit of the ICA from the venous lumen of the CavSin.[3]

Vascular Relationships

The ICA is classically divided into cervical, petrous, cavernous, and supraclinoid regions (**Fig. 7–2**). The ACP traditionally separates the cavernous (that portion of the ICA completely surrounded by the venous blood of the CavSin) from the ophthalmic segment of the supraclinoid region (the subarachnoid portion of the ICA).

1. ARTERIAL SEGMENTS
   The CavSin region of the ICA can be divided into five components: (1) posterior vertical segment, (2) posterior genu, (3) horizontal segment, (4) anterior genu, and (5) anterior vertical segment. The true cavernous segment (CavSeg) encompasses the first four of these divisions, all of which lie within the venous channels of the CavSin between the foramen lacerum and below the COM. True cavernous segment aneurysms are surrounded by venous blood in close proximity to cranial nerves III, IV, V, and VI and the ocular sympathetics.[10]

   The fifth division represents a transitional zone between the venous blood within the CavSin and the subarachnoid space, and is herein termed the clinoid segment (ClinSeg). The ClinSeg is that portion of the ICA lying medial to and below the ACP between the carotid–oculomotor membrane and the DR. This segment is neither within the venous lumen of the CavSin nor within the subarachnoid space, and essentially represents an "interdural" ICA segment.

   The ophthalmic segment (OphSeg) is the longest subarachnoid ICA segment. This segment begins at the DR as the ICA enters the subarachnoid space and ends at the origin of the posterior communicating artery. All

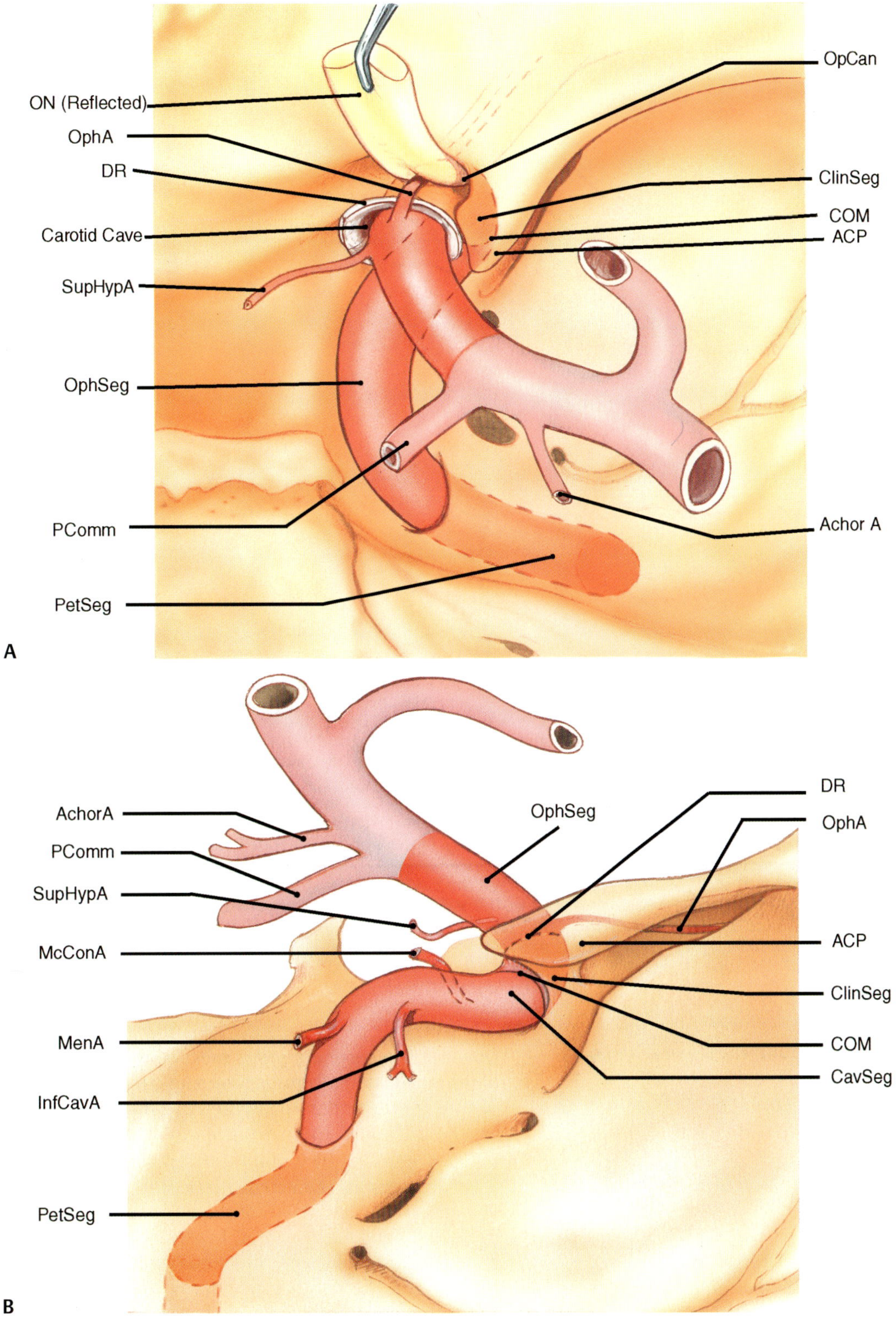

Figure 7–2 Paraclinoid osseous, dural, vascular, and neural anatomy. **(A)** Dorsal, **(B)** lateral, and

(Continued on page 120)

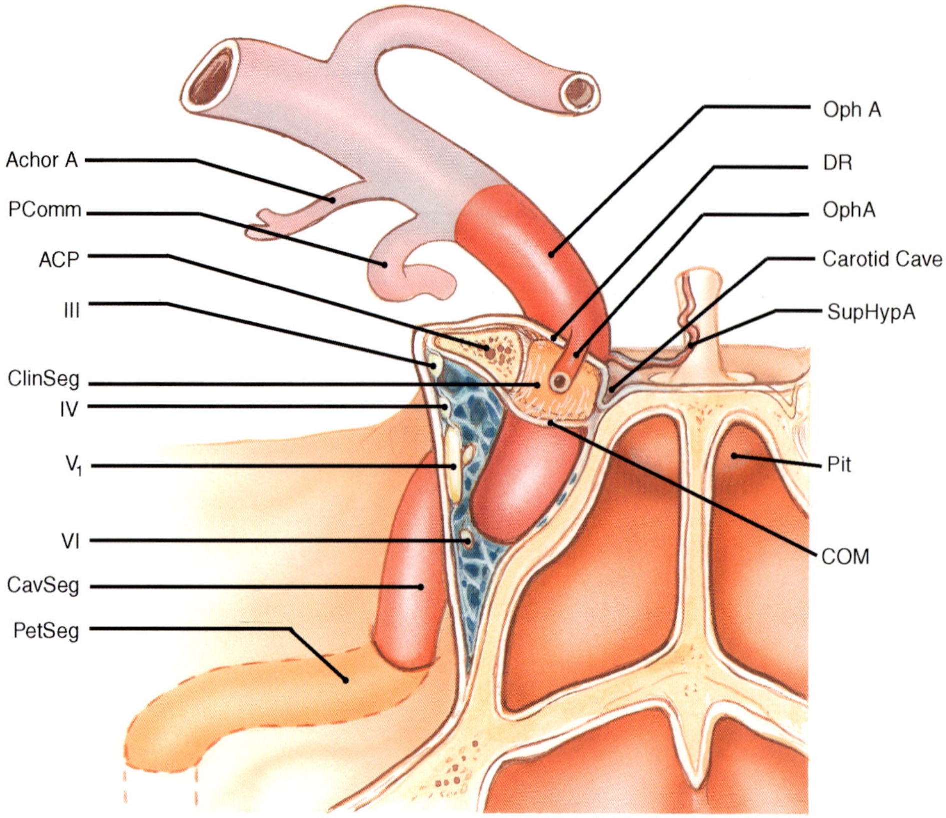

C

(*Continued*) **Figure 7–2 (C)** anteroposterior (AP) views. Note the three internal carotid artery (ICA) segments having proximity to the anterior clinoid process (ACP): cavernous segment (CavSeg), clinoid segment (ClinSeg), and ophthalmic segment (OphSeg). The CavSeg lies within the venous channels of the cavernous sinus (seen best on AP view), the ClinSeg has an interdural location between the dural ring (DR) and the carotid–oculomotor membrane (COM) (seen best on AP view), and the OphSeg is entirely subarachnoid. Also note the ICA bends: the prominent anterior bend (AntBend) and posterior bend (PostBend) (seen best on lateral view) and the more subtle medial bend (MedBend) (seen best on dorsal view). Also note the ICA branches: the ophthalmic artery (OphA) arises just past the DR and projects beneath the optic nerve (ON) as it travels to the orbit, the superior hypophyseal arteries (SupHypA) arise distal to the OphA from the medial OphSeg and supply the pituitary gland, the artery of the inferior cavernous sinus (InfCavA) arises from the inferolateral surface of the horizontal CavSeg to supply the cavernous sinus dura, and the meningohypophyseal artery (MenA) arises from the posterior genu of the CavSeg and splits into three branches. Finally, note the location of the oculomotor (III), trochlear (IV), first division of the trigeminal (V_1) nerves within the lateral sinus wall and the abducens nerve (VI) within the venous channels between the CavSeg and V_1. Care during ACP removal is critical because the oculomotor nerve exits the cavernous sinus just beneath the ACP (see AP view). PetSeg, petrous segment; PComm, posterior communicating artery; AchorA, anterior choroidal artery; Pit, pituitary gland.

OphSeg aneurysms originate within the subarachnoid space.

The cavernous, clinoidal, and ophthalmic ICA segments all have intimate involvement with the ACP, and lesions from each of these segments are often included whenever "paraclinoid" aneurysms are considered.[1–4] Only those arising from the clinoidal segment are discussed in this chapter.

2. BENDS AND BRANCHES

As noted by Rhoton,[8] aneurysm formation typically occurs along an arterial segment at two hemodynamic stress points—bends and branch sites. Two major bends and several prominent arterial branches along the proximal ICA predispose the paraclinoid region to aneurysm development. The first bend, seen best on a lateral projection angiogram, is a sharp, posteriorly projecting turn of the ICA as it ascends through the DR. This prominent bend places a superiorly directed hemodynamic force upon the dorsal wall of the ClinSeg and OphSeg. The second bend is most conspicuous on an anteroposterior (AP) projection angiogram, which reveals a gentle medial to lateral curve beginning at the anterior genu of the CavSeg and continuing as the artery approaches its terminal bifurcation.

Branch sites also contribute to turbulence and hemodynamic stress that may contribute to aneurysm formation. Two consistent arterial branches arise from the paraclinoid region, both of which typically arise from the OphSeg. The ophthalmic artery (OphA) is the most prominent and usually arises from the dorsomedial surface of the OphSeg to accompany the optic nerve through the optic canal to supply the retina and orbit. The superior hypophyseal artery(ies) (SupHypA) typically arise from the medial or inferomedial ICA surface just distal to the ophthalmic artery takeoff, along the medial to lateral ICA bend. This series of arterial perforators project medially and may supply portions of the superior aspect of the pituitary stalk and gland, the

CavSin dura, and the optic nerves and chiasm.[9] Occasionally, the ophthalmic and/or the superior hypophyseal arteries originate more proximally from the ClinSeg or CavSeg. In such cases, the OphA reaches the orbit through a foramen in the OS or by piercing the COM to enter the SOF, while the SupHypA may continue to supply the pituitary gland, CavSin dura, and optic nerve.

Neural Relationships

The oculomotor, trochlear, abducens, first and second divisions of the trigeminal, and sympathetic nerves are intimately associated with the paraclinoid region (**Fig. 7–2**). The oculomotor nerve (CN III) pierces the dura lateral to the posterior clinoid process and courses in the upper portion of the lateral wall of the CavSin. The nerve exits the sinus by passing just below the ACP to enter the SOF. Cognizance of this anatomical relationship is crucial to preserving ocular motility following the removal of the ACP when exposing the proximal ICA. The trochlear nerve (CN IV) enters the CavSin roof posterolateral to the oculomotor nerve and travels in the lateral sinus wall inferior to the oculomotor nerve. The first and second divisions of the trigeminal nerve (CN V_1, V_2) exit Meckel's cave to enter the lower portion of the lateral sinus wall and project anteriorly. The abducens nerve (CN VI) enters the CavSin through Dorello's canal, and courses within the venous plexus of the CavSin between the cavernous artery and the first division of the trigeminal nerve. Finally, sympathetic fiber bundles course along the surface of the cavernous carotid artery, passing to the abducens nerve and then to the trigeminal nerve.[3] Dissections of the ClinSeg can easily disturb these sympathetic fibers, leading to a mild postoperative ipsilateral ptosis or miosis.

Each of these nerves eventually passes through the SOF to enter the orbit. Aneurysms in this segment generally project away from these nerves traversing the CavSin because hemodynamic forces direct their growth superiorly toward the subarachnoid space or medially into the pituitary fossa.

Classification and Presentation

Aneurysms may originate anywhere along the cavernous carotid artery, but are particularly prevalent along the horizontal segment (**Fig. 7–3**).[5,6] Any hemorrhage risks attributed to CavSeg aneurysms (as high as 7% in some studies) are largely due to the inclusion of ClinSeg aneurysms within the series.[11] If one excludes ClinSeg, certain superiorly projecting posterior genu lesions and traumatic pseudoaneurysms from this analysis, the risk of subarachnoid hemorrhage from a true intracavernous aneurysm is virtually zero.[5,6,12–14] Because ClinSeg aneurysms are located interdurally, below the DR and subarachnoid space, the risk of hemorrhage associated with small lesions (< 1 cm) is extremely low. As the ClinSeg aneurysm enlarges and exceeds this size, however, it may erode through the dura adjacent to the DR and extend into the subarachnoid space, at which time they assume the same or greater hemorrhage risks as those of the

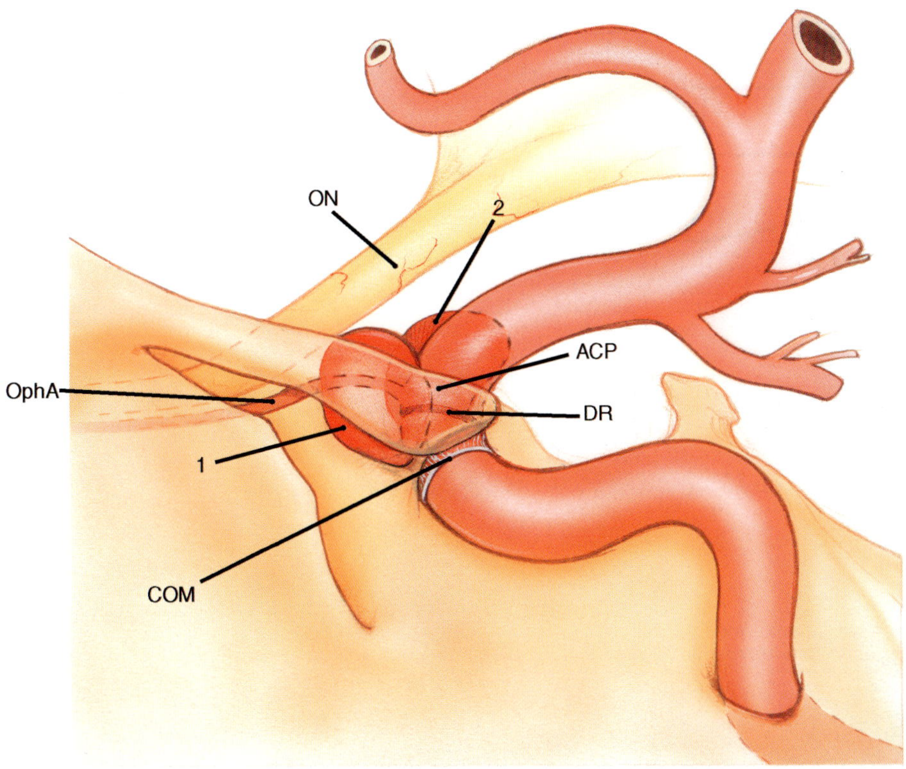

A

Figure 7–3 Clinoid segment aneurysm schematic. **(A)** Lateral view.

(*Continued on page 122*)

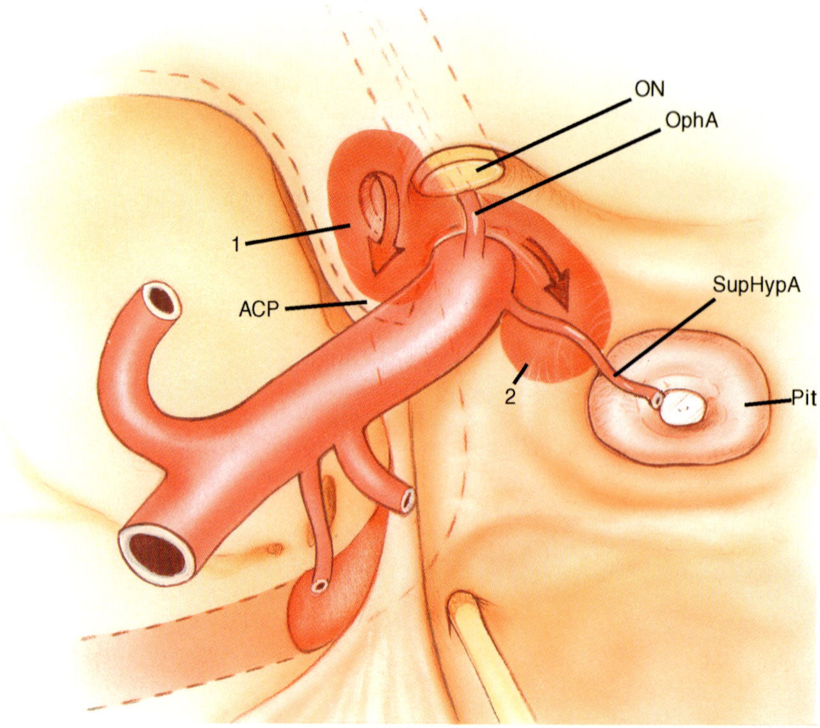

B

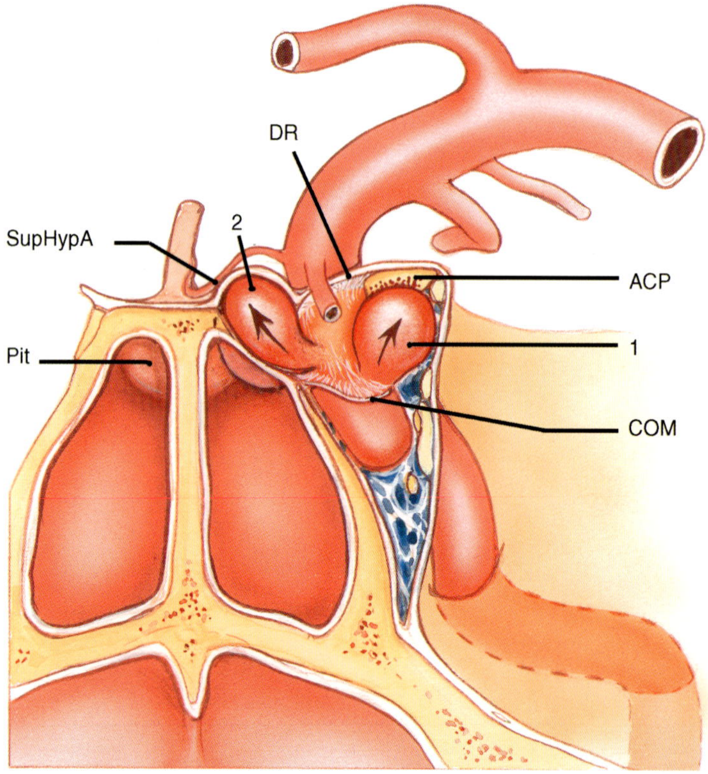

C

(Continued) **Figure 7–3** **(B)** Dorsal view. **(C)** Anteroposterior view. Aneurysm types (hatched areas): 1, anterolateral variant; 2, medial variant. ACP, anterior clinoid process; COM, carotid–oculomotor membrane; DR, dural ring; ON, optic nerve; OphA, ophthalmic artery; Pit, pituitary gland; SupHypA, superior hypophyseal artery.

OphSeg.[1,2,4] Headaches from ClinSeg aneurysms are infrequent, generally limited to the ipsilateral V_1 and retro-orbital regions, and are presumed due to pulsatile distortion of the dura overlying this segment. Much less commonly, ClinSeg lesions may produce facial numbness or diplopia, but a full-blown CavSin syndrome from these lesions is rare.

ClinSeg aneurysms are herein classified according to their site of origin and direction of projection, each influenced by the arterial bends and branches within the segment and any adjacent dural and osseous structures. This system allows for accurate diagnosis of the aneurysm type, offers prognostic information regarding propensity for subarachnoid hemorrhage or cranial nerve deficits, and helps direct the treatment plan into observation, endovascular intervention, or surgical obliteration arms. Two variants of this aneurysm subtype (and their clinical presentations) can be discerned.

1. *Anterolateral variant* This variant arises from the anterolateral surface of the ClinSeg as it obliquely ascends toward the DR medial to the ACP. The superiorly and slightly medially directed hemodynamic vector and the occasional presence of a proximal ophthalmic artery origin promote a superomedially projecting aneurysm that may on first glance mimic an ophthalmic artery OphSeg aneurysm. When small, the anterolateral variant may erode the OS and undersurface of the ACP to compress the ipsilateral optic nerve within the optic canal. Larger lesions may secondarily compress the visual system within the subarachnoid space after extension through the dura adjacent to the DR.
2. *Medial variant* This aneurysm variant extends from the medial surface of the ClinSeg and enlarges toward the sphenoid sinus and sella. The projection of these lesions arises from the more subtle, medially directed hemodynamic vector created as the ICA turns from lateral to medial to lateral during its ascent toward and through the DR. At least initially, this aneurysm type expands beneath the diaphragma sella, but differentiation from a superior hypophyseal artery aneurysm may prove difficult. Visual loss from this aneurysm type does not occur with small lesions, but patterns of visual loss resembling those of pituitary tumors may occur with large or giant lesions. Rarely, rupture within the gland itself may simulate pituitary apoplexy, or slow gradual enlargement may cause hypopituitarism.

◆ Indications for Intervention

With proper operative exposure and a firm grasp of the paraclinoid osseous, dural, vascular, and neural anatomy, direct surgical obliteration of most ClinSeg aneurysms can be accomplished with low brain or cranial nerve morbidity. Surgical treatment requires considerable experience and a broad exposure of the skull base and clinoidal segment, including extensive removal of the ACP and OS. Exposure of the cervical ICA is often required to assure proximal control.

The narrow constraints of these aneurysms' origins between the DR and COM (their neck is often quite small, particularly the medial variant) makes many of these lesions ideal candidates for attempted endovascular obliteration. Indirect surgical methods [i.e., proximal ICA or (common carotid arteryl) CCA ligation] may not provide optimal visual system decompression, however, and complete aneurysm thrombosis is not assured. In addition, the risk of hemispheric stroke following ICA sacrifice may be high. Proximal ICA ligation should be considered as a last alternative and is usually done in combination with simultaneous cerebral blood flow augmentation.

Small (< 1 cm) asymptomatic ClinSeg aneurysms carry a very low risk of subarachnoid hemorrhage, and isolated lesions should generally be treated conservatively with periodic follow-up imaging. Surgery or endovascular methods should be strongly considered for small, symptomatic ClinSeg aneurysms presenting with visual loss or focal headaches. If the ACP is removed to treat another aneurysm in the region (i.e., OphSeg), small asymptomatic ClinSeg lesions should be clipped during the same exposure because their dural protection has now been breached.

Most large (1.0–2.4 cm) or giant (2.5 cm) ClinSeg aneurysms have enlarged sufficiently to enter the subarachnoid space. Because the risk of hemorrhage now becomes significant, intervention should be considered even if the offending lesion is asymptomatic. Large or giant symptomatic unruptured and all ruptured ClinSeg aneurysms should be aggressively managed by an experienced cerebrovascular neurosurgeon.

◆ Preoperative Preparation

The preoperative management of patients harboring paraclinoid aneurysms is very similar to that of patients harboring aneurysms at other sites. Patients with unruptured paraclinoid aneurysms are evaluated and treated in an elective manner unless there is a rapid progression of compressive symptoms. The preoperative neurological assessment should place special emphasis on the extraocular movements, facial sensation, visual field/visual acuity, and endocrine status. Patients presenting with epistaxis or subarachnoid hemorrhage are admitted to the intensive care unit and treated in the same manner as those with ruptured aneurysms at other locations. The most appropriate method of treatment is selected after the patient is stabilized and the radiographic workup is complete, which may include a preoperative trial balloon occlusion test.

Imaging studies are extremely helpful in delineating ClinSeg aneurysms, in distinguishing them from OphSeg lesions, and in planning any required intervention.

Computed Tomography

Computed tomographic (CT) scan is often the initial imaging study obtained in patients with neurological complaints and is the best test for diagnosing subarachnoid hemorrhage. A ruptured ClinSeg aneurysm typically produces hemorrhage in the chiasmatic and parasellar cisterns. Due to the aneurysm's somewhat medial extension, any extension into the sylvian fissure is often worse opposite the aneurysm's origin.[1,15]

CT can also reveal thrombus or calcification within the aneurysm neck or fundus, indicating a more complicated lesion that will likely prove more difficult to obliterate and will dictate the need for prolonged proximal temporary clipping. Thin-section CT scanning with bone windows may also disclose other ACP anomalies such as pneumatization of the OS and ACP, ossification of the interclinoidal fold, or a caroticoclinoidal foramen. As the anterolateral variant enlarges, pressure on the OS and ACP may lead to erosion often demonstrable on CT, an abnormality not seen with typical OphSeg ophthalmic artery aneurysms. This finding confirms the diagnosis of a ClinSeg aneurysm, mandates careful intradural removal of the ACP and OS, and encourages preliminary cervical carotid exposure. Because they expand within the pituitary fossa below the diaphragma sella, giant medial variant ClinSeg aneurysms can expand the sella turcica in a pattern suggestive of a pituitary adenoma.

Magnetic Resonance Imaging

Magnetic resonance imaging (MRI) provides excellent anatomical detail that may help define the aneurysm's relationship to various soft tissue structures such as the visual apparatus and the pituitary gland. It is less useful than CT for delineating bony anatomy.

Angiography

Four-vessel transfemoral cerebral arteriogram is required as the primary study to determine the presence and type of all paraclinoid region aneurysms and to clarify treatment options. The cervical carotid artery should be carefully examined to determine if atherosclerotic plaques are present that would make proximal temporary clamping hazardous. The ipsilateral superficial temporal artery (STA) should be assessed for its applicability as a bypass conduit. An awake trial balloon occlusion test augmented with induced hypotension or cerebral blood flow studies (single-photon emission CT or xenon CT) should be considered in complex lesions, which could require longer temporary or permanent ICA ligation.

ClinSeg aneurysms are low-lying lesions that on lateral views invariably appear as a "double density" overlying the anterior vertical or proximal ophthalmic segments. The anterolateral variant often has a similar appearance to an ophthalmic artery OphSeg aneurysm. Close inspection of the study will usually reveal the subtle double density of the neck on the anterolateral ICA wall arising in proximity to the ophthalmic artery origin. The two aneurysm types can usually be easily differentiated on an anteroposterior view because the anterolateral ClinSeg variant projects lateral to the OphSeg toward the ACP, whereas the ophthalmic artery aneurysm projects superiorly and medially from the OphSeg. Larger aneurysms also often demonstrate a "waist," marking the point where the aneurysm has penetrated the dura to enter the subarachnoid space.

Medial ClinSeg variant aneurysms are often difficult to discern from superior hypophyseal artery or "carotid cave" aneurysms, especially when small, because each type may project medially and somewhat inferiorly. Large or giant medial variant ClinSeg aneurysms generally have surprisingly small necks, secondary to the confines of their origins between the COM and the DR (in contrast to the broad neck typically seen in superior hypophyseal artery aneurysms).

◆ Surgical Technique

Anesthesia

As with most aneurysm operations, prophylactic antibiotics, steroids, and mild hypothermia are routinely used throughout the procedure. An indwelling radial arterial line is used to monitor and maintain the desired blood pressure during the surgery. Continuous evoked potential and electroencephalographic (EEG) monitoring is also standard protocol. Typical brain relaxation techniques include modest $PaCO_2$ reduction and wide sylvian fissure splitting with generous cerebrospinal fluid (CSF) drainage. Spinal drainage is not routinely used. In patients presenting with a subarachnoid hemorrhage, mannitol is administered 20 minutes prior to dural opening to aid in brain relaxation and for its potential cerebral protectant effects. In cases where temporary ICA clamping is necessary, mild hypertension is induced, and intravenous barbiturates are titrated to EEG burst suppression.

Positioning

The patient is placed on the operating table in the supine position with a shoulder roll underneath the ipsilateral shoulder. The head is fixed in a radiolucent rigid fixation system (allowing for intraoperative angiography if needed), turned 45 degrees toward the contralateral side, and elevated above the heart (promoting venous drainage). The vertex is lowered so the maxilla is the highest bony landmark, thereby allowing gravity to gently retract the frontal and temporal lobes.

Cervical Internal Carotid Artery Exposure

The ipsilateral cervical carotid is prepped and sterilely draped into the operative field to allow access for proximal ICA control or for a saphenous vein bypass as needed. An incision is marked along the anterior margin of the sternocleidomastoid muscle overlying the carotid bifurcation. The cervical ICA is exposed for all giant, complicated, or ruptured ClinSeg aneurysms, and for simple unruptured ClinSeg aneurysms, the threshold for opening the neck should be low.

Scalp Flap and Craniotomy

The scalp incision extends from the midline to the zygoma just behind the hairline. Care should be taken to spare the major trunk of the STA because it may be needed for a bypass later in the procedure. A Yasargil-type temporalis muscle flap,[16] sparing the frontalis nerve, is used to allow a lower basal exposure to these proximal ICA lesions. A frontotemporal free bone flap is constructed and elevated, exposing low enough anteriorly to access 2 to 3 cm of the frontal fossa floor. Extensive extradural removal of the sphenoid ridge allows exposure of the orbital roof, the orbital lateral wall, and the anterior aspect of the middle cranial fossa to the SOF.

Anterior Clinoid Process Removal

Removal of the ACP and OS is mandatory for safe obliteration of ClinSeg aneurysms (**Fig. 7–4**). Anterolateral variant ClinSeg aneurysms have an intimate association with the ACP, and are often adherent to or eroding through this bony

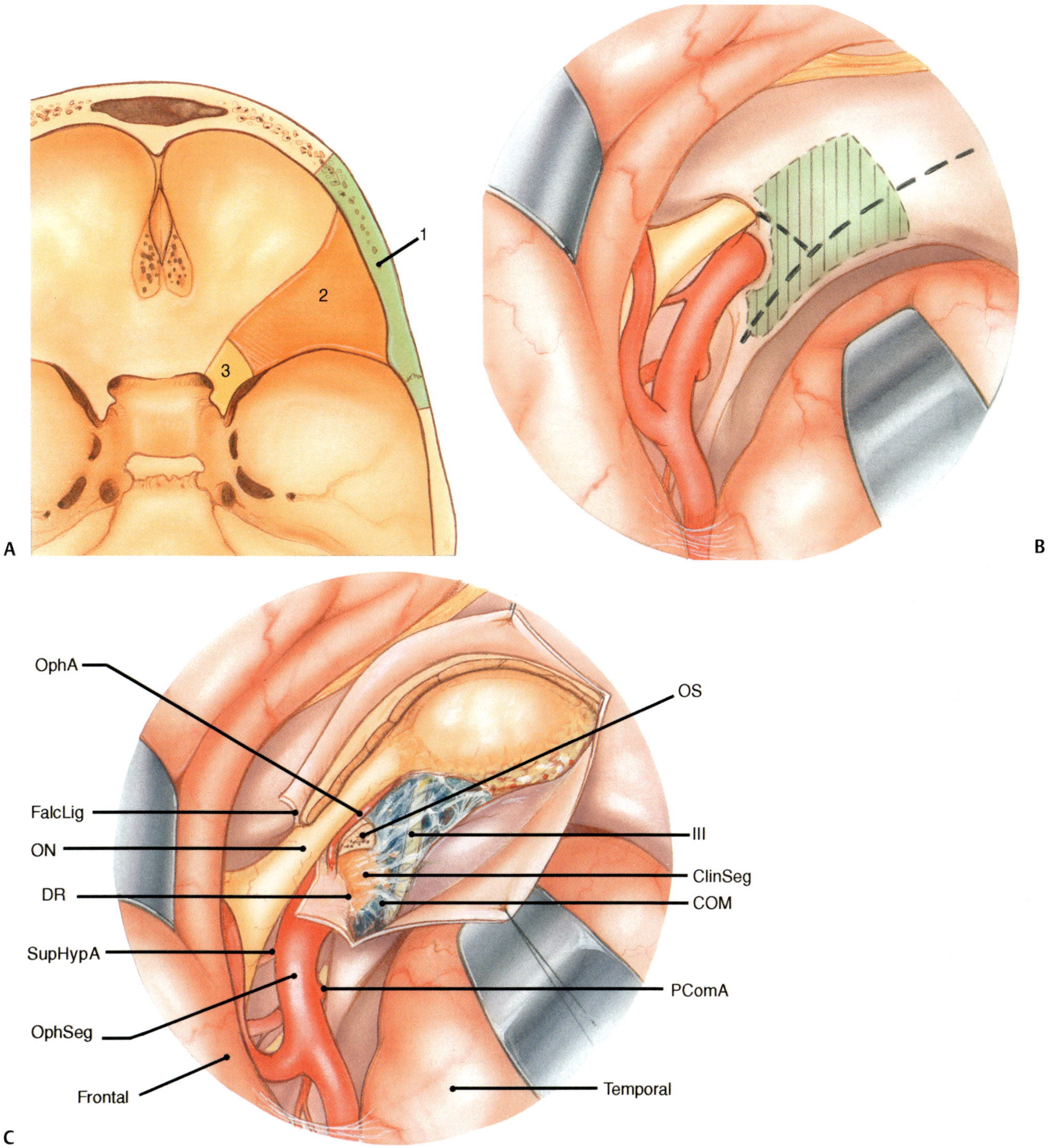

Figure 7–4 The bony resection for paraclinoid aneurysm surgery. **(A)** The extradural bone removal including the frontotemporal craniotomy (hatched area #1) and the sphenoid ridge, posterior orbital roof, and medial floor of the superior orbital fissure (SOF) (hatched area #2). The removal of the remaining medial sphenoid wing and anterior clinoid process (ACP) (#3) is generally performed intradurally to reduce the risk of operative aneurysm rupture. **(B)** The dural incisions for intradural ACP removal. The dashed lines represent the dural incision along the medial sphenoid wing and ACP. An extension of this incision is carried through the falciform ligament and optic nerve (ON) ensheathment to decompress and mobilize the ON. **(C)** Exposure following intradural ACP removal and optic strut (OS) drilling. This is the standard exposure for clinoid segment (ClinSeg) aneurysm clipping with excellent visualization of the ClinSeg portion of the internal carotid artery (ICA).

(*Continued on page 126*)

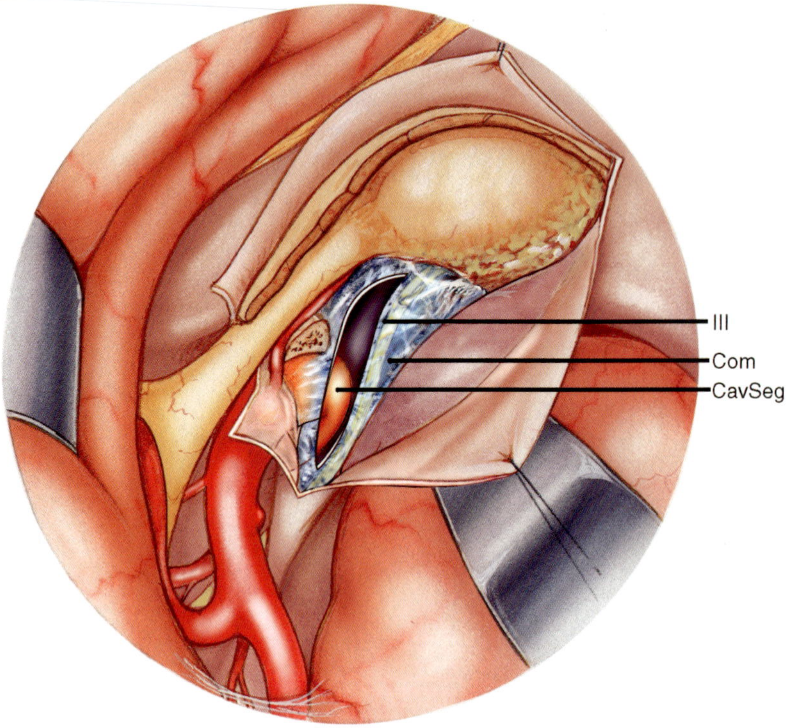

D

(*Continued*) **Figure 7–4** **(D)** Exposure following entry into the cavernous sinus. Opening of the carotid–oculomotor membrane (COM) between the ClinSeg and ON (III) allows excellent exposure to the anterior genu of the cavernous segment (CavSeg) of the internal carotid artery. This exposure allows for clipping of most anterior genu CavSeg aneurysms. OphA, ophthalmic artery; SupHypA, superior hypophyseal artery; PcomA, posterior communicating artery; DR, dural ring; FalcLig, falciform ligament; OphSeg, ophthalmic segment; Temporal, temporal lobe; Frontal, frontal lobe.

landmark. This association makes extradural removal of the ACP hazardous, and we routinely approach this portion of the procedure intradurally.

The dura is opened in a curvilinear fashion based on the sphenoid ridge, and the sylvian fissure is widely split from lateral to medial to expose the middle cerebral and internal carotid arteries down to the ACP. Once adequate brain relaxation is obtained, a 3 to 4 cm longitudinal dural incision is from the tip of the ACP laterally, well past the resected edge of the medial sphenoid ridge. The dura is stripped free from the underlying bone and tacked back with stay sutures. An additional relaxing incision is made through the falciform ligament, a crucial step that decompresses and mobilizes the optic nerve and allows identification of the ophthalmic artery. Utilizing a small, high-speed diamond drill, the ACP and the superior and lateral bony walls of the optic canal are carefully thinned and removed while simultaneously viewing the ICA and aneurysm. Finally, the OS is drilled away down to the body of the sphenoid bone to expose the medial surface of the ClinSeg.

Aneurysm Dissection and Clipping

Because these aneurysms are often burrowed into the ACP and adherent to adjacent dura and the CavSin, the decision whether to gain proximal control at the cervical ICA is made early in the dissection. Great care is taken to extensively remove the ACP and OS, followed by circumferential section of the DR to allow complete mobilization of the ICA and viewing of the entire clinoidal segment of the parent vessel. Sectioning the ring also allows for unimpeded clip blade passage from the proximal OphSeg to the distal CavSeg, thereby spanning the entire ClinSeg. Using these preparations, most premature aneurysm ruptures can be avoided.

The anterolateral variant lies on the anterolateral surface of the ClinSeg. To eliminate the proximal neck, the clip blades must be passed proximal to the COM, most frequently using a gently curved or side-angled clip that runs parallel to the ICA (**Fig. 7–5**). Opening the COM and gentle packing of the CavSin lumen with Gelfoam or Surgicel will achieve the desired meticulous hemostasis and gently displace the cranial nerves away from the plane of the advancing clip blade. The medial variant projects beneath the diaphragma sella into the pituitary fossa. Circumferential section of the DR allows placement of a fenestrated clip whose blades run parallel to the curvature of the ClinSeg medial wall (**Fig. 7–6**). Care must be taken to spare the ophthalmic and any superior hypophyseal or other perforating vessels that arise from either the ClinSeg or the OphSeg.

Closure

Following apparently successful clipping, it may be difficult to determine ICA patency with certainty through direct inspection alone. An intraoperative angiogram through a direct common carotid artery puncture (if the cervical

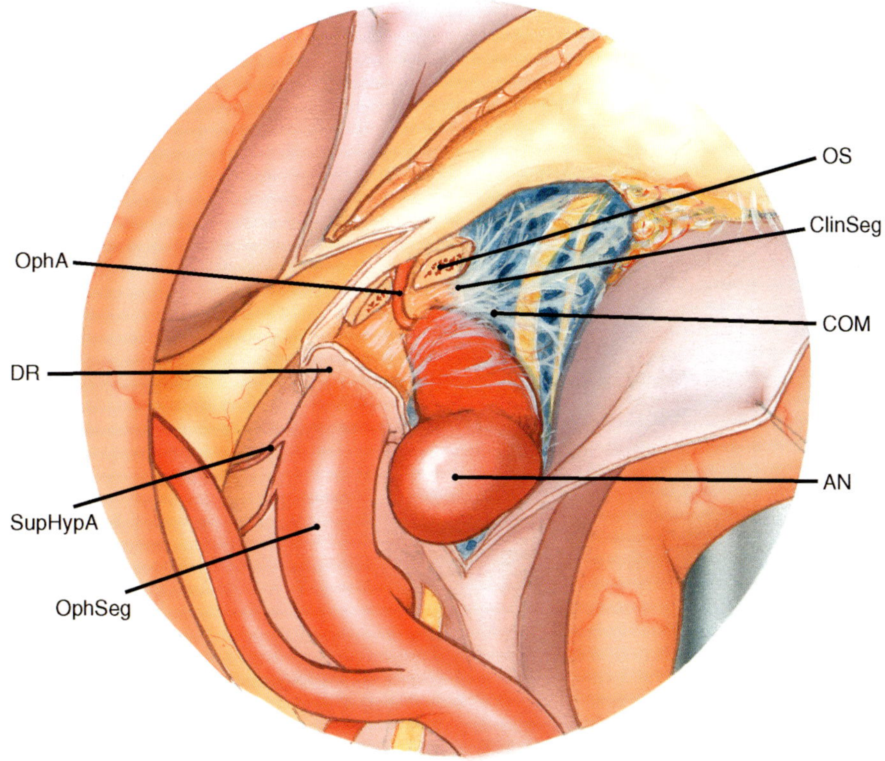

A

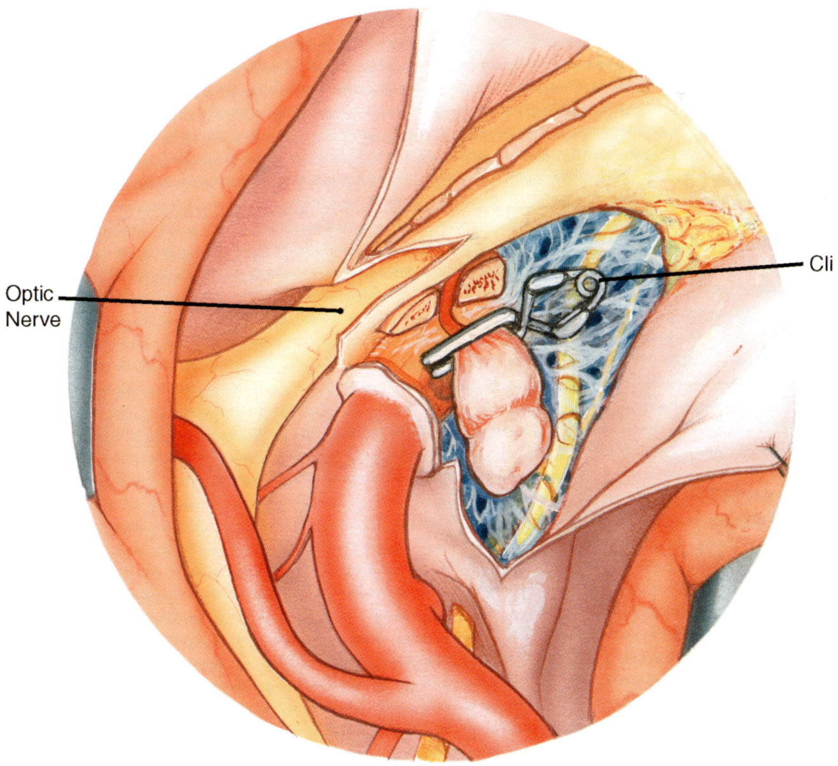

B

Figure 7–5 Clinoid segment (ClinSeg) aneurysm, anterolateral variant. **(A)** Operative view. The anterior clinoid process (ACP) has been carefully removed intradurally and the optic strut (OS) drilled to expose the ClinSeg of the internal carotid artery (ICA). The aneurysm originates from the ClinSeg, proximal to the dural ring (DR) but distal to the carotid–oculomotor membrane (COM), and projects from the lateral ICA superiorly toward the original location of the ACP. Note the constriction of the aneurysm at the point it entered the subarachnoid space. **(B)** A gently curved aneurysm clip was placed along the long axis of the ICA, paralleling the curve of the ICA. After adequate clip placement is assured, the aneurysm is aspirated and the ICA directly inspected for patency.

(Continued on page 128)

C

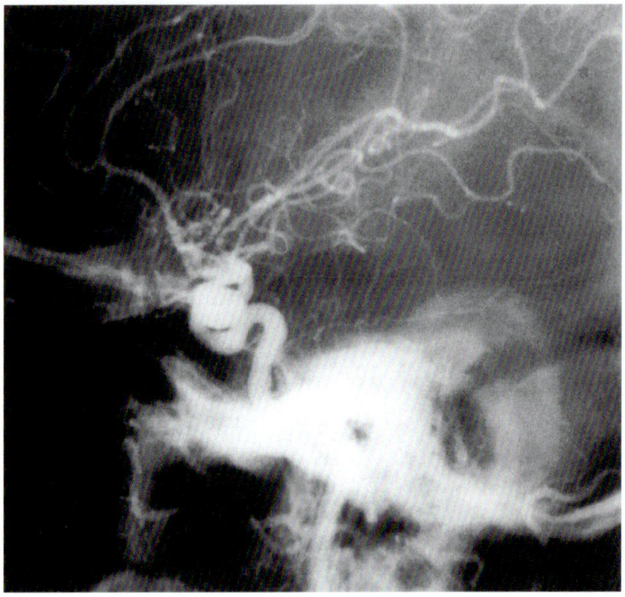

(*Continued*) **Figure 7–5** **(C)** Lateral angiogram. Note the superiorly projecting aneurysm originating along the ClinSeg proximal to the ophthalmic artery (OphA) and distal to the anterior genu of the cavernous segment (CavSeg) of the ICA. Note the large aneurysm's extension into the subarachnoid space. The direct operative approach should include cervical ICA exposure for proximal control and intradural removal of the ACP and OS.

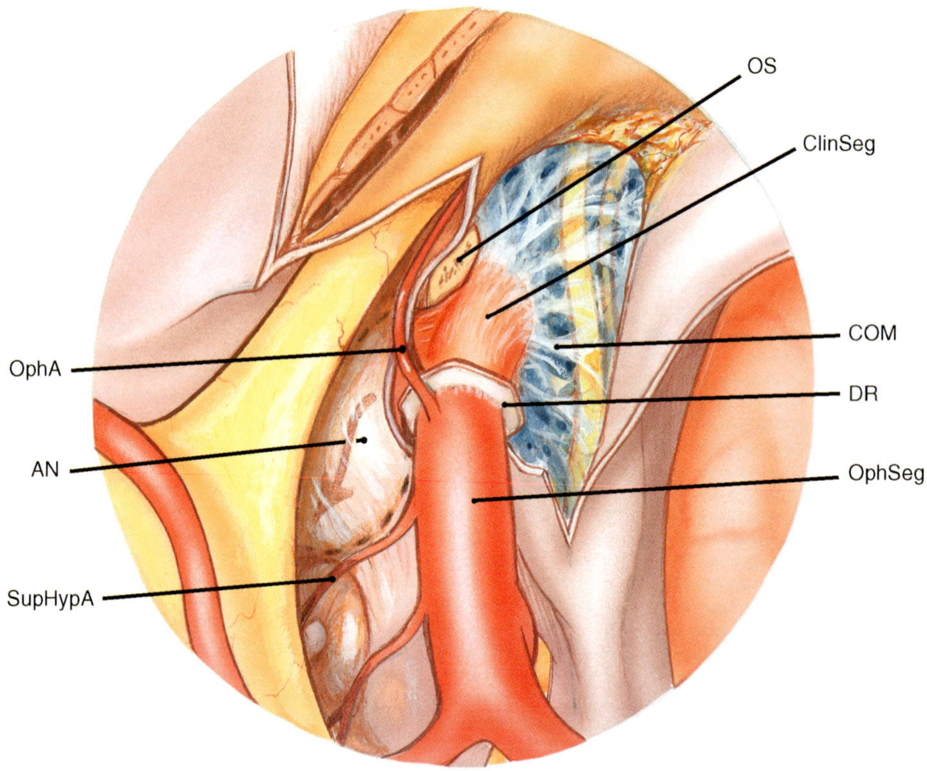

A

Figure 7–6 Clinoid segment (ClinSeg) aneurysm, medial variant. **(A)** Operative view. Note the aneurysm's origin from the medial aspect of the ClinSeg and its projection into the pituitary fossa beneath the diaphragma sella. Also note the close relationship of the aneurysm neck to the optic strut (OS).

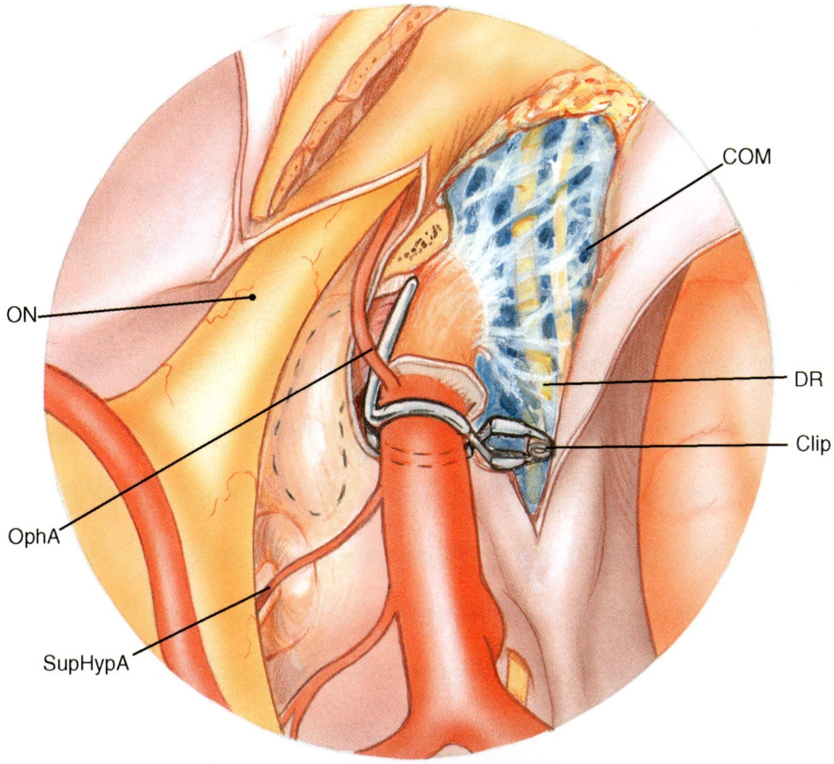

B

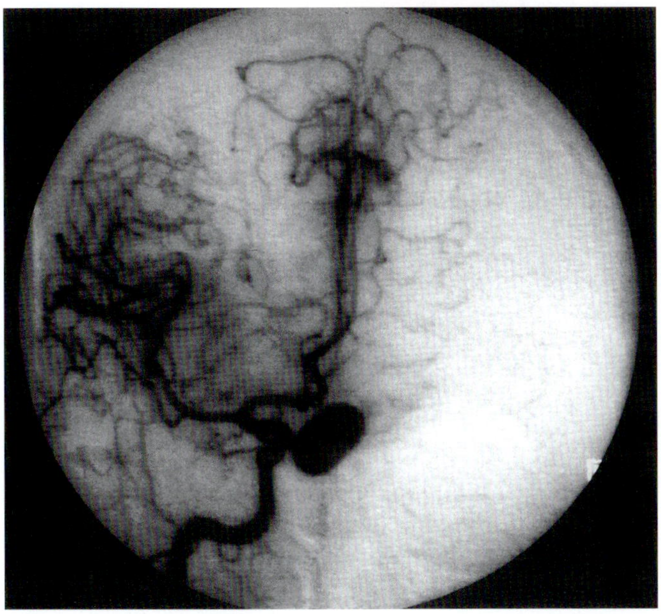

C

(*Continued*) **Figure 7–6** **(B)** The dural ring (DR) is sectioned circumferentially, allowing improved medial exposure and permitting the clip blades access to the ClinSeg. A fenestrated clip is placed parallel to the ICA with the tips abutting or extending past the carotid–oculomotor membrane (COM), taking care to spare the ophthalmic and superior hypophyseal arteries (OphA and SupHypA). The aneurysm is then aspirated, and internal carotid artery (ICA) and perforator patency is assured. **(C)** Anteroposterior angiogram. The medial variant originates from the medial ICA convexity, projects below the diaphragma sella, and enlarges within the sella in direct continuity with the pituitary gland. AN, aneurysm; OphSeg, ophthalmic segment.

carotid is already exposed) or through a preoperatively placed transfemoral catheter is invaluable in these circumstances. Once ICA patency is assured, dural closure begins. First, any communication between the OS and the sphenoid sinus is identified and sealed with muscle, Gelfoam, and methylmethacrylate. The dural leaves that covered the medial sphenoid wing are then closed primarily, followed by a watertight closure of the more superficial dural opening. Thereafter, the bone flap is returned and secured, the temporalis muscle reapproximated, a subgaleal drain placed, and the skin closed.

◆ Postoperative Care

The postoperative care for ClinSeg aneurysm patients follows the same guidelines for aneurysm patients in general. If the aneurysm was unruptured, the patient generally has a 1-day ICU stay followed by early mobilization and normalization of diet and medications. If the patient suffered a subarachnoid hemorrhage, aggressive hydration and monitoring for signs of vasospasm are critical during the window of risk. The delayed development of hydrocephalus, CSF leak through the ispilateral nostril, and subtle early signs of parent vessel stenosis or occlusion must be particularly closely monitored.

◆ Complications

Complications specific to paraclinoid aneurysms revolve around the structures encountered during the procedure. Compromise or occlusion of the ICA may occur or become evident early in the postoperative period, and any hemibody neurological deficits should be emergently addressed with CT scan and angiography. This complication is more frequently encountered in patients with large or giant calcified or partially thrombosed lesions and should generally be managed with emergent reexploration and clip adjustment. A low threshold for intraoperative angiography is the best route to avoiding this complication.

Postoperative visual deterioration is a potential complication in all paraclinoid aneurysm patients, especially in those with previous visual deficits. Intraoperative optic nerve manipulation or perforator compromise can lead to immediate or delayed optic nerve dysfunction. If intraoperative events do not adequately explain a postoperative visual deficit, reexploration should be entertained because the blood supply to the optic nerve or chiasm is likely embarrassed by the clip. Other cranial nerve deficits (oculomotor and abducens most commonly) are also potential complications and generally result from surgical trauma during ACP removal, clip blade advancement, excessive cranial nerve manipulation during dissection, or overzealous sinus packing. These deficits are usually partial and transient and are best avoided by careful bony removal and minimal dissection and retraction of the cranial nerves and their blood supply.

◆ Conclusion

The unique location of ClinSeg aneurysms dictates a more conservative approach to most lesions. Those aneurysms having a clear or likely communication with the subarachnoid space or those causing compressive symptoms or hemorrhage should be treated. The majority of ClinSeg aneurysms can be surgically obliterated with ICA preservation through a standard pterional craniotomy with extensive extradural sphenoid ridge resection and intradural ACP and OS removal. Endovascular techniques may be quite useful for some lesions, particularly those small aneurysms with narrow necks, and may also be used in combination with surgical intervention for more complicated lesions. Those lesions not amenable to direct surgical obliteration may be treated with proximal ICA ligation with or without cerebral blood flow augmentation, based on their trial balloon-occlusion test and other clinical features of the lesion in question.

References

1. Day AL. Aneurysms of the ophthalmic segment: a clinical and anatomic analysis. J Neurosurg 1990;72:677–691
2. Day AL, Masson RL, Knego RS. Surgical management of aneurysms and fistulas involving the cavernous sinus. In: Schmidek HH, Sweet WH, eds. Operative Neurosurgical Techniques. Philadelphia: WB Saunders; 1995:975–984
3. Inoue T, Rhoton AL, Theele D, et al. Surgical approaches to the cavernous sinus: a microsurgical study. Neurosurgery 1990;26:903–932
4. Cawley CM, Zipfel GJ, Day AL. Surgical treatment of paraclinoid and ophthalmic aneurysms. Neurosurg Clin N Am 1998;9:765–783
5. Al-Rhodan NRF, Piepgras DG, Sundt TM, et al. The microsurgical management of cavernous sinus aneurysms [abstract]. J Neurosurg 1991;75:170
6. Al-Rhodan N, Piepgras DG. Aneurysms within the cavernous sinus and transitional cavernous aneurysms. In: Wilkens RH, Rengachary SS, eds. Neurosurgery. New York: McGraw-Hill; 1996:2283–2289
7. Higashida RT, Halbach VV, Dowd C, et al. Endovascular detachable balloon embolization therapy of cavernous carotid artery aneurysms: results in 87 cases. J Neurosurg 1990;72:857–863
8. Rhoton AL Jr. Anatomy of saccular aneurysms. Surg Neurol 1980;43:59–66
9. McConnell EM. The arterial blood supply of the human hypophysis cerebri. Anat Rec 1953;115:175–203
10. Barr HWK, Blackwood W, Meadows SP. Intracavernous carotid aneurysm: a clinical pathological report. Brain 1971;94:607–622
11. Linskey ME, Sekhar LN, Hirsch W, et al. Aneurysms of the intracavernous carotid artery: clinical presentation, radiographic features, and pathogenesis. Neurosurgery 1990;26:71–79
12. Kupersmith MJ, Hurst R, Berenstein A, et al. The benign course of cavernous carotid artery aneurysms. J Neurosurg 1992;77:690–693
13. Ding MX. Traumatic aneurysm of the intracavernous part of the internal carotid artery presenting with epistaxis: case report. Surg Neurol 1988;30:65–67
14. McCormick WF, Beals JD. Severe epistaxis caused by ruptured aneurysm of the internal carotid artery. J Neurosurg 1964;21:678–686
15. Nishio S, Matsushima T, Fukui M, et al. Microsurgical anatomy around the origin of the ophthalmic artery with reference to contralateral pterional surgical approach to the carotid-ophthalmic aneurysm. Acta Neurochir (Wien) 1985;76:82–89
16. Yasargil MG, Gasser JC, Hodosh RM, et al. Carotid-ophthalmic aneurysms: direct microsurgical approach. Surg Neurol 1977;8:155–165

8

Middle Cerebral Artery Aneurysms

Michael R. Chicoine and Ralph G. Dacey Jr.

Middle cerebral artery (MCA) aneurysms constitute 20 to 30% of all intracranial berry aneurysms, occur at the MCA bifurcation in ~80%,[1,2] and are bilateral in 18 to 25% of cases.[3,4] MCA aneurysms are also the most common type in familial cases of cerebral aneurysms (47%).[5]

◆ Anatomy

The MCA and anterior cerebral artery (ACA) are the two branches at the termination of the internal carotid artery (ICA), the MCA being the larger of the two. The initial segment of the MCA (M1) begins at the ICA bifurcation in the proximal sylvian fissure and courses distally in the fissure deep to the lateral sphenoid wing. The M1 segment typically bifurcates into the M2 segment, which has a superior and an inferior trunk.[8,9] There are two main groups of branches from the M1 segment: (1) the superior lateral or temporal group and (2) the inferior medial or lenticulostriate group (**Fig. 8–1**).[8] The superior lateral group consists of the uncal, polar temporal, and anterior temporal arteries. Many variations of these arteries are described, including a single origin for the polar temporal, and anterior temporal arteries, and in 70% the uncal artery arises from the ICA.[8] The lenticulostriate group consists of two to 15 branches, which supply subcortical areas, and most commonly have a single origin but may have multiple origins.[10] The M1 segment typically bifurcates into two M2 branches but may have three or four branches, resulting in a so-called trifurcation or quadrification. More uncommon variants of the cerebral vasculature include the accessory MCA arising from the ACA.[8,11]

◆ Indications

Indications for treatment of MCA aneurysms can broadly be divided into (1) hemorrhage and (2) mass effect. Patients with MCA aneurysms most commonly (90%) present with subarachnoid hemorrhage[3] but may also have intraparenchymal, intraventricular, or subdural hemorrhages. Intraparenchymal hemorrhage occurs in up to 40% of patients with rupture of an MCA aneurysm as opposed to 10% of patients with other aneurysms.[3] Hemorrhage is an indication for early surgery. In the event of a large intraparenchymal or subdural hematoma, immediate surgery may be indicated, and angiography may have to be postponed until after evacuation of the hematoma. Intraoperative angiography in this situation may be appropriate to identify the aneurysm after the mass effect of the hemorrhage has been relieved if the anatomy of the aneurysm is not readily apparent by microsurgical dissection.

Large or giant MCA aneurysms can present with mass effect upon the frontal or temporal lobes, resulting in headaches, seizures, or other symptoms of neurological dysfunction. Smaller unruptured aneurysms may be incidental findings discovered in the workup of other diseases, including cervical carotid artery artherosclerotic disease, or any of a wide variety of intracranial pathologies. Because of the high rate of fatality from rupture of the aneurysms, surgical management has generally been advocated, particularly for aneurysms that have previously ruptured. Some newer data suggest that perhaps smaller aneurysms (< 1 cm in diameter) carry a reduced risk of hemorrhage if they have not previously ruptured and are not associated with other ruptured aneurysms.[12]

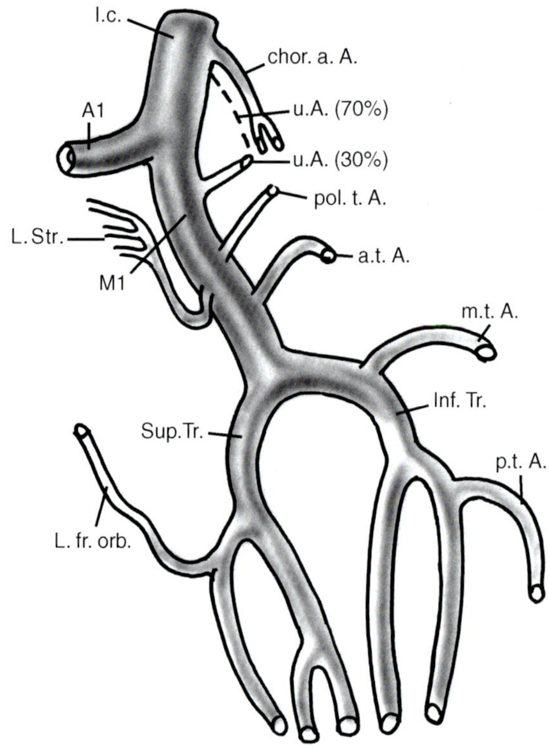

Figure 8–1 Typical origin and branching pattern of the middle cerebral artery (MCA); note many variations described in text. A1, first segment of anterior cerebral artery; i.c., internal carotid artery; M1, first segment of MCA; chor.a.A, anterior choroidal artery; u.A., uncal artery; pol. t. A, polar temporal artery; a.t.A., anterior temporal artery; Sup.Tr., superior trunk; Inf.Tr.; inferior trunk; p.t.A., posterior temporal artery; L.str., lateral striate arteries; m.t.A., middle temporal artery; L.fr.orb., lateral orbitofrontal artery. (From Yasargil MG. Microneurosurgery. Vol 1. Permission request submitted.)

The current gold standard for treatment of MCA aneurysms is surgery, although in certain situations, other therapies may be indicated. The endovascular technique of Guglielmi detachable coils (GDCs) is becoming a more viable technique for many aneurysms.[13–15] The utility of the GDC technique for these aneurysms remains limited because of the breadth of the aneurysm neck and complex relationship to the distal parent artery branches in the majority of MCA bifurcation aneurysms. External carotid to ICA bypass may be indicated for some larger and more complicated MCA aneurysms.[16]

◆ Preparation

Preoperative studies obtained in preparation for clipping of MCA aneurysms include computed tomographic (CT) scan of the head, as well as four-vessel cerebral angiography (**Fig. 8–2**). We do not feel that, at this point, magnetic resonance angiography (MRA) provides an adequate substitute to conventional angiography. In some cases, in particular in giant aneurysms or aneurysms in which there is thought to be a large thrombosed component, preoperative magnetic resonance imaging (MRI) may also be useful. The CT scan identifies the location of subarachnoid hemorrhage within the cisterns, evidence of calcification of the aneurysm wall, as well as the presence of hydrocephalus, cerebral infarcts, or other associated findings. In the case of multiple aneurysms, an attempt is made to identify which aneurysm is the source of hemorrhage based upon the distribution of subarachnoid blood in the cisterns. Additionally, preoperative CT scanning identifies intraparenchymal or subdural hematomas that may need to be addressed at the time of surgery.

A

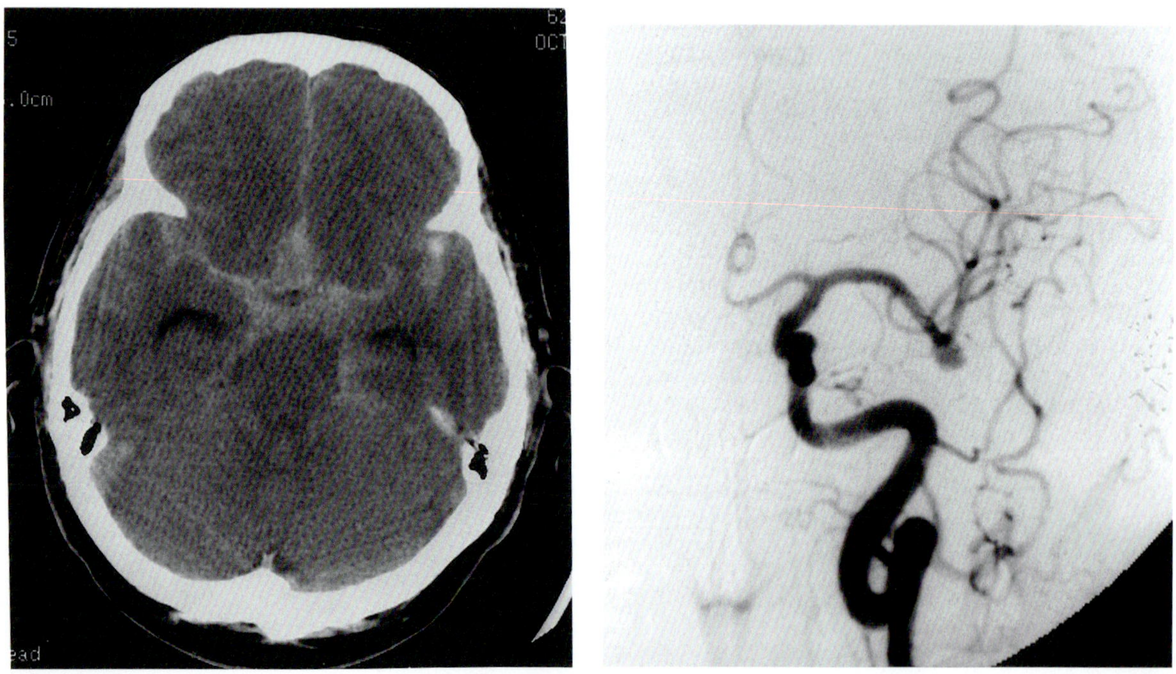

B

Figure 8–2 **(A)** Computed tomography of patient with diffuse subarachnoid hemorrhage; note enlarged temporal horns.

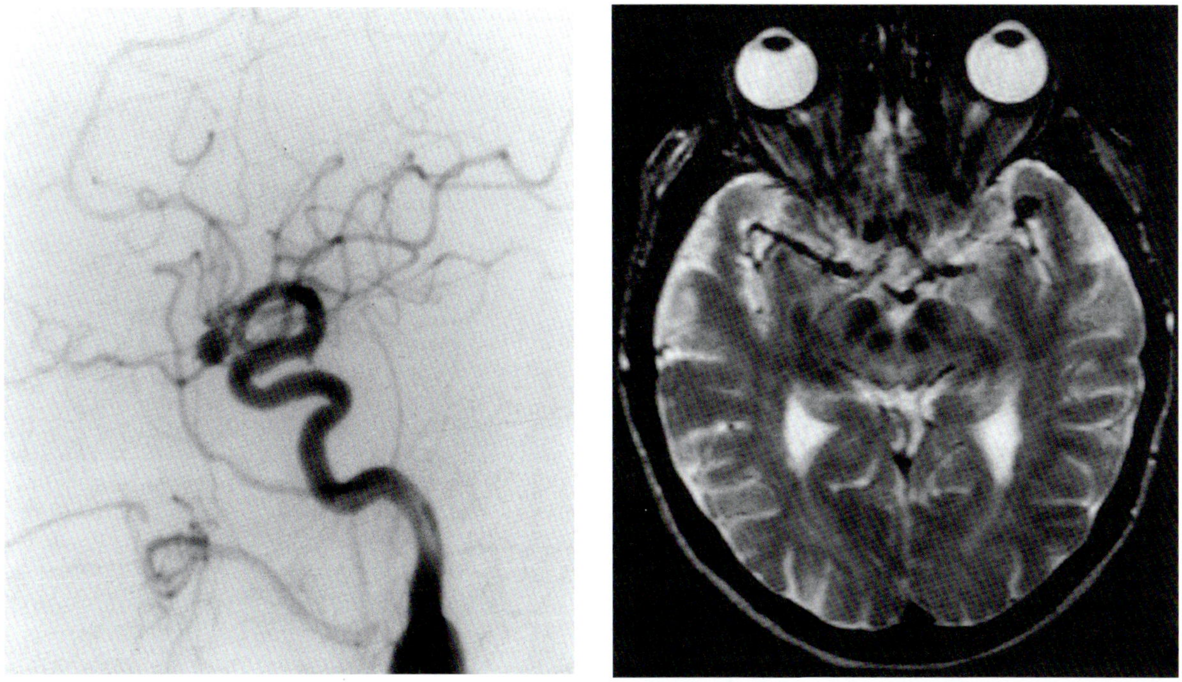

C D

(*Continued*) **Figure 8–2** **(B, C)** Anteroposterior and lateral angiography of different patient with left middle cerebral artery (MCA) bifurcation aneurysm. **(D)** Magnetic resonance imaging of same patient as **(B)** and **(C)** with left MCA aneurysm.

Cerebral angiography defines the site of origin of the aneurysm, relationship to and number of M2 branches (usually two or three), orientation of the fundus (projection into the temporal lobe vs the frontal lobe), and the breadth and shape of the neck of the fundus. A thorough search is also conducted for any additional aneurysms that might need to be addressed at the time of surgery. Venous drainage can also be assessed at the time of angiography, including anomalies of the vein of Labbé or of the superficial middle cerebral veins. If bypass is to be considered, the cervical carotid arteries are evaluated, and the size and course of the superficial temporal arteries are identified from the external carotid artery injection.

◆ Surgical Technique

Approach

We typically approach MCA aneurysms via a standard pterional craniotomy and proceed with opening of the sylvian fissure from distal to proximal. Two other common approaches to these aneurysms include (1) a transsylvian exposure with proximal to distal opening of the sylvian fissure, and (2) a superior temporal gyrus approach as advocated by Ojemann, Heros, Ogilvy, and others.[6,7] We feel that the transsylvian approach is the safest and most efficient route for identification of the MCA branches proximal and distal to the aneurysm to establish early vascular control of these lesions in preparation for possible intraoperative rupture. We favor the superior temporal gyrus approach for MCA aneurysms associated with a large intraparenchymal temporal hematoma. The craniotomy and initial exposure are the same for each of these approaches, and conversion can easily be made from one of these approaches to the other if dictated by the intraoperative findings.

Anesthesia and Intraoperative Monitoring

All patients undergoing craniotomy for clipping of aneurysms are placed under general anesthesia with oral intratracheal intubation, and an internal jugular or subclavian venous catheter is placed for intraoperative central venous pressure monitoring. Arterial lines are also placed for continuous blood pressure monitoring. A femoral arterial sheath is inserted during positioning of the patient in preparation for subsequent intraoperative angiography after clipping of the aneurysm. Scalp needle electrodes are applied for intraoperative electroencephalographic (EEG) monitoring. Asymmetry of the EEG generated intraoperatively serves as an indication that cerebral perfusion may be compromised, and efforts are made to correct this when including manipulation of the brain retractors or removal of temporary clips if possible. The EEG also serves as a guide for the establishment of pharmacological burst suppression when this is needed, as in the situation of intraoperative aneurysm rupture. The patient's volume status is maintained euvolemic to mildly hypervolemic with normotensive to slightly elevated blood pressures to optimize cerebral perfusion. For patients with cardiac dysfunction, intraoperative pulmonary arterial catheters are utilized as well. A microDoppler probe is also used intraoperatively to make gross assessments of patency of native vessels after clipping of the aneurysm.

Positioning

The patient is positioned supine with the head rigidly fixed in a radiolucent three-pin head holder. The head is rotated ~30 degrees to the side contralateral to the MCA aneurysm

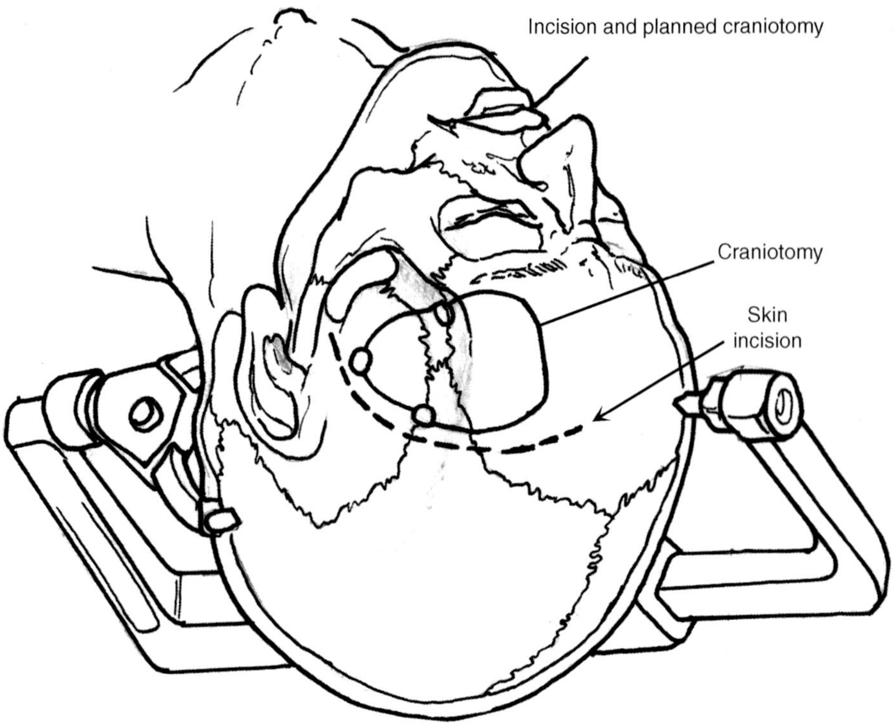

Figure 8–3 Initial patient positioning and skin incision.

being addressed (**Fig. 8–3**). The head is also extended so as to make the malar eminence the highest surface of the head. The back is elevated 10 to 15 degrees to promote venous drainage, with care to avoid constriction of the jugular veins by the tape of the endotracheal tube. If an external carotid to internal carotid (EC–IC) bypass is considered, then the ipsilateral cervical region is also prepped into the field. The frontotemporal area is shaved, scrubbed, and prepped with alcohol and Betadine and injected with local anesthetic.

Operative Procedure

The initial frontotemporal incision is taken down to the temporalis fascia and to the frontal pericranium. The incision extends from the level of zygoma at the temporal zygomatic process just anterior to the tragus to the anterior aspect of the hairline at the midline (**Fig. 8–3**). The cutaneous flap is reflected forward, and attention is paid to the temporalis fat pad to avoid injury to the branches of the facial nerve to the frontalis muscle. The temporalis muscle and fascia are incised with a monopolar cautery, leaving a small cuff of muscle on the portion of bone removed with the frontotemporal flap (**Fig. 8–4**). This will allow reapproximation of the temporalis muscle and fascia at the completion of the procedure. The temporalis is reflected so as to expose the frontal zygomatic process and McCarty's keyhole. The musculocutaneous flap is retracted with fishhooks on elasticized bands.

Bur holes are placed at the keyhole and in the squamous temporal bone just superior to the zygoma and at the superior temporal line posteriorly at the limits of the exposure, thus forming three points of a triangle. The underlying dura is stripped free with dural separators, and a craniotome is used to fashion a frontotemporal bone flap (**Fig. 8–5**). The dura is tacked to the margins of the craniotomy with sutures to reduce epidural venous bleeding. Further removal of the lateral sphenoid wing is accomplished with a high-speed drill and rongeurs. The dura is incised across the sylvian fissure, reflected anteriorly and inferiorly over the remnants of the sphenoid wing and orbit, and secured with additional sutures.

The exposed brain is covered with moistened, nonadherent Telfa strips, and a brain retraction system is brought into position. From this point forward, the operation is performed with the assistance of an operating microscope with a second binocular eyepiece for the assistant. Additionally, a video camera and monitor enable the scrub nurse to follow and anticipate operative maneuvers. Using a diamond-tipped arachnoid knife, the distal portion of the sylvian fissure is incised. The superficial sylvian veins are generally retracted to the temporal lobe side (**Fig. 8–6**). The opening of the sylvian fissure is expanded with bipolar forceps and a combination of sharp and blunt section. Distal MCA branches are traced from their superficial course on the lateral aspect of the frontal and temporal lobes to their deeper, more proximal locations at the M2 branches. It is more direct and efficient to open the sylvian fissure from distal to proximal and from "inside out" (i.e., to identify the M2 branches early in the depth of the fissure), and then to continue the proximal dissection of the more superficial aspect of the fissure, having identified these important vessels first.

In general, MCA aneurysms are directed anterior, inferior, and laterally into the temporal lobe. In light of this fact,

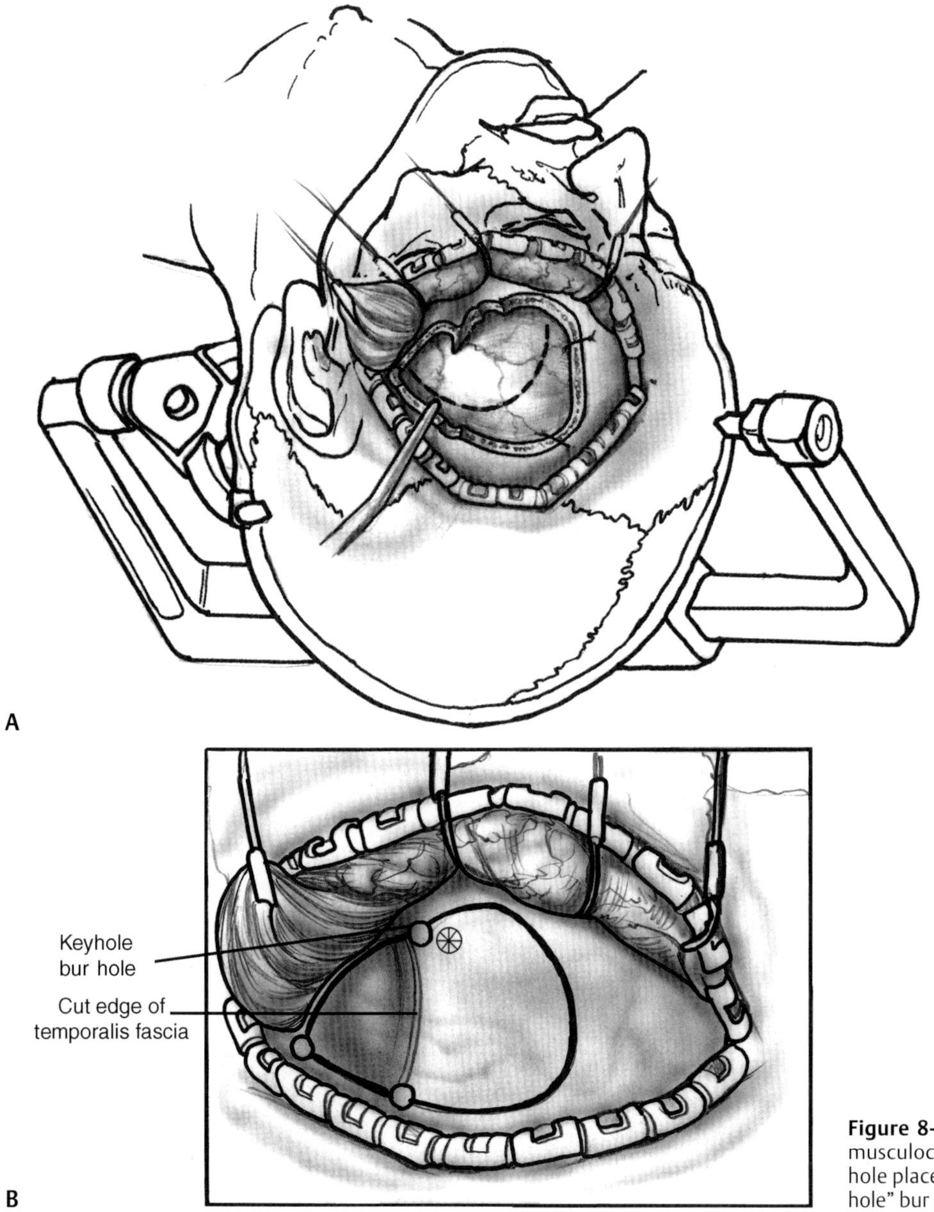

Figure 8–4A,B Elevation of left frontotemporal musculocutaneous flap. Asterisk denote site of bur hole placement. Asterisk with circle specifies "key-hole" bur hole.

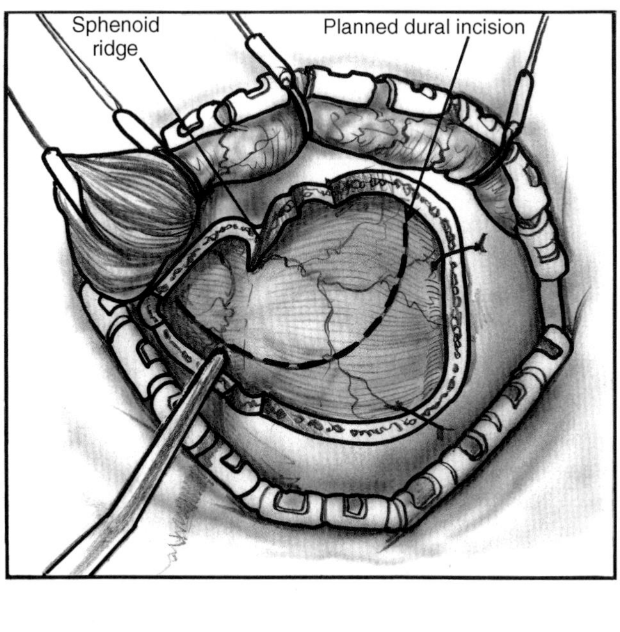

Figure 8–5 Exposed left frontal and temporal lobe dura after elevation of bone flap and drilling of lateral sphenoid wing. Dashed line indicates location of planned dural opening.

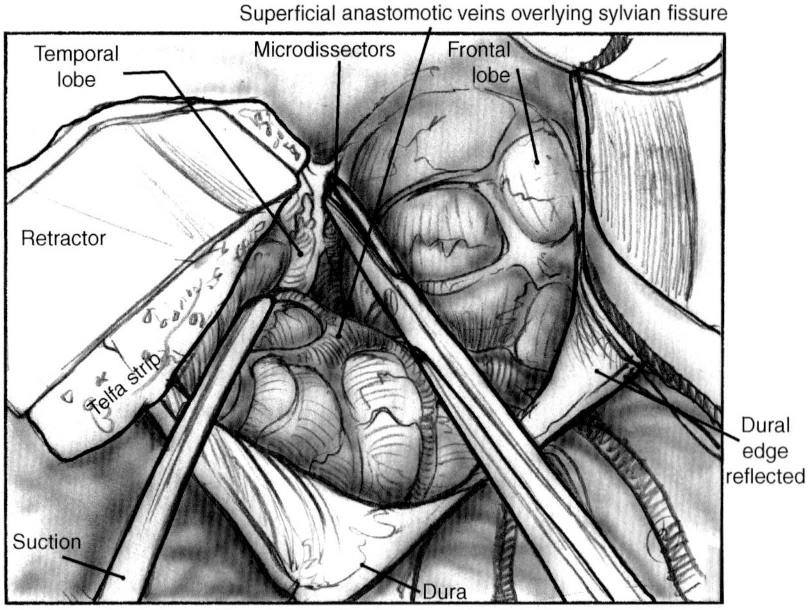

Figure 8–6 Initial microsurgical exposure of sylvian fissure after opening of the dura. Fissure is opened with careful sharp and blunt dissection of the arachnoid investments.

dissection along the MCA branches is performed on the frontal lobe side to trace the M2 branches back to their M1 origin at the bifurcation or trifurcation, avoiding disruption of the dome of the aneurysm (**Fig. 8–7**). This dissection route is altered as appropriate for the findings on the preoperative angiography. The initial focus is to identify the M1 and M2 branches to determine potential sites for placement of temporary clips in the event of intraoperative rupture of the aneurysm (**Fig. 8–8**).

Having achieved proximal and distal vascular control, the neck of the aneurysm is dissected and the anatomy of the lesion identified. Depending on the direction of projection of the predominant mass of the aneurysm, access to the M1 will be most practical either medial (i.e., toward the insular cortex) or lateral (i.e., toward the lateral sphenoid wing) to the aneurysm fundus. MCA aneurysms are often multilobulated and may incorporate the proximal portions of M2 branches of the bifurcation. Very often the long axis of the orientation of the aneurysm neck will parallel the origins of the predominant M2 branches. In this case the blades of the aneurysm clip must be parallel to the long axis. In other instances, reconstruction of the native vessels may be necessary and may require application of multiple aneurysm clips. Occasionally, the aneurysm clip blades will occlude one of the M2 branches. This complication may occur because the clip blades are passed too "low" on the fundus and neck, and the thick walls of the aneurysm are forced down on the luminal origin of the branch. To remedy such a situation, either the clip can be repositioned primarily or a second permanent clip can be placed in tandem to the first

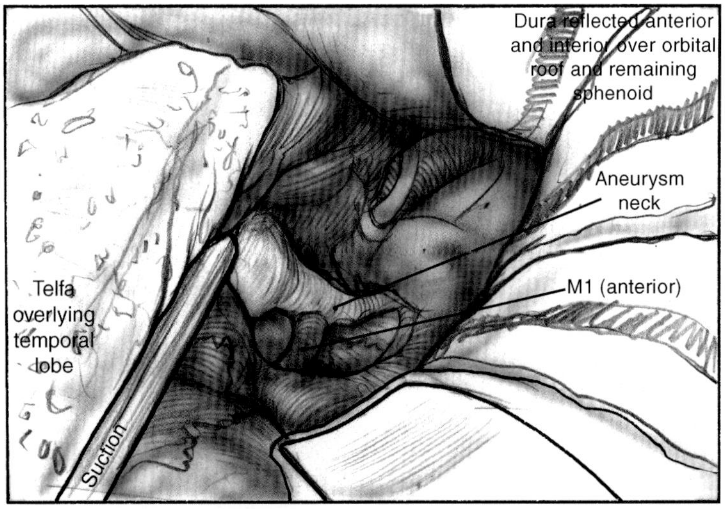

Figure 8–7 Dissection of sylvian fissure exposes distal portion of superior M2 segment, which is followed to the M1 segment, thus exposing the neck of the aneurysm at the middle cerebral artery (MCA) bifurcation.

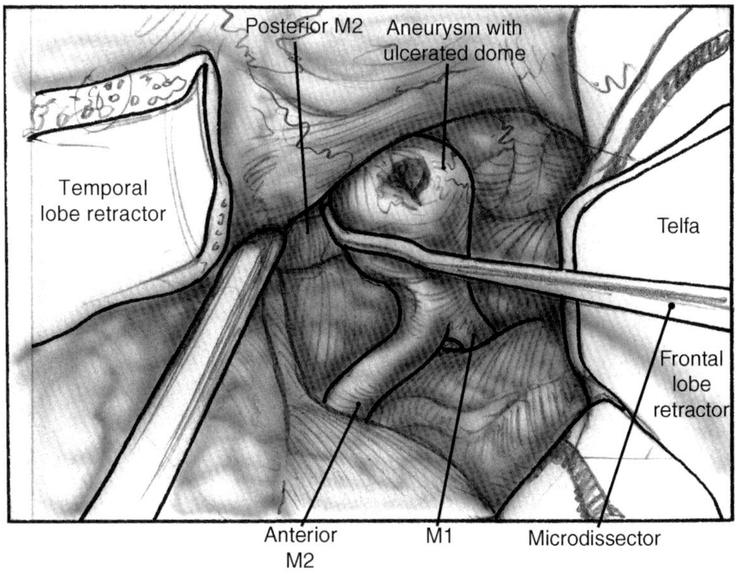

Figure 8–8 Further microsurgical dissection exposes the inferior M2 segment.

clip (i.e., parallel to the first clip immediately distal on the fundus), and then the first clip can be removed.

In the event of intraoperative rupture of the aneurysm, temporary clips are applied to the M1 branches and M2 branches to isolate the aneurysm from the cerebral circulation and stop the bleeding (**Fig. 8–9**). It is also sometimes desirable to decompress the aneurysm with a suction-needle device prior to clip application (**Fig. 8–10**) or to open the apex of the aneurysm fundus to remove atheroma or clot from a large partially thrombosed aneurysm (**Fig. 8–11**). Temporary clips are applied in these situations as well. Prior to application of temporary clips, the patient is placed in burst suppression as verified with the scalp EEG by the anesthesiologist, using barbiturates or propofol. A normal to mildly elevated arterial blood pressure is maintained so that cerebral perfusion can be optimized in this situation of local cerebral circulatory arrest. In the event of an intraoperative aneurysm rupture cottonoids and a suction tip are maintained over the site of rupture until hemostasis is obtained with the temporary clips. The circulating nurse monitors temporary occlusion time.

Surgical management of large or giant MCA aneurysms, particularly those with thrombosed or calcified elements, may require opening of the aneurysm to collapse its contents so that clip application can be performed (**Fig. 8–12**). Aneurysmorrhaphy is generally performed after temporary clips are applied (**Fig. 8–13**). Dense calcified material may even require the use of an ultrasonic aspirator to debulk the contents of the aneurysm (**Fig. 8–14**). In the event that a bypass procedure is indicated, the bypass is generally performed prior to addressing the aneurysm.

After final clip application on the MCA aneurysm neck, the aneurysm and the MCA vessels are thoroughly inspected. Intraoperative Doppler is used to confirm the

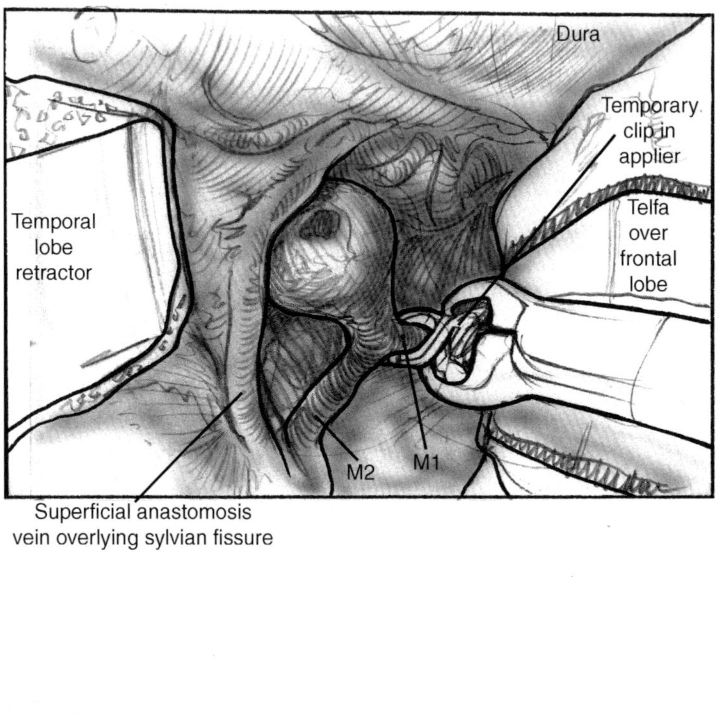

Figure 8–9 Application of a temporary clip to M1.

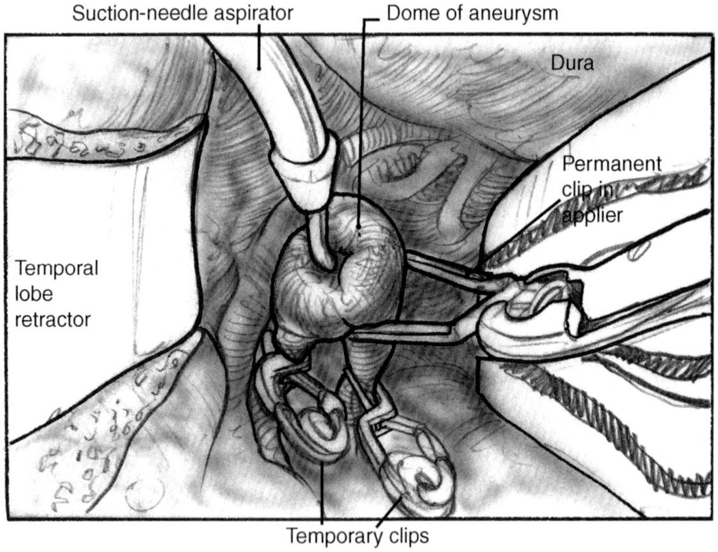

Figure 8–10 Suction-needle aspirator inserted into dome of aneurysm to collapse it while permanent clip is applied simultaneously. Proximal and distal control obtained with temporary clips on M1 and M2 segments.

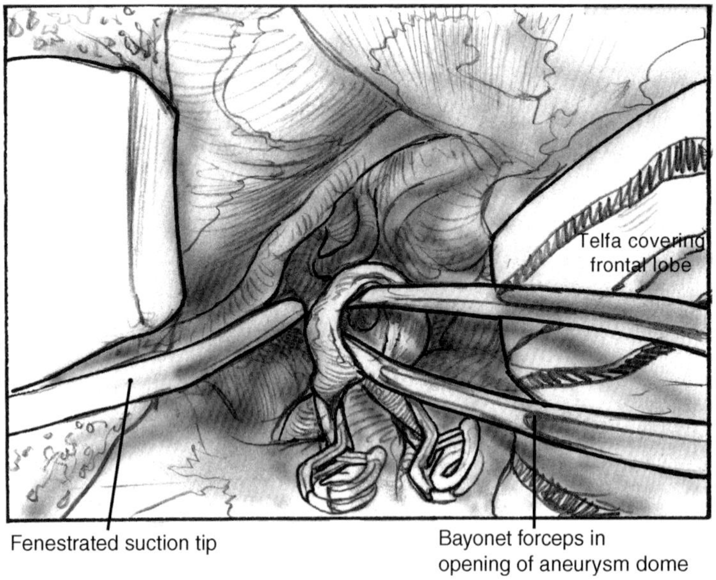

Figure 8–11 Firm nature of aneurysm prevented application of permanent clip, and, therefore, aneurysmorrhaphy is performed during period of temporary clipping to internally decompress aneurysm. Note the orifice of the aneurysm neck at the base of the aneurysm.

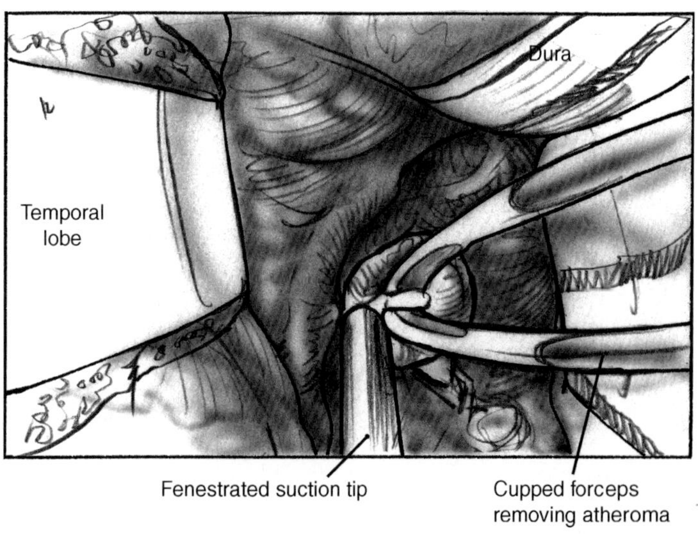

Figure 8–12 Atheroma is removed from within the aneurysm.

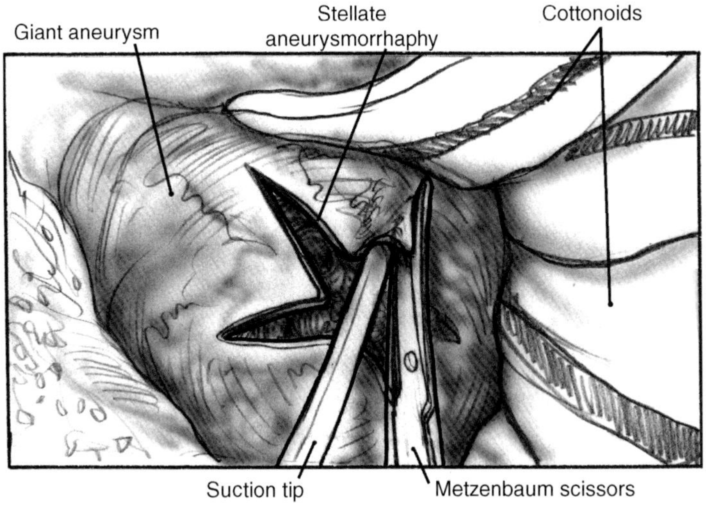

Figure 8–13 Giant middle cerebral artery aneurysm. After initial aneurysmorrhaphy with scalpel during period of temporary clipping, opening is expanded with Metzenbaum scissors.

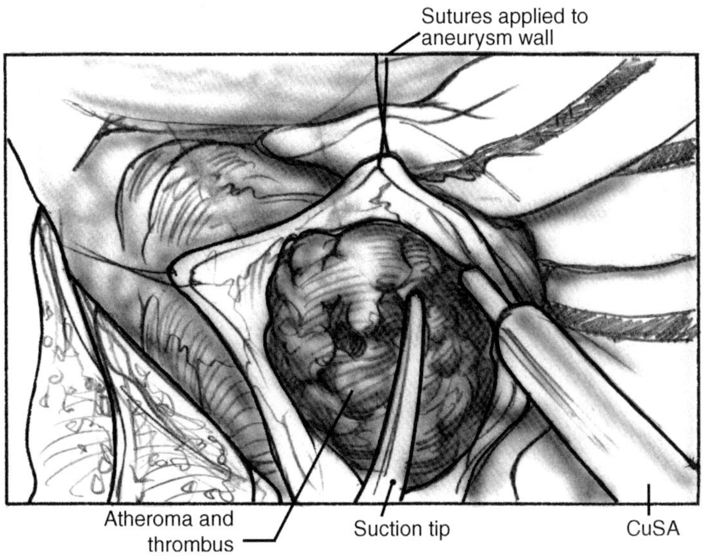

Figure 8–14 Internal decompression of giant middle cerebral artery aneurysm performed with ultrasonic aspiration of atheroma and thrombus.

patency of the native vessel, and if necessary, clips are adjusted. When an aneurysm has been completely obliterated with clips and all native vessels are felt to be patent, the dome of the aneurysm is punctured with a 25 gauge needle applied to suction. When the aneurysm has been clipped, and patency of the native vessels is confirmed visually, consideration is given to intraoperative angiography.[17]

Intraoperative angiography may be performed by removing the brain retraction system, covering the exposed brain with damp cottonoids from which the radiopaque markers have been removed, and covering the surgical exposure with a lactated Ringer's soaked lap sponge.

Intraoperative angiography is performed via the femoral arterial sheath placed at the time of patient positioning. If intraoperative angiography demonstrates obliteration of the aneurysm and good filling of the native vessels, the wound is closed (**Fig. 8–15**). If these criteria are not met, then the brain retractor and operating microscope are brought back into position and clip adjustments are performed as necessary until satisfactory clipping is achieved.

Closure

After intraoperative angiography is completed and obliteration of the aneurysm and patency of the native vessel are confirmed, closure is begun. Meticulous hemostasis is obtained with the bipolar cautery. Copious irrigation is applied to the wound, and the dura is closed with 4–0 sutures. The bone flap is secured into position with microplates and screws. The temporalis muscle and fascia are reapproximated with interrupted sutures, as is the galea. The skin is closed with surgical skin staples. A Jackson-Pratt drainage bulb and catheter are placed during the scalp closure for postoperative wound drainage, which is generally maintained for 24 hours.

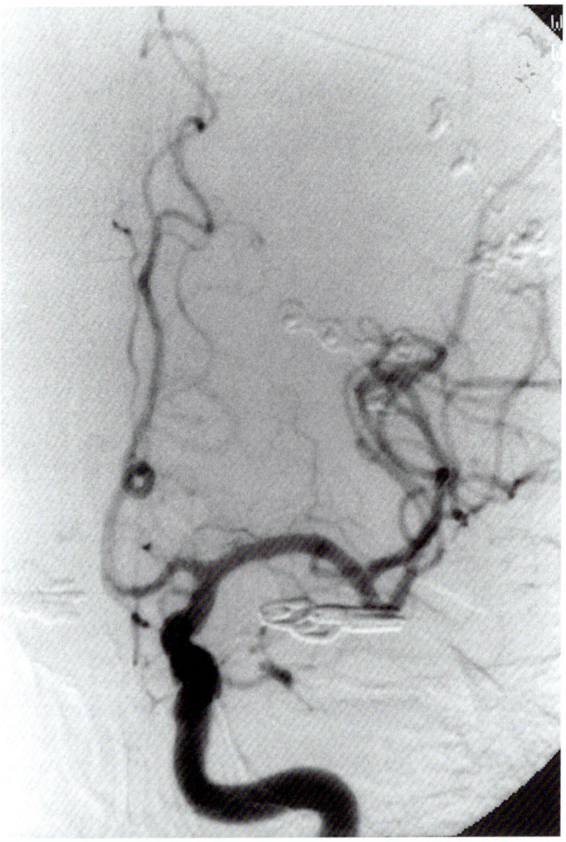

Figure 8–15 Final position of permanent aneurysm clip occluding neck of aneurysm and preserving patency of M1 and M2 branches demonstrated on angiography.

◆ Postoperative Care

Postoperatively, the patient is monitored in the intensive care unit. Strict attention is paid to the patient's serum electrolytes and cardiopulmonary status. If the patient has had a subarachnoid hemorrhage, hypervolemia and, if necessary, hypertensive therapy are administered. Perioperative antibiotics are generally administered for a 24-hour period beginning just prior to skin incision. Hydrocephalus resulting from subarachnoid hemorrhage is managed with ventricular drainage, and later, if necessary, placement of a cerebrospinal fluid shunt.

◆ Complications

Potential complications of MCA aneurysm and surgery for these lesions are multiple. In the face of a recent subarachnoid hemorrhage, prevention of rerupture of an untreated aneurysm is possible, and we therefore advocate early clipping of these lesions whenever feasible. Perioperative complications can be divided into intraoperative and postoperative complications.

Intraoperative rupture of an aneurysm is one of the potential risks of any aneurysm surgery. Careful examination of the preoperative angiogram enables appropriate dissection so as to avoid early exposure of the aneurysmal dome, and therefore minimize the risk of intraoperative rupture. Preparedness for the occurrence of intraoperative rupture is also important, including early identification of sites for appropriate placement of temporary clips. Maintenance of adequate blood pressure and the administration of cerebral protective agents by the anesthesiologist when appropriate are also important. Postoperative cerebral infarction can result from injury to the MCA vessels or their branches, including small perforating vessels. Meticulous dissection is therefore necessary to avoid hemiparesis, aphasia, or other postoperative neurological deficits.

Potential postoperative complications include the development of postoperative hemorrhage, either intraparenchymal, subdural, or epidural. Meticulous intraoperative hemostasis, of course, is an important component to this as well as tack-up sutures of the dura and tight regulation of postoperative blood pressure. In the event of a clinically significant postoperative hemorrhage, prompt identification with CT scan is vital. Immediate evacuation is indicated for hematomas of any significant size. Seizures are another potential complication, and preoperative initiation of prophylactic anticonvulsants is also a routine part of the procedure. Hyponatremia is common and must be treated aggressively. Patients are monitored for cardiopulmonary complications, including pul-monary emboli, pneumonia, and myocardial infarction, which are treated appropriately. Patients with subarachnoid hemorrhage must be monitored for neurological deterioration that can accompany vasospasm or hydrocephalus.

◆ Conclusion

MCA aneurysms represent a large percentage of the aneurysms encountered by vascular neurosurgeons. Optimal management of these lesions includes prompt recognition of the signs and symptoms associated with these aneurysms and verification with appropriate imaging studies, including CT scanning, angiography, and possibly MRI. Appropriate surgical management includes an understanding of the anatomy as demonstrated on the angiography. Precise microsurgical dissection is vital to surgical management of MCA aneurysms. Surgeons must have several techniques at their disposal as potential adjuncts to these operations, including methods of temporary clipping, EC–IC bypass, resection of thrombus and endarterectomy for larger lesions, and intraoperative angiography.

References

1. Kassell NF, Torner JC, Haley EC, Jane JA, Adams HP, Kongable GL. The international cooperative study on the timing of aneurysm surgery, I: Overall management results and, II: Surgical results. J Neurosurg 1990;73:18–47
2. Miyaoka M, Sato K, Ishii S. A clinical study of the relationship of timing to outcome of surgery for ruptured cerebral aneurysms. J Neurosurg 1993;79:373–378
3. Rinne J, Hernesniemi J, Niskanen M, Vapalahti M. Analysis of 561 patients with 690 middle cerebral artery aneurysms: anatomic and clinical features as correlated to management outcome. Neurosurgery 1996;38:2–11
4. Weir B. Aneurysms Affecting the Nervous System. Baltimore: Williams and Wilkins; 1987
5. Ronkainen A, Hernesniemi J, Ryynanen M. Familial subarachnoid hemorrhage in east Finland, 1977–1990. Neurosurgery 1993;33: 787–796
6. Heros RC, Ojemann RG, Crowell RM. Superior temporal gyrus approach to middle cerebral artery aneurysms: technique and results. Neurosurgery 1982;10:308–313
7. Ogilvy CS, Crowell RM, Heros RC. Surgical management of middle cerebral artery aneurysms: experience with transsylvian and superior temporal gyrus approaches. Surg Neurol 1995;43:15–22
8. Yasargil MG. Microneurosurgery. Vol 1: Microsurgical Anatomy of the Basal Cisterns and Vessels of the Brain: Diagnostic Studies, General Operative Techniques and Pathological Considerations of the Intracranial Aneurysms. New York: Thieme Stratton; 1984
9. Gibo H, Carver CC, Rhoton AL, et al. Microsurgical anatomy of the middle cerebral artery. J Neurosurg 1981;54:151–169
10. Aydin IH, Takci E, Kadioglu HH, Kayaoglu CR, Tuzun Y. The variations of lenticulostriate arteries in the middle cerebral artery aneurysms. Acta Neurochir (Wien) 1996;138:555–559
11. Watanabe T, Togo M. Accessory middle cerebral artery: report of four cases. J Neurosurg 1974;41:248–251
12. Unruptured intracranial aneurysms: risk of rupture and risks of surgical intervention. International Study of Unruptured Intracranial Aneurysms Investigators. N Engl J Med 1998;339:1725–1733
13. Guglielmi G, Vinuela F, Sepetka I, Macellari V. Electrothrombosis of saccular aneurysms via endovascular approach, I: Electrochemical basis, technique, and experimental results. J Neurosurg 1991; 75:1–7
14. Guglielmi G, Vinuela F, Dion J, Duckwiler G. Electrothrombosis of saccular aneurysms via endovascular approach, II: Preliminary clinical experience. J Neurosurg 1991;75:8–14
15. Malisch TW, Guglielmi G, Vinuela F, et al. Intracranial aneurysms treated with the Guglielmi detachable coil: midterm clinical results in a consecutive series of 100 patients. J Neurosurg 1997;87: 176–183
16. Spetzler RF, Selman W, Carter LP. Elective EC–IC bypass for unclippable intracranial aneurysms. Neurol Res 1984;6:64–68
17. Derdeyn CP, Moran CJ, Cross DT, Grubb RL Jr, Dacey RG Jr. Intraoperative angiography: a review of 112 consecutive examinations. AJNR Am J Neuroradiol 1995;16:307–318

9

Anterior Communicating Artery Aneurysms

Hirotoshi Sano

There are two main types of approaches for anterior communicating artery (AcomA) aneurysms, namely, a pterional approach and an interhemispheric approach.[2] A pterional approach is the most common for aneurysm surgery, not only for anterior circulation aneurysms but also for basilar tip aneurysms. There are some variations for the interhemispheric approach, including bifrontal, unifrontal, basal interhemispheric, and transcrista galli interfalcine approaches.

This chapter describes the pterional and transcrista galli interfalcine approaches because the usual interhemispheric approach is described in Chapter 10, and the transcrista galli approach can provide easy access to the prechiasmatic cistern.[1] If the space is too small for approaching the aneurysm, you can cut one side of the falx to enlarge the operative field as in a unilateral basal interhemispheric approach.

◆ Preparation

Preoperative imaging is important for deciding the approach. Three-dimensional computed tomography (3D-CT) is useful for these cases.[4] In the acute stage of subarachnoid hemorrhage (SAH), determining how to remove the hematoma takes precedence, and clipping is the second step. Therefore, an approach must be based on the location of the SAH and intracerebral hematoma (ICH). The approach that can cope with intraoperative difficulties should be selected. It must be minimally invasive if possible.

◆ Surgical Technique

Pterional Approach

The pterional approach has the following advantages:[3,5,6,7,10,11] the subarachnoid space is widely opened and the hematoma can be removed as much as possible in the acute stage of SAH; damage of the olfactory nerves is minimized; and the bilateral parent arteries on the proximal side can be secured in the early stage of the procedure. As a disadvantage, the brain must be compressed, and partial resection of the gyrus rectus is occasionally required in cases of high-positioned anterior cerebral artery (ACA) aneurysms.

Because this area is composed of five densely aggregated arteries, it can be difficult to visualize the aneurysm and blood vessels in cases of high-positioned and posterosuperiorly directed aneurysms.

The pterional approach to aneurysms of the AcomA is described from these viewpoints in this chapter.

Determinants of the Approaching Side

Determining factors include A1 predominance, the direction of the A2 fork, the direction of the aneurysm, the size of the aneurysm, and the multiplicity of aneurysms. The presence of fenestration of the AcomA is an important factor in determining the side of approach. In cases of acute-stage SAH, determining factors include the distribution of SAH and ICH.

In the case of small- to large-sized aneurysms directed anteriorly (**Fig. 9–1**), the A1 dominance should be the most important factor because it is sometimes difficult to secure the opposite side of A1. But there is no marked difference in surgical difficulty between the right and left approaches.

In the case of aneurysms directed superiorly, the A1 is bilaterally secured before approaching the aneurysm. Therefore, entry into the open part of the A2 fork (i.e., the side of A2 facing posteriorly) facilitates clipping (**Fig. 9–2**).

In the case of aneurysms directed posteroinferiorly and that are located at the back of the AcomA, entry into the side of the A2 located more anteriorly is recommended, as if the posterior surface of the A2, especially in cases with fenestration of the AcomA (**Fig. 9–3**).

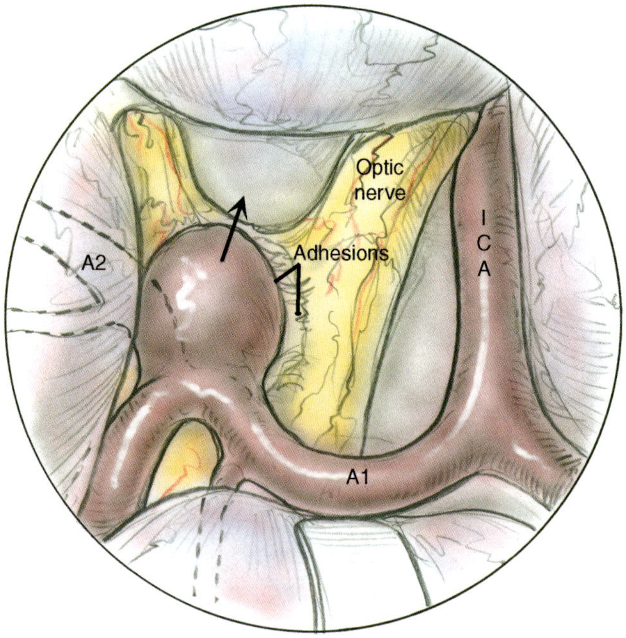

Figure 9–1 Aneurysm facing inferiorly and anteriorly. This type of aneurysm frequently adheres to or is embedded in the optic nerve. Premature rupture is most likely to occur during the retraction of the frontal lobe. Entry from the dominant A1 side is recommended. ICA, internal carotid artery.

Giant aneurysms are, as a rule, treated by the approach from the direction in which early arrival at the aneurysmal neck is accomplished. Approaching from the side of the dominant A1 is generally recommended, but for such an aneurysm that projects anteriorly, the interhemispheric approach is recommended. The interhemispheric approach is also recommended in high-positioned AcomA aneurysms.

Positioning[8,11]

The patient is placed in the supine position with the upper part of the body elevated at 20 degrees to control the venous pressure. The head is placed down ~0 to 10 degrees with the chin up and rotated to the contralateral side of the craniotomy, ~35 degrees on the right side and ~45 degrees on the left side (**Fig. 9–4A,B**).

Incision

A semicoronal incision is made along the hairline starting 5 mm anterior to the tragus in the superior zygomatic margin to the middle of the forehead.

Because the facial nerve runs between the skin and galea, the skin is reflected over the muscle sheath to avoid facial nerve injury. Especially around the orbit it is not necessary to dissect the skin, but instead to dissect the attachment of the temporalis muscle 1 cm under the zygoma (**Fig. 9–4C**).

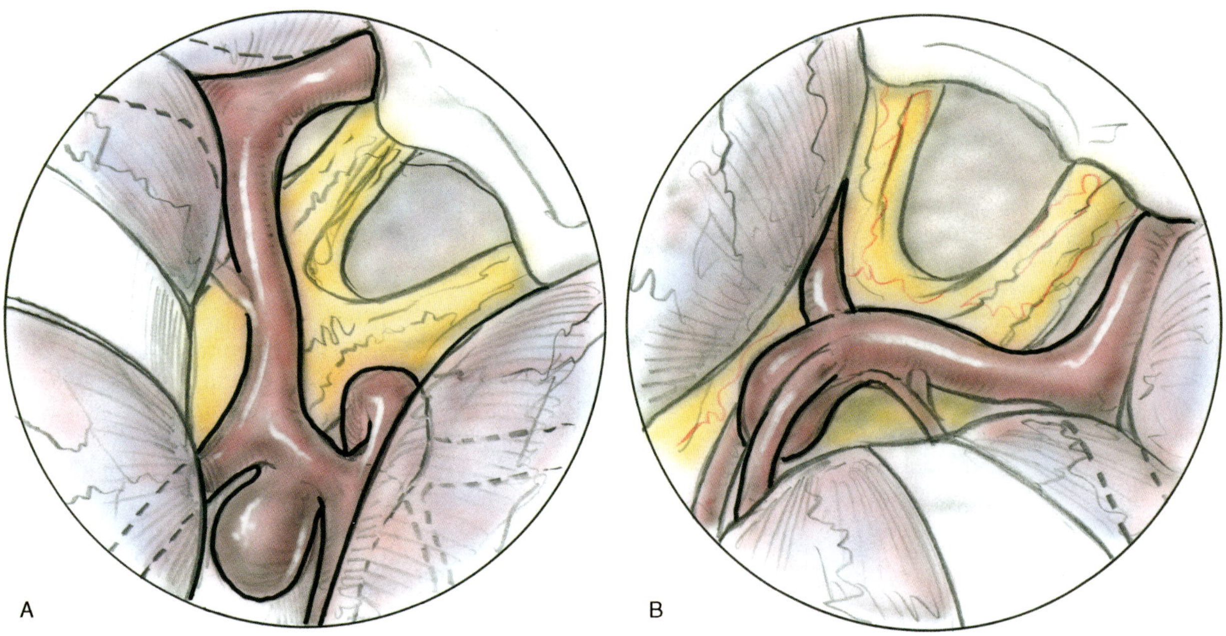

Figure 9–2 Aneurysm facing superiorly. **(A)** Entry into the closed side of the A2 fork makes the exposure of the neck difficult because the neck is behind the ipsilateral A2. **(B)** On the other hand, entry into the open part of the A2 fork (i.e., the side of the A2 located posteriorly) makes clipping easier.

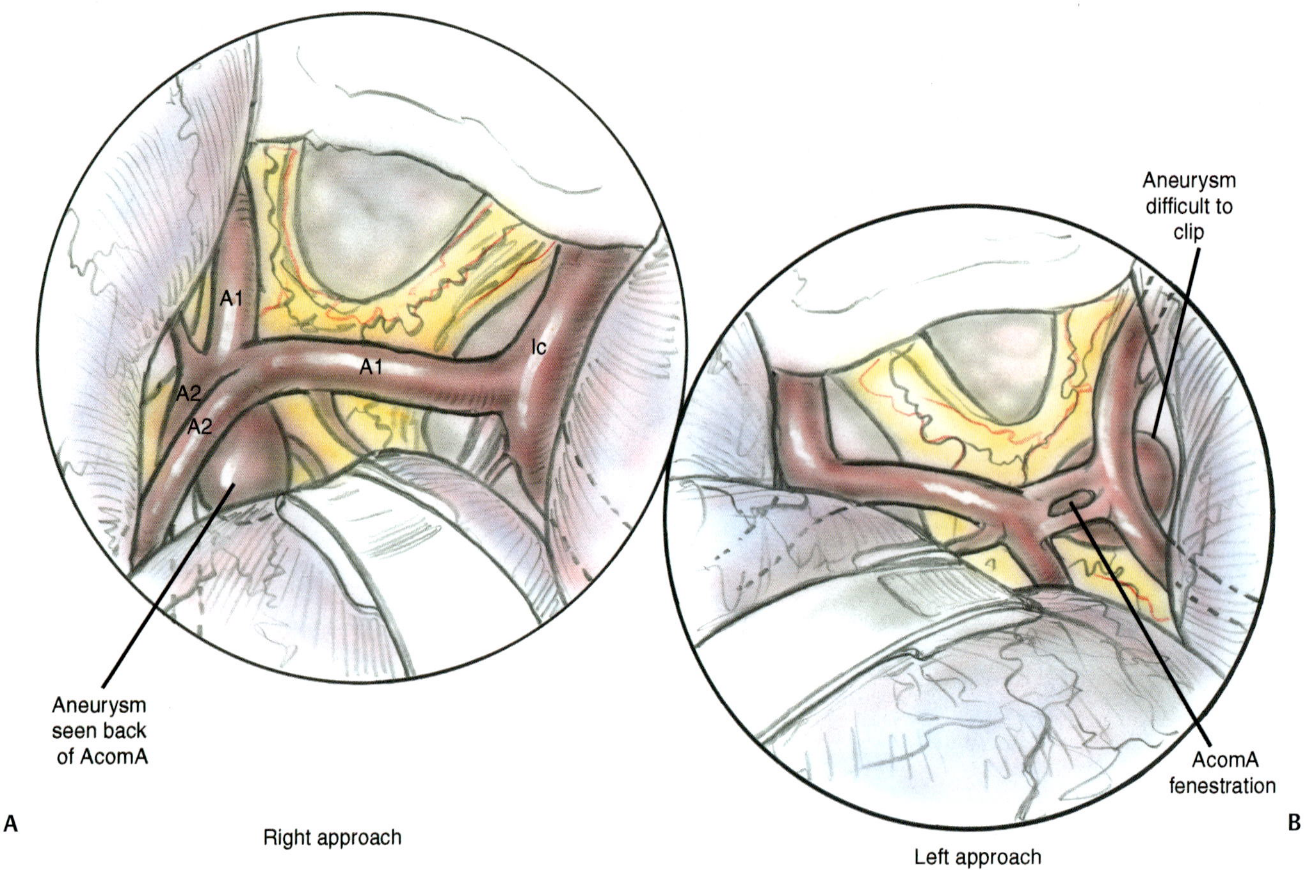

Figure 9–3 Aneurysm facing posteriorly, combined with fenestration of the AcomA. **(A)** In this case, entry into the part on which the A2 faces anteriorly is recommended because the mobility of the AcomA is poor. **(B)** With entry into the contralateral part, the aneurysmal neck cannot be confirmed because of interruption with the AcomA fenestration.

Incision of the Temporalis Muscle

A pedicle bone flap is recommended to be prepared for the following reasons: (1) the side of the head closure after craniotomy is cosmetically better with the pedicle flap, and (2) the pedicle flap is more resistant to infection than the free flap. With regard to subcutaneous dissection, part of the temporal fascia, particularly of the superior zygomatic margin near the orbit, should be separated carefully because of the facial nerve. It should be noted that transient facial palsy may be caused by the heat of electric cauterization.

If a free flap is selected, the temporalis muscle must be separated with the skin. The pterion is adequately exposed by posterior eversion after separation of the temporalis muscle on the orbital margin (**Fig. 9–4C**).

Craniotomy

Craniotomy should be performed so that the temporal and frontal lobes will be included in the visual field in an almost symmetrical pattern centering on the sylvian fissure. Bur holes are opened at the following three points (**Figs. 9–4C, 9–5**): (1) near the orbit beneath the temporalis muscle on the superior orbital margin, (2) the deep side of the temporal bone near the posterior part of the zygoma, and (3) beneath the temporalis muscle above the sylvian fissure. For cosmetic purposes, a titanium miniplate is positioned before bone separation. An airtome is used for bone separation, and the bur holes at points 1 and 2 may be omitted for cosmetic reasons.

On this occasion, it is important that the dura mater be adequately separated with a dural separator through the bur hole at point 3. The separation of the dura mater must be performed while the inner surface of the bone is in contact with the tip of the dural dissector. After bone flap separation, the bone flap is elevated and reflected. The pterion is eliminated with a Luer's rongeur or removed with an air drill, especially the inner surface. Bleeding is controlled with bone wax. Dural bleeding is controlled by coagulation, tenting of the dura with Gelfoam (Johnson & Johnson, New Brunswick, NJ) and oxidized cellulose with fibrin glue (**Figs. 9–4D, 9–5**).

Intradural Procedures

Dissection of the Sylvian Fissure

The sylvian fissure is, as a rule, separated on the side of the frontal lobe of the sylvian veins (**Fig. 9–6**). Because of the

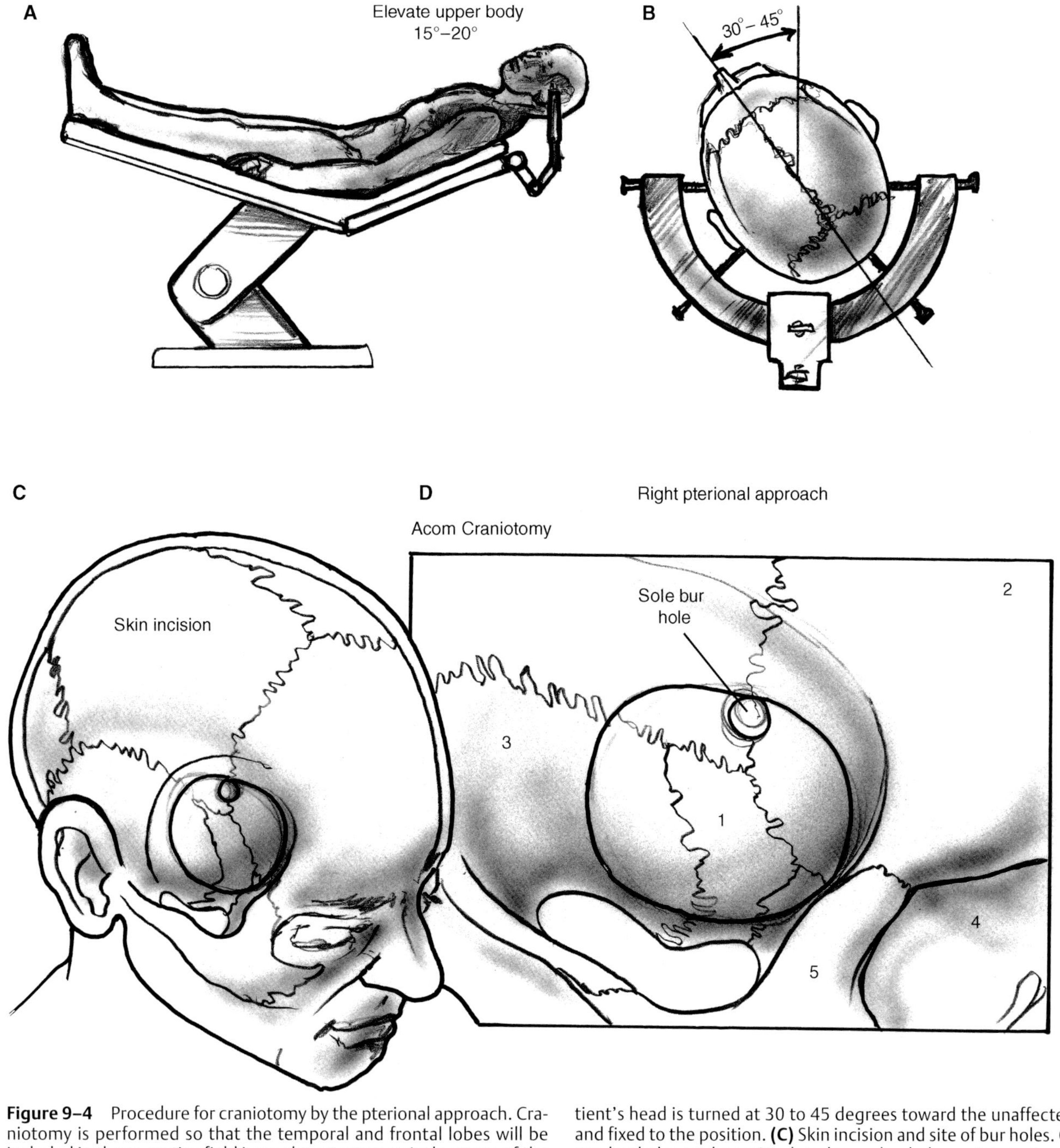

Figure 9–4 Procedure for craniotomy by the pterional approach. Craniotomy is performed so that the temporal and frontal lobes will be included in the operative field in an almost symmetrical pattern of the lobes centering on the sylvian fissure. **(A)** The upper body is elevated at 15 to 20 degrees so that the venous return will improve. **(B)** The patient's head is turned at 30 to 45 degrees toward the unaffected side and fixed to the position. **(C)** Skin incision and site of bur holes. One to two bur holes can be omitted, and a one bur hole craniotomy is enough. **(D)** Basic craniotomy by the right pterional approach. 1, sphenoid bone; 2, frontal bone; 3, temporal bone; 4, orbit; 5, zygomatic bone.

number of small veins enter the medial side of the sylvian vein from the frontal lobe, the lateral side of the veins is spared as long as possible, and particularly thick-walled large veins must be preserved. In cases where the vein must be cut, the venous circulation should be considered.

A microknife (disposable tuberculin syringe with 21–23 gauge disposable injection needle) is used for dissection of the arachnoid membrane of the sylvian fissure. For successful incision of the arachnoid membrane, the vein is protected with an aspirator in the surgeon's left hand, tension is added to the membrane, and the blade of the microknife is pulled toward the surgeon, being used like a knife rather than a needle. On this occasion, a neurosurgical spatula should be placed on the frontal lobe to give mild tension to the arachnoid membrane of the sylvian fissure.

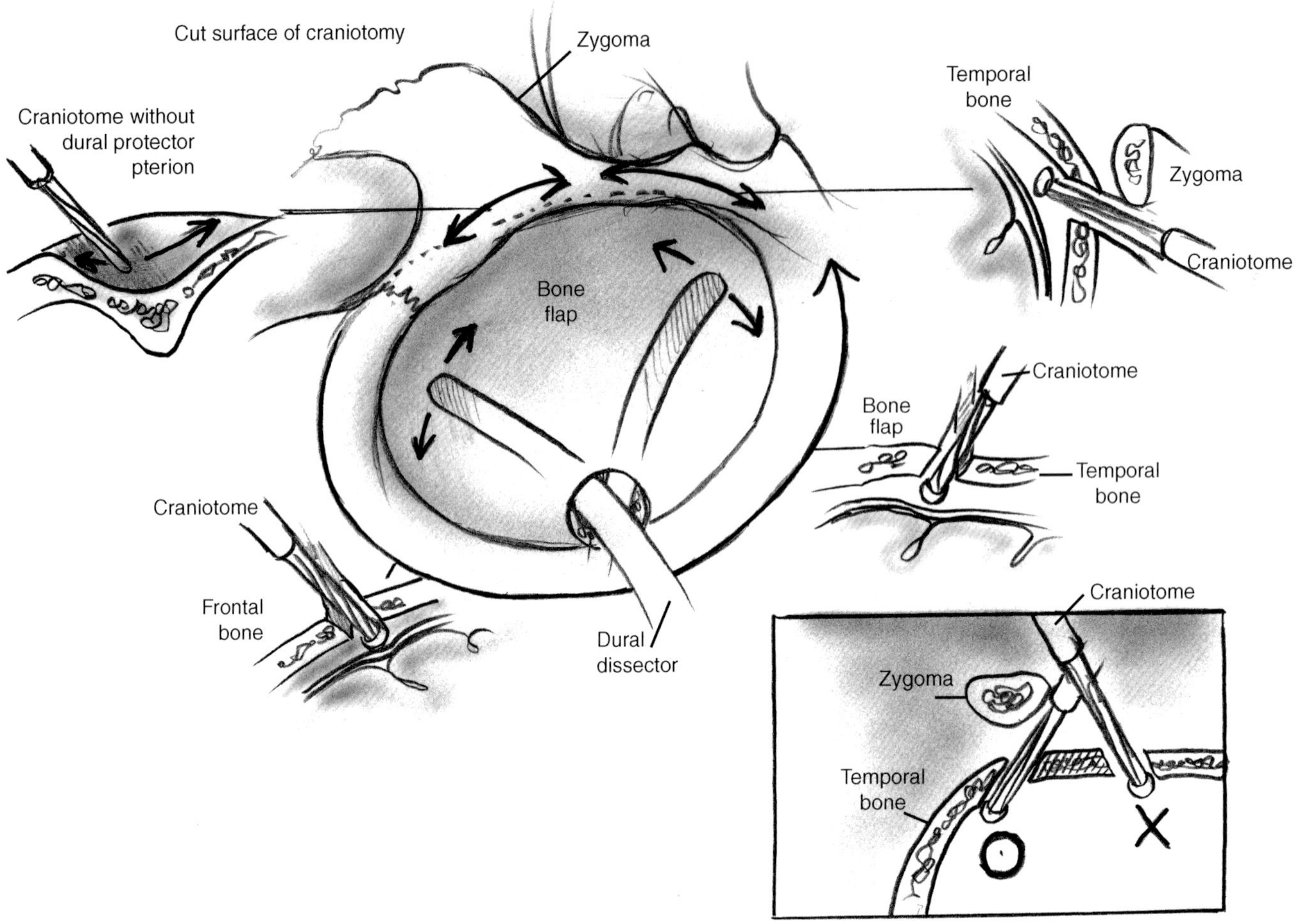

Figure 9–5 The craniotomy must be done in an oblique direction, making the outer table of the bone lateral and the inner table medial. But the basal port of the temporal bone under the zygoma is used for craniotomy. However, if the oblique direction is reversed, making the outer table medial and the inner table lateral, then the craniotomy will not be convenient. For the pterion only grooving of the outer table is necessary to facilitate reflection of the bone by bone elevators.

The arachnoid membrane is dissected with bipolar forceps or microscissors after it is incised with a microknife and the tight connective tissue is cut with a scissor. After the entry into the sylvian fissure, the arachnoid membrane is separated and raised from the inside of the sylvian fissure with an aspirator by the surgeon's left hand, and the arachnoid membrane is incised sharply with scissors.

The angle of the microscope and the position of the spatula should be changed to facilitate the surgical procedure. Retrograde dissection of the sylvian fissure leads toward the oculomotor nerve. Therefore, the parachiasmatic cistern may be opened by way of dissection of the sylvian fissure and be connected to the sylvian fissure. A tight ligament exists in the boundary between the frontal lobe and temporal lobe and also between the parachiasmatic cistern and the sylvian fissure as if it is connecting the frontal lobe with the temporal lobe. After the ligament is sharply dissected, the sylvian fissure is opened and the approach becomes possible by mild compression of the frontal lobe.

After the sylvian fissure is opened, the spatula is inserted to hold the frontal lobe and gradually retracted toward the parachiasma. The internal carotid artery (C2) is secured, then the arachnoid membrane is incised so that the contralateral optic nerve is exposed. The parent artery (A1) is secured and followed by the approach to the aneurysmal peduncle.

Approach to the Aneurysm[6,8,11]

The direction of the A1 is generally correlated with that of the aneurysm; in cases where the A1 takes an anterior bend in its the posterior part, the aneurysm will be present on the extension line (i.e., to face anteroinferiorly) (**Fig. 9–1**). In cases where the A1 extends straight toward the posterosuperior part, the aneurysm will be present on the extension line (i.e., to face posterosuperiorly) (**Fig. 9–2**). In case of the aneurysm facing on anteriorly or inferiorly (**Fig. 9–1**). A1 is directed anteriorly and posteriorly.

Many aneurysms may adhere to or be embedded in the optic nerve. Because this type of aneurysm is most likely to rupture prematurely during retraction of the frontal lobe, the surgeon should focus on gentle retraction so that the approach to the aneurysmal neck can be accomplished using temporary clipping to ipsilateral A1 and the aneurysm. Even in cases

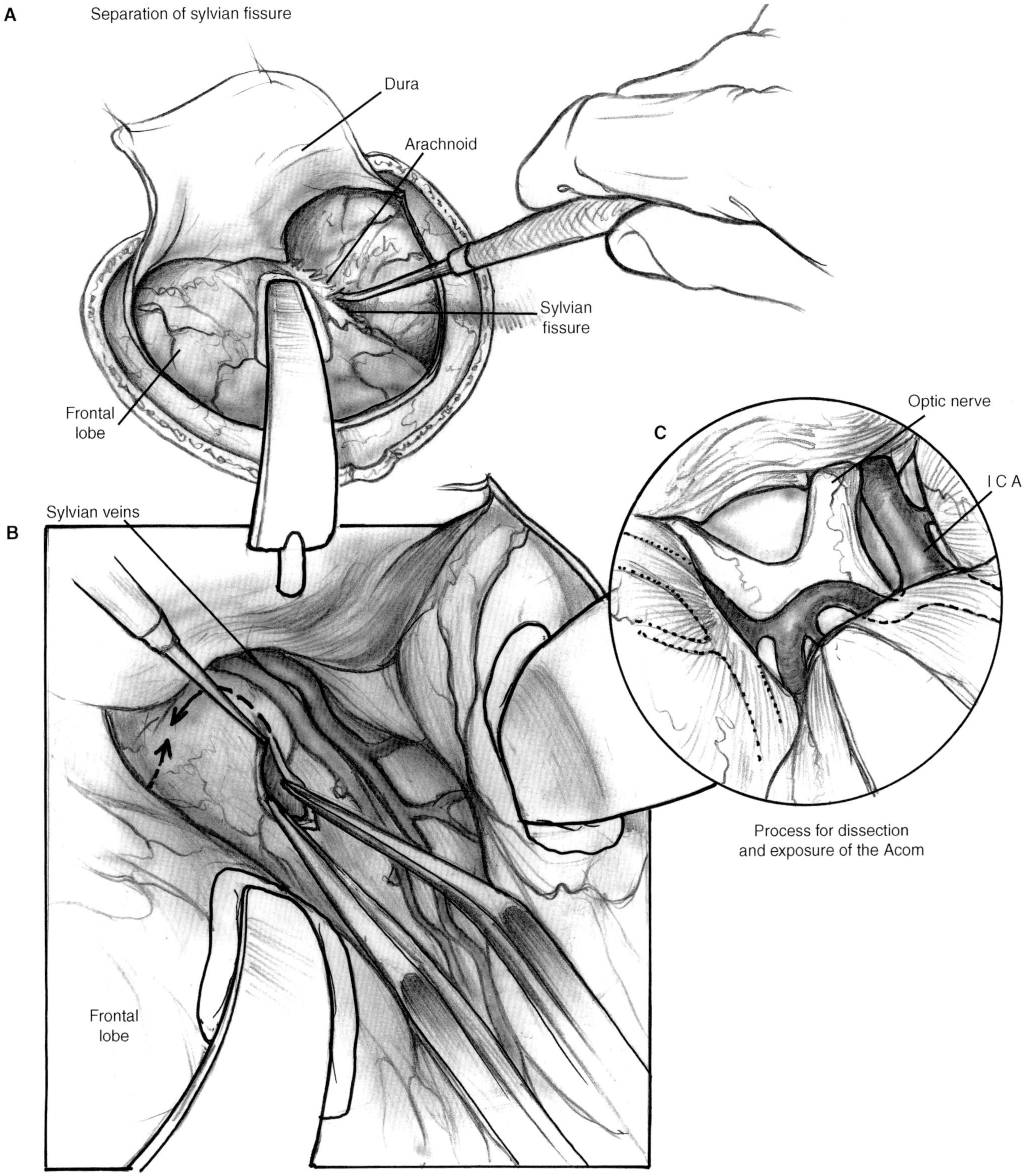

Figure 9–6 **(A)** Separation of the sylvian fissure. As a rule, the fissure is separated on the side of the frontal lobe of the sylvian veins. **(B)** Of the veins entering on the side of the frontal lobe, those of particular thickness should be preserved. **(C)** The process of dissection and exposure of the AcomA. The internal carotid artery and the optic nerve are exposed after preparation of the sylvian fissure, then the anterior part of the optic chiasma is dissected. After the contralateral A1 is secured beyond the inferior surface of the AcomA, the AcomA is separated.

where the aneurysm adheres to the optic chiasm, the adhesions can be dissected after tentative clipping of the aneurysms, and the contralateral A1 patency can be confirmed. Permanent clipping should then be reapplied if necessary.

Aneurysm Directed Laterally or Superiorly

The aneurysm may exist on the extension line of A1 (**Fig. 9–2**). This type of aneurysm projects to the contralateral side along the AcomA. The aneurysm is observed parallel to A2; if an approach from the side on which the A2 faces anteriorly (i.e., the side on which the A2 fork is closed), is selected, the aneurysm is covered by A2, and the contralateral A1–A2 junction is concealed behind the aneurysm. This situation makes it difficult not only to secure the contralateral A1 but also to dissect and clip the aneurysmal neck; therefore the approach must be selected from the open side of the A2 fork. Prior to clipping, the aneurysmal neck is dissected between the A2 and the AcomA.

Aneurysm Directed Posteriorly

The approach to posteriorly directed aneurysms must be selected to visualize the back side of the AcomA on which the aneurysm exists (**Fig. 9–3**). Usually it is the nondominant side of the A1. After the A1 is secured at the bifurcation of the internal carotid artery, the anterior part of the optic chiasma is dissected, when the A1 is located in the high position, and the contralateral A1 is easily secured beyond the anteroinferior surface of the AcomA. The gyrus rectus is sometimes partly aspirated and removed in the case of a high-positioned AcomA, and the distal A1 and proximal A2 are exposed. The proximal control site can also be secured, and the contralateral A1 is confirmed. Subsequently, the medial side of the A2 on the approaching side of the aneurysm approached. When the surrounding area of the aneurysmal neck is dissected, the origin of the contralateral A2 is exposed beyond the aneurysm.

Clipping

In this region, five blood vessels must be confirmed before neck clipping of the aneurysm, namely, the bilateral A1 and A2 and the AcomA. In some cases, it may be difficult to dissect the neck of the aneurysm completely. For such cases, a tentative clipping method is useful[7,8] (**Fig. 9–7**).

There are two types of tentative clipping methods: (1) dome clipping on the proximal side of the ruptured point to

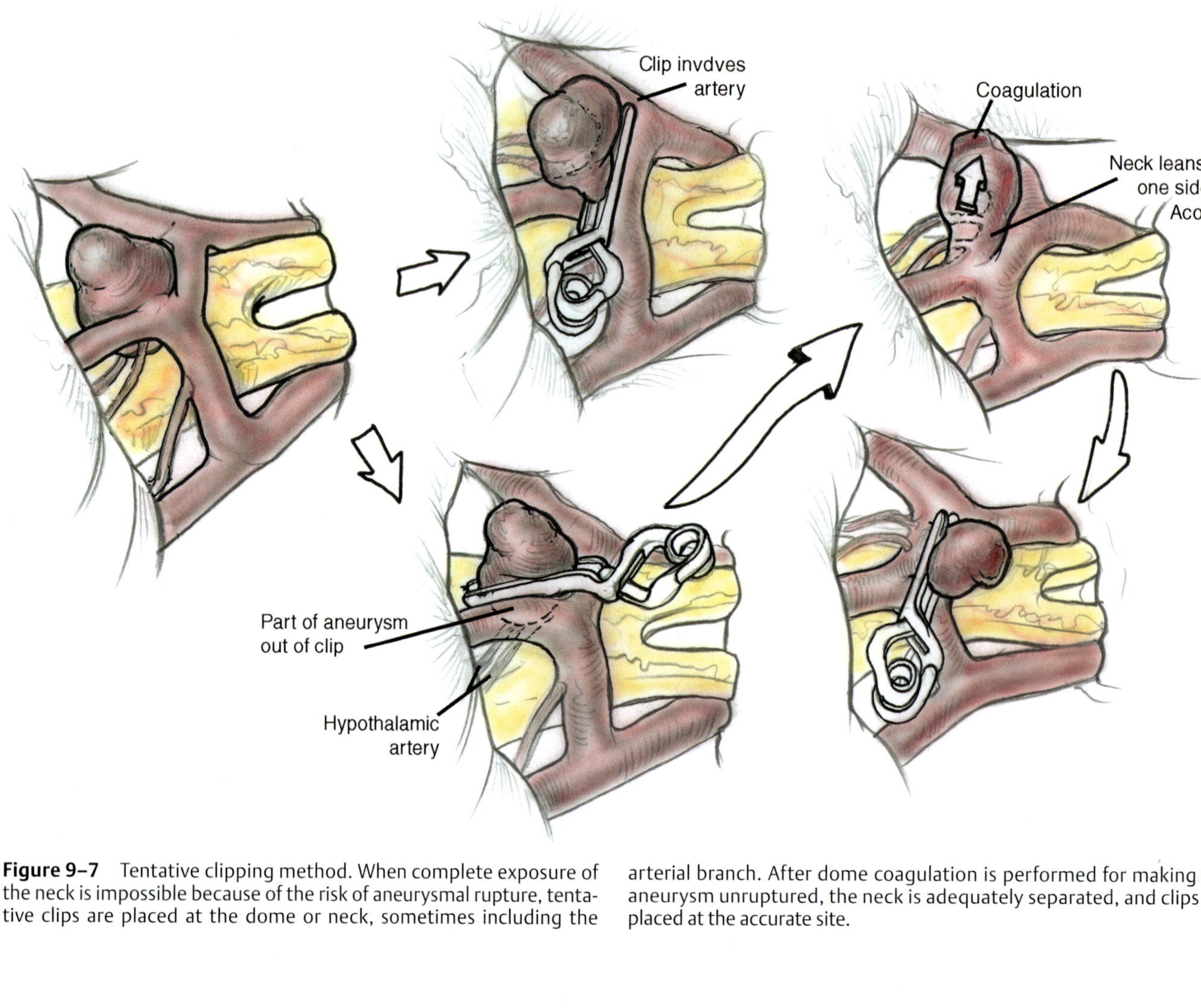

Figure 9–7 Tentative clipping method. When complete exposure of the neck is impossible because of the risk of aneurysmal rupture, tentative clips are placed at the dome or neck, sometimes including the arterial branch. After dome coagulation is performed for making the aneurysm unruptured, the neck is adequately separated, and clips are placed at the accurate site.

prevent further rupturing, and (2) aneurysmal neck clipping, sometimes including arterial branches behind the aneurysm. After tentative clipping the aneurysm can be dissected completely, then the ruptured point is coagulated with or without trimming of the aneurysm. This makes the aneurysm small, and accurate neck clipping becomes easy. For dissection bipolar forceps, silver dissector is useful. When the bipolar forceps is used as a dissector, the tip must be placed accurately at the dissecting point; otherwise it causes bleeding.

In the acute stage of SAH,[7] jet irrigation is very useful.[9] The surgeon can irrigate the blood clot to recognize blood vessels of the arachnoid membrane. Water itself raises the arachnoid membrane, so that the arachnoid membrane can be cut sharply, accurately, and safely. The point of dissection is dissected using bipolar forceps or a dissector, and then the strong adhesion is cut with microscissors. The dissection is performed toward the direction of the aneurysm, and the space for the clip blade is secured without tension to the aneurysm. Exposure of the whole aneurysm is not necessary and is avoided.

Before clipping, the area surrounding the aneurysm should be inspected for arterial branches and perforators. During clipping, the clip holder should be gradually inserted to allow visibility of blade tip during opening and closing of the clip. The clip is placed parallel to the parent artery as a rule.

It should be kept in mind that the natural morphology of the parent artery should remain for avoiding stenosis and kinking. Intraoperative rupture most frequently occurs at the time of aneurysmal preparation. Temporary or tentative clipping under the administration of a cerebral protective drug facilitates the surgical procedure. The full circumference of the A1 at the side of the temporary clip must be separated. Usually, an average of eight perforating arteries branch from the posterior surface of the A1.

Because disorders of the anterior hypothalamus cause emotional change, personality disorders, and intellectual deficit, damage to it must be avoided. The absence of involvement of branch by clipping or neck residual must be confirmed by dome puncture and coagulation following neck clipping. Attention must be paid to occlusion of the contralateral A2 in the case of an aneurysm facing superolaterally and that of the contralateral A1 in the case of an aneurysm facing anteroinferiorly. Care must be taken to prevent occlusion of those perforating arteries arising from the AcomA, particularly the hypothalamic artery, in the case of an aneurysm facing posteriorly. In this situation, trapping should be avoided as much as possible.

The recurrent artery of Heubner runs in the reverse direction along the A1 around the AcomA or from the origin of the A2. A large recurrent artery of Heubner may be confused with the A1. Care must also be taken to avoid confusing the fronto-orbital artery originating from the proximal side of the A2 with a recurrent artery because it also runs on the inferior surface of the frontal lobe.

Closure

The dura mater is sutured watertight. Sometimes fibrin glue with antibiotics may be sprayed over the dural closure to prevent cerebrospinal fluid (CSF) leakage.

A drain is kept extradurally, and the bone flap is fixed at several sites with titanium miniplates that were marked during craniotomy. The temporalis muscle and the fascia are sutured from the pterion, and the scalp is sutured in a bilayered pattern.

Because the pterional approach is a common craniotomy procedure to the anterior circulation and to the tip of the basilar artery, surgeons should become expert in the procedure, so that these operations will proceed smoothly.

Interhemispheric Approach

Another main approach for anterior communicating aneurysms is the interhemispheric approach. There are several kinds of interhemispheric approaches, such as the bifrontal interhemispheric, transcrista galli interfalcine approach,[1] and so on. The interhemispheric approach is advantageous in that it is a midline approach so that the bilateral A1 and A2 are visualized equally and long enough. The disadvantage of this is the possibility of venous injury and a slight difficulty in dissecting the interhemispheric fissure.

The usual unilateral interhemispheric approach is described in Chapter 10. The transcrista galli interfalcine approach is very unpopular; however, it is minimally invasive, because it avoids venous cutting or brain injury of the interhemispheric fissure, and it allows the operative field to be enlarged for a unilateral or bilateral interhemispheric approach by cutting the falx.

Procedure

The patient is placed in the supine position. A coronal skin incision is made behind the hairline. The skin flap is reflected to expose the craniotomy site down to the nasion. The periorbital bone is detached bilaterally from the superior margin of the orbital rim. Two bur holes are made paramedian, situated 4 cm above the nasion. The dura is gently dissected using a dural dissector or 5 mm spatula. The dural in the basal portion is thin and requires careful dissection. A 4 $\times$ 4 cm craniotomy is performed in the centrobasal portion of the bone. The upper portion of the lateral side of the craniotomy is performed with a craniotome. The lower part of the craniotomy involving the frontal air sinus is performed with a surgical saw. However, only the outer table of the sinus is dissected, and the inner table is fractured by the elevation of the bone flap. Titanium miniplates required for closure are placed at this time.

The mucous membrane of the frontal air sinus is completely dissected. It is trimmed and pushed into the frontonasal duct. The frontal air sinus region is subsequently sterilized with Betadine and packed with bone dust and fibrin glue several times. The crista galli and the inner table of the frontal sinus are removed with rongeurs, a bone punch, and an air drill (**Fig. 9–8**).

The basal portion of the falx, which is visible after the removal of the crista galli, is split into two leaves with the back side of a knife. Venous bleeding from the superior sagittal sinus is controlled by packing with oxidized cellulose and fibrin

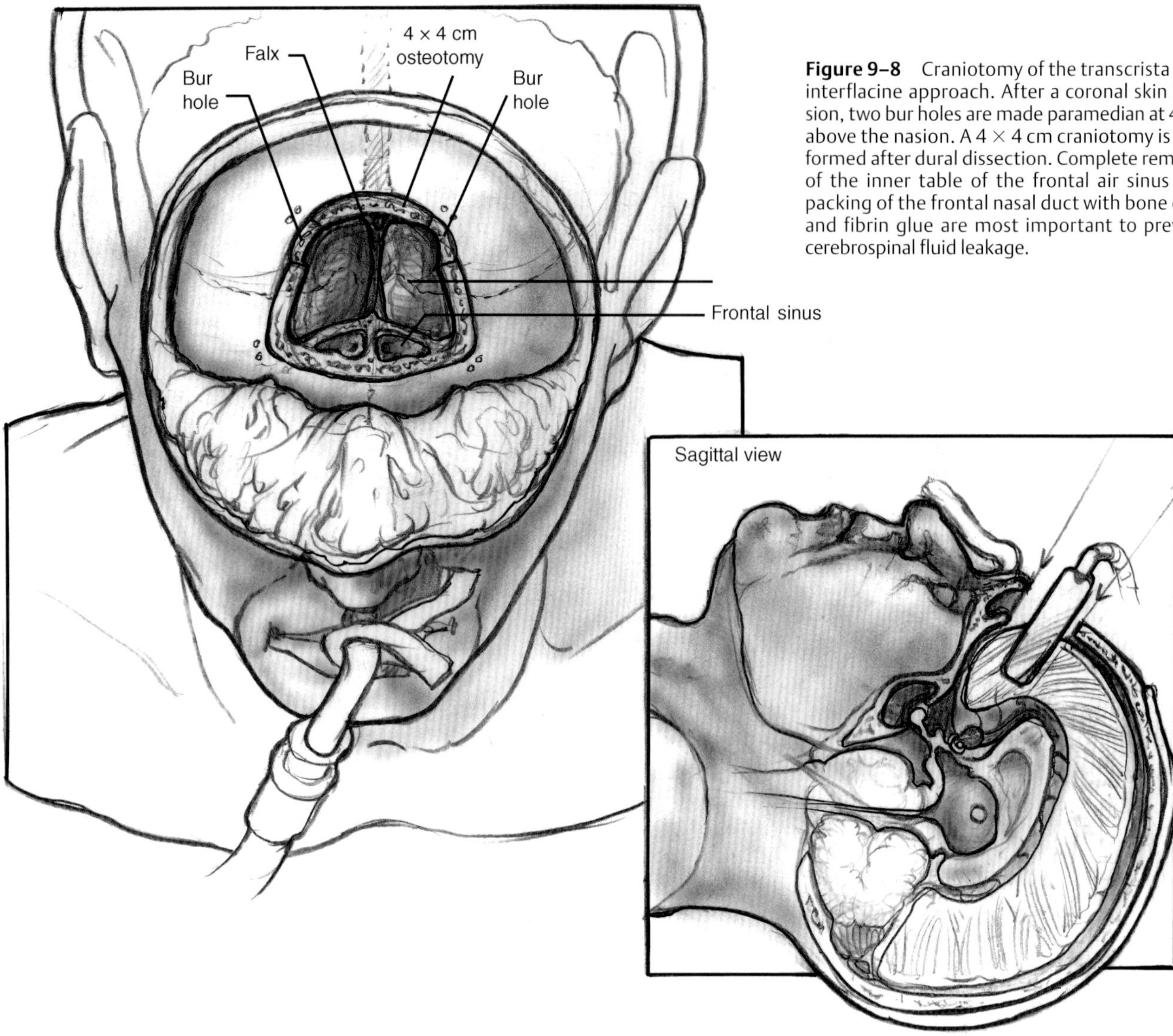

Figure 9–8 Craniotomy of the transcrista galli interflacine approach. After a coronal skin incision, two bur holes are made paramedian at 4 cm above the nasion. A 4 × 4 cm craniotomy is performed after dural dissection. Complete removal of the inner table of the frontal air sinus and packing of the frontal nasal duct with bone dust and fibrin glue are most important to prevent cerebrospinal fluid leakage.

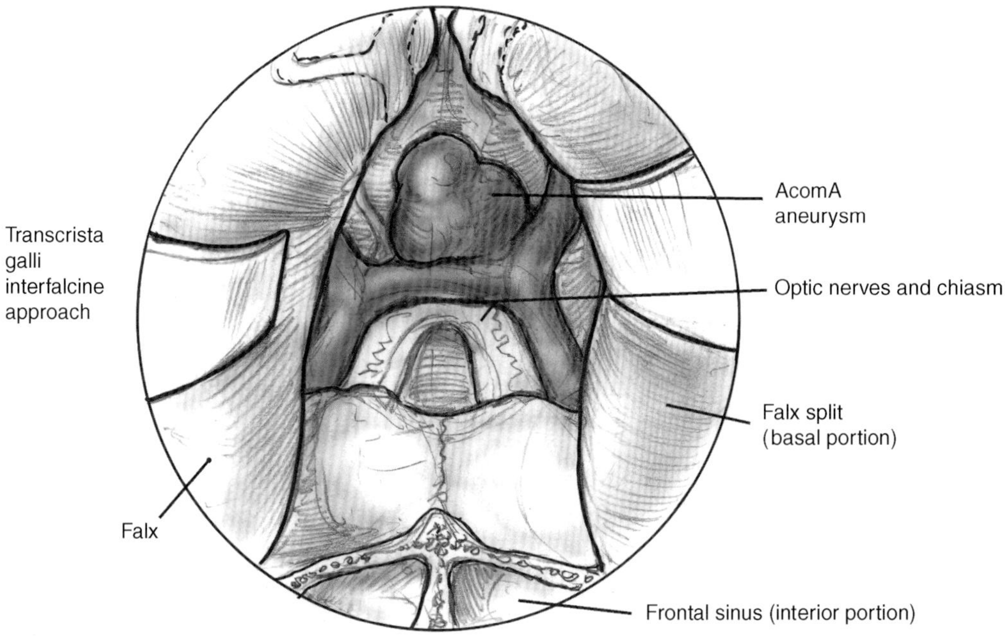

Figure 9–9 Enlargement of the operative field from the transcrista galli interflacine approach to a unilateral interhemispheric approach. Bilateral A1, A2, and AcomA with aneurysm are easily visible.

glue. Both the olfactory nerves and the bridging veins that lead into the sagittal sinus are protected by the split basal leaves of the falx.

After the basal interhemispheric fissure is opened, the optic chiasma and the AcomA are visible. The method of neck clipping and head closure is the same as for the pterional approach.

An important key point of the skull base approach is the repair of the frontal sinus. The complications associated with this are CSF leakage, pneumocele, and infection. Usually the frontal sinus is repaired with the temporalis fascia, fascia lata, or a packing of fat tissue. We recommend the defect be covered with bone; pack the frontal sinus with bone dust and fibrin glue mixed with antibiotics. This packing procedure is performed three times. We have performed this procedure many times to repair the frontal air sinus and have successfully prevented CSF leakage.

References

1. Fujitsu K, Sekino T, Sakata K, et al. Basal interflacine approach through a frontal sinusotomy with vein and nerve preservation. J Neurosurg 1994;80:575–579
2. Fukumitsu T. The points of aneurysm operation according to sites. In: Fukumitsu T, ed. Anterior Communicating Aneurysm: Cerebral Aneurysm. Tokyo: Bunko-do; 1987:110–122
3. Hashimoto N, Kikuchi H. Anterior communicating aneurysm. In: Takakura K, ed. Treatment of Cerebral Aneurysms. Tokyo: Gendai Iryo-sha; 1990:139–150
4. Kato Y, Sano H, Katada K, et al. The usefulness of helical scanning CT (HES-CT), particularly 3-dimensional (3-D) CT endoscopy, for the decision of aneurysm treatment. No Shinkei Geka 1995;23:685–691
5. Kikuchi H. Anterior communicating aneurysm: pterional approach. In: Kikuchi H, ed. Microsurgery in Neurosurgery. Tokyo: Igaku Shoin; 1988:13–20
6. Saito I. Anterior communicating aneurysm. In: Abe H, ed. Operation in Neurosurgical Disease and the Indication. Vol 2., Tokyo: Asakura Shoten; 1990:8–22
7. Sano H, Kanno T, Ishiyama N, Kato Y, Adachi K, Shinomiya Y. The points of operation for acute ruptured cerebral aneurysms. Collected Lectures of the 12th Meeting of Stroke Surgery. Cerebral aneurysms: various inoperative problems. 1993:237–241
8. Sano H. Middle cerebral aneurysms. In: Abe H, ed. Operation for Neurosurgical Disease and the Indication. Vol 2. Tokyo: Asakura Shoten; 1990:56–83
9. Sano H, Kato Y, Zhou J, et al. New jet irrigation bipolar system. Neurosurgery 1996;38:1251–1253
10. Sano H, Kato Y, Hayakawa M, Akashi K, Kanno T. A transcrista galli, translamina terminalis approach for highly placed basilar bifurcation aneurysms. Acta Neurochir (Wien) 1997;139:1020–1025
11. Yasargil MG. Microneurosurgery. Vol 2: Clinical Considerations: Surgery of the Intracranial Aneurysms and Result. Stuttgart: Georg Thieme; 1984

10

Distal Anterior Cerebral Artery and Distal Middle Cerebral Artery Aneurysms

Hirotoshi Sano

There is no alternative to the interhemispheric approach for distal anterior cerebral artery (ACA) aneurysms. The left or right side must be selected for the best position of the craniotomy. The site of the craniotomy is determined according to the size and direction of the aneurysm and bridging veins and the location of a hematoma in cases of an acute stage.

The only approach for distal middle cerebral artery (MCA) aneurysms is transsylvian. The location of the aneurysm will differ even in distal MCA aneurysms. The deeper variable posterior sylvian aneurysm is the most difficult to approach.

◆ Indications

Currently we consider indications for direct clipping surgery when we have:

- Hematoma associated with the aneurysm
- A broad aneurysmal neck
- Branches arising from the aneurysm
- Younger patients

◆ Distal Anterior Cerebral Artery Aneurysms

Preparation

Arterial and venous phase digital subtraction angiography (DSA) is essential. Presubtraction angiography is important to determine the relation between the skull and veins, and therefore to determine the best craniotomy site.

Three-dimensional computed tomographic (3D-CT) angiography shows the relationship of the aneurysm, parent artery, and skull (**Fig. 10–1**).

Obtaining the venous phase angiography, especially the lateral view, is important to determine the craniotomy site. Selection of the right or left side for craniotomy depends on the location, direction, and size of the aneurysm. The location of the bridging veins is an important factor in determining a right or left approach too.

As an example, angiography in a 57-year-old male with subarachnoid hemorrhage (SAH) grade III revealed a left A2–A3 aneurysm directed superiorly. The venous phase showed the right side had fewer bridging veins above the aneurysm than the left side. The aneurysm was located on the left A2 (**Fig. 10–2**). However, aneurysm clipping was not affected by the side of approach. Therefore, the right unilateral interhemispheric approach was selected (**Fig. 10–3**).

Another factor in choosing the craniotomy side is the location of the hematoma in the acute stage.

Anesthesia

We routinely use general anesthesia with endotracheal intubation, normotension, and normo- or hypothermia (35–36°C).

Neurophysiological Monitoring

We routinely use only an intraoperative Doppler probe to test the flow rate of intracranial vessels.

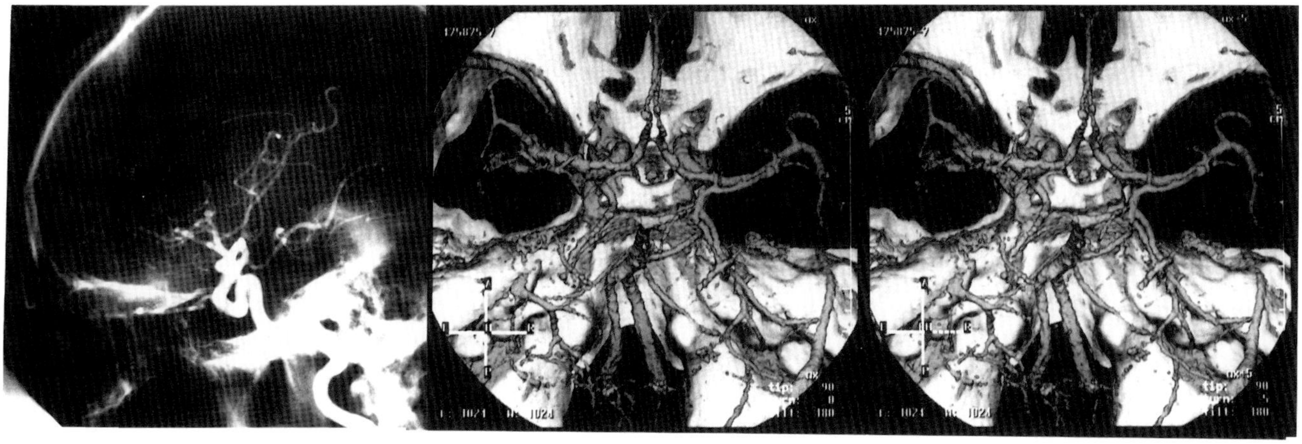

Figure 10–1 Preoperative examination using digital subtraction angiography and three-dimensional computed tomographic (3D-CT) angiography is useful in showing the aneurysm location and direction. In this case, the aneurysm is located under the corpus callosum. 3D-CT shows a stereoscopic view. For this case we approach through the transcrista galli or use the basal interhemispheric approach.

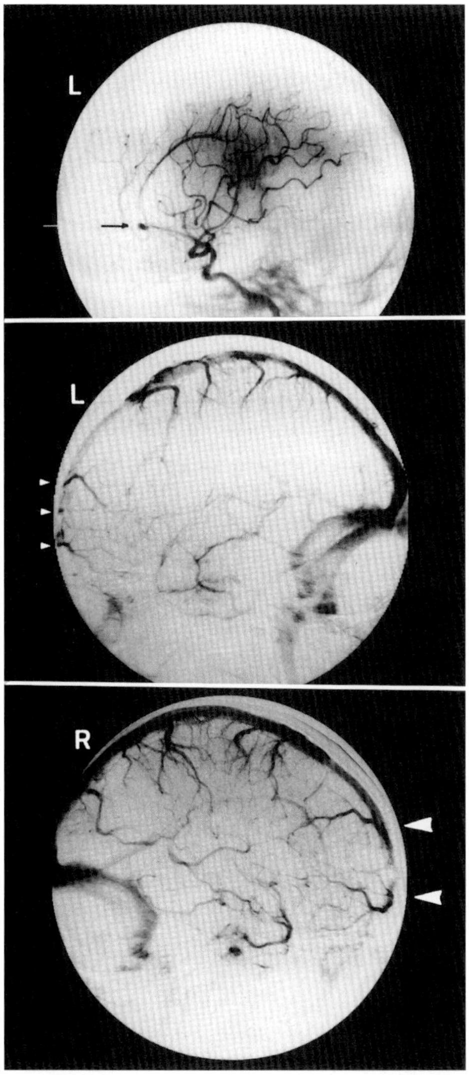

Figure 10–2 A 57-year-old male has a left A2–A3 aneurysm directed superiorly. Venous phase angiography shows there are three bridging veins in the left frontal area and two bridging veins in the right frontal area. The operative field is better with a right interhemispheric approach than with a left one.

Position

The patient is positioned supine with the upper body elevated ~30 degrees. The head is fixed at 0 to 10 degrees, with the chin up and rotated to the contralateral side of the craniotomy ~5 to 15 degrees.

Craniotomy

The craniotomy site must be decided by the location of the bridging veins above the aneurysm. The superficial veins

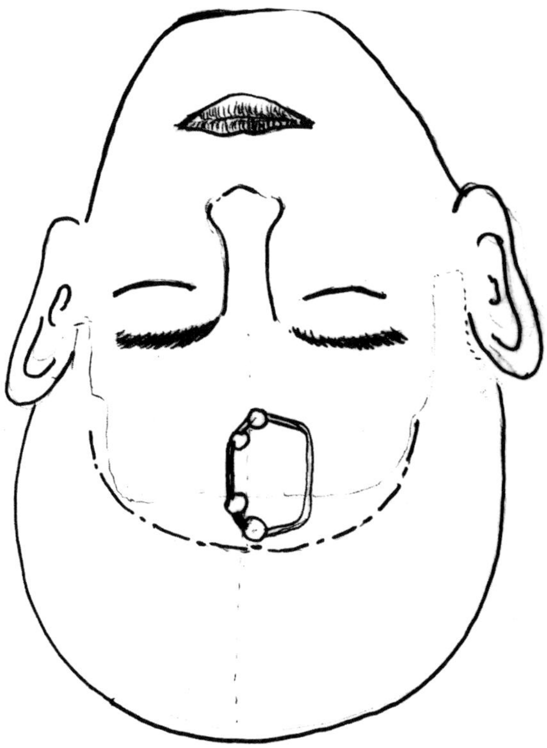

Figure 10–3 Skin incision and craniotomy for the transcrista galli interhemispheric approach.

indicate the surgeon's approach to the aneurysm. The surgeon must determine the direction and distance from the superficial vein to the aneurysm by using an angiogram.

The craniotomy must cross the midline so that the operative field can be enlarged medially 5 to 6 mm by retraction. This enlargement of the operative field is very important.

Four bur holes are drilled bilaterally on both sides of the superior sagittal sinus. Bur holes on the contralateral side must be opened close to each other and not parallel to the ipsilateral bur holes. This is essential not for the craniotomy but for retraction of the superior sagittal sinus (SSS). The short distance between contralateral bur holes minimizes the risk of lacerating the dura, the pacchionian granulations, and the SSS. Two anterior bur holes next to the SSS can be substituted with a bur hole over the SSS because the anterior part of the SSS is narrow and has low blood flow. One of the two lateral bur holes is made anteriorly and the second posteriorly. Only one lateral bur hole is needed for the dural dissection (**Fig. 10–4**).

Dural Dissection

It is important to perform adequate dural dissection via the bur holes. Craniotomy should begin with the safer lateral part followed by the contralateral part parallel to the SSS, and finally traversed over the SSS. Before the final craniotomy, titanium miniplates are fixed covering the bur holes. Each miniplate should be fixed on the bone flap with one screw to shorten the operative time. The bone flap is reflected during dissection of the dura, especially over the SSS.

To treat bleeding from the SSS, if the dura is not expanded and the bleeding point is small, the surgeon may coagulate with a weak monopolar or bipolar coagulation. When bleeding is not controlled by coagulation, or the bleeding point is large a small piece of Oxycel with fibrin glue should be put on the bleeding point covered by a large piece of Oxycel.

Tenting sutures must be done, especially around the meningeal arteries. Before the dural opening, complete hemostasis must be accomplished. The dural opening starts from the lateral side and progresses to the medial side close to the anteroposterior edge of the SSS. The surgeon must pay attention to the bridging veins, which may be attached to the dura. Dural sutures should be done to pull the dura up to prevent blood flow into the operative field.

Intradural Procedures

The surgeon must first check the location of veins to determine the direction of the aneurysm. Once the surgeon is oriented to the surface anatomy of the brain, a collagen sponge is placed on the surface of the brain for protection.

The interhemispheric fissure is retracted along the falx by spatula; sometimes small cortical vessels attached to the falx at that point can be cut. Beneath the falx edge, the interhemispheric fissure must be dissected by cutting the arachnoid membrane. The ipsilateral callosomarginal artery and cingulate gyrus are observed. When the interhemispheric fissure is dissected more deeply, the white-colored corpus callosum and bilateral pericallosal arteries are observed.

At the branching point of this pericallosal artery and callosomarginal artery, an A2–A3 aneurysm can be located. The parent artery of A2 comes up around the corpus callosum. To secure the A2 first, the aneurysm must be approached from the front.

Exposure and Clipping of the Aneurysm

A distal ACA aneurysm is usually located on the branching point of the pericallosal and callosomarginal arteries. The clip is usually applied parallel to the pericallosal artery (**Fig. 10–5**). The distal ACA is small, so maintaining blood flow is important. Blood flow must be checked with a Doppler flowmeter. If the artery is stenotic, the clip must be replaced by a temporary clip or a tentative clip.

In the case of an acute-stage aneurysm, the hematoma must be removed by suction and irrigation. Bipolar Jet irrigation is useful in this instance.

The hematoma is usually located in the cingulate gyrus, corpus callosum, and/or the ventricle. For removal of the hematoma, it is best to select the size of the suction probe according to the size of the hematoma. In the case of a large hematoma, a large suction probe is helpful.

After removing most of the hematoma, the suction probe must be exchanged for a smaller one for hemostasis to prevent injury of the small vessels. Hemostasis must be completed with irrigation of the bipolar system.

Closure

The dura mater is closed watertight. If there is a small defect in the dura, fascia is helpful. If there is a large defect in the dura, Gore-Tex membrane is used, which is sutured with Gore-Tex string and covered by Dexon mesh with fibrin glue. A mixture of either or both Betadine and antibiotic powder can be used to prevent infection. The flap is fixed using titanium miniplates, especially over the bur holes. The galea is sutured and the skin closed with skin staples.

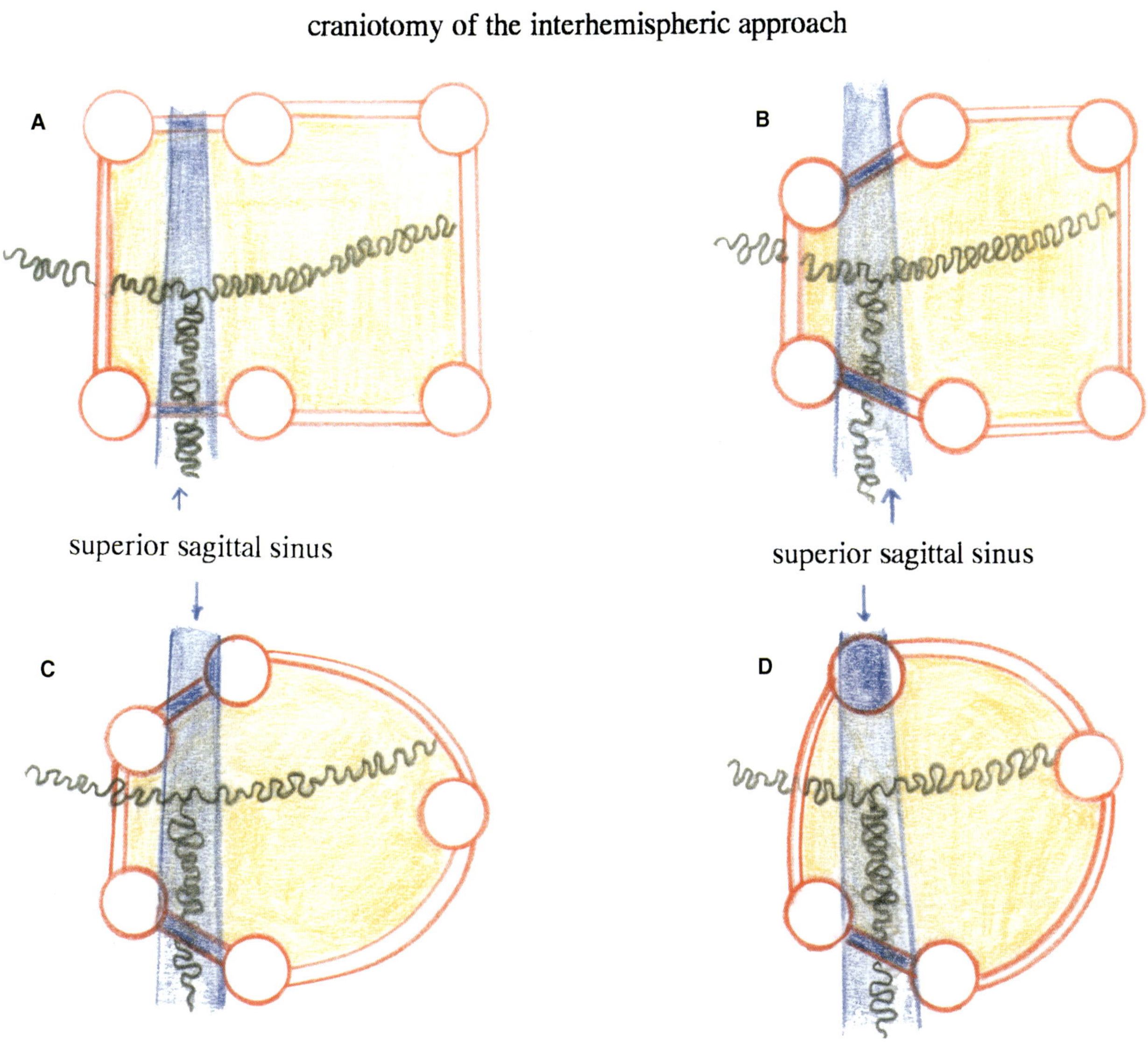

Figure 10–4 Craniotomy of the right interhemispheric approach. **(A)** The classic bur holes for an interhemispheric approach. **(B)** The approximation of the contralateral parasagittal bur holes to minimize the risk of injury of dural superior sagittal sinus. **(C)** After using the craniotome, the lateral two bur holes can be omitted into one bur hole. **(D)** The two anterior parasagittal bur holes can be joined into one because the anterior part of the sinus is narrow with low blood flow. **(C)** and **(D)** are recommended.

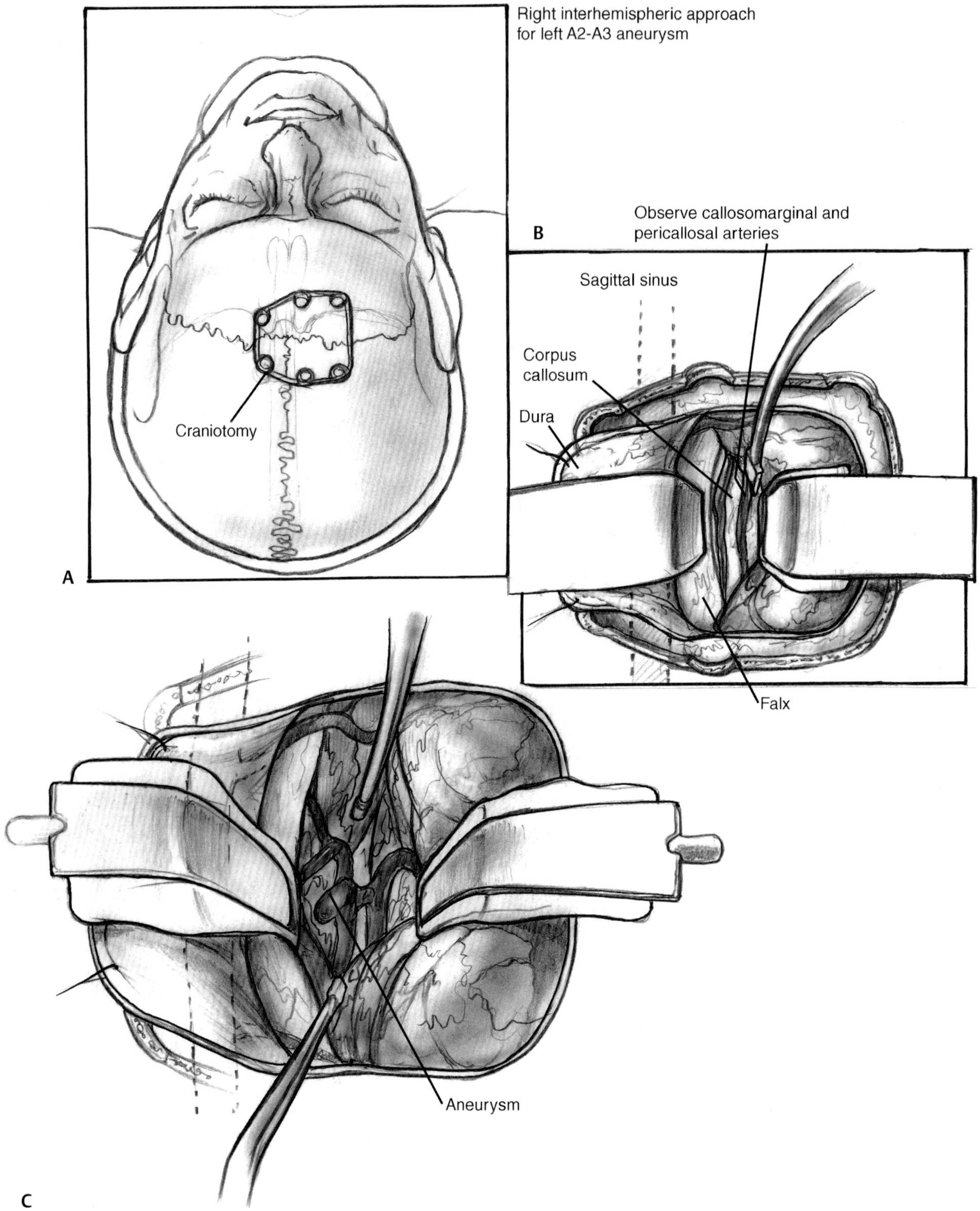

Figure 10–5 Right interhemispheric approach for left A2–A3 aneurysm. The callosomarginal and pericallosal arteries are observed. The parent artery comes up behind the corpus callosum. The aneurysm was clipped with a titanium slightly curved Yasargil miniclip (Aesculap; Tuttingen, Germany). Blood flow was examined by echosonography.

◆ Distal Middle Cerebral Artery Aneurysms

Preparation

DSA is an essential tool, not only in the arterial phase but also in the venous phase, especially with sylvian veins. Location must be decided by using anteroposterior, oblique, and lateral views of the angiography. 3D-CT angiography is useful to recognize the aneurysm location in anterior, middle, or posterior sylvian, Aneurysm size and direction are also important.

Position

We use the supine position with elevation of the upper body at ~30 degrees and the legs elevated to help venous return. The head is fixed at ~5 to 10 degrees with the chin up and rotated to the contralateral side of the cra-niotomy ~45 degrees.

The craniotomy must be done centering on the sylvian fissure. The posterosuperior end must be taken with enough length. The question mark skin incision starts at 5 mm anterior to the external auditory meatus and extends forward to the lateral forehead behind the hairline. One bur hole is opened above the sylvian fissure at the posterior end of the skin incision.

The dura is separated from the bone using a dural dissector or a 5 mm wide spatula. During the dissection of the dura, the surgeon can feel the inner surface of the bone at the tip of the dissector.

After the dissection of the dura, the craniotomy is done using a craniotome in an oval or long heart shape centering over the sylvian fissure. Before reflection of the craniotomy flap, one titanium miniplate is usually placed on the bur hole, and two are placed on the frontal and temporal end of the craniotomy. These miniplates are placed on the flap side so as not to disturb the operative field, and operative time is shortened (**Fig. 10–6**).

Hemostasis of the dura must be completed by coagulation of the meningeal arteries, Oxycel with fibrin glue, and tenting of the dura. After complete hemostasis, the dura is opened in a Y shape, and the edge of the dura is pulled up with sutures to prevent extradural blood flow into the operative field.

Intradural Procedure

To begin, the surgeon must watch the brain surface to establish orientation. In this type of aneurysm, the sylvian fissure must be separated widely. When opening the sylvian fissure, the surgeon must watch to know which part is less invasive for the veins. The arachnoid membrane is cut with a needle arachnoid knife, which is usually a 22 gauge needle in a holder. Mild coagulation of the arachnoid membrane is necessary to create tension because tensile tissues are easily cut by the needle arachnoid knife, but soft, loose tissues are not.

The posterior sylvian fissure is very deep, but the surgeon must separate the fissure as much as possible. When the sylvian fissure is widely opened, the operative field becomes shallow. To avoid injury to the pia mater, or if it is injured, apply Surgicel for protection. Temporal or frontal arteries can be followed to the main trunk of the MCA. Then the parent artery may be secured by comparing 3D-CT angiography or DSA.

Follow the parent artery distally to find the aneurysm; however, the main problem is that the operative field is deep, and the neck must be dissected (**Fig. 10–7**).

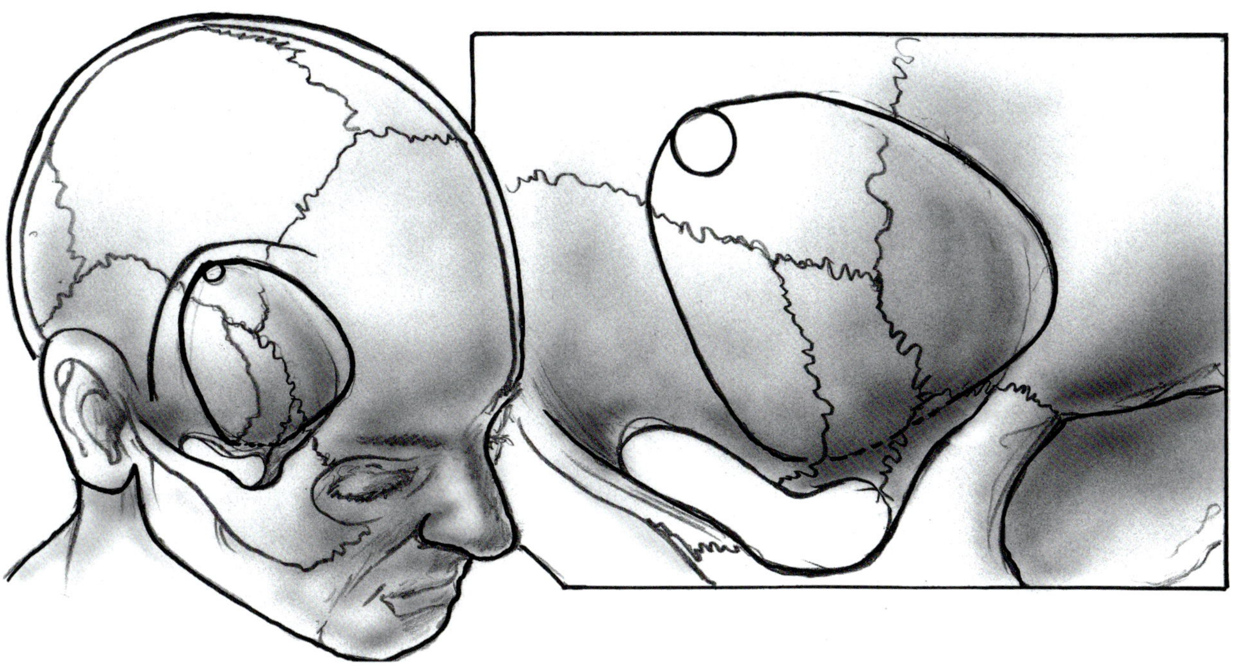

Figure 10–6 Craniotomy of a distal middle cerebral artery aneurysm. The craniotomy was centered over the sylvian fissure.

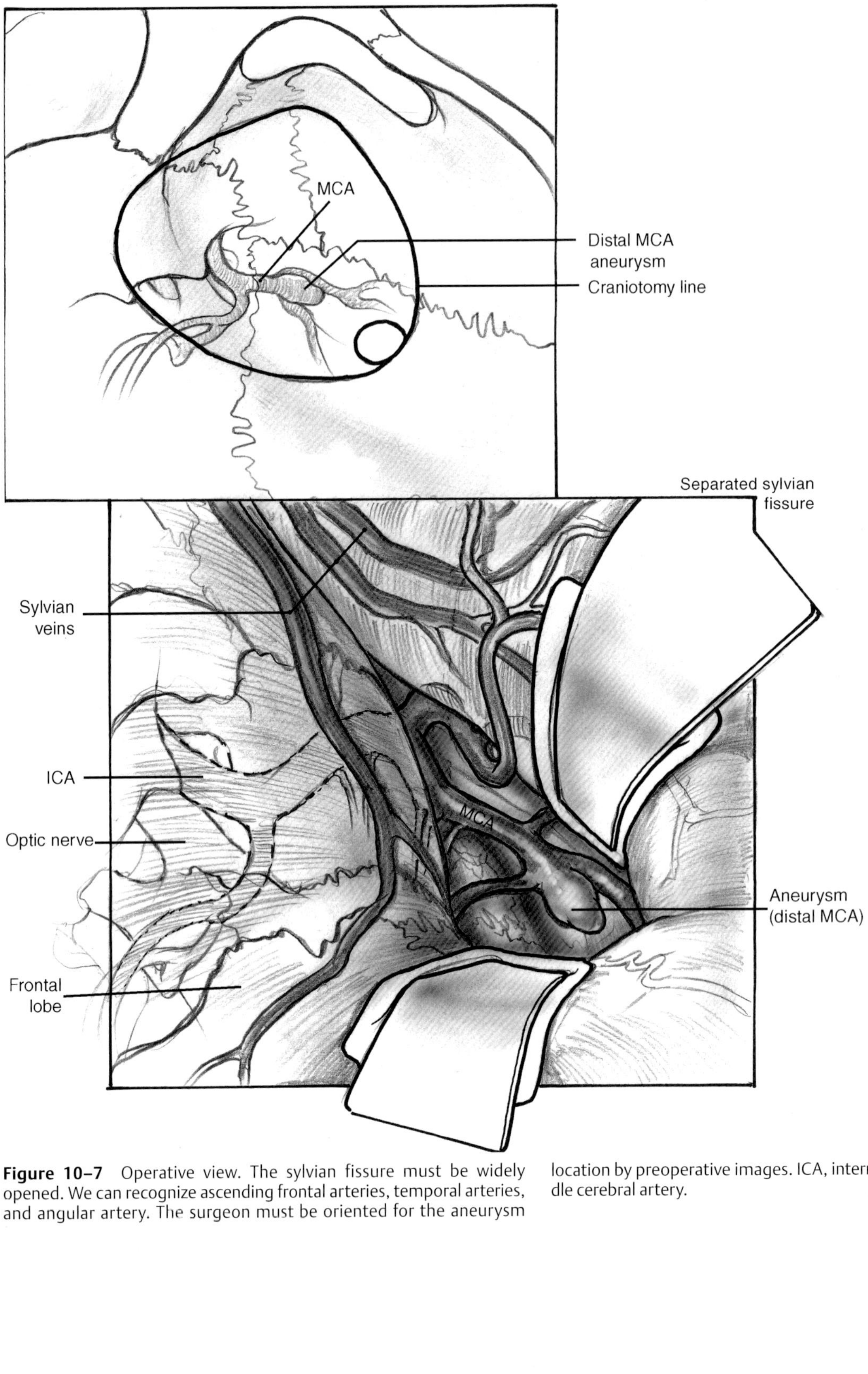

Figure 10–7 Operative view. The sylvian fissure must be widely opened. We can recognize ascending frontal arteries, temporal arteries, and angular artery. The surgeon must be oriented for the aneurysm location by preoperative images. ICA, internal carotid artery; MCA, middle cerebral artery.

Exposure and Clipping of the Aneurysm

The deep operative field creates the biggest problem in such a lesion. In cases of small-sized aneurysms, the clipping pattern depends on the direction of the aneurysm. If the aneurysm is located behind the arteries, a fenestrated clip is sometimes useful.

In cases of large aneurysms, reconstruction of the M3 artery is sometimes difficult because of the patency of the small artery. In such cases, an aneurysmectomy and anastomosis are two options.

Closure

The dura mater is closed watertight; if there is a dural defect, fascia is useful to obliterate the defect. The bone flap is fixed with a miniplate that is applied to the bone flap. The muscle and galea are sutured, and the skin is closed with skin staples.

◆ Postoperative Care

Our postoperative care is the usual for major intracranial surgery. In severe SAH cases, postoperative monitoring includes intracranial pressure and transcranial Doppler.

◆ Complications

The most serious complications can be intraoperative premature rupture and occlusion of arteries by the clip. These approaches can be inadvertently compromised by regional bridging veins or the superior sagittal sinus itself, or regular venous channels in the sylvian fissure. These complications are treated in the usual way. Arterial occlusions can be avoided by endovascular inspection after clipping because the operative field is usually deeper than that of the commonly located proximal aneurysms. In peripheral locations, before clipping is more important to gain good proximal control of the parent vessel.

Suggested Readings

Kato Y, Sano H, Katada K, et al. The usefulness of helical scanning CT (HES-CT), particularly 3-dimensional (3-D) CT endoscopy, for the decision of aneurysm treatment. No Shinkei Geka 1995;23:685–691

Sano H. Middle cerebral aneurysm. In: Abe H, ed. Operation for Neurosurgical Diseases and the Indication. Vol 2. , Tokyo: Asakura Shoten; 1990:56–83

Sano H, Hoshino M, Ishiyama N, Kato Y, Kanno T, Adachi K. Utility of dome coagulation technique at clipping of aneurysms. In: Proceedings of the 12th Conference of Surgical Treatment of Stroke. Tokyo: Nyuuronsya; 1983:237–241,

Sano H, Ishiyama N, Kato Y, et al. How to approach the cerebral aneurysms. In: Proceedings of the 12th Conference of Surgical Treatment of Stroke. Tokyo: Nyuuronsya; 1983:85–87

Sano H, Kato Y, Zhou J, et al. New jet irrigation bipolar system. Neurosurgery 1996;38:1251–1253

Sano H, Nagata J, Kato Y, Katada K, Kanno T, Adachi K. Operation of cerebral aneurysms in the acute stage. In: Proceedings of the 12th Conference of Surgical Treatment of Stroke. Tokyo: Nyuuronsya; 1983:105–110

Yasargil MG. Microneurosurgery. Vol 2 Clinical Considerations, Surgery of the Intracranial Aneurysms and Results. Stuttgart: Georg Thieme; 1984:124–164, 224–231

11

Basilar Tip Aneurysms

Michael Horowitz, Thomas Kopitnik, and Duke Samson

Basilar apex aneurysms represent only ~5 to 7% of all intracranial saccular aneurysms. Their deep location, complex surrounding vascular anatomy, and rarity make successful surgical treatment difficult.

◆ Anatomy

The basilar apex, located within the interpeduncular cistern, is a complex region with a variety of nomenclatures used to describe its anatomy. The portion of the basilar artery situated between the summit and the ostium of the posterior communicating artery (PCommA) is referred to as the P1 segment of the posterior cerebral artery (PCA), mesencephalic artery, or basilar communicating artery.[1] The portion of the PCA distal to the PCommA is referred to as the P2 segment or the PCA proper.[1] It lies within the peduncular and ambient cisterns and runs from the PCommA origin to the level of the posterior midbrain.[2]

The PCommA commonly gives rise to the polar or anterior thalamoperforating arteries, which supply portions of the optic chiasm, tuber cinereum, mammillary bodies, posterior hypothalamus, subthalamic nucleus, posterior internal capsule, cerebral peduncle, and ventral and paraventricular thalamic nuclei. In 30 to 75% of cases the PCommA does not contribute significantly to the thalamic circulation.[1] The basilar apex (P1) gives rise to the posterior thalamoperforating vessels of Foix and Hillemand that supply the thalamus, hypothalamus, subthalamic nucleus, and posterior limb of the internal capsule. These vessels may arise as a sheath of arteries, each taking its origin directly from the posterior P1 wall as a single vessel that initially exits the basilar apex and then arborizes into numerous arteries, or from an arterial arcade that connects the two P1s.[1] Often the number of anterior and posterior perforant vessels and the areas they supply have a reciprocal relationship in that the presence of numerous anterior perforators is accompanied by a paucity of posterior perforators and vice versa.

◆ Indications

The patients are assessed by the Hunt and Hess grading scale. In our practice, the majority of patients with Hunt and Hess scores I to IV are treated within 24 hours of admission using either surgical or endovascular techniques. More urgent treatment is reserved for those patients with a life-threatening intraparenchymal hematoma. Our choice of procedure depends upon the individual patient's vascular anatomy and neurological and medical condition.

◆ Treatment

Approach

Direct surgical repair of a basilar apex aneurysm was first described by Gillingham in 1958 and then by Drake in 1961.[3,4] Both surgeons used a subtemporal approach with modest initial success (50% mortality in Drake's initial series of four patients). Drake ultimately perfected his technique and reported excellent clinical results in the majority of treated patients. The actual procedure for subtemporal basilar apex aneurysm clipping is well described by Crowell and Ogilvy.[5] We favor the pterional (sylvian) or half-and-half approaches as opposed to the subtemporal approach. We feel such procedures afford us greater ability to control the basilar artery prior to aneurysm dissection, more working room, and better access to and visualization of the contralateral posterior cerebral and superior cerebellar arteries both to aid final aneurysm clipping and to allow for expedient afferent and efferent vessel temporary clipping should aneurysm rupture occur. Although visualization of the perforating vessels may be slightly hindered by the more frontal vector, we are able to identify and free the vessels by moving in a temporal direction as the case proceeds.

Alternative Therapies

Although direct surgical clipping remains the gold standard for aneurysm treatment and as such is the focus of this chapter, the reader must not forget that alternative therapies are available in the management of these difficult lesions. In 1993, Steinberg et al published the London, Ontario, experience with deliberate basilar or vertebral artery occlusion for the treatment of posterior circulation aneurysms. Eighty-three basilar apex and superior cerebellar artery aneurysms were treated in this manner, with 57% excellent and 7% good outcomes. Five percent and 31% of treated patients had poor outcomes or died, respectively.[6] As an alternative to open surgical clipping, endovascular embolization of basilar apex aneurysms using Guglielmi detachable coils (GDCs) is coming into vogue. Five series reporting the results of such treatments have demonstrated a 0 to 4.1% rebleeding rate over a follow-up period of less than 5 years.[7–11] Endovascular treatment has the advantages of a less invasive procedure with generally shorter treatment times. Disadvantages include aneurysm recurrence, especially with large and partially thrombosed lesions and an unknown long-term track record. Indications for endovascular therapy vary from institution to institution and from surgeon to surgeon even within the same center. As of yet, no hard-and-fast rules exist concerning which patients should undergo open surgery and which should undergo embolization.

◆ Preparation

Imaging

All patients at our institution undergo preoperative head computed tomography (CT) scanning and cerebral angiography. The former is performed to assess ventricular size (presence or absence of hydrocephalus), subarachnoid clot thickness (Fisher grade), aneurysm consistency (presence or absence of neck or fundal calcium, intra-aneurysmal thrombus), frontal sinus size and location, and presence or absence of an intraparenchymal hematoma. Cerebral angiography is generally performed using digital and biplanar technology. It is imperative to identify all anterior and posterior vessel bifurcations including both postero-inferior cerebellar arteries so that additional aneurysm can be identified. It is also critical to note the presence and size of the PCommAs as well as the existence of fetal PCAs. The common carotid bifurcations are filmed as well to identify those patients with significant cervical internal carotid artery hemodynamic lesions, which may put the patient at risk for embolic events or limit flow across a patent PCommA. The basilar apex is imaged and filmed using transfacial, Towne's, and Stenver's views so that the relationship of the aneurysm neck with the PCAs is clearly elucidated prior to beginning treatment. We are also cognizant of identifying the position of the aneurysm neck in relation to the dorsum sellae, the direction in which the aneurysm points, the relative heights of the PCAs (which side has the higher PCA), aneurysm size, and shape.

Preoperative magnetic resonance (MR) scanning can occasionally be useful. We tend to reserve MR scanning for the evaluation of large, complex lesions to better visualize an aneurysm's position relative to the brain stem as well as to identify the extent of intrafundal thrombus. MR can also be useful in evaluating the extent of brain stem injury in a patient with a poor neurological examination to help determine whether irreversible damage has occurred. Such findings can assist in the decision to withhold additional care.

Although three-dimensional CT angiography often provides impressive images, we have not found it to be particularly useful in the surgical management of basilar apex aneurysms. The rare cases where it has been helpful have been in giant lesions that we suspect have incorporated the PCA and possibly the superior cerebellar artery (SCA) origins into the fundus. Occasionally a CT angiogram will confirm our suspicions and help us determine whether the lesion is treatable.

Importance of Imaging Findings

The presence of particular findings on preoperative imaging is more than just of academic interest. Our particular concerns are listed here.

Aneurysm height relative to the dorsum sellae: When the aneurysm neck lies within 1 to 1.5 cm rostral or caudal to the dorsum sellae, it is generally accessible through a routine sylvian and half-and-half exposure, as will be described later. When the neck is located more than 1.5 cm caudal, it may require a transcavernous exposure of the basilar artery to obtain proximal basilar control and neck visualization. When located more than 1.5 cm rostral, resection of the zygoma may be required to allow the surgeon to look up at the neck. These techniques will be discussed later in the chapter.

Aneurysm projection: A posteriorly projecting basilar apex aneurysm is a more difficult operation because the fundus lies in close opposition to the posterior thalamoperforating vessels. The surgeon can therefore expect to spend more time freeing these vessels from the aneurysm wall prior to clipping and will generally have to hold the neck and fundus forward while applying the clip so that perforators are not inadvertently occluded.

Posterior cerebral artery heights: Although we generally prefer to operate from the right side for reasons that will be discussed later, it is important to note the PCAs' relative positions to one another. During clipping it is easier to visualize, control, and avoid occluding the opposite PCA if it is lower than the ipsilateral PCA. The chance of inadvertent clipping is reduced both due to better visualization of a lower contralateral PCA and due to the angle at which the clip blades approach the aneurysm neck using a sylvian approach. For these reasons, a significantly lower right PCA might persuade us to approach the aneurysm from the left.

PCommA condition: The presence or absence of PCommAs is important for several reasons. As we will discuss later, we tend to divide the ipsilateral PCommA, when necessary, to improve our exposure. When working lateral to the supraclinoid internal carotid artery (ICA), division of the PCommA allows the surgeon to move the ICA more medially and the ipsilateral PCA more posteriorly and laterally, thus providing more room at the bottom of the dissection to introduce scissors and clip appliers. The presence of an ipsilateral fetal PCA, however, makes such division impossible. The presence of a PCommA can also help salvage a case. If the aneurysm neck is torn at its contralateral base, for example, the contralateral P1 segment can be included in the clip blades to help close the rent, knowing that the contralateral PCA will continue to be irrigated by the contralateral PCommA. This converts the basilar quadrification into a trifurcation.

Intra-aneurysmal thrombus and neck/wall calcification: The presence of intrafundal thrombus indicates to the surgeon that complete temporary trapping and thrombectomy may well be necessary to permit clip occlusion of the neck. Without thrombectomy the surgeon risks being unable to completely occlude the aneurysm with the clip and risks having the clip slide down the fundus and occlude the PCAs and perforators. Calcium also makes clip application more problematic and neck damage more likely. The presence of either of these findings should raise a red flag. More than 20 minutes of temporary occlusion will likely be required to clip this lesion, making the option of hypothermic circulatory arrest a consideration. Although the presence of thrombus makes recanalization after GDC embolization more likely, the presence of neck calcification in a nonthrombotic aneurysm may make the surgeon consider this treatment option.

CT findings: The presence of hydrocephalus indicates that the patient may be better than the Hunt and Hess score indicates were the hydrocephalus to be treated. While this is not particularly important to us when dealing with a grade I to III patient, it is important with a grade IV to V patient whose score may be determining the type of therapy offered. The size of a patient's frontal sinuses does not affect our craniotomy but does determine whether we prepare the abdomen for a possible fat harvest. The presence of a large intraparenchymal hematoma, a rare occurrence with basilar aneurysms, makes accurate Hunt and Hess grading impossible. Emergent surgery may be performed in the face of a life-threatening hematoma. Coiling would not be offered.

Anesthesia

Although excellent anesthesia will not make up for shoddy surgical technique, it cannot be too overemphasized that the quality of the neuroanesthetic is directly related to the overall surgical result. The principal anesthetic management goals for aneurysm surgery are prevention of intraoperative rupture or rebleeding and protection against cerebral ischemia. Other goals include brain relaxation, continued management of the patient's ongoing medical problems, and rapid recovery from anesthesia for a timely postoperative neurological evaluation.

Premedication

In patients with Hunt and Hess grade 0 or I, premedication with a benzodiazepine anxiolytic (e.g., midazolam 1 to 2 mg IV) is reasonable. Hunt and Hess grade III patients are not further sedated for fear of depressing respiration. Grade IV or V patients are generally intubated, making respiratory depression a nonissue. Following sedation, blood pressure (BP), respiratory rate, and oxygenation are carefully monitored. Prophylaxes against pulmonary aspiration (ranitidine 150 mg PO or 50 mg IV; metoclopramide 10 mg PO or IV) are usually given.

Monitors

Routine intraoperative monitoring includes noninvasive BP device, five lead electrocardiogram (EKG), pulse oximeter, esophageal stethoscope, temperature probe, Foley catheter, capnograph, peripheral nerve stimulator, arterial catheter, and central venous catheter. A precordial Doppler and a multiport central venous catheter are used for detection and possible treatment of venous air embolism. A pulmonary artery catheter is warranted in patients with congestive heart failure or decreased left ventricular function, and those who are being treated for vasospasm. Defibrillator pads are placed in case of dysrhythmia during cooling, and leads for compressed spectral array electroencephalogram (EEG) are placed to monitor burst suppression.

Induction

The primary anesthetic goal at induction is minimization of the risk of intraoperative aneurysm rupture. Sudden increases in systemic arterial BP and sudden decreases in intracranial pressure must be avoided. Prolonged periods of hypotension are also avoided because they may lower cerebral perfusion in patients with increased intracranial pressure (ICP).

Induction proceeds with gradual increase in anesthetic depth. After monitors are placed, the awake patient is denitrogenated with 100% oxygen by face mask. (Denitrogenation is omitted if the patient is already intubated and ventilated.) Induction is accomplished with propofol (1–2 mg/kg IV). Etomidate (0.2–0.5 mg/kg IV) may be administered should the patient have any cardiac risk or be hemodynamically unstable. A small dose of sufentanil (10 µg IV) is given initially, followed by a low-dose infusion of alfentanil (0.25–0.5 µg/kg/min) or remifentanil (0.125 µg/kg/min) to blunt the hemodynamic response to laryngoscopy. Muscle paralysis is provided by one of many nondepolarizing muscle relaxants with stable cardiovascular profile such as rocuronium (0.8 mg/kg IV), vecuronium (0.1 mg/kg IV), pipecuronium (0.07 mg/kg IV), or cisatracurium (0.2 mg/Kg IV). The patient is then hyperventilated with oxygen, nitrous oxide (N_2O), and isoflurane [1 minimum alveolar concentration

(MAC) or less] until intubation. Boluses of short-acting opioids like alfentanil and remifentanil are used to temporarily increase the anesthetic depth to prevent the hypertensive response during laryngoscopy and intubation. Alternatively, short-acting [short-acting and renergic] adrenergic antagonists such as esmoo (10 mg increments IV) or vasodilators such as nitroprusside or nitroglycerin (50 μg increments IV) are also effective in blunting the sympathetic response. Longer-acting agents or high-concentration inhalational anesthetics are avoided because they can lead to prolonged periods of hypotension after the transient sympathetic response has subsided.

Maintenance

A balanced anesthetic technique using oxygen, N_2O, isoflurane, opioid, and a nondepolarizing muscle relaxant is used. Hemodynamic goals are to avoid wide swings in BP and to control ICP at periods of intense stimulation, which include head pinning, skin incision, craniotomy, dural incision, and skin closure. Short-acting opioids will allow for rapid deepening of anesthesia. Local anesthetic infiltration before head pinning and skin incision can reduce the hemodynamic response.

Other goals are directed at providing optimal surgical conditions and protection against brain ischemia. A relaxed brain is needed for maximal exposure of the surgical site and to minimize brain-retraction pressure. Diuresis, hyperventilation, and placing the patient in the head-up position (if appropriate) are employed. Diuresis is established with mannitol (0.5–1 mg/kg IV) given ~30 minutes prior to dural incision. A rapid infusion of mannitol may cause a transient but significant reduction in systemic vascular resistance and blood pressure and can produce acute volume overload in patients with impaired cardiac function. Anticipation of potential complications and immediate treatment of hemodynamic changes are warranted in these patients. Furosemide, which does not lead to transient increase in intravascular volume, can be substituted in these patients. Significant fluid and electrolyte abnormalities can occur; therefore, volume status and electrolyte values are closely monitored and treated appropriately. Hyperventilation is aimed at maintaining the $PaCO_2$ at 25 to 30 torr.

Intraoperative fluid administration is guided by the patient's maintenance requirement, blood loss, and urine output. Because patients are aggressively diuresed, the urine output is not a good indicator of their volume status. The central venous pressure and pulmonary capillary wedge pressure followed as trends and other hemodynamic parameters such as BP and heart rate provide better guides of the intravascular volume. Iso-osmolar crystalloid and colloid can be used to replenish fluid loss. Hypo-osmolar solutions are avoided to prevent cerebral edema. Glucose-containing solutions are also not used because hyperglycemia may potentiate brain injury following brain ischemia.

Temporary Occlusion and Cerebral Protection

Frequently temporary arterial occlusion is used to facilitate aneurysm clipping. Such steps, however, can create ischemia in territories distal to the temporary clips. Many different methods are empirically used for "ischemic brain protection." The end point is indicated by the burst suppression pattern on the EEG monitor. Unfortunately, no randomized clinical trials have been done to systematically prove and evaluate their individual efficacies.

Mild to moderate hypothermia has demonstrated protection, but the protective value of hypothermia is not proportional to cerebral metabolic rate (CMR) depression. An alternative hypothesis proposes that cerebral protection from hypothermia may be conferred by preventing the release of neuroexcitatory transmitters triggered by ischemia.

At our institution, all the methods discussed above are combined into a "formula" that is empirically employed during temporary occlusion. Cooling the patient to 32 or 33°C by using cooling blankets is instituted immediately after induction. Glucose is carefully monitored and kept between 80 to 120 mg/dL. When the neurosurgeon requests burst suppression prior to placing temporary clips, several additional steps are taken. Mannitol (0.25 g/dL) is given as a free radical scavenger. N_2O is discontinued, the patient is ventilated with 100% O_2, and a hematocrit of at least 30% is maintained for optimal oxygen delivery. The patient is kept normotensive and normovolemic. The $PaCO_2$ is normalized from 25 to 30 torr to 35 to 40 torr to decrease cerebral vasoconstriction. Etomidate, propofol, or low-dose pentothal is given until a burst suppression pattern is noted on the EEG monitor. The choice of agent depends on the patient's cardiovascular status and physician's personal preference. When the temporary aneurysm clips have been applied, the patient's BP is raised 20% above baseline to increase collateral flow. This increase in BP can be accomplished by decreasing the concentration of the inhalational anesthetic agent or by administering a vasopressor. After temporary occlusion is completed, burst suppression is terminated, and anesthetic maintenance is resumed as before.

Emergence

The main goal for emergence is to allow for a smooth and rapid wake-up, thus facilitating neurological assessment. Coughing and straining are avoided. Emergence hypertension can cause bleeding at the surgical site and cerebral edema. BP can be controlled with rapidly titratable agents such as nitroprusside, nitroglycerin, esmolol, or labetalol. Patients with poor preoperative grades, those that were given a large amount of medications intraoperatively for burst suppression, those suspected with brain stem injury and lower cranial nerves damage, or those with cardiovascular instability may require sedation and continued ventilatory support.

Positioning

The procedure described following here will assume a right-sided approach. We prefer a right-sided approach if possible for a number of reasons. As right-handed surgeons, we find our ability to dissect and clip enhanced by a right trajectory. Because most patients are left hemisphere dominant, we prefer working beneath the right frontal lobe and medial to the right temporal lobe. The patient is positioned supine with the head placed in rigid pin fixation. A single pin is placed in the right mastoid, and two pins are placed

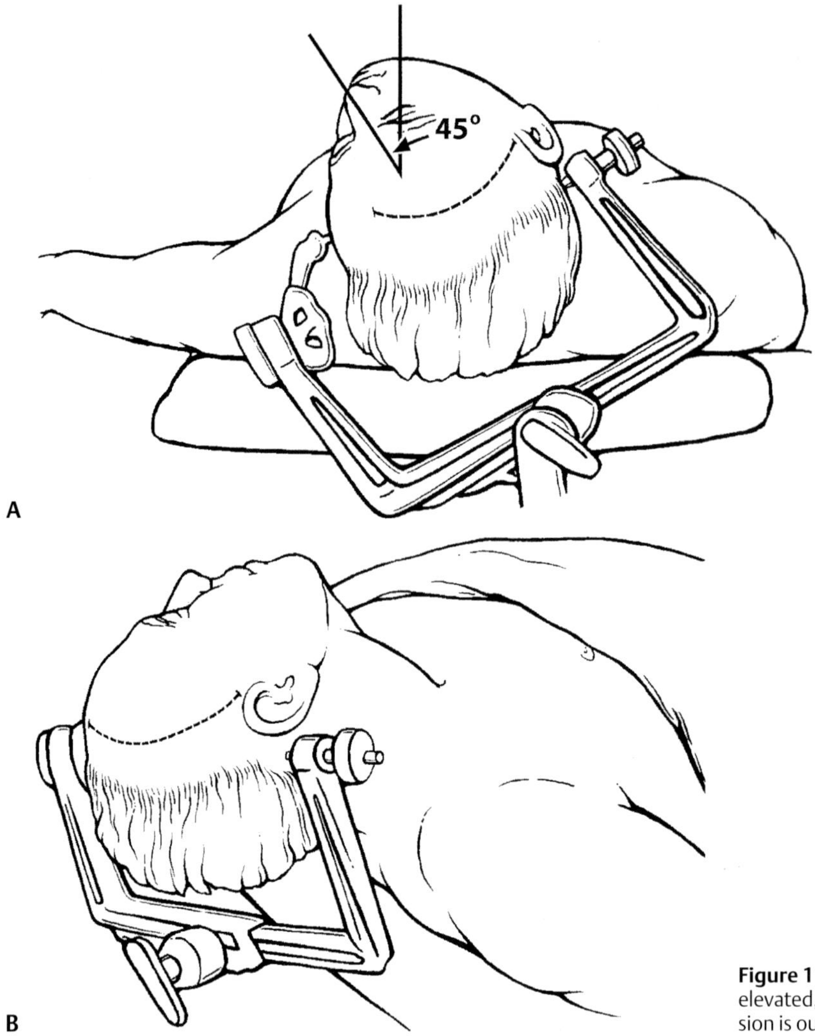

Figure 11–1 (A,B) The patient's head is positioned extended, elevated, and turned 45 degrees to the other side. The skin incision is outlined. Two views shown.

left frontally. The patient's head is rotated 45 degrees to the left, with the left ear flexed toward the left shoulder and the right malar eminence at the highest point of the operative field (**Fig. 11–1A,B**). Forty-five degrees of head rotation tends to rotate the posterior clinoids and clivus counterclockwise, making the basilar trunk more readily visible. Such rotation also provides the surgeon with the opportunity to approach the lesion from both a sylvian and a temporal direction. The right frontotemporal region is shaved and prepared with antiseptic and subsequently draped. Retractor arms and blades are connected to the table or head frame so they are ready in the advent of an early and unexpected aneurysm rupture. The microscope is draped prior to the skin incision so as to be ready at a moment's notice.

Incision

The skin is opened in a curvilinear fashion behind the hairline from a point 1 to 2 mm anterior to the tragus just above the zygoma to midline, and a single myocutaneous flap is reflected anteriorly to the level of the orbital rim. The flap is secured using fishhooks with a small sponge roll beneath the flap to avoid flap ischemia during prolonged inversion. Sponges are placed beneath the fishhook cables so that cable pressure on the face is avoided.

Craniotomy

Four bur holes—pterion, just above the zygoma, along the posterior temporal line, midfrontal at the level of the midpupillary line—are placed with the Midas Rex M8 bit (Medronic; Minneapolis, MN). The dura is freed from the inner surface of the skull using a Penfield no. 3 dissector, and the Midas Rex B1 foot plate bit is used to complete the craniotomy (**Fig. 11–2**).

The M8 is again used to generously drill the lateral sphenoid wing flat to the level of the superior orbital fissure. To assist with this, the meningo-orbital artery is coagulated and divided so that the temporal lobe dura can be retracted away from the wing. A moderate temporal craniectomy is performed using a Leksell rongeur to allow for temporal lobe retraction later in the case (**Fig. 11–3**). We have not found that orbital roof and rim resection improves our exposure.

Once the craniotomy is complete, hemostasis is achieved using bone wax and oxidized cellulose. A ¼ in. cottonoid strip is left with its tip near the superior orbital fissure and

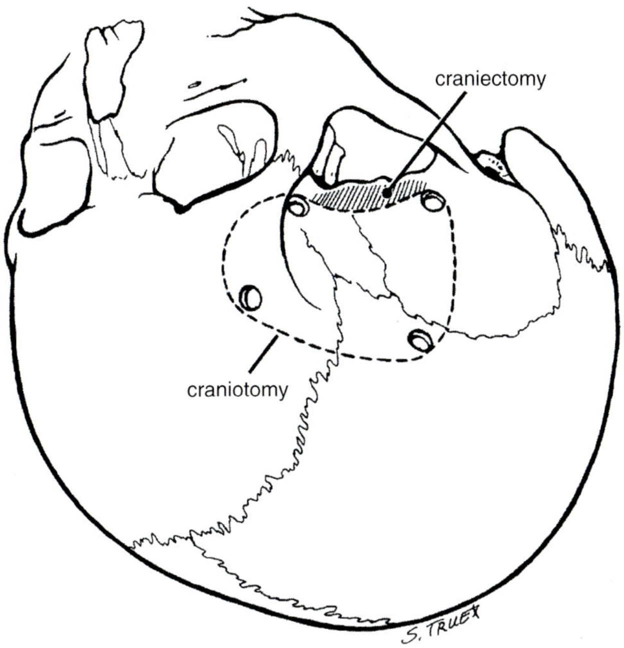

Figure 11–2 The extent of the craniotomy and craniectomy is shown.

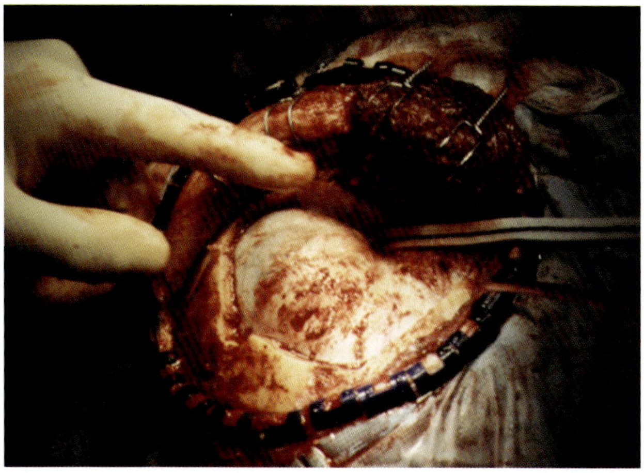

Figure 11–3 The exposure achieved after the craniotomy and craniectomy.

its distal end outside the incision at the base. This strip will wick any blood out of the space behind the dura when it is reflected anteriorly.

Dural Opening

The dura is opened widely in a curvilinear stellated fashion and reflected anteriorly and posteriorly with 4-0 tacking sutures attached to hemostats. Opening the dura and reflecting it posteriorly over the bone edge reduces epidural run-in during the case. Once the dura is opened, a ventriculostomy is inserted at Paine's point, and cere- brospinal fluid (CSF) is evacuated from the lateral ventricle[12] (**Fig. 11–4**). If possible we prefer to place our ventriculostomy at the time of surgery. We feel this provides superior brain relaxation as compared with drainage from a previously placed catheter and reduces the risk of preoperative aneurysm rerupture. If the brain is very full at the time of catheterization, the CSF can be evacuated slowly to avoid sudden brain shifting and intraoperative rupture.

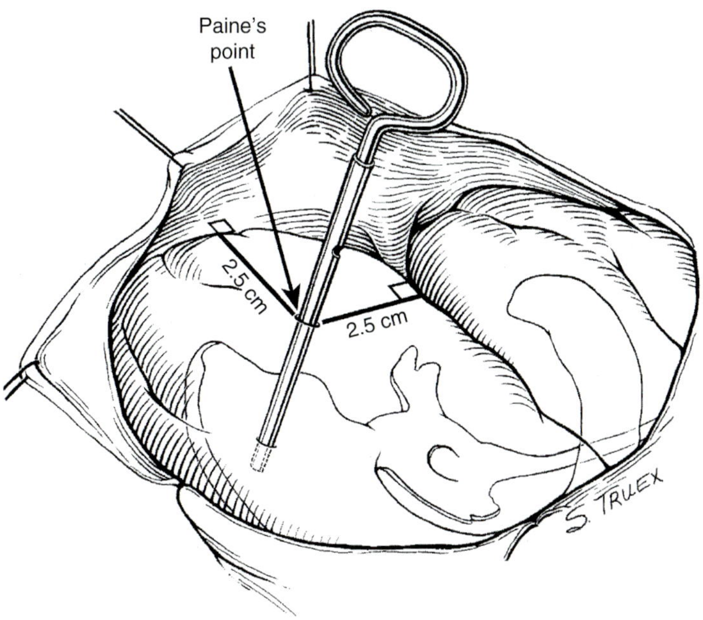

Figure 11–4 A ventriculostomy is placed into the frontal horn of the lateral ventricle, after incising the pia mater at Paine's point.

◆ Operative Procedure

Our approach to surgically clipping a basilar apex aneurysm is divided into a series of steps, one of which always follows the next in a regimented order. The ultimate goal is maximum exposure and working room deep at the level of the aneurysm neck and control of all afferent and efferent vessels.

Step1: The microscope is introduced to the operative field, the surgeon sits, and the table is left elevated. All bridging veins running from the sylvian fissure to the sphenoparietal sinus and anterior middle fossa dura are coagulated and divided so that the temporal lobe can be retracted later in the case without running the risk of avulsing the veins at their points of entry into the dura.

Step 2: The operating table is lowered. A self-retaining retractor blade is placed along the orbital frontal cortex at the level of the optic and carotid cisterns, and the cisterns are opened sharply using an arachnoid knife and microscissors.

Step 3: The sylvian fissure is opened in either a lateral to medial or medial to lateral direction until the anterior temporal branch of the middle cerebral artery (MCA) is identified. If the anterior choroidal artery and MCA anterior temporal branch are adherent to the uncus, they are sharply dissected free. At this point the supraclinoid ICA, PCommA origin anterior choroidal artery, ICA bifurcation, anterior temporal artery, and optic nerve are clearly visualized (**Fig. 11–5**).

Step 4: A self-retaining retractor is bent at 90 degrees, with its tip and blade gently retracting the temporal lobe laterally. The uncus bulges beneath the tip blade.

Step 5: The mesial temporal lobe and uncus are resected in a subpial fashion back to the level of the anterior temporal artery to completely expose the third cranial nerve (CN III). The pia is sharply dissected off CN III, and the retractor is placed with its tip against the anterior middle fossa dura so that the temporal lobe is gently retracted laterally, thus allowing the surgeon to visualize the arachnoid lateral to CN III (**Figs. 11–6** and **11–7**).

Step 6: The membrane of Lillequist is opened sharply with microscissors, as is the arachnoid lateral to CN III. All loose strands of arachnoid are cut so that exposure is maximized. The PCommA is now followed from its origin to its insertion into the PCA, which runs along the top surface of CN III. By looking lateral to and beneath CN III, one can locate the distal SCA and trace it to its origin with the basilar artery (**Fig 11–8**).

Step 7: Using sharp dissection along the PCA and SCA, the proximal basilar artery is identified. When operating on the right side, the artery, runs from 1 o'clock to 7 o'clock, and when working on the left side, it runs from 11 o'clock to 5 o'clock. The basilar trunk is dissected free and prepared for temporary clip application. Once the parent artery is sufficiently dissected, the surgeon practices placing the clip across the basilar from a vector lateral to and beneath CN III. When temporary clip application is made from this direction, the clip is completely out of the working area needed to clip the aneurysm.

Step 8: Proximal dissection along the basilar trunk permits identification of the contralateral SCA, which is prepared for temporary clipping. This can at times be difficult to distinguish from the contralateral PCA. Identification can be made easier both by reviewing the angiogram to better determine the projection of each vessel and by visu-

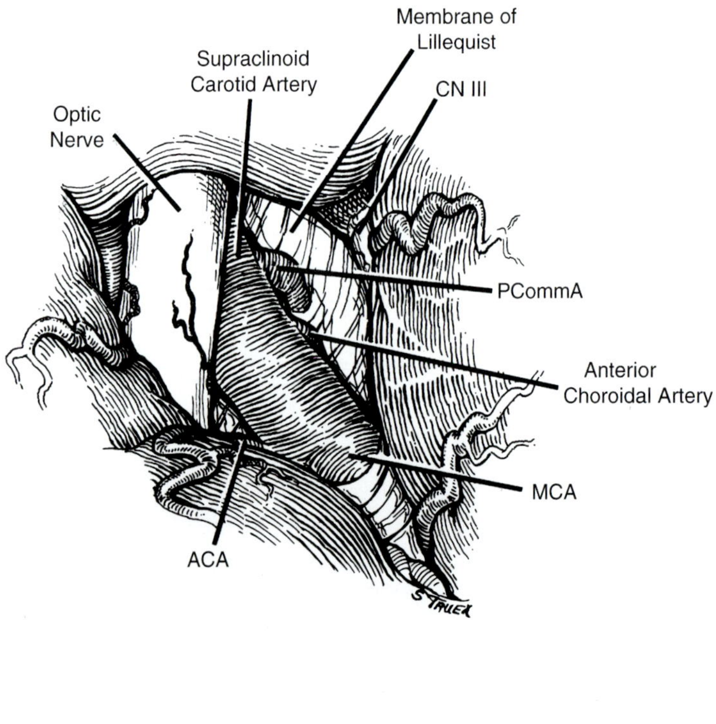

Figure 11–5 Opening carotid cistern.

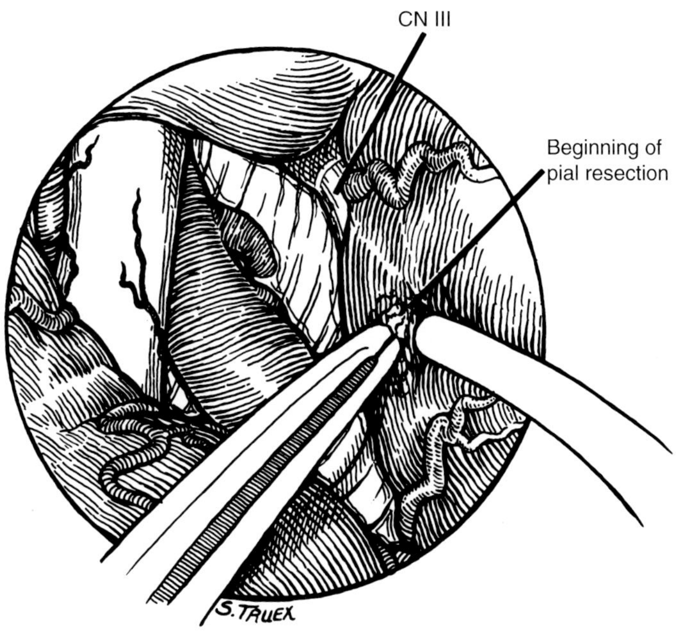

Figure 11–6 Resection of uncus.

alizing the contralateral CN III. The PCA runs above the nerve, while the SCA runs beneath it.

Step 9: If necessary for adequate visualization of the apex, the PCommA is now clipped at its insertion into the PCA using two small titanium vascular clips and divided. We prefer using vascular clips as opposed to bipolar cautery because the cautery often spreads to adjacent anterior thalamoperforators and inadvertently occludes them. Once the PCommA is divided, the ICA can be mobilized more medially, thus markedly improving access and visualization of the basilar apex and interpeduncular cistern (**Fig. 11–9**).

Step 10: At this point the anesthesiologist places the patient into burst suppression. While this is being achieved, the vessels are all auscultated using the microDoppler probe so that the surgeon knows what the patent vessel signals should sound like after the final clipping is achieved. As much dissection as is safely possible is done along the anterior and posterior aneurysm neck wall to identify the contralateral PCA and posterior thalamoperforators. When the surgeon feels the dissection is no longer safe, a temporary clip is introduced lateral to CN III and placed on the basilar trunk (**Fig. 11–10**). The fundus is palpated and decreased turgor should be felt. The dissection is completed by slowly reflecting the aneurysm anteriorly with the sucker while the perforators are displaced posteriorly away from the neck by gentle dissection with the microscissors or a fine dissector

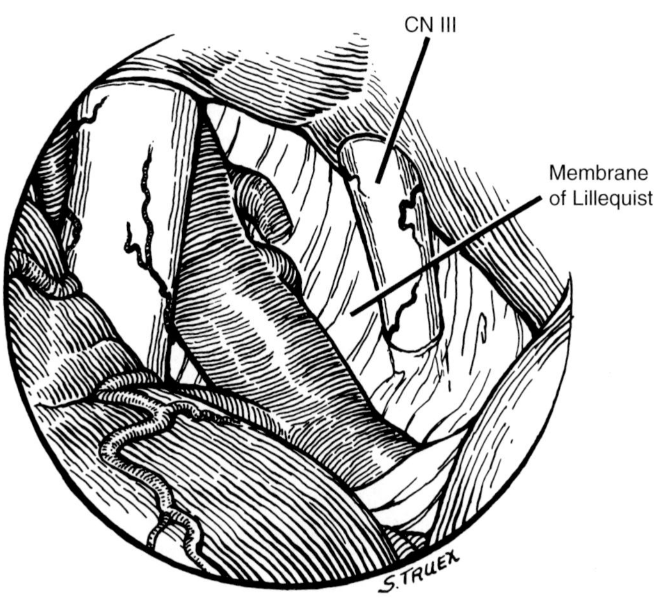

Figure 11–7 Exposure of Lillequist's membrane.

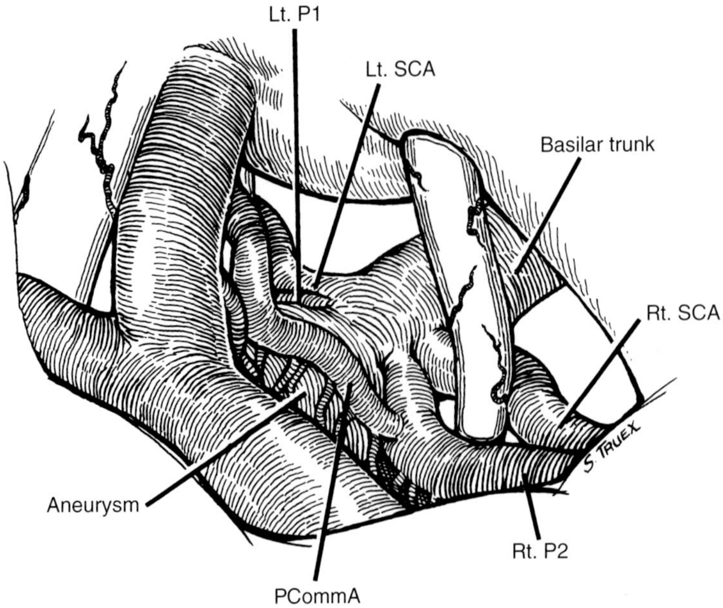

Figure 11–8 Exposure of interpeduncular cistern. SCA, superior cerebellar artery.

(**Fig 11–11**). The aneurysm is then usually clipped with a permanent bayoneted clip loaded upside down. It is common for the first clip placement to be across the contralateral P1 origin. Repositioning of the clip is then carried out until the PCAs are patent and the aneurysm is obliterated (**Fig. 11–12**). Tandem clip application using two or more clips in parallel is often necessary to completely occlude even relatively small aneurysm necks.

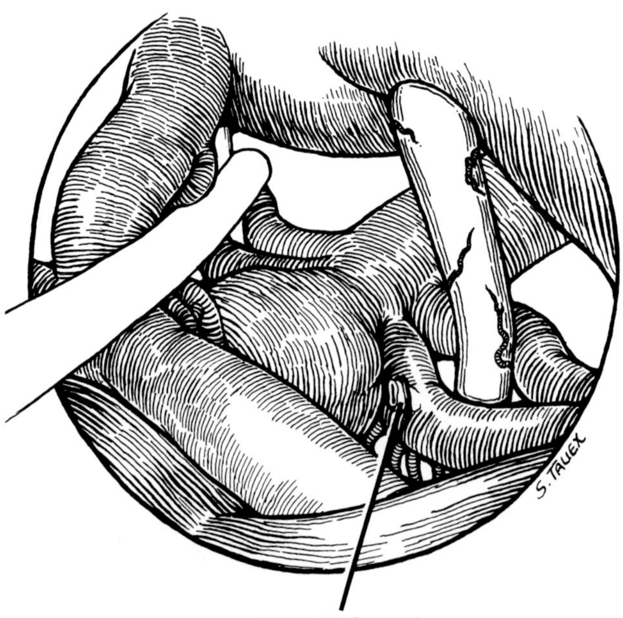

Figure 11–9 Sacrifice of posterior communicating artery.

Step 11: The aneurysm is carefully inspected to be sure the clip blades are completely across the neck and no perforators or efferent vessels are within the blades. If even the smallest perforator is within the blades, the clip must be removed, the perforator dissected free, and the clip replaced. If the aneurysm ruptures prematurely, the SCA and PCA vessels must be temporarily occluded with clips to allow the permanent clip to be removed and replaced satisfactorily. The surgeon will have more room to work if the ipsilateral temporary clips are placed on the SCA and PCA lateral to CN III. To achieve a dry field will often require that all SCA vessels (they are often paired) are temporarily occluded. This can often be achieved using a single clip.

Step 12: Once the aneurysm is satisfactorily clipped, the fundus is punctured with a spinal needle as far away from the clip as is possible in case a second clip needs to be placed or the first clip needs to be repositioned. If no refilling is seen, the temporary clips are removed with the basilar trunk clip removed last. The vessels are then auscultated with a microDoppler to assure patency.

Special Considerations

Low-lying basilar apex aneurysms (more than 1.5 cm below the dorsum sellae) may require a transcavernous approach (**Fig. 11–13**). For such lesions the cavernous sinus dura lateral and 3 mm posterior to the cavernous insertion of CN III is opened with the incision often transecting CN IV. As the dura is opened profuse bleeding occurs, which is controlled by stuffing the hole in the cavernous sinus with cotton or Surgicel. Ultimately sewing the cut corners back to the middle fossa dura and opening the underlying arachnoid provides exposure of the basilar trunk (**Fig. 11–14**). If the patient is properly positioned with the head rotated 45 degrees

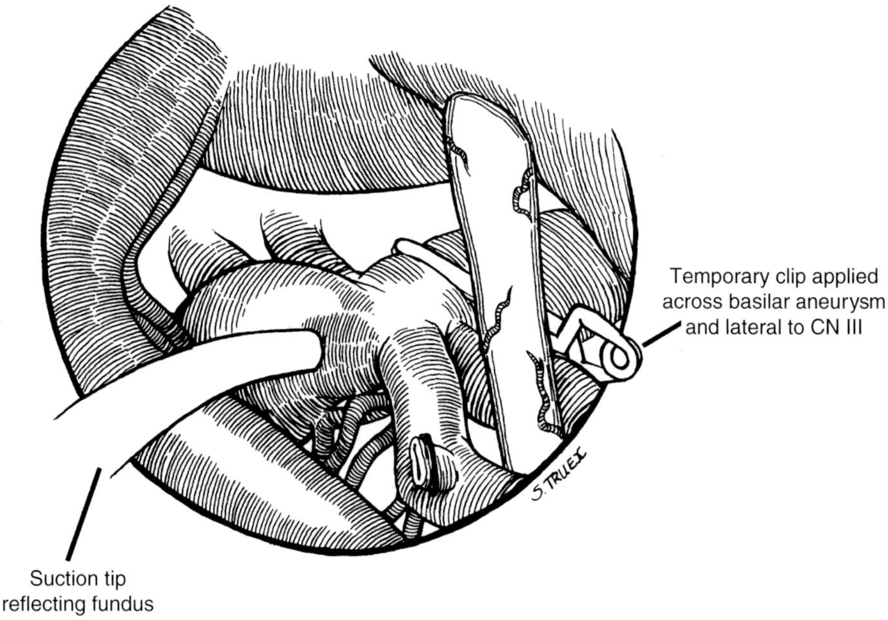

Figure 11–10 Temporary clip placement and initial elevation of fundus.

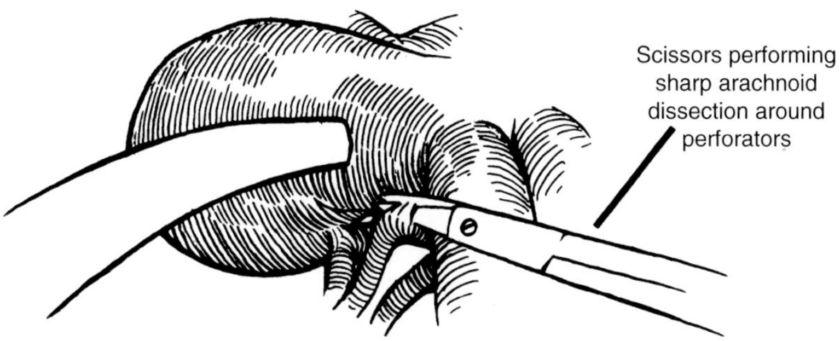

Figure 11–11 Perforator dissection.

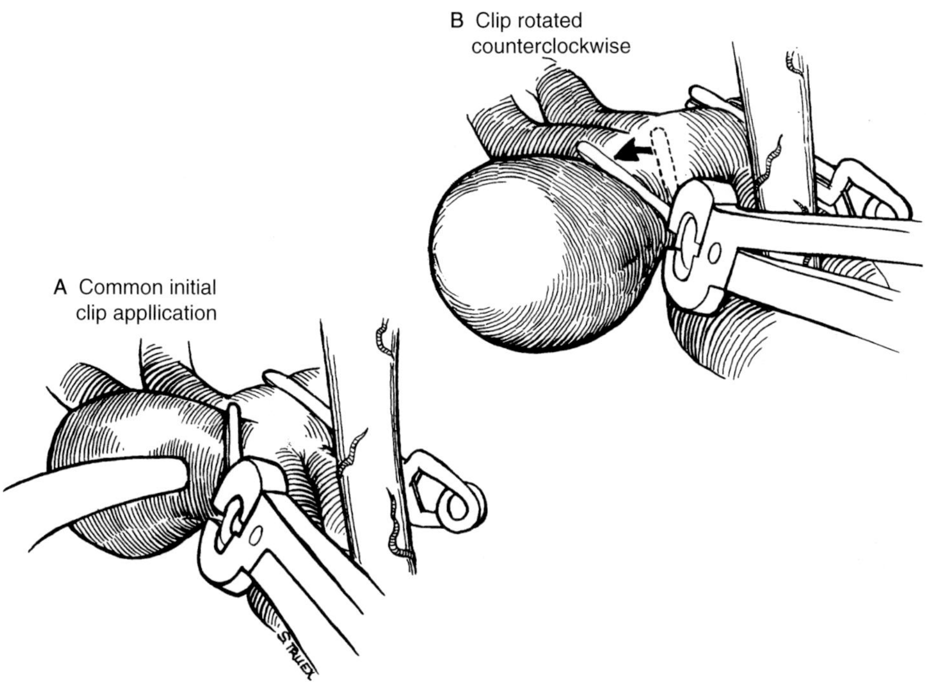

Figure 11–12 **(A–B)** Clip placement.

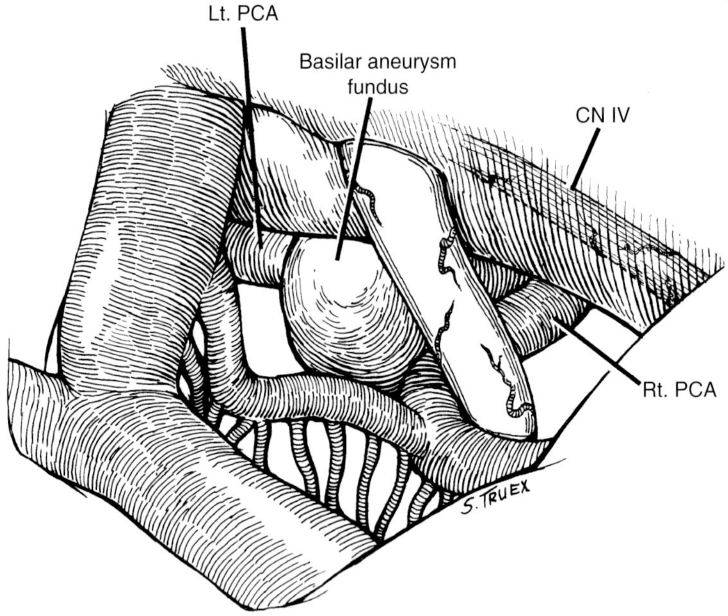

Figure 11–13 Initial exposure of low-lying apex aneurysm. PCA, posterior cerebral artery.

away from the operative side, removal of the posterior clinoid process is rarely necessary for visualization of the aneurysm itself. Posterior clinoid resection may on occasion assist the surgeon in identifying the contralateral P1 segment.

High-lying basilar apex aneurysms (more than 1.5 cm above the dorsum sellae) may best be visualized by performing an interfascial temporalis muscle opening and removing the zygomatic arch. This will permit the surgeon to more easily look up into the interpeduncular cistern from a temporal-temporopolar vector.

Closure

If the ventriculostomy is to remain, it is brought out through a separate stab incision in the scalp. The dura is then closed using 4–0 Neurilon suture in a watertight fashion, and any necessary tackup sutures are placed. The bone flap is then replaced using three miniplates with screws, and a partial methylmethacrylate cranioplasty is performed to fill in the drilled sphenoid wing and temporal bone defects. The temporalis muscle is closed with 2–0 Vicryl suture. A subgaleal drain is left if necessary. The galea is closed using inverted

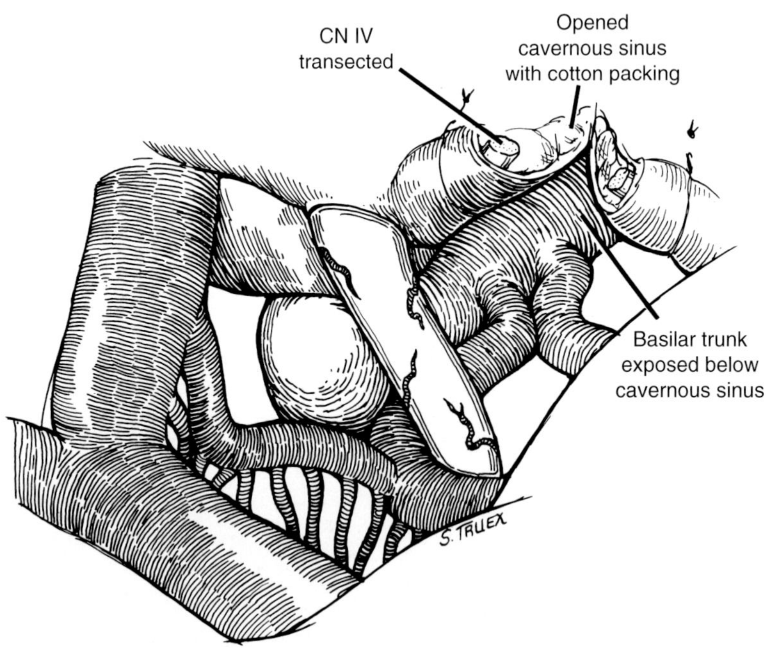

Figure 11–14 Opening cavernous sinus.

3–0 Vicryl sutures, and the skin is closed with staples or 4–0 nylon. Sterile dressings are applied, and the patient is returned to the intensive care unit either intubated or extubated, depending upon the neurological condition and respiratory status.

◆ Postoperative Care

Postoperative care is no different for basilar apex aneurysms than for aneurysms at other intracranial locations. The reader may refer to previously published excellent reviews of this topic.[13]

◆ Complications

All neurosurgeons are aware of the common complications of aneurysm surgery. These include entry into air sinuses with resultant CSF leakage and infection, frontalis nerve palsy, efferent and afferent vessel damage, aneurysm rupture, brain contusion and laceration, and perforator vessel occlusion. These complications are no less common with basilar aneurysms than with other lesions. Some complications, however, are specific to the approach just described and as such will be listed and discussed here.

1. *Anterior choroidal artery injury:* The anterior choroidal arteries most commonly arise from the posterior carotid wall just distal to the PCommA and just proximal to the ICA bifurcation. The vessels then travel medially along the uncus and enter the choroidal fissure. During uncal resection it is important to first dissect the choroidal vessel(s) free of the pia so that they are not inadvertently damaged while this portion of the temporal lobe is being removed.
2. *Third nerve injury:* The third nerve is well uncovered after uncal resection. Our approach utilizes the space lateral to and below the third nerve as a corridor for placement of the basilar artery temporary clip. Even without using this corridor the third nerve is often manipulated during aneurysm exposure, thus leading to postoperative third nerve palsy. The third nerve is quite resilient, and we have not noted long-term paralysis even when the patient awakens with total loss of function. Some patients have complained of mild sustained diplopia, which can often be managed with prism glasses or muscle shortening.
3. *Posterior communicating artery anterior thalamoperforator damage:* To mobilize the internal carotid artery medially so that the carotico-third nerve corridor is widened the PCommA is often sacrificed. We generally use Weck clips to ligate the vessel at the P1–P2 junction. The use of bipolar cautery risks thermal injury to small perforators that appear to be a safe distance from the instrument. Even if the vessel is sacrificed optimally, flow may be compromised through it such that the anterior thalamoperforators thrombose. Any of these complications can lead to hypothalamic, posterior internal capsule, and partial thalamic infarction.
4. *MCA laceration:* To adequately visualize the P1–P2 junction, we often find it useful to open the sylvian fissure widely at least as far as the anterior temporal branch of the MCA. Not only does this permit better exposure of the aneurysm and parent vessels but it also minimizes the risk of inadvertent MCA laceration. Such injury can occur when the clip applier is moved in and out of the operative field. The MCA can be torn if it is on excessive stretch. It may also be torn by the clip applier's proximal moving joint, which opens when the clip is opened and closes when the clip is closed. If the vessel gets caught in this joint, it can be torn when the clip applier is removed from the operative field.
5. *MCA occlusion:* Often a retractor blade is placed along the frontal lobe to elevate the lobe and move it medially. The surgeon must be careful that the blade is not placed into the sylvian fissure, inadvertently occluding the MCA. Prolonged occlusion will lead to MCA ischemia and stroke.
6. *Temporal lobe temporopolar vein avulsion:* Exposure of a basilar aneurysm often requires temporal lobe mobilization. During this mobilization the temporopolar veins draining into the sphenoparietal sinus are often placed on stretch. In order to avoid vein avulsion, we locate these veins early and cauterize and cut them. We have not had any instances of venous infarction from such a step.
7. *Retractor migration:* We commonly use a temporal lobe retractor placed on the anterior temporal lobe. It is important to place the tip of the retractor against the middle fossa floor's dura so that inadvertent bumping of the retractor does not advance it into the brain stem or aneurysm.

◆ Conclusion

Basilar apex aneurysms are difficult lesions to treat. By using a regimented stepwise approach, however, one can maximize exposure and vascular control, thus making good outcomes an expected rather than a hoped for result.

References

1. Castaigne P, Llernitte F, Buge A, Escourolle R, Hauw JJ, Lyon-Caen O. Paramedian and midbrain infarcts: clinical and neuropathological study. Ann Neurol 1981;10:127–148
2. de Oliveira E, Tedeschi H, Rhoton AL, Peace DA. Microsurgical anatomy of the posterior circulation: vertebral and basilar arteries. In: Carter LP, Spetzler RF, Hamilton MG, eds. Neurovascular Surgery. New York: McGraw-Hill; 1994:25–34

3. Gillingham FJ. The management of ruptured intracranial aneurysms. Ann R Coll Surg Engl 1958;23:89–117
4. Drake CG. Bleeding aneurysms of the basilar artery: direct surgical management in four cases. J Neurosurg 1961;18:230–238
5. Crowell RM, Ogilvy CS. Management of basilar and posterior cerebral artery aneurysms be subtemporal approaches. In: Rengachary SS, Wilkins RH, eds. Neurosurgical Operative Atlas. Vol 3. Philadelphia: Williams and Wilkins; 1993:379–394
6. Steinberg GK, Drake CG, Peerless SJ. Deliberate basilar or vertebral artery occlusion in the treatment of intracranial aneurysms. J Neurosurg 1993;89:161–173
7. Guglielmi G, Vinuela F, Duckwiler G, et al. Endovascular treatment of posterior circulation aneurysms by electrothrombosis using electrically detachable coils. J Neurosurg 1992;77:515–524
8. McDougall CG, Halbach VV, Dowd CF, Higashida RT, Larsen DW, Hieshima GB. Endovascular treatment of basilar tip aneurysms using electrolytically detachable coils. J Neurosurg 1996;84:393–399
9. Pierot L, Boulin A, Castaings L, Rey A, Moret J. Selective occlusion of basilar artery aneurysms using controlled detachable coils: report of 35 cases. Neurosurgery 1996;38:948–954
10. Raymond J, Roy D, Bojanowski M, Moumdjian R, L'Esperance G. Endovascular treatment of acutely ruptured and unruptured aneurysms of the basilar bifurcation. J Neurosurg 1997;86:211–219
11. Eskridge JM, Song JK. Endovascular embolization of 150 basilar tip aneurysms with Guglielmi detachable coils: results of the Food and Drug Administration multicenter clinical trial. J Neurosurg 1998;89:81–86
12. Paine JT, Batjer HH, Samson D. Intraoperative ventricular puncture. Neurosurgery 1988;22:1107–1109
13. Bederson J, ed. Subarachnoid Hemorrhage: Pathophysiology and Management. AANS Neurosurgical Topics. Chicago: AANS; 1997

12

Posterior Cerebral Artery and Mid-Basilar Aneurysms

Akira Yamamura

Mid-basilar aneurysms arise on the basilar artery at the region of the anterior inferior cerebellar artery (AICA). Because these lesions rarely occur in the basilar artery circulation, they have not been reported until recently. Drake reported his first case in 1963. In Drake and his colleagues' series, there were a similar number of aneurysms arising on the basilar trunk between the superior cerebellar artery (SCA) and the AICA, including fusiform aneurysms and dissecting types. Distal basilar trunk aneurysms, which are not related to SCA in origin, are much rarer.

It is difficult to describe the surgery for mid-basilar and posterior cerebral artery (PCA) aneurysms in the same chapter. In most cases both operations may begin with the subfrontal approach; however, these two aneurysms arise at different locations. A PCA aneurysm is obviously located above the tentorium and a mid-basilar aneurysm is located in the posterior fossa far below the tentorium incisura. Different techniques are required at the critical points. The deep location of a mid-basilar aneurysm requires much further retraction for exposure after reaching the tentorial hiatus. A vertebral union aneurysm can be managed with a technique similar to that of a mid-basilar aneurysm because these two aneurysms are often located at the same level in the posterior fossa.

◆ Indications

Indications for surgery are not different from those for aneurysms in other locations. However, all aneurysms of the mid-basilar artery are difficult to treat, and this is particularly true when they are large or giant in size, with or without thrombosis/calcification, or when they arise at the fenestration of the basilar artery. Unruptured large or giant aneurysms require very careful attention for surgical indication. Recent advances in endovascular surgery techniques may offer an alternative method for dealing with a mid-basilar aneurysm, if an excellent endovascular surgeon is available.

◆ Preparation

A good-quality cerebral arteriography is mandatory as a preoperative study. Magnetic resonance imaging (MRI) and three-dimensional computed tomography (3D-CT) will give additional information to enhance the three-dimensional understanding of the aneurysm and related structures. It is important to know the size and direction of the aneurysm axis, as with aneurysms at any location.

PCA aneurysms arise at four common sites: at the origin of the large perforating artery of P1, at the junction of the posterior communicating artery and the PCA, at the origin of the anterior temporal artery and internal occipital artery, and at the terminal branches of the PCA. The most common sites are the first three locations. Mycotic aneurysms can arise at the very distal PCA. The PCA aneurysms are often large or giant in size, and it is difficult to identify the aneurysm neck and the origin of related PCA branches. A large or giant aneurysm of PCA may be difficult to manage.

In the case of a mid-basilar aneurysm, arteriography will give information about the level of the aneurysm and the location in the posterior fossa in relation to such landmarks as the posterior clinoid process, sellar floor, internal auditory canal, and foramen magnum. Whether the aneurysm is located on or off the midline, as seen in anteroposterior views of arteriography, will help decide the side for the surgical approach. The side of approach is a matter of concern. It is recommended to select the side that allows a shorter approach even if the aneurysmal fundus is located on the opposite side. Drake's approach was from the side of aneurysm projection. These aneurysms tend to project laterally, and in Drake's series, one fourth projected anteriorly against the clivus or even posteriorly to indent the pons (three of 14 patients). Sometimes the differentiation between a basilar AICA aneurysm and a vertebral basilar junction is quite difficult, particularly when the aneurysm is large or giant in size.

◆ Anesthesia

Anesthesia and monitoring do not differ from that used for aneurysms of other locations. PCA and mid-basilar artery aneurysms are often quite difficult to treat, so hypothermic anesthesia and-or the deep hypothermic circulating arrest technique is recommended by some surgeons. This kind of anesthesia would be helpful, particularly when the aneurysm is large or giant, with or without thrombosis, or if it arises at the basilar artery fenestration, because these aneurysms require prolonged temporary clipping and complete decompression during manipulation at the critical point of surgery. Both aneurysms may require significant retraction of the temporal lobe, so monitoring of the retraction pressure may be advisable.

◆ Positioning

Both PCA and mid-basilar aneurysms are operated in a lateral head position (**Fig. 12–1**). The patient may be placed in a true lateral position (**Fig. 12–1A**) or in a supine position with a pillow beneath the shoulder (**Fig. 12–1B**). For a PCA aneurysm at P1–P2 or P2, the author prefers positioning the head with the face slightly rotated upward (**Fig. 12–1C**) rather than in the true lateral position (**Fig. 12–1A,B**) because the origin and proximal portion of the PCA can be more easily identified. This modification may be referred to as an anterior subtemporal approach or a half-and-half approach. Additionally, slightly tilting the head toward the floor would give some advantage. Surgeons have to pay careful attention to the patient's cervical spine and confirm that the patient can tolerate a long operation in the specific position under anesthesia and muscle relaxation. For an aneurysm located further distal on the PCA, an occipital interhemispheric approach is recommended in a prone position or modified lateral position.

The most common craniotomy for these aneurysms is illustrated in **Figs. 12–2** and **12–3. Figs. 12–2** and **12–3** show a typical temporal craniotomy with a very low margin. **Fig. 12–3** shows a craniotomy with extension to the mastoid region to expose the posterior fossa anterior to the sigmoid sinus. The superior petrosal sinus is divided and the supra- and infratentorial compartments are exposed (**Fig. 12–4**). The latter is used to obtain a wider exposure to treat a low or large/giant aneurysm of the mid-basilar artery.

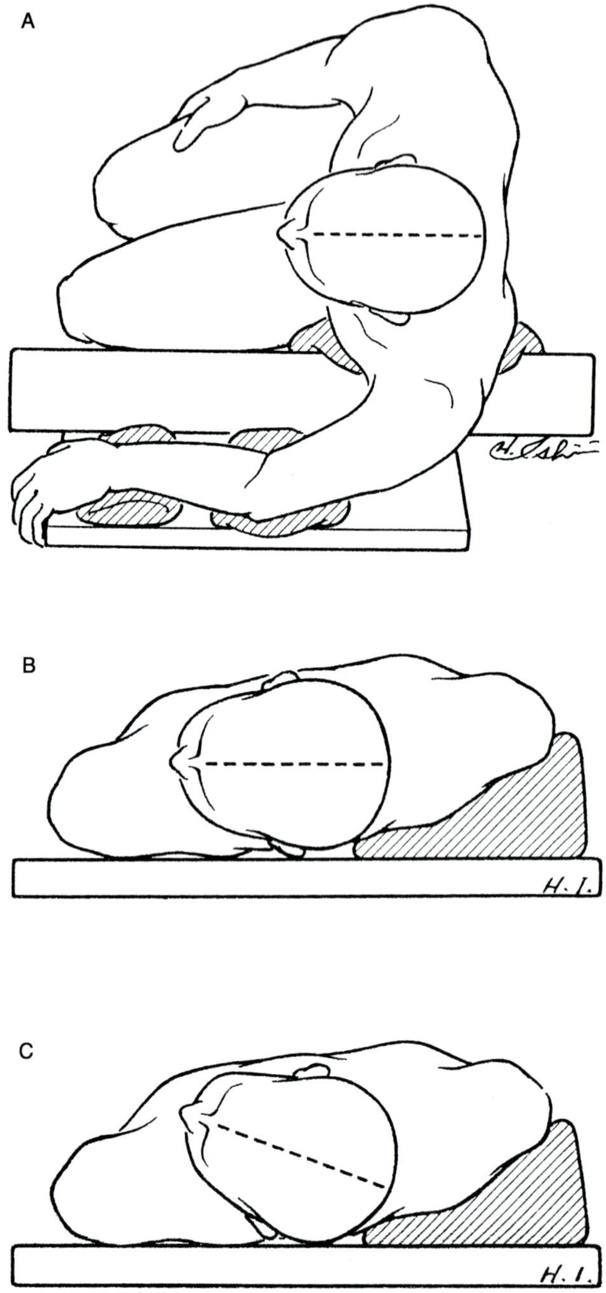

Figure 12–1 Positioning and head position. **(A)** Lateral position, head position—true lateral. **(B)** Supine position, head position—true lateral. **(C)** Supine position, head position oblique.

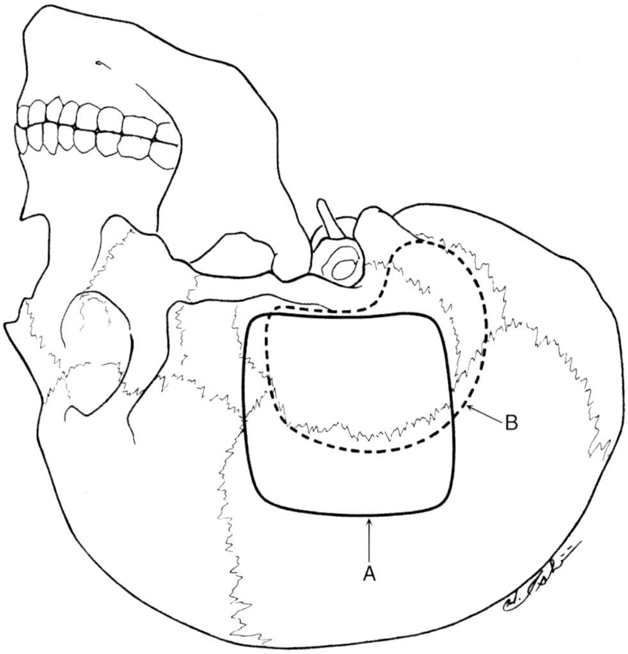

Figure 12–2 Temporal craniotomy.

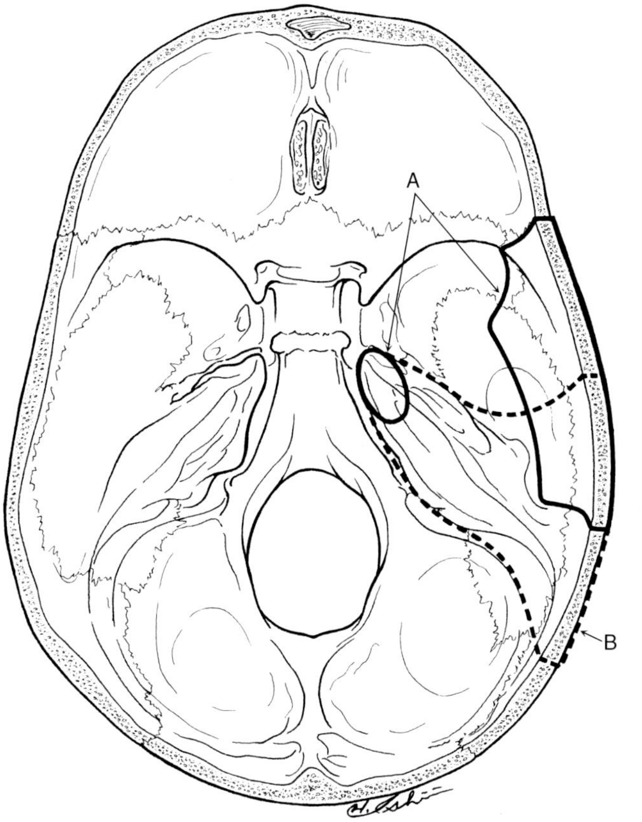

Figure 12–3 Temporal craniotomy with posterior extension for supra- and infratentorial opening.

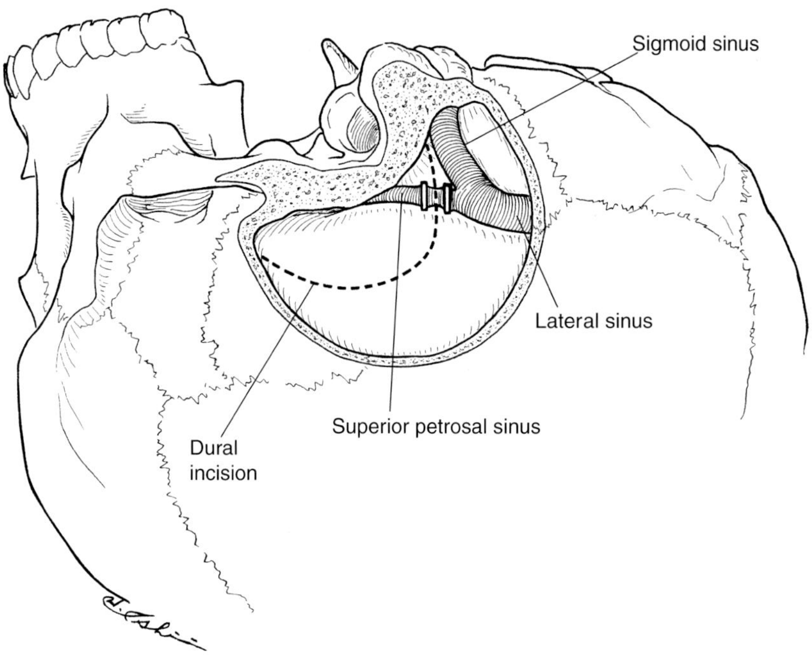

Figure 12–4 Wider exposure for a low or large/giant aneurysm of the mid-basilar artery. The superior petrosal sinus is divided, and the supra- and infratentorial compartments are exposed.

◆ Surgical Technique

Posterior Cerebral Artery Aneurysm

For proximal PCA aneurysms (P1 or P2 junction), a transsylvian or subtemporal approach is indicated similar to that for a basilar bifurcation aneurysm. An aneurysm at the junction of the posterior communicating artery, with the PCA on the right side (**Fig. 12–5**) is exposed by a transsylvian approach. The craniotomy for this lesion is frontotemporal with adequate drilling of the pterion and the sphenoid wing. The sylvian fissure is then widely opened, and the frontal and temporal lobes are retracted. If the surgeon is used to a transsylvian approach to basilar bifurcation aneurysms, PCA aneurysms are nearer to the surgeon, and hence easier to perform. When the aneurysm projects anteriorly, there is no problem in clipping the aneurysm, and the risk of damaging perforators or other structures is small.

PCA aneurysms at the origin of the anterior temporal artery or internal occipital artery (P2 segment) are located lateral to the midbrain and often hidden by the hippocampus. A low temporal craniotomy is made (**Figs. 12–2** and **12–3**), and then the temporal lobe is elevated. The surgeon must pay attention to the presence of the vein of Labbé, and every effort should be made to protect the draining vein. **Fig. 12–6** shows a typical PCA aneurysm located lateral to the midbrain. The first landmark is the trochlear nerve running along the tentorial hiatus. This nerve would be seen through an intact arachnoid. Unnecessary wide exposure is not recommended, and an alternative is cutting the arachnoid on the medial side of this cranial nerve. The nerve is then moved laterally past the intact arachnoid lateral to the nerve and is kept out of the working space. It is important to follow the PCA from the P1 region distally to avoid disorientation. Also, it is important to differentiate the SCA and PCA by their relation to the oculomotor nerve. The PCA runs superior to the oculomotor nerve and above the level of the tentorium, and the SCA runs inferior to the oculomotor nerve. Aneurysms at this location are often large or giant in size, and a special technique is required as for giant aneurysms of any location. Occlusion of the PCA, deliberately or inadvertently, may not cause significant neurological deficits because of rich collateral blood flow to the PCA territory.

PCA aneurysms located far distally (P3 segment) are managed by an occipital interhemispheric approach. The surgeon has to follow the distal branch of the PCA, and in the case of a ruptured aneurysm, subarachnoid or superficial intracerebral hematomas are marks of the aneurysm location.

Mid-Basilar Aneurysms

There are several options for managing mid-basilar aneurysms, depending on the level of the aneurysm's location (**Fig. 12–7**). When the aneurysm is located high and above the sellar floor level, the transsylvian approach using an anterior tentorium incision or subtemporal approach would be indicated, either with or without a tentorial incision. The subtemporal approach using a tentorial incision and drilling of the petrous bone is advisable for an aneurysm located at the level between the sellar floor and the internal auditory canal, namely, at the lower third of the clivus.

A transoral-transclival approach was once used, but this approach was abandoned by the author because of the risk of postoperative cerebrospinal fluid (CSF) leakage. Drake and colleagues also abandoned this approach for aneurysms because it is too narrow and confining and poses the risk of meningitis. A small and very low craniotomy for this aneurysm is not recommended. At the critical point, further retraction of the temporal lobe is required. If the superior bony margin is too low, the retractor will hit against the superior bony margin, causing sufficient retraction. The superior margin

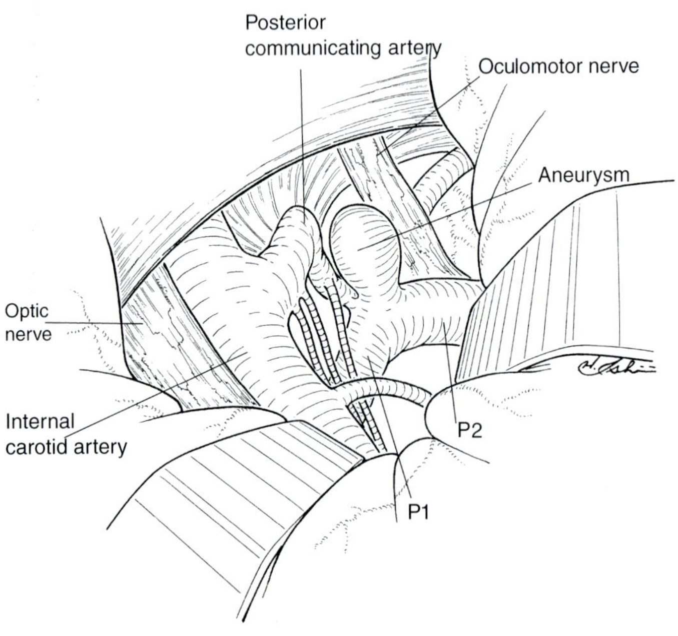

Figure 12–5 Proximal posterior cerebral artery aneurysm and related structures, right transsylvian approach.

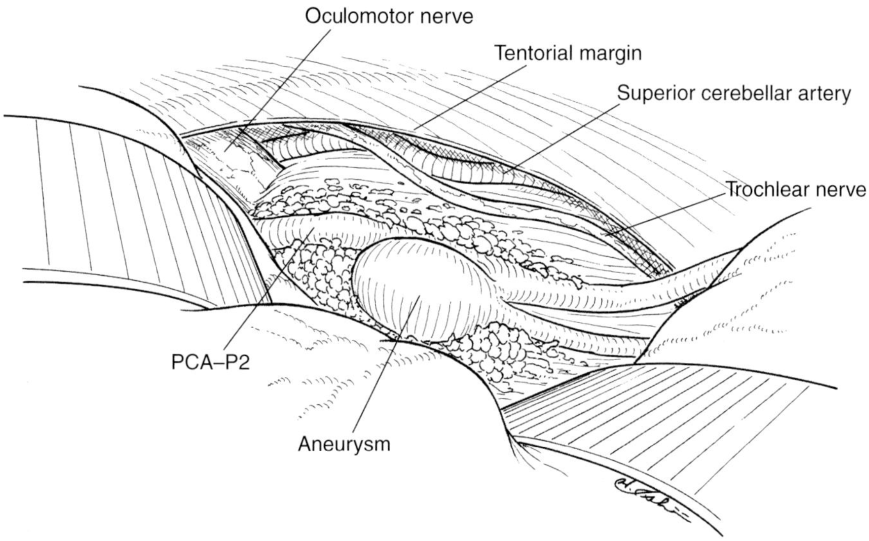

Figure 12–6 P2–P3 posterior cerebral artery (PCA) aneurysm, subtemporal approach.

of the craniotomy should be reasonably high, and the inferior margin should be maximally low. A large or giant aneurysm at the lower third of the clivus may require further exposure, including mastoid drilling and division of the superior petrosal sinus (**Fig. 12–4**).

A typical case of a mid-basilar aneurysm related with an origin of AICA is shown in **Fig. 12–8A-C.** After making a temporal craniotomy and opening the dura mater (**Fig. 12–3**), the surgeon should first observe the vein of Labbé. The arachnoid around this vein is dissected free at a certain distance. Then the vein will tolerate stretching during temporal lobe elevation. The vein is covered by a cottonoid and kept wet by an assistant until closure. By gentle elevation of the temporal lobe at its middle portion, the tentorial hiatus is reached (**Fig. 12–8A**). The first landmark to look for will be the trochlear nerve and the SCA under the arachnoid. The arachnoid lateral to the nerve is incised. The trochlear nerve will then move medially by natural shrinkage of the intact arachnoid medial to the nerve. The nerve is covered with a cottonoid. For the aneurysms located at the lower third of the clivus, a tentorial incision and a petrosectomy, or drilling, of the petrous bone is usually required. It is recommended to remove the tentorium along the superior petrosal sinus instead of making a simple incision perpendicular to the petrous margin. This procedure should be done 1 cm or more posterior to the exit of the trochlear nerve. When the tentorium is simply incised, the edge of the tentorium leaflet and the divided petrosal sinus stump are pulled away from the working space by stitches. The posterior aspect of the petrous bone between the trigeminal nerve and facial/acoustic nerves is exposed by peeling the overlying middle-fossa dura. A rubber dam is placed to protect the surrounding tissue during drilling. Careful drilling will make a good space for mid-basilar exposure. A crucial portion is first exposed by adequate drilling of the petrous bone (**Fig. 12–8 B,C**). The drilled

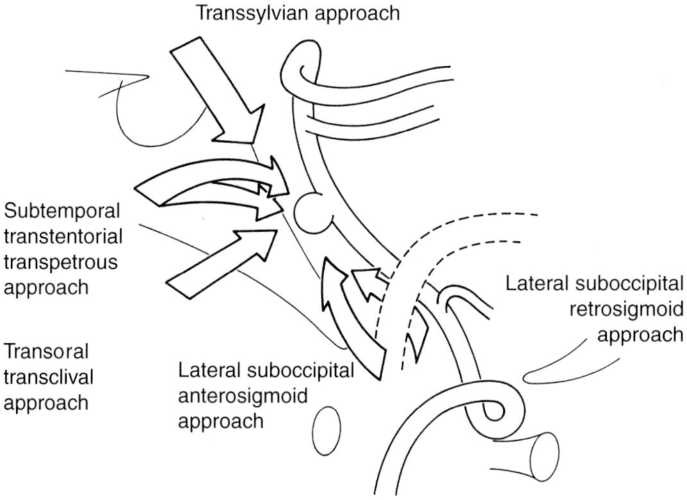

Figure 12–7 Schematic diagram for a variety of approaches to a mid-basilar aneurysm.

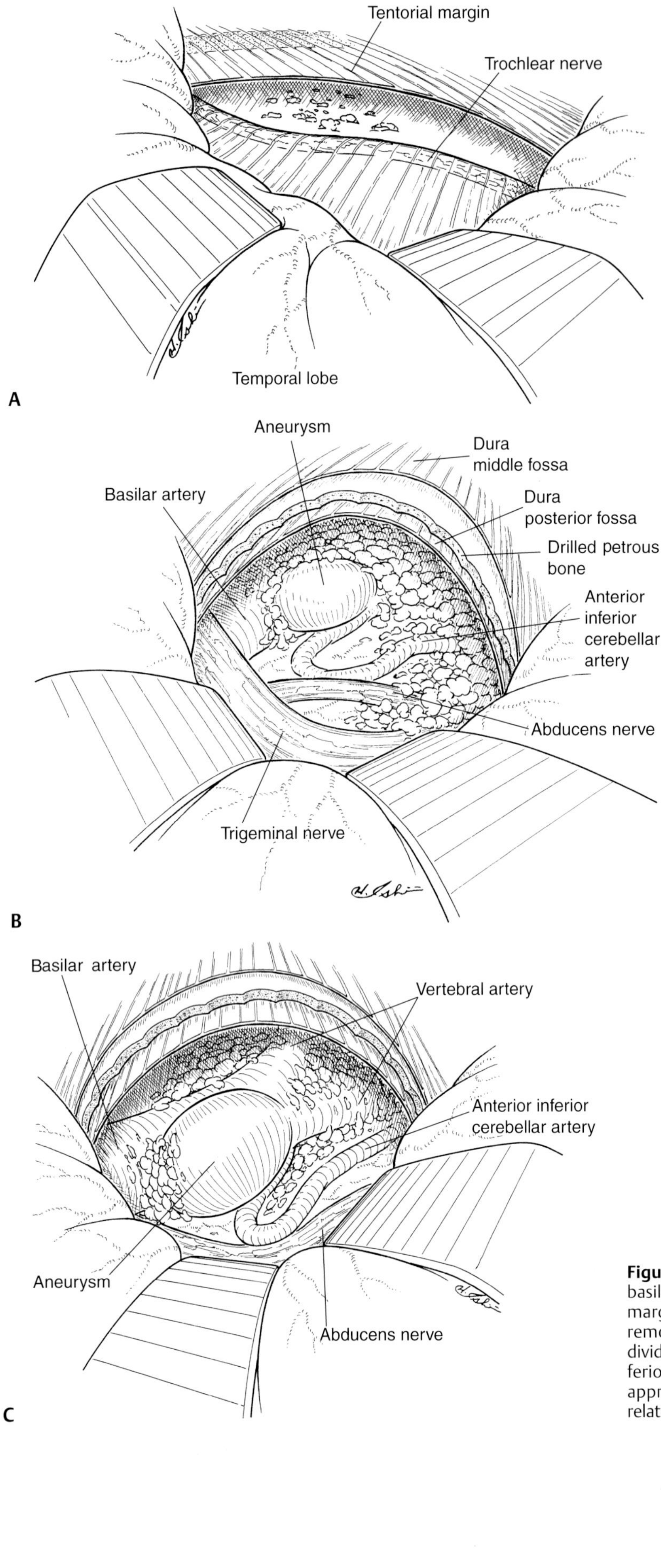

Figure 12–8 Subtemporal-transpetrosal approach to a mid-basilar aneurysm. **(A)** Elevation of the temporal lobe, tentorial margin, and trochlear nerve. **(B)** A part of the tentorium is removed, the petrous drilled, and the superior petrosal sinus divided. The trigeminal nerve, abducens nerve, and anterior inferior cerebellar artery (AICA) are shown. **(C)** Transoral approach. The aneurysm is exposed, and the aneurysm and related structures are shown.

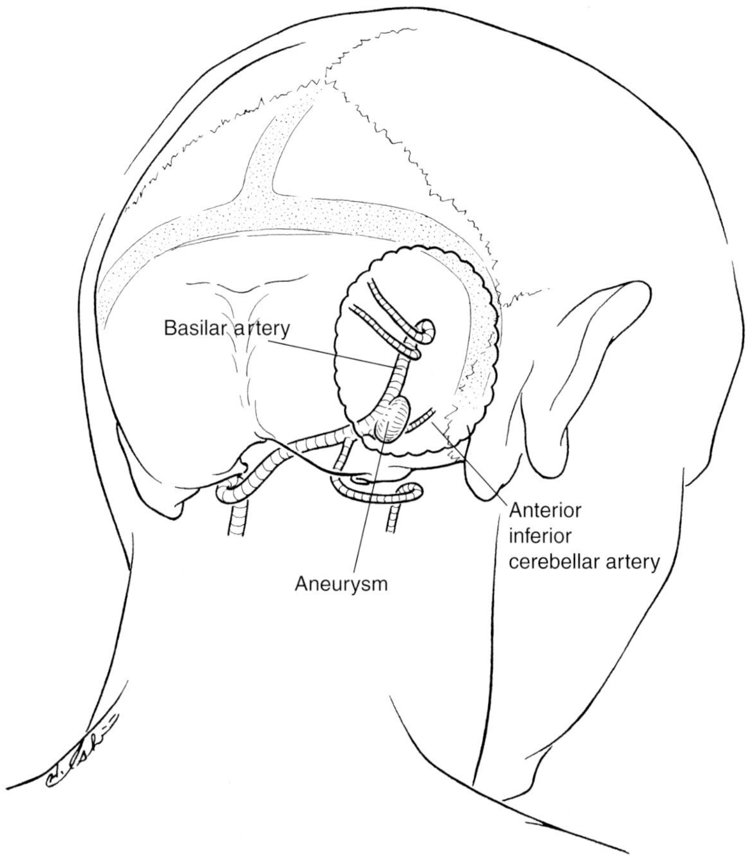

Figure 12–9 The lateral suboccipital approach for a low-set mid-basilar aneurysm located off the midline.

surface of the bone is carefully covered by bone wax. The trigeminal nerve may be retracted (**Fig. 12–8B**), because it can tolerate the manipulation and retraction.

The next important landmarks are the AICA and the abducens nerve. The abducens nerve runs along the basilar artery. The nerve is covered with a cottonoid and kept out of the working space. The abducens nerve has a remarkable propensity for complete recovery when handled gently. A loop of the AICA is a useful landmark for locating the basilar trunk (**Fig. 12–8B**). The surgeon is able to reach the basilar artery by simply following the AICA. Gentle dissection and removal of a clot in a direction away from the presumed position of the ruptured dome will expose the aneurysm. Sometimes tight adhesion of the AICA to the aneurysm requires painstaking dissection. Complete dissection of the aneurysm neck is necessary before placing a clip (**Fig. 12–8C**). An anteriorly projecting aneurysm is usually adherent to the clival dura. This adhesion should remain undissected. The working space for temporary clipping of the proximal basilar artery is usually very limited.

For aneurysms located below the internal auditory canal, a lateral suboccipital approach is indicated, and a retromastoid route is often adequate (**Fig. 12–9**). After the lateral suboccipital craniotomy and dural opening, the cerebellar hemisphere is retracted medially and posteriorly, and the lower cranial nerves are identified. The space between the vestibule and cochlear nerve and glossopharyngeal and vagus nerves is a common route to the aneurysm (**Fig. 12–10**).

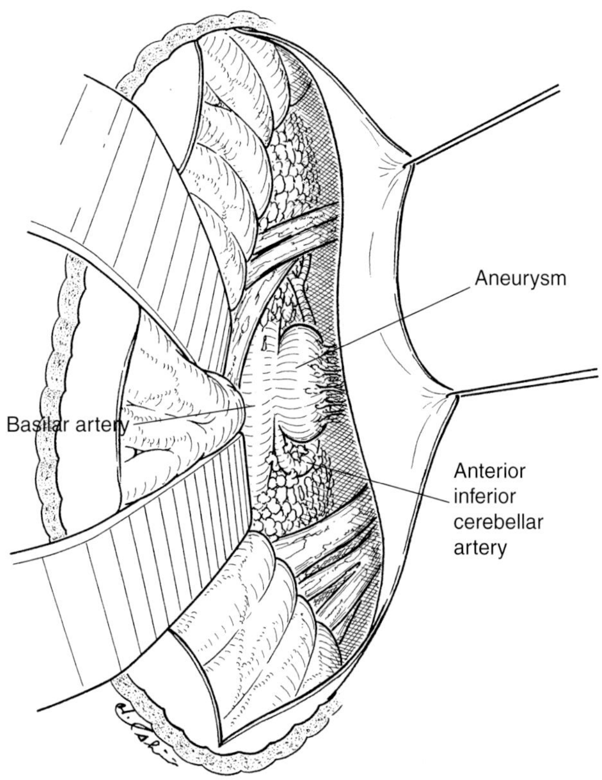

Figure 12–10 A low-set, off-midline mid-basilar aneurysm can be exposed between cranial nerves (CN) VII–VIII and CN V or between CN VII–VIII and IX–X.

Drake performed permanent basilar artery occlusion in 19 patients with mid-basilar aneurysms after a test occlusion with a "Drake tourniquet," and 15 of these did well. Only two patients suffered from brain stem infarcts. Drake was surprised about the good outcome despite the fact that in many patients pontine perforators were seen to be arising from that portion of the basilar artery involved in the aneurysm wall. This indicates that deep, unseen brain stem collaterals to these vital vessels were sufficient to prevent pontine infarction.

Closure

If a petrosectomy is done, it should be covered by bone wax and, if necessary, by a muscle piece with fibrin glue. The dura is closed, and a bone flap is placed in the usual manner.

◆ Postoperative Care

During a subtemporal approach, the most concern is directed toward avoiding damage to the temporal lobe. Injury to the vein of Labbé would be the most common cause of temporal lobe damage. With or without considerable and prolonged retraction to the base of the temporal lobe, a swelling of the temporal lobe is a matter of concern. Prompt postoperative images such as CT scan are indicated when the patient shows any delay of recovery or any deterioration. Generally conservative therapy would ameliorate the symptoms, but some permanent neurological deficits may occur.

◆ Complications

The cranial nerves are less often involved in these situations. The P1–P2 aneurysm is located near the oculomotor nerve; however, severe damage to this cranial nerve is less common when the aneurysm is anteriorly directed. The very thin trochlear nerve is the first cranial nerve to be observed in the suboccipital approach. The nerve should be covered with a cotton patty and protected until the end of surgery. The abducens nerve is routinely observed during surgery for a mid-basilar aneurysm. This nerve is also immediately covered with a cotton patty and protected, and severe damage is less common. To prevent the involvement of the vein of Labbé or other major draining venous systems, maximal caution should be exercised. Retraction of the temporal lobe may be severe and prolonged. The involvement of venous return and prolonged retraction of the brain are a major cause of postoperative temporal lobe swelling with or without intracerebral hemorrhage. Wide extradural dissection may avoid the involvement of the vein of Labbé.

◆ Conclusion

Attention to detail at every step is important to clip mid-basilar and PCA aneurysms successfully. Selection of the best option from several, including endovascular surgery, is also an important task, particularly for aneurysms arising at the midportion of the basilar artery.

Suggested Readings

Drake CG, Peerless SJ, Hernesniemi JA, eds. Surgery of Vertebrobasilar Aneurysms. New York: Springer-Verlag; 1996:119–132, 133–166, 221–229, 230–248

Hamilton MG, Spetzler RF. Surgical management of mid-basilar and lower basilar aneurysms. In: Schmidek HH and Sweet WH, eds. Operative Neurosurgical Techniques. 3rd ed. Vol 1. Philadelphia: WB Saunders; 1995:1087–1101

Peerless SJ, Hernesniemi JA, Drake CG. Surgical management of terminal basilar and posterior cerebral artery aneurysms. In: Schmidek HH and Sweet WH, eds. Operative Neurosurgical Techniques. 3rd ed. Vol 1. Philadelphia: WB Saunders; 1995:1071–1086

Piepgas DG. Posterior cerebral and superior cerebellar artery aneurysms. In: Apuzzo ML, ed. Brain Surgery. Vol 1. New York: Churchill Livingston; 1993:1082–1111

Tew JM Jr, Loveren HR, eds. Aneurysms of the distal posterior cerebral artery. In: Atlas of Operative Microneurosurgery. Vol 1. Philadelphia: WB Saunders; 1994:183–185

Tew JM Jr, Loveren HR, eds. Aneurysms of the mid-basilar trunk. In: Atlas of Operative Microneurosurgery. Vol 1. Philadelphia: WB Saunders; 1994:192–201

Weir B, ed. Posterior cerebral artery aneurysms. In: Aneurysms Affecting the Nervous System. Baltimore: Williams and Wilkins; 1987:484–485

13

Vertebrobasilar Junction and Vertebral Artery Aneurysms

Gabriel Gonzales-Portillo, Ernesto Coscarella, Roberto C. Heros, and Jacques J. Morcos

Aneurysms of the posterior circulation account for ~15% of all intracranial aneurysms. Aneurysms located on the basilar artery (BA) are the most common (50%),[1,2] followed by the vertebral artery (VA) in 20 to 30%.[1,2] VA aneurysms can arise anywhere along the intradural segment, although traumatic aneurysms have been reported between the first and second cervical vertebrae and close to the foramen transversarium. VA aneurysms may be midline or pointing laterally, depending on the direction and tortuosity of the VA. Most point superiorly and relate to the medulla.

The great majority of VA aneurysms are located at the distal crotch of origin of the posterior inferior cerebellar artery (PICA). Other common locations are along the PICA and at the carina of the VA–BA junction, particularly on the proximal angle of a fenestration. Less common locations are between the PICA and vertebrobasilar junction, and at the proximal crotch of origin of the PICA. Three distinct types of aneurysms have been described: saccular, dissecting, and atherosclerotic fusiform.[3] Saccular aneurysms are the most common (60%), followed by the dissecting type (28%), and the fusiform type (13%).[3] In Drake et al's series,[4] dissecting and fusiform aneurysms were seen less frequently (13% and 7%, respectively).

In most series a female preponderance was reported in VA aneurysms—80%,[4] 76%,[5] 65%,[6] and 86%.[7] Most of the time, VA aneurysms are located on the left side—66%,[4] 60%,[3] and 57%.[3] Mean age of presentation is in the sixth decade.[3,5–8] Conversely, the sex distribution in dissecting aneurysms is equal in both sexes,[4,8] and Yamaura[3] found that dissecting aneurysms were more common in men and in relatively young individuals.

The risk of rupture of a posterior circulation aneurysm has been found to be higher than anterior circulation aneurysms.[9] This is particularly true for the aneurysms less than 12 mm in size. The 5-year cumulative rupture rates for a 7 mm and for a 7 to 12 mm aneurysm located in the posterior circulation are 2.5 and 14.5%, respectively. Conversely, in the anterior circulation, those rupture rates are 0 and 2.6%, respectively.[9]

◆ Presentation

VA aneurysms present with an ictus anywhere between 67 and 100%.[3,5–8] Subarachnoid hemorrhage (SAH) caused by a ruptured posterior circulation aneurysm presents classically, mainly with severe sudden headache, nausea, and vomiting followed by altered level of consciousness in 65 to 95%.[3,6,8] Abrupt loss of consciousness is perhaps more common in posterior circulation aneurysms, and the headaches are invariably located in the occiput. It is also interesting to note that even with large aneurysmal sacs and significant distortion of the pons and medulla, patients harboring these aneurysms can remain asymptomatic.[1] Sixth nerve palsy was the most common but false localizing sign in

Drake et al's series.[4] They also found a very low incidence of lower cranial deficits and medullary signs such as cardiorespiratory arrest. The incidence of focal deficits such as monoparesis, lower extremity dysesthesia, oculomotor dysfunction, abducens palsy, and dysarthria has been reported as 35 to 50%.[5,6]

Occasionally (3–10%) VA aneurysms will present with mass effect or ischemic symptoms.[3,8] They have also been associated with multiple aneurysms and arteriovenous malformations.

In Andoh et al's series,[8] all fusiform aneurysms ruptured, saccular aneurysms ruptured in 90%, and dissecting aneurysms did so in 63%. Yamaura,[3] however, found that none of the 12 fusiform aneurysms in his series ruptured, and that dissecting aneurysms ruptured at a higher rate than saccular aneurysms (81 and 75%, respectively). Of the 12 fusiform aneurysms in Yamaura's series, six were associated with other aneurysms, five presented with mass effect, and one was an incidental finding.

◆ Imaging

Computed tomography may suggest a PICA aneurysm when there is little blood in the cisterns supratentorially compared with the cisterna magna, around the brain stem, and in the fourth ventricle. In Kallmes et al's retrospective series of 44 patients, [10] with PICA aneurysms in 70% of the cases, evidence of supratentorial SAH (25% sylvian and 23% anterior interhemispheric) was found. Intraventricular hemorrhage and hydrocephalus were seen individually in 95% of cases, and simultaneously in 93%. Isolated intraventricular hemorrhage was seen in only 5%. The high frequency of intraventricular hemorrhage in this type of aneurysm has been related to the close relationship of the PICA to the foramina of Luschka and Magendie.

In the same series, perimedullary subarachnoid hematomas large enough to displace the medulla were noted in 50% and always correlated with the side of the ruptured aneurysm. In series that include vertebrobasilar junction aneurysms, diffuse SAH in the basal cisterns with intraventricular extension was seen less frequently (41–85%).[6,8]

Software improvement has brought the sensitivity and specificity of the multislice helical computed tomographic (CT) angiogram closer to that of the cerebral angiogram.[11] It also allows the surgeon to rotate the aneurysm 360 degrees, see the relationship of the bony structures to the aneurysm, and place the aneurysm exactly as it will be seen after positioning the patient in a head holder.

Conventional cerebral angiography continues to be the test of choice. It not only will provide pertinent information concerning the aneurysm, it will also reveal the presence of other vascular anomalies in association with PICA aneurysms, including arteriovenous malformations and additional aneurysms at different locations.[3,5,12] The pattern of the collateral circulation and size of the ipsilateral anterior inferior cerebellar artery (AICA) should be noted in the event that the PICA or the VA needs to be sacrificed.

Previous reports have emphasized the importance of a truly four-vessel cerebral angiogram, unless there is adequate reflux of contrast material to fill the contralateral VA down to the origin of the PICA.[5] This technique proved not to be sufficient in seven cases of distal PICA aneurysms[13] and in one case in another series.[7] Therefore, when clinical suspicion is strong for a posterior fossa aneurysm, especially distal PICA, four-vessel cerebral angiography is mandatory because reflux from a contralateral vertebral injection rarely fills more than a small segment of the opposite proximal PICA. Special projections, such as the Huang view[7] or oblique views,[8] may be needed in addition. In Hidgins series,[8] two cases were reported initially as negative for PICA aneurysms. In one of these cases the PICA–VA junction from which the aneurysm arose was not studied, and in the other case the posterior circulation study was not done after a middle cerebral artery aneurysm was found on the carotid injections. In both patients subsequent angiograms revealed a PICA aneurysm. In Salcman et al's series,[6] two negative cerebral angiograms were reported. In both cases an aneurysm was found in the PICA distribution after a subsequent hemorrhage.

◆ Anesthesia

It is of paramount importance that a dedicated neuroanesthesiologist be part of the team. An arterial line to continuously monitor the systemic arterial pressure is inserted in the radial artery. A central venous line is inserted only in cases in which the assessment of the intravascular volume is in doubt. Swan-Ganz catheter insertion is reserved for patients with abnormal cardiac function or where the accurate assessment of the intravascular volume is necessary. An indwelling Foley catheter is inserted, and an accurate hourly account of urinary output is maintained. The patient should be kept euvolemic. Anesthesia is induced with thiopental and maintained with nitrous oxide and isoflurane. With the goal to decrease the amount of retraction of the cerebellum, the patient receives mannitol 20% (1 g/kg) at the time of skin incision. The end-tidal CO_2 is kept between 25 and 30 mm Hg. One dose of a broad-spectrum prophylactic antibiotic is routinely given. Occasionally a lumbar drain is inserted to aid intracranial relaxation. This is kept closed until the dura is open; afterward it is used to drain 30 to 50 mL of cerebrospinal fluid (CSF).

Careful attention to the systemic arterial pressure should be given during induction, head pinning, temporary clipping, and extubation. Routinely we will use intravenous neosynephrine to increase the systemic arterial pressure during temporary clipping. After removal of the temporary clips the systemic arterial blood pressure is returned to baseline values. At the end of the procedure the lumbar drain is removed, and the patient is extubated. If significant manipulation of the lower cranial nerves is suspected, we will keep the patient intubated until the next morning. That day the endotracheal tube is withdrawn slowly with an otolaryngologist in attendance to assess the movement of the vocal cords. Patients who cannot protect their airway are reintubated immediately. A second assessment of vocal cord mobility is performed in subsequent days, and if mobility is not regained, a tracheostomy is considered.

◆ Surgical Techniques: Vertebrobasilar Junction Aneurysms

Far Lateral Suboccipital Approach

The vertebrobasilar junction may be approached in several ways. The decision hinges primarily on the aneurysm height in relation to the clivus, side of vascular dominance, location of aneurysm neck with respect to the midline, and projection of the fundus. The far lateral approach is the workhorse for the exposure and handling of most aneurysms at or below the basilar origin. In view of the bony, dural, and parenchymal anatomical confines, it is, however, best suited for lesions of the lower third of the clivus. Higher lesions require different techniques to make clipping possible and safer. We prefer to approach most vertebrobasilar aneurysms from a far lateral suboccipital approach. This is a modified standard lateral suboccipital approach that has been previously described.[14] This section describes the general surgical principles as well as some of the newer modifications.

Positioning

The patient is placed in the straight lateral position, with a flat folded sheet under the axilla as padding. The head is maintained in the straight-ahead position (nose at 90 degree angle from the floor), with a 30 degree angle tilt toward the ipsilateral shoulder. With the patient in this position, the cerebellum tends to fall away, minimizing the need for retraction; in the same way, the CSF tends to drain actively due to gravity without the need for suction. A risk of air embolism is unlikely because the head is only slightly higher than the heart. The ipsilateral shoulder is gently pulled caudally with 2 in. silk tape applied to the bottom of the table to improve access to this region. Brachial plexus injury can occur with vigorous pulling of the shoulder.

It is noteworthy that one of us (JJM) prefers the three-quarter prone, with the vertex of the head tilted to the floor, the face rotated toward the floor, and the neck flexed. This significantly enlarges the shoulder–occiput space available to the surgeon and allows an angle of dissection that is more in line with the vertebral and basilar arteries, at the same time allowing a higher reach up the clivus.

Incision

We currently favor the hockey-stick incision over the original paramedian incision. The upper part of the incision is started at the top of the ear in a sagittal plane in line with the mastoid tip. It is carried medially and gently curved down into a midline incision down to the level of C2 (**Fig. 13–1**). Using the electrocautery, the cervical musculature is incised in the midline through an avascular plane down to the suboccipital bone and spinous processes of C1 and C2. At the superior nuchal line, the muscle attachment is incised in a "T" fashion, leaving a 1 cm wide cuff of muscle attached to the occipital bone, facilitating watertight fascial closure at the end of the procedure. Using subperiosteal dissection, the muscle mass is elevated from the suboccipital bone and from the lamina of C1 and C2. It is not necessary and rather undesirable to separate "anatomically" the individual muscle layers, given the risk of creating additional soft tissue trauma and encouraging dead space formation. The incision is held open with the help of fishhooks attached to a Leyla bar. Sharp dissection of the lamina of C1 is done to prevent injury to the VA. It is preferable to definitely identify the VA to avoid injuring it, but, with experience, this may not be necessary. A perivertebral venous plexus exists next to the VA at the level of the sulcus arteriosus (**Fig. 13–2**). It can become the source of troublesome bleeding, which can be easily controlled with bipolar coagulation or packing with powdered Gelfoam/thrombin paste or Surgicel. The foramen magnum is exposed with angled sharp curettes.

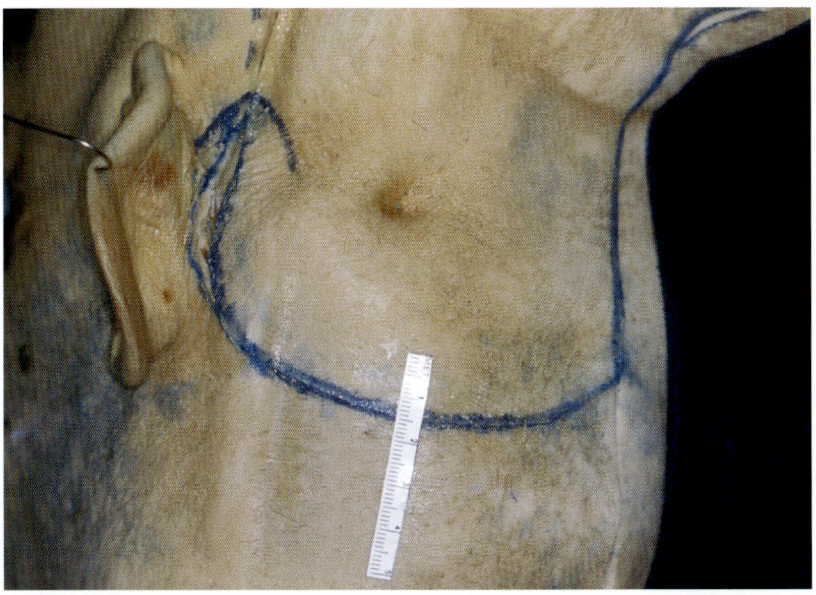

Figure 13–1 Hockey-stick incision for a right far lateral approach. The cadaver head is in the three-quarter prone position. The medial limb is exactly midline, and the lateral limb ends at the mastoid tip. The horizontal limb is 2 cm above the superior nuchal line.

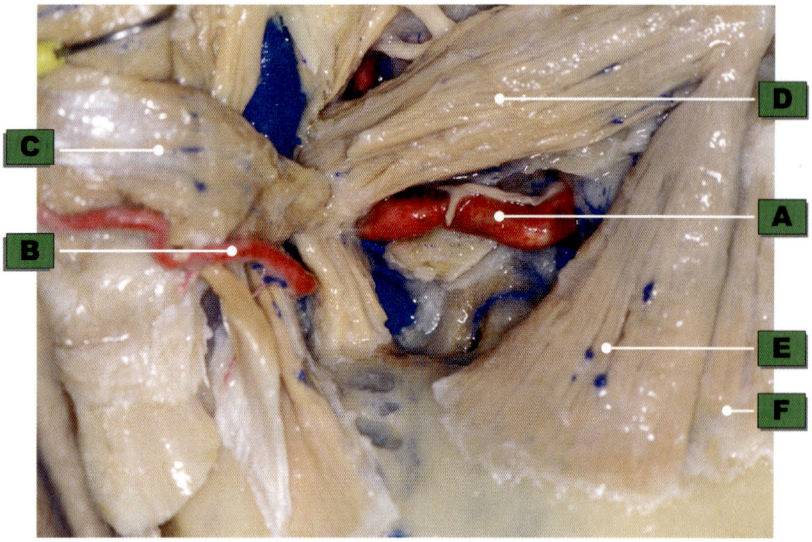

Figure 13–2 The right suboccipital vertebral triangle. **(A)** The right vertebral artery is seen coursing above the sulcus arteriosus. **(B)** Occipital artery emerging lateral to the rectus capitis lateralis. **(C)** Superior oblique muscle reflected laterally. **(D)** Inferior oblique muscle. **(E)** Rectus capitis major. **(F)** Rectus capitis minor.

Craniotomy

It is generally sufficient to place a small bur hole in the occipital bone and use the high-power drill to elevate a free bone flap. In the elderly, more than one bur hole might be necessary to avoid tearing a tightly adherent dura. The craniotomy may extend up to the junction of the transverse and sigmoid sinus superolaterally if necessary, to just beyond the midline through the foramen magnum inferiorly in a teardrop fashion with the wider opening superolaterally (**Fig. 13–3**). The height of the craniotomy varies from case to case; the more rostral one desires to expose intradurally, the closer to the transverse sinus the craniotomy needs to be made. Using a high-speed air drill with the foot plate attachment, the craniotomy can be started either at the level of the foramen magnum or through the bur hole. Bone is then drilled laterally until the area of the condylar fossa, just posterior to the occipital condyle and just above the dural entrance of the VA (**Fig. 13–3**). Here again it is helpful to have the VA exposed for orientation and to protect it from injury. This completes what is properly designated the "paracondylar" approach because no condylar bone has been drilled yet (**Fig. 13–4**). As the lip of the foramen magnum curves forward to become the occipital condyle, the bone becomes too "vertical" from the surgeon's point of view, and Kerrison rongeurs cannot be used. Therefore, a high-speed air drill with a cutting olive-shaped tip is very useful for the last 6 to 10 mm of the exposure, which includes drilling of the medial third of the condyle. A condylar emissary vein is almost always present and often needs to be sacrificed. This lateral removal of condylar bone is the key to being able to approach the front of the brain stem from an inferolateral angle with minimal or no brain stem retraction. Each extra millimeter removed from the

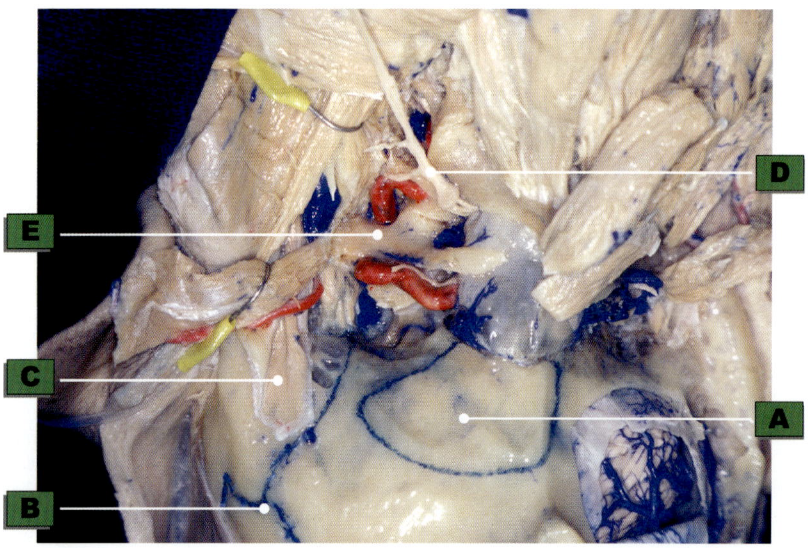

Figure 13–3 The bony exposure. **(A)** The outline of a "teardrop" suboccipital craniotomy. **(B)** The asterion. **(C)** Posterior belly of digastric muscle. **(D)** Dorsal ramus of C2 nerve root. **(E)** Posterior arch of C1.

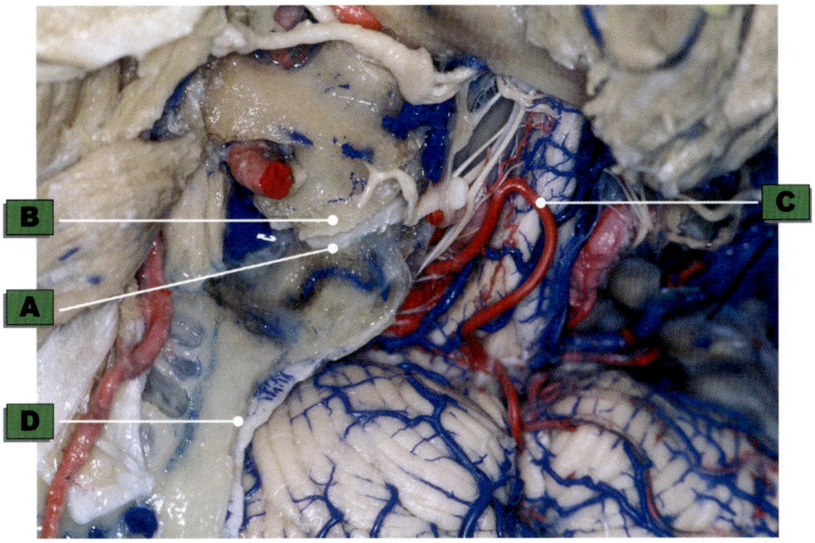

Figure 13–4 The paracondylar approach. This stage represents an intermediate step. The arch of C1 has been removed and the vertebral artery transected for anatomical clarity. **(A)** The occipital condyle, with its condylar emissary vein, can be seen and has not been drilled yet. With the dura open, one can appreciate that the condyle is an anatomical obstacle to the lower clivus and brain stem. **(B)** Lateral mass of C1. **(C)** Right posterior inferior cerebellar artery, coursing unusually caudally. **(D)** Level and position of the sigmoid sinus.

lateral rim of the foramen magnum provides the surgeon several additional millimeters of exposure at the depth. In this respect, the lateral rim of the foramen magnum and condyle represent to the suboccipital exposure what the pterion represents to the frontotemporal exposure. After the suboccipital craniectomy is accomplished, the hemiarch of C1 is removed from just beyond the midline on the opposite site to the sulcus arteriosus underlying the VA, at ~10 mm anterior to the dural entrance of the VA. Removing the arch of C1 allows an approach from a more inferior direction, below the cerebellar tonsil, without having to retract the cerebellar hemisphere medially (**Fig. 13–5**).

Intradural Dissection

The dura is opened in a gentle curve, starting superolaterally and coming down toward the midline in the area of the foramen magnum and then continuing straight down about the level of C1, where it turns again laterally, allowing the dural flap to be retracted inferolaterally. The lateral aspect of the dura is tented up tightly to the lateral muscle mass to maximize the lateral angle of exposure. After the dura is opened, the microscope is brought into the field, and the arachnoid is opened at the cisterna magna. The VA is encountered immediately. It is often necessary to cut the first dentate ligament to allow the medulla to fall away (**Fig. 13–5**). The cerebellar tonsil is gently lifted upward and medially with a self-retaining retractor. The origin of the PICA is found. We then prefer to continue the approach in the direction of the VA between the eleventh cranial nerve inferiorly and the ninth and tenth cranial nerves superiorly (**Fig. 13–6**). The vertebrobasilar junction can be reached through this space in the majority of cases. We have found that this space is wider than that between the ninth/tenth cranial nerves and the seventh/eighth cranial nerves more superiorly.

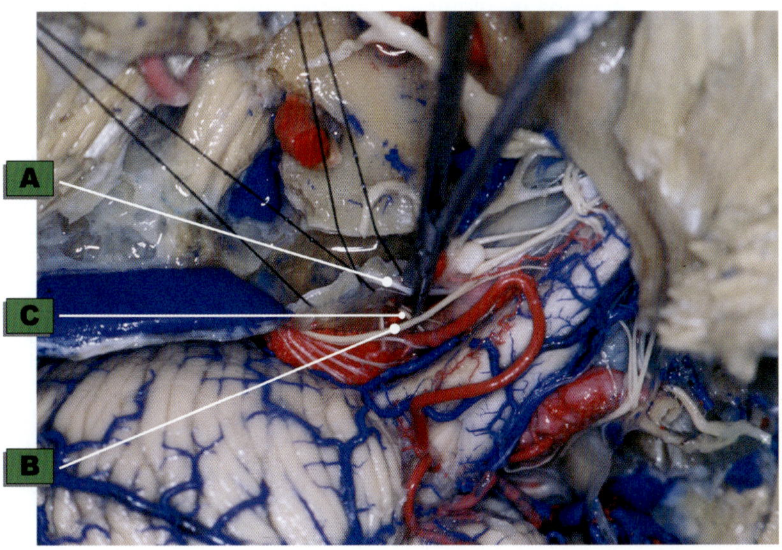

Figure 13–5 The partial transcondylar approach completed. With the condyle partially drilled, the intradural exposure is much more flat and direct. **(A)** The first dentate ligament is being divided to uncover the intradural vertebral artery. **(B)** Spinal accessory nerve. **(C)** Hypoglossal rootlets emerging anterior to the olive and coursing toward the hypoglossal canal, located just above the occipital condyle.

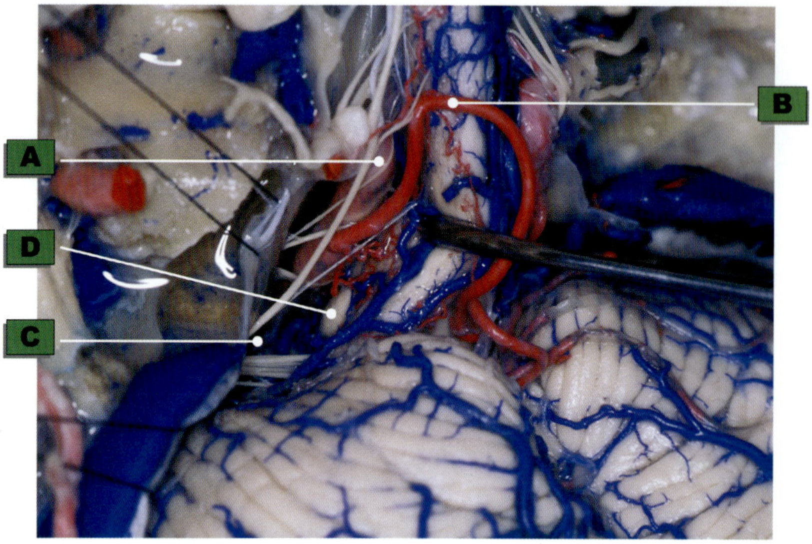

Figure 13–6 **(A)** Exposure of the vertebral artery and **(B)** posterior inferior cerebellar artery origin. **(C)** Note the wide triangular surgical space between the eleventh and ninth/tenth nerve complex. **(D)** The olive.

In cases of a high vertebrobasilar junction aneurysm, the surgeon must move the line of sight upward to the space above the ninth/tenth nerves. Another useful maneuver is to direct the line of vision through the upper space, between the seventh/eighth and ninth/tenth nerve complexes, but to apply the clip through the wider space below the ninth/tenth cranial nerves.

With this approach, the surgeon can usually see not only the ipsilateral vertebrobasilar junction but also the highest portion of the opposite VA, thus gaining complete control at the origin of the aneurysm. In cases of large aneurysms that may obscure the BA, the aneurysm must be retracted forward or backward to see the artery clearly. It is because of this confining intradural exposure that an appropriately generous extradural drilling needs to be accomplished to allow maximal maneuverability.

Closure

The dura is closed in a watertight fashion, and a pericranial graft is needed more often than not to achieve this. Exposed air cells are generously waxed. The bone flap is placed back and secured with a titanium osteosynthesis plating system, avoiding placing screws in the air cells. The muscles and fascia are closed in several layers with absorbable material, and the skin is closed with a running nylon suture.

Retrolabyrinthine Presigmoid and Transsigmoid Approaches

This approach was developed for the more medial vertebrobasilar junction aneurysms, low basilar trunk aneurysms, and high vertebral-PICA aneurysms.[15] It is best selected when the aneurysm is level with the midclivus. With this approach there is increased rostral exposure as well as shortening of the operative distance, decreasing cerebellar and brain stem retraction. The size and dominance of the sigmoid sinus will determine if the surgeon will be able to work through the sinus or on either side of it. This method may not be indicated for aneurysms located on the side of a dominant sinus.

The patient is positioned either supine or laterally. In the supine position the head is turned 60 degrees away from the side of entry, allowing the cerebellum to fall away. A C-shaped retroauricular incision exposes the bone from the root of the zygoma superoanteriorly, to the tip of the mastoid inferoposteriorly. A modified mastoidectomy is then made with a high-speed air drill removing air cells from an area bordered superiorly by the floor of the middle fossa and superior petrosal sinus, inferiorly by the jugular bulb, anteriorly by the posterior semicircular canal, and posteriorly by the sigmoid sinus. The sigmoid sinus is then skeletonized, and bone is removed behind the sinus for ~2 cm. For the transsigmoid variant, the dura posterior to the sinus is opened, and the sigmoid sinus is ligated and divided at its junction with the jugular bulb. It is often useful to confirm by intraoperative direct venous pressure measurements that the sinus is indeed unessential. Dural opening is completed, and the dura is reflected laterally, covering the intact labyrinth. The operative field is centered on the seventh and eighth complex (**Fig. 13–7**). Opening of the arachnoid exposes the VA as it meets its contralateral counterpart to form the vertebrobasilar junction. The aneurysm is then clipped in a standard fashion. Attention should be paid to the dural closure; generous bone waxing as well as a watertight dural closure must be obtained. A fat graft should also be placed to prevent CSF leakage.

We have needed to resort to transection of the sigmoid sinus in only a handful of cases, and those have generally been unplanned, resulting from insufficient intraoperative exposure (aneurysm and tumor cases alike). In an effort to prevent venous thrombotic complications, and when the retrosigmoid angle is insufficient for exposure, we greatly favor the "presigmoid" approach, which lends itself easily to a combination if necessary with the "retrosigmoid" approach.

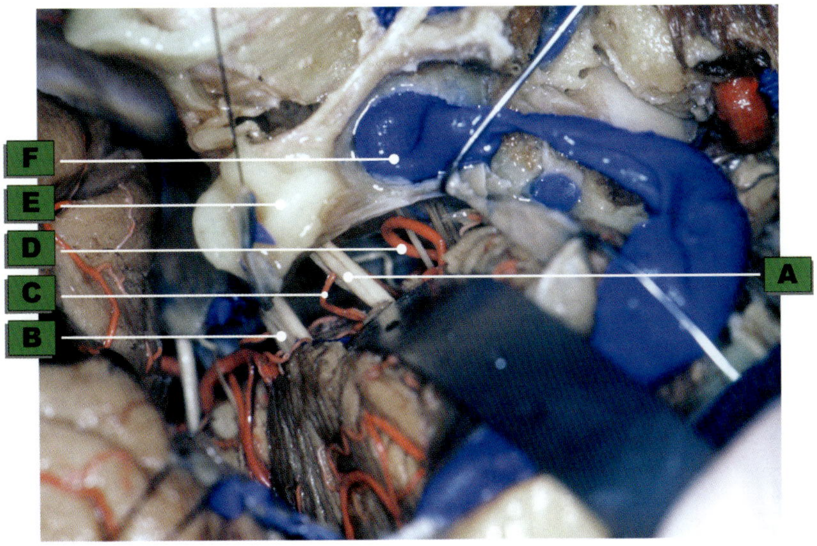

Figure 13–7 The presigmoid retrolabyrinthine exposure. A retractor is placed on the right cerebellar hemisphere, exposing **(A)** seventh/eighth nerve complex, **(B)** fifth nerve, **(C)** anterior inferior cerebellar artery, and **(D)** posterior inferior cerebellar artery. **(E)** The intact otic capsule with its three semicircular canals is plainly seen. **(F)** The jugular bulb poses a caudal limit to the drilling. In this specimen, a combined subtemporal approach, division of the tentorium, as well as an anterior petrosectomy were also done.

Anterior Transpetrosal Approach

Kawase et al[16] was the first to use and describe this approach for aneurysms of the vertebrobasilar junction and AICA. This approach allows the surgeon to reach the midfrontal portion of the pons and the cerebellopontine angle within a minimal distance and with no brain stem retraction.

In the middle fossa transpetrous approach originally described by House et al[17] for lesions in the anterosuperior cerebellopontine angle, hearing is preserved because drilling of the pyramidal bone is confined to its anterior part, leaving the cochlea and labyrinth intact. This is in contradistinction with the translabyrinthine approach (one of the variants of the "posterior transpetrous approaches"), where there is an extensive resection of the posterior aspect of the pyramidal bone.

The patient is positioned supine with the head turned maximally. The scalp incision is shaped as a question mark, as for a standard subtemporal approach. The craniotomy is centered low over the petrous ridge and flush with the floor of the middle fossa (**Fig. 13–8**). After peeling the dura from the middle fossa, the petrous ridge is identified. This peeling is performed from posterior to anterior to avoid avulsing the greater superficial petrosal nerve (GSPN) as it emerges forward from the facial hiatus. Lumbar drainage is utilized routinely. The middle meningeal artery in the foramen spinosum is coagulated. The posterior edge of V3 is identified extradurally. The so-called Kawase's rhomboid is thus uncovered (**Fig. 13–9**). It is an area limited by V3 anteriorly, the position of the internal auditory canal posteriorly, the sphenopetrosal groove containing GSPN laterally, and the petrous ridge medially. The

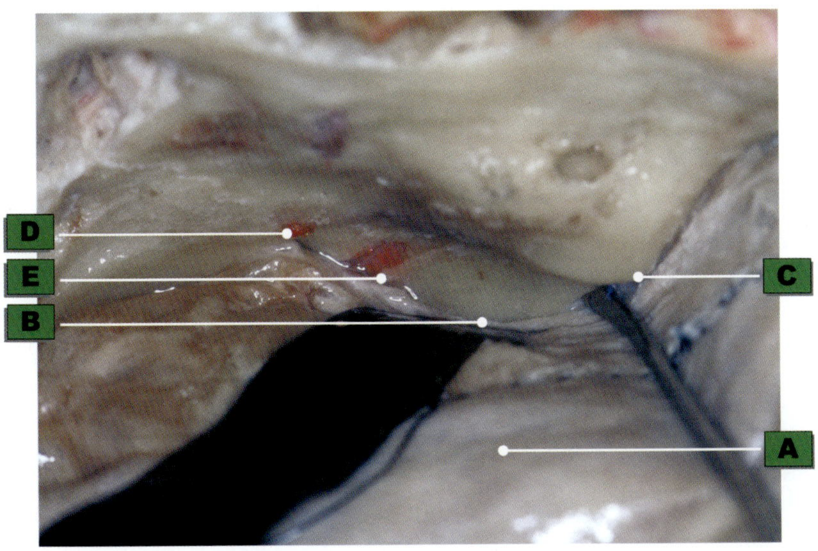

Figure 13–8 The right middle fossa approach. **(A)** The right temporal lobe is retracted extradurally, and the dural dissection performed from posterior to anterior, until **(B)** the petrous ridge is defined. **(C)** Landmarks include the arcuate eminence, **(D)** foramen spinosum, and **(E)** the greater superficial petrosal nerve.

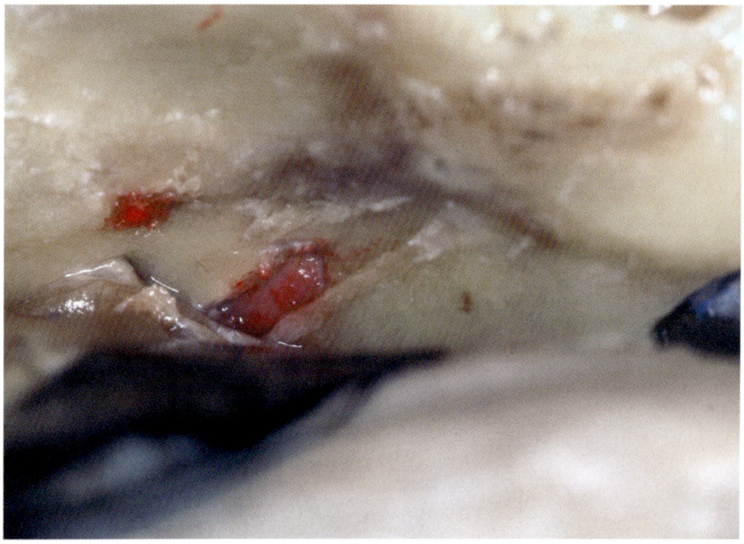

Figure 13–9 The right middle fossa approach. A magnified view of "Kawase's rhomboid."

two primary structures to preserve while drilling this bone are the horizontal petrous carotid laterally and the basal turn of the cochlea in the posterolateral corner. When drilling the internal auditory canal, special precaution must be taken to preserve the dura to avoid damage to the seventh and eighth cranial nerves. The deepest limit of the drilling is the inferior petrosal sinus, at the petroclival fissure. At the completion of the bony drilling, the convexity temporal dura is opened, an intradural subtemporal approach is achieved, and the tentorium is incised transversely behind the fourth nerve entrance, leading to coagulation/clipping and division of the superior petrosal sinus, leading in turn to an incision of the presigmoid dura toward the clivus. The anterolateral pons is thus exposed (**Fig. 13–10**). The vertebrobasilar junction aneurysm is then approached between the fifth and seventh cranial nerves and clipped in a standard fashion.

We limit this approach to lesions that are rostral to the midclivus (i.e., the level of the porus acusticus). With respect to vertebrobasilar aneurysms, it is therefore more typical to use this modified Kawase approach for low basilar bifurcation, basilar trunk, or high vertebrobasilar junction aneurysms.

Extreme Lateral Approach

Sen and Sekhar[18] described this approach, a more extensive variation of the far lateral approach, for VA aneurysms and for tumors located ventral or ventrolateral to the spinal cord and medulla. In this approach, the condyle is almost completely drilled, the sigmoid sinus and jugular bulb are skeletonized, and the VA is mobilized and translocated medially. We have not found this extra bone removal necessary or particularly useful in the case of aneurysms.

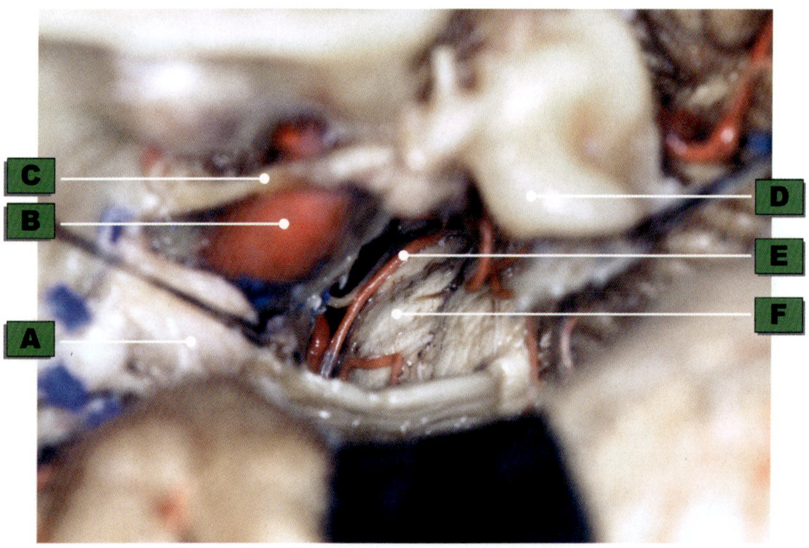

Figure 13–10 The right anterior transpetrous approach (Kawase's approach). This view is obtained after the completion of drilling of the pyramidal petrous apex, going intradurally subtemporally and dividing the tentorium and presigmoid dura. **(A)** V3 is retracted anteromedially. **(B)** The horizontal petrous carotid is covered by **(C)** the greater superficial petrosal nerve. **(D)** The superior semicircular canal is preserved. **(E)** The anterior inferior cerebellar artery and **(F)** the anterolateral pons are well seen.

Transoral-Transclival Approach

The transoral approach has been used by several authors for the treatment of extradural lesions confined to the midline of the lower third of the clivus, the craniocervical junction, and the upper two cervical vertebrae. The use of this approach for intradural lesions has been less frequent and for good reason. Drake initially, and a few other surgeons based on Drake's single case report, started using the transclival approach for vertebrobasilar junction aneurysms and middle third basilar aneurysms.[19] Due to the high incidence of CSF leakage and meningitis, it was abandoned and condemned by Drake. Lately, with the use of fibrinogen-based tissue adhesives in Europe, and of autologous preparation of fibrin glue in the United States, a significant decrease in the incidence of CSF leakage has being observed, and some authors have been using this approach successfully, especially when combined with prolonged lumbar drainage.[19]

Oral endotracheal intubation is required in these cases, although some prefer to perform a tracheostomy at the beginning of the procedure. For lesions below the foramen magnum, patients are nasotracheally intubated. A lumbar drain is inserted routinely. The authors who utilize this approach propose either the supine or the left lateral decubitus position. The advantage of the left lateral decubitus position is that blood, drilled fragments, and irrigation fluids will flow down to the tonsillar fauces and thus allow continuous visibility. The disadvantage is that the surgeon must "relearn" the anatomy of the region rotated through 90 degrees.[20] The transoral approach to this region requires division of the soft and hard palate. A special retractor (Crockard self-retaining retractor) is needed to improve the exposure. The clival window obtained after drilling is ~2 cm in width and 2 to 3 cm in length. The depth of the working area in an adult from the incisor teeth is more than 10 cm.[20]

While we routinely utilize this approach and modifications of it for extradural lower clival tumors, we strongly discourage its use for primarily intradural tumors and vertebrobasilar aneurysms. The access is long and narrow, the exposed target is small, and the risk of intraoperative rupture and postoperative meningitis is high.

Translabyrinthine and Transcochlear Approaches

Progressively more drilling of the temporal bone in a forward and medial direction produces, respectively, the retrolabyrinthine (**Fig. 13–7**), the partial translabyrinthine (**Fig. 13–11**), the "translabyrinthine" (**Fig. 13–12**), and the "transcochlear" (**Figs. 13–13** and **13–14**) approaches. House and Hitselberger[21] described the transcochlear approach for the resection of tumors located in front of the brain stem arising from the clivus or the petrous tip. In this approach, after drilling of the mastoid and bony labyrinth (the end of the translabyrinthine approach), the facial nerve is mobilized posteriorly out of its fallopian canal (**Fig. 13–13**). This involves skeletonization of the facial nerve and geniculate ganglion in the temporal bone from the stylomastoid foramen to the internal auditory canal, sacrificing the chorda tympani, and transecting the greater superficial petrosal nerve at its origin from the geniculate ganglion. This allows the uncovering and drilling of the cochlea, with the vertical petrous carotid forming the deep limit. Bone removal is performed medially to the inferior petrosal sinus, clivus, and jugular bulb, and superiorly to the superior petrosal sinus and middle fossa floor dura, thus creating a large triangular window (**Fig. 13–14**).

These variants of the posterior transpetrous route are only useful for the exposure of the vertebrobasilar aneurysms when combined with a temporal craniotomy and a tentorial incision, unifying the middle and posterior fossa compartments. These, along with the retrolabyrinthine variant, form the family of so-called combined subtemporal/presigmoid approaches. A detailed anatomical exposition of the temporal bone is beyond the scope of this chapter, but **Fig. 13–15** shows the surface surgical landmarks of the temporal bone in relation to the sigmoid sinus and otic capsule, after a retrolabyrinthine drilling was accomplished.

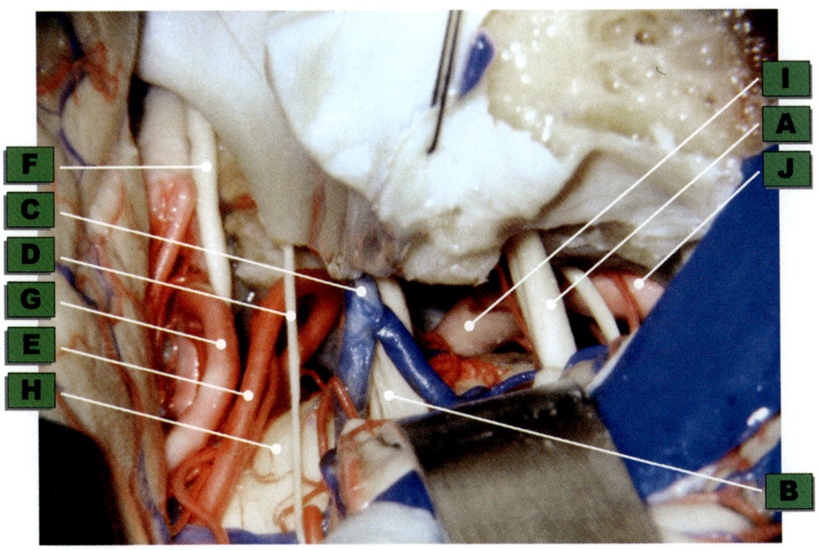

Figure 13–11 The right "partial" translabyrinthine/combined subtemporal approach. The superior semicircular canal has been drilled and the dura reflected laterally, exposing **(A)** seventh/eighth nerves, **(B)** fifth nerve, **(C)** petrosal vein, **(D)** fourth nerve, **(E)** superior cerebellar artery, **(F)** third nerve, **(G)** posterior cerebral artery, **(H)** pons, **(I)** basilar artery, **(J)** vertebral artery and posterior inferior cerebellar artery, among others.

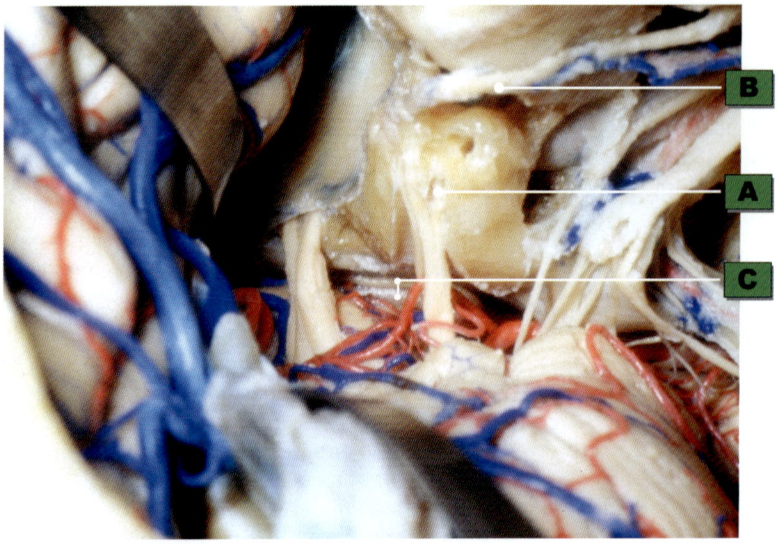

Figure 13–12 The right translabyrinthine/combined subtemporal approach. **(A)** All three semicircular canals have been drilled down to the cochlea. **(B)** The descending portion of the seventh nerve is exposed. A much flatter view of the clivus is obtained, compared with **Fig. 13–11.** **(C)** The basilar artery and adjoining sixth nerve are well seen.

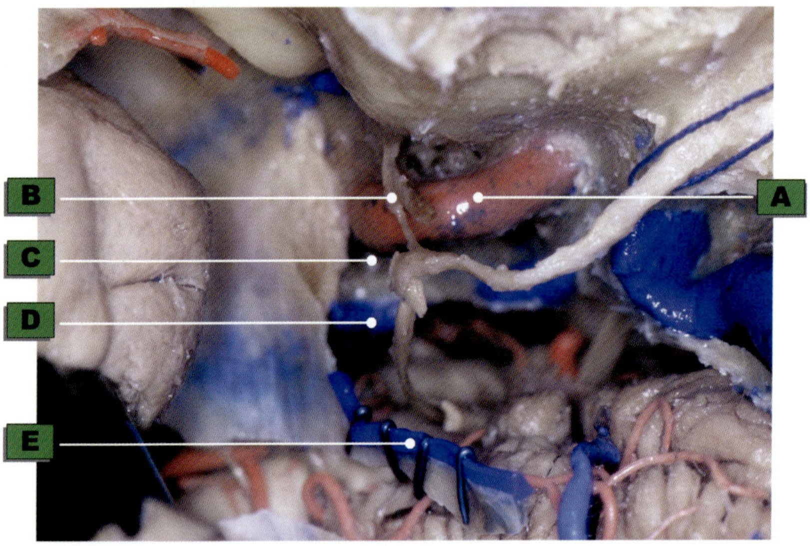

Figure 13–13 The right transcochlear/combined subtemporal approach. **(A)** The vertical carotid artery is exposed. **(B)** The greater superficial petrosal nerve is ready to be transected, **(C)** to allow the geniculate ganglion and the rest of the facial nerve to be transposed posteriorly, allowing unimpeded view of the clivus. **(D)** The inferior and **(E)** superior petrosal sinuses were preserved for anatomical clarity.

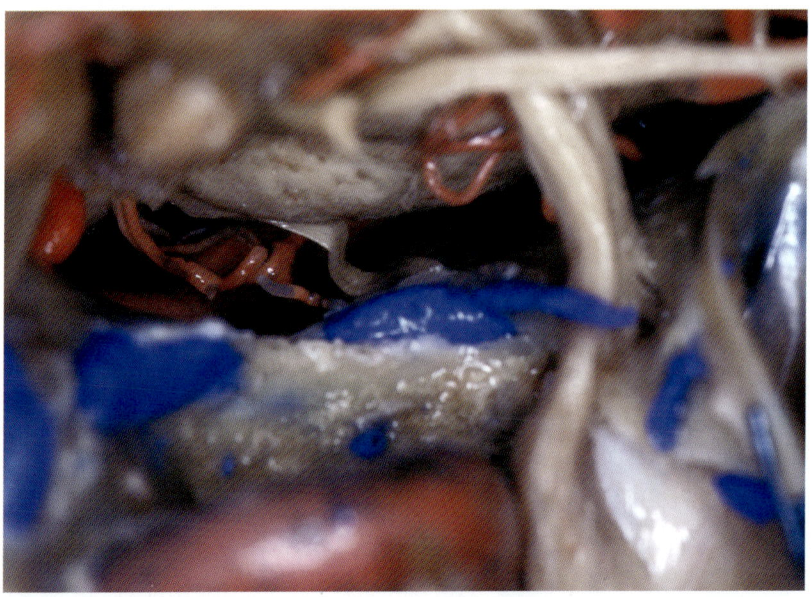

Figure 13–14 The right transcochlear/combined subtemporal approach, magnified view. The pons, basilar artery, and sixth nerve are well exposed.

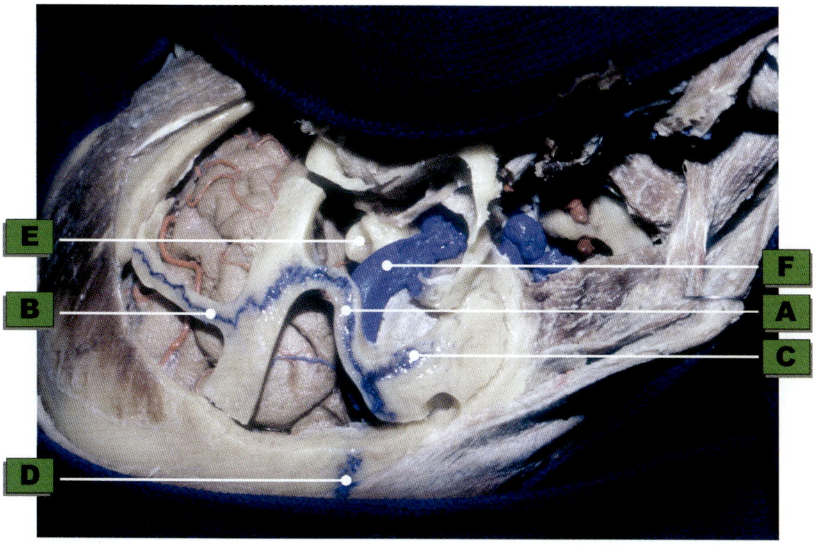

Figure 13–15 Surface landmarks of the posterior petrosectomy approaches. **(A)** The parietomastoid suture crosses the sigmoid sinus. It joins **(B)** the squamosal suture to **(C)** the occipitomastoid and **(D)** lambdoid sutures, the latter two meeting at the asterion. **(E)** Otic capsule. **(F)** Sigmoid sinus.

◆ Vertebral-Posterior Inferior Cerebellar Artery Aneurysms

These aneurysms can be approached through a unilateral suboccipital craniotomy.[3,4,6] We, however, prefer to use the far lateral suboccipital approach already described for vertebrobasilar junction aneurysms; the degree of condylar drilling necessary is usually less than for the more medially placed vertebrobasilar junction aneurysm. Likewise, depending on the location of the aneurysm, the surgeon may choose not to remove the arch of C1, although we prefer to do it routinely to achieve early intradural VA control.

More proximally located VA aneurysms are immediately seen after the dura is opened through a simple unilateral suboccipital craniotomy that is carried to the foramen magnum. The intradural dissection is identical to that of the far lateral approach and includes a thorough division of the tela of the tonsillomedullary fissure. After this step, the cerebellum is lifted off the medulla with a narrow retractor blade placed on the base of the tonsil. The eleventh cranial nerve is exposed. The VA is identified emerging from under the dentate ligament, and the loop of the PICA is seen. The VA is traced distally. The origin of the PICA is almost always just proximal to the aneurysm and serves as a good landmark. Exposure is gained with gentle dissection. The access to the aneurysm is between the filaments of the tenth and eleventh cranial nerves, which must be protected meticulously against the possibility of injury and consequent disabling hoarseness and dysphagia. All perforators to the medulla should be spared. As the rest of the aneurysm is brought into view, it is best to work on either side of the PICA and up to the sides of the VA beyond the neck. Usually, the portion of the dome of the aneurysm adherent to the medulla can be left undisturbed, and only the neck is isolated. Occasionally, depending on the projection of the aneurysm, it may be necessary to dissect the dome out of the medullary indentation. Bipolar coagulation of the aneurysm may be needed to define the neck, and that should always be done under the protection of temporary clipping and adequate irrigation to avoid tissue sticking. Care should be exercised to avoid injury to the twelfth cranial nerve in the depth of the exposure, medial to the olive. With aneurysms intimately involved with the PICA origin, a small, straight, fenestrated clip encircling the PICA is often the best strategy.

◆ Distal Posterior Inferior Cerebellar Artery Aneurysms

The surgical approach to these aneurysms must be based on a good understanding of the anatomy of the PICA. This artery can be divided into five segments.

Anterior Medullary and Lateral Medullary Segments

The first two segments (anterior medullary and lateral medullary) lie anterior and lateral to the medulla, respectively. Aneurysms in these locations can be approached inferolaterally by gentle elevation and medial retraction of the tonsil, as already described for vertebral PICA aneurysms.

Tonsillomedullary Segment

The next segment, the tonsillomedullary segment, courses behind the medulla in front of the tonsil. For aneurysms in this location, we would use a combined lateral and medial suboccipital craniotomy, essentially as described for vertebral PICA aneurysms but with bone removal extending well past the midline in the inferior aspect of the occipital bone and the foramen magnum as well as the arch of C1. It is not necessary to drill the occipital condyle. Control of the PICA is then gained from the lateral angle. The tonsil is then retracted upward, medially, or laterally, based on the exact aneurysm location. We again rely heavily on temporary clipping to soften the aneurysmal sac and reconstruct the neck while preserving patency of the PICA. A modest subpial resection of part of the tonsil might be necessary with an adherent dome.

Telovelotonsillar and Cortical Segments

Aneurysms of the PICA distal to its cranial loop (telovelotonsillar and cortical segments) can be approached by a standard midline suboccipital craniotomy extending through the foramen magnum.[12] The aneurysm can be approached between the tonsils by gently retracting them laterally or, if adherent to the tonsil, by subpial dissection.

Aneurysms located more peripherally on a cortical branch are almost always mycotic in etiology and should be treated by resection rather than clipping. This seems to be almost always well tolerated at this far distal arterial level because the last important branches to the deep cerebellar nuclei are given at about the level of the "choroidal point" in the cranial loop (telovelotonsillar segment).[22]

◆ Dissecting Aneurysms

SAH from dissecting aneurysms of the VA is not as unusual as it was previously thought.[23] In recent series of VA aneurysms it has been reported in 21 to 28%.[3,8] Most commonly they are distally located and usually present with sudden, severe suboccipital headache in a known hypertensive patient.

Multiple descriptions have been given to the angiographic findings of dissecting aneurysms such as "pearl and string sign," linear defects, true and false lumen (double lumen), and retention of contrast medium in the venous phase. In spite of all these descriptions, it is difficult at times to differentiate among saccular, dissecting, and fusiform aneurysms. Magnetic resonance imaging may occasionally demonstrate a false lumen or intramural thrombus (an eccentric target sign). Andoh et al[8] reported five cases that were brought to the operating room with the diagnosis of saccular aneurysms. Three proved fusiform, and the other two were dissecting aneurysms. Yamaura[3] described that the angiographic characteristics of dissecting aneurysms—in relatively young patients with no other responsible lesions for an SAH—may merely be a "narrowed segment" proximal and/or distal to a "fusiform dilatation" of the affected artery, and the persistence of contrast medium in an intramural false lumen at the late phase.

The risk of rebleeding from dissecting aneurysms seems to be as high as for saccular aneurysms, and it can be as high as 40% within several hours;[8] therefore, their treatment should not be delayed. Dissecting VA aneurysms are best treated by trapping the VA either distally to the PICA origin or in certain cases as high as the origin of the BA. Several authors have previously attempted to clip the aneurysm without success because there is no clear neck. The state of the art today, however, involves the role played by endovascular trapping with balloons or coils. The challenge is in the preservation of the PICA origin. In dissections that involve this origin, particularly if the involved PICA is large with a poor prospect for collaterals, it may be necessary to consider combining a PICA revascularization with the trapping (occipital artery to PICA, or PICA to PICA).[24] Andoh et al[8] suggested a balloon test occlusion to assess the collateral circulation, even though this test may increase the risk of rebleeding when performed in the acute stage. An alternative technique is to reimplant the PICA in the VA in an end-to-end fashion.[24,25]

References

1. Peerless SJ, Hernesniemi JA, Drake CG. Posterior circulation aneurysms. In: Wilkins RH, Rengachary SS, eds. Neurosurgery. 2nd ed. New York: McGraw-Hill; 1996:2341–2356
2. Pia HW. Classification of vertebrobasilar aneurysms. Acta Neurochir (Wien) 1979;47:3–30
3. Yamaura A. Diagnosis and treatment of vertebral aneurysms. J Neurosurg 1990;72:183–188
4. Drake CG, Peerless SJ, Hernesniemi JA. Surgery of Vertebrobasilar Aneurysms. New York: Springer; 1996:167–203
5. Hudgins RJ, Day AL, Quisling RG, et al. Aneurysms of the posterior inferior cerebellar artery: a clinical anatomical analysis. J Neurosurg 1983;58:381–387
6. Salcman M, Rigamonti D, Numaguchi Y, et al. Aneurysms of the posterior inferior cerebellar artery-vertebral artery complex: variations on a theme. Neurosurgery 1990;27:12–21
7. Lee KS, Gower DJ, Branch CL Jr, et al. Surgical repair of aneurysms of the posterior inferior cerebellar artery: a clinical series. Surg Neurol 1989;21:85–91
8. Andoh T, Shirakami S, Nakashima T, et al. Clinical analysis of a series of vertebral aneurysms cases. Neurosurgery 1992;31:987–993
9. Wiebers DO, Whisnant JP, Huston J 3rd et al, and the International Study of Unruptured Aneurysms Investigators. Unruptured intracranial aneurysms: natural history, clinical outcome, and risks of surgical and endovascular treatment. Lancet 2003;362:103–110
10. Kallmes DF, Lanzino G, Dix JE, et al. Patterns of hemorrhage with ruptured posterior inferior cerebellar artery aneurysms: CT findings in 44 cases. AJR Am J Roentgenol 1997;169:1169–1171
11. Hoh BL, Cheung AC, Pryor JC, Carter BS, et al. Results of a prospective protocol of computed tomographic angiography in place of catheter angiography as the only diagnostic and pretreatment planning study for cerebral aneurysms by a combined neurovascular team. Neurosurgery 2004;54:1329–1342
12. Beyerl BD, Heros RC. Multiple peripheral aneurysms of the posterior inferior cerebellar artery. Neurosurgery 1986;19:285–289
13. Sutton D, Trickey SE. Subarachnoid hemorrhage and total cerebral angiography. Clin Radiol 1966;13:297–303
14. Heros RC. Lateral suboccipital approach for vertebral and vertebrobasilar artery lesions. J Neurosurg 1986;64:559–562
15. Giannotta SL, Maceri DR. Retrolabyrinthine transsigmoid approach to basilar trunk and vertebrobasilar artery junction aneurysms: technical note. J Neurosurg 1988;69:461–466
16. Kawase T, Toya S, Shiobara R, et al. Transpetrosal approach for aneurysms of the lower basilar artery. J Neurosurg 1985;63:857–861
17. House WF, Hitselberger WE, Horn KL. The middle fossa transpetrous approach to the anterior-superior cerebellopontine angle. Am J Otol 1986;7:1–4
18. Sen CN, Sekhar LN. An extreme lateral approach to intradural lesions of the cervical spine and foramen magnum. Neurosurgery 1990;27:197–204
19. Crockard HA, Sen CN. The transoral approach for the management of intradural lesions at the craniovertebral junction: a review of 7 cases. Neurosurgery 1991;28:88–98
20. Crockard HA. The transoral approach. In: Sekhar LN, Janecka IP, eds. Surgery of Cranial Base Tumors. New York: Raven; 1993:225–234
21. House WF, Hitselberger WE. The transcochlear approach to the skull base. Arch Otolaryngol 1976;102:334–342
22. Friedman AH, Drake CG. Subarachnoid hemorrhage from intracranial dissecting aneurysms. J Neurosurg 1984;60:325–334
23. Madsen JR, Heros RC. Giant peripheral aneurysm of the posterior inferior cerebellar artery treated with excision and end-to-end anastomosis. Surg Neurol 1988;30:140–143
24. Durward QJ. Treatment of vertebral artery aneurysm by aneurysm trapping and posterior inferior cerebellar artery implantation. J Neurosurg 1995;82:137–139
25. Ausman JI, Diaz FG, Mullan S, et al. Posterior inferior to posterior inferior cerebellar artery anastomosis combined with trapping for vertebral artery aneurysm: case report. J Neurosurg 1990;73: 462–465

14

Cranial Base Approaches to Aneurysms

Laligam N. Sekhar and Chandrasekar Kalavakonda

Skull base approaches are very useful during aneurysm surgery for a variety of reasons. The removal of basal cranial bones improves the working space and exposure of aneurysms while reducing brain retraction, especially when the brain is tense after aneurysmal rupture. The placement of saphenous vein or other grafts and the deep hypothermic circulatory arrest technique can be facilitated by the use of skull base approaches. The disadvantages of the use of skull base approaches are the increased time taken to perform the approach and the slightly increased risk of cerebrospinal fluid (CSF) leakage through any communications that may be created with paranasal sinuses or the middle ear cavity, especially in the presence of hydrocephalus. These risks have to be weighed against the advantages in selecting the approach.

◆ Indications

The use of a skull base approach is dependent upon the location, size, and other anatomical features of the aneurysm and the tightness of the brain. It also depends upon the surgeon's experience with the use of skull base approaches. In general, orbital and orbitozygomatic osteotomies required for anterior circulation aneurysms can be performed with a minimal increase of the operative time (about 1 hour). Temporal bone and extreme lateral approaches used for some posterior circulation aneurysms do add about 2 to 3 hours. However, the benefits of these approaches are greatest with posterior circulation aneurysms. When a giant aneurysm or an aneurysm requiring a vascular reconstruction is operated upon, a skull base approach is essential.

◆ Preparation

In addition to the standard preoperative studies that may include computed tomographic (CT) scan, magnetic resonance imaging (MRI), and a cerebral angiography, the following studies may be of value. A three-dimensional CT (3D-CT) angiogram often displays the aneurysm in relation to the basal skull bones, and this can help select the type and side of approach. The venous phase of the cerebral angiogram is important in planning transtemporal approaches and in evaluating the dominance and collateralization of the sigmoid sinuses and the anatomy of the vein(s) of Labbé.

◆ Anesthesia

The anesthetic technique is the same as with all aneurysms. However, when a transpetrosal approach is employed, neuromuscular blockade should be short acting or avoided to allow the facial nerve to be identified and dissected.

Neurophysiological monitoring is employed in all aneurysm operations and may consist of electroencephalogram (EEG), somatosensory evoked potential (SEP), and brain stem auditory evoked response. Facial nerve monitoring is added during transtemporal approaches.

◆ Positioning

Patient position will vary according to the type of approach and is usually a supine position with varying degrees of head turn or a lateral (park bench) position. At the time of initial positioning, a femoral artery sheath is usually placed by the radiologist for intraoperative angiography (5 French sheath connected to a heparinized saline flush bag), and an area is prepared for the extraction of fat or fascia, either the abdomen or the thigh.

◆ Approaches

The different types of approaches used will be described first, along with pitfalls and complications of each approach. The selection of the approach to match the aneurysm will be described later. The operative approaches to be described include orbital osteotomy, middle fossa petrous apex resection, anterior and posterior clinoidectomy, petrosal approaches with varying degrees of petrosectomy, and the extreme lateral approach, with or without excision of the jugular tubercle.

Orbital Osteotomy

An orbital osteotomy is used in the management of anterior circulation aneurysms, including anterior communicating complex aneurysms, internal carotid artery aneurysms, and some middle cerebral artery (MCA) aneurysms. The extent of the osteotomy should be tailored according to the aneurysm. The senior author prefers to perform an orbital osteotomy for anterior communicating artery (ACommA) and internal carotid artery aneurysms to reduce brain retraction and provide for improved operating space. But for posterior communicating artery (PCommA) and MCA bifurcation aneurysms, it is sufficient to perform a posterior orbitectomy to obtain more operating space.

The skin incision is started just below the zygoma in the preauricular area very close to the pinna and extended into the frontotemporal area, reaching the hairline near the midline. It can be extended bicoronally in patients with a receding hairline. The skin, subcutaneous tissue, and pericranium are dissected away from the temporal fascia after making an incision in the temporal fascia just lateral to the orbital rim. The periorbita is then dissected away from the orbital rim, roof, and lateral wall. If the supraorbital nerve and vessels are in a foramen, they will need to be released with a small bone drill or by a chisel and mallet. The periorbita should be dissected for a distance of at least 3 cm posterior to the orbital rim. After a frontotemporal craniotomy is performed, the frontal and temporal dura are separated from the roof and lateral walls of the orbit. If the brain is very tense, a ventriculostomy or the opening of the basal cisterns may be needed to perform this dissection.

A self-retaining retractor is placed on the basifrontal dura. The periorbita is protected by a broad ribbon retractor held by the assistant, and the osteotomies are performed. The medial extent of the osteotomy will depend upon the aneurysm. For anterior communicating complex aneurysms, it is made at or just medial to the supraorbital notch. For internal carotid artery (ICA) or MCA aneurysms, it is made lateral to the supraorbital notch. The osteotomy cuts are made with a reciprocating saw from the cranial to the orbital side. The first cut is sagittal, extending at least 3 cm posterior to the orbital rim. The second cut is coronal, extending laterally along the roof, and then vertically along the lateral wall. The orbital retractor must be moved ahead of the saw to protect the periorbita. The third cut is made horizontally through the lateral wall. The osteotomized orbit is loosened up, if necessary, with a chisel and mallet, and removed. The frontal sinus may be exposed by the medial osteotomy, depending upon the size and lateral extension of the sinus (**Fig. 14–1**).

After the osteotomy piece is removed, the surgeon starts to work under the microscope. Further dissection of the periorbita is performed. The superior orbital fissure is unroofed by the removal of the lateral portion of the lesser wing of the sphenoid bone and a part of the greater wing of the sphenoid bone. The anterior clinoid process and the optic nerve canal are not removed during this process. At the end of the bone removal, the orbit will be seen to be continuous with the frontotemporal dura (superior orbital fissure unroofed).

At the end of the operation, the frontal sinus must be closed, if it was exposed, to prevent a CSF leak. Under microscopic or endoscopic vision, the frontal sinus mucosa is removed as completely as possible. The frontonasal duct is plugged with a large roll of Surgicel (Johnson & Johnson, Arlington, TX). Fat obtained from the abdominal wall or thigh is packed into the sinus, and the sinus is covered with a pedicled flap of pericranium, which is then sutured to the frontal dura. The orbital osteotomy piece is then reattached with titanium miniplates. The frontotemporal bone flap is anchored as usual.

Anterior Clinoidectomy and Optic Canal Unroofing

The removal of the anterior clinoid process (ACP) and the optic canal is necessary for ICA–paraclinoid aneurysms and for basilar quadrification aneurysms. This can be done intradurally or extradurally. Intradural removal of the last portion of the clinoid process is preferred for aneurysms adjacent to the clinoid, and when the clinoid process is very long or fused to the sphenoid bone, forming a caroticoclinoid foramen. Extradural resection can be performed when

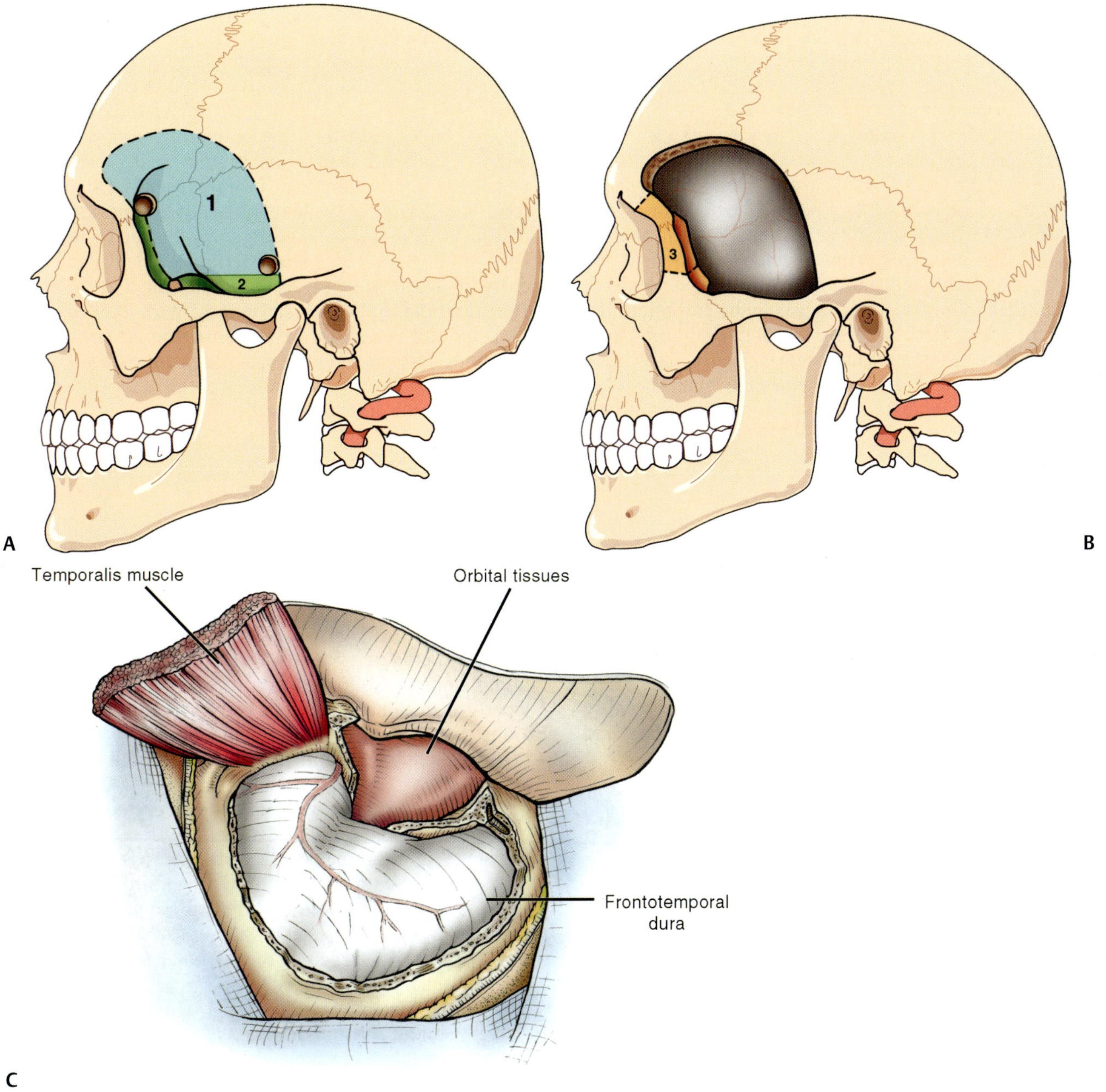

Figure 14–1 **(A)** Frontotemporal craniotomy and orbital osteotomy. Shaded areas 1 and 2 represent the frontotemporal craniotomy and the craniectomy down to the base of the skull, respectively. **(B)** Shaded area 3 represents the osteotomy. **(C)** The final exposure obtained after the craniotomy, osteotomy, and orbital decompression. (Courtesy of Laligam N. Sekhar.)

the clinoid process is short or normal in size and when the aneurysm is at a distance from the clinoid process (e.g., basilar tip aneurysms).

For extradural resection, after unroofing the superior orbital fissure, the lateral end of the superior orbital fissure is divided for a distance of ~5 mm. This contains the orbital meningeal artery and possibly a vein. Once this is done, the dura mater of the lateral wall of the cavernous sinus can be further peeled away from the ACP if necessary. Using a high-speed drill, the ACP is cored out, and then the bone of the optic canal is thinned. An inexperienced surgeon should use a diamond drill bit, but the experienced surgeon may use a small cutting bur. The last part of the clinoid process and the optic strut are removed with fine rongeurs after separation of the dura mater. Any venous bleeding from the cavernous sinus is stopped by gently packing with Surgicel or Gelfoam.

Before intradural removal, a part of the optic nerve canal and the distal portion of the ACP can be removed extradurally. After opening the dura mater and displaying the aneurysm, a small dural flap is created around the ACP and the optic nerve canal. This flap is retracted toward the aneurysm with sutures, and bone drilling is performed with the aneurysm under direct vision. If the aneurysm is thin walled and large or giant, it is wise to temporarily occlude the cervical ICA during the drilling and bone removal in an intermittent fashion. After the bone removal, for paraclinoid aneurysms, the optic nerve dural sheath is opened completely to allow the nerve to be mobilized.

The sphenoid or ethmoid sinuses frequently extend into the optic strut and sometimes into the ACP. This must be looked for. At the end of the aneurysm operation, any such opening must be packed with a piece of temporalis fascia and fat. This is followed by a dural closure that is performed as well as possible. If there is an opening into the sphenoid, any defect in the clinoidal dura must be closed, using if necessary a small dural graft. The graft can usually be sutured to the dura of the optic sheath and to the fold of the tentorium joining the orbital apex. Watertight closure is often not possible. If there is no opening into the sphenoid sinus, then the dural defect in the anterior fossa can be sutured circumferentially to the periorbita.

Pitfalls

1. Cutting the orbital roof too far anteriorly. At least two thirds of the orbital roof must be included in the osteotomy; otherwise, too much bone is discarded by rongeuring, and enophthalmos could result.
2. In addition to the sphenoid sinus, the frontal sinus may extend into the orbit. This sinus will need to be exenterated, and the frontonasal duct occluded with a plug of Surgicel. The frontal sinus is then packed with fat and covered with a pericranial flap.
3. During the dissection of the periorbita, orbital fat may extrude through holes in the periorbita. However, if any muscles of the orbit herniate through holes in the periorbita, these should be pushed in and held in place with sutures in the periorbita.

Orbitozygomatic Osteotomy

A frontotemporal craniotomy is performed. Bone is rongeured to the anterior limit and floor of the middle fossa. The frontal and the temporal dura are separated off the bony floor and the periorbita separated off the roof and the lateral wall of the orbit. The periorbita is separated at least 3 cm posteriorly from the orbital rim. The frontal dura is elevated and protected with a retractor. Similarly, the periorbita is protected with a retractor, advancing the retractor as the cut is being made. A sagittal cut is made through the roof of the orbit for a distance of 3 cm, with the cut being made from the cranial to the orbital side. A horizontal cut is made extending across the roof of the orbit down the lateral orbital wall to the inferior orbital fissure.

Anteriorly, the zygoma is cut just lateral to the zygomaticomaxillary suture. The external landmark for this is a small foramen through which a small nerve and an accompanying artery emerge. The cut is made just posterior and behind this foramen, and this avoids entry into the maxillary sinus. The cut is extended posteriorly to the inferior orbital fissure. Posteriorly, the zygoma is cut at the junction of its root with the squamous portion of the temporal bone (**Figs. 14–2E** and **14–3**).

If the condylar fossa is to be included in the osteotomy, the temporomandibular joint will need to be opened and the meniscus depressed. The dura is dissected off the middle fossa floor, exposing the foramen spinosum with the middle meningeal artery, mandibular nerve, and arcuate eminence. The cuts are made in a V-shaped fashion just anterior and posterior to the confines of the fossa, both the cuts meeting medially. The surgeon will need to be careful not to make the cuts too far posteriorly or medially to avoid entry into the middle ear or the carotid canal, respectively. Transilluminating the condylar fossa with light does this best, and this will allow the surgeon to define the limits of the condylar fossa. After the osteotomy, unroofing of the superior orbital fissure with drilling of the ACP and the optic canal is done as mentioned earlier.

Presigmoid Petrosal Approaches

The patient is positioned supine, with a heavy roll placed under the ipsilateral shoulder. The head is rotated 70 degrees to the contralateral side and fixed in the Mayfield head clamp.

The incision will depend on whether the presigmoid approach is being performed alone or in combination with a frontotemporal orbitozygomatic osteotomy (OZO) approach. If performed alone, a C-shaped incision is done that extends along the superior temporal line down the retroauricular region ~3 cm behind the mastoid and into the upper neck area along a skin crease. The skin, subcutaneous tissue, galea, and pericranium are incised and elevated. The posterior part of the temporalis muscle is elevated and reflected forward. The sternomastoid fascia and muscle are reflected forward along with the skin to improve the vascularity of the scalp flap. The splenius and semispinalis muscles are detached from their insertions and reflected posteroinferiorly. The root of the zygoma the temporal and mastoid, and occipital squama are exposed.

The mastoidectomy will be performed by a neuro-otologist, and, under the microscope, the sigmoid sinus and the basitemporal dura are skeletonized. About 1 cm of the retrosigmoid dura may also be skeletonized during this drilling. The neurosurgical team then performs the temporal craniotomy.

The neuro-otologist, working under the surgical microscope, skeletonizes the posterior aspect of the vertical segment of the facial nerve; exposes the lateral, posterior, and superior semicircular canals; and skeletonizes the sigmoid sinus and the jugular bulb. The surgeon takes care not to damage the endolymphatic sac, located in the lower half of the presigmoid dura.

For a partial labyrinthectomy, petrous apicectomy (PLPA) approach, the ampullae of the superior and the lateral canals and the common crus are fenestrated. The membranous labyrinth is occluded with bone wax or bone dust, and the bony and membranous portions of these canals are excised. This step avoids loss of any endolymph. The petrous apicectomy is now performed. The removal of the petrous apex extends anteriorly from the region of the horizontal

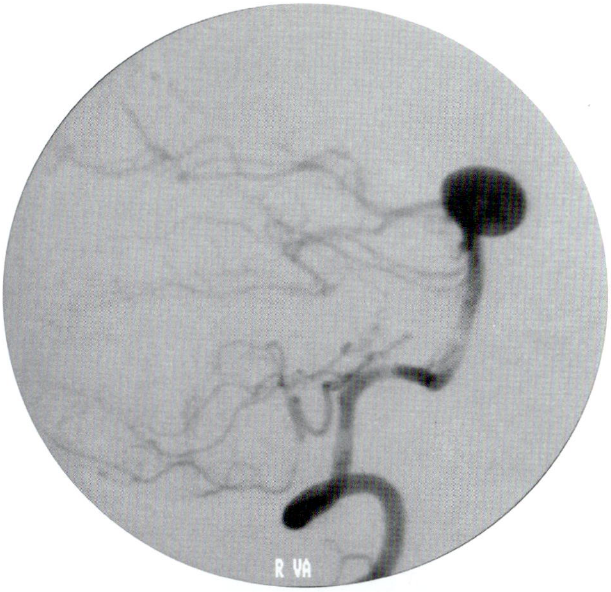

A

Figure 14–2 **(A)** The lateral view of the right vertebral angiogram and **(B,C)** the three-dimensional computed tomographic angiogram show a large basilar tip aneurysm with a broad neck and tilted to the right. **(D)** The intraoperative angiogram shows complete occlusion of the aneurysm. **(E)** Schematic representation of the frontotemporal craniotomy with the orbitozygomatic osteotomy and the approach to the aneurysm (arrows). (Copyright to **Fig. 14–2E** belongs to Laligam N. Sekhar.)

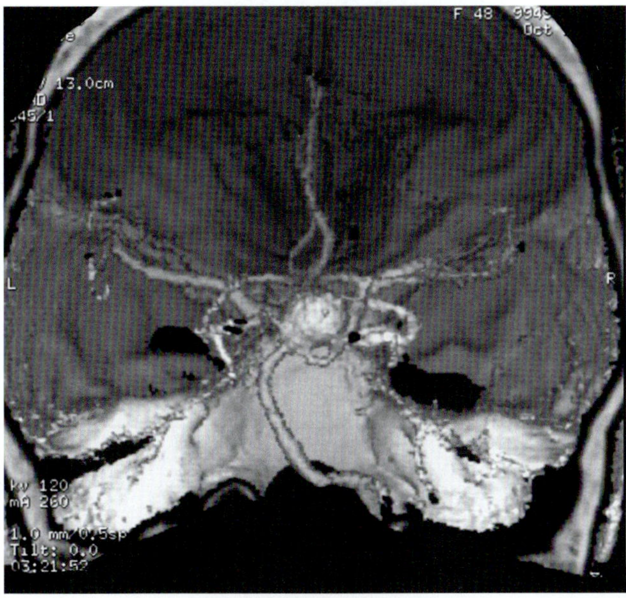

B

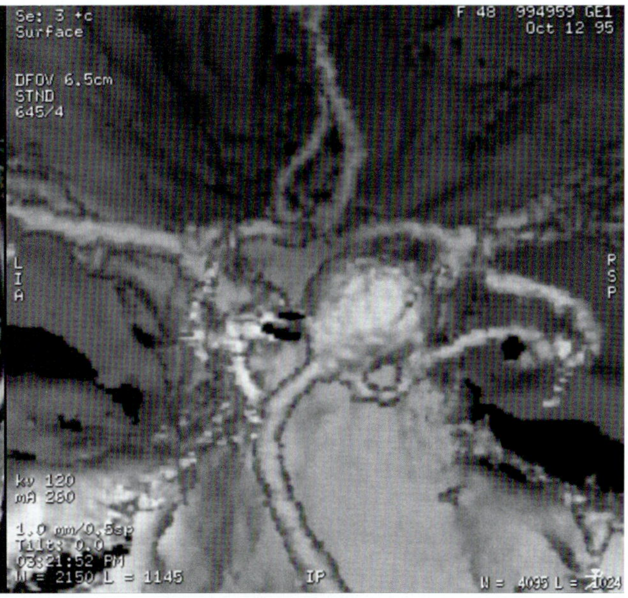

C

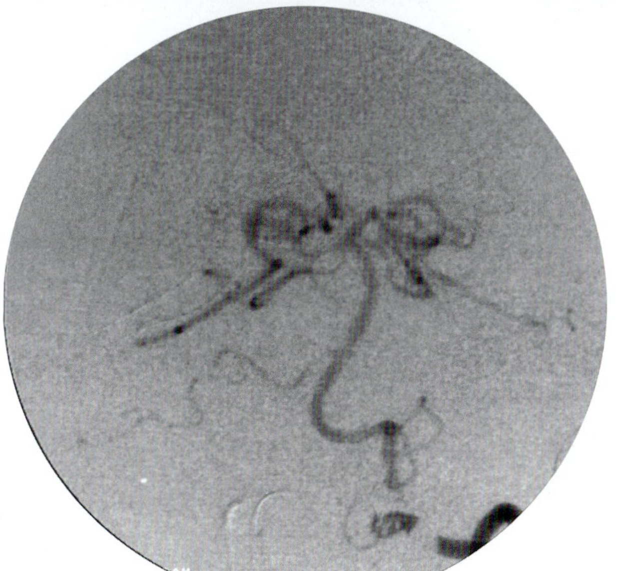

D

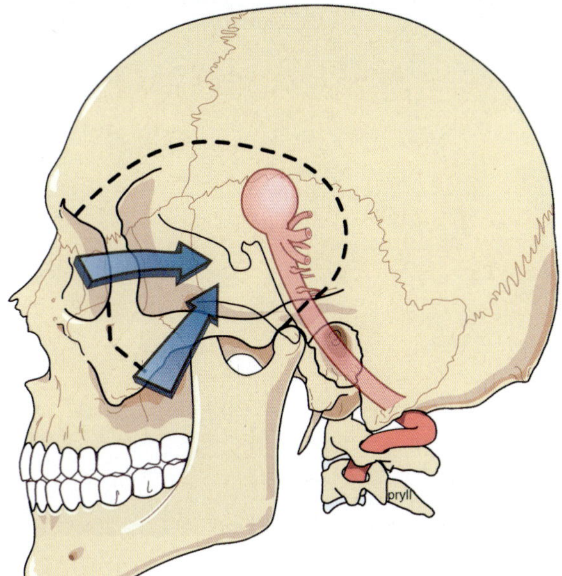

E

(*Continued on pages 198 and 199*)

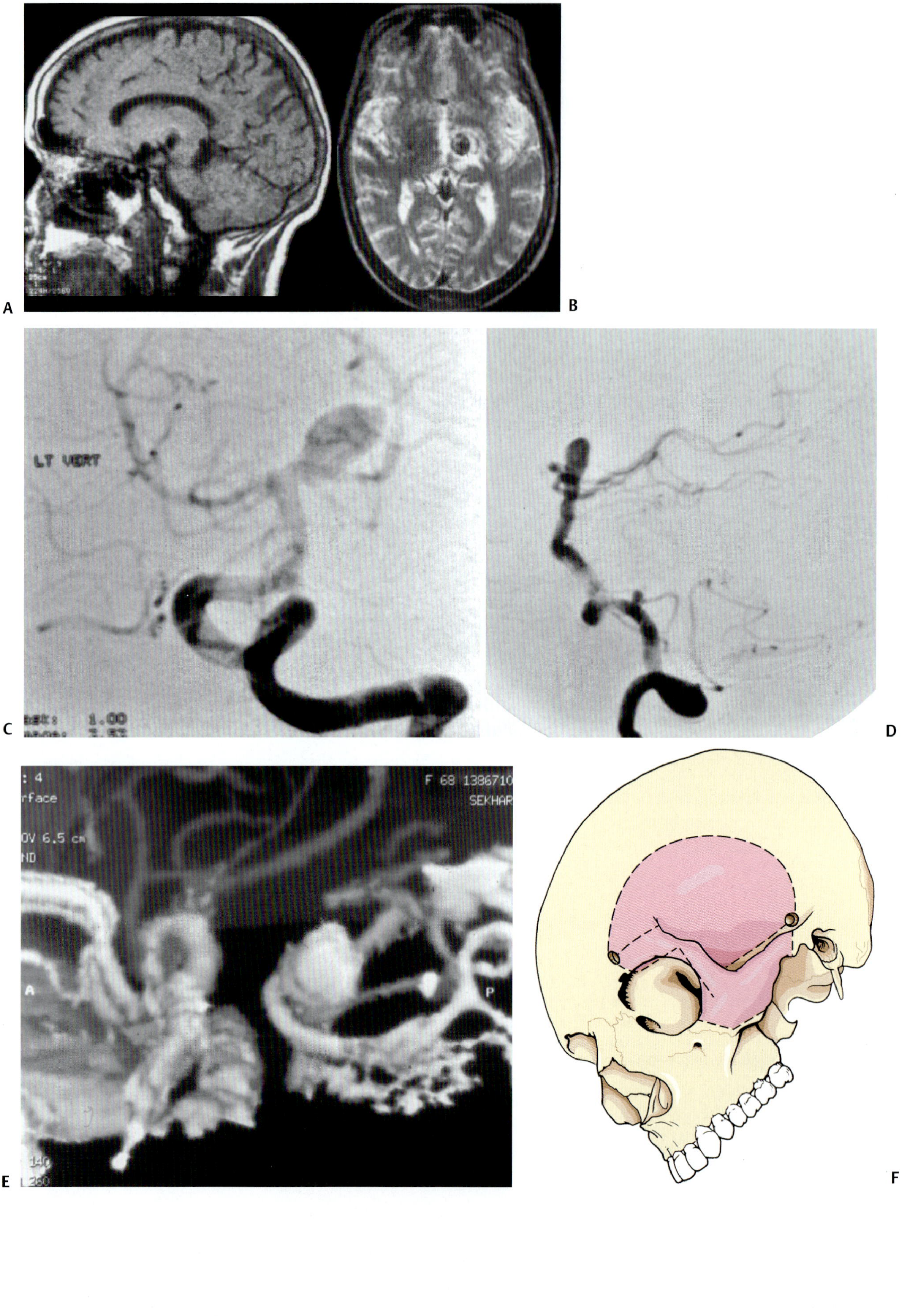
LT VERT
F 68 1386710
SEKHAR

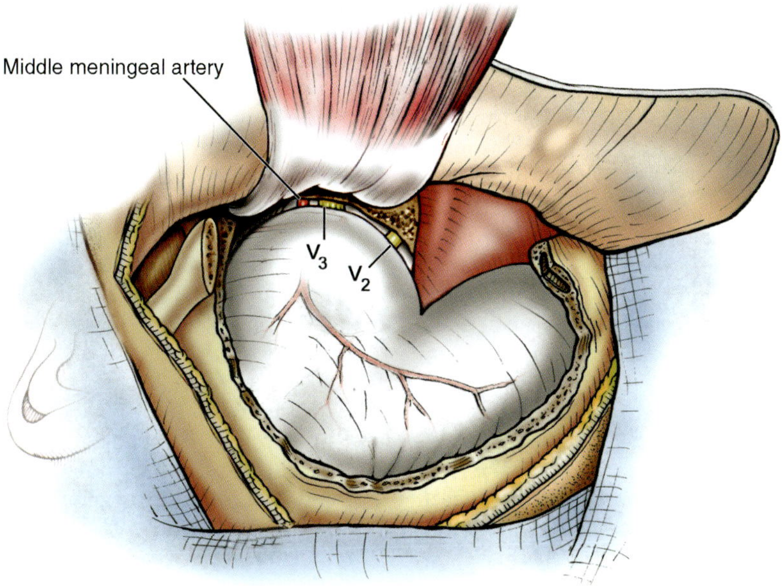

G

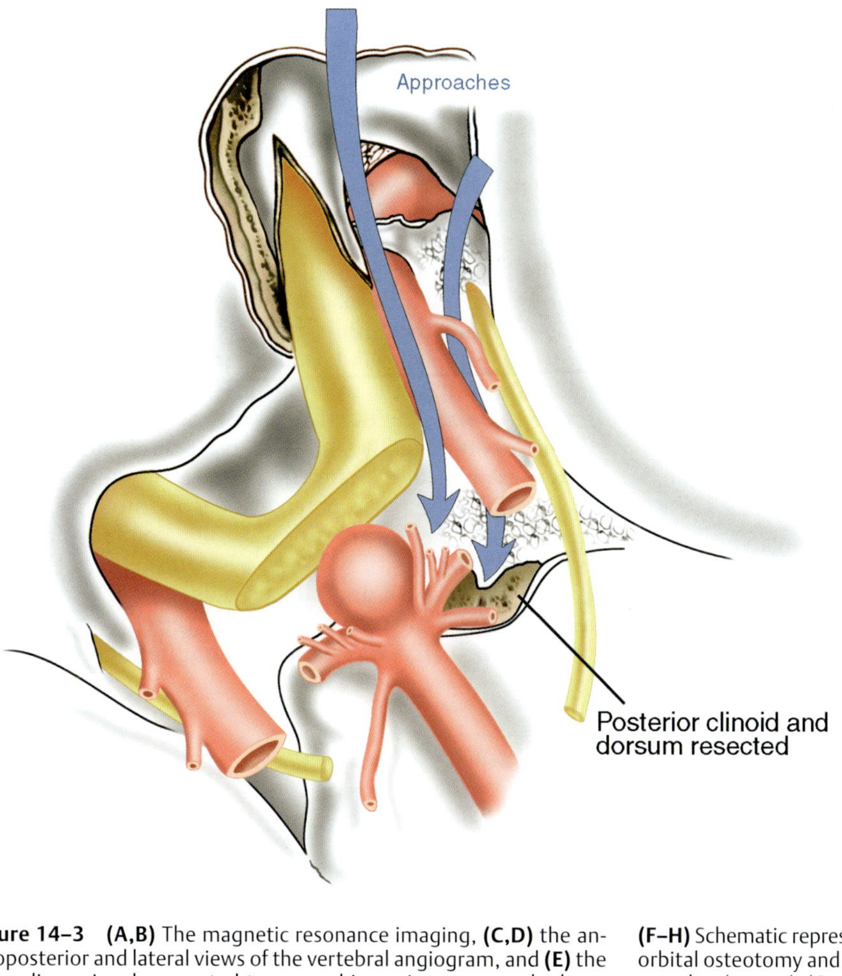

H

Figure 14–3 **(A,B)** The magnetic resonance imaging, **(C,D)** the anteroposterior and lateral views of the vertebral angiogram, and **(E)** the three-dimensional computed tomographic angiogram reveal a large basilar artery–superior cerebellar artery aneurysm on the left side. **(F–H)** Schematic representation of the frontotemporal craniotomy with orbital osteotomy and the transclinoid with extended transsylvian approaches (arrows). (Courtesy of Laligam N. Sekhar.)

portion of the petrous ICA, around the superior aspect of the internal auditory canal (IAC), and inferiorly down to the level of the endolymphatic sac. Hyperventilation and intravenous mannitol may be used to relax the brain to achieve an adequate petrous apicectomy. The posterior aspect of the root of the zygoma and the superior aspect of the external auditory canal are also drilled away for a flat exposure.

For a total petrosectomy, the facial nerve will need to be completely skeletonized, from the IAC down to the stylomastoid foramen. The greater superficial petrosal nerve is sectioned just anterior to the geniculate ganglion, and the facial nerve is mobilized posteriorly. Damage to the facial nerve during the operation may result in facial paralysis with a prolonged and incomplete recovery. The most important part of the procedure is the exposure and mobilization of the facial nerve; hence it is well worth the time spent to achieve this. The blood supply from the anterior inferior cerebellar artery (AICA) and the stylomastoid branch of the ascending pharyngeal artery must be preserved to maintain optimal facial nerve function. Neurophysiological monitoring is used during the facial nerve mobilization, and this also is useful. We often perform the total petrosectomy approach on one day and operate the aneurysm the next day. After the facial nerve has been mobilized posteriorly, the petrous ICA is exposed in its entirety and mobilized anteriorly. The petrous bone superior to the jugular foramen and the parts of the lateral clivus are drilled away. This approach provides a very wide exposure of the anterolateral brain stem and the petroclival region. The eustachian tube is packed with fat and closed with suture to prevent CSF leakage.

Complications

1. Temporal lobe retraction–related injury
2. Damage of the vein of Labbé
3. Damage to the semicircular canals; may affect hearing
4. Facial nerve injury during exposure and mobilization, being most common with total petrosectomy
5. Vestibular symptoms may be observed and are usually transient.
6. The risk of postoperative CSF leakage, more so with the PLPA approach, will need to be kept in mind and adequate precautions taken to pack the middle ear and the eustachian tube.

Far Lateral Retrosigmoid Approach

The patient is positioned in a lateral or park bench position. Some surgeons prefer to position the patient supine with the head rotated to the opposite side, but this can produce kinking of the vertebral artery (VA) and also obstruct venous outflow.

We use a C-shaped skin incision in the retroauricular area. The incision starts just above the pinna, curving posteriorly and medially to the planned limit of the craniotomy and continued inferiorly into the upper neck area, confining to the hairline. The skin, subcutaneous tissue, and galea are reflected forward, along with the sternomastoid fascia and muscle. The splenius capitis, semispinalis capitis, and suboccipital muscles are reflected inferiorly. This layered elevation of the muscles has reduced our incidence of CSF leakage and also the occurrence of persistent postoperative headaches.

We prefer to do a craniotomy in younger patients and a craniectomy in the elderly. Two bur holes are first placed. The first bur hole is placed at a point just posteroinferior to the intersection of the following two imaginary lines. The first line is drawn along the base of the mastoid, with the second extending horizontally from the external occipital protuberance to intersect the first. The second bur hole is placed at an inferior and medial corner of the planned bone flap. The dura is completely separated off the overlying bone at these bur hole sites, and the holes are connected to raise the bone flap. In elderly patients we perform a craniectomy because the dura is usually densely adherent to the overlying bone. In most cases, the foramen magnum will need to be unroofed to allow the surgeon to obtain proximal control of the VA.

If there is accidental laceration of the sigmoid sinus, it can be repaired with one or two 5–0 Prolene sutures if the opening is small. Larger ones may require temporary packing with dural tack-up sutures but carry the risk of occlusion. On the dominant side, this could result in either cerebellar swelling or delayed hydrocephalus. If a larger laceration occurs, the sigmoid sinus is exposed under the microscope and repaired with 5–0 Prolene sutures, using a dural flap or a vein patch.

Intravenous mannitol and furosemide administered at the time of skin incision facilitates brain relaxation. A lumbar drain is frequently used, but care must be taken to avoid overdrainage, which may result in the development of a subdural hematoma. Dura mater is opened under the microscope just medial and parallel to the sigmoid sinus, curving posteriorly at the inferior corner. The sigmoid sinus is rotated laterally by dural sutures. The cerebellum is elevated superomedially, and the lateral cerebellomedullary cistern is opened to drain CSF. The cerebellum is gently retracted to expose the lower cranial nerves initially. Once the lower cranial nerves are exposed, the VA and the posterior inferior cerebellar artery (PICA) are identified and exposed. Cranial nerves IX, X, and XII have a very close relationship to the VA-PICA aneurysms. Therefore, the clips must be positioned in such a way as not to compress or kink these nerves.

Complications

1. CSF leakage—Usually responds to lumbar spinal drainage done for 3 to 5 days. If persistent, reexploration may be needed—adequate dural closure and resealing of the mastoid air cells with bone wax are performed. Communicating hydrocephalus is often present, which may be the cause of the leakage—this will warrant a ventriculoperitoneal (VP) shunt.
2. Facial paralysis and hearing loss are possibilities.
3. The patient should be observed for lower cranial nerve paralysis. If suspected, the patient should have a swallowing evaluation before being fed. Further confirmation of the paralysis should be obtained from a larynx

specialist, using endoscopy. Mild weakness will resolve in time, and nasogastric feeding will be necessary for a short time. An arytenoid and vocal cord medialization procedure will be necessary to resolve a significant paralysis, and the patient may also require a feeding jejunostomy or gastrostomy for ~2 to 3 months.

Extreme Lateral Retrocondylar and Partial Transcondylar Approach

We prefer to place the patient in a lateral position. The lateral position, however, makes intraoperative angiography and vein graft extraction more difficult. If the extreme lateral approach is combined with a presigmoid petrosal approach, it is easier to place the patient supine with the head rotated to the opposite side. Besides the disadvantages of the VA kinking and venous outlet obstruction due to neck rotation, a greater than 60 degree rotation to the opposite side will move the transverse process and foramen of C1 medial and inferior to the mastoid tip, making exposure of the VA in the C1 transverse foramen more difficult.

We prefer to make a C-shaped skin incision, which commences in the retroauricular region and extends into the cervical area along a skin crease. The sternomastoid fascia and muscle are reflected forward, along with the skin. The spinal accessory nerve, which leaves the posterior border of the sternomastoid muscle, could be injured if the exposure extends below the level of C1. The splenius muscle that forms the next layer is reflected inferomedially. The third layer of muscles consists of the semispinalis capitis and the longissimus capitis. Between these two layers runs the occipital artery. This could be either preserved for use at a later time or ligated at the digastric groove. The fourth layer is formed by the suboccipital muscles and the levator scapulae. The levator scapulae attaches to the lateral aspect of the transverse process of C1–C2 and the occipital bone. The VA lies in the suboccipital triangle, the boundaries of which are formed by the suboccipital muscles. The VA is surrounded by a venous plexus that extends along the artery from the dural entrance of the artery down to the C6 transverse foramen. This venous plexus connects the condylar emissary vein to the epidural venous plexus.

The levator, superior, and inferior oblique muscles are detached from the C1 transverse process and reflected inferiorly and medially, exposing the arch of C1. The rectus capitis muscle is detached from the suboccipital bone and reflected inferiorly. The surgeon ought to take great care not to damage the VA between the C1 and C2, where it has a tortuous course. The venous plexus around the artery and the ventral ramus of C2, which runs posterior to the artery, serve as a guide to the artery. The artery and the venous plexus are dissected off the posterior arch of C1. The bony foramen of C1 through which the artery runs is unroofed. The artery can then be mobilized from the C2 ramus up to its entry into the dura.

A low mastoidectomy is performed, unroofing the sigmoid sinus and the posterior aspect of the jugular bulb. The portion of mastoid overhanging the occipital condyle is removed by this mastoidectomy. It is not necessary to unroof the facial nerve completely in its mastoid segment. A small suboccipital craniotomy is performed, extending ~3 cm posteriorly from the sigmoid sinus, and the lateral third of the foramen magnum is removed. The lateral half to one third of the posterior arch of C1 is removed along with the fibrofatty tissue between the C1 and foramen magnum. This completes the retrocondylar approach and is used for laterally placed aneurysms.

The *partial transcondylar approach* is used for intradural lesions lying anterior to the brain stem. The VA is unroofed and mobilized medially from the C2 to its dural entry. During drilling of the condyle, care must be taken not to damage the VA, usually protecting the artery with the suction held in the surgeon's hand. The atlanto-occipital joint is identified and the capsule incised to open the joint. The lateral mass of the C1 and the posterior one third to half of the condyle are drilled away. The condyle is initially cored out, and fine rongeurs are used to remove the remaining pieces of bone. Epidural venous oozing can be controlled with Gelfoam packing, or by injecting fibrin glue in the epidural space.

In the *transtubercular approach*, a complete mastoidectomy is performed with anterior mobilization of the facial nerve and the digastric muscle. The lateral mass of the C1 is drilled away, mobilizing the VA medially. The posterolateral one third of the condyle is drilled. Extradurally, a part of the jugular process is drilled. Complete excision of the jugular tubercle is possible only with intradural drilling. This usually has to be done by working inferior to cranial nerves IX and X, or between fascicles, with a thin diamond drill bit. The dura is opened retrosigmoid. The sigmoid sinus can be divided if it is nondominant or well collateralized. After measuring the intrasinus pressure, the sinus can be divided between temporary clips and resutured with 6–0 Prolene at the completion of the procedure. If the sinus is dominant, the tubercle can still be drilled through the intradural approach. This approach gives a good exposure to manage aneurysms located on the distal vertebral artery and vertebrobasilar junction.

Complications

1. VA injuries are generally due to the surgeon's inexperience. Therefore, adequate experience with cadaver dissection is a must before using this approach on patients.
2. Injury to the sigmoid sinus and jugular bulb can have devastating consequences if it is dominant. This can be avoided by performing the drilling carefully. The bone must be carefully separated from the sinus dura, and in older patients a thin layer of bone may need to be left on the venous sinus.
3. CSF leakage can be avoided by a meticulous dural closure, using a dural graft if needed. If communicating hydrocephalus is present, then lumbar spinal fluid drainage may be used.
4. Patients will need to be observed for lower cranial paresis, and if present, treatment is provided, as stated previously.

◆ Posterior Circulation Aneurysms

Cranial base approaches are particularly important for posterior circulation aneurysms because of the difficult access to these aneurysms with standard approaches. These approaches can also be nicely combined with the deep hypothermic circulatory arrest technique for complex aneurysms. The choice of approach will be discussed first, followed by some details of each approach.

Approach

The choice of approach for *anterior circulation aneurysms* is relatively straightforward. An orbital osteotomy is combined with the craniotomy for ICA aneurysms below the PCommA origin, with the ACP being removed intradurally if the aneurysm is adjacent, giant ICA aneurysm at any location, giant MCA aneurysm. This allows a tangential view of the ACommA aneurysm with the sagittal cut of the osteotomy being more medial.

The choice of approach to *posterior circulation aneurysms* depends upon the position of the aneurysm in relation to the bony anatomy rather than the vessel of origin. The size of the aneurysm and the branches at the bifurcation also play a role. The side of the approach will be determined by the position of the neck in relation to the midline, with the aneurysm being usually approached from the side of the neck. The use of a deep hypothermic circulatory arrest technique also plays a role in the choice of the side of the approach because the ability to decompress a large or giant aneurysm sac early in the operation allows the surgeon to approach the aneurysm from the same side rather than from the side of the aneurysm neck.

Basilar tip aneurysms may be the most difficult to expose surgically. The choice of the skull base approach depends upon the position of the neck in relation to the tip of the dorsum sellae; those that are just below (within 5 mm) or above (within 5 mm) the dorsum sellae are considered to be intermediate in position, those that are lower than 5 mm from the tip of the dorsum are considered low in position, and those more than 5 mm above the tip are considered high in position. Intermediate-position basilar tip aneurysms are the easiest to expose and are reached via a frontotemporal, orbitozygomatic approach using a combination of trans-sylvian and anterior subtemporal approaches. High-position basilar tip aneurysms are approached by the same technique; however, certain aneurysms that are extraordinarily high in their location may be difficult to expose by any approach. An endovascular technique for occlusion must be strongly considered in such cases. If microsurgery is elected, the combination of an orbitozygomatic and a lamina terminalis approach may be considered to expose the aneurysm. Such an aneurysm may have to be pushed inferiorly to adequately expose the neck and the perforators. Low-position basilar tip aneurysms are difficult to expose via an orbitozygomatic approach. Either a subtemporal, transpetrous apex, transcavernous, or petrosal approach is preferred for such aneurysms. The senior author prefers the petrosal approach.

Upper third and midbasilar aneurysms require a petrosal approach. For upper third basilar artery (BA) aneurysms, a transzygomatic, subtemporal approach may be adequate, depending upon the exact location of the aneurysm along with the presence and orientation of branches. A 3D-CT scan and the arteriogram are reviewed to make the decision between a subtemporal approach and the petrosal approach. When a midbasilar aneurysm is placed lower along the clivus, the retrolabyrinthine petrosal approach may not provide adequate room for working, but a PLPA petrosal approach can provide the necessary space. In rare cases of giant midbasilar aneurysms, a total petrosectomy approach is needed. In such patients, it is better to perform the approach on one day and the aneurysm surgery on another day.

Vertebrobasilar junction (VBJ) aneurysms can be very difficult to expose, especially if they are located in the midline and if the brain stem is swollen. The position of the VBJ is variable in relation to the clivus and will determine the approach used, based on the appearance on a 3D-CT scan. The combination of a presigmoid and retrosigmoid approach with the displacement or division of the sigmoid sinus is appropriate for high-position VBJ aneurysms. For others, a very lateral retrosigmoid approach with unroofing of the sigmoid sinus, and if possible its division, is adequate. To be divided, the sigmoid sinus must be nondominant or equidominant and connected with the one on the contralateral side through the torcula and visible on the preoperative angiogram. At surgery, the intrasinus pressure is measured before and after temporary occlusion, and the sinus is not divided unless the increase of pressure is less than 5 mm Hg. The cerebellum is also observed for swelling, and evoked potentials during surgery are observed for any deterioration. The senior author prefers to occlude the sinus between temporary clips and reconstruct it at the end with 6–0 Prolene sutures. The removal of the jugular tubercle intradurally can be very helpful with the exposure of VBJ aneurysms. Occasionally, the senior author has also used the subtemporal-infratemporal approach for the exposure of VBJ aneurysms.

VA aneurysms may arise at the origin of the PICA, or may be dissecting or fusiform aneurysms arising from the main trunk of the artery, not specifically at the origin of a branch but incorporating one of the branches. Most vertebral-PICA aneurysms may be dealt with by a far lateral retrosigmoid approach. Depending upon the level of origin of the PICA, the craniotomy may have to be extended inferiorly to include the foramen magnum. Fusiform and dissecting VA aneurysms may require a very lateral retrosigmoid approach, an extreme lateral partial transcondylar approach with jugular tubercle resection, or a presigmoid and retrosigmoid approach with sigmoid sinus division. Either or both vein graft reconstruction and reimplantation of branches may need to be performed in such patients. The following cases will be used to illustrate the surgical approaches, pitfalls, and complications to be avoided.

◆ Illustrative Cases

Case 1—Large Basilar Tip Aneurysm—Orbitozygomatic Approach with Deep Hypothermic Cardiac Arrest

This 48-year-old woman presented with severe headaches and a family history of aneurysms (**Fig. 14–2**). The preoperative angiogram and 3D-CT scan revealed a large BA tip aneurysm with a very broad neck and slightly tilted toward the right. A small MCA bifurcation aneurysm was also present. The aneurysm was approached via a right frontotemporal craniotomy and orbitozygomatic osteotomy. An anterior clinoidectomy was necessary because of the short length of the supraclinoid ICA. The large aneurysm was exposed, without the proximal BA being visible. By transfemoral cannulation, deep hypothermia with cardiac arrest was induced to a core temperature of 18°C. The PCommA was divided close to its junction with the posterior cerebral artery (PCA), allowing for slight retraction of the ICA. The aneurysm could now be dissected from the perforators, shrunk down with bipolar cautery with a brief period of circulatory arrest of 8 minutes. Adequate clipping of the aneurysm was confirmed by intraoperative angiography. After rewarming, a platelet transfusion was necessary to correct a coagulopathy. The patient did well postoperatively, with resolution of a transient oculomotor palsy, and returned to work.

Case 2—Basilar–Superior Cerebellar Artery Aneurysm

This 68-year-old woman was discovered to have a large basilar artery–superior cerebellar artery (BA-SCA) aneurysm (**Fig. 14–3**) and a small VA-PICA aneurysm after she had presented with headaches. The BA-SCA aneurysm was approached via a left frontotemporal craniotomy and OZO; using an extended transsylvian approach, it was clipped uneventfully. The VA-PICA aneurysm was exposed and clipped via a standard retrosigmoid approach.

Case 3—Low Neck Basilar–Superior Cerebellar Artery Aneurysm

This 10-year-old boy presented with a history of subarachnoid hemorrhage. Angiography revealed a complex aneurysm of the basilar quadrification, and the left SCA was not seen (**Fig. 14–4**). Preoperative 3D-CT scan revealed a very broad and low neck. The aneurysm was exposed by a petrosal approach. With proximal occlusion of the BA and trapping of the branches, the broad-necked heavily thrombosed aneurysm was emptied of clot and clipped. The clip occluded the PCA arising from the aneurysmal neck; however, it was well collateralized by distal branches of the MCA. The patient recovered without any deficit.

Case 4—Upper Third Basilar Aneurysm

This 46-year-old woman had had an ICA-PCommA aneurysm clipped many years previously. She was known to have an upper third BA aneurysm at that time. Upon routine follow-up angiography several years later, the aneurysm was found to have enlarged (**Fig. 14–5**). Although the aneurysm was accessible by a subtemporal transzygomatic approach, a retrolabyrinthine petrosal approach was chosen because a large artery (the AICA) originated from the neck of the aneurysm and proceeded inferiorly. The fourth cranial nerve was divided to improve the exposure but could not be reconstructed. The aneurysm was occluded by the tandem application of clips in such a way as to preserve the AICA. Her postoperative course was complicated by CSF leakage through the eustachian tube, which required packing of the middle ear, and a lumboperitoneal shunt because of the presence of communicating hydrocephalus. The patient suffered persistent diplopia, but this was corrected by strabismus surgery.

Case 5—Giant Midbasilar Aneurysm

This 58-year-old patient presented with a giant midbasilar aneurysm that ruptured and rebled. The aneurysm severely indented the pons to the left of the midline and had a very broad neck (**Fig. 14–6**). It was managed by deep hypothermic cardiac arrest technique. Because of the size of the aneurysm and its location, a partial labyrinthectomy, petrous apicectomy, petrosal approach was employed. As soon as the aneurysm was exposed, it started to leak, but this was controlled with hypotension and gentle pressure with a cottonoid patty. The patient was placed under deep hypothermic cardiac arrest, and with a circulatory arrest time of 28 minutes, the aneurysm was dissected and clipped with two clips. Small remnants of the neck were left on either side because of the origin of perforating arteries. The patient had a protracted postoperative course because of hydrocephalus and residual hemiparesis but made a good recovery after ~3 months and returned to independent living with a near complete resolution of the hemiparesis.

Case 6—Giant, Thrombosed Vertebral Artery Aneurysm

This 49-year-old patient presented with neck pain and was discovered to have a thrombosed, giant aneurysm arising from a dominant VA just proximal to the origin of the PICA (**Fig. 14–7**). The aneurysm was very high in position, extending from the jugular foramen to just above the level of the internal auditory canal. The contralateral VA was small, and the ipsilateral sigmoid sinus was dominant. The aneurysm was exposed via a combination of a presigmoid approach, which allowed distal control of the VA near the VBJ, a lateral retrosigmoid approach to expose the aneurysm, and the exposure of the VA at the C1 level extradurally. Under induced hypertension, mild hypothermia, and systemic heparinization, trapping of the aneurysm with removal of clot and aneurysmorraphy was attempted. However, this was not successful; therefore a saphenous vein graft was placed from the extradural VA (end to side), to the intradural VA and PICA (end to end). The patient suffered a small distal cerebellar infarct but recovered with a hearing loss as his only permanent complication.

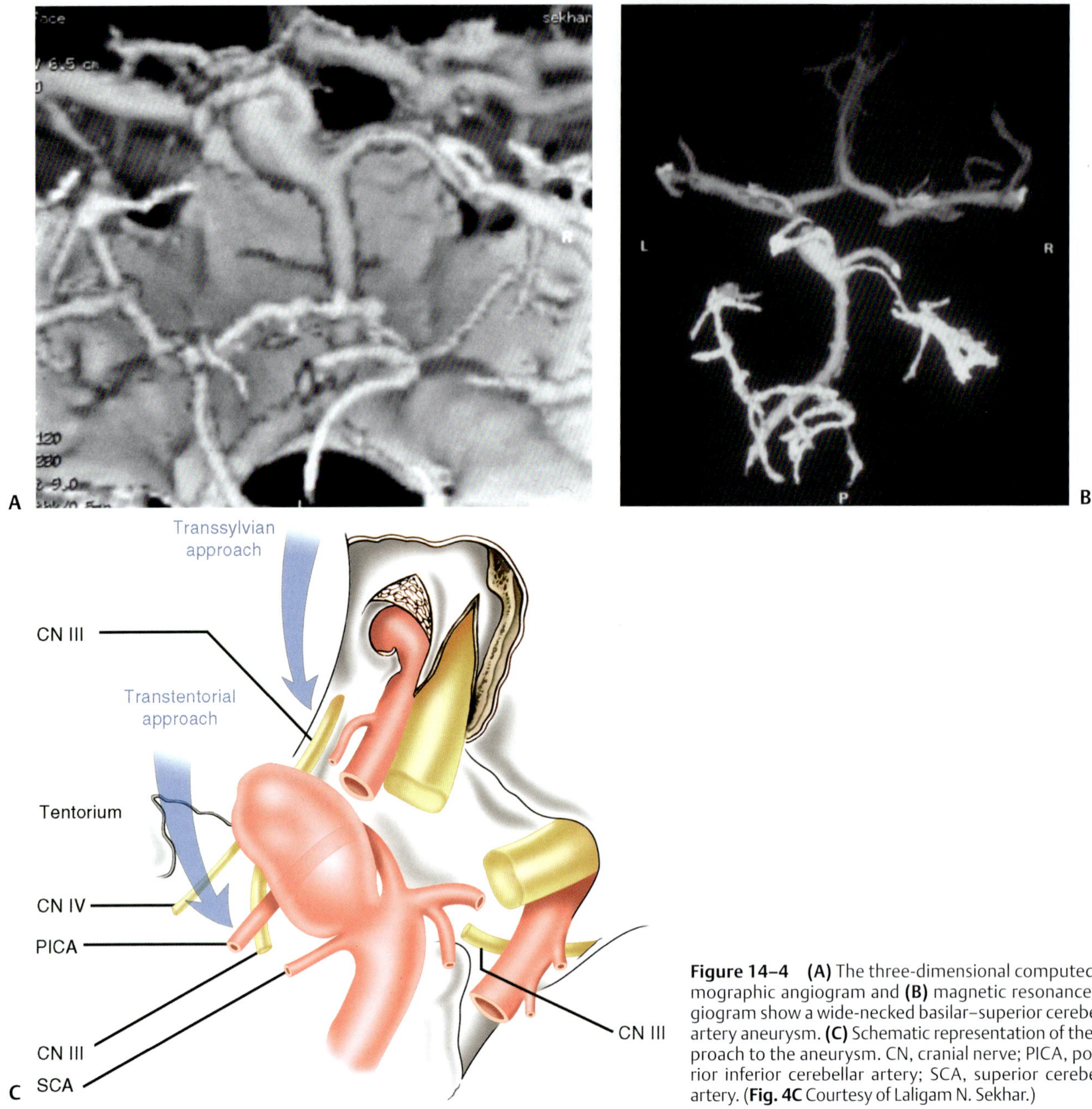

Figure 14–4 **(A)** The three-dimensional computed tomographic angiogram and **(B)** magnetic resonance angiogram show a wide-necked basilar–superior cerebellar artery aneurysm. **(C)** Schematic representation of the approach to the aneurysm. CN, cranial nerve; PICA, posterior inferior cerebellar artery; SCA, superior cerebellar artery. (**Fig. 4C** Courtesy of Laligam N. Sekhar.)

Case 7—Vertebrobasilar Junction Aneurysm

This 39-year-old patient presented with subarachnoid hemorrhage secondary to a VBJ aneurysm (**Fig. 14–8**). The aneurysm arose at a fenestration of the BA and was located directly anterior to the pontomedullary junction. The lesion was exposed by a transmastoid and a retrosigmoid approach, with complete unroofing of the sigmoid sinus. The sinus was equidominant, with good connection with the contralateral side. After a test occlusion, the sinus was divided between temporary clips. Exposure of the aneurysm was still difficult because the brain stem was swollen. However, the VA and BA were dissected free and occluded temporarily. The aneurysm was clipped without any residual neck. The sigmoid sinus was then resutured with 6–0 Prolene. Postoperative angiography demonstrated the patency of the sinus and the occlusion of the aneurysm. The patient did well postoperatively, with transient deficits of CN IX and X, recovering without any problems.

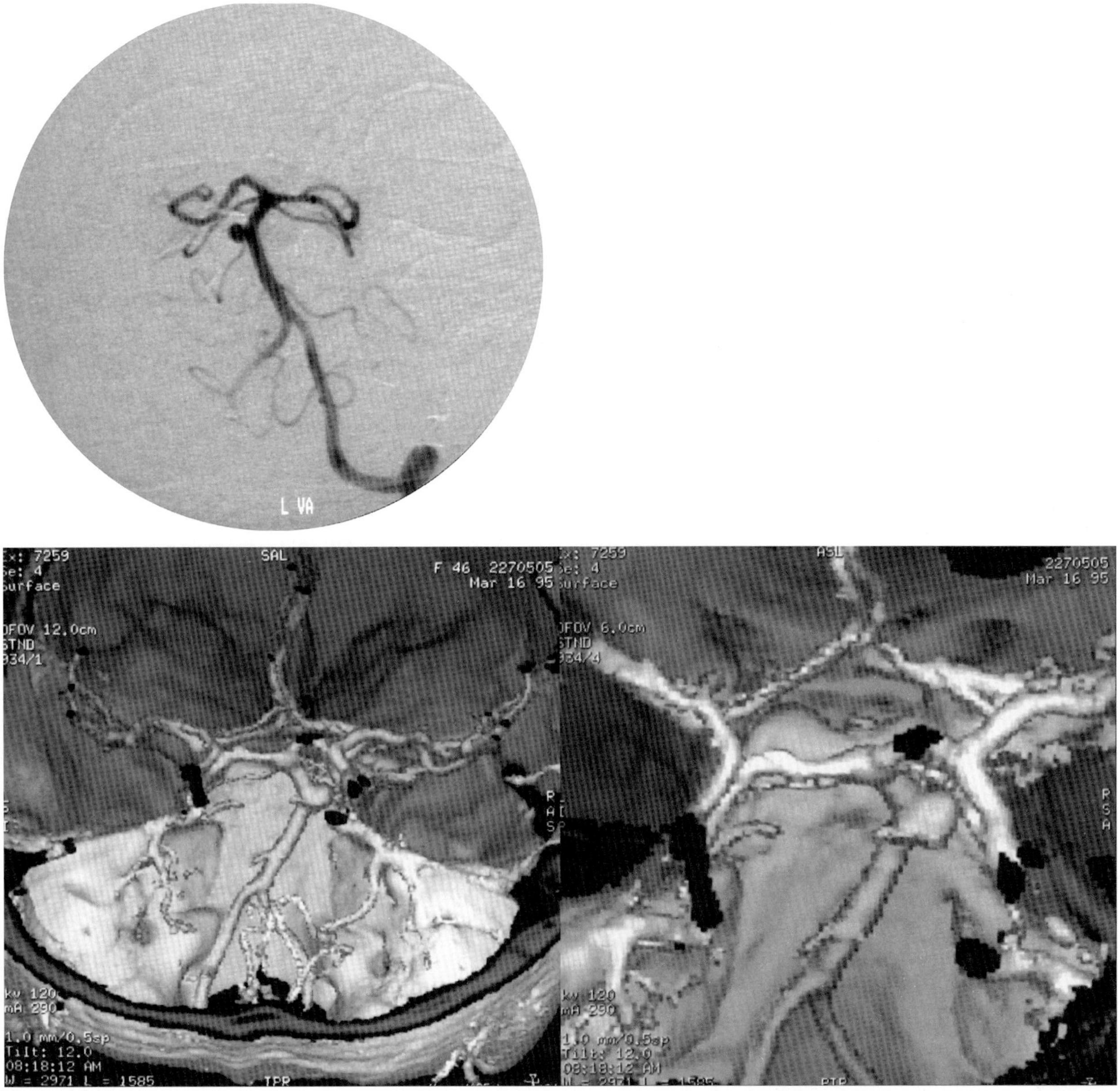

A B C

Figure 14–5 **(A)** The vertebral angiogram and **(B,C)** the three-dimensional computed tomographic scan show an upper third basilar trunk aneurysm projecting to the right. The anterior inferior cerebellar artery is seen originating from the neck of the aneurysm.

Case 8—Vertebral Artery Dissecting Aneurysm

This 38-year-old man presented with subarachnoid hemorrhage. Initial unilateral angiography did not reveal any abnormality. He had a rebleed, which led to a repeat angiogram (**Fig. 14–9**). This demonstrated a dissecting aneurysm of the right VA, but because of the horizontal course of the vessel, it was located directly anterior to the medulla. The PICA was originating directly from the dissecting aneurysm. Because of this, endovascular occlusion of the VA was not preferred. Because the aneurysm was directly anterior to the medulla, it was approached via an extreme lateral partial transcondylar approach, with the removal of the jugular tubercle. The PICA was sectioned and reimplanted into the AICA, and the aneurysm was trapped. The patient made a good recovery from a preoperative hemiparesis and was able to return to work.

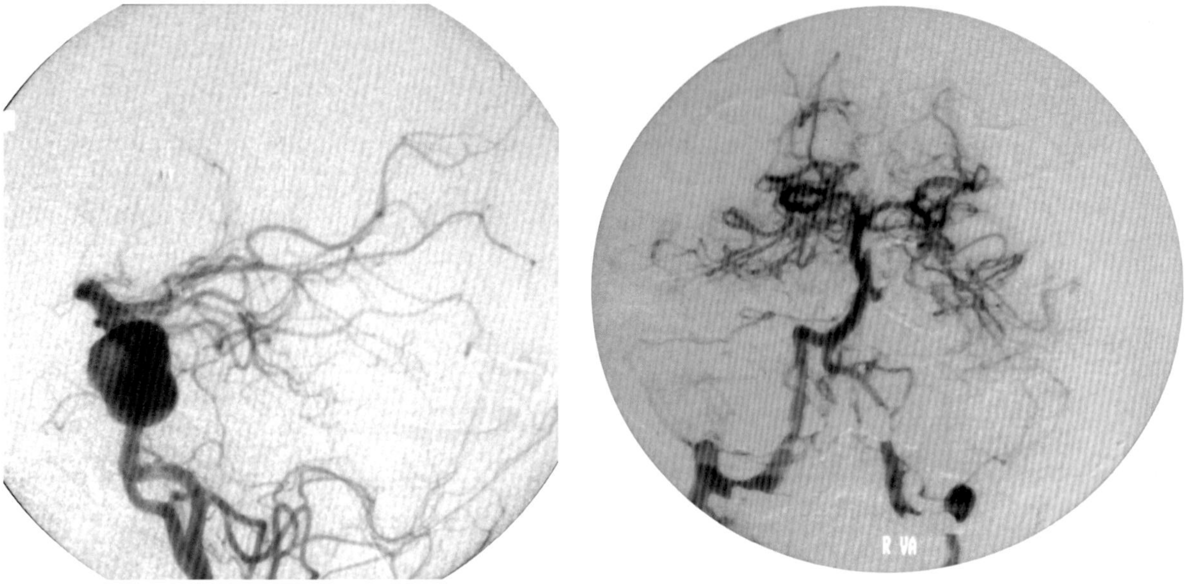

A B

Figure 14–6 **(A)** The lateral view of the vertebral angiogram shows a giant midbasilar artery aneurysm. **(B)** The postoperative angiogram shows no residual aneurysm.

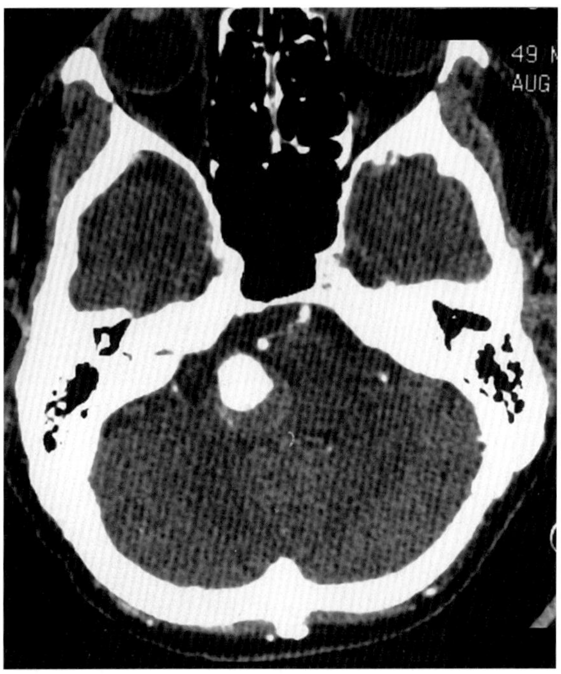

A

Figure 14–7 **(A)** The computed tomographic scan shows a well-circumscribed, rounded, hyperdense lesion in the posterior fossa on the right side and abutting the brain stem.

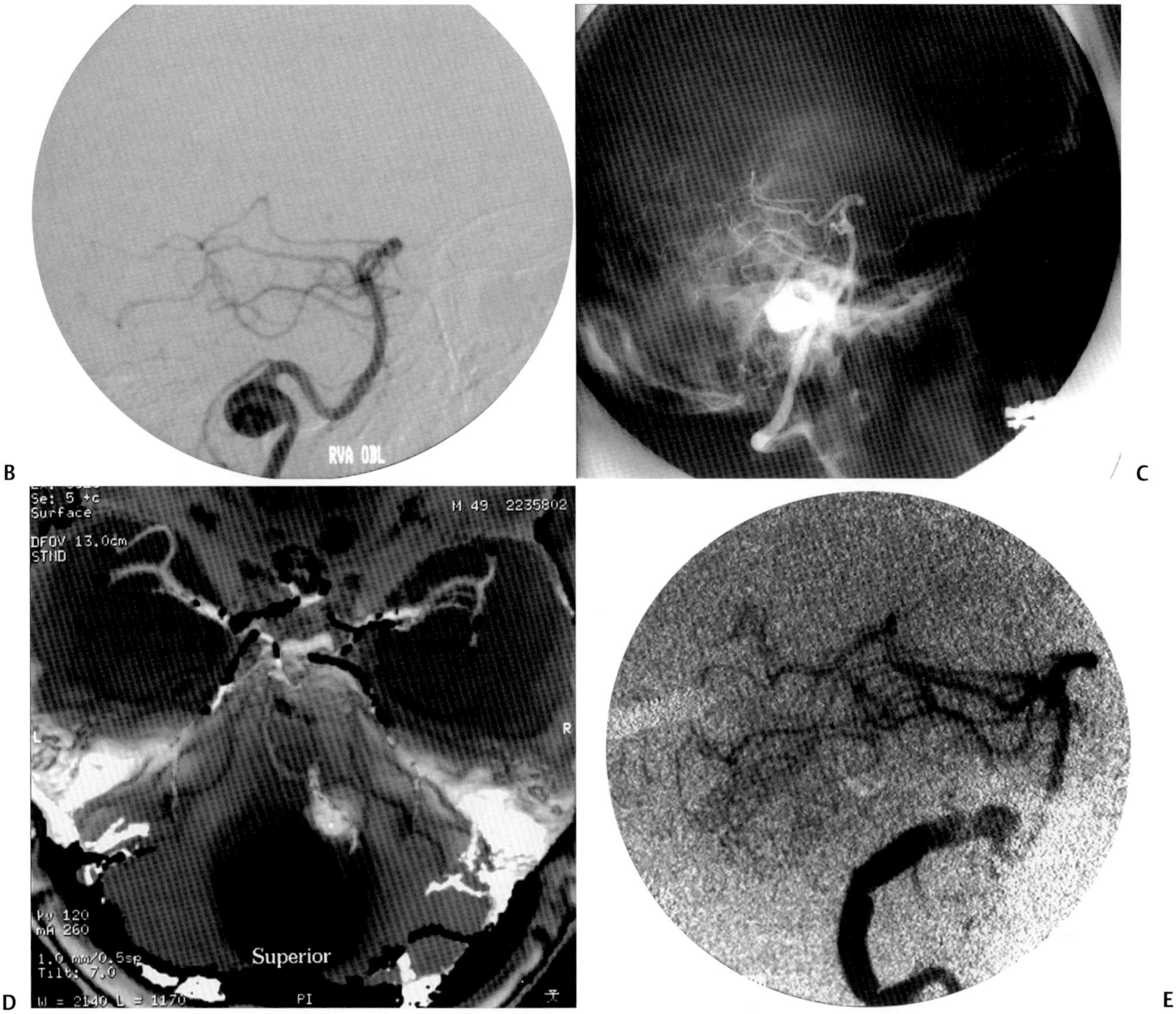

(*Continued*) **Figure 14–7** **(B,C)** The vertebral angiogram and **(D)** the three-dimensional computed tomographic angiogram show a giant aneurysm arising from the vertebral artery. The posterior inferior cerebellar artery is seen to arise from the vertebral artery just distal to the aneurysm. **(E)** The postoperative angiogram shows a widely patent graft with no evidence of the aneurysm.

(*Continued on page 208*)

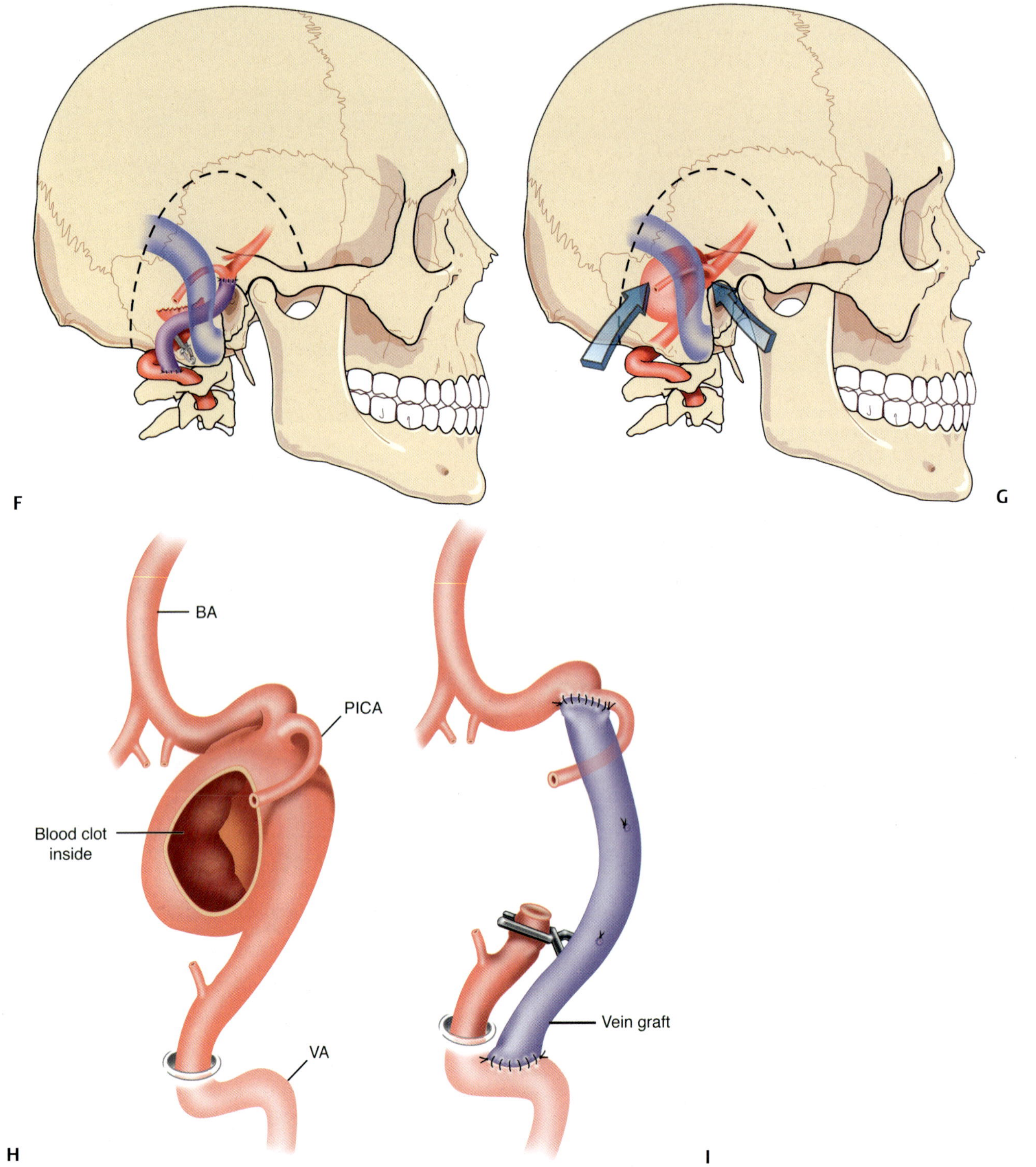

(*Continued*) **Figure 14–7 (F–I)** Schematic illustration of the approach used to access the aneurysm and the bypass with a saphenous vein graft from the extradural to intradural vertebral artery with trapping of the aneurysm. BA, basilar artery; PICA, posterior inferior cerebellar artery; VA, vertebral artery. (**Figs. F–I** courtesy of Laligam N. Sekhar.)

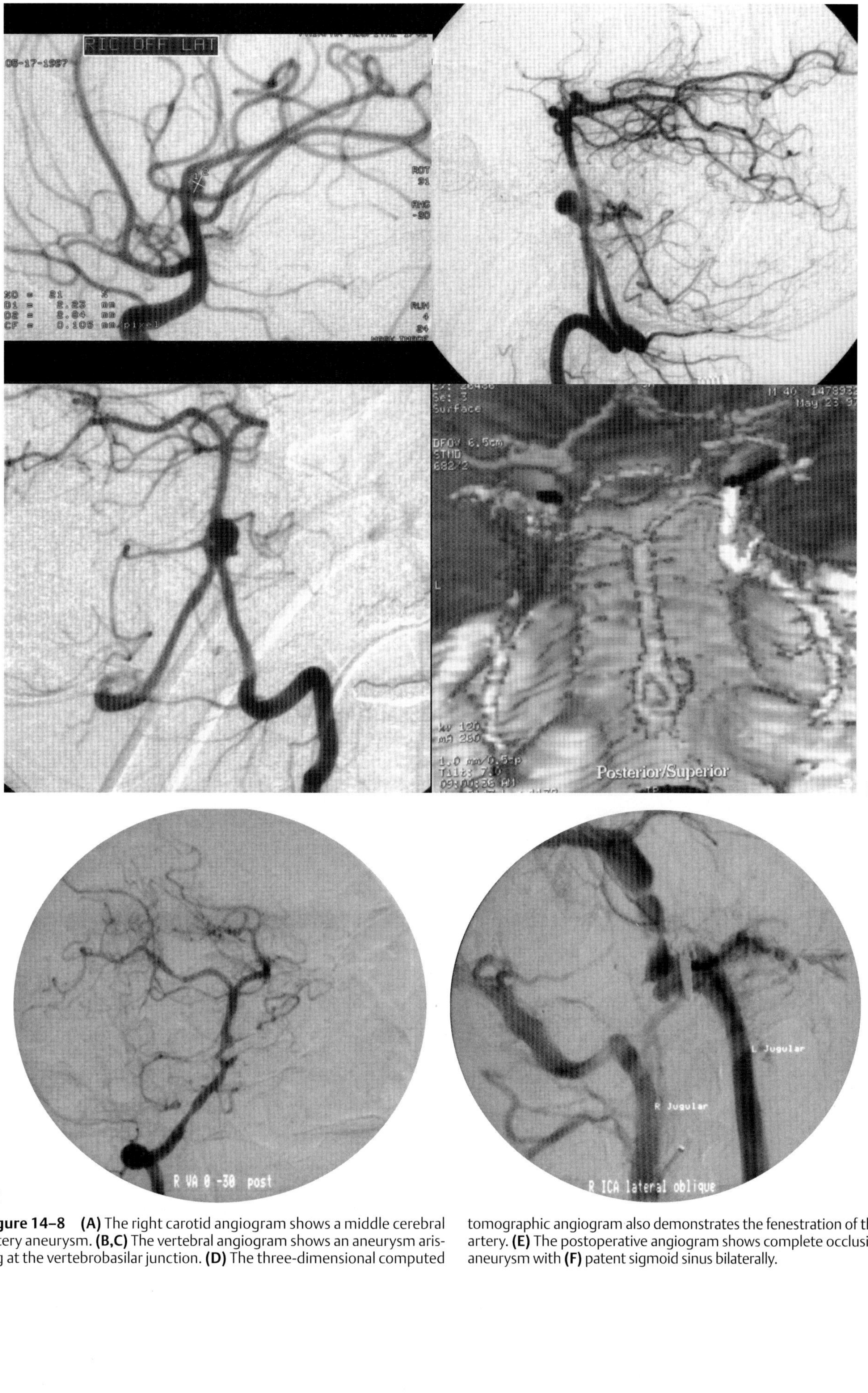

Figure 14–8 **(A)** The right carotid angiogram shows a middle cerebral artery aneurysm. **(B,C)** The vertebral angiogram shows an aneurysm arising at the vertebrobasilar junction. **(D)** The three-dimensional computed tomographic angiogram also demonstrates the fenestration of the basilar artery. **(E)** The postoperative angiogram shows complete occlusion of the aneurysm with **(F)** patent sigmoid sinus bilaterally.

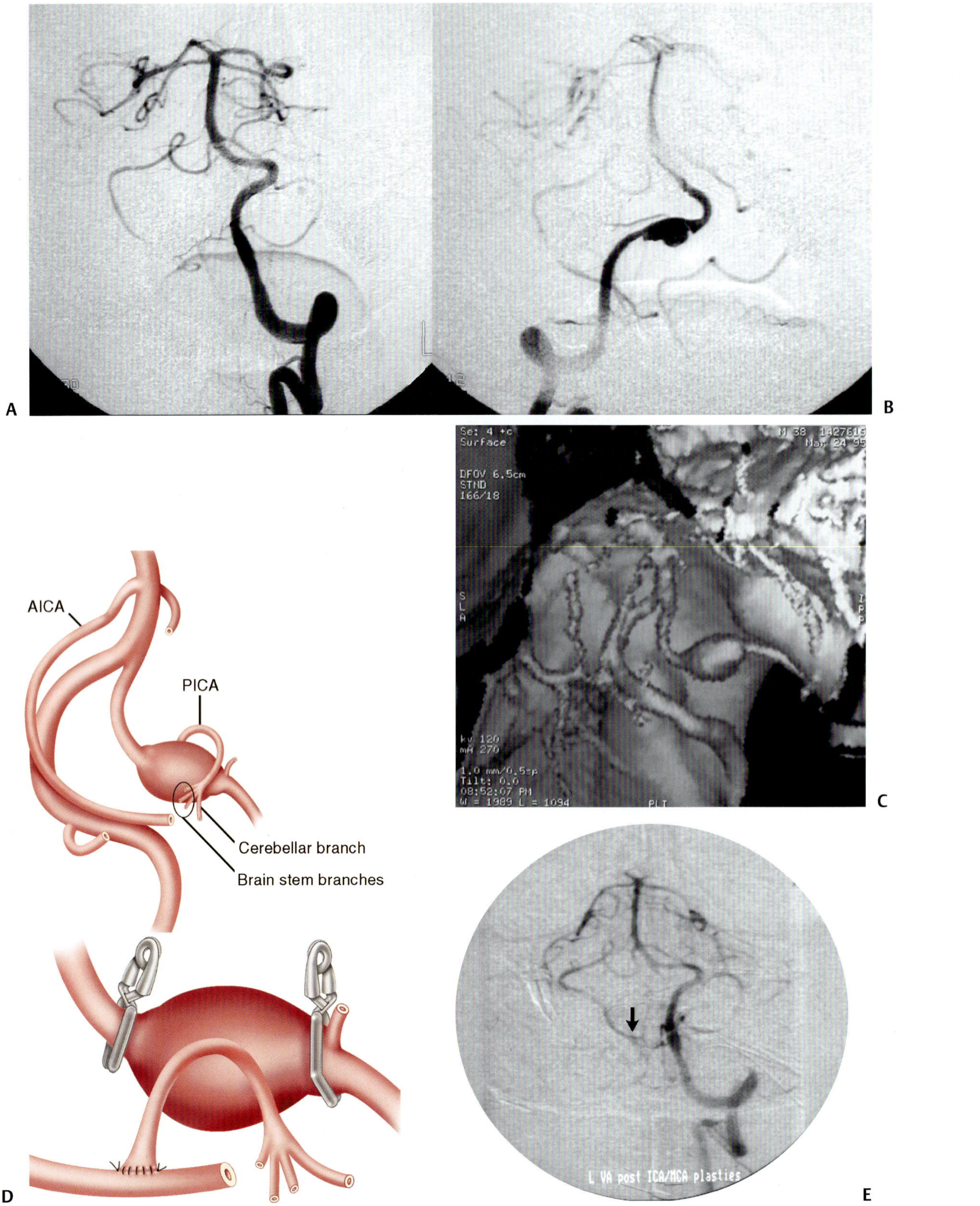

Figure 14–9 **(A,B)** The vertebral angiogram and **(C)** the three-dimensional computed tomographic angiogram show an irregular aneurysm arising from the right vertebral artery, with the posterior inferior cerebellar artery (PICA) originating from the dome of the aneurysm. **(D)** Schematic representation of the trapping of the aneurysm followed by reimplantation of the PICA into the anterior inferior cerebellar artery (AICA). **(E)** Postoperative angiogram shows filling of the branches of the PICA from the AICA with no resid-ual aneurysm. (**Fig. 14–9D** courtesy of Laligam N. Sekhar.)

◆ Reconstruction

Reconstruction after basal approaches to aneurysms is very crucial to prevent CSF leakage and a cosmetic deformity. The dura mater should be closed as tightly as possible, often necessitating a dural graft. Fibrin glue is used to supplement the closure. Any air-containing cavities will need to be packed to prevent extension of CSF through them. In case of orbital osteotomy and orbitozygomatic approaches, any exposed frontal sinus, ethmoidal sinus, and the sphenoid sinus extension into the anterior clinoid process or the optic strut will have to be packed with fascia and fat and, if possible, covered with a pericranial flap.

After petrosal approaches, the mastoid antrum is closed with bone wax if it is small. If it is large, especially after a partial labyrinthectomy, petrous apicectomy approach, the eustachian tube is exposed directly by a facial recess approach, and it is packed with Surgicel, which provides a temporary seal against CSF leakage until the dural opening is healed. The mastoid and any petrous apex defect are packed with abdominal fat and covered with a split calvarial graft or a titanium mesh and BoneSource (Stryker Corporation, Leibinger Micro Implants, Portage, MI) to prevent a cosmetic deformity.

Because many patients with ruptured aneurysms have hydrocephalus, CSF leakage may occur postoperatively despite an adequate closure. A shunt procedure may be needed in such patients to prevent CSF leakage.

15

Giant Aneurysms

A. Giancarlo Vishteh, Carlos A. David, and Robert F. Spetzler

- Diagnostic Evaluation
- Indications
- Preparation
- Surgical Strategies
- Direct and Indirect Obliteration Techniques
- Conclusion

Few other lesions are as challenging to neurovascular surgeons as giant aneurysms. To be designated as giant, an aneurysm must measure more than 2.5 cm at its largest diameter.[1] Saccular, fusiform, or dolichoectatic aneurysms can reach giant proportions. Historically, however, fusiform and dolichoectatic aneurysms have been classified separately from saccular giant aneurysms.[2]

The natural history of giant aneurysms is dismal. The mortality rate 2 and 5 years after diagnosis is 68% and 85%, respectively.[3,4] Furthermore, patients who survive after their initial presentation are left with or eventually develop significant neurological dysfunction. Although some giant aneurysms are discovered incidentally, most cause symptoms as the result of compression (i.e., brain, brain stem, or cranial nerves), irritation of neural tissue (seizures), thromboembolism (aneurysm nidus), or subarachnoid hemorrhage (SAH). A small number cause obstructive hydrocephalus by direct or indirect compression of cerebrospinal fluid (CSF) pathways. The rupture of giant aneurysms in the cavernous segment of the internal carotid artery (ICA) can lead to carotid-cavernous fistulae or fatal epistaxis if the rupture is uncontained and extends into the sphenoid or ethmoid sinus.

Giant aneurysms tend to occur mostly in females, and the peak age of diagnosis is 40 to 60 years of age.[1,3–10] Most giant aneurysms occur in the anterior circulation along the ICA (including cavernous, ophthalmic, and paraclinoid segments), middle cerebral artery (MCA), and anterior cerebral artery [anterior communicating (ACommA) segment]. In the posterior circulation, giant aneurysms most often involve the basilar artery apex, followed by the vertebrobasilar junction, peripheral segments of the posterior cerebral artery (PCA), posterior inferior cerebellar artery (PICA), and the trunk of the basilar artery. Multiple giant aneurysms are seldom encountered in a single patient based on Fox's series of 693 patients (7% had multiple giant aneurysms).[6]

Early attempts to exclude these formidable lesions surgically from the circulation were fraught with complications. Several of these lesions were misdiagnosed as tumors and surgically approached as such, with disastrous results.[11] Consequently, the practice of sacrificing the parent vessel proximally (Hunterian ligation) evolved as an option in the management of giant aneurysms, especially those of the anterior circulation.[5] With advances in microneurosurgery and bypass techniques, however, these lesions became more amenable to direct surgical approach. Isolated parent-vessel sacrifice (i.e., ICA) for giant aneurysms of the anterior circulation is usually performed after sophisticated testing, such as the balloon occlusion test (BOT), to confirm that patients can tolerate sacrifice of the ICA. Parent-vessel sacrifice can also be used as an adjunct when combined with distal revascularization.

With advances in the field of endovascular neurosurgery in the past 3 decades, the management of aneurysms has continued to evolve. Although endovascular treatment is an effective option in the treatment of aneurysms with small necks, giant aneurysms are recalcitrant to endovascular treatment, even at the most experienced centers. Furthermore, the long-term angiographic follow-up and outcome of endovascularly treated giant aneurysms have yet to be reported. Coils and stents have been used in combination to obliterate giant aneurysms. After endovascular coiling of the aneurysm, a stent is placed along the aneurysm orifice to prevent the coils from protruding into the parent vessel to encourage thrombosis of the aneurysm and to further reduce the incidence of remodeling at the internal aneurysm orifice. The reverse strategy (i.e., stenting across the aneurysm orifice, followed by coiling through a stent window) has also been performed. In other instances, balloons have been used to help compact coils into an aneurysm sac. Ultimately, smaller, more flexible "pored" stents alone may represent a better alternative, one that may obviate the need for coils. Theoretically, the smaller pores would allow blood to flow through small perforators and branches of the parent vessel while significantly altering flow within the aneurysmal sac and leading ultimately to thrombosis of the aneurysm.

◆ Diagnostic Evaluation

A complete diagnostic evaluation of giant aneurysms is crucial to formulating an appropriate treatment plan. Conventional selective cerebral catheter angiography (with cross - compression and Allcock's test,[4,12,13] where indicated) is the gold standard. Review of time-sequenced angiograms (with all appropriate views) and the angiographic video (when available) reveals crucial information regarding the morphology of the aneurysm and its neck (if present), as well as the anatomy of adjacent vessels and its exact location, luminal size, filling pattern, and inflow-outflow sites (fusiform or dolichoectatic aneurysm).

Magnetic resonance (MR) angiography and computed tomographic (CT) angiography are useful adjuncts to angiography. Three-dimensional CT (3D-CT) angiography can help determine the lobularity and three-dimensional conformation of aneurysms. CT angiography, however, usually requires large loads of contrast dye administered intravenously with the attendant risk of an allergic reaction compared with the intra-arterial route. Although catheter angiography is the gold standard, thrombosed portions of giant aneurysms are not well visualized by this modality. Therefore, brain MR imaging or CT can provide important information about the actual size of an aneurysm.

Preoperatively, the BOT along with adjuncts [xenon cerebral blood flow test (Xe CT-CBF) and induced hypotension] can be used to help select patients who may tolerate sacrifice of the parent vessel. The BOT, however, is not consistently reliable, and the test itself has inherent risks. Furthermore, permanent occlusion of the parent vessel has both short- and long-term risks. We reserve the BOT and parent-vessel occlusion for patients for whom surgery is too risky (i.e., elderly patients or those who lack the proper medical reserve to undergo surgical therapy) and when endosaccular aneurysm occlusion is impossible. Overall, therefore, we are not strong proponents of the BOT for the ICA because in experienced centers the risks of revascularization may be less than the combined risks of the BOT and parent-vessel sacrifice.[14]

In contrast, our philosophy about BOT for the basilar artery is different, especially for complex symptomatic dolichoectatic aneurysms of the posterior circulation where effective obliteration of the aneurysm may be impossible and bypass and trapping schemes are too risky. If such patients have the appropriate circle of Willis vascular interconnections (i.e., PCA), we have used the BOT to determine their tolerance for occlusion of the basilar artery. The inherent risks of this test and those of parent-vessel sacrifice also apply to the posterior circulation but may be outweighed by the risk of surgery (clipping or revascularization, and trapping).

Before a patient is scheduled for a BOT and permanent parent-vessel sacrifice, an experienced neurovascular surgeon must be consulted. Contralateral ICA and ACommA aneurysms, the presence of vasospasm (after aneurysmal SAH), and significant atherosclerosis of the contralateral ICA or common carotid artery are contraindications to ICA occlusion. Furthermore, the basilar artery should not be occluded electively if aneurysms are present on the posterior communicating arteries (PCommAs).

◆ Indications

Because their prognosis is so poor, an effective treatment strategy should be devised, if possible, once a giant aneurysm is diagnosed. With the rare exception of the completely asymptomatic intracavernous ICA aneurysm (which we choose to observe), our posture toward most other giant aneurysms is aggressive but not cavalier.

The goals of surgery (open or endovascular) are threefold: (1) exclusion of the aneurysm from the circulation, (2) preservation of distal blood flow, and (3) decompression of neural structures where indicated. In general, we prefer to treat aneurysms that present with SAH in the early phase. Early treatment, however, does not imply surgery without a complete diagnostic evaluation and careful consideration of all options. Emergency surgery is reserved for intraparenchymal extension of a hemorrhage, which creates a mass lesion that threatens a patient's life. If CSF must be diverted, a ventriculostomy catheter is placed early, before surgery.

The impetus to recommend treatment of these lesions is based on their dismal natural history. Aneurysmal endosaccular coiling can be considered to temporize ruptured giant aneurysms. Based on studies by Guglielmi et al[15] and Gobin et al,[16] it appears that endovascular coil occlusion is most effective for aneurysms with small necks or those with favorable neck to fundus ratios. But without the long-term angiographic follow-up of endovascularly treated aneurysms, we prefer to use endosaccular coil occlusion of giant aneurysms as a first-line therapy only in patients who require treatment but who are too unstable to undergo open surgery and for patients who require medical stabilization after an SAH before definitive surgical therapy. Coiling of such aneurysms offers some protection against repeated rupture in patients who require hypervolemic-hemodilutional hypertensive therapy for vasospasm. Although overlooked by many surgeons, endovascular therapy usually requires general anesthesia. Therefore, the risks of anesthesia and the additional angiographic dye loads must also be considered in unstable patients. As already discussed, proximal sacrifice of the parent vessel is yet another option that can be performed endovascularly.

◆ Preparation

Detailed preoperative planning is essential to minimize complications. The completed angiographic and diagnostic imaging should be reviewed by a neurovascular team (neurovascular surgeon, endovascular specialist, neuroradiologist), and appropriate intraoperative adjuncts should be planned at this stage. Adjuncts such as hypothermic circulatory arrest, intraoperative angiography, and neurophysiological monitoring (somatosensory evoked potentials, specific cranial nerve monitoring) may be scheduled. If a temporal bone-based approach is needed (i.e., transcochlear) for more complex posterior circulation aneurysms, a neuro-otologist should also be consulted. Other intraoperative instrumentation and equipment (i.e., radiolucent head holder, appropriate aneurysm clips, microDoppler ultrasonography) are also procured during this phase.

When approaching a handful of cavernous or ophthalmic ICA aneurysms surgically, we have used an endovascular balloon for proximal control instead of exposing the cervical ICA. In such cases, an intravascular femoral artery access sheath is placed in the operating room before surgery, and a catheter is passed transarterially to the level of the cervical ICA. When needed, the balloon is inflated for proximal control. Blood distal to the balloon can also be suctioned, effectively deflating the aneurysm after distal control of the parent vessel. Again, however, this strategy requires the appropriate preoperative planning.

Finally, patients undergoing elective surgery should have any coexisting medical conditions stabilized and should receive clearance from the appropriate specialist before surgery, especially patients undergoing hypothermic circulatory arrest.

◆ Surgical Strategies

Aneurysm surgery is governed by the need for proximal and distal vascular control. Furthermore, complete exposure of the entire aneurysm is crucial, especially in the case of giant aneurysms, because debulking may be needed. If trapping and bypass are planned, exposure is limited to the vessel segment chosen for revascularization and to the proximal portion of the vessel chosen for sacrifice. Alternatively, the parent vessel can be sacrificed endovascularly at a different setting.

Approach

Surgical exposure must be considered separately from aneurysm obliteration techniques. Several surgical approaches are available for exposing these lesions based on their location. Step-by-step descriptions of each surgical exposures are discussed elsewhere in this text.

In general, aneurysms arising from the anterior circulation can be approached adequately via the classic pterional approach. Aneurysms of the A3 segment of the anterior cerebral artery (ACA) and beyond require an interhemispheric approach. The addition of orbitozygomatic osteotomies facilitates exposure of aneurysms of the cavernous, clinoidal, and ophthalmic segments of the ICA aneurysms. Furthermore, resection of the anterior clinoid (either extradurally or intradurally) is facilitated, and an upward angle of view for high and posteriorly directed giant aneurysms of the ACommA is obtained. This approach also provides additional working space when the distal ICA must be revascularized. During the pterional exposure, in cases involving complex anterior circulation aneurysms, we make every effort to preserve either the frontal or the temporal branch of the superficial temporal artery should a bypass pedicle be needed.

For most subarachnoid ICA, ACA, or MCA aneurysms, proximal and distal control is obtained via the intracra-nial exposure itself. For clinoidal and cavernous ICA aneurysms, proximal control can be obtained by exposing the extracranial ICA at the neck or by using a previously positioned endovascular catheter with a temporary balloon. For aneurysms of the ophthalmic segment, drill resection of the clinoid may provide some measure of proximal control. In the case of giant aneurysms, however, this exposure may not suffice. Furthermore, because of limited proximal ICA exposure, placement of a temporary clip may preclude effective placement of permanent aneurysm clips. It therefore may also become necessary to expose the cervical ICA in the case of giant ophthalmic segment ICA aneurysms. In the rare case of a completely intracranial bypass (i.e., petrous to supraclinoid ICA bypass) planned to treat an aneurysm of the cavernous ICA, exposure of the petrous carotid within Glasscock's triangle provides proximal control. Based on the surgeon's experience and comfort level, however, control of the ICA at the cervical level may still be needed during the actual drilling of the petrous ICA.

In the posterior circulation, exposure of aneurysms arising from the basilar apex or the superior cerebellar arteries is facilitated by using skull base approaches. Classical approaches to the region of the basilar apex include the subtemporal (popularized by Drake) and the pterional-transsylvian (popularized by Yasargil). We favor the transsylvian approach with the addition of orbitozygomatic osteotomies (**Fig. 15–1**). The orbitozygomatic osteotomies provide an upward angle of view of basilar apex aneurysms whose necks project well above the level of the posterior clinoid. If the neck of the aneurysm is below the level of the posterior clinoid, we still use the orbitozygomatic osteotomies. Additional working space is gained for drill resection of the posterior clinoid and a portion of the superolateral clivus, thereby obtaining exposure of the neck of lower-lying basilar apex aneurysms. Effective exclusion of giant aneurysms from this locale, however, remains a true challenge. The dissection of multiple small brain stem and thalamic perforating arteries from the aneurysm sac is particularly difficult.

Hypothermic circulatory arrest (**Fig. 15–1**) has added yet another dimension to the concept of temporary proximal-vessel occlusion, especially in the case of basilar apex aneurysms. Cardiac standstill can also be considered for complex aneurysms of the basilar trunk or ICA bifurcation. Circulatory arrest "softens" the aneurysm sac for manipulation, thereby facilitating dissection of the perforating arteries from the dome of the aneurysm, effective clipping of the aneurysmal neck, or clip reconstruction of the parent vessel.[17] Although aneurysms with "soft" walls may be amenable to circulatory arrest, giant aneurysms with hard

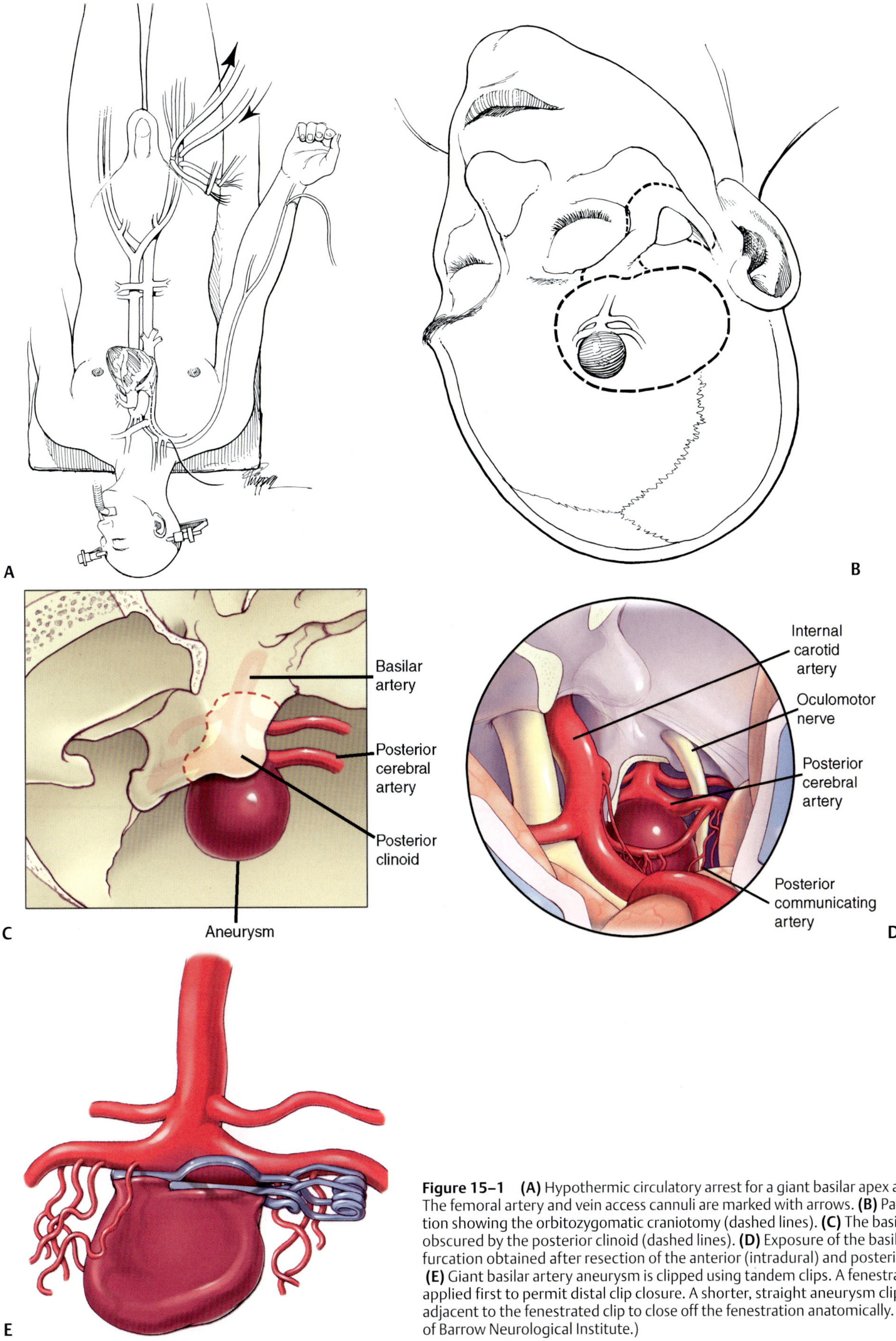

Figure 15–1 **(A)** Hypothermic circulatory arrest for a giant basilar apex aneurysm. The femoral artery and vein access cannuli are marked with arrows. **(B)** Patient position showing the orbitozygomatic craniotomy (dashed lines). **(C)** The basilar apex is obscured by the posterior clinoid (dashed lines). **(D)** Exposure of the basilar quadrifurcation obtained after resection of the anterior (intradural) and posterior clinoid. **(E)** Giant basilar artery aneurysm is clipped using tandem clips. A fenestrated clip is applied first to permit distal clip closure. A shorter, straight aneurysm clip is placed adjacent to the fenestrated clip to close off the fenestration anatomically. (Courtesy of Barrow Neurological Institute.)

atherosclerotic shells are inappropriate because they are not rendered malleable by circulatory arrest.

For giant, especially partially thrombosed serpentine or fusiform aneurysms, partial internal debulking may improve visualization of the neck or allow parent-vessel clip reconstruction (**Fig. 15–2**). This strategy, however, is rather risky, and the surgeon must be prepared to perform a distal bypass during the same setting. If aneurysmal debulking becomes necessary after temporary proximal and distal occlusion of the parent vessel, the aneurysm is opened and the thrombus is evacuated. We prefer to use ultrasonic aspiration. Using forceps or pituitary rongeurs to remove the thrombus is discouraged because tugging can cause the parent vessel to avulse, with disastrous complications. In the case of complex dolichoectatic aneurysms, proximal and distal control may not be readily attained because of

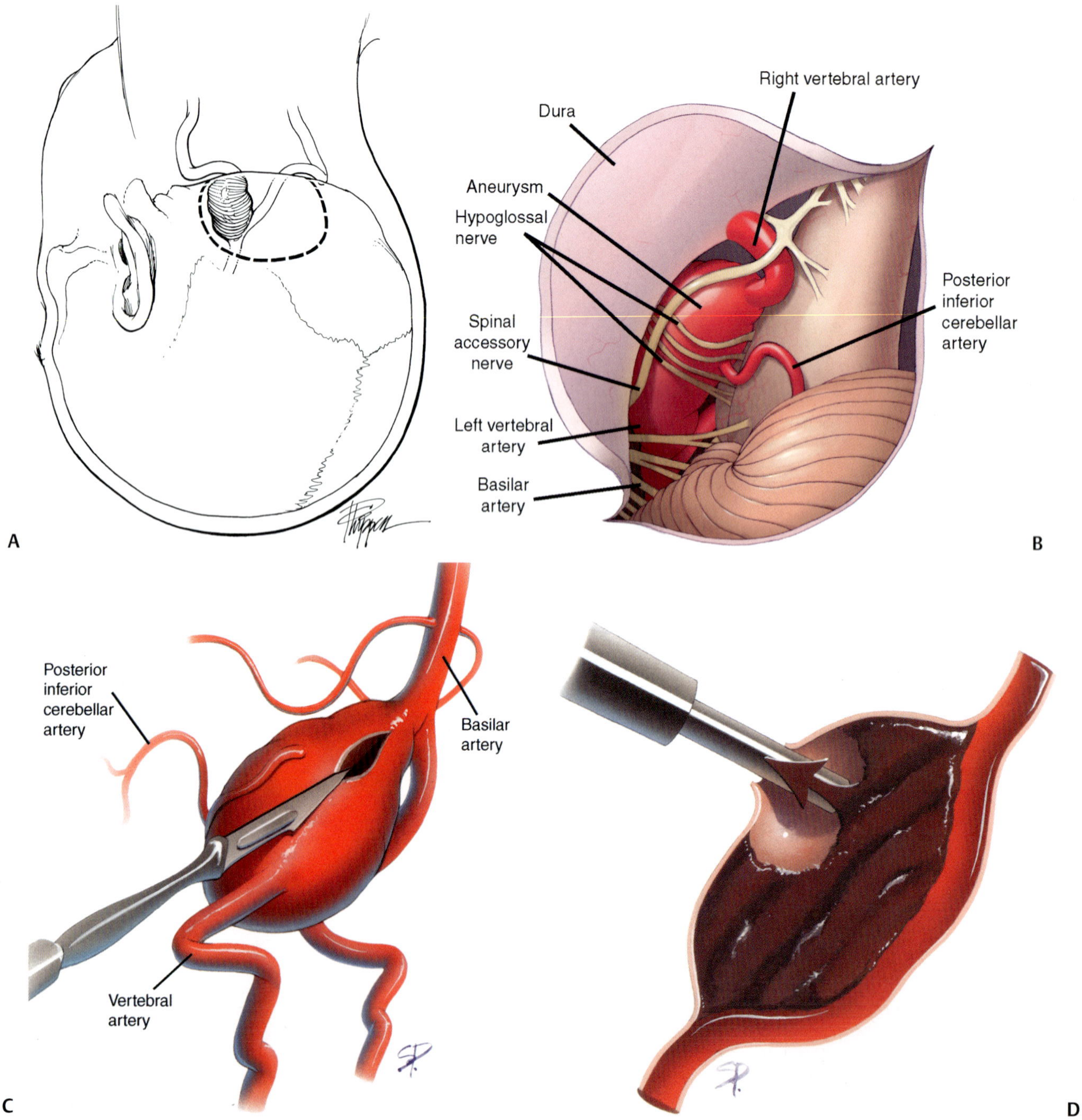

Figure 15–2 **(A)** Patient position showing the far-lateral craniotomy (dashed line) used to approach a giant vertebrobasilar junction aneurysm. **(B)** Intradural exposure of the craniovertebral junction and regional surgical anatomy of this approach. Treatment consists of **(C)** aneurysmorrhaphy with **(D)** debulking of layered thrombus (using ultrasonic aspiration) until the

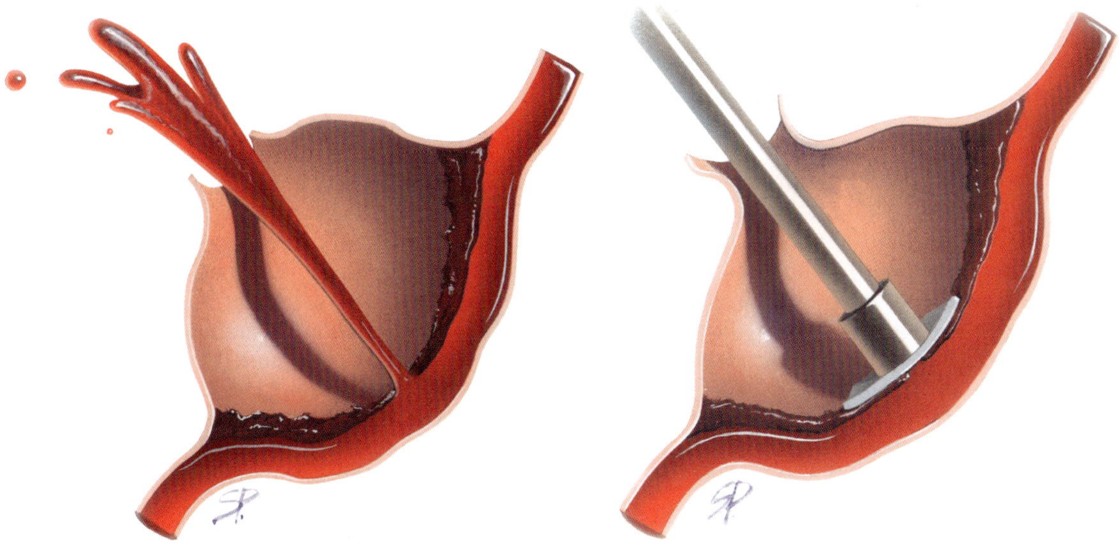

E

F

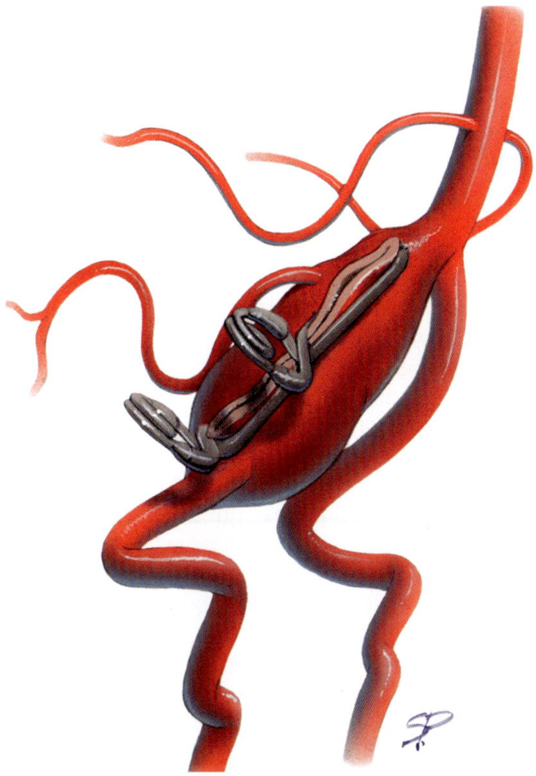

G

(Continued) **Figure 15–2** **(E)** parent-vessel flow channel is found. **(F)** Tamponade of the bleeding channel ensues with **(G)** clip reconstruction of the parent vessel using tandem, right-angled aneurysm clips. (With permission from Barrow Neurological Institute.)

the aneurysm's bulk and morphology. Very rarely in such cases, we have opened the aneurysm and removed thrombus until a channel of free-flowing blood was encountered. After this channel is packed, proximal and distal temporary occlusion typically becomes available, and clip reconstruction of the parent vessel can be attempted.[2] For softer, blood-filled giant aneurysms, a needle suction technique can help deflate a "soft" aneurysm, thereby allowing identification of the aneurysm neck as well as local neurovascular anatomy.[18]

Aneurysms of the basilar artery located below the superior cerebellar artery and above the vertebrobasilar junction are usually referred to as *basilar trunk* aneurysms. Despite recent advances in surgical techniques, exposure of these aneurysms remains challenging. Historically, the classic subtemporal transtentorial approach, popularized by Drake, is one of the most helpful for exposing these lesions. The addition of temporal bone–based approaches has greatly assisted in gaining a more optimal exposure. The subtemporal (middle fossa) approach with the addition of partial petrous apicectomy (Kawase's approach), for example, improves the exposure of basilar trunk aneurysms. Lateral suboccipital (i.e., the retrosigmoid) and posterior petrosal approaches (i.e., the retrolabyrinthine approach), with or without division of the sigmoid sinus, have assisted with gaining exposure along the midportion of the basilar artery. The transcochlear approach offers the most panoramic view of this segment of the basilar artery but sacrifices hearing and leads to transient seventh nerve paresis (the seventh nerve is rerouted). Transsigmoid approaches sacrifice the sigmoid sinus to provide adequate exposure. The sacrifice of the sigmoid sinus can lead to posterior fossa venous hypertension and hemorrhage and risks the delayed formation of a dural arteriovenous fistula. If this approach is chosen, preoperative angiograms (venous phase) must be reviewed carefully to ascertain communication between the transverse sinuses and the patency of the contralateral sigmoid sinus. Intraoperative test occlusion of the sinus with pressure measurements before and after occlusion further helps determine the safety of sacrificing the sigmoid sinus.

We do not routinely recommend transsigmoid approaches. Furthermore, we have moved away from the posterior petrosal approaches (i.e., transcochlear, transotic, translabyrinthine) for approaching basilar trunk aneurysms. Instead, we attempt to reach more superiorly situated basilar aneurysms from above (via a pterional/ orbitozygomatic craniotomy and posterior clinoid/clivus drilling) or to approach more caudal lesions from below using the far-lateral combined with the retrosigmoid approach. In a few cases these strategies may not provide adequate exposure. Petrosal approaches are then used. A strictly retrolabyrinthine approach for basilar trunk aneurysms is inappropriate because it provides only a very narrow working corridor, and a "knuckle" of bone formed by the drilled-out semicircular canals obstructs the surgeon's view. Although a partial labyrinthectomy that preserves hearing has been used to approach this area, long-term hearing outcomes have yet to be determined.

For aneurysms of the vertebrobasilar junction and PICA, we routinely use the far-lateral approach (**Fig. 15–2**). This approach provides both excellent exposure and proximal and distal vascular control. Aneurysms extending along the axis of the basilar artery from the vertebrobasilar junction to the basilar apex may be approached via combination exposures (i.e., far-lateral, combined with a petrosal approach, the so-called combined-combined approach).

◆ Direct and Indirect

Obliteration Techniques

Surgical options for exclusion of giant aneurysms from the circulation fall into two general categories: direct and indirect. Direct techniques include clipping (single or tandem) the neck of an aneurysm, aneurysmal excision with or without primary reanastomosis of the vessel, and aneurysmorrhaphy. Indirect techniques include aneurysm "trapping" with extracranial–intracranial or in situ bypasses and parent-vessel sacrifice (Hunterian ligation) without bypass. For the most part, previous indirect techniques of wrapping and coating aneurysms have been abandoned. More esoteric techniques (i.e., "muslin/ clip sling combination") have also been reported.[19] In extremely complex cases, we have reversed the flow through a parent vessel to help thrombose and effectively exclude an aneurysm from the circulation. For example, in a patient with patent PCommAs and a giant fusiform aneurysm of the basilar trunk, occlusion of one vertebral artery proximal to the PICA and the other distal to the PICA (1) irrigates the PCA territories via the PCommAs, (2) supplies one PICA territory via the ipsilateral vertebral artery, and (3) irrigates the contralateral PICA via reversed blood flow down the trunk of the basilar artery (via PCommAs). In effect, a "sump" that reverses blood flow down the basilar artery is created, leading to thrombosis of the aneurysm while preventing thrombosis of the lower basilar and anterior spinal arteries.

Clip obliteration is appropriate if the neck of an aneurysm can be appreciated during intraoperative inspection. Tandem clipping techniques can be used for aneurysms with broad-based necks or to reconstruct the aneurysmal part of the parent-vessel wall. Extreme caution must be exercised to avoid parent-vessel occlusion in such cases. Although intraoperative microDoppler ultrasonography is quite useful to confirm distal flow after tandem clipping of giant aneurysms (especially MCA aneurysms), we find that intraoperative angiography is the more reliable option for assessing clipping and distal blood flow within a vessel.

When the neck of a giant aneurysm is calcified, the distal tip of a long aneurysm clip may not close the lesion effectively. In such cases, booster clips have been used to help close the distal portion of the aneurysm clips. Because it is difficult to apply booster clips in tight spaces, it may be more practical to use a fenestrated clip (so that the distal tips of the fenestrated clip are together) in conjunction with a shorter adjacent straight clip that occludes the portion of the aneurysm protruding through the fenestration of the first clip (**Fig. 15–1E**). "Crushing" the neck of a calcified aneurysm with forceps as first described by Drake permits better seating of an aneurysm clip.[4] This maneuver, however, is best left for the most experienced neurovascular surgeons.

When a fusiform aneurysm is encountered on a perforator-free segment of a vessel, vessel excision and primary reanastomosis of the cut ends of the vessel may suffice (**Fig. 15–3**). This approach is usually adequate for aneurysms of the peripheral MCA. Mycotic aneurysms, however, seldom reach giant dimensions. Simple excision is another option for treating such aneurysms, especially if they arise from the side wall of a vessel.

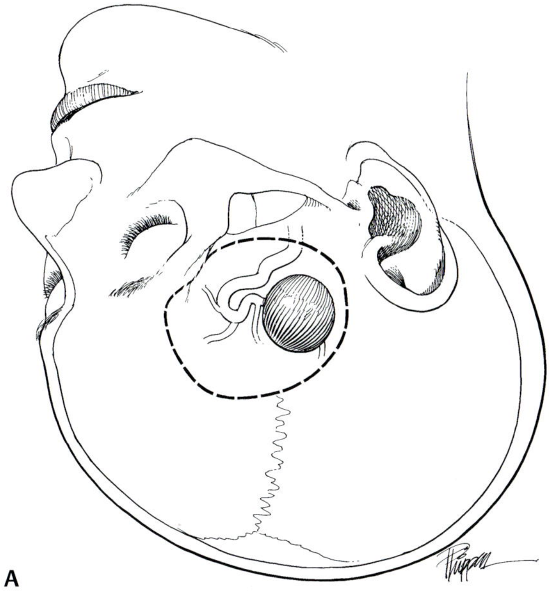

A

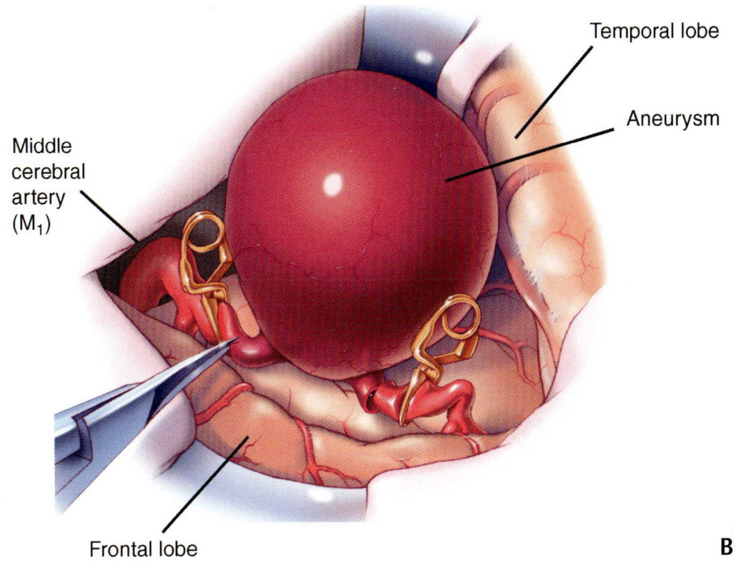

B

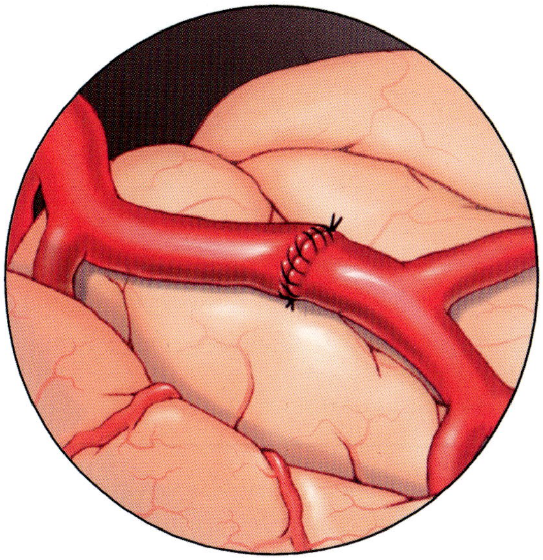

C

Figure 15–3 **(A)** Pterional craniotomy (dashed line) used to approach a giant middle cerebral artery (MCA) aneurysm. **(B)** Temporary clips are positioned for primary excision of the aneurysm. **(C)** End-to-end anastomosis of the MCA. (With permission from Barrow Neurological Institute.)

When revascularization and trapping combinations are considered, bypass pedicles are available from a variety of vessels, depending on the volume of blood flow needed. High-flow vein bypass conduits are recommended when de novo sacrifice of the ICA is planned (**Fig. 15–4**). Although Xe CT-CBF can help determine the volume of blood flow needed, we favor high-volume bypasses when the ICA is to be sacrificed acutely. More distal MCA, PCA, PICA, and superior cerebellar arteries can be revascularized with lower flow pedicles from the superficial temporal or occipital arteries. In situ bypasses use vessels available at the operative site (intradural) to provide distal flow to the domain of the parent vessel being sacrificed. For example, an anterior temporal artery can be anastomosed to a more distal segment of the MCA trunk to trap a more proximal aneurysmal segment of the MCA.[20] Other examples of in situ bypasses include a distal A3 to A3 (side-to-side) bypass for giant aneurysms of the pericallosal artery or a PICA–PICA bypass for aneurysms of the vertebrobasi-lar junction or PICA in preparation for parent-vessel sacrifice.

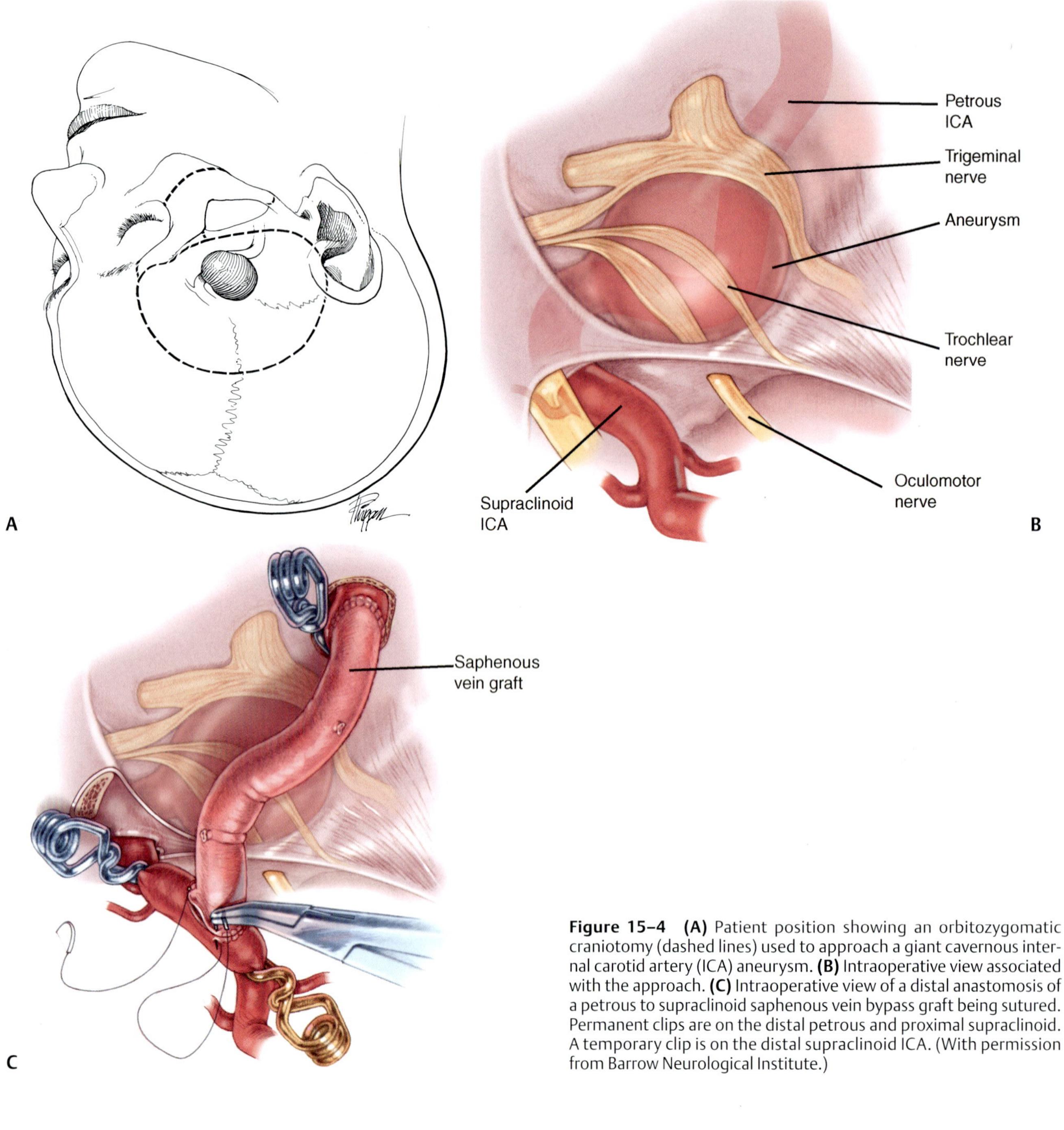

Figure 15–4 **(A)** Patient position showing an orbitozygomatic craniotomy (dashed lines) used to approach a giant cavernous internal carotid artery (ICA) aneurysm. **(B)** Intraoperative view associated with the approach. **(C)** Intraoperative view of a distal anastomosis of a petrous to supraclinoid saphenous vein bypass graft being sutured. Permanent clips are on the distal petrous and proximal supraclinoid. A temporary clip is on the distal supraclinoid ICA. (With permission from Barrow Neurological Institute.)

◆ Conclusion

Surgical management of giant aneurysms has evolved greatly over the past 3 decades. The advent of microneurosurgery, bypass techniques, and skull base approaches has revolutionized the management of these formidable lesions. Advances in the field of endovascular neurosurgery have added yet another valuable dimension to the armamentarium of neurovascular surgeons. Despite these advances, however, surgery on giant aneurysms remains extremely challenging. Effective treatment of these lesions requires a team effort that includes a complete preoperative diagnostic evaluation, appropriate preoperative planning, and the formulation of an appropriate treatment scheme based on the type and location of the aneurysm.

References

1. Morley TP, Barr HWK. Giant intracranial aneurysms: diagnosis, course, and management. Clin Neurosurg 1969;16:73–94
2. Anson JA, Lawton MT, Spetzler RF. Characteristics and surgical treatment of dolichoectatic and fusiform aneurysms. J Neurosurg 1996;84:185–193
3. Kodama N, Suzuki J. Surgical treatment of giant aneurysms. Neurosurg Rev 1982;5:155–160
4. Peerless SJ, Wallace MC, Drake CG. Giant intracranial aneurysms. In: Youmans JR, ed. Neurological Surgery: A Comprehensive Reference Guide to the Diagnosis and Management of Neurosurgical Problems. 3rd ed. Philadelphia: WB Saunders; 1990:1742–1763
5. Drake CG, Peerless SJ, Ferguson GG. Hunterian proximal arterial occlusion for giant aneurysms of the carotid circulation. J Neurosurg 1994;81:656–665
6. Fox JL. Giant aneurysms. In: Fox JL, ed. Intracranial Aneurysms. New York: Springer-Verlag; 1983:149–154
7. Hosobuchi Y. Direct surgical treatment of giant intracranial aneurysms. J Neurosurg 1979;51:743–756
8. Lawton MT, Spetzler RF. Surgical management of giant intracranial aneurysms: experience with 171 patients. Clin Neurosurg 1995;42: 245–266
9. Shibuya M, Sugita K. Intracranial giant aneurysms. In: Youmans JR, ed. Neurological Surgery: A Comprehensive Reference Guide to the Diagnosis and Management of Neurosurgical Problems. 4th ed. Philadelphia: WB Saunders; 1996:1310–1319
10. Sundt TM Jr, Piepgras DG. Surgical approach to giant intracranial aneurysms: operative experience with 80 cases. J Neurosurg 1979;51: 731–742
11. Michael WF. Posterior fossa aneurysms simulating tumours. J Neurol Neurosurg Psychiatry 1974;37:218–223
12. Allcock JM, Drake CG. Postoperative angiography in cases of ruptured intracranial aneurysm. J Neurosurg 1963;20:752–759
13. Pelz DM, Viñuela F, Fox AJ, et al. Vertebrobasilar occlusion therapy of giant aneurysms: significance of angiographic morphology of the posterior communicating arteries. J Neurosurg 1984;60:560–565
14. Lawton MT, Hamilton MG, Morcos JJ, et al. Revascularization and aneurysm surgery: current techniques, indications, and outcome. Neurosurgery 1996;38:83–94
15. Guglielmi G, Viñuela F, Duckwiler G. Coil-induced thrombosis of intracranial aneurysms. In: Maciunas RJ, ed. Endovascular Neurological Intervention. Park Ridge, IL: American Association of Neurological Surgeons; 1995:179–187
16. Gobin YP, Viñuela F, Gurian JH, et al. Treatment of large and giant fusiform intracranial aneurysms with Guglielmi detachable coils. J Neurosurg 1996;84:55–62
17. Lawton MT, Raudzens PA, Zabramski JM, et al. Hypothermic circulatory arrest in neurovascular surgery: evolving indications and predictors of patient outcome. Neurosurgery 1998;43:10–21
18. Flamm ES. Suction decompression of aneurysms: technical note. J Neurosurg 1981;54:275–276
19. Bederson JB, Zabramski JM, Spetzler RF. Treatment of fusiform intracranial aneurysms by circumferential wrapping with clip reinforcement: technical note. J Neurosurg 1992;77:478–480
20. Bederson JB, Spetzler RF. Anastomosis of the anterior temporal artery to a secondary trunk of the middle cerebral artery for treatment of a giant M_1 segment aneurysm: case report. J Neurosurg 1992;76:863–866

16

Endovascular Technique of Treating Aneurysms

Harry J. Cloft and Jacques E. Dion

Endovascular therapy for intracranial aneurysms began in the early 1970s with the pioneering work of Serbinenko, who used detachable latex balloons.[1] Endovascular techniques have evolved considerably since that time. Although balloons still have a place in the treatment of aneurysms as a parent artery occlusion device, embolization with retrievable coils has become the primary endovascular technique for the treatment of intracranial saccular aneurysms. The Guglielmi detachable coil (GDC, Target Therapeutics/Boston Scientific Corporation, Natick, MA) was approved by the United States Food and Drug Administration for cerebral aneurysm therapy in September 1995. Other retrievable coil systems such as the tungsten Spirales (Balt, Montmorency, France) and the interlocking detachable coil (IDC, Target Therapeutics/Boston Scientific Corporation, Natick, MA)[2] are available outside the United States. We will limit our discussion to the endovascular treatment of aneurysms with the GDC, though many of the same principles apply to the treatment of aneurysms with other detachable coils.

The GDC consists of a platinum coil soldered to a stainless steel delivery wire (**Fig. 16–1**). The coil is delivered into an aneurysm percutaneously through a microcatheter. The platinum coil is electrolytically detached from the delivery wire when the operator is satisfied with its deposition in the aneurysm. If the GDC does not deposit properly, it can be retrieved instead of being detached. The platinum coil is radiopaque and can be clearly distinguished from the less radiopaque delivery wire on fluoroscopy. The GDCs are platinum coils that are relatively soft and therefore will adapt to the size and shape of the aneurysm wall during deposition with only minimal increase in wall tension. Coil embolization has been shown to reduce the risk of rebleeding of ruptured aneurysms over 6 months from ~30 to 4%.[3,4] The long-term efficacy of GDC embolization of human cerebral aneurysms is still largely unknown. In 100 patients followed for 2 to 6 years (mean = 3.5 years), the rehemorrhage rate was 0% for small aneurysms, 4% for large aneurysms, and 33% for giant aneurysms.[5] The principal advantage of coil embolization of intracranial aneurysms is that it is less invasive than surgical clipping. The principal disadvantages of coil embolization are that it does not work well for aneurysms that are large or have a wide neck, and the long-term efficacy remains unclear.

◆ Indications

The indications for coil embolization of intracranial aneurysms continue to evolve and vary somewhat between institutions. In our practice, surgical clipping remains the primary mode of therapy for intracranial aneurysms. Indications for endovascular therapy include (1) an aneurysm deemed unclippable by a neurosurgeon, (2) incomplete aneurysm clipping, (3) a patient who refuses surgery, (4) poor condition of the patient due to subarachnoid hemorrhage (e.g., Hunt and Hess grade IV or V), and (5) the patient cannot tolerate surgery for other medical reasons. A neurosurgeon with adequate vascular experience should be available for backup, in the event of coil maldeployment requiring surgical retrieval or perforation (however, one may be able to finish embolization despite perforation).

The size of the aneurysm neck has been found to correlate well with treatment success and can therefore be useful in selecting patients for coil embolization. Complete aneurysm thrombosis can be achieved in 85% of aneurysms with a neck < 4 mm, and in only 15% of aneurysms with a neck ≥ 4 mm.[6] Balloon assistance (see later discussion) may

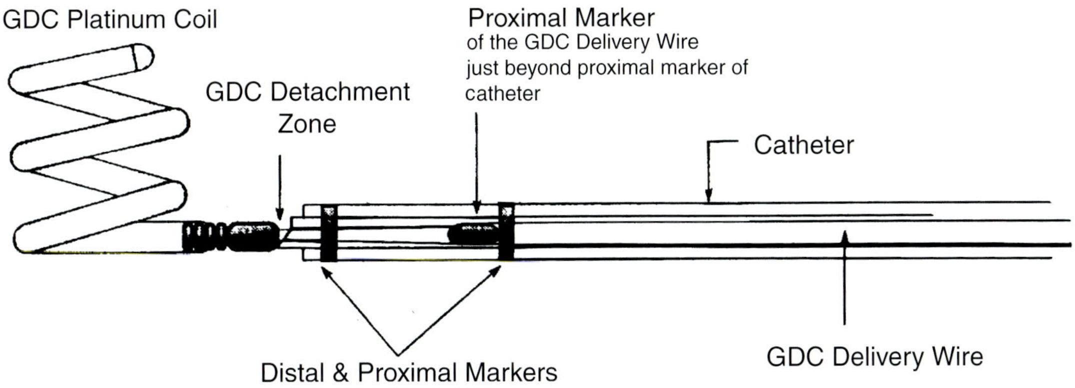

Figure 16–1 Schematic diagram of the Guglielmi detachable coil (GDC).

be necessary if the aneurysm neck is wide.[7] Permanent balloon occlusion of the carotid or vertebral artery may be needed if it is not feasible to preserve the parent vessel with coil embolization or if the aneurysm is too large for complete coil embolization.

◆ Procedural Assessment

Cerebral aneurysms are generally diagnosed with catheter cerebral angiography. However, an increasing number are being recognized with noninvasive magnetic resonance imaging and computed tomographic techniques. Regardless of how an aneurysm was initially diagnosed, a conventional catheter angiogram is generally necessary to clearly assess the anatomy of an aneurysm and to assess the entire intracranial circulation for additional aneurysms. The angiogram provides essential information about the relationship of the aneurysm neck to parent vessel, the size and shape of the aneurysm body and fundus, and the size of the aneurysm neck. This information allows the team of physicians treating the patient to decide if the aneurysm is best treated with an endovascular procedure or surgery. If angiography fails to clearly display the neck of an aneurysm and the relationship of the aneurysm to the parent artery branches, computed tomographic angiography (CTA) is often helpful. When coil embolization is performed, a working projection that optimally demonstrates the relationship of the aneurysm to the parent artery branches is necessary. Sometimes the neck can be better visualized if angiography is performed with injection of a microcatheter with its tip in the aneurysm (i.e., an intra-aneurysmal injection). Digital road map fluoroscopy is extremely useful for depositing the first coil. Subsequent coils can usually then be delivered using standard fluoroscopy, with the first coil acting as a landmark delineating the aneurysm.

A head CT may be needed to assess the degree of subarachnoid hemorrhage, intracerebral hemorrhage, intraventricular hemorrhage, hydrocephalus, or infarction from vasospasm.

◆ Surgical Technique

Anesthesia

Coil embolization of intracranial aneurysms can be performed with intravenous conscious sedation or general anesthesia. The decision is based upon considerations about the patient's condition and the personal preferences of the treating physician. Some physicians prefer to always use general anesthesia when performing coil embolization of aneurysms. If general anesthesia is not used, the patient must be able to reliably remain relatively motionless throughout the procedure with only the assistance of intravenous sedation. The advantages of general anesthesia include (1) patient comfort, (2) improved visualization due to decreased patient movement, (3) improved control of endovascular devices due to decreased patient motion, and (4) controlled manipulation of cardiopulmonary status. The disadvantages of general anesthesia include (1) cost, (2) added risk of general anesthesia, and (3) loss of the physician's ability to immediately assess the patient's neurological status. The treating physician must consider all of these factors in light of the particular patient's condition and make a decision about the type of anesthesia to be used.

Endovascular Procedure

The catheter system used for endovascular aneurysm therapy is shown schematically in **Fig. 16–2.** A sheath is placed percutaneously in the common femoral artery. A large-bore guide catheter (usually 6 French), which allows digital road mapping and angiography, is placed next. The guiding catheter may be placed primarily in the carotid or vertebral artery, or via exchange technique following initial catheterization with a diagnostic angiography catheter. The guiding catheter is placed as high in the cervical segment of the artery as safety will allow.

Finding a working projection that shows the neck and parent vessel clearly is essential. The working projection

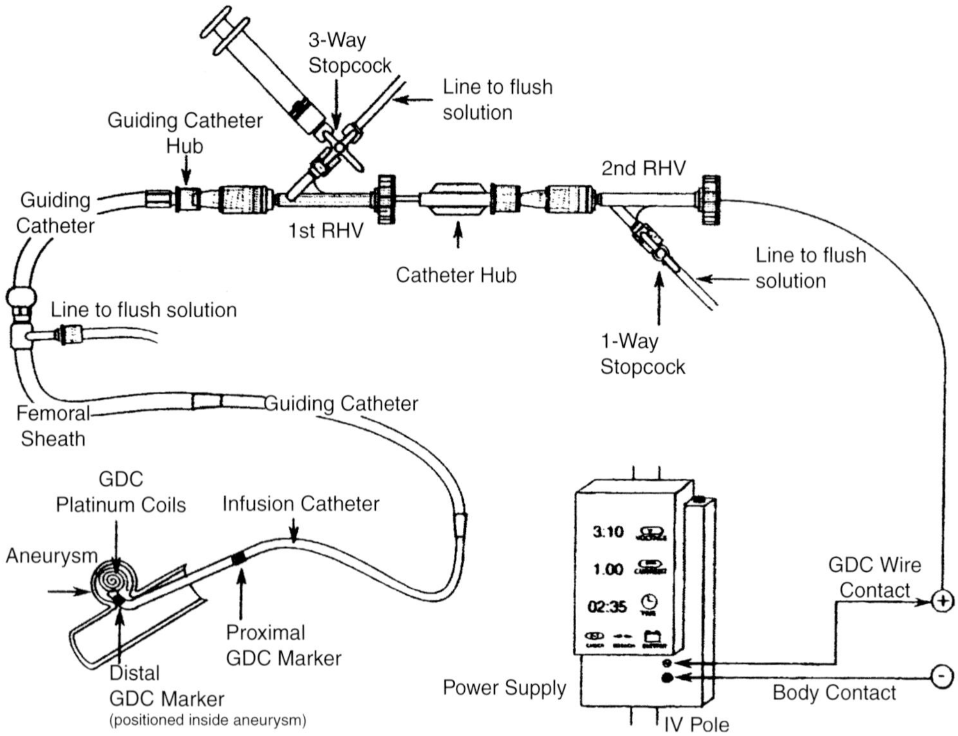

Figure 16–2 Schematic diagram of catheter system used for endovascular aneurysm therapy.

should also allow visualization of the proximal marker on the microcatheter. The microguidewire tip is directed into the aneurysm. The microcatheter is advanced over the microguidewire until the microcatheter tip is in the center of the aneurysm. Contacting the walls of the aneurysm with the microguidewire or microcatheter tip must be minimized, especially in a ruptured aneurysm, because perforation can occur. In very small aneurysms, the microcatheter may be placed at the aneurysm ostium rather than in the aneurysm.

Several commercially available microcatheters can be used. The microcatheter must have two distal markers specifically designed for coil embolization. The presence of the second marker, which is located 3 cm proximal to the microcatheter tip, allows the operator to know that a coil is fully deployed when the marker on the stainless steel pusher is aligned with the proximal microcatheter marker (**Fig. 16–1**). This system is necessary because, after detachment of the first coil, it is generally difficult to see the platinum–stainless steel junction of the second and subsequent coils within the intra-aneurysmal coil mesh.[8] Such careful, reliable alignment is necessary because the stainless steel delivery wire is relatively stiff and sharp and could potentially perforate the aneurysm after detachment if it extends beyond the microcatheter tip.

Braided catheters are often extremely useful because they will not kink and their Teflon lining substantially reduces friction. Hydrophilic catheters can make access easier, but they may also be more likely to kick out of the aneurysm during coil deployment. Some operators will shape the microcatheter with steam to make access easier and to prevent the microcatheter tip from pointing into a wall. However, one must use caution when steam-shaping a microcatheter because heat-shrinking may result in friction and unraveling with coil deposition and retrieval, and the curved catheter may hook onto coils in the aneurysm and dislodge the coils when the microcatheter is removed.

The guide catheter and microcatheter must be continuously flushed with heparinized saline (4000 U/L) to prevent blood from entering the catheters. Blood in microcatheters causes friction, which can lead to unraveling of the GDC. Continuous flushing eliminates static blood in the catheters, which can result in thromboembolism.

There are currently 80 different GDCs available to choose from (Jonathan Leyman, Target Therapeutics/Boston Scientific Corporation, personal communication). The coils are available in two main versions: coils with a 0.010 in. nominal diameter (the GDC-10) and coils with an 0.018 in. nominal diameter (the GDC-18). Both the GDC-18 and GDC-10 coils are available in a variety of lengths and diameters. The GDC-18 and GDC-10 coils are also available in soft versions, which are more deformable during deployment.

The first coil is often the most difficult to deposit. The appropriate-size coil should be chosen based upon angiographic assessment of the diameter of the aneurysm dome and ostium. The first coil should have a diameter similar to the aneurysm diameter (**Fig. 16–3**). The diameter of the first coil should never be less than the width of the ostium, given the potential for the coil to extend out of the aneurysm and into the parent artery. The size of the aneurysm can be estimated by comparing it to the parent artery, comparing it to metal sizing standards placed on the patient during angiographic filming, a guess based on experience, behavior of a test coil during a deployment attempt,

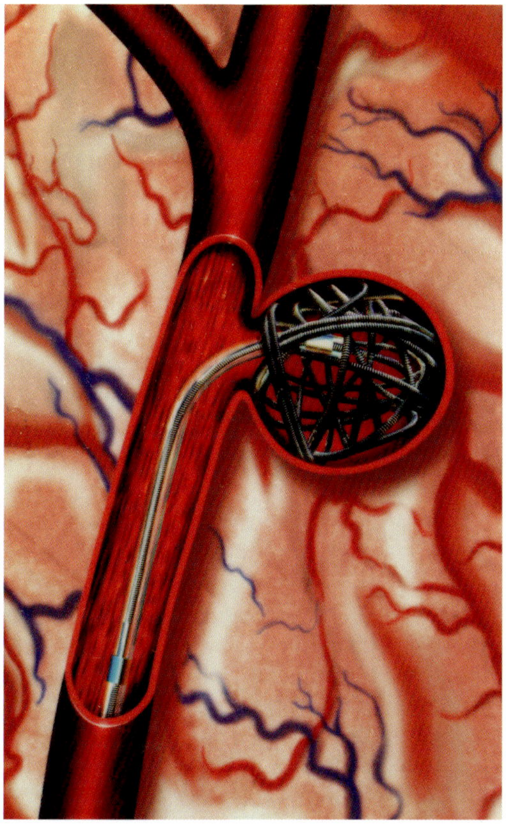

Figure 16–3 The first coil should have a diameter similar to the aneurysm diameter but not less than the width of the ostium.

or some combination of the above. A first coil of appropriate size and softness should form a complex basket in which the subsequent coils can be deposited. Some operators use only GDC-10s and soft GDC-18s in ruptured aneurysms to minimize wall tension. The speed of coil deposition affects the shape of the basket. Gently changing the catheter position back and forth can also change the shape of the basket formed. It is essential that some of the loops of the first coil extend across the neck with your first coil. The coil can be retrieved and redeposited until the operator is satisfied with the coil configuration or is convinced that the coil will not work in the aneurysm.

Coils that are too small will usually deploy as a helix ("coin-stacking") rather than assume a complex pattern. Sometimes in a small aneurysm, you can start with a smaller-diameter coil that will coin-stack initially and then will no longer coin-stack due to "dynamic volume" (e.g., use a long 3 mm coil in a 4 mm aneurysm; after part of the aneurysm volume is filled with the first several loops of coil, the coil will begin to pack tightly into the smaller remaining aneurysm volume and generate enough wall tension to stabilize the coil). Coils that are too large in diameter may herniate into the parent vessel, kick the catheter out, or be difficult to push. If the coil is too short, you will use more coils (which is more expensive). If the catheter kicks out when a coil is being deployed, try one of the following: (1) try advancing the catheter further into the aneurysm, (2) use a smaller coil, (3) use a softer coil, or (4) put forward tension on the catheter. If a coil will not advance, sometimes pulling back the microcatheter slightly will help. Pulling back the microcatheter can also help in coil retrieval by reducing curves and kinks, which can cause friction.

Advance the coil until the radiopaque proximal marker on the delivery wire is exactly aligned with the proximal marker on the microcatheter (**Fig. 16–1**). An angiogram may be performed at this time by injecting the guide catheter to confirm satisfactory coil deployment. Once a coil has been properly deployed in an aneurysm, it is detached by applying current from the GDC Power Supply (Target Therapeutics/Boston Scientific Corporation). The negative ground electrode from the power supply is connected either to a hypodermic needle placed in the patient's skin near the arterial sheath or to a skin patch placed on the patient's shoulder. The positive electrode is clipped to the proximal end of the GDC delivery wire. The power supply is then turned on to initiate detachment. When the power supply indicates that the coil has detached, the delivery wire is removed under fluoroscopy to confirm that the coil has detached. Tungsten Spirales and the IDC become detached when the proximal end of the coil exits the catheter. New detachment systems are currently being developed and will probably be available in the near future.

Repeat the foregoing steps if additional coils are required. Additional GDCs should be placed into the aneurysm until the operator is satisfied that the aneurysm has been filled as completely and as densely as can safely be achieved (**Fig. 16–4**). After the first coil, use progressively smaller and

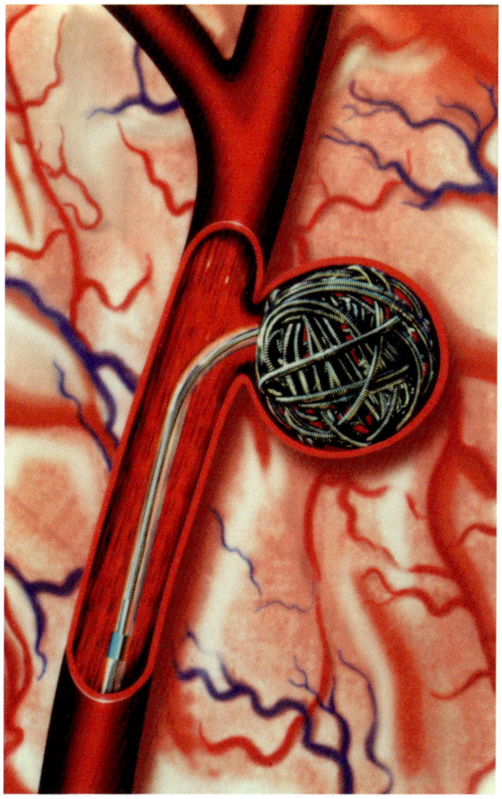

Figure 16–4 Additional Guglielmi detachable coils are placed into the aneurysm until the operator is satisfied that the aneurysm has been filled as completely as can safely be achieved.

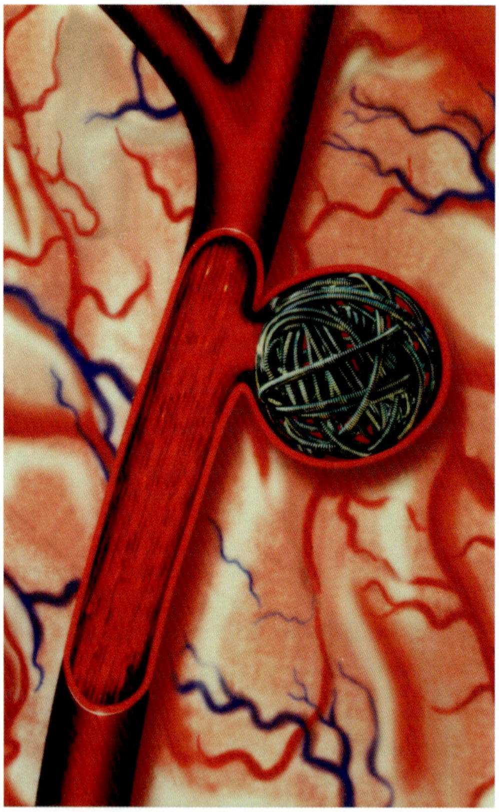

Figure 16–5 After the aneurysm has been completely coiled, the microcatheter is withdrawn from the aneurysm.

possibly softer coils. Softer coils with small diameters can be used to pack the aneurysm tightly after the basket has been formed with bigger coils. GDC-18 coils have more metal in them per centimeter of coil than GDC-10 coils, so more aneurysm filling per centimeter of coil is achieved with GDC-18 coils. Some aneurysms require compartmental coiling, sometimes creating a "snowman" appearance of coils.

After the aneurysm has been completely coiled, the microcatheter is slowly withdrawn from the aneurysm under fluoroscopic monitoring, with care not to dislodge the previously placed coils (**Fig. 16–5**). A final angiogram is obtained to assess the degree of occlusion of the aneurysm, the patency of the parent artery, and the distal vascular tree for possible thromboembolic complication.

The remodeling technique may be useful in wide-necked aneurysms.[9] Two guiding catheters (usually both 6 French) or a single, large guide catheter (at least 7 French) that can accept both the microcatheter and the balloon catheter are needed. The balloon catheter is positioned first because it can more easily dislodge the microcatheter if it is placed second. The technique works best with softer coils (GDC-18 soft, GDC-10, and GDC-10 soft). The balloon is only inflated during coil deposition. It should be deflated before detachment to confirm stability of the coil in the aneurysm. Risks of the balloon remodeling technique include vessel rupture and additional risk of thromboembolic complications by adding a second catheter system.

◆ Postoperative Care

Until Discharge

Patients are always transferred to the neurological intensive care unit for bed rest and close monitoring for 24 hours following coil embolization of an aneurysm. They are then generally kept in the hospital for one additional day in a regular hospital bed. In patients with recent subarachnoid hemorrhage or other complications, a longer stay in the intensive care unit may be indicated. Some operators administer intravenous heparin for 24 to 48 hours if a coil loop extends into the parent artery or if a large number of coil loops bridge a wide aneurysm neck. Aspirin may also be administered to these patients. Some operators always administer intravenous heparin for 24 to 48 hours following coil embolization.

After Discharge

No strenuous activity is allowed for 2 weeks following endovascular therapy. A follow-up angiogram should be performed at 6 months following embolization to assess for changes in coil configuration that could result in aneurysm recanalization. The timing of follow-up angiograms beyond 6 months varies among operators, but long-term follow-up angiography, perhaps every 1 or 2 years, is probably prudent because late aneurysm recurrence can occur.[10]

◆ Complications

The overall procedural morbidity and mortality has been reported to be 6 to 9%.[4,9,11]

Thromboembolic Complications

Thromboembolic complications are a primary consideration because they occur in 2.5% of cases.[11] Continuous flushing of the catheters with heparinized saline eliminates static blood in the catheters, which can clot and embolize. Patients should generally be systemically anticoagulated with heparin during the procedure. If the aneurysm has not ruptured, they should be fully anticoagulated (partial thromboplastin time > 2 times normal) from the time the sheath is placed until the time the catheters are removed. How to anticoagulate patients with ruptured aneurysms is more controversial. Some operators will anticoagulate patients with ruptured aneurysms at the beginning of the procedure as in unruptured aneurysms, whereas others wait until at least one coil is in place in a ruptured aneurysm before giving heparin. Some operators use a lower dose of heparin for ruptured aneurysms than for unruptured aneurysms. The risk of anticoagulation and rebleeding forming a ruptured aneurysm is likely to be considerably lower than the risk of thromboembolic complications in a patient who is not anticoagulated. However, it is important to have protamine sulfate immediately available to reverse heparin if a rupture does occur during the procedure.

Thromboembolic complications can also occur after the embolization is complete. If coils extend into the parent vessel or if there is a large surface area of coils exposed to the parent vessel at the neck, anticoagulation for 24 to 48 hours after the procedure may be warranted.

Fortunately, many thromboembolic events that occur during embolization of aneurysms will be asymptomatic or only transiently symptomatic. However, disability and even death can occur. Intra-arterial thrombolysis is a reasonable treatment of thromboembolic complications for patients with unruptured aneurysms. However, in patients with ruptured aneurysms, thrombolysis must be considered to be extremely hazardous, even with a completely coiled aneurysm, because the coils themselves are not a mechanical barrier that prevents bleeding. If thrombolysis dissolves the clot in the aneurysm and at the rupture site, subarachnoid hemorrhage will occur.

Coil Damage

Coil damage can be caused by (1) excessive pulling or pushing force when deploying or retrieving the coil, (2) torquing the pusher wire, (3) entrapment of the coil in the aneurysm or microcatheter, (4) withdrawing the coil too fast, and (5) blood in the microcatheter resulting in increased friction, which can lead to unraveling. If the coil is difficult to both push and pull, it indicates that there may be blood in the catheter or the coil may be damaged. If the coil ravels, a fading of radiopacity in the portion of the coil that is raveling (almost always the most proximal portion) can be seen. More subtle damage may be seen as irregularity of part of the coil. GDC-10 coils may become damaged in microcatheters with a larger lumen diameter because the coil has more space in which to move, and one segment of the coil can actually override another segment if excessive force is applied. Increased friction occurs with smaller diameter coils, especially if they are long, because they have more contact points in the microcatheter lumen.

If a coil becomes raveled, several solutions can be attempted. If possible, the coil should simply be removed and discarded. If the coil continues to ravel when retrieval is attempted, it may be possible to remove both the microcatheter and the coil together. This necessitates reaccessing the aneurysm with a microcatheter if further treatment is desired, but it may be the safest option in many cases. If the GDC fractures during attempted removal, it may be possible to remove it by wedging two 0.010 in. wires in the microcatheter against the fractured coil and pulling the entire system out.[7] The fractured coil can potentially be retrieved with a snare, though this is usually quite technically challenging.[12] A new device, the Attractor (Target Therapeutics/Boston Scientific Corporation, Natick, MA), promises less challenging removal of the fractured coil by ensnaring the coil in a cluster of filaments at the end of the device. If the fractured coil cannot be removed by endovascular means and its location is seriously threatening to vital arterial supply to the brain, surgical removal may be necessary.

All operators must be aware that coils can become knotted together when retrieving a coil. GDC-10s and soft coils become knotted together more easily than standard GDC-18 coils. If they are knotted together, an attempt should be made to deploy the knotted coil because attempts at retrieval might dislodge all or some of the intra-aneurysmal coil mass into the parent artery.

Coil Malpositioning and Unintended Parent Artery Occlusion

The GDC is designed to be retrievable in the event of malpositioning. However, sometimes the coil becomes malpositioned after detachment, or it cannot be completely retrieved because it has become damaged. Permanent occlusion of the parent artery is a potential option if adequate collateral circulation exists. If some coil loops are left extending into the parent artery, they can be a source of delayed thromboemboli. To avoid delayed thromboembolic complications, these patients can be treated with a short course of intravenous heparin or aspirin or both. Malpositioned coils may be retrieved with endovascular techniques or surgery (see earlier discussion).

Aneurysm Perforation

Aneurysm perforation has been reported to occur in 2.7% of ruptured aneurysms embolized with GDCs.[11] The microcatheter or microguidewire is much more often the cause of aneurysm perforation than is the GDC itself. Be very careful to minimize contact of the aneurysm wall with the wire and microcatheter, especially in a ruptured aneurysm. Heparin should be reversed immediately with intravenous protamine sulfate to prevent further subarachnoid hemorrhage. Aneurysm perforation can usually be treated by continuing to embolize the aneurysm.

Failure to Treat the Aneurysm Completely

If an aneurysm cannot be completely embolized with GDC, surgical clipping may still be an option.[13,14] Permanent balloon occlusion of the carotid or vertebral artery is another potential option if an aneurysm cannot be adequately treated with GDCs.[15]

Aneurysm Recurrence

If an aneurysm recurs, it may be technically feasible to cure the aneurysm with a second GDC embolization procedure. If an aneurysm recurs a second time, it is probably not wise to embolize it with GDCs any further because it will likely recur.

Puncture Site Complications

Small hematomas are common and generally inconsequential. Expanding hematomas, arterial occlusions, and pseudoaneurysms can be serious problems and are fortunately much less common. For these more serious puncture site complications, a vascular surgeon should be consulted promptly.

Aneurysm Rebleeding

Aneurysm rebleeding is a potential delayed complication and represents a form of treatment failure. In 100 patients followed for 2 to 6 years (mean = 3.5 years) after GDC embolization, the rehemorrhage rate was 0% for small aneurysms (< 15 mm), 4% for large aneurysms (15–25 mm), and 33% for giant aneurysms (> 25 mm).[5] Rebleeding requires an angiogram to assess the status of the previously coiled aneurysm and to look for additional aneurysms. It may be technically feasible to treat the aneurysm if there is a large enough remnant or if significant regrowth has occurred. Depending on the patient's condition and the anatomy of the aneurysm, surgical clipping or permanent balloon occlusion may also be options.[13–15]

References

1. Serbinenko FA. Balloon catheterization and occlusion of major cerebral vessels. J Neurosurg 1974;41:125–145
2. Manabe H, Fujita S, Hatayama T, Ohkuma H, Suzuki S, Yagihashi S. Embolisation of ruptured cerebral aneurysms with interlocking detachable coils in acute stage. Interventional Neuroradiology 1997;3: 49–63
3. Graves VB, Strother CM, Duff TA, Perl J. Early treatment of ruptured aneurysms with Guglielmi detachable coils: effect on subsequent bleeding. Neurosurgery 1995;37:640–648
4. Raymond J, Roy D. Safety and efficacy of endovascular treatment of acutely ruptured aneurysms. Neurosurgery 1997;41:1235–1246
5. Malisch TW, Guglielmi G, Vinuela F, et al. Intracranial aneurysms treated with Guglielmi detachable coil: midterm clinical results in a consecutive series of 100 patients. J Neurosurg 1997;87:176–183
6. Zubillaga AF, Guglielmi G, Vinuela F, Duckwiler GR. Endovascular occlusion of intracranial aneurysms with electrolytically detachable coils: correlation of aneurysm neck size and treatment results. AJNR Am J Neuroradiol 1994;15:815–820
7. Standard SC, Chavis TD, Wakhloo AK, Ahuja A, Guterman LR, Hopkins LN. Retrieval of a Guglielmi detachable coil after unraveling and fracture: case report and experimental results. Neurosurgery 1994;35: 994–999
8. Guglielmi G, Vinuela F. Intracranial aneurysms: Guglielmi electrothrombotic coils. Neurosurg Clin N Am 1994;5:427–435
9. Moret J, Cognard C, Weill A, Castaings L, Rey A. The "remodelling technique" in the treatment of wide neck intracranial aneurysms: angiographic results and clinical follow-up in 56 cases. Interventional Neuroradiology 1997;3:21–35
10. Mericle RA, Wakhloo AK, Lopes DK, Lanzino G, Guterman LR, Hopkins LN. Delayed aneurysm regrowth and recanalization after Guglielmi detachable coil treatment: case report. J Neurosurg 1998;89:142–145
11. Vinuela F, Duckwiler G, Mawad M. Guglielmi detachable coil embolization of acute intracranial aneurysm: perioperative anatomical and clinical outcome in 403 patients. J Neurosurg 1997;86:475–482
12. Zoarski GH, Bear HM, Clouston JC, Ragheb J. Endovascular extraction of malpositioned fibered platinum microcoils from the aneurysm sac during endovascular therapy. AJNR Am J Neuroradiol 1997;18: 691–695
13. Gurian JH, Martin NA, King WA, Duckwiler GR, Guglielmi G, Vinuela F. Neurosurgical management of cerebral aneurysms following unsuccessful or incompletely endovascular embolization. J Neurosurg 1995;83:843–853
14. Civit T, Augue J, Marchal JC, Bracard S, Picard L, Hepner H. Aneurysm clipping after endovascular treatment with coils: a report of eight patients. Neurosurgery 1996;38:955–961
15. Mathis JM, Barr JD, Horton JA. Therapeutic occlusion of major vessels, test occlusion and techniques. Neurosurg Clin N Am 1994;5:393–402

Section III

Arteriovenous Malformations

17

Classification, Evaluation, and General Principles of Treatment of Arteriovenous Malformations

Ram Prasad (Robin) Sengupta

Management of arteriovenous malformations (AVMs) has been a continuing challenge for neurosurgeons. Early surgical attempts reported by Cushing and Dandy[21,22] were discouraging due to difficulty in appreciating the intricate angioarchitecture of AVMs. However, with the advent of cerebral angiography, Olivecrona and Riives[23] demonstrated in 1948 that surgical resection of AVMs is feasible with good outcome. In the last 2 decades sophisticated radiological investigations, preoperative embolization, microsurgical techniques, and a better understanding of the pathophysiology of AVMs have greatly improved surgical results. On the other hand, radiosurgery offers a real alternative for a select group of AVMs. In spite of all these advances, controversy remains concerning the optimal management of some AVM patients, including those having very large lesions, lesions with a complex blood supply, lesions that are deep and located in critical areas of the brain, and lesions that have never bled.[1–3,6,9] Where feasible, surgery is the gold standard for the treatment of AVMs, which ensures immediate protection from hemorrhage. However, surgery requires meticulous attention to detail.

◆ Classification

Vascular malformations are congenital, nonneoplastic lesions of the brain that are the effect of developmental anomaly. The various forms of malformations, each with

Table 17–1 Practical Classification of Cerebral Vascular Malformations

Parenchymal
Arteriovenous malformations (AVMs)
Cavernous
Venous
Capillary (telangiectases)
Occult lesions
Cryptic
Thrombosed
Dural
Involving lateral sinus
Involving cavernous sinus
Remote from sinus

their own angioarchitecture and distinct natural history, are often confused with AVMs.[4,19] A practical classification of cerebral malformations is given in **Table 17–1.**

Arteriovenous Malformations

AVMs are masses of dilated tortuous vessels characterized by a direct connection between arteries and veins (shunt) without the interposition of a capillary network. Morphologically, AVMs are composed of feeding arteries, draining veins, and a nidus (which is composed of an abnormal vascular network, more like veins). The arteriovenous shunts are mainly located in the nidus of the AVM. They have a very low resistance to blood flow, causing increased venous pressure. A large AVM with high flow can steal blood from the surrounding brain tissue, causing hypoperfusion. No functional neural tissue is found within the malformation, which is often surrounded by gliotic tissue. The brain surrounding the AVM does not have normal autoregulation, which is responsible for some of the problems after successful excision of AVMs. Saccular aneurysms can sometimes be seen either at the main feeding artery (flow aneurysms) or at the nidus.

Cavernous Malformations

Cavernous malformations are well circumscribed, compact masses composed of enlarged vascular channels and septae. The lesion has low flow, and no cerebral tissue is found within it. They are more common in cerebral hemispheres in the subcortical tissue. Cavernous malformations have frequent minor local extravasation of blood, whereas the annual rate of symptomatic hemorrhage is ~1%.[5] Angiographically, they are occult and best diagnosed with magnetic resonance imaging (MRI) scan. They are not sensitive to radiosurgery. Surgical excision does not involve the usual difficulties encountered with AVMs.

Venous Malformations

Venous malformations consist of a collection of medullary veins that converge in a dilated central vein, assuming the characteristic shape of caput medusae. The lesion is located in the white matter and is more frequently found in the frontal lobe and cerebellum. Normal brain tissue is present between the anomalous veins. The natural history is benign, and patients rarely present with any symptoms.

Capillary Telangiectases

Patients with capillary telangiectases are rarely seen by neurosurgeons. They are a collection of dilated abnormal capillaries that resemble microscopically petechial hemorrhage. Capillary telangiectases are separated by normal nervous tissue and are mostly found in the pons. They are usually clinically silent.

Occult Arteriovenous Malformations

Occult malformations are not visualized by angiography. Although cavernous angiomas are also angiographically occult, they have distinct morphological characteristics. When the commoner AVMs are thrombosed, they become angiographically occult as well. There is a specific group of malformations known as cryptic lesions, which present with massive hemorrhage. They are more common in the young and in the cerebral hemispheres. In the wall of the hematoma cavity, a small tangle of blood vessels histologically similar to the capillary type can be found.

Arteriovenous Malformations Involving the Dura

Dural malformations have feeding arteries mainly from the external carotid, but the internal carotid and vertebral arteries may also contribute. The predominant symptom is noise in the head. They are difficult to diagnose and surgically excise because of major venous sinus involvement. Embolization procedures can be very effective.

◆ Preparation

The advancement of diagnostic imaging in the last 10 to 15 years has permitted extensive study of the features of AVMs and of the related neurovascular structures. A complete understanding of anatomical and physiological characteristics of the malformation is a key factor for correct management and surgical planning.

Computed Tomography

The role of computed tomography (CT) in studying the anatomical details of the AVM and the surrounding neurovascular structures is limited. However, it is usually the first radiological investigation performed after the onset of symptoms, and it is used for the evaluation of post-treatment complications. The diagnostic CT scan should be performed with and without contrast. A noncontrast study can show intracerebral hemorrhage, its mass effect, and any other brain abnormalities. Calcification of the AVM can be found in 25% of patients.[6] The enhanced CT scan is usually able to distinguish the AVM from the other types of vascular malformations and from an associated intracerebral hematoma.

Magnetic Resonance Imaging

MRI has the advantage of noninvasively defining the anatomical details of the lesion. Its multiple imaging planes with high resolution delineate accurately the relationship between the AVM and the related neural structures. Involvement of eloquent regions, the distance from the brain surface to the lesion, and the surgical corridor available to reach the AVM are invaluable information obtained from the MRI to decide if surgery is feasible and to plan its resection.

MR angiography (MRA) is a simple technique that may provide additional details of the vascular anatomy. However, it cannot substitute for conventional angiography in the diagnostic workup, nor can it be used postoperatively to evaluate if the lesion is completely resected.

Digital Subtraction Angiography

Angiographic evaluation includes the study of both carotid and vertebral arteries. Superficial AVMs require selective study of the external carotid artery to identify the dural feeders to the AVM and its collateral circulation. The angiographic findings that help the management of malformations are summarized in **Table 17–2.**

Superselective angiography using flow-guided microcatheters allows visualization of the feeders to the AVM and distinguishes them from those that supply the normal brain.

Table 17–2 Angiographic Findings of the Arteriovenous Malformation and of the Cerebral Circulation

Arterial Feeders
Location: superficial versus deep
Size
Length
Number
Dural supply
Aneurysms
Nidus
Location
Size
Compactness
Shunt speed
Daughter nidus
Aneurysms
Venous Drainage
Location: deep versus superficial
Number
Ectasia/varices
Stenosis/occlusion
Cerebral Circulation
Transit or en passage artery
Hypoperfusion normal brain
Collateral circulation
Venous sinus stenosis/occlusion
Vasospasm
Aneurysms

The arteries that are close to the malformation can be divided into three types (**Fig. 17–1**).

1. Terminal arteries that exclusively feed the AVM without any collaterals to the normal brain
2. Arteries en passage, which have branches to the AVM but end in the cerebral tissue
3. Transit arteries that pass close to the AVM but perfuse only the brain parenchyma

Functional information about the arteries surrounding the AVM can be obtained by injecting Amytal in an awake patient. If the artery studied is supplying eloquent brain tissue, the patient will develop temporary neurological deficit. This test is used to minimize ischemic complications from embolization or surgery.

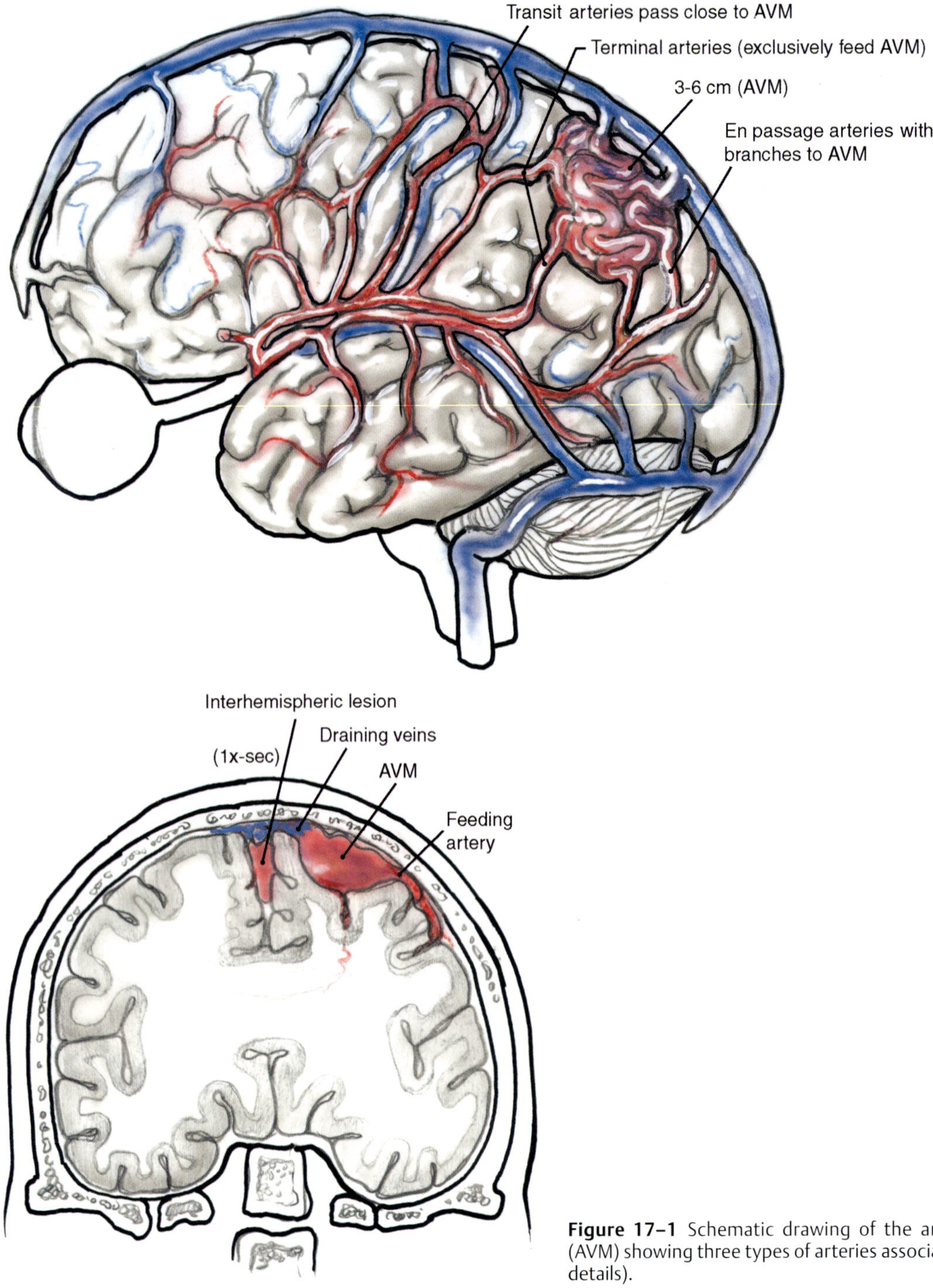

A

B

Figure 17–1 Schematic drawing of the arteriovenous malformation (AVM) showing three types of arteries associated with AVMs (see text for details).

◆ Arteriovenous Malformation Management

The decision process for the management of AVMs is more complex than any other in neurosurgery. Once an AVM is diagnosed either by its clinical manifestation or incidentally while investigating another condition, the purpose of any form of treatment is a balance between the risk of future hemorrhage (with consequent neurological deficit or death) and the risk of treatment itself. The factors that formulate this balance are risk of hemorrhage from the AVM, age of the patient, size of the lesion, morphological features of the AVM, location of the lesion, presenting symptoms, and treatment options.[3,7]

Age of the Patient

The highest incidence of AVMs is between the second and fifth decade of life. It is obvious that younger patients have a longer exposure to the devastating natural history. On the other hand, young patients also have a better chance of withstanding the surgical manipulation for excision. No specific relationship exists between pregnancy and AVM hemorrhage.

Size of the Lesion

At presentation 30% of AVMs are less than 3 cm, 60% are between 3 and 6 cm, and 10% are above 6 cm in maximum diameter.[8] Smaller AVMs have a higher tendency to bleed, probably due to higher pressure in the feeding arteries. Some AVMs have a sharp, well-circumscribed margin, allowing comfortable and accurate excision, whereas others have diffuse, ill-defined margins, making excision difficult.

Morphological Features

Complicating factors in surgical excision include number and size of shunts, dilated deep feeders of the thalamostriate and choroidal arteries, extensive venous drainage, and the nature of the surrounding major arteries.

Location of the Lesion

Obviously, excision of an AVM from some areas of the brain carries a greater risk of poorer outcome than other areas with similar lesions. In this regard, the sensorimotor, language, and visual cortex, the hypothalamus and thalamus, the internal capsule, the brain stem, the cerebellar peduncle, and the deep cerebellar nuclei are regarded as hazardous areas for surgical excision.

Presentation

Sixty-five percent of AVMs present with hemorrhage, 26% with seizures, and 9% with other complaints, including progressive neurological deficit from steal phenomena and headache.[9] Although the overriding problem associated with an AVM is the risk of future bleeding, there is no evidence that treatment is beneficial for headache, and it is doubtful if there is any indication to treat for seizures alone.

Treatment Options

After considering the natural history of AVMs, the morphological characteristics of a given AVM, the status of the patient, and the risk:benefit ratio of a particular procedure, a decision can be taken on the optimal treatment option.

The options include embolization, radiosurgery, surgery, combined therapy, and observation alone with encouragement and expectation of possible future treatment.

Role of Embolization

Embolization has had a profound influence on the management of AVMs. The purpose of embolization is to occlude the feeding arteries and the nidus of the AVM while arteries supplying the normal, brain, and draining veins are preserved. However, as a therapeutic option its role is limited because complete obliteration of the lesion is possible in only 5% of patients.[10] The benefit of preoperative embolization, on the other hand, is considerable. It can reduce the size and flow of the AVM in two thirds of patients.[11] With gradual reduction in the number and size of shunts, perfusion problems can be avoided. With interruption of deep feeders, some inoperable AVMs can become operable. The flow aneurysms can also be obliterated. Surgery should be scheduled within 2 weeks of final embolization to prevent recanalization or development of collateral feeders.

Because embolization often cannot cure the lesion completely, there is no point in embarking on this procedure if further treatment with surgery or radiosurgery is contraindi- cated.

Role of Radiosurgery

Stereotactic radiosurgery is an attractive alternative treatment for AVM in selected cases. Focused small-beam, high-energy radiation delivered through a gamma knife, linear accelerator, or proton beam and directed to cerebral blood vessels causes a progressive endarteritis obliterans. The angiographically verified obliteration rate after 3 years is ~70%.[12] The effectiveness of radiosurgery decreases in medium or large malformations. It has the disadvantage of leaving the patient at risk of bleeding until complete thrombosis is achieved. However, this modality of treatment has the distinct advantage of avoiding demanding surgery in less skilled hands. Radiosurgery can be used to eliminate residual AVMs after surgery or embolization procedures.

Indications for Surgery

Surgical excision is the ideal treatment for AVM. However, it cannot be advocated in every case. It must be stressed that any residual AVM left after operation has an unchanged risk of bleeding. The classification of Spetzler and Martin[13] given in **Table 17–3** is a practical method of estimating surgical risk and can be adopted with some modification in choosing the surgical option.[12,14]

Table 17–3 Spetzler-Martin Classification of the Arteriovenous Malformation

Graded Feature*	Points Assigned
Size of AVM	
Small (< 3 cm)	1
Medium (3–6 cm)	2
Large (> 6 cm)	3
Eloquence of Adjacent Brain	
Noneloquent	0
Eloquent	1
Pattern of Venous Drainage	
Superficial only	0
Deep	1

*Grade = size + eloquence + venous drainage.

Brain eloquent regions are sensorimotor, language, and visual cortex; hypothalamus and thalamus; internal capsule; brain stem; cerebellar peduncle; and deep cerebellar nuclei.

Indications for Radiosurgery

1. AVMs under 3 cm with multiple small feeding vessels are deemed inoperable.
2. Small AVMs in critical areas, as discussed earlier
3. Small residual AVMs after embolization or surgery
4. Small operable AVMs where surgery is hazardous because of age or associated medical problems

Indications for Observation Only

1. Patients over the age of 55 where radiosurgery is not feasible
2. Symptomatic grades IV and V where combined therapy is not feasible
3. Asymptomatic grades IV and V

Anesthesia

Skill and knowledge of the anesthesiologist contribute to no less than 50% of the success or otherwise of surgical outcome. Brain relaxation is achieved with mild hyperventilation, diuretics, and cerebrospinal fluid (CSF) drainage. Mannitol 40 to 60 g, depending on the body weight, is given as a brain protector. The patient is maintained on normal or modestly low blood pressure at mean 60 to 80 mm Hg. Extensive hypotension may cause ischemic complications to the brain adjacent to the AVM that may have compromised autoregulation.

Anticonvulsants, steroids, and antibiotics are administered preoperatively.

◆ Surgical Technique

Neurophysiological Monitoring

Various forms of monitoring techniques have been advocated to assess physiological and neurological changes in the brain during AVM resection. These include:

1. Intravascular pressure measurement. This is extremely helpful during surgery to assess the pressure at various stages of surgery.
2. Corticography with stimulation mapping under local anesthesia has been used to delineate the eloquent areas of the brain.
3. Somatosensory evoked potential (SEP)
4. Intravascular pressure measurement of feeding artery along with regional cerebral blood flow (CBF) measurement with laser Doppler flow meter to assess the risk of hyperperfusion breakthrough following excision of a large AVM[15,16]
5. Intraoperative angiography is very helpful in assessing completeness of AVM excision.

It must be stressed that there is no substitute for proper understanding of the hemodynamic changes associated with AVM excision and careful and skilful surgical technique.

Positioning

The ideal head position promotes venous drainage, provides perpendicular access to the AVM, and facilitates brain retraction. This is achieved by raising the chest piece of the operating table to a 30 degree angle and making the surface of the AVM parallel to the floor (**Fig. 17–2**). When the AVM is located on the medial surface and an interhemispheric approach is indicated, a lateral position with the ipsilateral side down is appropriate. Most of the malformations in the posterior fossa can be approached with the patient in a prone position. Rarer midline deep-seated posterior fossa AVMs need to be explored with the patient in a lounging position. It must be remembered that in this position deliberate hypotension can lead to spontaneous thrombosis of veins, resulting in venous infarction.

Craniotomy and Exposure

The craniotomy should be generous and centered on the projected AVM. A large craniotomy not only can reveal unexpected extension of the AVM, it can also help in overcoming the postoperative brain swelling. For midline lesions the medial bur holes should be placed over the sagittal sinus itself, where the dura is thicker and can be easily stripped away. While planning the craniotomy, normal brain around the AVM and location of the major draining veins should be considered (**Fig. 17–3**).

Brain relaxation helps dural opening. Care must be taken not to damage any draining veins while opening and reflecting the dura. Even a small subarachnoid bleed can obscure the landmarks and preclude accurate dissection of the AVM.

After elevating the dural flap, the surgeon should get oriented with the angioarchitecture through analysis of the MRI and the angiogram by inspection of the cortical surface. A large cortical vein is an excellent landmark, whereas the feeding arteries are serpentine and lie deep in the sulci as they approach the AVM. They cannot be easily seen until the sulci are open.

Dissection of the AVM

The dissection of the malformation is started after opening the thickened arachnoid at the periphery of the lesion. A plane of cleavage must be found between the AVM and the brain. Subcortical components of the AVM may be exposed through opening of one or more sulci (**Fig. 17–4**). If this is not possible due to the presence of cortical bridging vessels, resection of nonfunctioning brain tissue is necessary. The dissection of the malformation should be performed circumferentially around the AVM and gradually deepened (**Fig. 17–5**). Sometimes a glial plane or a clot cavity will help the separation of the AVM from the brain. During dissection small vessels on the way to the AVM are coagulated and divided. Two concepts are important at this stage of the operation.

1. The feeding arteries should be occluded at their point of entry to the nidus to preserve the arteries supplying normal brain tissue.

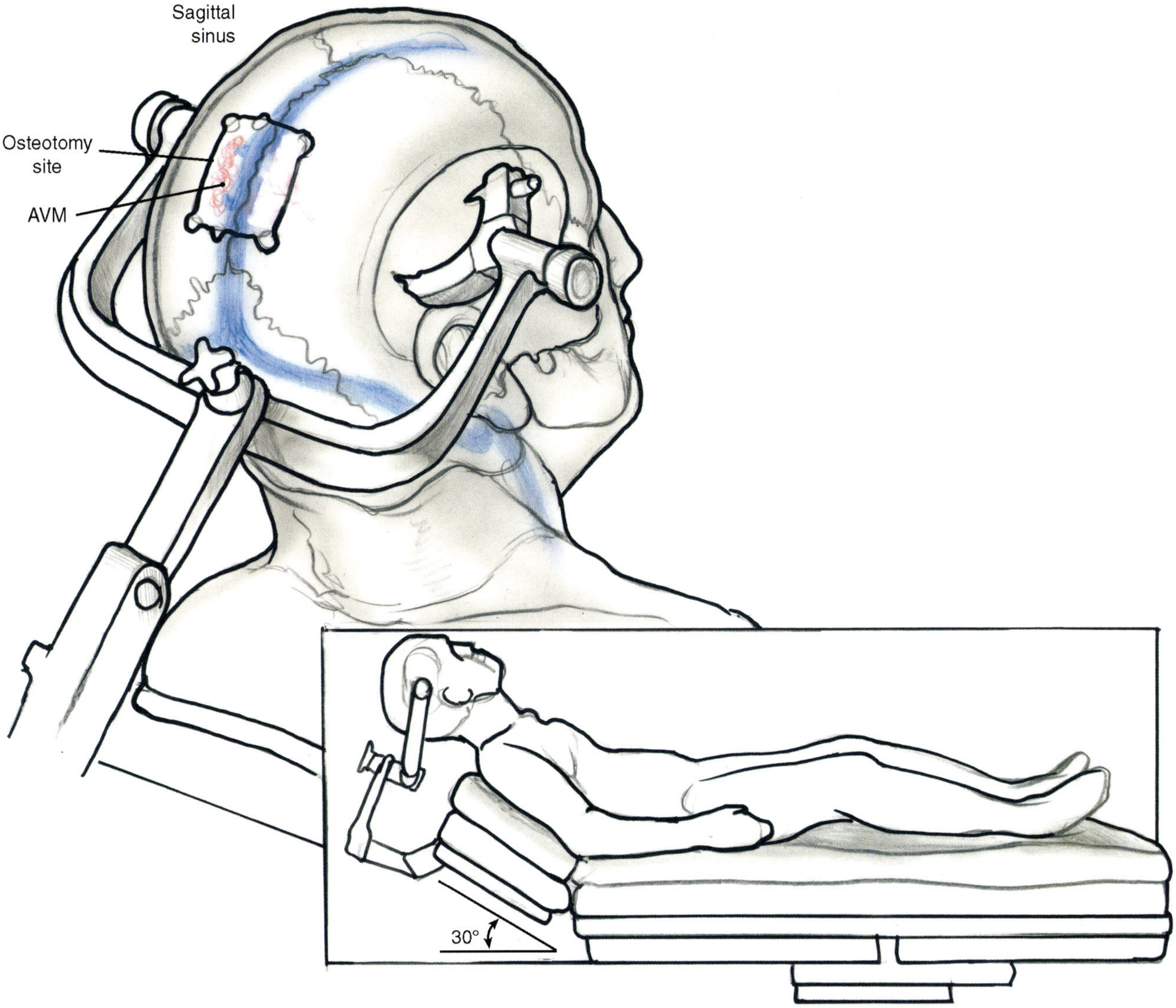

Figure 17–2 Position of the patient on the table (see text for details).

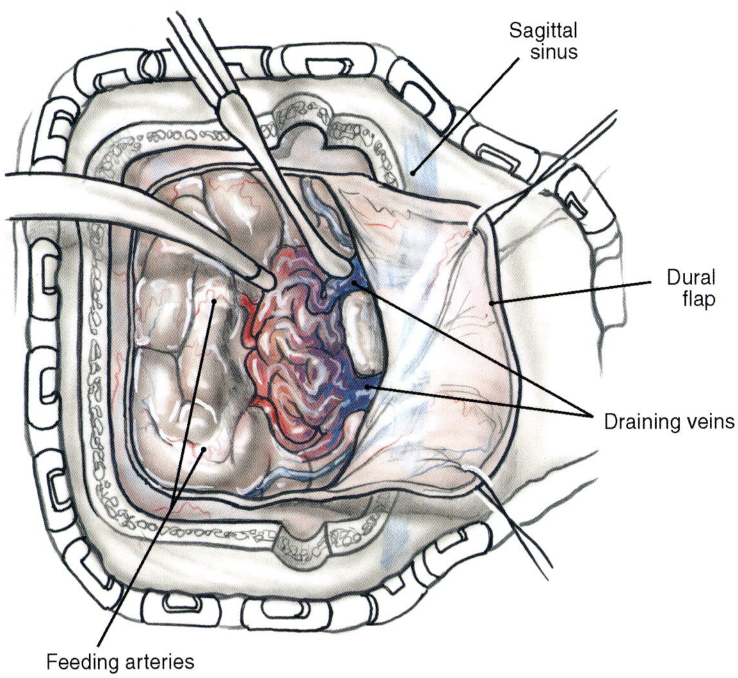

Figure 17–3 A left convexity arteriovenous malformation close to the midline has been exposed. Two large veins of the malformation can be seen draining into the sagittal sinus. The feeding arteries are hidden by the cortex. The brain surface is left exposed for clarity.

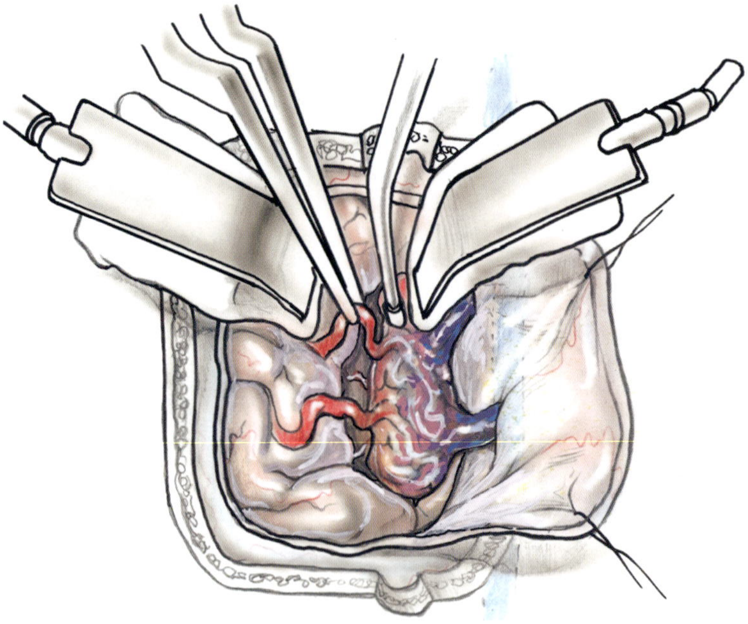

Figure 17–4 Two feeding arteries have been exposed by cortical dissection.

2. The major draining veins should be preserved until the end of the AVM resection to avoid swelling of the lesion. Sometimes it is necessary to sacrifice a draining vein to continue the dissection all around the malformation. It is harmless to do so provided temporary occlusion of the vein with microclip does not cause swelling of the AVM. Temporary occlusion can also be used to distinguish a feeding artery from a red draining vein.

Coagulation of the vessels is performed under gentle irrigation to prevent sticking of the bipolar forceps. Coagulation should be done over a long segment of the vessel before dividing it. Continuous coagulation in one point may result in the rupture of the vessel. Titanium vascular clips as designed by Sundt should be used to occlude feeding arteries. The cleavage plane should be maintained with a layer of Surgicel and cottonoid on the normal brain while proceeding with the dissection toward the white matter. Multiple self-retaining retractors are very useful at this stage. The brain tissue surrounding the AVM may have lost its autoregulatory mechanism; therefore, the retraction should be very gentle to avoid ischemic injury. It is important to advance the dissection progressively all around the AVM rather than making a small hole where bleeders are much more difficult to control (**Fig. 17–6**).

The resection of the periventricular component of the AVM is the most difficult part of the operation (**Fig. 17–7**). The reason is that many small, thin-walled arteries that are friable and difficult to coagulate feed the apical portion of the lesion. These deep arteries frequently burst during coagulation. Once the dissection of the AVM has been completed, the remaining draining veins, which should be blue and collapsed by now, can be coagulated and divided (**Fig. 17–8**). Occasionally a feeding artery is found on the undersurface of the major draining veins, and this must not be neglected.

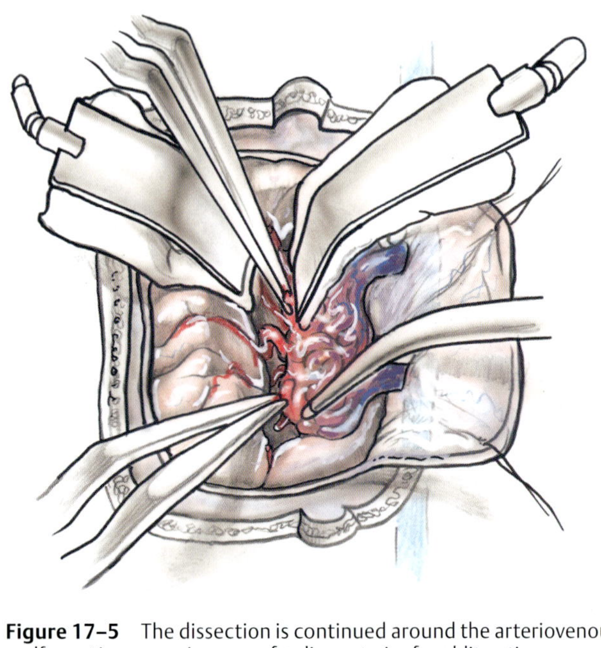

Figure 17–5 The dissection is continued around the arteriovenous malformation, exposing more feeding arteries for obliteration.

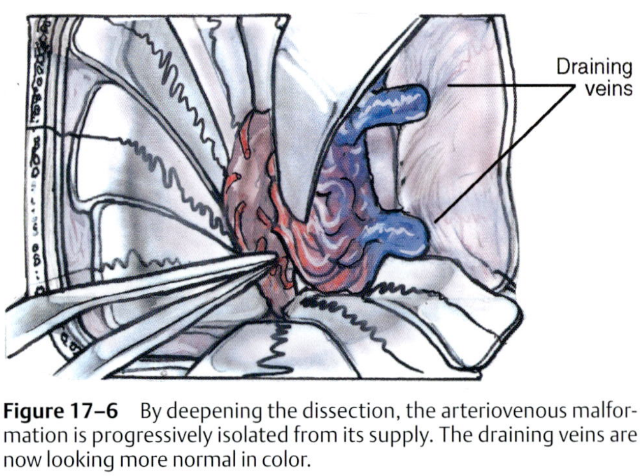

Figure 17–6 By deepening the dissection, the arteriovenous malformation is progressively isolated from its supply. The draining veins are now looking more normal in color.

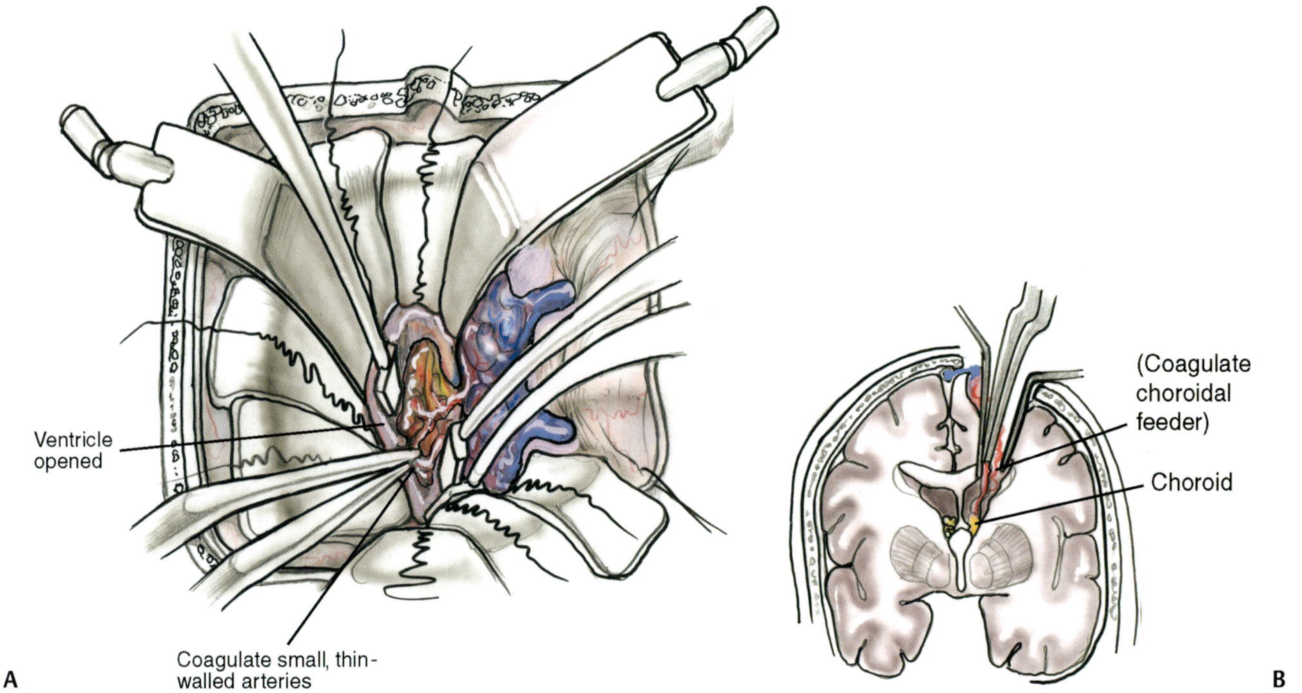

Figure 17–7 (A, B) Toward the end of the dissection, the feeders from choroidal vessels are exposed by opening the ventricle. (A) Intra-operative view. (B) Coronal orientation of AVM dissection.

Intraoperative Angiography

Intraoperative angiography is very important to verify a complete resection of the AVM. Occasionally it can be used during the dissection of the malformation to distinguish between feeders to the AVM from a transit artery supplying the normal brain. A metallic marker can be used for this purpose. If the films are of good quality, a postoperative check angiogram is not necessary.

Closure

Hemostasis after completion of an AVM excision is the single most important factor for avoiding postoperative hematoma. During hemostasis the blood pressure is slightly elevated to a systolic pressure of 120 mm Hg. The bed of the malformation must be carefully inspected to verify if the lesion has been completely resected. All the bleeding points should be coagulated until the bed is absolutely dry. Small clots on the wall of the

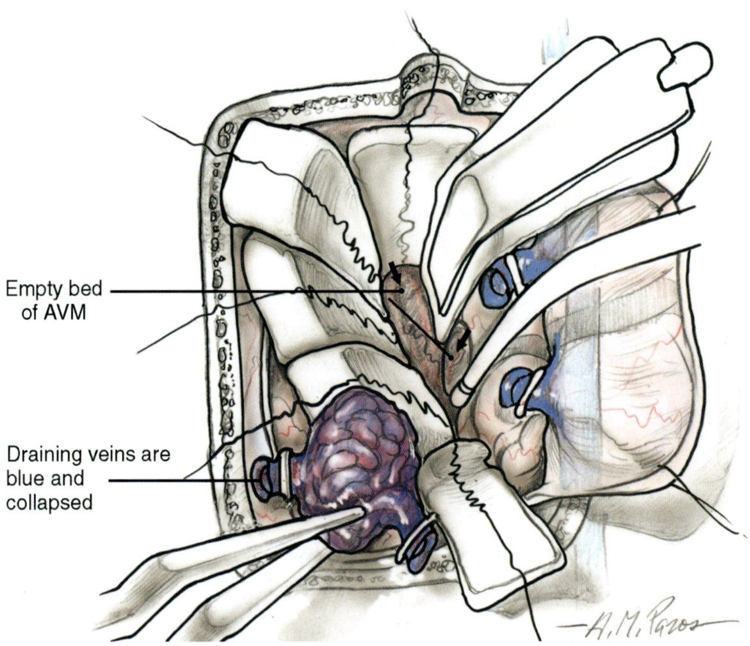

Figure 17–8 Appearance of the cortical bed after removal of the arteriovenous malformation. The excised AVM is illustrated.

cavity should be evacuated and inspected. Then small pieces of Surgicel are used to line the wall of the cavity. Once hemostasis has been adequately obtained, it is our practice to wait for 10 to15 minutes before closing the dura. A subdural intracranial pressure (ICP) monitor of CAMINO type (Integra Neurosciences, Plainsboro, New Jersey) is inserted for postoperative monitoring of ICP. The craniotomy is then closed in a routine manner.

◆ Postoperative Care

It is advisable to keep the patient ventilated overnight. In spite of diligent searching, some of the vessels can retract within the wall of the cavity and later open up when the patient becomes restless during extubation. In addition, elective ventilation mitigates against postoperative brain swelling, and the physiological parameters are better controlled. Although neurological status or subsequent deterioration cannot be assessed clinically with the patient asleep, a rise in ICP will indicate the need for urgent CT scan to exclude hematoma or brain swelling.

Strict fluid control is essential to avoid brain swelling. A total fluid intake of 1500 mL per 24 hours is adequate for the first 48 to 72 hours.

◆ Complications

Intraoperative Hemorrhage

Troublesome intraoperative hemorrhage may be encountered in one of the following situations:

1. Failure to control the bleeding from the deep feeding arteries
2. Inadvertent tearing of the lesion
3. Rupture of the AVM from premature occlusion of the draining veins
4. Normal perfusion pressure breakthrough (NPPB)

Independent of any of the above causes, the bleeding can be better controlled by reducing the blood pressure. Broad-tipped bipolar forceps are very useful for the fragile arteries. If cauterization is unsuccessful, packing the bleeding source with Gelfoam and cottonoids for a few minutes should be the next move. Coagulation and packing may be used several times alternatively. Packing is particularly useful if the bleeding is from multiple sources when the AVM ruptures. Microclips or even aneurysm clips may be necessary if the bleeders are of larger size. Sometimes the dissection has to be advanced into the brain parenchyma to expose the bleeding vessels more adequately. The surgeon must always try to avoid dissecting through the AVM because more vessels can be injured, making the bleeding worse. If the hemorrhage is still extensive despite all these measures, a fast resection of the AVM under most unfavorable circumstances may be the last resort.

Postoperative Hemorrhage

The incidence of postoperative hemorrhage varies between 0 and 34%.[17,18] The surgeon's skill and experience are crucial to reduce this complication. Inadequate hemostasis and incomplete resection of the malformation are the main causes of intracerebral hematoma after surgery. While evaluating a postoperative hemorrhage, it is advisable to perform an angiographic study to exclude a residual AVM.

Normal Perfusion Pressure Breakthrough

Normal perfusion pressure breakthrough is an abrupt change in the hemodynamic status of the cerebral circulation caused by resection of a large high-flow AVM, which can occur during or after surgery, culminating in severe brain edema and multifocal bleeding. Before making a diagnosis of NPPB, other causes of brain edema or hematoma must be excluded. The cause of NPPB is unknown, but an attractive theory is that it is due to chronic low flow in the cerebral circulation surrounding the AVM that has lost its autoregulatory mechanism and is not able to receive a sudden increase of blood flow following resection of a large malformation. The prevention of NPPB can be achieved with staged embolization of the AVM to allow a gradual change in the hemodynamic state. NPPB is treated with mannitol, hyperventilation, and, rarely, barbiturate coma. Surgical decompression must be considered for significant mass effect if other treatment modalities are ineffective.

Brain Injury

The most common cause of brain injury is occlusion of any of the normal vessels around the AVM. The brain can also be injured during attempts to expose or dissect the malformation in eloquent regions. A safer trajectory to reach subcortical or deep AVMs has to be carefully studied preoperatively, particularly on MRI scan, and the anatomical routes through cortical sulci, ventricles, or cisterns should be preferentially used. During dissection the surgeon must remain within the cleavage plane at the border of the AVM, avoiding the brain parenchyma. In selected cases the dissection adjacent to eloquent areas can be performed using cortical stimulation, as previously mentioned.

Seizures

Postoperative epileptic seizures can be a frequent complication, reported in as many as 50% of cases in some of the literature.[19] It is therefore important to maintain an adequate blood level of anticonvulsants during the entire hospital course and subsequently for a seizure-free year. Seizures in the immediate postoperative period may be extremely dangerous because they can cause intracerebral hemorrhage. Elective hyperventilation can overcome this problem as well.

Retrograde Thrombosis of Parent Arteries

This is a rare complication in the acute postoperative period. Its pathophysiological process is unknown, but it has been suggested that resection of a high-flow AVM causes an abrupt reduction of blood flow in the feeding arteries, leading to thrombosis. Risk factors for this complication are advanced age, large AVMs with long feeding vessels, and atherosclerotic vessels. Preoperative staged embolization may reduce this complication, as in NPPB. Successful treatment of retrograde thrombosis with intra-arterial urokinase has been reported.[20]

References

1. Brown RD Jr, Wiebers DO, Forbes G, et al. The natural history of unruptured intracranial arteriovenous malformations. J Neurosurg 1988;68:352–357
2. Heros RC, T Y-K. Is surgical therapy needed for unruptured arteriovenous malformations. Neurology 1987;37:279–286
3. Ondra SL, Troupp H, George ED. The natural history of symptomatic arteriovenous malformations of the brain: a 24-year follow-up assessment. J Neurosurg 1990;73:387–391
4. Wilkins RH. Natural history of intracranial vascular malformations: a review. Neurosurgery 1985;16:421–430
5. Robinson JR, Awad IA, Little JR. Natural history of the cavernous angioma. J Neurosurg 1991;75:709–714
6. Kumar AJ, Fox AJ, Vinuela F, et al. Revisited old and new CT findings in unruptured larger arteriovenous malformations of the brain. J Comput Assist Tomogr 1984;8:648–655
7. Graf CJ, Perret GE, Torner JC. Bleeding from cerebral arteriovenous malformations as part of their natural history. J Neurosurg 1983;58: 331–337
8. Spetzler RF, Zabramski JM. Grading and staged resection of cerebral arteriovenous malformations. Clin Neurosurg 1990;36:318–337
9. Stein BM, Kader A. Intracranial arteriovenous malformations. Clin Neurosurg 1992;39:76–113
10. Frizzel RT, Fisher WS. Cure, morbidity, and mortality associated with embolisation of brain arteriovenous malformations: a review of 1246 patients in 32 series over a 35 year period. Neurosurgery 1995;37: 1031–1040
11. Vinuela F, Dion J, Duckwiler G, et al. Combined endovascular embolisation and surgery in the management of cerebral arteriovenous malformations: experience with 101 cases. J Neurosurg 1991;75: 856–864
12. Heffez DS, Osterdock RJ, Alderete L, et al. The effect of incomplete patient follow-up on the reported results of AVM radiosurgery. Surg Neurol 1998;49:373–384
13. Spetzler RF, Martin NA. A proposed grading system for arteriovenous malformations. J Neurosurg 1986;65:476–483
14. Samson D, Batjer HH. Preoperative evolution of the risk/benefit ratio for arteriovenous malformations of the brain. In: Wilkins RH, Rengachary SS, eds. Neurosurgery Update II, New York: McGraw-Hill; 1991:129–133
15. Spetzler RF, Martin NA, Carter LP, et al. Surgical management of large AVMs by staged embolisation and operative excision. J Neurosurg 1987;67:17–28
16. Young WL, Prohvnik I, Ornstein I, et al. The effect of arteriovenous malformation resection on cerebrovascular reactivity to carbon dioxide. Neurosurgery 1990;27:257–267
17. Hamilton MG, Spetzler RF. The prospective application of a grading system for arteriovenous malformations. Neurosurgery 1994;34: 2–7
18. Pasqualin A, Scienza R, Cioffi F, et al. Treatment of cerebral arteriovenous malformations with a combination of preoperative embolization and surgery. Neurosurgery 1991;29:358–368
19. Korouse K, Heros RC. Complications of complete surgical resection of AVMs of the brain. In: Barrow DL, ed. Intracranial Vascular Malformations. Park Ridge, IL: American Association of Neurological Surgeons; 1990:157–168
20. Sipos EP, Kirsch JR, Nauta HJW, et al. Intra-arterial urokinase for treatment of retrograde thrombosis following resection of an arteriovenous malformation: case report. J Neurosurg 1992;76: 1004–1007
21. Dandy WE. Venous abnormalities and angiomas of the brain. Arch Surg 1928; (Chicago) 17:715–93
22. Cushing HP, Bailey P. Tumors arising from blood vessels of the brain: vol. 3. Angiomalous malformations and hemangioblastomas. 1928; Springfield, IL
23. Olivecrona H, Riives S. Anterionemous aneurysms of the brain: their diagnosis and treatment. Arch Neurol Psychiatry 1968; 59:567–602

18

Preoperative and Therapeutic Embolization of Cerebral Arteriovenous Malformations

Anton Valavanis and Greg Christoforidis

Cerebral arteriovenous malformations (AVMs) encompass a variety of lesions whose mutual features are abnormal arteriovenous communications. They are regarded as congenital errors of cerebrovascular embryogenesis within the capillary bed. Recent evidence suggests that they represent the phenotypic expression of a group of biological dysfunctions that involve the endothelial remodeling process at the level of the capillarovenous junction.[1,2] The first operative description was by Cushing and Bailey in 1921, who together with Dandy were the first to recognize the presence of arteriovenous shunting within these lesions. Dott is credited with the first angiographic description of an AVM in 1929. Olivecrona performed the first successful removal of a cerebral AVM in 1932.[3] Surgical techniques were considerably refined with the introduction of microneurosurgical techniques by Yasargil.[3] Despite the progress in surgical techniques, AVM surgery remains complex and associated with several complications primarily consisting of postsurgical cerebral edema and bleeding. Spetzler and Martin deduced that surgical outcome correlated to AVM size, location, relationship to "eloquent brain," and venous drainage pattern.[4] Attempts to circumvent complications led to the development of various adjunct techniques to improve surgical results. These have included preoperative partial embolization and radiation therapy. Advances and refinements in neuroendovascular techniques and the development of gamma knife surgery have made these newer techniques viable alternatives to surgical resection.

Endovascular embolization of brain AVMs was first described by Luessenhop and Spence in 1960, who introduced methylmethacrylate-covered steel particles into the surgically exposed internal carotid artery to block the feeding arteries to brain AVMs.[5] A variety of embolic agents have been introduced that included various microparticles, alcohol, suture material, and acrylics. With the introduction of variable-stiffness microcatheters and microguidewires in 1987 and flow-guided microcatheter systems, a safer and more effective endovascular approach was possible.

Besides conservative treatment, there are currently three generally accepted modalities for the treatment of AVMs: microneurosurgical resection, radiosurgery, and endovascular embolization. Treatment approach ultimately depends on the experience available at a given institution, as well as the relative risk of active treatment versus the natural history of the disease. Surgical removal historically is the most common treatment approach. According to the Spetzler-Martin grading system, surgical risks depend predominantly on size, location, and venous drainage pattern.[4] Successful removal is counterbalanced by postsurgical hemorrhagic events and neurological deficits. Complete removal is not always possible. Radiosurgical ablation of AVMs is most effective when the nidus is less than 2 to 3 cm in size and requires a latency period of up to 3 years.[6] Radiosurgery failures have been correlated to multiple isocenters, high Spetzler-Martin grades, increasing AVM volume, and a history of hemorrhage.[7] The role of radiosurgery is predominantly for small lesions with difficult endovascular or surgical access.[8]

Transcatheter embolization possesses potential advantages over surgical and radiosurgical techniques. The endovascular approach forgoes the craniotomy and thus any necessary care or associated complications. It also avoids direct contact with the brain and cranial nerves, which may potentially damage the brain. More importantly, it provides the operator with a more detailed and readily available visualization of the AVM angioar-chitecture during the procedure. This allows the operator to adjust treatment planning according to any hemodynamic changes and allows for the identification of angioarchitecturally weak elements. In addition, a hemorrhagic or a thromboembolic complication occurring during the procedure can be identified and treated during the procedure.

Endovascular techniques are often limited by unfavorable AVM angioarchitectural features such as the caliber of the feeding arteries, the length and tortuosity of feeders, and the flow conditions as they relate to microcatheter construction. The smallest microcatheter available today is ~330 microns (μ) in size, and catheter flexibility and ability to take advantage of flow are counterbalanced by navigational control. Feeders that are not accessible with microcatheters are of course more difficult to embolize. Other limiting angioarchitectural features include concomitant arterial feeder supply to normal brain and extensive vascular tortuosity. Potential complications introduced with endovascular techniques include contrast reaction and catheter-related complications such as arterial dissection, thromboembolic event, hemorrhage, inguinal hematoma, and pseudoaneurysm formation.

◆ Indications

The decision to actively treat an AVM depends on the expected natural history of the disease, the patient's neurological and medical condition, and the anticipated risks incurred with the various treatment modalities. The primary goal of AVM treatment is to prevent intracranial hemorrhage. In addition, AVM treatment may help improve or stabilize neurological deficits, epilepsy, or headaches. Each treatment modality attempts to achieve these goals by completely excluding the AVM from the cerebrovascular circulation.

Ondra et al prospectively followed patients with untreated cerebral AVMs who presented without hemorrhage over a 24-year period. They reported a constant annual bleeding rate of 4%.[11] Crawford et al followed 217 patients over 10 to 20 years and found a 42% risk of hemorrhage, 18% risk of seizures, and 27% risk of neurological deterioration.[12] Angioarchitectural features such as flow-related aneurysms, stenosis or occlusion of a draining vein, deep location, or posterior fossa location have a higher incidence of hemorrhage, whereas AVM size has not been clearly found to predispose toward hemorrhagic events.[1] Seizures have been associated with temporal lobe and motor–sensory strip locations and are thought to result from rerouting of venous drainage.[13,14] When not due to hemorrhage, neurological deficits are thought to result from a hemodynamic steal effect by the AVM, arterial stenosis, venous hypertension, or mass effect from venous ectasia or varices.[14] Patients with AVM frequently complain of headache. This has been correlated with the angiographic demonstration of dilated vessels near the meninges or the presence of dural supply to the AVM.[14]

Although various grading systems have been developed to predict the outcome of surgical removal of an AVM, it should be emphasized that these grading schemes fail to effectively predict outcome from endovascular treatment. Successful endovascular treatment of AVMs depends on the angioarchitecture of the lesion and the topographical relationship of the AVM to its vascular supply. Morbidity relates to the operator's ability to safely reach the nidus and remain within it during embolization. The identification of angioarchitecturally weak elements (see later discussion), which place the patient at a higher risk for a hemorrhagic complication, should be taken into account when deciding to treat an AVM.

The most frequent indication for the endovascular occlusion of AVMs described in the literature is as an adjunct to either or both surgical removal and radiosurgical obliteration. The strategy for embolization prior to surgery or radiation therapy differs from that of embolotherapy alone. The primary goal of presurgical embolization is to reduce the overall nidus size and to occlude the nidal components corresponding to arterial feeders, which are difficult to access surgically. Vinuela et al found that surgical dissection and control of fragile, deep-feeding arteries is significantly improved following embolization of 75% of the nidus volume.[9] If embolization of the nidus is less than 50% of the nidal volume, the surgeon will not notice a significant benefit of the procedure unless surgically inaccessible components are embolized. Other factors that affect the postembolization resectability of an AVM include the remaining degree of hemodynamic shunting, the number of nonembolized perforators, and the recruitment of pial collaterals following the embolization.[1]

The goal of preradiosurgical embolization is also to reduce the overall nidus volume because the overall volume of irradiation is thought to be directly related to the incidence of postradiosurgical complications.[10]

The systematic analysis of brain AVMs on the basis of angioarchitectural features with the intention of cure via endovascular means has been routinely applied at the University of Zurich. This has resulted in a complete obliteration rate of 40% over the past 10 years. After the initial session the patient can return for additional transcatheter treatments. Therefore, endovascular cure of brain AVMs can play an important role in the overall management of brain AVMs.[1] In cases where complete embolization is not possible in otherwise untreatable AVMs, the ability to analyze AVM angioarchitecture in detail during embolization allows the operator to target embolic treatment toward angioarchitecturally weak elements responsible for symptoms such as bleeding (palliative embolization).

◆ Preparation

The preembolization evaluation for AVMs demands an understanding of the angioarchitecture of AVMs to decide how to approach the AVM, how to avoid potential complications, and what to expect from the embolization. This preprocedural evaluation intuitively differs from presurgical consideration in that the therapeutic access is endovascular. The experience at the University of Zurich has thus led to a critical evaluation of the angioarchitectural features of AVMs as they relate to the embolization.[15] This concept is a modification of the Yasargil[3] classification of brain AVMs, which divides AVMs into convexial and deep types and takes into consideration the intrinsic arterial supply and the pattern of venous drainage. It additionally incorporates an evaluation of the AVM arterial feeders as they relate to the specific location of the AVM nidus as identified on magnetic resonance imaging (MRI). At the University of Zurich, typical MR protocol for AVMs includes triplanar T1-weighted imaging with and without gadolinium using 3 mm cuts and four excitation pulses, T2 and proton density–weighted imaging, as well as postgadolinium three-dimensional time-of-flight (3D-TOF) and phase contrast MR angiographic sequences displayed using surface rendering postprocessing technique. These sequences provide a good appreciation of the topographic location and overall size and geometry of the AVM, as well as a 3D display of most vessels involved (**Figs. 18–1** and **18–2**). In addition, some information can be obtained regarding angioarchitecturally weak elements of the AVM.

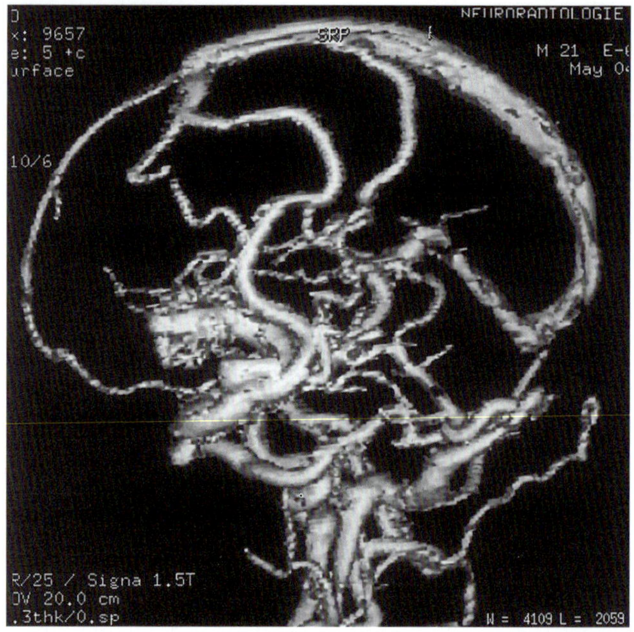

Figure 18–2 Lateral view of magnetic resonance angiogram (three-dimensional time-of-flight technique with surface rendering) showing the nidus of the arteriovenous malformation, the exiting draining vein, and its connections to multiple cortical veins.

◆ Classification

Because the endovascular route of AVM access is via the arterial system, a detailed analysis of the arterial supply to AVMs is necessary to predict appropriate access to these lesions prior to isolating a compartment of an AVM for the purpose of treatment. Thus both convexial and deep AVMs are further subdivided into subtypes with respect to gyral and sulcal anatomy in the case of convexity AVMs, and with respect to the basal fissures, cisterns, ventricular system, deep gray matter nuclei, and white matter tracts in the case of deep AVMs.[1] **Table 18–1** summarizes the topographic classification of cerebral AVMs developed and used at the University of Zurich.

An understanding of the microscopic vascularization of the pial surface of the brain, the cortex, and the subcortical white matter when applied to the topographic location of the AVM nidus results in the distinction of three subtypes of cortical AVMs: (1) sulcal AVM, (2) gyral AVM, and (3) mixed sulcal-gyral AVM. This analysis leads to a better appreciation of the predominant arterial supply to an AVM. Sulcal AVMs are located primarily in a specific sulcus within the subpial space. They therefore conform to the shape of the sulcus, generally obtaining a pyramidal shape. They often extend into the underlying brain, becoming sulcal with subcortical extension and even sulcal with subcortical and ventricular extension. Arterial supply to a sulcal AVM is predominantly via pial arteries. In the case of sulcal AVMs, the pial arteries directly terminate into the nidus after contributing cortical, medullary, and corticomedullary branches to the adjacent brain parenchyma with no additional supply to normal brain distal to the AVM. This direct type of termination of the feeding supply implies that there is no risk of damage to normal

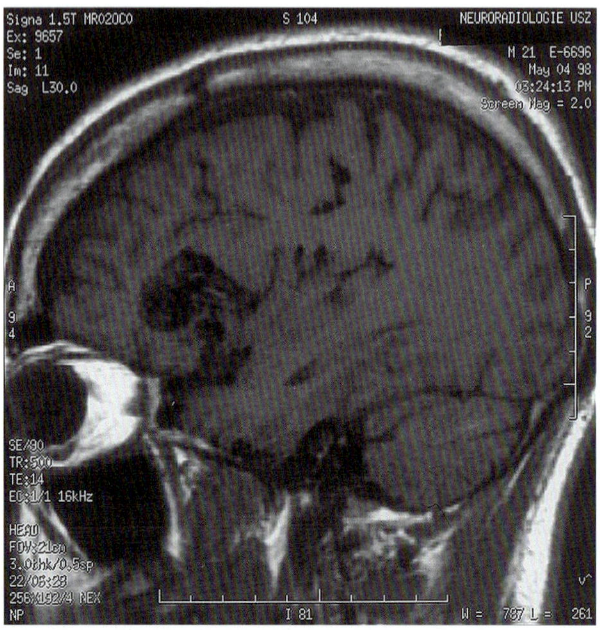

Figure 18–1 Sagittal T1-weighted magnetic resonance image showing a middle-sized arteriovenous malformation with compact appearance located in the left inferior frontal gyrus.

Table 18–1 Topographic Classification of Cerebral Arteriovenous Malformations

Convexity (pallial) AVMs
Sulcal
Pure sulcal
With subcortical extension
With ventricular extension
Gyral
Pure gyral
With subcortical extension
With ventricular extension
Mixed sulcal-gyral
Pure sulcal-gyral
With subcortical extension
With ventricular extension
Subcortical AVMs
Pure subcortical
With gyral and ventricular extension
Deep (central) AVMs
Subarachnoid (fissural, cisternal)
Small
Moderate
Large
Parenchymal
Small
Moderate
Large
Intraventricular (plexal)
Small
Moderate
Large
Mixed (complex)
1+2
2+3
1+3
1+2+3

brain tissue if one embolizes distal to the last normal feeder but proximal to the AVM. Deeper portions of a large sulcal AVM may receive supply from short and long medullary and corticomedullary arteries arising from the pial arterial system as well as from basal perforating arteries.

One must also consider that, unlike short and long medullary arterial feeders, short and long corticomedullary as well as basal perforating arteries also participate in the supply of normal brain. In the case of sulcal AVMs these feeders can provide supplementary supply to the AVM; the dominant supply, as already stated, is via pial feeders. Furthermore, because sulcal AVMs are covered by arachnoid layers and not brain along their superficial aspect, meningeal arteries have the opportunity to participate as additional feeders.

In contradistinction to sulcal AVMs, gyral AVMs are located within a specific gyrus and are completely covered by cortex. They tend to conform to a rounded shape. The gyrus tends to expand with larger AVMs, and adjacent sulci are found to be effaced on MR. The nidus may extend into the subjacent subcortical white matter and even the ventricle. Gyral AVMs are predominantly supplied by cortical, corticomedullary, and medullary branches of the pial arteries. After contributing supply to the AVM these pial feeders continue their course distally to supply normal brain. Additional supply may be recruited from the basal perforating arteries. Because they are not in contact with arachnoid layers, they do not receive meningeal supply.

As the name implies, mixed sulcal-gyral AVMs contain both gyral and sulcal elements. They are typically larger AVMs involving both adjacent sulci and gyri and usually extend to involve subcortical white matter and ventricular wall. Dominant arterial supply is derived from a combination of cortical, corticomedullary, and subcortical branches as well as terminal supply from the pial arteries. Basal perforators and meningeal arteries often provide a supplementary supply.

The term *subcortical AVM* characterizes the location of a rare group of AVMs, which are usually classified as deep AVMs and account for 1% of cases in our material. They are located within the arterial territory belonging to the long medullary and corticomedullary arteries arising from the pial system and the venous territory of the deep transmedullary veins draining to the deep subependymal system. Concomitant venous drainage to the cortical system may also be present.

Analysis of deep brain AVM topography results in four subtypes: subarachnoid, parenchymal, intraventricular (plexal), and mixed. Much like sulcal cortical AVMs, subarachnoid deep AVMs are located outside the brain parenchyma. They are within the basal cisterns and fissures receiving supply from the subarachnoid segment of basal perforators and of choroidal arteries. Parenchymal deep AVMs are encountered within the deep brain structures and are predominantly supplied by basal perforators. Auxiliary supply can be derived from long medullary or corticomedullary branches of the pial arterial system. As the name implies, plexal AVMs originate from the choroid and as such derive their supply from the terminal portion of the choroidal arteries. Additional supply can potentially arise from the subependymal branches of the circle of Willis. Finally, mixed deep AVMs are usually large and contain elements of parenchymal, subarachnoid, and sometimes plexal AVMs.

◆ Angioarchitecture

After identifying the topography of the AVM, an analysis of the angioarchitectural features should be made on the basis of various angiographic studies available. This analysis is confirmed and further explored as the initial stage of the procedure prior to embolization. This analysis should include identification of the feeding arteries, the nidus, the draining veins, and any associated vascular anomalies, as well as secondary vascular changes such as high-flow angiopathy.

Once an artery is identified as a feeding vessel to an AVM, an analysis of the vessel prior to endovascular treatment is made. Successful obliteration of the nidus clearly depends on the operator's ability to catheterize the distal (prenidal) portion of the feeding arteries and on identifying the extent of the hemodynamic contribution to the nidus, its relationship to the nidus and normal brain, and the presence of arterial high-flow angiopathy.

If the hemodynamic contribution of an arterial feeder involves a large vascular compartment of the nidus, it is referred to as a dominant feeder; otherwise it is considered a supplementary feeder. Dominant feeders tend to be larger in diameter and of higher flow than supplementary type feeding arteries. Most AVMs are supplied by both dominant and supplementary type feeders in various combinations. Usually supplementary feeders outnumber dominant feeders. In general, AVMs with exclusively dominant feeders or those fed by more dominant than supplementary feeders have a higher chance of complete obliteration.

Identifying the geometric relationship of AVM feeders to the nidus and the normal brain is critical in determining accessibility and approach to endovascular treatment of an AVM. On this geometric basis direct (terminal) and indirect feeders can be distinguished.

Direct-type feeding arteries terminate directly into the nidus without continuing on to normal brain distal to the nidus. Direct feeders can end as a single monoterminal feeder or may divide into two or more branches as a multiterminal feeder. Proximal to its termination to the nidus the feeder may supply normal brain or give off indirect or other direct feeders. These other branches, particularly the branches to normal brain, may not be apparent on selective internal carotid or vertebral angiography and may only reveal themselves on superselective injections.

Pseudoterminal feeders represent vessels that hemodynamically and angiographically may appear as terminal feeders; however, anatomically they are identical to indirect feeders and continue distal to the AVM nidus into the territory of normal brain. This phenomenon results from the hemodynamic sump effect that an AVM can cause. The AVM sumps blood not only from the proximal portion of the feeding artery but also from the dilated distal portion of the parent vessel via collateral supply. The pseudoterminal appearance can also be temporarily induced by vasospasm of an indirect feeder or by wedging the microcatheter into a feeding artery. It is important to be aware of pseudoterminal feeders because they carry a risk for ischemic complications in the territory immediately distal to the AVM. As one injects liquid embolic material into a feeder, the hemodynamic conditions change during the injection. If the injection is into a pseudoterminal feeder, the embolic agent can readily enter the angiographically occult segments of the feeder and occlude supply to normal brain tissue. Furthermore, amobarbital testing will give a false sense of security in this situation because amobarbital injection into a pseudoterminal feeder will not test the distal territory.

Indirect feeders are arteries that predominantly supply normal brain tissue but also contribute supply to an AVM nidus. Subtypes of indirect feeders include the transit subtype and the retrograde collateral subtype. Transit arteries are arterial trunks that give off one or more nidal side branches as they course by the AVM nidus and then continue on distally to supply normal brain. These side branches emanate from their parent artery, usually at a sharp angle, are smaller than direct feeders, act as supplementary feeders, and usually terminate in the nidus. A nidal feeder may also branch more distally from a transit artery but will have a longer and recurrent course. The transit artery is usually dilated proximal to its nidal branches. Although the branches from transit arteries are notoriously difficult to catheterize, recent improvements in microcatheter systems have made safe catheterization of these vessels possible in certain cases.

The retrograde collateral subtypes of indirect feeding arteries are usually found adjacent to a watershed area between territories of major cerebral arteries. These arteries are found in the same anatomical territory as the AVM, but because the AVM sumps blood flow toward the nidus, these are supplied by dilated collateral arteries from the adjacent cerebral arterial system. This phenomenon has been referred to as watershed transfer by Berenstein and Lasjaunias and represents a manifestation of high-flow angiopathy.[14]

The AVM nidus can be defined by the vascular components interposed between the arterial feeders and the venous drainage of the AVM. Any brain tissue within a nidus is gliotic and functionless. It is the location of the AVM shunt pathways and is the therapeutic target of AVM treatment. AVM nidal sizes have a broad range from 0.5 mm (micro-AVM) to over 6 cm (giant AVM). Although the size is of critical importance in determining surgical resectability, it does not directly affect endovascular accessibility. It is the angioarchitectural and topographical features that will ultimately determine endovascular accessibility and endovascular treatment. On the other hand, embolization of larger AVMs usually requires more time and more sessions than smaller AVMs.

Angiographically, three basic nidal shunt patterns exist: plexiform (36%), fistulous (11%), and mixed (53%). Plexiform AVMs consist of multiple arteriovenous microcommunications, whereas fistulous AVMs consist of dilated arterial feeders ending directly into venous channels. Most AVMs, however, are composed of a mixture of these two types of communications.

Almost all patients with AVMs have a single nidus; however, rarely, multifocal nidi may be present with normal brain between these foci. Furthermore, the term *diffuse AVM* has been applied to rare cases in which a niduslike network of vessels without clearly defined borders is situated within normal brain tissue. This type of diffuse pattern of AVM may involve one or a few gyri or may involve one or multiple lobes or even an entire hemisphere. Recent evidence suggests that these diffuse-type AVMs probably represent a proliferative form of angiopathy that should not be considered with AVMs.

We have identified a subgroup of AVMs (23%) that do not have a single compact nidus but rather a nidus surrounded by loosely arranged, abnormal-appearing vessels that do not belong to the nidus. These abnormal vessels, when studied superselectively, do not necessarily supply the AVM and furthermore regress after embolization of the AVM nidus. Most likely these vessels represent an angiogenic response to chronic hypoperfusion or ischemia in normal brain induced by the arteriovenous shunt, which may eventually be recruited as supplementary supply to the AVM. This concept of perinidal angiogenesis is important to keep in mind so as not to overestimate AVM nidal size. Furthermore, embolization of perinidal angiogenesis may result in infarction of normal brain tissue.[1]

Nidal compartmentalization of an AVM refers to an angiographic description of subunits of an AVM nidus with one or more feeding arteries and a single draining vein. An AVM may have a single compartment (14%) or multiple compartments (86%). Draining veins may diverge into more than one vein, or draining veins from more than one compartment may converge into a single vein. Furthermore, intercompartmental communications are frequent. This concept of intercompartmental communication is a feature that may be used to reach otherwise inaccessible portions of an AVM nidus during embolization.

Vascular cavities often exist within an AVM nidus and can represent intranidal arterial aneurysms, arterial pseudoaneurysms, venous pseudoaneurysms, or intranidal venous ectasias.[1] The walls of these aneurysms and pseudoaneurysms are thin and thus are thought to represent weak angioarchitectural elements and a risk factor for rupture. This hemorrhagic risk is felt to be exacerbated by the presence of venous hypertension, which may occur as a result of downstream venous stenosis or obstruction. Intranidal venous ectasias and varices represent focal venous dilations with either a narrowed exit or a closed exit. A closed exit to a venous ectasia is caused by thrombosis of a draining vein and is associated with acute hemorrhage and likely associated with venous hypertension. It is therefore felt to represent one of the few indications for urgent treatment.[16]

Venous drainage for an AVM may be deep or superficial. Expected drainage for topographically deep AVMs is via the deep venous system and that of superficial AVMs via the superficial cortical veins. Superficial AVMs with subcortical extension may drain via both superficial and deep venous systems. Unexpected venous drainage (deep drainage to a superficially located AVM or superficial drainage to a deep AVM) can occur in up to 30% of cases. This unexpected venous drainage pattern probably represents an alternate venous drainage following thrombosis of the original venous drainage.

High-flow angiopathy refers to arterial and venous changes that occur in the presence of the high rates of blood flow attending AVMs. This includes both arterial and venous enlargement, arterial (20%) and venous stenoses or occlusions, arterial aneurysm (2.7–58%) or variceal formation, arterial and venous collateral recruitment, reversal of flow, and an increased incidence of variants, especially venous, in patients with AVMs.[14] High-flow angiopathic changes may account for many of the complications seen with AVMs such as intraparenchymal or subarachnoid hemorrhage from aneurysm rupture or venous occlusion or thrombosis, venous infarction, arterial ischemia from vessel occlusion, symptoms of mass effect from enlarging venous varices or arterial aneurysms, venous congestion, and rupture of the AVM nidus from progressive venous hypertension. High-flow angiopathic changes often represent impending complications and may be an indication for more expeditious treatment.

Infants and children with AVMs may suffer from what is referred to as a hydrovenous disorder in which high flow rates within a dural sinus may impair cerebrospinal fluid (CSF) reabsorption and lead to hydrocephalus. This eventually can lead to subependymal atrophy. Patients with hydrocephalus as a result of hydrovenous disorders will respond poorly to shunting. Hydrocephalus in these cases responds better to treatment of the underlying AVM.[14]

◆ Premedication

Prior to embolization, Decadron 4 mg PO qid is started the day before the procedure and tapered after the third postprocedural day. Antiepileptic medication is continued in those patients suffering from seizures or patients with recent intracranial bleed.

◆ Surgical Technique

Anesthesia

At the University of Zurich, general anesthesia is routinely used in patients undergoing cerebral AVM embolization. By reducing patient motion, general anesthesia allows for better digitally subtracted imaging. It also eliminates patient anxiety and associated cardiovascular and neurovegetative reactions. In case of a complication it allows for better and more immediate treatment delivery.

Patients are premedicated 45 to 60 minutes prior to induction of anesthesia with a hypnotic agent (midazolam). General anesthesia is typically induced with propofol. In general, atracurium is the typical muscle relaxant, and remifentanil is administered for analgesia and narcosis. Ventilation is performed with air and O_2. Systemic blood pressure, electrocardiogram (ECG), O_2 saturations, and degree of muscle paralysis are continually monitored during the procedure. Nitroprusside drip infusion for induced hypotension is rarely reserved for embolization of high-flow fistulas.

Neurophysiological Monitoring

The predominant sources of neurophysiological information are the angiographic images obtained during the procedure. Familiarity with cerebrovascular anatomy and angioarchitecture of brain AVMs should form the basis for decision making during AVM embolization. Electroencephalographic (EEG) studies, Amytal studies, and intraoperative cortical stimulation mapping have demonstrated the functional plasticity of language and to a lesser degree sensorimotor cortex in patients with AVMs.[14] The identification of such plasticity in an individual patient may influence the treatment strategy for an AVM. Although many centers employ a combination of Amytal testing (30 mg intra-arterial) and EEG testing administered following superselective catheterization,[17] in our experience the flow dynamics of an AVM, as we described earlier, can give a false sense of security prior to embolization and should be regarded with great caution.

Surgical Procedure

The neurangiographic investigation and the endovascular treatment of cerebral AVMs is performed on a biplane digital subtraction angiography unit equipped with high-resolution imaging, simultaneous live fluoroscopic and roadmapping capabilities, capacity for high-frame rate image acquisition, and rapid postprocessing capabilities. These features allow for high-contrast resolution, reduced volume of contrast use, reduced radiation exposure, reduced study time, and enhanced imaging. Nonionic contrast agents are exclusively used for endovascular work to reduce toxicity to the patient. All injections, including carotid and vertebral injections, are performed by hand to reduce the chances for vessel injury. Initial catheterization is performed using a 5.5F Valavanis cerebral catheter (Cook), which can also act as a guiding catheter for superselective neuroangiography (**Figs. 18–3** and **18–4**).

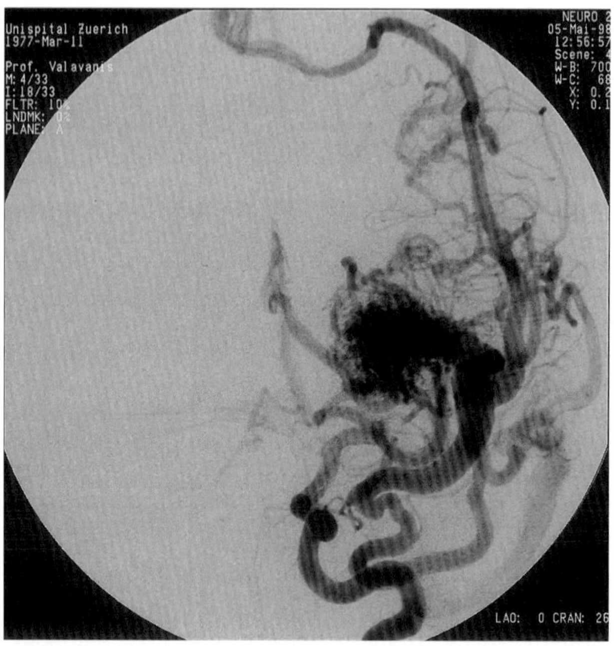

Figure 18–3 Left internal carotid angiogram in frontal projection showing the compact-appearing nidus of the arteriovenous malformation in the left inferior frontal gyrus, being fed by fronto-opercular branches of the left middle cerebral artery and draining in a dominant fashion in superficial cortical veins and in an accessory fashion into the deep venous system (basal vein of Rosenthal).

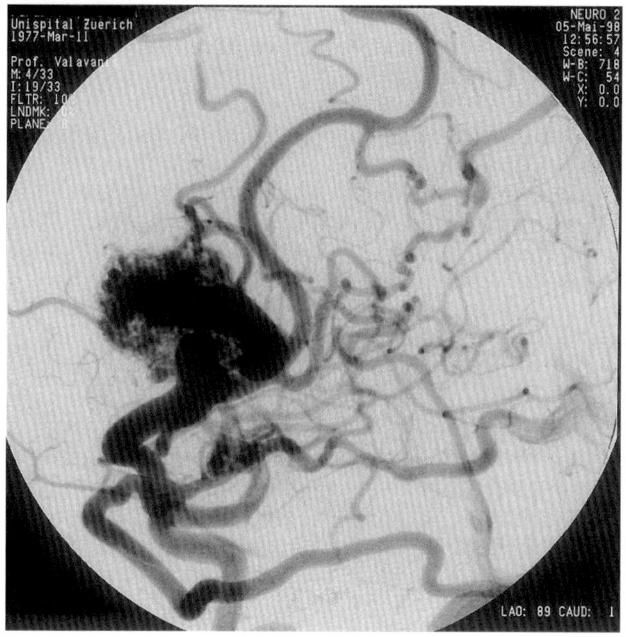

Figure 18–4 Left internal carotid angiogram in lateral projection showing the nidus of the arteriovenous malformation and the draining veins involved.

Once the patient is catheterized, a thorough analysis of the angioarchitecture of the AVM can begin. This includes a confirmation of the features predicted from the preprocedural studies such as identification and assessment of the vascular territories involved, the feeding arteries, draining veins, nidus size and shape, nidal hemodynamic features, weak elements within the nidus, any associated vascular anomalies as well as high-flow angiopathy, and the supply and drainage of normal brain.

Priorities for endovascular embolization of AVMs include the occlusion of angioarchitecturally weak elements and the occlusion of dominant and direct feeders followed by occlusion of supplementary feeders. Vascular accessibility and any potential risks that may be encountered during catheterization play a significant role in further individualizing strategies for embolization. Obviously, catheterization of vessels corresponding to already damaged brain are lower risk than those corresponding to perforating arteries. Catheter manipulation within a vessel in vasospasm may result in damage to that vessel. Operators must also be familiar with their capacity to catheterize certain vessels to avoid prolonged catheterization and inadvertent thromboembolic complications. If such is the case, systemic anticoagulation may be an option. On the basis of analysis the operator should choose the first nidal region to explore for potential embolization and the appropriate vessel to place the guiding catheter. The guiding catheter should be kept within either the cervical segment of the internal carotid artery or the vertebral artery. If access into the external carotid is needed, placing the guiding catheter at the origin of the external carotid and not beyond this point will help avoid vasospasm.

A large variety of variable-stiffness microcatheters are available for superselective endovascular work. They are coaxially entered into a guiding catheter, and their distal outer diameters generally range from 1.0F to 2.5F. These microcatheters are relatively stiff proximally, flexible in their midportion, and soft distally. The variable-stiffness design allows for torque control of the catheter via its stiffer components while preventing vessel damage with its softer portions. Their caliber tapers as one goes distally, allowing for better torque control. These microcatheters are often hydrophilically coated, reducing friction between catheter and vessel. Most microcatheters have a steam-shapable tip, which allows the operator to better steer the catheter and engage vessels that are more difficult to catheterize. Microguidewires are used to direct the catheter into an appropriate vessel and to atraumatically advance the catheter in these vessels. Flow-directed microcatheters have also been developed. A slightly broadened and specially shaped distal tip allows the microcatheter to take advantage of the high flow rates present in AVMs and can more readily enter distal vessels with high flow while forgoing some control over which the vessel is cannulated. Newer flow-directed catheter designs allow for the choice of flow directed over the guidewire navigation, thus offering the advantages of flow directionality as well as some of the control one receives with an over-the-guidewire system. New distal tip braiding catheter designs allow for better catheter control and steerability.[17]

Superselective evaluation of a cerebral AVM allows a better appreciation of AVM features not readily identified on selective angiography (**Figs. 18–5** and **18–6**). Because of the lack of overprojection from multiple opacified structures and the individual analysis of the AVM components, a better appreciation for the AVM can be obtained. The types of arterial feeders and draining veins are more readily apparent, the angioarchitectural elements are better evaluated, the compartmentalization of the AVM is better analyzed, and the hemodynamic features of each element of the AVM are appreciated. It is not unusual to identify elements not seen on the selective injections, such as deep venous drainage, where none was seen on the selective injection. The same analysis applied during selective angiographic evaluation should be

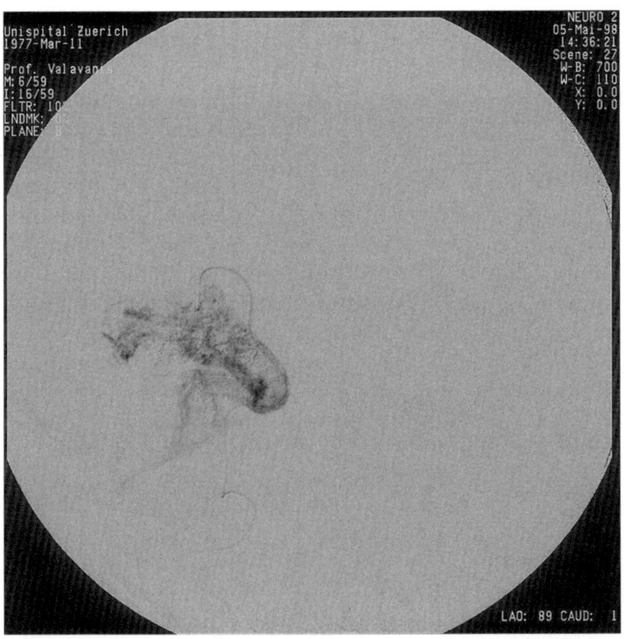

Figure 18–5 Superselective angiogram of a medullary branch of the left prefrontal artery supplying a central compartment of the nidus.

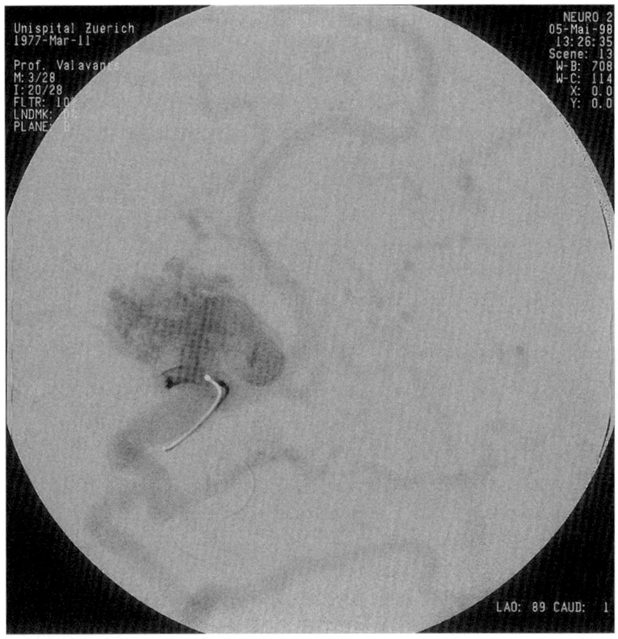

Figure 18–6 Superselective angiogram of the left frontobasal lateral artery supplying the inferior compartment of the nidus through medullary branches.

reapplied with each superselective injection. It is preferred to first embolize the dominant and direct-type feeders and then proceed to a supplementary supply. However, feeders to angioarchitecturally weak elements and feeders with flow-related aneurysms also represent priorities.

If an AVM receives supply from two different vascular territories, simultaneous catheterization of both territories may allow for a better appreciation of an AVM. Furthermore, concomitant embolization of two such territories may allow for a more effective embolization, especially if compartments are shared. This may help prevent glue dilution via inflow from different feeders during embolization.

Currently, cyanoacrylates represent the most effective material for AVM embolization and have been employed to this end for over 15 years. Cyanoacrylates are adhesive liquid embolic agents that polymerize upon contact with an ionic solution. Although isobutyl-2-cyanoacrylate (IBCA) was the first such agent for the purpose of AVM nidal embolization, it eventually was replaced with N-butyl-2-cyanoacrylate (NBCA), which has a higher surface tension and viscosity, creating a more uniform embolic cast with less fragmentation. The polymerization time of NBCA can be adjusted by the addition of a retarding agent such as Pantopaque or glacial acetic acid. NBCA polymerization time can thus be varied from 0.2 to 5.0 seconds. Increasing the polymerization time with a retarding agent allows for better penetration of NBCA into an AVM nidus. In general, the polymerization time is adjusted to approximate the time it would take for the agent to be injected into the nidus without penetrating into the draining veins. This requires experience because underestimation of the flow rate can result in penetration of glue beyond the nidus and well into draining veins, with their subsequent occlusion and attendant risk for AVM rupture. Overestimation of the flow rate may result in underpenetration of the AVM nidus with suboptimal results of embolization. Fine tantalum powder, a biologically inert substance, is added to increase the fluoroscopic visualization of the NBCA mixture. In this way the operator is able to clearly visualize the acrylic mixture as it penetrates the AVM nidus and is better able to avoid any reflux into arterial feeders or prevent excess glue from penetrating into the venous system. Prior to the injection of glue through a microcatheter, the microcatheter should be flushed with 5% dextrose solution to avoid premature polymerization.

The goal of AVM embolization is an intranidal glue deposition through the identified feeding arteries to ultimately form a complete cast of glue of the entire nidus (**Figs. 18–7** and **18–8**).

Two basic methods for glue injection are commonly used: the continuous column method and the sandwich technique. In the continuous column method, glue is injected continuously while its nidal penetration is observed under fluoroscopy. The volumes of the acrylic mixture employed can vary from less than 0.1 mL to over 1 mL, depending on the volume of the nidus and its penetration. Glue is injected in a continuous fashion without an intermission because this may result in inappropriately early polymerization. A syringe of glucose may be used to push glue farther out into the nidus if deemed necessary. The rate of glue injection should attempt to match the acceptance rate of the vessel. A low injection rate leads to the admixture of blood within or around the cast of glue left behind, which may result in reabsorption of the blood products with subsequent recanalization of the nidus. Too high an injection rate can result in damage to the vessel or reflux of the embolic agent proximal to the catheter tip into normal territories. The sandwich technique involves deposition of a small amount of the acrylic mixture (0.1.–0.3 mL) into the microcatheter after

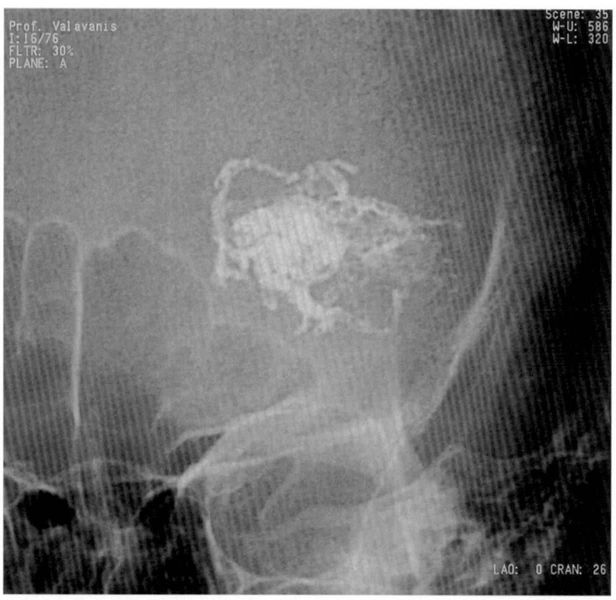

Figure 18–7 Plain x-ray in anteroposterior view showing the cast of glue within the nidus of the arteriovenous malformation.

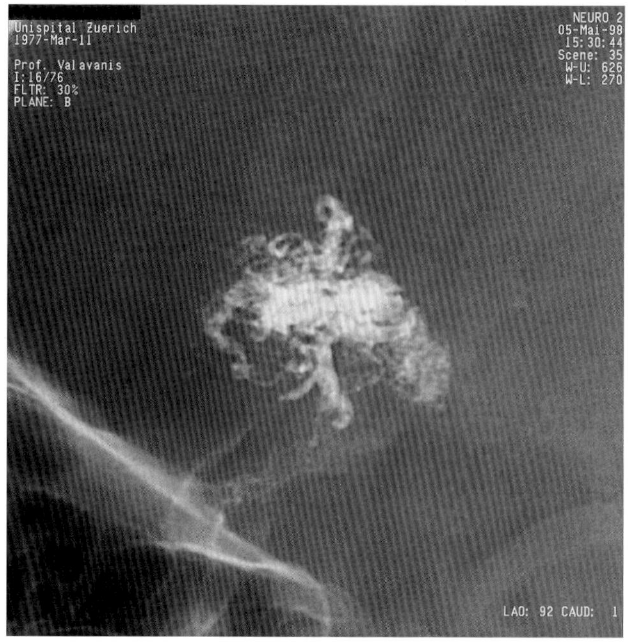

Figure 18–8 Plain x-ray in lateral view showing the cast of glue within the nidus of the arteriovenous malformation.

flushing the microcatheter with glucose. A syringe filled with glucose is then used to quickly eject the glue out of the microcatheter. The acrylic then courses throughout the vascular matrix until it polymerizes. In this way glue can be applied to regions of the nidus beyond the microcatheter tip. Following any glue injection, the microcatheter should be immediately withdrawn in one swift gesture to avoid gluing the microcatheter in place and to reduce the chance that glue inadvertently escapes from the tip of the microcatheter. The guiding catheter must then be suctioned with a hand syringe to prevent embolization of glue particles that may have adhered to the guiding catheter hub or be exchanged for a new guiding catheter. Histologic examination of post-NBCA injection AVM specimens has demonstrated that NBCA provokes a foreign-body reaction, which may be accompanied by focal necrosis of the vessel wall and occasionally migration of NBCA into the extravascular space.

Polyvinyl alcohol particles are another embolic agent that may be used as an adjunct to acrylic embolization of AVMs. This particulate form of embolization is injected as a suspension of particles that mix with blood and cause it to stagnate and subsequently coagulate. A high rate of recanalization accompanies embolization with this agent. Foreign-body reaction and focal angionecrosis have been observed using this agent. Particle sizes range from 45 to 1250 µ. Larger particles have greater efficacy in occluding higher-flow lesions, whereas smaller particles can be used to supplement larger particles for a more effective embolization. Choice of particles also depends on the size of the feeding vessels relative to vessels feeding normal brain and the inner luminal diameter at the tip of the microcatheter.

Platinum microcoils and Guglielmi detachable coils may also be used as an embolic agent. They are available in varying sizes and shapes. Dacron fibers attached to microcoils have increased thrombogenicity but are usually deployed with greater difficulty. Coils are especially useful in high-flow arteriovenous fistulae such as vein of Galen malformations or fistulous AVMs. They can be used to slow the shunt flow for a safer injection of glue in high-flow situations.

◆ Procedural Care

At the end of the endovascular procedure a final angiogram is performed through the guiding catheter to confirm the degree of AVM obliteration and to check the vascularization of the normal brain (**Figs. 18–9** and **18–10**).

Unless there is reason to suspect that the patient is at an unusually high risk for a thromboembolic event following the procedure, all catheters are withdrawn at the end of the procedure, and the patient is monitored for potential hemorrhage, pseudoaneurysm formation, or vessel occlusion at the site of puncture, as well as potential postanesthesia complications.

Following all embolization procedures, the patient should be closely monitored for neurological complications over the next 72 hours with regular evaluations of the neurological status and vital signs. The sudden onset of headache, acute neurological deficit, mental status change, or significant change in vital signs should be regarded with suspicion in considering the possibility of a complication. Transient neurological deficits may occasionally be observed within the first week of the procedure. These complications are probably a result of changing hemodynamic supply to the normal brain following AVM embolization. If there is reason to believe that the patient is at very high risk for a thromboembolic event, the operator has to weigh this risk against the risk of postprocedural hemorrhagic complication before anticoagulating the patient. In such a case a sheath is left in place at the puncture site for 24 hours following the procedure. It should be kept in mind that a minor hemorrhagic complication can be converted into a deadly hemorrhagic complication if the patient is kept anticoagulated.

A follow-up MRI and MR angiography are routinely performed 2 to 3 days following the embolization to assess nidus obliteration and the state of normal brain (**Figs. 18–11** and **18–12**).

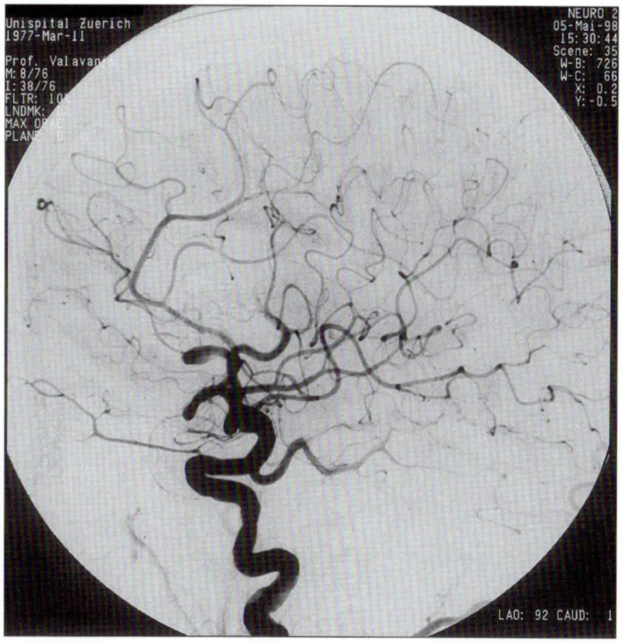

Figure 18–10 Left internal carotid angiogram in lateral projection showing complete obliteration of the arteriovenous malformation.

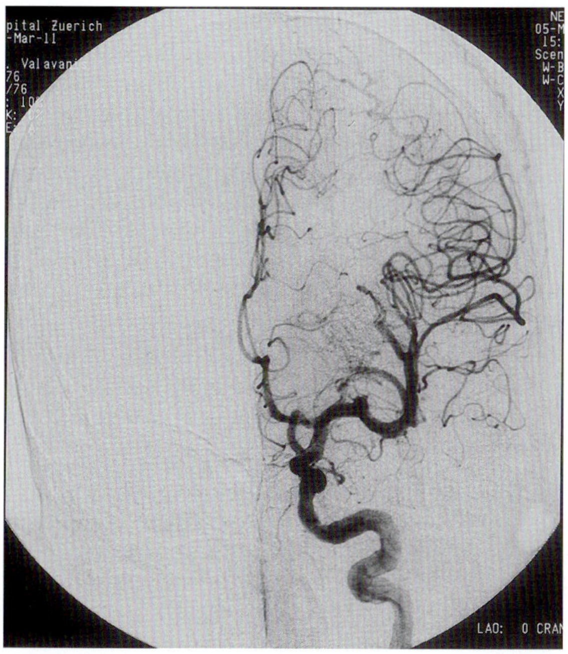

Figure 18–9 Left internal carotid angiogram in frontal projection showing complete obliteration of the arteriovenous malformation.

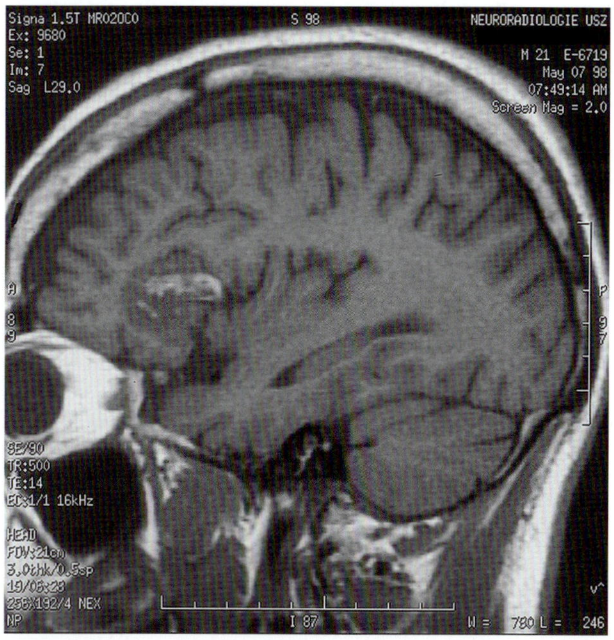

Figure 18–11 Sagittal T1-weighted magnetic resonance imaging following embolization showing the completely obliterated nidus of the arteriovenous malformation.

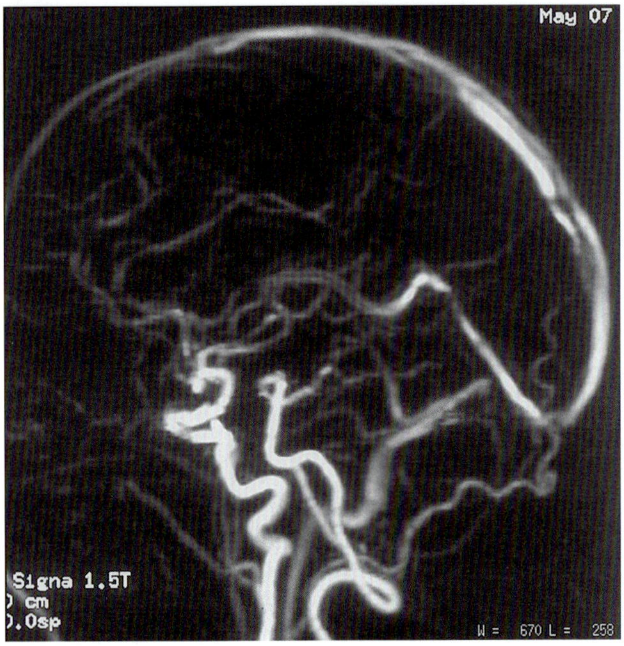

Figure 18–12 Follow-up magnetic resonance angiogram at 6 months showing the persisting obliteration of the embolized arteriovenous malformation.

◆ Complications

The majority of intraprocedural complications resulting from endovascular treatment of AVMs are either ischemic or hemorrhagic. Ischemic complications may occur during catheter manipulation or during the delivery of embolic material. Attention to meticulous technique helps avoid iatrogenic complications.[1]

Hemorrhagic complications may result from microcatheter- and guidewire-related vessel-wall trauma, from flow-related aneurysm perforation, or following venous occlusion; however, sometimes the cause is unclear. An intraprocedural hemorrhagic complication may be identified immediately on the basis of contrast extravasation. With such an occurrence the microcatheter should be left in position so as to have immediate access for potential endovascular treatment. If extravasation continues, the site should be immediately accessed for delivery of embolic material. Following successful occlusion of the hemorrhagic source, an angiographic evaluation should take place to confirm that the extravasation has ceased and to identify any significant mass effect, herniation, hydrocephalus, or new vascular compromise that may require endovascular or surgical treatment. In our experience intraprocedural extravasation occurred in eight of 387 patients (2.0%) who underwent 710 embolization sessions, 3550 superselective catheterizations, and 2985 embolic injections. Of these, 3 (0.7%) were related to arterial perforation and were contained without embolization. The other five resulted from other causes such as venous occlusion or aneurysm rupture. Postprocedural hemorrhagic complications are rare but usually occur within 72 hours of the procedure. Rapid neurological deterioration following AVM embolization is a strong sign of a hemorrhagic complication and an indication for emergency noncontrast computed tomography. If hemorrhage is determined to be the cause of the patient's symptoms, the patient should be administered an intravenous bolus of 100 mg mannitol followed by emergency craniotomy and evacuation of the hematoma. Following hematoma evacuation, the patient is placed in a pentobarbital-induced coma with close hemodynamic and intracranial pressure monitoring until the intracranial pressure returns to normal. In our experience with 387 patients, 11 hemorrhagic complications (2.8%) were identified within 72 hours postembolization. Four were asymptomatic and were identified only on routine early postembolization MR. Of six patients who underwent emergency craniotomy following either intraprocedural or early postprocedural intracerebral hemorrhage, five had a moderate to good outcome. These five patients were treated within 45 minutes of onset of neurological deterioration. The one patient with a poor outcome was treated more than 1 hour after the onset of symptoms. Mortality from hemorrhagic complication within 72 hours was 0.7%. Postembolization angiographic analysis of the 16 hemorrhagic complications not due to arterial perforation revealed that none had been completely embolized; however, 12 (75%) were subtotally embolized. The predominant causes are most likely an inability to compensate for venous outflow restriction and the rupture of flow-related aneurysms.[1,18] Factors that may contribute to venous outflow compromise include the deposition of embolic agent into veins that drained nonembolized portions of the AVM, the occlusion of AVM compartments, which results in the exclusion of major drainage routes from the AVM, and the thrombosis or embolic occlusion of the majority of venous drainage to normal brain. Furthermore, the occlusion of one portion of an AVM may result in increased hemodynamic stress in another compartment to the point of aneurysm rupture.

Intraprocedural ischemic complications can result from a thromboembolic event or inadvertent deposition of embolic material into normal vascular territories. If determined to be thromboembolic, rapid administration of thrombolytic agents may help avoid infarction. There is currently no known method of dissolving embolic material. In our experience ischemic complications detected on postembolization MRI occurred in 36 (9.3%) patients. Five were asymptomatic, and 18 had an associated transient neurological deficit lasting 24 hours to several weeks. Thirteen (3.3%) had a permanent neurological deficit, which included one death, two severe deficits, four moderate deficits, and six mild deficits.

◆ Conclusion

Present microcatheter techniques allow for a unique form of cerebral AVM treatment during which angioarchitectural and hemodynamic changes can be evaluated. The treatment demands a firm understanding of cerebrovascular anatomy, AVM angioarchitecture, and topography. In most centers it is used as an adjunct to radiosurgical ablation or microneurosurgical removal. Our experience is that 40% of patients with brain AVMs can be cured with embolization alone, with a severe morbidity rate of 1.3% and a mortality rate of 1.3%. Endovascular treatment of AVMs is ideally administered under general anesthesia. The primary embolic agent is N-butyl-2-cyanoacrylate; however, particulate agents and coils can be used to supplement its effectiveness. Because of hemodynamic alterations, surveillance for hemorrhagic and to a lesser extent ischemic complications should follow the procedure. Further advances in microcatheter systems and embolic agents are needed to further improve the endovascular obliteration of cerebral AVMs.

References

1. Valavanis A, Yasargil MG. The endovascular treatment of brain arteriovenous malformations. Adv Tech Stand Neurosurg 1998;24:131–214
2. Rhoton RL, Comair YG, Shedid D, Chyatte D, Simonson MS. Specific repression of the preproendothelin-1 gene in intracranial arteriovenous malformations. J Neurosurg 1996;86:101–108
3. Yasargil MG. Microneurosurgery: IIIA. New York: Thieme; 1987
4. Spetzler RF, Martin NA. A proposed grading system for arteriovenous malformations. J Neurosurg 1986;65:476–483
5. Luessenhop AJ, Spence WT. Artificial embolization of cerebral arteries: report of use in a case of arteriovenous malformation. JAMA 1960;172:1153–1155
6. Friedman WA, Bova FJ, Mendenhall WM. Linear accelerator radiosurgery for arteriovenous malformations: the relationship of size to outcome. J Neurosurg 1995;82:180–189
7. Ellis TL, Friedman WA, Bova FJ, Kubilis PS, Buatti JM. Analysis of treatment failure after radiosurgery for arteriovenous malformations. J Neurosurg 1998;89:104–110
8. Wallace RC, Bourekas EC. Brain arteriovenous malformations. Neuroimaging Clin N Am 1998;8:383–400
9. Vinuela F, Dion JE, Duckwiler G, et al. Combined endovascular embolization and surgery in the management of cerebral arteriovenous malformations: experience with 101 cases. J Neurosurg 1991;75: 856–864
10. Gobin YP, Laurent A, Merienne L, et al. The treatment of brain arteriovenous malformations by embolization and radiosurgery. J Neurosurg 1996;85:19–28
11. Ondra SL, Troupp H, George ED, et al. The natural history of symptomatic arteriovenous malformations of the brain: a 24-year follow-up assessment. J Neurosurg 1990;73:387–391
12. Crawford PM, West CR, Chadwick DW, et al. Arteriovenous malformations of the brain: natural history in unoperated patients. J Neurol Neurosurg Psychiatry 1986;49:1–10
13. Crawford PM, West CR, Shaw MD, Chadwick DW. Cerebral arteriovenous malformations and epilepsy: factors in the development of epilepsy. Epilepsia 1986;27:270–275
14. Berenstein A, Lasjaunias P. Surgical Neuroangiography. Vol 4. New York: Springer; 1991
15. Valavanis A. The role of angiography in the evaluation of cerebral vascular malformations. Neuroimaging Clin N Am 1996;6:679–704
16. Garcia-Monaco R, Rodesch G, Alvarez H, et al. Pseudoaneurysms within ruptured intracranial arteriovenous malformations: diagnosis and early endovascular management. AJNR Am J Neuroradiol 1993; 14:315-321
17. Deveikis JP. Endovascular therapy of intracranial arteriovenous malformations: Materials and techniques. Neuroimaging Clin N Am 1998; 8:401–424
18. al-Rodhan NR, Sundt TM Jr, Piepgras DG, et al. Occlusive hyperemia: a theory for the hemodynamic complications following resection of intracerebral arteriovenous malformations. J Neurosurg 1993; 78: 167–175

19

Frontal, Occipital, and Temporal Arteriovenous Malformations

Allan Friedman and Ketan Bulsara

Optimal treatment of cerebral arteriovenous malformations (AVMs) remains a challenging undertaking for neurosurgeons. Cerebral AVMs come to clinical attention because of a seizure, persistent headaches, an intracranial hemorrhage, or an incidental finding on a cerebral imaging study. Rarely, an AVM will present as a slowly progressive neurological deficit secondary to ischemia of adjacent brain. The danger of an AVM is masked by its good short-term prognosis. Even AVMs that have hemorrhaged have a rebleed rate of 6% over the ensuing 6 months and 4% per year thereafter.[6,11] Unfortunately, long-term follow-up studies demonstrate that patients harboring an intracranial AVM have a major morbidity or mortality risk of at least 1% per year. These are not benign lesions.

Small AVMs can be treated with focused radiation therapy. The surgeon should be familiar with the success rate, complications, and limitations of that form of therapy. Knowing the statistical probabilities of the lesion's natural history, the results of alternative therapy, and the realistic estimation of morbidity and mortality of operating on a particular AVM in a given surgeon's hands, the surgeon can advise the patient on the most appropriate therapy.

An interventional radiologist can significantly reduce the blood flow to an intracerebral AVM, facilitating surgical resection. At this writing, it is unusual for an AVM to be completely obliterated by the interventional radiologist. As with surgery, the risks of catheter-directed intervention vary with the anatomy of the AVM and the skills of the interventionalist. It is important for the surgeon and interventionalist to design a treatment plan that minimizes the risks to the patient.

Anesthesia for intracerebral AVM excision is not passive. The anesthesiologist and surgeon must plan the use of cerebral protective agents, intraoperative physiological monitoring, and modulation of the patient's blood pressure as indicated. When larger AVMs are being approached, the anesthesiologist must be prepared to replace intravascular volume at short notice.

◆ Preparation

Magnetic resonance imaging (MRI) is the best study to delineate the relationship of the AVM to the surrounding brain. The surgeon should know the relationship between the AVM and potentially "eloquent" areas of brain, the ventricles, and major feeding arteries.

◆ Arteries

The preoperative angiogram reveals the course of feeding arteries and arteries passing by the AVM. Because the veins are more apparent on the surface of the brain at the time of surgery than the arteries, which are often buried deep in the sulci, the surgeon should be oriented to the relationship of the feeding arteries to the cortical veins. A feeding artery may distribute branches to the normal brain parenchyma prior to entering the AVM or may run adjacent to the malformation, sending several branches to the AVM before continuing on to nourish normal brain (**Fig. 19–1**). Feeding vessels are often hidden by draining veins. Most insidious are the perforating arteries that enter the deep surface of an AVM after taking a long course through the white matter.

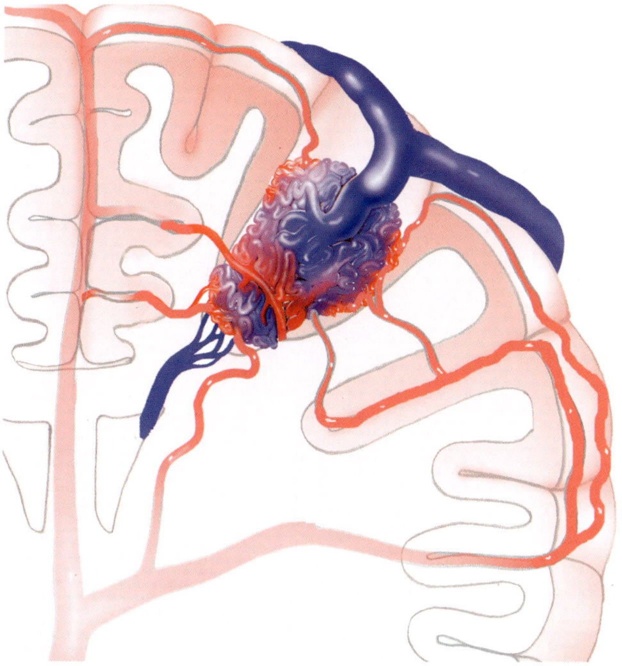

Figure 19–1 Arteries may end in the arteriovenous malformation (AVM), pass by the AVM without contributing to the malformation, or send branches to the AVM prior to supplying normal cortex. Only the arteries entering the AVM should be taken.

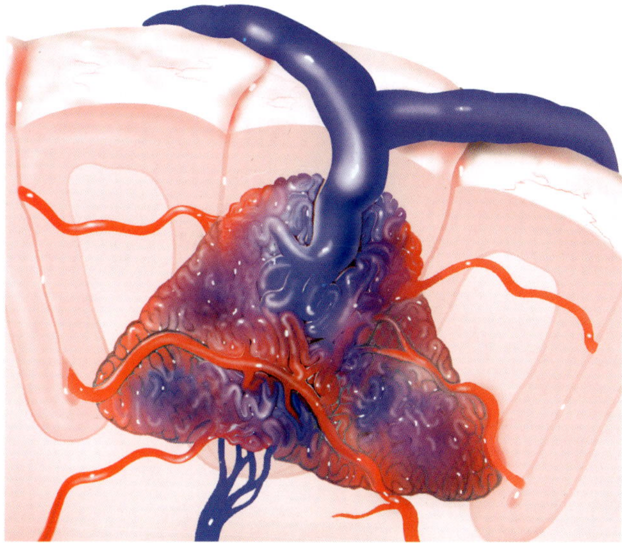

Figure 19–2 Although the gyri surrounding an arteriovenous malformation may appear normal on the surface, feeding vessels may pass to the AVM from adjacent gyri.

◆ Veins

Veins are the most reliable surgical landmark because, unlike the feeding arteries, the draining veins are usually lying on the cortical surface visible to the operating surgeon.[13] Large veins decompress the malformation and should be preserved throughout the resection. Smaller veins may be sacrificed to gain exposure as long as the malformation remains decompressed through large venous channels. Veins should be reversibly occluded with a temporary clip prior to ligation to assess their importance in decompression of the AVM.

◆ Surgical Technique

The technique for removing an AVM is easy to articulate but difficult to execute. Surgeons agree on the basic steps taken to remove an AVM but disagree on the details of execution. The basic steps are occlusion of large feeding arteries, circumferential dissection of the AVM from the cortex, systematic separation of the AVM from the white matter, and coagulation of the vessels entering the deep or periventricular surface of the malformation. As written by Yasargil, the surgery should be an exercise of anticipation, not just reaction.[14] Large feeding arteries are often buried deep in sulci, and the exact anatomy of the deep, distended, thin-walled vessels is not seen on an angiogram (**Fig. 19–2**).

Most surgeons recommend that the AVM should be approached through the large cranial flap, allowing feeding arteries to be ferreted out of deep sulci at a distance from the AVM and keeping the surgeon from chasing troublesome bleeding vessels under a bone edge. The surgeon should never be confined by the bony opening.

Care must be taken in raising the bone flap so as not to tear a bulbous dural-based draining vein that has burrowed into the inner table of the skull, or a dural artery that feeds the AVM. The dura is lifted cautiously, coagulating the dural arterial supply to the AVM and sharply severing adhesions between the thickened arachnoid of the AVM and the dura.

Most lobar AVMS are present on the cortical surface. The surgeon should orient a mental picture of the AVM to the large draining veins seen on the cortical surface. Although some malformations have a classic cone shape based on a cortical surface, most AVMs have an irregular shape, receiving feeding vessels from the depth of adjacent sulci. Dissecting around the visible surface of the AVM will isolate important segments of the AVM fed but not drained from adjacent sulci. These isolated segments of AVM will cause troublesome bleeding late in the dissection.

The surgeon's first maneuver is to secure the large feeding arteries to the malformation. The operating microscope facilitates an accurate dissection. If the malformation presents on the surface, the surgeon should begin by opening the arachnoid adjacent to a large draining vein to deliver an edge on the malformation. Frequently, the malformation will involve the cortex on one side of the sulci. The sulci extend deep within the brain and offer the surgeon a natural plane in which the feeding arteries can be delineated. Large AVMs almost invariably are supplied by feeding arteries that originate in the sulci adjacent to the cortical surface of the AVM (**Fig. 19–3**). The surgeon should be suspicious that this anatomy exists when the anatomy of feeding vessels displayed on the angiogram does not coincide with the anatomy encountered at surgery. Once the sulci are opened, cortical feeding vessels are followed to their terminus in the AVM or to where they have thrombosed from prior endovascular intervention (**Fig. 19–4**). Vessels passing to parenchyma beyond the malformation should be spared. It is not unusual

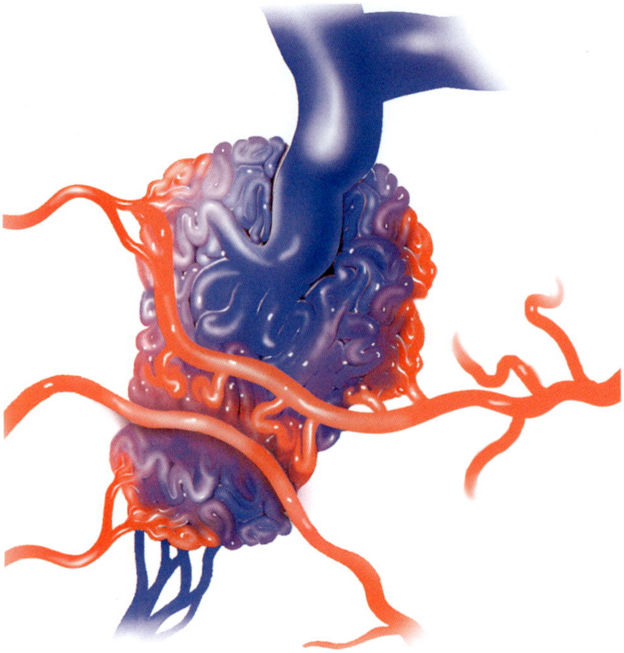

Figure 19–3 Large arteriovenous malformations may receive feeding arteries from vessels passing over several cortical surfaces.

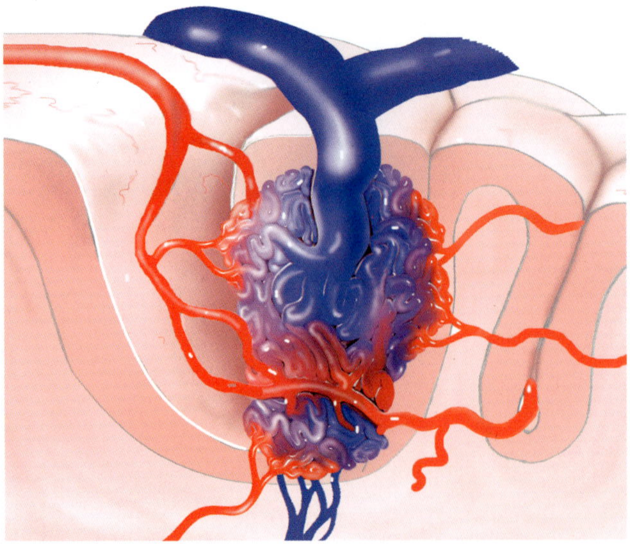

Figure 19–4 Sulci in the vicinity of the arteriovenous malformation should be opened and inspected for positions of the malformation or feeding arteries in their depths.

for an artery to give multiple branches to the AVM and other branches to important viable cerebral cortex, a point regularly demonstrated by endovascular therapists. Special care should be taken to search the arachnoid around the large draining vein, which often hides a feeding vessel. The vessel should not be grasped and coagulated at a single point but rather gently held between the tips of a very smooth or silver alloy bipolar cautery and coagulated over a 5 to 10 mm length (**Fig. 19–5**). Tightly grasping the vessel with the bipolar forceps or coagulating the vessel with pitted bipolar tips is likely to result in laceration or tearing of the vessel wall. If a length of vessel cannot be freed between the parent artery and the AVM, a temporary clip may be applied to the parent vessel to reduce the turgor of the vessel being coagulated.

Once the large feeding vessels have been ligated, the AVM should be freed from the cortex in a circumferential fashion

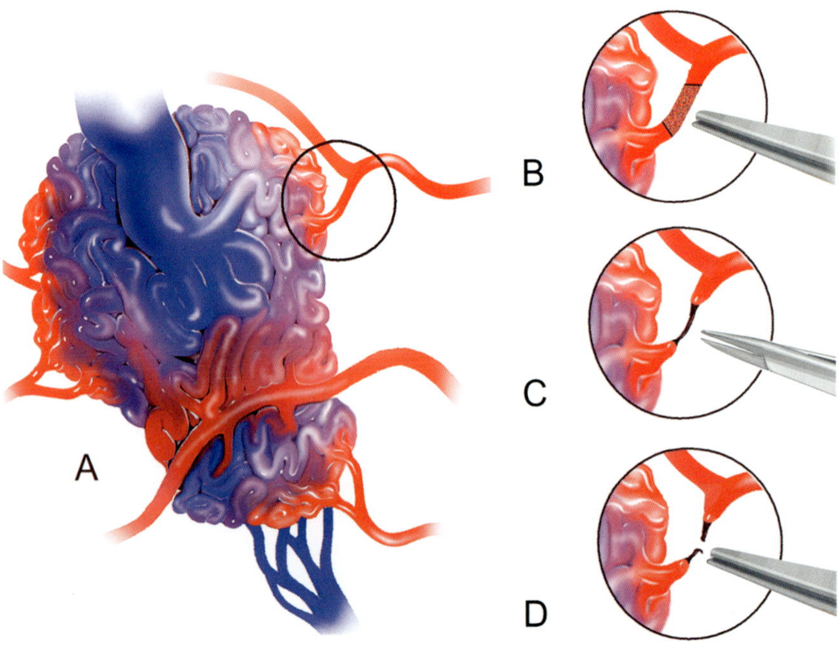

Figure 19–5 Only arteries entering the malformation should be occluded. They should be coagulated over a broad length prior to being divided. Perfect hemostasis must be maintained.

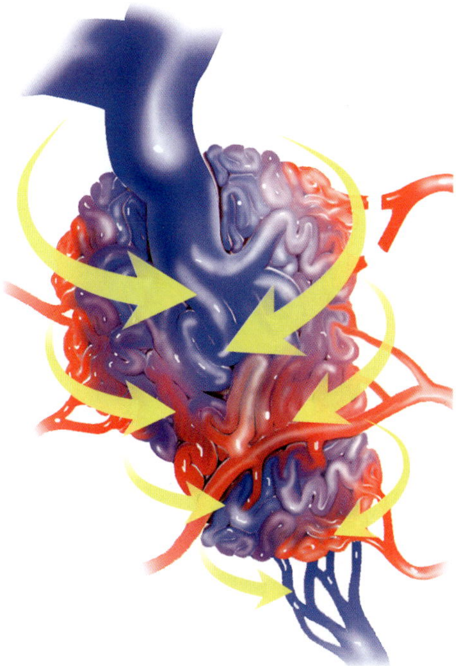

Figure 19–6 Once the large feeding vessels have been divided, the malformation should be dissected from the adjacent white matter in a circumferential fashion. The surgeon must avoid the temptation of following an avascular plane into a deep hole.

(**Fig. 19–6**). Large draining veins should be kept intact. Smaller veins can be ligated if their temporary occlusion does not affect the turgor of the malformation. The temptation to dissect the less vascular white matter prior to separating the malformation from the cortex must be resisted. The thin-walled, engorged vessels of the white matter will be easier to control after the malformation has been partially decompressed.

The white matter is then dissected from the malformation in a circumferential fashion spiraling down to the base at the malformation. The surgeon must avoid working in a narrow channel down one side at the malformation where bleeding will be difficult to control

The most challenging step of the AVM excision is the division of the thin-walled, engorged feeding vessels that pass through the white matter to feed the deep surface of the AVM. These vessels should not be attacked until the large cortical arteries to the AVM have been ligated, and the AVM is decompressed. It is easiest to coagulate these thin-walled vessels prior to their rupture. The surgeon should work around the tufts of thin-walled vessels and coagulate the solitary vessels that pass through the white matter to feed the malformation. The vessels should be coagulated with a broad, smooth-tipped, or silver alloy-tipped bipolar forceps, which is less likely to stick to the vessel wall. The vessel is grasped, but not squeezed, and coagulated over a long segment, gradually shrinking the vessel's lumen with short bursts of low-power coagulation. Several methods have been described to stem the bleeding from a thin-walled vessel that has burst and retracted into the white matter. Some surgeons prefer occluding the vessel's lumen with a temporary or microaneurysm clip. Although this method is usually effective, the clip can tear the thin wall of the vessel or get in the way of further dissection. Other surgeons dissect a length of the vessel from the surrounding white matter, aspirate the bleeding end of the vessel into a low-power suction tip, occlude the neck of the vessel with the bipolar forceps, and attempt to cauterize the vessel. This author prefers to compress the bleeding site with a small cotton patty at the end at a suction tip and dissect into the white matter behind the bleeding vessel. Sometimes the bleeding point will be found to emanate from an amputated tuft of AVM, and the bleeding will best be controlled by dissecting around the residual AVM, coagulating the feeding vessels as they leave the white matter. If dissecting behind the bleeding site reveals only a solitary vessel, that vessel is coagulated along with some adjacent white matter in the same fashion described for nonhemorrhaging, thin-walled, distended vessels. In difficult situations, lowering the patient's arterial pressure will facilitate occlusion of recalcitrant bleeding vessels. If the ventricular wall is opened, a cotton ball is placed in the ventricle to mark the opening and block the flow of blood into the ventricle. Coagulating vessels passing between the falx cerebri and through the ependyma are a good way to occlude the deep feeding vessels.

If the skeletonized AVM remains red, there is probably a small artery running along the wall of a draining vein. Prior to ligating the large draining veins at the end of the procedure, the effect of occluding these veins with a temporary clip should be observed. The surgeon should then inspect the walls of the resection cavity to be certain that no residual tufts of AVM remain. The patient's systolic blood pressure should be raised 10 to 15 mm Hg to be certain that all occlusions are secure. Absolute hemostasis is mandatory.

◆ Frontal AVMs

Cortically based frontal AVMs (**Fig. 19–7**) can arise from the mesial, lateral, or orbital surface of the frontal lobe. AVMs based on the mesial surface receive their predominant arterial supply from branches at the anterior cerebral artery.[7,15] The superficial venous drainage is predominantly into the superior sagittal sinus.[5] Malformations involving the cingulate gyrus drain inferiorly into the interior sagittal sinus or the anterior cerebral vein, which runs anteriorly along its corpus callosum and drains into the basal vein. Large malformations receive additional blood supply of the lenticulostriate arteries or branches of the distal middle cerebral artery, which travel in the sulci over the apex of the hemisphere. The anatomy of mesial frontal AVMs is problematic in that the surgeon is working parallel and not perpendicular to the cortical surface of the AVMs, the draining veins are closer to the surgeon than the feeding arteries, and the draining veins tether the brain to the midline.

When the anatomy is favorable and the draining veins run posteriorly, the frontal lobe can be retracted from the midline, allowing the surgeon to dissect around the periphery of the malformation. Care should be taken to separate the adhesion and coagulate dural-based feeding arteries between the falx, cerebrum, and mesial surface at the frontal lobe.

Very small AVMs of the cingulate gyrus and adjacent cortex supplied solely from the anterior cerebral artery can be approached from the contralateral side, providing the surgeon with access to the branches at the anterior cerebral

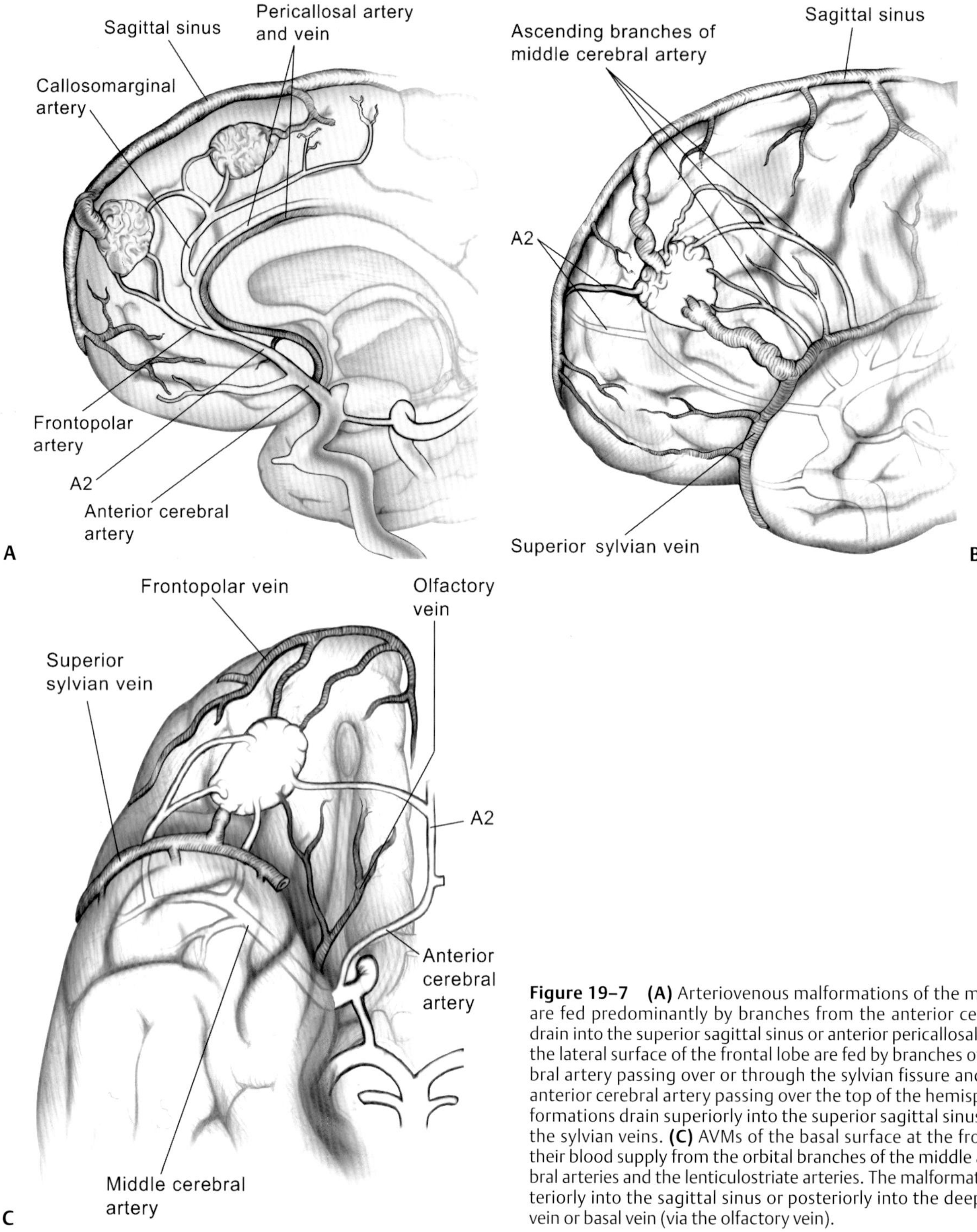

Figure 19–7 **(A)** Arteriovenous malformations of the mesial frontal lobe are fed predominantly by branches from the anterior cerebral artery and drain into the superior sagittal sinus or anterior pericallosal vein. **(B)** AVMs of the lateral surface of the frontal lobe are fed by branches of the middle cerebral artery passing over or through the sylvian fissure and branches of the anterior cerebral artery passing over the top of the hemisphere. These malformations drain superiorly into the superior sagittal sinus or inferiorly into the sylvian veins. **(C)** AVMs of the basal surface at the frontal lobe receive their blood supply from the orbital branches of the middle and anterior cerebral arteries and the lenticulostriate arteries. The malformation may drain anteriorly into the sagittal sinus or posteriorly into the deep middle cerebral vein or basal vein (via the olfactory vein).

artery while protecting the draining veins on the side opposite the falx cerebri.

A large, tortuous vein sitting squarely between the surgeon and the vascular malformation can sometimes be freed by dividing its pial attachments to the mesial hemisphere, allowing the hemisphere to be retracted from under the vein. In recalcitrant situations a subpial dissection of the mesial superior frontal lobe will afford the surgeon access to the AVM.

Arteries not feeding the AVM must be spared. Branches of the anterior cerebral artery may provide feeding vessels to the malformation and then continue to supply the mesial motor, sensory, and supplementary motor areas. AVMs close to the corpus callosum may be adherent to contralateral A2 branches even though these contralateral vessels do not supply the malformation.

Blood supply from the thalamostriate vessels is problematic. These vessels cannot be occluded at their origin from the middle cerebral artery where they are providing blood to the subcostal structure as well as the malformation. The AVM should be dissected circumferentially from the mesial frontal cortical surface and the supply from the lenticulostriate vessels is cauterized and ligated as the surgeon spirals around the malformation toward the ventricles.

Convexity-based frontal AVMs are supplied mainly by arterial branches of the middle cerebral artery and secondarily by lenticulostriate and anterior cerebral artery branches.[8] The veins of the malformation may drain into superficial or deep sylvian veins or into the sagittal sinus.[5,16] AVMs based posteriorly in the frontal convexity may receive branches from the same arteries that supply the motor cortex and on the dominant-side speech-related cortex. Inferior frontal convexity AVMs involve the frontal operculum and even the insular cortex.[1] Middle cerebral artery branches looping under the frontal operculum may appear to enter the AVM or give a branch to the AVM at the apex of their upward course.[12,16] The sylvian fissure must be widely opened so that MCA branches directly feeding the AVM can be distinguished from vessels passing over the AVM's surface.

Frontal convexity AVMs are resected in the classical fashion of isolating the large feeding vessels in the sulci of the cortical surface, ligating branches of these vessels as they pass into the malformation, disconnecting the AVM from the adjacent white matter in a spiral fashion, and finally disconnecting the small, deep AVM feeding and draining vessels.

AVMs of the orbital surface of the frontal lobe are fed by orbital frontal branches of the anterior and middle cerebral arteries, lenticulostriate branches, and occasionally dural branches from the ethmoid artery.[8] The surgeon must be aware that lateral lenticulostriate arteries may arise from a lateral frontal orbital branch of the middle cerebral artery, and the medial lenticulostriate arteries and recurrent artery of Heubner may originate from the frontal orbital artery of the anterior cerebral artery.[12] Therefore, only the arteries should be occluded as they enter the malformation.

Venous drainage of orbital surface AVMs may be anterior into the sagittal sinus, or posteriorly toward the anterior perforating substance draining into the deep middle cerebral or basal veins.[5]

Most often these malformations are exposed by a pterional craniotomy, including a variable amount of medial frontal exposure. The inferior sylvian fissure is opened, allowing the surgeon to trace feeding branches from the middle cerebral artery to the malformation. Because the lateral and medial striate vessels often originate from the middle or anterior cerebral arteries, respectively, as a single trunk, it is important to occlude only those arteries that enter the malformation and not the enlarged trunks at their origins. Once the cortical feeding arteries have been occluded, the malformation is removed in the usual fashion.

◆ Temporal AVMs

AVMs of the temporal lobe (**Fig. 19–8**) receive their arterial supply from the temporal branches of the middle cerebral artery, the anterior choroidal artery, and the temporal branch of the posterior cerebral artery.

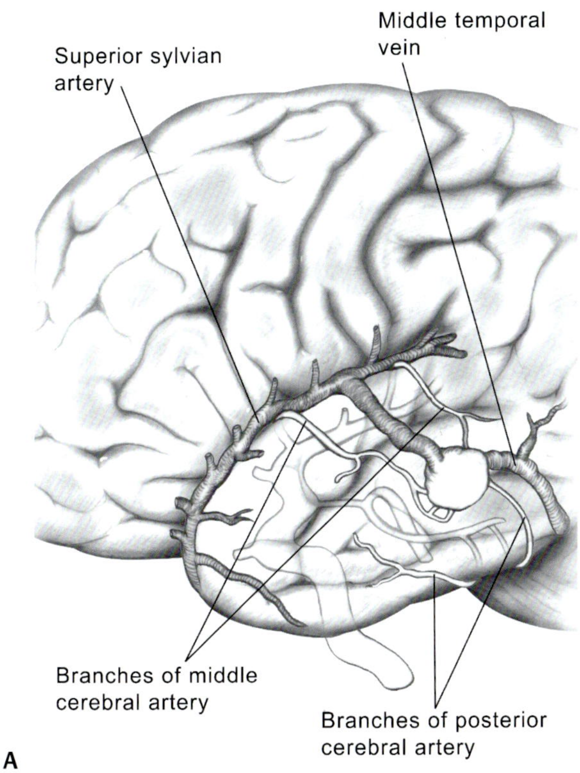

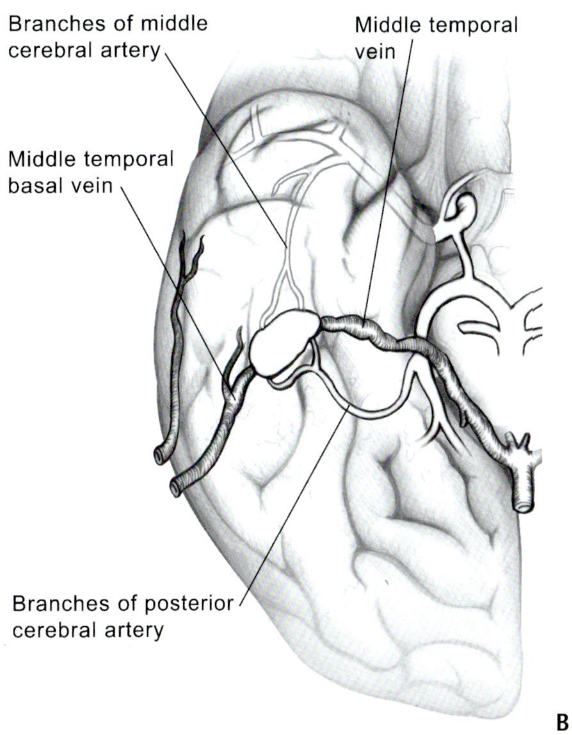

Figure 19–8 **(A)** Lateral temporal arteriovenous malformations receive branches from the middle and posterior cerebral arteries. The superior temporal gyrus drain into the superficial sylvian veins and the middle and inferior temporal gyri drain into the sigmoid sinus. **(B)** AVMs of the interior surface of the temporal lobe receive branches from the middle and posterior cerebral arteries. (AVM involving the uncus and hippocampus also receive anterior choroidal artery branches.) They drain into the basal vein of Rosenthal and the sigmoid sinus.

The lateral temporal surface drains venous blood superiorly into the superficial sylvian veins and inferiorly into veins that terminate in the tentorial dura close to the transverse sinus or the vein of Labbé. The lateral inferior temporal surface drains posteriorly into an anterolateral tentorial sinus. The mesial inferior temporal lobe drains into the basal vein, and temporal poles can drain into the sphenoparietal and cavernous sinuses.[5]

In planning a surgical resection the surgeon must be aware of the optic radiations that pass lateral to the atrium and temporal horn of the lateral ventricle and the possibility of encountering important speech cortex.

Lateral Surface

Malformations of the lateral surface of the temporal lobe are best approached by first opening the sylvian fissure and identifying the feeding arteries to the malformation. Branches may pass through the circular sulcus to AVMs residing in the superior and middle temporal gyri. Important arteries such as the posterior temporal or angular arteries may pass over a malformation embedded in the superior temporal gyrus to supply normal parenchyma distally. Malformations of the temporal operculum must be separated from middle cerebral artery branches passing through the insula. Once the middle cerebral artery's contribution to the malformation is eliminated, the malformation is freed from the cortical surface circumferentially, thereby obliterating cortical feeding vessels from the posterior cerebral artery. Dissection down to the temporal horn of the lateral ventricle will provide the neurosurgeon with an excellent opportunity to coagulate branches from the choroidal arteries that are passing from the ventricle to the deep surface of the AVM.

Interior Surface

AVMs confined to the interior surface at the temporal lobe are approached in a subtemporal fashion.[9] Care must be taken not to disrupt the drainage at the inferior or lateral temporal veins into the lateral tentorium. The lateral bridging veins can be separated from the lateral cortex by opening the arachnoid, which binds the veins to the cortex. Entering the cortex through the occipitotemporal gyrus has the best chance of sparing the optic radiations, which travel along the lateral side of the ventricle. Large feeding branches from the posterior cerebral artery should be sought out and coagulated as they enter the AVM. If the malformation extends to the temporal horn or inferior atrium of the lateral ventricle, feeding branches from the anterior and posterior choroidal arteries can be coagulated as they pass through the ventricle to the malformation.

Anterior Mesial

Anterior mesial temporal AVMs, which involve the uncus amygdala and anterior hippocampus, derive their blood supply from the uncal branch of the middle cerebral artery, the anterior temporal branch of the posterior cerebral artery, and predominantly from the anterior choroidal artery.[2,10] These malformations drain through the basal vein. Traditionally, these lesions have been approached through a small anterior temporal lobectomy, but, in fact, they may better be approached through the anterior sylvian fissure.[3,10] After the sylvian fissure is opened, the surgeon has an excellent view of the anterior choroidal artery giving branches laterally to the uncus, the medial temporal lobe, and the temporal choroidal fissure, and giving branches medially to the optic tract and posterior perforating substance. The branches passing to the temporal lobe and choroidal fissure can be occluded as they enter the choroidal fissure. Branches from the interior temporal artery and parietal occipital branch of the posterior cerebral artery may also enter the choroidal fissure. The temporal horn is entered along the inferior insular sulcus as has been described for resection of the amygdala and anterior hippocampus. Opening the choroidal fissure exposes feeding vessels from the posterior lateral choroidal artery and from the P2 and P3 segments of the posterior cerebral artery. This approach is not suitable for larger, more posteriorly situated malformations where a significant blood supply is derived from the temporal branches of the posterior cerebral artery.

◆ Occipital AVMs

The arterial supply to AVMs at the occipital pole (**Fig. 19–9**) is varied. Laterally placed lesions are supplied by branches from the middle cerebral artery and the posterior temporal artery and parieto-occipital and calcarine branches of the posterior cerebral artery.[16] Medial lesions may also be fed by distal branches at the anterior cerebral artery. Transdural feeding vessels are commonly seen in occipital AVMs.

The lateral surface at the occipital lobe is usually drained by the occipital vein into the sagittal sinus. The occipital vein may run anteriorly along the sagittal sinus, entering that sinus 16 to 24 cm anterior to the torcula. This leaves the occipital pole free to be retracted away from the falx cerebri. Occasionally, the occipital vein drains inferiorly into the transverse sinus. The mesial surface of the occipital lobe is drained by the internal occipital vein into the deep galenic system and by the posterior calcarine vein, which enters the sagittal sinus at approximately the same level as the occipital vein. The inferior surface of the occipital lobe drains into the lateral tentorium via the occipitobasal vein. All of these veins drain away from the occipital pole, so the pole can be mobilized without injury to the venous drainage.

The surgical approach must take into account the position of the visual cortex and the optic radiations. The dura is opened with attention to transdural feeding arteries.

The technique for resection of AVMs of the lateral occipital cortex is the same as that for AVMs of the lateral cortex of the temporal or frontal lobes.

Resection of AVMs of the mesial occipital lobe is facilitated by the lack of draining veins at the occipital pole. Resection begins by the coagulation of branches at the middle cerebral artery as they pass over the superior ridge of the hemisphere.[4] Because the parieto-occipital and calcarine branches at the posterior cerebral artery are buried deep

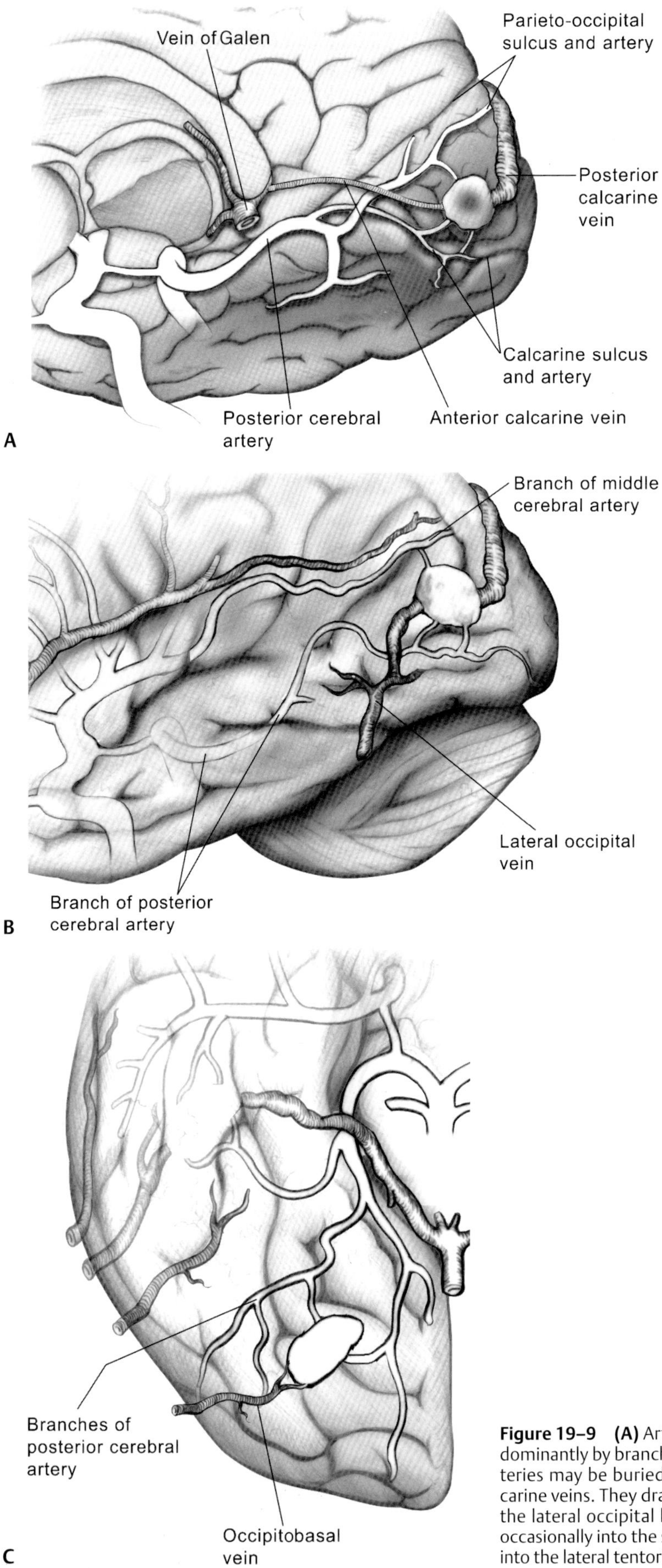

Figure 19–9 **(A)** Arteriovenous malformations of the medial surface are fed predominantly by branches of the medial posterior and anterior cerebral arteries. Arteries may be buried deep within the parieto-occipital sinus and posterior calcarine veins. They drain via the anterior and posterior calcarine veins. **(B)** AVMs of the lateral occipital lobe drain via the occipital vein into the sagittal sinus and occasionally into the sigmoid sinus. **(C)** AVMs of the inferior occipital surface drain into the lateral tentorium via the occipitobasal vein.

within the calcarine and parieto-occipital sulci, some authors have advocated localization of the posterior cerebral artery as it passes over the edge of the tentorium and following the branches into the AVM. The parieto-occipital branch of the posterior cerebral artery is often buried within the deep parieto-occipital sulcus. Opening this deep sulcus affords the surgeon a surprisingly good view of the anterior face of the AVM. The calcarine artery travels in the calcarine fissure, giving off branches to the lingual gyrus inferiorly and inferior cuneus gyrus superiorly. Opening these two sulci will facilitate the occlusion of the large cortical feeding arteries to the AVM.

References

1. Varnavas GG, Grand W. The insular cortex: morphological and vascular anatomic characteristics. Neurosurgery 1999;44:127–138
2. Fujii K, Lenkey C, Rhoton AL Jr. Microsurgical anatomy of the choroidal arteries: fourth ventricle and cerebellopontine angles. J Neurosurg 1980;52:504–524
3. Heros RC. Arteriovenous malformations of the medial temporal lobe: surgical approach and neuroradiological characterization. J Neurosurg 1982;56:44–52
4. Martin NA, Wilson CB. Medial occipital arteriovenous malformations: surgical treatment. J Neurosurg 1982;56:798–802
5. Oka K, Rhoton AL Jr, Barry M, Rodriguez R. Microsurgical anatomy of the superficial veins of the cerebrum. Neurosurgery 1985;17:711–748
6. Ondra SL, Troupp H, George ED, Schwab K. The natural history of symptomatic arteriovenous malformations of the brain: a 24-year follow-up assessment. J Neurosurg 1990;73:387–391
7. Perlmutter D, Rhoton AL Jr. Microsurgical anatomy of the distal anterior cerebral artery. J Neurosurg 1978;49:204–228
8. Rosner SS, Rhoton AL Jr, Ono M, Barry M. Microsurgical anatomy of the anterior perforating arteries. J Neurosurg 1984;61:468–485
9. Solomon RA, Stein BM. Surgical management of arteriovenous malformations that follow the tentorial ring. Neurosurgery 1986;18:708–715
10. Stein BM. Arteriovenous malformations of the medial cerebral hemisphere and the limbic system. J Neurosurg 1984;60:23–31
11. Wilkins RH. Natural history of intracranial vascular malformations: a review. Neurosurgery 1985;16:421–430
12. Yasargil MG. Microsurgery. Vol 1. Microsurgical Anatomy of the Oncal Arteries and Vessels of the Brain: Diagnostic Studies, General Operative Techniques and Pathological Considerations of Intercranial Arteries. New York: Thieme; 1984
13. Yasargil MG. Microsurgery. Vol 3A. AVM of the Brain: History, Embryology, Pathological Considerations, Hemodynamics: Diagnostic Studies, Microsurgical Anatomy. New York: Thieme; 1987
14. Yasargil MG. Microneurosurgery. Vol 3B. AVM of the Brain: Clinical Considerations, General and Special Operative Techniques, Surgical Results, Nonoperative Cases, Cavernous and Venous Angiomas, Neuroanethesia. New York: Thieme; 1987
15. Yasargil MG, Jain KK, Antic J, Laciga R, Kletter G. Arteriovenous malformations of the anterior and the middle portions of the corpus callosum: microsurgical treatment. Surg Neurol 1976;5:67–80
16. Zeal AA, Rhoton AL Jr. Microsurgical anatomy of the posterior cerebral artery. J Neurosurg 1978;48:534–559

20

Sylvian and Perimotor Arteriovenous Malformations: Rationale for Surgical Management

Feres E. A. Chaddad, Fábio L. F. Godinho, Rodrigo F. F. Naufal, Helder Tedeschi, and Evandro de Oliveira

Surgical indications for sylvian (also called insular) and perimotor arteriovenous malformations (AVMs) are questionable due to the increased risk of producing sensory and motor deficits or speech disorders. The majority of cases are thus treated conservatively. When treatment is indicated, the choice is usually radiosurgery for small lesions and embolization plus radiosurgery for larger lesions.[1] Nevertheless, some lesions may be amenable to surgical resection. It is our belief that surgical excision of AVMs in the region of the insula, frontal and parietal opercula, and superior temporal region, and even in the area of the precentral and postcentral sulcus can be performed with low morbidity in selected cases.

This chapter discusses in detail the rationale for the management of AVMs arising in the sylvian region.

The anatomical knowledge and the precise topographic localization of the AVM through the aid of neuroimaging studies has provided the means to classify these AVMs and plan operative strategies for some selected cases with relatively low morbidity.[1–3]

◆ Anatomy

The neural, arterial, and venous relationships of the AVMs arising in the sylvian region important to the surgical decision-making process are presented in the following sections.

Neural Relationships

The stem of the sylvian fissure is related medially to the basal cisterns (chiasmatic, lamina terminalis, interpeduncular, and carotid), to the anteromedial surface of the uncus and the planum polare of the temporal lobe inferiorly, to the anterior perforated substance and the limen insulae superiorly, to the lesser wing of the sphenoid anteriorly, and to the anteromedial surface of the uncus and the limen insulae posteriorly.

The part of the sylvian fissure that is located on the lateral surface of the brain is related to the frontal and parietal opercula superiorly, to the temporal operculum inferiorly, and to the insula and its circular sulci medially. In the depths of the sylvian fissure, situated deep to the frontoparietal and temporal opercula lies the insula.[1,3] The insula has a pyramidal shape and its anterior part is located in the most anterior portion of the sylvian cistern, lateral to the limen insulae and between the frontal and temporal opercula. The middle part of the insula is located in the middle portion of the sylvian cistern. At the posteriormost extension of the sylvian cistern the surface of the insula lies very deep, as the insular cleft and the space between the temporal and parietal lobes are almost virtual.

The deep cerebral structures located directly adjacent to the insular cortex are the extreme capsule, the claustrum, the external capsule, and the putamen.

Arterial Relationships

The arterial supply to the sylvian region is predominantly by branches of the middle cerebral artery. Large AVMs, those located in the depths of the sylvian fissure, or those on the insular cortex may recruit supply from choroidal vessels and from the lenticulostriate arteries.

Venous Relationships

The part of the sylvian fissure that is located on the lateral surface of the brain is drained by the superficial cortical veins bordering the sylvian fissure (i.e., sylvian vein, vein of Labbé, and vein of Trolard). The veins of the cortex of the insula predominantly drain through connections between the deep sylvian vein and the superficial cortical veins bordering the sylvian fissure. Sometimes they may also drain into the basal vein of Rosenthal.

◆ Indications

Surgery of lesions such as sylvian and perimotor AVMs still represents one of the most challenging tasks confronting neurosurgeons. Surgical indication for patients harboring AVMs in that location is still a controversial matter.

Although surgical excision is the best therapeutic option, the surgeon must always consider the location, the size, the form of the AVM's nidus (diffuse or compact), the eloquence of the area, and the patient's neurological status.[2,3] In many instances, when these factors are combined the majority of cases are either followed conservatively or are referred to alternative methods of treatment such as radiosurgery. In our view a team approach is the ideal for some selected lesions, with the neurosurgeon, neuroradiologist, and radiosurgeon working together.

Based on our own clinical experience, it became clear to us that surgery has a place in some cases. To aid the decision process of surgical indication and the best surgical approach, we have divided the AVMs in that region into anterior, middle, and posterior taking into account the location in the sylvian region in relation to the insula. Also, the size of the lesion, the eloquence of the area, and the patient's clinical and neurological condition are determinants for the surgical indication.

◆ Preparation

A cerebral angiogram is necessary to display the arterial and venous anatomy, the size, the location, and the AVM's arterial supply and venous drainage pattern. A magnetic resonance imaging (MRI) scan is necessary to display the AVM adequately and to determine its relationship to the other neural structures.[2,3]

◆ Surgical Technique

Anesthesia

There are several goals of anesthesia during surgery of AVMs. The induction of anesthesia should be smooth and profound. Hypotension should be treated whenever it occurs because it may produce ischemic changes in hypoperfused areas. In choosing the induction agent one has to consider the ability to readily correct the hemodynamic changes. Midazolam may prove helpful for this during the induction period.

Anesthesia is maintained with isoflurane and intravenous agents. In general, both nitrous oxide/narcotic (particularly fentanyl) and volatile anesthetic (usually isoflurane) techniques have been used successfully in these patients. In our experience surgical exposure is usually facilitated by normal ventilation ($PaCO_2$ of 40–45 mm Hg). Cerebrospinal fluid (CSF) drains may be necessary for surgical access to AVMs located deep in the brain or large AVMs, or in patients with brain swelling secondary to intracerebral hemorrhage (ICH). The use of crystalloids for fluid replacement should be monitored according to the intrajugular venous pressure (venous pressure should be kept at normal levels). Replacement with colloids rather than crystalloids is preferred to maintain intravascular volume and to decrease the risk of intracerebral swelling from increased brain intracellular water.

After the AVM has been resected, the arterial pressure should be maintained at lower levels than those of the induction period of anesthesia.

Position

The position varies depending on location of the lesion. The head is fastened in a Mayfield or Sugita device. Brain retraction should be minimal and aided by gravity whenever possible. Compression of the neck veins, which could significantly impede venous drainage, should be avoided. The knowledge of the cisternal and sulcal anatomy must be used to reduce the amount of cerebral tissue that should be transgressed.

A generous craniotomy and dural opening with enough exposure of brain tissue around the AVM nidus is the rule. It allows easier orientation of the position of the arterial feeders, draining veins, and other cortical landmarks.

Approach

We have treated AVMs of this region basically through a combination of approaches: the pterional transsylvian, the pretemporal, or a temporal craniotomy.

Those AVMs located in the sylvian region can be subdivided into anterior, middle, and posterior types. These AVMs are usually approached through the transsylvian route.

Anterior sylvian AVMs are located in the most anterior portion of the region, between the frontal and temporal opercula, just posterior to the limen insulae. They may project to the frontal or the temporal opercula or to the anterior perforated substance and are usually supplied by perforating branches originating from the M1 or M2 segments of the middle cerebral artery and at times by perforating branches from the A1 segment of the anterior cerebral artery. The venous drainage is done through the deep sylvian vein into the basal vein of Rosenthal or through a superficial sylvian vein into the sphenoparietal sinus. These AVMs are located in a usually wide cisternal space and can be surgically approached in cases were there is no extension into the anterior perforated substance (**Fig. 20–1**).

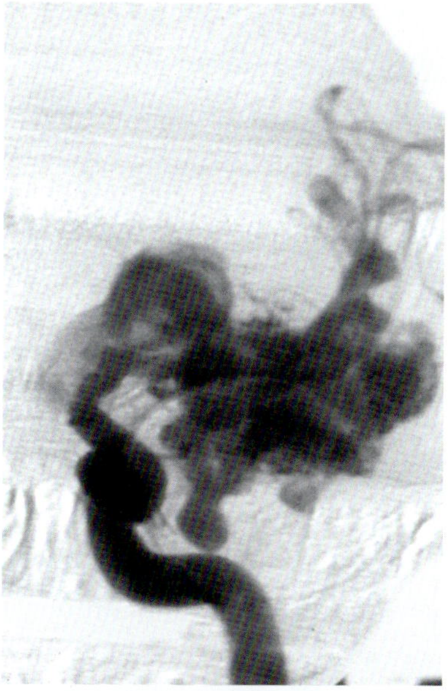
A

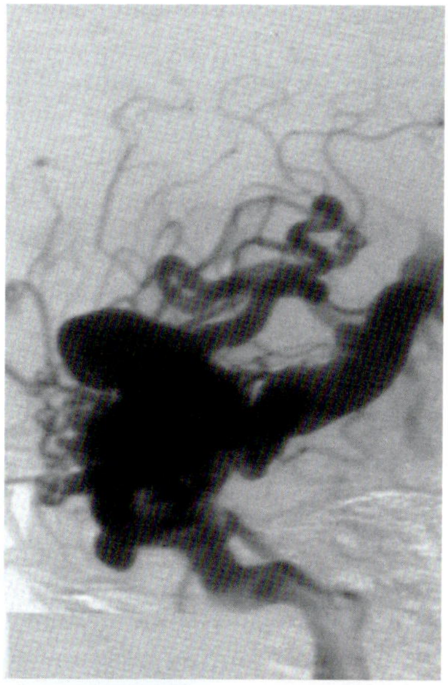
B

Figure 20–1 Arteriovenous malformation (AVM) involving the left superior temporal gyrus. **(A)** Left carotid digital subtraction angiogram disclosing the AVM (anteroposterior view) and **(B)** lateral view of the same case. **(C)** Anatomical specimen showing the location of the AVM. **(D)** Operative view of the AVM after opening the sylvian fissure; the AVM was dissected and the arterial feeders coagulated. **(E)** Operative view after complete removal of the AVM. **(F)** Postoperative left carotid digital subtraction angiogram showing complete removal of the AVM (anteroposterior view).

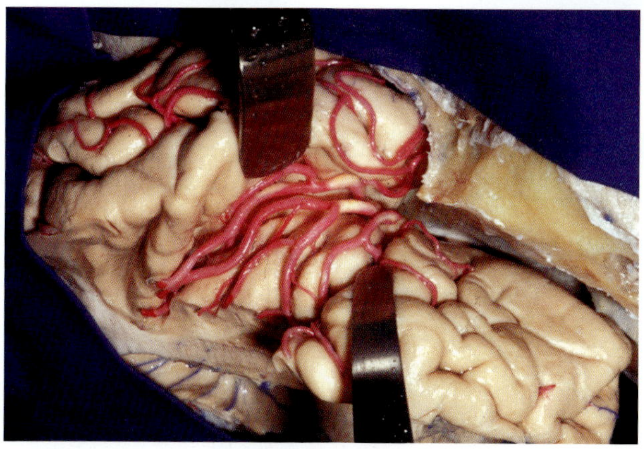
C

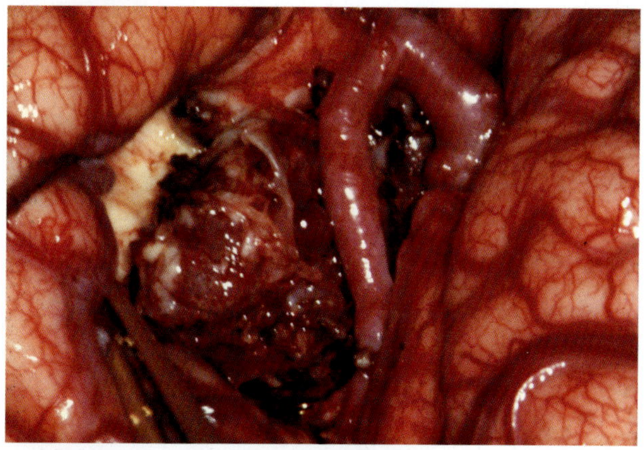
D

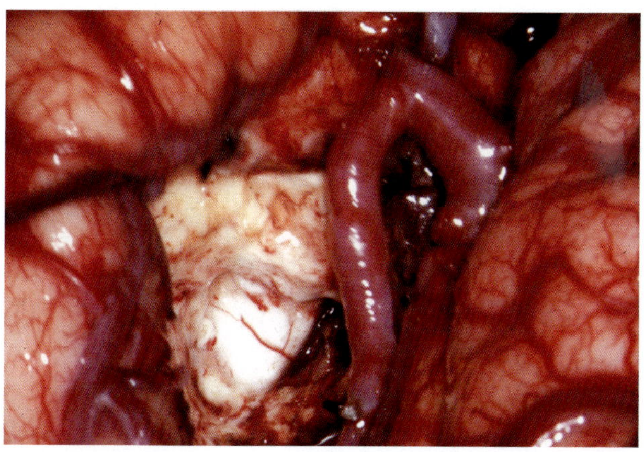
E

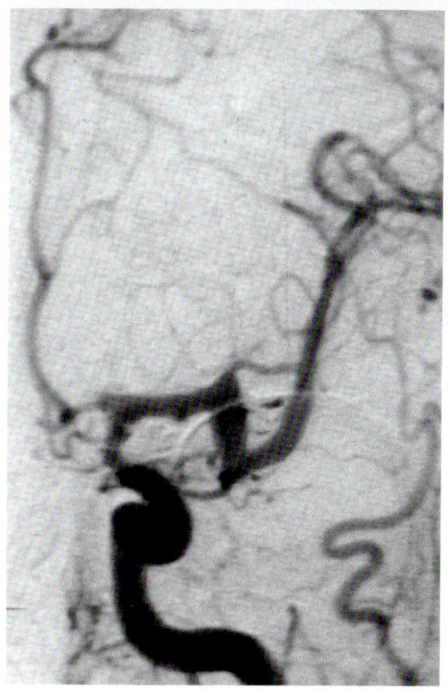
F

Middle sylvian AVMs may arise either at the fronto-parietal or temporal opercula and extend to the middle portion of the insula (**Fig. 20–2**). They may also originate over the cortex of the insula medial to the M2 branches of the middle cerebral artery and lateral to the internal capsule, in the middle portion of the sylvian cistern. They are supplied by branches of the M2 segment of the middle cerebral artery and, depending on their extension and size, can

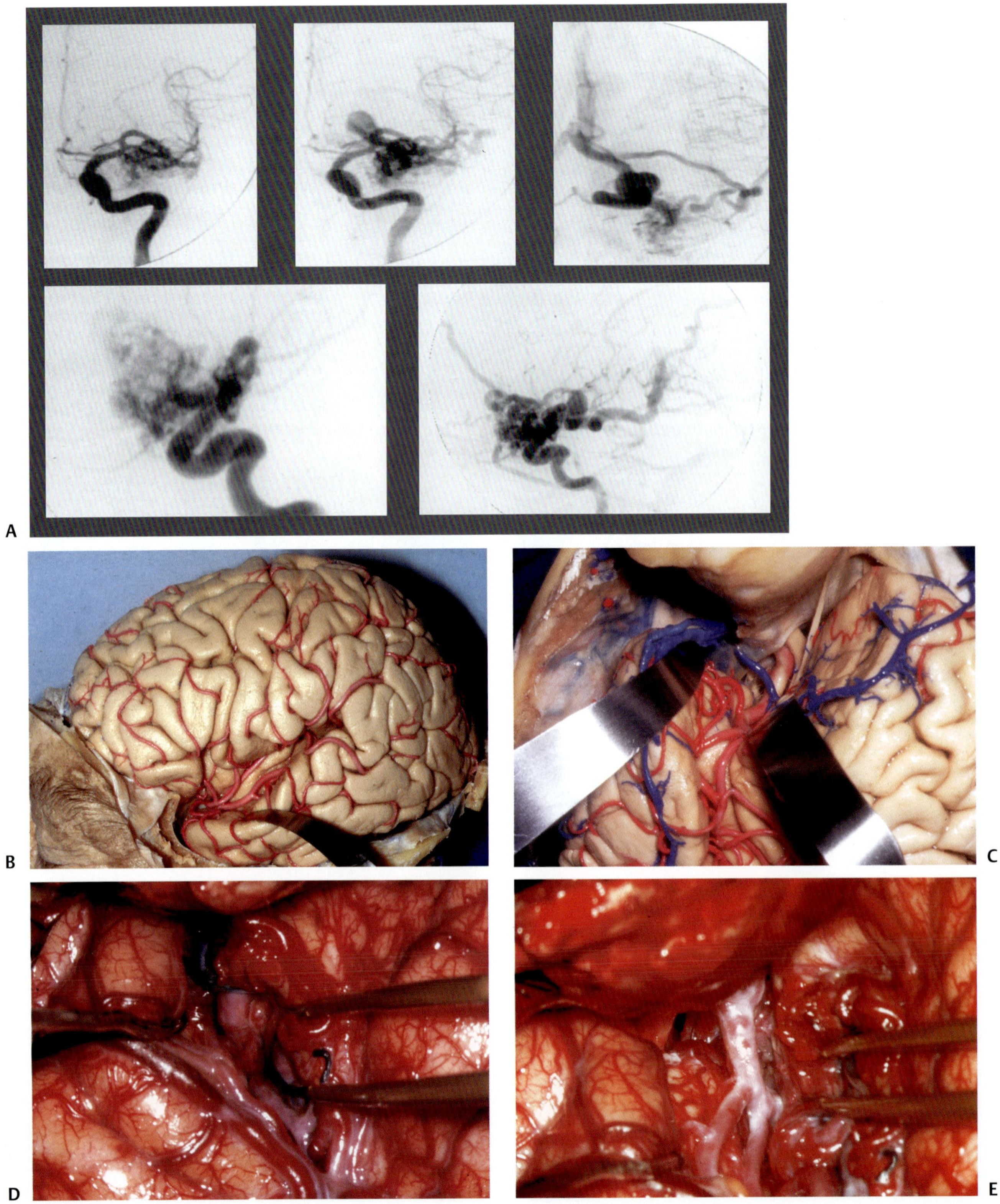

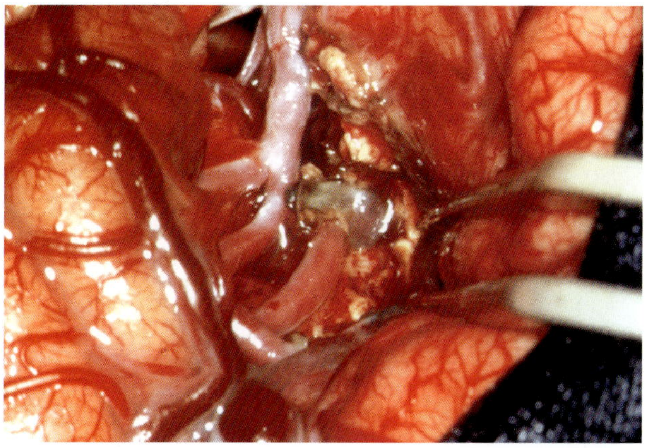
F

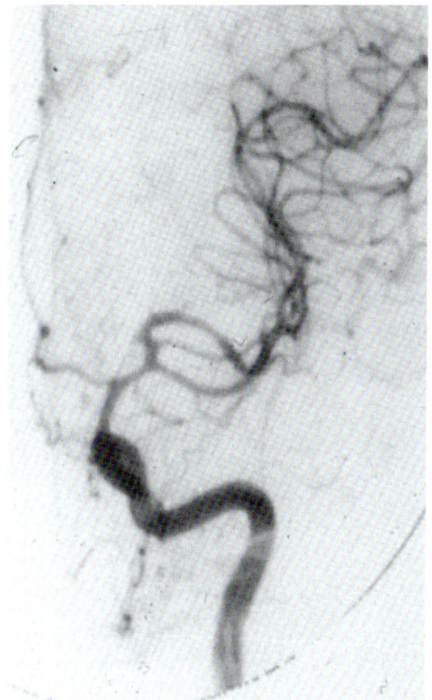
G

Figure 20–2 Arteriovenous malformation involving the left superior temporal gyrus. **(A)** Left carotid digital subtraction angiogram disclosing the AVM (anteroposterior and lateral views). The AVM is supplied by branches of the middle cerebral artery and drained through the superficial sylvian vein and through the deep sylvian vein into the basal vein of Rosenthal. **(B)** Anatomical specimen showing the location of the AVM. **(C)** Anatomical specimen mimicking the actual surgical exposure through a left pterional craniotomy. **(D)** Operative view of the AVM after opening the sylvian fissure. **(E)** The AVM was dissected and the arterial feeders coagulated. **(F)** Operative view after complete removal of the AVM. **(G)** Postoperative left carotid digital subtraction angiogram showing complete removal of the AVM (anteroposterior view).

receive perforators from the M1 segment of the middle cerebral artery and at times also from the A1 segment of the anterior cerebral artery. The venous drainage is usually superficial through the superficial sylvian vein, through the vein of Labbé, or through the vein of Trolard. Surgical indications for these malformations depend on the depth of the lesion, and surgery is always more difficult because one has to work between the branches of the middle cerebral artery.

Posterior sylvian AVMs are situated in the most posterior extension of the sylvian cistern. At this point the space between the temporal and parietal lobes is almost virtual and the sylvian cistern is very deep and in close proximity to the lateral ventricle. The vascular supply to these AVMs is through the M2 and M3 branches of the middle cerebral artery and at times from ventricular branches of the lateral posterior choroidal artery. The venous drainage is through the superficial system. In larger cases where the vascular supply has contribution from branches of the lateral posterior choroidal artery, the venous drainage may be done through the deep system.

Due to their location and vascular supply the posterior sylvian AVMs, especially those located on the left side, are sometimes technically very difficult lesions to approach.

◆ Postoperative Care

The blood pressure must be kept below the level that was tested after the resection for 24 to 48 hours. We usually perform a computed tomographic scan on the first postoperative day to assess for postoperative clots. No patient is discharged without first undergoing cerebral angiography to demonstrate complete obliteration of the AVM. Intraoperative angiography in complicated AVMs could also be done.

◆ Complications

Avoidance of complications should start with the selection of cases amenable for surgical resection. AVMs that are deeply situated and receive blood supply from deep perforators, those of a large size related to eloquent areas, and those whose nidus is not compact should not be candidates for surgery.

Apart from mistaken surgical indication the major potential complication is due to postoperative hemorrhage. Residual AVM is the most common cause of hemorrhage in the postoperative period.[1,2] For this reason, careful inspection of the resection wall is advisable. Also, blood pressure should be kept at low levels after the resection for 24 to 48 hours.

◆ Conclusion

Arteriovenous malformations arising at the sylvian and perimotor areas are complex lesions whose therapeutic approach is somewhat controversial. The precise localization of such lesions through the aid of neuroimaging studies allied with a thorough knowledge of the relevant anatomy has made definitive surgical treatment possible for some selected AVMs in the vicinity of such structures, with minor or even no postoperative morbidity.

References

1. de Oliveira E, Tedeschi H, Siqueira MG, Ono M, Rhoton AL Jr. Arteriovenous malformations of the basal ganglia region: rationale for surgical management. Acta Neurochir (Wien) 1997;139:487–506
2. de Oliveira E, Tedeschi H, Raso J. Comprehensive management of arteriovenous malformations. Neurol Res 1998;20:673–683
3. Yasargil MG. Microneurosurgery. Vol 3B. AVM of the Brain. Stuttgart: Georg Thieme Verlag; 1988:293–357

21

Interhemispheric Region Arteriovenous Malformations

Fernando C. G. Pinto, Fabrizio R. F. Porro, Feres E. A. Chaddad Neto, Helder Tedeschi, and Evandro de Oliveira

Arteriovenous malformations (AVMs) arising along the interhemispheric fissure can compromise the medial cortical surface of the cerebral hemispheres, the corpus callosum, and the midline structures related to the walls of the cerebral ventricles.[1] These AVMs can present different anatomical and surgical features according to their location along the interhemispheric fissure. To aid the location of AVMs, we have divided the interhemispheric fissure into thirds: the anterior third comprises the medial surface of the frontal lobe up to the level of the genu of the corpus callosum; the middle third includes the medial surface of the frontal and parietal lobes related to the body of the corpus callosum; and the posterior third is composed of the medial surface of the parietal and occipital lobes related to the splenium of the corpus callosum.

◆ Indications

The treatment of AVMs must be preceded by a cautious radiological study, where some crucial characteristics that may guide the surgeon through treatment choices are evaluated. In addition to the neurosurgeon's experience, the selection criteria are based on the characteristics of the AVM itself.[1,2] The indications for each specific lesion are discussed in the Anatomy section.

◆ Imaging

Magnetic resonance imaging of the brain demonstrates anatomical features in greater detail than other modalities. It is the best neuroimaging exam for evaluating the precise anatomical location and the relationships with surrounding structures, and for selecting the best surgical approach.

The "gold standard" investigation is digital subtraction four-vessel angiography. It shows with precision the three-dimensional relation between the AVM and its feeders and drainage veins. It is, consequently, the definitive study for diagnosis and operative planning and decision making.[3]

◆ Surgical Technique

Anesthesia

There are several goals of anesthesia during surgery of AVMs. The induction of anesthesia should be smooth and profound. Hypotension should be treated whenever it occurs because it may produce ischemic changes in hypoperfused areas. In choosing the induction agent, one has to consider the ability to readily correct the hemodynamic changes. Midazolam may prove helpful during the induction period.

Anesthesia is maintained with isoflurane and intravenous agents. In general, both nitrous oxide/narcotic (particu- larly fentanyl) and volatile anesthetic (usually isoflurane) techniques have been used successfully in these patients. In our experience surgical exposure is usually facilitated by normal ventilation ($PaCO_2$ of 40–45 mm Hg). Cerebrospinal fluid drains may be necessary for surgical access to AVMs located deep in the brain or for large AVMs, or in patients with brain swelling secondary to intracerebral hemorrhage (ICH). The use of crystalloids for fluid replacement should be monitored according to the intrajugular venous pressure (venous pressure should be kept at normal levels). Replacement with colloids rather than crystalloids is preferred to maintain intravascular volume and to decrease the risk of intracerebral swelling from increased brain intracellular water.

After the AVM has been resected, the arterial pressure should be maintained at lower levels than those of the induction period of the anesthesia.

Approach

The AVM's surgical treatment is based on the following concepts[3]:

- The AVM's nidus must be positioned such that its surface is parallel to the floor.
- Feeder vessels must be as perpendicular to the surgeon as possible, and readily accessible.

The surgical positioning for interhemispheric AVMs varies according to the location of the nidus, as follows:

- Anterior and middle interhemispheric AVM: supine position and anterior interhemispheric approach
- Posterior interhemispheric AVM: sitting, prone, lateral, or three-quarter prone position, according to surgeon's experience

The craniotomy and the dural opening must be generous to allow the surgeon to adjust the microscope and to expose a large portion of brain tissue next to the probable nidus of the malformation for easier location and orientation to the brain's landmarks. The key to the AVM's surgical treatment is the approach to arterial feeders. The subsequent steps are the same as those for surgical removal of a well-vascularized tumor.

◆ Surgical strategies

Superficial AVMs located in the interhemispheric fissure, above the pericallosal arteries, that may have either a compact or a diffuse nidus are usually amenable for treatment with minor morbidity. Exception is made for those located in eloquent areas (like the posterior frontal lobe). Some small, compact AVMs located in eloquent areas may also at times be surgically excised with good results.[1,3]

AVMs that compromise the medial cortical surface of the cerebral hemispheres in the anterior third of the interhemispheric fissure are usually supplied by branches of the proximal A2 segment of the anterior cerebral artery and drain into the anterior third of the superior sagittal sinus. Those interhemispheric malformations located in proximity to the gyrus rectus (i.e., to the basal surface of the frontal lobe) can also receive supply from branches of the A1 segment of the anterior cerebral artery.

AVMs located in the anterior third of the interhemispheric fissure in the posterior part of the frontal lobe in the area below the rostrum of the corpus callosum (paraterminal and paraolfactory gyri) may extend posteriorly to involve the walls of the third ventricle and the hypothalamic area. These are lesions in which surgery should be avoided because the morbidity is exceedingly high.

Anterior third interhemispheric AVMs can involve portions of the cingulated gyrus. These AVMs may extend laterally and recruit vessels either from choroidal arteries or from perforating branches of the middle cerebral artery, the lenticulostriate arteries. In such cases, due to the depth of the exposure and to the lateral extension, coagulation of the feeding vessels is more difficult, and resection of the AVM may require excessive cerebral retraction.

Pure midline callosal AVMs are rare but in general are less difficult lesions to approach. The pericallosal arteries run on top of the AVM, sending branches to the lesion along their way in the interhemispheric fissure. The AVM can be excised with little difficulty after careful coagulation of its feeding vessels while sparing the pericallosal artery. Callosal AVMs nevertheless may extend laterally and also recruit vessels from the ventricles. In such cases resection is more troublesome due to the difficult control of bleeding from small vessels in a deep surgical field.

These lesions usually involve portions of the cingulate gyrus and sometimes may extend inferiorly to include the midline structures of the lateral and third ventricles. Those AVMs that involve the anterior third of the corpus callosum are supplied by branches of the anterior cerebral artery (**Fig. 21–1**). They may have a superficial drainage into the superior sagittal sinus or may drain into the septal and thalamostriate veins in the ventricles.

AVMs arising in the middle third of the interhemispheric fissure are usually difficult to approach. The exposure is usually hampered by the veins that drain either the malformation or the normal brain. The proximity of the sensorimotor cortex also prohibits any excessive retraction. These malformations are usually supplied by branches of the pericallosal or callosomarginal arteries. When the malformation extends to the ventricles, it is also supplied by branches of the posterior choroidal arteries. The venous drainage is through the superficial system via bridging veins to the superior or inferior sagittal sinuses, and at times, to the deep venous system through ependymal veins and the internal cerebral veins (**Figs. 21–2** and **21–3**).

AVMs that arise in the posterior third of the interhemispheric fissure comprise those located in the posterior parietal and mesial occipital regions that are related to the posterior third of the falx cerebri.

The medial surface of the occipital lobe is separated from the parietal lobe by the parieto-occipital sulcus. The calcarine fissure extends forward from the occipital pole toward the splenium, dividing this surface into an upper part, the cuneus, between the parieto-occipital and the calcarine sulci, and into a lower part, the lingula.

Parafalcine AVMs of the posterior third of the interhemispheric fissure may involve the cuneus, the precuneus (adjacent to the parieto-occipital sulcus), the isthmus of the cingulate gyrus, as well as the lingula. These AVMs are usually supplied by branches of the posterior cerebral artery and the parieto-occipital and calcarine arteries, and occasionally by branches of the middle cerebral artery and posterior branches of the anterior cerebral artery. Depending on the extension of the AVM, these lesions can reach the ventricular trigone and receive supply from branches of

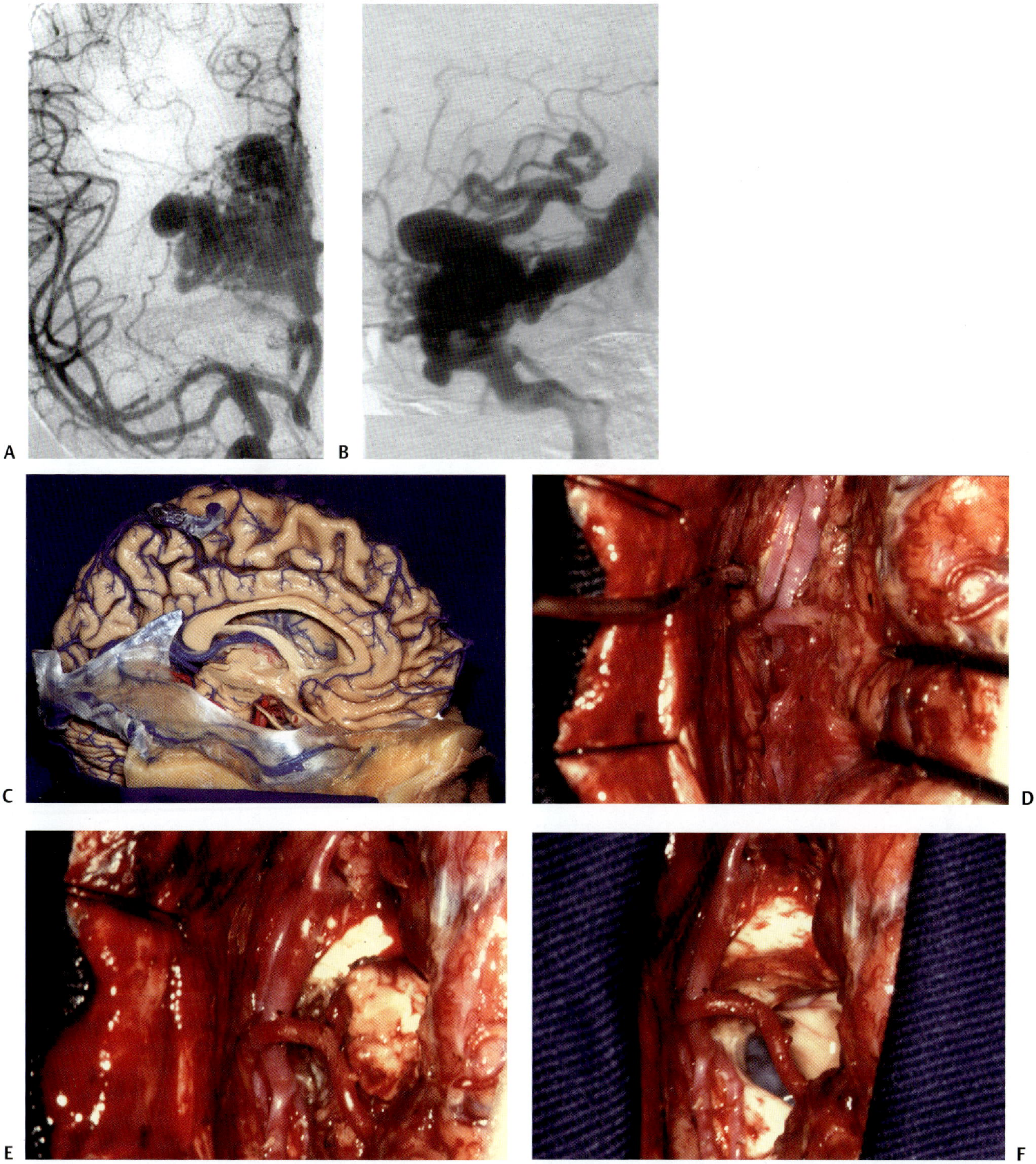

Figure 21–1 Arteriovenous malformation (AVM) involving the anterior part of the right cingulate gyrus and corpus callosum. **(A)** Right carotid digital subtraction angiogram disclosing the AVM (anteroposterior view). **(B)** Lateral view of the same case showing the arterial supply through the anterior cerebral artery and the venous drainage through the septal vein into the internal cerebral vein. **(C)** Anatomical specimen showing the location of the AVM and the pattern of the venous drainage. **(D)** Operative view of the AVM after opening of the interhemispheric fissure. **(E)** The AVM was dissected and the arterial feeders coagulated. **(F)** Operative view after complete removal of the AVM.

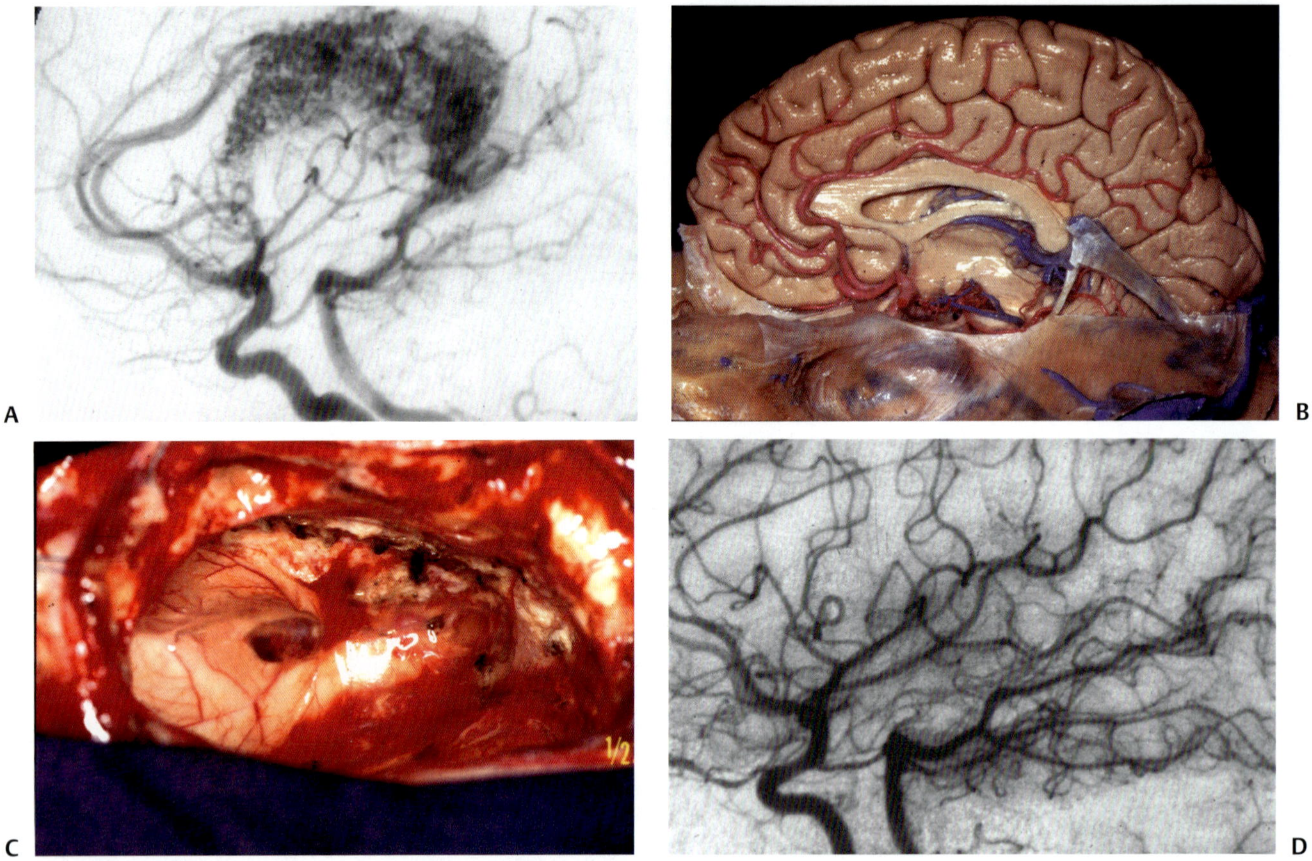

Figure 21–2 Arteriovenous malformation involving the middle and posterior part of the corpus callosum. **(A)** Digital subtraction angiogram of the carotid and vertebral arteries (displayed together for the purpose of visual effect only) showing an AVM involving the middle and posterior part of the corpus callosum supplied by branches of the anterior cerebral artery and branches of the posterior cerebral artery. **(B)** Anatomical specimen showing the location of the AVM and the pattern of the arterial supply. **(C)** Intraoperative view after complete removal of the AVM. **(D)** Postoperative digital subtraction angiogram of the carotid and vertebral arteries (again, displayed together for the purpose of visual effect only) after complete removal of the AVM.

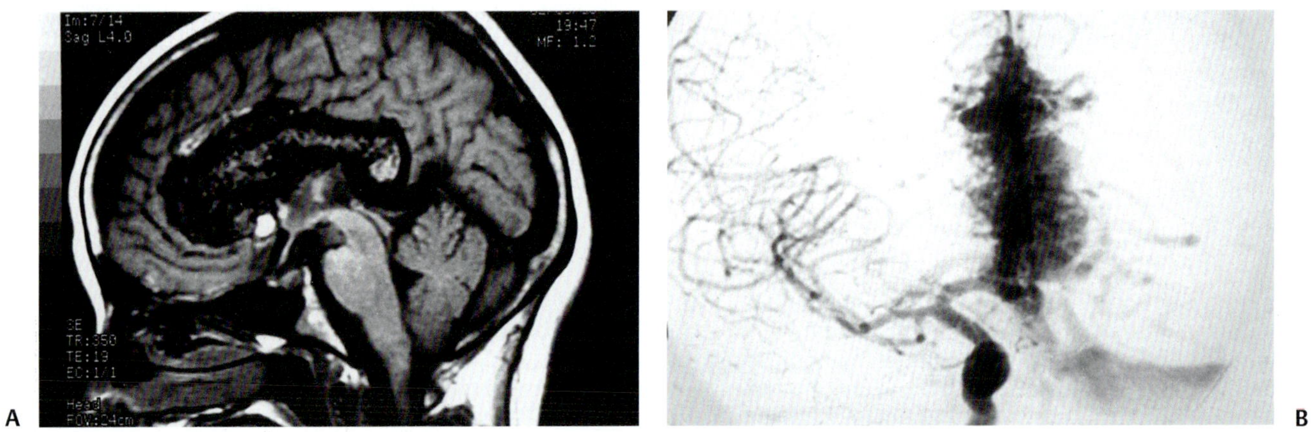

Figure 21–3 Arteriovenous malformation involving the entire corpus callosum, the septum, the fornix, and the velum interpositum. **(A)** T1-weighted magnetic resonance imaging sagittal view of the AVM. **(B)** Right carotid digital subtraction angiogram disclosing the AVM (anteroposterior view) supplied by both anterior cerebral arteries.

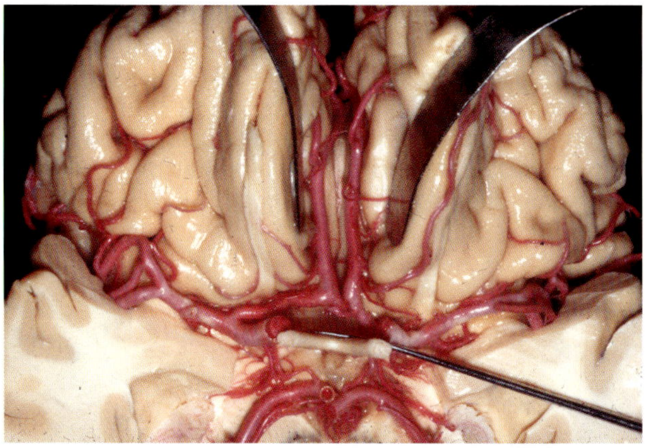

C

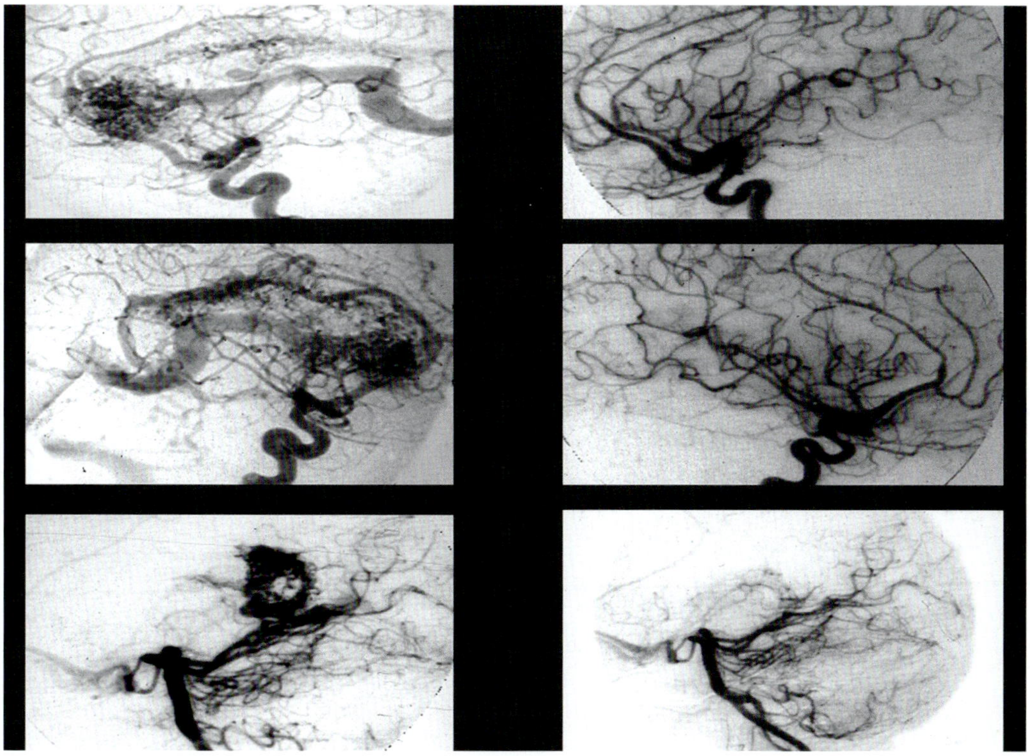

D

(*Continued*) **Figure 21–3** **(C)** Anatomical specimen showing the location of the AVM and the pattern of the arterial supply. **(D)** Intraoperative view after complete resection of the AVM.

the lateral posterior choroidal arteries. The venous drainage is through cortical veins into the superior sagittal sinus or through the group of veins that drain into the vein of Galen.

AVMs that involve the splenium of the corpus callosum are supplied by branches of the posterior pericallosal artery and lateral posterior and medial posterior choroidal arteries, and by branches directly from the posterior cerebral artery. In cases where the AVM extends to the ventricles, it may drain through subependymal veins into the basal vein of Rosenthal and then into the vein of Galen.

The surgical approach to these AVMs is as difficult as that to AVMs of the mesial temporal lobe because they tend to be buried in the depths of the sulci and are surrounded by delicate elements.

◆ Postoperative Care

The resection of an AVM demands a smooth awakening, without blood pressure elevations, Valsalva maneuvers, or strain that could raise intracranial pressure.[2,3]

The blood pressure is kept under the initial anesthesia induction value for 24 to 48 hours after the resection.

The patient undergoes cerebral arteriography to demonstrate complete obliteration of the AVM before discharging.

◆ Complications

Judicious evaluation of the patient and of the preoperative exams, correct surgical strategy, and surgical experience are mandatory to avoid surgical complications.

The avoidance of potential complications includes a preoperative clinical evaluation of pulmonary and cardiovascular systems because the patient must be able to withstand a prolonged time under anesthesia, blood loss, and hemodynamic alterations.[2,3]

Retraction tissue injury next to the AVM and its consequent edema can result in transient or even permanent postoperative deficits and thus should be avoided.

Postoperative hemorrhage can result from incomplete resection. Careful inspection of the resection area is necessary. Intraoperative angiography might prove helpful in preventing such complications.[2,3]

References

1. Tedeschi H, de Oliveira E, Rhoton AL Jr. Microsurgical Anatomy of Arteriovenous Malformations: Vascular Malformations of the Central Nervous System. 1999:253
2. de Oliveira E, Tedeschi H, Raso J. Comprehensive management of arteriovenous malformations. Neurol Res 1998;20:673–683
3. Yasargil MG. Microneurosurgery. Vol 3B. AVM of the Brain. Stuttgart: Georg Thieme Verlag; 1988:293–357

22

Posterior Fossa Arteriovenous Malformations

James P. Chandler, Yannick Grenier, Christopher C. Getch, Eric J. Russell, and H. Hunt Batjer

- Cerebellar Arteriovenous Malformations
- Cerebellopontine Angle Arteriovenous Malformations
- Brain Stem Arteriovenous Malformations
- Radiosurgery of Posterior Fossa Arteriovenous Malformations
- Conclusion

Infratentorial arteriovenous malformations (AVMs) of the vertebrobasilar system include cerebellar and brain stem AVMs. Estimates of the prevalence of posterior fossa AVMs range from 7%[1] to 18 to 20%[2,3] of all intracranial AVMs. Although cerebellar and brain stem AVMs share a close anatomical relationship, they have distinct natural histories, clinical presentations, and operative risks.

According to Yasargil, the first clinical description of a cerebellar AVM was made by Clingenstein in 1908.[4] The landmark technological advances that have made the treatment of such lesions possible include the advent of vertebral angiography. This technique remains the gold standard for diagnosis both of the feeding arteries to the AVM nidus and of the draining veins of the malformation, as well as for the documentation of total AVM nidus obliteration after treatment of the malformation. Magnetic resonance imaging (MRI) has become invaluable for defining the anatomical relationship of the AVM to the brain stem and cranial nerves as well as for planning surgical removal of the AVM. More recently, MRI has been used to noninvasively follow the patency of the AVM nidus after stereotactic radiosurgery.[5] Superselective catheterization of AVM feeders now allows a better preoperative understanding of the exact number and size of arterial feeders in more complex lesions and has contributed the tool of embolization to treatment strategies for these lesions.[6] Additionally, continued efforts are being made to develop improved three-dimensional planning and dosimetry for the stereotactic radiosurgical treatment of the AVM nidus; a technique with unique and often delayed complications.[6] A final technological advance that should be mentioned in this context concerns functional imaging. It is now becoming possible to precisely localize supratentorial functions that can be critical in patient selection as well as intraoperative strategy. The same may apply to posterior fossa lesions.

The most common presentation of patients with posterior fossa AVMs is hemorrhage, often associated with hydrocephalus (headache, nausea, vomiting, diplopia, ataxia, dysmetria), although a somewhat older population also presents with symptoms of progressive brain stem or cerebellar dysfunction, which can be attributed to vertebrobasilar insufficiency related to AVM steal.[7] The natural history risk of the posterior AVMs is apparently similar to that of AVMs in other anatomical locations (i.e. 3-4% of risk of bleeding per year).[8] These data, however, do not address issues inapparent in the Troupp experience, which may increase risks such as intranidal aneurysms and compromise of venous outflow.

The reported surgical experience in treating these lesions is best described by several key series: Yasargil reported on 82 patients with infratentorial AVMs. Of the 68 patients who underwent surgery, complete AVM excision was achieved in 67 (58 cerebellar, five mesencephalic, four pontine).[4] Drake et al presented a series of 66 patients with posterior fossa AVMs; 47 AVMs were completely resected, with an overall operative mortality of 15%, mostly secondary to sudden postoperative hemorrhage, and a morbidity of 14%.[2] More recently, Samson et al reported a series of 103 AVMs of the posterior fossa, 23 of which were located in the brain stem. They were able to completely resect 100 of these lesions with 6% mortality and 8% morbidity.[3] Based on their surgical experience, they identified subgroups of brain stem AVMs: subpial or deep. Of the 23 brain stem AVMs treated surgically, the parenchymal or deep lesions ($n = 10$) were completely resected with a 30% mortality and a 40% morbidity. In contrast the superficial or pial lesions ($n = 13$) were completely resected with a 0% mortality and a 14% morbidity.[9]

◆ Cerebellar Arteriovenous Malformations

Cerebellar AVMs are the most common type of posterior fossa AVM encountered in clinical practice. They tend to occur four to five times more commonly than brain stem AVMs.[3] Yasargil described several types of cerebellar AVMs: hemispheric, vermian (superior and inferior), cerebellopontine (extrinsic in the subarachnoid space of the cerebellopontine angle or intrinsic), and giant.[4] The majority of cerebellar AVMs present with intraparenchymal hemorrhage with or without intraventricular extension or subarachnoid extension. When life-threatening hemorrhage is present at the time of initial presentation, surgery to reduce a mass effect of the clot and treat intracranial pressure should be performed. Commonly, a subtotal resection of the clot may be necessary, with definitive treatment of the AVM performed in a delayed fashion 4 to 8 weeks later to allow for a significant resolution of the effect of hemorrhage and recovery from the initial bleed. At the time of definitive AVM resection, a repeat angiogram and MRI are recommended to obtain a better understanding of the specific anatomy of the lesion because acute hematoma can compress and obscure important components of the lesion. At the time of surgery, the anesthetic technique employed should allow for tight control of systemic blood pressure, with care being taken to avoid any periods of hypertension or hypotension. Additionally, appropriate agents should be utilized to minimize any rises in intracranial pressure. Large volumes of colloid, crystalloids, and blood should be available in the event of a significant hemorrhage. Should massive hemorrhage occur, prior to inducing any degree of hypertension, burst-suppressive doses of cerebroprotective agents, such as pentobarbital or etomidate, should be administered.

In general, the Concorde, prone, or park bench position will provide adequate access to most cerebellar AVMs. Although the sitting position is an option for superiorly located cerebellar AVMs, the risk of air embolism and surgeon upper extremity fatigue are considerations that may make selection of an alternate position more desirable. A midline or perimedian exposure is made, extending from the inion superiorly to the foramen magnum inferiorly. A large suboccipital craniotomy is performed with a single bur hole just inferior to the mastoid and the Midas Rex (Medtronic; Minneapolis, MN) with a B1 footplate. This exposure should allow for clear visualization of the transverse and sigmoid sinuses superolaterally and the dura of the cervical medullary junction inferiorly. Following the opening of the dura, the cisterna magna can be dissected to allow cerebrospinal fluid drainage and cerebellar relaxation, especially if significant cerebellar swelling or distension is present. Once the cerebellum is relaxed, careful identification and dissection of arterial feeders and the arterialized venous drainage of the malformation are performed. The arterial feeders are most often branches from the superior cerebellar artery (SCA) or posterior inferior cerebellar artery (PICA). When anterior inferior cerebellar artery (AICA) feeders are present, they may be most reliably identified at or near the foramen of Luschka. The arterial feeders are followed into the cerebellar parenchyma to the AVM nidus. The nidus is then sharply dissected circumferentially from medial to lateral to allow for the gentle elevation of the malformation away from normal cerebellar tissue. The arterial feeders are coagulated with the bipolar cautery and cut with microscissors. The fourth ventricle should only be entered in situations where the AVM extends into the periependymal area. The draining veins are the superior cerebellar, precentral cerebellar, vermian, and lateral mesencephalic veins. The paramedian veins may enter the dura of the tentorium lateral to the straight sinus but have not been seen to enter the transverse sinus directly.[4] When the arterial supply to the AVM has been appropriately eliminated, the venous drainage takes on a more typical venous coloration and flow pattern. The draining vein or veins then should be coagulated and cut or occluded with microaneurysm clips.

Vermian AVMs will commonly extend into the fourth ventricle (**Fig. 22–1A**). The surgical principles described above apply to these lesions as well. The relevant arterial feeders are most commonly from PICA or SCA and are often bilateral (**Fig. 22–1B**). They most often drain via the superior or inferior vermian veins, then to the galenic system medially or to the petrosal vein laterally. We prefer the Concorde position for these lesions. As previously described, a large bony exposure allows for opening of the arachnoid over the cisterna magna and significant cerebellar relaxation, thereby minimizing the need for retraction. After all arterial feeders have been carefully exposed, they are followed into the vermis, where the nidus of the AVM can be clearly identified, prior to their sacrifice. The nidus is then dissected and coagulated in a circumferential manner. If the AVM remains turgid, the contralateral PICA should be examined at the medial margin of the tonsils because they frequently may contribute branches to the AVM. In many instances, the anatomy of the malformation necessitates entry into the fourth ventricle. Upon exposure of the fourth ventricle, a small cottonoid strip should be placed along the floor for protective purposes during the course of the dissection. A diligent inspection of the periependymal surface for any evidence of AVM should follow. It is imperative that complete, careful hemostasis be achieved in this periependymal area to lessen the risk of postoperative obstructive hydrocephalus. As with any surgical procedure for an AVM, an immediate intraoperative or postoperative angiogram while the patient is maintained under general anesthesia is strongly recommended to rule out the presence of residual AVM (**Fig. 22–1C**). In the event that residual AVM is detected, the patient should be taken back to surgery immediately and that residual lesion resected. Potential sacrifice of important venous drainage with persisting arterialization can set the stage for early postoperative hemorrhage if immediate resection is not performed.

Caudal cerebellar AVMs, also referred to as tonsillar AVMs, are generally approachable from a midline and a lateral or far-lateral perspective (**Fig. 22–2A,B**). The specific approach implemented will be a function of the anatomy of the arterial supply and the venous drainage. Most commonly, the arterial supply of these malformations arises from PICA and venous drainage into the inferior vermian and the perimesencephalic veins. The dorsal- or ventral-based midline tonsillar AVMs are well suited for midline approaches. Options for patient positioning include prone, Concorde, or sitting, with the neck maximally flexed. The bony exposure should include the foramen magnum and the posterior ring of C1. After completion of an opening, which should extend

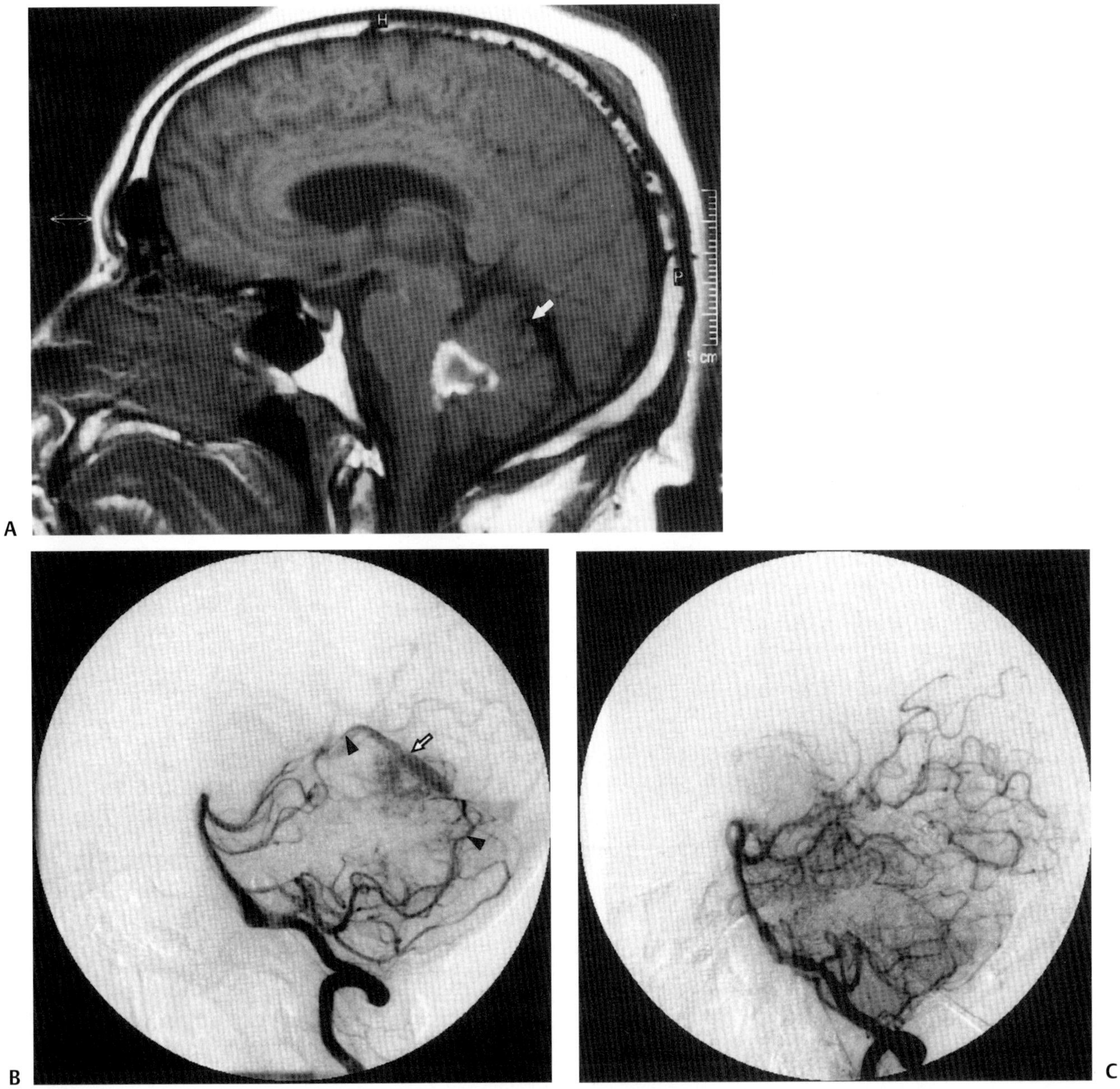

Figure 22–1 Vermian arteriovenous malformation (AVM). Forty-three–year-old male with a history of hypertension and multiple substance abuse presented with headache, nausea, vomiting, and diplopia. Head computed tomography documented an intraventricular hemorrhage. A cerebral angiogram revealed a small vermian AVM, which was completely resected. He recovered with only residual imbalance of his gait. **(A)** Preoperative magnetic resonance, T1-weighted image showing subacute blood in the fourth ventricle and some prominent flow voids in the declive (arrow) of the vermis. **(B)** Preoperative cerebral angiogram, left vertebral artery injection, showing the left posterior inferior cerebellar artery and left superior cerebellar artery feeders (arrowheads) to the AVM nidus (arrowheads) and the enlarged superior vermian draining vein (white arrow). **(C)** Postoperative angiogram showing no residual AVM.

from the level of the transverse sinus superiorly to the level of the arch of C1 inferiorly, the cisterna magna may be punctured to allow for cerebellar relaxation and maximization of corridors available for surgical maneuvering. The fourth ventricle may be entered through the obex, and, as with vermian lesions, a cottonoid strip should be placed along the ependymal floor for protective purposes. The lateral and posterior medullary components of PICA are identified and the arachnoidal bands are sharply dissected to allow progressive dissection along the flocculus and ventral surface of the tonsils. Arterial feeders are followed to the nidus and then progressively coagulated and cut or clipped. The involved tonsil may be reflected laterally and resected to expose the inferior vermian draining vein.

More laterally located tonsillar AVMs may require a more lateral exposure for adequate visualization for feeding arteries and draining veins. A far lateral approach with or without mobilization of the vertebral artery for partial condylectomy is ideal for such lesions. In such instances, the surgeon should anticipate the presence of venous

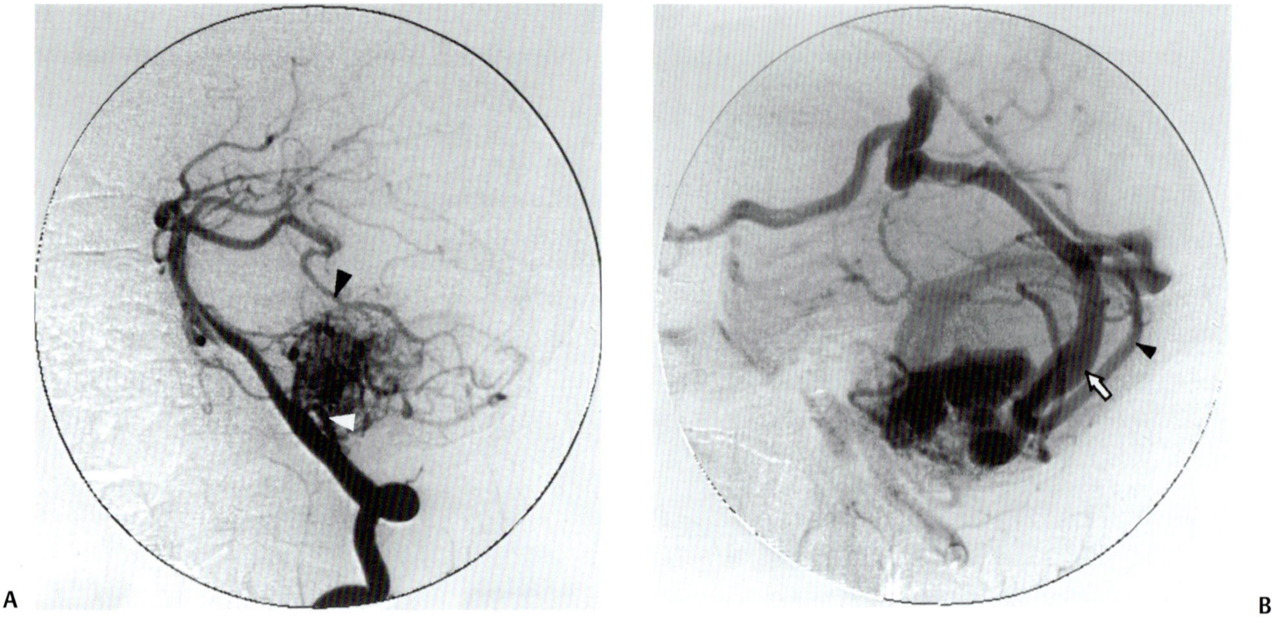

Figure 22–2 Tonsillar arteriovenous malformation. **(A)** Cerebral angiogram, oblique view of arterial phase of a left vertebral artery injection, showing the left posterior inferior cerebellar artery (white arrowhead) and superior cerebellar artery feeders (black arrowhead) to a left tonsillar AVM. **(B)** The venous phase demonstrates a large vein draining to the vermian vein and galenic system (white arrow), as well as a hemispheric vein draining to the transverse sinus (arrowhead).

hypertension and the risk of difficult or uncontrollable blood loss emanating from the dissection of the perivertebral venous plexus and the condylar vein.

◆ Cerebellopontine Angle Arteriovenous Malformations

Cerebellopontine angle AVMs may be completely extrinsic to the brain stem and cerebellum, anatomically confined to the subarachnoid space, where intimate relationships with multiple cranial nerves may exist (**Fig 22–3A**). Usually, however, some pial representation is present. These lesions are most often supplied by the AICA, but may include PICA and SCA feeding branches (**Fig. 22–3B**). The drainage tends to occur initially through lateral pontine veins, then later to the petrosal vein or the galenic system. Additionally, preoperative superselective catheterization of arterial feeders and embolization can successfully reduce the size of the nidus.

Fig. 22–4 demonstrates a case in which preoperative embolization was part of the treatment strategy of large hemispheric AVMs. In the first case **(Fig. 22–4A–J)**, selective catheterization of the right SCA and PICA successfully reduced the AVM nidus size by an estimated 40%.

Many positioning options exist for approaches to the cerebellopontine angle. We prefer a modified park bench position with the head turned 90 degrees opposite the surgeon and the contralateral arm supported in a sling. A paramedian skin incision originating 2 cm posterior to the most superior aspect of the auricle and continuing inferiorly to approximately 2 cm inferior to the mastoid tip is performed, allowing for excellent exposure of both the posterior aspect of the mastoid and the lip of the foramen magnum. Through a single bur hole at the level of the asterion, a generous craniotomy that includes the foramen magnum should be performed. The dural exposure should include the transverse sigmoid sinus junction laterally, the inferior cerebellar sinus medially, and the marginal sinus inferiorly. The dural opening should optimize the superolateral exposure of the transverse sigmoid junction and additionally expose the lateral aspect of the cisterna magna. As previously described, the cisterna magna is opened to facilitate cerebellar relaxation and generous opening of the pontocerebellar cisterns laterally. A sharp dissection of the AVM's arterial supply follows. With adequate drainage of spinal fluid and manipulation of the operative table rotation, the critical vascular anatomy can be well visualized without brain retraction. Meticulous microdissection of the feeding arteries as they course through the cerebellopontine angle and across the brain stem and into the cerebellum is necessary to prevent inadvertent sacrifice of vessels critical to blood supply of the brain stem. A sequential elevation of the AVM nidus with circumferential cauterization and clipping of entering arteries is then performed. Elimination of the preserved venous drainage is the terminal maneuver in excising this lesion. Care must be taken to avoid injury of peripheral vessels en passage and excessive manipulation of adjacent or attached cranial nerves. Cranial nerve palsies are a frequent occurrence in the resection of such lesions but are most often transient and related to vascular insult.[2–4]

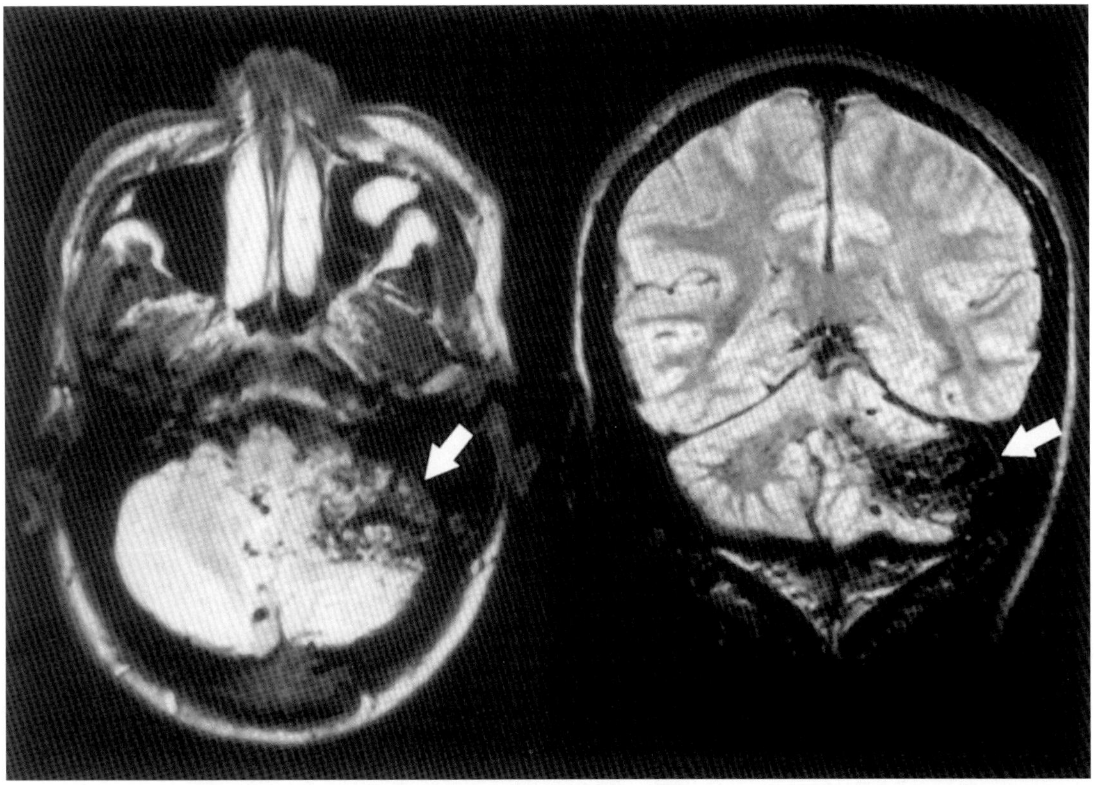

A

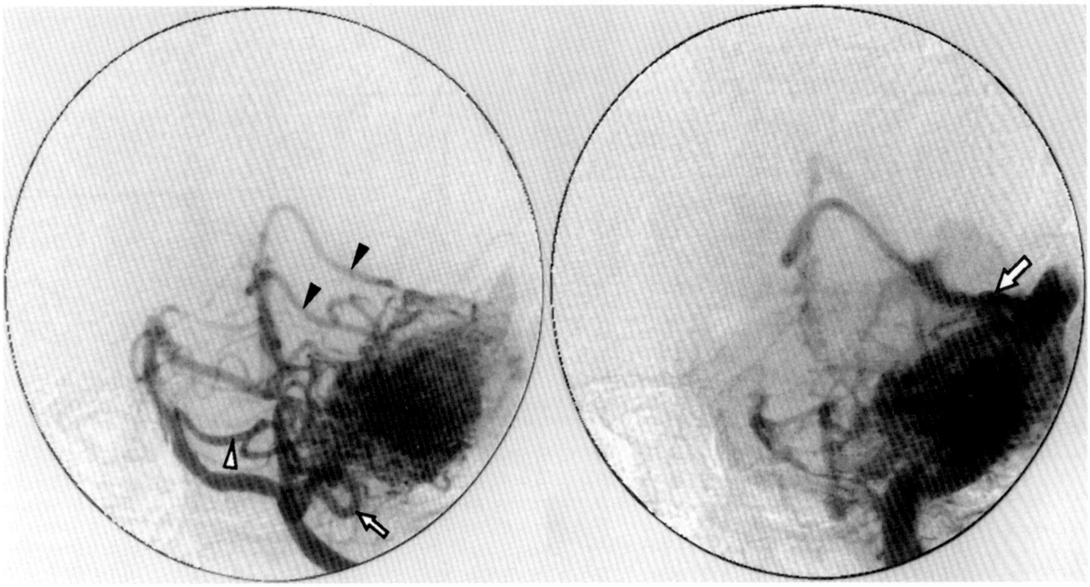

B

Figure 22–3 Cerebellopontine arteriovenous malformation. Thirty-two–year-old male presented with a 6-year history of atypical left trigeminal neuralgia and a more recent history of left glossopharyngeal neuralgia. **(A)** Axial magnetic resonance imaging, T2-weighted, showing a large left cerebellar hemispheric AVM with prominent flow voids extending to the left cerebellopontine angle cisterns (arrow). Note also the coronal view (to the right). **(B)** Cerebral angiogram, left vertebral artery injection. The arterial phase on the left shows the left posterior inferior cerebellar artery (white arrow), the left anterior inferior cerebellar artery (white arrowhead), and branches of the left superior cerebellar artery (black arrowheads) feeding the AVM nidus. The venous phase on the right shows an enlarged hemispheric vein draining into the superior vermian vein and galenic system (White arrow).

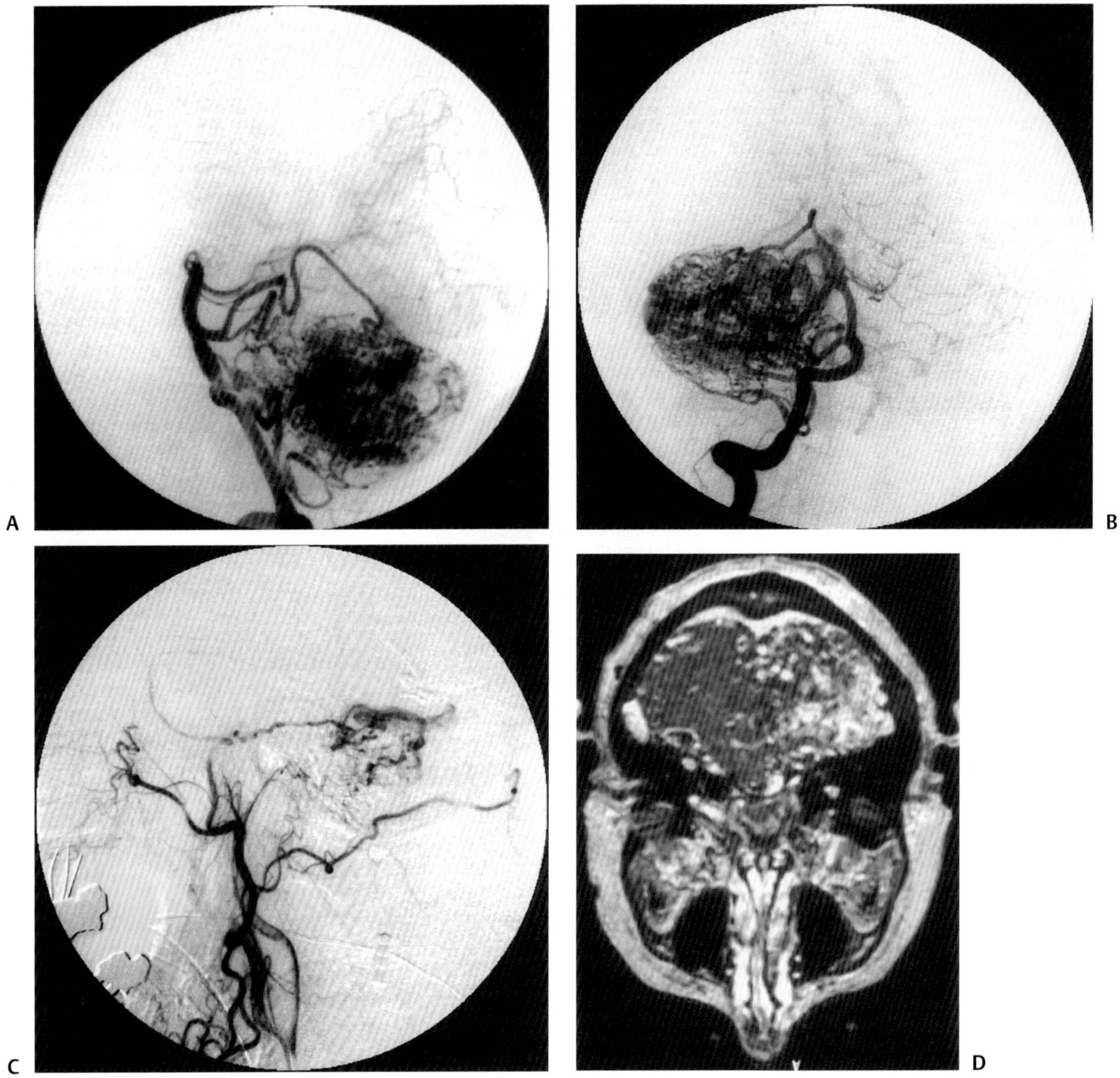

Figure 22–4 Embolization of hemispheric arteriovenous malformation. Sixty-one–year-old female initially presented with headaches and mild tandem gait ataxia. Evaluation with cerebral angiogram demonstrated a large right cerebellar AVM. She was neurologically stable for several years but then developed a nystagmus, hemiataxia, and left fourth nerve palsy. Computed tomographic scan revealed obstructive hydrocephalus requiring shunting. **(A)** Anteroposterior and **(B)** lateral right vertebral artery injection demonstrating a large right cerebellar AVM with arterial supply from the right superior cerebellar, anterior inferior cerebellar, and posterior inferior cerebellar vessels. **(C)** Right common carotid injection demonstrating external carotid contribution through an accessory middle meningeal artery to the AVM nidus. **(D)** Axial and **(E)** sagittal gradient echo volume acquisition magnetic resonance imaging revealing a large cerebellar panhemispheric AVM. **(F)** Lateral view of a right vertebral artery injection demonstrating the remaining patent AVM nidus after four staged embolizations with N-butyl-2-cyanoacrylate, and **(G)** Anteroposterior and **(H)** Common carotid injection demonstrating the remaining external carotid supply to the AVM nidus, and **(I)** Lateral and **(J)** anteroposterior view of a right vertebral artery injection demonstrating no early arteriovenous shunting following surgical removal of the AVM utilizing an extensive suboccipital craniectomy.

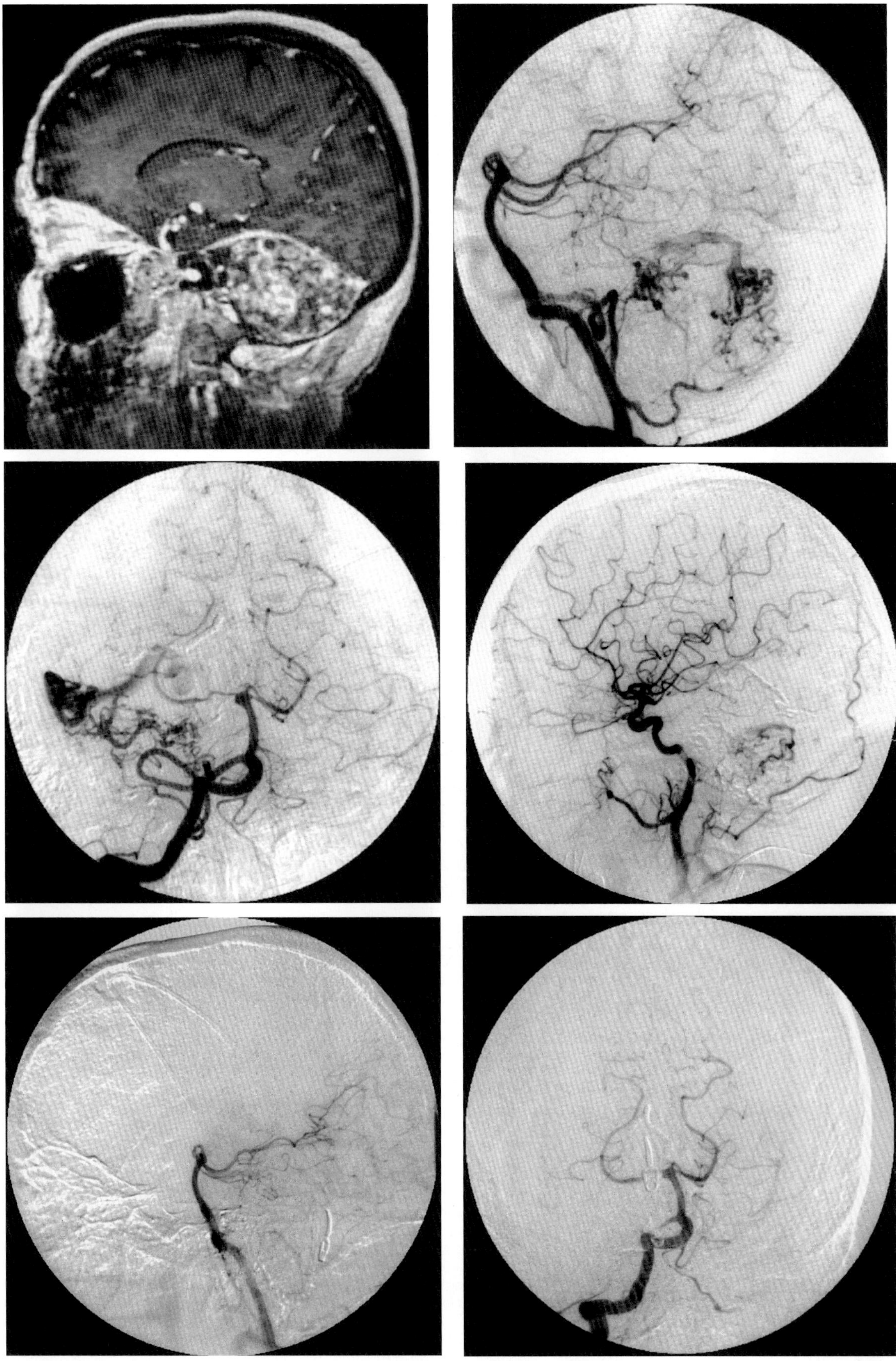

E F

G H

I J

◆ Brain Stem Arteriovenous Malformations

The intrinsic or subpial brain stem AVMs are fortunately rare but carry a distinct natural history and prognosis. Although superficial and lateral lesions located in the mid to upper pons may be successfully approached in a similar fashion, as described previously, a petrosal or far lateral approach in combination with suboccipital craniotomy may provide enhanced visualization of the pontomedullary surface with less need for cerebellar or brain stem retraction. In general, the only brain stem AVMs that are considered for open surgery are those presenting to the pial surface. The subpial brain stem AVMs carry a prohibitively high and unacceptable operative risk. These lesions commonly present with intraparenchymal hemorrhage or with progressive neurological deficits. Their clinical presentation may mimic a neoplasm or a demyelinating process. **Fig. 22–5A,B** shows the clinical case of a patient with a brain stem AVM that presented with hemorrhage. The pial representation of the AVM is exemplified in **Fig. 22–5A**. The right AICA and multiple small basilar perforating arteries that contributed to the AVM nidus are shown in **Fig. 22–5C.**

In addition to standard cerebral angiography, an MRI is mandatory for radiographic evaluation of these lesions.

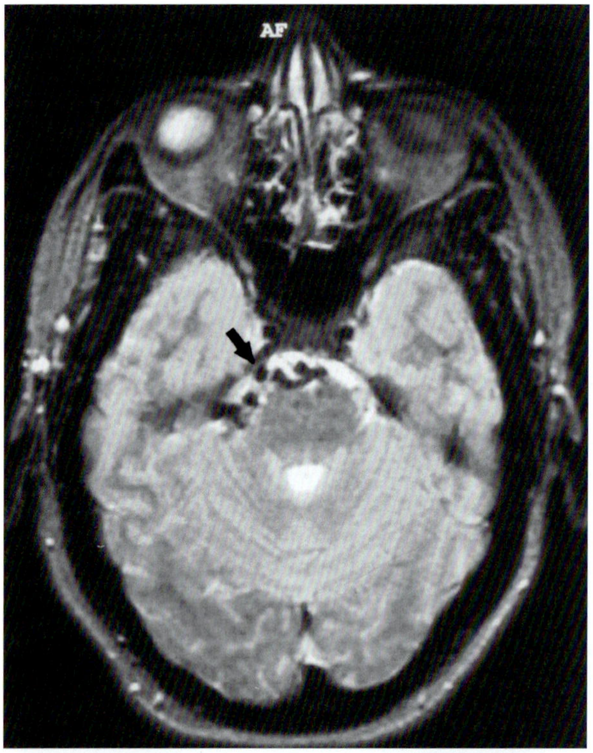

A

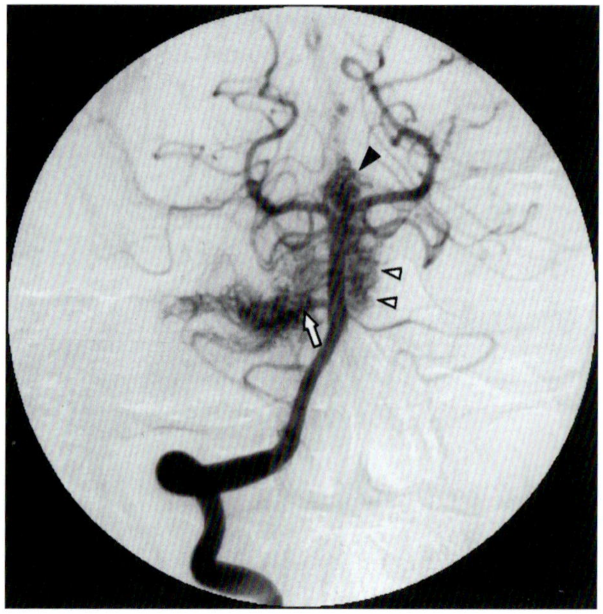
B

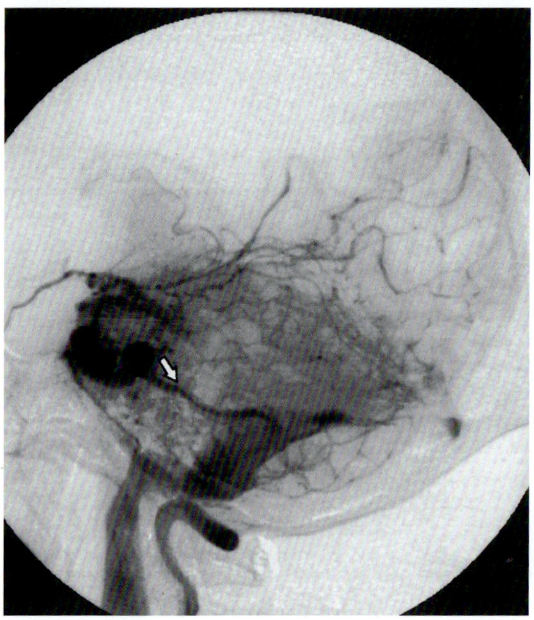
C

Figure 22–5 Brain stem arteriovenous malformation. Thirty-year-old female sustained a hemorrhage in the brain stem, resulting in a left hemiparesis, diplopia, and hearing loss. A cerebral angiogram demonstrated an anterior pontine AVM. She was referred for stereotactic radiosurgery. **(A)** Axial magnetic resonance imaging, T2-weighted, showing enlarged flow voids in the prepontine cistern (arrow). **(B)** Cerebral angiogram, right vertebral artery injection, anteroposterior view, showing a nidus fed primarily by the right anterior inferior cerebellar artery (white arrow), and a second nidus fed by multiple small basilar trunk (white arrowheads) and basilar apex (black arrowhead) perforators. **(C)** Venous phase, lateral view, showing drainage of the AVM via an enlarged right transverse pontine vein (white arrow) to the right sigmoid sinus.

Specifically, the MRI can give information as to the degree of pial representation and AVM nidus. The main challenge of these lesions is that their arterial supply involves penetrating feeders from the basilar artery (as shown in **Fig. 22–5B**), which cannot be safely dissected or embolized due to the substantial risk of ischemia or hemorrhage.[3,4]

Even radiosurgery in this location carries a higher risk of ischemic changes. A recent series of 304 patients who received gamma knife radiosurgery reported a 3.24 times increased risk of symptomatic T2-weighted changes on MRI, as compared with AVMs in other locations at 24- to 96 month follow-up (median 44-month follow-up).[10]

Hence the surgical goal of complete AVM excision in this location has been associated with a high price. In Drake et al's surgical series, only two of seven brain stem AVMs could be excised safely.[2] Samson et al report a 30% mortality with resection of deep brain stem AVMs. An exception, however, to intrinsic brain stem lesions are the perimesencephalic AVMs. Anecdotal resection of lesions within the quadrigeminal plate with good postoperative results was documented by Drake et al[2] and Yasargil.[4] In both reports, the lesions resected were described as minimally visible angiographically and were diagnosed predominantly by the early appearance of a dorsal mesencephalic vein.

◆ Radiosurgery of Posterior Fossa Arteriovenous Malformations

Stereotactic radiosurgery, using the linear accelerator or the 201-source cobalt-60 gamma knife unit, has an evolving role in the treatment of select posterior fossa AVMs. Specifically, small lesions within the cerebellar peduncle, pons, and medulla may be amenable to treatment with radiosurgery. Although long-term data on the radiosurgical treatment of brain stem AVMs does not exist, overall 2-year complete obliteration rates between 75 and 80% have been reported following the treatment of small-volume intraparenchymal AVMs with the linear accelerator and the gamma knife.[11,12]

The primary hazards of radiosurgery for brain stem lesions include incomplete nidus obliteration, radiation-induced injury to surrounding tissue, and increased postradiosurgical hemorrhage rate. As previously stated, there have been several studies to suggest that radiosurgery is effective in obliterating 80% of AVMs less than 3 cm in diameter with a latency interval of 2 to 3 years. During the latency interval, hemorrhage rates between 4.8 and 16% have been reported within the first 12 months following treatment. This hemorrhage rate exceeds the 2 to 4% annual hemorrhage rate determined in natural history studies.[8] The issue of radiation injury is a function of dosimetry and the specific location of the lesion.

Given the high operative morbidity of posterior fossa AVMs, in particular, those within the brain stem, radiosurgery is an option that must be considered. Improvements in integration of MRI and angiographic data as they relate to enhanced lesion localization and more optimal dose planning may result in improved results with this form of treatment.

◆ Conclusion

Posterior fossa AVMs, with the important exception of intrinsic brain stem lesions, may be safely resected using the available modern microsurgical techniques. A preoperative high-quality angiogram and an MRI are generally recommended, and safe embolization of arterial feeders is generally thought to be useful. Cranial base approaches may dramatically enhance the surgeon's visualization of the AVM and allow greater working room with less brain retraction. A postoperative angiogram is mandatory to document the absence of residual AVM. The most feared complication remains postoperative hemorrhage from suboptimal hemostasis or from unrecognized residual AVM. Postoperatively, tight hemodynamic control is crucial for the prevention of cerebellar ischemia.

Both arterial and venous anomalies associated with posterior fossa AVMs have been described, the most common of which is the presence of aneurysms. In Drake et al's series of 66 patients, 12 patients had concomitant aneurysms, all related to feeding arteries, and nine had ruptured.[2] In Batjer and Samson's series of 32 patients, six patients had aneurysms, and a total of 10 aneurysms were counted. Eight of 10 were in the vertebrobasilar system, and four of eight were located on feeding arteries. Two aneurysms presented with subarachnoid hemorrhage.[7] Other anomalies include a case of bilateral occlusion of both transverse and sigmoid sinuses and drainage of arterial blood from a cerebellar artery feeder to the cavernous and sphenopalatine venous systems.[4] Preoperative imaging studies must be very carefully screened to detect these anomalies because treatment strategies may be impacted.

Acknowledgment The authors wish to thank Keri Kramer for her keen editorial eye and invaluable assistance in the preparation of this manuscript.

References

1. Perret G, Nishioka H. Report on the cooperative study of intracranial aneurysms and subarachnoid hemorrhage, VI: Arteriovenous malformations: an analysis of 545 cases of craniocerebral arteriovenous malformations and fistulae reported to the cooperative study. J Neurosurg 1966;25:467–490
2. Drake C, Friedman A, Peerless S. Posterior fossa arteriovenous malformations. J Neurosurg 1986;64:1–10
3. Samson D, et al. Technical features of the management of arteriovenous malformation of the brainstem and cerebellum. In: B. HH, ed. Cerebrovascular Diseases., Philadelphia: Lippincott-Raven; 1997
4. Yasargil M. Infratentorial AVMs: AVM of the Brain, Clinical Consideration, General and Special Operative Techniques, Surgical Results, Non-operated Cases, Cavernous and Venous Angiomas, Neuroanesthesia. Vol 3B. New York: Thieme; 1988
5. Pollock BE, Kondziolka D, Flickinger JC, Patel AK, Bissonette DJ, Lunsford LD. Magnetic resonance imaging: an accurate method to evaluate arteriovenous malformations after stereotactic radiosurgery. J. Neurosurg 1996;85:1044–1049
6. Yamamoto M, Jimbo M, Hara M, Saito I, Mori K. Gamma knife radiosurgery for arteriovenous malformations: long-term follow-up results

focusing on complications occurring more than 5 years after irradiation. Neurosurgery 1996;38:906–914
7. Batjer H, Samson D. Arteriovenous malformations of the posterior fossa. J Neurosurg 1986;64:849–856
8. Ondra S, Troupp H, George E. The natural history of symptomatic arteriovenous malformations of the brain: a 24-year follow-up assessment. J Neurosurg 1990;73:387–391
9. Samson D, Batjer H, Kopitnik T. Arteriovenous malformations of the brainstem: surgical management and classification. J Neurosurg 1996;84:365
10. Flickinger JC, Kondziolka D, Pollock BE, Maitz AH, Lunsford LD. Complications from arteriovenous malformation radiosurgery: multivariate analysis and risk modeling. Int J Radiat Oncol Biol Phys 1997;38:485–490
11. Lunsford LD, Kondziolka D, Flickinger JC, et al. Stereotactic radiosurgery for arteriovenous malformations of the brain. J Neurosurg 1991;75:512–524
12. Colombo F, Pozza F, Chierego G, Casentini L, De Luca G, Francescon P. Linear accelerator radiosurgery of cerebral arteriovenous malformations: an update. Neurosurgery 1994;34:14–21

Suggested Readings

Friedman W, Bova F. Linear accelerator radiosurgery for arteriovenous malformations. J Neurosurg 1992;77:832–841

Friedman W, Bova F, Mendenhall W. Linear accelerator radiosurgery for arteriovenous malformations: the relationship of size to outcome. J Neurosurg 1995;82:180–189

Kjellberg R. Proton beam therapy for arteriovenous malformations of the brain. In: Schmidek H, Sweet W, eds. Operative Neurosurgical Techniques: Indications, Methods, and Results. Philadelphia: WB Saunders; ; 1988:911–915

Kondziolka D, Lunsford LD, Flickinger JC. Intraparenchymal brain stem radiosurgery. Neurosurg Clin N Am 1993;4:469–479

Pollock BE, Lunsford LD, Kondziolka D, Maitz A, Flickinger JC. Patient outcomes after stereotactic radiosurgery for "operable" arteriovenous malformations. Neurosurgery 1994;35:1–8

Steiner L, Lindquist C, Adler JR, Torner JC, Alves W, Steiner M. Clinical outcome of radiosurgery for cerebral arteriovenous malformations. J Neurosurg 1992;77:1–8

23

Cavernous Malformations of the Brain

Robert C. Rostomily, Laligam N. Sekhar, and Foad Elahi

Classification

The cavernous malformation (CM) is also known as cavernoma, cavernous angioma, or cavernous hemangioma. It is one of a larger group of vascular lesions collectively known as the angiographically occult vascular malformations (AOVMs). AOVMs consist of CMs, arteriovenous malformations (AVMs), capillary telangiectasias, developmental venous anomalies (also referred to as venous angiomas or venous malformations), and mixed types. An increase in detection by magnetic resonance imaging (MRI) has renewed interest in these lesions and fostered a better understanding of their distinct pathological and clinical characteristics and natural history as well as the role of surgery in their management.

Each of these pathological subtypes of AOVMs has a distinct natural history and clinical significance. Capillary telangiectasias are rarely symptomatic and consist of capillaries with intervening normal neural tissue. They are usually found incidentally at autopsy and thus are not considered surgical lesions. Developmental venous anomalies (DVAs) are variants of normal venous drainage; their historical inclusion in the AOVM group is technically incorrect because most can be visualized with angiography.[1] DVAs are rarely considered for surgery because they represent normal venous drainage, they rarely bleed, and in the setting of hemorrhage they are associated with CMs in as many as 20 to 30% of cases.[2] In a recent series of patients with CMs of the brain stem, all 86 patients who underwent resection had an associated DVA found at operation.[3] Angiographically occult true AVMs are rare and represent small "micro-AVMs" or AVMs that are thrombosed or compressed by hemorrhage and are managed as any AVM would be.[4] This chapter focuses on the surgical management of adult cerebral and brain stem cavernomas. The general features of the different AOVMs are summarized in **Table 23–1.**

CMs are benign AOVMs with an estimated prevalence of 0.4–0.8%[5] that represent ~5–13% of all intracranial vascular lesions.[6] They occur equally in men and women and present between the ages of 20 and 40.[5] The location of CMs seems to be distributed in proportion to tissue volume such that about three quarters of the lesions are supratentorial,[7,8] 15% are in the posterior fossa and 5% spinal. Of the supratentorial lesions, ~5% are located deep in the diencephalon or septal area.[8] In the posterior fossa, lesions in the cerebellum and brain stem occur with equal frequency and the pons is the most common brain stem location for a CM. Other rarer sites for CMs include

Table 23–1 Angiographically Occult Vascular Malformations (AOVMs)

Type	Histology	Risk for Hemorrhage?	Potential Surgical Lesion?
Capillary telangiectasia	Normal capillaries Intervening brain	No	No
Developmental venous anomaly (DVA)	Variant drainage of normal veins	Low (majority due to another associated AOVM)	Rare
Arteriovenous malformation (AVM)	Collection of abnormal arteries and veins	Yes	Yes
Cavernous malformation (CM)	Compact epithelial sinusoids	Yes	Yes
Mixed	Variable	Yes	Only AVM or CM component

Table 23–2 General Features of Cavernous Malformations

Location	Proportional to tissue volume ~ 75% supratentorial
Sex predilection	Male = Female
Age	Majority between 10–40 years
Familial	30–50%
Multiple	50–80% familial; 20% sporadic
Presentation	Incidental (11–44%)
	Headache (6–50%)
	Overt bleed (8–37%)
	Seizure/epilepsy (20–50%)
	Neurological deficit (20–50%)
Hemorrhage risk (annualized)	0.6–0.7%
Rehemorrhage risk (annualized)	4.5%
Risk factors for hemorrhage	Female, pregnancy, brain stem, prior bleed, associated developmental venous anomaly
Factors not associated with hemorrhage	Size, multiplicity, familial

the optic nerves and chiasm,[9,10] cranial nerves,[11] cerebellopontine angle,[12] and cavernous sinus.[13] **Table 23–2** displays a summary of the general clinical features of CMs.

◆ Pathology

CMs are slow-flow AOVMs that consist of thin-walled, single-cell layer epithelial sinusoids devoid of elastic or muscular tissue arranged in a compact trabecular architecture fed by a varying number of small blood vessels.[2,14] A discrete gliotic border separates CMs from adjacent brain tissue. Neural tissue is generally only apparent at the periphery of lesions, although intervening neural tissue has been described in a "racemose" type.[15] Within the CM are varying degrees of thrombosis, cyst formation, hyalinization, hemorrhage, and calcification, whereas hemosiderin-laden macrophages line the gliotic capsule. Grossly, they vary in size from millimeters to several centimeters and resemble a cluster of small grapes or a raspberry with multiple lobules. The adjacent brain is stained yellow or green from blood breakdown products. The presence of mixed types of AOVMs (most commonly CM and DVA) suggests that these lesions may be part of a clinical spectrum of vascular malformations with similar pathogenesis, or that they can arise independently in close proximity.[2,16,17]

CMs are familial in ~30 to 50% of cases.[18] Multiple lesions occur in 50 to 80% of familial cases but in only ~20% of sporadic cases.[5,19] The majority of familial cases investigated to date have been traced to a founder mutation on chromosome 7[20] but in some cases other genetic loci appear to be involved.[21] CMs have been considered congenital lesions and most studies of their natural history have calculated hemorrhage risks based on this assumption. However, documentation of de novo lesions in patients with a familial syndrome,[22,23] the sporadic form,[24] or who have undergone irradiation for an unrelated reason,[25] suggests that mechanisms for the development of acquired lesions exist. Although cavernomas are not considered neoplastic, they can enlarge, sometimes dramatically, and become symptomatic, presumably through a process of repeated hemorrhage, thrombosis, hyalinization, and recanalization.[26–30] Recent studies of CMs that have reported proliferative activity[31] and expression of angiogenic growth factors such as vascular endothelial growth factors (VEGFs)[32] additionally suggest that the biology of these lesions is more complex and dynamic than was previously appreciated.

◆ Natural History

Patients with CMs can present with seizures, headache, hemorrhage, and neurological deficits related to hemorrhage or mass effect or as asymptomatic incidental findings. The incidence of each presentation ranges from 11 to 44% for asymptomatic patients, 6 to 50% with headache, 20 to 50% for seizures, overt hemorrhage in 8 to 37% versus any form of hemorrhage in up to 50% of patients, whereas neurological deficits are seen in ~20 to 50% of patients.[5,19] Hemorrhage from CMs is generally not catastrophic because these are slow-flow lesions unless they are in a crucial location such as the brain stem.

The determination of CM natural history is important to devising rational management protocols. Natural history studies have focused on hemorrhage rates, but the evolution of seizure disorders or other patient events must be considered as well when weighing the role of surgery. In addition, the natural history of special subgroups such as brain stem or deep cortical lesions and assessment of predictors of CMs that display particularly aggressive courses are also relevant when selecting surgical candidates.

In retrospective studies based on identification of patients from large databases of MRI images and assumptions that lesions are all congenital, Robinson et al reported an annualized bleeding rate of 0.7% with a significantly greater risk of overt hemorrhage in females.[8] In a similar study by Del Curling et al the estimated risk of hemorrhage was 0.25%/person-year of exposure and the estimated risk of seizure development was 1.51%/person-year.[33] In a prospective study by Kondziolka et al, the retrospective annual hemorrhage rate (61 bleeds/4550.6 patient-years of life) was 1.3%. In patients without a prior bleed, the prospective annual rate of hemorrhage was 0.6%, whereas patients with prior hemorrhage had an annual bleed rate of 4.5%.[34] A comprehensive literature review of factors affecting natural history by Maraire and Awad identified female sex, pregnancy, age (bimodal; pediatric population and > 30 years of age), brain stem location, and prior bleed as factors that seem to increase the risks of hemorrhage.[19] Not all studies have confirmed these generalizations, however, and Kondziolka et al could not demonstrate a correlation between hemorrhage and gender or location.[34] A recent analysis found an association in CM patients between the presence of DVAs and symptomatic bleeds, repeated symptomatic bleeds, posterior fossa location, and female sex.[35] Factors that do not seem to be associated with increased hemorrhage risk include lesion size,[19] multiplicity, or familial forms.[19,22,34]

The increased hemorrhage risk of brain stem CMs is supported by data from two large retrospective studies. Fritschi et al published the largest analysis of brain stem CMs, which includes a series of 41 patients treated by the authors and an additional 98 abstracted from the literature.[36] This retrospective series estimates a minimum bleeding rate of 2.7% per year and an average rebleeding rate of 21% per year and per lesion. Of the 138 patients, 88% had evidence of recent or previous bleeds with 55% having had one, two, and three or more bleeds in 55%, 17%, and 17%, respectively. Of 12 patients who died from a bleed, five expired after the first hemorrhage and seven after subsequent bleeds.[36] In another recent, large study of 100 patients, the retrospective annual hemorrhage rate was estimated at 5% per lesion per year.[3] Thus, brain stem CMs appear to behave in a manner distinct from cerebral CMs, and their propensity to rebleed and produce catastrophic neurological deficits or death must be factored into management decisions.

Most of the available natural history data relates to the incidence of overt hemorrhage without consideration of the clinical significance of an overt hemorrhage. Because the functional impact of a bleed is dependent on multiple factors such as lesion location, hemorrhage size, and patient condition, the decision to operate must be individualized using current natural history data as a guideline. Although one study reports a 1.5% rate of seizure development per patient-year,[33] the precise natural history of epilepsy in CM patients is not well understood. Another unanswered question relates to the natural history of asymptomatic lesions found to enlarge on serial imaging studies.

◆ Indications

The indications for surgery and the type of surgery are individualized based on the patient's symptoms, lesion location, patient condition, and consideration of the natural history when untreated. The main indications for resection are symptomatic rupture and hemorrhage, seizures or medically intractable epilepsy, and the presence of neurological deficits produced from mass effect. Most patients with incidental CMs or those who present with headache alone should be followed clinically and with serial imaging studies. The indications for surgical resection of CMs is outlined in **Table 23–3** and discussed in more detail following here.

Hemorrhage

In cases of frank symptomatic hemorrhage, surgery is indicated if the lesion is accessible or is likely to produce a permanent deficit upon rebleeding. In noneloquent cortical

Table 23–3 Cavernous Malformations: Indications for Surgery

Hemorrhage
Seizure/epilepsy
Mass effect
Neurological deficit
Anticipated pregnancy

areas a routine excision is performed, whereas lesions near speech, language, motor, sensory, or memory areas, or deeper cortical or subcortical lesions can be resected with the aid of pre- or intraoperative functional localization, frameless stereotactic navigation, stereotactic craniotomy, or ultrasound localization.

Seizure/Epilepsy

Patients with medically intractable epilepsy or seizures and CMs should be considered for surgery. Although good prospective data are not available, medical management alone is often unable to provide adequate seizure control for patients with CM.[37] In one study of CM natural history, 50% of patients had seizures, of which ~60% were controlled on medication and 40% were refractory to medication.[34] However, whether this profile changes over time is not known.

For CM patients with epilepsy, it is controversial whether a formal epilepsy evaluation and surgical resection aimed at identifying and resecting specific epileptic foci significantly improves seizure control versus lesionectomy alone. The controversy is based on the following observations: (1) independent seizure foci can disappear after lesionectomy, (2) seizures can be cured after lesionectomy despite the persistence of electroencephalographic (EEG) abnormalities, and (3) seizures can persist after successful lesionectomy. This latter situation has been hypothesized to be due to the presence of a persistent independent seizure focus, "dual pathology" such as concurrent CM with mesial temporal sclerosis, residual CM, or postoperative scar.[37] However, based on recent surgical series there is an emerging consensus as to the best approach.

The surgical options for patients with CM and epilepsy include lesionectomy alone, lesionectomy with resection of glial scar, or concurrent lesion and epileptic focus resection. The latter option requires some form of extra- or intraoperative electrophysiological evaluation to identify the seizure focus. Lesionectomy alone is most effective when performed prior to the development of an established chronic or medically intractable epileptic condition. For patients operated on "early" (generally within the first 12 months of seizure onset or before the occurrence of five seizures), 80 to 100% of cases who had lesionectomy had seizure-free outcomes, whereas those operated on "later" (some with medically intractable epilepsy) were seizure-free in only ~50 to 70% of cases.[38–41] In two of these series, no additional benefit for seizure control was found by resecting the glial scar surrounding the CM.[39,41] The reported results of lesionectomy alone for seizure control are summarized in **Table 23–4**.

Thus, lesionectomy alone is a reasonable option for patients with a short duration and small number of seizures. A more extensive seizure evaluation with monitoring and resection of epileptic cortex should be considered for those patients with longer histories, medically intractable epilepsy, or lack of concordance between localization of seizure onset (by semiology or EEG findings) and CM location. In a meta-analysis by Weber et al, of patients with medically intractable epilepsy and structural lesions, seizure focus resection in addition to lesionectomy increased seizure-free rates at 2 years.[42] Thus the decision to operate and choice of surgical approach remain somewhat controversial and must be tailored to each patient.

Mass Effect

Although most cavernomas are less than 2 cm, some can attain large size (4–5 cm) and produce symptoms through mass effect on adjacent neural tissue. In addition, a small percentage of cavernomas enlarge over time and become symptomatic.[27,29] Symptomatic lesions producing mass effect should be resected if possible, whereas asymptomatic lesions that enlarge on serial imaging studies provide a relative indication for surgical resection.

Neurological Deficits

Patients who present with neurological deficits should be considered for CM resection because the deficits improve in many cases and the risk of permanent worsening from

Table 23–4 Lesionectomy Alone and Seizure Outcome

Study	Follow-up	Grouping	% Seizure-Free
Cappabianca et al, 1997[38]	2 years	< 5 seizures and/or < 12 months' duration	100
		> 5 seizures and/or > 12 months' duration	62.5
Cohen et al, 1995[40]	> 1 year	1 seizure; < 2 months' duration	100
		2–5 seizures; 2–12 months' duration	75–80
		> 5 seizures; duration > 12 months	50–55
Casazza et al, 1996[39]*	> 2 years	"Sporadic seizures" Mean duration1.5 years	88.5
		"Chronic epilepsy" Mean duration 5.3 years	62
Zevgaridis et al, 1996[41]*	1–9 years	< 2 years' duration	95.8
		> 2 years' duration	76.7

*Resection of glial scar did not improve outcome.

surgery is relatively low.[43,44] Chaskis and Brotchi reported 26 of 34 patients with preoperative neurological deficits were improved after surgery; 12 totally, five moderately, and nine slightly.[43] In another study by Amin-Hanjani et al, the neurological outcome was greatly influenced by lesion location, but overall 16.5% of patients improved whereas 5.2% worsened.[44]

Anticipated Pregnancy

Women under the age of 40 seem to present more often with hemorrhage, whereas men are more likely to have seizures. Aiba et al found an increased risk of hemorrhage in females and hypothesized that a hormonal factor is related to lesion expansion and hemorrhage.[45] Two studies have demonstrated a marked predilection not only for hemorrhage presenting in women (75% and 86%), but also for pregnancy in these patients (66% and 33%, respectively).[8,46] Thus the resection of known lesions in women contemplating pregnancy may be relatively indicated, particularly for lesions near eloquent brain that are likely to produce significant morbidity with hemorrhage or growth.

◆ Treatment

Aside from surgery, radiotherapy is the only other potential treatment option for patients with CMs. Stereotactic radiosurgery (SRS) has been used at several centers for surgically inaccessible or risky lesions.[47–49] Some recent data suggest a significant reduction in annual rebleed rates from ~30 to 35% to ~9% after the first 2 to 3 years and 1 to 2% thereafter.[48,49] However, other reports question whether this reduction in bleeding rate is due to a true protective effect of radiosurgery or simply a reflection of the CM natural history.[50] In one series, this improvement in rebleed rate was not accompanied by reduction in lesion size.[48] Worsening neurological status related to perilesional edema that responded to steroids was reported in 12% of patients in one series[49] and symptomatic radiation edema or necrosis in 9% of patients in another series.[48] However, in another study the permanent complication rate for radiosurgery of deep inoperable CMs was 41%.[50] This rate was significantly higher than that for AVMs of similar size and location that were treated with radiosurgery at the same institution. Clearly, longer-term follow-up and additional studies of CM natural history are needed to assess the efficacy and usefulness of SRS in treating CM.

◆ Imaging

Prior to surgery every patient should have an MRI study. This study not only confirms the diagnosis of CM, it also provides the anatomical detail necessary to assess the potential for involvement of eloquent cortex, important subcortical structures, unrecognized additional lesions, and the presence of other associated vascular anomalies. In most cases it is sufficient to evaluate the anatomy of associated DVAs that must be preserved during resection of CMs. These anatomical relationships are particularly important in the brain stem where one series has reported a 100% incidence of DVAs in association with CMs.[3] Specific MRI characteristics have also been associated with the presence of angiographically occult AVMs[51] and the probability of rehemorrhage.[52]

Computed tomographic scans are useful for planning skull base approaches to deep cortical lesions or brain stem lesions but add little to the evaluation of cortical CMs. Preoperative angiography can be useful to rule out an associated AVM, better define venous drainage patterns around CMs with associated DVAs, or assist in surgical planning for skull base approaches where the location and dominance of major draining veins or sinuses is crucial. It can also be used in conjunction with a Wada evaluation to confirm cerebral dominance for language. The use of functional MRI (fMRI) can help confirm the relationship of the CM to sensorimotor or language cortex and thus alert the surgeon to the need for specialized intraoperative monitoring or specific surgical approaches to spare vital structures.

◆ Surgical Technique

There are no special considerations in positioning for patients with cavernomas other than what is considered standard for the approach of choice for a particular lesion. Anesthetic plans should allow for appropriate neurophysiological monitoring. Cortical lesions in noneloquent brain do not require monitoring unless the lesion is large or prolonged retraction is required, in which case, cortical somatosensory evoked potential (SEP) monitoring can be helpful in assessing the effects of brain retraction and alter surgical technique to minimize injury. Resection of cortical lesions near eloquent brain can be assisted by identification and monitoring of motor/sensory or speech/language sites. Additional sensitivity can be gained by performing the resection with the patient awake using propofol sedation.[53] Various centers have different protocols and techniques for accomplishing this type of mapping and monitoring, and it is beyond the scope of this chapter to detail these techniques; the reader is referred to the review by Mueller and Morris.[54] Brain stem resections should be monitored during surgery for brain stem auditory evoked responses (BAERs), SEPs, directed cranial function with electromyographs (EMGs), and, occasionally, monopolar stimulation to identify adjacent motor nuclei.

Approach

The choice of approach should provide a generous exposure that allows adequate direct visualization of the lesion and associated venous malformations as well as the course of nearby vessels that must occasionally be extensively dissected to ensure that they are either en passage or contributing to the malformation.

Dissection

The dissection of the cavernoma, which grossly resembles a cluster of grapes, begins at its most superficial location. If the lesion is subcortical, the most direct path with the smallest corticectomy is preferred unless this path transgresses functional brain. Frameless stereotaxis is used in most patients with subcortical lesions. The gliotic capsule is identified and a plane is developed between the lesion and capsule with blunt dissection. The lesion is gently retracted toward its center and coagulated with bipolar cautery to reduce its mass and aid in the dissection. There are usually several small feeding vessels that can be coagulated and divided as the dissection continues. Large lesions, particularly those in critical areas such as the brain stem, can be removed piecemeal (3–4 pieces). This technique can provide central debulking and reduce the amount of manipulation of adjacent normal tissue.

Complete removal of the CM is the goal of surgery. Small amoebalike extensions or associated lobules can be difficult to detect and account for a significant number of cases where rehemorrhage occurs. Although not necessary, the removal of the capsule can help ensure that removal is complete. Capsular resection of hemosiderin-stained tissue has been advocated in lesionectomy for seizures because of the presumed irritant effect of the hemoglobin breakdown products on the surrounding cortex. However, some studies have not found that this necessarily leads to improved seizure control.[39,41] Resection of the capsule is absolutely contraindicated for brain stem lesions or cavernomas in eloquent cortex and relatively contraindicated for lesions adjacent to eloquent cortex. A recent study has demonstrated the utility of color-flow Doppler ultrasonography to assist in lesion localization and identification of DVAs and to determine completeness of resection intraoperatively.[55] The general principles of surgical technique for resection of CMs are outlined in **Table 23–5**.

Table 23–5 Cavernous Malformations: Principles of Surgical Resection

General
Complete resection (may be facilitated by capsule removal)
Lesion localization (intraoperative navigation or ultrasound for deep lesions)
Careful Inspection of resection cavity for remnants or associated lobules
Preservation of associated developmental venous anomalies
Small corticectomy (transgyral or transsulcal), short path length
Piecemeal debulking (3–4 fragments) if large
Brain Stem
Only resect exophytic or rarely intrinsic lesions with thin rim of overlying tissue
Do not resect gliotic capsule
Use cranial base approaches to maximize exposure
Intraoperative brain stem and cranial nerve monitoring

Brain Stem Cavernous Malformations

Approximately 15 to 20% of all pathologically proven CMs are localized in the brain stem. The treatment of brain stem CMs is controversial, but the success reported in several recent surgical series[3,6,44] supports the rationale for surgical resection to avoid recurrent hemorrhage, regrowth, severe disability, or even death.[56] The indications for surgery include a single or repetitive hemorrhage, presence of neurological signs or symptoms, documentation of lesion growth (relative), or need for prophylactic measures (controversial). In addition, the lesion must be accessible through one of the brain stem pial surfaces. Contraindications for surgery include asymptomatic lesions, particularly those that are small ($\leq$ 1 cm), and in a deep location. Although patients with CMs that are candidates for treatment but not surgery due to general health or lesion location can be considered for SRS (see earlier discussion in the Alternative Treatment section), there is no proven benefit for this approach and there is a significant risk of treatment-related morbidity.

The preoperative evaluation must include careful neurological evaluation of cranial nerve (CN), long tract, and cerebellar function. Patients with preexisting deficits of the lower CNs may be candidates for either or both tracheostomy and feeding jejunostomies prior to or at the time of surgery. All patients should have preoperative testing to determine their suitability for specialized monitoring. Intraoperative monitoring includes bilateral SEPs, BAERs, and CNs III, VI, VII, and XII with electromyography and direct stimulation as needed.[57] The surgical approaches used for resection of brain stem cavernomas are outlined in **Table 23–6** and illustrated in **Fig. 23–1**.

Table 23–6 Surgical Approaches to the Brain Stem

Posterior
Supracerebellar
Combined supra- and infratentorial transsinus
Subtonsillar-transcerebellomedullary
Midline transvermian
Posterolateral
Retrosigmoid
Transsigmoid
Extreme lateral, transcondylar
Lateral
Subtemporal-transzygomatic
Petrosal
Partial labyrinthectomy
Retrolabyrinthine
Translabyrinthine
Anterolateral
Orbitozygomatic-transsylvian
Anterior
Transmaxillary-transoral

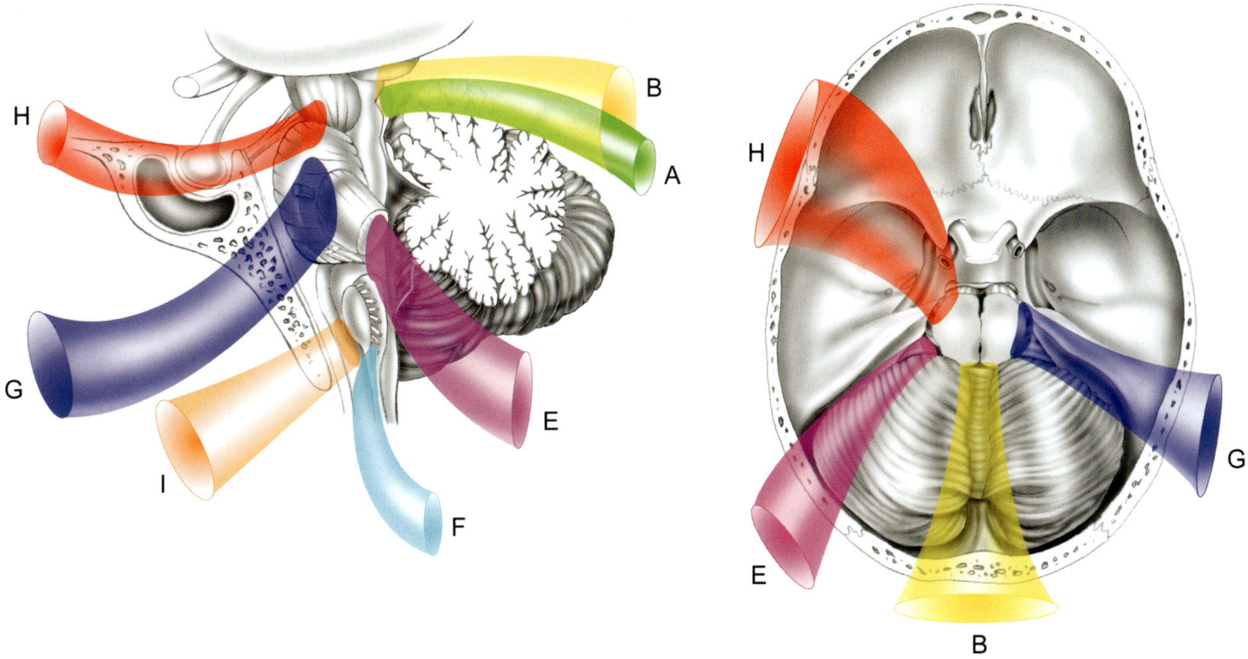

Figure 23–1 Artist's drawing summarizing surgical approaches to the brain stem cavernoma in sagittal (left) and axial (right) orientations. A, supracerebellar infratentorial; B, combined supra- and infratentorial-trans-sinus; C, subtonsillar-transcerebellomedullary; D, midline transvermian; E, retrosigmoid; F, extreme lateral, transcondylar; G, petrosal; H, orbitozygomatic-transsylvian; I, transmaxillary-transoral. (Adapted from Ziyal IM, et al. Surgical management of cavernous malformations of the brain stem. Br J Neurosurg 1999;13:366–375 with permission).

Posterior Approaches

The posterior approaches to the brain stem are used for collicular plate or fourth ventricular lesions that are exophytic or immediately subpial. The supracerebellar or combined supra- and infratentorial trans-sinus approaches are appropriate for collicular lesions. A transvermian approach is necessary for midline fourth ventricular lesions. Excessive splitting of the vermis is avoided to prevent permanent truncal ataxia. Pontomedullary junction and medullary lesions in the lateral aspect of the fourth ventricle can be resected with a subtonsillar-transcerebellomedullary approach. In this approach, the cerebellar tonsil is mobilized and the cerebellomedullary fissure is opened without splitting the cerebellar vermis.

Posterolateral Approaches

A far lateral retrosigmoid approach is indicated for pontomedullary lesions that present in the middle or inferior cerebellar peduncles or in the olivary area. The extreme-lateral transcondylar or retrocondylar approach provides access to the lateral and anterolateral surface of the medulla, as well as the cervicomedullary junction. Some medullary lesions may be accessed by combining the retro- and presigmoid approach with the section of a nondominant sigmoid sinus. However, when the lesion is located in the cervicomedullary area and presents anteriorly in the midline, the exposure provided may still be inadequate.

Lateral and Anterolateral Approaches

The petrosal approach, either retrolabyrinthine, partial labyrinthine, or translabyrinthine, can be used to expose lesions of the anterior or anterolateral pons or lateral midbrain.

Lesions that present close to the anterior surface of the midbrain are best removed by a frontotemporal, orbitozygomatic, trans-sylvian, or anterior subtemporal approach.

Anterior Approaches

Both transmaxillary and transoral approaches can be utilized for CMs in the anterior and midline brain stem, but these approaches should be used sparingly because of the great risk of cerebrospinal fluid (CSF) leakage and infection. Careful intraoperative repair and protracted lumbar CSF drainage are essential to promote healing.

Operative Strategy

Upon exposing the brain stem, the normal anatomical structures should be localized. In the floor of the fourth ventricle, it is useful to stimulate the CN nuclei (especially the facial) while observing EMG recordings. However, the normal anatomy of brain stem structures may be distorted or even involved by the lesion, which compromises the usefulness of this technique for subpial lesions under the floor of the fourth ventricle.[3] Usually a slight discoloration on the pial surface will lead to the lesion. A small opening (≤ 1 cm) is then created in the brain stem, through which the lesion is initially debulked and then removed completely. When approaching the lesion through the anterior or lateral surface of the brain stem, perforating arteries that run through or adjoin the lesion must be carefully preserved. In addition, "safe" zones for ventral entry through the medullary anterolateral sulcus and paramedian sagittal pons have been outlined for CMs.[58] Many CMs in the posterior fossa are associated with DVAs that must be carefully preserved. CMs appear like a cluster of grapes, with amoebalike extensions into different areas of the adjoining brain stem. A hemorrhagic, gliotic plane around the cavernoma enables its safe removal, but it is not present in all cases. Therefore, the surgeon must strike a balance between complete removal of the lesion and avoidance of permanent neurological deficits. This trade-off is guided in part by intraoperative monitoring. Changes in the SEP or BAER signal the surgeon to stop manipulation of the lesion, further debulk it, or change the working area. Such deterioration is usually due to the compression of normal brain stem structures. At the conclusion of the resection, hemostatic material is left in the resection cavity only if necessary because it may confound the interpretation of postoperative MRI.

◆ Postoperative Care

All patients are monitored in the intensive care unit for airway, respiratory, and cardiac rhythm abnormalities. Dysfunction of CNs IX, X, or the medulla may impair swallowing and coughing. An arytenoid adduction procedure and a percutaneous jejunostomy are performed for unilateral paralysis of CNs IX and X, and a tracheostomy and a jejunostomy are performed for bilateral problems. Dysfunction of the cranial nerves is usually temporary, allowing for removal of tubes after several months. A postoperative CT scan is performed to rule out a hematoma or hydrocephalus, and a follow-up MRI at 3 months helps ensure that the resection is complete.

◆ Results

In the senior author's (LNS) personal series of 10 patients with brain stem cavernomas (nine reported by Ziyal et al[6]), six different surgical approaches were employed depending on the location and the extension of the lesion in the brain stem. In eight patients there was complete resection with excellent or good outcome. One patient with an incompletely resected large medullary cavernoma had asymptomatic recurrence after 1 year. In the absence of symptoms the patient will be followed conservatively. In contrast, another patient deteriorated after rebleeding and attempted resection of an initially subtotally resected large pontomesencephalic CM. The patient's poor outcome may be related to the size and location of the lesion, and injury to the cerebellar vermis or nuclei and tracts in the dorsal midbrain. These results point out the aggressive nature of many brain stem CMs and the importance of complete resection when possible.

Cases

Case 1

This 46-year-old female had four previous bleeds and presented with ataxia, left hemiparesis, and ptosis. The lesion primarily involved the pons and midbrain and was dorsally exophytic (**Fig. 23–2A,B**) Resection was performed through a midline transvermian approach. Residual cavernoma is present in the left cerebral peduncle (**Fig. 23–2C,D**). The patient had one clinically significant postoperative bleed and has persistent hemiparesis, urinary incontinence, and swallowing difficulty. This case points out the importance of achieving a total resection if possible. This was also a patient with the largest brain stem cavernoma treated by the senior author, and may have been impossible to excise totally without morbidity.

Case 2

This 62-year-old male presented at the time of his initial bleed with imbalance, dysphagia, diplopia, and right foot drop. Preoperative MRI showed a pontomedullary junction, dorsally situated cavernoma (**Fig. 23–3A**). Of note, the lesion presented at the pial surface posteriorly and thus could be approached surgically. A subtonsillar transcerebellomedullary approach was used to resect the lesion totally (**Fig. 23–3B**). Postoperative images show a complete excision of the lesion. Some residual enhancement is thought to be scar tissue. He has had no further bleeds and made a near total recovery except for mild ataxia, diplopia, and sexual dysfunction.

Case 3

This 46-year-old male had suffered two prior bleeds and presented with left-sided pain, numbness, and weakness. MRI showed a cavernoma of the right lateral medulla that presented at the pial surface (**Fig. 23–4A–C**). A far lateral retrosigmoid approach was used to achieve a total resection (**Fig. 23–4D**). He has had no further bleeds and has made a full recovery except for slight swallowing difficulty and persistent body and face pain.

Case 4

This 55-year-old female presented with two prior bleeds and had a left hemiparesis and right third nerve palsy. A large cavernoma was demonstrated on MRI in the right cerebral peduncle (**Fig. 23–5A–D**). This was completely resected through

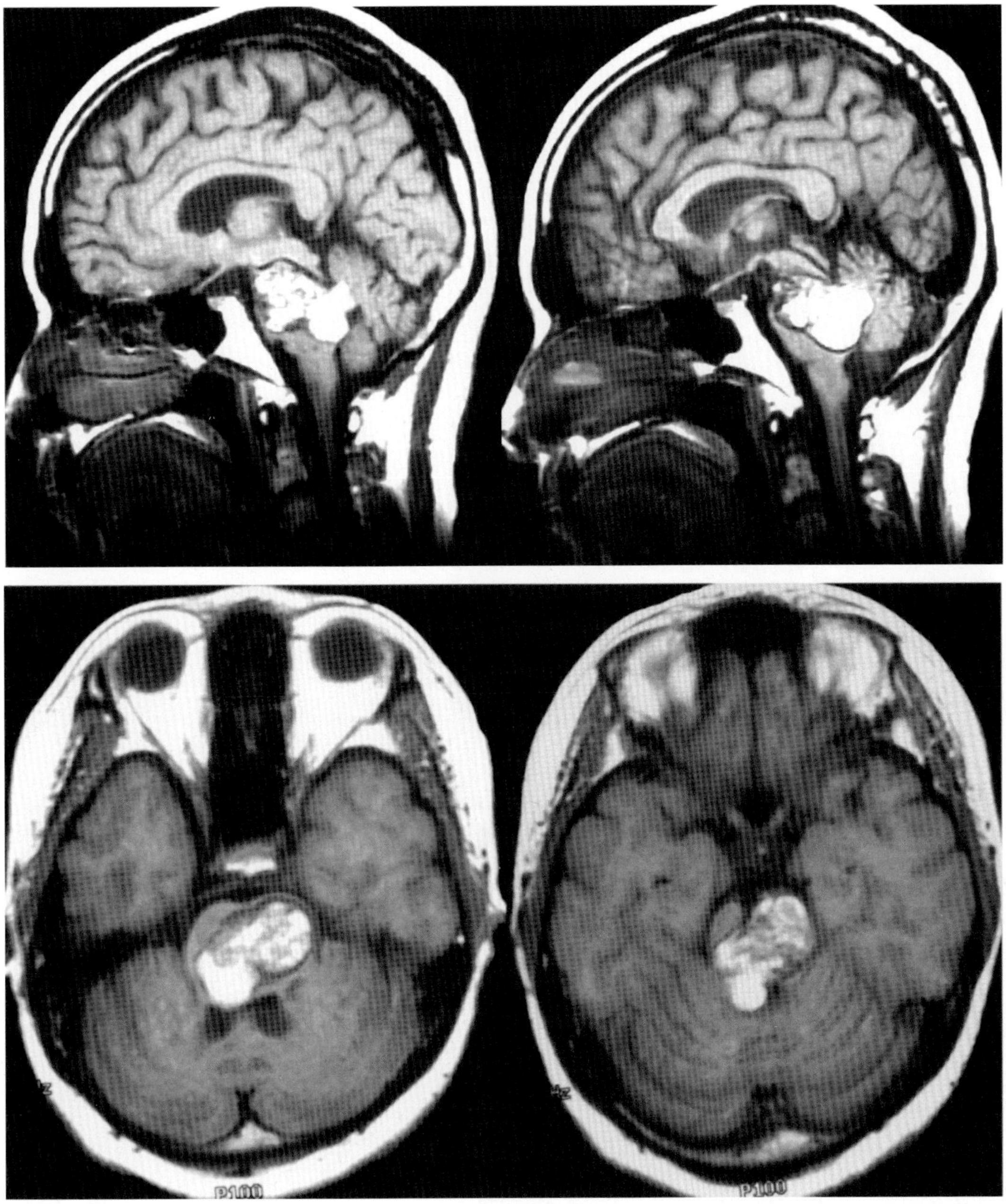

A

B

Figure 23–2 Case 1. **(A,B)** A giant midbrain and pontine cavernous hemangioma.

(*Continued on page 294*)

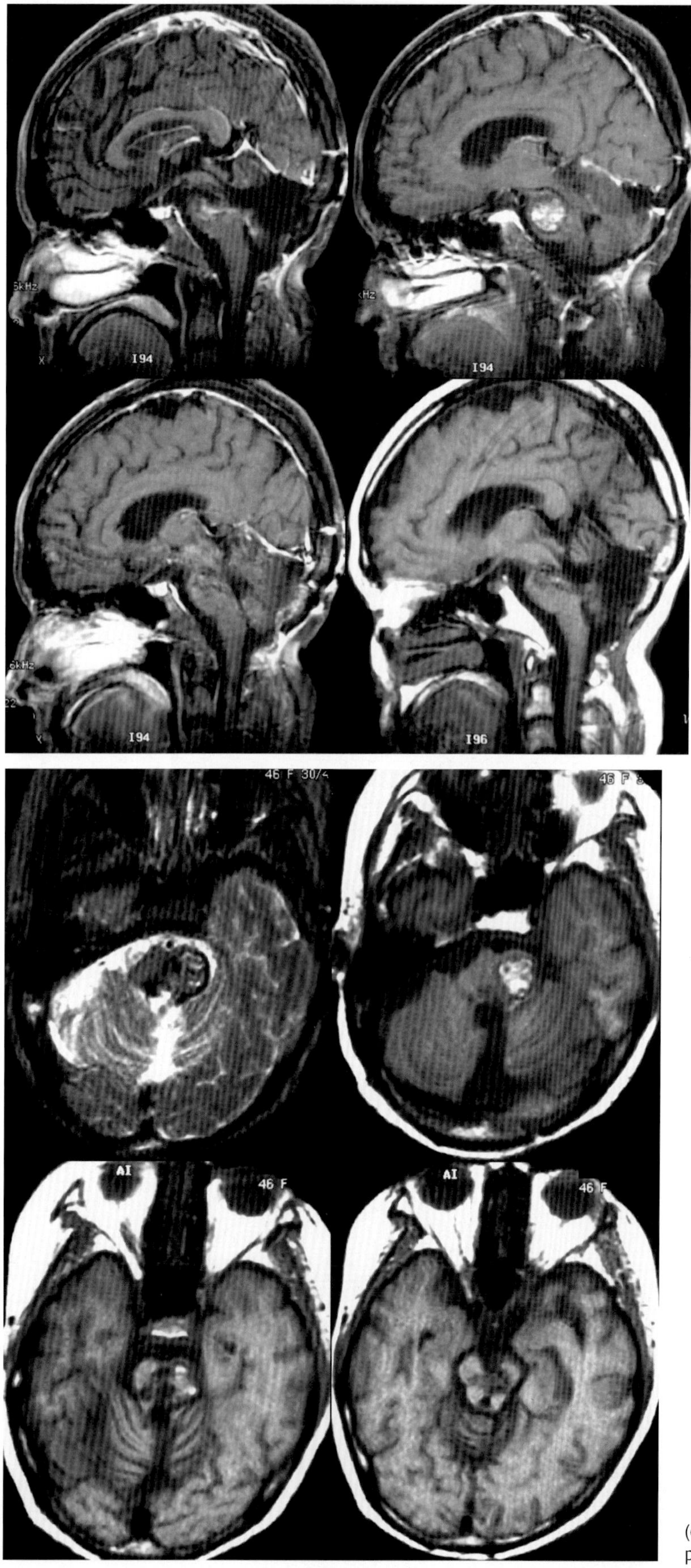

C

D

(*Continued*) **Figure 23–2 (C,D)** After two operations in this patient, postoperative images show residual cavernoma.

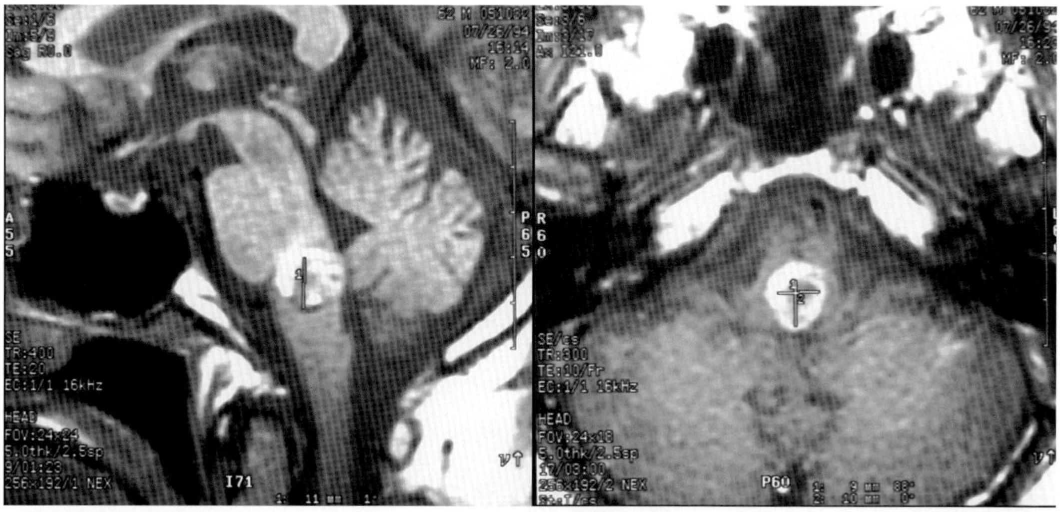

A

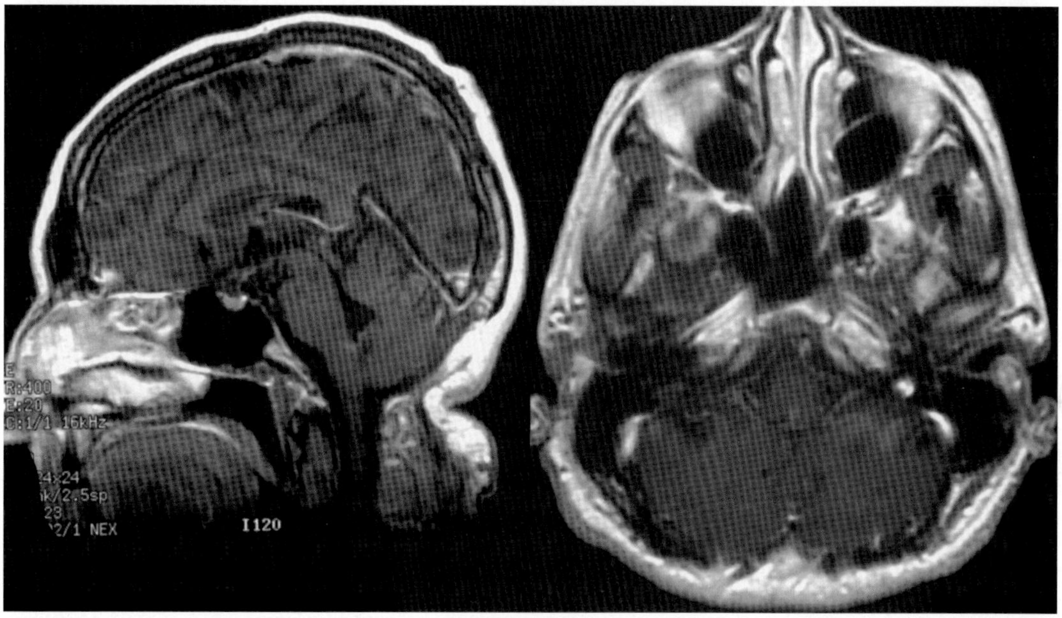

B

Figure 23–3 Case 2. **(A)** A dorsally situated pontomedullary junction cavernoma, approachable through the fourth ventricle. **(B)** Postoperative images show complete resection.

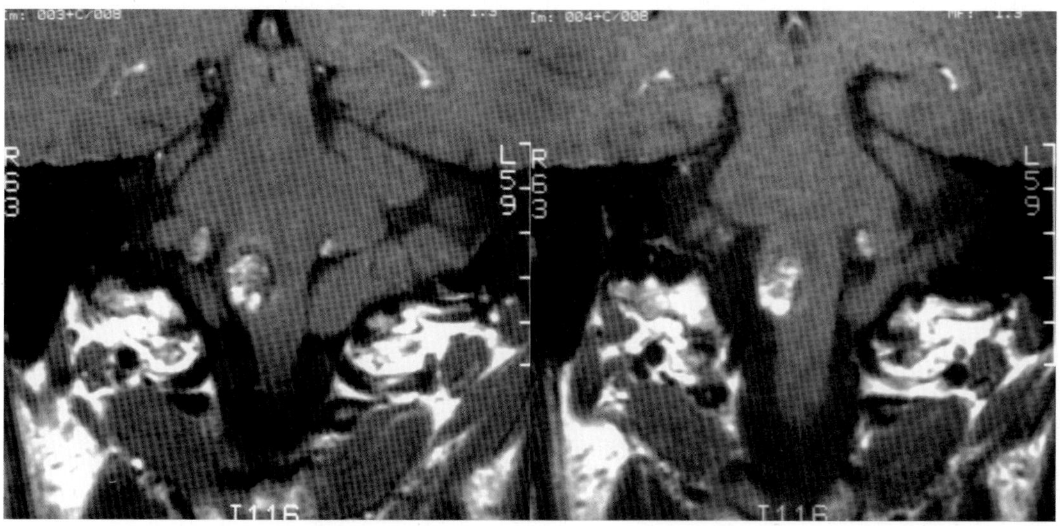

A

(*Continued on page 296*)

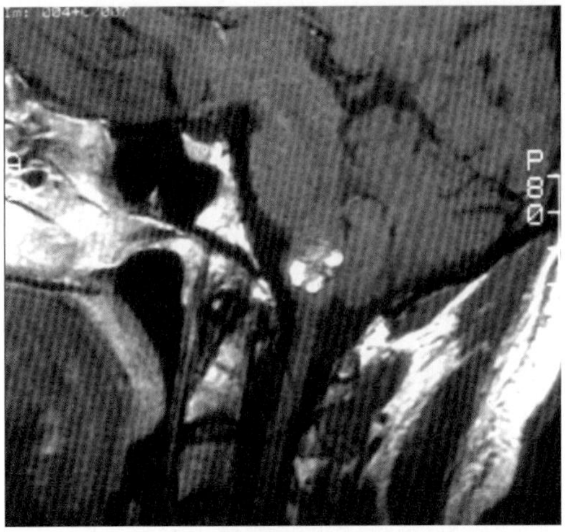

B

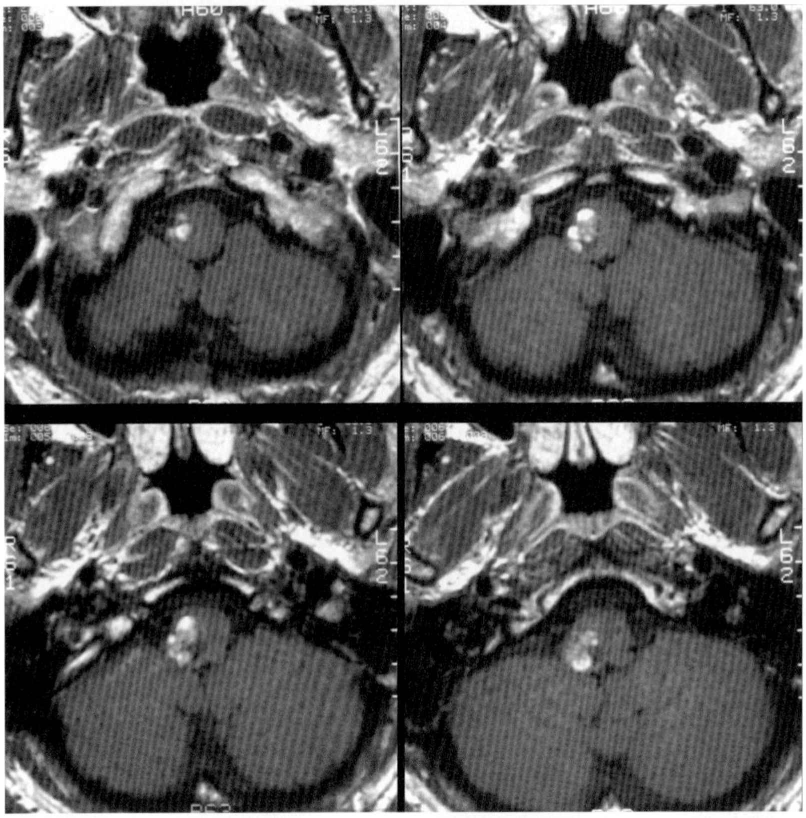

C

(*Continued*) **Figure 23–4** Case 3. **(A–C)** Patient with a lateral medullary cavernoma. **(D)** Postoperative images after excision by a far lateral retrosigmoid approach.

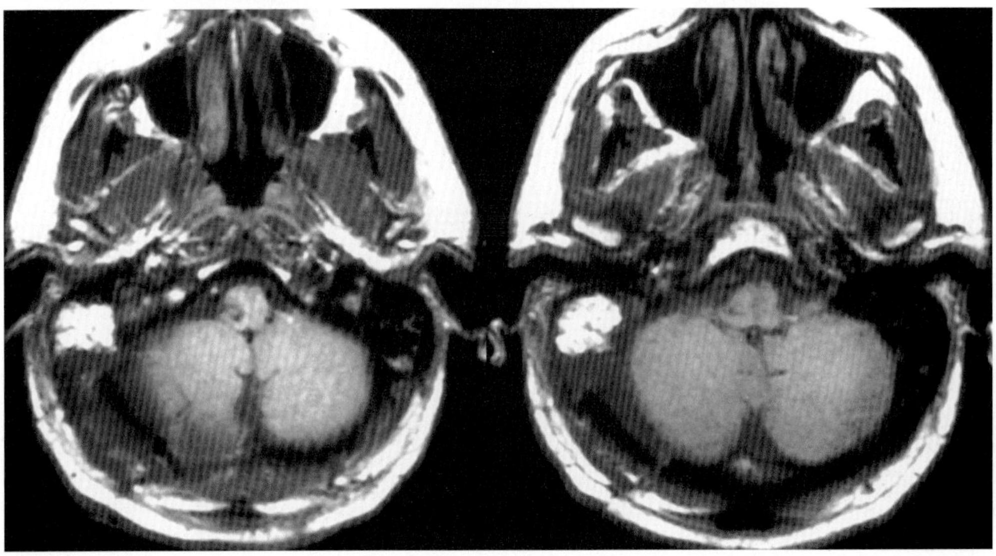

D

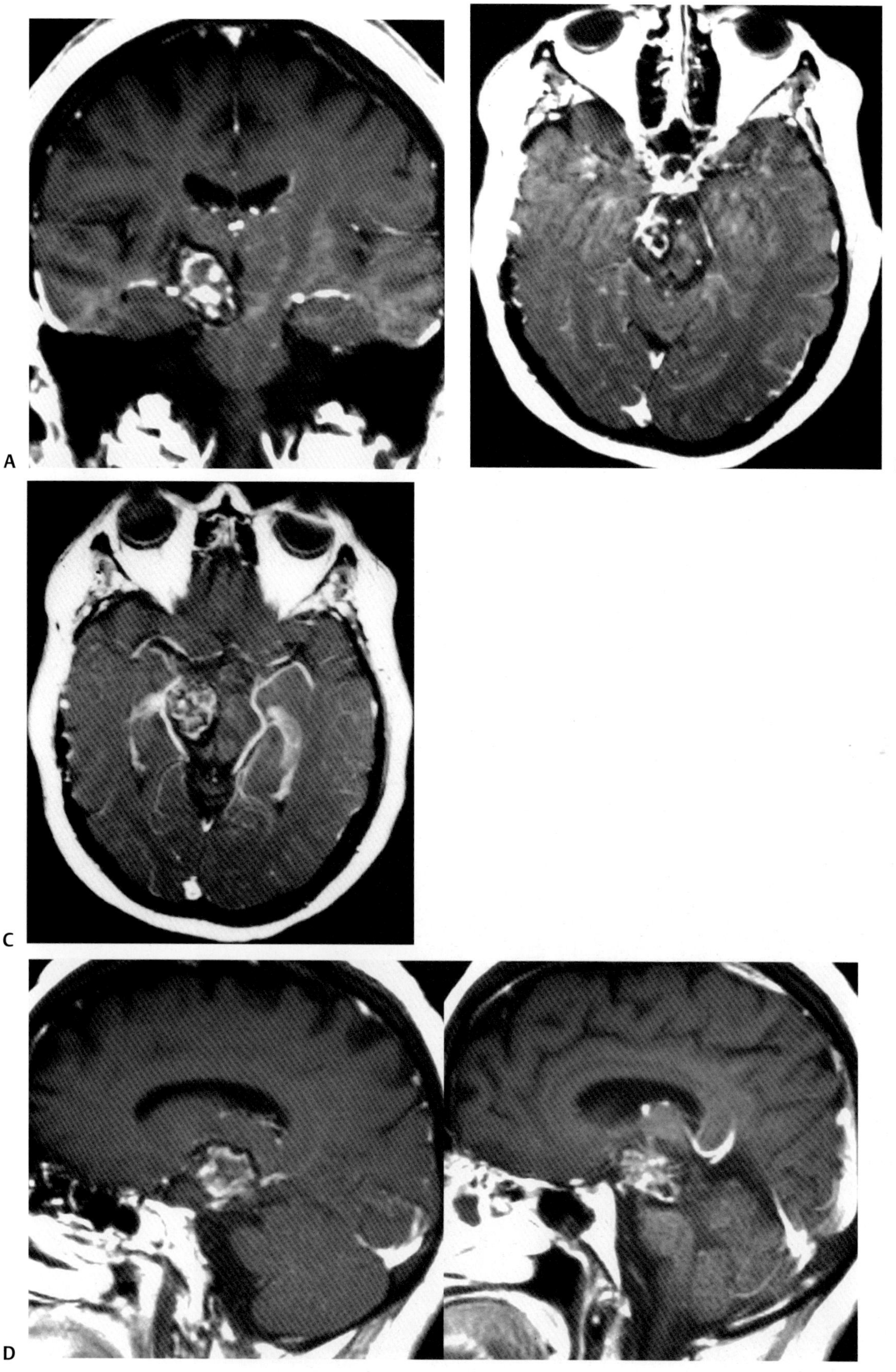

Figure 23–5 Case 4. **(A–D)** Cavernoma of the right cerebral peduncle.

(*Continued on page 298*)

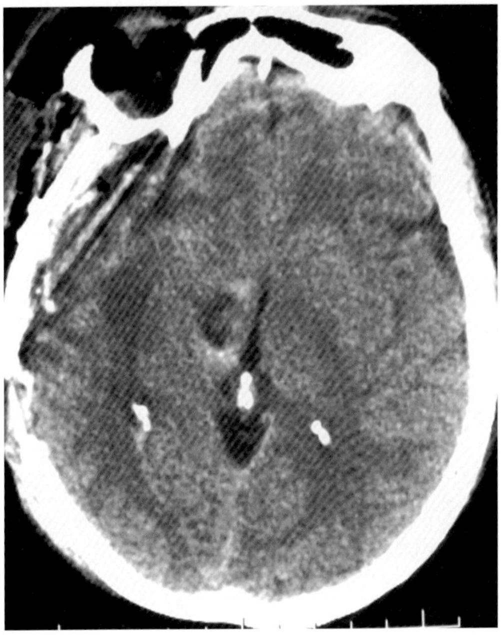
E

(*Continued*) **Figure 23–5** **(E)** The lesion was completely removed by a transsylvian orbitozygomatic approach.

an orbitozygomatic transsylvian approach (**Fig. 23–5E**). The patient has not rebled and is neurologically unchanged.

Case 5

This 34-year-old woman presented with a 3-week history of severe, daily headaches and nausea. Imaging studies revealed a CM in the deep left cerebellar hemisphere adjacent to the dentate nucleus (**Fig. 23–6A**). The lesion was approached via a posterior fossa craniotomy and totally resected through an incision in the fissure between the vermis and cerebellar hemisphere (**Fig. 23–6B**). Gait and balance were normal postoperatively.

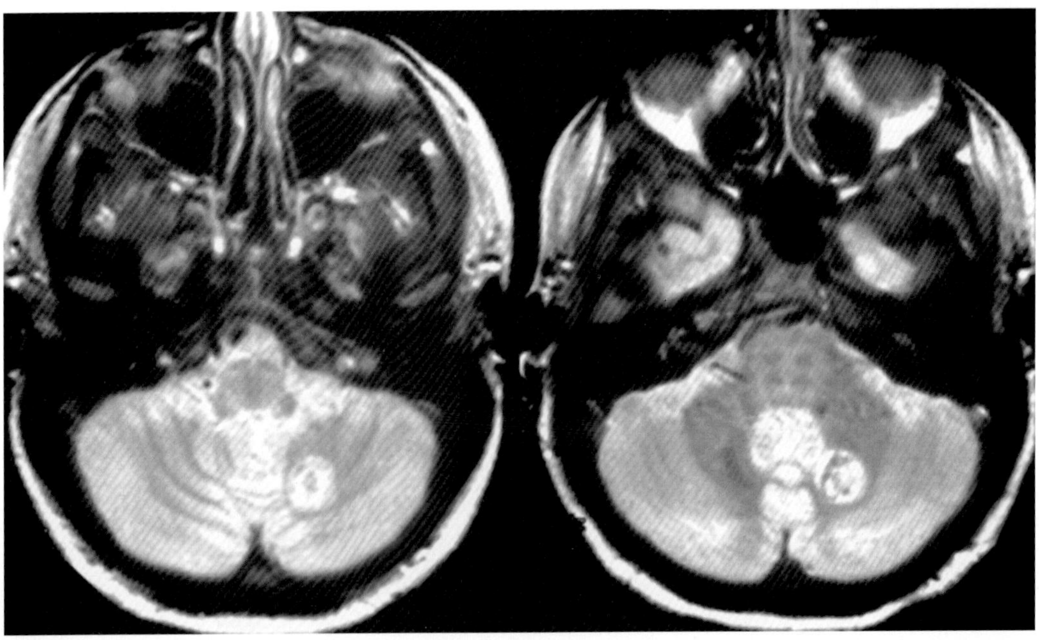
A

Figure 23–6 **(A)** Cavernoma involving the dentate nucleus area of the cerebellum,

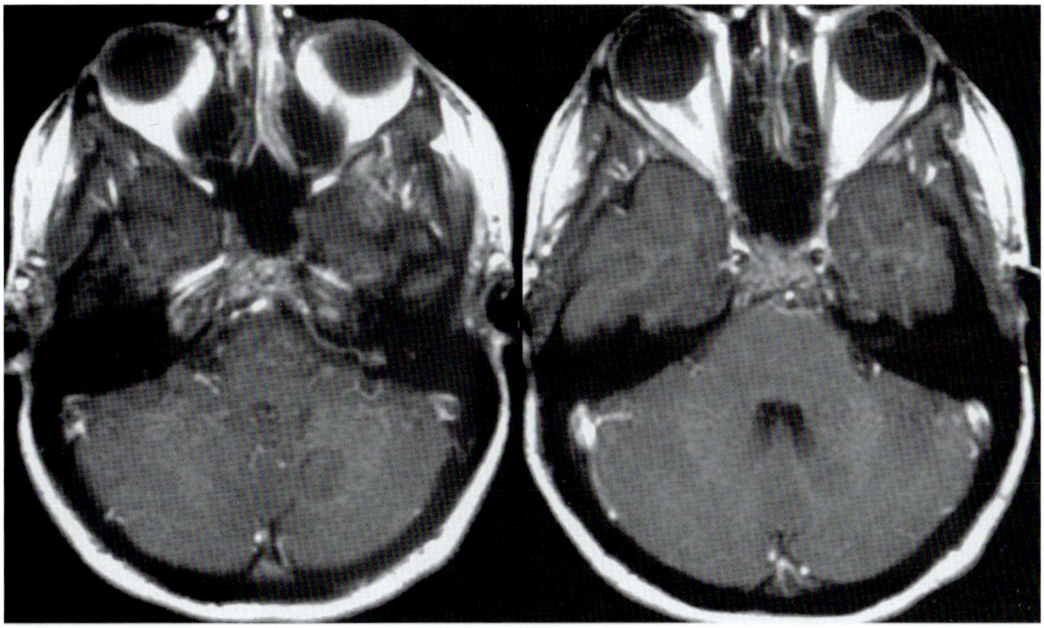

B

Figure 23–6 **(B)** resected totally, without deficits.

◆ Deep-Seated Parieto-occipital Cavernomas

For deep-seated or subcortical parieto-occipital CMs, one must choose an approach with the least likelihood of producing neurological morbidity while providing adequate exposure to ensure a complete resection. The choice of cortical trajectory must factor in both the path length and CM location. Generally, the shortest path length is chosen. Because a deep-seated lesion will not be evident at the cortical surface, it is helpful to employ some form of intraoperative localization technique. Either intraoperative ultrasound or a frameless navigation system (or both) can be used. Ultrasound provides "real-time" information, helps evaluate the completeness of resection, and, with color duplex sonography, can detect associated DVAs. Frameless stereotaxic systems can be used to formulate preop plans and guide intraoperative localization and trajectory. The neurological functions that can be affected by surgical intervention in deep lesions in these locations include visual field loss and one or more of the parietal lobe syndromes.

Case

Case 6

This 40-year-old female presented with headaches. MRI showed a deep-seated left parieto-occipital cavernoma, posterosuperior to the atrium of the lateral ventricle (**Fig. 23–7A**). A left parieto-occipital craniotomy was performed after the lesion was localized with a stereotactically placed catheter. The catheter was used as a guide to minimize brain resection and traction and the CM was totally resected with no neurological morbidity (**Fig. 23–7B**).

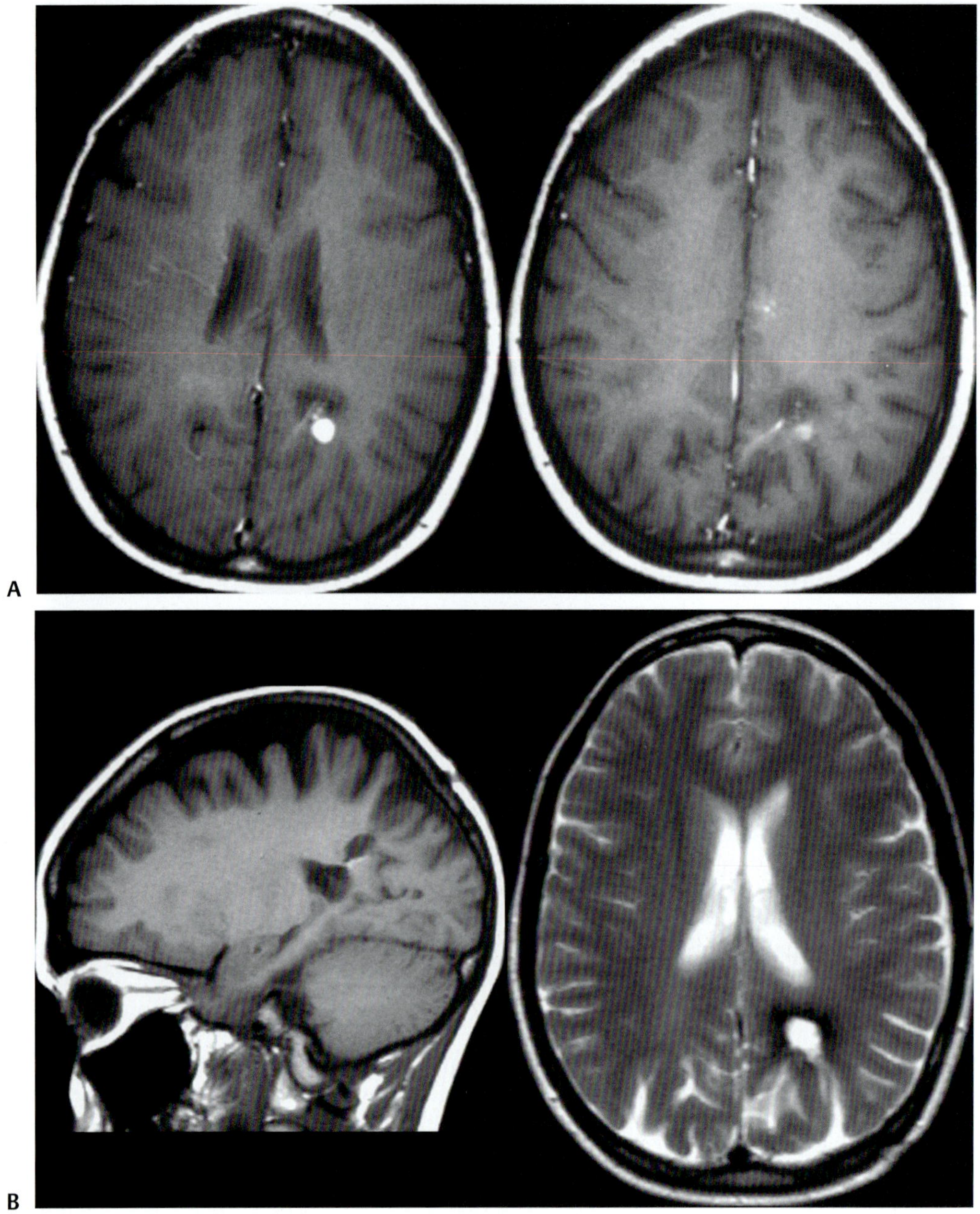

Figure 23–7 Case 6. **(A)** Deep-seated parieto-occipital cavernoma. **(B)** It was resected by a microsurgical stereotactic approach.

◆ Mesial Temporal/Basal Frontal Cavernoma

Lesions in the mesial temporal and basal frontal region can be resected with a minimum of retraction and excellent exposure with the use of orbital or orbitozygomatic osteotomy (OZO). The orbital osteotomy is used to augment exposure to lesions in the basal frontal lobe and anterior frontal operculum. After a pterional craniotomy is completed, an orbital osteotomy that contains at least two thirds of the orbital roof (to prevent enophthalmos postop) is performed. Lateral basal lesions (orbitofrontal gyrus) can be easily accessed by splitting the sylvian fissure, whereas more medial lesions (gyrus rectus) are accessed from a subfrontal approach. If the lesion is subcortical, a frameless navigational system or intraoperative ultrasound is useful to precisely localize the lesion and plan the corticectomy with the least amount of tissue disruption.

Lesions in the mesial temporal lobe can be reached with a frontotemporal craniotomy and OZO or subtemporal transzygomatic approach. The cortical approach to the lesion depends on its anatomical location and the surgical goals. If an epilepsy operation is incorporated into the surgery then the lesion is accessed as part of the resection. For lesionectomy alone, the mesial temporal lobe (parahippocampus, uncus, amygdala, and hippocampus) can be reached by several methods, including temporal tip (2–3 cm of inferior and middle temporal gyrus) resection with entry into the temporal horn, an inferior temporal and fusiform gyrus resection subtemporally; a slot corticectomy in the middle temporal gyrus at the level of the anterior tip of the temporal horn; or a trans-sylvian approach as described for selective amygdalohippocampectomies. In all these approaches one must be cognizant of the proximity of the anterior choroidal artery in the choroidal fissure, posterior cerebral artery, third nerve, fourth nerve, cerebral peduncle, and optic tract on the medial side of the deep temporal lobe. Although damage to these structures can be avoided by respecting the arachnoid plane on the mesial side of the temporal lobe, bleeding from the cavernoma may obscure these planes and resection above the choroidal fissure (i.e., above the superior aspect of the plane) can disrupt Meyer's loop, leading to a superior quadrantic visual field loss.

Cases

Case 7

This 42-year-old female presented with a sudden left superior quadrant visual field loss. MRI showed a right mesial temporal lobe CM involving the uncus and amygdala (**Fig. 23–8A–D**). This lesion was gross totally resected by a frontotemporal craniotomy with an OZO and trans-sylvian intracranial approach.

Case 8

This 49-year-old female presented with a 3-year history of headache. Her MRI showed a right basal frontal cavernoma with extension to the hypothalamus (**Fig. 23–9A,B**). The lesion was totally resected via a frontotemporal craniotomy and orbital osteotomy with subfrontal and trans-sylvian intracranial approaches and frameless stereotactic navigation. The skull base approach and stereotactic navigation aid in reducing surgical morbidity.

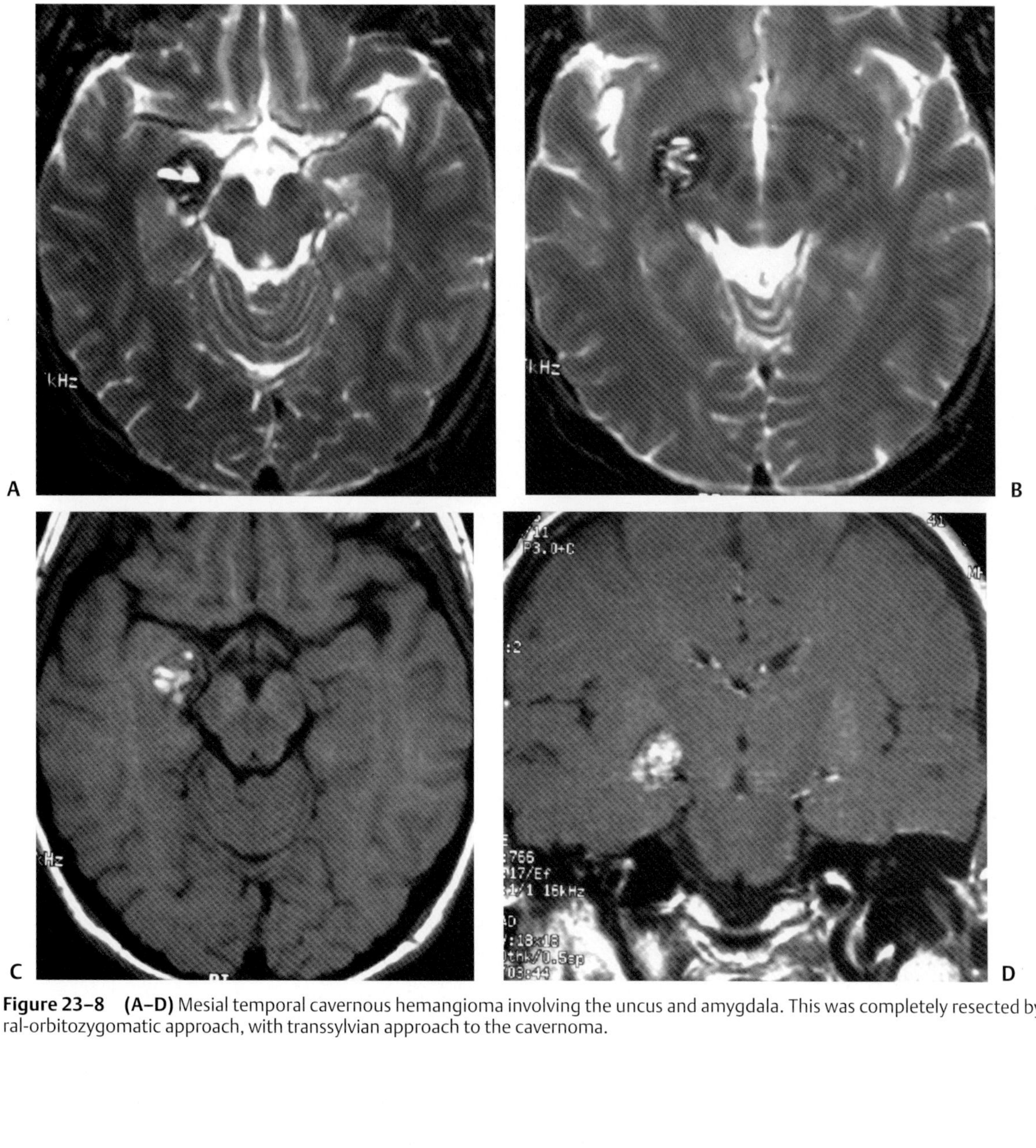

Figure 23–8 (A–D) Mesial temporal cavernous hemangioma involving the uncus and amygdala. This was completely resected by a frontotemporal-orbitozygomatic approach, with transsylvian approach to the cavernoma.

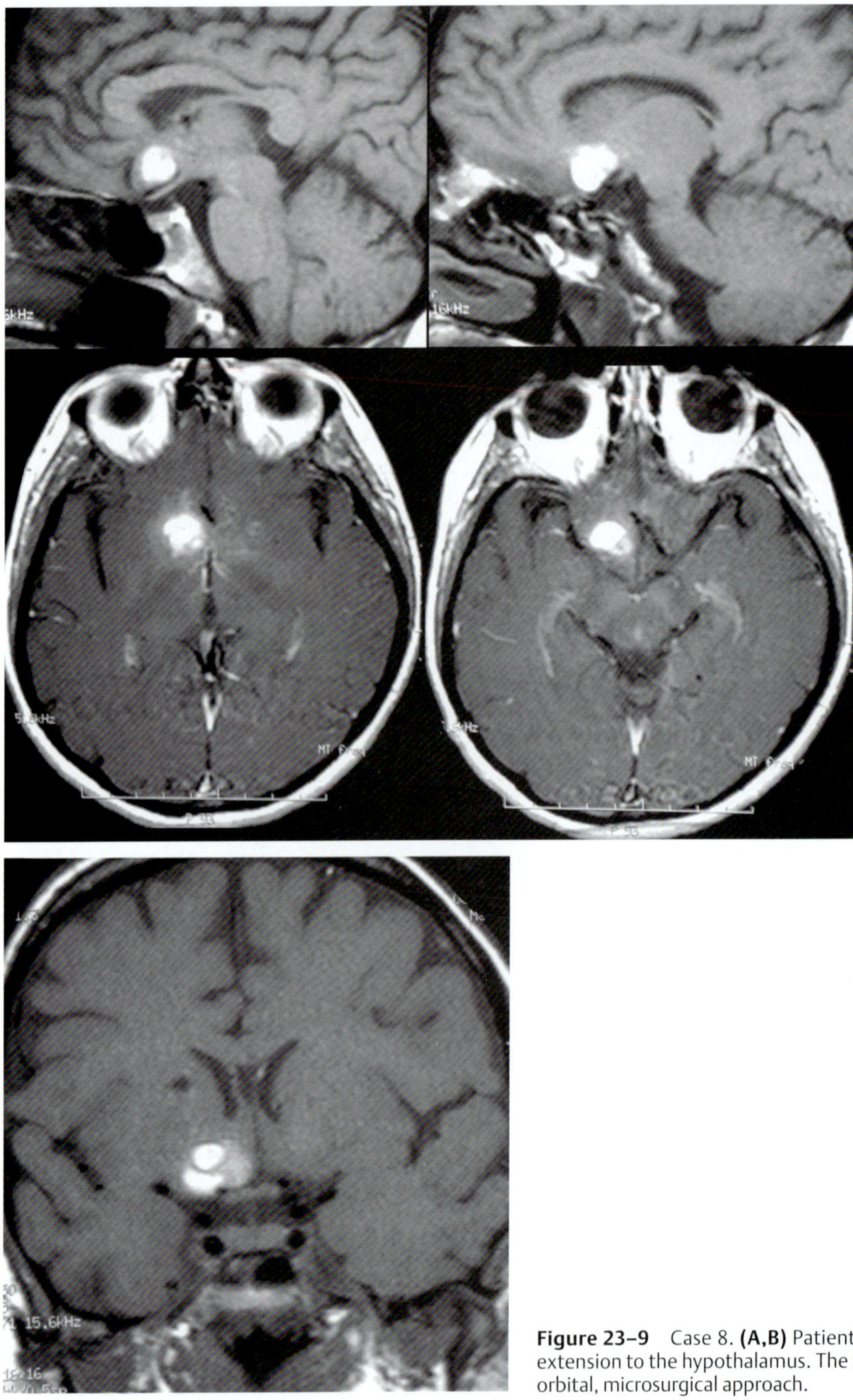

A

B

Figure 23–9 Case 8. **(A,B)** Patient with a right basal frontal cavernoma with extension to the hypothalamus. The lesion was completely removed by a fronto-orbital, microsurgical approach.

◆ Epilepsy and Cavernous Malformations

The majority of patients with CM and seizures can be treated surgically with lesionectomy alone. The surgical technique for these cases is no different than for cortical lesions at similar locations that present with other signs or symptoms. There are no data that support the resection of the gliotic capsule to improve seizure control, but in noneloquent cortical areas this additional resection does not increase morbidity and can reduce the likelihood of leaving residual malformation. For the smaller number of patients who fail to achieve seizure control after lesionectomy or in whom there is a high chance of failure to achieve control with lesionectomy alone (see earlier in Indications) a more extensive epilepsy evaluation and resection should be considered. The details of such evaluations and surgical strategies are beyond the scope of this chapter, and the reader is referred to a more comprehensive review.[59] Currently there are no data that compare the costs and benefits of lesionectomy versus epilepsy resection stratified by prognostic factors. Because these evaluations are labor intensive and costly, and seizure control is achieved in the majority of "poor-risk" surgical patients, some authors advocate an initial lesionectomy with more intensive epilepsy evaluation and surgery for those patients who fail.[37] However, in the setting of epilepsy where the EEG or semiology does not correlate with the CM location, a formal epilepsy evaluation must be undertaken.

Illustrative Case

Case 9

This 47-year-old female presented with a generalized seizure in the setting of several years of intermittent spells of numbness and weakness involving the left upper and lower extremity. A preoperative MRI showed a superficially located right parietal lesion (**Fig. 23–10A**). The lesion and surrounding gliotic capsule were totally resected (**Fig. 23–10B**). Postoperatively, the patient has been free of any "spells" or generalized seizures. For

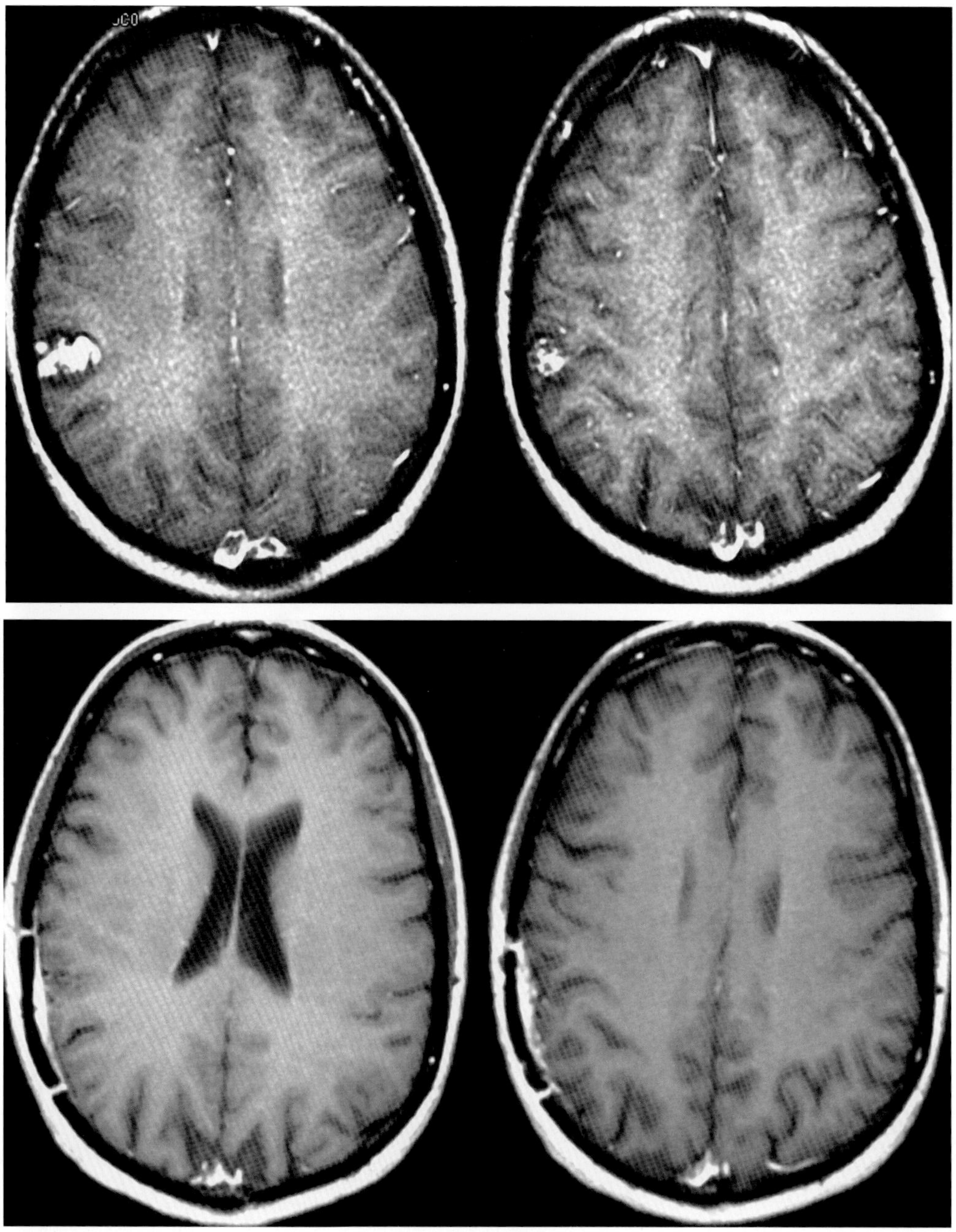

A

B

Figure 23–10 Case 9. **(A)** A perirolandic parietal cavernoma. **(B)** The postoperative image.

this patient with a short history of seizure activity (< 12 months), lesionectomy alone is expected to result in a high chance of long-term seizure control.

Results of Surgical Intervention

Surgical results must be interpreted based on preoperative indications and lesion location. The results of surgery for epilepsy have been discussed at length in the preceding text (see Indications, Seizure/Epilepsy). The goal of any surgery is to achieve complete resection because any residual CM can rebleed. The completeness of resection is dependent on lesion location and operative technique. It is often difficult to achieve a complete resection in eloquent cortical areas or in the brain stem, but the majority of cortical lesions should be completely resected. In rare instances where rebleeding occurs after resection, some residual CM is found.[60] Unfortunately, there is no detailed analysis of surgical resection with MRI documentation of resection and outcome. Most patients with neurological deficits will either improve or stabilize.[43,44]

Overall, most series of CMs report either a significant improvement or stabilization in patient condition rather than worsening.[19,43,44] The morbidity for CM surgery has been detailed in a recent report by Amin-Hanjani et al.[44] Not unexpectedly, the greatest morbidity occurs in surgery of brain stem CMs where neurological worsening was seen in 14.3% of patients compared with 4.8% of cerebral CM surgeries.[44] Porter et al report that of brain stem CM patients, 87% were better or unchanged, about 10% were worse, and 4% died after surgery.[3]

◆ Complications

The specific causes of complications and their avoidance are not discussed in detail in the literature. For patients with cerebral CMs, the cause of postoperative morbidity relates to multiple factors that are not unique to CMs. Thus the general medical condition of the patient, lesion location, operative approach, and technique (cortical access, retraction, method of resection) all contribute to complications. For brain stem CMs one must adhere to general neurosurgical principles of working in the posterior fossa. In addition, the selection of patients is critical. Only those patients with exophytic lesions or intrinsic lesions with an extremely thin rim of overlying tissue should be considered for surgery. During surgery any associated DVAs (which were reported to occur in all cases in one report[3]) must be carefully preserved. This principle applies to CM resection in all regions. The "safe" entry points for intrinsic brain stem lesions must be carefully considered because the CM can distort normal anatomy such that anatomical or physiological landmarks are misleading. Because of these concerns, Porter et al recommend that intrinsic lesions in the paramedian floor of the fourth ventricle not be removed unless the patient is rapidly deteriorating.[3]

◆ Conclusion

CMs should be considered for resection in the setting of overt hemorrhage, seizures or epilepsy, mass effect, or neurological deficits. Resection in an anticipated pregnancy should also be considered because of the apparent increased risk of hemorrhage and aggressive lesion behavior. CMs present unique surgical considerations because of their frequent deep subcortical locations and association with DVAs. The goals of surgery are complete resection with alleviation or stabilization of signs or symptoms related to the CM. Even in brain stem lesions, good results are achieved with microneurosurgical techniques.

Acknowledgment The authors would like to acknowledge Jennifer Pryll for her work on the Figure 23–1 and illustrative cases in this chapter.

References

1. Pryor J, Setton A, Berenstein A. Venous anomalies and associated lesions. Neurosurg Clin N Am 1999;10:519–525
2. Zabramski JM, Henn JS, Coons S. Pathology of cerebral vascular malformations. Neurosurg Clin N Am 1999;10:395–410
3. Porter RW, et al. Cavernous malformations of the brainstem: experience with 100 patients. J Neurosurg 1999;90:50–58
4. Stiver S. Microarteriovenous malformations. Neurosurg Clin N Am 1999;10:485–501
5. Moriarity JL, Clatterbuck RE, Rigamonti D. The natural history of cavernous malformations. Neurosurg Clin N Am 1999;10:411–417
6. Ziyal IM, et al. Surgical management of cavernous malformations of the brain stem. Br J Neurosurg 1999;13: 366–375
7. Robinson J, Awad I. Clinical spectrum and natural course. In: Awad I, Barrow D, eds. Cavernous Malformations. Vol 1. Park Ridge: American Association of Neurological Surgeons; 1993:25–36
8. Robinson JR, Awad IA, Little JR. Natural history of the cavernous angioma. J Neurosurg 1991;75:709–714
9. Arrue P, et al. Cavernous hemangioma of the intracranial optic pathways: CT and MRI. J Comput Assist Tomogr 1999;23:357–361
10. Steinberg GK, et al. Occult vascular malformations of the optic chiasm: magnetic resonance imaging diagnosis and surgical laser resection. Neurosurgery 1990;27:466–470
11. Ogilvy CS, Pakzaban P, Lee JM. Oculomotor nerve cavernous angioma in a patient with Roberts' syndrome. [see comments] Surg Neurol 1993;40:39–42
12. Kim M, et al. Cavernous malformation presenting as an extra-axial cerebellopontine angle mass: case report. Neurosurgery 1997;40: 187–190
13. Linskey ME, Sekhar LN. Cavernous sinus hemangiomas: a series, a review, and an hypothesis. [see comments] Neurosurgery 1992;30: 101–108
14. Johnson P, et al. Definition and pathologic features. In: Awad I, Barrow D, eds. Cavernous Malformations. Park Ridge: American Association of Neurological Surgeons; 1993:1–11
15. Tomlinson FH, et al. Angiographically occult vascular malformations: a correlative study of features on magnetic resonance imaging and histological examination. Neurosurgery 1994;34:792–799 discussion 799–800
16. Van Roost D, et al. Intracerebral capillary telangiectasia and venous malformation: a rare association. Surg Neurol 1997;48:175–183
17. Rigamonti D, et al. Cerebral venous malformations. J Neurosurg 1990;73:560–564
18. Rigamonti D, et al. Cerebral cavernous malformations: incidence and familial occurrence. N Engl J Med 1988;319:343–347
19. Maraire JN, Awad IA. Intracranial cavernous malformations: lesion behavior and management strategies. Neurosurgery 1995;37: 591–605

20. Gunel M, et al. A founder mutation as a cause of cerebral cavernous malformation in Hispanic Americans. N Engl J Med 1996;334: 946–951
21. Gunel M, et al. Genetic heterogeneity of inherited cerebral cavernous malformation. Neurosurgery 1996;38:1265–1271
22. Zabramski JM, et al. The natural history of familial cavernous malformations: results of an ongoing study. J Neurosurg 1994;80:422–432
23. Tekkok IH, Ventureyra EC. De novo familial cavernous malformation presenting with hemorrhage 12.5 years after the initial hemorrhagic ictus: natural history of an infantile form. Pediatr Neurosurg 1996;25:151–155
24. Detwiler PW, et al. De novo formation of a central nervous system cavernous malformation: implications for predicting risk of hemorrhage: case report and review of the literature. [see comments] J Neurosurg 1997;87:629–632
25. Larson JJ, et al. Formation of intracerebral cavernous malformations after radiation treatment for central nervous system neoplasia in children. [see comments] J Neurosurg 1998;88:51–56
26. Gangemi M, et al. Rapid growth of a brain-stem cavernous angioma. Acta Neurol (Napoli) 1993;15:132–137
27. Pozzati E, et al. The growth of cerebral cavernous angiomas. Neurosurgery 1989;25:92–97
28. Frim DM, et al. Immunohistochemically identifiable tissue plasminogen activator in cavernous angioma: mechanism for re-hemorrhage and lesion growth. Pediatr Neurosurg 1996;25:137–141 discussion 141–142
29. Houtteville JP. Brain cavernoma: a dynamic lesion. Surg Neurol 1997;48:610–614
30. Pozzati E, et al. Growth, subsequent bleeding, and de novo appearance of cerebral cavernous angiomas. Neurosurgery 1996;38: 662–669 discussion 669–670
31. Notelet L, et al. Proliferating cell nuclear antigen (PCNA) in cerebral cavernomas: an immunocytochemical study of 42 cases. Surg Neurol 1997;47:364–370
32. Rothbart D, et al. Expression of angiogenic factors and structural proteins in central nervous system vascular malformations. Neurosurgery 1996;38:915–924 discussion 924–925
33. Del Curling O Jr, et al. An analysis of the natural history of cavernous angiomas. J Neurosurg 1991;75:702–708
34. Kondziolka D, Lunsford LD, Kestle JR. The natural history of cerebral cavernous malformations. J Neurosurg 1995;83:820–824
35. Abdulrauf SI, Kaynar MY, Awad IA. A comparison of the clinical profile of cavernous malformations with and without associated venous malformations. Neurosurgery 1999;44:41–46 discussion 46–47
36. Fritschi JA, et al. Cavernous malformations of the brain stem: a review of 139 cases. Acta Neurochir (Wien) 1994;130:35–46
37. Cosgrove GR. Occult vascular malformations and seizures. Neurosurg Clin N Am 1999;10:527–535
38. Cappabianca P, et al. Supratentorial cavernous malformations and epilepsy: seizure outcome after lesionectomy on a series of 35 patients. Clin Neurol Neurosurg 1997;99:179–183
39. Casazza M, et al. Supratentorial cavernous angiomas and epileptic seizures: preoperative course and postoperative outcome. [see comments] Neurosurgery 1996;39:26–32 discussion 32–34
40. Cohen DS, Zubay GP, Goodman RR. Seizure outcome after lesionectomy for cavernous malformations. J Neurosurg 1995;83:237–242
41. Zevgaridis D, et al. Seizure control following surgery in supratentorial cavernous malformations: a retrospective study in 77 patients. Acta Neurochir (Wien) 1996;138:672–677
42. Weber JP, Silbergeld DL, Winn HR. Surgical resection of epileptogenic cortex associated with structural lesions. Neurosurg Clin N Am 1993;4:327–336
43. Chaskis C, Brotchi J. The surgical management of cerebral cavernous angiomas. Neurol Res 1998;20:597–606
44. Amin-Hanjani S, et al. Risks of surgical management for cavernous malformations of the nervous system. Neurosurgery 1998;42:1220–1227 discussion 1227–1228
45. Aiba T, et al. Natural history of intracranial cavernous malformations. J Neurosurg 1995;83:56–59
46. Sage MR, et al. Cavernous haemangiomas (angiomas) of the brain: clinically significant lesions. Australas Radiol 1993;37:147–155
47. Kondziolka D, et al. Reduction of hemorrhage risk after stereotactic radiosurgery for cavernous malformations [see comments]. J Neurosurg 1995;83:825–831
48. Chang SD, et al. Stereotactic radiosurgery of angiographically occult vascular malformations: 14-year experience. Neurosurgery 1998;43:213–220 discussion 220–221
49. Maesawa S, Kondziolka D, Lunsford LD. Stereotactic radiosurgery for management of deep brain cavernous malformations. Neurosurg Clin N Am 1999;10:503–511
50. Pollock BE, et al. Stereotactic radiosurgery for cavernous malformations. J Neurosurg 2000;93:987–991
51. Vanefsky MA, et al. Correlation of magnetic resonance characteristics and histopathological type of angiographically occult vascular malformations Neurosurgery 1999;44:1174–1180 discussion 1180–1181
52. Yoon PH, et al. Cerebral cavernous malformations: serial magnetic resonance imaging findings in patients with and without gamma knife surgery. Neurol Med Chir (Tokyo) 1998;38(Suppl):255–261
53. Silbergeld DL, et al. Use of propofol (Diprivan) for awake craniotomies: technical note. Surg Neurol 1992;38:271–272
54. Mueller WM, Morris GL III. Intraoperative and extraoperative identification of eloquent brain using stimulation mapping. Neurosurg Clin N Am 1993;4:217–222
55. Woydt M, et al. Localization and characterization of intracerebral cavernous angiomas by intra-operative high-resolution colour-duplex-sonography. Acta Neurochir (Wien) 1999;141:143–151
56. Moro M, et al. Growing patterns of cavernous angioma in the fourth ventricle: case report. J Neurosurg Sci 1998;42:221–225
57. Eisner W, et al. The mapping and continuous monitoring of the intrinsic motor nuclei during brain stem surgery. Neurosurgery 1995;37: 255–265
58. Cantore G, Missori P, Santoro A. Cavernous angiomas of the brain stem: intra-axial anatomical pitfalls and surgical strategies. Surg Neurol 1999;52:84–93 discussion 93–94
59. Silbergeld DL, Ojemann GA. Epilepsy surgery. In: Winn HR, Mayberg MR, eds. Neurosurgery Clinics of North America. Vol 4. Philadelphia: WB Saunders; 1993; 193–356.
60. Duffau H, et al. Early radiologically proven rebleeding from intracranial cavernous angiomas: report of 6 cases and review of the literature. Acta Neurochir (Wien) 1997;139:914–922

24

Carotid Cavernous Fistula

Gerard M. Debrun

A carotid cavernous fistula (CCF) is an abnormal communication between the internal carotid artery (ICA) and the cavernous sinus (CS). There are two types of CCFs: Type I are the direct fistulas, which are usually high flow and will be treated through the endoarterial route with detachable balloons, rarely with coils or acrylic glue. Type II are the indirect CCFs, which are usually slow flow and will be treated with coils through the endovenous route, sometimes with balloons and rarely with acrylic glue.

◆ Historical Review

The first autopsy, which clearly demonstrated that the post-traumatic pulsating exophthalmos was associated with a tear of the carotid siphon communicating with the CS, is due to Nelaton,[1] in 1876.

The first surgical treatments consisted of ligation of the common carotid artery or ICA, usually with incomplete or no cure of the fistula.

The next progress consisted of ligating the ICA intracranially and in the neck but also plugging the CS with pieces of muscle.

In 1971, Prolo and Hanberry occluded the ICA and the fistula with their nondetachable balloon catheter.[2]

In 1973, Black et al[3] elegantly cured a CCF with a plug of muscle attached to a thread, which blocked the fistula with preservation of the ICA.

In 1974, I treated a traumatic CCF with a Prolo's catheter. I occluded both the ICA and the fistula. The proptosis and chemosis subsided within a few days. When I repeated the angiogram 1 week later to demonstrate the cure of the fistula, I found that the balloon, still inflated, had migrated into the CS, and the ICA was well open. I realized that we desperately needed detachable balloons.

Serbinenko[4] in 1974 published his first article in the English literature. He had successfully treated a CCF with his latex detachable balloon. In fact, he had published his technique in the Russian literature in 1972.[5]

Debrun and colleagues, in 1975, developed a tied latex balloon and showed successful treatments of fistulas in animals and in humans.[6,7]

Surgical direct repair of the fistula in the CS is rarely done today but has been supported by the works of Parkinson,[8] Mullan,[9] and Isamat et al.[10]

The reader who seeks all the available knowledge on the subject of CCFs is referred elsewhere.[11]

◆ Etiology

Fast Flow Direct Fistulas

A fast flow direct CCF can be due to:

- Head trauma or gun shot
- Direct orbital trauma and penetrating injuries
- Iatrogenic complication during thrombectomy with Fogarty catheter or during rhizotomy
- Dissection of the ICA
- Ruptured cavernous aneurysm
- Collagen vascular disease, like Ehlers-Danlos syndrome, Marfan, or fibromuscular dysplasia

Slow Flow Indirect Fistulas

A slow flow indirect CCF can be due to:

- Sinus infection
- Phlebitis of the CS or draining veins
- Pregnancy and postpartum
- No etiology found

◆ Pathophysiology

Fast Flow Carotid Cavernous Fistulas

The fast flow CCFs arterialize the CS and generate retrograde flow in veins that normally drain into the CS. Two of these veins must be considered: the superior ophthalmic vein (SOV) and the sylvian vein (SV). Arterialization of the SOV is responsible for increased intraorbital venous pressure, proptosis, chemosis, glaucoma, and potential sudden loss of monocular vision. Arterialization of the SV may cause a subarachnoid or intraparenchymal hemorrhage.

The steal can be complete and induce ischemic complications in patients who have poor collateral circulation through the circle of Willis.

These fistulas must be treated as soon as possible because their spontaneous cure cannot be expected.

Slow Flow Indirect Carotid Cavernous Fistulas

The elevation of the intraocular pressure (IOP) is usually less severe in this type of CCF. The cortical venous drainage is rarer than in direct CCFs. The spontaneous closure of the fistula is more frequent than in direct CCFs with fast flow.

We will consider the clinical presentation, radiological workup, and treatment with its results for each type of CCF.

◆ Direct Fast Flow Fistulas

We will consider the traumatic CCFs, and we will see at the end how other etiologies may change the therapeutic strategy.

Presentation

The patient typically presents with proptosis and chemosis. However, the direct fistulas, which drain posteriorly through the petrosal sinuses and very little anteriorly through the SOV, may present without proptosis.

Diplopia is frequent because of oculomotor nerve deficit; the abducens is more frequently affected than the third nerve.

The elevation of the IOP is responsible for glaucoma. These patients should always be examined by a neuro-ophthalmologist who will establish baseline findings and will determine whether the treatment should be done emergently.[12]

The patient usually hears a swishing noise, and auscultation of the temporal region and over the eyelid will record a loud, pulsatile bruit.

In a patient comatose with multiple injuries, auscultation over the eye is the best way to make the clinical diagnosis.

Radiological Workup

Computed tomography (CT), magnetic resonance imaging (MRI), and magnetic resonance angiography (MRA) play a role, but the angiographic workup only helps in defining the therapeutic strategy.

- CT with contrast will show the proptosis and the dilation of both the SOV and the CS. It is very useful for analyzing the bony structures and showing any brain damage.
- MRI and MRA play a similar role but will not show the bony structures as well as CT.
- Angiographic workup will determine (**Fig. 24–1**):
  - ◇ Anatomy of the common carotid artery and ICA in the cervical area

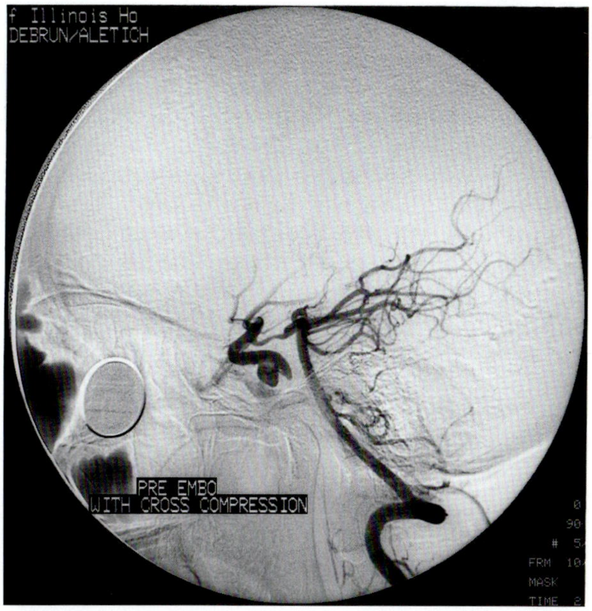

Figure 24–1 Localizing the fistula on the siphon. Vertebral angiography with ipsilateral occlusion of the internal carotid artery.

- ◇ Location of the fistula on the carotid siphon
- ◇ Size of the CS and its relationship with the dura and the sphenoid sinus
- ◇ Type of venous drainage of the CS
- ◇ Existence of a partial or complete steal
- ◇ Quality of the circle of Willis

This information is easily obtained with:

- ◆ Ipsilateral common carotid angiography
- ◆ Ipsilateral internal carotid angiography
- ◆ Contralateral internal carotid angiography to demonstrate the patency of the communicating artery
- ◆ Vertebral angiography with compression of the ipsilateral carotid artery.

This maneuver is the best way to demonstrate the location of the fistula. It precludes a patent posterior communicating artery (PCommA) on the side of the fistula. When this artery does not fill, other techniques can be used like a double lumen balloon catheter with slow injection of contrast distal to the balloon inflated in the ipsilateral ICA, proximal to the fistula.

- ◆ Selective external angiography will almost always be normal in this type of CCF.

An analysis of the information already mentioned will provide crucial data for treatment:

Anatomy of the Common Carotid Artery and ICA in the Cervical Area

We postulate that the ICA is patent and will allow access to the carotid siphon through the arterial route. In the case of gunshots the ICA cannot be used. In this situation we will have access to the CS either through the PCommA[13] or through the venous route: SOV or inferior petrosal sinus (IPS).[14–16]

The origin of the ICA may present with severe atheromatous stenosis with or without ulcers. It is wise to keep the guiding catheter in the common carotid artery (CCA) and to advance only the balloon through the stenosis. Angioplasty and stenting of the ICA may be necessary before treating the CCF.

The origin of the ICA may present with a very large bulb originating at a right angle from the CCA. Usually the ICA makes a sharp kink distal to this large bulb. The advancement of the guiding catheter into the ICA may induce vasospasm or dissection and it is preferable to keep the guiding catheter in the CCA or at the origin of the ICA.

When the ICA presents with a 360 degree loop in the cervical region or with a double kink, we will also keep the guiding catheter below the loops.

Location of the Fistula on the Carotid Siphon

The fistula is usually found on the horizontal C3 portion of the siphon, on the C4 posterior curve, or on the C5 vertical posterior intracavernous portion of the siphon. It is rarer to find the fistula on the C2 or C1 portion of the siphon. Vertebral angiography with compression of the ICA below the fistula stops the antegrade flow in the ICA and the fistula now steals blood from the distal ICA and PCommA. A double-lumen balloon catheter will give the same information but increases the complexity of the technique and should be used only when the PCommA is not large enough for retrograde filling of the siphon. During the balloon treatment, it is possible to inflate the balloon in different segments of the siphon and to know exactly where the fistula is.

Size of the CS and Its Relationship with the Dura and the Sphenoid Sinus

The septations of the CS are more or less preserved by the trauma and therefore the CS may be large. Great attention should be paid to any bulging of the CS through the dura intracranially because the risk of subarachnoid hemorrhage (SAH) or intraparenchymal hemorrhage is higher. It is also critical to note whether the CS does not fill the sphenoid sinus, with the risk of lethal rupture in the rhinopharynx.

It is usually in CCFs that have not been treated for years that the CS can reach a gigantic size (up to 5 cm).

Type of Venous Drainage of the CS

The CS drains anteriorly through the orbital veins and facial veins, posteriorly through the petrosal sinuses, inferiorly through the pterygoid plexus, and superiorly through the sylvian and cortical veins.

Massive cortical venous drainage would indicate that the treatment is urgent.

We look at the size of the SOV and the IPS, which will be used if the arterial route fails.

Existence of a Partial or Complete Steal

Most of the time the steal is partial and the distal ICA and its branches fill. However, 5% of traumatic CCFs present with a complete steal. This subgroup of CCFs provides interesting clinical information. A patient who has a complete steal and no contralateral neurological deficit has excellent collateral circulation through the circle of Willis, and we know that ischemic complications will not develop if we cannot preserve the carotid blood flow. However, we must be very careful during the treatment to not only occlude the ICA proximal to the fistula but also to not leave the fistula partially open, because the fistula would then steal blood from the intracranial circulation, and ischemic complications may occur. It is not rare to see at bedside that such patients do not tolerate compression of the ICA in the neck. This also demonstrates that a balloon occlusion test (BOT) done proximal to the fistula must be very carefully interpreted. Negative, it clearly shows that the patient would tolerate permanent occlusion of the ICA. Positive, it does not mean for certain that the ICA cannot be occluded, and we must complete the test by inflating the balloon distal to the fistula. In this case, a positive test tells us that we cannot permanently occlude the ICA.

Such information must be collected before definitive treatment of the fistula.

Quality of the Circle of Willis

Most patients have a patent anterior communicating artery and PCommA. But a few patients have an isolated hemisphere. These patients cannot tolerate a complete steal and are at risk of developing ischemic complications. The ICA cannot be permanently occluded in these patients.

Indications for Treatment of a Traumatic Carotid Cavernous Fistula [11,17]

The treatment of a traumatic CCF is an emergency when:

- There is rapid or acute deterioration of vision with very high IOP.
- There is massive cortical venous drainage.
- The CS bulges upward in the subarachnoid space or in the sphenoid sinus anteriorly and inferiorly.
- There is transection of dissection of the cervical portion of the ICA with a pseudoaneurysm after a gunshot.
- The fistula is caused by an object penetrating through the orbit and still present.

Aside from these particular situations, the treatment should be done within a few days.

The route of choice is the arterial route. The embolic material of choice is a detachable balloon. The venous route through the SOV or the IPS is reserved for failures of the arterial route.

Treatment of a Fast Flow Direct Carotid Cavernous Fistula through the Arterial Route

Treatment through the arterial route (**Fig. 24–2**) is done under general anesthesia, which improves the quality of the images and the comfort of the patient, although the treatment can be done under sedation, provided that the patient is fully cooperative.

A 9F or 10F sheath is inserted into one femoral artery. A 5F sheath is inserted in the contralateral femoral artery to give access to the vertebral artery and contralateral carotid artery during the treatment of the fistula.

A 9F or 10F guiding catheter is positioned in the ipsilateral ICA or at the origin of the ICA or even in the CCA, depending on the anatomy of the ICA as already described.

Detachable Balloon Technique

There is no Food and Drug Administration (FDA) approved detachable balloon at the present time, although the technique has been used efficiently for more than 20 years. The silicone detachable balloon made many years ago by International Therapeutics Corporation should be approved soon by the FDA and is marketed by Target Therapeutics Inc. (Freemont, CA). The latex detachable balloons are made by Nycomed France (Paris), and sold all over the world but are not FDA approved.

I use exclusively the latex detachable balloons made by Nycomed. I used them as a compassionate procedure approved by our chief staff and by the University of Illinois hospital administrators and attorneys.

There are two types of latex balloons available. The type I is a latex sleeve that the user must ligate over a microcatheter before using it. The steps necessary to learn how to ligate this type of balloon have been described many times in the literature.[11,17]

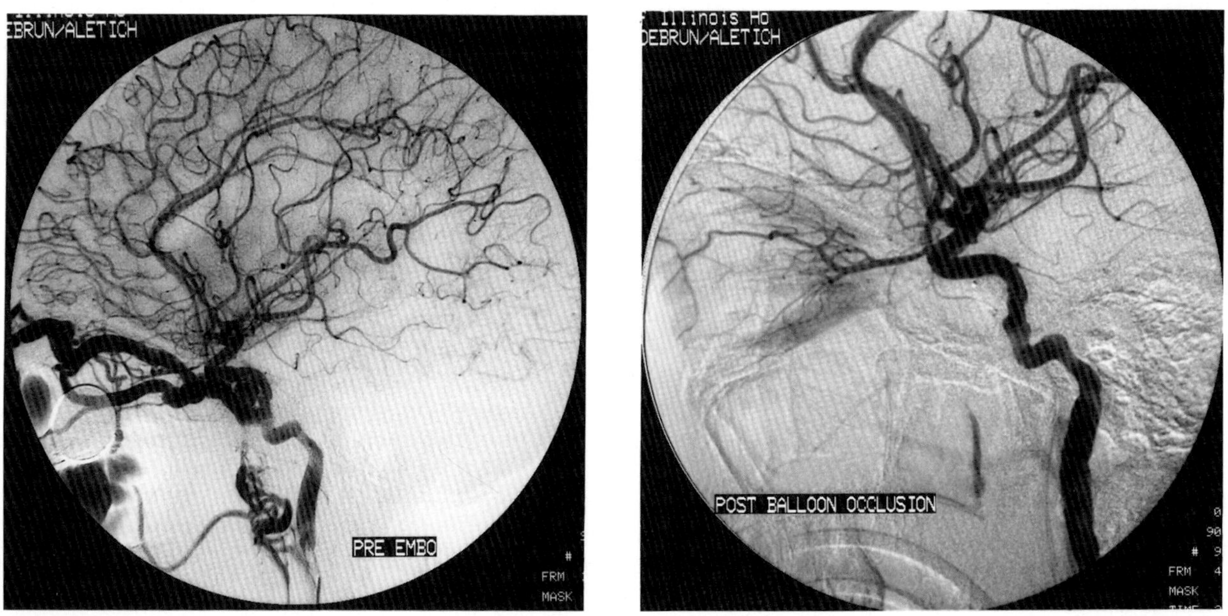

A B

Figure 24–2 Successful treatment of a direct carotid cavernous fistula with a detachable balloon. The fistula is closed and the carotid artery patent. **(A)** Pre and **(B)** postballoon occlusion.

The advantages are the almost total safety of the balloon, which is strongly attached without risk of premature detachment. The detachment of the balloon can hardly be done without the use of a coaxial microcatheter, which anchors the balloon while we pull out the microcatheter to which the balloon is tied.

The disadvantage is the necessity to learn how to tie the balloon, a tedious learning process that requires a lot of skill. The young generation of interventionalists do not have the appropriate training and are not comfortable in using this technique

The type II detachable balloon is the gold valve balloon made by Nycomed France. The balloon is ready for use and sterile. Valve function can be tested by entering the valve and the balloon with the microcatheter. The advantage is the facility of preparing the material.

The inconvenience is the higher risk of premature detachment because the balloon is not held over the microcatheter as strongly as the ligated type I balloon.

These latex balloons come in four sizes and volumes (of more than 20 sizes, only four have been commercialized).

The number 12 is the biggest and can be inflated with 2 mL of contrast. Its optimal advancement requires a 10F guiding catheter, although it advances through a 9F with some friction.

- The number 9 is smaller and contains 1 mL of contrast.
- The number 16 is smaller than the no. 9 and contains 0.7 mL.
- The number 17 is even smaller and contains only 0.5 mL.

When the CS is of moderate size (< 2 cm) I start with a no. 9 balloon. If the CS is bigger than 2 cm or if the first no. 9 balloon does not occlude the fistula, I use a no. 12 balloon.

The balloon, uninflated, is advanced into the ICA by pushing the microcatheter. If the balloon does not pass a curve of the ICA, gentle inflation will propel the balloon further. With the gold valve balloon (and this is true for any balloon with a valve mechanism) the risk of premature detachment is maximum when the size of the balloon approximates the size of the artery.

When the balloon has advanced to the level of the fistula, it is suction from the flow draws it into the CS. The balloon is inflated until the fistula is occluded. The balloon may overlap the ICA in one view. It is crucial to check from another plane of view at a 90 degree angle that the balloon is totally inside the CS and not occluding the fistula but still inside the ICA.[18]

The balloon is detached by pulling the microcatheter with or without the help of its coaxial catheter.

In a large CS it may be necessary to detach more than one balloon to close the fistula.

Results

The fistula is closed and the ICA is well patent in 85% of the cases. The remaining 15% of cases include CCFs with such a large tear that the balloon bulges through the tear and occludes or severely narrows the lumen of the ICA. Also included are the rare cases where no balloon enters the CS because the tear is too small. Permanent occlusion of the ICA should not be considered a bad result provided that the patient has excellent collateral circulation through the circle of Willis and the fistula is completely closed.

Complications

- Premature detachment of the balloon is theoretically possible although it did not happen in my experience with more than 150 cases.
- Recurrence of the fistula occurs in 5% of cases due to slight displacement or deflation of the balloon. A second treatment completes the closure of the fistula.
- Incomplete closure of the fistula and inability to reenter the CS with any type of balloon. By waiting 1 week and repeating the angiogram, a certain number of these cases evolve to complete closure and all the symptoms subside. If the fistula is still open, it will usually be possible to complete the closure with another balloon.
- Up to 30% of patients will develop an oculomotor nerve deficit post-treatment, usually a sixth more often than a third nerve. These paralyses are transient in the majority of cases and it is rare to see a patient at 6 months post-treatment who has a permanent nerve deficit.
- Venous pouch or false aneurysm post-treatment. The quality of healing of the tear can be appreciated only if the patient has angiographic follow-up. It is frequent to see at 6 months follow-up that there is some irregularity of the siphon at the level of the fistula with some outpouching into the CS. It is rare that this pouch is large and pseudoaneurysmal and needs a new treatment. Today, we would probably not treat this pseudo cavernous aneurysm with a balloon but with coils, with or without the help of a balloon inflated in the siphon during the deployment of the coil to keep it from bulging into the siphon (Jacques Moret's so-called remodeling technique).
- Normal pressure breakthrough phenomenon. This is exceptional but has occurred in a fast flow fistula where it was necessary to stage the closure of the fistula when the acute closure was not tolerated.[19]
- Rupture of the CS by the balloon. This is exceptional but has occurred in one case of CCF with complete steal, a gigantic CS, which had not been treated for 25 years. This CS was in contact with the subarachnoid space and the patient died from massive hemorrhage. Retrospectively, it would have been wise simply to occlude the ICA permanently.
- Complete occlusion of the ICA but incomplete closure of the fistula, which fills from retrograde flow into the ICA distal to the fistula. If the patient is asymptomatic we can wait and see whether the fistula closes spontaneously. If the patient is symptomatic because of the steal, either the ICA should be clipped surgically, ideally below the ophthalmic artery, or we can try to reach the ICA from the posterior circulation through the PCommA and seal the remaining leak with coils.

- The balloon in the CS does not completely occlude the fistula but occludes the posterior venous drainage through the IPS. This situation usually increases the anterior venous drainage through the SOV, increases the IOP, and dramatically increases the proptosis and chemosis. It is urgent to complete the closure of the fistula through the arterial route whenever possible, or through the venous route, which has to be the SOV approach in this scenario.

Treatment of a Fast Flow Direct CCF through the Venous Route[14–17]

When we do not succeed in entering the CS with a balloon through the ICA or when we do not have access to the ICA (after a gunshot or after previous surgical ligation), we still have the option to reach the CS through the vertebral artery, basilar artery, PCommA, ICA, and CS.[13]

If the PCommA is absent or too small, the venous route becomes the first choice of access to the CS.

The IPS is usually easy to catheterize. Although I have treated a few CCFs through the IPS with ligated latex balloons, the retrograde navigation into the IPS with balloons is difficult. Also, we cannot always reach the compartment of the CS, which is in direct communication with the tear of the ICA. Therefore it is easier, faster, and safer to use a microcatheter and to plug this compartment of the CS with coils. The fact that the CS does not drain into the IPS does not mean it is not functional, and catheterization should be attempted even if we do not see it opacified on the angiogram. However, if we cannot position the tip of the microcatheter in the compartment of the fistula, the SOV approach becomes the best option.

The SOV approach is an excellent technique. Its success depends on the experience of the neuro-ophthalmologist and vascular surgeon in generously exposing the vein at the medial angle of the orbit, installing two vessel loops, which allow a perfect puncture or venotomy and control any bleed. It is possible to directly advance the balloon catheter through the venotomy or to advance a microcatheter with a wire that will reach the CS. As with the IPS, it is easier to reach the CS with a microcatheter and to use coils than to reach the CS with a balloon.

Halbach et al[14] have shown that it is possible to reach the CS through the femoral vein, external jugular vein, angular vein, and SOV. I have used this technique in a couple of cases. It is more complicated than the direct exposure of the SOV and it precludes the use of balloons. Only coils can be used. Liquid embolic agents can be used but are very risky.

I discourage the direct puncture of SOV without surgical exposure. I think that the potential risks of trauma to the vein, of dissection, and of orbital hematoma are too high.

Special Situations

A direct fast flow CCF can be due to causes that warrant special attention.

Ruptured Cavernous Aneurysms

The classical treatment of giant unruptured cavernous aneurysms with a wide neck is the permanent occlusion of the ICA when the patient passes the BOT.

When the same aneurysm has ruptured in the CS and induced a CCF the treatment is much more complex because it is sometimes difficult to advance the balloon distal to the fistula, which is the prerequisite for doing a valuable BOT. Therefore, it is probably simpler to occlude the fistula with a balloon and leave the neck of the aneurysm open (**Fig. 24–3**). The BOT and the final treatment of the aneurysm will be

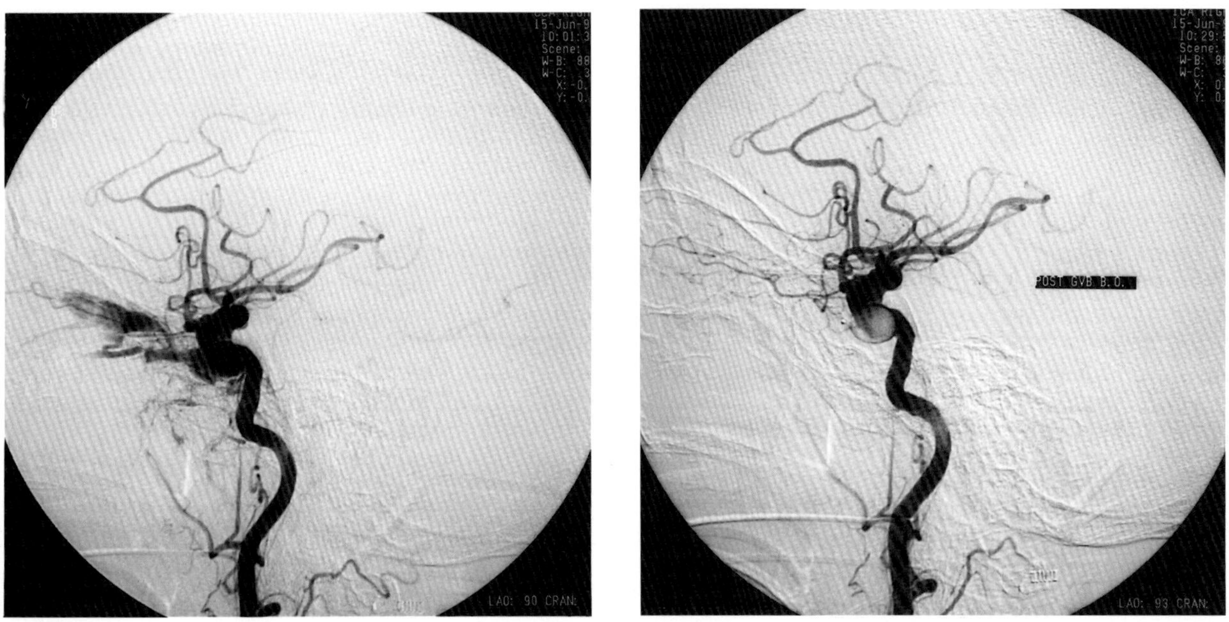

A B

Figure 24–3 Successful treatment with balloon of a direct carotid cavernous fistula due to a ruptured cavernous aneurysm in a 79-year-old female. The aneurysm is only partially occluded and may need further treatment. **(A)** Pre-(lateral view) and **(B)** postballoon occlusion (lateral views).

done later. This choice presents some risk of migration of the balloon after detachment.

Collagen Vascular Diseases

The CCF is frequently associated with dissection of the ICA or with a preexisting aneurysm. The tissues, particularly in patients with Ehlers-Danlos type IV disease,[20,21] are very friable. Even the puncture of the femoral artery can be complicated with dissection or false aneurysm. It may be wiser to use coils rather than detachable balloons and to use the venous rather than the arterial route.

CCF Caused by Gunshot

It is rarely possible to preserve the ICA because the artery is often transected and the tear large and irregular.

◆ Indirect Slow Flow Carotid Cavernous Fistulas

Classification

The Barrow's classification[22] is widely accepted, which refers to the direct fast flow CCFs as type A and the slow flow indirect CCFs as types B, C, and D.

- Type B, C, D—CCFs are exclusively dural AVMs of the CS.
- Type B are dural fistulas supplied solely by branches of the ICA.
- Type C are dural fistulas supplied exclusively by external artery branches (ECA).
- Type D are dural fistulas fed by branches of both the ICA and the ECA without precising whether both ICAs and both ECAs are involved.

Although there are a few cases of type B dural CCFs fed solely by the ICA, I am not convinced that this dural CCF exists. Most of the cases classified as type B were investigated many years ago when the resolution of the images was less optimal than today and when superselective catheterization of the branches of the internal maxillary artery was not done. It should also be noted that these dural fistulas heal spontaneously in 30% or more according to some statistics. Therefore they evolve with time and I have patients with dural CCFs who presented initially with feeders from the ECA and ICA but, at some point in later follow-up, with feeders only from the ICA. For these two reasons, the percentage of type B CCFs is overstated, even if it is extremely low (2 or 3%).

The type C dural CCF is also rare and I have found a traumatic origin to most of these fistulas. Therefore we are left essentially with the type D dural fistulas. Barrow's classification does not distinguish two different subgroups: the first including the cases of unilateral CCF where feeders from one or two ICAs and one or two ECAs converge to the ipsilateral CS. In this situation, the fistula is only on one side, even if this CS drains into the contralateral CS through coronal veins.

The second subgroup includes the cases of true bilateral dural CCFs where ICA and ECA branches on one side communicate with the ipsilateral CS while the contralateral ICA and ECA branches communicate with the contralateral CS. These are true bilateral dural CCFs, which may need bilateral treatment.

Presentation

It is sometimes possible to ascertain by questioning that the patient has a history of previous sinusitis, injury, or inflammatory episodes consistent with a phlebitis of the facial angular vein or SOV. It is probably not fortuitous that some young females develop the symptomatology of a CCF during their pregnancy or in the postpartum period.

The proptosis and chemosis are not as prominent as they are in type A direct CCFs. The IOP is not as high as in type A. It is a disease that affects more females than males and often elderly females. Eye redness is not usually what bothers these patients the most, but they are very disturbed by the double vision, almost always present and associated with a sixth nerve deficit.

Radiological Workup

CT and MRI are useful to rule out other neurological conditions such as atrophy, previous infarctions, or hydrocephalus.

The angiographic workup must include:

- Both common carotid arteries
- Both internal carotid arteries
- Both external carotid arteries and ideally bilateral selective angiography of the ascending cervical artery, of the internal maxillary artery, and of the meningeal arteries
- At least one vertebral artery, usually the left

Patient Selection and Treatment

The screening and treatment of patients is more selective than with the direct type of CCF (**Fig. 24–4**). There are wide discrepancies in the percentage of spontaneous cures published in different series, from 10% to 90%, but the highest percentages usually refer to the group of patients who had minor symptoms and who were treated conservatively. Therefore, considering all cases, with minor symptoms and those with severe symptoms, it is fair to consider that 30% of these dural fistulas will improve spontaneously with time and will finally heal spontaneously.

The peak of chemosis and proptosis should be correlated with the angiographic findings because some of these patients are in fact in the process of thrombosing their SOV and healing spontaneously.

The age of the patient and the existence of multiorgan failure must be considered before embarking on any aggressive treatment.

Patients who do not improve with medical treatment, who have persistent increased ocular pressure, who are greatly disturbed by their sixth nerve deficit and double vision, who continue to have intractable retro-orbital pain, who are found to have cortical venous drainage on the

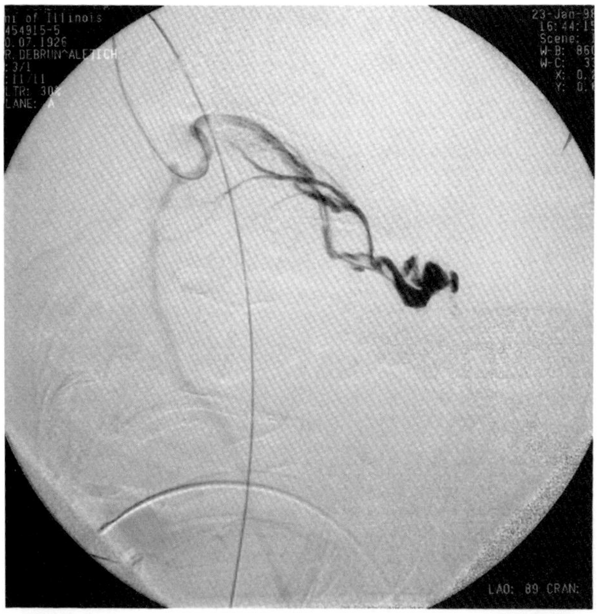

A

Figure 24–4 Successful treatment of a dural carotid cavernous fistula through the superior ophthalmic vein with coils. **(A)** Tip of the microcatheter in the cavernous sinus. **(B)** Closure of the fistula postcoiling from external carotid artery and **(C)** internal carotid artery.

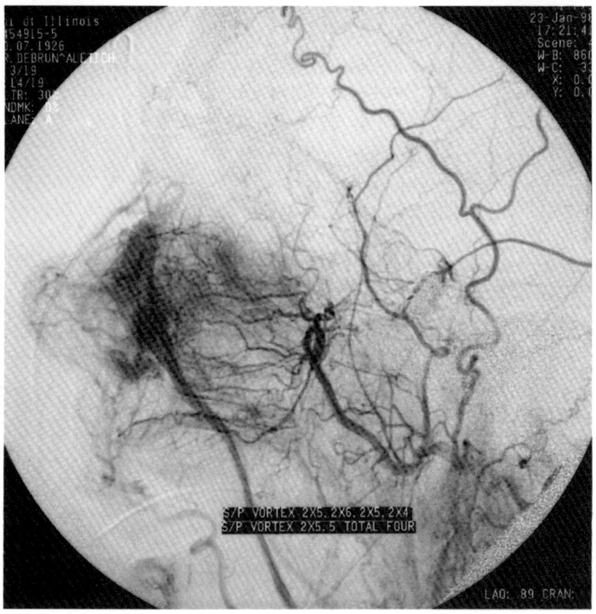

B

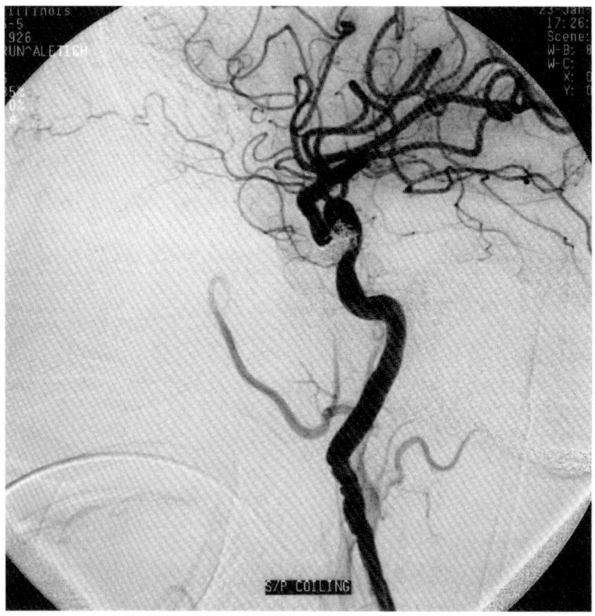

C

angiogram (10% of the dural CCFs), or who are noted to have progressive loss of vision, should be treated. This decision needs to be taken with the neuro-ophthalmologist who follows these patients from day 1.

Treatment Options

Assuming that the decision to treat has been taken, several alternatives of treatment are available and they have evolved with the rapid development of new microcatheters and devices.

Several years ago, the gold standard was the embolization of all the feeders from external carotid arteries, usually with particles, more rarely with acrylic glue. It was not rare to do three or four embolizations over a 6-month period. Most patients were improved clinically, but a substantial number remained incompletely cured anatomically and clinically. The morbidity, which was very low in institutions with broad experience and a large volume of patients, was not always negligible.

Embolization of the ICA branches has been done but remains difficult and risky because the tip of the microcatheter cannot be advanced very far into the CS, and the margin of safety for avoiding reflux of any embolic material into the ICA is limited. The use of acrylic glue bears the risk of reflux of glue into the ICA. The use of coils should be limited to retrievable coils because of the risk of migration or partial deployment of the coil in the ICA.

Today, there is a consensus that the venous route is easier, safer, faster, and more efficient than arterial embolization. The choices are the same as those for the treatment of direct fistulas through the venous route. The techniques are the same

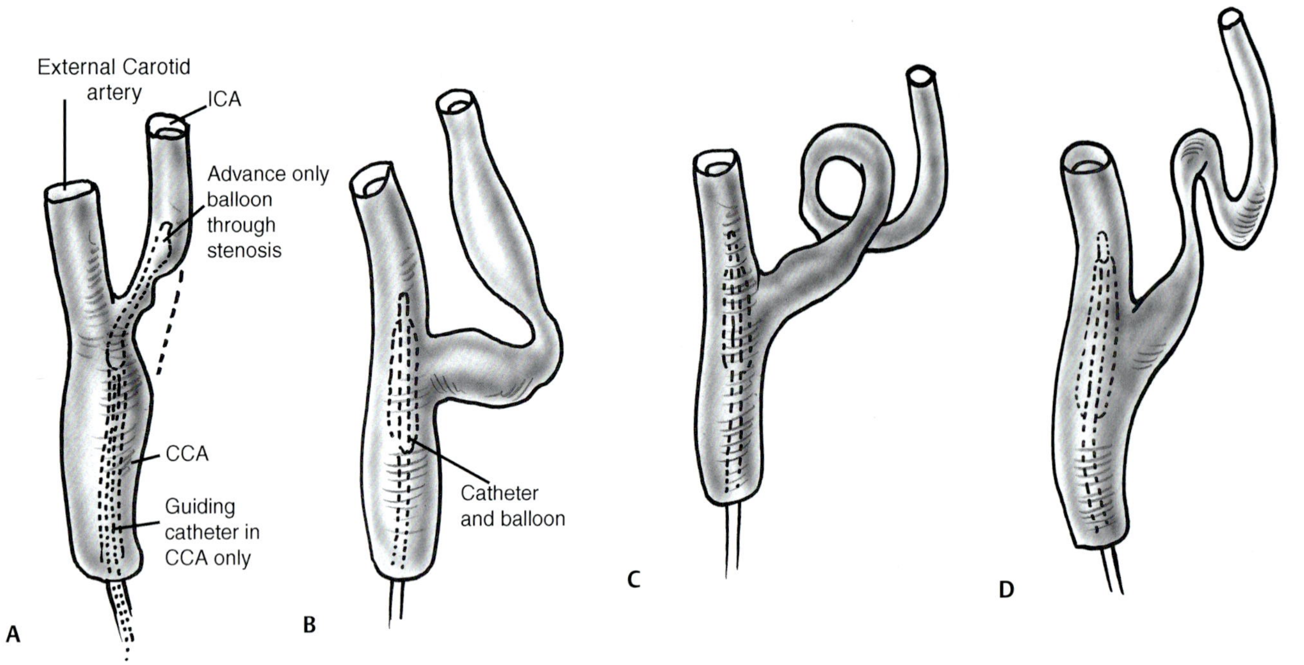

Figure 24–5 **(A)** Severe atheromatous stenosis with ulcer at the origin of the internal carotid artery (ICA). The guiding catheter will stay in the common carotid artery (CCA), and only the balloon will be advanced through the stenosis. Angioplasty plus stent or endarterectomy may be considered before treating the fistula. **(B–D)** The guiding catheter will stay in the CCA or at the origin of the ICA without trying to advance beyond the kink or looping of the ICA.

and the results are similar with a very high yield of complete clinical and anatomical cure and very low morbidity.

Finally, radiation of the CS is an option that has rarely been used. It should be reserved for patients who are not amenable to any type of embolization. Because it takes 2 years for the radiation to be effective in 70% of cases, this treatment option is not very attractive.

◆ Conclusion

Endovascular therapy is the treatment of choice for CCFs. The elegance and the simplicity of the concept of closure of a CCF with detachable balloon, coils, or acrylic glue is only apparent because in fact these techniques need skill, judgment, and experience.

References

1. Nelaton H. Carotid cavernous fistula. Lancet 1876;2:142
2. Prolo DJ, Hanberry JW. Intraluminal occlusion of the carotid cavernous fistula with a balloon catheter. J Neurosurg 1971;35:237–242
3. Black P, Uematsu S, Perovic M, et al. Carotid cavernous fistula: a controlled embolus technique for occlusion of the fistula with preservation of carotid blood flow: technical note. J Neurosurg 1973;38:113–118
4. Serbinenko FA. Balloon catheterization and occlusion of major cerebral vessels. J Neurosurg 1974;41:125–145
5. Serbinenko FA. Reconstruction of the cavernous section of the carotid artery in carotid-cavernous anastomosis. Vopr Neirokhir 1972;36:3–8
6. Debrun G, Lacour P, Caron J, et al. Inflatable and released balloon technique: experimentation in dogs. Neuroradiology 1975;9:267–271
7. Debrun G, Lacour P Cavon P, et al. Experimental approach of treatment of carotid-cavernous fistulas with an inflatable and isolated balloon. Neuroradiology 1975;9:9–12
8. Parkinson D. Carotid cavernous fistula: direct repair with preservation of the carotid artery: technical note. J Neurosurg 1973;38:99–106
9. Mullan S. Treatment of carotid cavernous fistulas by cavernous sinus occlusion. J Neurosurg 1979;50:131–144
10. Isamat F, Ferrer E, Twose J. Direct intracavernous obliteration of high flow CCFs. J Neurosurg 1986;65:770–775
11. Tomsick TA. Carotid Cavernous Fistula. Digital Educational Publishing; 1997
12. Kupersmith MJ, Berenstein A, Flamm E, et al. Neuroophthalmologic abnormalities and intravascular therapy of traumatic carotid cavernous fistulas. Ophthalmology 1986;93:906–912
13. Debrun GM, Ausman JI, Charbel FT, et al. Access to the cavernous sinus through the vertebral artery: technical case report. Neurosurgery 1995;37:144–147
14. Halbach VV, Higashida RT, Hieshima GB, et al. Transvenous embolization of direct carotid cavernous fistulas. AJNR Am J Neuroradiol 1988;9:741–747
15. Uflacker R, Lima S, Ribas G, et al. Carotid-cavernous fistulas: embolization through the superior ophthalmic vein approach. Radiology 1986;159:175–179
16. Monsein LH, Debrun GM, Miller NR, et al. Treatment of dural carotid cavernous fistulas via the superior ophthalmic vein. AJNR Am J Neuroradiol 1991;12:435–439
17. Debrun G, Viñuela F, Fox A, et al. Indications for treatment and classification of 132 carotid-cavernous fistulas. Neurosurgery 1988;22: 285–289
18. Graeb D, Robertson WD, Lapointe JS, et al. Avoiding intraarterial balloon detachment in the treatment of posttraumatic carotid-cavernous fistulae with detachable balloons. AJNR Am J Neuroradiol 1985;6: 602–605
19. Halbach VV, Higashida RT, Hieshima GB, et al. Normal perfusion pressure breakthrough occurring during treatment of carotid and vertebral fistulas. AJNR Am J Neuroradiol 1987;8:751–756
20. Halbach VV, Higashida RT, Dowd CF, et al. Treatment of carotid-cavernous fistulas associated with Ehlers-Danlos syndrome. Neurosurgery 1990;26:1021–1027
21. Debrun G, Aletich V, Neil R, et al. Three cases of spontaneous direct carotid cavernous fistulas associated with Ehlers Danlos type IV syndrome. Surg Neurol 1996;46:247–252
22. Barrow DL, Spector RH, Braun IF, et al. Classification and treatment of spontaneous carotid-cavernous fistulas. J Neurosurg 1985;62: 248–256

25

Vein of Galen Aneurysms

J. Parker Mickle

With rapid advances in imaging and interventional technologies, the neurosurgery for vein of Galen aneurysms has evolved rapidly into a technically demanding exercise with a high chance of success.[1] Prior to the 1980s, as all neurosurgeons remember, this disease entity was well defined clinically and angiographically and was rarely cured by the standard therapies available at that time. Occasional anecdotal reports gave hope to better outcomes with more refined technique and a better definition of the individuals successfully responsive to those techniques. Rarely, individuals were found harboring essentially asymptomatic lesions in the adult years. However, the natural history of this entity in its myriad of clinical presentations remained progressive injury to the nervous system and other organ systems and, therefore, often demanded therapy, albeit risky.[2] Since 1984 in this institution, we have evolved therapies for vein of Galen aneurysms that have tended toward transvenous and transarterial interventional techniques, reserving surgery for the rare individual with progressive disease no longer amenable to interventional approaches. There are Yasargil type I lesions, which can be effectively treated with open surgery, but which can also be just as effectively, and with less risk, eliminated with transarterial embolization. The armamentarium available to the neurosurgeon in treating vein of Galen aneurysms is large and encompasses multiple subspecialties. For optimum outcome, these lesions are best treated at a multispecialty center, but life-saving initial therapies can be performed by virtually any neurosurgeon until the patient can be globally treated at a tertiary care center.

◆ Contraindications to Treatment

Severe brain injury due to ischemia and venous hypertension.

◆ Surgical Technique

Approaches

Para-occipital Approach

The surgical exposure of the vein of Galen and its malformations can be accomplished in a three quarter prone position via a paraoccipital approach with opening of the tentorial incisor and the posterior corpus callosum (**Fig. 25–1**). The small arterial feeders are then taken in turn with small vascular clips and bipolar coagulation.[3] The thickened wall of the vein of Galen in this location can be easily displaced so that more feeders can be reached toward the anterior margin of the malformation. Also, at this point, the aneurysm can be punctured, and thrombosing wires, silk, or glue can be injected. Anteroinferiorly, the vein of Galen is thin walled and easily broken.

Interventional Approach

The interventional approach is the most common therapy today because it offers the best opportunity to rid the patient of the malformation while protecting cardiac and neurological function.[4] Hydrocephalus remains a not uncommon complication of this syndrome and probably results from increased venous pressure deep within the neurovascular bed. Aqueductal stenosis may also contribute to the incidence of this entity. We have treated hydrocephalus early in this group of patients and ultimately shunt around 50% of them.

Transarterial Approach

The transarterial approach to vein of Galen malformations is performed in neuroradiology through a transfemoral puncture

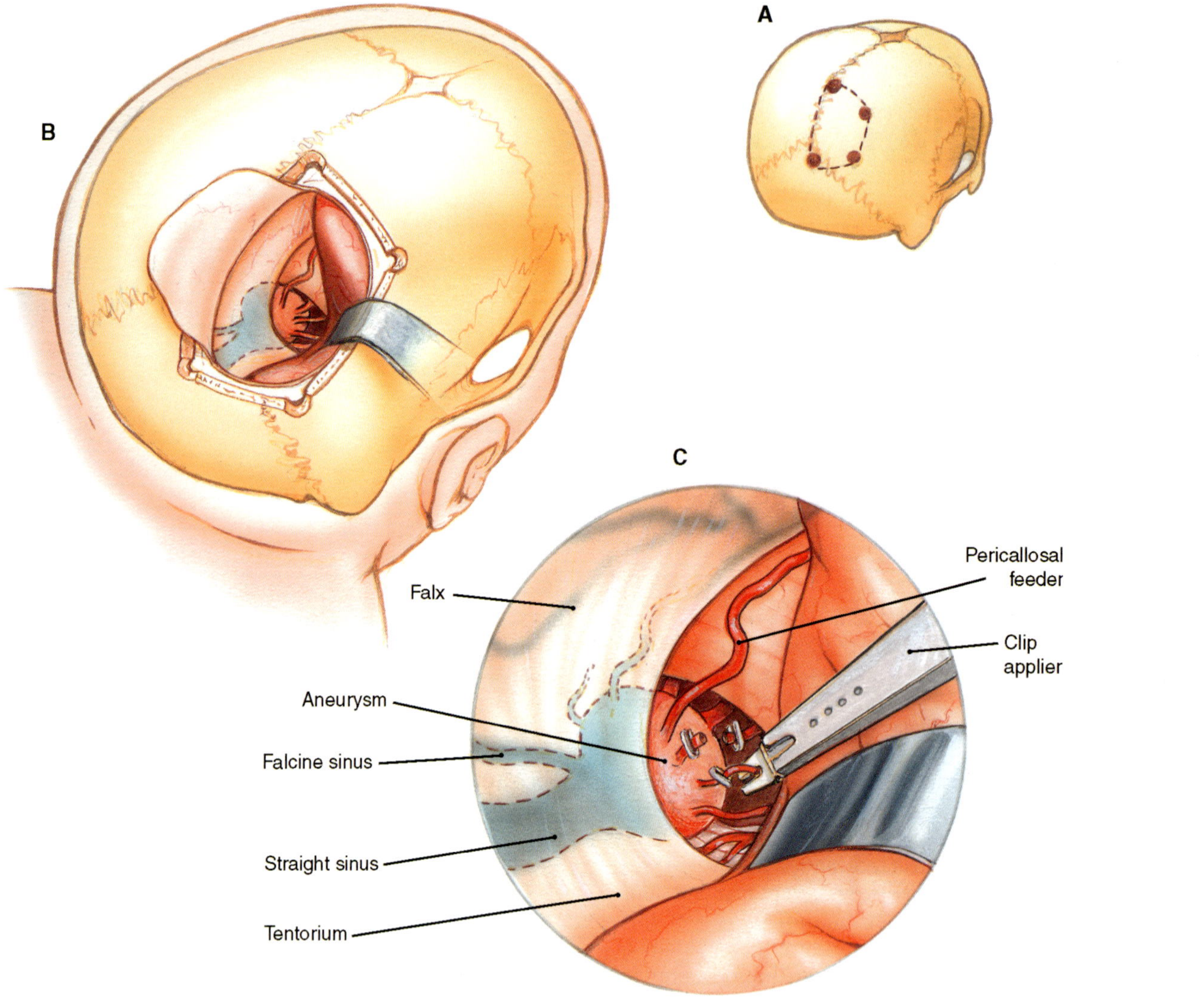

Figure 25–1 These diagrams show the general position and surgical technique for a craniotomy to expose a typical vein of Galen aneurysm. It is critical to retract as little as possible and to use gravity as much as possible in the exposure.

and flow-directed microcatheters, depending on the pedicular supply to the aneurysm. The general principle is to get as close to the fistulous connection as possible so that small arterial feeders to the brain stem are protected in the embolic process. In the newborn, the transarterial approach can be difficult because of tortuous feeding vessels in the thorax and neck and the very small amount of dye tolerated by the small child already compromised in somatic perfusion. Several pedicles are usually chosen and embolized very distally with either silk, polyvinyl alcohol, or glue. Rarely have we required a cutdown in the neck to access the transarterial approach. The transvenous approach popularized by Mullan in his treatment of carotid cavernous fistulas[5] became our standard initial therapy for vein of Galen aneurysms in 1984. We have subsequently evolved toward a transvenous/transarterial technique because we feel the retarding vein of Galen aneurysm basket so deposited gives us the best opportunity to positively affect cardiac function rapidly and allows for safer transarterial therapy in the subsequent efforts to rid the patient of the lesion entirely.[4]

On occasion, we have been able to rid the patient of the lesion completely with transvenous embolization only. The technique we use in the transvenous approach is the same in all age groups in vein of Galen aneurysms. The only variable is the degree to which we push as defined by the clinical demand. In an individual with massive progressive heart failure, an immediate and dramatic effect must be obtained in the operating room with the transtorcular approach or the therapy will fail rapidly.

Technical Steps in the Transtorcular Embolization Procedure

The relationship of the vein of Galen malformation with the straight sinus or accessory straight sinus is identified on

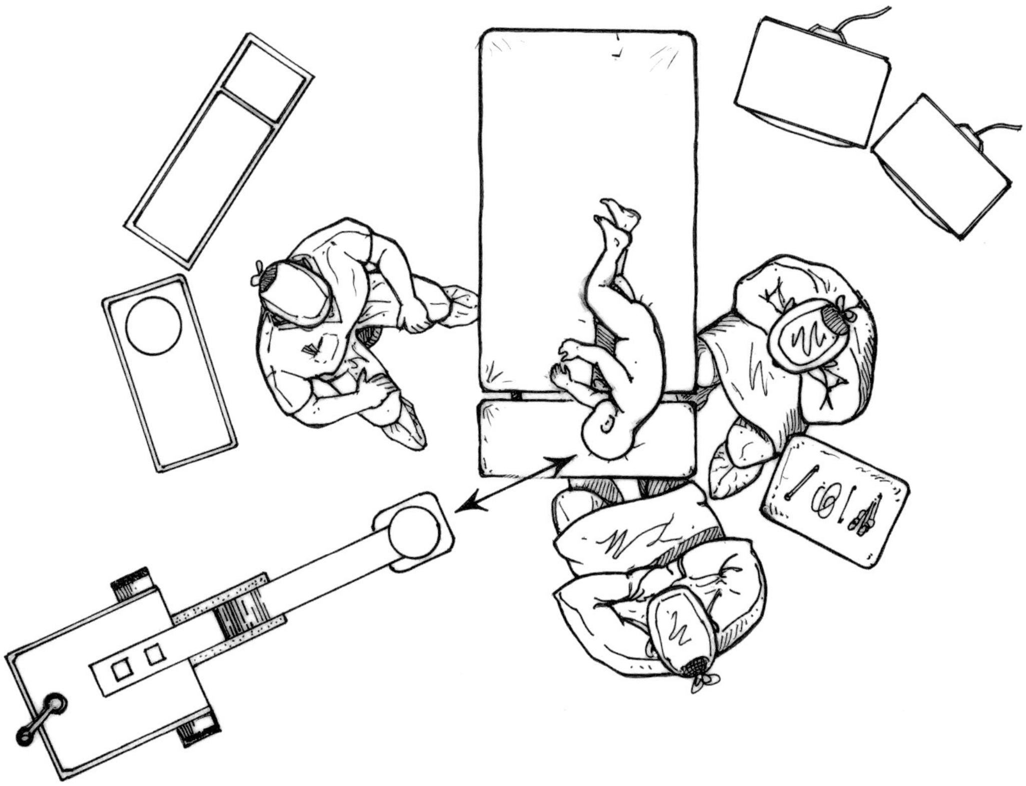

Figure 25–2 This cartoon is self-explanatory but critical for the intraoperative transvenous delivery of embolic materials. The fluoroscopic control of the progress of the procedure is vital, and the procedure must be deliberate and unhurried.

preoperative studies, usually a computed tomographic (CT) scan, a magnetic resonance imaging (MRI) scan, or an angiogram. In an operating room with the capability of doing intraoperative angiography and venography, the patient is placed in a supine position with a bump under the right or left shoulder (**Fig. 25–2**). The head is turned so that the sagittal suture is parallel with the floor. Fluoroscopy is brought in to identify major landmarks, including the approximate positions of the torcula and the aneurysm. A small but generous craniectomy is performed over the torcula and this can be accomplished with virtually no blood loss.

The general and detailed steps in the transtorcular treatment of these high-flow fistulae are depicted in **Figs. 25–3** and **25–4A–E**. The greatest danger in this procedure is the inadvertent puncture of the thin anteroventral wall of the aneurysm with the tip of the coil. The careful placement of the coil under x-ray control utilizing the "push-pull" technique minimizes this risk.

Intraoperative ultrasound is useful for identifying torcula, straight sinus, and aneurysm, and the area of puncture is entered with a 25 gauge needle to ensure that brisk arterial bleeding is obtained. A small needle, or angiocath, is used to puncture this same dural hole, and a very soft guidewire is advanced into the torcula, straight sinus, and aneurysm. Over this guidewire, a coaxial catheter system is twisted through the dura while maintaining a stable guidewire position under fluoroscopic control. The coaxial system is advanced into the aneurysm and a venogram is obtained. At this point, intra-aneurysmal straight sinus and torcula pressures can be measured and compared for therapeutic purposes. A demandreled 018 angiographic guidewire is then carefully, and without resistance, folded into the aneurysm cavity forming a basket to change the flow characteristics in the aneurysm and to act as a lattice onto which other embolic agents, including coils, balloons, or glue can be deposited (**Fig. 25–3**). If the patient is suffering from heart failure, a significant reduction in intra-aneurysmal pressure is essential for significant benefit. The guideline should be to reduce the intra-aneurysmal mean arterial pressure to about half. The great risk in this part of the operation is the inappropriate forcing of the wire through the thin-walled anteroinferior portion of the aneurysm. This will lead to subarachnoid and intraventricular hemorrhage and can result in death. We have had this unfortunate circumstance occur three times. In two of these patients delay in therapy for the intraventricular hemorrhage resulted in death. In one patient we immediately realized that an intraventricular hemorrhage had occurred (as identified by extravasation of dye on the venogram) and we performed an immediate ventriculostomy; this patient survived with a good quality of life. The deposition of the 018 demandreled guidewire is of special importance because it may require a coordinated push-pull technique, which works very well but requires some technical development to master (**Fig. 25–4A–E**). Although this technique

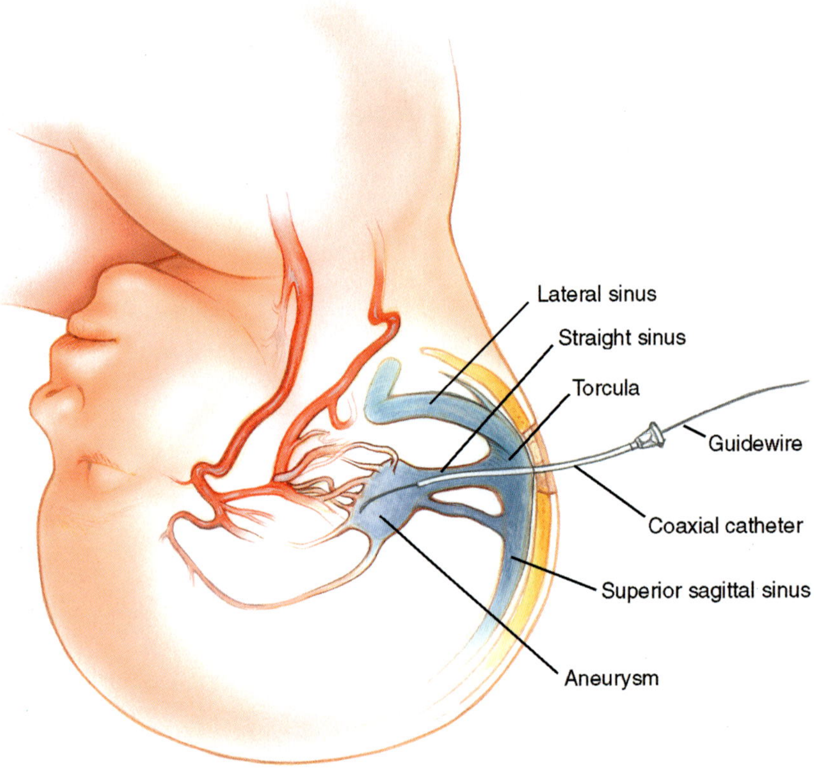

Figure 25–3 An overall schematic of the positioning and general technical steps in the transtorcular deposition of a coil basket into a typical vein of Galen aneurysm.

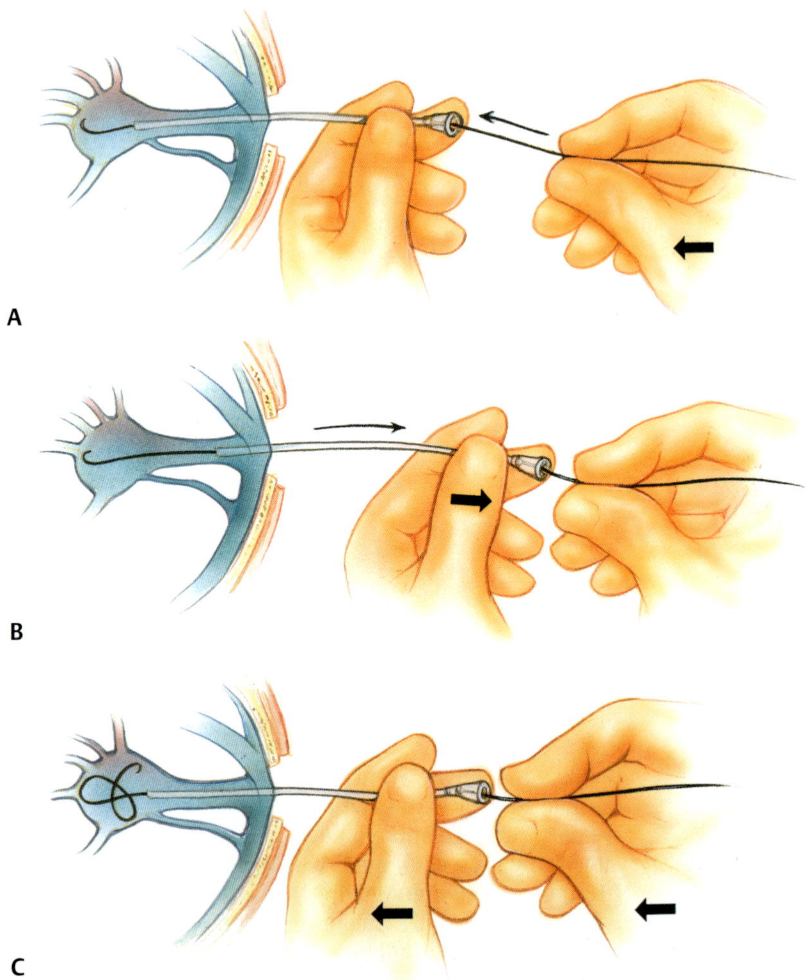

Figure 25–4 The manipulative deposition of a coil in an aneurysm may require a push-pull technique for optimal safety. **(A)** If the initial attempt at safely depositing the coil is unsuccessful, **(B)** the catheter is slowly and smoothly withdrawn as the coil-wire is advanced under x-ray control. This allows the initial coiling to occur without force being applied at the tip of the coil. **(C)** The entire construct can then be advanced with both hands simultaneously.

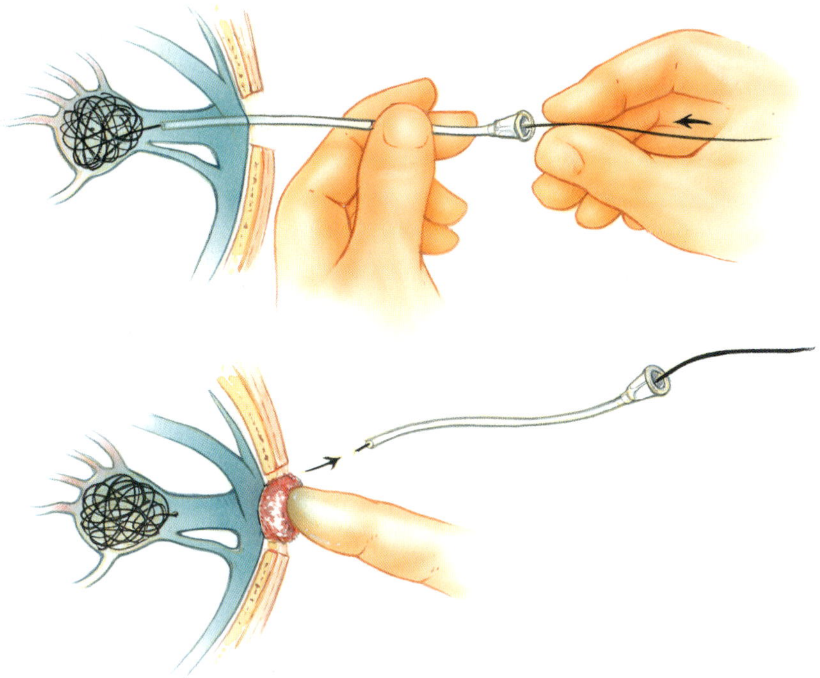

D

E

(*Continued*) **Figure 25–4** **(D)** The folding process progresses well from this point, and **(E)** the entire construct is removed, with bleeding being controlled with Gelfoam under a supporting finger.

is not frequently required, it is essential where the wire will not fold on itself effortlessly. Once the operating surgeons have accomplished their goal, a postembolization venogram is obtained and pressures recorded. The coaxial catheter system is removed, and a piece of Gelfoam or other material is placed over the exit hole, which usually bleeds quite briskly. A finger holding pressure on the Gelfoam for 5 minutes suffices to control this bleeding and the wound is closed in layers.

◆ Conclusion

The intervention treatment (transvenous, transarterial, and radiosurgical) of vein of Galen malformations is still evolving. This team approach, however, is the treatment of choice today and offers the best chance for cure. The role of surgery in this entity is utilized to treat resulting hydrocephalus and to gain access to those lesions no longer treatable with interventional technologies.

References

1. Mickle JP, Quisling RG. The transtorcular embolization of the vein of Galen aneurysms. J Neurosurg 1986;64:731–735
2. Hoffman HJ, Chang S, Hendricks EB. Experience at the Hospital for Sick Children, Toronto. J Neurosurg 1982;57:316–322
3. Amacher AL, Shillito J Jr. The syndromes of surgical treatment of aneurysms of the great vein of Galen. J Neurosurg 1973;39:89–98
4. Mickle JP, Hubert A. Vein of Galen and dural malformations in childhood. In: Albright AL, Pollack IF, Adelson PD, eds. Principles and Practices of Pediatric Neurosurgery. New York: Thieme; 1999: 1033–1051
5. Mullan S. Treatment of carotid cavernous fistulas by cavernous sinus occlusion. J Neurosurg 1979;50:131–144

Section IV

Occlusive and Hemorrhagic Vascular Diseases

26

Carotid Endarterectomy: Vascular Surgery Perspective

Dipankar Mukherjee

Stroke is the third leading cause of death in the United States. Randomized clinical trials have demonstrated the efficacy of carotid endarterectomy (CEA) in the prevention of stroke when performed in centers of surgical excellence.[1,2] First described in 1954, the procedure saw rising popularity until the mid-1980s, when several reports published very high rates of perioperative complications (stroke and death),[3,4,5] raising concerns about its benefits in stroke prevention. In a subsequent randomized controlled trial (North American Symptomatic Endarterectomy Trial), it was unequivocally demonstrated that CEA is effective to prevent stroke in symptomatic patients with carotid stenosis of 70% or more if the procedure is performed in high-volume centers with low complication rates.[1] Similar results were published from European trial enrolling patients with high-grade stenosis and in the Veterans Affairs Cooperative Symptomatic Carotid Stenosis Trial.[2,6]

The results of the Asymptomatic Carotid Atherosclerosis Study (ACAS) in 1994 suggested that even asymptomatic patients with a stenosis of as little as 60% could benefit with regard to prevention of stroke from an operative procedure.[7]

Percentage of stenosis is determined by comparing the narrowest portion of the lumen with the diameter of the distal noninvolved internal carotid artery (ICA): a 50% diameter reduction corresponds to a 75% reduction in cross-sectional area and becomes hemodynamically significant. There is a positive correlation between a stenosis of > 70% and the incidence of neurological events.

Risk factors for cerebrovascular disease are age > 60, hypertension, tobacco use, diabetes, coronary artery disease/ arrhythmias/history of congestive heart failure, peripheral vascular disease, and hyperlipidemia. Other factors to be considered include morphology of the plaque as seen on imaging studies, the incidence of silent stroke as confirmed by computed tomography (CT), and the status of the contralateral and vertebral circulation. A comprehensive algorithm for CEA addressing all aspects of perioperative management as described following here results in improved outcome with decreased resource utilization.

◆ Indications

- Hemodynamically significant carotid artery stenosis of > 60% in asymptomatic good risk candidates
    - Hemodynamically significant stenosis in patients symptomatic with
    - Transient ischemic attacks (TIA)
    - Transient monocular blindness
    - Stroke with minimal neurological deficit or stroke with subsequent neurological recovery
- Large ulcerated plaque in symptomatic patients independent of degree of stenosis may be an indication in selected cases.

◆ Preoperative Studies

Noninvasive preoperative evaluation is preferred. All patients undergo duplex ultrasonography (DU) in a laboratory accredited by the Intersocietal Commission for Accreditation of Vascular

Laboratories (ICAVL). For confirmation of findings and for precise anatomical definition of the arterial vessels proximal and distal to the lesion that may influence the indication for operation, magnetic resonance angiography (MRA) is indicated as the second study. Conventional angiography (CA) is reserved for patients in whom MRA is contraindicated (e.g., pacemaker implant), technically not feasible (e.g., uncooperative patient, motion artifact), or if there is a significant discrepancy between findings obtained by DU and MRA.

Operation is performed based on duplex findings alone only in the presence of an appropriate lesion on DU in combination with a history of the classic symptoms and if there is severe contrast allergy.

If a lesion progresses in severity on serial follow-up DU after the performance of appropriate imaging and CEA on the one side in the past, the second CEA can be performed based on DU alone.

MRA less severely overestimates stenosis and CA underestimates it.[8]

In most series, CA has an incidence of procedure-related combined stroke and death rate up to ~0.5%. In two studies, CA was associated with a higher probability of an inaccurate diagnosis than MRA and DU. Kuntz et al demonstrated a significantly smaller 5-year risk for stroke for MRA and DU.[8,9]

◆ Surgical Technique

Anesthesia

A combination of locoregional anesthesia (LRA) and light intravenous sedation, when indicated, is used whenever feasible. This allows awake mental status monitoring. The patient is given a squeaking toy in the contralateral hand and is instructed to squeeze it every 30 to 60 seconds during cross-clamping of the carotid artery. The patient also has to respond to simple questions.

Standard, or general, endotracheal anesthesia (GET) induced with thiopental, etomidate, or propofol is reserved for patients not able to perform these tasks and patients who refused LRA. LRA can be converted to GET in the setting of an unstable or uncooperative patient.

Positioning

The patient is positioned with the head raised 30 to 45 degrees and the neck extended and turned to the contralateral side. A crossbar fixed to the operating room (OR) table is placed at the level of the patient's forehead. A sterile towel draped over the bar allows the patient's face to stay clear and hence prevents a sensation of claustrophobia or feeling smoth-

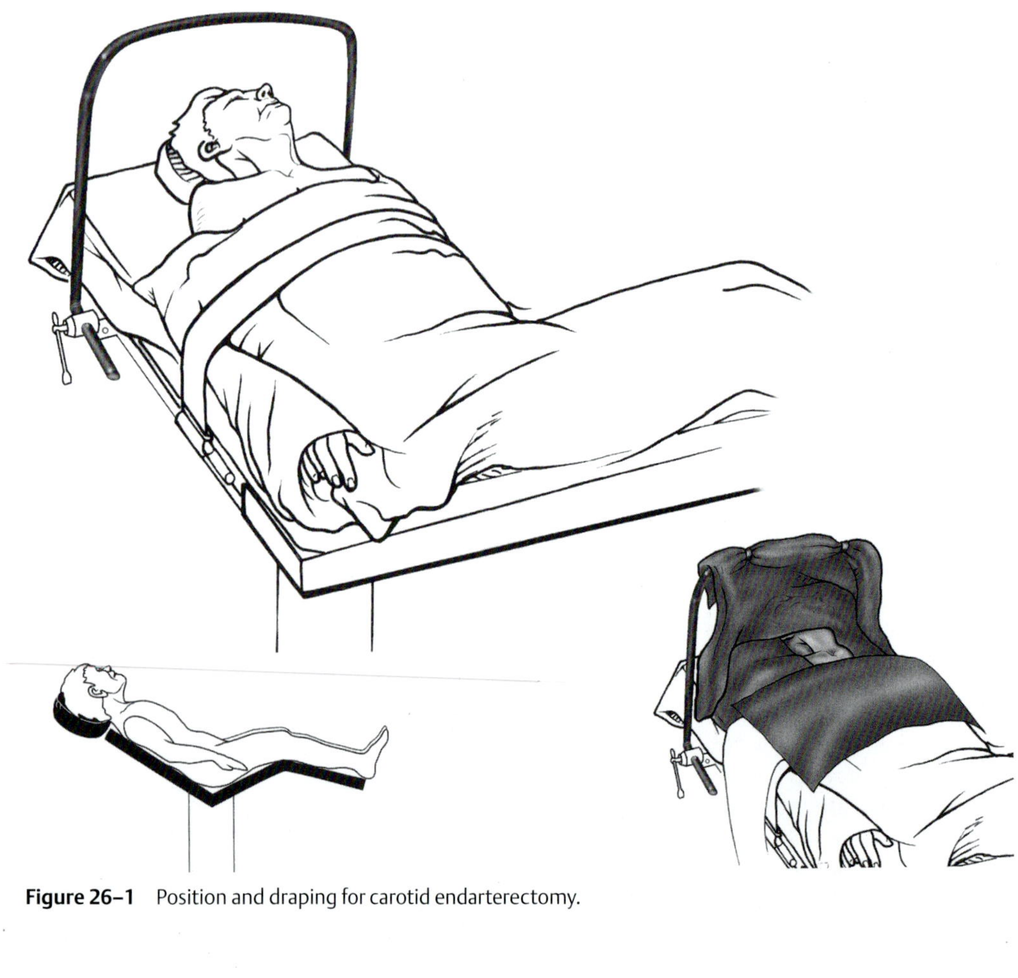

Figure 26–1 Position and draping for carotid endarterectomy.

ered. The surgeon is standing to the right of the patient regardless of the operative side (**Fig. 26–1**).

Initial Exposure

The skin incision is placed along the anterior border of the sternocleidomastoid muscle (SCM). The platysma and investing layer of the deep cervical fascia are divided. Dissecting medially to the SCM, the vascular sheath is exposed. Self-retaining Weitlaner retractors are placed. Small vessel branches are ligated with 4–0 silk ties. Care should be taken not to injure the accessory nerve, which crosses the superior aspect of the wound to innervate the SCM. The vascular sheath is opened, dividing the omohyoid muscle crossing the inferior aspect of the field if needed. To dissect and retract posteriorly the internal jugular vein, the common facial vein has to be divided. This immediately exposes the carotid artery, most commonly at the level of the bifurcation. The vagus nerve is identified and protected from trauma.

With precision, sharp arterial mobilization is performed using Metzenbaum scissors, taking care to prevent dislodgement of emboli from the diseased vessel. This is achieved by minimizing dissection around the bulb of the ICA. Elastic rubber loops are placed around the common carotid artery (CCA) and the external carotid artery (ECA) as well as the ICA. The superior thyroid artery is encircled with a 0 silk tie in a double loop.

Dissection at the bifurcation in the area of the carotid body is kept to a minimum. Instillation of local anesthetic into this area (nerve of Herring) is used only if bradycardia or hemodynamic instability is encountered.

The ansa cervicalis nerve is divided as necessary in the course of clearing tissues from the anterior surface of the carotid arteries (**Fig. 26–2**).

The hypoglossal nerve trunk crossing the ICA at a variable distance superior to the bifurcation is carefully preserved. The usual posterior and lateral location of the ICA in relation to the ECA can be distorted on account of tortuosity or variance in anatomy. The lower edge of the submandibular and parotid gland is retracted anteriorly and superiorly if necessary. Division of a branch of the ECA, which passes over the 12th nerve to supply the SCM, allows superior mobilization of the 12th nerve and distal exposure of the ICA for an additional 2 to 3 cm.

Currently our technique involves preoperative DU to mark the carotid bifurcation on the skin surface with the patient positioned for surgery. This allows the anesthesiologist to place a regional block limited to the surgical site. The incision is usually 5 to 7 cm in length, with more of the incision given to expose the ICA than the CCA. If extent of disease mandates a more generous exposure, then such is provided. The benefits of a limited regional block have translated into

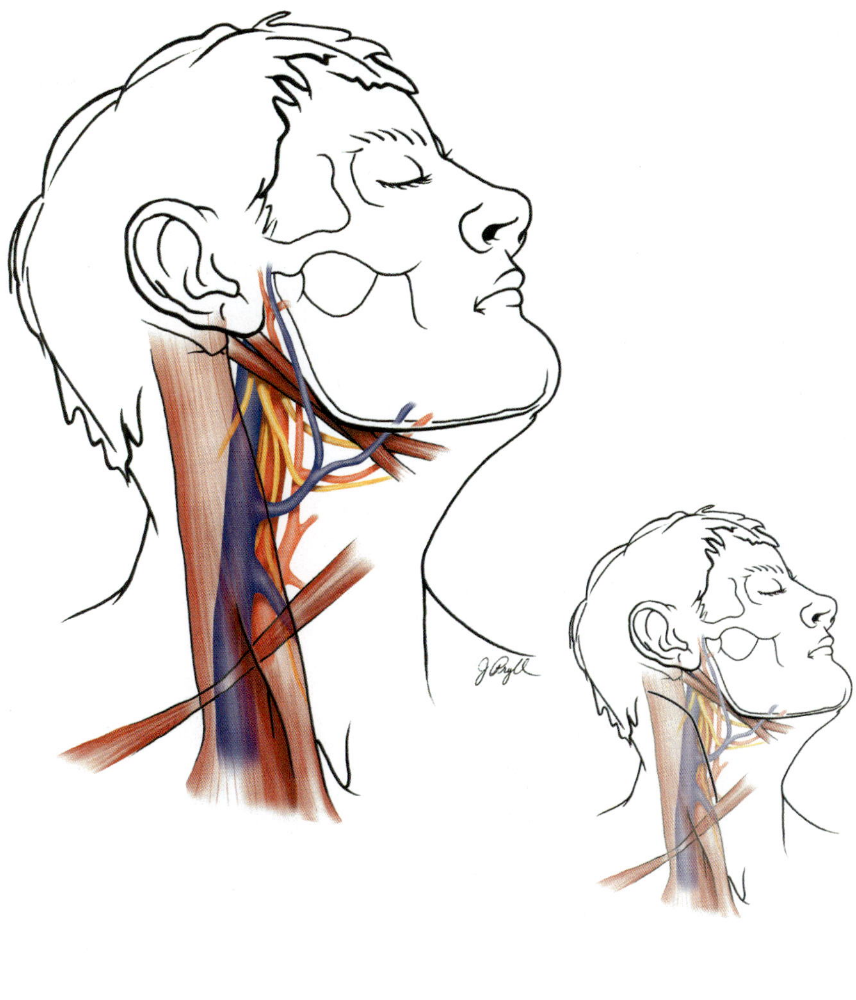

Figure 26–2 Anatomical illustration of structures surrounding the carotid bifurcation.

use of a third less volume of local anesthesia compared with the previous extensive cervical block. This also resulted in absence of hematoma formation and freedom from swallowing problems because vagus nerve function is usually maintained. From the surgical perspective, the limited incision contributes to decreased morbidity from the procedure. Apart from the obvious benefits of patient comfort and cosmetic considerations, there is usually no need to traumatize the parotid gland, decreasing the possibility of seventh nerve injury.

Indications for Shunt

Under condition of LRA and awake mental status monitoring, the carotid is cross-clamped, and the patient is asked to squeeze a squeaking toy with the contralateral hand every 30 seconds as well as answer simple questions while flow is interrupted.

An Inahara-Pruitt 200/20 (LeMaitre Vascular, Burlington, MA) indwelling shunt is placed if there is

- High-grade stenosis or complete occlusion of the contralateral ICA regardless of anesthesia regimen chosen
- Deterioration in mental status observed during LRA
- General endotracheal anesthesia

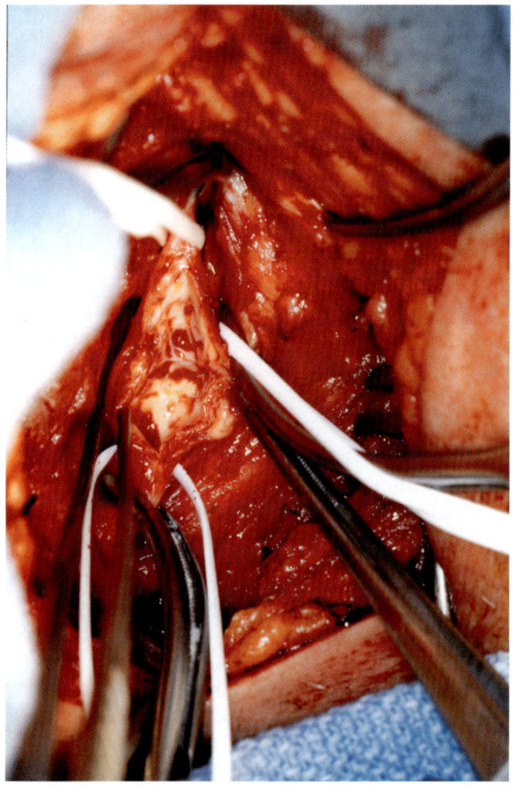

Figure 26–3 Arteriotomy extends beyond the limit of the disease into normal vessel. Internal carotid artery is at the top of the picture, and common carotid artery is at the bottom.

Plaque Removal

The carotid artery is opened along the lateral wall of the CCA with a no. 11 scalpel blade, and the incision is extended using Pott's scissors through the plaque in the middle of the ICA. The arteriotomy should be extended beyond the limits of the plaque into the normal vessel (**Fig. 26–3**). With a dissector, the plaque is gently elevated. Utmost care is taken to achieve a perfect distal end point in the ICA. Generally, there is tapering of the plaque at its distal limit, which makes tacking of the intima to the adventitia with 7–0 interrupted monofilament sutures usually unnecessary. The latter is performed infrequently, if after extension of the arteriotomy onto the distal ICA an imperfect end point is noted (i.e., mildly diseased, thickened intima is noted at the distal end).

Eversion endarterectomy of the ECA is performed by pushing out the luminal aspect of the ECA by advancing the adventitial aspect of the ECA toward the arteriotomy.

If the intima or the plaque in the CCA is bulky, it is tacked down to prevent infolding and creation of a new site of prolific neointimal hyperplasia (**Fig. 26–4**).

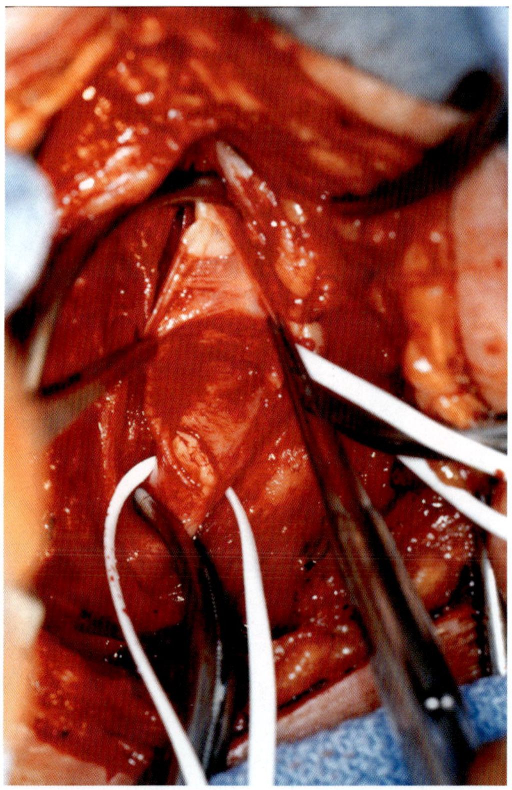

Figure 26–4 Plaque in common carotid artery (CCA) is tacked down. End point in internal carotid artery (ICA) is normal intima. ICA is at the top of the picture. CCA is at the bottom.

Closure

The artery is routinely patched using prosthetic material (Gore-Tex Acuseal Cardiovascular Patch; W.L. Gore & Associates, Inc. Flagstaff, AZ). Autogenous vein can be used alternatively but may be more time consuming without conferring measurable benefit. A monofilament nonabsorbable 6–0 single running suture is used (**Fig. 26–5**). The

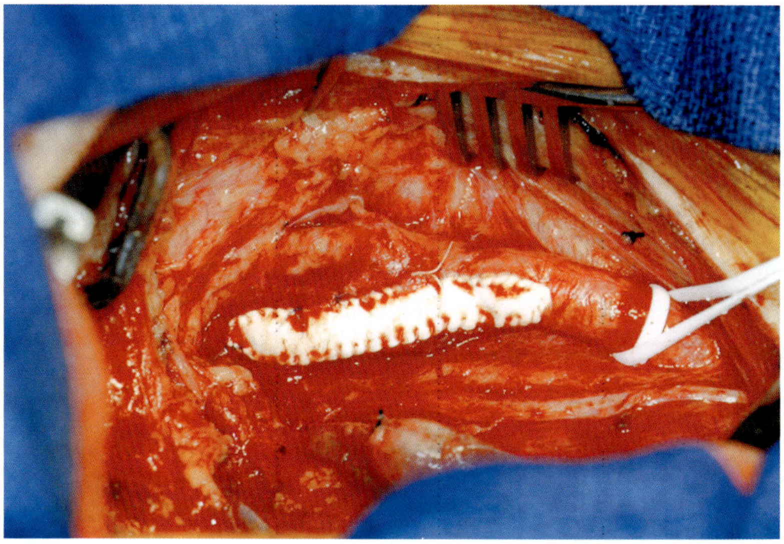

Figure 26–5 Patch repair of carotid arteriotomy using Hemashield Finesse (Boston Scientific, Natick, MA) patch. Internal carotid artery is at the top of the picture, common carotid artery is at the bottom.

CCA and ECA, then the ICA clamps, are briefly released for flushing prior to completion of closure. In this fashion, flow is restored in the ECA before the ICA. After clamp removal, all patients undergo intraoperative Doppler examination of ECA and ICA distal to repair for documentation of a triphasic signal.

A small closed-suction drain is routinely placed through a separate stab incision inferomedially. The wound is closed in three layers, with approximation of tissues about the neurovascular sheath, followed by a running closure of the platysma and skin.

◆ Postoperative Care

All patients are monitored in the recovery room for 4 hours postoperatively. If not requiring intravenous medication for blood pressure regulation and remaining in their preoperative cardiac rhythm, patients are then transferred to the general ward. If requiring inotropic or vasodilator therapy intravenously or treatment of cardiac rhythm disturbances, patients are admitted to the intensive care unit (ICU) after 4 hours. Drain removal and discharge on postoperative day 1 is the rule if off intravenous medications and tolerating regular diet. Patients are discharged on enteric-coated aspirin 81 mg once a day and clapidogrel 75 mg once a day for 30 days, after which aspirin alone is continued indefinitely unless gastrointestinal problems preclude the use of aspirin.

All patients are seen in the office within 1 week. They are then followed by serial DU annually.

◆ Results

Utilizing the previously outlined integrated management algorithm in a series of 128 consecutive patients between 1997 and 1998, there were two perioperative strokes with subsequent recovery and one death following a myocardial infarction, for a mortality rate of 0.8% and a stroke rate of 1.5%. Hospital stay was < 24 hours (discharge on postoperative day 1) in 89.8% of patients; 93.8% were discharged by day 2.

Eight patients required admission to the ICU after the monitoring period; no patients required admission to the ICU after being transferred to the floor. There were no hospital readmissions for postoperative complications.

Generally accepted limits for combined incidence of stroke and death for CEA performed for asymptomatic stenosis is < 3%; CEA performed for TIA is < 5%; for stroke with fixed deficit < 7%, for restenosis < 10%; accepted mortality is up to 2 or 3%.

Long-term significant restenosis (i.e., > 50% stenosis) of the ICA or the CCA at the site of previous endarterectomy as detected by serial DU examination was ~3% in the present series, and the intervention for the recurrent high-grade restenosis was 1.5%.

◆ Complications

Postoperative Stroke

In the event of a postoperative neurological deficit noted in the operating room, immediate reexploration of the endarterectomy site is warranted. Technical problems such as a distal arterial flap leading to thrombosis of the endarterectomy site need immediate correction. If the endarterectomy site is technically perfect, then one may need to perform angiography in the interventional radiology suite where availability of tracker catheters, thrombolytic agents, and balloon angioplasty catheters in the hands of a competent neuroradiologist can limit the size of the cerebral infarct and salvage an acceptable result as opposed to a disastrous one without the aforementioned aids.

If the neurological deficit is noted in the recovery room, immediate DU of the endarterectomy site is performed. If technical problems such as a thrombus or intimal flap are detected, the patient is immediately returned to the operating room for reexploration. If the endarterectomy site is noted to be without problems, angiography is recommended for major neurological deficit.

Neck Hematoma

Use of a closed suction drain is routine following CEA. Nevertheless, one may encounter a nonfunctioning drain and accumulation of a significant hematoma in the neck. If the hematoma is substantial or compromises the airway in any manner, evacuation in the operating room is advised. Anything less than perfectly sterile conditions would place the prosthetic patch angioplasty at risk for infection.

Carotid Restenosis

Serial postoperative DU follow-up examinations of the CEA sites at 6 months and annually thereafter will reveal an incidence of significant restenosis in the 2 to 5% range.[10] Carotid repair without the use of patches leads to a much higher incidence of restenosis, particularly in women.[11]

Fortunately, carotid restenosis has proven to be a more benign entity compared with the primary disease process.[12] Reoperation for carotid restenosis is therefore reserved for symptomatic patients or those with extremely high-grade restenosis (80–99%) that show no regression on serial ultrasound scans 3 and 6 months apart. Operations for recurrent carotid stenosis are performed under general anesthesia, and patients will be counseled regarding a higher incidence of possible complications, particularly cranial nerve injuries, usually transient in nature.

Cranial Nerve Palsy

It is not unusual to see temporary weakness in the distribution of the seventh cranial nerve, usually as a result of the local anesthetic block. More profound block of the ipsilateral brachial plexus with motor weakness of the upper extremity can be seen but is uncommon. Patient anxiety is easily relieved when the temporary nature of the weakness is pointed out. Injury related to traction of the seventh or 12th nerve can be longer lasting. By avoiding incising the parotid gland or placing undue traction on the glands, the incidence of seventh nerve injury can be minimized. Injury to the recurrent laryngeal nerve is very uncommon unless there is an unrecognized anatomical variation.

Management of the high carotid bifurcation requires division of the posterior belly of the digastric muscle and careful mobilization of the 12th nerve after ligating and dividing the arterial branch of the ECA to the SCM, which courses cephalad to the nerve and usually tethers it down. This maneuver alone will allow an additional 2 cm of distal mobilization of the ICA. Mobilization of the parotid gland may be necessary, and temporary traction on the seventh nerve may be unavoidable. In our experience with carotid surgery, temporary mandibular subluxation to gain an additional length of distal ICA has not been necessary, although this technique is well described in the literature.[13]

◆ Conclusion

Alternative treatment strategies for carotid stenosis, most notably percutaneous carotid angioplasty and stent placement, may compare favorably in patient outcome but not so with cost.[14,15] Long-term follow-up and specific stent-related complications are at present insufficiently investigated. The Carotid Revascularization Endarterectomy versus Stenting Trial (CREST) trial is being launched to answer the much sought after question as to whether carotid stenting is an equivalent alternative to CEA.

Use of GET seems to be responsible for many of the postoperative hemodynamic alterations. LRA results in significantly shorter duration of operation as well as hospital stay and a decreased incidence of cardiopulmonary events .

In conclusion, noninvasive preoperative evaluation in combination with LRA, precise surgical technique with diligent attention to the end point of the endarterectomy in the ICA, and efficient postoperative monitoring with selective ICU observation is a safe and cost-efficient approach with a low complication rate.

References

1. North American Symptomatic Carotid Endarterectomy Trial Collaborateurs. Beneficial effect of carotid endarterectomy in symptomatic patients with high-grade carotid stenosis. N Engl J Med 1991; 325: 445–453
2. European Carotid Surgery Trialists Collaborative Group. MRC European carotid surgery trial: interim results for symptomatic patients with severe (70–99%) or with mild (0–29%) carotid stenosis. Lancet 1991;337:1235–1243
3. Eastcott HH, Pickering GW, Rog CG. Reconstruction of internal carotid artery in a patient with intermittent attacks of hemiplegia. Lancet 1954;267:994–996
4. Muuronen A. Outcome of surgical treatment of 110 patients with transient ischemic attack. Stroke 1984;15:959–964
5. Allen BT, Anderson CB, Rubin BG, et al. The influence of anesthetic technique on perioperative complications after carotid endarterectomy. J Vasc Surg 1994;19:834–843
6. Mayberg MR, Wilson SE, Yatsu F, et al. Carotid endarterectomy and prevention of cerebral ischemia in symptomatic carotid stenosis. JAMA 1991;266:3289–3294
7. Executive Committee for the Asymptomatic Carotid Atherosclerosis Study. Endarterectomy for asymptomatic carotid artery stenosis. JAMA 1995;273:1421–1428
8. Pan XM, Saloner D, Reilly, LM, et al. Assessment of carotid artery stenosis by ultrasonography, conventional angiography, and magnetic resonance angiography: correlation with ex vivo measurement of plaque stenosis. J Vasc Surg 1995;21:82–89
9. Kuntz KM, Skillman JJ, Whittemore, AD, et al. Carotid endarterectomy in asymptomatic patients—is contrast angiography necessary? A morbidity analysis. J Vasc Surg 1995;22:706–716
10. O'Donnell TF Jr, Rodriguez AA, Fortunato JE, et al. Management of carotid stenosis: should asymptomatic lesions be treated surgically? J Vasc Surg 1996;24:207–212

11. Eiekelboom BC, Ackerstaff RG, Hoenveld H, et al. Benefits of carotid patching: a randomized study. J Vasc Surg 1988;7:240–247
12. Healy DA, Zierler RE, Nicholls SC, et al. Long-term follow-up and clinical outcome of carotid restenosis. J Vasc Surg 1989;10:662–669
13. Dossa C, Shepard AD, Wolford DG, et al. Distal internal carotid exposure: a simplified technique for temporary mandibular subluxation. J Vasc Surg 1990;12:319–325
14. Jordan WD Jr, Roye GD, Fisher WS III, et al. A cost comparison of balloon angioplasty and stenting versus endarterectomy for the treatment of carotid artery stenosis. J Vasc Surg 1998;27:16–24
15. Ouriel K, Yadav JS, Wholey M, et al. The SAPPHIRE randomized trial of carotid stenting versus endarterectomy: a subgroup analysis. American Association of Vascular Surgeons Annual Meeting, Chicago, IL June, 2003; Abstract 16:88

27

Carotid Endarterectomy: Neurological Perspective

Sumon Bhattacharjee and Christopher Loftus

Embolization from or occlusion of carotid vessels accounts for a significant number of ischemic strokes. Improved prophylactic measures and surveillance of those at risk are essential in decreasing the morbidity and cost associated with stroke. Until relatively recently controversies existed in the benefits of medical management versus surgical management of carotid stenosis. The availability of evidence-based cooperative trial data has been a major advance in the science of carotid reconstruction and has validated the benefit of carotid reconstruction in qualified hands.

◆ Indications

Symptomatic Carotid Stenosis

Carotid endarterectomy (CEA) is beneficial for symptomatic patients with recent nondisabling carotid artery ischemic events and ipsilateral 50 to 99% carotid artery stenosis. It is not beneficial for symptomatic patients with 0 to 49% stenosis. "Best" medical therapy (customarily antiplatelet agents and management of hypertension) is recommended for these < 50% stenosis patients. The surgical benefit was unanimous in the North American Symptomatic Endarterectomy Trial (NASCET),[1] the Department of Veterans Affairs Cooperative Study Program (VACSP),[2] and European Carotid Surgery Trialists (ECST)[3] trials.

Asymptomatic Carotid Stenosis

The evidence is not unanimous for asymptomatic trials. Prophylactic CEA for asymptomatic disease was reviewed in four prospective controlled and randomized studies, which differ substantially in trial design, patient selection, and methodology. The Carotid Artery Stenosis with Asymptomatic Narrowing Operation Versus Aspirin (CASANOVA) trial of asymptomatic lesions of the carotid tree concluded that endarterectomy was not helpful in preventing stroke or death in 410 patients with 50 to 90% carotid artery stenosis. Patients with greater than 90% stenosis, however, were excluded from the trial (and had surgery) on the basis of presumed surgical benefit. This methodological flaw severely limits the applicability of the CASANOVA data.[4]

The Mayo Asymptomatic Carotid Endarterectomy (MACE) study randomized patients to 80 mg per day of aspirin versus endarterectomy.[5] No conclusions could be obtained because the trial was discontinued due to increased cardiac mortality in the surgical group.

The Veterans Affairs (VA) Cooperative Study of asymptomatic carotid artery disease showed no benefits in stroke prevention from CEA or medical therapy in patients with 50 to 99% asymptomatic stenosis. There was a demonstrable and significant benefit of CEA in preventing transient ischemic attacks (TIAs) in asymptomatic patients.[6]

The largest of all these studies was the Asymptomatic Carotid Atherosclerosis Study (ACAS) study.[7] The trialists randomized 1659 patients, with 834 treated medically and 825 treated surgically, between ages 40 and 79 years with 60 to 99% internal carotid artery (ICA) stenosis to 325 mg of aspirin plus risk factor management, or endarterectomy plus medical therapy. The trial was stopped prematurely because of a demonstrated benefit for surgery in all patients with > 60% linear stenosis. (It was considered unethical to continue randomization of patients in the face of a known surgical benefit.) After median follow-up of 2.7 years, the aggregate estimated risk over 5 years for ipsilateral stroke or perioperative stroke or death was 5.1% for patients who underwent surgery and 11% for patients treated medically. CEA reduced the estimated 5-year risk of ipsilateral stroke by 1% per year. The benefit did not extend to major stroke alone and could not be demonstrated for women as a subgroup, probably because of the small numbers and premature closure of the trial. The success of the ACAS trial and of the operative procedure depended on maintenance of a perioperative morbidity and mortality of less than 3%.

◆ Other Factors in Decision Analysis

Contralateral Stenosis

The presence of bilateral significant disease in asymptomatic or symptomatic patients is common. Results from the VA asymptomatic trial showed that bilateral stenosis > 50% significantly increased the risk of both stroke and death in surgical groups.[6] The NASCET symptomatic trial showed no such difference. Our policy is to operate on appropriate lesions regardless of the status of the contralateral system.

Contralateral Occlusion

The presence of contralateral carotid occlusion increased both the natural history and the surgical risk. The NASCET trial found that for such patients over 2 years the risk of stroke in the medical group was 69% and in the surgical group 22%. The perioperative risk of stroke or death was 4%. We operate without hesitation for patients with appropriate lesions and contralateral carotid occlusion. The likelihood of placing a shunt in such cases increased from 15% without to 25% with contralateral carotid occlusion in our series.

Recurrent Carotid Stenosis

There is a small but finite incidence of recurrent carotid stenosis after CEA. Both technical inadequacies in surgery and continued patient smoking habits appear to be two of the primary reasons for restenosis. The reoperation of carotid stenosis has always been associated with a higher risk:benefit ration but is felt to be justifiable at our institution for patients with angiographically proven disease meeting NASCET criteria and neurological symptoms related to the same vessel distribution. Surgery is also considered when there is documented asymptomatic severe stenosis in patients being followed with annual serial duplex examination.

Acute Stroke

Operation in the face of recent stroke is a complex issue. Certainly patients who have documented in-hospital occlusion deserve immediate exploration. Such cases are extremely rare. More commonly patients with small strokes are heparinized and then found to have surgical carotid disease. We do not delay operation for these patients if they have a normal level on consciousness and no major mass effect on brain computed tomography (CT) or magnetic resonance imaging (MRI). We also do not hesitate to operate with full systemic heparinization and have stopped the practice of discontinuing heparin at some time point before surgery.

◆ Preparation

Patients with acute ischemic strokes or TIAs undergoing workup for their stroke etiology should have bilateral carotid duplex studies or magnetic resonance angiography (MRA). Asymptomatic patients who on clinical evaluation are noted to have a carotid bruit or significant atherosclerotic disease should undergo similar evaluation. The population of patients with a documented lesion in either study should proceed to a tailored arteriogram (arch and both carotids, cervical and cranial), which at our institution still remains the gold standard for preoperative evaluation for CEA. The stenosis is defined from the NASCET criteria, where N is the linear diameter at the area of greatest narrowing, and D is the greatest diameter of the normal artery distal to the carotid bulb.

$$\text{Percent (\%) stenosis} = (\text{I} - \text{N/D}) \times 100$$

Preoperative evaluation also involved aggressive workup of any patients with cardiac symptoms before CEA. If procedures for both circulations are indicated, staged procedures (carotid first always for symptomatic patients, sometimes coronary first for asymptomatic patients—"reverse staged") are preferable unless coronary circulation disease makes anesthesia for symptomatic CEA a difficult proposition. In such cases a combined procedure may be acceptable but at a significantly higher risk.

Patients on anticoagulation therapy other than aspirin (e.g., Coumadin), for artificial heart valves, TIAs, and other indications should be preoperatively admitted to the hospital and have their coagulopathy corrected with concurrent institution of IV heparin therapy. The heparin should be continued to the operating room and is stopped when the arterial closure is complete. We do not use protamine, and we restart daily American Society of Anesthesiologists (ASA) treatment immediately postop.

◆ Surgical Technique

Anesthesia

Local/regional and general anesthesia are both acceptable techniques for CEA. Although less popular than general anesthesia, local anesthesia has a loyal following of surgeons who argue that patient evaluation during the time of cross-clamping is far superior to electroencephalographic (EEG) monitoring in the assessment of cerebral ischemia. Harbaugh was shown excellent results in a large series of CEA patients with local anesthesia and point out that the technique is suitable for high-risk cases. In their hands local anesthesia reduces complications from cardiac, pulmonary, and urinary systems, and facilitates early postoperative hospital discharge.[8] Other proponents of local or regional anesthesia point to a 2 to 5% rate of shunt malfunction (either from migration of the distal end of the shunt with eventual abutment against the internal carotid artery wall with subsequent occlusion, or through thrombosis of the shunt itself)[9] and argue that monitoring the awake patient is more sensitive than other methods in detecting early ischemia.

General anesthesia remains the technique of choice in our center. There are several benefits to this technique. It provides a more controlled environment and a theoretical advantage of brain protection by reduction of cerebral metabolic rate for oxygen ($CMRO_2$) with the use of inhalation anesthetic and intravenous use of barbiturates. Use of general anesthesia also facilitates rapid manipulation of arterial $PaCO_2$ and blood pressure. In practice, however, little manipulation of CO_2 is used for carotid surgery, with most patients being maintained as either normocapneic or under mild hyperventilation.

There is a significant increase in regional cerebral blood flow (rCBF) and stump pressure with pharmacologically induced hypertension. Current anesthetic management should be directed at normotensive blood pressure with tolerance of systolic blood pressure up to 20% higher before antihypertensive measures are instituted. Intraoperative hypotension should be avoided.

Neurophysiological Monitoring

Monitoring (aside from direct observation in awake patients) is directed toward reducing morbidity and mortality from carotid surgery under general anesthesia. Vascular integrity can be monitored by measuring stump pressure, xenon (Xe) rCBF, transcranial Doppler (TCD) monitoring, ocular pneumoplethysmography, Doppler/duplex scanning, angiography, and near infrared spectroscopy (NIRS). EEG and somatosensory evoked potential (SEP) tests allow direct monitoring of cerebral function.

Measurement of residual "stump" pressure is proposed as a simple and reliable indicator for intraluminal shunting. However, stump pressure measurements are often eclipsed by intraoperative evaluation of physiological function in the need for shunting. The once recommended minimum carotid stump pressure of 25 mm Hg has often been shown to be inadequate because patients with greater than 50 mm Hg of stump pressure may undergo intraoperative ischemic EEG changes.

In several centers carotid artery injection of Xe is used to perform intraoperative rCBF analysis. Stoneham's extensive experience places the critical threshold of rCBF at 18 to 20 mL/100 gm/min.[10] In most series, good correlation existed between failure of ipsilateral rCBF and slowing and flattening of EEG, but several authors have stressed the lack of such correlation between rCBF and ipsilateral EEG changes. This technique has limited use for the majority of carotid surgeons, primarily from lack of availability.

Transcranial Doppler Monitoring

Continuous online recording of systolic and mean TCD velocity in the ipsilateral middle cerebral artery (MCA) during CEA is gaining increasing favor in the neurovascular surgical community. TCD predicts the need for shunting by virtue of measuring decrement in MCA velocities. It also provides the ability to assess function of the shunt after insertion (with increase in MCA velocity) and during arterial repair (where presumably a shunt malfunction would manifest a profound decrease in MCA velocity). Audible TCD monitoring allows detection of particulate embolization.

Other Vascular Assessments

Sundt and colleagues showed that a pre- versus postoperative discrepancy in retinal arterial pressure was a marker for acute carotid artery thrombosis and the need for immediate reexploration of the carotid system. Perioperative retinal pressure monitoring is not, however, in common use. In intraoperative angiography a single intraoperative common carotid artery (CCA) angiogram is obtained after arterial closure with hand injection of contrast. Radiographic changes leading to revision of arterial sutures are demonstrated in 2.5 to 8% of procedures, depending on the series. Proponents of the technique stress that the benefit of completion angiography is in recognizing technical errors that might otherwise go undetected. Arguments against intraoperative angiography are issues of time and convenience, and a case can be made that the risk of subintimal injection (and potential dissection) outweighs the benefit from the procedure. Intraoperative Doppler scanning and the informal use of sterilized Doppler probes applied to all vessels in the arterial tree are commonly used as qualitative measures of patency after arteriotomy. The senior author (CL) used this method routinely to demonstrate audible patency after carotid reconstruction. We also use the Doppler probe to auscultate flow through an indwelling shunt.

Functional Evaluation

Electroencephalographic Monitoring

Intraoperative EEG has withstood the test of time as a popular, readily available, and reliable method of determining cross-clamping-dependent ischemia and the need for indwelling shunt. EEG monitoring gained favor because several groups showed that EEG changes correlated well with the need for shunting in both awake and anesthetized patients. The number of patients showing EEG changes during carotid clamping has varied from 8.5 to 31%. Curiously, patients with contralateral carotid occlusion (who appear to require more shunting) still have shown EEG changes in only 17% and 42% in two series.

The EEG changes associated with intraoperative ischemia are well documented and consist most often of generalized slowing and decreased amplitude of the involved hemisphere. Trojaborg and Boysen[11] have documented EEG slowing corresponding to rCBF values of 16 to 22 mL/100 g/min, whereas flattening of EEG waves occurred with values of 11 to 19 mL/100 g/min. Several groups have documented EEG changes developing with intraoperative hypotension and have stressed the avoidance of this complication. There is an inclination of many surgeons, including our senior author, to use shunts in those with moderate EEG changes. Blume et al[12] have studied 176 patients undergoing CEA without shunting. In their group 19% had moderate and 22% had major EEG changes. No shunts were used and no postoperative changes were noted in the unchanged and moderately changed EEG groups. Postoperative strokes developed in 9% of the patients with major clamp-associated EEG changes. We recognize that by shunting for moderate changes the shunt may be overused, but the gratifying results and low (nonexistent) complication rate in our hands make us continue to use this method of cerebral protection.

Positioning

Two surgeons trained in the procedure are always present during carotid surgery.[13] Both stand on the operative side, the primary surgeon standing below the assistant and facing cephalad. The operative nurse may stand either behind or across the table from the primary surgeon. The patient's head is placed on a foam donut, and five to six towels are placed between the patient's shoulder blades, thereby permitting the shoulders to drop back, away from the surgical field. The patient is positioned with the head extending and turned somewhat toward the opposite side from the proposed surgical incision (**Fig. 27–1**). The degree of head turning is dependent upon the relationship of the external carotid artery (ECA) to the ICA. The head is turned radically to the contralateral side when the ICA is hidden and tucked underneath the ECA. Two anatomical landmarks are used from radiographic studies to provide clues to the high extent of the exposure. The first includes the angle of the mandible, which is palpated and marked before skin incision. The second anatomical landmark is the position of the bifurcation and the distal extent of the cervical plaque in relationship to the cervical section of the spine. The senior author believes that the surgeon needs to be prepared for high exposure with every carotid surgery. The cardinal principle mandating exposure is to obtain distal control well beyond the top of the plaque prior to cross-clamping.

A vertical incision is made along the palpable anterior border of the sternocleidomastoid muscle. The incision can be placed higher or lower, depending on the height of the carotid bifurcation. The incision can be made as low as the sternal notch or can go well up behind the ear in cases in which a high bifurcation is anticipated. The vertical incision is preferred at our institution; however, for routine exposures a transverse incision can also be made that falls along the skin lines. The third incision as proposed by Sundt[13] for a very high exposure goes anterior to the ear, up along the side of the face. We have not had occasion to use this technique.

Operative Procedure

The skin is infiltrated with 1% Xylocaine with 1:200,000 parts of epinephrine to reduce bleeding. The skin incision along the anterior border of the sternocleidomastoid is opened to the level of the platysma.[14] The platysmal layer is opened sharply. The edge of the sternocleidomastoid is identified and retracted laterally. A blunt Wietlaner retractor is used to spread the skin cephalad and caudally. The retractors are left superficial on the medial side to prevent injury to laryngeal nerves, but laterally they may be placed more deeply. The retraction of the sternocleidomastoid and underlying fat dissection expose the internal jugular vein underneath the muscle. The superficial dissection along the jugular vein exposes the common facial vein, which is identified and secured with 2–0 silk ties and weck clips, then divided. The dissection is continued along the medial border of the jugular vein to open the carotid sheath and identify the underlying CCA. In case of low-lying bifurcation of the CCA, the omohyoid muscle is split with bipolar coagulation. A stitch is placed at the muscle edges to be reapproximated at the end of the procedure.

A "no-touch" technique is applied to prevent any atheromatous material from dislodging in the carotid artery. Upon first visualization of the CCA, 5000 units of intravenous heparin is administered. The dissection of the carotid complex isolates the CCA, ECA, and ICA, which are then encircled with 0 silk ties passed with right-angle clamps. The superior thyroid artery is also dissected out and controlled with an encircling Potts tie of 2–0 silk. The CCA is prepared for proximal control by placement of a Rummel tourniquet that

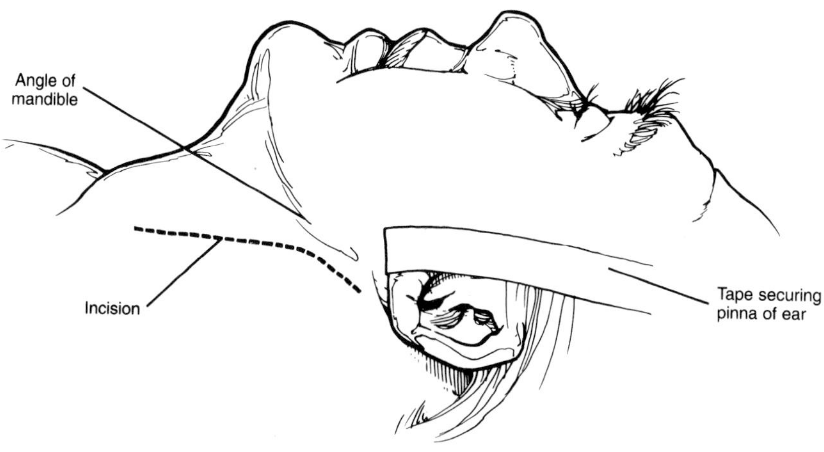

Figure 27–1 A vertically oriented incision is made along the anterior border of the sternocleidomastoid muscle, and it tails off toward the mastoid process. Note the relationship with the angle of the mandible.

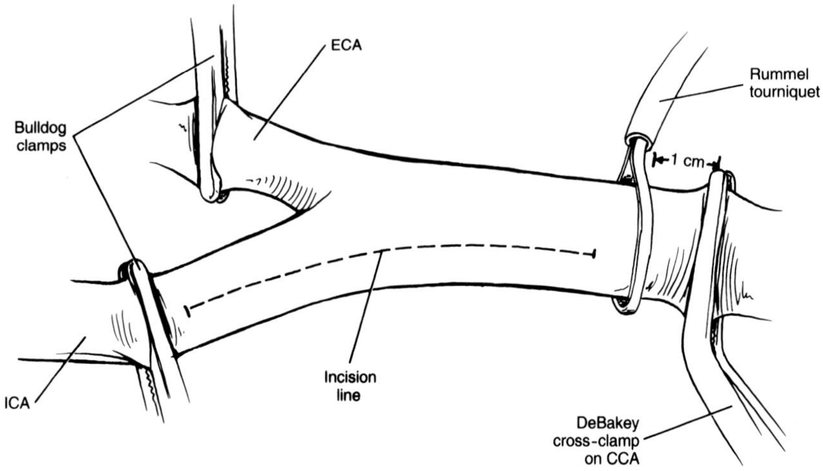

Figure 27–2 The carotid vessels are prepared for arteriotomy. Sufficient internal carotid artery has to be exposed to ensure the arteriotomy will extend well above the end of the plaque. A blue line is useful to prevent a jagged arteriotomy, which would be difficult to close. The Rummel tourniquet is in place to secure the shunt if it is needed during surgery. CCA, common carotid artery; ECA, external carotid artery; ICA, internal carotid artery.

facilitates constriction of the vessel around an intraluminal shunt if such is necessary.

The plaque in the artery is appreciated by visual cues as well as by tactile sensation. The yellowish atherosclerotic carotid wall turns a pink/blue hue beyond the atheroma. Distal control must be obtained beyond this plaque. During high exposure of the ICA a silk suture is passed around it, and a Loftus encircling shunt clamp (Scanlan International, St. Paul, MN) is tested to clamp around the ICA if shunting is necessary. Adequate proximal exposure of the CCA is necessary because the vessel loops are placed 1 cm distal to the area of the DeBakey cross-clamp. The clamp must be far down the CCA to facilitate bloodless shunt placement. After appropriate control proximally and distally, a sterile pen is used to mark on the vessel wall the intended line of arteriotomy (**Fig. 27–2**). After notifying the encephalographer, a bulldog clamp is used to close the ICA first, followed by DeBakey cross-clamping of the CCA and with a second bulldog applied to the ECA below the level of any branches except for the superior thyroid artery. This pattern of clamping (protecting the ICA first) prevents dislodging any plaque to the intracranial circulation. Following cross-clamping, a stab incision is made with a no. 11 blade in the proximal CCA. Potts scissors are used to extend the incision along the previously drawn blue line (**Fig. 27–3**).

The decision is made at this time as to whether a shunt is to be placed. Changes in the EEG mandate a rapid trial of hypertension. If there is no immediate change, an intraluminal shunt is placed. We use a custom shunt of our own design (Loftus Shunt, Integra NeuroCare, Plainfield, NJ). A fat black marking band is included in the middle of the tubing to monitor the positioning of the shunt at all times intraoperatively. The shunt is first inserted in the CCA and

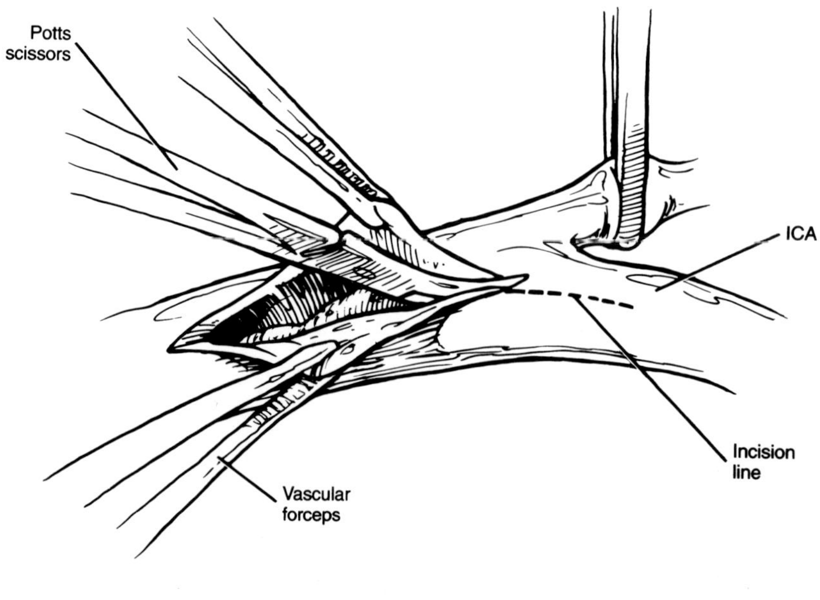

Figure 27–3 The Potts scissors are used to cut directly up the center of the vessel wall, following the blue line drawn previously. ICA, internal carotid artery.

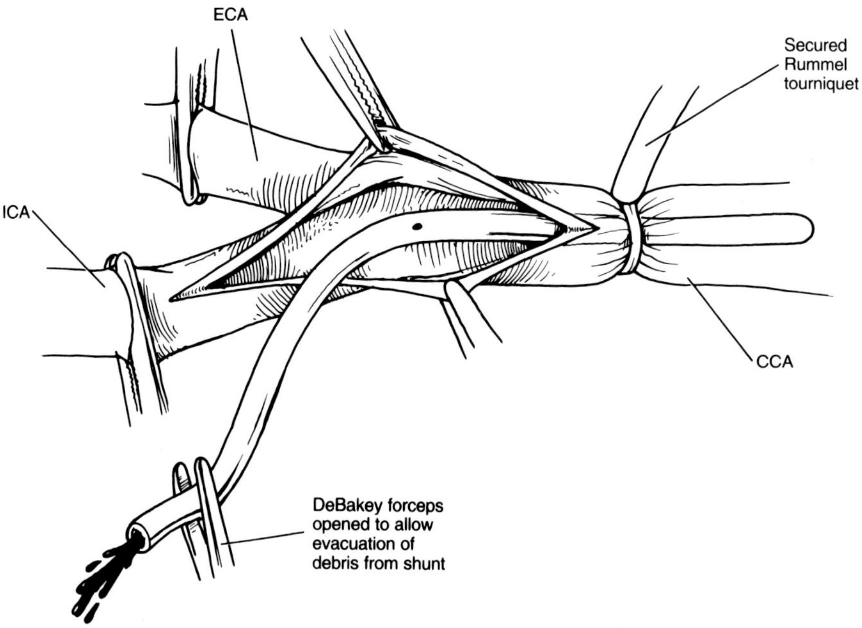

Figure 27–4 The shunt is secured in place at the common carotid artery (CCA) end by the Rummel tourniquet. Prior to its insertion into the internal carotid artery, the shunt is opened and bled for evacuation of debris.

secured with the Rummel tourniquet. The distal end is opened to confirm blood flow and evacuate any debris from the tubing. The shunt is then inserted in the ICA, bled to confirm flow and evacuating air, and secured in position by the Loftus shunt clamp (**Fig. 27–4**). The mark in the tubing is always placed in the center of the arteriotomy to confirm its positioning. Handheld Doppler is applied to the tubing to confirm flow.

The plaque removal begins with a Penfield no. 4 microdissector, which is rubbed gently back and forth against the lateral vessel wall. This generates a cleavage plane along the vessel wall between the plaque and intimal layer. Dissection is carried from a rostral to caudal direction and in a circumferential pattern. Attention must be paid so no buttonholing or transection of the vessel wall takes place. If the plaque extends into the common carotid and no feathered edges are present, a sharp transection is made proximally with a no. 15 blade or fine tenotomy scissors. If the dissection is taken high enough, the atheromatous plaque usually feathers nicely distally into the ICA and can be easily removed. However, at times it may leave a "shelf" with tattered edges that needs to be cleaned and the edges tacked down with 6–0 Prolene sutures to prevent dissection. After the separation of the plaque from the ICA and the CCA, the remaining plaque is grabbed by vascular forceps and pulled down from the ECA. We free the plaque in the ECA by sweeping around it with a small dissector or with a curved mosquito clamp passed up to the first major branch. If there is any question of residual plaque, a separate arteriotomy and repair of the ECA should be done.

After gross plaque removal a careful search is made for remaining fragments adherent to the arterial wall (**Fig. 27–5**). These can best be removed with microscopic ring-tipped forceps from the Scanlan Loftus set. If tacking sutures are required in the distal ICA, double-armed sutures of 6–0 Prolene are placed vertically from the inside of the vessel out so they transverse the intimal edge and are tied outside to the adventitial layer (**Fig. 27–6**). The arteriotomy closure is now always performed by us with synthetic patch grafting under 3.5 × loupe magnification. We prefer the Hemashield patch (Meadox Medicals, Inc, Oakland, NJ), a vascular graft of collagen-impregnated Dacron. This patch has several advantages over other synthetic materials: (1) It is easily shaped with scissors. (2) It does not require preclotting or special handling. (3) There is little or no leakage from the suture holes. (4) Standard needles and sutures can be used (6–0 Prolene, BV-1 needle).

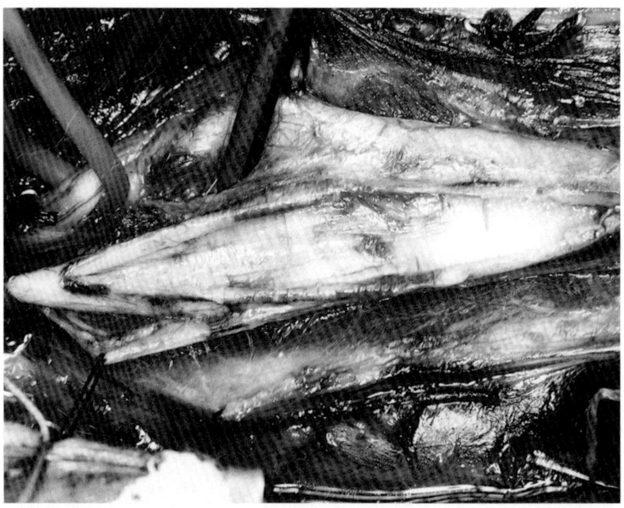

Figure 27–5 The plaque is removed with a Freer dissector or Penfield no. 4 from the lateral edge of the arteriotomy. The plaque-free segment of the carotid artery is shown following removal of the atherosclerotic plaque.

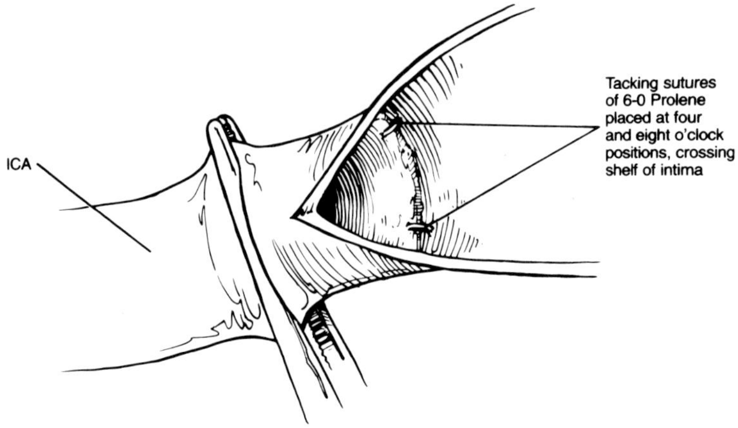

Figure 27–6 Tacking sutures are placed where there is a shelf of normal intima from removal of the plaque. Excessive thinning where only an adventitial layer is present is also plicated with tacking sutures to avoid untoward consequences. ICA, internal carotid artery.

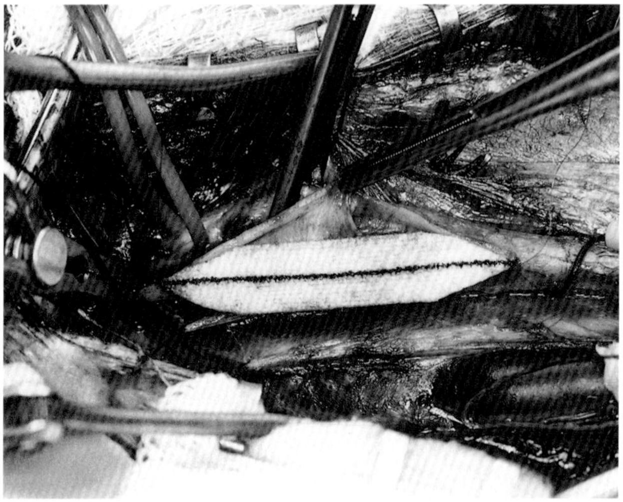

Figure 27–7 A Dacron patch graft is measured and cut to cover the entire length of the arteriotomy defect. The ends are trimmed and tapered to a fine point and anchored with double-armed 6–0 Prolene sutures.

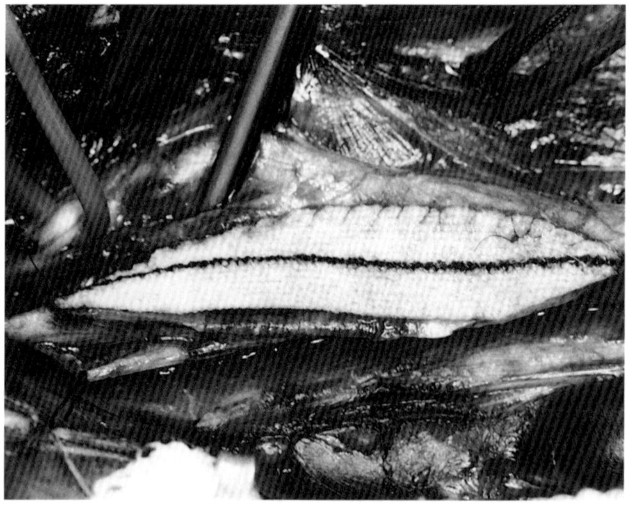

Figure 27–8 The medial wall of the arteriotomy is closed first with a running nonlocking stitch.

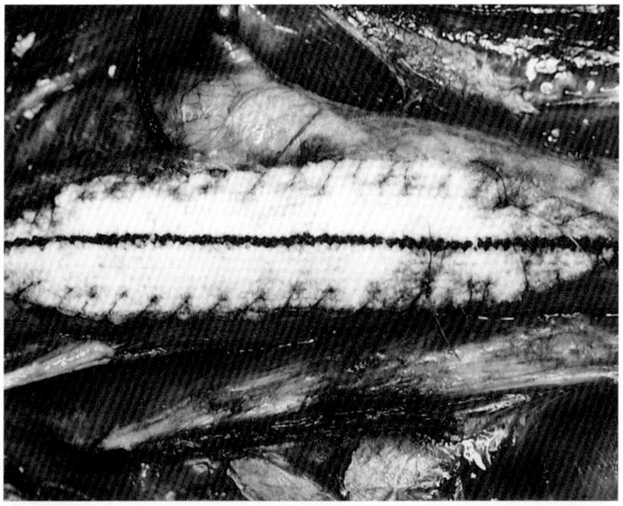

Figure 27–9 The lateral wall is closed with two arms of the suture, from the top and the bottom, meeting in the center of the arteriotomy.

The patch material is placed over the arteriotomy and cut to the exact length of the opening. After removal from the field, the ends are trimmed and tapered to a point with fine Metzenbaum scissors. Each end of the patch is anchored to the arteriotomy with double-armed 6–0 Prolene sutures (**Fig. 27–7**). The medial wall suture line is closed first with a running nonlocking stitch (**Fig. 27–8**). The lateral wall is closed next in two arms from the top and bottom of the repair, meeting in the center of the arteriotomy (**Fig. 27–9**). Small, evenly spaced bites are taken close to the arterial edge throughout, and sutures are placed relatively close together to prevent leaks. Several millimeters of the vessel are left unsewn on the lateral wall, ensuring room for removal of the shunt if one is being used. When shunt extraction is necessary, it is removed by initially double clamping with two parallel straight mosquitoes, cutting straight in between them, and removing in two sections.

Closure

The final closure of the arteriotomy is performed with opening and closing in sequence of the ICA, ECA, and CCA to ensure back bleeding. Heparinized saline is introduced into the arterial lumen to evacuate air prior to the final surgeon's knot on the free end of the sutures. When the vessel has been closed, a prescribed sequence of declamping is followed. The clamps are removed first from the ECA, then the CCA, and finally 10 seconds later from the ICA. This sequence of clamp removal ensures that any loose debris or air is flushed into the ECA rather than up into the cerebral circulation. Following clamp removal, the suture lines are inspected for any leaks, which are customarily controlled with pressure, patience, and surgical gauze. In occasional cases a single throw of 6–0 Prolene is needed to close persistent hemorrhage. The repair is lined with Surgicel, and the handheld Doppler is used to check the vessel patency. The retractors are removed, and the wound is closed in layers. The carotid sheath is first closed to provide a barrier against infection. The platysma is closed in separate layers to give a good cosmetic result. Either running or interrupted subcuticular stitches are applied to the skin, which are then apposed with Steri-Strips. A hemovac drain is placed in the carotid sheath and is routinely removed 1 day after surgery.

◆ Postoperative Care

Immediately postoperatively, patients are monitored in the recovery room and then transferred to the intensive care unit (ICU). The ICU management of patients is primarily for control of blood pressure and reduction of the risk of myocardial infarction. The goal is to support systolic blood pressure at 100 mm Hg and to use antihypertensives if pressure exceeds 160 mm Hg. It is especially important to control hypertension in patients who have had tight stenosis reopening because the ipsilateral cerebral hemisphere is dysautoregulated, and hypertension may predispose these patients to intracerebral hemorrhage.

Any postoperative neurological deficit, including TIAs, is addressed with immediate angiography. Any occluded carotid artery postop is reexplored and repatched immediately, but since we adopted the primary Hemashield patch repair our incidence of postop occlusion has dropped to zero. Patients are transferred to the floor after 24 hours of ICU monitoring and discharged home the following day. Postoperative follow-up is in 4 weeks for wound check and then at 3 months with a duplex study. Patients are maintained on 325 mg of aspirin daily indefinitely.

◆ Conclusion

The current data clearly document the superiority of surgery in the management of asymptomatic (> 60%) and symptomatic (> 50%) carotid artery stenosis, and carotid artery reconstruction has been refined to a safe and reproducible procedure. Although angioplasty and the new advent of carotid artery stenting are appealing to patients, there is no evidence that they produce superior or even equivalent results to open surgery. We recommend endovascular treatment for a small subset of patients, including those with extremely high ICA stenosis (beyond surgical reach) or those with recent myocardial infarctions. These are rare occasions in our experience.

The surgical methods presented here have been successful in producing acceptable postoperative results in the broad spectrum of carotid patients. Minor technical details that may vary among surgeons are probably of little consequence. However, subtleties of technique (such as extensive exposure) that may add operative time to the "routine" carotid assume greater importance when difficult lesions or high exposures are encountered or when the patient is unstable. The importance of a good outcome under these more difficult circumstances leads the senior author to use the same technical approach for all carotid surgery, no matter how simple it may seem. Perhaps the most important factor in ensuring acceptable carotid surgery is the availability of a skilled cerebrovascular surgeon with demonstrable morbidity and mortality below 3% and proper understanding of both vascular principles and cerebral physiology.

References

1. NASCET. Beneficial effect of carotid endarterectomy in symptomatic patients with high-grade carotid stenosis. North American Symptomatic Carotid Endarterectomy Trial Collaborators. N Engl J Med 1991;325:445–453
2. Mayberg MR, Wilson SE, Yatsu F, et al. Carotid endarterectomy and prevention of cerebral ischemia in symptomatic carotid stenosis. Veterans Affairs Cooperative Studies Program 309 Trialist Group. JAMA 1991;266:3289–3294
3. ECST. MRC European Carotid Surgery Trial: interim results for symptomatic patients with severe (70–99%) or with mild (0–29%) carotid stenosis. European Carotid Surgery Trialists' Collaborative Group. Lancet 1991;337:1235–1243
4. CASANOVA. Carotid surgery versus medical therapy in asymptomatic carotid stenosis. The CASANOVA Study Group. Stroke 1991;22:1229–1235
5. MACE. Results of a randomized controlled trial of carotid endarterectomy for asymptomatic carotid stenosis. Mayo Asymptomatic Carotid Endarterectomy Study Group. Mayo Clin Proc 1992;67:513–518
6. Hobson RW II, Weiss DG, Fields WS, et al. Efficacy of carotid endarterectomy for asymptomatic carotid stenosis. The Veterans Affairs Cooperative Study Group. N Engl J Med 1993;328:221–227
7. ACAS. Endarterectomy for asymptomatic carotid artery stenosis. Executive Committee for the Asymptomatic Carotid Atherosclerosis Study. JAMA 1995;273:1421–1428
8. Harbaugh RE. Outcomes analysis of the treatment of carotid artery disease. Neurosurg Clin N Am 2000;11:377–388
9. Stoneham MD, Knighton JD. Regional anaesthesia for carotid endarterectomy. Br J Anaesth 1999;82:910–919

10. Messick JM Jr, Casement B, Sharbrough FW, et al. Correlation of regional cerebral blood flow (rCBF) with EEG changes during isoflurane anesthesia for carotid endarterectomy: critical rCBF. Anesthesiology 1987;66:344–349

11. Trojaborg W, Boysen G. Relation between EEG, regional cerebral blood flow and internal carotid artery pressure during carotid endarterectomy. Electroencephalogr Clin Neurophysiol 1973;34: 61–69

12. Blume WT, Ferguson GG, McNeill DK. Significance of EEG changes at carotid endarterectomy. Stroke 1986;17:891–897

13. Sundt TM Jr, Whisnant JP, Houser OW, Ford NC. Prospective study of effectiveness and durability of carotid endarterectomy. May. Clinic Proc. 1990 May; 65(5): 625–635

14. Honeycutt JH Jr, Loftus CM. Carotid endarterectomy: general principles and surgical technique. Neurosurg Clin N Am 2000;11: 279–297

28

Cerebral Revascularization

Laligam N. Sekhar, Chandrasekar Kalavakonda, and Foad Elahi

The brain represents only 2% of the total body weight, but it receives ~20% of the cardiac output and uses 20% of the oxygen supply.[1] The normal cerebral blood flow ranges between 45 and 60 mL/100 g of brain tissue per minute.[2] The brain is dependent on a regular and adequate blood supply in view of its high metabolic demand and the absence of any significant energy reserves. Alterations in blood supply can make the brain vulnerable to ischemia. A state of inadequate cerebral blood flow is known as cerebral ischemia, which could be either focal or global. If it is significantly severe and prolonged, it will lead to cell death, producing what is known as cerebral infarction.

Cerebral revascularization is an important tool in the neurosurgeon's armamentarium. It has an important role in the treatment of a select group of patients with cerebral ischemia, and in patients with involvement of arteries by tumor or complex aneurysms. Cerebral revascularization broadly includes a variety of surgical procedures such as embolectomy, endarterectomy, procedures to establish a collateral blood supply (encephalomyosynangiosis), and the various procedures under the category of extracranial-intracranial (EC-IC) bypass surgery, or intracranial vascular reconstructive operations.

◆ History of Extracranial-Intracranial Bypass

Fisher in 1951 suggested the possibility of treating cerebrovascular occlusive disease with an extracranial to intracranial bypass procedure.[3] Pool and Potts[4] in 1964 reported using a plastic tube as a shunt between the superficial temporal artery (STA) and distal anterior cerebral artery (ACA) during the surgical treatment of an ACA aneurysm. However, the shunt thrombosed and did not function postoperatively.[3] Story et al used a Gore-Tex tube graft for the bypass from the common carotid artery (CCA) to a cortical branch of the middle cerebral artery (MCA).[5] Jacobson and his colleagues were the first to describe the microsurgical anastomosis of blood vessels and also the use of microsurgery as an aid to endarterectomy of the MCA.[3] Yasargil in 1966[6a,6b] performed the first successful STA-MCA bypass on a dog[7] and published his first patient series in 1970.[8] Spetzler and colleagues described the use of the occipital artery (OA) or the middle meningeal artery (MMA) as a donor vessel as an alternative to the STA if it is diseased by atherosclerotic changes.[9,10] Woringer and Kunlin[11] in 1963 performed the first saphenous vein interposition graft from the CCA to the intracranial internal carotid artery (ICA) in a patient with ICA occlusion. The patient died of a pulmonary embolus, but the graft was found to be patent at autopsy. In 1971, Lougheed and colleagues reported performing a CCA to intracranial ICA anastomosis using a saphenous vein graft, with the graft being demonstrated to be patent on postoperative angiogram.[12] A right CCA to distal MCA bypass with a saphenous vein graft was performed in a patient with episodic cerebral ischemia and reversible ischemic neurological deficit by Story and colleagues.[13] Ausman and colleagues used a saphenous vein graft bypass from the ipsilateral subclavian artery to the external carotid artery (ECA) and combined this with an STA-MCA bypass.[14] Spetzler and colleagues used a saphenous vein graft from the subclavian to a branch of the MCA.[15] Sundt and colleagues reported experience with vein grafts in treating patients with cerebrovascular occlusive disease in the posterior circulation, and giant aneurysms.[16] Little and colleagues used a short saphenous vein graft bypass from the preauricular STA to a branch of the MCA and from the proximal OA to the posterior temporal or angular branch of the MCA.[17] The first vein graft bypass from the petrous ICA to the supraclinoid ICA was performed in cadavers by Sekhar et al[18] and in patients by Fukushima (personal communication) and Sekhar et al.[19] Sekhar et al reported the first case of MCA reconstruction using a vein graft,[20] extracranial to intracranial vertebral reconstruction with vein graft,[21] and the only reported case of a saphenous vein graft from the ICA to the basilar artery under deep hypothermic cardiac arrest.[22] Radial artery grafts (RAGs) have also been used for intracranial revascularization, and their use was perfected by the "pressure distention technique,"[23,24] which prevents the occurrence of postoperative vasospasm. In addition, the superior thyroid artery has been used as an interposition graft.[25]

◆ Indications

Symptomatic Cerebral Ischemia

Patients with vascular occlusive disease will have to meet the following criteria before being considered for revascularization: (1) neurological symptoms are unresponsive to maximal medical therapy including blood pressure (BP) adjustment, treatment with aspirin, or clopidogrel bisulfate (Plavix, Sanofi-Aventis, Bridgewater, NJ) and in case of posterior circulation ischemia, a trial of Coumadin for a period of 3 months; (2) the cause of ischemia is a lesion such as atherosclerotic carotid occlusion, stenosis of the carotid siphon, occlusion or stenosis of a major cerebral artery that is not amenable to direct repair, younger patients with MCA occlusion as in moyamoya disease, traumatic ICA injuries with ischemia, and spontaneous ICA or vertebral artery (VA) dissection; and (3) reduced cerebral perfusion documented by measurement of regional cerebral blood flow or metabolic studies. This group of patients is now the focus of a National Institutes of Health (NIH)-funded randomized study (Carotid Occlusion Surgery Study).

Unclippable, Uncoilable Aneurysms

These may be unclippable due to their (1) size—giant aneurysms, (2) shape—fusiform dilatation of the parent vessel, (3) location—intracavernous, (4) content—organized intramural thrombus with a serpentine vascular channel, (5) wall—presence of calcification at the neck or atherosclerotic plaques, or (6) symptomatic dissecting aneurysms. The origin of a major artery from the aneurysmal neck or sac may also necessitate a revascularization procedure. Such aneurysms are also frequently untreatable by endovascular procedures, such as coiling. However, balloon- or stent-assisted coiling should be considered as treatment options before making the final decision about revascularization.

Cranial Base Tumors

Tumor involvement of the ICA or VA may require resection of part of these vessels along with tumor removal because the tumor cannot be dissected free in case of benign tumors. In case of malignant tumors such as squamous cell carcinoma, it may be necessary to resect the encased ICA or VA for oncological purposes, or it is necessary to reroute the ICA because of potential of infection from the nasopharynx, with the likelihood of pseudoaneurysm and rupture of the ICA.

◆ Preparation

Patients undergo computed tomographic (CT) scan, magnetic resonance imaging (MRI), and magnetic resonance angiography (MRA) to evaluate the original disease. Selective four-vessel angiography is very important in assessing the anatomy of the involved artery, the collateral circulation, and the potential collateral channels. A cerebral blood flow (CBF) study using Xe_{133}, stable xenon-CT, or single photon emission computed tomography (SPECT) may be performed in patients with occluded arteries. In most patients, the need for a bypass procedure is established with these preoperative studies. In a small percentage of patients the necessity of a bypass procedure may only be apparent intraoperatively but can be anticipated preoperatively (e.g., large or giant aneurysm found to be unclippable during surgery). Preparation of the donor site will have to be made taking this fact into consideration.

In patients with ICA aneurysms or tumors involving the ICA, to assess the collateral circulation in the event of ICA occlusion, we perform a 15-minute balloon occlusion test (BOT) with clinical examination followed by an ICA-occluded SPECT study. If possible, the patient's systolic blood pressure is electively lowered to 70 torr. The occlusion test carries a slight risk (0.1%) of intimal dissection and thromboembolic complications. The patient is placed on aspirin prior to the test, and a low-pressure balloon must be used. At present, we use the test mainly to assess the collaterals in the event of temporary occlusion, except in patients with petrous or cavernous aneurysms in whom permanent intravascular ICA occlusion is being considered.

Prolonged test occlusion of the VA carries a much higher risk of arterial dissection. A positive clinical BOT of the cervical VA is considered significant but provides little information about the effects of occlusion distal to the vertebrobasilar junction. Clinical BOT distal to the origin of the posterior inferior cerebellar artery (PICA) is hazardous because it can lead to brain stem and cerebellar strokes as a result of occlusion of perforators. A four-vessel angiogram to evaluate the presence, size, and dominance of both VAs, the size and anatomy of both posterior communicating arteries, and any atherosclerotic occlusive disease in the cervical VAs and basilar artery (BA) is still preferred to evaluate the adequacy of posterior circulation collateral flow distal to the PICA.

General medical evaluation, especially a thorough cardiac evaluation, is very important because the agents used for temporary metabolic suppression and those used to induce temporary hypertension can affect cardiac function. Clopidogrel is stopped 5 days prior to surgery; however, aspirin is usually continued through the surgical period.

◆ Surgical Technique

Anesthesia

The patient is started on steroids on the morning of surgery or 24 hours before surgery and continued postoperatively as needed for the primary disease (e.g., tumor). A prophylactic antibiotic, usually ceftriaxone 1 g, is administered intravenously just prior to surgery and continued for 48 hours postoperatively. The patient is loaded with 1 g of phenytoin or another anticonvulsant, and this is usually continued for a period of 3 months. It is usually stopped after checking a sleep-deprived electroencephalogram (EEG) to make sure that there is no seizure activity.

A balanced anesthetic technique is used. The patient is maintained normocapneic through the procedure except in the case of skull base tumors in which mild hyperventilation ($PaCO_2 > 30$ torr) is employed. Mannitol and Lasix are used if the intracranial pressure (ICP) is elevated. In patients with chronic ischemia, adequate care is taken to load the patient with fluids and not to drop the BP during induction to prevent further ischemia. In aneurysm and tumor patients, during the arterial occlusion, the patient is cooled to 34°C, the blood pressure is raised 20% above the baseline, and the patient is placed in EEG burst suppression using barbiturates. These are maneuvers to reduce the brain metabolism and increase the collateral blood flow and greatly reduce or eliminate ischemic damage from the temporary vascular occlusion. Before the extraction of the vein graft, 1 g of methylprednisolone is administered intravenously to provide protection to the venous endothelium upon its exposure to the arterial blood flow. The patient is also given 2000 units of heparin intravenously, which is usually not reversed at the end of the procedure. In patients with tumors, the tumor may be explored and partially resected, followed by the revascularization procedure and resection of the tumor.

Intraoperatively, cerebral hemispheric function is monitored continuously with EEG and somatosensory evoked potentials (SEPs), and brain stem function is monitored with SEP and brain stem auditory evoked response (BAER). EEG is also used to achieve the burst suppression with barbiturates to protect the brain. Autoregulation of CBF may be impaired or absent in the high-flow vein grafts used for revascularization. Hence systemic hypertension must be avoided after the graft is completed.

Intraoperative angiography has become important for vein and radial artery (RA) grafting procedures. It provides an opportunity to identify and correct any technical problems related to the grafting. With the use of intraoperative angiography, our graft patency rate has improved to 98% (from 86% before its use).[23] Currently we also use an intraoperative microDoppler to check the graft flow; it provides a very fast, qualitative means of flow measurement, and quantitative Doppler flow measurements are also possible (Flowmeter BLF21A Laser Doppler; Transonic Systems, Inc., Ithaca, NY). For smaller vessels (e.g., interposition arterial grafts), intraoperative Doppler may be combined with a postoperative angiogram.

Postoperatively, we maintain the patients on heparin administered subcutaneously, 5000 units three times daily for a period of 5 to 7 days. The patients with vein grafts are subsequently placed on aspirin, 325 mg, once daily for life. RAGs and other types of arterial grafts may not require any antiplatelet therapy unless the patient has evidence of atherosclerotic disease.

Choice of Graft Vessel

The choice of graft (**Table 28–1**) depends upon four factors: (1) size of the recipient vessel, which is the major determinant, (2) availability of donor vessel, (3) availability of graft material, and (4) extent of blood flow augmentation required. The measured blood flow immediately after anastomosis in STA-MCA anastomosis is 20 to 60 mL/min. In RAGs it is 40 to 70 mL/min, and in saphenous vein grafts (SVGs) it is 70 to 140 mL/min.[23–27]

SVGs provide maximal flow, but the potential for turbulence leading to occlusion at the anastomotic sites (especially recipient) and for hyperemia and hemorrhage in chronically ischemic patients is a potential drawback. On the other hand, the STA-MCA anastomosis and RAGs may not provide flow adequate to prevent a stroke in cases of acute ICA occlusion with poor or no collaterals. In addition to flow-related problems, the potential for thromboembolism and vasospasm (in arterial grafts) must be considered.

In general, direct reconstruction is performed for unexpected vascular injuries during aneurysm or tumor surgery and during the excision of distally placed aneurysms. Examples include MCA branch reimplantation, MCA branch repair, ACA to ACA or PICA to opposite PICA side-to-side anastomosis, and PICA to (ipsilateral) anterior inferior cerebellar artery (AICA) anastomosis. For similar circumstances, if direct repair is not possible because the gap is too long, then a short interposition graft using the STA, occipital artery (OA), or even the superior thyroid artery (SThyA) can be utilized.

STA-MCA or OA-MCA anastomosis is employed if some collaterals are present and blood flow augmentation requirement is small, or if only distal arteries are available for anastomosis. Examples include revascularization for ischemia not

Table 28–1 Revascularization Procedures—March 1985 to January 2005*

Type of Graft:	Aneurysm (71)	Ischemia (37)	Tumor (70)**
RAG	28	24 (three revisions)	14
SVG	34 (one revision)	15 (one revision)	85 (two revisions)
Other	11	4 (two revisions)	0
Total grafts	73	43	99
Graft patency	87%	98%	95.2%

RAG, radial artery graft; SVG, saphenous vein graft.

*Death occurred in three patients due to (1) systemic sepsis, (2) pneumonia and cardiac arrest during bronchoscopy, (3) rupture of abdominal aortic aneurysm (Marfan's syndrome). Superficial temporal artery–middle cerebral artery bypasses for ischemia performed 1984–1988 are excluded.

**Numbers in parentheses indicate number of patients.

responsive to medical therapy and tumor patients with chronic arterial occlusion of the MCA. As the graft matures with time, the flow will increase in several patients.

RAG is used when some collateral circulation is present, the recipient vessel is not large enough (= 2 mm), it is desired to provide moderate amount of flow in ischemic patients, or in cases of failure of SVG.

SVG provides a high flow rate. Therefore, it is preferred in patients in whom acute ICA replacement is needed or in patients with posterior circulation aneurysms or tumors where acute VA or BA occlusion is needed for treatment.

Operative Procedure: General Steps

Patient positioning takes into account the location of pathology, the donor and recipient vessel, and the site of graft extraction. Intraoperative angiography should be considered for the large grafts, although for smaller vessels a microDoppler probe will be adequate. For SVG and RAG, intraoperative angiography is mandatory; the patient's head is fixed in a radiolucent head holder, the groin and thigh are prepared, and a femoral artery sheath is placed at the beginning for intraoperative angiogram. The graft extraction site should be prepared at the beginning, but in situations of unexpected emergency, preparation can also be done during the case.

A craniotomy alone may be adequate in some patients, but in most patients with basal tumors or aneurysms, a skull base approach is added to improve the exposure and to reduce brain retraction. Recipient vessel(s), donor vessel, and the graft are exposed, and a wide tunnel is created for the graft. The graft is extracted just before the anastomosis. As mentioned earlier, the patient is placed in electroencephalographic burst suppression with pharmacological agents, and the systolic pressure is elevated 20% above baseline during vascular occlusion. For vein grafts and RAGs, 2000 units of intravenous heparin, and for vein grafts 1 g of methylprednisolone is administered intravenously. For patients with arterial grafts, we also administer 325 mg of aspirin by mouth prior to the operation.

The recipient vessel is isolated, and the segment where the anastomosis is planned should be free of any major perforators. The graft is adequately prepared and thoroughly flushed with heparinized saline. The distal anastomosis is performed first. Temporary clips of appropriate size are placed on the recipient vessel. Generally, the anastomosis time should be less than 45 minutes, and preferably less than 30 minutes, but for the posterior cerebral artery (PCA) and superior cerebellar artery (SCA) it can be as long as 50 minutes. The suture thickness is chosen according to the thickness of the vessel wall. Usually 8–0 to 10–0 nylon is used for the intracranial vessels, but it can be 7–0 Prolene for the supraclinoid ICA. After the anastomosis is complete, the graft is flushed with heparinized saline before the last suture is tied. A temporary clip is placed on the graft, followed by the release of temporary clips on the recipient vessel. The graft is brought through the tunnel previously created and anastomosed to the donor artery. The anastomosis is either end to end or end (graft) to side (donor artery). The temporary clips are opened proximally, followed by the distal one, while the operator inspects for leaks and any kinking. Flow in the graft and the recipient vessel is confirmed with microDoppler. Half of the heparin may be reversed if excessive epidural oozing is encountered after vein grafts. The dura mater is slit in a cruciate fashion to allow the free entry of the graft. Intraoperative angiogram is usually done after dural closure to rule out the possibility of obstruction from dural closure. An appropriate opening is fashioned in the bone flap to accommodate the entry of graft freely without any kink or tension. The graft is checked again with Doppler after the affixation of the bone flap.

Postoperative monitoring of graft patency usually consists of palpation of the graft and Doppler evaluation. If there is any doubt regarding the functioning of the graft, a cerebral angiography or MRA is performed. Patients are maintained on subcutaneous heparin, 5000 U every eight hours for 1 week, and then switched over to aspirin, 325 mg once daily.

Long-term follow-up is performed annually with MRA or three-dimensional (3D)-CT angiography.

Superficial Temporal Artery to Middle Cerebral Artery Anastomosis

The patient is placed supine, the head is rotated 70 degrees to the opposite side, and a roll is placed under the ipsilateral shoulder. The angiogram is carefully reviewed; at least one STA branch must be large enough to be used. The temporoparietal branch is usually preferred over the frontal branch, but the frontal branch can be used if it is the larger of the two. The recipient MCA vessel can be chosen on the basis of the preoperative angiogram, and the site of the craniotomy can be precisely determined. If the MCA branches are not clearly seen on the angiogram, the craniotomy site is determined by Chater's landmark (see later discussion).[28] The STA is exposed by the cut-down technique. The course of the vessel is traced by palpation and Doppler and drawn with a marking pencil or a fine needle on the scalp. Dissection is started distally, and the vessel is traced proximally, working under the microscope. Incision is limited to the skin and subcutaneous tissue because the STA lies superficial to the galea initially and then penetrates the galea to lie just deep to it. The vessel is dissected with fine microscissors and jeweler's forceps; the artery should be traced to the zygoma. The superficial temporal vein accompanies the artery near the zygoma. A small cuff of connective tissue is left around the artery. Small branches are coagulated with bipolar cautery, and the larger ones are ligated with 6–0 Prolene and divided.

If the bypass is planned into a distal cortical branch of the MCA, a small craniotomy, ~4 cm in diameter, is performed 6 cm above the external auditory canal (Chater's point). If the STA is larger, then anastomosis is performed onto an M3–MCA branch (these are 1.5 to 2.0 mm in diameter) in the sylvian fissure through a routine pterional craniotomy.

If the parietal branch of the STA is being used, it is divided distally, and the temporalis muscle is split along the line of incision and the craniotomy is done. If the frontal branch is used, then a separate incision is used for the craniotomy, and the STA is brought to the anastomotic site without twisting (**Fig. 28–1A,B**). The dura is tacked up all around to prevent any epidural collection of blood. A cruciate dural opening is made. A middle cerebral branch in the distal sylvian fissure, the largest temporal or parietal cortical branch relatively free of perforators, is used for anastomosis. Tiny perforators can be divided. Ideally, the recipient vessel has to be 1.5 mm in diameter but can be as narrow as 1.0 mm. The recipient vessel is dissected free of its arachnoidal covering, and a small rubber dam (a piece of rubber glove) is placed under the artery. A Spetzler micromalleable suction (NMT Medical, Inc., Boston, MA) is positioned near the vessel to aspirate fluids, and periodic intermittent irrigation is done to keep the field clean of blood. Prior to dividing the STA, a temporary clip is applied proximally. The terminal 1 cm of the STA is denuded of its adventitial covering (**Fig. 28–2**). It is cannulated with a blunt needle and irrigated with heparinized saline; the temporary clip on the STA is opened, then closed, so as to fill the segment of the artery with heparinized saline. An oblique arteriotomy with slight fish-mouthing of the STA is done. Temporary clips are placed on the MCA branch on either side of the site of anastomosis, and a small arteriotomy, 3 to 4 mm in length, is performed with microscissors. It is irrigated with heparinized saline to clear any blood. End stitches are placed with 10–0 nylon, initially at the heel and then at the opposite end to anchor the graft for an appropriate fit. One side is anastomosed with continuous sutures, leaving the loops long and tightening at the end of the anastomosis on this side. The vessel is reflected, and the opposite side is anastomosed with

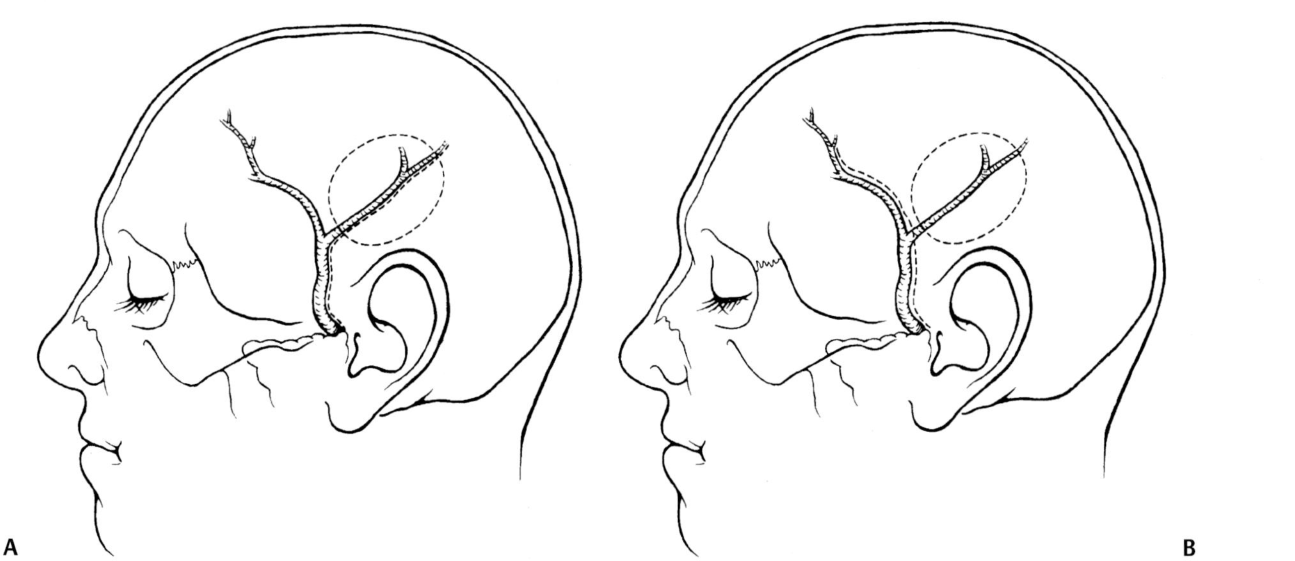

Figure 28–1 **(A)** This figure illustrates the use of the parietal branch of the middle meningeal artery for the superficial temporal artery–middle cerebral artery anastomosis. The heavy dotted line indicates the line of skin incision. Also shown is the site of craniotomy. **(B)** This figure illustrates the skin incision for exposure of the frontal branch of the middle meningeal artery for the anastomosis. (Courtesy of Laligam N. Sekhar.)

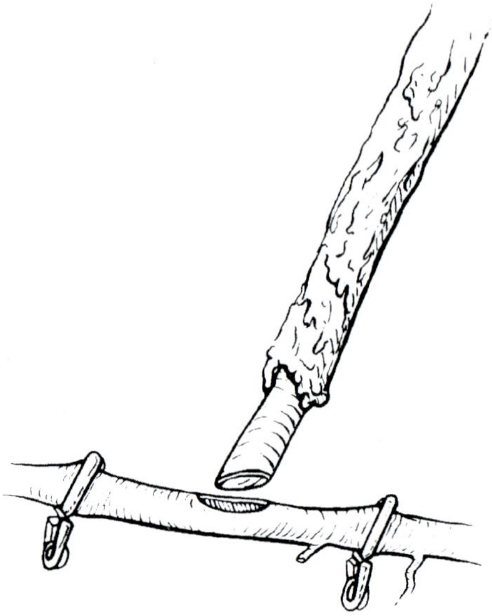

Figure 28–2 The terminal 1 cm of the superficial temporal artery is denuded of its adventitial covering. (Courtesy of Laligam N. Sekhar.)

interrupted sutures, which are tied after all the sutures are placed (**Fig. 28–3**). Prior to tying the last suture, the lumen is flushed with heparinized saline and the suture tightened. The temporary clips on the MCA branch (distal followed by proximal) are released first, followed by the temporary clip on the STA. Small leaks usually stop with small pieces of Gelfoam. Flow through the STA is checked with a Doppler probe.

The vascular edges must be handled very delicately with the forceps, either directly or with a counterpressure technique. The suture needle is passed through the vessel wall and pushed through, then grasped on the other side. Near the corners of the anastomosis, it is better to suture the walls individually, whereas in the remainder, both walls can be sutured with one motion (**Fig. 28–4**).

Occipital Artery to Posterior Inferior Cerebellar Artery Bypass

The OA can be used for OA to MCA branch bypass if the STA is too narrow or diseased or is absent due to prior surgery. OA to AICA or PICA anastomosis is performed for ischemia or aneurysms in the posterior circulation. Dissection of the OA is relatively difficult, and a clear knowledge of its anatomical course is necessary. The OA runs horizontally deep to the mastoid tip and digastric muscle, medial to the splenius capitis muscle, medial or lateral to the longissimus capitis muscle, and lateral to the semispinalis capitis muscle. It then perforates the muscular fascia to enter the subcutaneous tissue and turns to run vertically at the level of the superior nuchal line. It has a very tortuous course and gives off multiple muscular branches.

An inverted U-shaped incision is made and the skin and subcutaneous flap are reflected. The course of the OA is marked with a Doppler sonogram. The artery is dissected carefully and troublesome venous oozing can be encountered from accompanying veins or muscular arterial branches (**Fig. 28–5**). Tortuosity makes the dissection difficult. Smaller branches are coagulated and the larger ones ligated. A cuff of periadventitial tissue is left around the artery. The dissection of the OA is more difficult than that of the STA. For posterior fossa anastomoses, it is adequate to dissect the OA until it penetrates the muscular fascia and turns vertically upward.

A retrosigmoid craniotomy is then performed, followed by the removal of the rim of the foramen magnum. If the PICA is the vessel selected for the anastomosis, it is isolated in its tonsillar loop and dissected free off its arachnoid. The technique of anastomosis is similar to that of the STA-MCA bypass. If the AICA is the recipient vessel, the lateral branch of the AICA posterior to the eighth cranial nerve is isolated and used for the anastomosis. A watertight dural closure is usually not possible, but Gelfoam is placed in the dural opening and reinforced with fibrin glue. This is followed by a good muscle and skin closure to prevent cerebrospinal fluid (CSF) leakage. A Spetzler micromalleable suction (NMT Instruments, Boston, MA) is very useful for aspirating CSF and blood from the wound during the anastomosis.

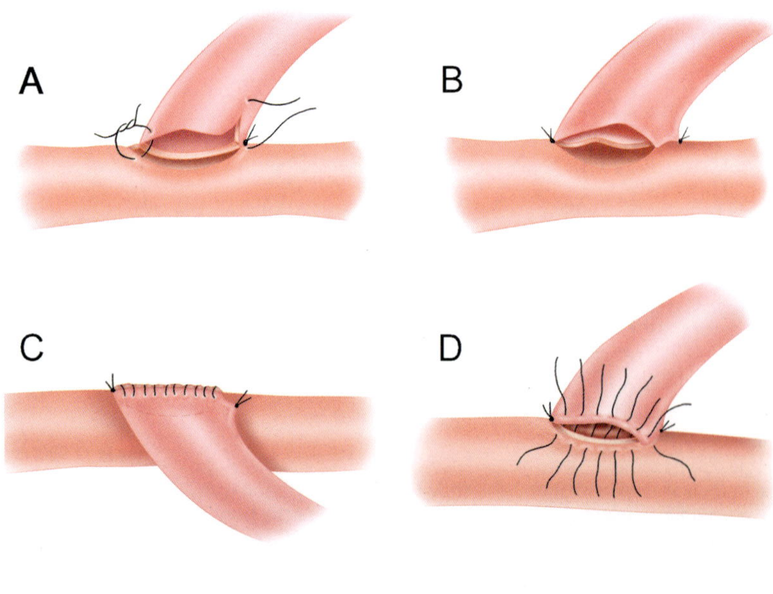

Figure 28–3 **(A,B)** Terminal stitches are placed at the heel and the diametrically opposite ends. Also note the fish-mouthing of the graft. **(C)** One side is anastomosed with continuous sutures and **(D)** the opposite side with interrupted sutures. (Courtesy of Laligam N. Sekhar.)

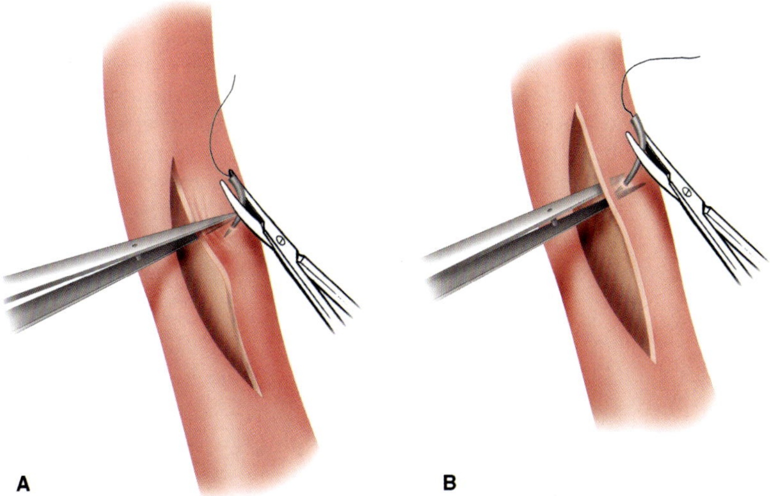

Figure 28–4 The technique of handling the vessel wall while passing the needle. **(A)** Either the edge of the vessel wall is held gently or **(B)** a counterpressure technique is used. (Courtesy of Laligam N. Sekhar.)

Superficial Temporal Artery–Superior Cerebellar Artery Bypass

This is a rare procedure used for upper basilar ischemia or aneurysms. A relatively large and long STA is needed. It is dissected as far distally as possible. Lumbar spinal drainage is instituted, and the SCA is approached subtemporally with division of the tentorium just posterior to the entrance of the fourth cranial nerve. A transpetrosal approach may also be utilized. The superior side of the anastomosis is performed first, then the STA is placed under the retractor gently and the inferior side of the anastomosis is completed. Alternatively, the inferior side can be sutured first by an inside-out suturing technique (see later discussion).

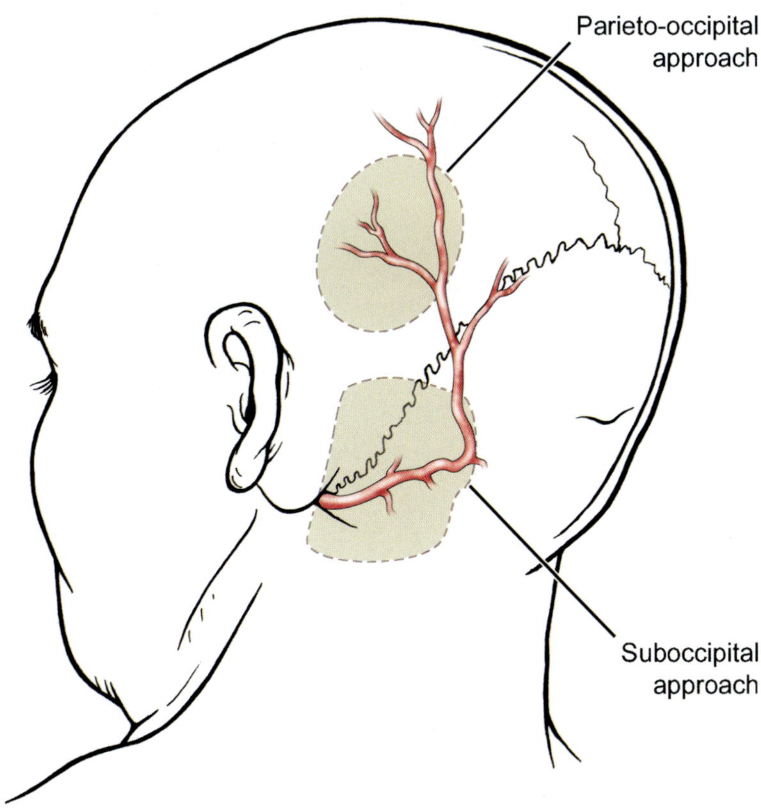

Figure 28–5 The course of the occipital artery, which is usually more tortuous in the elderly. The sites of parieto-occipital and suboccipital craniotomies are indicated. (Courtesy of Laligam N. Sekhar.)

Side-to-Side Anastomosis

This procedure is usually done between the ACA and ACA or PICA and PICA. It can also be done between the AICA and PICA. The vessels must be naturally close to each other or able to be mobilized to lie close to each other. For an A3-to-A3 anastomosis (pericallosal to pericallosal) or A2-to-A2 anastomosis, a bifrontal craniotomy with interhemispheric dissection is performed. This procedure may be necessary during the treatment of a complex anterior communicating artery (ACommA) aneurysm, wherein one A2 has to be occluded electively or because of a tear in the aneurysm neck (**Fig. 28–6**). Both the vessels are dissected, and a rubber dam is placed under both the vessels. Induced hypertension with brain protection is instituted. Temporary clips are placed on either side of each vessel. A linear arteriotomy, ~5 mm long, is made on the superior-medial aspect of either vessel. The superficial wall may be excised partly to enlarge the orifice.

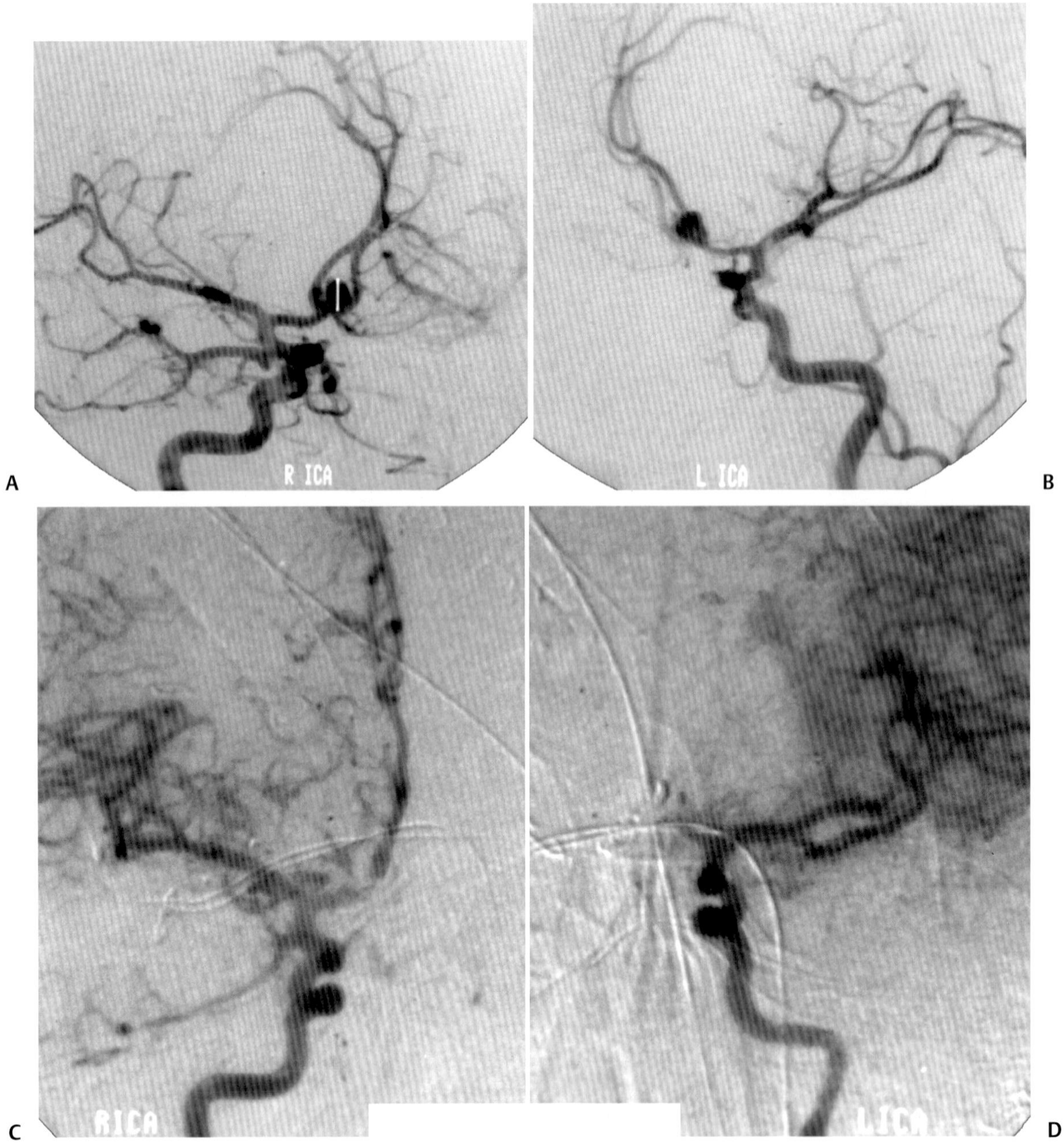

Figure 28–6 This 55-year-old woman presented with subarachnoid hemorrhage. She had no neurological deficit. **(A,B)** Her angiogram revealed an anterior communicating artery aneurysm. The anterior cerebral arteries and the aneurysm were filling from both sides. **(C,D)** She underwent surgery for attempted clipping but suffered a tear at the neck. Consequently, the aneurysm could only be trapped along with occlusion of the left A2 segment of the anterior cerebral artery (ACA), as evident on the intraoperative angiogram. Because there was no deterioration of the evoked potentials despite dropping the systolic blood pressure to 70 mm Hg and because she was not prepared for a revascularization procedure, the same was not attempted. She recovered with no neurological deficit. She was managed with hypervolemia and induced hypertension. About 8 hours following surgery, she developed significant right hemiparesis and dysphasia, which showed improvement with further elevation of her blood pressure, only to worsen again.

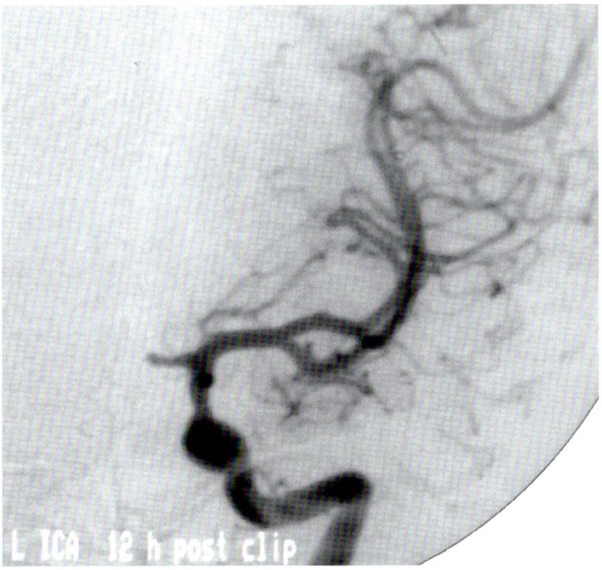

E

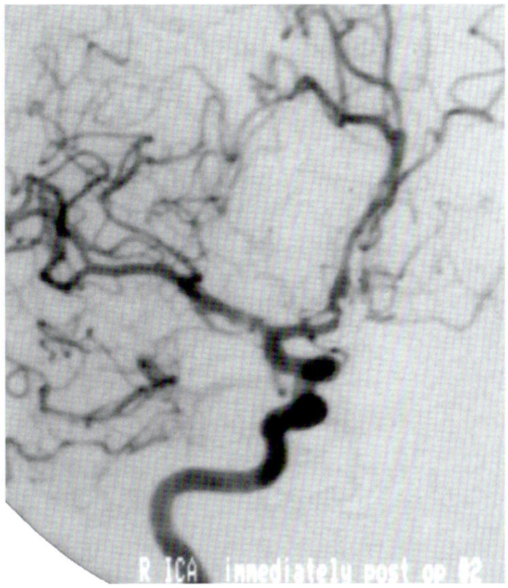

F

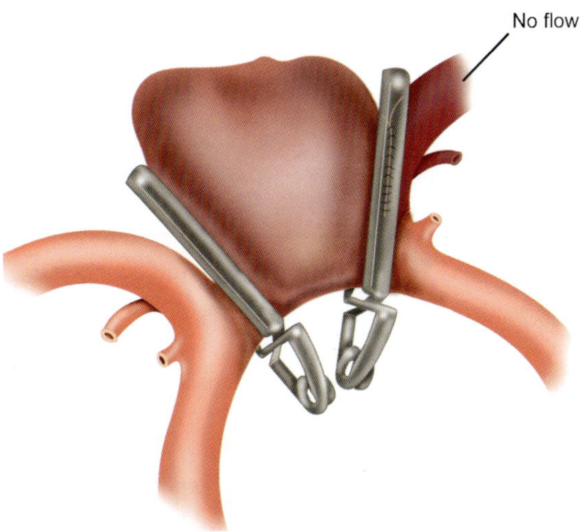

G

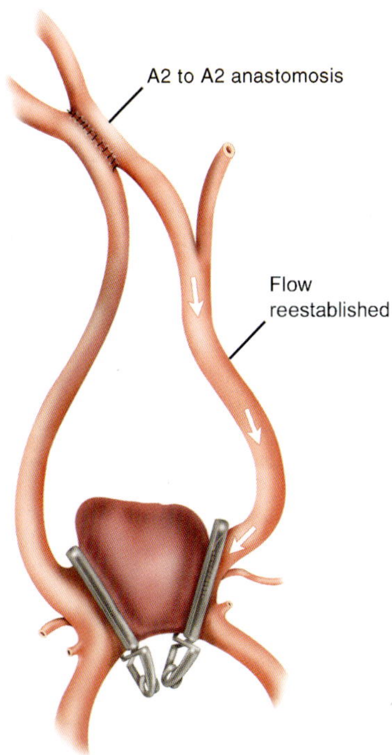

H

(*Continued*) **Figure 28–6** **(E)** An angiogram repeated ~12 hours after surgery confirmed the intraoperative angiogram findings. At this stage it was decided to perform a side-to-side ACA-to-ACA bypass procedure. Her postoperative scan obtained 24 hours after the second surgery showed evidence of a small ACA territory infarct. **(F)** An angiogram done after the second surgery shows filling of both the A2 segments of the ACAs and the recurrent artery of Heubner on the left side. **(G)** Schematic representation of clips with no blood flow before A2-to-A2 anastomosis. **(H)** Blood flow restored to the no-flow territory. (Fig 28–6G,H courtesy of Laligam N. Sekhar.)

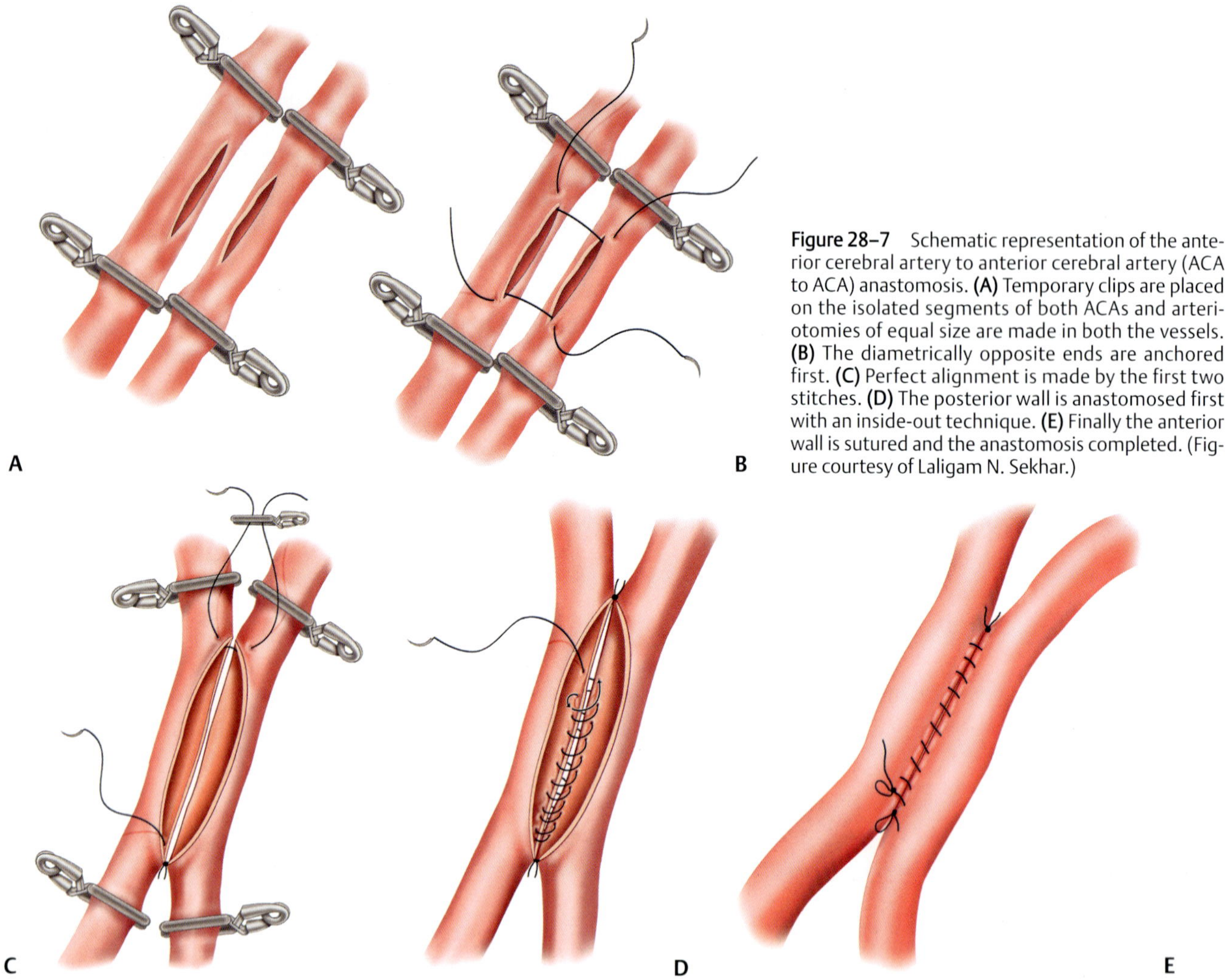

Figure 28–7 Schematic representation of the anterior cerebral artery to anterior cerebral artery (ACA to ACA) anastomosis. **(A)** Temporary clips are placed on the isolated segments of both ACAs and arteriotomies of equal size are made in both the vessels. **(B)** The diametrically opposite ends are anchored first. **(C)** Perfect alignment is made by the first two stitches. **(D)** The posterior wall is anastomosed first with an inside-out technique. **(E)** Finally the anterior wall is sutured and the anastomosis completed. (Figure courtesy of Laligam N. Sekhar.)

The ends are anchored with 9–0 or 10–0 nylon. The deeper or posterior wall is sutured first by an inside-out technique, and the superficial or anterior wall is then sutured (**Fig. 28–7**). Temporary clips are removed. This is a very effective technique and, although rarely needed, is quite successful.

Direct Reconstruction/Interposition Graft

The reconstruction of cerebral arteries is usually performed after the excision of an aneurysm or after an inadvertent tear of a vessel wall. When the artery cannot be mobilized and sutured without tension, then a short interposition graft can be used. In some patients (e.g., MCA aneurysms), section and reimplantation of a branch may be done. In all of these situations, the operative technique is similar.

For direct reconstruction, the two arterial ends to be reconstructed are sharply sectioned obliquely and slightly fish-mouthed at the opposing ends (**Fig. 28–8**). A rubber dam is placed beneath the vessels, and temporary clips are positioned on both the vessels. The diametrically opposed ends are anchored with 9–0 or 10–0 nylon suture. Continuous sutures are placed on one side, and then continuous or interrupted sutures on the other side. Before the last suture is tied, the lumen is flushed with heparinized saline.

When the gap between the two ends of the artery is such that they cannot be approximated without tension, then an arterial interposition graft is used. The grafts available for this purpose include the STA, OA, and superior thyroid artery (SThyA). The technique of suturing is similar to direct reconstruction (**Figs. 28–9, 28–10**).

The reimplantation of an artery into a branch vessel is usually performed in cases where the branch cannot be preserved during aneurysm clipping, usually encountered with MCA aneurysms. Reimplantation may be performed either directly or with an interposition graft, as shown in **Fig. 28–11.**

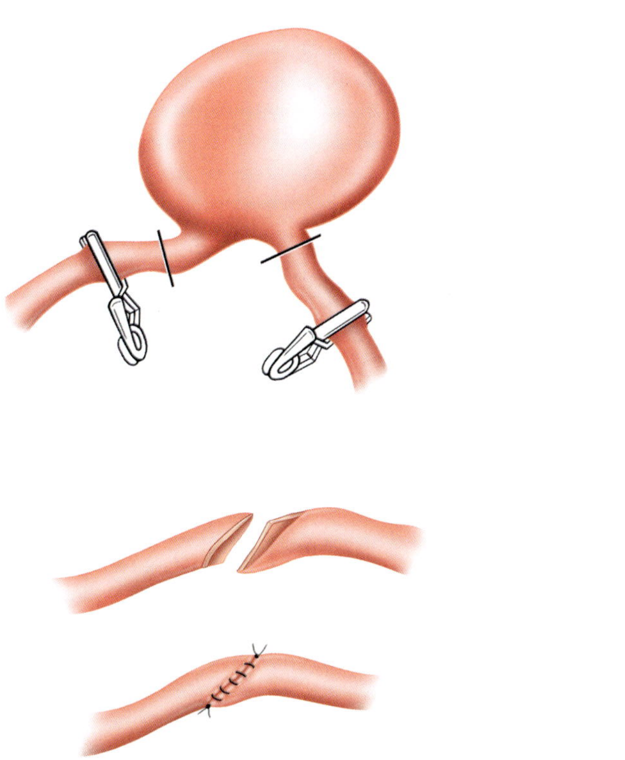

Figure 28–8 After excision of the aneurysmal sac, either arterial end is sharply sectioned obliquely, slightly fish-mouthed, and sutured. (Figure courtesy of Laligam N. Sekhar.)

Radial Artery Graft

The RAG can be anastomosed into smaller recipient vessels and carries a moderate volume of flow. The problem of postoperative vasospasm has been solved by the use of the pressure distension technique.

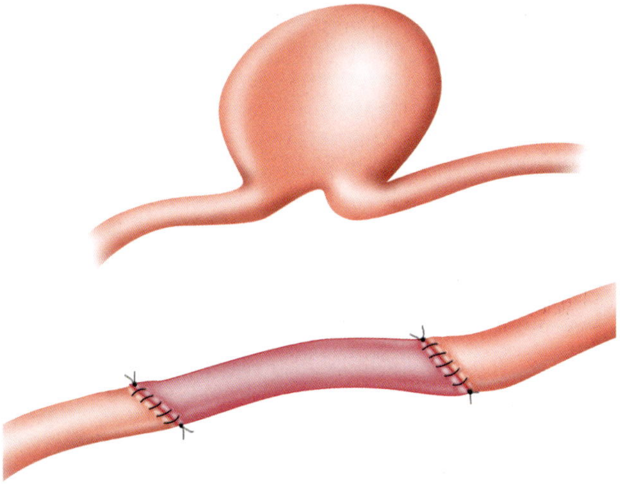

Figure 28–9 If the parent artery cannot be adequately mobilized to suture the ends without tension, then a short interposition graft is used. (Figure courtesy of Laligam N. Sekhar.)

Rarely, the RA may be the dominant or the only supply to the hand. The presence of adequate perfusion to the hand must be confirmed by the Allen test preoperatively, prior to the extraction of the RA. The Allen test is performed as follows: The hands of the patient are held out in front. The RA and the ulnar artery are located by their pulsations. With a good view of the hand, the RA and the ulnar artery are occluded tightly just above the wrist. The patient closes and opens the hands repeatedly for a period of 1 minute to squeeze the blood out of the hand. When the hand is blanched, the pressure on the ulnar artery is released, and the hand color is carefully observed. In individuals with an intact palmar arch, the pallor is quickly replaced by rubor of a higher degree than normal, which gradually fades to normal color. If the ulnar artery is occluded or atreitic, or if the palmar arch is inadequate, the hand remains pale until the pressure on the RA is released.[29] At the time of surgery, the RAG is exposed, and adequacy of perfusion of the fingers must be confirmed again by using a temporary clip on the vessel, with a pulse oximeter on the finger, to check distal perfusion.

A gently curved longitudinal incision is made on the ventral aspect of the forearm. The artery is identified distally on the volar aspect of the forearm between the tendons of the flexor carpi radialis and brachioradialis muscles. It is then traced proximally, where it lies under the brachioradialis. The entire length can be used if required. Its branches are coagulated or ligated and cut at least 2 mm away from the artery, but the venae comitantes are left attached to the artery except near the ends. The venae comitantes and periadventitial tissue are stripped away from the vessel for 2 cm near the sites of the anastomosis. The artery is left in situ and harvested just prior to the anastomosis. After the graft is harvested, the incision is closed in two or three layers, and a soft bulky dressing is applied. The graft surface is marked longitudinally with methylene blue to prevent torsion during its application.

Pressure Distention Technique

After extraction of the graft, a small blunt needle (an angiocath needle) is introduced into the RA, and after pinching the artery shut with the fingers near the needle and ~4 cm beyond, it is forcefully distended with pressure using heparinized saline until the artery is visualized to "pop" and distend. The artery is then plicated over the blunt needle, and the procedure is repeated. The same procedure is also performed from the other end of the graft (**Fig. 28–12**). This procedure prevents the occurrence of postoperative vasospasm.

Through an oblique cervical skin crease incision, the ECA and its branches and the ICA are dissected. The craniotomy and any skull base exposures needed are performed. The recipient vessel is isolated for a 1 cm segment, and a rubber dam is inserted under it. The patient's blood pressure is raised 20% above baseline, and brain protection with barbiturates is instituted to achieve burst suppression of monitored EEG. Intravenous heparin at a dose of 2000 U is administered. The RAG is extracted, the distal end denuded of periadventitial tissue for ~1 cm, and an oblique

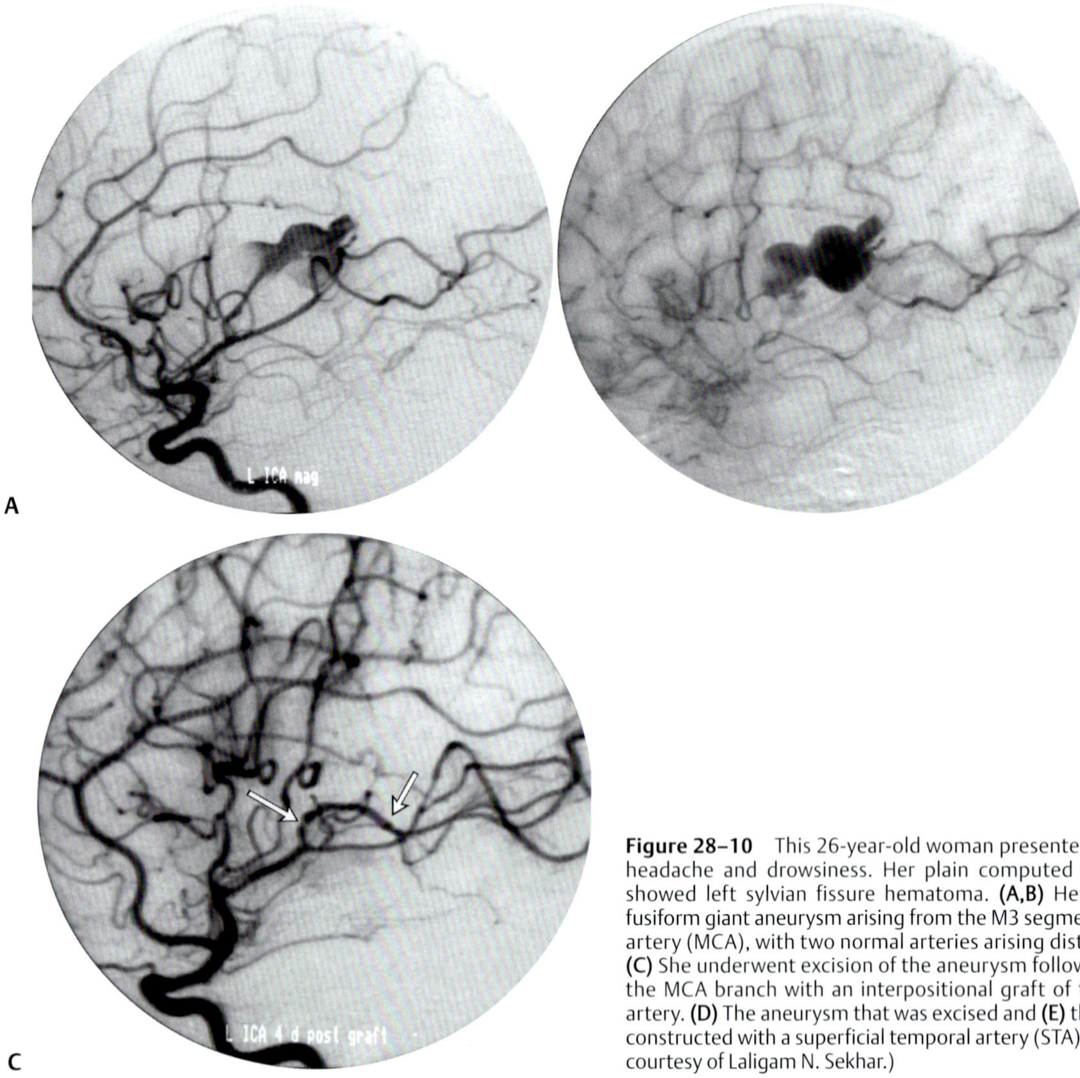

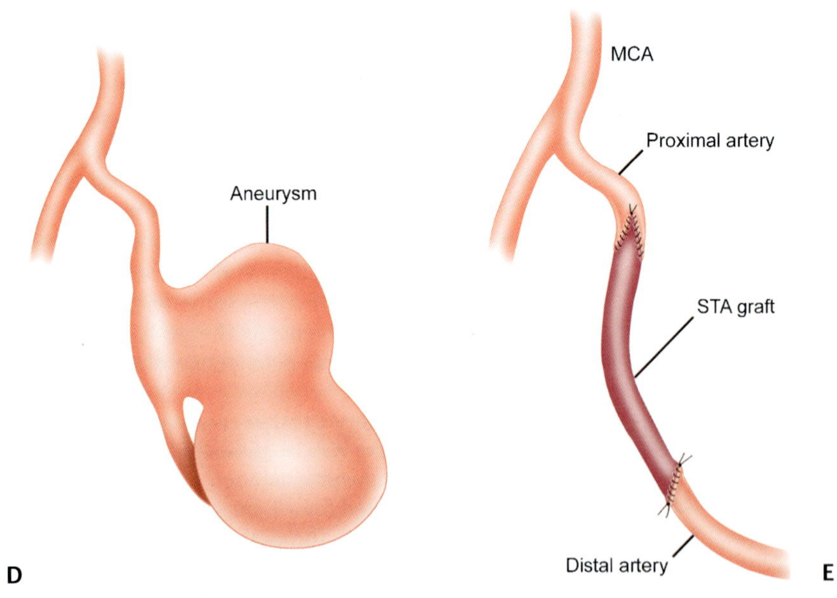

Figure 28–10 This 26-year-old woman presented with a 2-day history of headache and drowsiness. Her plain computed tomographic (CT) scan showed left sylvian fissure hematoma. **(A,B)** Her angiogram revealed a fusiform giant aneurysm arising from the M3 segment of the middle cerebral artery (MCA), with two normal arteries arising distally from the aneurysm. **(C)** She underwent excision of the aneurysm followed by reconstruction of the MCA branch with an interpositional graft of the superficial temporal artery. **(D)** The aneurysm that was excised and **(E)** the MCA branch vessel reconstructed with a superficial temporal artery (STA) graft. (Figures 28–10D,E courtesy of Laligam N. Sekhar.)

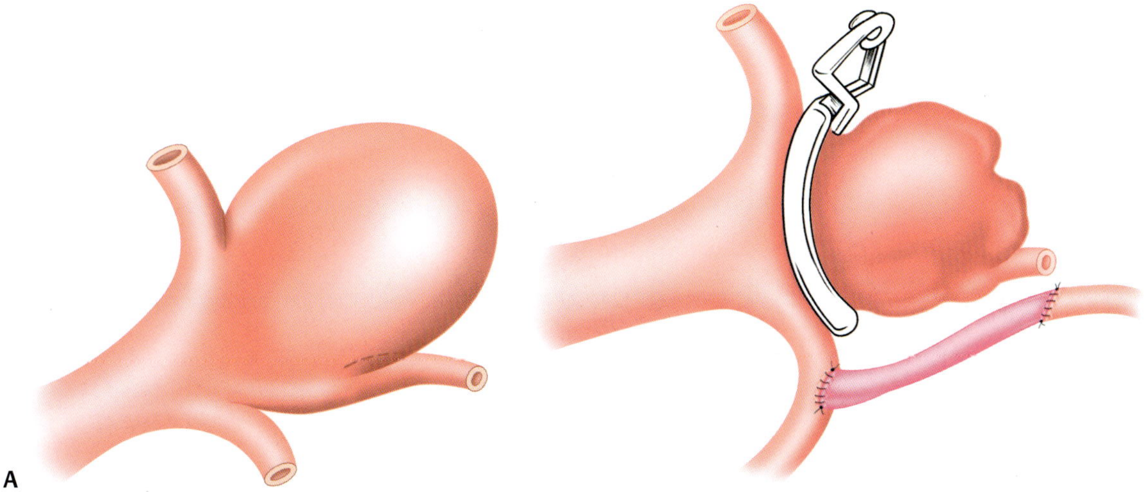

Figure 28–11 **(A,B)** An artery can be reimplanted into a branch vessel when it cannot be preserved during aneurysm clipping with or without an interposition graft. (Courtesy of Laligam N. Sekhar.)

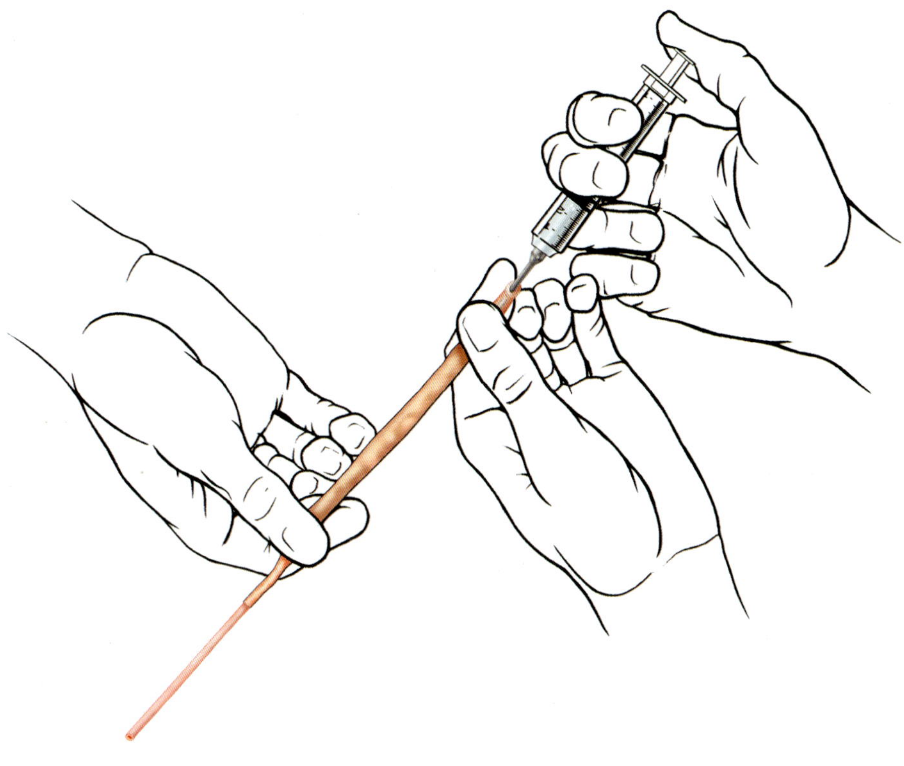

Figure 28–12 The pressure distention technique to perform a hydrostatic angioplasty of the radial artery.

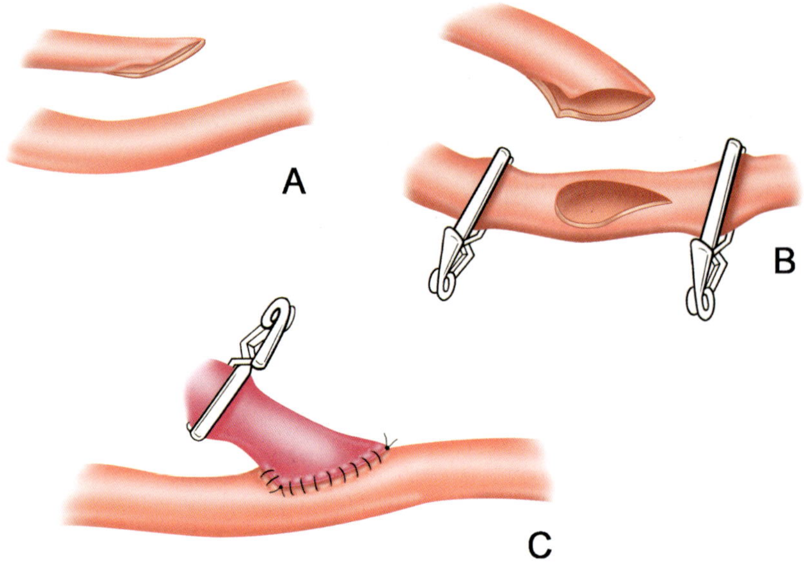

Figure 28–13 The sequence of radial artery grafting. **(A)** The graft is fish-mouthed. **(B)** A teardrop-shaped arteriotomy is made in the recipient vessel. **(C)** The completed anastomosis. (Courtesy of Laligam N. Sekhar.)

arteriotomy is made with a single fish-mouth incision. After placing temporary clips on the recipient artery, a teardrop-shaped arteriotomy is made in the recipient vessel, ~5 to 6 mm in length. The heel and the opposite end of the RAG are anchored with 8–0 nylon. One side of the RAG is anastomosed with continuous sutures and the opposite side with two continuous sutures, starting from the ends of the anastomosis and working toward the middle. Prior to tying the last suture, the lumen of both arteries is flushed with heparinized saline. A temporary clip is placed on the RAG ~1 to 2 cm from the anastomotic site, and temporary clips are released from the recipient artery to check for any leakage from the suture line. Leaks may require additional stitching (**Fig. 28–13**).

A retroauricular or preauricular tunnel is created for the passage of the RAG with a large curved scissor and a chest tube. The RAG may be passed through the tunnel through a chest tube. Prior to passing, the RAG is distended with heparinized saline to check for leaks from branch sites, and if found, closed with 8–0 nylon or 7–0 Prolene. Caution must be exercised to avoid twisting of the vessel.

The donor vessel (usually the ICA or ECA) is occluded with clips; usually proximally, a permanent aneurysm clip is needed because of the large pressure head and the thickness and large diameter of the vessel. Distally, a temporary clip will be adequate.

The RAG is shortened adequately, to be slack but not tortuous. The graft expands after revascularization. If the length is too short, anastomosis may be difficult and can be under tension. The arteriotomy of the ECA is similar to the cranial end, but a larger opening is created, usually 8 to 10 mm in length. If the vessel is small, an end-to-end anastomosis can be created. The anastomosis is performed using 7–0 nylon. The clips are released from the donor artery, and the anastomotic site and the RAG are inspected for spasm or leaks. Spastic areas can be dilated with gentle massage or by sharply dissecting adventitial bands.

A Sugita or Transonic (Transonic Systems Inc., Ithaca, NY) Doppler probe is used to check the flow. If quantitative flow is measured with the Transonic Doppler probe, it is usually in the range of 40 to 70 mL/min. When the RAG is anastomosed to smaller vessels (e.g., fetal posterior communicating artery), the flow may be as low as 20 mL/min. The dura is closed, but a cruciate incision must be made at the site of entry of the RAG. Half of the heparin administered may be reversed if there is excessive epidural bleeding. A subgaleal drain may be needed. An intraoperative angiogram is performed after the dural closure. The graft must be checked with Doppler again after affixing the bone flap.

Postoperatively, the graft is palpated and checked with Doppler every 2 hours for 24 hours and then thrice daily. On the second or third postoperative day, a 3D-CT angiogram, or an MRA is performed. If any narrowing is observed, an intra-arterial digital subtraction angiogram is obtained. Many types of RA bypasses have been used by the senior author (**Figs. 28–14, 28–15**).

Saphenous Vein Graft

The SVG provides a high flow rate but is prone to thrombosis because of technical problems. Such thrombosis may be caused by inadequate flow due to a poor proximal anastomosis, turbulence or kinking at the distal anastomosis, or injury to venous endothelium due to poor handling technique or storage. Every step during the operation is important, as is the performance of intraoperative angiography, which allows the recognition and immediate correction of the problem.

For anterior circulation bypass grafting, the vein is exposed in the thigh from the groin inferiorly for ~20 to 25 cm, and for posterior circulation grafting, the vein is exposed in the lower thigh or upper leg (**Fig. 28–16**). For exposure in the thigh, the femoral arterial pulse is palpated at the inguinal

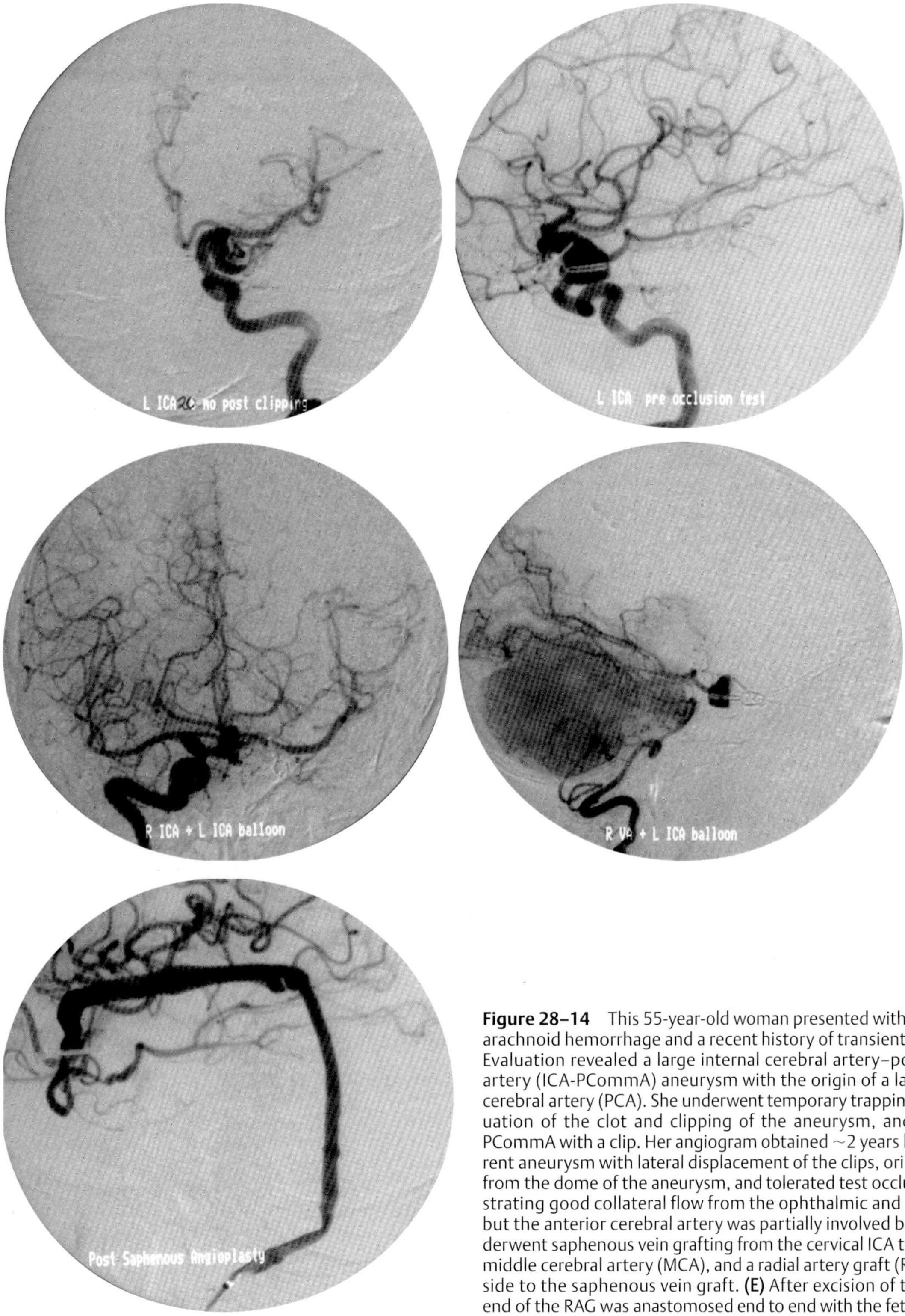

A B C D E

Figure 28–14 This 55-year-old woman presented with a remote history of subarachnoid hemorrhage and a recent history of transient ischemic attacks. **(A–D)** Evaluation revealed a large internal cerebral artery–posterior communicating artery (ICA-PCommA) aneurysm with the origin of a large fetal-type posterior cerebral artery (PCA). She underwent temporary trapping of the aneurysm, evacuation of the clot and clipping of the aneurysm, and reconstruction of the PCommA with a clip. Her angiogram obtained ~2 years later shows a large recurrent aneurysm with lateral displacement of the clips, origin of the fetal-type PCA from the dome of the aneurysm, and tolerated test occlusion of the ICA, demonstrating good collateral flow from the ophthalmic and anterior cerebral artery, but the anterior cerebral artery was partially involved by the aneurysm. She underwent saphenous vein grafting from the cervical ICA to the M2 segment of the middle cerebral artery (MCA), and a radial artery graft (RAG) was inserted end to side to the saphenous vein graft. **(E)** After excision of the aneurysm, the other end of the RAG was anastomosed end to end with the fetal PCommA.

(*Continued on page 354*)

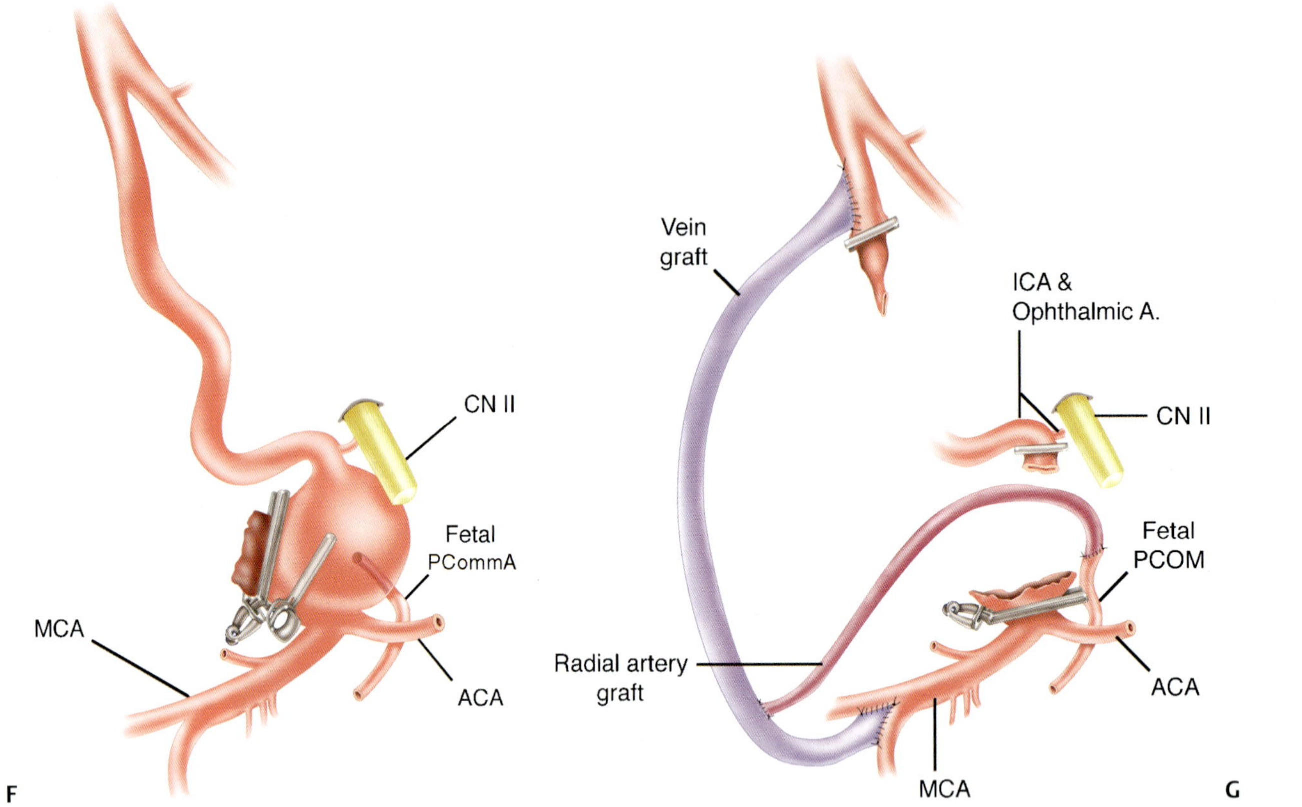

(*Continued*) **Figure 28–14** **(F)** Schematic representation of the recurrent aneurysm, its excision along with the saphenous vein graft (SVG) and **(G)** RAG is shown. (Figures 28–14F,G courtesy of Laligam N. Sekhar.)

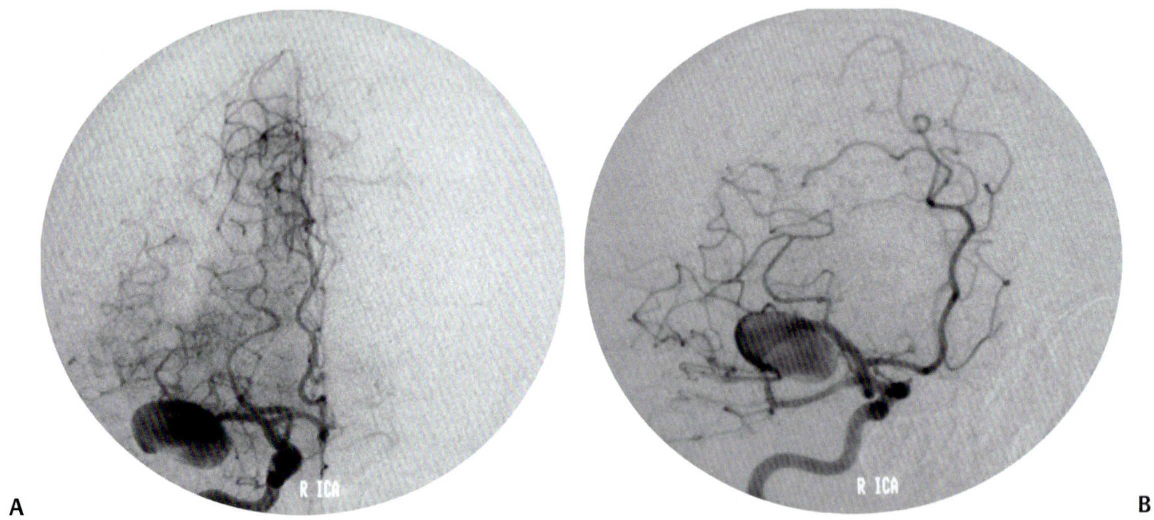

Figure 28–15 This 72-year-old woman presented with a history of persistent bifrontal headaches with recent increase in severity. **(A,B)** Her angiogram

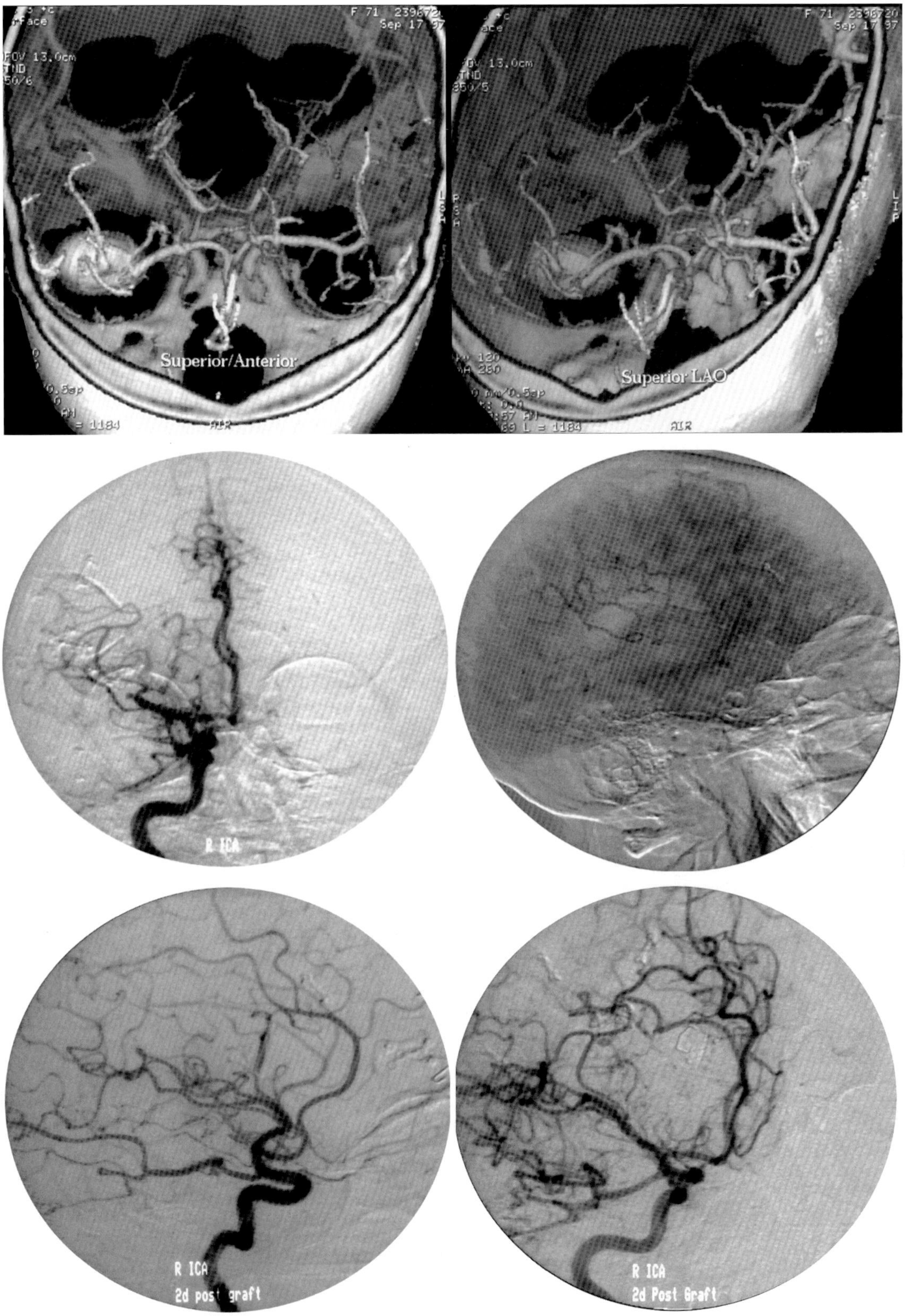

C D E F G H

Figure 28–15 **(C,D)** and three-dimensional computed tomographic (3D–CT) scan revealed a giant M2 segment aneurysm, with the main distal branch arising from the dome of the aneurysm. An aneurysmorraphy was performed. Her intraoperative angiogram showed good flow through the aneurysmorraphy segment and also distally, although there was some irregularity of the lumen. **(E,F)** The postoperative angiogram obtained the next day showed an asymptomatic MCA occlusion with distal perfusion defect. She was immediately taken up for surgery. At surgery there was complete thrombosis of the aneurysmorraphy segment. She underwent excision of this segment, and a 3 cm long radial artery graft was interposed between the middle cerebral artery (MCA) trunk and its major branch. **(G)** Her postoperative CT scan revealed no evidence of infarct, and **(H)** the angiogram revealed good flow through the graft and distal branches.

(*Continued on page 356*)

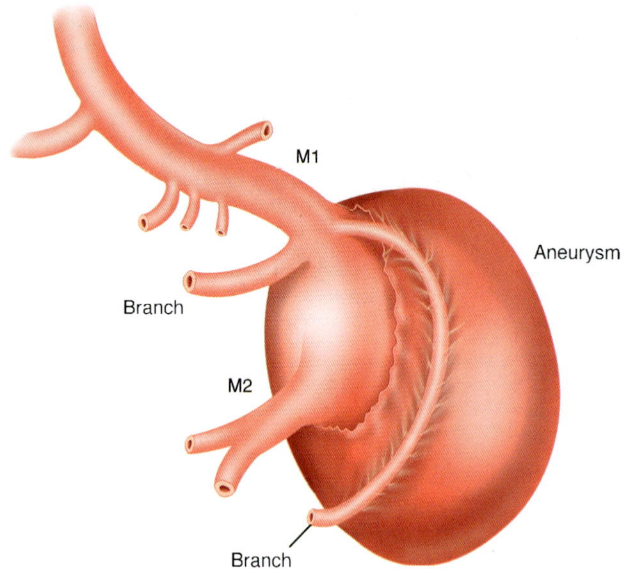

I

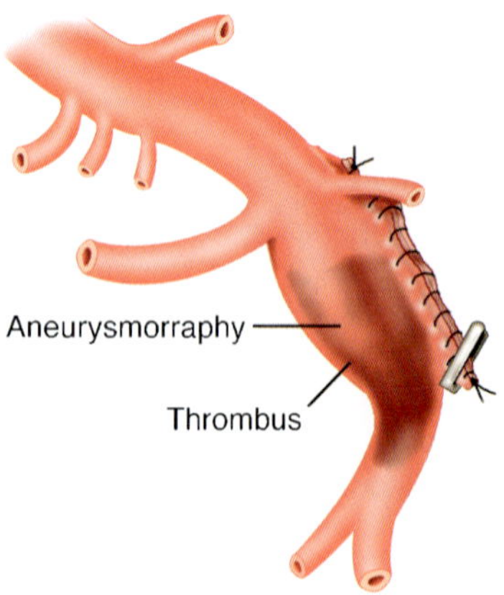

J

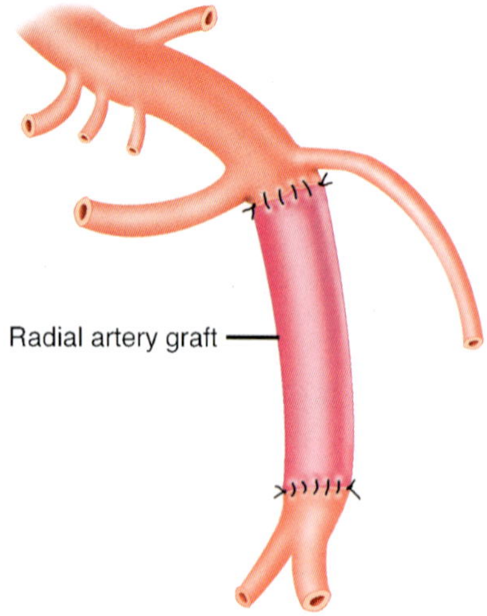

K

(*Continued*) **Figure 28–15** **(I)** Schematic representation of the location of the aneurysm with the branches in relation to it, **(J)** the aneurysmorraphy performed preserving the branches, and **(K)** subsequently the interposition radial artery graft. (Figures 28–15I–K Courtesy of Laligam N. Sekhar.)

ligament, and the femoral vein lies just medial to this. This spot is marked. Another spot is marked at the middle of the medial aspect of the knee. A line connecting these two points indicates the course of the saphenous vein in the thigh. The patient is preferably positioned supine with the hip externally rotated and pillows placed under the knee and ankle. When the surgeon stands on one side of the patient, it is easier to extract the vein from the opposite leg. The ipsilateral groin and thigh must also be prepared, and a sheath placed in the femoral artery for performance of an intraoperative angiogram. The patient's head is placed in a radiolucent head holder.

A longitudinal incision is started at the upper portion of the marked skin incision. Dissection is performed through the subcutaneous tissues, and the vein is identified. It is traced superiorly to the femoral ring where it pierces the cribriform fascia and traced inferiorly for a length of ~25 cm. The vein should be at least 3 mm in diameter, preferably 4 mm. The branches are ligated with 4–0 Neurolon or with titanium hemoclips about a millimeter from the vein. The vein is sharply dissected along the periadventitial tissue, care being taken to handle the vein gently. It is left in situ until just prior to anastomosis. After the vein has been completely dissected, cottonoids soaked in 3% papaverine are first placed on the medial side and then on the lateral aspect. This relaxes any spasm of the vein. If the vein is not large enough, then the dissection was far too lateral, and the surgeon will need to look for a more medial vein. Careful hemostasis is essential. At extraction, both the ends are ligated, and the vein is sectioned and removed. The lumen is flushed out with heparinized saline by pinching different areas and is distended with heparinized saline to release spasm and check for leaks. Any leaks detected are closed with 6–0 Prolene. The graft is marked on the anterior surface with methylene blue to prevent any torsion during its placement. Methylprednisolone, 20 mg/kg, is given 30 to

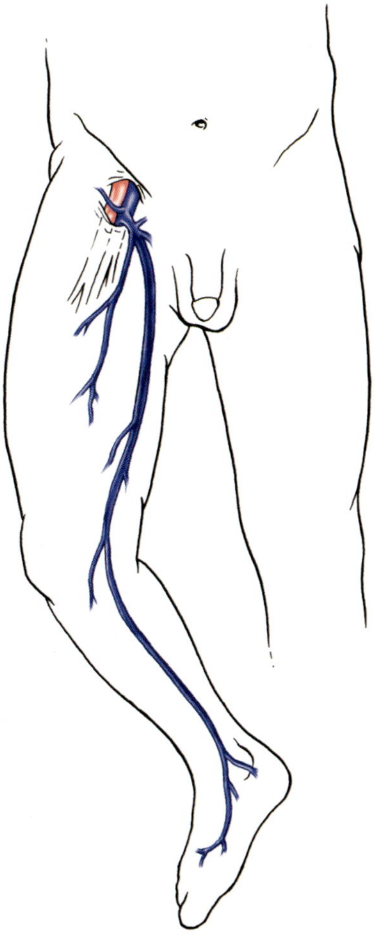

Figure 28–16 The course of the saphenous vein from the foot to its termination in the femoral vein. (Figure courtesy of Laligam N. Sekhar.)

60 minutes before the extraction of the graft. This appears to protect the venous endothelium from shedding when it is exposed to arterial blood flow. At the end of the operation, the vein graft extraction site must be carefully checked for hemostasis and closed with a suction drain to prevent a hematoma.

The saphenous vein in the leg can be found on the tibia anterior to the medial malleolus. It may be difficult to find the vein on the medial aspect of the thigh, and it may be necessary to trace it superiorly from the leg. After the graft extraction, careful hemostasis is obtained and the incision closed with a drain to prevent any hematoma formation.

Vein-Grafting Procedure

The ICA to MCA graft will be described first, followed by other types of grafts. A frontotemporal craniotomy is done, and an orbital osteotomy is also usually performed for exposure of aneurysm or tumor. The sylvian fissure is widely opened, and the MCA is carefully inspected. The ideal place to anastomose the graft is at the MCA bifurcation beyond the lenticulostriate vessels. Sometimes, when the bifurcation is very proximal, the graft can be inserted into a large M2 branch, preferably distal to the perforators (**Fig. 28–17**). Rarely, the presence of a very proximal MCA bifurcation with the origin of a large perforator from an MCA branch vessel may necessitate temporary occlusion of the perforator. An alternative arrangement could be the anastomosis of the SVG to the supraclinoid ICA, or the insertion of a RAG into the MCA branch beyond the perforating vessel. Insertion of the graft into the bifurcation minimizes turbulence by orienting the jet of the blood flow along the long axis of the vessel rather than onto a wall of the vessel.

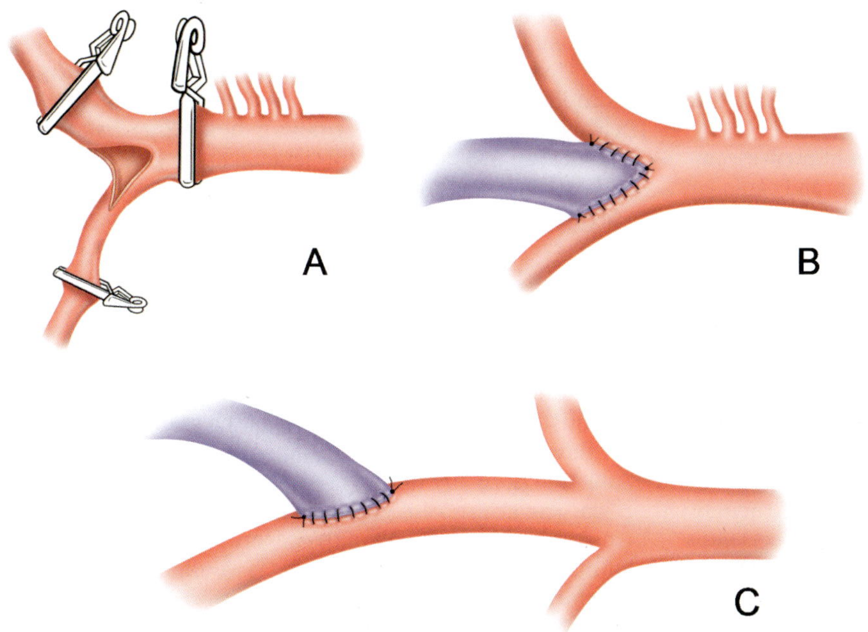

Figure 28–17 **(A)** An arteriotomy is made at the middle cerebral artery (MCA) bifurcation to match the venotomy opening. **(B)** Saphenous ventomy matched the artery opening. The ideal location to place the saphenous vein graft is the MCA bifurcation. **(C)** In the presence of a very proximal bifurcation, the graft can be inserted into a large M2 branch. (Figure courtesy of Laligam N. Sekhar.)

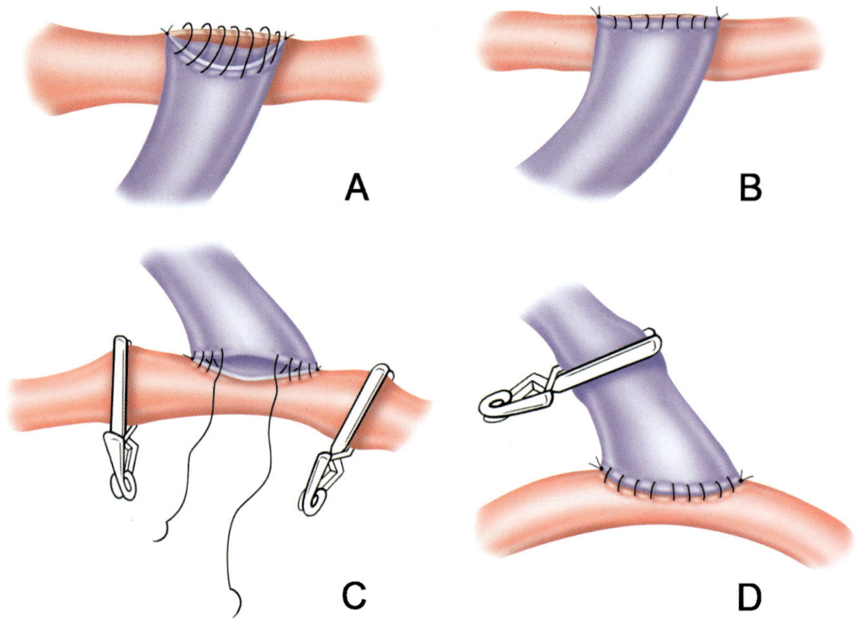

Figure 28–18 **(A,B)** The medial side of the middle cerebral artery–saphenous vein graft (MCA-SVG) is anastomosed first, with a continuous suture starting from the more difficult corner. The loops are left loose to be tightened and tied at the end. **(C)** On the lateral side two sutures are run from either end to meet in the middle. **(D)** At the completion of the anastomosis, a temporary clip is placed on the vein graft ~1 cm from the site of the anastomosis. (Figure courtesy of Laligam N. Sekhar.)

The patient's blood pressure is raised 20% above the baseline, and burst suppression is induced with barbiturates. Heparin (2000 U) is administered intravenously. The vein graft is harvested and used without reversal. It is denuded off its periadventitial tissue near the ends, and an oblique venotomy is made. Temporary clips are placed on the MCA and branches beyond the perforators. An arteriotomy at the MCA bifurcation is made to match the venotomy. The heel and the diametrically opposite ends, of the vessels are anchored with 8–0 nylon. The medial side is anastomosed with a continuous suture starting at the more difficult corner. The loops are left loose and tightened and tied at the end. On the lateral side, two sutures are run from the ends of the arteriotomy to meet in the middle. The loops are similarly tightened, and, before they are tied in the middle, the lumen is irrigated with heparinized saline. The vein graft is also irrigated with heparinized saline, and a temporary clip is placed on the vein ~1 cm from the anastomotic site (**Fig. 28–18**).

The cervical incision is made along a skin crease commencing ~1 cm inferior to the angle of the jaw and extended toward the mastoid process. The sternomastoid muscle is dissected from the skin and is retracted posteriorly with suture and rubber bands. If anastomosis is planned to the ICA, the ICA must be dissected as high as possible, up to the level of the 12th nerve. If desired, it can be traced further superiorly by dividing the digastric muscle. If grafting is into the ECA, the dissection is performed near the bifurcation of the CCA and the ECA branches. Generally it is preferable to anastomose end (vein) to side (artery) because of the discrepancy in size between the artery and vein (**Fig. 28–19**). But end to end anastomosis can also be done if the vein graft is large in size (**Fig. 28–20**).

The temporary clips on the MCA are released and the suture line inspected for any leaks. If any leaks are detected, an additional stitch or two may be necessary. Ideally the duration of anastomosis should be less than 30 to 45 minutes, with a maximum of 50 minutes. When the vein graft is placed into the MCA, it is usually passed through a retroauricular tunnel because it has a parallel orientation to the MCA in the sylvian fissure. The tunnel is created prior to the anastomosis with a large, curved scissor and chest tube. The graft is passed into the neck area without twisting or turning. If the graft is placed into the supraclinoid ICA, it is passed through a preauricular tunnel.

The arteriotomy in the ECA or ICA should be at least 8 mm long. Because the vein graft expands considerably upon reflow, it should be under slight tension for the inferior anastomosis. The anastomotic technique is similar to the radial graft, as described earlier. For anastomosis, 6–0 or 7–0 is used. Upon completion of anastomosis, temporary clips are gradually released, and the anastomotic site is checked for leaks, which are repaired if present. The patency of the graft is confirmed by intraoperative Doppler studies, and the cervical ICA is occluded with titanium hemoclips distal to the cervical anastomosis. For intracranial aneurysms with mass effect, a distal clip is placed on the clinoidal or ophthalmic segment of the ICA, but the aneurysms frequently thrombose even without the distal clip. In the case of tumors, a temporary clip is mandatory, and the ophthalmic artery can usually be sacrificed without visual compromise because of collaterals from the ECA.

A cruciate incision is made at the site of entry of the vein graft and the dura closed. An intraoperative angiogram is mandatory to ensure the patency of the graft and the speed of flow, which is very important. The intracranial arteries must fill normally through the graft before the ECA circulation. The entire vein graft and both the anastomotic sites must be visualized. Half of the heparin can be reversed with protamine, but if epidural oozing is minimal, no reversal is performed. If the extradural oozing is excessive, occasionally the bone flap can be left out, with subgaleal drainage

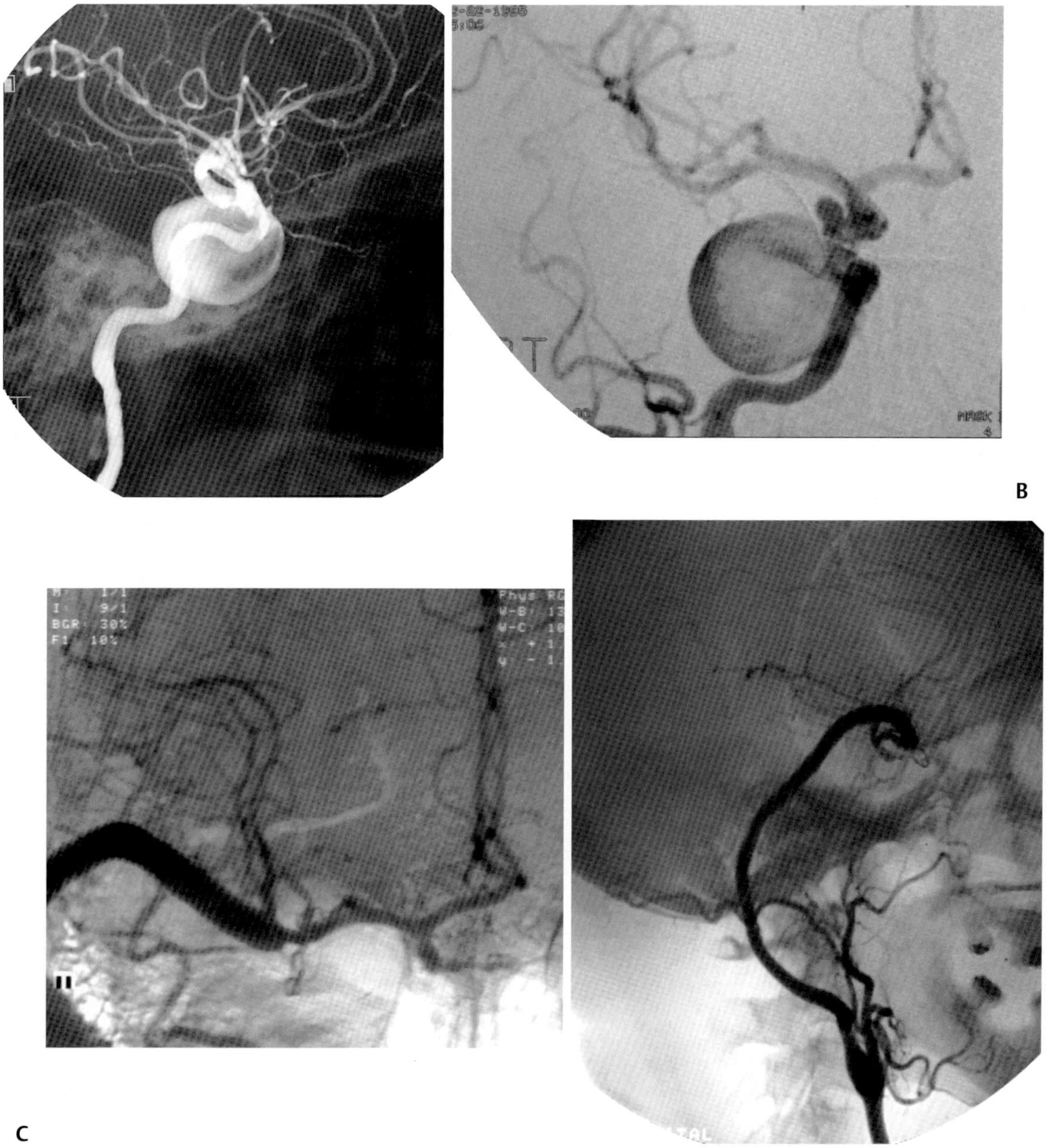

A B C D

Figure 28–19 This 48-year-old woman presented with diplopia on right lateral gaze. **(A,B)** On evaluation she had multiple intracranial aneurysms, with the prominent among them being the giant intracavernous internal cerebral artery (ICA) aneurysm. **(C,D)** She underwent saphenous vein grafting from the cervical ICA to the M2 segment of the middle cerebral artery with trapping of the cavernous ICA aneurysm and clipping of the other aneurysms.

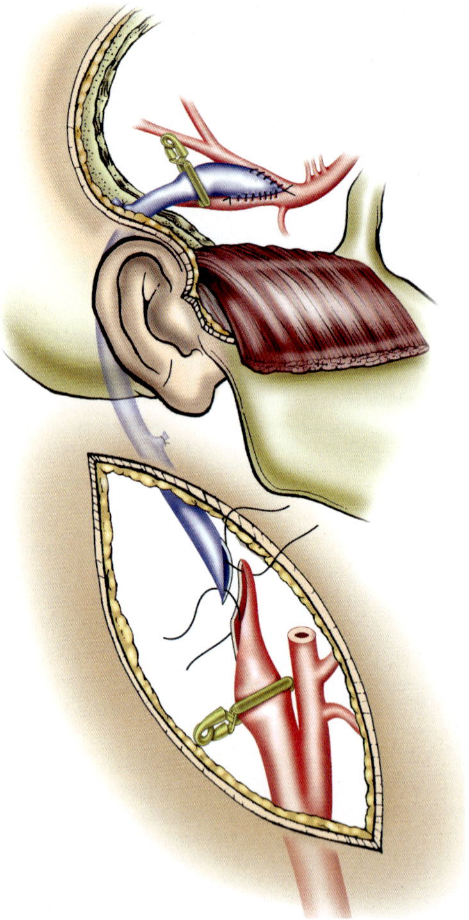

Figure 28–20 After completion of the graft to middle cerebral artery (MCA) anastomosis, a temporary clip is placed on the vein graft ~1 cm from the anastomotic site. The graft is then tunneled through a retroauricular tunnel into the cervical area, and an end-to-end anastomosis of the graft to the internal cerebral artery is performed. Also note the oblique arteriotomy and venotomy along with fish-mouthing of both vessels. (Figure courtesy of Laligam N. Sekhar.)

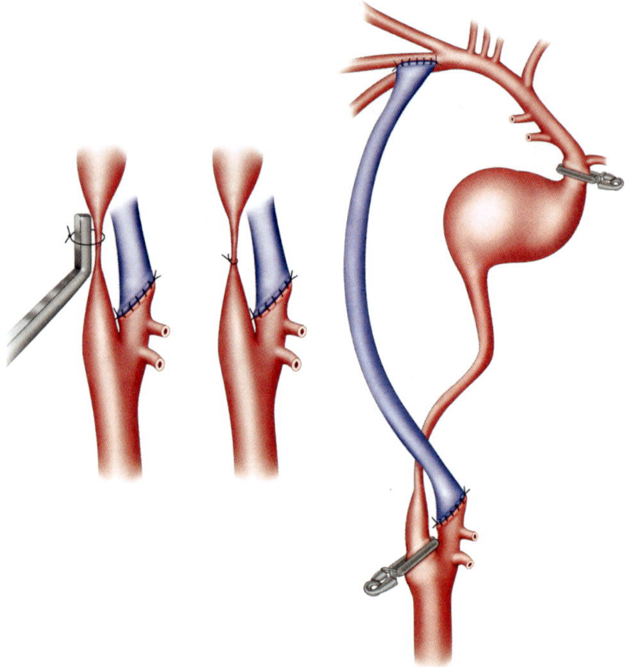

Figure 28–21 Following external carotid artery to middle cerebral artery grafting, an artificial stenosis may have to be created by placing a Mixter clamp as shown here to promote flow through the graft. The clamp is then withdrawn after the successful creation of a stenosis. At this stage, an intraoperative angiogram is obtained to confirm good flow through the graft. If the somatosensory evoked potentials show no change upon test occlusion of the internal cerebral artery (ICA) along with demonstration of good flow through the ICA, then the ICA can be trapped during the same operation. Alternatively, the graft can be allowed to mature further, and the ICA can be occluded at a later time with an intraluminal balloon. (Figure courtesy of Laligam N. Sekhar.)

for 72 hours. The patient is monitored postoperatively with periodic neurological evaluation, palpation of the graft, and Doppler study performed every hour on the first day and thrice daily thereafter. A 3D-CT angiogram is obtained on the first postoperative day to check for the graft function. Graft failure is very rare after 24 hours.

Cervical ECA as Donor Vessel

The ECA is used as a donor when collateral circulation is very poor. In this instance, after the graft is opened, the ICA is occluded with a temporary clip, with monitoring of neurophysiological function, Doppler study of graft flow, and intraoperative angiogram. If the flow is tenuous, the graft may need to be revised. Alternatively, the ICA can be artificially narrowed as shown (**Fig. 28–21**), and the patient is slightly anticoagulated. The graft function is checked by an angiogram a few days later, and the ICA can be permanently occluded with an intraluminal balloon if graft flow is good.

The various other techniques of anastomosis used by the senior author are illustrated in **Figs. 28–22** through **28–26.**

Cervical ICA (or ECA) to Supraclinoid ICA

When the MCA branches early and the branches are small, the supraclinoid ICA is used for anastomosis. An orbital osteotomy with clinoid resection and optic canal decompression is necessary. The ICA is generally divided superior to the ophthalmic artery for end-to-end anastomosis. The optic nerve is mobilized by opening the dural sheath to avoid injury to the nerve. The anastomosis to the ICA is usually performed end to end using 8–0 nylon or 7–0 Prolene suture. The graft is then passed through the dural opening in the clinoid space and brought extradurally. The graft is passed through a preauricular tunnel because it is a more direct and shorter path to the neck. The cervical anastomosis is as described earlier. This type of graft can provide more blood flow than an ICA to MCA

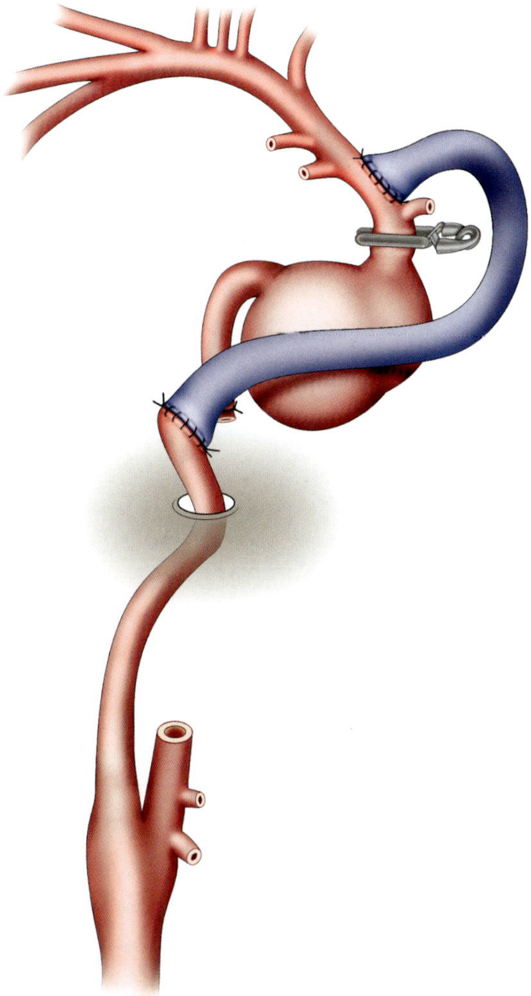

Figure 28–22 Intracavernous aneurysms can be managed by a petrous to supraclinoid internal cerebral artery anastomosis with a short segment of vein graft and trapping of the aneurysm. (Figure courtesy of Laligam N. Sekhar.)

graft. The distal anastomosis can also be done end to end, with sacrifice of the ophthalmic artery. The vein graft expands upon reflow and may kink the distal anastomotic site. If this occurs, the patient may need a pexy procedure; that is, the vein is pulled back and sutured to the dura mater to reduce any kinking at the anastomotic site.

External Carotid Artery or Vertebral Artery to Posterior Cerebral Artery Anastomosis

This type of anastomosis is performed for midbasilar aneurysms. A temporal craniotomy with a zygomatic osteotomy or a petrosal approach is used for the exposure of the PCA. If temporal craniotomy is used, a spinal drain is needed to relax the brain. The P2 segment of the PCA is isolated for about 1.5 cm, and a rubber dam is placed under it. An arteriotomy to match the size of the graft is performed. The ends of the graft are anchored with 8–0 nylon. The superior edge is anastomosed first, then the graft is placed under the retractor and the inferior side of the anastomosis is completed. This is a difficult anastomosis due to the depth and usually takes about 50 to 60 minutes, but the temporary occlusion is usually well tolerated. The graft is tunneled to the ECA or VA proximally and anastomosed. It is preferable to use vein from the lower thigh or upper leg for grafting.

Vertebral Artery to Vertebral Artery Grafting

This type of anastomosis is performed for tumors or giant aneurysms of the VA when collateral flow is poor. If the anastomosis is planned as a prelude to tumor or aneurysm excision, an extreme lateral retrocondylar or partial transcondylar approach is used. Resection of the jugular tubercle may be needed to expose the aneurysm. The distal anastomosis, whether proximal or distal to the PICA, is dependent on the aneurysm anatomy. Proximal anastomosis to the VA is done

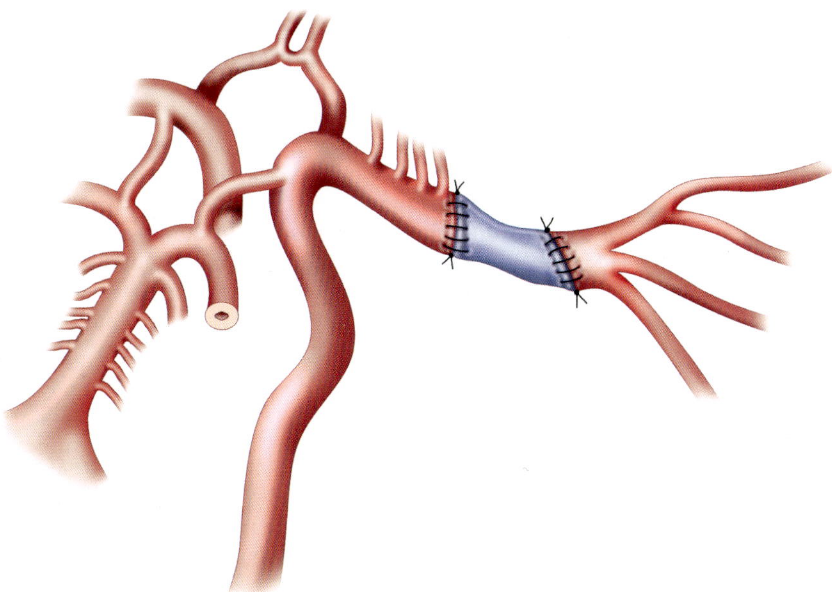

Figure 28–23 The M2 segment of the middle cerebral artery can be replaced with a short saphenous vein graft. We used this in a patient who failed embolectomy. The distal flow was successfully reestablished following this procedure. (Copyright belongs to Laligam N. Sekhar.)

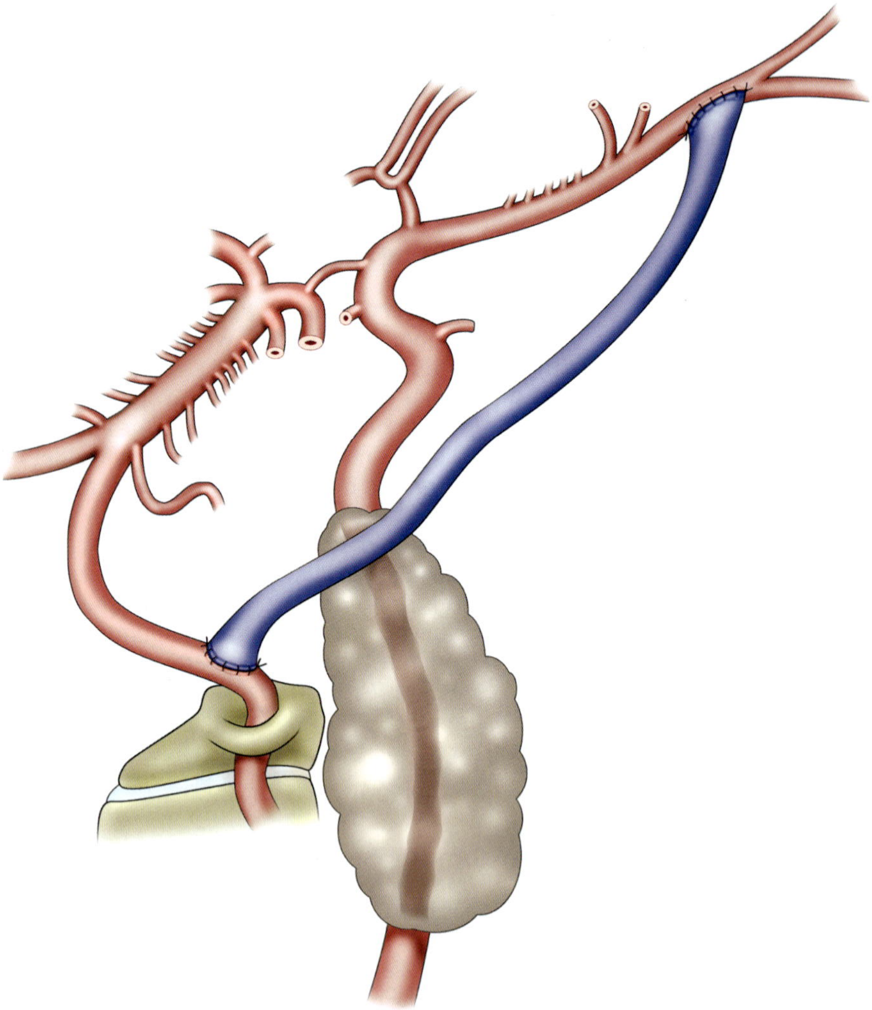

Figure 28–24 The vertebral artery can be used as a donor vessel if either the internal cerebral artery or the external cerebral artery is not available for the proximal anastomosis. (Copyright belongs to Laligam N. Sekhar.)

at the level of C1–C2. If the distal anastomosis is distal to the PICA, then the PICA may be reimplanted or a PICA to PICA anastomosis performed, or the PICA may be occluded if there is good collateral flow from the distal vessel. The vein graft is obtained from the distal thigh or upper leg, and usually a length of ~6 cm is adequate (**Fig. 28–27**).

Vertebral Artery or Internal Cerebral Artery to Basilar Artery Grafting

VA or ICA to BA grafting is used for a very special situation in the presence of a giant midbasilar aneurysm. The distal anastomosis is performed under deep hypothermic circulatory arrest. This is technically a very difficult and demanding procedure[22] (**Figs. 28–28, 28–29**).

Troubleshooting

If the flow through the vein graft is poor, it should be corrected before the surgeon leaves the operating room. Angiography will usually reveal the cause, but if the flow is very poor and sluggish, the problem may not be evident on the angiogram. The patient must be reheparinized. Initially, reexploration with a small venotomy near the distal anastomosis is done to check the flow, which can be checked from the distal and proximal ends of the graft. If the flow from the proximal end of the graft is poor, the problem is either at the proximal anastomosis or along the tunnel. Proximal anastomotic problems may require a pexy procedure or a revision of the proximal anastomosis. If the retrograde flow through the graft is good, the most common problem is a kink of the recipient artery through the vein caused by excessive flow. The graft is pulled back to the dura with traction sutures to relive the kink. If there is a constriction along the tunnel, it can be released by making a small skin incision and directly releasing the constriction.

If the graft clots in the first 24 hours (this is rare if flow was good), then it will be necessary to do another anastomosis with a fresh graft. It is not possible to use the same graft if it is clotted. Either a fresh saphenous vein or RAG will have to be used.

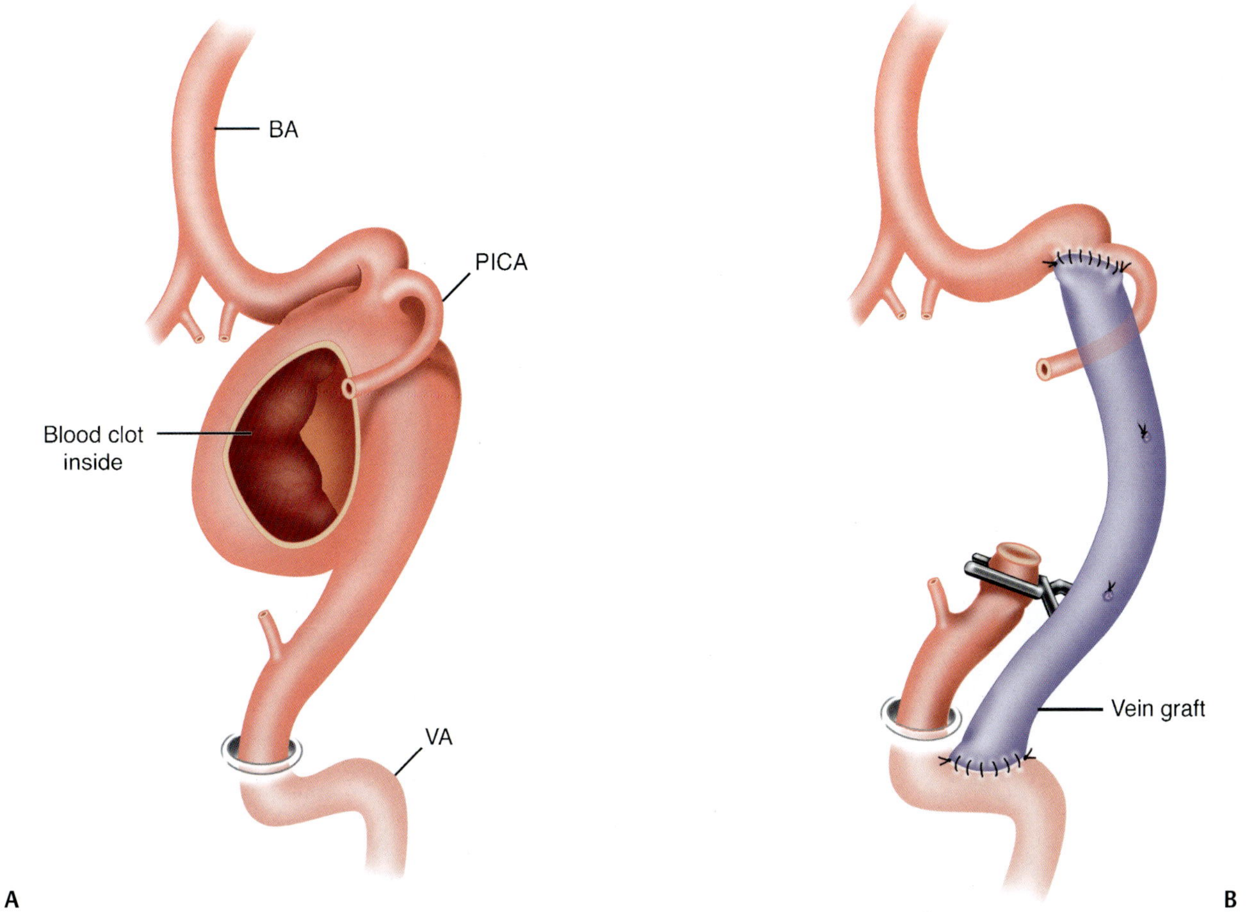

Figure 28–25 **(A)** This patient with a large thrombosed vertebral artery aneurysm was managed with **(B)** a vein graft from the proximal to the distal vertebral artery. BA, basilar artery; PICA, posterior inferior cerebellar artery; VA, vertebral artery. (Copyright belongs to Laligam N. Sekhar.)

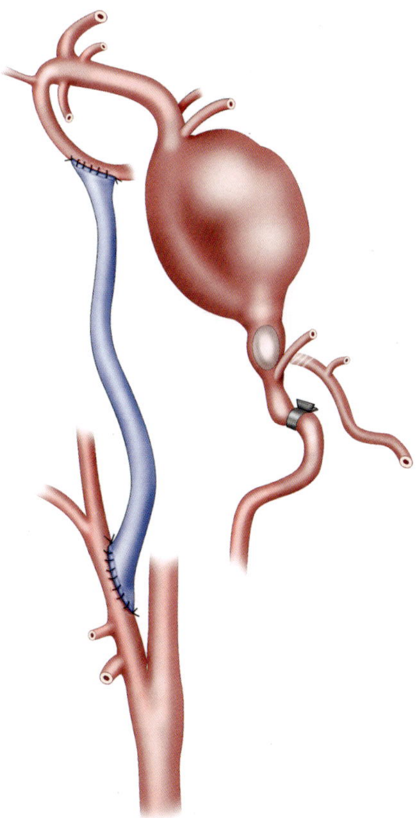

Figure 28–26 An external carotid artery to P2 segment of the posterior cerebral artery anastomosis using the radial artery or a saphenous vein graft is used to manage a giant midbasilar aneurysm. A Sundt-Kees clip is placed around the vertebral artery (VA) to produce artificial stenosis of the vessel to promote flow through the graft. In this patient the opposite VA was hypoplastic and ended primarily in the posterior inferior cerebellar artery. (Copyright belongs to Laligam N. Sekhar.)

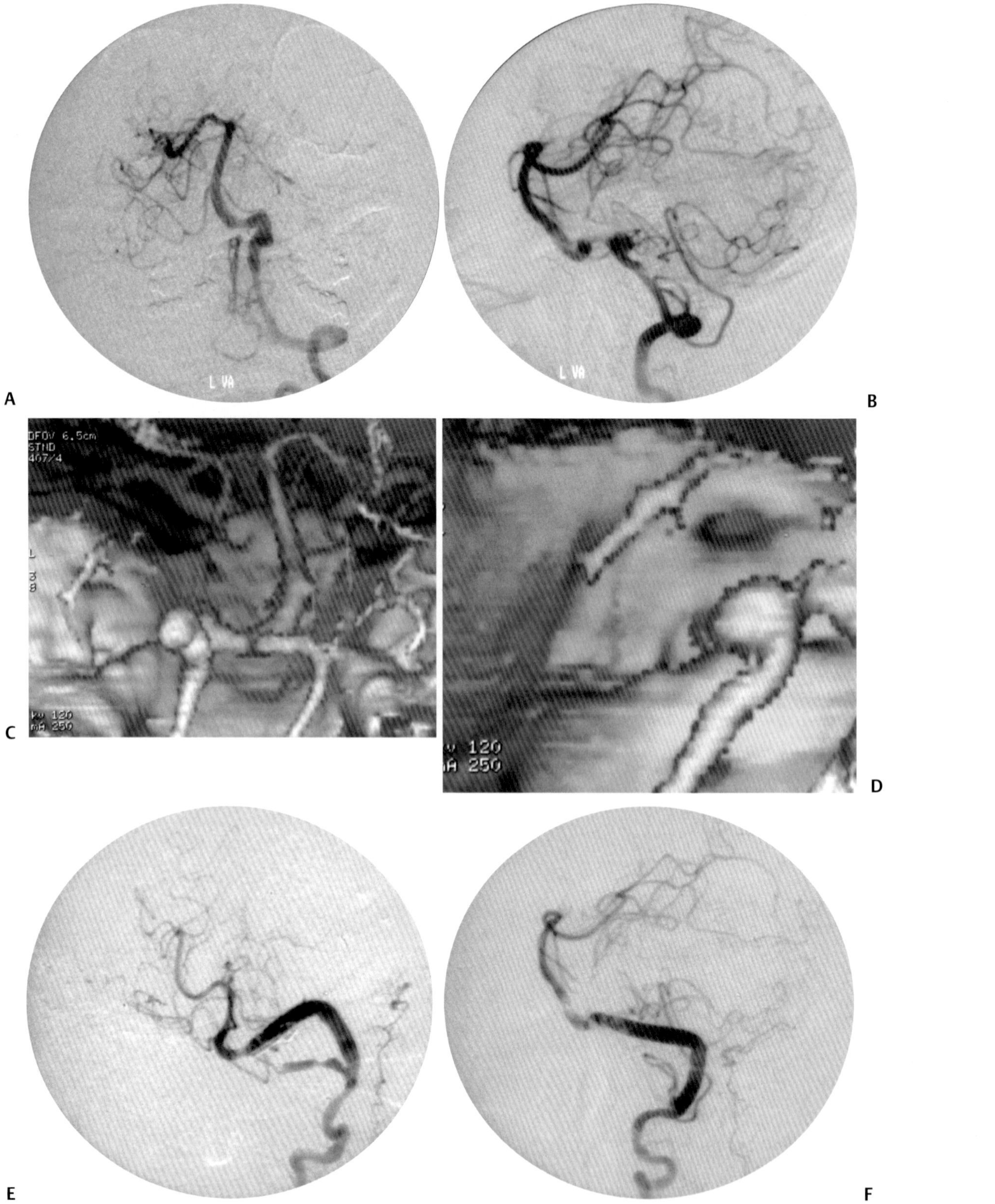

Figure 28–27 **(A–D)** This 60-year-old man was evaluated for headaches. His preoperative angiogram and three-dimensional computed tomographic (3D–CT) scan showed evidence of a fusiform aneurysm of the left vertebral artery. He underwent saphenous vein grafting from the distal extracranial vertebral artery to the distal intracranial vertebral artery. **(E,F)** His intraoperative angiogram and

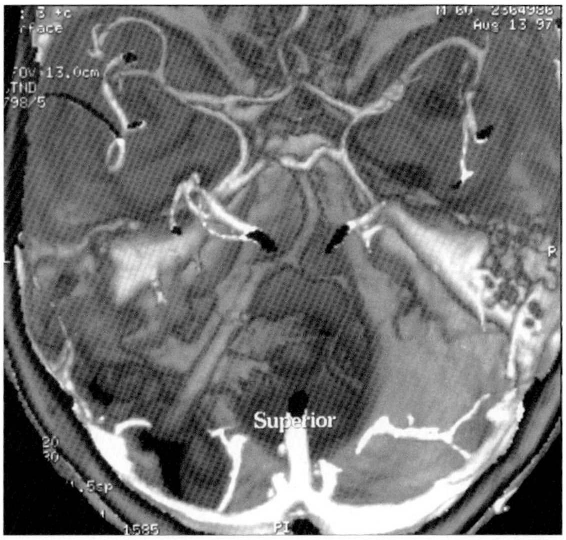

G

(*Continued*) **Figure 28–27** **(G)** postoperative 3D-CT scan shows a patent graft.

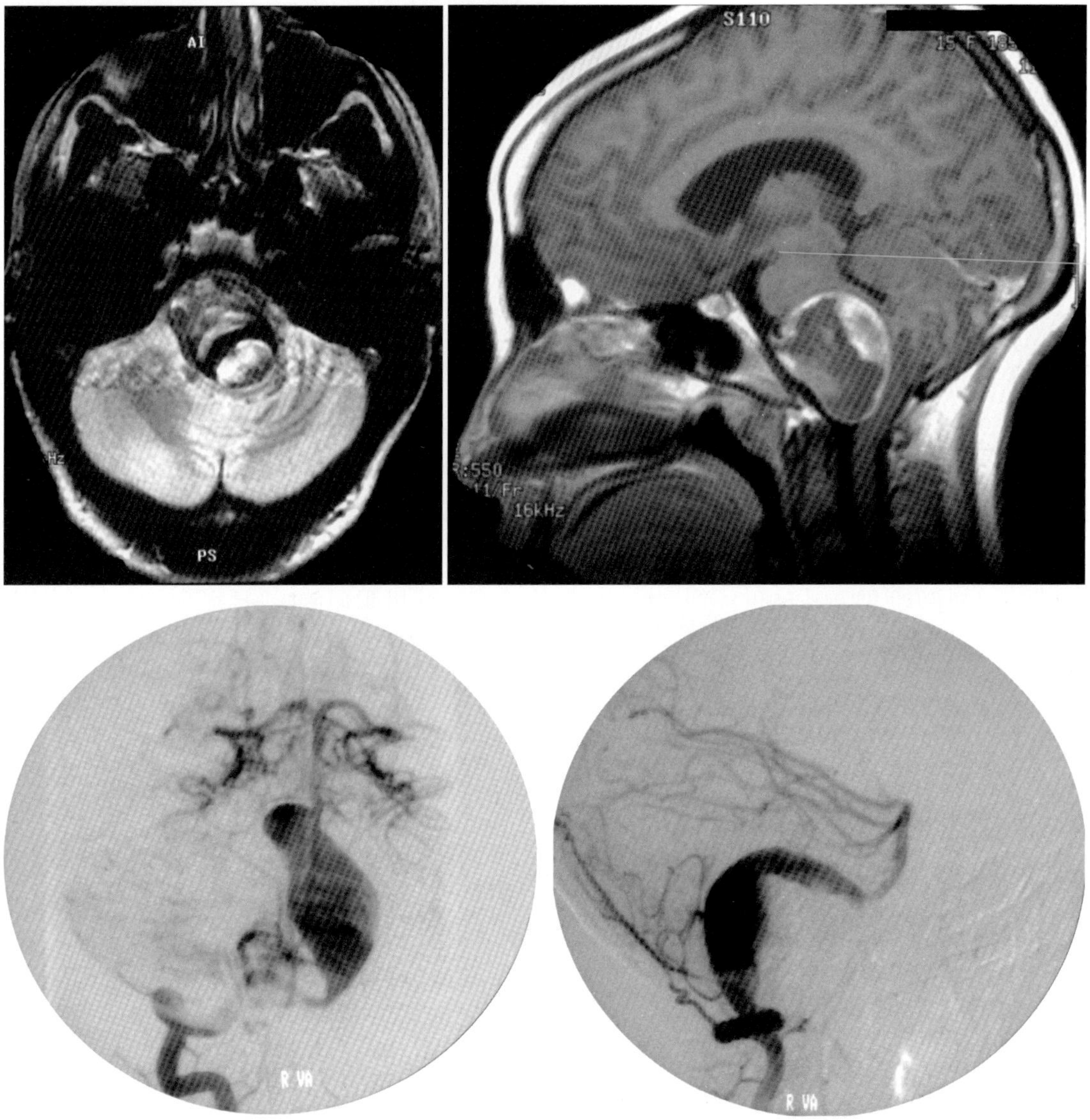

A B C D

Figure 28–28 This 15-year-old girl presented with features of progressive brain stem compression. **(A,B)** Magnetic resonance imaging revealed a giant vertebrobasilar aneurysm, partially thrombosed with gross compression and distortion of the brain stem. **(C,D)** Her angiogram and

(*Continued on page 366*)

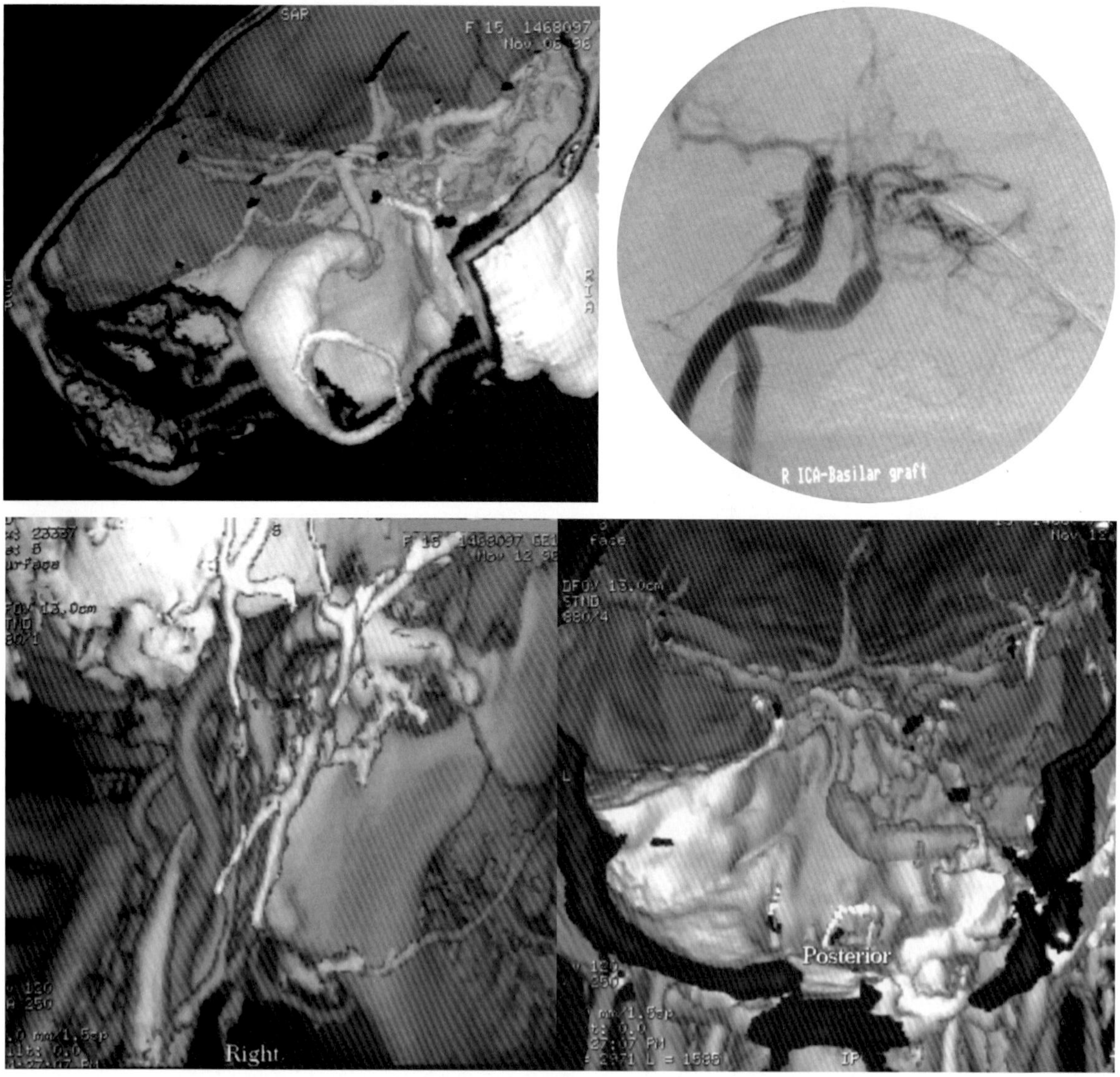

E F G H

(*Continued*) **Figure 28–28** **(E)** three-dimensional computed tomographic (3D-CT) scan revealed a giant fusiform aneurysm involving the left vertebral and the most proximal part of the basilar artery, and arising distal to the posterior inferior cerebellar artery. She underwent saphenous vein grafting from the cervical internal cerebral artery to the basilar artery followed by trapping of the aneurysm. **(F)** Her postoperative angiogram and **(G,H)** 3D-CT scan.

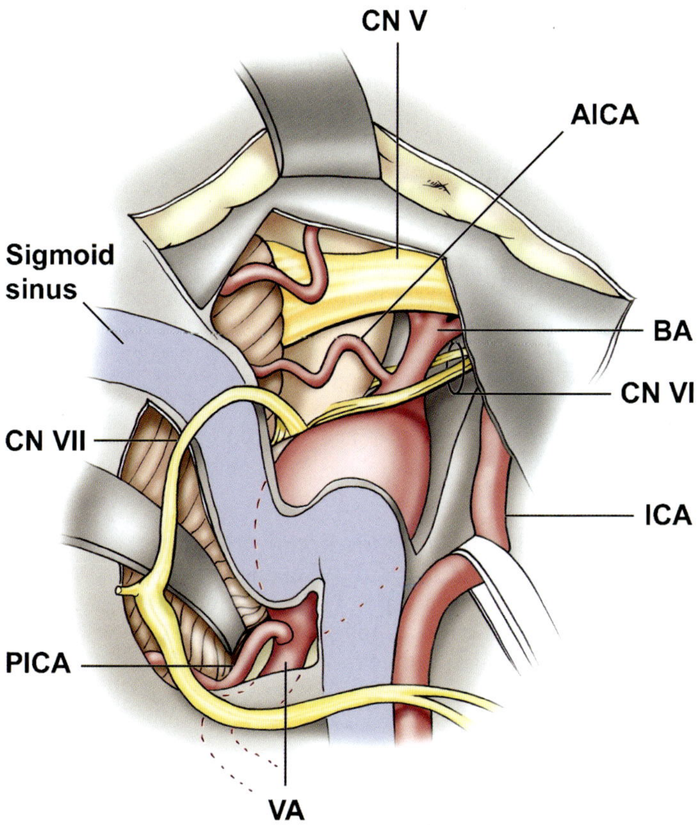

A

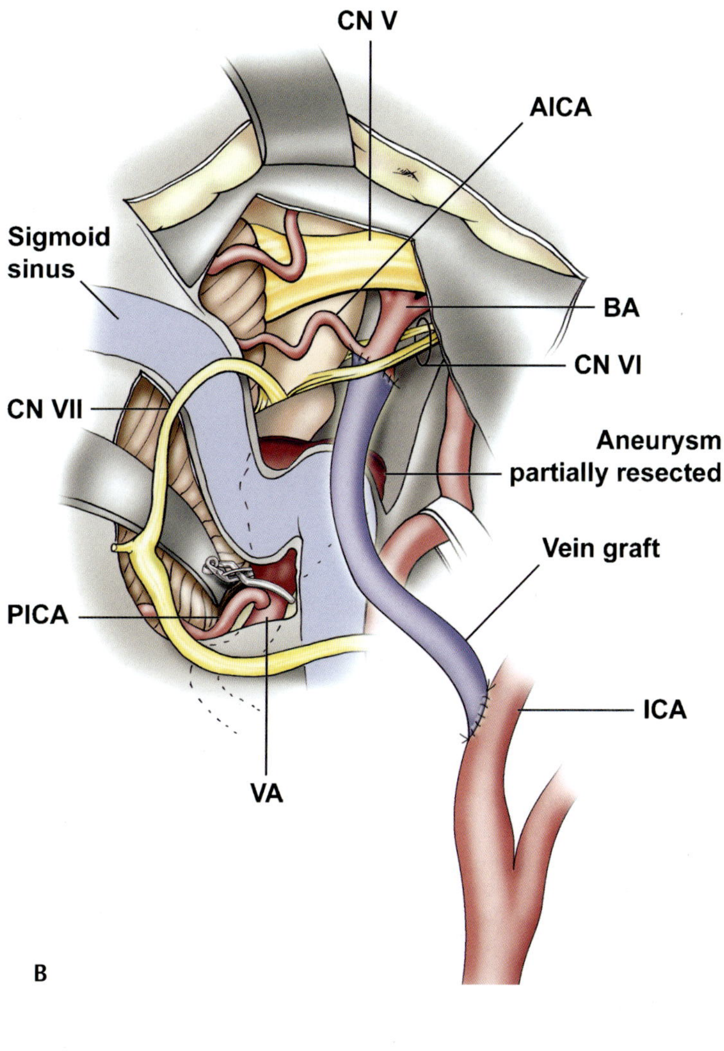

B

Figure 28–29 **(A)** Schematic representation of the patient discussed in **Fig. 28–28** showing the aneurysm location and its excision, with **(B)** the saphenous vein graft from the cervical internal carotid artery to the basilar artery. AICA, anterior inferior cerebellar artery; BA, basilar artery; CN, cranial nerve; PICA, posterior inferior cerebellar artery; VA, vertebral artery. (Courtesy of Laligam N. Sekhar.)

◆ Complications

1. *Ischemic injury:* This is a rare complication with good technique and short anastomotic time. If the ischemic injury is not in the perforator territory, the patient will recover.
2. *Epidural hematoma:* This usually occurs in a setting of excessive oozing and partial reversal of heparin. The bone flap can be left out temporarily for 48 to 72 hours, and a subgaleal drain is placed. The bone flap is replaced when the patient is stable 3 to 5 days later.
3. *Reperfusion hemorrhage:* This rare but possible complication must be kept in mind when treating patients who have suffered a recent stroke. In such patients, the BP must be kept below normal levels for several weeks.
4. *Vasospasm:* For tumor removal, if a second-stage surgery is planned, we perform the operation either before 72 hours or after the second postoperative week to minimize the risk of vasospasm of the MCA branches. If significant vasospasm is observed angiographically, angioplasty may be performed carefully.
5. *Graft extraction site:* The complications include infection, seroma, hematoma, and lymphocele. If they occur, a wound revision will be needed.

◆ Follow-up

Following discharge (7–10 days), the patients are kept on aspirin, 325 mg PO once daily for life. A yearly MRA or 3D-CT angiogram is obtained to check for graft function. The patient must wear a medical alert bracelet stating that "the pulse behind (or in front of) the ear is my carotid artery," if the graft is subcutaneous.

◆ Results

A total of 215 revascularization procedures were performed in 178 patients for cerebral aneurysms, tumors, and cerebral ischemia. A summary of the procedures and related complications is seen in **Tables 28–1** and **28–2.** The classification of revascularization procedures is seen in **Table 28–3.**

Table 28–2 Graft-related Complications

Complication	RAG	SVG
Kinking	1	11
Tear in the ICA	–	1
ICA, bypass origin stenosis	–	1
Thrombosis	4	9
Pressure on cranial nerve	1	2
Vasospasm	4	–
Compression in the tunnel	–	1
Intraoperative Fogarty angioplasty	1	–
Initial poor flow	1	5
Rupture of the graft (Marfan's syndrome)	–	1
Hyperemia	2	–
Graft-related stroke/deficit* (14%)	9 (5%)	19
Non–Graft-related Complications		
Death**	–	3

*Majority of deficits cleared partially or completely at 3 months follow-up.

**Death occurred in three patients due to (1) systemic sepsis, (2) pneumonia and cardiac arrest during bronchoscopy, (3) rupture of abdominal aortic aneurysm (Marfan's syndrome).

ICA, internal cerebral artery; RAG, radial artery graft; SVG, saphenous vein graft.

Table 28–3 Bypass Grafts and Other Procedures

Saphenous vein grafts	127
Radial artery grafts	70
Total	**197**
Others	
STA interposition	1
ACA-ACA anastomosis	1
Anterior temporal artery reimplant	1
MCA patch-RAG	1
SThyA graft	1
ICA direct reanastomosis	1
PICA reimplant	1
PICA reanastomosis	1
SCA-SCA anastomosis	1
PICA-AICA	1
Total	**10**
Total of all procedures	**207**

ACA, anterior cerebral artery; AICA, anterior inferior cerebellar artery; ICA, internal cerebral artery; MCA, middle cerebral artery; PICA, posterior inferior cerebellar artery; RAG, radial artery graft; SCA, superior cerebellar artery; STA, superficial temporal artery; SThyA, superior thyroid artery.

References

1. Selman WR, Lust WD, Ratcheson RA. Cerebral blood flow. In: Wilkins RH, Rengachary SS, eds. Neurosurgery. Vol 2. 2nd ed. New York: McGraw-Hill; 1996:1997–2006
2. Osterholm JL, Frazer GD. Pathophysiologic consequences of brain ischemia. In: Wilkins RH, Rengachary SS, eds. Neurosurgery. Vol 2. 2nd ed. New York: McGraw-Hill; 1996:2033–2037
3. Carter LP, Temeltas O, Guthkelch. Cerebral revascularization. In: Carter LP, Spetzler RF, eds. Neurovascular Surgery. New York: McGraw-Hill; 1995:441–456
4. Pool JL, Potts DG. Aneursyms and arteriovenous anomalies of the brain. New York: Hoeber; 1964:221–222
5. Story JL, Brown WE, Eidelberg E, Arom KV, Stewart JR. Cerebral revascularization: proximal external carotid to distal middle cerebral artery bypass with a synthetic tube graft. Neurosurgery 1978; 3(1):61–65

6a. Jacobson JH 2nd Suarez EL. Microsurgery in anastomosis of small vessels. Surg Forum 1960;11:243

6b. Jacobson JH 2nd, Wallman L J, Schumacher GA, Flauaganm, Suarez EL, Donaghy RM. Microsurgery as an aid to middle cerebral artery endarterectomy. Microsurgery 1992;13(3):112–117; discussion 117–118

7. Yasargil MG. History of microsurgery. In: Spetzler RF, Carter LP, Selman WR, Martin NA, eds. Cerebral Revascularisation for Stroke. New York: Thieme-Stratton; 1985:28–33
8. Yasargil MG, Krayenbuhl HA, Jacobson JH. Microneurosurgical arterial reconstruction. Surgery 1970;67:221–233
9. Spetzler R, Chater N. Occipital artery–middle cerebral artery anastomosis for cerebral artery occlusive disease. Surg Neurol 1974;2:235–238
10. Miller CF, Spetzler RF, Kopaniky DJ. Middle meningeal to middle cerebral artery bypass for cerebral revascularisation: case report. J Neurosurg 1979;50:802–804
11. Woringer E, Kunlin J. Anastomosis between the common carotid and the intracranial carotid or the sylvian artery by a graft using the suspended suture technique. Neurochirugie 1963;200:181–188
12. Lougheed WM, Marshall BM, Hunter M, Michel ER, Smyth HR. Common carotid to internal carotid bypass venous graft: technical note. J Neurosurg 1971;34:114–118
13. Story JL, Brown WE, Eidelberg E, et al. Cerebral revascularization: common carotid to distal middle cerebral artery bypass. Neurosurgery 1978;2:131–135
14. Ausman JI, Lindsay W, Ramsay RC, Chou SN. Ipsilateral subclavian to external carotid and STA-MCA bypasses for retinal ischemia. Surg Neurol 1978;9:5–8
15. Spetzler RF, Rhodes RF, Roski RA, Likavec MJ. Subclavian to middle cerebral artery saphenous vein bypass. J Neurosurg 1980;53: 465–469
16. Sundt TM, Pipegras DG, Houser OW, Campbell JK. Interposition saphenous vein grafts for advanced occlusive disease and large aneurysms in the posterior circulation. J Neurosurg 1982;56: 205–215
17. Little JR, Furlan AJ, Bryerton B. Short vein grafts of cerebral revascularisation. J Neurosurg 1983;59:384–388
18. Sekhar LN, Burgess J, Akin O. Anatomical study of the cavernous sinus emphasizing operative approaches and related vascular and neural reconstruction. Neurosurgery 1987;21:806–816
19. Sekhar LN, Sen CN, Jho HD. Saphenous vein graft bypass of the cavernous internal carotid artery. J Neurosurg 1990;72:35–41
20. Sekhar LN, Iwai Y, Wright DC, Bloom M. Vein graft replacement of the middle cerebral artery after unsuccessful embolectomy: case report. Neurosurgery 1993;33:723–727

21 Iwai Y, Sekhar LN, Goel A, Cass S. Vein graft replacement of the distal vertebral artery. Acta Neurochir (Wien) 1993;120:81–87

22. Sekhar LN, Chandler JP, Alyono D. Saphenous vein graft reconstruction of an unclippable giant basilar artery aneurysm under deep hypothermic circulatory arrest: case report. Neurosurgery 1998;42: 667–673
23. Sekhar LN, Bucur SD, Bank WO, Wright DC. Venous and arterial bypass grafts for difficult tumors, aneurysms and occlusive vascular lesions: evolution of operative management and improved results. Neurosurgery 1999;44:1207–1224
24. Sekhar LN, Kalavakonda C. Saphenous vein and radial artery grafts in the management of skull base tumors and aneurysms. Operative Techniques in Neurosurgery 1999;2:129–141
25. Sekhar LN, Stimac D, Bakir A, Rak R. Reconstruction options for complex middle cerebral artery aneurysms. Neurosurgery 2005;56(Suppl 1):66–74
26. Evans JJ, Sekhar LN, Rak R, Stimac D. Bypass grafting and revascularization in the management of posterior circulation aneurysms. Neurosurgery 2004;55:1036–1049
27. Sekhar LN, Duff TM, Kalavakonda C, Olding M. Cerebral revascularization using radial artery graft in the treatment of complex aneurysms; techniques and outcome in 17 patients. Neurosurgery 2001;44: 646–659
28. Spetzler RF, Carter LP. Revascularization and aneurysm surgery: current status. Neurosurgery 1985;16:111–116
29. Sundt TM, Piepgras DG, Marsh WR, Fode NC. Saphenous vein bypass grafts for giant aneurysms and intracranial occlusive disease. J Neurosurg 1986;65:439–450

29

Cerebral Revascularization: Superficial Temporal Middle Cerebral Artery Anastomosis

Fady T. Charbel, Kern H. Guppy, and James I. Ausman

Cerebral revascularization encompasses a vast range of surgical techniques used to increase cerebral perfusion by allowing additional blood flow to reach the brain.[1–9] For many years cerebral revascularization had been noted to occur spontaneously with the formation of collateral blood supplies from external sources. The first reported study of surgical cerebral revascularization was done in animals in 1939.[10]

In most cases of surgical cerebral revascularization, the source of the new blood supply is from the external carotid artery, and the vessel to which the anastomosis is made is the internal carotid artery or a branch of the vessel (**Fig. 29–1**). The procedure is called the external carotid to internal carotid (EC-IC) bypass. The persons most acknowledged for pioneering the use of the EC-IC bypass for cerebral revascularization were Yasargil[11] and Donaghy[12]. The procedure was used widely for the treatment of patients with cerebral ischemia caused by cerebro-occlusive disease. Yasargil and Yonekawa's initial work consisted of 86 patients who underwent the bypass procedure for ischemia and were followed over a 3- to 9-month period.[13] In the years to follow the procedure became widely accepted, with several thousand operations performed annually in the United States and with studies showing patency rates ranging from 90 to 100%.[14–16]

The effectiveness of the bypass procedure for cerebral ischemia was examined in the International Cooperative Study of Extracranial-Intracranial Arterial Anastomosis in 1985. The study was a multicenter, 5-year follow-up of over 1500 patients and studied the effectiveness of cerebral revascularization versus aspirin for the treatment of strokes or transient ischemic attacks (TIAs).[17,18] The authors concluded that the EC-IC bypass surgery was no more effective than the best medical care in reducing the risk of strokes. This paper was highly criticized[19–26] and was found flawed for many reasons, including biased selection of the patients as well as inclusion of a large number of patients with carotid occlusions who probably did not require bypass surgery because their collateral circulation was in most cases adequate. Moreover, the conclusions by the authors were far more detailed than the data supported and should have been limited to the population studied.

Over the last 15 years, several diagnostic techniques have been developed to improve selection of patients with cerebro-occlusive disease who would benefit from the bypass procedure. In addition to the standard angiographic studies, it is now possible to determine if patients have impaired cerebral perfusion by estimating their cerebrovascular reserve capacity.[27,28] In particular, xenon computed tomography (CT) and positron emission tomography (PET) have made this possible. A new EC-IC bypass study (Carotid Occlusion Surgery Study, Coss) sponsored by the National Institutes of Health (NIH) is currently under way to identify a group of patients who would benefit from cerebral revascularization. This study involves 30 centers across the United States and uses PET data for choosing patients with impaired cerebral hypoprofusion.

This chapter focuses on the EC-IC bypass technique and in particular the superficial temporal artery to the middle cerebral artery (STA-MCA) anastomosis.

◆ Indications

The indications for cerebral revascularization can be divided into two main categories:

1. *Preservation of cerebral blood flow (CBF):* This involves replacement of the current blood flow from a vessel that will be sacrificed, for example, carotid occlusion for a skull base tumor that has invaded the artery or an inoperable aneurysm requiring occlusion of its arterial supply.
2. *Augmentation of CBF:* In these cases there exists critical cerebral perfusion that has resulted from some disease process. For example, in cases of patients with atherosclerosis, stenosis, or occlusion of intracranial or extracranial arteries, the blood flow is compromised, and augmentation of the CBF may be required. In moyamoya disease, additional collateral CBF is needed to prevent cerebral ischemia. In all cases it must be proven that CBF is critical and there is a loss of cerebrovascular reserve ("misery perfusion"). The EC-IC bypass is used to increase collateral blood flow to the brain with the expectation of restoring cerebrovascular reserve capacity.[28]

◆ Preparation

Medical Workup

Patients undergoing cerebral revascularization must undergo a thorough medical workup. Preoperative evaluation consists of a physical examination with chest x-rays, electrocardiogram, and routine laboratory work. Any patients with known heart disease should have clearance from a cardiology consultation before surgery. All patients undergoing bypass surgery are placed on antiseizure medication.

Diagnostic Studies

All patients should have a magnetic resonance imaging (MRI) scan of the brain to identify parts of the brain that may show irreversible ischemia or "border zone infarction." Patients with evidence of major MCA territory infarction or areas that are to be considered for revascularization that have infarction are excluded.

Cerebral Blood Flow Measurements

As we have noted previously, there must be evidence of CBF compromise before the patient is considered for revascularization. Several forms of imaging can be used, including positron emission tomography, xenon-enhanced CT, SPECT, transcranial Doppler sonography, and magnetic resonance imaging.

At our institution xenon-enhanced CT[27,28] is routinuely used for evaluating patients for revascularization. The technique uses 1 to 2 minutes of inhalation of 28% xenon gas mixed with oxygen. The CBF is detected by the increase in Hounsfield units as measured by CT. The hemisphere is divided into arterial flow regions and the mean regional CBF (rCBF), measured in cc/100 g/min, is determined for both hemispheres. The patient is given acetazolamide (1 g IV) and the CBF is repeated in 20 minutes. The difference between the two studies can give information about the cerebrovascular reserve. The patients that are considered for bypass are those with severely impaired, absent, or paradoxically decreased ("steal phenomenon") flow.

Another method for estimating hemodynamic failure was demonstrated in the St. Louis Carotid Occlusion Study using PET.[29] Using ^{15}O isotope, impaired cerebral perfusion was measured by increased oxygen-extraction fraction (OEF, stage II hemodynamic failure). The disadvantage of this method, however, is the half-life of the isotope is only two minutes and it requires on-site production, which is available at only a limited number of centers. At the time this chapter is being written, the Carotid Occlusion Surgery Study is under way and uses PET for identifying candidates for surgery. New methods for cerebral blood flow are currently being developed.

Angiographic Studies

Angiographic studies, especially selective injections of the external carotid artery, will also aid in the selection of the STA, which is further divided into an anterior and posterior branch. The anterior branch is more commonly used since the posterior branch has limited choice of cortical vessels for anastomosis. Selection of the donor vessel will be based on finding a branch with a diameter greater than 1 mm.

Other Tests

In cases in which the bypass is used to supplement the sacrifice of a major artery, it is appropriate to do a balloon occlusion test of the vessel to determine the clinical outcome if the artery is sacrificed. The procedure consists of placing via a femoral catheter a deflated balloon, which is subsequently inflated in the selected artery. A cerebral oximeter or electroencephalographic (EEG) recording is used to monitor the cerebral perfusion and hence the effect of the temporary occlusion of the prospective artery. Single photon emission computed tomography (SPECT) scans before and after balloon occlusion can also be used to monitor cerebral perfusion.

The most reliable method is to note changes in the neurological examination in the awake patient before and after temporary occlusion of the prospective artery as well as after the hypotensive challenge. The neurological examination is done every 5 minutes for a total of 30 minutes. The patient is made hypotensive by pharmacologically decreasing the systolic blood pressure by 20%. Development of any neurological deficit means the end of the examination with the patient having failed the test. Failure of the test will mean any sacrifice of the artery will require revascularization.

At our institution, phase contrast MRI is used to estimate flow rates in the extracranial and intracranial vessels.[30] Over 200 such studies have been done and used to identify normal values for these vessels, which aids in determining the severity of the hypoperfusion. Numerical modeling techniques have been used to model each patient's CBF and therefore can simulate different bypass schemes.[31,32] These techniques are helpful in designing and planning the bypass surgery.

◆ Surgical Technique

Anesthesia and Positioning

General anesthesia is induced by an endotracheal tube, and the standard monitoring devices are applied. Depending on the age and cardiac status of the patient, a pulmonary arterial catheter (Swan-Ganz) can be placed. The mean arterial blood pressure is kept 10 to 20 mm Hg above the baseline preop level (average 100–130 mm Hg during the surgery).

The patient is placed in a supine position, with a roll placed behind the shoulder. The head is turned to the opposite side, taking care to avoid compromising flow in the contralateral carotid artery. The shoulder roll allows the head to be horizontal, exposing the side of interest. The head can be anchored in a pin fixation device (**Fig. 29–1**).

Exposure of the Superficial Temporal Artery

Once the head is shaved and scrubbed with alcohol and Betadine, under semisterile conditions a handheld Doppler is used to trace the STA as it follows the path chosen from the angiogram (**Fig. 29–1**). The artery is traced out using a permanent marking pen, and crosshatch marks are made for the closure. The head is now cleaned with Betadine and draped in the usual fashion. Using a Colorado microneedle-tip monopolar cautery (Stryker Leibinger, Kalamazoo, MI) at a low setting of 8, an incision is made over the outline of the STA. The incision is carefully deepened through the epidermis and dermis until loose areolar tissue is reached. Using a pointed hemostat, the soft tissue is dissected, exposing the surface of the artery, which overlies the temporalis fascia or periosteum (**Fig. 29–2**). The artery is exposed from its origin anterior to the tragus of the ear. A 0.5 cm pedicle, lateral to the artery on each side, is isolated by cutting the galea down to the temporalis fascia or periosteum (**Fig. 29–3**). At the proximal end of the STA the pedicle is cleared off the artery to allow easy application of the artery for temporary clips. Side branches are coagulated at a safe distance from the artery using a Bovie electrocautery (Bovie Medical Corp., St. Petersburg, FL) with a coated shaft at a setting of 25 to 30. It is important to keep the operative field dry (this can be accomplished by using an irrigating suction). Once isolated, over a desired length, the STA is wrapped in papaverine-soaked cottonoids.

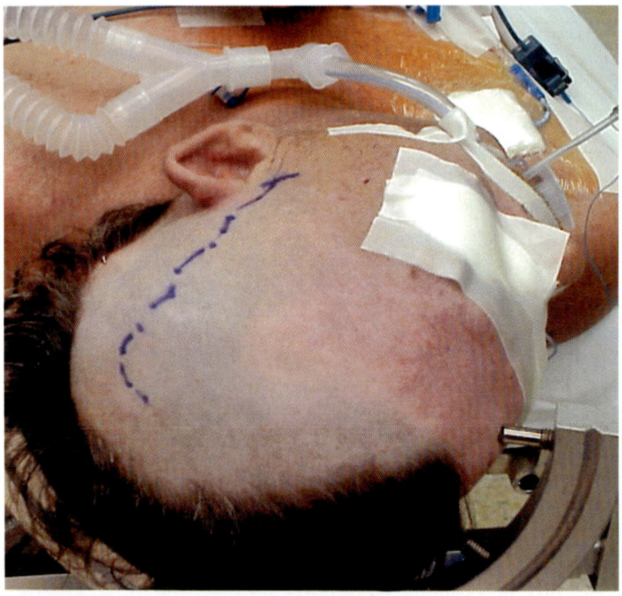

Figure 29–1 Placement of patient's head in three-pin fixation device with outline of superficial temporal artery.

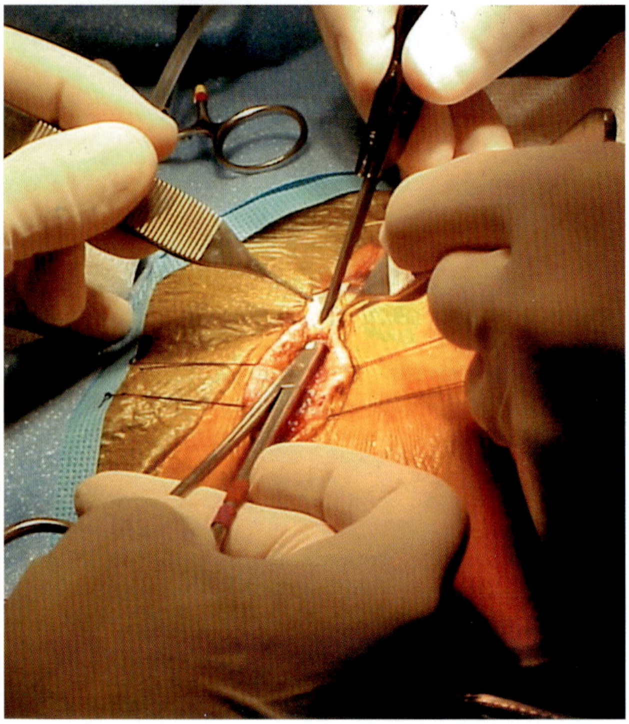

Figure 29–2 Exposure of superficial temporal artery below skin.

Skin and Cranial Flap

Depending on the branch of the STA that is chosen, the appropriate skin flap is made. In most cases the incision generated by exposure of the STA will suffice to create a large

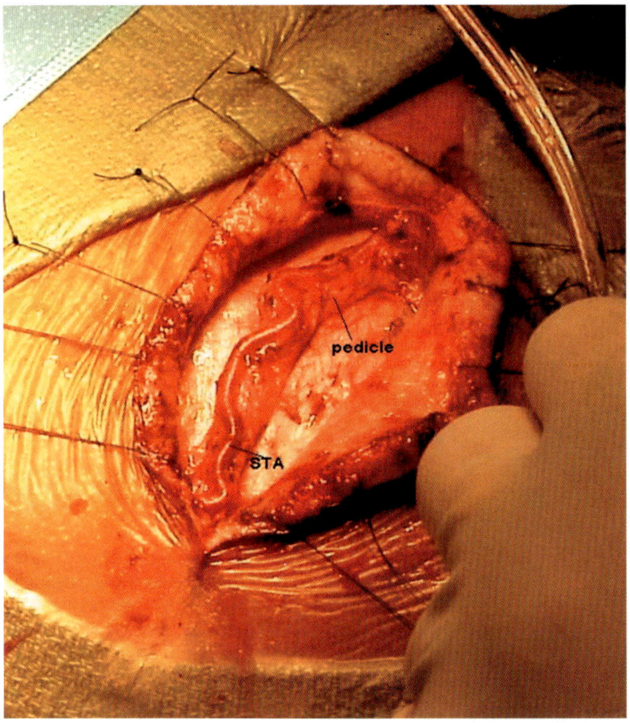

Figure 29–3 Isolation of superficial temporal artery with its pedicle.

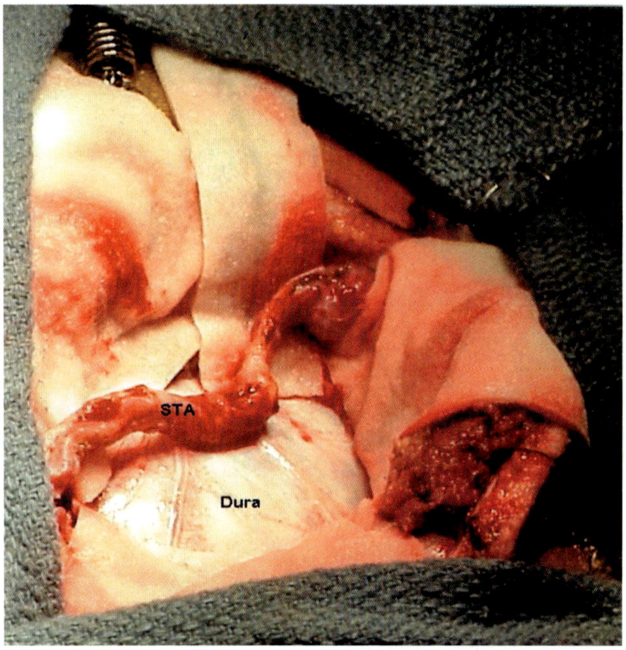

Figure 29–4 Superficial temporal artery dissected and lying on dura.

enough skin flap: Using monopolar cautery, the temporalis muscle is incised down to the periosteum in the same direction as the STA. The muscle is then retracted bilaterally with spring hooks, exposing the skull. A temporal or pterional craniotomy is selected, depending on whether a superficial cortical or deep sylvian bypass is needed. Two bur holes are made, one at each end of the STA, allowing the craniotomy to be done away from the STA.

The dura is tacked up using 4–0 Neurolon (Ethicon, Somerville, NJ), and the STA is brought onto the dura (**Fig. 29–4**). The dura is opened, and the microscope is used to identify the recipient vessel. A cortical vessel of good caliber, usually a temporal branch, is selected. If one is not found, then the sylvian fissure can be dissected using an arachnoid knife and bipolar cautery. Retractors are best avoided, but if needed, must be used with the greatest of care. The donor vessel is freed from the cortical surface with microdissecting scissors and an arachnoid knife (**Fig. 29–6**). A latex strip is placed below the cortical vessel over a small piece of Gelfoam to elevate the recipient vessel (**Fig. 29–7**). It is then covered with one or two papaverine-soaked cotton balls, which are left undisturbed until the donor vessel preparation is completed.

Anastomosis

The cottonoids are removed from the pedicle and the distal end of the STA is tied off. A temporary clip is placed at the proximal end of the STA. The tied-off end of the STA is transected using a tenotomy scissor. The distal end of the cut STA is dissected off the pedicle and is beveled and "fish-mouthed" at the free end (**Fig. 29–5**). The artery is unclamped and flushed retrograde using a blunt 25 gauge needle with a syringe with heparinized saline.

A critical step at this point is to measure the free "cut flow" of the STA. This number is used as an important benchmark to assess the technical success of the bypass (34). The temporary clip is removed and a microvascular ultrasonic flow probe (Charbel Micro-Flowprobe; Transonics Systems, Inc., Ithaca, NY) is used to measure the uninhibited flow of the STA(**Fig. 29–6**). The temporary clip is replaced after the measurement.

Using the same probe, baseline flow measurements are made in the cortical vessel. Temporary occlusion of a small segment of the vessel is made using 15 g temporary clips. A longitudinal incision is made in the isolated segment approximately the same size as the donor diameter. A small Silastic stent (Dow Corning, Auburn, MI), the diameter of the cortical vessel, is placed in the lumen of the opened cortical vessel to prevent accidental suturing of the opposite wall of the vessel. Using 10–0 nylon (Ethicon), sutures are placed between the STA and cortical vessel at the superior and inferior edges of these vessels. Multiple sutures are placed in an interrupted fashion except for the final two sutures. The stent is removed and the vessels are flushed with heparinized saline. The final sutures are placed securely. The temporary clips are removed, first the cortical, then the STA. Bleeders from the anastomosis line are not coagulated because to do so may injure and weaken the sutures. If needed, Gelfoam or additional sutures are placed for complete homeostasis. It is best to have the first attempt at closing the anastomosis be as complete as possible. Once the entire bypass is secure and homeostasis is reached, the flow

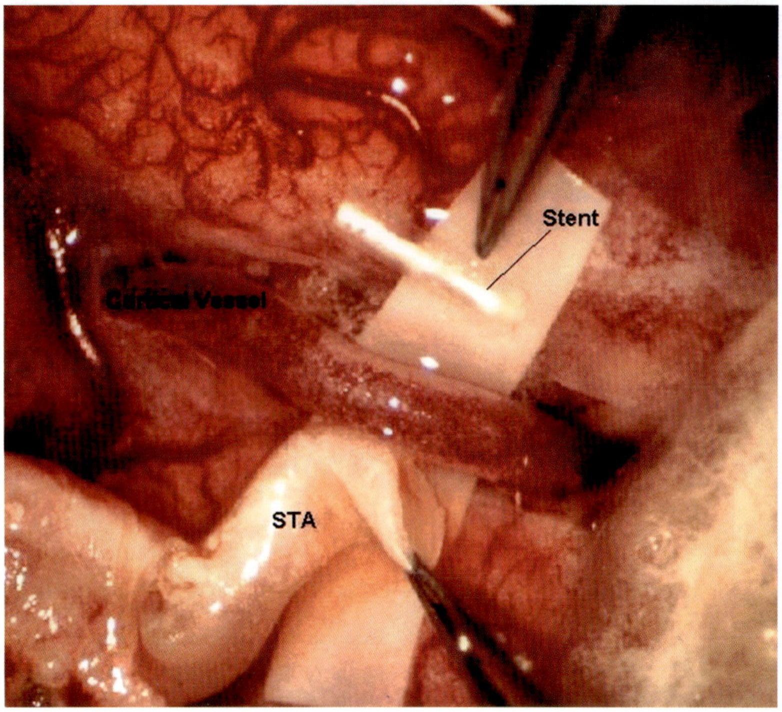

Figure 29–5 The recipient vessel is freed from the cortical surface with microdissecting scissors and an arachnoid knife. A latex strip is placed below the cortical vessel over a small piece of Gelfoam to elevate the recipient vessel. It is then covered with one or two papaverine-soaked cotton balls, which are left undisturbed until the STA vessel preparation is completed.

probe is used to determine flow rate measurements in the STA and the cortical vessel (**Fig. 29–7** and **Fig. 29–8**).

Using the same probe, baseline flow measurements are made in the cortical vessel. Once completed, temporary occlusion is made to the vessel using 15 g temporary clips. A longitudinal incision is made in the cortical vessel approximately the same size as the donor, and a stent is inserted. Using 10–0 nylon (Ethicon), sutures are placed between the STA and cortical vessel at the superior and inferior edges of these vessels. Multiple sutures are placed in an interrupted fashion except for the final two sutures. The stent is removed, and the vessels are flushed with heparinized saline. The final sutures are placed securely.

At this time, the temporary clips are removed, first the cortical, then the STA. Bleeders from the anastomosis line are not coagulated because to do so may injure and weaken

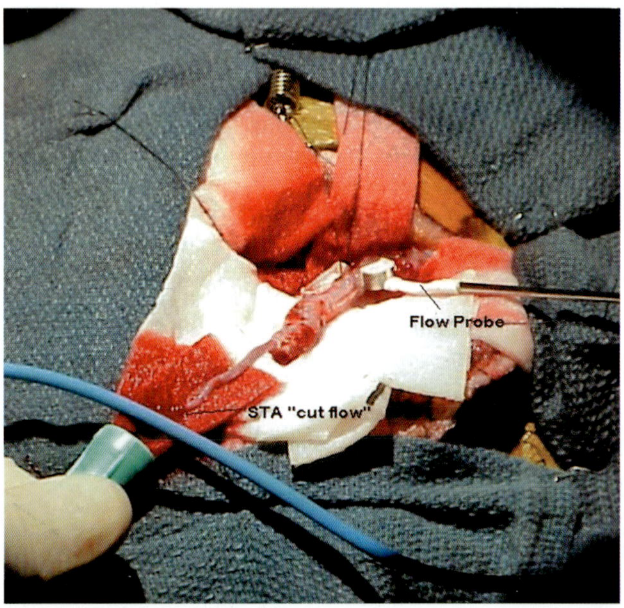

Figure 29–6 Measurement of "cut flow" from superficial temporal artery using flowmeter probe.

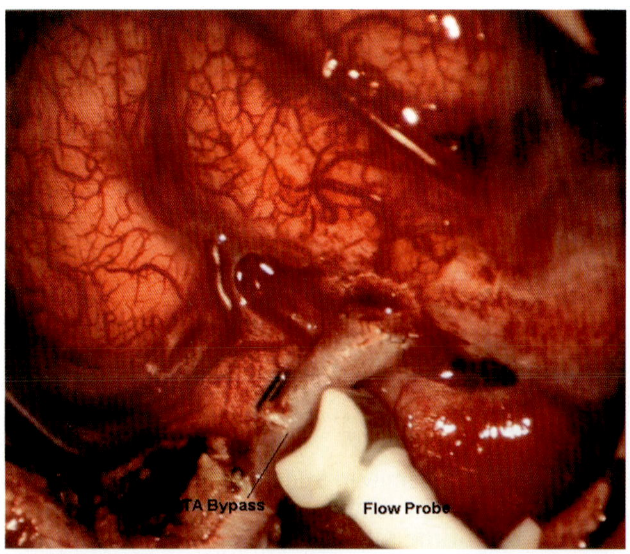

Figure 29–7 Completed superficial temporal artery bypass and the use of the flowmeter for estimating flow rates in the bypass vessel.

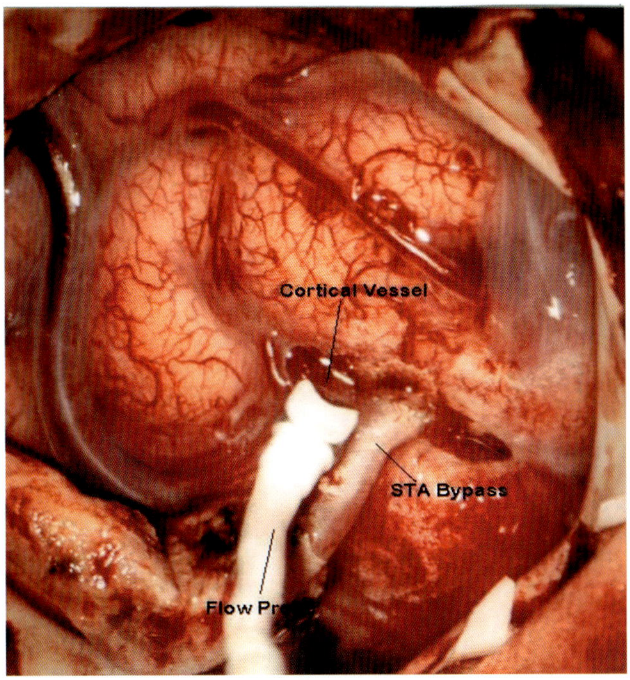

Figure 29–8 Flowmeter measuring flow rate in cortical vessel.

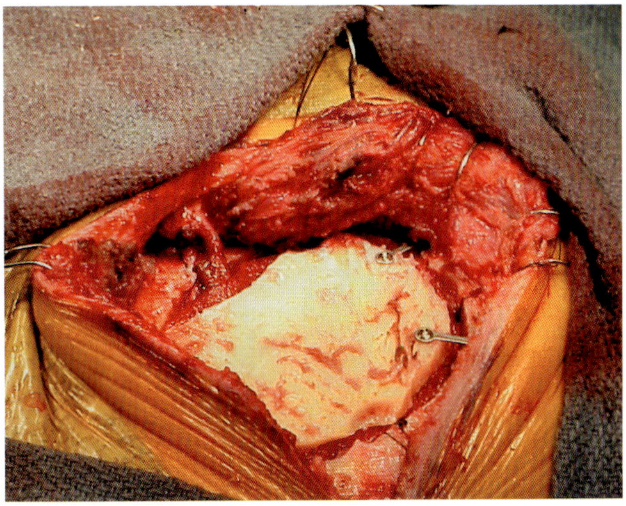

Figure 29–9 If the artery appears compromised a rongeur can be used to widen the bur hole, or a new one is made.

the sutures. If needed, Gelfoam or additional sutures are placed for complete homeostasis. It is best to have the first attempt at closing the anastomosis be as complete as possible. Once the entire bypass is secure and homeostasis is reached, the flow probe is used to determine flow rate measurements in the STA and the cortical vessel (**Figs. 29–7, 29–8**).

Intraoperative Studies

Several surgeons have advocated the use of intraoperative angiography to evaluate the caliber of the bypass. For small cortical vessels it is difficult to visualize the patency and to estimate the volume of flow through the bypass. The authors have instead used flowmeter probes for evaluation of bypass patency.[34,35] The flowmeter gives an actual value of the flow rate in mL/min. Hence the actual flow rates pre- and postanastomosis of the STA and cortical vessels are determined. The cortical bypass flow rates should be greater than the preanastomosis cortical flows. If there is any discrepancy, the graft must be reexamined. This method also allows the surgeon to decide if the bypass flow rate is too high for the cortical vessel so as to avoid breakthrough bleeding.

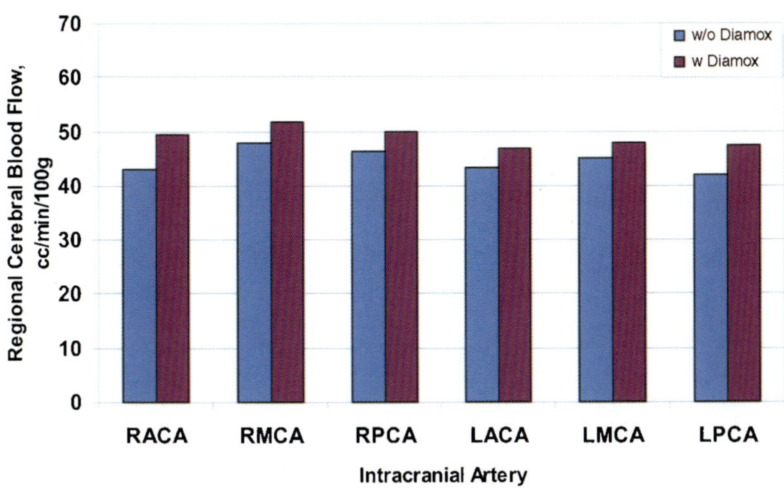

Figure 29–10 Regional cerebral blood flow (rCBF) in different arterial distributions before surgery with and without Diamox. (RACA, right anterior cerebral artery; RMCA, right middle cerebral artery; RPCA, right posterior cerebral artery; LACA, left anterior cerebral artery; LMCA, left middle cerebral artery; LPCA, left posterior cerebral artery)

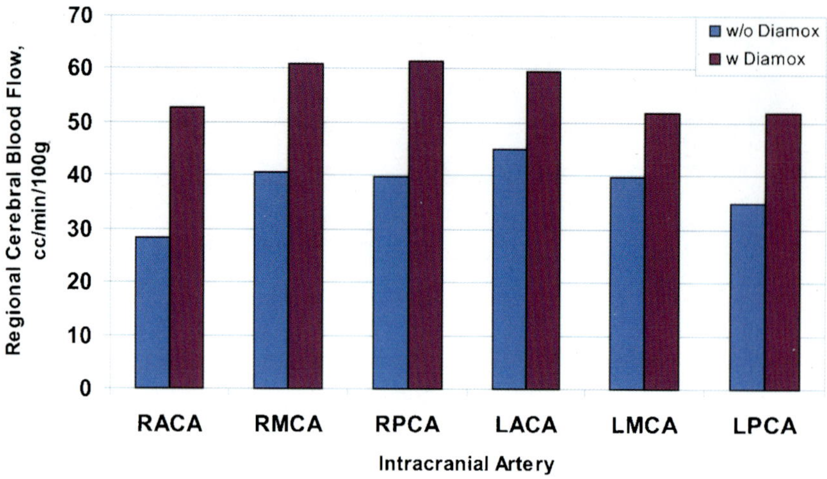

Figure 29–11 Regional cerebral blood flow (rCBF) in different arterial distributions after left superficial temporal artery to middle cerebral artery (STA-MCA) bypass. (RACA, right anterior cerebral artery; RMCA, right middle cerebral artery; RPCA, right posterior cerebral artery; LACA, left anterior cerebral artery; LMCA, left middle cerebral artery; LPCA, left posterior cerebral artery)

Closure

The dura is partially closed around the STA with 4–0 Neurolon, care being taken not to strangulate it. The bone flap is replaced, allowing the STA to enter through an already created bur hole that was opened using the craniotome. If the artery appears compromised, a rongeur can be used to widen the bur hole, or a new one is made (**Fig. 29–9**). The galea and muscle are reattached with 3–0 Vicryl (Ethicon). Care should be taken in placement of the sutures not to include the STA. The skin is closed using a watertight closure with 4–0 Dermalon (Ethicon). Care should be taken not to necrose the skin in view of its now limited vascular supply.

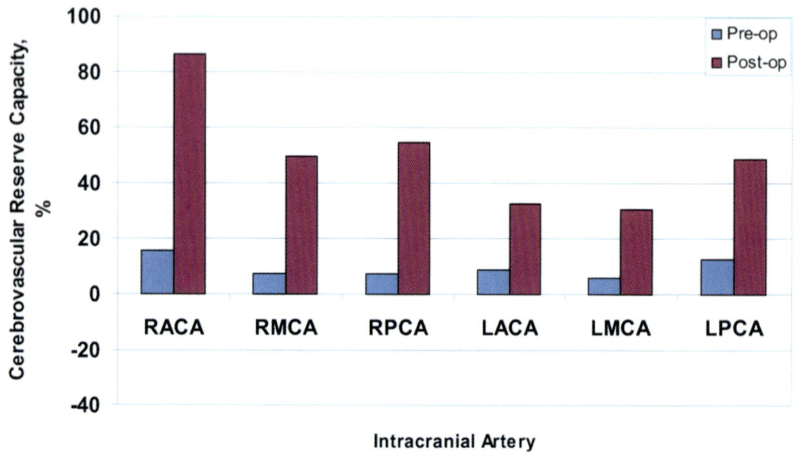

Figure 29–12 Cerebrovascular reserve capacity before and after left superficial temporal artery to middle cerebral artery (STA-MCA) bypass surgery. (RACA, right anterior cerebral artery; RMCA, right middle cerebral artery; RPCA, right posterior cerebral artery; LACA, left anterior cerebral artery; LMCA, left middle cerebral artery; LPCA, left posterior cerebral artery)

◆ Postoperative Care

The postoperative care is just as important as the procedure itself. Antibiotics are given before and 24 hours after the procedure. The wound should be kept clean and dry and the sutures left in place for at least 3 weeks to allow skin healing in the devascularized tissue. Immediately postoperative, the patient is continued on antiepileptic medication. The mean arterial blood pressure is maintained 10 to 20 mm Hg below the preoperative range. Some patients may require long-acting antihypertensive agents.

Postoperative studies include an angiogram on postop day 1 or 2. A repeated PET or xenon CT with and without acetazolamide (Diamox; Wyeth Pharmaceuticals, Collegeville, PN) is recommended a few days after surgery. This is also repeated in 3 and 6 months. We now routinely utilize quantitative phase contrast magnetic resonance flow rate measurements to noninvasively monitor the progression of the bypass and compare it to intraoperative measurements.

◆ Complications

The most common complication of this procedure is having a bypass with a low flow rate. Patency rates over the years have increased, with many large series reporting rates between 96 and 100%. Other complications can include breakthrough bleeding, infections, skin flap necrosis, subdural hematomas, and seizures.[13,36,37]

◆ Case Illustration

Mr. B is a 45-year-old, right-handed male who for 1 year has had TIA symptoms, resulting in right upper extremity numbness with episodes of speech disturbances. He has had increased frequency of these symptoms even though he was placed on Coumadin for the past year. The patient had a 30-pack smoking history. His neurological examination was normal.

Angiogram studies showed moderate stenosis in the right internal carotid artery with severe left internal carotid/middle cerebral artery stenosis. The collateral to his left hemisphere comes primarily from the left posterior cerebral artery. The rCBF using xenon CT showed baseline low values of perfusion bilaterally, with no improvement of rCBF with Diamox, indicating absence of cerebrovascular reserve capacity (**Fig. 29–10**).

The conclusion from these studies was that Mr. B had limited flow to his left hemisphere with very little reserve. Any further increase in his left MCA stenosis could result in a left hemispheric infarction. Angioplasty was considered high risk in view of the location of the close proximity of the stenosis to several perforators of the MCA, hence the indication for a left STA-MCA bypass in view of the evidence of hypoperfusion in a patient refractory to anticoagulation.

The patient underwent a left STA-MCA bypass to the M2 level without any difficulty. **Fig. 29–11** shows the xenon CT results of rCBF after the left STA-MCA bypass. It is evident that the rCBF increased significantly from levels prior to surgery, and the effect of vasodilation showed the presence of a new cerebrovascular reserve capacity. **Fig. 29–12** shows the increase in cerebrovascular reserve (rCVR) after surgery. The patient showed maintenance of this newly acquired rCBF in follow-up studies.

The foregoing case illustrates the methodology that is required for choosing patients who can benefit from this type of procedure. The planning, however, for bypass surgery is still in its infancy. At our institution, we have developed mathematical models and have used phase contrast MRI to better understand the hemodynamic changes that occur in these patients. Presently, it is possible to design the size of the bypass needed to meet each patient's specific hemodynamic needs. Further advances in cerebral revascularization are still forthcoming.

References

1. Day AL. EC/IC bypass for MCA obstruction. In: Spetzler RF, Selman WR, Carter LP, Martin NA, eds. Cerebral Revascularization for Stroke. New York: Thieme Stratton; 1985:458–566
2. Ausman JI, Diaz FG, Sadasivan B, Gonzeles-Portillo M, Malik GM, Deopujari CE. Giant intracranial aneurysm surgery: the role of microvascular reconstruction. Surg Neurol 1990;34:8–15
3. Yokoh A, Ausman JI, Dujovny M, Diaz FG, Berman SK, Sanders J, et al. Anterior cerebral artery reconstruction. Neurosurgery 1986;19:26–35
4. Andrews BT, Charter NL, Weinstein PR. Extracranial-intracranial arterial bypass for middle cerebral artery stenosis and occlusion. J Neurosurg 1985;62:831–838
5. Ausman JI, Pearce JE, de los Reyes RA, Schanz G. Treatment of a high extracranial carotid artery aneurysm with CCA-MCA bypass and carotid ligation: case report. J Neurosurg 1983;58:421–424
6. Ausman JI, Diaz FG, Vacca DF, Sadasivan B. Superficial temporal and occipital artery bypass pedicles to superior, anterior inferior and posterior inferior cerebellar arteries for vertebrobasilar insufficiency. J Neurosurg 1990;72:554–558
7. Morgan JK, Sadasivan B, Ausman JI, Mehta B. Thrombolytic therapy and posterior circulation extracranial bypass for acute basilar artery thrombosis: case report. Surg Neurol 1990;33:43–47
8. Olds MV, Griebel RW, Hoffman HJ, et al. The surgical treatment of childhood moyamoya disease: operative technique for refractory cases. J Neurosurg 1987;66:675–680
9. Sundt TM Jr, Piepgras DG, Marsh WR, et al. Saphenous vein bypass grafts for giant aneurysms and intracranial occlusive disease. J Neurosurg 1986;65:439–450
10. German WJ, Taffel M. Surgical production of collateral intracranial circulation. Proc Soc Exp Biol Med 1939;42:349–353
11. Yasargil MG. Microsurgery, Applied to Neurosurgery. Stuttgart: Georg Thieme; 1969
12. Donaghy RM. What's new in surgery: neurologic surgery. Surg Gynecol Obstet 1972;134:269–271
13. Yasargil MG, Yonekawa Y. Results of microsurgical extra-intracranial arterial bypass in the treatment of cerebral ischemia. Neurosurgery 1977;1:22–24
14. Chater N, Popp J. Microsurgical vascular bypass for occlusive cerebral disease: review of 100 cases. Surg Neurol 1976;6:115–118
15. Piepgras DG. Factors influencing postoperative vascular patency. Clin Neurosurg 1976;23:310–317

16. Latchaw RE, Ausman JI, Lee MC. Superficial temporal–middle cerebral artery bypass: a detailed analysis of multiple pre- and postoperative angiograms in 40 consecutive patients. J Neurosurg 1979;51: 455–465
17. The EC/IC Bypass Study Group. Failure of extracranial-intracranial arterial bypass to reduce the risk of ischemic stroke: results of an international randomized trial. N Engl J Med 1985;313:1191–1200
18. The EC/IC Bypass Study Group. The international cooperative study of extracranial/intracranial arterial anastomosis (EC/IC bypass study): methodology and entry characteristics. Stroke 1985;16: 397–406
19. Ausman JI, Diaz FG. Critique of the extracranial-intracranial bypass study. Surg Neurol 1986;26:218–221
20. Barnett HJM, Fox A, Hachinski V, et al. Further conclusions from the extracranial-intracranial bypass trial. Surg Neurol 1986;26:227–235
21. Day AL, Rhoton AL, Little JR. The Extracranial-Intracranial Bypass Study. Surg Neurol 1986;26:222–226
22. Awad IA, Spetzler RF. Extracranial-intracranial bypass surgery: a critical analysis in light of the international co-operative study. Neurosurgery 1986;19:655–664
23. Sundt TM. Was the international randomized trial of extracranial-intracranial arterial bypass representative of the population at risk? N Engl J Med 1987;316:814–816
24. Gratzl O, Schmiedek P, Spetzler R, Steinhoff H, Marguth F. Clinical experience with extra-intracranial arterial anastomosis in 65 cases. J Neurosurg 1976;44:313–324
25. Chater N. Neurosurgical extracranial-intracranial bypass for stroke with 400 cases. Neurol Res 1983;5:1–9
26. Weinstein PR, Rodriguez y Baena R, Chater NL. Results of extracranial-intracranial bypass for intracranial internal carotid artery stenosis: review of 105 cases. Neurosurgery 1984;15:787–794
27. Celsis P, Goldman T, Henrisken L, et al. A method of calculating regional cerebral blood flow from emission computer tomography of inert gas concentrations. J Comput Assist Tomogr 1981;5:641–645
28. Schmiedek P, Piepgras A, Leinsinger G, Kirsch CM, Einhaupl K. Improvement of cerebrovascular reserve capacity by EC-IC arterial bypass surgery in patients with ICA occlusion and hemodynamic ischemia. J Neurosurg 1994;81:236–244
29. Grubb RL Jr, Powers WJ, Derdeyn CP, Adams HP, Clarke WR, The Carotid Occlusion Surgery Study. Neurosurg Focus 2003;14:Article 9.
30. Zhao M, Charbel FT, Alperin, N, Loth F, Clark ME. Improved phase-contrast flow quantification by three-dimensional vessel localization. Magn Reson Imaging. 2000;18(6):697–706
31. Charbel FT, Guppy KH, Zhao M, Clark ME. Computerized hemodynamic evaluation of the cerebral circulation for bypass. Neurosurg Clin N Am. 2001;12(3):499–508
32. Charbel F, Shi J, Quek F, Zhao M, Misra M.. Neurovascular flow simulation review. Neurol Res 1998;20:107–115
33. Clark ME, Zhao M, Loth F, et al. A patient-specific computer model for prediction of clinical outcomes in the cerebral circulation using MR flow measurements. Proceedings of MICCCI (Medical Image Computing and Computer-Assisted Intervention), 2nd International Conference. Cambridge Sept. 19 – 22, 1999
34. Amin-Hanjani S, Du X, Mlinarevich N, Meglio G, Zhao M, Charbel FT. The cut flow index: an intraoperative predictor of the success of extracranial-intracranial bypass for occlusive cerebrovascular disease. Neurosurgery. 2005;56(1 Suppl):75–85
35. Charbel FT, Hoffman WE, Misra M, Ostergren L. Ultrasonic perivascular flow probe: technique and application in neurosurgery. Neurol Res 1998;20:439–442
36. Reichman OH. Complications of cerebral neurovascularization. Clin Neurosurg 1976;23:318–335
37. Whisnant JP, Sundt RM Jr, Fode NC. Long-term mortality and stroke morbidity after superficial temporal artery–middle cerebral artery bypass operation. Mayo Clin Proc 1985;60:241–246

30

Cerebral Veins and Dural Sinuses: Preservation and Reconstruction

Laligam N. Sekhar, Amitabha Chanda, and Akio Morita

Cerebral veins and venous sinuses have received adequate attention only recently, although they are very important to the neurosurgeon. When the venous outflow is compromised due to a lack of adequate collateral circulation, venous infarction follows, with swelling, hemorrhage, and neuronal death. The clinical consequences, which can often be disastrous, will depend upon the region of involvement of the brain and size of the venous structure occluded. The symptoms may include seizures, hemiplegia, aphasia, coma, and death. The consequences of cerebral venous sinus occlusion also depend upon the availability of collateral circulation. When such collaterals are not available, papilledema and visual loss and a pseudotumor cerebri syndrome are observed in milder cases, whereas severe diffuse brain swelling, coma, and death may be observed in severe cases.

Acute venous or venous sinus occlusion is potentially very dangerous, whereas slow and chronic venous or venous sinus occlusion is better tolerated. Even in such patients, some neurological manifestations may follow when the collaterals are poor.

◆ Venous Anatomy and Structures at Risk

Several publications[1–6] have discussed the venous anatomy (**Fig. 30–1**) in exquisite detail. Venous sinuses are at risk whenever a pathological process directly involves them, or when they are divided to approach a deep-seated lesion. Similarly, major cerebral veins are usually at risk during operations that involve the displacement of the brain from the fixed drainage sites of the veins (e.g., transcallosal approach, subtemporal approach, or supracerebellar approach) (**Table 30–1**). This chapter first discusses the cerebral veins and then the dural venous sinuses.

◆ Imaging

Although it is uncommon nowadays to obtain cerebral angiography before operation on convexity lesions, it is prudent to do so before operating on parasagittal and falx lesions. In some patients magnetic resonance angiography will be adequate to show the details. Magnetic resonance venography (MRV) is useful to observe the size of the sinus but is inadequate to discriminate between slow flow and

Table 30–1 Approaches Where the Veins Can Be in Jeopardy

Interhemispheric approach
Transcallosal approach
Subtemporal approach
Petrosal approaches
Supracerebellar infratentorial approach

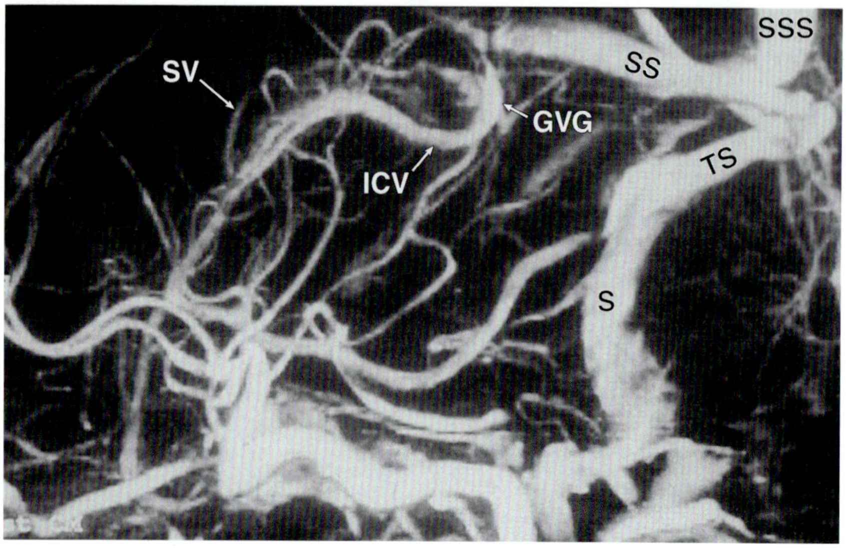

Figure 30–1 Magnetic resonance venogram showing the different major intracranial veins. SSS, superior sagittal sinus; SS, straight sinus; SV, septal vein; ICV, internal cerebral vein; GVG, great vein of Galen; TS, transverse sinus; S, sigmoid sinus. (With permission from Morita A, Sekhar LN. Reconstruction of the vein of Labbé by using short saphenous vein bypass graft. J Neurosurgery 1998;89:671–675, 672.)

complete occlusion (**Fig. 30–1**). Before operating on parasagittal meningiomas invading the sagittal sinus, angiography with bilateral internal carotid artery injection is necessary to determine if the sinus is occluded or patent. Before operating on large basal or deep lesions, particularly near the torcula, transverse and sigmoid sinuses, vein of Labbé, straight sinus, or deep venous system, angiography with venous phase filming is equally important to provide imaging of the adjacent venous anatomy and collaterals.

◆ Cerebral Veins—Avoidance of Injury

Cerebral veins may be damaged by three mechanisms during operations: intentional coagulation and division to prevent their rupture, traction during an operation from their fixed drainage sites (into a dural sinus) causing their rupture, or damage during their dissection in the brain. Veins have thinner walls and are not as tortuous as arteries, allowing them less ability to be manipulated before rupture. These factors make the veins more liable to be damaged than arteries. Moreover, both basal and convexity operations stretch the veins and put them at risk for rupture, whereas arteries are stretched mainly during basal operations.

To avoid its rupture, a cerebral vein should be stretched minimally either by minimizing the extent of brain retraction or by releasing it from adhesions to allow its lengthening. With convexity operations, the dura mater must always be opened from a lateral to medial direction because a vein may drain into a dural venous lake in the paramedian area, or be densely adherent to the convexity dura. In such cases, a small strip of dura mater is cut on either side initially along the vein to allow its preservation (**Fig. 30–2A,B**).

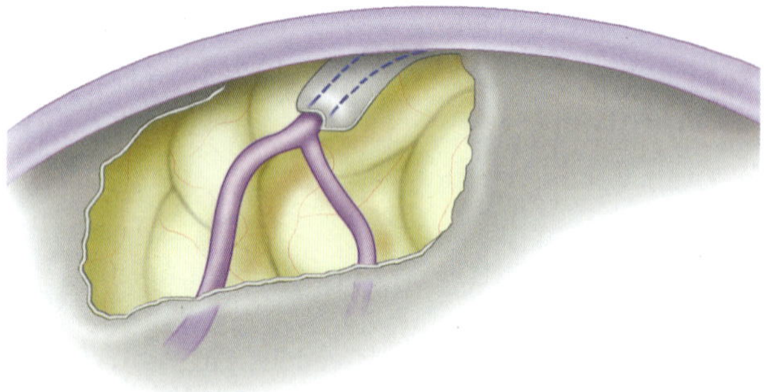

A

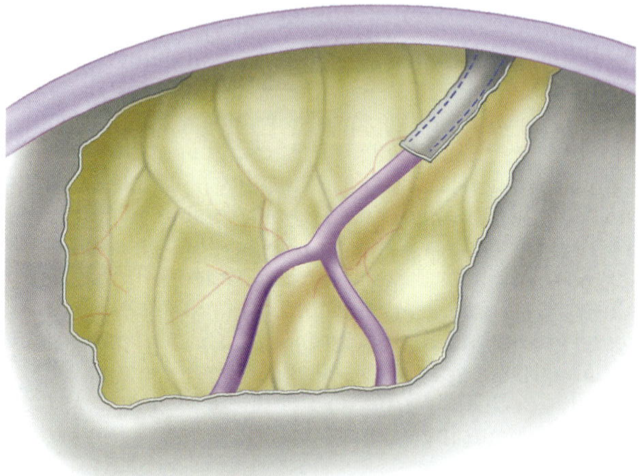

B

Figure 30–2 **(A)** Dura has been opened, leaving a small leaf attached to an adherent or early draining vein. **(B)** Further dissection of the vein has been performed, leaving some dura around the dural sinus. (With permission from Morita A, Sekhar LN. Reconstruction of the vein of Labbé by using short saphenous vein bypass graft. J Neurosurgery 1998;89: 671–675, 672.)

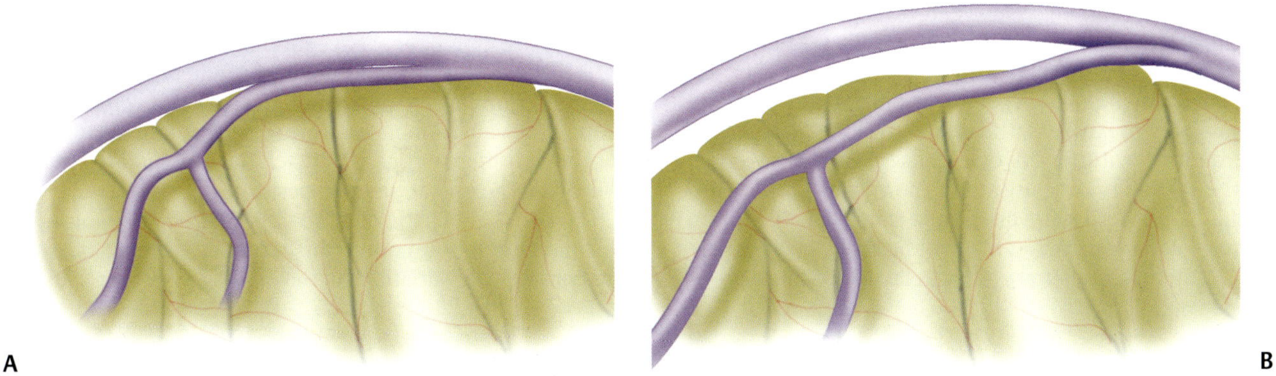

A B

Figure 30–3 **(A)** Illustrating how the convexity vein runs along the sinus before emptying into it. **(B)** Demonstrating the dissection of the vein away from the sinus, allowing its stretching. (With permission from Morita A, Sekhar LN. Reconstruction of the vein of Labbé by using short saphenous vein bypass graft. J Neurosurgery 1998;89:671–675, 673.)

Subsequently, it is possible to dissect some of the veins away from the dura mater under the microscope. Many convexity veins turn forward and are densely attached to the dura near the sagittal sinus for a short distance before they drain into the sinus (**Fig. 30–3A**). In such cases, the vein can be dissected away from the dura mater to allow its lengthening. In a similar fashion, the vein can be dissected away from the arachnoidal adhesions, and a small branch/tributary can be sacrificed to allow its lengthening (**Fig. 30–3B**).

In convexity parasagittal approaches, the brain retraction and the venous stretching must be kept to a minimum to prevent venous injury. In some cases when the target is at a greater depth (e.g., a deep-seated tumor or arteriovenous malformation), the approach trajectory may have to be changed (**Fig. 30–4A**) to be distant from a major vein to prevent its damage. Other potential strategies include changing the approach side (e.g., right to left) and a small corticectomy (**Fig. 30–4B–D**).

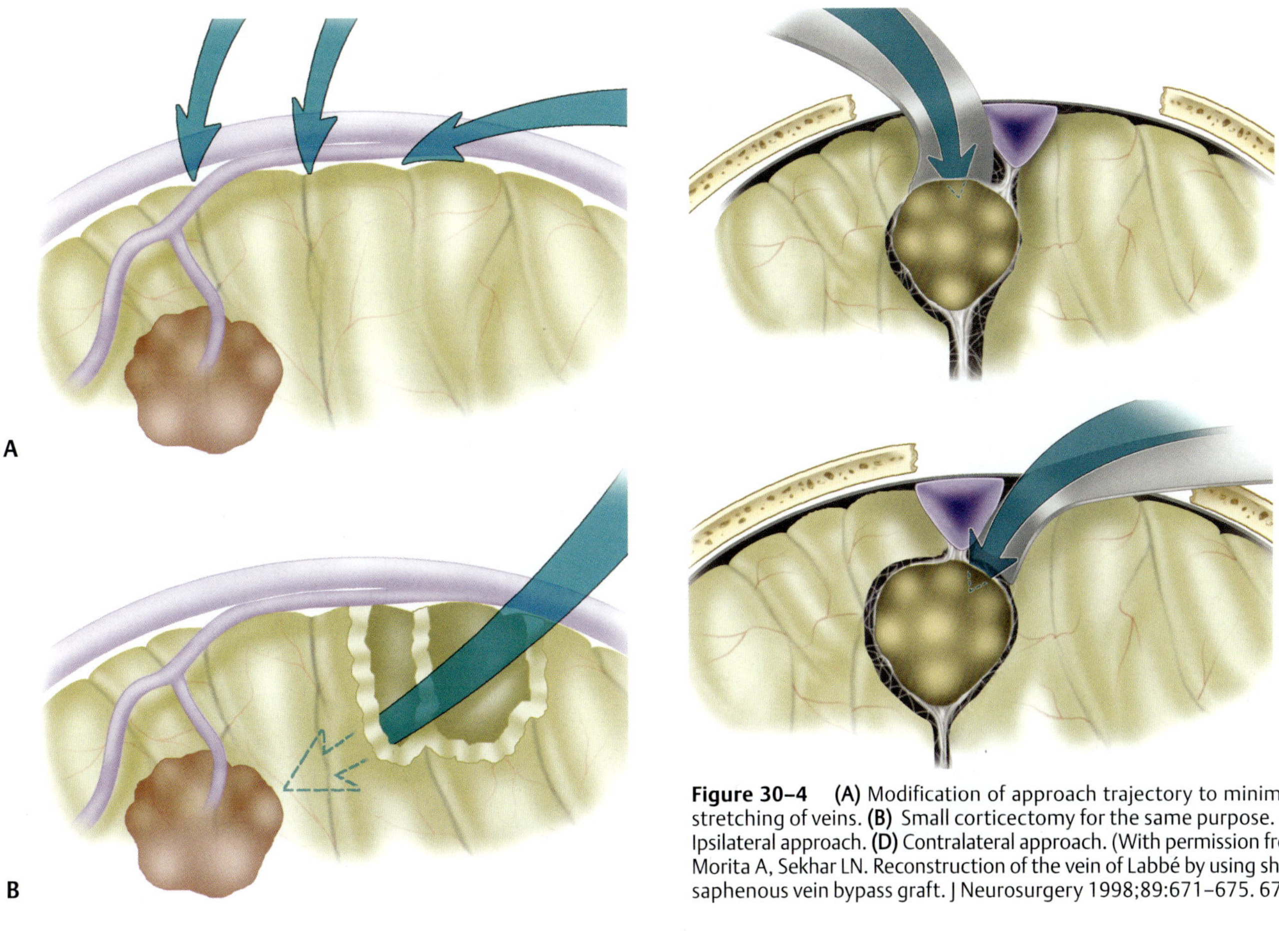

A B C D

Figure 30–4 **(A)** Modification of approach trajectory to minimize stretching of veins. **(B)** Small corticectomy for the same purpose. **(C)** Ipsilateral approach. **(D)** Contralateral approach. (With permission from Morita A, Sekhar LN. Reconstruction of the vein of Labbé by using short saphenous vein bypass graft. J Neurosurgery 1998;89:671–675. 673.)

With basal lesions, veins at greatest risk for rupture are the temporal tip draining veins, and the vein(s) of Labbé. In these instances, the surgeon must be aware of any aberrant venous anatomy before surgery to avoid major problems. In the majority of patients, the temporal tip draining veins can be divided without adverse consequences. However, when the sylvian is very large, or if the vein of Labbé is absent due to prior surgery or is very small because of an anatomical variation, then it may not be safely occluded. In such a situation, a temporary clip can be placed on the concerned vein, and the brain is observed for swelling for 5 to 10 minutes. Kanno[7] et al have measured regional blood flow by a thermodilution clearance technique before the occlusion of major veins to determine the safety of venous occlusion. If the vein cannot be safely occluded, in many patients a change in the surgical approach or a small corticectomy will allow the operation to be performed.

The vein(s) of Labbé (**Fig. 30–5A–D**) are at risk for injury during subtemporal and transpetrosal approaches. There are considerable variations in the drainage site of the vein(s).

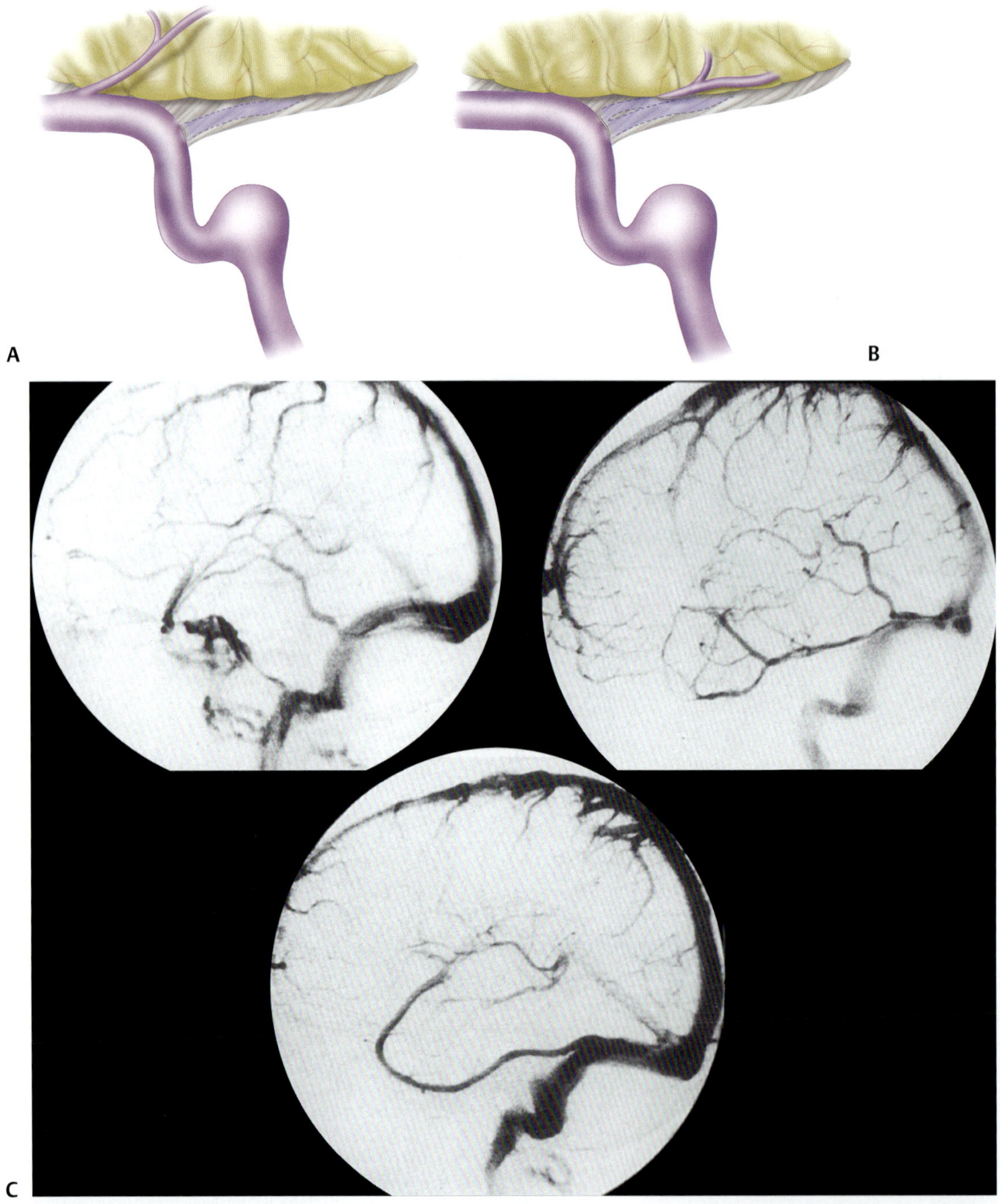

Figure 30–5 **(A)** Normal type of vein of Labbé. **(B)** Very anteriorly draining vein of Labbé into a tentorial sinus. **(C)** Variation of anatomy of vein of Labbé seen in angiogram.

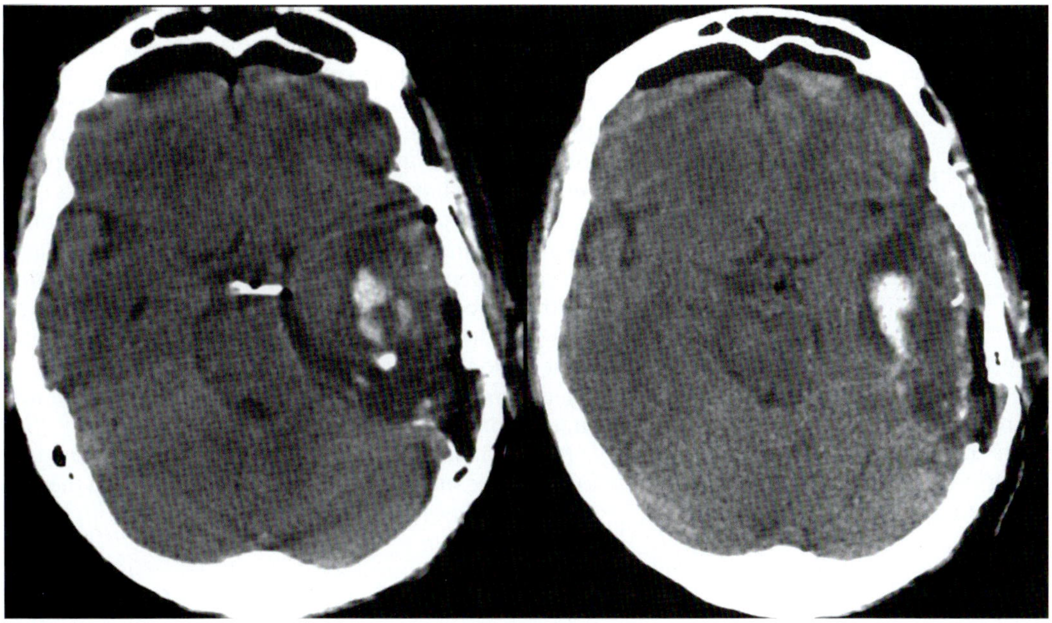

D

Figure 30–5 **(D)** Postoperative venous infarction of the temporal lobe.

In some patients, the vein may drain into the tentorium or the dura mater before draining into the transverse sinus. The partial labyrinthectomy petrous apicectomy transpetrosal approach, the translabyrinthine approach, and the total petrosectomy approach all move the surgeon anteriorly from the drainage point of the vein of Labbé. However, in some patients, these strategies may not be enough to prevent excessive stretching of the vein. In some patients, the tentorium may be divided with minimal brain retraction, and then the retractor can be placed on the tentorium rather than the temporal lobe to prevent venous stretching. When the vein is very large and dominant with a very anterior drainage site (**Fig. 30–5B**), then the surgical approach may have to be changed to the retrosigmoid (or retrosigmoid + orbitozygomatic with frontotemporal craniotomy) to prevent venous injury, especially on the dominant side.

◆ Venous Reconstruction

In cases of accidental injury to large veins, if brain swelling is noted after the occlusion of a vein, or after the injury to any deep vein, venous reconstruction is indicated. In such patients, the easiest reconstruction may be by direct suture, using 8–0 nylon sutures (**Table 30–2**). If the anastomosis is under tension, some of the tension can be released by dural mobilization. Direct repair is usually successful, even if the repaired vein is slightly stenotic.

Table 30–2 Indications of Reconstruction of Cerebral Veins

Damage to large superficial or deep vein
Brain swelling observed after venous occlusion

A segment of the vein may be missing in many patients, however, and the repair may be difficult without using a graft. In such patients, a segment of saphenous vein from the leg, or a vein from the forearm or the neck, or the radial artery may be used as an interposition graft.[3] Postoperative thrombosis is the main problem with venous reconstruction and may occur because of injury to the endothelium of the transplanted vein, and the slow blood flow through the vein in general. To prevent this, we give the patients 2000 U of intravenous heparin during the reconstruction procedure, subcutaneous heparin during the first 7 postoperative days (5000 U q8h), and aspirin 325 mg daily thereafter for 2 to 3 months.

◆ Preservation of Cerebral Venous Sinuses

Because they transmit a large volume of venous blood from the brain, the patency of the venous sinuses is very important to preserve the functional integrity of the brain. The outcome of venous sinus occlusion depends upon the presence of collateral channels (**Table 30–3**) and the rapidity of occlusion. It is commonly believed that the anterior third of the sagittal sinus can be occluded without any significant damaging effect. But, in an occasional patient, such an occlusion may result in venous infarction in one or both frontal lobes. The only venous sinuses that may safely be occluded in most patients are the cavernous sinuses, the superior petrosal sinuses, and the nondominant collateralized transverse and sigmoid sinuses. Occlusion of the cavernous sinus can usually be performed without adverse effects on vision and the orbit due to the presence of many collateral drainage channels from the orbit.

Table 30–3 Indication of Reconstruction of Cerebral Venous Sinuses

Status of Collaterals	Decision
Excellent collaterals	Reconstruction unnecessary; practice for surgeons
Marginal collaterals	Reconstruction recommended
Poor or no collateral	Occlusin dangerous; reconstruction only if accidental injury

During surgery, before occluding a sinus, a test occlusion must be performed (**Fig. 30–6**). To do this, the intrasinus pressure is measured by inserting a 20 gauge butterfly needle connected to a pressure transducer. The normal venous sinus pressure should be less than 15 mm Hg, depending upon the position of the head. After a stable reading has been obtained, a temporary clip is applied on the venous sinus at the appropriate period of expected occlusion. Observation of the brain or cerebellum for swelling and of the evoked potentials and intrasinus pressure is performed for at least 5 minutes. Intrasinus pressure is the most sensitive indicator of the three, but cerebellar swelling may occur very quickly. If brain swelling occurs, evoked potentials change, or intrasinus pressure increases by more than 5 mm Hg, then the temporary clip is removed, and the sinus cannot be occluded. If the initial intrasinus pressure was above 15 mm Hg but there is not a significant increase in the pressure, the sinus may be occluded, but continuous monitoring of the pressure must be done during the rest of the operation because a delayed increase in intrasinus pressure may occur and necessitate reconstruction.

Preoperative occlusion tests of the venous sinuses are not safe because the clinical response is delayed, and the effects are not fully reversible.[7]

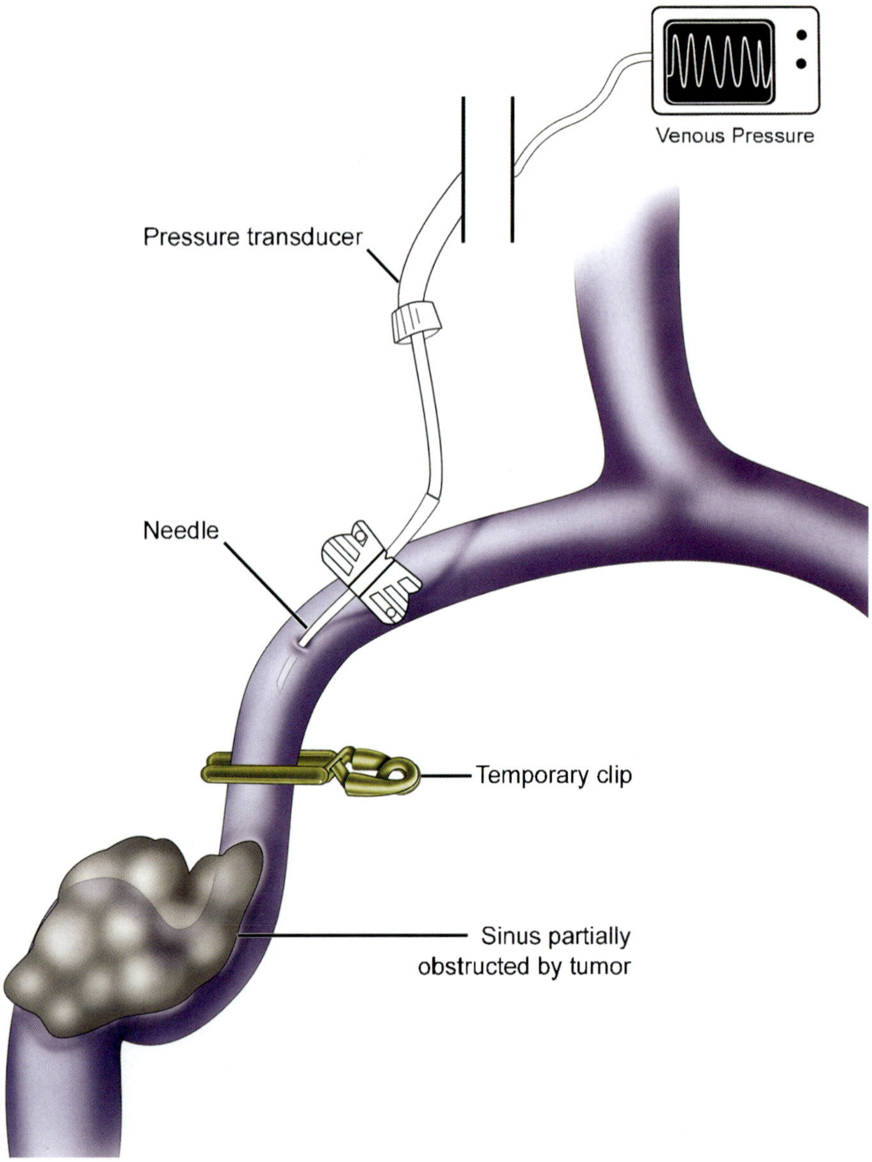

Figure 30–6 Technique of inserting a butterfly needle into the sinus following placement of temporary clip to occlude the sinus.

◆ Reconstruction of Venous Sinuses

Direct Repair

When a small portion of the circumference of a venous sinus is involved by a tumor such as meningioma, paraganglioma, or schwannoma, direct repair is desirable. The repair of sinuses after tumor excision is done either by direct suturing with 5–0 Prolene (**Fig. 30–7A,B**) or with a dural or venous graft.

In cases of sagittal sinus repair, the graft is sutured onto some of the sinus wall before removal of the tumor (**Fig. 30–8A,B**). After removal of the tumor, the sinus may be allowed to bleed if it is a small rent, occluded by finger pressure or temporary clips if some collaterals exist, or occluded with a balloon shunt if high flow exists through the sinus (**Fig. 30–8C**). If the repair is likely to take more than 10 minutes, then the patient must be heparinized.

Direct repair of the sigmoid sinus with 6–0 Prolene sutures may be done when the sinus is divided to improve the exposure of a tumor or an aneurysm (Cases 3 and 4).

Graft Reconstruction

When there is a segmental defect[8] that cannot be repaired directly as already described, graft reconstruction of the sinus is performed. Such a repair is redundant in patients with excellent collaterals and mainly provides practice for the surgeons. Sinus resection followed by repair is recommended for patients with marginal collaterals. In patients with poor or no collaterals, the sinus should be left open with residual tumor. In such cases repair is only indicated in cases of accidental injury.

When the sinus to be repaired is large (≥ 1 cm diameter), the saphenous vein, extracted from the thigh, is used

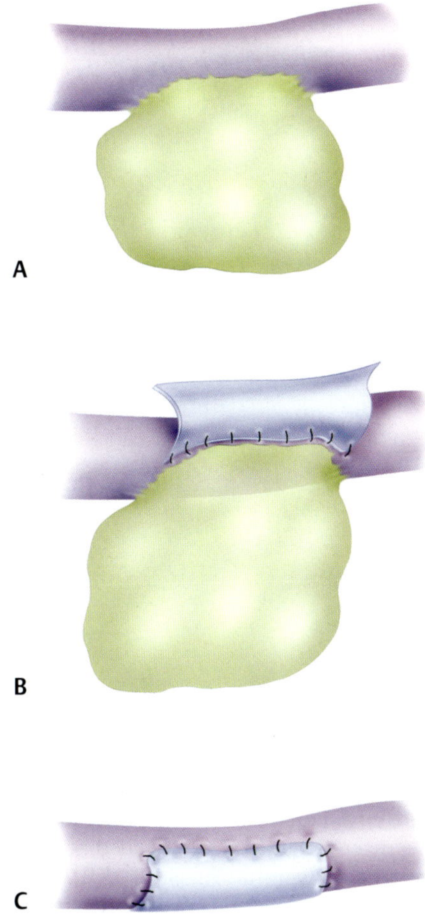

Figure 30–8 Repair of a superior sagittal sinus by graft. **(A)** Tumor invading the sinus. **(B)** Part of the patch graft is sutured to the sinus wall with tumor in situ. **(C)** Patch graft sutured after tumor excision.

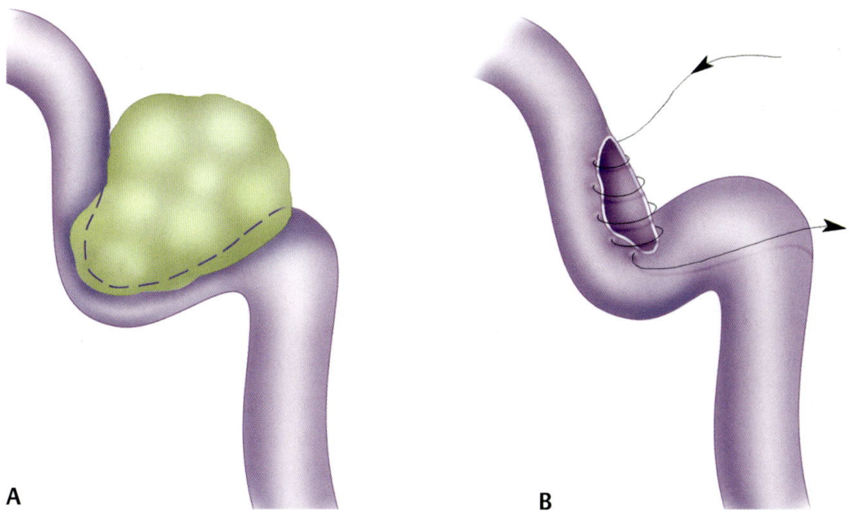

Figure 30–7 **(A,B)** Direct repair of the sigmoid sinus after resection of a schwannoma, which had encased the sinus.

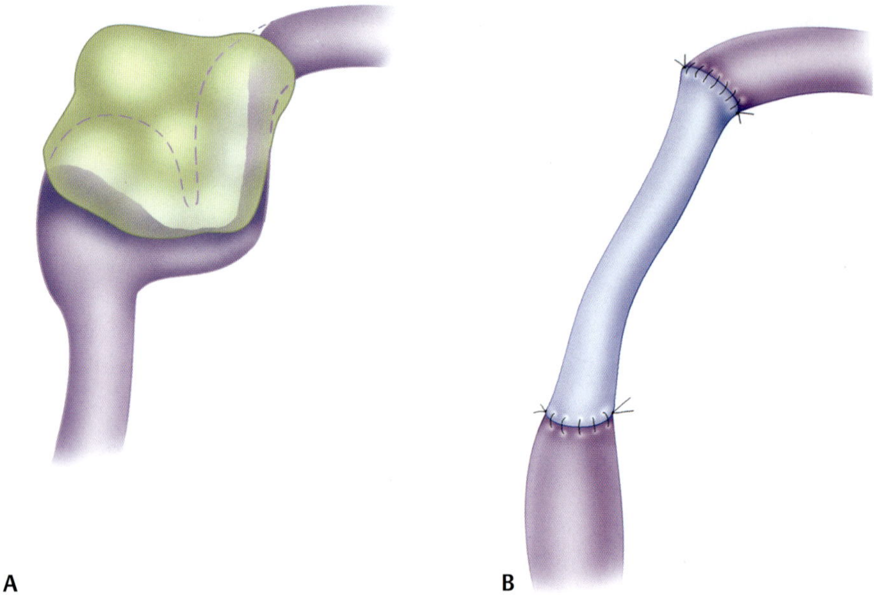

Figure 30–9 **(A)** Tumor encased and invaded the sigmoid sinus to narrow the sinus. **(B)** Part of the sinus was resected along with the tumor, and an interposition graft (saphenous vein) was placed (end-to-end anastomosis).

(**Fig. 30–9A,B**). When the sinus has been previously partially occluded by the tumor, the radial artery is used because it tends to stay open even when the flow rate is low. To prevent vasospasm, the artery should be distended under pressure with heparinized saline (unpublished data). Because of the discrepancy in size, an end-to-side technique is used for radial artery grafts (**Fig. 30–10A,B**), whereas an end-to-end technique is used for saphenous vein grafts (Cases 1 and 2).

Results of vein and sinus reconstruction in the 6 years from 1993 to 1999 are shown in **Table 30–4.**

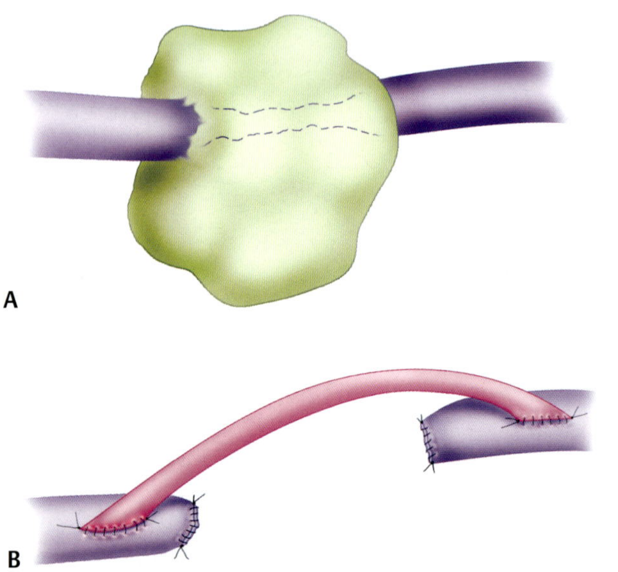

Figure 30–10 **(A)** Tumor invading sinus. **(B)** Tumor resected with sinus and interposition graft (radial artery) placed (end-to-side anastomosis).

Table 30–4 Results of Venous Reconstruction from 1993 to 1999

Type of Vein/Venous Sinus Reconstructed	No. of Patients	No. of Patients in Which They Are Patent Finally
Cortical vein		
Resuture graft	1	1
SVG	1	1
RAG	1	1
Superior sagittal sinus		
SVG	2	2
Transverse sinus (pineal region)		
Division only	5	NA
Division + SVG	1	1
Sigmoid sinus–jugular vein		
Division + resuture	4	4
Repair after tumor excision	2	1
SVG	2	2

RAG, radial artery graft; SVG, saphenous vein graft.

◆ Case Illustrations

Case 1

A 58-year-old woman presented with facial pain and numbness caused by a right petroclival meningioma [tumor equivalent diameter (TED) = 2.17 cm] extending into the Meckel's cave and the cavernous sinus. There was mild brain stem compression (**Fig. 30–11**). The venous phase of

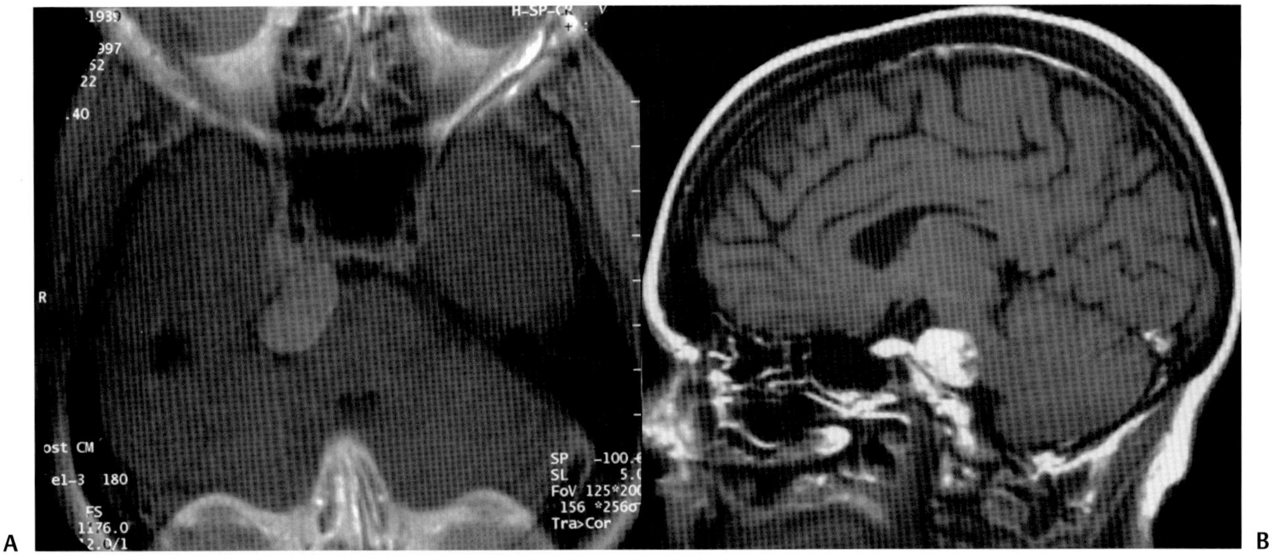

Figure 30–11 (**A**) Axial and (**B**) sagittal contrast-enhanced T1 image of a magnetic resonance imaging scan showing the petroclival meningioma in Case 1.

the angiogram showed a prominent vein of Labbé (**Fig. 30–12**). The tumor was removed by a transpetrosal retrolabyrinthine approach. However, early in the operation, an aberrant vein of Labbé, draining the entire temporal lobe and draining into a dural sinus anterior to the transverse sinus, was damaged. Because significant temporal lobe swelling was noted, the vein of Labbé was reconstructed with a short saphenous vein graft from the vein to the sigmoid sinus (**Fig. 30–13**). A special technique of venous attachment to the sigmoid sinus was used without significant flow interruption by placing the attaching sutures first and then cutting the hole into the sinus before tying the sutures (**Figs. 30–14** and **30–15**). The tumor was seen to involve the trigeminal fascicles severely. The temporal lobe swelling resolved postoperatively, and the patient recovered well. Postoperatively, the patient had partial sixth cranial nerve palsy and diminished sensation in the V1 and V2 region and absent corneal reflex. Postoperative MRV and three-dimensional computed tomographic (CT) angiogram showed patency of the graft (**Fig. 30–16**). After a follow-up of 2 years there was no tumor recurrence. The sixth cranial nerve palsy has disappeared totally, but trigeminal loss persisted. The venous reconstruction was felt to be important in this patient in avoiding major problems.

Case 2

A 62-year-old man presented with a history of recurrent seizure with prickly tongue, distorted speech, and numbness in 1976, 1983, and 1995. During an airplane flight he

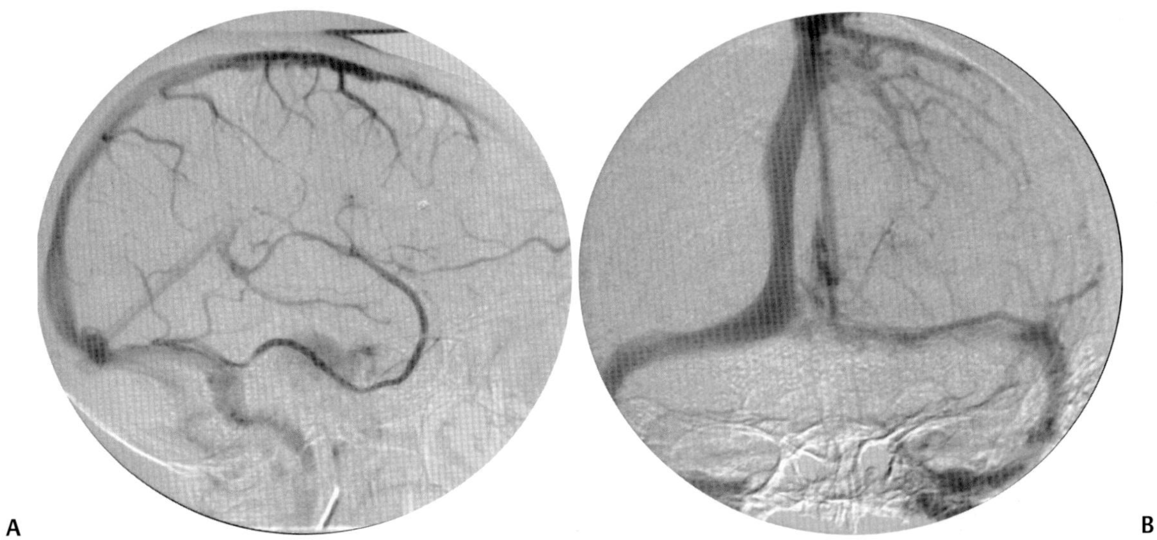

Figure 30–12 (**A,B**) Venous phase of angiogram showing prominent vein of Labbé and dominance of the right lateral sinus.

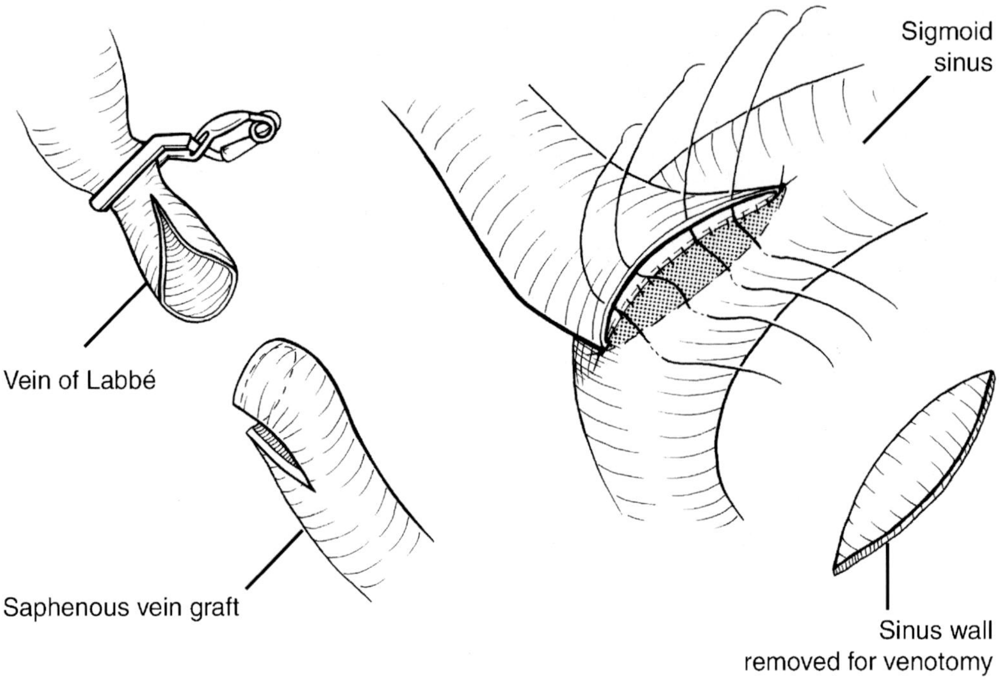

Figure 30–13 Diagrammatic representation of the vein graft technique. Fish-mouth opening is made in the vein as well as in the graft to reduce the amount of stenosis later on. Also, a part of the sinus wall was removed.

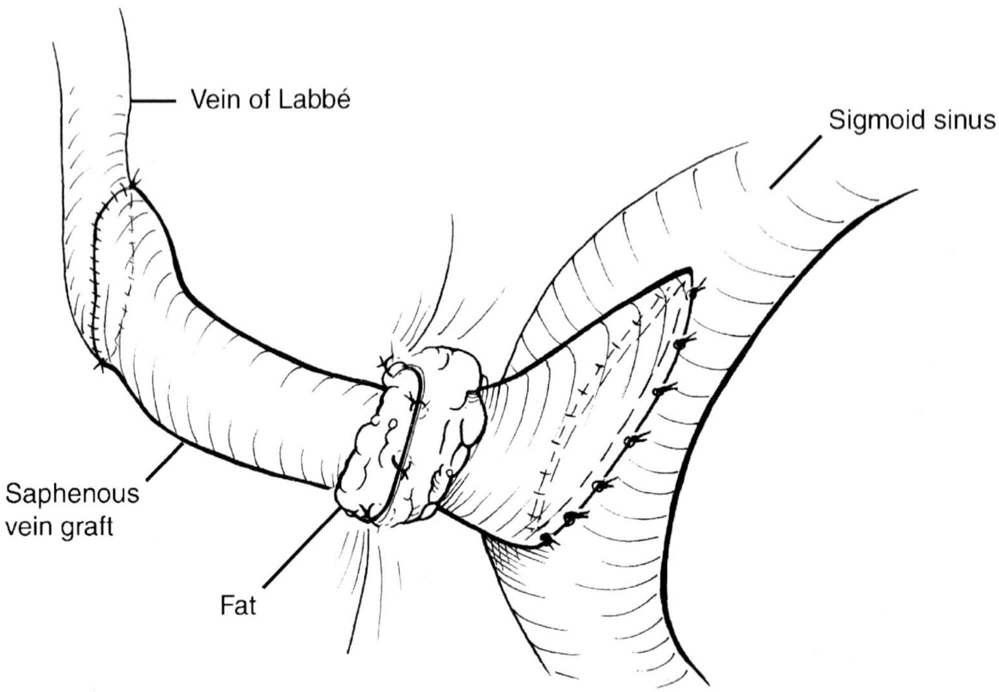

Figure 30–14 Diagrammatic representation of the vein graft technique (continued). The anastomosis is completed, and a pad of fat supports the graft.

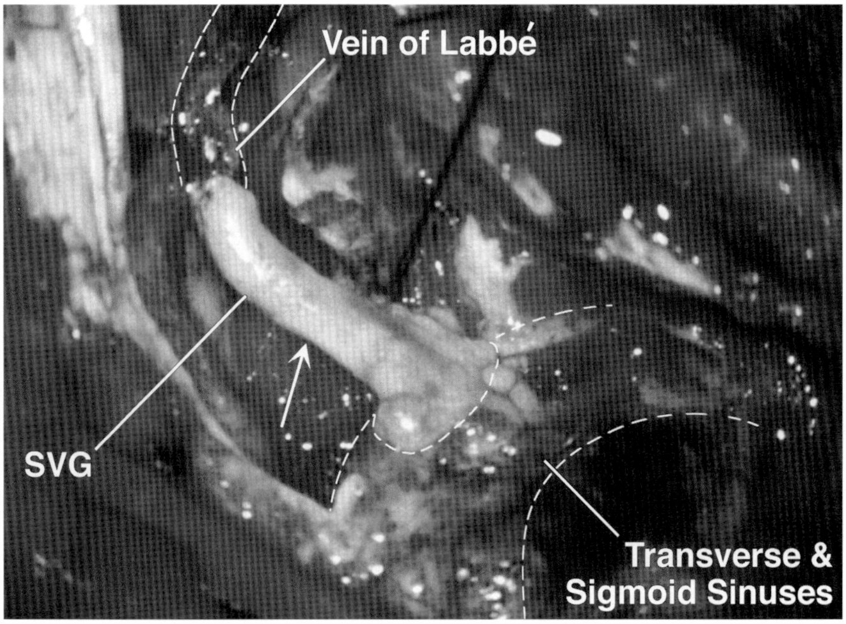

Figure 30–15 Operative picture of the completed anastomosis. The arrow points to the saphenous vein graft (SVG).

had severe dizziness and loss of hearing, which resolved spontaneously. He also had pulsatile tinnitus. On examination he had 20% hearing loss in his right ear and was unable to perform tandem walk. He had nystagmus. Magnetic resonance imaging (MRI) scan showed a highly vascular glomus jugulare tumor (TED = 2.42 cm) in the jugular foramen (JF) filling the region of the right jugular bulb (**Fig. 30–17**) without occluding the sigmoid sinus (SS) and internal jugular vein (IJV). The tumor encased the petrosal segment of the internal carotid artery (ICA), bowing it forward. The cerebral angiography showed that the tumor was supplied by an enlarged right ascending pharyngeal artery with additional supply arising from the meningodural branch of the right occipital artery, a small branch of the right posterior auricular artery, and the meningohypophyseal trunk. The sigmoid and transverse sinuses were larger on the right side but were subtotally occluded by the tumor. There was a good communication between the two sinuses at the torcular Herophili (**Fig. 30–18**). Therefore, it was felt to be safe to occlude the

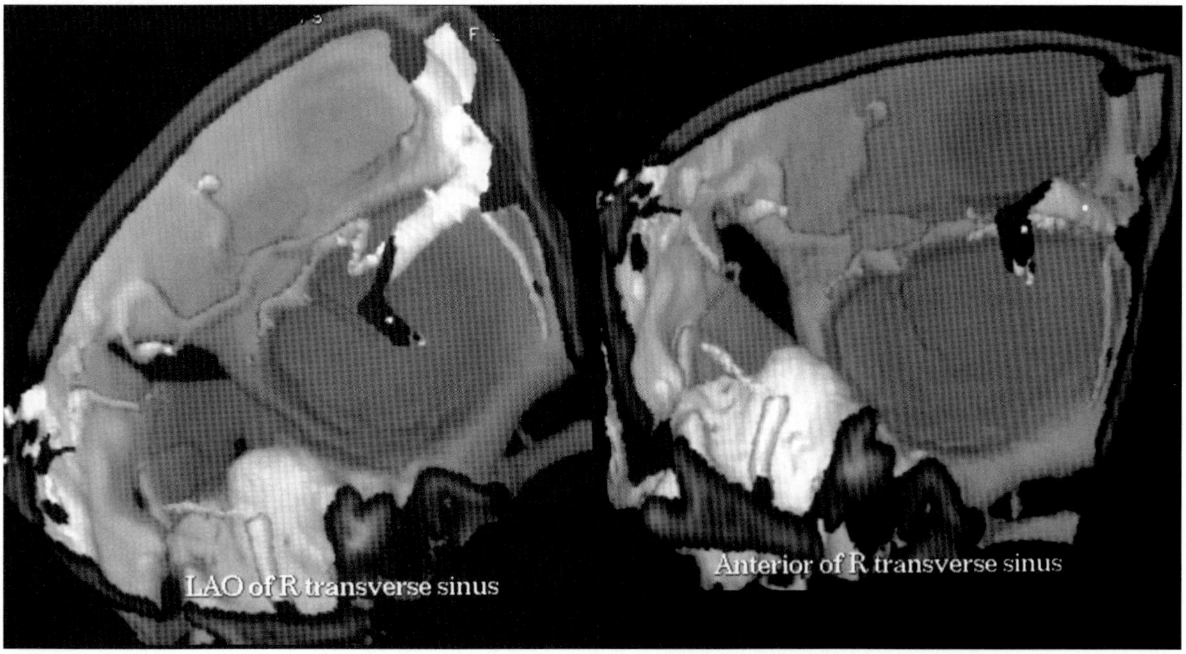

Figure 30–16 **(A,B)** Three-dimensional computed tomographic angiogram of Case 1 showing a patent graft and sinus.

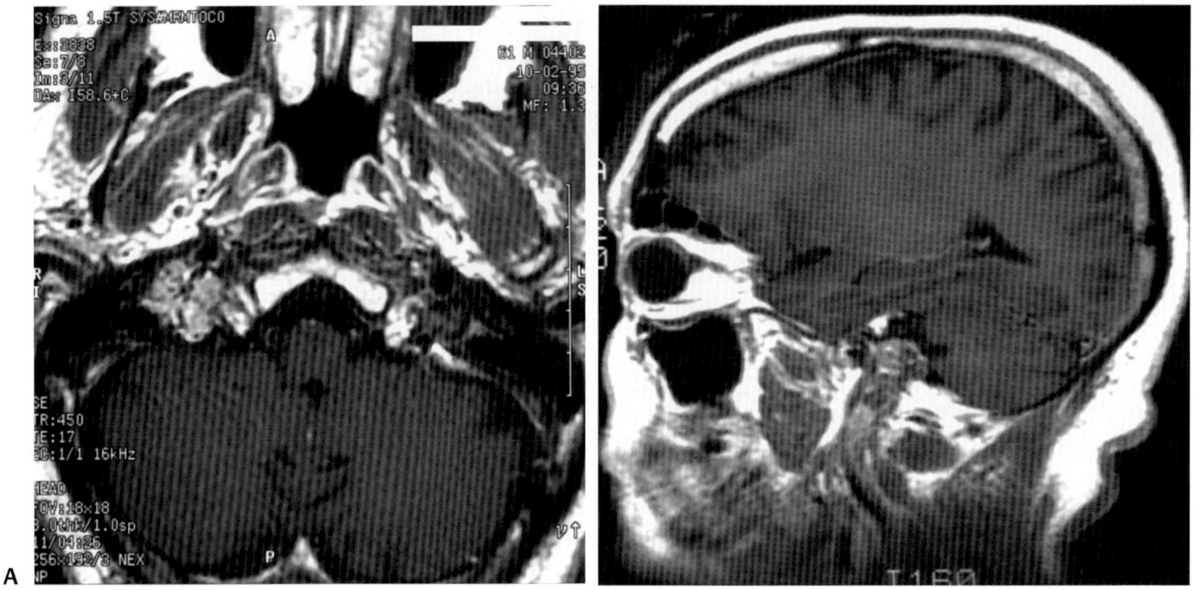

A B

Figure 30–17 **(A)** Contrast-enhanced axial and **(B)** sagittal T1 image of magnetic resonance imaging of Case 2 showing a glomus jugulare tumor.

sinus during tumor resection. At operation, the intrasinus pressure was measured prior to sinus occlusion and excision of the tumor (**Fig. 30–6**). Although the intrasinus pressure was initially unchanged after occlusion, the pressure increased steadily during the operation in the range of 35 to 40 torr. Because of this, reconstruction of the sinus was elected and was performed with a saphenous vein graft (**Fig. 30–19**). A 5 cm long vein graft was sutured from the sigmoid sinus to the internal jugular vein. Patency of the graft was verified by intra-arterial and magnetic resonance angiography (**Fig. 30–20**). Postoperatively, the patient had communicating hydrocephalus, for which a

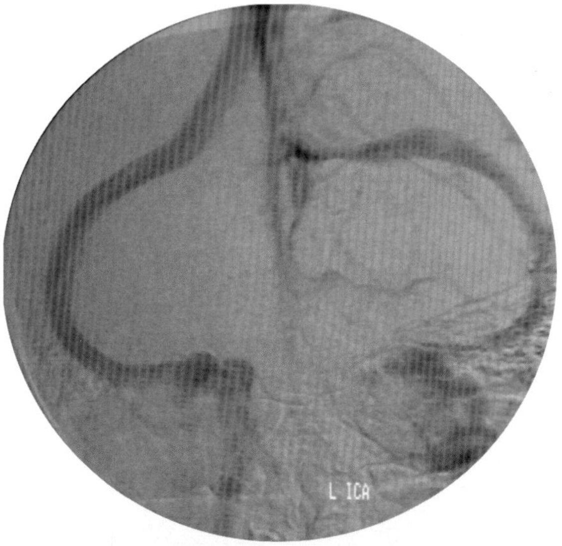

Figure 30–18 Angiogram of patient (Case 2) showing good cross-circulation and patent torcular Herophili and dominant right lateral sinus.

lumboperitoneal shunt was done. The patient had transient postoperative facial nerve palsy, which recovered completely. After a follow-up of 21 months, the patient was seen to have very mild impairment of the tandem gait. There was no recurrence of the tumor, and there was no other neurological deficit.

Case 3

This 40-year-old man presented at another institution with subarachnoid hemorrhage. He rebled and deteriorated. He was in Hunt and Hess grade IV and Fisher grade 4 at admission. Cerebral angiogram revealed aneurysms at the vertebrobasilar junction (VBJ) and at the middle cerebral artery (MCA) bifurcation (**Fig. 30–21**). Because the aneurysm at the VBJ had bled, it was operated by a retrosigmoid and transmastoid presigmoid approach performed for exposure. To enhance the exposure, it was planned to section the sigmoid sinus (**Fig. 30–22**). The left sigmoid sinus was slightly larger than the right sigmoid sinus. Intrasinus pressure was measured to be 12 to 13 mm Hg before occlusion. With occlusion, sinus pressure increased to 18 mm Hg, and the sinus was sectioned. During surgery, the sinus pressure was transiently elevated to 20 mm Hg. Both vertebral arteries were occluded temporarily for 31 minutes, and mild hypotension was also used. The somatosensory evoked potential (SEP) deteriorated initially and then improved after blood pressure was raised to normal and when the temporary clip was removed from the vertebral artery. The aneurysm neck was at the vertebrobasilar (**Fig. 30–23**) fenestration, and the aneurysm was occluded with two long clips. A minor intraoperative rupture was managed uneventfully. The sigmoid sinus was resutured directly with 5–0 and 6–0 Prolene. Postoperative angiogram showed patency of the sinus (**Fig. 30–24**). The patient had a stormy postoperative period

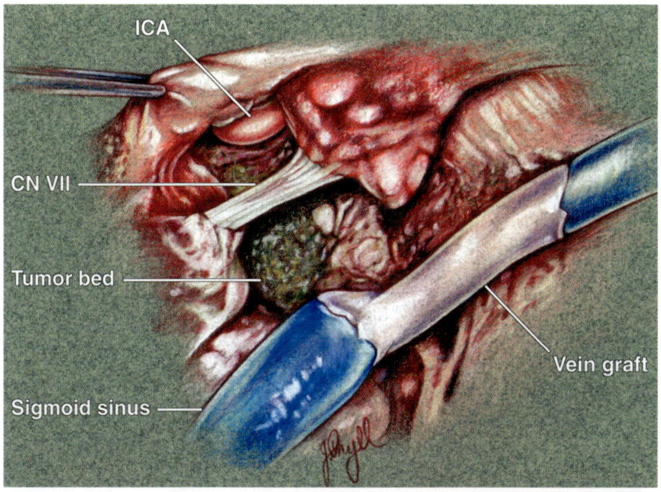

A

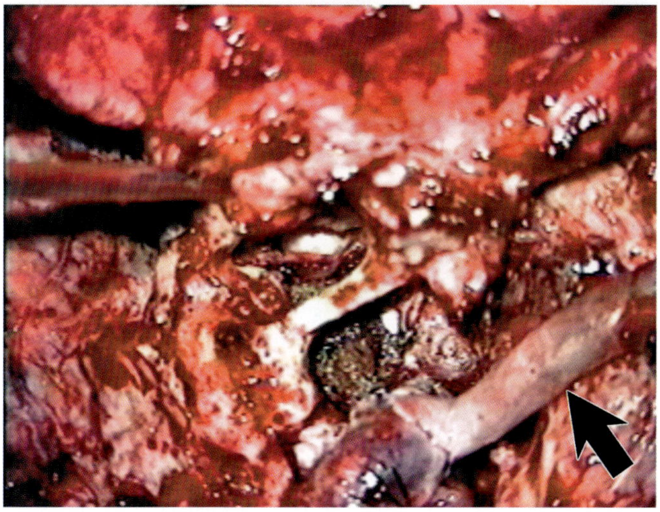

B

Figure 30–19 **(A)** Diagrammatic representation of the vein graft done to reconstruct the sigmoid sinus. **(B)** Operative picture showing the vein graft (black arrow).

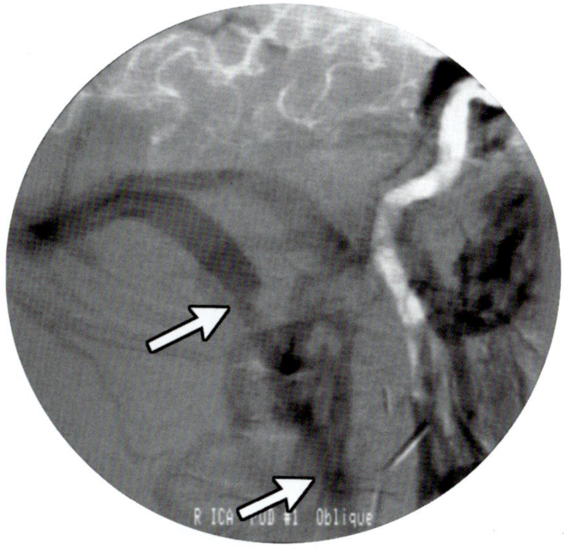

Figure 30–20 Postoperative angiogram showing patent graft (arrows) in Case 2.

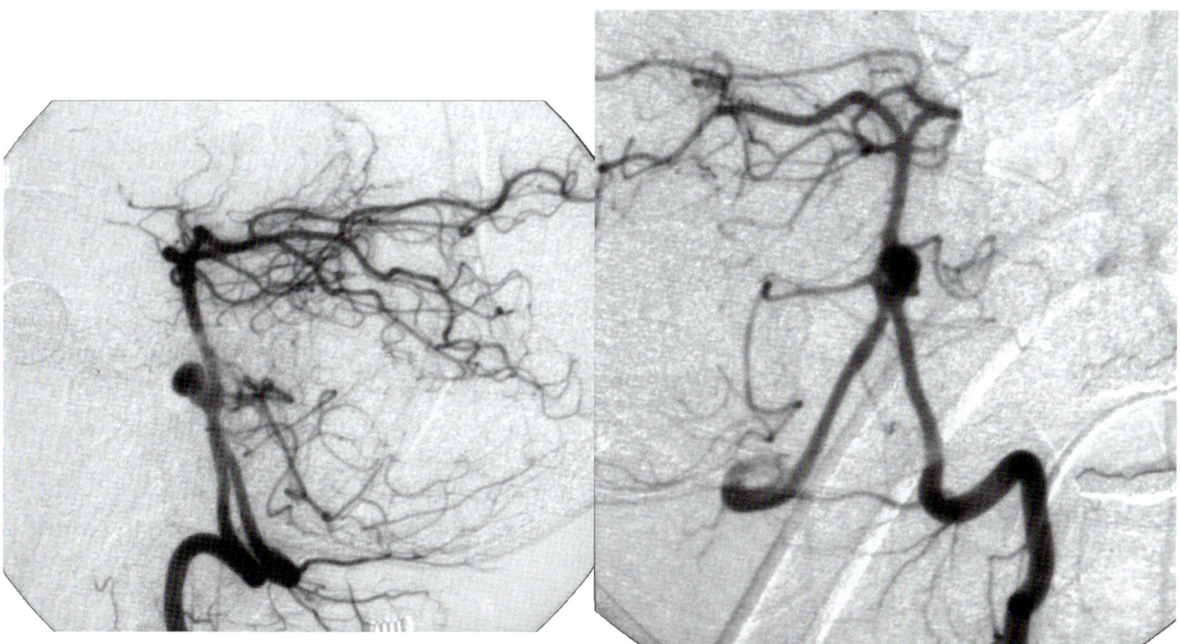

A

B

Figure 30–21 **(A, B)** Angiogram of Case 3 showing the aneurysm at the vertebrobasilar junction.

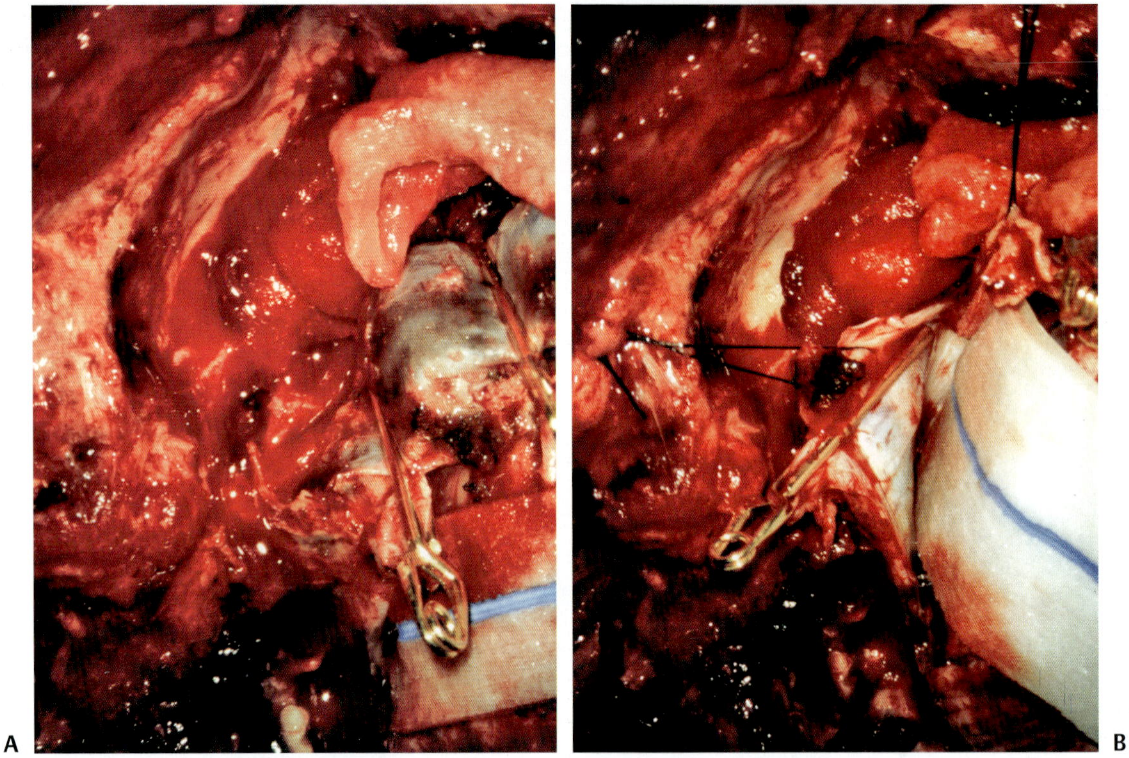

Figure 30–22 (A,B) Operative picture of Case 3 showing temporary clips are placed on the lateral sinus and then cut in between the clips.

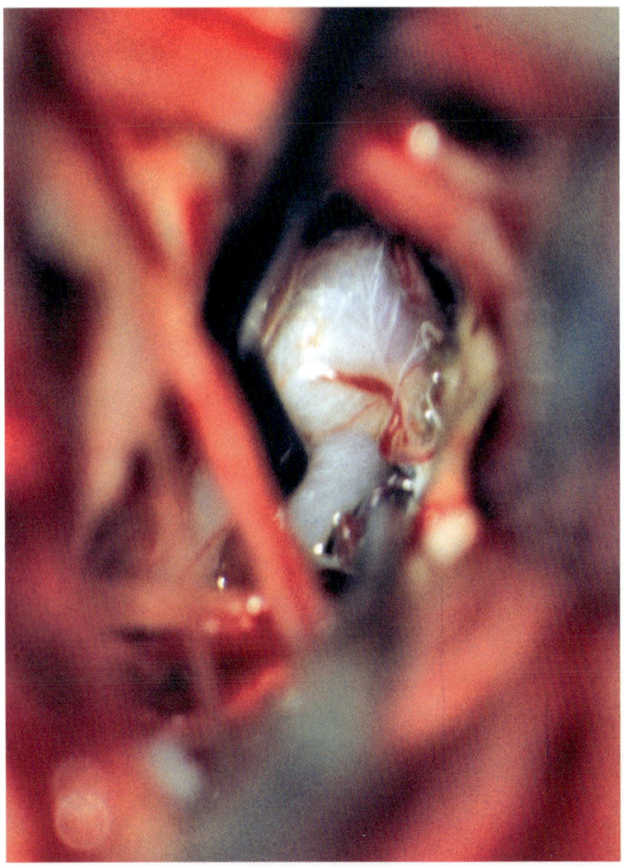

Figure 30–23 Intraoperative picture of Case 3 showing the aneurysm.

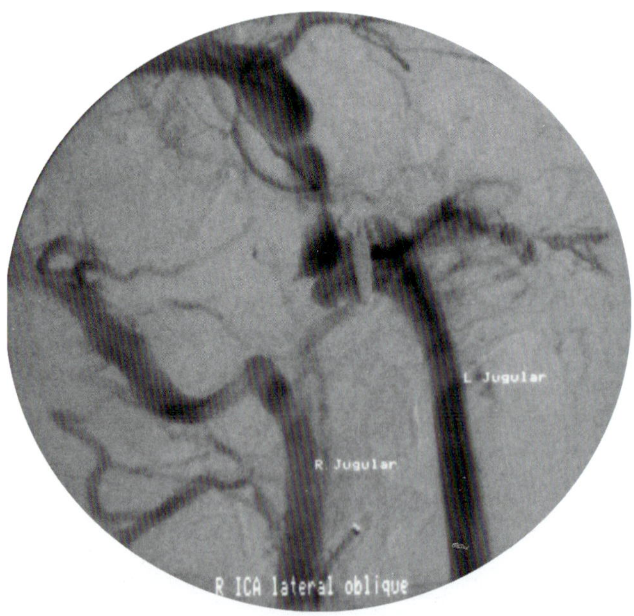

Figure 30–24 Postoperative angiogram of Case 3 showing the patent sinus.

with meningitis and pneumonia. He also had postoperative vasospasm and underwent angioplasty. However, he recovered well and subsequently underwent elective clipping of the unruptured MCA aneurysm. At follow-up 6 months postoperatively, he was found to be neurologically intact and had returned to work.

Case 4

A 46-year-old man presented with a history of mental deterioration and gait ataxia. MRI scan showed a giant pineal region meningioma (TED = 4.08 cm) compressing the brain stem severely and producing hydrocephalus (**Fig. 30–25**). An arteriogram (**Fig. 30–26**) in the venous phase showed good collateralization of the two transverse sinuses and the nondominance of the left side. The lesion was initially approached by a supracerebellar infratentorial approach, with the patient in a sitting position, but this was difficult and found to be inadequate for tumor resection. The patient was reoperated on by a combined approach (occipital, transtentorial, supracerebellar, transsinus approach) in a semiprone position. The transverse sinus was clipped, and the pressure was measured. The intrasinus pressure before clipping was 8 mm Hg and after clipping was 9 mm Hg. The sinus was transected between two temporary clips. The tumor was debulked, and the capsule of the tumor was dissected away from the brain stem and the encased veins. The transverse sinus was resutured with 5–0 Prolene. The postoperative recovery was good, and after a follow-up of 61 months the patient had no neurological deficits, and there was no recurrence of the tumor (**Fig. 30–27**). (Note: In this patient, as in Case 3, the reconstruction of the sinus was mainly to preserve both sinuses for the future and was not mandatory.)

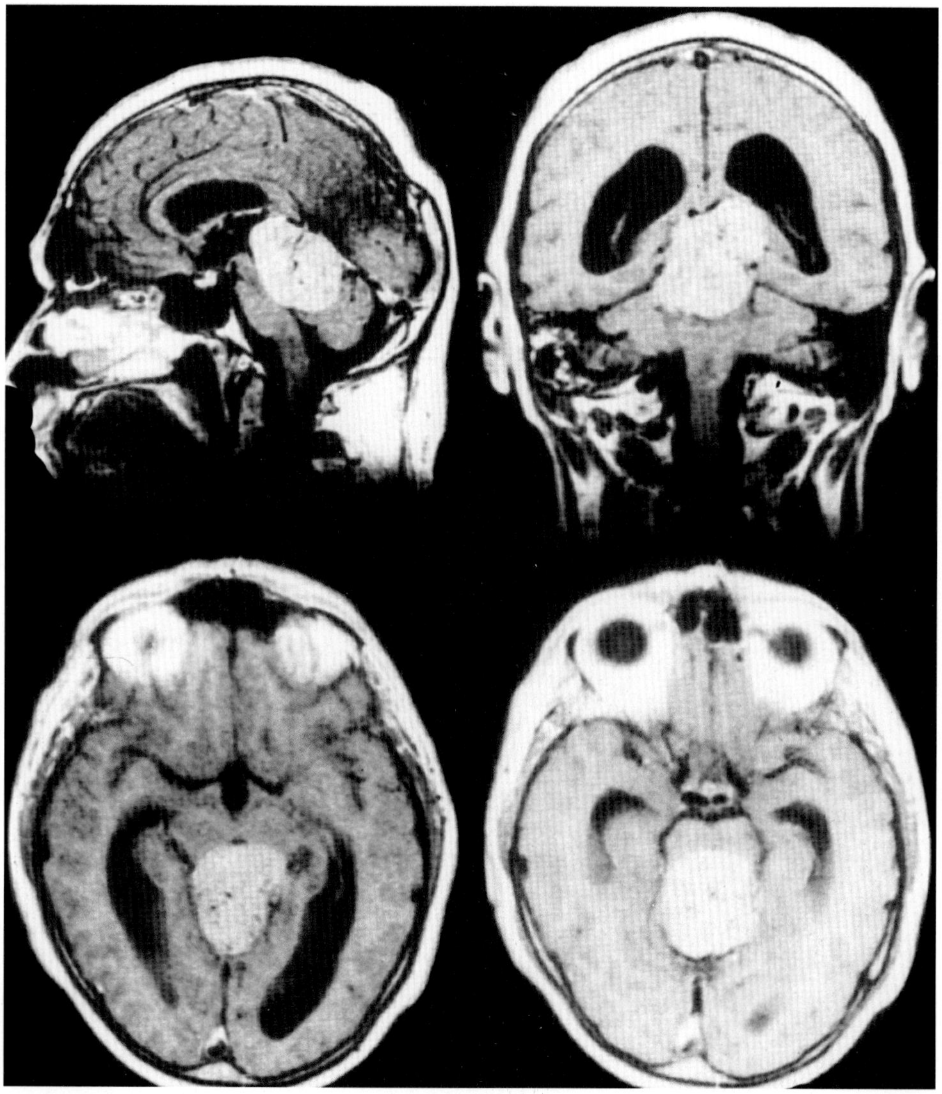

Figure 30–25 Preoperative sagittal, coronal, and axial enhanced T1 magnetic resonance imaging scans of Case 4 showing a pineal region tumor compressing the brain stem, producing hydrocephalus.

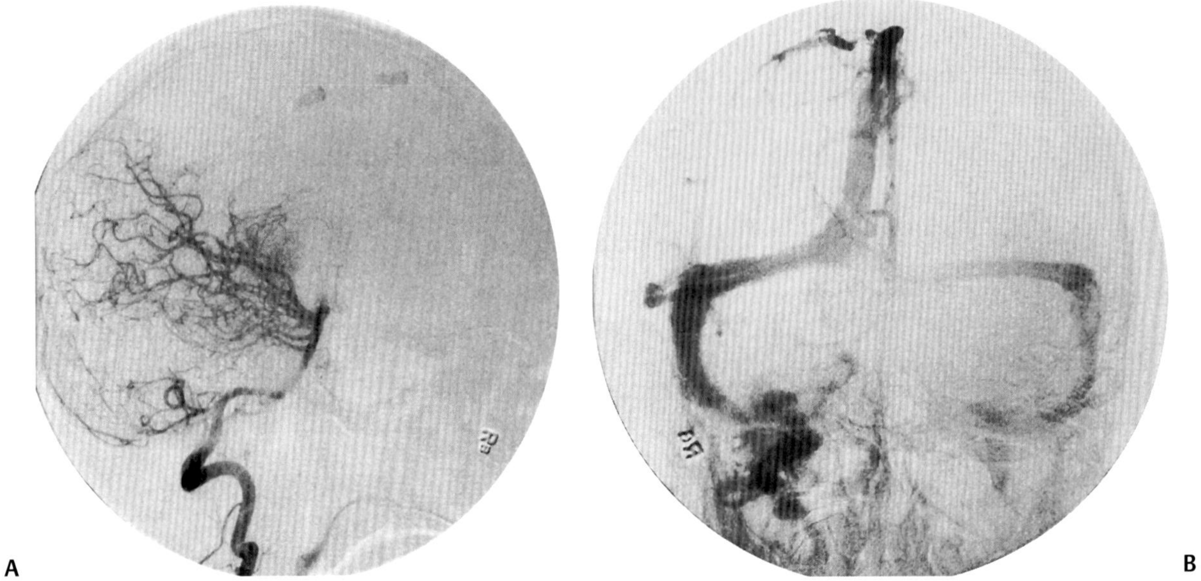

Figure 30–26 Preoperative angiogram of Case 4. **(A)** Tumor blush, although no major supplies from the posterior cerebral artery (PCA). **(B)** Venous phase showing good collateralization of the two lateral sinuses and the dominance of the right sinus.

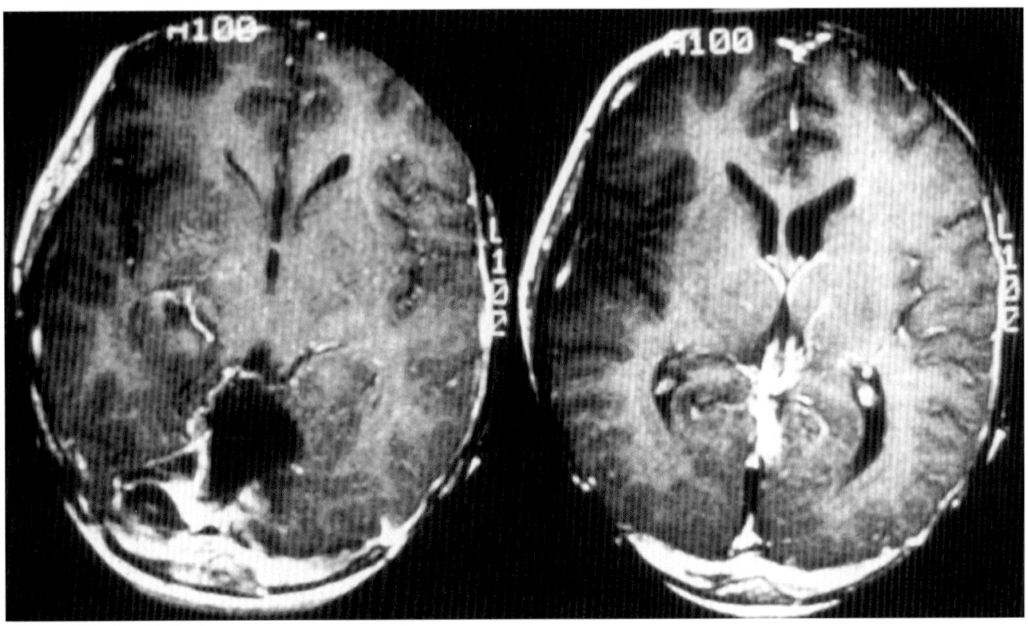

Figure 30–27 Postoperative enhanced axial T1 image of magnetic resonance imaging scan showing complete tumor removal of Case 4.

◆ Conclusion

To ensure an optimal postoperative outcome for the patient, the neurosurgeons must pay attention to cerebral veins and venous sinuses. Further research in this area is necessary.

References

1. Krayenbuhl H, Yasargil MG. Radiological anatomy and topography of the cerebral veins. In: Vinken PJ, Bruyn GW, eds. Handbook of Clinical Neurology. Vascular Diseases of the Nervous System. Part 1. Vol 2. Amsterdam: North-Holland; 1972:102–117
2. Matsushima T, Rhoton AL Jr, De Oliveira E, Peace D. Microsurgical anatomy of the veins of posterior fossa. J Neurosurg 1983;59: 63–105
3. Morita A, Sekhar LN. Reconstruction of the vein of Labbé by using a short saphenous vein bypass graft: technical note. J Neurosurg 1998; 89:671–675
4. Oka K, Rhoton AL Jr, Barry M, Rodriguez R. Microsurgical anatomy of the superficial veins of the cerebrum. Neurosurgery 1985;17: 711–748
5. Sakata K, Al-Mefty O, Yamamoto I. Venous consideration in petrosal approach: microsurgical anatomy of the temporal bridging vein. Neurosurgery 2000;47:153–161
6. Schmidek HH, Auer LM, Kapp JP. The cerebral venous system. Neurosurgery 1985;17:663–678
7. Kano I, Iida H, Muira 5. A system for cerebral flow measurement using $H_2(15)O$ intravenous injection and PET. J Cereb Blood flow Metab 1987; 7:143–153
8. Sekhar LN, Tzortzidis FN, Bejjani GK, Schessel DA. Saphenous vein graft bypass of the sigmoid sinus and jugular bulb during the removal of glomus jugulare tumors: report of two cases. J Neurosurg 1997;86: 1036–1041

31

Vertebral Artery Surgery

Bernard George

The vertebral artery (VA) is a vessel that is generally considered difficult and dangerous to expose. The first surgical exposure was achieved by Maisonneuve in 1852. The first endarterectomy was performed in 1959 by Cate and Scott.[2] However, since then, very few cases of surgery around the VA have been reported.[3–6] In fact, pathologies involving this vessel are numerous and various. Moreover, the VA control increases the possibilities of access to some regions such as the anterior foramen magnum (FM), the jugular foramen (JF), and the intervertebral foramen (IF) areas.

The VA is divided into four segments: (1) proximal (or ostial), (2) transversary (from C6 to C2), (3) suboccipital (from C2 to FM), and (4) intracranial.

There are two main surgical approaches to the VA[7–9]: (1) the anterolateral approach, which permits the surgeon to expose any segment or the whole length of the VA, including the intracranial segment; and (2) the posterolateral approach, which is essentially applied to expose the distal part of the VA from C1 to the vertebrobasilar junction.

Alternative approaches are the anterior cervical approach, which is much less comfortable, especially above C3, and the interscalenic approach, which gives a narrow access between the scalenius muscles following the nerve roots. In these two approaches, the VA control is an extension of the standard technique, which is basically designed for another exposure; the anterior approach leads to the anterior aspect of the cervical spine and the interscalenic approach to the brachial plexus. Conversely, the anterolateral approach leads directly to the transverse processes and the VA.

◆ Indications

Lesions Involving the Vertebral Artery

Any lesion involving the VA may need either or both a surgical exposure and control of the VA.[7,10–12] Lesions for which

Table 31–1 Vertebral Artery Surgery (December 2003)

Intrinsic lesions	152 (137 distal bypass)
External compression	137 (103 tumors)
Oblique corpectomy	356
Tumors V1–V2	193 (142 neurinomas)
Foramen magnum	159 (98 meningiomas)
Craniocervical junction	194
Jugular foramen	91
TOTAL	1282

VA surgery was indicated are listed in **Table 31–1.** These lesions may be intrinsic pathologies, most commonly atheriosclerosis, but also fibromuscular dysplasia, dissecting hematoma, neurofibromatosis, radiation-induced lesions, and many others responsible for arterial stenosis or aneurysm. Arteriovenous fistulae are generally treated by endovascular techniques but may occasionally require surgical treatment, and exposure of the VA.

There are also extrinsic pathologies inducing a variable degree of compression of the VA. Extrinsic compression may be divided into two categories: (1) intermittent compression, generally produced by osteophytes or fibrous bands and more rarely by nerves or other elements and for which surgery is required only when symptoms occur during the same movement of the neck as the one producing the VA compression on angiography; and (2) permanent compression, which is generally due to space-occupying lesions such as tumors.

Intrinsic lesions are usually observed at both ends of the VA (ostial and intracranial), whereas extrinsic lesions most commonly develop at the level of the transversary and suboccipital segments.

◆ Improvement of Surgical Access

Control of the VA may also be helpful to reach a lesion located at some distance from this vessel.[9,13–17] This control is essential in several surgical techniques, including oblique corpectomy, the FM anterolateral approach, the juxtacondylar approach to the JF, and the FM posterolateral approach.

Oblique Corpectomy

Through the anterolateral approach (**Fig. 31–1A–C**), the lateral aspect of the cervical vertebral bodies can be exposed completely, including the intervertebral foramina and the transverse processes with the VA. Drilling of the lateral aspect of the vertebral bodies permits an oblique corpectomy, which exposes the anterior aspect of the spinal cord. This technique is mainly applied to treat spondylotic myelopathy and hour-glass tumors.[10,13]

Foramen Magnum Anterolateral Approach

The anterolateral approach at the level of C1 and C2 gives access to the lateral wall of the craniocervical junction, including the jugular tubercle, the occipital condyle (C0), and the lateral mass of the atlas with the two joints C0–C1 and C1–C2. This approach can be extended anteriorly to the odontoïd process, the anterior arch of the atlas, and the inferior aspect of the clivus. This technique needs the mobilization or the transposition of the VA out of the C1 transverse foramen[7,9,14] (**Fig. 31–1**).

Juxtacondylar Approach to the Jugular Foramen

Running along the atlas and condyle after VA transposition leads to the inferior aspect of the JF.[16] The juxtacondylar approach permits exposure and resection of any tumor

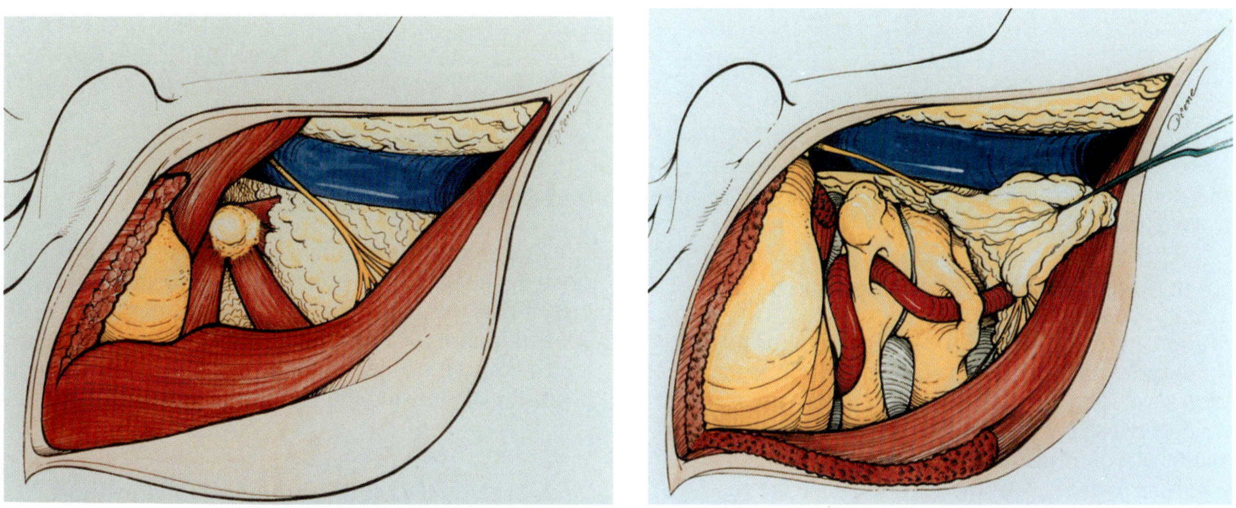
A B

Figure 31–1 **(A)** Anterolateral approach to the vertebral artery (VA) suboccipital segment (C2–FM). Sternomastoid muscle has been detached from the mastoïd process. Accessory nerve is identified and dissected free from the lymphatic and fatty sheath covering the transverse process of C1 and deep muscles. **(B)** The fatty sheath is rolled around the accessory nerve so as to protect it during retraction. Deep muscles are detached from the transverse process of C1 with exposure of the C1–C2 and the above C1 segments of the VA.

(*Continued on page 398*)

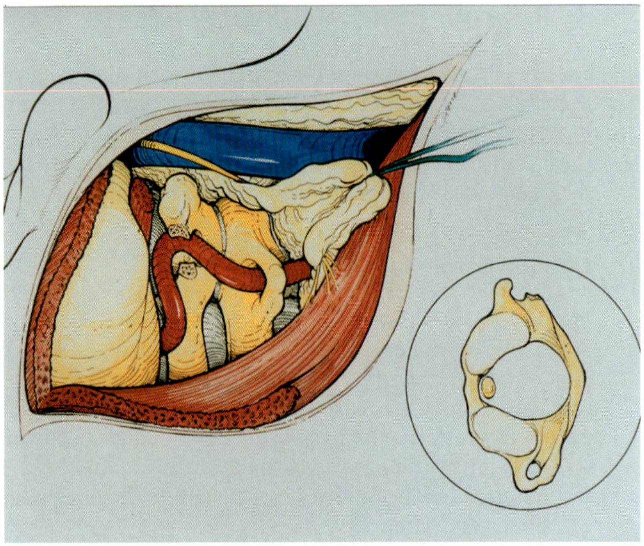

C

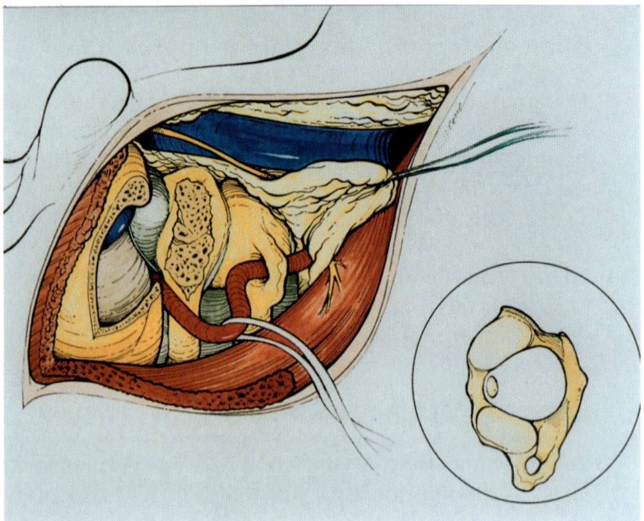

D

(*Continued*) **Figure 31–1** **(C)** Transverse process of C1 is unroofed subperiosteally. **(D)** VA is transposed inferiorly and medially out of the transverse foramen of C1. Partial mastoidectomy exposes the sigmoid sinus. Inferolateral part of the occipital bone is resected as well as the C1 transverse process. (With permission from George B. Management of the vertebral artery. In: Donald PJ, ed. Surgery of the Skull Base. New York: Lippincott-Raven; 1998:533–553.)

located in the JF without any petrous bone drilling. In tumors like paraganglioma extending out of the JF toward the petrous bone, it helps reduce the petrous bone drilling and often avoids facial nerve transposition.

Foramen Magnum Posterolateral Approach

The posterolateral approach (**Fig. 31–2**) exposes the posterior arch of the atlas up to the transverse process and so includes the VA groove. Then the posterior aspect of the lateral wall of the craniocervical junction is brought into view by mobilization of the VA. For intradural lesions, the posterior arch of the atlas and the lower part of the occipital bone are resected. For lesions located below the intracranial VA, the medial third of the lateral mass of the atlas is drilled off, whereas for lesions located above the intracranial VA, the medial third of the condyle and the jugular tubercle are resected.[9,14,15,17]

◆ Surgical Technique

Vertebral Artery Control

The first step is always the control of the VA out of the periosteal sheath in the transversary and suboccipital segments (C6 to FM). Then the periosteal sheath may be opened if necessary (intrinsic lesions). This requires bipolar coagulation or packing of the perivertebral venous plexus located inside the periosteal sheath around the VA.

Vertebral Artery Mobilization or Transposition

Either or both VA mobilization and transposition are performed with the VA enclosed in the periosteal sheath. They need to open one or several transverse foramina. Therefore,

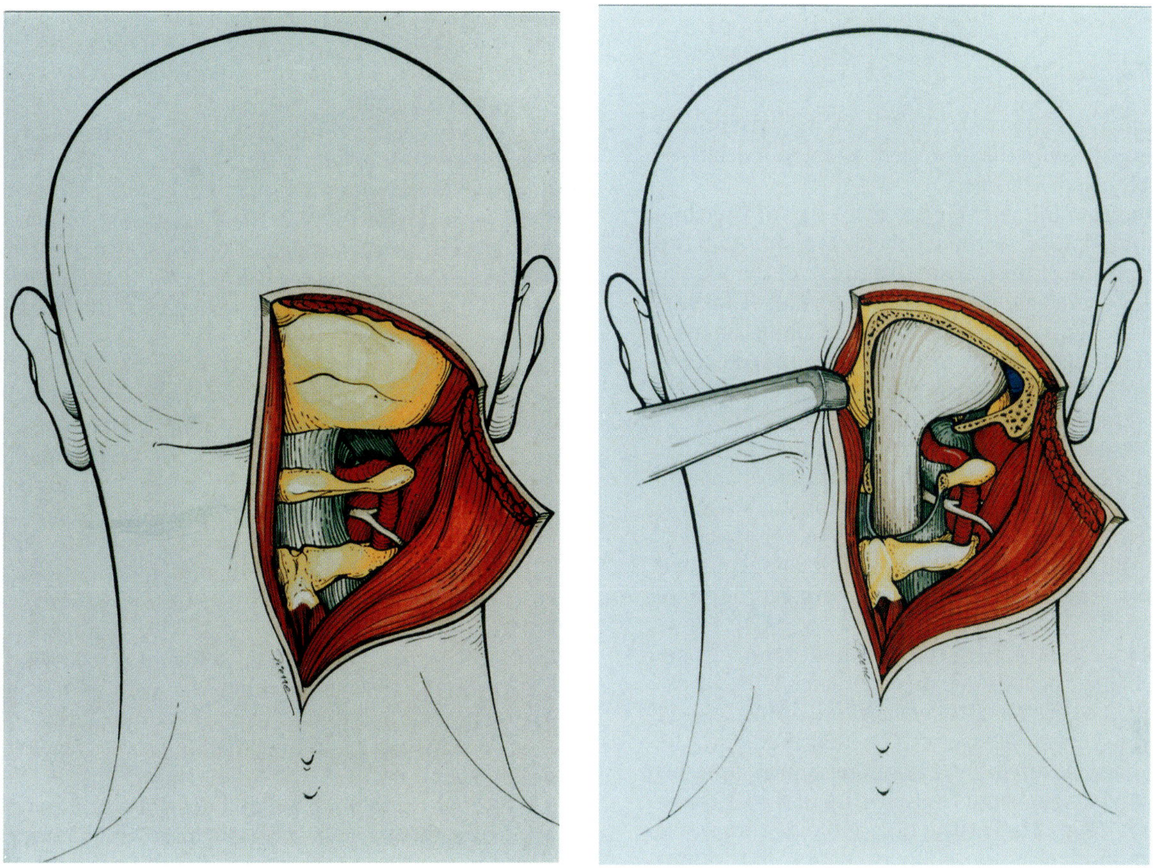

Figure 31–2 **(A)** Posterolateral approach to the above C1 and intracranial segments of the vertebral artery (VA). Exposure of the inferior part of the occipital bone and posterior arch of atlas with subperiosteal control of the VA in its groove. **(B)** Resection of the occipital bone and of the posterior arch of atlas. AP, aponeurosis; DA longus capitis muscle; IT, intertransversary muscle; LC, longus colli muscle; RN, nerve root; Σ, sympathetic nerve. (With permission from George B. Management of the vertebral artery. In: Donald PJ, ed. Surgery of the Skull Base. New York: Lippincott-Raven; 1998:533–553.)

the periosteal sheath must have been previously separated from the bone inside each foramen.

Revascularization

Endarterectomy is not an effective treatment for atherosclerotic stenosis. The VA is a small, thin-walled vessel, which explains technical difficulties of direct suture and the high risk of restenosis. A carotid to VA artery bypass is certainly more efficient.[7,11] Bypass is also indicated in some cases of occlusion, regardless of the cause, which may be intrinsic, extrinsic, or therapeutic. However, revascularization is only necessary in case of a dominant or single VA, or after a failed balloon occlusion test.

For proximal lesions, the VA may be reimplanted directly or with an interposed venous graft on the posterior aspect of the common carotid artery (CCA).

For distal lesions, a venous graft is implanted proximally on the CCA and distally on the C1–C2 VA segment. In a few cases of more distal lesions, the distal implantation may be performed onto the VA above the C1 or onto the intracranial segment. In any case, the venous graft must run as vertical as possible so as to avoid stretching or compression during rotation of the head.

◆ Surgical Approaches

The preoperative workup includes different studies depending on the pathology. For intrinsic lesions, and for extrinsic lesions producing intermittent compression, angiography is mandatory. For the other pathologies, magnetic resonance imaging (MRI) and MR angiography may be sufficient to provide the necessary information about size and course of both VAs. For instance, an abnormal level of entrance of the VA into the transverse canal is a rare condition that must be identified preoperatively because it may lead to VA injury.[18] Angiography in these cases is only performed when high tumoral vascularization is suspected and embolization is contemplated. A balloon occlusion test may also be useful, especially in the case of invasive tumors in which one may need to sacrifice the VA.

Anesthesia

No drug affecting the neuromuscular junction (curare-like drugs) must be used so that nerve functions (accessory nerve and spinal nerve roots) can be intraoperatively tested.

Intraoperative Doppler monitoring may be helpful to check the patency of the VA or of a venous graft.

Approach

Anterolateral Approach

For the anterolateral approach (**Fig. 31–1**), the patient is in the supine position with the head slightly extended and rotated toward the opposite side.

The skin incision follows the anterior edge of the sternomastoïd muscle (SM) at the level corresponding to the lesion. For exposure of the proximal segment of the VA, the skin incision is curved along the clavicle; for the distal segments of the VA, the skin incision is curved along the mastoïd process and then variably extended toward the occipital protuberance along the superior occipital line. The SM is cut along its attachment on the mastoïd process.

The area between the lateral side of the internal jugular vein (IJV) and the medial aspect of the SM muscle is opened. In the depth of this area, a fatty and lymphatic sheath is found. Above the C3 level, the accessory nerve must be identified inside this fatty sheath; the sheath is dissected and rolled around the accessory nerve so as to protect the nerve during retraction.

All the great vessels, nerves, trachea, and esophagus are retracted medially. The fatty sheath is retracted laterally except above C3, where it is rolled around the accessory nerve. The transverse processes can be identified with the finger. They are covered by the prevertebral muscles (longus colli and longus capitis muscles) up to the C2 transverse process (**Fig. 31–3**). The C1 and C2 transverse processes are hidden by the oblique, rectus, and levator scapulae muscles. To expose the transverse processes of C1 and C2 and control the VA suboccipital segment, all these small muscles must be divided. The exposure of the VA transversary segment and of the transverse processes from C6 to C2 needs the resection of the longus colli muscle. The longus capitis is usually preserved except if the spinal nerve roots lateral to the VA have to be exposed. Before cutting the muscle, the sympathetic chain must be identified under the aponeurosis and then gently displaced laterally so as to preserve its connections with the nerve roots.

The transverse processes are exposed subperiosteally on their anterior aspects, then inside the transverse foramina so that the periosteal sheath around the VA is separated.

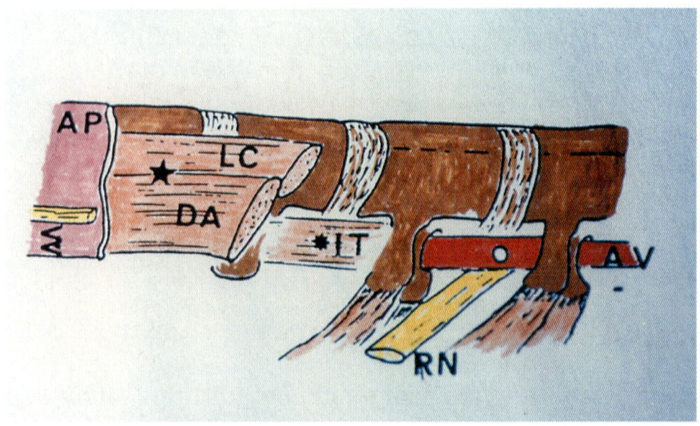

Figure 31–3 Schematic drawing of exposure of the vertebral artery (VA) transversary segment (C6–C2). AV, vertebral artery; RN, nerve root; Σ sympathetic nerve; AP, aponeurosis; LC, longus colli muscle; DA, longus capitis muscle; IT, intertransversary muscle.

Therefore, the VA is controlled within the periosteal sheath, which also encloses the perivertebral venous plexus. Control of the VA is achieved for the required length with opening of as many foramina as necessary.

The VA is crossing anterior to the nerve roots, which run over the intervertebral joints (**Fig. 31–2**). At the C1–C2 level, the C2 nerve root divides into two branches crossing anterior and posterior to the VA. The C2 anterior branch is a good landmark in the exposure of the VA at this level. The C1 nerve root runs underneath the VA in the groove of the posterior arch of the atlas and emerges at the middle of the groove.

The proximal segment (from the VA origin to C6) is exposed through the same approach. However, it is sometimes easier to pass between the IJV and the internal carotid artery. At this level, the VA is not in the transverse canal and has no periosteal sheath. There are usually two vertebral veins anterior and posterior to the VA. The inferior thyroid artery crosses the field horizontally anterior to the VA. The lymphatic duct and a variable number of lymphatic vessels are running in the fatty sheath. They must be carefully controlled and ligated to avoid postoperative lymphocele or leakage. To control the proximal segment of the VA, one way is to go directly to it; another way is to go to the C6 transverse process and to start by the exposure of the VA inside the C6 transverse foramen, then to progress inferiorly toward the VA origin.

The anterolateral approach is not designed to expose the intracranial segment. However, it can be achieved after having exposed the VA in the groove of the atlas and having opened the inferolateral part of the occipital bone up to the mastoïd process and to the occipital condyle. The dura is then opened in a horizontal T-shaped fashion, giving two triangles, one based on the sigmoid sinus and the other one based on the condyle. In the supine operative position, the cerebellum falls away by gravity, and the VA is easily seen in the depth. It is crossed posteriorly by the medullary root of cranial nerve (CN) XI and CN XII rootlets. The exposure is not very comfortable because the occipital condyle is in the way. This is why many authors propose to drill off the condyle. However, there is no reason to destroy the condyle and the C0–C1 joint if they are intact because the posterolateral approach can be used instead of the anterolateral one and permits the surgeon to preserve these structures.

Posterolateral Approach

For the posterolateral approach (**Fig. 31–3**) the patient is in a sitting (or occasionally in the prone or lateral) position.

The skin incision is vertical in the midline up to the occipital protuberance and then curved laterally along the occipital line.

The occipital bone, posterior arch of the atlas, and laminae of C2 are subperiosteally exposed. Then the periosteum of the posterior arch is elevated from its medial to lateral and inferior to superior parts. So progressing, the groove of the atlas is reached, and the VA within the periosteal sheath is exposed. The inferior aspect of the VA is easily visible by elevation of the periosteal sheath. Conversely, the superior aspect is more difficult to expose because the periosteal sheath must be separated from the occipitoatlantal membrane and the C0–C1 joint capsule. In some cases, this membrane may be calcified or even ossified, turning the VA groove into a tunnel, which makes the VA exposure even more difficult. At this point, the posterior aspect of the lateral wall of the FM is visible, including, from superior to inferior, the jugular tubercle, condyle, lateral mass of the atlas with the VA groove, and C1–C2 joint crossed by the C2 nerve root. The exposure can be extended laterally as far as the transverse foramen of C1 and the VA C1–C2 segment. However, the posterolateral approach is basically designed for the segment of the VA above C1 and the intracranial segment.

To expose the intracranial segment of the artery, the inferior part of the occipital bone and the posterior arch of the atlas are resected. Then, according to which space, the superior, inferior, or both sides of the VA have to be opened, and a part of the condyle or the lateral mass of the atlas or both are drilled away. This drilling is always very limited and never exceeds the medial third of these structures. Then the dura is opened by a vertical paramedian incision curved laterally at both extremities. A horizontal dural incision is made toward the VA running either superior or inferior or on both sides of the VA according to the space that needs to be opened. The VA passes under the first arch of the dentate ligament, which is cut. The medullary root of CN XI runs posterior to the dentate ligament; it is connected to the first nerve root and then crosses the posterior aspect of the VA. Next, as one follows the VA up to the vertebrobasilar junction, the rootlets of CN XII and then of the lower cranial nerves (IX, X, XI) are encountered crossing the posterior aspect of the VA. To go up to the vertebrobasilar junction, the jugular tubercle must have been drilled away extradurally as much as possible. So doing, instruments are passing easily in an axis parallel to the VA without any retraction of the medulla oblongata.

Oblique Corpectomy from C7 to C3

For an oblique corpectomy (**Figs. 31–4 and 31–5**), after the exposure of the VA and of the lateral aspect of the chosen vertebral bodies, the posterolateral corners of the vertebral bodies are drilled off.[13] At the maximum extent of the drilling, the opposite pedicle is reached, thus giving access to the anterior aspect of the spinal cord (**Fig. 31–4**). At the minimum extent of the drilling, it enlarges the intervertebral foramen (IF), giving exposure of the proximal part of the nerve roots from its junction with the dural sac to the VA and then if necessary lateral to the VA up to the brachial plexus.

Juxtacondylar Approach to the Jugular Foramen

After an anterolateral approach to the suboccipital VA segment (C2 to FM), the VA is transposed medially out of the C1 transverse foramen. Then a partial mastoidectomy gives exposure of the distal part of the sigmoid sinus. Next, the bone remaining between the end of the sigmoid sinus and the origin of the IJV is resected. This bone corresponds to the jugular tubercle and to the posteroinferior wall of the JF[16] (**Fig. 31–1D**).

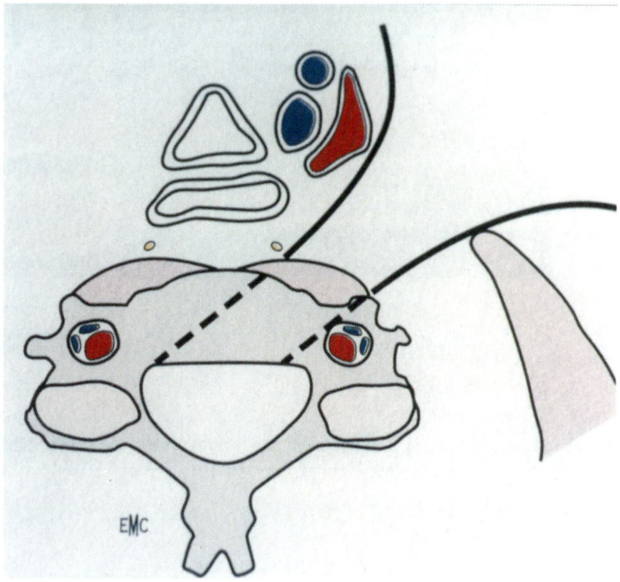

Figure 31–4 Oblique corpectomy technique. Schematic drawing showing the surgical route lateral to the vascular nervous elements and between the dotted lines, the extent of bone drilling for a complete exposure of the anterior aspect of the spinal cord. (With permission from George B. Myélopathie cervicarthrosique. In: Encyclopédie pratique de Médecine 5-0990 . Paris: Elsevier; 1998:1–4.)

Lateral Bone Grafting

Through the anterolateral approach, tumors invading the condyle, lateral mass of the atlas, anterior arch, and odontoid can be removed. Therefore, the stability of the craniocervical junction may be compromised and may require a fusion procedure. This fusion is usually realized by a posterior plating between the occipital bone and the first cervical vertebrae through a posterior approach in a second stage. However, in some cases, an iliac bone graft can be impacted between C2 and what is remaining of the condyle through the same anterolateral approach. No plating is necessary.

Vertebral Artery Revascularization

Proximal Reimplantation

The lower cervical part of the CCA and the proximal segment of the VA are controlled. Then the VA is divided distal to the lesion (generally atherosclerotic plaque); the VA is mobilized up to the posterior aspect of the CCA. The CCA is clamped with a U-shaped clamp, and a longitudinal opening (6 × 4 mm on average) is made on its posterior wall. The proximal end of the VA is cut obliquely to match the CCA wall opening. An end-to-side anastomosis is achieved using monofilament 7-0 sutures.

Distal Anastomosis

The VA is fully controlled with opening of the periosteal sheath between the C1 and C2 transverse foramina. Occasionally, one

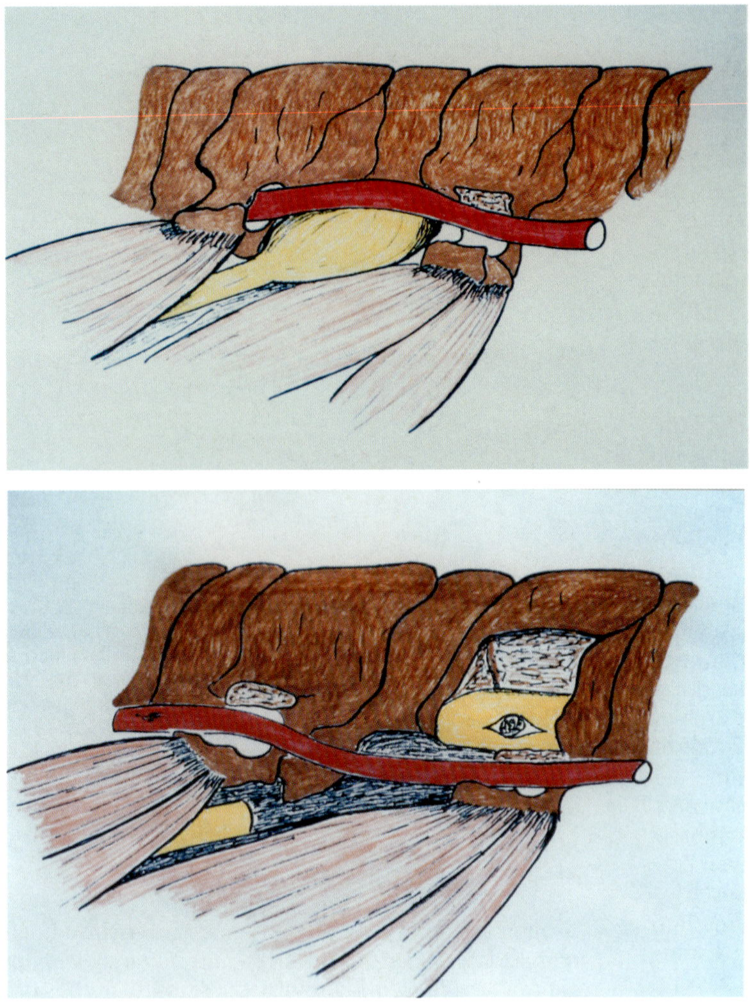

A

B

Figure 31–5 Oblique corpectomy technique to remove an hourglass neurinoma. **(A)** Exposure of the vertebral artery, distal nerve root, and tumor through an anterolateral approach. **(B)** Operative view after tumoral resection. The nerve root has been cut distally and proximally at the junction with the dural sac. (With permission from Lot G, George B. Cervical neuromas with extradural components: surgical management in a series of 57 patients. Neurosurgery 1997;41:813–822.)

or both of these foramina are opened so as to increase the available length. Then the CCA is exposed 4 cm inferior to the carotid bifurcation. A saphenous vein graft is harvested in the thigh. Distal implantation of the vein graft on the C1–C2 VA segment is performed end to side using 7–0 sutures. Proximal implantation is then achieved on the CCA end to side using 6–0 sutures.

Whatever the level of anastomosis, Heifetz or temporary aneurysmal clips are very efficient for clamping the VA. They occupy very limited space, so they leave enough room for suturing.

Closure

For the anterolateral approach, closure is very simple because only the platysma muscle and the skin have to be sutured. However, after the exposure of the suboccipital segment of the VA, the SM muscle must be very tightly reattached to the mastoid process.

After the posterolateral approach, the muscles are sutured in two or three layers similar to a standard midline approach to the posterior fossa.

◆ Complications

Related to the Exposure of the Vertebral Artery

The main risk is VA injury during exposure if an abnormal VA course has not been recognized[18] (VA entrance into the transverse canal at the C5, C4, or even C3 level; intradural course of the VA from the C2 level; displacement of the VA by a tumoral compression).

Horner's syndrome is sometimes observed postoperatively after VA exposure of the proximal and transversary segment. If the main trunk of the sympathetic chain has been preserved, Horner's syndrome is mild and recovers rapidly.

Lymph oozing must be avoided by careful ligation of every lymphatic vessel.

Accessory nerve stretching due to excessive retraction of the SM muscle may produce pain, stiffness, or even palsy of the trapezius muscle.

Related to the Pathology of Foramen Magnum Tumors

Obviously, in the case of FM tumors, there is a potential risk of injury of the lower cranial nerves, the brain stem, the intracranial VA, and VA branches. Using the lateral approach, these complications must be very limited. In our series of 117 cases, all the patients improved except one, who retained some preoperative swallowing difficulties and three who died from pulmonary embolism, air embolism, and poor preoperative condition with coma and tetraplegia, respectively.

Related to Jugular Foramen Tumors

Using the juxtacondylar approach, the petrous bone drilling is avoided or limited. The facial nerve is not to be transposed and is kept in its fallopian canal, so the risk of facial nerve palsy is very reduced. This approach also permits very good control of the lower cranial nerves. For schwannomas, only the rootlets involved in the tumor have to be divided.

◆ Conclusion

Exposure of the VA is possible at any level from its origin to the vertebrobasilar junction. The anterolateral approach permits the surgeon to expose any segment, including the intracranial one. The posterolateral approach gives access to the suboccipital and intracranial segments. Being able to expose and control the VA offers many possibilities: removal of tumors, release of VA compression by osteophytes, fibrous bands, and other factors; revascularization of VA stenosis and occlusion; oblique corpectomy for spinal decompression (spondylotic myelopathy, tumors, etc.); removal of FM and JF tumors. In most cases, the VA flow may be preserved or restored, and the morbidity related to exposure and control of the VA is very limited.

◆ Illustrative Cases

Case 1: C3 Dumbbell Neurinoma with Intradural Extension—Anterolateral Approach without Fusion

A 30-year-old man presented with a 2-year history of neck pain, mostly at night, then paresthesia and hypesthesia of the right hand, and finally difficulty with walking and writing over the last 2 months. Neurological exam showed pyramidal signs on the four limbs, with motor deficit of the right hand and the right leg and sensory disturbances on both hands. Computed tomographic (CT) scan and MRI demonstrated features of a dumbbell tumor at the C2–C3 level, most likely suggesting a neurinoma with intradural, foraminal, and extraspinal components (**Fig. 31–6**).

In another institution, a posterior approach had only removed a small part of the intradural component. The patient was referred to us, and complete surgical resection was achieved 10 days later using an anterolateral approach. The distal C3 root was divided after its stimulation showed no response. The VA was exposed on both sides of the tumor by unroofing the C2 and C3 transverse foramina. Then the foraminal tumoral part was resected. Next, after having enlarged the foramen by drilling the adjacent vertebral bodies, the intraspinal intradural tumoral component was removed through a small vertical opening of the dura. Finally, the proximal nerve root was cut ~3 mm from the spinal cord. Dural defect was occluded by packing the fatty sheath with its vascular pedicles still in the IF. Follow-up was uneventful except for some cerebrospinal fluid (CSF) subcutaneous accumulation, which spontaneously resolved in 2 weeks (**Fig. 31–7**).

Case 2: Osteoblastoma of C2—Anterolateral Approach, Oblique Drilling without Fusion

A 20-year-old man presented with a 2-year history of pain and stiffness of the neck not improved by medical treatment and physiotherapy. CT scan (**Fig. 31–8**) and MRI showed a bone lesion within the right lateral part of the C2 vertebral body. Complete surgical resection was achieved using the anterolateral approach. The VA was exposed at the C3 and C2 levels with opening of the transverse foramina. A vascular tumor infiltrating the posterolateral corner of the C2 vertebral body was resected. To ensure radical resection, the peripheral bone was drilled out (**Fig. 31–9**). Histological diagnosis was osteoblastoma. Follow-up was uneventful.

A

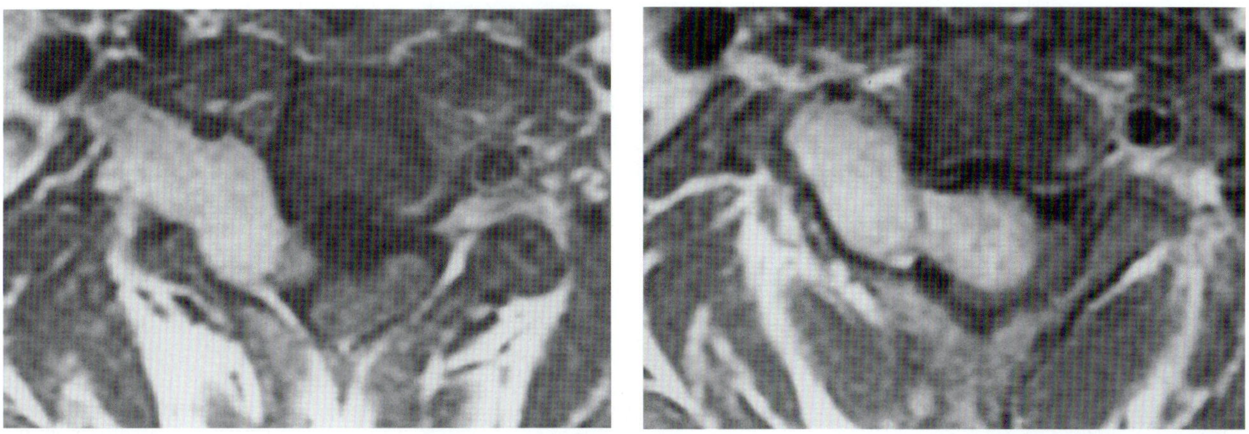

B

Figure 31–6 **(A,B)** Preoperative magnetic resonance imaging axial views.

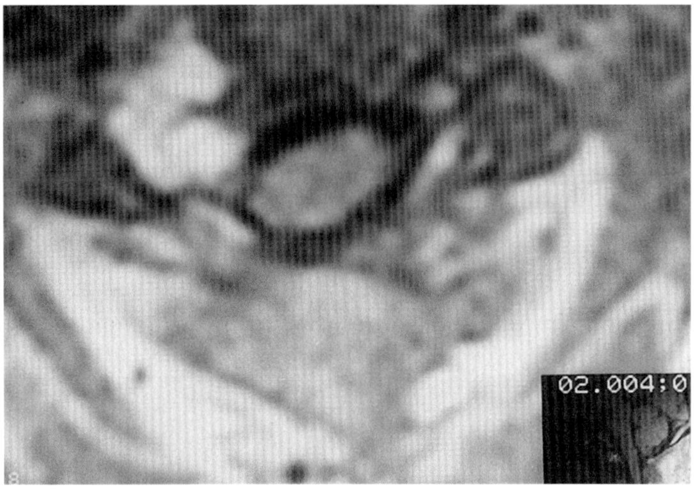

A

Figure 31–7 Postoperative magnetic resonance imaging axial view. **(A)** The fat filling the space after tumoral resection and computed tomographic coronal views. **(B)** The bone defects after drilling of the foramen edges.

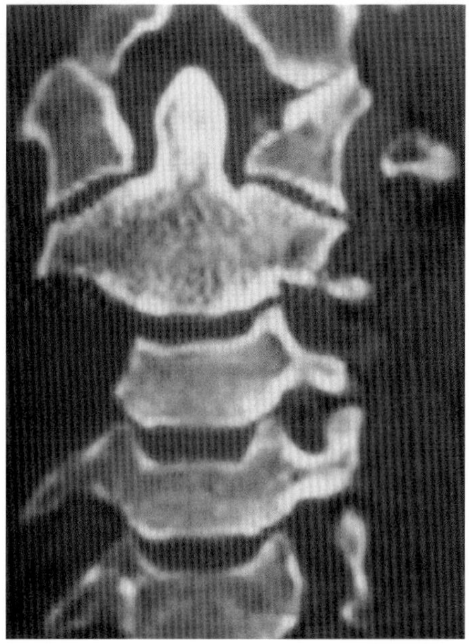

B

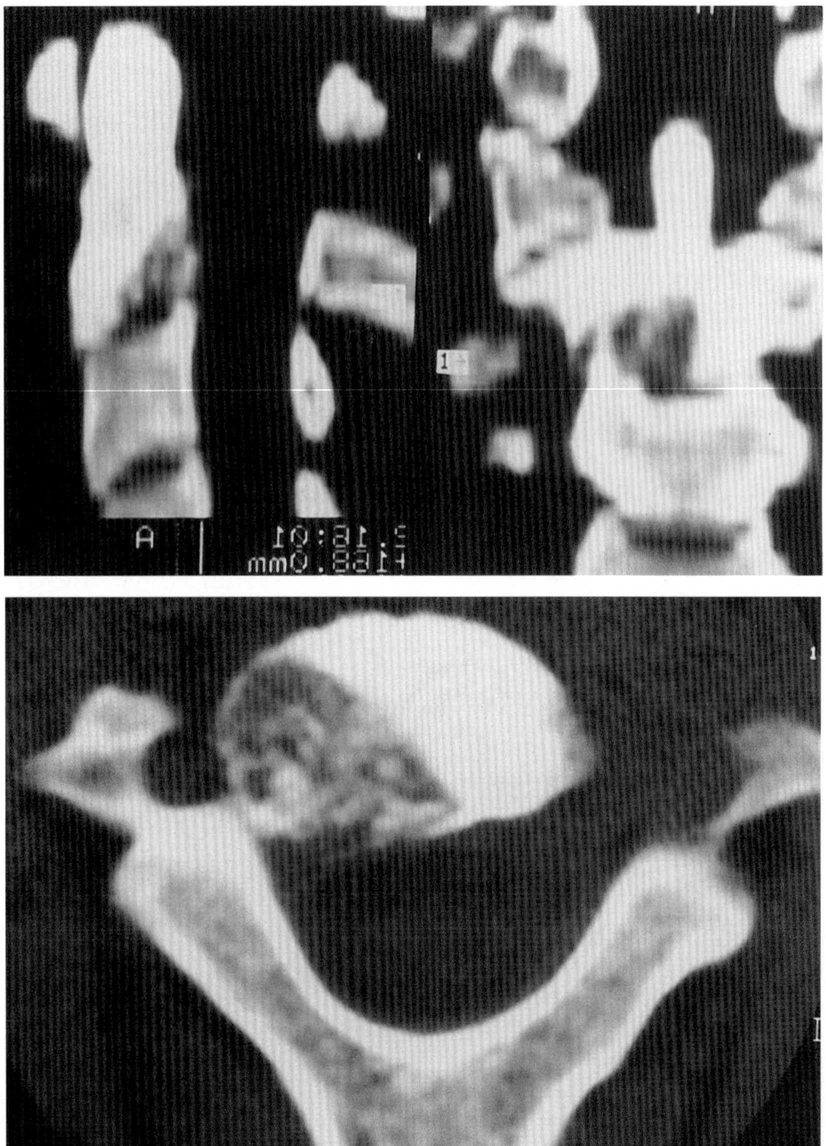

A B C

Figure 31–8 Preoperative computed tomographic scan. **(A)** Sagittal, **(B)** coronal, and **(C)** axial views.

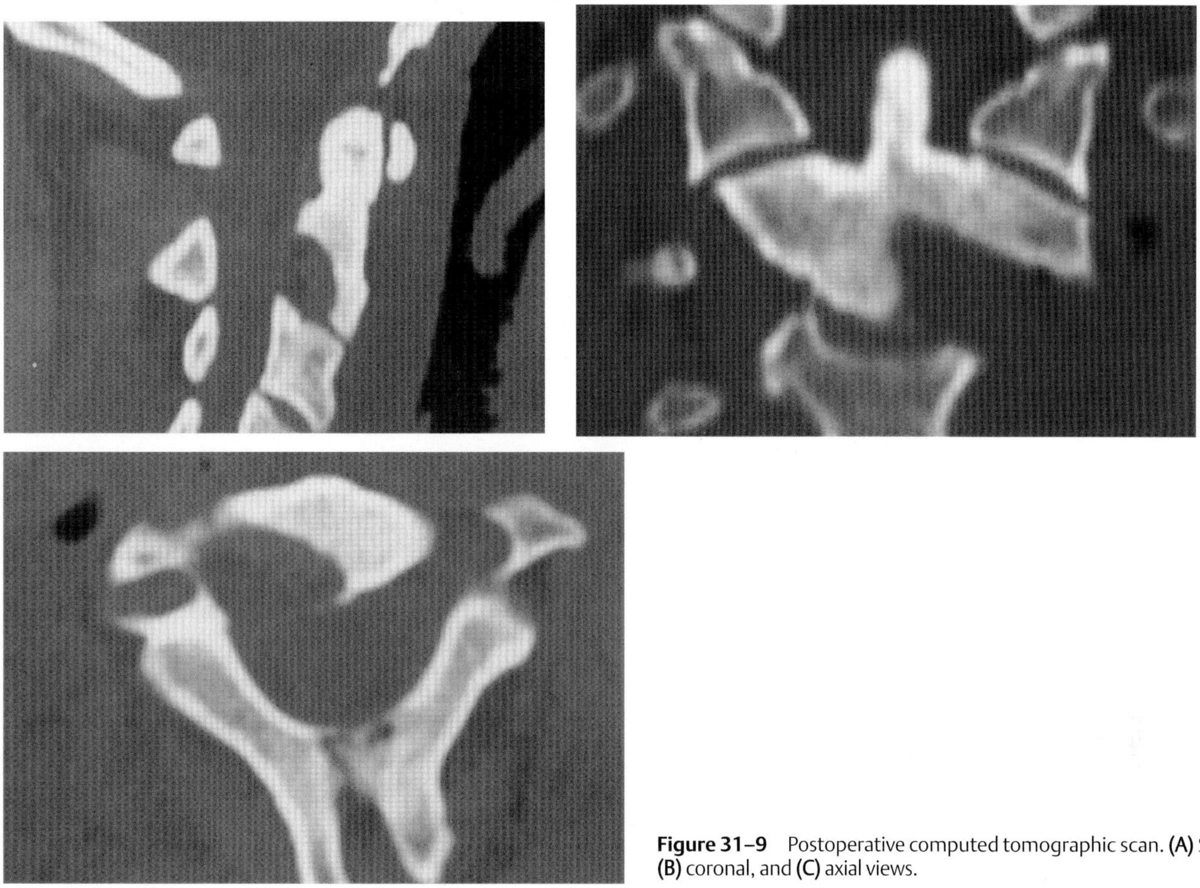

A B C

Figure 31–9 Postoperative computed tomographic scan. **(A)** Sagittal, **(B)** coronal, and **(C)** axial views.

Case 3: Osteoid Osteoma of the Lateral Mass of the Atlas—Anterolateral Approach without Fusion

A 27-year-old woman presented with a 10-year history of suboccipital pain, mostly on the right side. In another institution surgical removal of a bony lesion of the lateral mass of the atlas had failed with use of a posterior approach. Persisting pain led to referral to our department. CT demonstrated a heterogeneous bony lesion surrounded by hyperdense bone reaction located in the medial part of the lateral mass of the atlas (**Fig. 31–10**). Complete resection including part of the peripheral bone was achieved through an anterolateral approach with exposure and medial transposition of the VA from the C2 transverse process to the FM dura (**Fig. 31–11**). Histological diagnosis was osteoid osteoma. Follow-up was uneventful.

Case 4: Anterior Foramen Magnum Meningioma—Posterolateral Approach

A 38-year-old woman presented with a long history of neck pain following a cervical injury, with 4 years of neuralgia in the right arm. Over the last 5 months, she had developed weakness and sensory loss in the right arm and walking difficulties. MRI demonstrated an anterior meningioma with predominant right lateral extension and location below the VA (**Fig. 31–12**). Complete surgical removal was achieved through a right posterolateral approach with control of the VA above the arch of the atlas. No drilling of the condyle and lateral mass of the atlas was realized (**Fig. 31–13**). Follow-up was uneventful.

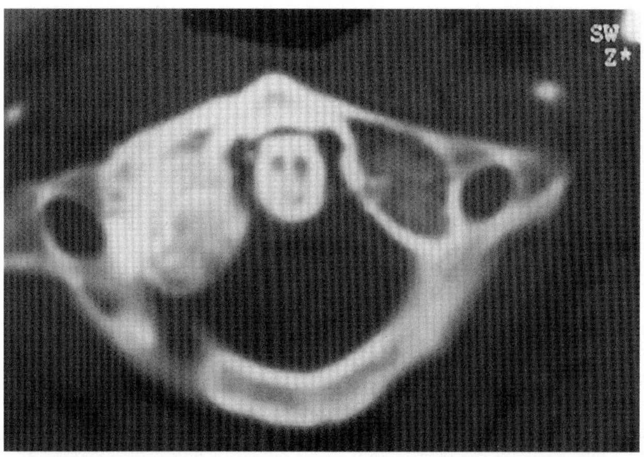

Figure 31–10 Preoperative computed tomographic scan, axial view.

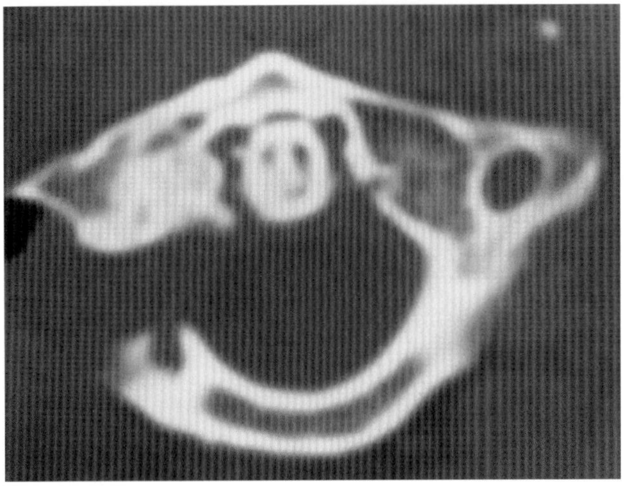

Figure 31–11 Postoperative computed tomographic scan, axial view.

Case 5: Paraganglioma of the Jugular Foramen—Combined Juxtacondylar and Infratemporal Approach without Facial Nerve Transposition

A 60-year-old woman presented with a 2-year history of pulsatile tinnitus and decreased hearing. Neurological exam showed symptoms of CN IX and X dysfunction. CT and MRI demonstrated a JF tumor with foraminal and intracranial intradural extension up to the internal auditory canal (**Fig. 31–14**). Angiography showed typical features of a paraganglioma with vascular supply from the ascending pharyngeal and stylomastoidian arteries. Microparticle embolization was realized preoperatively. Complete resection could be achieved in one stage using a combined infratemporal and juxtacondylar approach. The VA was controlled from C2 to the FM dura, with complete resection of the C1 transverse process. The JF was first opened inferiorly by drilling out the jugular tubercle, then superiorly by petrous

A 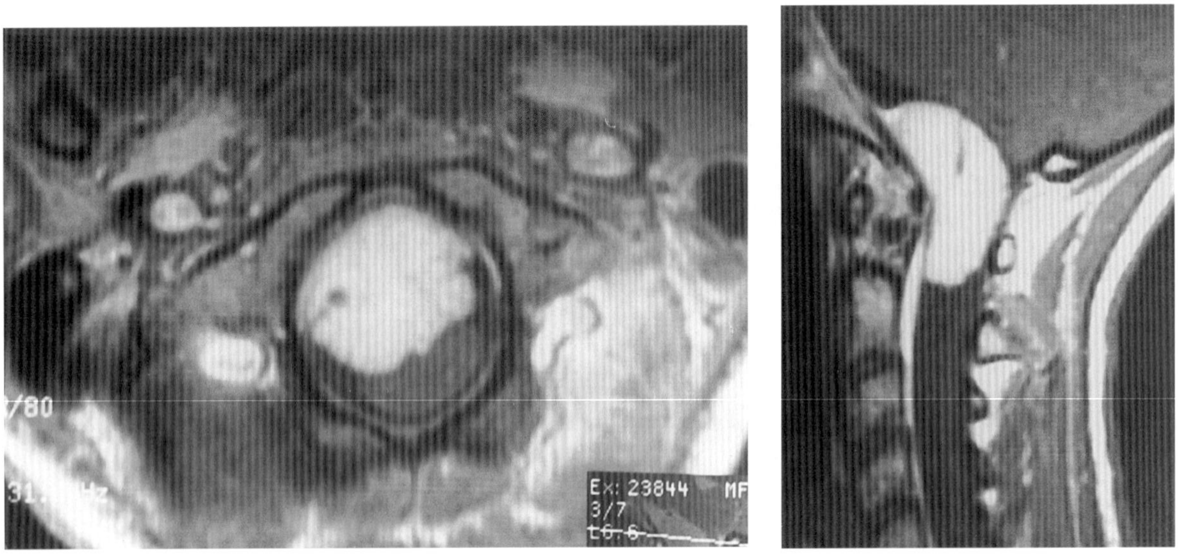

B

Figure 31–12 Preoperative magnetic resonance (**A**) axial and (**B**) sagittal views.

A 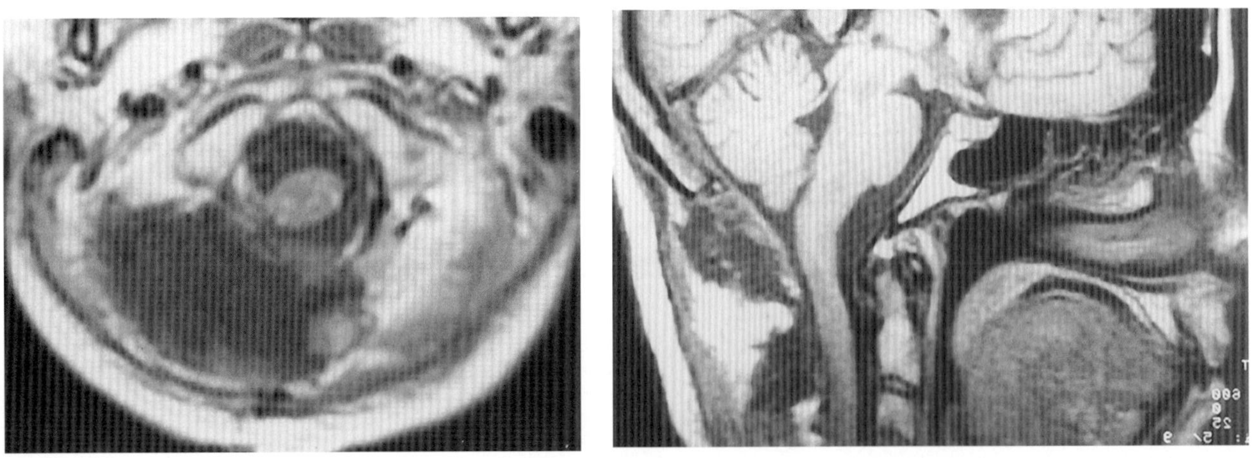 B

Figure 31–13 Postoperative magnetic resonance imaging (**A**) axial and (**B**) sagittal views. Notice the integrity of the occipital condyle and lateral mass of the atlas.

A
B
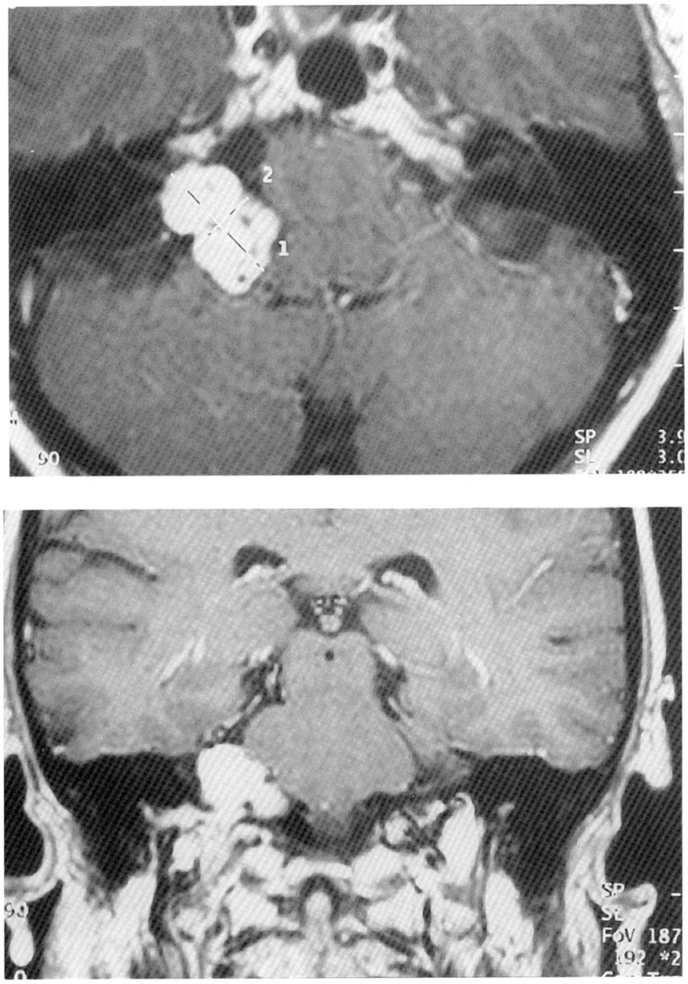

Figure 31–14 Preoperative magnetic resonance imaging **(A)** axial and **(B)** coronal views.

bone drilling. The vertical petrosal segment of the internal carotid artery was exposed as well as the facial nerve in its second and third portion while keeping a bony shell around the nerve and preserving the integrity of the labyrinthine bloc (**Fig. 31–15**). Only CN X and XII could be kept intact because CN IX and XI were infiltrated by the tumor. External lumbar drainage was placed at the beginning of surgery and removed on the fourth postoperative day. Follow-up was uneventful except for mild and transient swallowing difficulties.

A
B
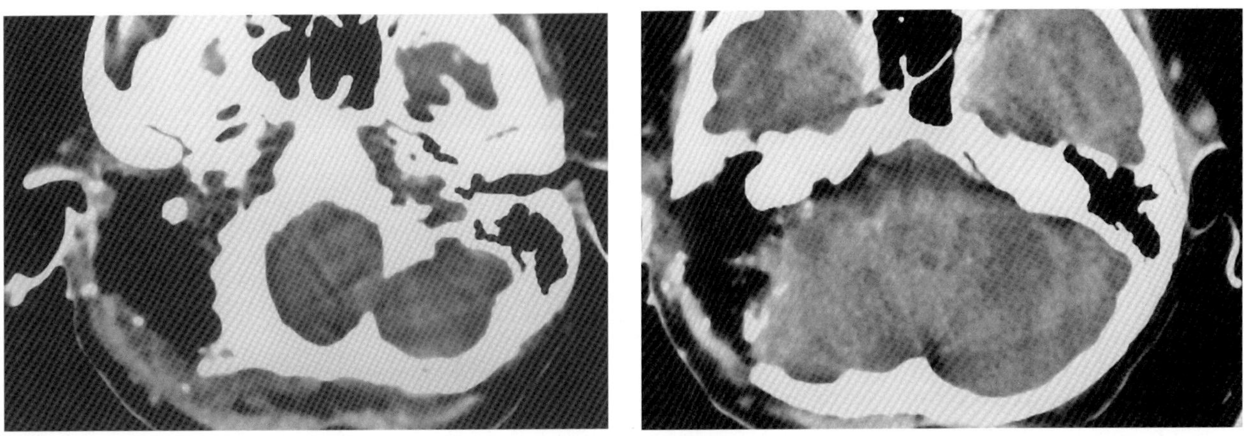

Figure 31–15 **(A,B)** Postoperative computed tomographic scan axial views at two different levels. Notice the integrity of the labyrinthine bloc.

References

1. Maisonneuve JG, Favrot A. Observation de ligature de l'artère vertébrale. Journal des Connaissances médico-chirurgicales 1852;11:181
2. Cate WR, Scott HN. Cerebral ischemia of central origin: relief by subclavian vertebral artery thrombo-endarterectomy. Surgery 1959;45:19–31
3. Matas R. Traumatisms and traumatic aneurysms of the vertebral artery, and their surgical treatment with report of a cured case. Ann Surg 1893;18:477–516
4. Elkin DC, Harris MH. Arteriovenous aneurysm of the vertebral vessels: report of ten cases. Ann Surg 1946;124:934–951
5. Henry AK. Exposures of long bones and other surgical methods. Cited in the author's book: Extensile Exposures (Wright 1927). Edinburgh, London: Livingstone; 1966:58–66
6. Corkill G, French BH, Michas C, Cobb GA 3rd, Mims TJ. External carotid vertebral artery anastomosis for vertebro-basilar insufficiency. Surg Neurol 1977;7:109–115
7. George B, Laurian C. The Vertebral Artery: Pathology and Surgery. Berlin: Springer Verlag; 1987
8. George B, Laurian C. Surgical approach to the whole length of the vertebral artery with special reference to the third portion. (Acta Neurochir) New York: Wien; j1980;51:259–272
9. George B, Lot G. Anterolateral and posterolateral approaches to the foramen magnum: technical description and experience from 97 cases. Skull Base Surg 1995;5:9–19
10. George B, Laurian C, Keravel Y, et al. Extra-dural and hourglass cervical neurinomas: the vertebral artery problem. Neurosurgery 1985;16: 591–594
11. George B, Laurian C. Indications for revascularization of the distal cervical vertebral artery [in French]. Ann Med Interne (Paris) 1986;137: 108–111
12. George B, Laurian C. Impairment of vertebral artery flow caused by extrinsic lesions. Neurosurgery 1989;24:206–214
13. George B, Zerah M, Lot G, et al. Oblique transcorporeal approach to anteriorly located lesions in the cervical spinal canal. Acta Neurochir (Wien) 1993;121:187–190
14. George B, Lot G, Velut S, et al. Tumors of the foramen magnum [in French]. French Speaking Society of Neurosurgery. 44th Annual Congress. Brussels, 8–12 June 1993. Neurochirurgie 1993;39(Suppl 1): 1–89
15. George B, Lot G. Neurinomas of the first two cervical nerve roots: a series of 42 cases. J Neurosurg 1995;82:917–923
16. George B, Lot G, Tran Ba Huy P. The juxtacondylar approach to the jugular foramen (without petrous bone drilling). Surg Neurol 1995; 44:279–284
17. George B, Lot G. Foramen magnum meningiomas: a review from personal experience of 37 cases and from a cooperative study of 106 cases. Neurosurgery Quarterly 1995;5:149–161
18. Francke JP, Dimarino V, Pannier M, et al. Les artères vertébrales: segments atlanto-axoïdiens V3 et intra-crânien V4 collatéraux. Anat Clin 1980;2:229–242

Section V

Brain Tumors

- 32. General Principles of Brain Tumor Surgery
- 33. Stereotactic Biopsy
- 34. The Surgical Management of High-Grade Astrocytomas
- 35A. Oligodendroglioma
- 35B. Ganglion Cell Tumors
- 35C. Cerebellar Astrocytomas
- 36. Brain Stem and Cervicomedullary Tumors
- 37. Metastatic Brain Tumors
- 38. Tumors in Eloquent Areas
- 39. Convexity Meningiomas
- 40. Torcular and Peritorcular Meningiomas

32

General Principles of Brain Tumor Surgery

Raymond Sawaya

The performance of a craniotomy has greatly evolved since the pioneering work of neurosurgical giants such as Cushing and Dandy in the first half of the twentieth century.[1,2] This is largely due to improved diagnostic imaging studies, enhanced physiological understanding of the nervous system, and great advancements in the creation and design of surgical adjuncts such as the operating microscope, intraoperative ultrasonography, cortical mapping, and image guidance devices, to name just a few.[3] These advances have enhanced the ability of the surgeon to completely resect benign as well as malignant brain tumors with preservation of neurological function in the majority of patients. The introduction of new or improved surgical adjuncts, however, is only intended to be coupled with meticulous techniques and the judgment and wisdom that come with experience and practice. The limits of operability of a brain tumor have been expanded to include all but a few exceptions, and the role of surgery has assumed increasing importance as the alternative therapies have reached the plateau of their effectiveness.[4–6] For surgical excision to be beneficial, strict adherence to basic principles and techniques cannot be overemphasized. This chapter reviews our current understanding and approach employed in performing a craniotomy for a brain tumor.

◆ Strategy

Regardless of the symptomatology, a patient requiring a craniotomy typically presents with a computed tomographic (CT) or magnetic resonance imaging (MRI) scan showing a mass lesion. The decision-making process at this point must take into consideration the necessity and the feasibility of performing a craniotomy and removing the mass. To this end, a careful history taking, physical examination, and detailed assessment of the diagnostic images are essential to arrive at the appropriate decision. For instance, having a patient present with a past history of cancer and a symptomatology that does not correspond anatomically to the location of an intracranial mass lesion might suggest the presence of leptomeningeal disease in that patient and may lead to a lumbar puncture instead of a craniotomy for the establishment of a diagnosis.

The evaluation of the diagnostic images is the next most critical step in decision making. As a rule, high-resolution MRI is preferred to CT scans unless the bony structures at the base of the skull are involved, in which case both CT and MRI are required. In analyzing the images, the first consideration is directed toward a differential diagnosis. Could the lesion be nonneoplastic, such as an inflammatory mass as seen in sarcoidosis; vascular, representing an evolving infarction; or autoimmune, as in multiple sclerosis? Each of these conditions will require a specific diagnostic workup that will probably not include a craniotomy. Within the neoplastic categories, the main consideration lies in the benefit of the craniotomy over other treatment modalities, including watchful follow-up and no intervention whatsoever, as in the case of an asymptomatic calcified lesion that is not exerting any mass effect on the surrounding brain parenchyma. For the majority of lesions that do require an intervention, careful attention must be given to conditions that are less likely to benefit from a resection and that are predominantly treated by medical means. Examples of such conditions are lymphoma, germinoma, and small-cell lung carcinoma. If one is in doubt, the diagnosis of these conditions is usually best made via a stereotactic biopsy.[7,8]

At this point in the decision whether to perform a craniotomy, the benefit to the patient from the resection is weighed against the risk to the patient's quality of life. Having excluded the relatively rare conditions already highlighted, the majority of brain neoplasms are best controlled following a gross-total resection. This includes gliomas of all grades, metastases, and meningiomas. Together, these categories represent approximately 90% of all intracranial neoplasms. The role of alternative therapies is beyond the scope

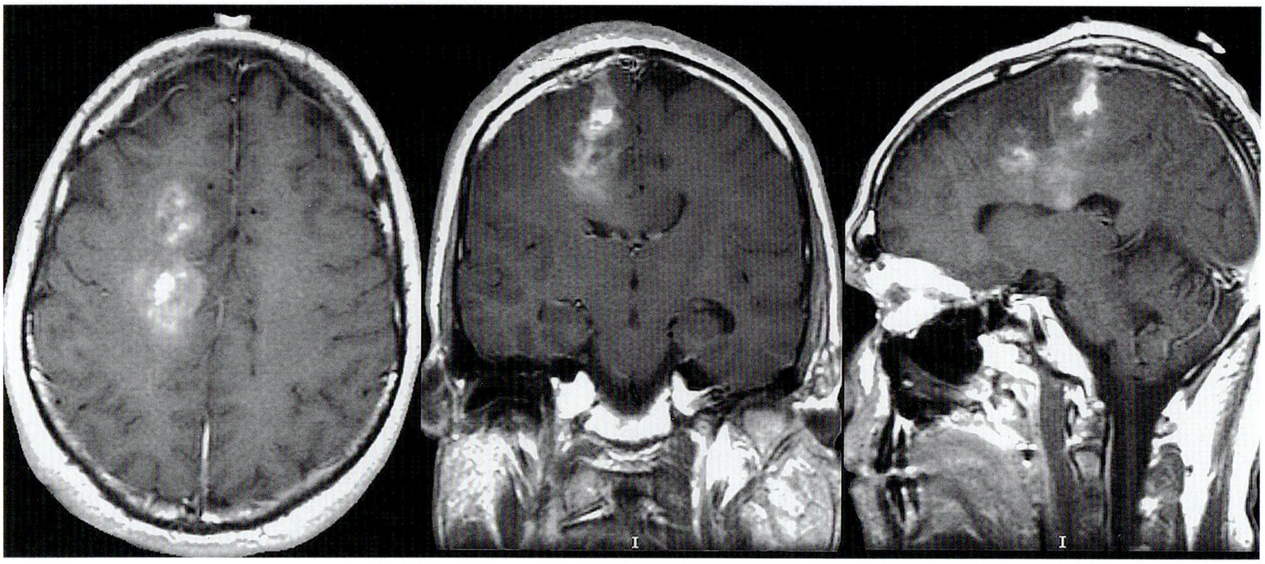

Figure 32–1 Gadolinium contrast-enhanced, T1-weighted magnetic resonance images showing a right posterior frontal irregularly enhancing mass in the axial (left), coronal (middle), and sagittal (right) planes. Note the extension of the tumor into the corpus callosum. A fiducial marker for the image-guided surgery is seen in the middle of the patient's forehead in the axial view.

of this chapter and is covered in the references cited as well as in other chapters that discuss the specific diseases in question. The benefit expected from the resection is also based on its feasibility. To this end, MRI provides a clear sense of the size, location, proximity to eloquent brain, and boundaries of the mass, or masses if more than one lesion is present (**Fig. 32–1**). Each of these characteristics presents special issues. For instance, a mass that is less than 5 mm in diameter will most likely be followed with a repeat MRI at a later date. A mass in the center of the pons that does not reach the surface of the brain stem will be considered inoperable. However, proximity to eloquent brain is no longer a contraindication to resection because the majority of patients (85% or more) will not sustain a major neurological deficit as a result of the operation.[9] The feature of an intracranial mass that is the most discouraging to surgical intervention is the presence of boundaries that are ill-defined, especially if the mass is multicentric, is near eloquent brain, or traverses critical anatomical structures such as the sylvian fissure or the basal ganglia.

Throughout this assessment, the surgeon must consider the overall physical and psychological health of the patient and the level of skill and expertise available to tackle the tumor. An honest and open discussion will help the patient and the family understand all the issues that are necessary for making the decision and for building trust. In complex situations, second opinions from other centers of excellence in the field should be encouraged.

◆ Preparation

As highlighted in the previous paragraph, a careful history and high-quality MRI provide the essentials for a preoperative evaluation. Depending on the age and medical condition of the patient, a chest x-ray and an electrocardiogram (ECG) might be required. Typically, the former is done for patients over 40 years old and the latter in patients over 60 years old. Laboratory tests are limited to a complete blood count (CBC) with a platelet count and electrolytes. A blood typing and screen is ordered only for patients who are likely to require a transfusion perioperatively. A prothrombin time (PT), partial thromboplastin time (PTT), bleeding time, and other hemostatic tests are ordered only if the history suggests a bleeding disorder. A systemic radiographic workup is frequently completed in patients known to have cancer and includes CT scans of the chest and abdomen and sometimes a bone scan. Cerebral angiography is not required for intrinsic brain tumors but is an important adjunct to surgery in many basal tumors.

Medications prescribed prior to the operation are primarily those needed to prevent seizures in patients who have had seizures as a presenting symptom. Phenytoin is among those most commonly used, at a dose of 100 mg tid. Antiepileptic drugs are otherwise not recommended for routine use unless the operation involves the temporal lobe or will result in extensive cortical scarring. Steroids are also not routinely prescribed unless the tumor is surrounded by vasogenic edema, in which case dexamethasone is given at a dose of 4 mg every 6 hours along with Pepcid, an H_2 blocker, at a dose of 20 mg every 12 hours.

The operative consent form is explained in detail and is signed by the patient or caregiver in the presence of a witness. In addition, consent by the patient to receive blood transfusions may also be required. It is only after all questions have been answered that the patient is referred to the preoperative anesthesia area for further assessment by the anesthesia staff. To facilitate communication with the operating room (OR) team, a form that describes the patient's medical condition and surgical requirements is sent with the patient for review by the anesthesiologist. A second form is faxed to the OR nursing team to inform them of the specific positioning of the patient and the needs for instruments that will be used during surgery. Whether cortical mapping or image-guided surgery or both will be used and the type of retractor, power drill, and bipolar cautery apparatus needed by the surgeon are typical examples of things that need to be communicated to the OR personnel.

◆ Surgical Technique

Anesthesia

The main goals of anesthetic management in patients with intracranial pathology are to (1) maintain stable cerebral perfusion pressure (CPP), (2) maintain neuronal homeostasis, (3) achieve optimal brain relaxation, and (4) provide a smooth transition into the postoperative period. Hemodynamic variables are monitored with beat to beat arterial blood pressure to rapidly detect any changes in CPP. In addition, continuous intraoperative ECG monitoring is used to detect early ischemia and dysrhythmias. Hemodynamic monitoring with central venous pressure or pulmonary artery catheterization is performed if the patient's medical condition warrants it. Core temperature can be monitored conveniently with the esophageal stethoscope. Pulse oximetry and capnography are now routinely monitored, along with urine output.

Induction of anesthesia is usually achieved with a combination of intravenous short-acting benzodiazepines (midazolam), hypnotic agents, and nondepolarizing muscle relaxants. Barbiturates (thiopental 3–5 mg/kg) are most frequently used in neurosurgical patients because of their beneficial effects on reducing cerebral metabolic rate of oxygen ($CMRO_2$) and intracranial pressure (ICP). Narcotics (fentanyl, sufentanil) are best administered after the neuromuscular blockade is complete because chest rigidity associated with even small doses of these drugs can markedly increase ICP. Dexamethasone (10 mg, IV) is administered prior to induction of anesthesia. Once the induction is complete and the patient's condition is stable, 1 g of cefazolin is administered IV, or if the patient is allergic to penicillin, vancomycin (1 g) is used. Anticonvulsants can also be given IV if required. A Foley catheter is inserted at this time, and compression stockings and pneumatic compression boots are applied to both calves.

Anesthesia is maintained with a combination of volatile agents, small doses of narcotics, and muscle relaxants. Isoflurane is the agent of choice in neurosurgery because it produces a much smaller, if any, increase in cerebral blood flow (CBF), while at the same time decreasing $CMRO_2$ to a much greater degree than halothane and enflurane, thus offering cerebral protective effects similar to thiopental. In addition, isoflurane increases ICP only slightly.

In the past, it was common practice to limit fluid administration in the neurosurgical patient to what was absolutely necessary to maintain hemodynamic stability. However, in view of the current understanding of the mechanisms responsible for water transfer across the intact or pathologically altered blood–brain barrier, fluid management has changed. Only iso-osmolar fluids are now used in these patients to provide a hemodynamically stable intraoperative course, to maintain adequate cerebral perfusion, and to preserve neuronal homeostasis. Glucose-containing solutions and hyperglycemia are avoided because of their negative effect on neurological outcome in ischemic cerebral injury.[10]

Smooth emergence of the patient from anesthesia is probably one of the most important and challenging goals in neuroanesthetic practice. Hypertension, bucking, and coughing on the endotracheal tube can threaten the delicate hemostasis achieved in the operative bed at the conclusion of the surgery and cause hemorrhaging and all its associated consequences. Intravenous lidocaine and small doses of barbiturates or propofol are useful adjuncts to help patients have a smooth emergence.[11] Hemodynamic stability can be achieved with minimal effect on cerebral circulation by the judicious use of β-blockers or calcium channel blockers.

Positioning

Once the intubation is completed, attention is directed toward positioning the patient. The overriding principle guiding this step is that of enhancing the exposure to the tumor while maintaining the patient's comfort and safety. A Mayfield clamp is firmly attached to the patient's head with the three points of fixation placed as far away from the incision as possible and with the vertical arms of the clamp kept perpendicular to the floor regardless of whether the head is straight or rotated to either side (**Fig. 32–2**). Prior to the attachment of the head to the table, the body is adjusted to maintain a physiological neck position. The patient's head can be turned as far as 45 degrees to one side with the body

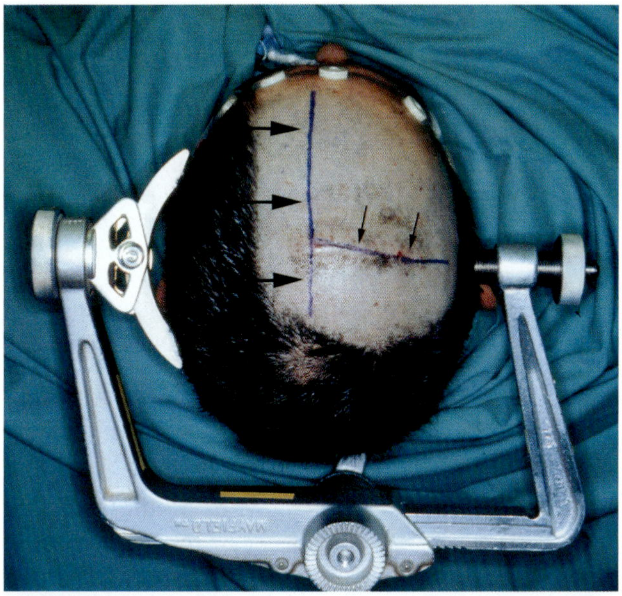

Figure 32–2 The patient's head is firmly fixed in the Mayfield head holder. After taking into consideration the location of the scar from a previous craniotomy (small arrows), the outline of the incision is drawn on the scalp (large arrows).

in the supine position as long as a cushioning roll is placed under the opposite shoulder. To expose the posterior half of the scalp, it is preferable to place the body in a lateral or park-bench position. This will then require the head clamp to be rotated so that the clamp arm with the single pin is placed around the forehead and the arm with two pins is placed around the occiput. Attention should be paid to whether any shunt device is present that might be crushed by the pin. The patient's body is then secured with the necessary padding to protect the elbows and the axillas, where peripheral nerve injuries can occur. The back and the extremities are flexed moderately with the help of pillows. If the body is in the lateral position, it is advisable to place a beanbag that can be molded to shape and then deflated of its air once the body position is satisfactory.

At this point, the patient and the OR table become one fixed unit that can be moved and centered as needed. It is critical at this moment to visualize the placement of all surgical adjuncts around the table so that ample room is left for the OR personnel to move about the room. It is equally important to position the various monitors such that the surgeon can view them without excessive head turning. Now the table can be locked and the scalp prepared for surgery. Shaving of the head is normally kept to a minimum; however, this includes the entire wound exposure with a small margin around it. The planned incision is then drawn on the scalp after great care has been given to studying the precise location of the intracranial tumor. This step typically requires measurements, with a ruler in hand, of the projections of the tumor on all three MRI planes. Knowing the proximity of the mass to external landmarks, such as the external auditory canal, as seen on a coronal MRI, adds greatly to the accuracy of the localization.

The use of surgical adjuncts such as image-guided systems and electrophysiological monitoring can proceed at this time. The patient's head is then prepped while the surgeon is scrubbing and being gowned.

Procedure

The head is draped with towels that are placed around the surface to be exposed and secured to the scalp with staples. A transparent adhesive cover impregnated with a disinfectant is then applied to the scalp. The table that holds the surgical instruments is then positioned next to the patient, with its upper edge maintained below the top of the patient's shoulder. A large craniotomy sheet is then wrapped over the entire surgical field and is used to separate the anesthesiologist from the surgical arena. The craniotomy drape has a plastic bag incorporated within it at one end for the collection of irrigation fluids. Any additional equipment placed within reach of the surgeon is draped as necessary. The image-guided arm shown in **Fig. 32–3** is first covered with its own plastic bag and is then surrounded by the craniotomy sheet. Two suction tubes and a Bovie and a bipolar coagulator are then placed within reach of the surgeon and the assistant.

The incision is then made with a no. 10 scalpel blade, and Raney clips are applied along the cut edges. The scalp is reflected away from the exposed skull with the help of Fisch microhooks. In the example shown in **Figs. 32–2** and **32–4**, the incision was T-shaped because of the existence of a prior linear incision that alone would not have sufficed to provide the necessary exposure. The craniotomy can now be performed. The number and placement of bur holes depend on the proximity of the planned bone flap to any of the major venous sinuses. In the parasagittal location, it is typically necessary to make two bur holes over, or immediately next to, the superior sagittal sinus. If none of the sinuses is in proximity, then a single bur hole will suffice. A high-powered drill is used to drill the holes to the depth at which the dura is exposed. The dura is then separated from the undersurface of the skull using any appropriately sized instrument. This step is particularly important if the craniotomy is near or crosses a venous sinus. The skull is then cut with the craniotome to a size and shape that will provide adequate exposure for the surgeon. Frequent irrigation should be used whenever the bone is being drilled or cut to cool the cutting tool and minimize the spread of the bone dust that typically results from this action. Because the number of bur holes is kept to a minimum, it is important to cut the skull by moving in a direction away from the sinus. This entails carrying the cut from the first bur hole only halfway through, sliding the craniotome back, and starting again from the second bur hole. The cut directly above the sinus is saved for last, as is shown in **Fig. 32–4**.

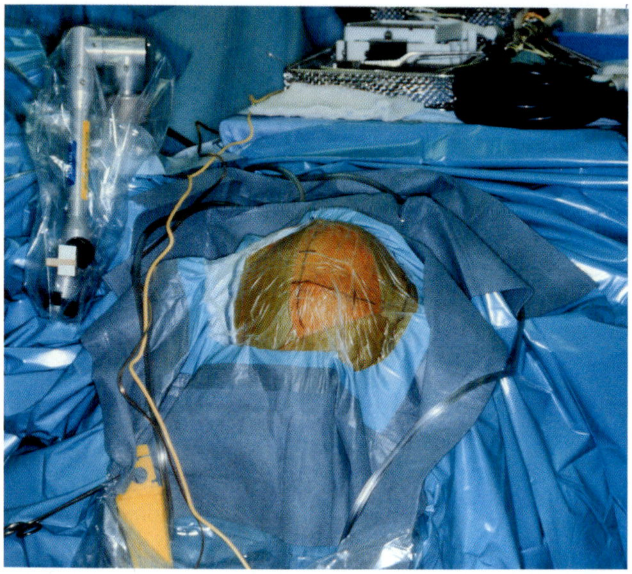

Figure 32–3 The operating field is fully draped showing the relative positions of the suction tubes, electrocautery, image-guided arm, and surgical table.

The skull flap can now be elevated by gently separating the dura from the inner table of the skull. A combination of Penfield instruments and periosteal elevators is used for this purpose. The bone is carefully handed over to the scrub nurse, who then wraps it with a wet sponge and places it in a basin. With the dura exposed, it is possible to use the intraoperative ultrasound (IOUS) probe to verify the location of the intracranial mass and the adequacy of the bony exposure (**Fig. 32–5**). If it is judged that the tumor will not be properly exposed, then the craniotomy should be expanded in the appropriate direction. This sometimes means extending the scalp incision as well. Prior to opening the dura, its

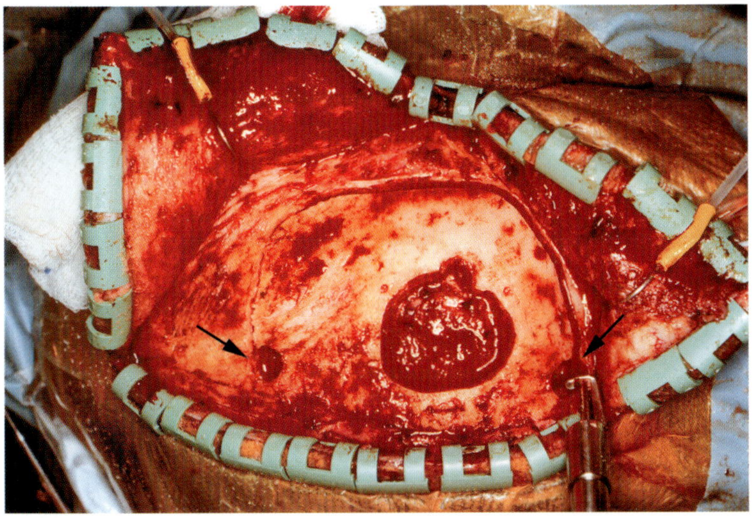

Figure 32–4 The scalp flaps with Raney clips attached are shown reflected using Fisch microhooks and exposing the skull. The central defect in the skull is from a previous craniotomy for biopsy of the tumor. A larger craniotomy flap is being created after drilling two bur holes (arrows) at the midline. The craniotome is shown over the posterior bur hole and is being used to complete the craniotomy over the midline.

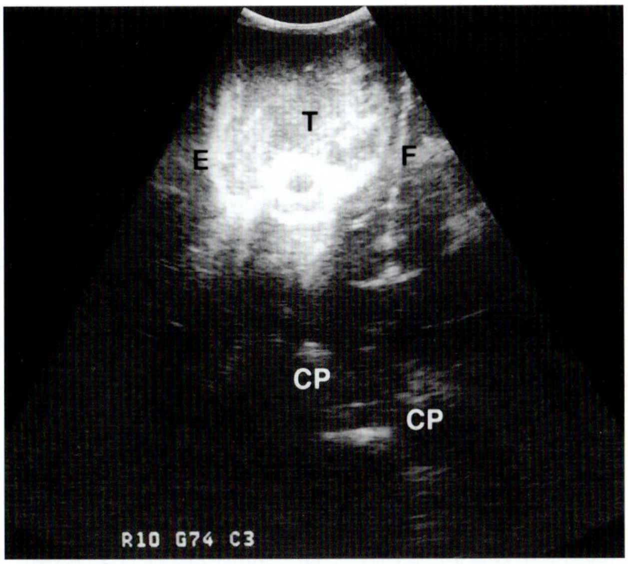

Figure 32–5 Intraoperative ultrasound image taken in the coronal plane and showing the tumor (T), the falx (F), surrounding edema (E), and choroid plexus (CP) in the lateral ventricles, bilaterally. Notice the well-defined margin of the tumor.

tenseness is assessed to determine whether head elevation is necessary. The use of diuretics can be avoided in most circumstances. The dura is then opened circumferentially as a flap with its base against the sinus. The initial cut in the dura is performed with a sharp no. 15 blade while the dura is being tented upward with the help of a dural stitch that was placed near the site of incision. Once the arachnoid is exposed, the dura is cut with Metzenbaum scissors along the edge of the craniotomy, with care to maintain enough distance from the bone to facilitate the closure of the dura at the end of the operation. When the dura is being cut, great attention must be given to veins traversing or attaching to its undersurface. Also, in patients who have previously undergone a craniotomy at the same site, adhesions are commonly encountered and must be separated gently and tediously, especially if the underlying parenchymal regions represent areas of eloquent brain such as the motor cortex or the speech centers. Once cut, the dura is reflected over the sinus and onto a wet cottonoid patty to prevent it from drying out over the course of the operation. Dural stitches are then placed wherever necessary to maintain adequate exposure (**Fig. 32–6**). All means of tumor and functional localization that are necessary for this operation can be used at this point. Visual inspection will determine the surface extension of the mass, if applicable. The ultrasound probe is again placed directly on the surface of the brain. Frequently, this provides better images than those obtained through the dura because its thickness can interfere with the penetration and reflection of the ultrasonic waves.[12] To reach subcortical lesions, it is critical to avoid areas of functional anatomy. Either or both cortical mapping and direct electrical stimulation of the brain surface are employed as described in chapter 3 this volume. The use of image guidance is also detailed elsewhere in this atlas.

The specific techniques applied in the removal of a given tumor depend largely on the nature and biology of the tumor. In general, and particularly for intrinsic tumors, an en bloc resection is desirable, especially if the tumor's boundaries can be distinguished from the surrounding, and potentially eloquent, brain. These techniques are outlined within the chapters of this atlas that describe each specific tumor type. The example shown in **Fig. 32–7** demonstrates the technique used to circumferentially isolate the area of resection by performing a corticectomy and then proceeding through the deeper zones of the brain parenchyma until the bottom of the tumor is reached. For large resections and for tumors that reach deeper into the brain, it is helpful and desirable to rely on a versatile self-retaining retraction system. There are a variety of fixed-blade retractor systems available to the neurosurgeon, including the Leyla (Medicon eG., Tuttlingen, Germany), Greenberg (Codman Inc., Raynham, MA), Sugita (Mizuho. Ikakogyo Co., Ltd., Tokyo, Japan), and Budde Halo (Ohio Medical Instruments Co., Cincinnati, OH) systems. The advantage of these systems is that they are capable of providing steady, untiring exposure while allowing nearly unencumbered access to the mass. Once the resection is completed, much attention is given to meticulous and thorough control of hemostasis. This process is

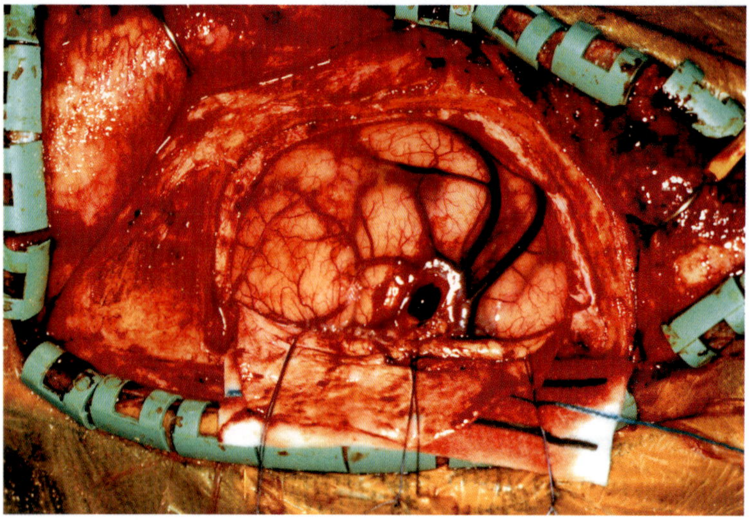

Figure 32–6 The cortical surface is exposed after the dural flap is cut and reflected medially over the sagittal sinus. The defect in the frontal lobe represents the site of a recent biopsy.

facilitated by performing a resection that surrounds the tumor instead of going through it. In the latter case, residual tumor tissue can present considerable difficulties in assuring total and durable control of bleeding in the OR and beyond. The most useful tool toward implementation of a secure hemostasis is the bipolar coagulator. Every attempt must be made to stop the bleeding with the bipolar, and, if this proves difficult, then the use of hemostatic agents may provide temporary relief.[13] The best choice of a resorbable chemical agent depends on the nature of the bleeding, but for most intrinsic tumors, oxidized cellulose (Oxycel) provides the most satisfying results. If brisk bleeding persists, it is most likely due to the presence of residual tumor; this should lead to further tumor resection with guidance from the ultrasound and knowledge of the functional and anatomical landmarks. Hemostasis is not assured unless some form of positive respiratory pressure has been applied for 30 seconds without encountering further bleeding. At this point, the surgical cavity within the brain should be clean and dry (**Fig. 32–8**).

The dural closure is done in a watertight fashion. If necessary, pericranium or allograft dura mater is used (**Fig. 32–9**).[14,15] To prevent cerebrospinal fluid (CSF) leaks, dural closure is especially important when the ventricular cavity is entered or when working in a reoperative irradiated field. The dura is tacked to bone edges to maintain epidural hemostasis. After dural closure, the IOUS may be used to ensure that no hematoma is forming in the resection bed prior to replacing and securing the bone flap. The bone is wired or plated in place depending on the location of the flap and the unevenness of the bony defects. Craniotomy flaps involving the anterior half of the skull are usually repaired and secured with miniplates to provide the most aesthetically desirable results (**Fig. 32–10**). The Raney clips are then removed, and brisk bleeding points are coagulated with the bipolar coagulator. The scalp is closed in two layers. The galea is closed with a 3–0 resorbable stitch and the skin edge approximated with staples (**Fig. 32–11**). If the scalp flap is thin or irradiated, sutures are used to meticulously approximate and tightly close the wound. Lastly, the wound is dressed locally. Closed drainage systems and large head wraps are generally avoided.

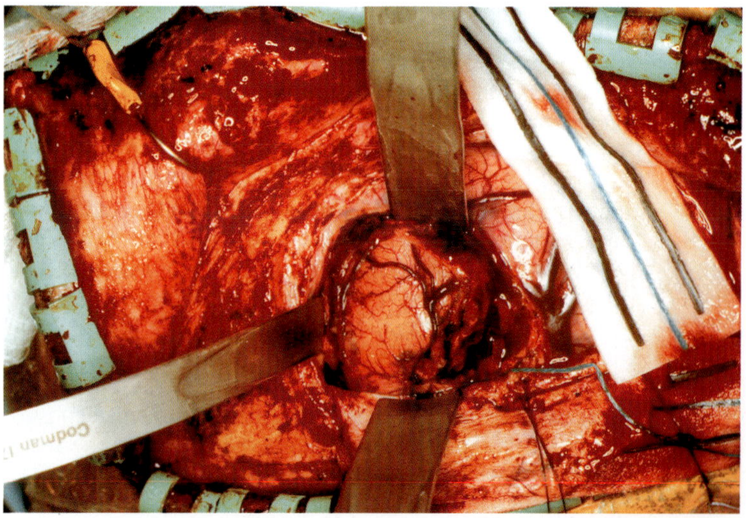

Figure 32–7 The cortical incision is shown encircling the mass. Three self-retaining retractor blades are shown at the periphery of the resection. These are advanced gradually as the margin of the mass is separated from the surrounding white matter.

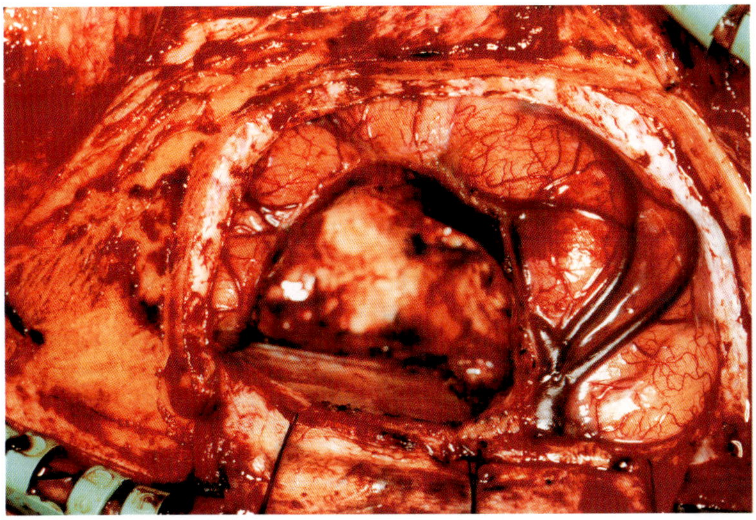

Figure 32–8 A large cavity has been created following the en bloc removal of the mass. The edge of the cortical incision is sharp, and the bed of the resection is clean. The large cortical vein posterior to the resection has been preserved.

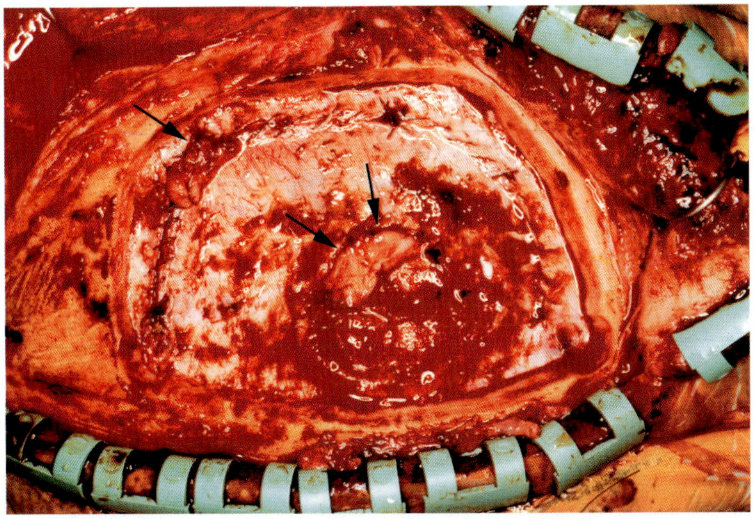

Figure 32–9 The dural flap is meticulously closed using running stitches. Gaps in the closure are approximated with pieces of periosteal tissue (arrows).

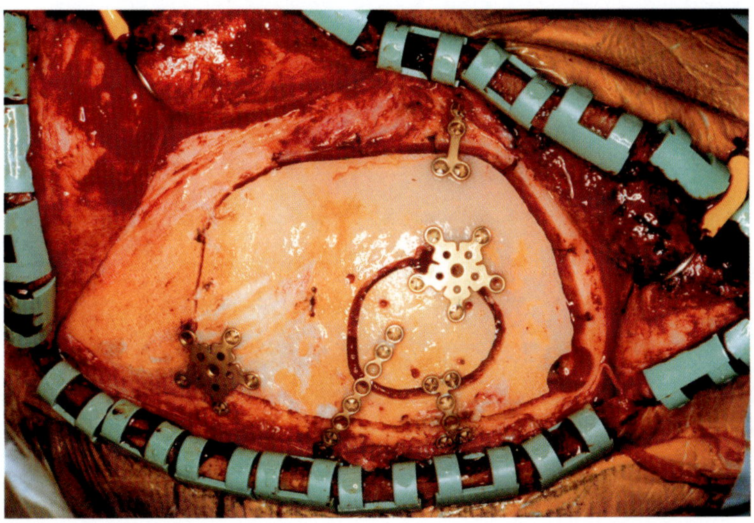

Figure 32–10 The bone flaps are secured in place using titanium plates, screws, and bur hole grids to provide an efficient and cosmetically acceptable reconstruction of the skull.

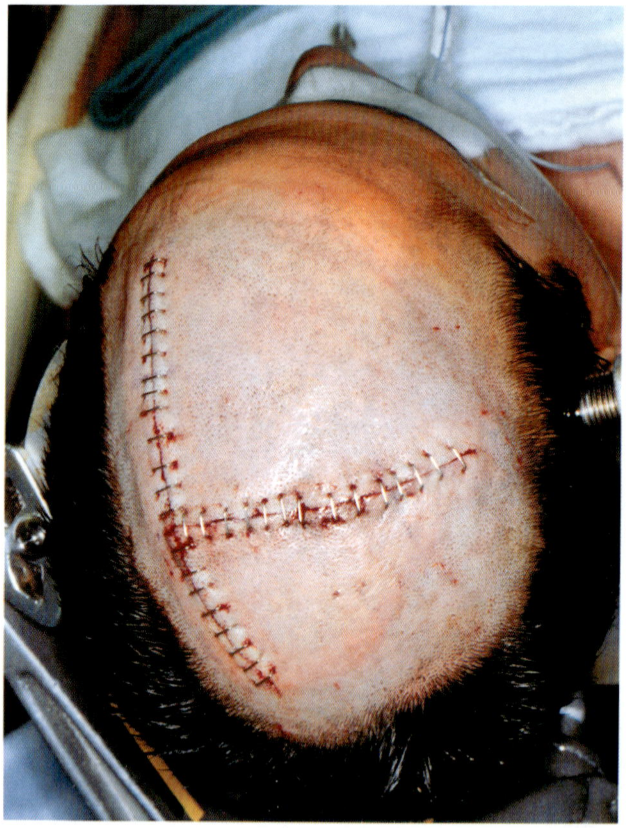

Figure 32–11 The wound closure is completed with the use of staples to approximate the skin edges.

◆ Postoperative Care

The patient should be awakened in the OR and assessed neurologically. It is not uncommon after resections adjacent to eloquent brain for the patient to exhibit a neurological decline when compared with preoperative status. If the deficit is focal and could be anticipated, close observation and timely improvement in neurological function may obviate the need for an urgent CT scan. However, if the patient is difficult to arouse or has a fixed, unexpected deficit, immediate CT scanning is warranted.

Patients are closely observed for the first night in a monitored bed, most typically in a step-down unit. Intravenous fluids consist of iso-osmolar glucose-free solutions given at the rate of 60 to 80 mL/hr. Medications include steroids, anticonvulsants, antibiotics, codeine-based pain killers, and other medications used as necessary, depending on the patient's complaints and vital signs. Oral intake is restricted to ice chips and small sips of water as needed. Pneumatic compression boots are applied to the calves, and the neurological and vital signs are recorded on an hourly basis.

The next morning, the patient is transferred to the ward where ambulation can begin. The Foley catheter is discontinued, and the diet is advanced as tolerated. Antibiotics are administered for a total of 24 hours, and steroids are maintained at a dose of 4 mg every 6 hours. The compression boots remain applied as long as the patient is in bed. They are easily disconnected when the patient is getting out of bed. An MRI scan is obtained within 48 hours to assess the extent of resection and any unexpected occurrences (**Fig. 32–12**). If the patient has any speech, motor, or sensory deficits, speech, physical, and occupational therapists are consulted early, and if appropriate, the patient is transferred to the physical medicine and rehabilitation service.

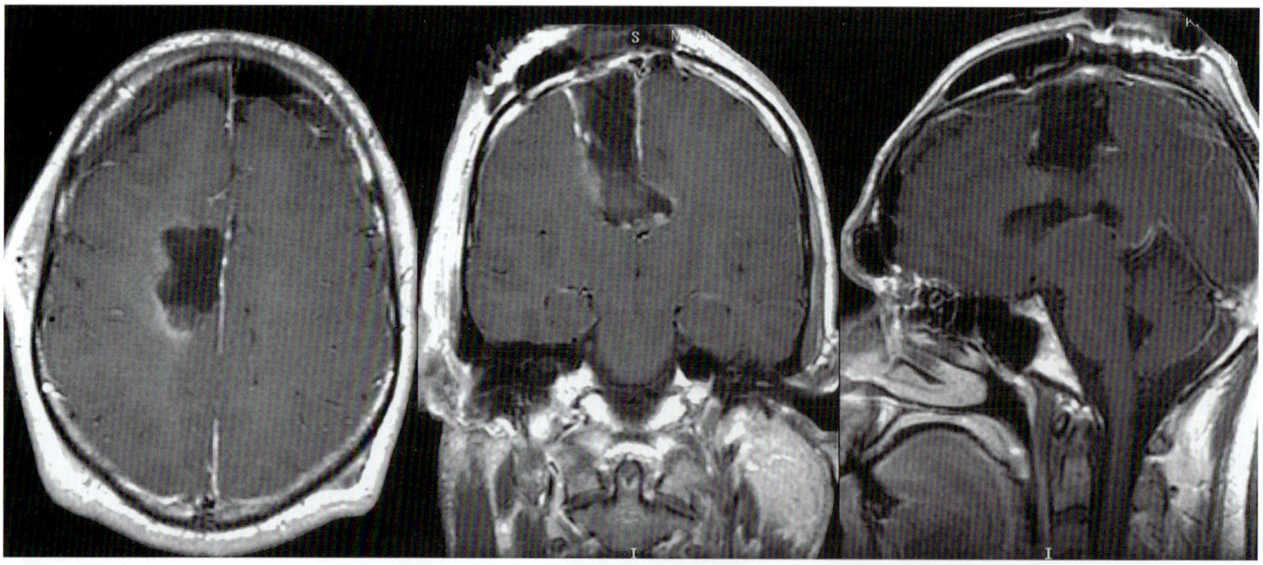

Figure 32–12 Postoperative gadolinium-enhanced, T1-weighted magnetic resonance images showing a gross-total resection of the mass seen in **Fig. 32–1** (axial, coronal, and sagittal scans are denoted as in **Fig. 32–1**). The large cavity created is filled with cerebrospinal fluid. The defect is seen extending into the corpus callosum.

Most hospital stays last approximately 3 days following the craniotomy. Discharge planning includes instructions on care of the wound at home, a description of restricted activities, and information on support groups and other social resources of importance to the patient and the family. A return appointment is made corresponding to the time for removal of the wound staples and stitches, and that will permit a review of the results from the pathologists and from postoperative MRI scanning, which will dictate further treatments or follow-up visits.

◆ Complications

In general, there are three types of complications that can occur following a craniotomy for a brain tumor: neurological, wound-related (regional), and systemic complications.[9] Neurological complications are the most common of the three and are due to the direct effects of the surgery on the brain or its blood supply, or are caused indirectly by cerebral edema. On average, they occur at a rate of 5 to 8%. Gentle techniques and the use of surgical adjuncts such as cortical mapping are intended to assist the surgeon in protecting eloquent areas of the brain while the tumor is being resected. It should be noted, however, that judgment and experience remain the most important factors in favorably maximizing the extent of resection and its consequent benefit while minimizing the risk of a permanent neurological deficit. As shown in **Fig. 32–13**, neurological complications are more likely to occur among patients who have tumors of high functional grade (located within or close to eloquent brain regions). Nevertheless, it can be seen from **Fig. 32–14** that gross total resections can be performed in eloquent brain areas with an acceptable level of neurological impairment, which suggests that the mere presence of a tumor in eloquent brain is not an automatic contraindication for surgery. As explained earlier, patients can be made aware prior to surgery of the likelihood that a certain type of deficit may occur and the fact that most deficits will improve with time and with rehabilitation.

Wound-related complications include mostly infections, dehiscences, and CSF leaks and occur at a rate of 2 to 3%. These complications are related to the surgical technique used and to the effects of prior radiation therapy and scarring. Infections tend to be superficial, and only rarely do they affect the bone. The use of antibiotics has had a strong prophylactic effect by maintaining the rate of wound infection at around 1%. A CSF leak is a potentially more serious problem because it entails the risk of meningitis. Frequently, additional stitches placed at the site of the leak will correct the problem. However, if this fails, it is necessary to place a lumbar drain for 3 to 5 days to give the wound time to heal completely. CSF leaks can be the result of a sluggish CSF circulation, in which case, a ventriculoperitoneal shunt might be required if the lumbar drain has not eliminated the problem.

Systemic complications can be minor, such as a urinary tract infection or a superficial vein thrombosis; however, in rare instances, these complications can be life threatening, such as with septicemia, pulmonary embolism, and pneumonia in an elderly emaciated patient. Fortunately, these complications are exceedingly rare, occurring at a rate of only 1 to 2%. Most complications in this category are treated with standard noncontroversial therapies, except in the case of deep venous thrombosis and pulmonary embolism. In general, the use of properly monitored anticoagulation therapy is safe in neurosurgical patients 5 days after a craniotomy.[16] The alternative to such therapy is the placement of a vena cava filter.[17] In general, use of anticoagulation therapy is preferred to using a vascular filter because of the effect this therapy has on the propagation of blood clots and the problems related to blood stasis in the lower extremities.

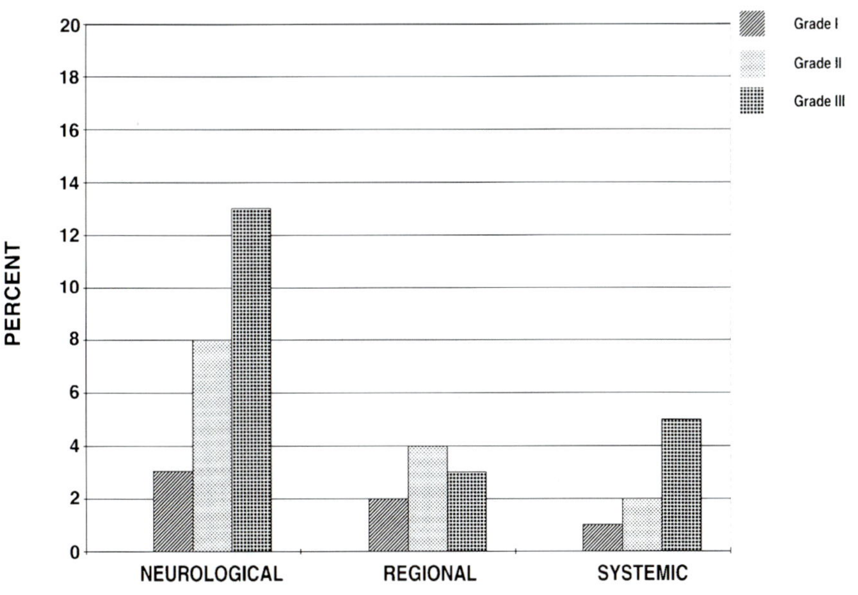

Figure 32–13 Bar graph showing effect of brain tumor functional grade on major complication incidences. Tumors were graded I, II, or III based on their location relative to brain function. Major neurological, regional, and systemic complication percentages are plotted against this functional grade. Twenty-six, 36, and 38% of patients had tumors of grade I (in noneloquent brain), II (in near-eloquent brain), and III (in eloquent brain), respectively. (With permission from Sawaya R, Hammoud M, Schoppa D, et al. Neurosurgical outcomes in a modern series of 400 craniotomies for treatment of parenchymal tumors. Neurosurgery 1998;42:1044–1056.)

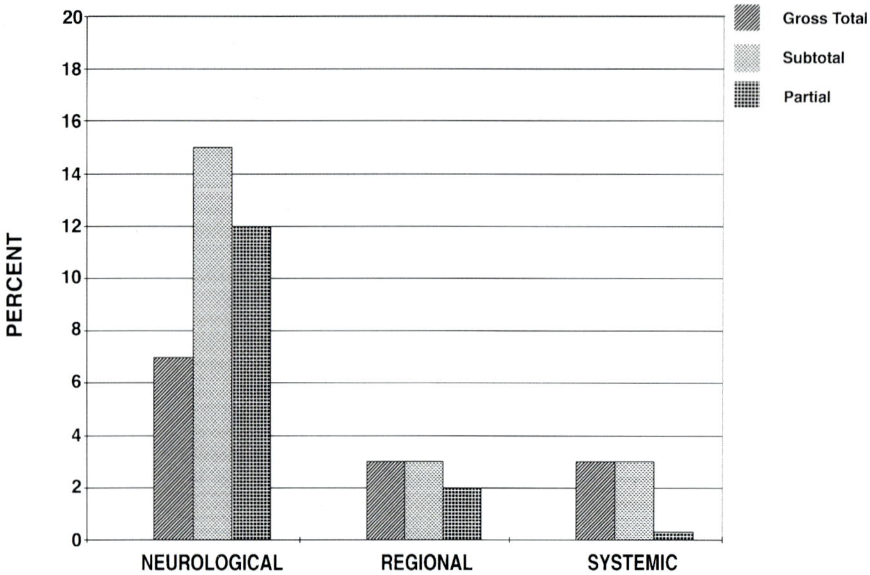

Figure 32–14. Bar graph showing effect of extent of surgery for extirpation of intra-axial brain tumors on major complication incidences. Major neurological, major regional, and major systemic complication percentages are plotted for each category of resection: gross total, subtotal, and partial resection. (With permission from Sawaya R, Hammoud M, Schoppa D, et al. Neurosurgical outcomes in a modern series of 400 craniotomies for treatment of parenchymal tumors. Neurosurgery 1998;42:1044–1056.)

◆ Conclusion

Neurosurgery is a highly technical specialty. This is particularly true when surgery is applied to the management of brain tumors. This chapter describes a step-by-step approach to the performance of a craniotomy for removal of a brain tumor. The initial evaluation with review of the MRI is the most critical step in selecting the appropriate patient and the correct approach for the craniotomy. A review of the differential diagnosis could help avoid unnecessary and inappropriate operations, and careful consideration of the neurological and functional anatomy will place the likelihood of a successful operation in a proper and realistic perspective. A variety of tools and instruments can be used to accomplish the task at hand, and the example given in this chapter is a description of just one approach. However, many of the principles detailed here can be generally applied to many, if not most, patients with intrinsic brain tumors. The rapport that the surgeon establishes with the patient and family is critical to building the necessary trust and can influence the speed of recovery. Similarly, development of excellence in communication with the anesthesiologist and the OR team will pay off in terms of cooperation, availability of instruments, correct room layout, and overall mood in the surgical suite. Lastly, strict adherence to details will avoid errors and complications and will also facilitate the patient's speed of recovery. This applies in particular to placement of the craniotomy in relation to the site of the tumor, to gentle handling of the brain surrounding the tumor, and to techniques of hemostasis and wound closure. Finally, the provision of continued care and the availability of the surgical team in the postoperative period will enhance the quality and timeliness of the recovery, especially if complications have occurred.

Acknowledgments I thank David M. Wildrick, Ph.D., for editorial assistance in the preparation of this manuscript; Edward Davis, Medical Photographer, for taking the intraoperative photographs; and Weiming Shi, M.D., for assistance with figure preparation.

References

1. Kaye AH, Laws ER Jr. Historical perspective. In: Kaye AH, Laws ER Jr, eds. Brain Tumors: An Encyclopedic Approach. Edinburgh: Churchill-Livingstone; 1995:3–8
2. Greenblatt SH, Dagi TF, Epstein MH, eds. A History of Neurosurgery. Park Ridge, IL: American Association of Neurological Surgeons; 1997:600
3. Sawaya R, Rambo WM, Jr., Hammoud MA, Ligon BL. Advances in surgery for brain tumors. Neurol Clin 1995;13:757–771
4. Ciric I, Ammirati M, Vick N, Mikhael M. Supratentorial gliomas: surgical considerations and immediate postoperative results. Gross total resection versus partial resection. Neurosurgery 1987;21:21–26
5. Curran WJ, Scott CB, Horton J, et al. Recursive partitioning analysis of prognostic factors in three radiation therapy oncology group malignant glioma trials. J Natl Cancer Inst 1993;85:704–710
6. Salcman M. The role of surgery in brain tumor management: malignant glioma management. Neurosurg Clin N Am 1990;1:49–63
7. Bernstein M, Parrent AG. Complications of CT-guided stereotactic biopsy of intra-axial brain lesions. J Neurosurg 1994;81:165–168
8. Apuzzo ML, Chandrasoma PT, Cohen D, Zee CS, Zelman V. Computed imaging stereotaxy: experience and perspective related to 500 procedures applied to brain masses. Neurosurgery 1987;20:930–937
9. Sawaya R, Hammoud M, Schoppa D, et al. Neurosurgical outcomes in a modern series of 400 craniotomies for treatment of parenchymal tumors. Neurosurgery 1998;42:1044–1056
10. Warner DS, Boehland LA. Effects of iso-osmolar intravenous fluid therapy on post-ischemic brain water content in the rat. Anesthesiology 1988;68:86–91
11. Van Hemelrijack J, Van Aken H, Plets C, Goffin J, Vermaut G. The effects of propofol on intracranial pressure and cerebral perfusion pressure in patients with brain tumors. Acta Anaesthesiol Belg 1989;40: 95–100
12. Hammoud MA, Ligon BL, ElSouki R, Shi WM, Schomer DF, Sawaya R. Use of intraoperative ultrasound for localizing tumors and determining the extent of resection: a comparative study with magnetic resonance imaging. J Neurosurg 1996;84:737–741
13. Arand AG, Sawaya R. Intraoperative chemical hemostasis in neurosurgery. Neurosurgery 1986;18:223–233

14. Rosomoff HL, Malinin TI. Freeze-dried allografts of dura mater: 20 years experience. Transplant Proc 1976;8:133–138

15. Cantore G, Guidetti B, Delfini R. Neurosurgical use of human dura mater sterilized by gamma rays and stored in alcohol: long-term results. J Neurosurg 1987;66:93–95

16. Sawaya R, Zuccarello M, Elkalliny M, Nishiyama H. Postoperative venous thromboembolism and brain tumors: Part I. Clinical profile. J Neurooncol 1992;14:119–125

17. Olin JW, Young JR, Graor RA, Ruschhaupt WF, Beven EG, Bay JW. Treatment of deep vein thrombosis and pulmonary emboli in patients with primary and metastatic brain tumors. Anticoagulants or inferior vena cava filter? Arch Intern Med 1987;147:2177–2179

33

Stereotactic Biopsy

Theodore H. Schwartz and Michael B. Sisti

The foundations of stereotactic surgery can be traced to the work of Horsley and Clarke, who developed a system for use in animals based on Cartesian coordinates.[1] The first practical stereotactic apparatus for use in humans was designed by Spiegel and Wycis in 1946.[2] Their device was based upon the relationship between a given anatomical target and specific internal brain landmarks defined by pneumoencephalography. With the development of computed tomographic (CT)- and magnetic resonance imaging (MRI)-based, frame-based and frameless computer-assisted systems, stereotactic localization has rapidly become a standard technique in the armamentarium of the modern neurosurgeon and the preferred minimally invasive method for biopsy of certain intracranial mass lesions. Several commercially available systems currently exist, most of which rely on common principles of frame or fiducial placement, entry site, trajectory, target identification, and patient positioning, all of which are covered in this chapter. The specifics of each individual system are beyond the scope of this work.

◆ Indications

Brain biopsies, in general, are indicated to determine the diagnosis of an intracranial lesion in a patient best treated without an open surgical resection. For example, some pathological processes that clinically and radiographically resemble a neoplasm are best managed with either medical therapy, as in an infectious lesion, or no therapy, as in an ischemic insult. Likewise, the outcome of certain neoplastic processes, such as a glioblastoma, lymphoma, germinoma, or metastases with advanced primary disease, may not be altered by surgical resection and should rather be managed strictly with radiation or chemotherapy. Patients who are medically unsuited for open surgery, on account of old age or poor medical condition, often require less invasive therapy despite indications for surgery. Finally, some regions deep in the brain such as the internal capsule, basal ganglia, or pons often cannot be reached safely with open surgery and require stereotactic biopsy for diagnosis.

Because stereotaxis is the least invasive way to obtain tissue, it is usually the technique of choice unless there is significant risk of hemorrhage. For this reason, closed stereotactic biopsy is contraindicated in the cases of suspected vascular pathology such as an arteriovenous malformation (AVM), aneurysm, cavernous malformation, or hemorrhagic tumor; in vascular territories such as the circle of Willis and sylvian fissure; or in juxtaposition to pial and ependymal surfaces. We do not recommend biopsy of the medulla due to both the concentration of critical nuclei in this area and the difficulty in coordinating an adequate entry site and trajectory. Biopsies in the pineal region are controversial because tumors in this location are known to be heterogeneous and prone to sampling error and can often be approached for biopsy utilizing an endoscopic transventricular approach. The decision to choose stereotactic over open biopsy is institutionally dependent and rests upon the experience and comfort of the operating surgeon. Open biopsy allows sampling of the leptomeninges and cortical vessels in suspected cases of central nervous system (CNS) vasculitis, a distinct advantage over closed stereotactic biopsy. Stereotactic biopsy and aspiration of colloid cysts are also controversial. We favor open surgical resection because the recurrence rate following partial treatment is high.[3] Finally, children under 2 years of age do not usually have thick enough skulls for adequate rigid frame fixation.

◆ Preparation

Prior to performing a stereotactic biopsy it is critical to know that the lesion will be visible with the radiographic technique upon which the localization is based. Some low-grade gliomas that are obvious on MRI scans will be nonenhancing, isointense lesions on CT. Several systems for MRI/CT coregistration or MRI-based stereotaxis exist to circumvent this problem.[4] Another important issue is the determination of hemorrhagic potential. Any lesion resembling an AVM or aneurysm should have an angiogram, CT angiography (CTA), or MR angiography (MRA) prior to a closed stereotactic biopsy. Likewise, special MR sequences sensitive to blood products such as the gradient-echo can help identify residual blood products associated with prior hemorrhagic events.

Communication with the primary medical or neurological physicians is important prior to proceeding with a biopsy. If any special cultures or stains are required, these should be determined and communicated to the pathologist. Similarly, if stereotactic biopsies are infrequently performed at an institution, a designated pathologist with experience processing the small stereotactic biopsy specimens should be available.

◆ Frame-based versus Frameless Stereotaxy

With the development of commercially available frameless stereotactic systems with rigid arms to hold biopsy probes, frameless stereotactic biopsies are now becoming the standard of care in many institutions. Many of the same principles apply to both frame-based and frameless systems with the following exceptions. Frame-based systems generally require placement of a skull-mounted frame and the acquisition of guidance images in the middle of the procedure. Frameless systems permit image acquisition the day prior to the procedure, saving time on the day of the operation. Frame positioning requires four points of skull fixation, which can limit the possible approaches as well as restrict conversion to a craniotomy in the case of a hemorrhage. Frame-based systems often require complex calculations in the operating room (OR), which can take valuable OR time and often limit the number of entry points and targets. Frameless systems permit real-time upgrading of entry points and targets and provide the ability to follow the probe into the target if the system can track the biopsy needle.

Frame-based systems offer a slightly higher degree of accuracy, although the frameless systems have a reported error of 1.1 $\pm$ 0.5 for CT and 1.3 $\pm$ 1.7 for MRI in phantom studies.[5] Although some authors have recommended using frame-based stereotaxy for lesions less than 1.5 mm or in the brain stem,[6] others have reported excellent results with such lesions using frameless stereotaxy.[7,8]

◆ Surgical Technique

Anesthesia

Stereotactic biopsies can be performed with the patients awake under mild sedation. If a frame is being placed, an intravenous line is placed beforehand, and patients are given oxygen by nasal cannula. Oxygen saturation is monitored, and if there is any cardiac history, continuous electrocardiogram (ECG) and blood pressure cuff monitoring are performed. Midazolam and fentanyl are administered and titrated for light sedation and patient comfort. Once in the operating room, end-expiratory pCO_2 is additionally monitored to ensure adequate flow of air under the drapes and avert possible air emboli.[9] During the surgical procedure, the addition of IV propofol is often useful for further sedation. However, patients must be adequately alert for periodic neurological examination and in most cases are able to calmly converse during the entire course of the procedure. A laryngeal mask airway should be kept nearby in case resuscitation is required. If patients are unable to tolerate awake surgery due to anxiety or neurological compromise, they can be intubated and maintained with standard neuroanesthesia during the procedure as well as during frame placement, CT/MRI scanning, and surgery. The frame is then removed prior to extubation.

Frame Placement

The base ring can be placed either in the operating room or in a nearby holding area prior to OR availability. Placement of the frame and image localization can be performed any time prior to surgery as long as the frame is not dislodged in the interim. In general, four pins are placed after age 5 years. Children between ages 2 and 5 may require six pins depending on the thickness of their skull, and below age 2 years, six pins are mandatory, although there is still significant risk of skull fracture, and stereotactic ring placement should be avoided in these patients.

Correct frame placement ensures that the stereotactic target and expected entry site are not obstructed by the stereotactic posts and pins. Additionally, there should be sufficient clearance between the stereotactic arc and the entry site so that preparation of the surgical site can be accomplished. The stereotactic surgical arc may be applied to the head frame prior to imaging to confirm that no obstructions, collisions, or interference from the stereotactic frame or its attachments will restrict the exposure of the surgical site.

Frame placement is performed with the patient in the sitting position and requires two sets of hands, one to maintain the frame position and another to insert the pins. No hair need be shaved. Two pins are placed frontally, at least 1 cm above the eyebrow and 1 cm medial to the insertion of the temporalis muscle. Care must be taken to avoid placing the pins over the frontal sinus because the bone is thin and can easily fracture. Pins placed too high on the forehead may slip over the convexity. The posterior pins are generally placed in the parietal bone and can be shifted depending on the target (**Fig. 33–1**). It is important that the four carbon posts are advanced equally until they are lightly touching the skin so

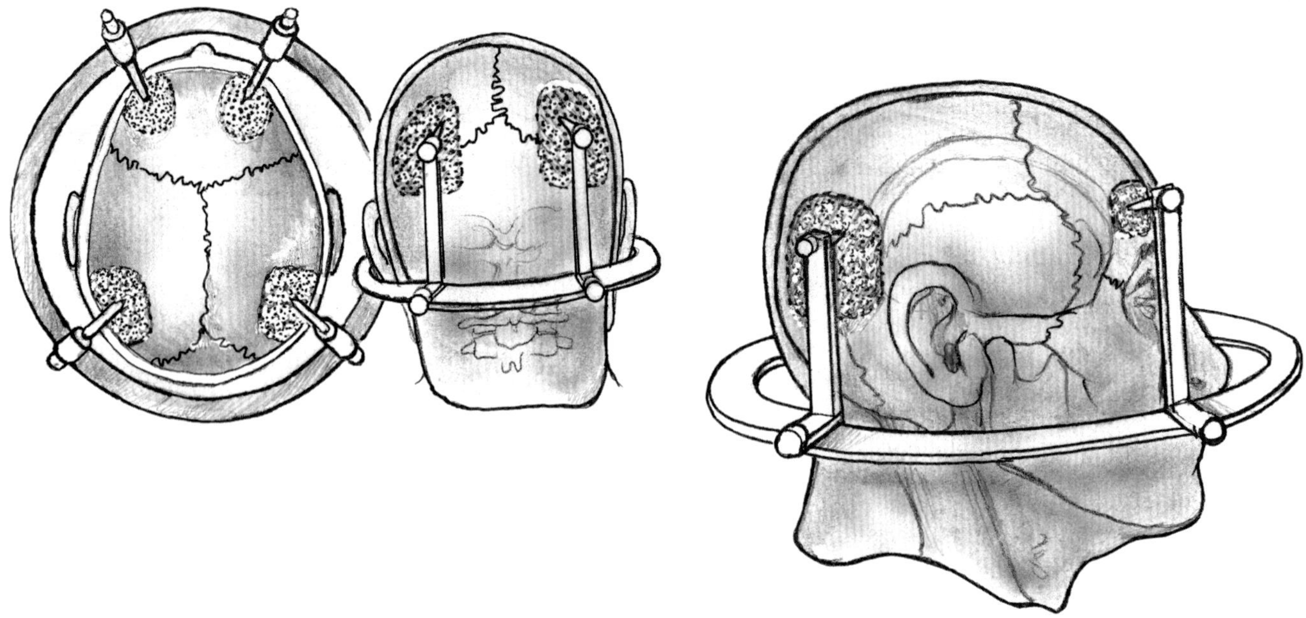

Figure 33–1 The grainy areas indicate safe areas for pin application for frame-based stereotactic procedures.

that the length of the pins is adequate to achieved the desired force. This will also ensure that the patient is centered in the ring. The skin is infiltrated with a mixture of 7 mL of 1% lidocaine with 1:100,000 U of epinephrine and 3 mL of bicarbonate. The pins are advanced into the cranium until fingertight. Care must be taken so that blood and local anesthetic do not run into the patient's eyes.

Skin Fiducial Placement

For frameless stereotactic biopsies, skin fiducials can be placed at any time prior to imaging; however, the shorter the latency to imaging, the less likely that the fiducials will be dislodged. Fiducials should be placed around the area of interest, with care taken to avoid mobile skin surfaces. At least five fiducials are required, but it is wise to place many more for the sake of redundancy and the inevitable possibility of fiducial movement. In general, fiducials can be placed bilaterally on the mastoid and zygoma in front of the tragus as well as in a zigzag pattern over the forehead, without shaving any hair (**Fig. 33–2**). It is helpful to place one or two fiducials over the convexity on the side of the procedure as well as on the contralateral side to increase accuracy; this can be done with minimal hair shaving. A fiducial can also be placed on the inion for procedures in the posterior fossa. To avoid mishaps related to fiducial movement between the time of the scan and the operation, we use a skin marker to outline the circumference and center of each fiducial as well as a headwrap to prevent dislodgment, particularly if the fiducials are placed the day before surgery.

Imaging

For frame-based procedures, once the frame is affixed to the head, the fiducial-localizing ring is secured to the base ring, and the anesthesiologist and neurosurgeon accompany the patient to the scanner. The patient is placed flat on the table in a comfortable position. For most biopsies the orientation of the head is not important as long as all the fiducials can be seen in the image. Patients are given a bolus of IV contrast to maximize visualization of abnormal tissue

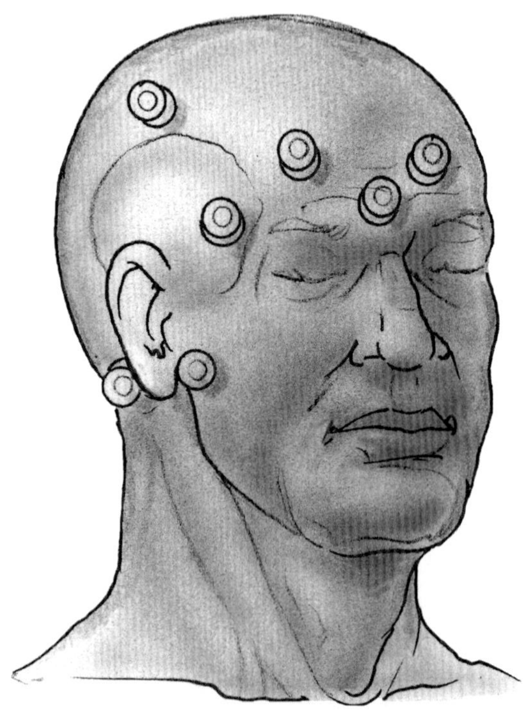

Figure 33–2 Location of skin fiducials for a frameless stereotactic biopsy.

and nearby blood vessels and to differentiate enhancing from nonenhancing areas. Serial axial sections are performed parallel to the plane of the base ring to maximize fiducial visualization. The neurosurgeon then records the pixel coordinates of the fiducials and the target sites in the relevant image or transfers the images over a network to a workstation for the entry site and trajectory calculations. For frame-based procedures, fine (1.0–1.5 mm) cuts can be obtained though the area of interest, whereas for frameless systems it is important to image the entire head for adequate three-dimensional (3D) reconstruction of the skin and skin fiducials.

Choosing a Target

One of the advantages of closed stereotactic biopsy over open biopsy unaided by stereotaxis is that tissue can be obtained from specific regions with known radiographic features. The diagnostic yield of a biopsy is greater if tissue is acquired from an area of enhancement. A biopsy from the necrotic center of a high-grade neoplasm will frequently be nondiagnostic. Similarly, if an area of necrosis is not included in the sampled tissue, the degree of malignancy will be underestimated. Multiple targets are often required if tumor heterogeneity is suspected either by location (e.g., pineal region) or radiographic appearance. If a lesion lies adjacent to a vascular structure or a ventricular surface, the target must be chosen to avoid these regions.

Entry Site and Trajectory

There are six major entry sites used for stereotactic biopsy. All lie along the midpupillary line, ~3 cm off the midline. Safe passage can be achieved on both sides of the brain through the first frontal convolution, the superior parietal lobule, and the cerebellar hemisphere into the middle cerebellar peduncle (**Fig. 33–3**). The frontal entry site is chosen 1 to 2 cm anterior to the coronal suture. The parietal entry

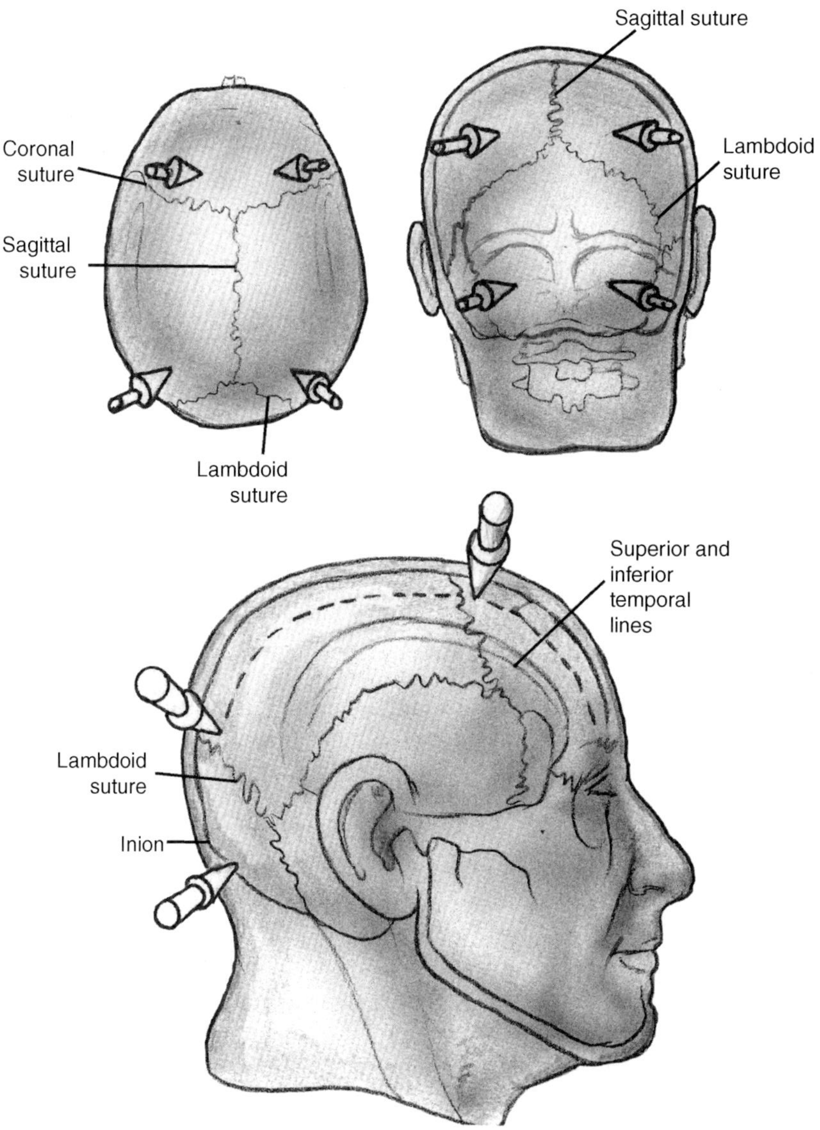

Figure 33–3 Arrows indicate safe entry points to obtain specimens from most intracranial locations.

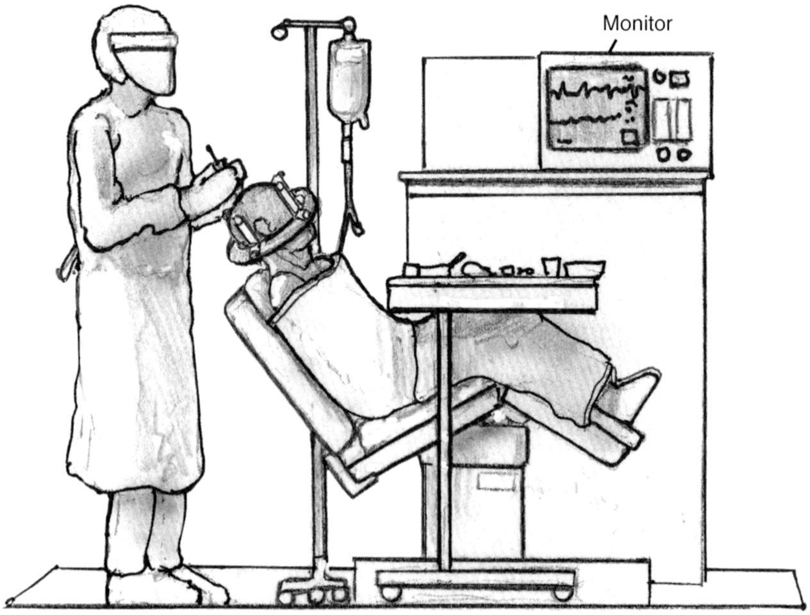

Figure 33–4 Operating room setup for awake stereotactic biopsy. The elevated table in front of the patient prevents the drapes from impairing ventilation and allows the anesthesiologist easy access to the naso- and oropharynx.

site is 7 cm above the inion or just above the lambdoid suture, and the posterior fossa entry site is 2 cm below the inion. Care must be taken to serially examine the axial sections of the chosen trajectory to avoid passing through a pial or ependymal surface that might cause bleeding. In general, if a blunt-tipped biopsy needle is slowly advanced through the brain, there is little damage to parenchymal tissue. Current stereotactic planning software permits a trajectory to be chosen to avoid passing through a sulcus, which can reduce the risk of hemorrhage.

Positioning, Prepping, and Draping

Most biopsies are performed with patients in the sitting or semisitting position with slight neck flexion for patient and surgeon comfort. Posterior fossa biopsies require a full sitting position, or they can be performed with the patient intubated in the lateral position. No Foley is placed. The knees are slightly bent, and all sensitive areas are padded. For frameless procedures, the patient is placed in the Mayfield head holder. Care must be taken not to move the skin fiducials during cranial fixation prior to registration. It is critical that the reference arm be locked into place to prevent localization error during the biopsy. Once the entry site is chosen, a small area is shaved (2 × 2 cm), primarily to fix a bandage after closing. Extreme care must be taken when draping the patient not to cover the face and interfere with the exchange of air. We drape with four sponges fixed in place with a clear self-adhesive surgical drape. For frame-based cases, a C-arm drape is cut and fashioned to fit over the base ring and extends forward onto a Mayo stand, which is placed at eye level in front of the patient to keep the drapes off the face and the airway clear. A window is cut out of the C-arm drape over the operative site, and another self-adhesive fixes this in place. After attaching the stereotactic arc to the base ring a split sheet is then used with the tails extending onto the Mayo stand in front of the patient (**Fig. 33–4**). The skin over the entry site is then infiltrated with 1% lidocaine and 1:100,000 epinephrine. For the frameless cases, after registration is performed, we leave the fiducials on the skin during the procedure in case reregistration is required.

Operative Procedure and Instrumentation

Once the draping is complete, prior to making an incision, all numbers and calculations are double-checked. For frame-based procedures, the phantom is set at the target point to ensure the accuracy of the calculated trajectory. For frameless procedures, the entry site and trajectory are checked to make sure there has been no movement of the reference arm. For frame-based procedures, a 5 mm incision is made with a no. 11 blade, and the arc is brought into position. The stereotactic outer sleeve is advanced through the block until it is firmly pressing on the cranium. The distance between the block and the end of the sleeve (S) is measured and added to the calculated depth to the target (T) and the width of the block (B; generally 10 mm) to arrive at a final distance (D) (**Fig. 33–5**). The biopsy needle is then placed through the outer cannula, and a fixed marker is attached to the cannula at distance (D) from the tip. As an additional fail-safe, we also measure the distance between the marker and the end of the cannula to recheck our position intermittently during the procedure in case of movement (D) (**Fig. 33–5**). A 2.7 mm drill is used to perforate the skull and dura in a controlled fashion. The inner blunt-tipped trocar is placed inside the cannula and advanced through the dura. If any resistance is encountered, the drill is used to complete the perforation of the inner table and dura. The probe is advanced to the desired depth, and the inner blunt-tipped

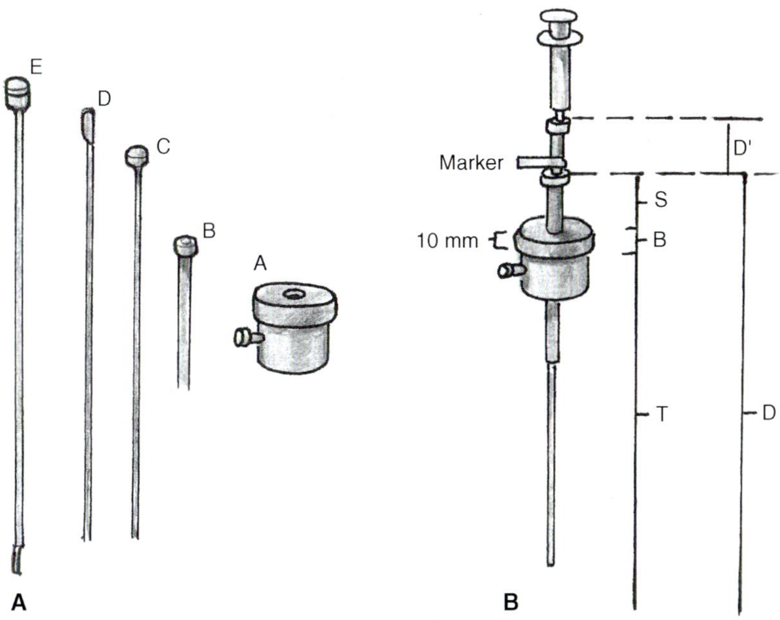

Figure 33–5 **(A)** The most commonly used instruments include the (a) block, (b) sleeve, (c) outer cannula, (d) blunt-tipped trocar, and (e) biopsy needle. **(B)** To accurately obtain the proper depth to the target, several measurements must be made and recorded for constant reference throughout the procedure. T, calculated depth to target; B, width of the block (generally 10 mm); S, distance between block and end of sleeve; D, final distance to target (= T + S + B); D′, distance between marker and end of cannula to ensure stability of the marker.

trocar is removed and replaced with the biopsy needle. For frameless procedures, a slightly larger incision and bur hole are utilized, and the rigid arm is brought into position and aligned prior to incising the dura to avoid leakage of cerebrospinal fluid. The pia is cauterized and incised with a no. 11 blade, and the biopsy needle is advanced using real-time frameless navigation.

We use a 3 mL syringe containing 1 mL of saline to produce the desired amount of negative pressure at the needle tip. One to two specimens are withdrawn, depending on the location of the tumor, and the process is repeated for each calculated target. Specimens are placed on a Petri dish in a few drops of saline for pathology or in culture tubes for microbiology.

Delivering the Specimen and Interpreting the Results

It is important to take an active rather than a passive role in the fate of the specimen to increase the diagnostic yield. The specimens are either directly presented to the pathologist in the operating room or delivered by hand to the laboratory. Providing a history and reviewing films with the pathologist are ideal. The slides should be reviewed by a member of the neurosurgical team as well. Nondiagnostic results such as inflammation or necrosis may require additional specimens. We will not infrequently change the depth of the target by a few millimeters to obtain tissue from a new location. With experience, both frame-based and frameless biopsies have diagnostic yield approaching 95%.[10]

Closure

Closure must be delayed until an adequate diagnosis has been made. One reabsorbable stitch is usually all that is required. Band-Aids are placed over the incision and the anterior pin sites after the frame is removed. Bleeding from pin sites can be controlled with either compression or a suture. Don't forget to remove the skin fiducials at the end of the case.

◆ Postoperative Care

Patients are brought to the recovery room and spend one night in the hospital for observation but do not require intensive care unit care. No anticonvulsants or steroids are administered. We routinely give perioperative antibiotics. It is possible to perform stereotactic biopsies as an outpatient procedure, but a postoperative CT is mandatory to ensure there is no hemorrhage, and patients should be observed for at least 6 hours.

◆ Complications

The literature reports an average morbidity of 2 to 4% and a mortality of 1% for both frame-based and frameless biopsies,[8,11] but with experience some groups achieve values of 1% and 0.2%, respectively. Epidural hematomas can occur if the dura is not penetrated with the drill and is stripped off the inner table with the blunt-tipped trocar. Subdural hematomas are more frequent in patients with cerebral atrophy, and special care should be taken in this population. Intraparenchymal hemorrhages also occur and can be avoided by ensuring normal preoperative coagulation, preventing postoperative hypertension, and avoiding known vascular structures. Patients should be instructed to stop taking aspirin or other nonsteroidal anti-inflammatory agents 7 days prior to the scheduled procedure. Biopsies adjacent to a ventricle are also dangerous because there is no tissue to tamponade a bleed should it occur. Infections are rare, and skull fracture can be avoided by placing extra pins in patients with thin skull and by careful inspection of the location of the sinuses on the preoperative CT scans.

References

1. Horsley V, Clarke RH. The structure and functions of the cerebellum examined by a new method. Brain 1908;31:45–124
2. Spiegel EA, Wycis HT, Marks M, Lee AJ. Stereotactic apparatus for operations on the human brain. Science 1947;106:349–350
3. Mathiesen T, Grane P, Lindgren L, Lindquist C. Third ventricular colloid cysts: a consecutive 12 year series. J Neurosurg 1997;86:5–12
4. Cohen DS, Lustgarten JH, Miller E, Khandji AG, Goodman RR. Effects of coregistration of MR to CT images on MR stereotactic accuracy. J Neurosurg 1995;82:772–779
5. Dorward NL, Alberti O, Palmer JD, Kitchen ND, Thomas DG. Accuracy of true frameless stereotaxy: in vivo measurements and laboratory phantom studies: technical note. J Neurosurg 1999;90:160–168
6. Grunert P, Espinosa J, Busert C, et al. Stereotactic biopsies guided by an optical navigation system: technique and clinical experience. Minim Invasive Neurosurg 2002;45:11–15
7. Paleologos TS, Dorward NL, Wadley JP, Thomas DG. Clinical validation of true frameless stereotactic biopsy: analysis of the first 125 consecutive cases. Neurosurgery 2001;49:830–837
8. Barnett GH, Miller DW, Weisenberger J. Frameless stereotaxy with scalp-applied fiducial markers for brain biopsy procedures: experience in 218 cases. J Neurosurg 1999;91:569–576
9. Stone JG, Schwartz AE, Berman MF, et al. Air embolization in seated, sedated, spontaneously breathing, neurosurgical patients. Anesthesiology 1997;87:1244–1247
10. Apuzzo ML, Chandrasoma PT, Cohen D, Zee CS, Zelman V. Computed imaging stereotaxy: experience and perspective related to 500 procedures applied to brain masses. Neurosurgery 1987;20:930–937
11. Neal JH, Apuzzo MLJ. History, instrumentation, and utility of stereotactic surgery. In: Chandrasoma PT, Apuzzo MLJ, eds. Stereotactic Brain Biopsy. New York: Igaku-Shoin; 1989:1–22

34

The Surgical Management of High-Grade Astrocytomas

Jack P. Rock and Mark L. Rosenblum

In 1985 Bucy et al drew attention to comments made by Percival Bailey in 1933, who, in his book entitled *Intracranial Tumors,* stated that it was futile to remove most glioblastomas. Bucy added that Dr. Bailey frequently mentioned that if he could be certain of the diagnosis of a glioblastoma, he would never operate on one.[1,2] This somewhat glib attitude can still be found today despite the positive impact surgery for malignant gliomas may have on survival and quality of life for many patients presenting with larger lesions. The fact is that removal of a significant mass lesion can extend survival and may provide time for adjuvant therapies to play their roles. No one working with patients with malignant glioma would deny these important and positive considerations. Whether or not surgery plays as critical a role for those patients with smaller lesions is yet to be determined. Therefore, even though when one considers the 5-year survival figures in isolation, we have extended survival by only a slight degree in the last 30 years by various new approaches to treatment, surgery remains an integral part of the overall management considerations for patients with newly diagnosed brain lesions suspected to be malignant glioma.

Because tissue diagnosis still remains the standard upon which treatment should be based, surgery for biopsy remains an important consideration in most patients. This chapter discusses the issues relevant to surgery for resection of tumor as opposed to biopsy alone, and it should also be noted that the designation "malignant glioma" will refer to both anaplastic glioma and glioblastoma multiforme.

◆ Indications

There are two categories of indications for surgery on lesions thought to be malignant gliomas: practical and theoretical (**Table 34–1**). There are four practical reasons for surgical intervention in patients with a brain tumor. The first indication is to obtain histologic diagnosis given the lack of absolute specificity of modern radiographic imaging. The second surgical indication is to improve neurological symptoms or signs in patients for whom the mass effect of their tumor and its surrounding edema is a direct cause of their disability. Third, surgery can be prescribed to delay the onset of new symptoms or signs when radiographic tumor growth has been documented, and, lastly, surgery can improve survival

Table 34–1 Indications for Surgery

Practical	Theoretical
Tissue diagnosis	Removal of poorly oxygenated, radiation-resistant tumor cells
Improve symptoms/signs	Removal of poorly vascularized and sequestered tumor regions
Delay onset of new symptoms/signs	Removal and decrease of tumor cells that are resistant to adjuvant therapy
Increase survival with life-threatening mass lesions	

by removing immediately life-threatening mass lesions. Theoretical indications for surgical intervention are always controversial but are generally thought to improve the patient's response to therapy. These indications include the removal of poorly oxygenated, radiation-resistant tumor cells, the removal of poorly vascularized regions of the tumors that on a basis of marginal blood supply are sequestered from systemic intravenous and intra-arterial therapies, and the removal of tumor cells that are or will become resistant to adjuvant therapies. The controversy surrounding these latter indications is based on the relative lack of scientific evidence directly correlating these indications with patient survival. These controversies are of less concern in treatment of lesions associated with mass effect than when brought to bear for treatment of small, asymptomatic lesions detected radiographically in the process of patient follow-up (**Table 34–1**).

All surgeons who frequently treat patients with malignant gliomas are exquisitely aware of what is perhaps the greatest surgical controversy, and this is whether to pursue a limited versus a more thorough attempt to remove the tumor. The basis for the controversy derives from the literature on malignant glioma, which until recently was inconclusive as to the relative efficacy of radical versus limited tumor removal with regard to prolongation of survival. Recent evidence[3] indicates that a significant survival advantage follows resection of 98% or more of the tumor volume, but because a majority of conclusions from this literature are based on retrospective, uncontrolled studies and can rightfully be contested from opposite ends of the argument, it necessarily remains the surgeon's bias as to the value of radical versus limited resections. Those who recommend limited removal of tumor usually proclaim the lack of information supporting radical resection, the increased morbidity associated with its performance, and the likelihood that adjuvant therapies are actually the primary source of increased patient survival. Those who advocate radical removal of tumor usually feel that the arguments noted in **Table 34–1** justify the risk of increased morbidity, but only when radical resection is performed in the hands of surgeons employing the latest techniques for brain mapping and intraoperative imaging, thereby implying decreased risk of these morbidities. At the present time, it is unclear which approach is optimal and treatment plans remain with the surgeons, their patients, and their biases.

Despite Dr. Bailey's schooled remarks, and in view of our still limited ability to predict the histology of a given lesion on the basis of the radiographic imaging data, most but not all contemporary surgeons would advocate radical or bulk removal for those large lesions with or without mass effect located on the surface of the brain or in "silent" regions of the brain (i.e., anterior two thirds of the right and left frontal lobes and the entire right nondominant temporal but limited left temporal lobes) for tissue confirmation and resection of tumor mass despite the controversies already mentioned. It must be recalled that the invasive nature of gliomas may disguise functional cortex lying within the perceived lesion even when the lesion is located on the surface of the brain.[4] For all other brain regions (i.e., those areas considered eloquent in that they contain neural tissue critical to the maintenance of a high quality of life such as vision, speech, understanding, muscle control, and sensory perception), the controversial issues would lead to varying approaches.

◆ Surgical Technique

Preparation

The study that is first and foremost for the assessment of patients with presumed malignant glioma is magnetic resonance brain imaging (MRI) with and without contrast. Although computed tomography (CT) is still a practical surrogate, the additional information generated by MRI can be especially helpful for differential diagnostic considerations. CT remains helpful in differential diagnosis for demonstrating calcium and blood within a lesion.

Cerebral angiography may occasionally prove helpful for differential diagnosis and for assessment of lesion vascularity; however, MRI and to a lesser degree magnetic resonance angiography (MRA) will serve both purposes in the majority of cases.

MRI spectroscopic imaging and positron emission tomography (PET) are working their way forward to greater utility for the diagnosis of malignant glioma but currently lack the necessary specificity to supplant biopsy for precise diagnosis.

Functional MRI technology allows the surgeon to preoperatively estimate the relationship of functional neurological tissues to tumor tissues and, thereby, gain greater appreciation of potential operative risks. However, this technology should not be considered an alternative to intraoperative brain mapping.

In terms of preparation for operation, it has been our experience that the administration of steroids (e.g., dexamethasone 4 mg q6h) for at least 48 hours prior to surgery may decrease the amount of brain swelling encountered upon opening the dura. Based on the literature, anticonvulsants may or may not be prescribed in patients without a history of seizures, but at our institution they are prescribed.

Anesthesia

Anesthesia should be administered by an experienced team familiar with neurophysiological monitoring. When preparing for intraoperative brain mapping, we generally begin with short-acting muscle paralysis and maintain the patient asleep with a combined low concentration of isoflurane (halogenated compounds can interfere with the mapping process) for amnesia and fentanyl for analgesia. Because halogenated anesthetics in higher concentration and nitrous oxide may lower electroencephalographic (EEG) and electromyographic (EMG) amplitudes, the isoflurane concentration is reduced to 0.5 minimum alveolar concentration (MAC) prior to mapping, and nitrous oxide is not used. After mapping is completed, standard concentrations and combinations of anesthetics are reinstituted.

Positioning

The details of preparation in the operating room are common to most approaches and include the following issues:

1. Venous pressure—the head should be maintained higher than the heart and oriented in a way to maximize blood return through the jugular veins.
2. Pressure points and stretch injuries—a visibly "comfortable" position for the patient will minimize the chance of pressure ulceration (e.g., padding under the heels, ankles, fibular heads, and wrists) and stretch injuries that may occur during lengthy procedures. Stretch injuries can occur as a result of taping the extremities, which, while optimizing surgeon comfort and thereby operative dissection, may lead to peripheral nerve injury. Examples of these considerations include careful taping of the shoulder to avoid traction on the brachial plexus, placement of pillows under the knees in the supine position to relieve tension on the sciatic nerves, use of extensions for the shoulder placed several inches below the table for lateral positions to relax the brachial plexus, and the use of soft towels under the axilla to prevent distortion of the shoulder and injury to the plexus.
3. Fluid balance—intravenous access by either or both peripheral line and central venous lines is required depending on the expected need for fluid replacement and the cardiovascular status of the patient. Urinary catheters are necessary for most intracranial procedures because of the time involved, the high volumes of urine expected after administration of osmotic diuretics, and the need to adequately assess the cardiovascular status throughout the procedure. Right atrial access is recommended for sitting and other positions that place the patient's head well above the heart during which the risk of air embolism is considered significant.
4. Medications and miscellaneous—Pre-, intra-, and postoperative steroids to limit brain edema, antibiotics, and anticonvulsants are always administered. Type and cross-matches are considered for procedures in which major vascular manipulation during approach and dissection is anticipated (e.g., hemangioblastoma).
5. Venous stasis is minimized by application of elastic stockings from the upper thigh to the ankles along with pneumatic compression wraps.
6. Patient positioning and operative procedure—the tumor should be at the "top" (e.g., the highest point anatomically to facilitate intraoperative dissection and promote venous return) of the patient, and the head should be oriented to most closely approximate standard anatomical position, thereby decreasing the chance of the surgeon becoming disoriented during the dissection. There are numerous publications that describe the elements of positioning for the various approaches involved for removal of brain tumors, and we will not discuss these issues. The following sections will overview the main concepts of the "standard procedure" as they relate specifically to surgery for malignant gliomas[5] (**Fig. 34–1**).

Incision

One of the considerations unique and common in glioma surgery is the placement and intraoperative care of the surgical incision (**Fig. 34–2**). The uniqueness of this aspect of the surgical procedure is derived from the fact that, for practical purposes, malignant gliomas are not curable, and sooner or later virtually all patients will at least have to consider second and subsequent operative interventions whether these be for stereotactic differential diagnosis (e.g., radiation necrosis vs recurrent glioma) or reoperation for recurrent mass effect from tumor, infection, or radiation necrosis. These realities will be superimposed on others relating to radiation therapy and other adjuvant therapies, which will all potentially compromise scalp healing. Although small incisions may be enticing to the surgeon and the patient, one would do well to anticipate future patterns of recurrence and be aware that the tumor is going to regrow from the anatomical point where the surgeon is least able to gain access during the first operation, whether this be as a result of adjacent eloquent tissues or depth. Attention to scalp blood supply relative to the length and width of the flap is critical, and generally the length of the flap should not be more than 30% greater than the width.

Cranial and Dural Opening

Small bone plates can severely limit tumor dissection when tumor extends beyond the edges of the plate, but perhaps more importantly when preoperative brain swelling is present (**Fig. 34–3**). In the latter case, the cortical tissue may swell into the cranial opening, obscuring tissue boundaries and possibly leading to infarction and hemorrhage along the bone edges, which may seriously complicate the resection, especially when done in proximity to eloquent tissue. With these considerations noted, it may be concluded that the cranial opening does not differ in consideration from openings for most other tumor types. The dural opening and more specifically its closure, however, may be more critical. Because the patient will ultimately have postoperative radiation therapy and chemotherapy or other adjuvant therapy, it is important that the dura be closed in a watertight fashion if at all possible. Pericranial grafts are optimal and can almost always be obtained if the need is properly anticipated at the time of the incision planning. Artificial grafts are less optimal but may suffice, although the incidence of meningocele or cerebrospinal fluid leak or both has been higher in our experience, especially for lesions in the posterior fossa.

Neurophysiological Monitoring

Although many surgeons may choose to avoid operation altogether when lesions are located in close proximity to eloquent regions or assume that simply "remaining within the center" of the enhancing or necrotic-appearing mass will preclude morbidity (a potentially misleading concept), techniques have been developed to decrease the morbidity of radical resection even when lesions abut, displace, or undercut these regions. The localization of the motor strip can

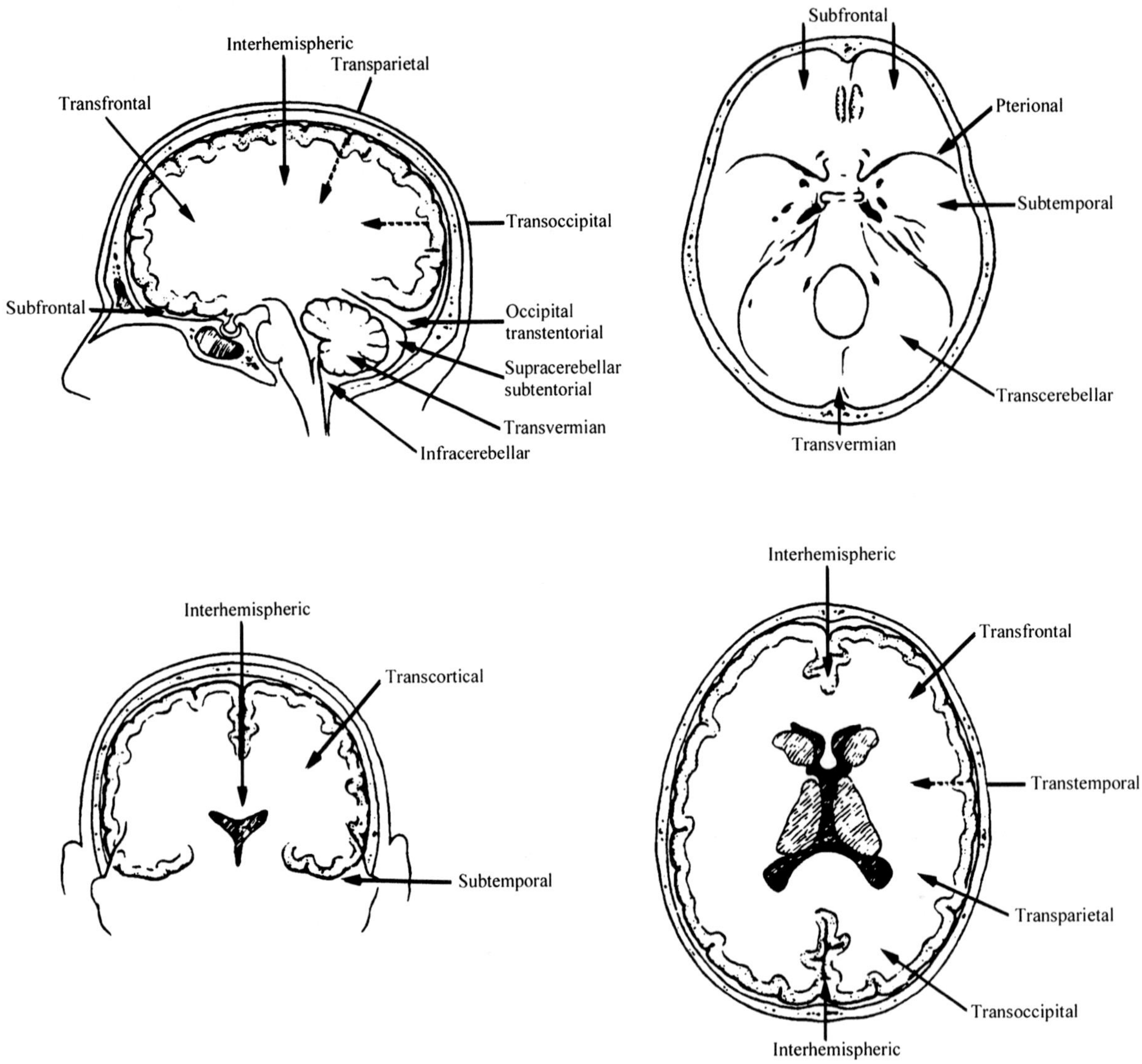

Figure 34–1 Surgical approaches employed for the treatment of patients with malignant glioma.

be estimated reliably in an anesthetized patient by cortical motor mapping. This technique involves neurophysiological methods to stimulate the cortex, causing the patient's face and limbs to move, thereby indicating the precise location of functional brain (**Fig. 34–4**). Similar technology is employed in the awake patient to localize the speech areas, in which case speech will be altered or halted when eloquent cortex is stimulated. For intraoperative speech mapping, electroencephalography (EEG) is used to indicate the occurrence of subclinical seizure activity and the length of the refractory period after suprathreshold stimulation.

Generally, a bipolar electrode with 5 mm spacing is used to stimulate the cortex. A constant current generator produces biphasic waves at a frequency of 50 Hz. For the anesthetized patient, anesthetic agent is maintained at ~0.5 MAC, and stimulatory currents range from 2 to 20 mA; for the awake patient the cortex will frequently stimulate with less than 6 mA. When the visible cortex does not stimulate, strip electrodes can be placed under the edge of the bone flap to determine whether eloquent cortex is nearby and its relation to the exposed surface, but, in general, larger craniotomies are better. Additionally, body temperature greater than 36.5°C, absence of paralytics, and charged batteries in the stimulator are required to assure successful mapping. Focal seizures resulting from cortical stimulation can be controlled by short-acting barbiturates, but iced Ringer's lactate solution[6] applied to the cortex will also control this activity, and, in some cases, the barbiturates will interfere with the mapping process. Although electrocorticography is not absolutely required for mapping cortical function in tumor surgery, its use, when indicated, may aid in locating a seizure focus and will allow the surgeon to determine the relative refractory period of the cortex after stimulation. This knowledge indicates the level of current below which to carry out the remainder of the mapping process to avoid further seizure activity. However, for practical reasons, the surgeon may assume that the stimulating current can be increased until a seizure occurs.

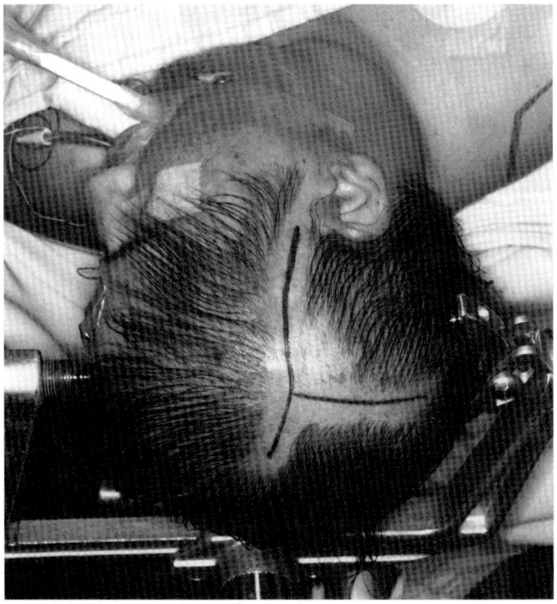

Figure 34–2 The original incision for this anteriorly positioned temporal glioma was linear, extending from the zygoma to the midline. At the time, this easily allowed subtotal resection. The remaining portion of the lesion, however, was located at the posterior temporal extent, and, predictably, the epicenter of the recurrence was positioned posteriorly. This required modification of the original incision, possibly compromising wound healing. A larger standard reverse question mark incision initially would have decreased the potential morbidity of the incision at the time of recurrence.

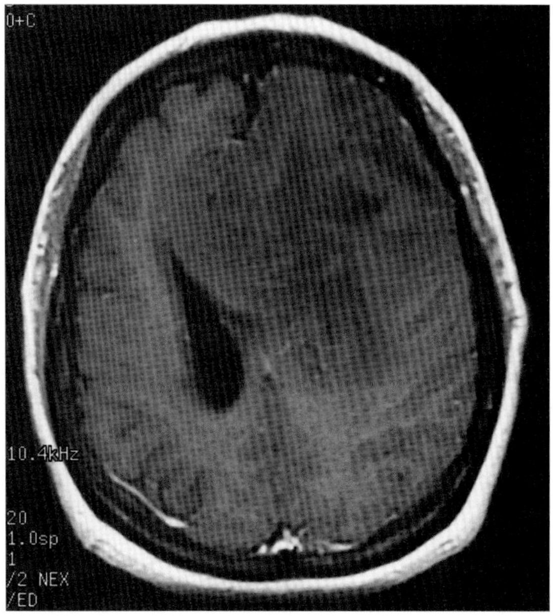

Figure 34–3 Operation on this large glioma would require a large bone plate because the brain will swell at opening.

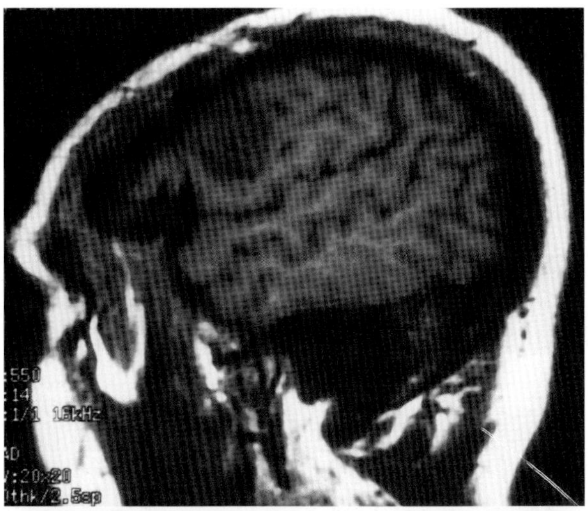

A

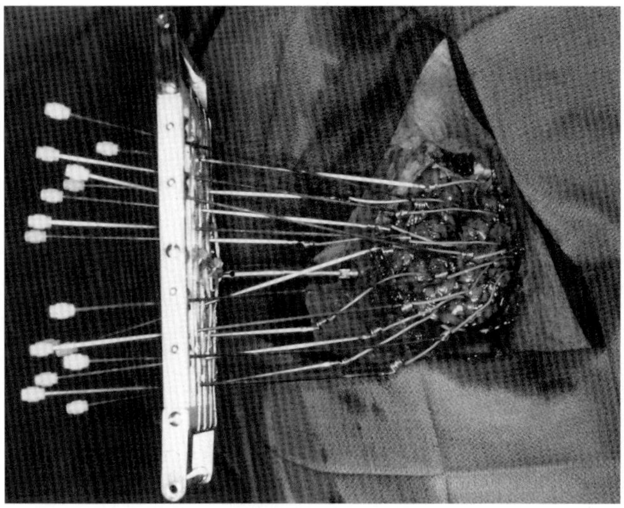

B

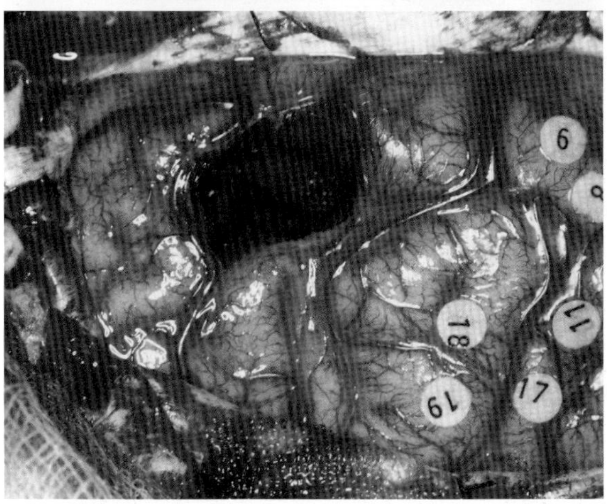

C

Figure 34–4 **(A)** Right-sided posterior frontal glioma. **(B)** Electrocorticography array in place. **(C)** Resection cavity noted anterior to precentral gyrus.

At that point, the seizure can be managed with iced lactate solution, and the surgeon can consider that the current utilized throughout the remainder of the procedure must be maintained below that level. In most situations, careful use of cortical and subcortical mapping will decrease the morbidity of the surgical procedure.

Tumor Removal

While the primary goal of tumor surgery should be to completely remove the pathological tissue, the invasive nature of malignant gliomas precludes curative resection, and, therefore, the first priority of the surgeon is to remove as much of the tumor as possible while preserving or improving neurological function.

Once the surgeon has determined the relationship of functional brain to tumor tissue, the resection can be undertaken. Although dissection around the perimeter of the tumor can be an effective technique for benign and vascular lesions, this approach will frequently not be useful with malignant gliomas because of the relative lack of a true tumor border. However, even though these lesions do not have a true boundary, there is an anatomical point at which the main body of the more necrotic and vascular tumor begins to blend almost imperceptibly with the surrounding white mater (**Fig. 34–5**). This pseudoplane will be infiltrated by microscopic tumor cells but is relatively bloodless. More commonly, a direct attack on the grossly abnormal central body of the tumor is performed by either or both suction and ultrasonic aspiration, thereby quickly debulking the mass. In this case the surgeon must be prepared for a brief period of brisk bleeding, which can usually be controlled by gentle compression with Gelfoam and cotton. Bipolar coagulation may be effective but will slow the procedure and invariably the vessels, which at this point in the dissection are being coagulated and will invariably bleed again in the latter points of the dissection.

In some glioblastomas the necrotic and vascular portions of the tumor may extend into less accessible brain regions deep within the operative exposure or into areas that the surgeon feels could contain functional brain tissue. In these instances, it is best to obtain hemostasis without “chasing” the tumor further than necessary. Some combination of bipolar coagulation, oxidized cellulose, Gelfoam soaked in thrombin, compression with cotton, and patience will, for practical purposes, always control the bleeding. Not uncommonly, chasing the tumor will lead to bleeding that can only be controlled by dissecting into areas that the surgeon had hoped to avoid altogether.

Preservation of arterial structures should always be attempted. Vessels that appear interwoven with the tumor capsule at the beginning of the dissection will usually become freed and more easily separable after internal decompression of the tumor.

Realizing that surgery cannot remove all the cells of a malignant glioma, the surgeon must have an end point in mind for the intervention, and this is usually gross tumor debulking. However, in attempting to more precisely define the extent of resection, the surgeon has recourse to intraoperative imaging technology. Three-dimensional image guidance allows the surgeon to achieve resection up to the peripheral borders of contrast enhancement and T2 signal abnormality when indicated (**Fig. 34–6**). More recent developments also suggest that magnetic resonance spectroscopy may act as an additional and possibly more thorough guide to surgical resection in the future.

Closure

After perfect hemostasis has been obtained, a single layer of oxidized cellulose may be left covering the surface of the operated tumor and brain. The dura is closed in a watertight fashion either primarily or secondarily. If the dural flaps are maintained moist throughout the procedure, primary closure is more likely, but grafting would be preferred to stretching the dry dural edges to the point that they just barely approximate one another, thereby falling short of watertight closure.

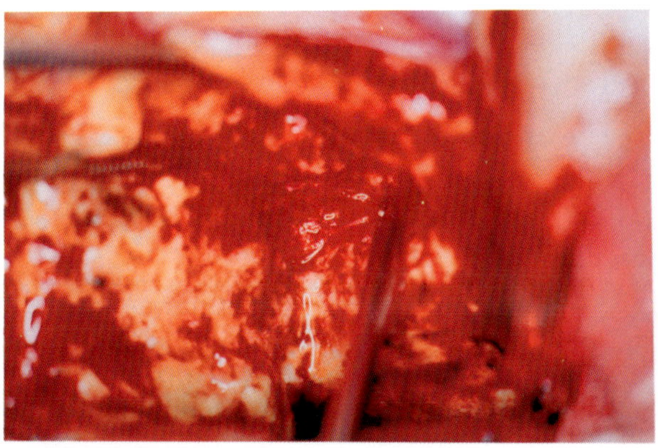
A

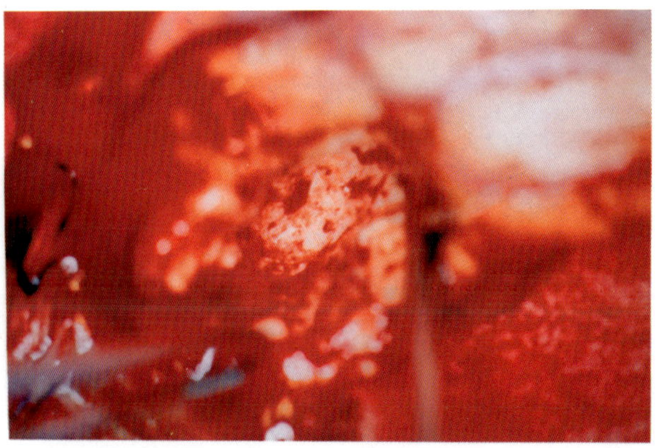
B

Figure 34–5 **(A)** As the bulk of the necrotic tumor is removed, one can appreciate the lack of defining border. **(B)** Although there still is no clear-cut border at the margins of the lesion, one can appreciate the relatively “avascular plane” beyond which resection may proceed with intraoperative guidance.

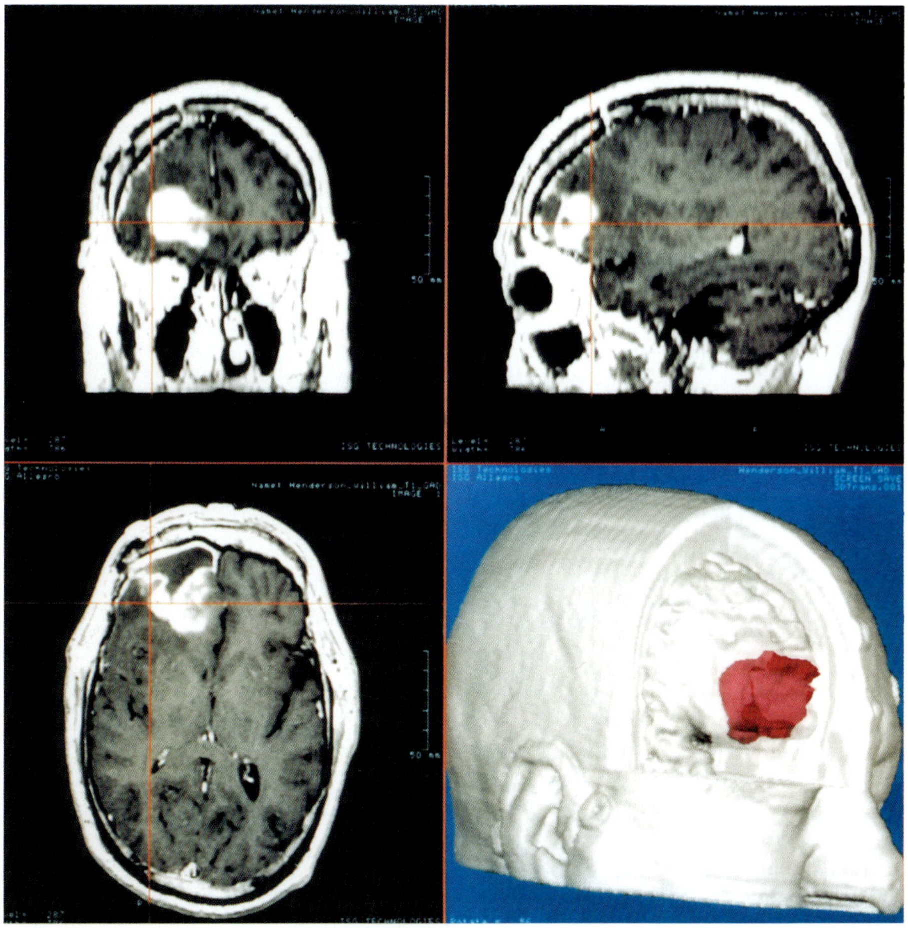

Figure 34–6 The cursors overlie the posterior margins of the tumor, and further resection of this particular lesion could proceed safely, but lesions in or adjacent to eloquent cortex would better be guided by intraoperative mapping or image guidance or both.

◆ Postoperative Care

In the immediate postoperative period, attention to blood pressure is paramount but is certainly not a substitute for absolute intraoperative hemostasis. If the patient does not awaken to some degree within the first 2 hours, CT scanning should be considered to assess for hematoma, hydrocephalus, or pneumocephalus. Within the first 2 days postoperative MRI should be considered to serve as a baseline upon which to determine and follow subsequent treatment initiatives.

◆ Conclusions

"Do no harm" is never more apt than when treating patients with malignant glioma. Life expectancy is limited, treatment alone will take its toll, and quality of life is critical. The discerning use of standard and newly developing technologies is essential to helping our patients live with their disease.

References

1. Bailey P. Intracranial Tumors. Springfield, IL: Charles C Thomas; 1933
2. Bucy PC, Oberhill HR, Siqueira EB, Zimmerman HM, Jelsma RK. Cerebral glioblastomas can be cured! Neurosurgery 1985;16: 714–717
3. Lacroix M, Abi-Said D, Fourney DR, Gokaslan ZL, Shi W, DeMonte F, et al. A multivariate analysis of 416 patients with glioblastoma multiferme: prognosis, extent of resection, and survival. J Neurosurg 2001; 95:190–198
4. Ojemann RG. Surgical principles in the management of brain tumors. In: Kaye AH, Laws ER, eds. Brain Surgery in Brain Tumors: Churchill Livingstone; 1995:293–303
5. Sartorius CJ, Berger MS. Rapid termination of intraoperative stimulation-evoked seizures with application of cold Ringer's lactate to the cortex. J Neurosurg 1998;88:349–351

35A

Oligodendroglioma

Ghassan K. Bejjani, Constantinos G. Hadjipanayis, and Marta Couce

Oligodendrogliomas are well-differentiated, diffusely infiltrating tumors of adults, typically located in the cerebral hemispheres and composed predominantly of cells morphologically resembling oligodendroglia. Sir Percival Bailey played an important role in laying the foundation of knowledge of this tumor and its behavior. In 1924, along with Hiller, he suggested that oligodendrocytes may be involved in brain tumors. In 1926, he was the first to describe oligodendrogliomas in a series of nine patients he published with Harvey Cushing. A subsequent paper by Bailey and Bucy in 1929 in which they described 13 cases of oligodendrogliomas correlated the tumor's histologic description and clinical behavior.

◆ Incidence

Oligodendrogliomas represent around 5% of all intracranial gliomas. They are the third most common intracranial glioma following glioblastoma multiforme and anaplastic astrocytoma.

The majority of oligodendrogliomas arise in adults, with a peak incidence in the fourth and fifth decades. About 6% of oligodendrogliomas arise during infancy and childhood, where they represent 1% of pediatric brain tumors.

◆ Localization

Oligodendrogliomas arise preferentially in the cortex and white matter of the cerebral hemispheres, where their distribution follows that of oligodendrocytes and the mass of the white matter. The frontal lobe is involved most commonly, followed by the temporal and parietal lobes and lastly the occipital lobe. Intraventricular, cerebellar, brain stem, spinal cord, and primary leptomeningeal tumors have been reported. Intraventricular oligodendrogliomas must be differentiated from central neurocytomas, which express neuronal cell markers. Oligodendrogliomas have rarely been noted to metastasize. Multiple intracranial lesions have been reported.

◆ Clinical Presentation

Most patients with oligodendrogliomas present with a several-year history of seizures. Seizures are the presenting symptom in 50% of patients and eventually occur in 70 to 90% of patients. In the pre-computed tomography (CT) era, the seizures were usually present for 5 years on average before the diagnosis was made, with some being present for an even longer period. These periods are becoming shorter with the use of CT and magnetic resonance imaging (MRI). Patients typically have generalized tonic–clonic seizures. The high incidence of seizures in patients with oligodendrogliomas may be related to the tendency of these tumors to diffusely infiltrate the cerebral cortex. Patients may also present with headache and focal neurological deficit.

◆ Imaging

Oligodendrogliomas are avascular or faintly vascular on angiography. They are readily demonstrated by CT and MRI (**Fig. 35A–1**). On CT, these tumors appear as hypodense, well-demarcated mass lesions located in the cortex and subcortical white matter. Enhancement is mild to moderate. Calcifications are hyperdense on CT and may appear ribbon-like or gyriform in pattern. They are seen in 70 to 90% of cases. Scalloping of the skull may be seen.

On MRI, T1-weighted images demonstrate a mixed hypo- and isointense lesion, and T2-weighted images demonstrate a hyperintense lesion, with patchy and moderate enhancement. These lesions appear very similar on MRI to other low-grade gliomas (low-grade fibrillary astrocytomas and

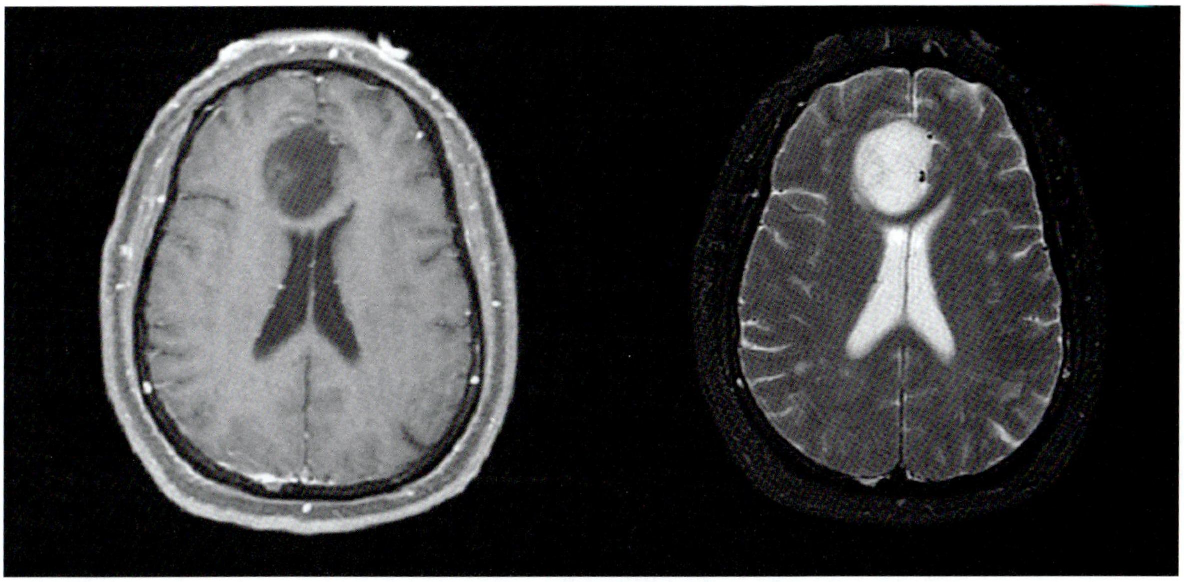

Figure 35A–1 Magnetic resonance imaging axial view, T1 with contrast and T2.

oligoastrocytomas). Some tumors may demonstrate heterogeneous signal intensities due to intratumoral hemorrhage and areas of cystic degeneration (**Fig. 35A–2**).

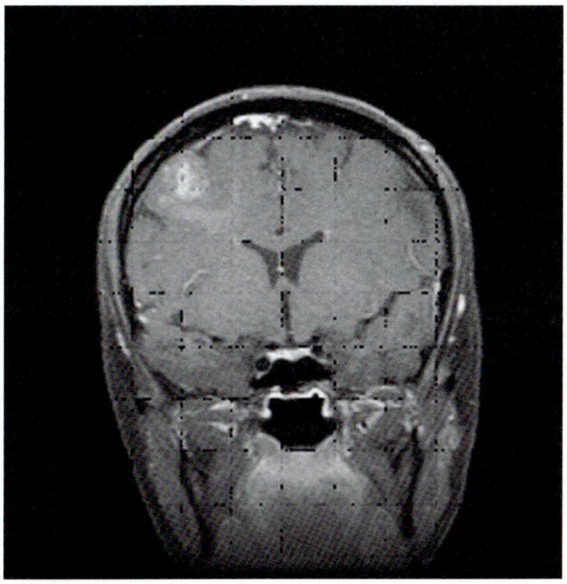

Figure 35A–2 Magnetic resonance imaging coronal view, T1 with contrast.

◆ Histopathology and Grading

These tumors are moderately cellular and composed of tumor cells with rounded, homogeneous nuclei. The "fried egg" artifact is a distinctive feature of many oligodendrogliomas on paraffin sections created by autolytic imbibition of water accompanying delayed fixation. This process forms clear perinuclear halos, which produce the "honeycomb" appearance characteristic of this tumor. Additional features include microcalcifications, mucoid/cystic degeneration, and a dense network of branching capillaries (**Fig. 35A–3**).

The World Health Organization (WHO) grading system recognizes two malignancy grades for oligodendroglial tumors: WHO grade II for well-differentiated tumors, and WHO grade III for anaplastic oligodendroglioma. Marked nuclear atypia and an occasional mitosis are compatible with the diagnosis of WHO grade II oligodendroglioma, but significant mitotic activity, prominent microvascular proliferation, or conspicuous necrosis indicates progression to anaplastic oligodendroglioma WHO grade III (**Fig. 35A–4**).

Oligodendrogliomas grow diffusely in the cortex and white matter. Within the cortex, tumor cells form secondary structures such as perineuronal satellitosis, perivascular aggregations, and subpial accumulations. The Ki67/Mib-1 index is usually below 5%.

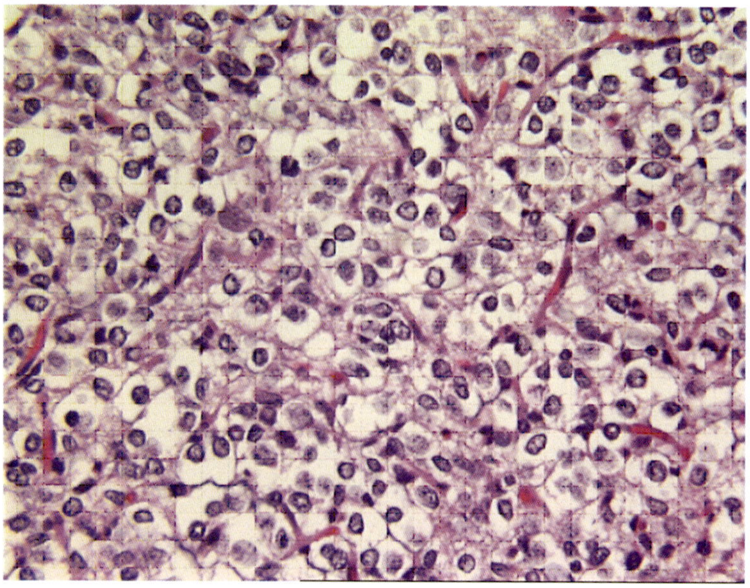

Figure 35A–3 Tumor cells with clear cytoplasm and well-defined plasma membrane. Note the typical dense network of branching capillaries.

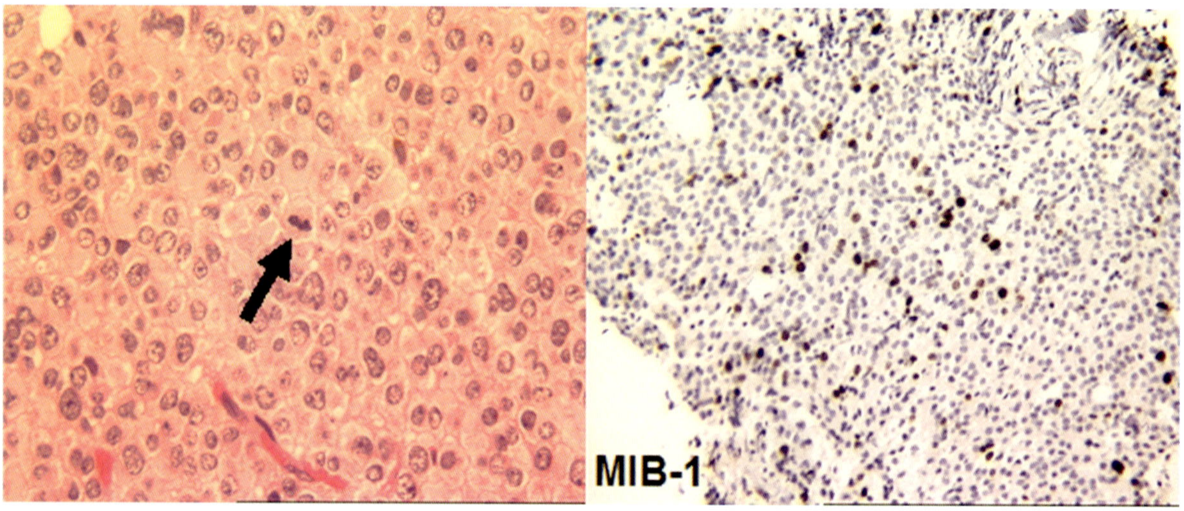

Figure 35A–4 Anaplastic oligodendroglioma **(A)** showing mitotic figures (arrow), and **(B)** focally increased Mib-1 proliferation index.

◆ Molecular Genetics

The most frequent genetic alteration in oligodendrogliomas is loss of heterozygosity (LOH) on the long arm of chromosome 19. The incidence of LOH on 19q varies between 50 and 80%. The second most frequent genetic alteration in oligodendrogliomas is LOH on the short arm of chromosome 1. Virtually all oligodendrogliomas with LOH on 1p have also lost alleles on 19q.

Anaplastic oligodendrogliomas share with low grade oligodendrogliomas the frequent loss of alleles on 1p and 19q, but additionally show an increased incidence of deletions on the short arm of chromosome 9 or on chromosome 10 or both. These additional alterations are also frequently seen in malignant astrocytomas.

◆ Treatment

Surgery

The goal of surgery is to provide the maximum volumetric reduction with the minimum functional loss. Although there are various opinions when it comes to the correlation between resection and survival, most series report a positive correlation between extent of resection and increased survival. The location of some lesions in the eloquent cortex makes surgery with minimal loss of function challenging. During surgery, a plane can be occasionally identified using the microscope where the difference in color and consistency between the tumor and adjacent brain can be seen. Calcifications are encountered during resection; they provide a gritty feel and are occasionally seen macroscopically. The vascularity is another differentiating feature between normal and tumoral tissues. Cortical and subcortical mapping, the operating microscope, neuronavigational techniques, and intraoperative ultrasound are useful adjuncts in this setting.

Radiation Therapy

Various series have been published with some showing a clear advantage for radiation therapy and others the opposite. In the lack of large, prospective, controlled series, the risk of radiation therapy has to be weighed against its benefit in the management of oligodendrogliomas.

Chemotherapy

Chemotherapy has been shown to be of benefit in the treatment of oligodendrogliomas, including procarbazine, CCNU (lomustine), and vincristine. Adjuvant chemotherapy should be considered in the treatment of residual or recurrent anaplastic oligodendrogliomas, as well as oligodendrogliomas with more aggressive clinical and radiological behavior. Chromosomal deletion 1p19q has been shown to predict chemosensitivity in these tumors.

Suggested Readings

Bailey DL, Cushing H. A Classification of Tumors of the Glioma Group on a Histogenetic Basis with a Correlation Study of Prognosis. Lippincott: Philadelphia; 1926

Lee YY, Van Tassel P. Intracranial oligodendrogliomas: imaging findings in 35 untreated cases. AJR Am J Roentgenol 1989;152:1263–1270

Mork SJ, Lindegaard KF, Lalvorsen TB, et al. Oligodendroglioma incidence and biological behavior in a defined population. J Neurosurg 1985;63: 881–889

Nijjar TS, Simpson WJ, Gadalla T, McCartney M. Oligodendroglioma: the princess Margaret Hospital experience. Cancer 1993;71:4002–4006

Reifenberger J, Reifenberger G, Liu L, James CD, Wechler W, Collins VP. Molecular genetic analysis of oligodendroglial tumors shows preferential allelic deletions on 19q and 1p. Am J Pathol 1994;145:1175–1190

World Health Organization Classification of Tumours. Pathology and Genetics. Tumours of the Nervous System. Paul Kleihues and Webster K Cavenee, eds. Lyon: IARC Press; 2000

35B

Ganglion Cell Tumors

Ghassan K. Bejjani and Marta Couce

The World Health Organization (WHO) categorizes central nervous system (CNS) tumors with neuronal and mixed neuronal–glial composition as follows:

1.7 Neuronal and mixed neuronal–glial tumors:
- 1.7.1 Gangliocytomas and gangliogliomas
- 1.7.2 Dysplastic gangliocytoma of the cerebellum (Lhermitte-Duclos)
- 1.7.3 Desmoplastic infantile ganglioglioma (DIG)
- 1.7.4 Dysembryoplastic neuroepithelial tumors (DNETs)
- 1.7.5 Neurocytoma

This chapter discusses these lesions, the majority of which fall in the *gangliocytoma/ganglioglioma* group, which will be the main focus. These lesions are a continuum between lesions with a predominant neuronal component (gangliocytomas) and those with a predominant glial component (ganglioglioma). The dysplastic gangliocytoma of the cerebellum or Lhermitte-Duclos disease may be considered a hamartomatous lesion more than it is a true tumor, rarely coming to the surgeon's attention, and will not be discussed here. *Desmoplastic infantile ganglioglioma* (DIG) is a very large, superficially located, glioneuronal tumor rich in collagen occurring in infancy. *Dysembryoplastic neuroepithelial tumors* (DNETs) consist of a quasi hamartomatous, multinodular, intracortical mass, with a mostly glial component mixed with neuronal elements. They frequently come to the surgeon's attention in patients with a history of temporal seizure. *Neurocytomas* are small-cell tumors occurring in the cerebral ventricles, resembling oligodendroglioma on optic microscopy.

◆ Gangliocytoma/Ganglioglioma

Epidemiology

These represent 0.5 to 7.6% of tumors of the CNS: the higher percentages are in pediatric series, whereas the overall incidence is around 1% in adult series with no sex predilection. Sixty to eighty percent occur in the initial 3 decades of life, with tumors encountered at both extremes of life. They represent 1% of intramedullary spinal cord tumors.

Location

Gangliocytomas and gangliogliomas occur throughout the CNS, including the spinal cord, but are mostly in the cerebral hemisphere, especially the temporal lobe. They can also occur along the midline: third and fourth ventricles, hypothalamus, thalamus, optic nerve and chiasm, and pineal area. They have been reported in the posterior fossa also (brain stem and cerebellum).

Clinical Manifestations

These are slow-growing tumors, with the duration of symptoms 4 to 8 years prior to diagnosis. Centrally located tumors present earlier than hemispheric lesions.

Usually they present with seizures or headaches, although focal deficits may be seen. Seizures are the most common presenting symptom (60 to 100%) in patients with hemispheric lesions present, whereas focal deficits are the most common presenting symptom (60%) in those with centrally located tumors.

Imaging

Computed Tomographic Scan

The appearance of these lesions is extremely variable, although classically they present as a cyst with an iso- or hypodense mural nodule that is frequently calcified. Hemispheric lesions close to the surface can cause scalloping of the skull because of the slow growth rate.

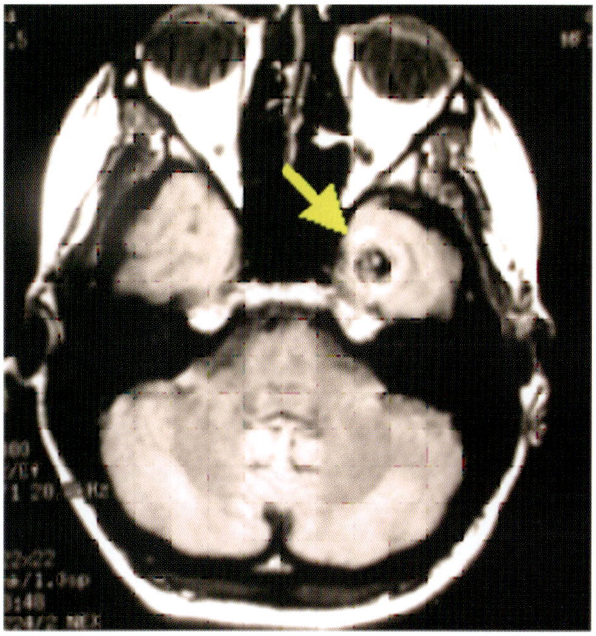

Figure 35B–1 Magnetic resonance imaging of a ganglioglioma.

Magnetic Resonance Imaging Scans

Magnetic resonance imaging (MRI) appearance is also variable. Lesions are mostly hypointense on T1 and hyperintense on T2, with a variable degree (from none to marked) and pattern (rim, solid, nodular) of enhancement **(Fig. 35B–1)**.

Angiography

Angiography is of limited use showing an avascular mass.

Pathology

These tumors are usually well circumscribed, but gangliogliomas may extend locally into leptomeninges. They are well-differentiated neuroepithelial tumors composed of neoplastic, mature ganglion cells, either alone (gangliocytomas) or in combination with neoplastic glial cells (gangliogliomas). Gangliocytomas are grade I under the WHO classification. Gangliogliomas can be WHO grade I, II, II, and, rarely, IV, when changes in the glial component are consistent with a glioblastoma.

Histopathologically, these tumors are commonly composed of neurons showing dysplastic features. In gangliocytomas, the stroma is composed of non-neoplastic glial elements. Gangliogliomas demonstrate an additional glial neoplastic element. The glial component can undergo malignant change. Other features commonly seen include perivascular lymphocytic infiltration, eosinophilic granular bodies, microcysts, and calcification **(Fig. 35B–2)**.

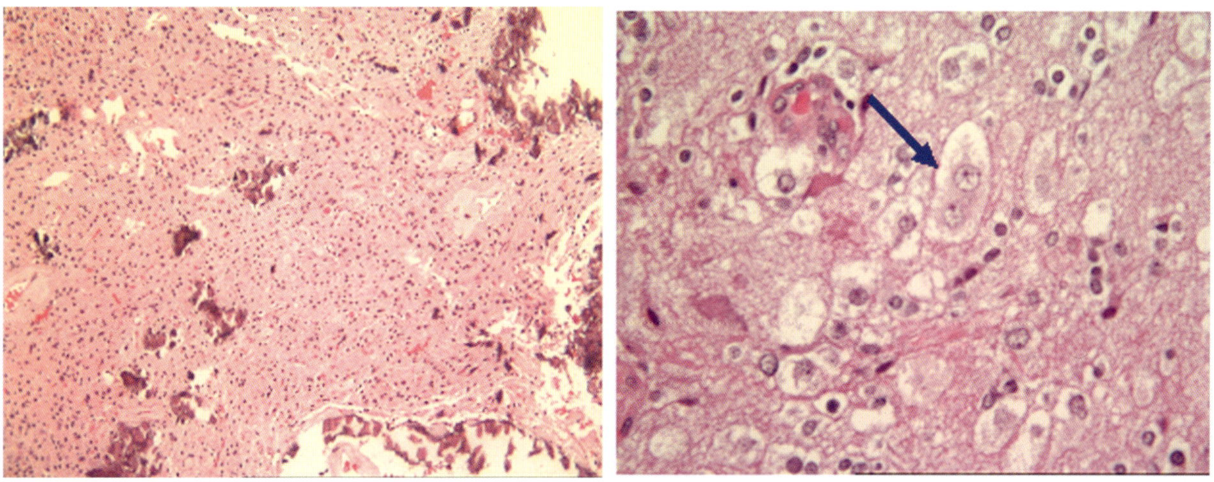

Figure 35B–2 Microscopic image of a ganglioglioma, demonstrating multiple foci of calcification and a hypercellular background composed of glial and ganglion cells. Dysplastic neurons are part of this tumor (arrow points to binucleate neuron).

Treatment and Prognosis

Gangliocytomas and gangliogliomas grow very slowly. Treatment is surgical for accessible lesions. Complete excision carries an excellent long-term outcome and recurrence is infrequent. The likelihood of recurrence is higher with partial excision. Seizure control improves with surgery. There is a very small potential for malignant transformation of the glial component.

◆ Neurocytoma

Incidence

Neurocytomas account for 0.5% of brain tumors, occurring mostly in young adults (second and third decades).

Location

They occur mostly in the lateral ventricle, adjacent to the foramen of Monro. This explains the frequent occurrence of increased intracranial pressure from obstruction of the flow of cerebrospinal fluid (CSF). Cases of hemispheric tumors have been reported, as well as cases arising from the corpus callosum, hypothalamus, spinal cord, or retina.

Clinical Presentation

The duration of symptoms is under 6 months. Neurocytomas commonly present with headaches and other signs of increased intracranial pressure like nausea, memory loss, and mental disturbance.

Imaging

Computed Tomographic Scan

Neurocytomas present as iso- to slightly hyperdense lesions in the body of the lateral ventricle close to the foramen of Monro, containing multiple small cysts. There is mild to moderate contrast enhancement, with frequent calcification. Hydrocephalus is also present.

Magnetic Resonance Imaging Scan

They are isointense on T1, although inhomogeneous, with the low signal areas corresponding to calcifications or tumor vessels. Appearance on T2 is variable from iso- to hyperintense. Contrast enhancement is variable and inhomogeneous (**Fig. 35B–3**).

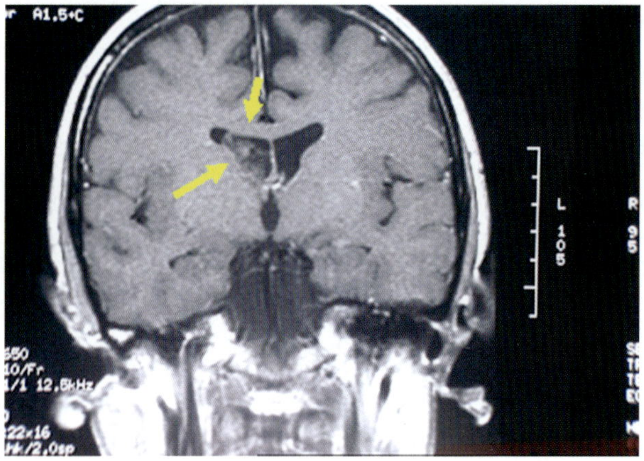

Figure 35B–3 Magnetic resonance imaging of a central neurocytoma.

Angiography

Most neurocytomas are avascular, although there have been reported vascular cases.

Pathology

Microscopically, this tumor shows a benign histologic appearance. It is composed of round, "oligolike" cells that demonstrate neuronal differentiation ultrastructurally and by immunohistochemistry. The background is usually fine fibrillary, and the tumor might contain foci of calcification and hemorrhage. Irregular rosettes, perivascular rosettes, and, rarely, Homer-Wright rosettes can be seen. Immunohistochemical stains for synaptophysin and other neuronal markers such as neuron specific enolase (NSE), class II B-tubulin, tau, or MAP2 are commonly positive. Electron microscopy demonstrates round nuclei with finely dispersed chromatin,. The cytoplasm contains cisternae of rough endoplasmic reticulum arranged in concentric lamellae, microtubules, dense cores, and clear vesicles. Proliferation as measured by K_i-67 labeling usually demonstrates a low proliferation index. Few reports on molecular genetics describe gains on chromosome 7 in some, and isochromosome 17 in others. The differential diagnosis includes oligodendroglioma, ependymoma, pineocytoma, and dysembryoblastic neuroepithelial tumor (DNET) (**Fig. 35B–4**).

Treatment and Prognosis

Complete resection is curative; however, due to the intraventricular location of the lesion there may be some residual tumor, but the residual grows very slowly.

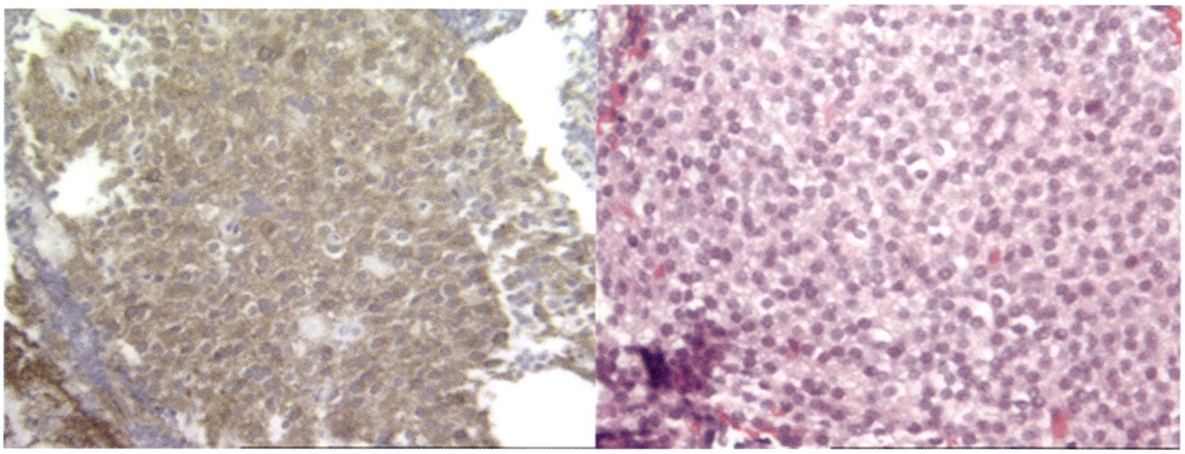

Figure 35B–4 Microscopic image of a central neurocytoma depicting a tumor composed of uniform round cells, with immunohistochemical features of neuronal differentiation (synaptophysin).

◆ Dysembryoplastic Neuroepithelial Tumors

These are among the most recent comers of the brain tumors. They were initially described by Daumas-Duport et al in 1988.

Incidence

They are common in the first 2 decades of life, with a mean age of 9 years. The male:female ratio is 1.5:1.

Location

Most tumors are hemispheric, occurring mostly in the temporal lobe, followed by the frontal lobe. They are located in the gray–white junction or in the gray matter.

Pathology

These tumors are graded as WHO grade I. They are characterized by a heterogeneous appearance, formed by so-called glioneuronal elements. These are composed of columns of oligodendroglia-like cells with intermixed, cytologically normal neurons that appear to "float" in a pale, eosinophilic matrix. Scattered astrocytic cells are usually found. The complex form of DNET has a typical multinodular architecture. The glial component is variable. Typically, they form nodules, but they may also show a diffuse pattern of growth. Largely, the glial component is of low grade; however, they may show atypia, rare mitosis, necrosis, or microvascular proliferation (**Fig. 35B–5**).

Clinical Presentation

Due to their location in the temporal lobe, a prolonged history of complex partial seizures is common. Headaches come in second after seizures.

Imaging

Magnetic Resonance Imaging

DNETs present as focal cortical lesions hypointense on T1 and hyperintense on T2, with variable enhancement making it difficult to differentiate them from low-grade gliomas and gangliogliomas. On proton-density images the signal is higher than that of CSF. They can be multinodular with microcysts and calcifications and may be associated with cortical dysplasia and bony scalloping.

Treatment and Prognosis

DNETs are very slow growing lesions. Treatment is surgical excision. Prognosis is good whether total or subtotal resection is achieved. Subtotal resection has been reported to provide good seizure control. Adjuvant radiotherapy does not appear to be of benefit.

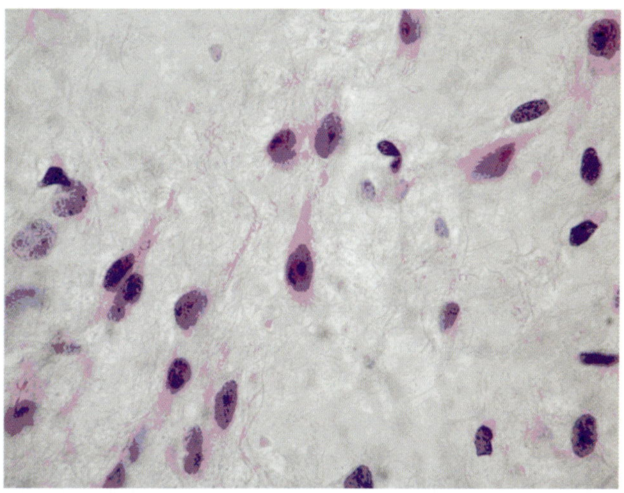

Figure 35B–5 Microscopic image of a dysembryoplastic neuroepithelial tumor showing the typical "floating neurons" in a pale matrix.

◆ Desmoplastic Infantile Ganglioglioma

Incidence

DIGs occur mostly in infants 4 to 6 months old, although cases have been reported in older patients. There is no sex predilection.

Location

These are massive, supratentorial, superficially located tumors.

Imaging

They appear as massive, multicystic, heterogeneously enhancing, calcified, hemispheric lesions.

Pathology

The predominant histopathologic feature is striking desmoplasia characterized by a dense stroma incorporating glial, neuronal, and fibroblastic elements. Most of the tumor consists of highly desmoplastic spindle cell or storiform patterns showing abundant collagen with a trichrome stain. The superficially situated neoplasm usually fills the subarachnoid space and can extend along perivascular (Virchow-Robin) spaces.

Within the densely fibrous tumor are heterogeneously distributed astrocytic and neuronal elements best demonstrated with glial fibrillary acidic protein (GFAP) and synaptophysin immunohistochemistry. The glial components can vary from elongate straplike cells to polygonal forms, but all are intensely GFAP positive. The neuronal constituents are similarly heterogeneous and can appear as small clusters of atypical ganglion-like forms to less distinctly neuronal cells with plump eosinophilic cytoplasm and peripherally displaced nuclei with prominent nucleoli. Nissl substance is only rarely conspicuous. Although the bulk of the DIG is superficial and seemingly well demarcated, some lesions include densely cellular focally infiltrative regions resembling a primitive neuroectodermal tumor, complete with mitotic figures. Some fascicular spindle cell components can also be densely cellular and mitotically active. The presence of a synaptophysin positive neuronal component distinguishes the DIG from the closely related desmoplastic cerebral astrocytoma of infancy, whereas both synaptophysin and GFAP positivity serve to exclude the fibrous histiocytoma and leptomeningeal fibromatosis from further consideration. The more common classic gangliogliomas and pure ganglion cell tumors typically contain more overtly ganglionic cells, including binucleate

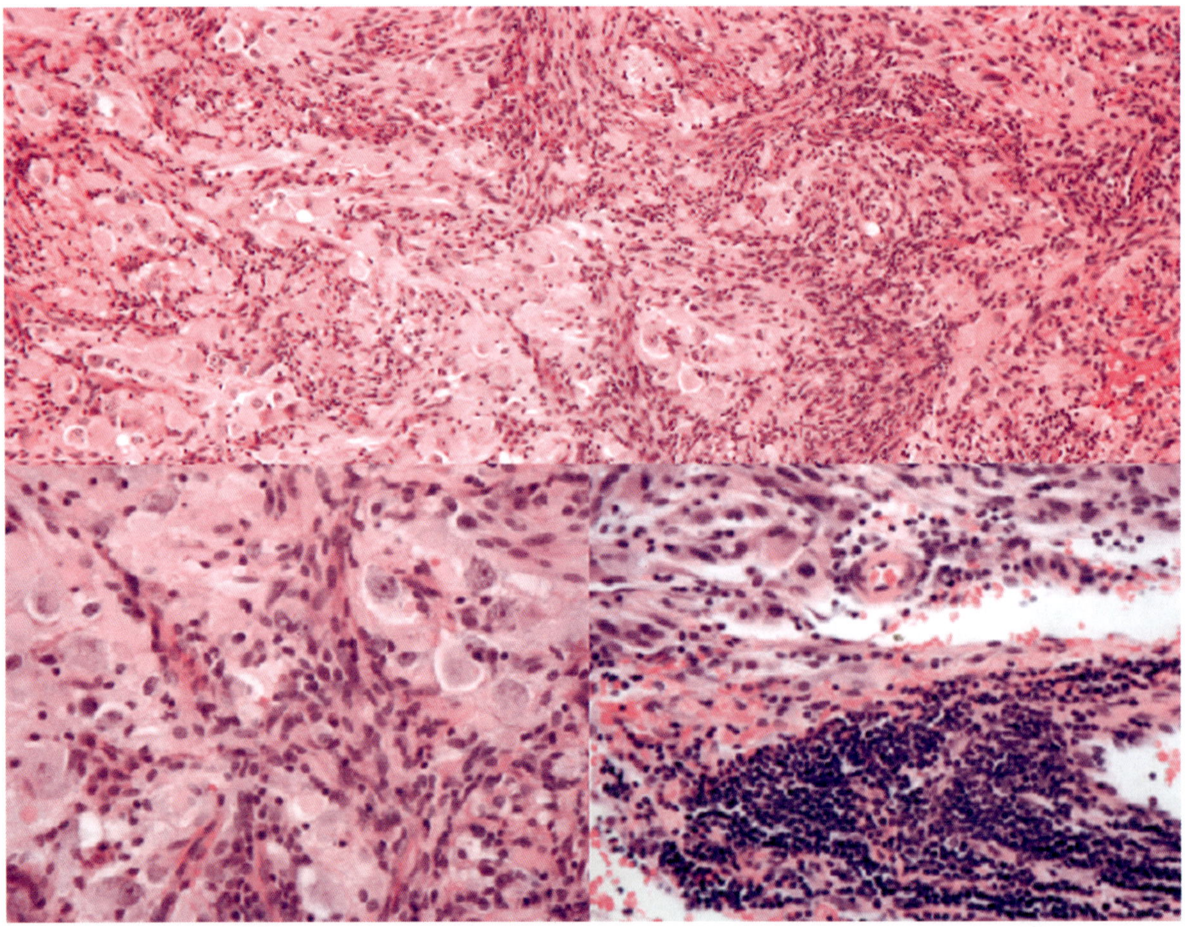

Figure 35B–6 Desmoplastic infantile ganglioglioma showing neoplastic astrocytes arranged in streams with a marked desmoplastic component. Scattered ganglion cells are depicted in the left lower corners. Prominent perivascular lymphocytic infiltrate, also characteristic of this lesion, is seen in the right lower corner.

neurons, and show perivascular lymphocytic cuffs and calcification. Mixed and overlapping forms of DIG and ganglioglioma do occur, however. Cortical tubers are entirely intraparenchymal, do not enhance, contain large, atypical neuronlike cells, and lack a fibrous component (**Fig. 35B–6**).

Treatment and Prognosis

Most patients have prolonged survival and some are even cured; however, the biological behavior has not been fully characterized.

Suggested Readings

Assoun J, Soylemezoglu F, Gambarelli D, Figarella B, von Ammon K, Kleihues P. Central neurocytoma: a synopsis of clinical and histological features. Brain Pathol 1993;3:297–306

Dash RC, Provenzale JM, McComb RD, Perry DA, Longee D, McLendon RE. Malignant supratentorial ganglioglioma: a case report and review of the literature. Arch Pathol Lab Med 1999;123:342–345

Daumas-Duport C. Dysembryoplastic neuroepithelial tumours. Brain Pathol 1993;3:283–295

Honavar M, Janota I. 73 cases of dysembryoplastic neuroepithelial tumour: the range of histologic appearances. Brain Pathol 1994;4:428

Jay V, Edwards V, Hoving E, et al. Central neurocytoma: morphological, flow cytometric, polymerase chain reaction, fluorescence in situ hybridization, and karyotypic analysis. J Neurosurg 1999;90:348–354

Prayson RA, Khajavi K, Comair YG. Cortical architectural abnormalities and MIB-1 immunnoreactivity in gangliogliomas: a study of 60 patients with intracranial tumors. J Neuropathol Exp Neurol 1995;54:513–520

Taratuto AL, Pomata H, Sevlever G, Gallo G, Monges J. Dysembryoplastic neuroepithelial tumor: morphological, immunocytochemical, and deoxyribonucleic acid analyses in a pediatric series. Neurosurgery 1995;36:474–481

VandenBerg SR. Desmoplastic infantile ganglioglioma: a clinicopathologic review of 16 cases. Brain Tumor Pathol 1991;8:25–31

VandenBerg SR. Desmoplastic infantile ganglioglioma and desmoplastic infantile astrocytoma of infancy. Brain Pathol 1993;3:275–281

World Health Organization classification of tumours. Pathology and genetics. Tumours of the nervous system. Lyon: IARC Press; 2000

35C

Cerebellar Astrocytomas

Ian F. Pollack

Cerebellar astrocytomas constitute 10 to 20% of intracranial tumors in children.[1] These neoplasms carry a more favorable prognosis than most other brain tumors because the majority are histologically benign and amenable to extensive resection.[1–7] Cushing first reported on his experience with these tumors in 1931;[8] subsequently, numerous authors have published their results with these common lesions.[1–7,9–13] Despite the large number of cases that have been reported, several issues concerning these tumors remain unresolved. First, the correlation between histology and prognosis among patients with low-grade cerebellar astrocytomas is uncertain: in some series, pilocytic [World Health Organization (WHO) grade 1] astrocytomas have had a better prognosis than nonpilocytic (WHO grade 2) tumors, but in other studies, no such relationship has been observed. Second, the role of radiotherapy after incomplete resection of a low-grade cerebellar astrocytoma remains problematic. In view of the lack of convincing data in this regard, many groups, including our own, defer radiotherapy until there is evidence of progressive disease that is surgically unresectable. Finally, the frequency of follow-up in patients with cerebellar astrocytomas remains largely empirical. Although most recurrences are detected within a few years after initial surgery, late recurrences are well known.[14,15]

Notwithstanding these areas of controversy, a point of uniform agreement among neurosurgeons is that resection extent has a strong impact on progression-free survival: patients undergoing gross total resection have a substantially better prognosis than those undergoing incomplete resection. Although certain biological characteristics, such as extensive brain stem invasion and disease dissemination, may preclude obtaining a complete resection in a small percentage of tumors, the vast majority of cerebellar astrocytomas are amenable to gross total resection.

A small percentage of cerebellar astrocytomas resemble high-grade gliomas (anaplastic astrocytoma or glioblastoma multiforme) that are more commonly seen supratentorially. In most reports, these lesions constitute only 5 to 10% of all cerebellar astrocytomas.[1,6] The biological behavior of cerebellar malignant gliomas is similar to that of high-grade astrocytomas found elsewhere with a very poor prognosis for long-term survival. Such lesions are invasive and biologically aggressive and often exhibit leptomeningeal dissemination at either diagnosis or progression. These tumors are currently treated with maximal resection, postoperative irradiation, and chemotherapy (although the optimal combination of agents remains uncertain). Despite these measures, median survival among affected children is only about 1 year.

◆ Presentation

Cerebellar astrocytomas are generally slow-growing tumors, and symptoms often progress insidiously during a period of months or, in some cases, years before diagnosis. This protracted course contrasts with the more rapid symptom progression characteristic of medulloblastoma, ependymoma, and brain stem glioma.

Presenting symptoms and signs usually reflect increased intracranial pressure and include headache, vomiting, and papilledema. Cerebellar dysfunction, such as ataxia and dysmetria, and brain stem impairment are also observed in some children. Cerebellar astrocytomas that arise in the vermis typically manifest with truncal ataxia, whereas those arising from the hemisphere often produce appendicular ataxia.

◆ Indications

Because most symptomatic cerebellar astrocytomas are large mass lesions, operative intervention for tumor resection is almost always indicated. Details regarding preoperative preparation, and technical caveats regarding the actual tumor resection are discussed in subsequent sections.

◆ Preparation

Imaging

Computed tomography (CT) or magnetic resonance imaging (MRI) can each establish the diagnosis of a posterior fossa tumor. No single feature is diagnostic of an astrocytoma, but certain imaging characteristics are commonly observed. CT typically reveals a lesion that is hypodense or isodense to the brain on unenhanced images. After administration of intravenous contrast, most tumors exhibit enhancement, which may be uniform, ringlike, or nodular (**Fig. 35C–1**). Foci of calcification are seen in 10 to 20% of cases, and cysts are seen in ~70%. MRI typically reveals a mass that is hypo- or isointense to brain on T1-weighted images (**Fig. 35C–2**) and hyperintense on T2-weighted images. Cerebellar astrocytomas involve the vermis and cerebellar hemispheres with approximately equal frequency. Hydrocephalus is apparent with most vermian and large hemispheric astrocytomas. In addition, compression or actual invasion of the cerebellar peduncles and brain stem is seen most commonly with vermian tumors; it is sometimes difficult to distinguish between these patterns of growth preoperatively.

Preoperative Preparation

Most children diagnosed with a posterior fossa tumor can be stabilized sufficiently by the administration of steroids (e.g., dexamethasone 0.1 mg/kg q6h) to allow surgery to be performed semielectively on the next operating day. We generally administer an H_2 blocker in conjunction with the steroid because of the known risk of perioperative stress ulceration in these patients.

Rarely, patients present in an obtunded state and urgent intervention is required. Because the depressed level of consciousness usually reflects severe hydrocephalus, symptomatic improvement can often be obtained by cerebrospinal fluid (CSF) diversion. However, we generally do not wait to see if the patient "wakes up" after this maneuver, but instead proceed directly with tumor removal. Although in the past, CSF shunting was advocated as a temporizing measure before resection of a posterior fossa tumor with associated hydrocephalus, it is clear that the majority of patients do not require long-term CSF diversion and can be spared the potential morbidity of shunting. In

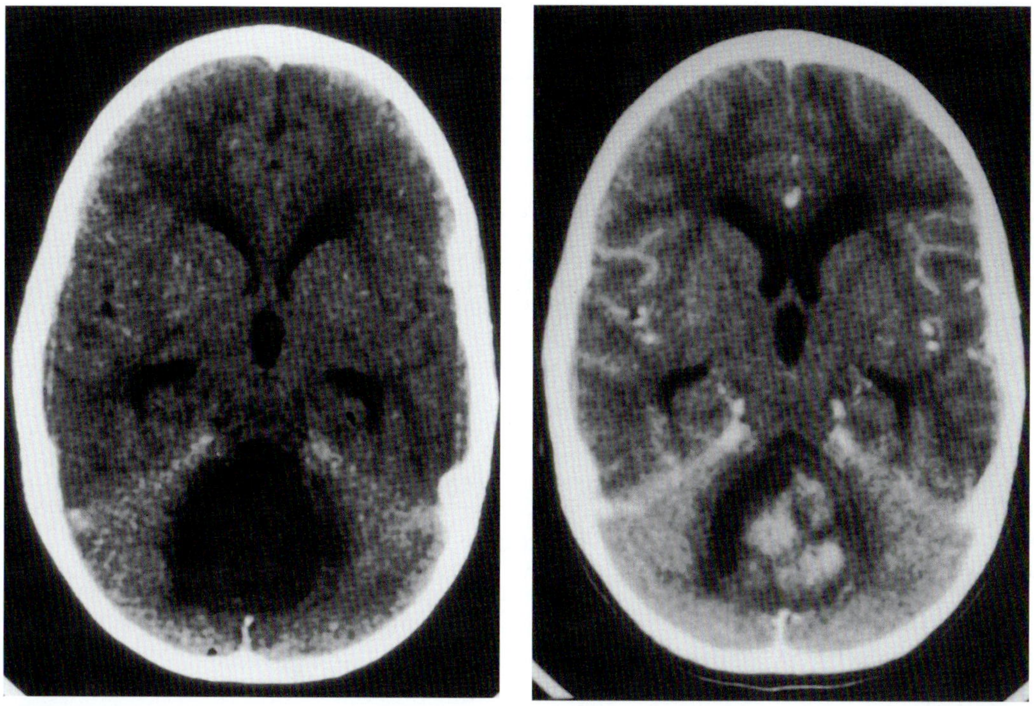

A B

Figure 35C–1 **(A)** This axial computed tomographic image shows a hypodense vermian astrocytoma, which is characterized by a large solid component in association with a small surrounding cyst. **(B)** After administration of intravenous contrast, the lesion shows moderate enhancement. Ventrally on the left, a plane is apparent between the tumor nodule and the surrounding brain tissue.

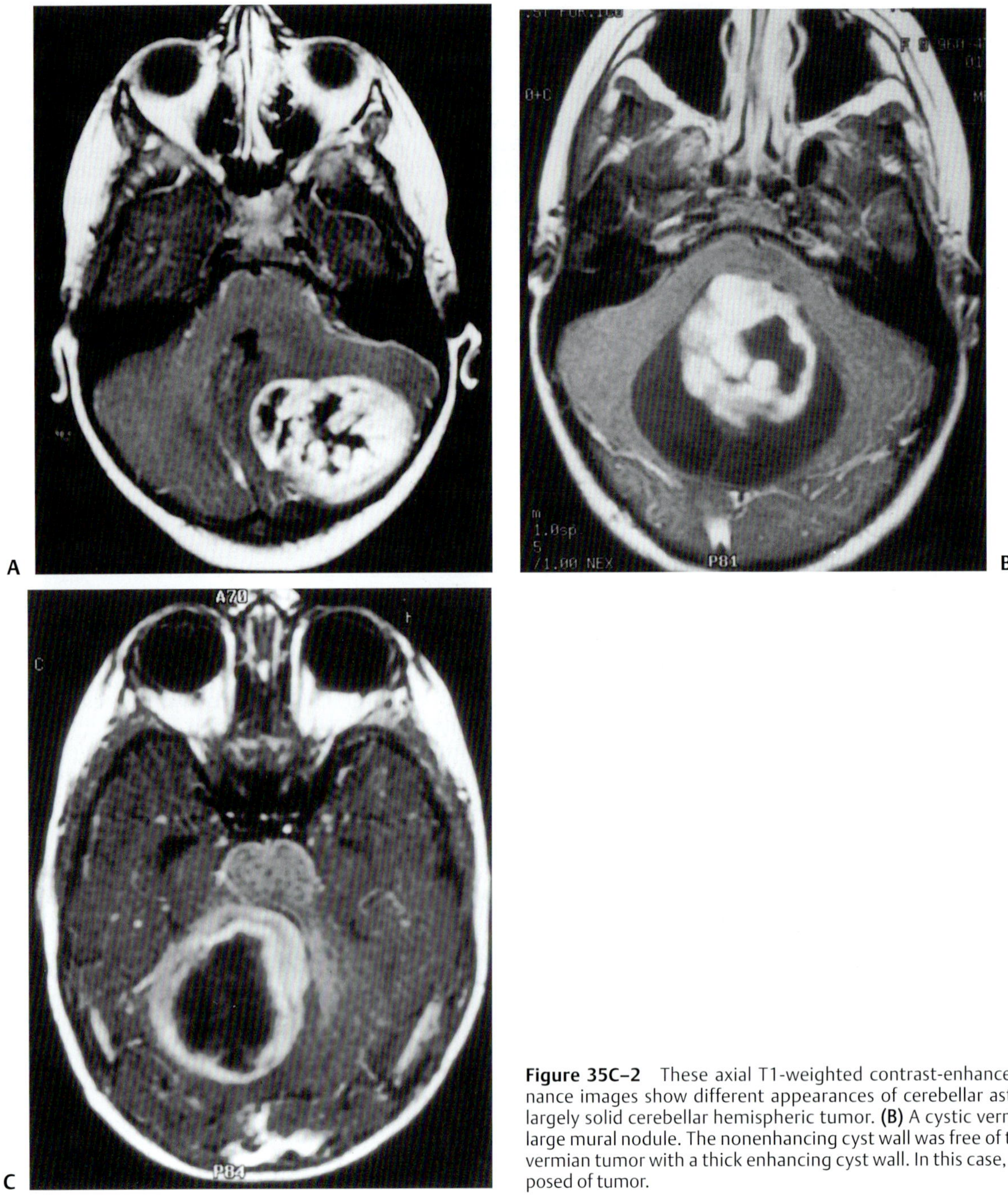

Figure 35C–2 These axial T1-weighted contrast-enhanced magnetic resonance images show different appearances of cerebellar astrocytomas. **(A)** A largely solid cerebellar hemispheric tumor. **(B)** A cystic vermian tumor with a large mural nodule. The nonenhancing cyst wall was free of tumor. **(C)** A cystic vermian tumor with a thick enhancing cyst wall. In this case, the wall was composed of tumor.

addition, shunted patients are at risk for catastrophic deterioration from upward herniation while awaiting definitive resection. Thus our preference is to insert an external ventricular drain immediately before beginning the tumor resection and, if possible, remove the drain several days postoperatively.

Rarely, for small or deep-seated cerebellar astrocytomas, image guidance techniques may be useful in facilitating the identification and resection of the tumor. The need for this modality should be anticipated preoperatively to ensure that a localizing scan of adequate quality is available.

◆ Surgical Technique

Anesthesia

The anesthetic technique generally consists of a mixture of fentanyl, vecuronium, nitrous oxide, and isoflurane, with the doses adjusted if monitoring of somatosensory and brain stem auditory evoked potentials and cranial nerve electromyography is planned. We often monitor sixth and seventh nerve function for vermian tumors and incorporate monitoring of other cranial nerves if we suspect that their sites of origin from the brain stem may be involved by the tumor, as typified by the lesions in **Fig. 35C–2B,C.** Achieving reliable monitoring while keeping the patient adequately anesthetized requires that the anesthesiologist be aware of the surgeon's plans preoperatively.

Other features of the surgical preparation include insertion of a urinary drainage catheter, an arterial line, and, in most cases, a central line, and placement of sizeable peripheral intravenous lines to facilitate blood replacement if needed. Prophylactic antibiotics are administered during the skin preparation and every 6 to 8 hours during the procedure. Steroids are also continued intraoperatively. A precordial Doppler monitor is often applied to detect air embolism. This problem, which is uncommon with the operative positioning that will be described here, is treated by attempting to aspirate the air through the central line, rewaxing the craniotomy bone edges, filling the field with saline, and lowering the head.

Cerebrospinal Fluid Diversion

An external ventricular drain is placed immediately before the tumor removal if the patient has hydrocephalus or is at high risk for developing hydrocephalus postoperatively. This situation is typically observed with vermian and large hemispheric astrocytomas. The author prefers to place the ventriculostomy via a frontal entry site immediately after anesthetic preparations are completed, using a bur hole at the junction of the coronal suture and the midpupillary line and a catheter trajectory aimed 1 cm in front of the tragus in the sagittal plane and at the inner canthus in the coronal plane. Catheter length is calculated, based on imaging data, to place the tip within the frontal horn. Other surgeons insert the drain from an occipital trajectory after the patient is placed in the prone position, using a bur hole ~6 cm above the inion and 2.5 cm lateral to the midline and aiming toward the glabella. After insertion, the drain is initially clamped to avoid the risk of upward herniation from rapid decompression of the ventricular system.

Approach

For most vermian and large hemispheric astrocytomas, we use a modified prone (Concorde) position (**Fig. 35C–3A,B**) with the head flexed forward 20 degrees and angled laterally ~30 degrees away from the surgeon, and the back of the operating table elevated ~20 degrees (which keeps the occipital region parallel with the floor). Chest rolls are placed from the shoulders to the iliac crests bilaterally to avoid abdominal compression. Care must also be taken to pad points of dependency and avoid excessive flexion of the neck, which can compromise jugular venous return. The head is held in position using a horseshoe headrest in children younger than 2 years, pediatric pin fixation in children between 2 and 5 years of age, and "adult" pins in older children.

As an alternative to the Concorde position, some surgeons prefer a sitting position. The advantages of this position are its allowance of a true midline orientation of the surgeon and drainage of blood and CSF by gravity out of the operative field. The disadvantages include a higher risk of air embolism, traction on bridging veins between the cerebellum and tentorium, increased risk of subdural hematoma formation, and fatigue of the surgeon's elevated arms. In the author's view, the disadvantages outweigh the advantages in most cases.

Occasionally, other approaches may be indicated to treat lesions in atypical locations. For example, a lateral hemispheric tumor may be best approached using a "park bench" (lateral) position, with a roll under the axilla and the head fixed in the Mayfield head holder (**Fig. 35C–3C**).

Vermian and medial hemispheric lesions are approached using a midline incision from the inion to the C1–C2 interspace (**Fig. 35C–4A**). The muscles are divided in the midline plane using a needle-tip electrocautery. A Weitlaner retractor is inserted to facilitate reflection of the muscles, which are dissected subperiosteally off the occipital bone. Bleeding from emissary veins is common and is controlled using bone wax. For vermian lesions, the muscles are elevated laterally for 3 to 4 cm off the midline. For medial hemispheric lesions, this extent of exposure is obtained on the side of the tumor, and only ~2 cm of exposure is obtained contralaterally. The interspace between the foramen magnum and C1 is then defined and cleared of tissue, and the dura is dissected from around the edge of the foramen magnum.

For lateral hemispheric tumors, a vertical paramedian incision is used, centered over the tumor (**Fig. 35C–3C**). The muscles are incised along the direction of the skin incision until the occipital bone is visualized. The bone is exposed sufficiently to permit a craniectomy or craniotomy that is adequate in size for thorough exposure of the tumor. Exposure of the foramen magnum is generally not required.

A craniectomy or craniotomy is then performed (**Fig. 35C–4A,B**). For vermian lesions, two bur holes are made in the occipital bone 3 cm lateral to midline and just below the transverse sinus on each side. Through the bur hole, dura is dissected from the undersurface of the bone medially and inferiorly. For a craniotomy (my preference), osteotomies are made from the lateral bur holes to the foramen magnum using a high-speed drill with a foot plate (e.g., a Midas Rex B5 bit and attachment, Midas Rex Pneumatic Tools, Inc., Fort Worth, TX). Bone cuts are then made toward the midline, but because the midline ridge is often quite thick, I sometimes thin this down using the B5 bit with the B (non-foot-plated) attachment and then crack this bone piece off by elevating the bone flap off the dura with an Adson dissector. Removal of the arch of C1 is rarely required. For hemispheric lesions, two bur holes are made at the margins of the anticipated craniotomy, and the bur holes are then connected using a Midas B5 bit.

If the dura is full, the anesthesiologist is asked to drain off 10 to 20 mL of CSF at this point. If there is a large superficially located cyst, this can also be aspirated through the dura to relieve pressure. The dura is then opened in a V-shaped fashion beginning over the cerebellar hemispheres and extending toward the midline at the occipitocervical junction (**Fig. 35C–4B,C**). Large dural venous channels at the foramen magnum region should be anticipated and occluded using either clips or sutures to avoid major bleeding. The incision is then carried inferiorly in the midline to the caudal margin of the tumor.

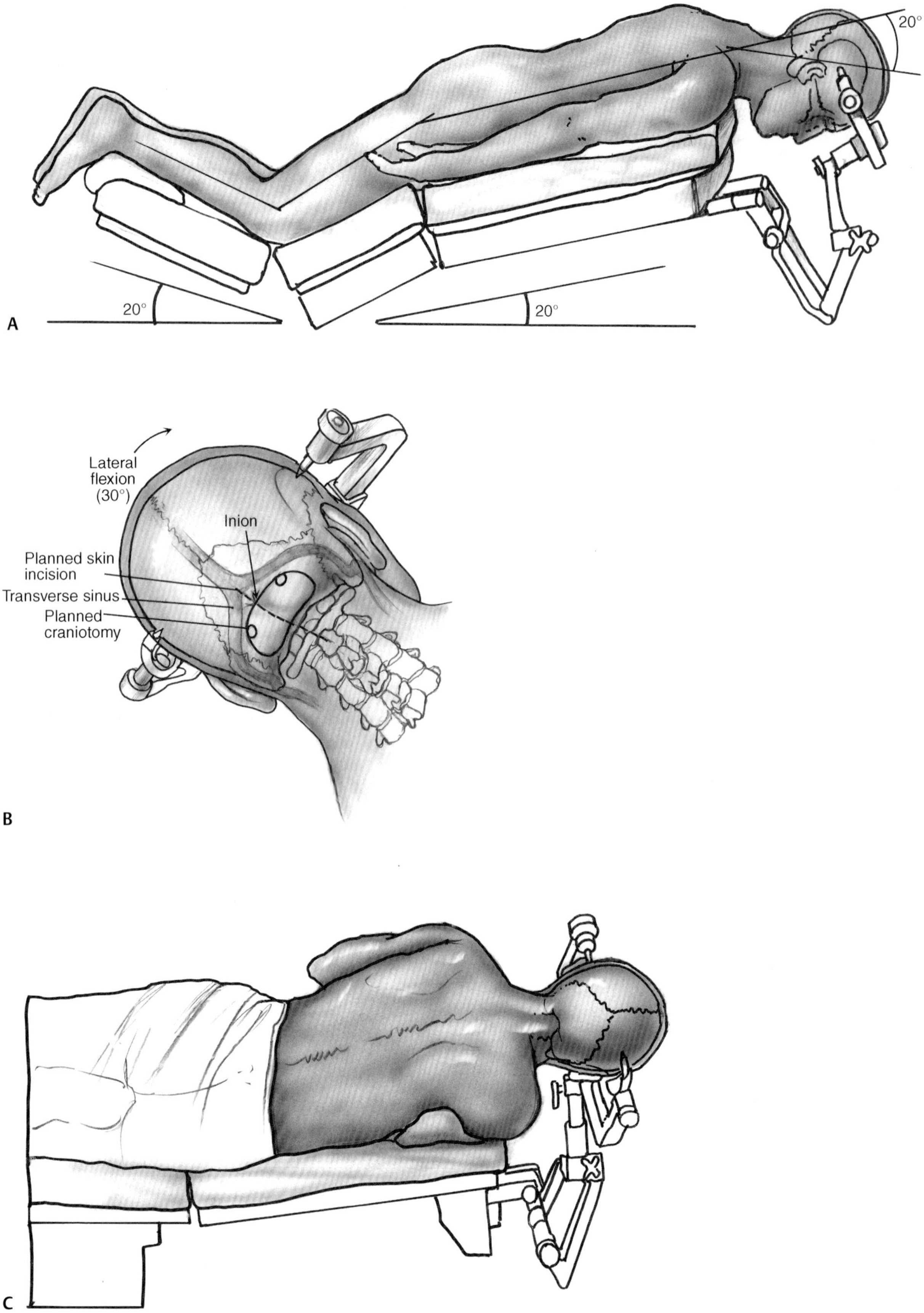

Figure 35C–3 **(A)** A side view of the modified prone position used for resection of vermian and medial hemispheric cerebellar astrocytomas. **(B)** A dorsal view of the planned approach. **(C)** For lateral hemispheric tumors, a "park bench" position is preferred.

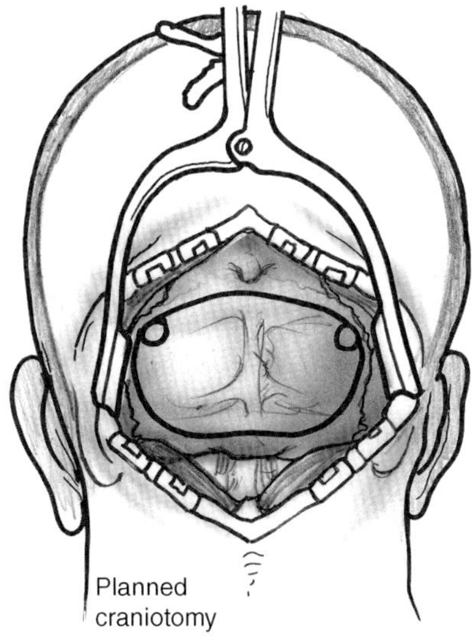

A

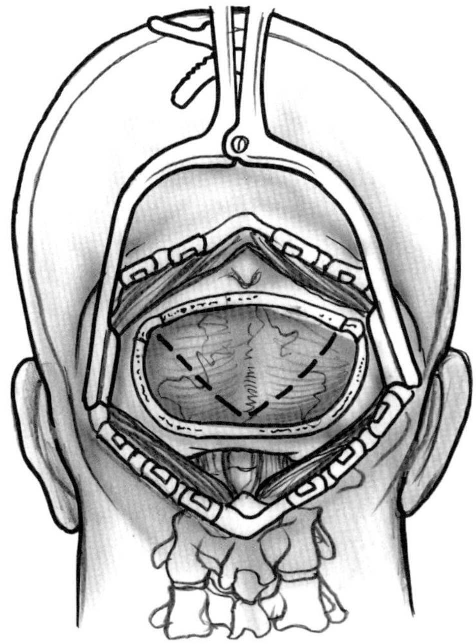

B

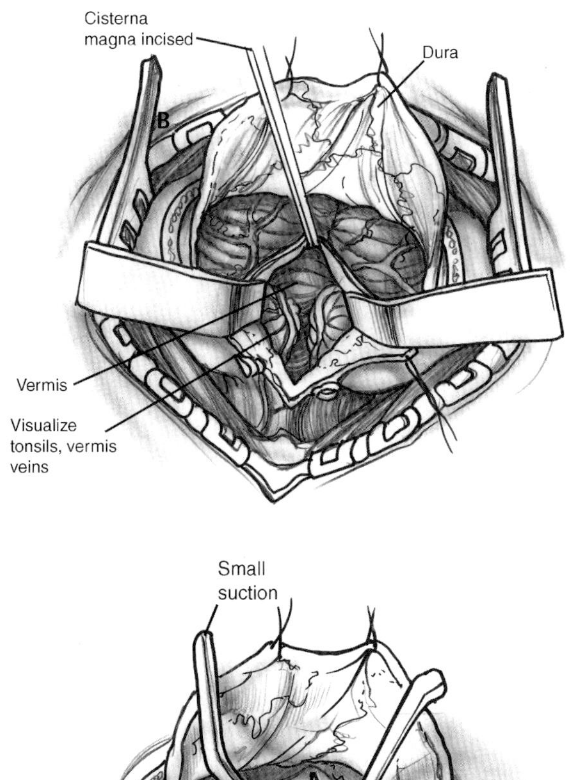

C

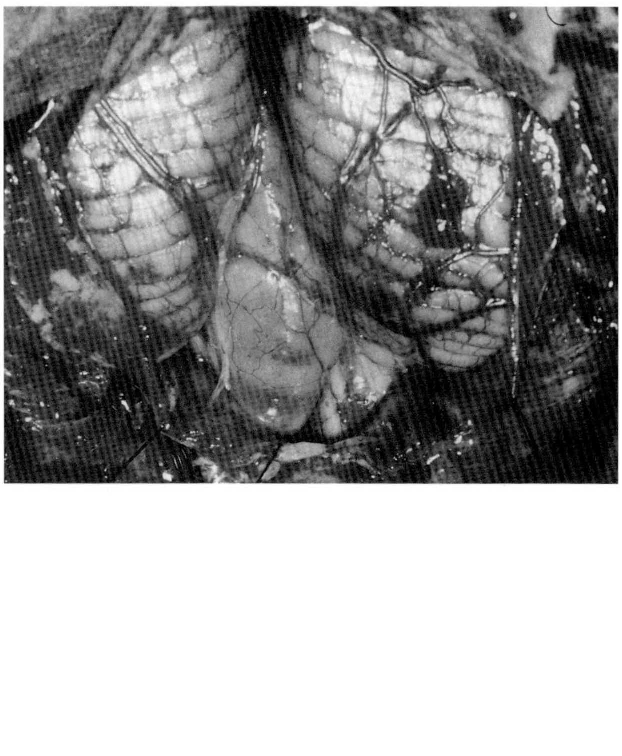

D

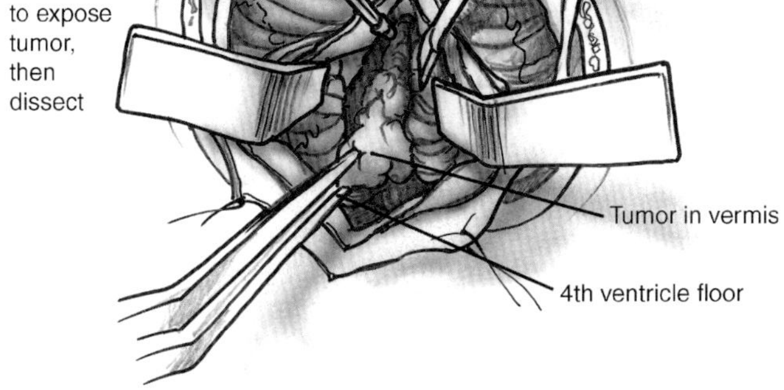

E

Figure 35C–4 **(A)** The planned craniotomy for a vermian or medial hemispheric tumor. **(B)** After the bone has been removed, the dura is opened in a V-shaped fashion over the cerebellar hemispheres. The occipital sinus is then controlled, and the apex of the incision is extended inferiorly toward the top of C1. **(C)** Once the dura is fully opened, the cerebellar vermis, hemispheres, and tonsils are visualized. **(D)** This operative photograph demonstrates the gliotic capsule of a pilocytic astrocytoma within the cisterna magna. **(E)** If the vermian tumor is not initially apparent, the inferior vermis is divided in the midline, exposing the tumor, which is then dissected from the surrounding cerebellum and resected.

In some vermian astrocytomas, the lesion is immediately apparent within the cisterna magna (**Fig. 35C–4D**) and is exposed simply by opening the overlying arachnoid. If the tumor is not initially visible, the cerebellar tonsils are gently separated using self-retaining retractors, which exposes the inferior pole of the vermis and, in some cases, a small nubbin of tumor protruding through the foramen of Magendie. The main component of the tumor is readily visualized upon dividing the inferior vermis (**Fig. 35C–4E**), which is first coagulated in the midline over the tumor and then "incised" using a small suction.

In many cerebellar hemispheric astrocytomas, the lesion is visible on the surface as an area of yellow or pink amorphous tissue that differs in appearance from the surrounding folia (**Fig. 35C–5A**). If the lesion is not apparent, the localization can usually be inferred by observing widened cerebellar folia overlying the lesion (**Fig. 35C–5B**). Rarely, for deep-seated or small lesions, intraoperative ultrasound or stereotactic localization techniques may be required to plan an appropriate pial opening. The pia is then coagulated transversely (parallel to the folia) over the tumor, and incised with a microscissors, and the

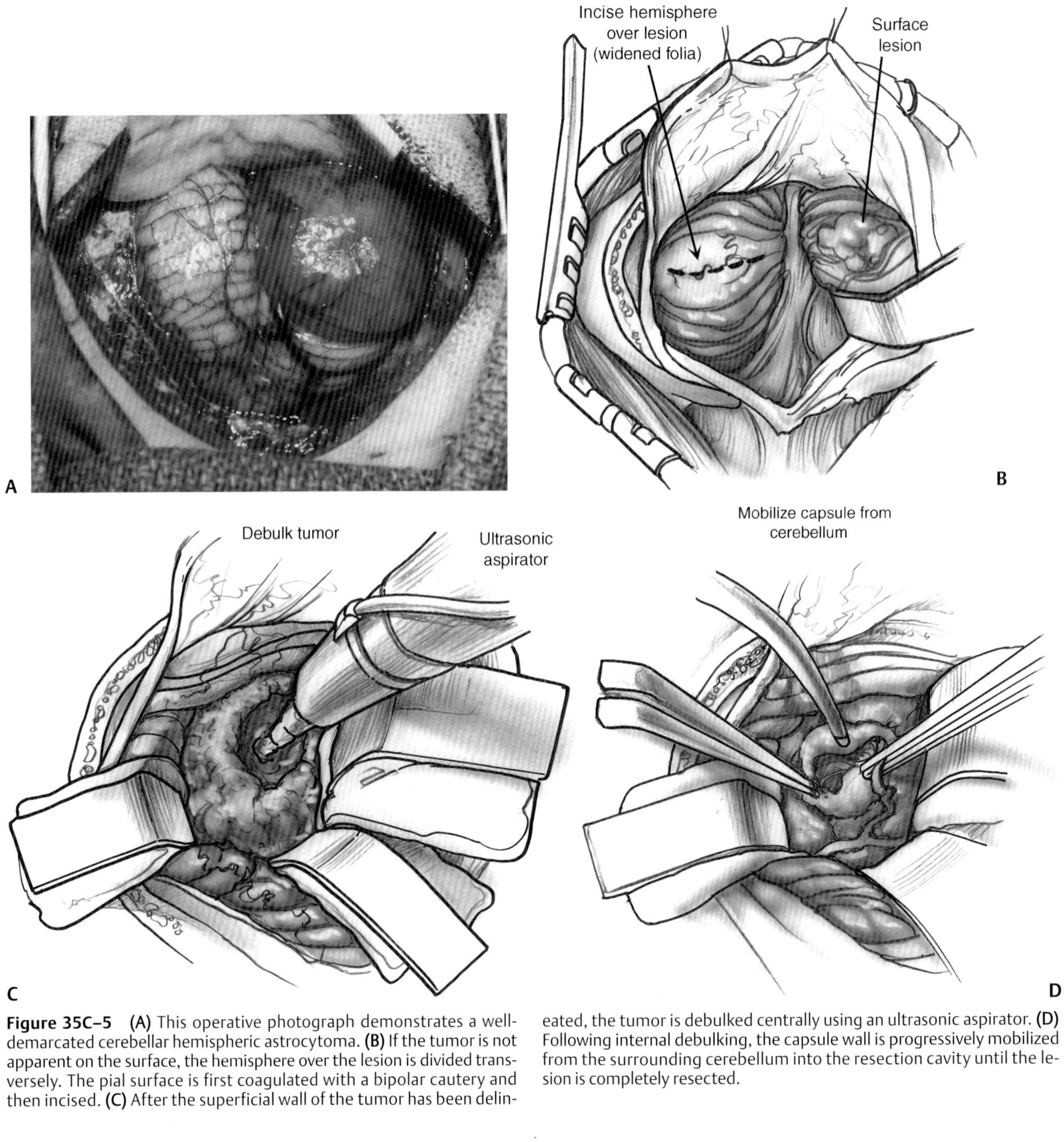

Figure 35C–5 **(A)** This operative photograph demonstrates a well-demarcated cerebellar hemispheric astrocytoma. **(B)** If the tumor is not apparent on the surface, the hemisphere over the lesion is divided transversely. The pial surface is first coagulated with a bipolar cautery and then incised. **(C)** After the superficial wall of the tumor has been delineated, the tumor is debulked centrally using an ultrasonic aspirator. **(D)** Following internal debulking, the capsule wall is progressively mobilized from the surrounding cerebellum into the resection cavity until the lesion is completely resected.

cerebellum overlying the tumor is opened with a small suction.

Once the lesion is visualized, self-retaining retractors are inserted over cottonoid patties. Care is taken to keep retraction to a minimum to avoid injury to the surrounding brain.

Tumor Resection

After the superficial surface of the tumor is delineated, a frozen section is often obtained to confirm the histopathological diagnosis. The microscope is then brought into the field for the resection. In astrocytomas with a sizeable associated cyst, the cyst is often encountered early in the tumor resection. Management of the cyst wall is influenced both by the imaging characteristics of the wall and by its appearance on direct inspection. Cyst walls that are translucent and nonenhancing are generally nonneoplastic and need not be resected. In such cases, simple removal of an intracystic mural nodule may be curative. Conversely, walls that are thick and enhance brightly are invariably neoplastic and should be resected to improve the likelihood of long-term disease control. If the nature of the cyst wall is in question, a frozen section can be obtained. Unfortunately, distinction of peritumoral gliosis from a benign astrocytoma is often difficult, and surgeons are frequently left to rely on their judgment.

The techniques used to remove the solid tumor component are influenced by the growth characteristics of the neoplasm. Juvenile pilocytic astrocytomas sometimes have a distinct pseudocapsule that facilitates their dissection from the surrounding cerebellum, and smaller lesions can often be removed as a single specimen. Larger, well-circumscribed lesions are removed in stages, with the superficial capsule first dissected from the surrounding cerebellum, followed by internal debulking of the tumor using an ultrasonic aspirator (**Fig. 35C–5C**), and reflection of the walls of the tumor into the resection cavity. Additional capsule is then separated from surrounding cerebellum, and the process is repeated until the tumor is completely removed (**Fig. 35C–5D**). For pilocytic and nonpilocytic astrocytomas that initially appear to have indistinct margins, the resection begins from the inside out. After the central component of the tumor is debulked using the ultrasonic aspirator, an attempt is again made to define distinct borders using a microdissector and bipolar cautery. In some cases, focal areas of such tumors will exhibit a discernible tumor–brain interface, which can be traced around the lesion to facilitate resection.

For lesions that are highly infiltrative into the surrounding brain, the resection is entirely performed using the ultrasonic aspirator, removing the tumor until a transition between tumor and normal-appearing tissue is visualized. This approach is particularly challenging for large vermian tumors that infiltrate into the dorsal brain stem surface. After debulking the center of the lesion and visualizing the fourth ventricular floor caudally, the author will follow the plane of transition between tumor and cerebellum rostrally until the roof of the fourth ventricle is identified. This yields a burst of CSF from the aqueduct, which is covered with a small cottonoid patty to prevent inflow of blood and tumor cells. With the fourth ventricular floor exposed well beneath the residual tumor, the lesion is then debulked in a rostral to caudal direction until the foramen of Magendie has been reached. Areas in which the tumor has clearly invaded the cerebellar peduncles and brain stem are resected last. To minimize the risk of postoperative neurological impairment, I generally avoid "chasing" the tumor into these structures because microscopic residual disease does not always progress, and instead resect the lesion flush with the surrounding brain stem surface. For lesions with potential brain stem infiltration, monitoring of brain stem auditory and somatosensory evoked potentials and cranial nerve electromyography are often helpful in identifying early evidence of neural compromise so that the operative approach can be modified accordingly.

Closure

Upon completion of the tumor resection, meticulous hemostasis is achieved. The walls of the resection cavity are sometimes lined with a single layer of Surgicel. Several Valsalva maneuvers are then performed to confirm hemostasis. The dura is closed in a watertight fashion, usually with a graft of pericranium, biocompatible dural substitute, or xenograft pericardium. The bone flap is replaced (if a craniotomy has been performed) and secured to the surrounding bone edges using 2–0 Vicryl or Neurilon sutures. The wound is then closed in layers using absorbable sutures.

◆ Postoperative Care

Patients are observed overnight in the intensive care unit and, if stable, are then transferred to the neurosurgical ward. If the patient fails to awaken promptly after surgery, an urgent CT scan is obtained to rule out intracranial hemorrhage or infarction. A postoperative MRI is performed electively during the first 24 hours after surgery to determine the extent of residual disease.

During the first 2 days after surgery, the drip chamber of the external ventricular drain is kept at a height of 5 cm to facilitate drainage of bloody CSF. The drain is then weaned by elevating the drip chamber by 5 to 10 cm/day during the ensuing 3 to 5 days. Steroids are tapered concurrently. Patients who continue to have high CSF outputs at chamber heights above 30 cm, develop a large pseudomeningocele, or exhibit progressive lethargy in conjunction with ventriculomegaly during weaning attempts generally require permanent CSF diversion. Although a third ventriculostomy may avoid the need for a shunt in some patients, this approach is not applicable in the majority, who need CSF diversion because of communicating rather than obstructive hydrocephalus.

◆ Complications

The frequency of complications from tumor removal is influenced by the location of the tumor and its pattern of growth. Meticulous microsurgical technique is essential for keeping morbidity to a minimum. Superficial hemispheric lesions can generally be removed with minimal neurological sequelae. In contrast, the resection of large hemispheric and vermian lesions is often associated with transient worsening of preoperative ataxia. Although ~15% of such patients experience either or both permanent residual ataxia and dysmetria, they are often mild and do not interfere with routine activities. Patients with large vermian tumors are also at risk for brain stem and cranial nerve dysfunction. Fortunately, this problem is encountered in less than 5% of patients and may perhaps be minimized by monitoring appropriate neurophysiological parameters during the course of the tumor resection.

A more common but less ominous complication is the development of mutism and pseudobulbar dysfunction, which occurs in at least 10% of children with vermian tumors[16,17] usually manifesting 24 to 72 hours after surgery, often after a period of relatively normal functioning. This syndrome is thought to result from injury to the dentate-rubrothalamic connections to the supplementary motor cortex.[17] Such deficits are generally seen after excision of large vermian tumors that involve the cerebellar peduncles bilaterally. Although we do not believe that involvement of the cerebellar peduncles by tumor is a contraindication to attempting a complete resection, such cases clearly require meticulous microsurgical technique to minimize peduncular injury and trauma to the adjacent brain stem. In contrast, frank infiltration of the brain stem by tumor, which is seen in ~10% of cerebellar astrocytomas, does constitute a practical limit to complete resection in certain cases. Generally, symptoms of cerebellar mutism begin to resolve within several weeks after operation; however, some deficits persist for several months, and a small percentage of patients exhibit persistent impairments.

Another syndrome of delayed onset is aseptic meningitis, which is characterized by fever, photophobia, and nuchal rigidity, usually occurring 5 to 7 days after operation. This syndrome must be distinguished from bacterial meningitis by examination of the CSF Gram stain and culture. Whereas aseptic meningitis is treated using corticosteroids, bacterial meningitis requires appropriately selected antibiotics, which may be instituted empirically until the culture results are reported.

◆ Tumor Recurrence and Adjuvant Management

The majority of cerebellar astrocytomas are histologically benign and amenable to gross total resection, which should be the operative goal. If the postoperative MRI shows that a radiologically complete resection has been obtained, patients are managed with periodic follow-up MRIs. Recent studies report survivals of more than 90% at 10 years after gross total resection.[2–4,11,12,18] Given these results, radiation therapy and chemotherapy are not indicated after radiologically confirmed gross total removal of a benign cerebellar astrocytoma. Although a small percentage of patients do exhibit disease progression after an apparently complete resection, most such cases are amenable to repeat resection. If a radiographically complete resection can again be achieved, adjuvant therapy may not be required. Because these tumors grow extremely slowly, recurrences may occur many years after the original operation.[14,15] Therefore, patients need long-term follow-up and cannot be regarded as "cured" at a standard interval after resection. The author typically obtains subsequent scans at 3 months, 9 months, 18 months, 3 years, 5 years, 7 years, and 10 years postoperatively, but this is admittedly somewhat arbitrary.

If the postoperative scan after an attempted complete resection shows resectable residual tumor, it is reasonable to consider reoperation to obtain a complete resection because the likelihood of long-term progression-free survival is adversely affected by the presence of residual disease, with as many as 80% of patients experiencing disease progression within 10 years.[2,3,6,11,18] However, in cases for which a gross total resection would result in unacceptable morbidity, an aggressive subtotal resection is a reasonable alternative. This approach is indicated when there is extensive infiltration of the brain stem or in rare instances of leptomeningeal spread.[19,20] Numerous studies have shown that long-term survival is still possible, despite the presence of small amounts of residual tumor.[2,7,14] Schneider et al[7] noted that only four of 12 patients with radiographically apparent residual tumor had disease progression, with a mean follow-up of 4.9 years. It is presently unknown why certain tumors remain quiescent for extended periods of time after a subtotal resection. This may reflect alterations in blood supply resulting from the resection or decelerating growth kinetics within the tumor over time. However, it is clear that incompletely resected tumors may recur many years after an initial operation.[14,15] In the University of California, San Francisco (UCSF) experience,[11] progression-free survival was 74% at 10 years, but only 41% at 20 years, which calls attention to the importance of maintaining close long-term follow-up in patients with known residual disease. Fortunately, most recurrences are amenable to reexploration and resection and, in many reports, overall survival has been as high as 80% at 10 years after an initial subtotal resection.

Thus, although a substantial percentage of incompletely resected tumors ultimately progress, not all lesions do so. If a postoperative scan shows small amounts of unresectable disease (i.e., within the brain stem), it is appropriate to follow this expectantly. The potential risks and uncertain benefits of radiotherapy for these tumors have complicated attempts to define the indications for irradiation after a subtotal resection. In view of this uncertainty, one goal of the original Children's Cancer Group and Pediatric Oncology Group low-grade glioma study (CCG-9891/POG-9130) was to address the role of radiotherapy in the management of these tumors using a prospective, randomized format. Unfortunately, difficulties in entering randomized patients precluded completion of this phase of the study. Patients who experience postoperative disease progression that is amenable to resection should undergo reoperation, and, if a complete or nearly complete resection can be achieved, adjuvant therapy may again be deferred. The chance to avoid the use of irradiation in some children and to delay its use for several years in others may constitute a significant benefit in terms of improving overall functional outcome.

In the absence of convincing evidence favoring the use of any form of adjuvant therapy as a routine measure for cerebellar astrocytomas, we currently advocate such intervention only for the small percentage of tumors that progress after two presumed total excisions or for those that exhibit progressive growth after an initial operation and cannot be completely resected. Children younger than 10 may be treated with chemotherapy, such as carboplatin and vincristine, and older children are managed with involved field irradiation. Early experience at our institution and elsewhere with stereotactic radiosurgery and radiotherapy for the treatment of focal areas of tumor recurrence suggests that these modalities may prove useful in managing small areas of unresectable disease in critical locations, such as the brain stem.

◆ The Effect of Histology on Outcome in Low-Grade Cerebellar Astrocytomas

Although it is generally agreed that lesions with histological features of malignancy, such as frequent mitotic figures and necrosis, carry a worse prognosis than low-grade lesions[6,12] and should be managed differently, it remains uncertain whether the large group of low-grade tumors can be further divided based on histology into prognostically meaningful subgroups. Winston et al identified clusters of features that correlated with survival of patients with cerebellar gliomas.[12] Glioma A tumors displayed microcysts, leptomeningeal deposits, Rosenthal fibers, or foci of oligodendroglia. Glioma B tumors displayed a combination of perivascular pseudorosettes, hypercellularity, mitosis, necrosis, and/or calcification in the absence of any glioma A feature. Glioma C tumors consisted of the remaining neoplasms that did not fit into these categories. Ten-year survivals in patients treated since 1948 with glioma A, B, and C tumors were 94%, 29%, and 69%, respectively.[12] Although this classification system provided a significant correlation between histology and prognosis, this schema did not directly address the issue of whether prognostically useful subgroups of low-grade gliomas, which are largely encompassed by the glioma A group, could be identified.

An alternative classification scheme that was popularized by Russell and Rubinstein and largely adopted by WHO[21] subdivides low-grade cerebellar astrocytomas into pilocytic and nonpilocytic groups. Pilocytic tumors exhibit a biphasic appearance, with compact areas of bipolar cells associated with Rosenthal fibers interposed with areas of loosely aggregated astrocytes associated with granular bodies and microcysts; these lesions correspond to WHO grade I tumors. So-called diffuse or nonpilocytic astrocytomas are essentially identical in appearance to low-grade astrocytomas found within the central nervous system in adults and correspond to WHO grade II tumors. These lesions typically display a monotonous proliferation of fibrillary or protoplasmic astrocytes with or without microcysts and characteristically exhibit poorly circumscribed borders with invasion of neoplastic cells into the surrounding parenchyma.[4,5]

Although it is assumed that the distinction between these two groups of astrocytomas is of prognostic value, this has yet to be proven conclusively. In support of this separation, Gjerris and Klinken[4] noted a 25-year survival rate of 94% in 31 children with "juvenile" (pilocytic) cerebellar astrocytomas versus only 38% in 13 children with diffuse (nonpilocytic) tumors. Similarly, Hayostek et al[5] found a substantial difference in survival between these variants. However, in both studies, other differences between the pilocytic and nonpilocytic groups may have also contributed to the disparities that were noted in their outcomes. For example, in the study of Hayostek et al, the median age of patients with pilocytic tumors was 12 years versus 52 years for those with diffuse tumors, and gross total resection was achieved in 53% of the pilocytic tumors as compared with only 19% of nonpilocytic tumors. Both age and extent of resection are known to have strong correlations with survival.

In contrast to the above results, several recent studies have suggested that childhood pilocytic and nonpilocytic astrocytomas have similar prognoses[6,7,9] and that the only predictor of outcome is whether or not a complete resection is obtained. In an attempt to more conclusively address the issue of whether histology is associated with outcome, a multi-institutional study of the Children's Cancer Group and the Pediatric Oncology Group is following the natural history of both completely and incompletely resected low-grade gliomas, using consistent histological criteria to separate pilocytic and nonpilocytic tumors, in the hope of identifying distinctions in the long-term progression-free survival of these two groups. At present, in the absence of any definitive differences in prognosis between grade I and grade II cerebellar astrocytomas, there is no compelling reason to manage these lesions differently. Thus extent of residual disease remains the only factor that currently guides therapeutic intervention.

◆ Conclusion

Low-grade cerebellar astrocytomas are associated with a better prognosis than most other central nervous system tumors. Gross total resection of the lesion provides the greatest likelihood of long-term progression-free survival. When this is not possible, subtotal resection may allow an extended period of disease control; however, a significant percentage of incompletely resected lesions ultimately progress and require additional therapy. At present, the role of radiation therapy after an incomplete resection remains uncertain. We currently reserve this modality for patients who have progressive disease after two apparently complete resections and those with unresectable residual disease after a single episode of disease progression. In view of the generally indolent growth of these lesions, long-term follow-up is needed because disease progression may occur many years after an initial operation. In contrast to the favorable results achieved with low-grade cerebellar astrocytomas, the prognosis for patients with high-grade lesions remains poor after conventional surgery, radiotherapy, and chemotherapy.

Acknowledgment This work was supported in part by NIH grant NS01810.

References

1. Pollack IF. Current concepts: brain tumors in children N Engl J Med 1994;331:1500–1507
2. Campbell JW, Pollack IF. Cerebellar astrocytomas in children. J Neurooncol 1996;28:223–231
3. Garcia DM, Latifi HR, Simpson JR, Picker S. Astrocytomas of the cerebellum in children. J Neurosurg 1989;71:661–664
4. Gjerris F, Klinken L. Long-term prognosis in children with benign cerebellar astrocytoma. J Neurosurg 1978;49:179–184
5. Hayostek CJ, Shaw EG, Scheithauer B, et al. Astrocytomas of the cerebellum: a comparative clinicopathologic study of pilocytic and diffuse astrocytomas. Cancer 1993;72:856–869
6. Ilgren EB, Stiller CA. Cerebellar astrocytomas. Clin Neuropathol 1987; 6:185–214
7. Schneider JH Jr, Raffel C, McComb JG. Benign cerebellar astrocytomas of childhood. Neurosurgery 1992;30:58–63
8. Cushing H. Experiences with the cerebellar astrocytomas. Surg Gynecol Obstet 1931;52:129–205
9. Palma L, Russo A, Celli P. Prognosis of the so-called "diffuse" cerebellar astrocytoma. Neurosurgery 1984;15:315–317
10. Undjian S, Marinov M, Georgiev K. Long-term follow-up after surgical treatment of cerebellar astrocytomas in 100 children. Childs Nerv Syst 1989;5:99–101
11. Wallner KE, Gonzales MF, Edwards MSB, Wara WM, Sheline GF. Treatment results of juvenile pilocytic astrocytoma. J Neurosurg 1988;69:171–176
12. Winston K, Gilles FH, Leviton A, et al. Cerebellar gliomas in children. J Natl Cancer Inst 1977;58:833–838
13. Larson DA, Wara WM, Edwards MS. Management of childhood cerebellar astrocytoma. Int J Radiat Oncol Biol Phys1990;18:971–973
14. Austin EJ, Alvord EC. Recurrences of cerebellar astrocytomas: a violation of Collins' Law. J Neurosurg 1988;68:41–47
15. Pagni CA, Giordana MT, Canavero S. Benign recurrence of a pilocytic cerebellar astrocytoma 36 years after radical removal: case report. Neurosurgery 1991;28:606–609
16. Cochrane DD, Gustavsson B, Poskitt KP, Steinbok P, Kestle JR. The surgical and natural morbidity of aggressive resection for posterior fossa tumors in childhood. Pediatr Neurosurg 1994;20:19–29
17. Pollack IF, Polinko P, Pang D, Albright AL, Towbin R, Fitz C. Mutism and pseudobulbar symptoms after resection of posterior fossa tumors in children. Neurosurgery 1995;37:885–893
18. Abdollahzadeh M, Hoffman HJ, Blazer SI, et al. Benign cerebellar astrocytoma in childhood: experience at the Hospital for Sick Children 1980–1992. Childs Nerv Syst 1994;10:380–383
19. Auer RN, Rice GP, Hinton GG, Amacher AC, Gilbert JJ. Cerebellar astrocytoma with benign histology and malignant clinical course. J Neurosurg 1981;54: 128–132
20. Pollack IF, Hurtt M, Pang D, Albright AL. Dissemination of low-grade intracranial astrocytomas in children. Cancer 1994;73: 2869–2878
21. Kleihues P, Burger PC, Scheithauer BW, et al. World Health Organization Histological Typing of Tumours of the Central Nervous System. New York: Springer-Verlag; 1993

36

Brain Stem and Cervicomedullary Tumors

George I. Jallo, Keith Y. C. Goh, and Fred Epstein

Sir Byrom Bramwell wrote that "the following appear to be the most important conditions for successful operative interference in the treatment of intracranial tumors: (1) satisfactory localization, (2) the tumor must be accessible, and (3) the tumor must be single and of such a pathological character as to permit complete enucleation or removal."[1] A century on, these basic tenets still hold true and have particular relevance to the problem of brain stem tumors.

In this respect, several advances in the 1970–'80s have contributed significantly to the surgical treatment of these once inoperable tumors; namely, magnetic resonance imaging (MRI), microsurgical techniques, and neurophysiological monitoring. Although there is a 10-fold higher overall incidence of primary brain tumors in adults, of which the majority of gliomas arise in the supratentorial compartment, ~75% of pediatric gliomas involve the cerebellum, brain stem, or diencephalon, making this predominantly a disease of childhood.[2] Thus there is a need to strive for improved treatments because these tumors afflict predominantly children under 15 years of age.

Brain stem tumors may now be reliably classified into subgroups based on their imaging characteristics and clinical presentation. These subgroups have relevance with respect to histology and prognosis, and they help to separate patients who may benefit from surgery from those in whom surgery is best avoided. Hoffman et al, in 1980, described a subgroup of brain stem gliomas that behaved in a clinically benign fashion in which an exophytic component could be surgically resected.[3] Shortly thereafter, Epstein and then Stroink et al proposed classification schemes based on the computed tomographic (CT) appearances of these brain stem tumors. The classifications basically described surgically treatable subgroups of brain stem gliomas.[4,5]

With the advent of MRI technology, which represented a significant improvement over CT imaging, the diagnosis and evaluation of brain stem tumors were revolutionized, which resulted in a classification scheme that allowed prognostication and surgical decision making.[5,6] Four subgroups are now generally accepted: diffuse intrinsic tumor, focal intrinsic tumor (solid or cystic), exophytic tumor (dorsal or lateral), and cervicomedullary tumor.[7] It should be noted, however, that the majority of cervicomedullary tumors do not actually involve the brain stem, instead behaving in the same manner as high cervical spinal cord tumors.

◆ Indications

Diffuse Tumors

The present consensus is that these are all malignant astrocytomas and carry a poor prognosis, with a mean survival of 12 months. This tumor typically arises in the pons. As such, there is no justification for surgical biopsy or resection for these tumors. The only therapeutic option consists of radiation and possibly adjuvant chemotherapy.[8] Unfortunately, the majority of brain stem gliomas fall into this subgroup.[9]

Focal Tumors

These tumors can arise in the midbrain, pons, or medulla. The tumor can be solid or have a cystic component. Children may present with symptoms of hydrocephalus because of the tumor or cyst. In particular, focal midbrain tumors are often indolent, and patients present with obstructive hydrocephalus. These children can be safely managed with cerebrospinal fluid (CSF) diversion. We prefer an endoscopic third ventriculostomy to a shunting procedure.

Exophytic Tumors

The majority of exophytic tumors arise in the medulla and have a dorsal exophytic portion protruding into the fourth ventricle. These tumors are typically juvenile pilocytic astrocytomas or gangliogliomas. Surgery is the preferred management strategy for these tumors because resection of the exophytic portion can be safely accomplished. Many children may present with hydrocephalus because of fourth ventricle obstruction. The hydrocephalus can be treated with the removal of exophytic tumor component.

Cervicomedullary Tumors

Surgery is beneficial in these tumors because they are usually low-grade astrocytomas or gangliogliomas.[10] This tumor involves the lower two thirds of the medulla and rostral segments of the cervical spinal cord. Children tend to present with either lower cranial nerve dysfunction or hemiparesis, depending upon the tumor epicenter in the medulla or cervical spinal cord.

◆ Preparation

Prior to surgery, gadolinium-enhanced MRI is the essential study to demonstrate the tumor, the presence of associated cysts, the relationship to vascular structures, and ventricular size. This information is very important for surgical planning, especially given that cyst decompression and CSF diversion may have to be considered.

Several of these patients will have significant bulbar dysfunction at the time of presentation, and it is prudent to assess the need for tracheostomy and feeding gastrostomy prior to brain stem surgery.

◆ Surgical Technique

Anesthesia

Endotracheal anesthesia is required, preferably by the nasal route if significant postoperative bulbar dysfunction already exists or is anticipated. This allows for a longer and more comfortable period of postoperative mechanical ventilation. The assessment for either or both a tracheostomy and feeding gastrostomy can then be performed in a less urgent manner. Large-bore intravenous access and an arterial line for blood pressure monitoring are required because surgical manipulation in the medulla can cause bradycardia, hypertension, and cardiac arrhythmias.

Especially in the prone position, care must be taken to ensure that the endotracheal tube is not kinked and that all lines and monitoring electrodes are free and easily accessible. If the sitting position is adopted, precordial Doppler monitoring is essential to detect air embolism, and central venous pressure should be monitored with a right atrial catheter.[11]

Neurophysiological Monitoring

Although there is currently no reliable method of continuously monitoring the visceral motor function of the lower cranial nerves, “mapping” techniques have recently been developed to identify cranial nerve motor nuclei in the floor of the fourth ventricle.[12–15] A monopolar electrode is used to stimulate the floor of the fourth ventricle with 1- to 2-second trains of electrical stimuli (maximum intensity, 2 mA; stimulus duration, 0.2 msec; repetition rate, 4 Hz). The evoked electromyographic activity is then recorded in the orbicularis oris and oculi muscles for cranial nerve motor nuclei (CN) VII, the posterior pharyngeal wall for CN IX/X, and the lateral aspect of the tongue for CN XII. This mapping method allows for a safe myelotomy in the floor of the fourth ventricle to approach subependymal lesions without damaging cranial nerve nuclei.[12] The incision in this setting is not always in the area that appears the thinnest.[15] A similar technique has also been used to identify the limits of the cerebral peduncle when lesions are approached on the ventrolateral surface of the brain stem.

In the case of cervicomedullary tumors, electrophysiological monitoring assumes greater importance because these tumors behave in a similar manner to high cervical spinal cord tumors with rostral extension and displacement of the medulla. Although both sensory (SEP) and motor evoked potentials (MEP) are monitored, MEPs have been found to be more reliable. Epidural electrodes placed caudal to the tumor can detect motor potentials evoked by transcranial stimulation of the motor cortex, and faster updating of the averaged signals can be achieved, approaching a real-time monitoring situation. Thus, if tumor resection disrupts these motor pathways, the drop in these potentials will alert the surgeon to the danger of causing permanent neurological damage. In most cases, the appropriate step is to stop further resection and to irrigate the tumor cavity with warm saline. If there is a return of potentials, resection can continue; if not, the surgeon should probably abandon the procedure.

Positioning

Because the majority of brain stem tumors involve the pons, medulla, or upper cervical cord, our preferred surgical approach is the prone position with the head of the patient securely fixed in pins, the neck flexed, and the trunk supported on adequately sized chest rolls (**Fig. 36–1**). In children and young infants we prefer the Sugita head holder (Mizuho Ikakogyo Co., Tokyo) with six pins. The abdomen should be resting freely between the rolls with no compression, with all pressure points carefully protected, especially in pediatric patients. For certain tumors involving the anterior and lateral midbrain and cerebral peduncle, a subtemporal approach is sometimes used.

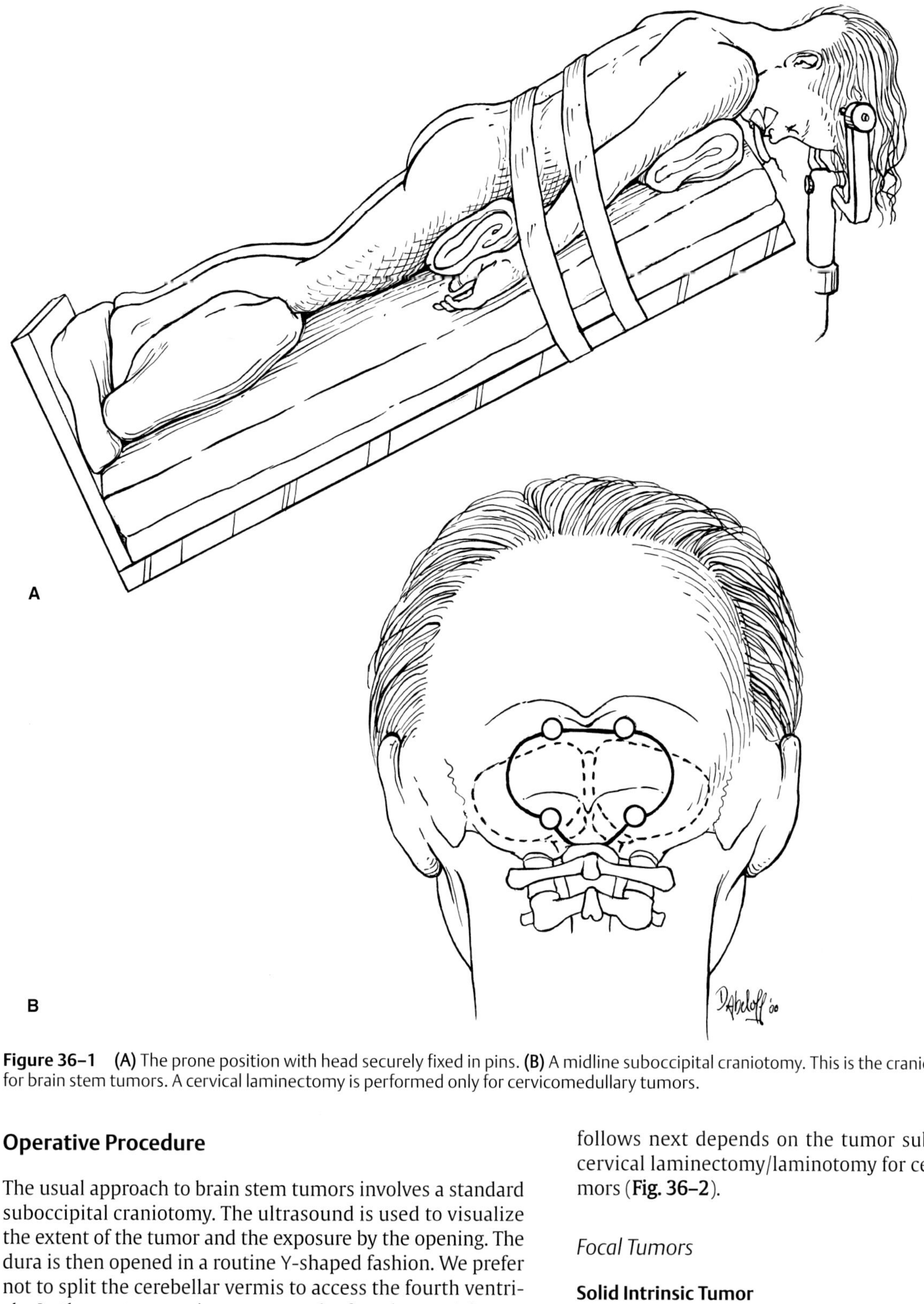

Figure 36–1 **(A)** The prone position with head securely fixed in pins. **(B)** A midline suboccipital craniotomy. This is the craniotomy most often used for brain stem tumors. A cervical laminectomy is performed only for cervicomedullary tumors.

Operative Procedure

The usual approach to brain stem tumors involves a standard suboccipital craniotomy. The ultrasound is used to visualize the extent of the tumor and the exposure by the opening. The dura is then opened in a routine Y-shaped fashion. We prefer not to split the cerebellar vermis to access the fourth ventricle. In the past, operative access to the fourth ventricle was obtained by splitting the vermis or resecting portions of the cerebellar hemisphere. Complications of these approaches included cerebellar mutism, ataxia, hypotonia, adiadochokinesia, and nystagmus. We prefer to access the fourth ventricle by opening the tela and inferior medullary velum at the cerebellomedullary fissure or telovelar junction. Recently this approach has been described in detailed prosections.[16,17] What follows next depends on the tumor subtype, for example, cervical laminectomy/laminotomy for cervicomedullary tumors (**Fig. 36–2**).

Focal Tumors

Solid Intrinsic Tumor

In general, the approach to a solid intrinsic tumor of the brain stem is along the shortest path, identified by intraoperative ultrasound. This point of entry is often marked by a small area of discoloration seen through the ependyma or pia-arachnoid. This area should be stimulated so as to localize the cranial nerve motor nuclei before making the myelotomy (**Fig. 36–3**). The safe area of the ependyma or pia is

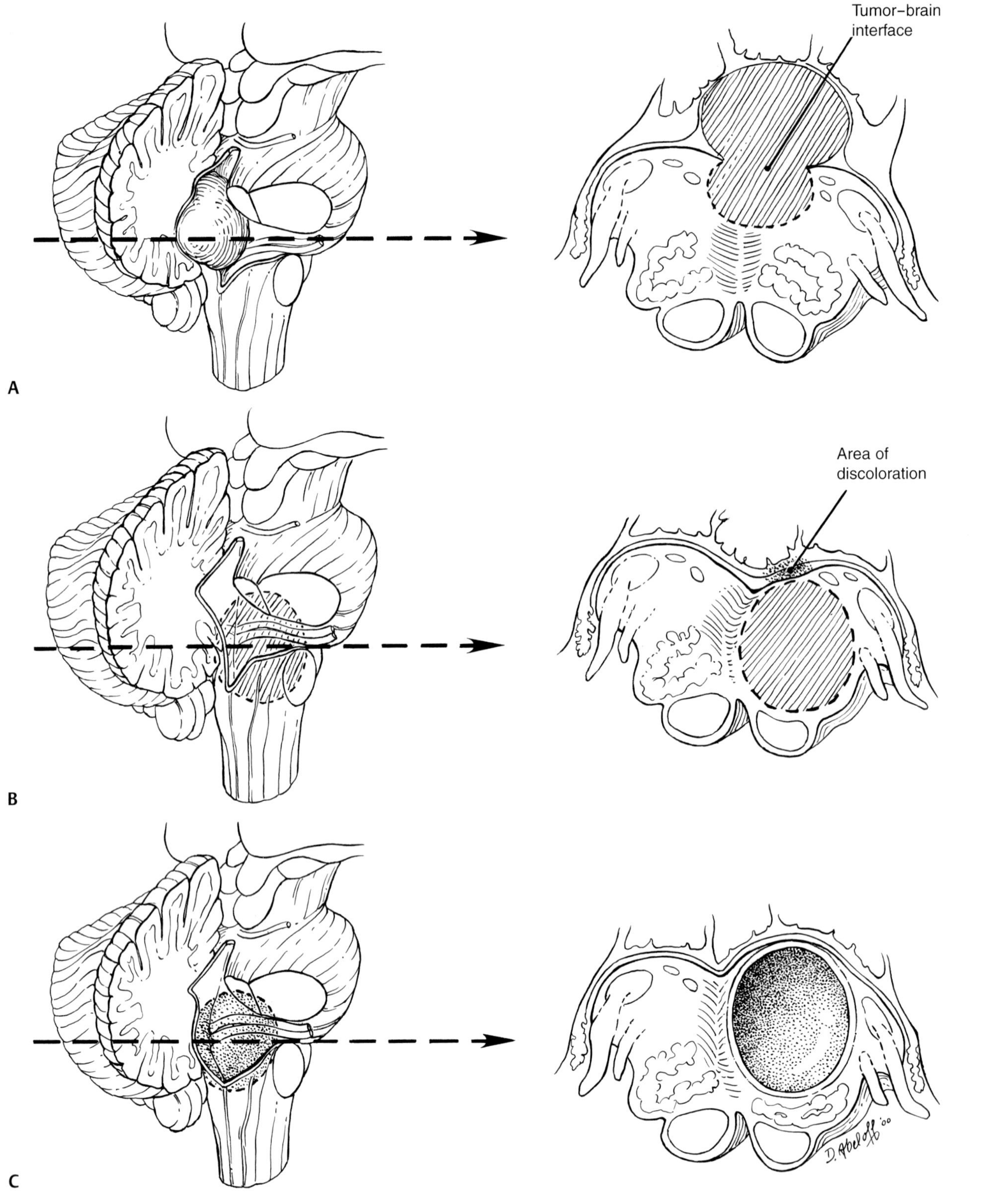

Figure 36–2 Several types of brain stem tumors. **(A)** Dorsal exophytic brain stem tumor. **(B)** Focal medullary tumor with discoloration seen on the floor of the fourth ventricle. **(C)** Focal tumor, which elevates the floor of the fourth ventricle.

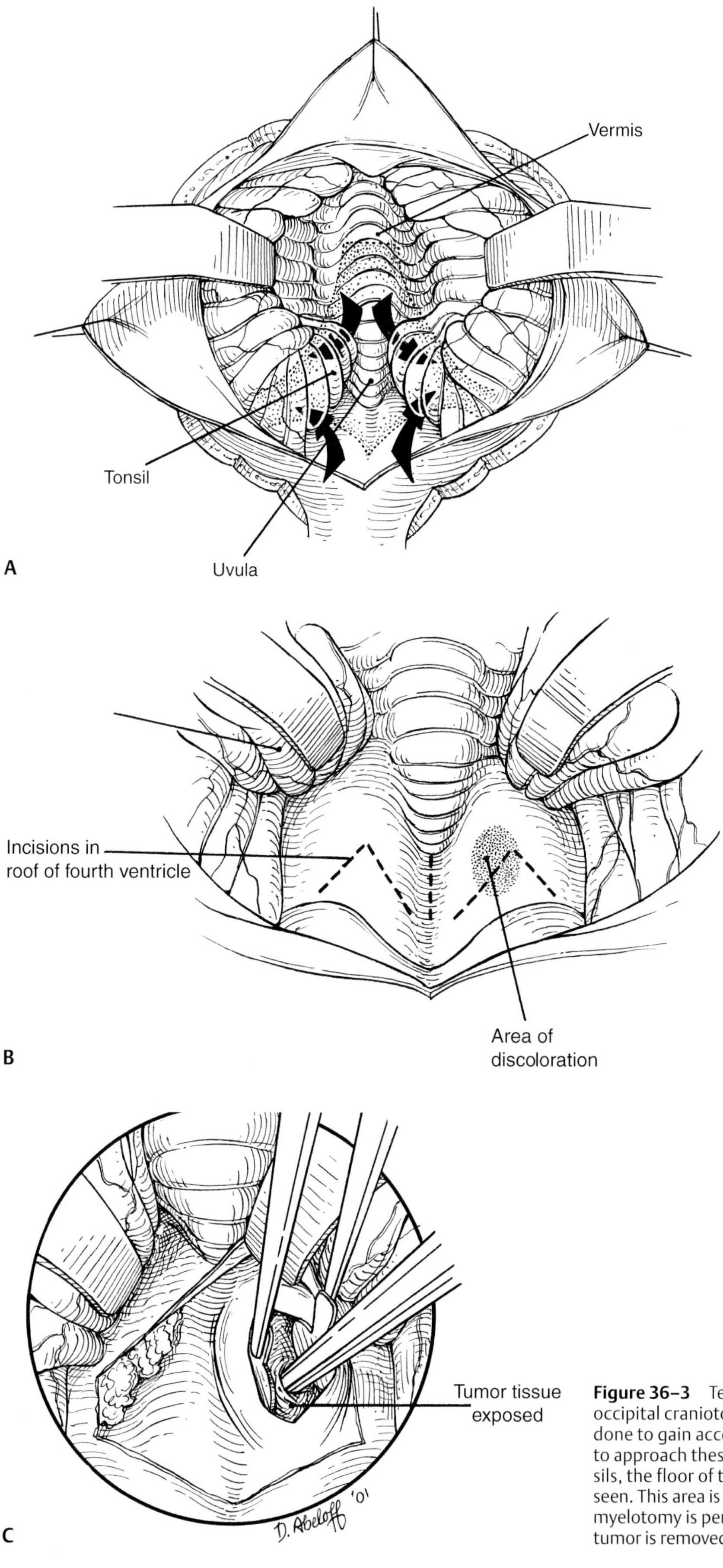

Figure 36–3 Technique for a focal medullary tumor. A standard suboccipital craniotomy is performed. **(A)** The telovelar approach is then done to gain access to the fourth ventricle. There are several avenues to approach these focal tumors. **(B)** After lateral retraction of the tonsils, the floor of the ventricle is identified. The area of discoloration is seen. This area is then stimulated to map the cranial nerve nuclei. **(C)** A myelotomy is performed in the discolored area with the laser, and the tumor is removed with the suction or ultrasonic aspirator.

then incised with the contact laser (SLT Technologies, Montgomeryville, PA), and the white matter is spread bluntly until discolored tumor tissue is encountered. This laser has a contact probe the shape of the scalpel, which can incise and obtain hemostasis. The use of this laser does not interfere with electrophysiological monitoring. Tissue for histological examination should be obtained immediately before applying suction or the ultrasonic aspirator. Aggressive surgical resection is not indicated in cases where the frozen histology is malignant.

The central portion of the tumor is resected using simple suction or the Cavitron Ultrasonic Surgical Aspirator (CUSA –Cavitron Corp., New York, New York) (CUSA). To minimize the extent of the incision through the normal white matter, the assistant exposes the lateral aspects of the tumor by gently retracting first in one direction and then the other as the surgeon works on the lateral aspects. The resection is halted when the consistency of the tissue begins to change toward normal or when significant hemodynamic instability develops.

A subtemporal approach is used for tumors that involve the anterior or lateral cerebral peduncle. Following opening of the arachnoid covering the upper midbrain cisterns, a bulging peduncle is usually obvious. The pia, as with the dorsal surface of the brain stem electrophysiological mapping is used to choose a safe entry site, is incised at the point of maximal bulging. Blunt dissection is used until the tumor is encountered. The pial incision is then lengthened parallel to the fiber tracts so as to expose the length of the tumor. Internal debulking is then performed until the normal white matter is seen.

Focal Cystic Tumors

These are clinically analogous to cystic cerebellar astrocytomas and are surgically treated in a similar fashion. The cyst is usually approached via the most direct route; once entered, little effort is needed to expose the margins of the tumor, and the solid portion can easily be resected. Mural nodules lend themselves to a more radical resection than diffuse infiltrative tumors.

Exophytic Tumors

Dorsal exophytic tumors can be approached as midline cerebellar neoplasms. Not infrequently, the provisional diagnosis is primitive neuroectodermal tumor (PNET) or a vermian astrocytoma. As the tumor is debulked, the origin from the subependymal surface of the fourth ventricle becomes apparent. It is for this reason that all midline tumors filling the fourth ventricle must be approached with caution. The floor of the fourth ventricle must be identified prior to debulking the more ventral portions of the tumor. We prefer not to split the vermis, which has been implicated with a postoperative cerebellar mutism syndrome. We approach these tumors through the telovelar or transcerebellomedullary approach. This provides the necessary exposure of the rostral portion of the tumor and the aqueduct. The tumor is then rolled gently in a caudal direction and the rostral floor of the fourth ventricle protected with a cottonoid. In this manner, the floor is identified both rostrally and caudally prior to tumor resection. The goal of tumor resection is to shave the tumor flush with the surrounding floor of the ventricle and not to proceed ventral to this plane (**Fig. 36–4**). No effort must be made to excise that part of the tumor within the brain stem because normal brain stem structures that are easily damaged lie just anterior to it.

Lateral exophytic tumors can be approached either via the cerebellopontine (CP) angle or a subtemporal-transtentorial route. In some cases, these tumors are erroneously diagnosed on MRI to have exophytic components but are found at surgery to be intrinsic. When confronted with this situation, the surgeon must decide whether to reorient the approach to a dorsal one or to persist with the approach through the lateral wall of the brain stem. In our experience, the lateral approach presents more difficulties in achieving a radical resection simply because the cranial nerves limit the surgical corridor.

Cervicomedullary Tumors

Tumors arising within the upper cervical cord and medulla are more appropriately thought of as spinal cord tumors. Their growth pattern reflects their benign biology with no infiltration. Consequently, when these tumors encounter the decussating fibers of the pyramidal tracts and dorsal columns, the tumor grows exophytically into the caudal fourth ventricle. If this pattern of growth is not observed, the probability is that the tumor is a high-grade infiltrating glioma or a tumor that has arisen within the medulla.

The surgical approach to this subtype of tumor is similar to that for a cervical spinal cord tumor. An osteoplastic laminotomy may be performed to expose the caudal limits of the tumor. The tonsils can be gently elevated or a telovelar approach performed to expose the rostral portion of the tumor. Again, we do not split the vermis to expose these tumors. In these cases, intraoperative electrophysiological monitoring can be useful, as mentioned previously. Because the spinal cord portion of the tumor is typically intramedullary, a midline myelotomy has to be made and the dorsal columns separated to expose the tumor. Central debulking can be performed with the ultrasonic aspirator, followed by suction or laser. The extent of the resection is carried rostrally to the medulla, where the surgeon should be more conservative. The exophytic component of the tumor is carefully removed to avoid injury to the posterior inferior cerebellar artery (PICA), which typically lies wedged between the tumor, inferior cerebellar hemisphere, and medulla. The medullary component of the tumor is addressed again by using the ultrasonic aspirator in the central bulk and then gentle aspiration at the periphery.

Closure

Once adequate hemostasis is obtained, the dura is closed in a watertight fashion, supplemented with an artificial duraplasty if necessary. We prefer Gore-Tex (W.L. Gore & Associates, Inc., Flagstaff, AZ) because it prevents adhesions

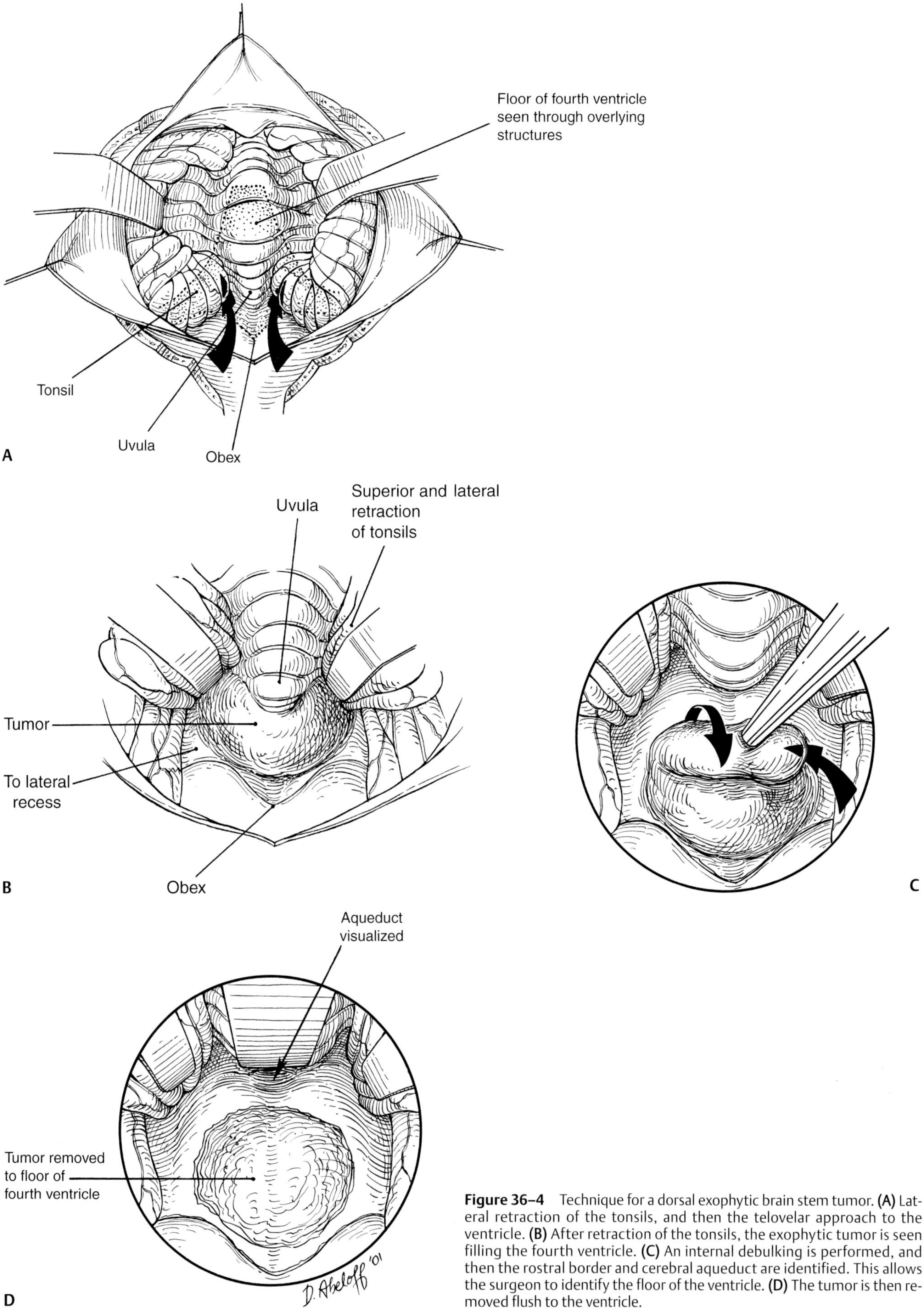

Figure 36–4 Technique for a dorsal exophytic brain stem tumor. **(A)** Lateral retraction of the tonsils, and then the telovelar approach to the ventricle. **(B)** After retraction of the tonsils, the exophytic tumor is seen filling the fourth ventricle. **(C)** An internal debulking is performed, and then the rostral border and cerebral aqueduct are identified. This allows the surgeon to identify the floor of the ventricle. **(D)** The tumor is then removed flush to the ventricle.

as compared with other dural substitutes. We use fibrin glue to seal the suture line. The bone flap is always returned with sutures. In young children and infants we do not routinely use titanium plates. The craniotomy not only improves the cosmetic result but more importantly facilitates reopening in the event of repeat surgery by restoring anatomical layers and eliminating the risk of inadvertently incising the dura during subsequent muscle dissection. We prefer to return the lamina if an osteoplastic laminotomy was performed for the cervicomedullary tumor. The overlying muscle and fascia are then closed in a multilayer fashion, with particular attention to the fascial layer so as to reduce the incidence of postoperative CSF leakage.

◆ Postoperative Care

One of the most important issues in the postoperative management of intrinsic tumors, and in particular tumors of the medulla, is the risk of progressive CO_2 retention, followed by respiratory collapse.[18,19] Although patients may not exhibit signs of lower cranial nerve dysfunction after surgery, respiratory collapse can occur within the first 48 hours postsurgery, with associated evidence of injury to a portion of the medulla. Tracheostomies and feeding gastrostomies are often required in children with preoperative cranial nerve dysfunction because of inability to protect the airway and to swallow. For this reason, we routinely keep all patients with intrinsic tumors of the medulla and cervicomedullary junction intubated for a minimum of 24 hours. Patients with tumors of the pons, midbrain, or dorsal exophytic tumors are not as vulnerable and usually do not require this level of ventilatory support. In pontine tumors however, diplopia from internuclear ophthalmoplegia as well as sixth and seventh nerve weakness can occur. Although these functions generally recover over a period of months, this is not always guaranteed.

◆ Complications

First, and most importantly, the surgeon must recognize that it is impossible to completely excise a glioma from the brain stem without potentially catastrophic consequences. The goal of surgery should be to obtain adequate tissue for histological diagnosis, to reduce tumor burden, and, when possible, to reestablish cerebrospinal fluid flow. The focal tumors, which lend themselves to resection, tend to displace functioning neural structures while invading only at their margin. In contrast, diffuse tumors aggressively infiltrate adjacent functioning structures, thereby providing no "bulk" to remove (with perhaps the exception of a large necrotic core). The success of surgery and the ultimate outcome of the patients are therefore dependent on tumor biology. A subtotally excised malignant tumor will rapidly regrow, negating any palliative benefit of the debulking procedure, especially when there is a risk for significant neurological deficits.

Second, there is never a cleavage plane between the glioma and the brain stem. For this reason, the surgeon must not attempt to define a tumor–brain interface. To do so in an aggressive surgical fashion will result in permanent cranial nerve deficits. These tumors may be removed with relative safety only if the resection proceeds from the core of the tumor outward until normal white matter begins to appear at the tumor margins. At this point, the resection is suspended, the extent of surgery evaluated by intraoperative ultrasound, and the electrophysiological monitoring reassessed. Such a technique will avoid permanent injury to neural tissue, especially in the case of low-grade gliomas that displace functioning neural elements and are minimally infiltrative by nature.

Third, bleeding vessels must not be chased into the brain parenchyma with the bipolar cautery but should be controlled with warm irrigation and hemostatic agents such as Avitene. The resection bed should be irrigated to clear any blood and cell debris prior to closure.

Lastly, when resecting cervicomedullary astrocytomas, the PICA is vulnerable because it typically lies wedged between the tumor and inferior cerebellar hemispheres. It is worthwhile to identify the PICA by examining the lateral aspect of the lower medulla where it branches off from the vertebral artery and passes toward the cerebellum.

◆ Conclusion

Until recently, the surgical management of brain stem astrocytomas was limited to biopsy and radiotherapy, with a generally accepted hopeless prognosis. Although the majority of these tumors are diffuse malignant astrocytomas, we now know that surgery can achieve acceptable results in certain subgroups. Surgery alone for these indolent tumors results in a long progression-free survival and outcome.

References

1. Bramwell B. Prognosis—duration, course, and termination—treatment. In: Critchley M, Flamm ES, Goodrich JT, eds. Intracranial Tumours. The Classics of Neurology & Neurosurgery Library. New York: Gryphon Editions; 1988:244–253
2. Packer RJ, Nicholson HS, Johnson DL, Vezina LG. Dilemmas in the management of childhood brain tumors: brainstem gliomas. Pediatr Neurosurg 1991;17:37–43
3. Hoffman HJ, Becker L, Craven MA. A clinically distinct group of benign brain stem gliomas. Neurosurgery 1980;7:243–248
4. Epstein F. A staging system for brain stem gliomas. Cancer 1985;56: 1804–1806
5. Stroink AR, Hoffman HJ, Hendrick EB, Humphreys RP. Diagnosis and management of pediatric brain-stem gliomas. J Neurosurg 1986;65:745–750

6. Barkovich AJ, Krischer J, Kun LE, Packer R, Zimmerman RA, Freeman CR, et al. Brain stem gliomas: a classification system based on magnetic resonance imaging. Pediatr Neurosurg 1990–91;16:73–83
7. Choux M, Lena G, Do L. Brainstem tumors. In: Choux M, Di Rocco C, Hockley AD, Walker ML, eds. Pediatric Neurosurgery. New York: Churchill Livingstone; 1999:471–491
8. Golden GS, Ghatak NR, Hirano A, et al. Malignant glioma of the brainstem: a clinicopathological analysis of 13 cases. J Neurol Neurosurg Psychiatry 1972;35:732–736
9. Smith RR, Zimmerman RA, Packer RJ, et al. Pediatric brainstem glioma: postradiation clinical and MR follow-up. Neuroradiology 1990;32:265–272
10. Jallo GI, Kothbauer KF, Epstein FJ. Surgical management of cervicomedullary and dorsally exophytic brain stem tumors. Operative Techniques in Neurosurgery 2000;3:131–136
11. Procaccio F, Gottin L, Arrighi L, et al. Anesthesia for brain stem surgery. Operative Techniques in Neurosurgery 2000;3:106–108
12. Deletis V, Sala F, Morota N. Intraoperative neurophysiological monitoring and mapping during brain stem surgery: a modern approach. Operative Techniques in Neurosurgery 2000;3:109–113
13. Eisner W, Urs SD, Reulen H-J, et al. The mapping and continuous monitoring of the intrinsic motor nuclei during brainstem surgery. Neurosurgery 1995;37:255–265
14. Morota N, Deletis V, Epstein FJ, et al. Brain stem mapping: neurophysiological localization of motor nuclei on the floor of the fourth ventricle. Neurosurgery 1995;37:922–930
15. Morota N, Deletis V, Lee M, Epstein FJ. Functional anatomic relationship between brain stem tumors and cranial motor nuclei. Neurosurgery 1996;39:787–794
16. Matsushima T, Inoue T, Inamura T, et al. Transcerebellomedullary fissure approach with special reference to methods of dissecting the fissure. J Neurosurg 2001;94:257–264
17. Rhoton AL. Cerebellum and fourth ventricle. Neurosurgery 2000; 47(Suppl):S7–S27
18. Abbott R, Shiminski-Maher T, Wisoff JH, Epstein FJ. Intrinsic tumors of the medulla: surgical complications. Pediatr Neurosurg 1991;17: 239–243
19. Abbott R, Shiminski-Maher T, Epstein FJ. Intrinsic tumors of the medulla: predicting outcome after surgery. Pediatr Neurosurg 1996;25:41–44

37

Metastatic Brain Tumors

Scott R. Shepard and Philip H. Gutin

The role of surgery in the treatment of metastatic brain tumors has been a source of controversy for most of this century. Until recently, there was a pessimistic attitude among neurosurgeons with respect to surgery for metastatic brain tumors. Previously, neurosurgeons were reluctant to operate on patients with systemic cancer. Also, before the development of modern brain imaging and refinements in neurosurgical technique, surgery for metastatic brain tumors was associated with a high complication rate. In series published before 1960, there was an operative mortality rate of between 25 and 38%.[10] Historically, metastatic brain tumors were not treated, and the survival was dismal, averaging 4 to 6 weeks following diagnosis.[4] During the mid-twentieth century, there were two major advances in the treatment of brain metastases—corticosteroids and whole brain radiation. These measures quickly became the standard of care because they significantly increased the survival of patients with metastatic tumors.[1] With the development of new methods of brain imaging and the refinement of neurosurgical techniques, surgery for metastatic brain tumors became more common. Although surgery for metastatic tumors became safer, this did not mean that it was beneficial in the treatment of metastatic brain tumors. In the early 1990s, two randomized, prospective trials demonstrated that surgery plus radiation therapy improved survival in patients with metastatic brain tumors versus radiation therapy alone and defined a role for surgery in the treatment of metastatic brain tumors.[15,19]

Traditionally, metastatic brain tumors were estimated to constitute 10% of all intracranial tumors. This was undoubtedly an underestimate because many of the initial estimates of the distribution of specific tumor types in intracranial tumors came from early surgical series in which metastatic tumors were clearly underrepresented.[23] This was the result of the reluctance of many neurosurgeons to operate on patients with intracranial metastases. Given recent advances in brain imaging and the increasing incidence of cancer in the United States, there has been an increase in the absolute number of brain metastases diagnosed. Also, there is strong evidence that the incidence of intracranial metastases is increasing.[1] Consequently, there has been an increase in the number of metastatic brain tumors the typical neurosurgeon encounters.

A discussion of brain metastases is not complete without highlighting their basic epidemiology. According to Posner's latest estimates from Memorial Sloan Kettering Cancer Center autopsy data, ~24% of all cancer patients have intracranial metastases present at the time of death. With an annual cancer death rate of 500,000 people in the United States, roughly 125,000 people per year have metastatic intracranial tumors present at the time of death.[1] This is the minimum number of intracranial metastases present in the United States annually. The systemic cancers that most frequently spread to the brain are lung, breast, renal cell, and melanoma.[1] Of these cancers melanoma has the highest propensity to metastasize to the brain, but lung cancer is the most common source for intracranial metastases because of its higher prevalence than melanoma.[1] Most metastatic brain tumors are supratentorial (80–85%), whereas 10 to 15% of metastatic tumors are located in the cerebellum and less than 5% of metastatic tumors are located in the brain stem.[6]

A metastatic brain tumor may be defined as the secondary spread to the intracranial structures of a primary tumor that has arisen outside of the central nervous system or its coverings. This may include intraparenchymal metastases, dural metastases, cranial metastases (calvarial or skull base), and leptomeningeal metastases. This discussion focuses on the surgical treatment of intraparenchymal metastatic tumors.

◆ Indications

There are many possible treatments for metastatic brain tumors, including surgery, radiation therapy, chemotherapy, and molecular therapies. Surgery for metastatic brain tumors includes craniotomy, stereotactic biopsy, stereotactic radiosurgery, or brachytherapy. The success of any of these treatments lies not only in the technical expertise they demand but also in proper patient selection. There are many considerations when evaluating the potential treatments for a patient with intracranial metastases, including cancer type, degree and control of systemic disease, patient life expectancy, responsiveness of the primary tumor type to different treatment modalities, and the extent of central nervous system (CNS) disease. When considering the extent of CNS disease, there are three general categories of patients: those patients with a single intracranial metastasis, patients with two or three intracranial metastases, and patients with diffuse disease, either more than three intracranial metastases or patients with intraparenchymal metastases and concomitant leptomeningeal disease. Approximately 25% of all patients with intracranial metastases will have a single metastasis, whereas roughly 50% will have two or three intraparenchymal metastases.[6]

When evaluating patients with metastatic brain tumors for possible surgical therapy, there are three general categories of patients. The first category includes patients for whom surgery is strongly indicated. This category includes patients who have a single, intracranial metastasis from a primary cancer that is not highly radiosensitive and stable or controlled systemic disease, or patients with intracranial lesions in whom a diagnosis has not been established. There is not universal agreement, however, that patients with a single intracranial metastasis and stable systemic disease should undergo surgery. There are many studies that demonstrate increased survival for surgery plus radiation versus radiation therapy alone, including the randomized prospective studies of Patchell et al and Vecht et al.[15,19] There are also some studies that do not demonstrate an increased survival for surgery plus radiation, including one randomized prospective study.[14] Nonetheless, the available data currently favor surgery plus radiation versus external beam radiation alone.[1,10,12,15,17–19,21,23] However, with the widespread application of stereotactic radiosurgery in the treatment of CNS metastases, several new issues have arisen. Currently, the role of radiosurgery in the treatment of CNS metastases is being evaluated, comparing the efficacy of radiosurgery with both external beam radiotherapy and surgery.[2,5,7–9,13]

The relative contraindications to surgery in patients with metastatic brain tumors are the presence of more than three intraparenchymal metastases or concomitant intraparenchymal and leptomeningeal disease. The issue is not as clear for patients with two or three intracranial metastases. Some authors advocate surgery in these patients and have shown increased survival for the resection of all metastatic lesions plus radiotherapy in these patients over radiation therapy alone.[3] Unfortunately, there is a relative lack of rigorous data regarding the benefit of resection of multiple CNS metastases. There are certain circumstances in which patients with multiple metastases may undergo resection of one or more of their metastases. For patients with intracranial metastases that are unlikely to respond to radiation (radiation insensitive tumors, highly cystic tumors, very large tumors), one or more of several intracranial metastases are sometimes resected to allow for treatment of remaining small metastases with either external beam radiation or stereotactic radiosurgery.[16,20]

◆ Imaging

In the evaluation of patients with suspected CNS metastases, there are three critical functions of preoperative imaging. First, an accurate diagnosis must be established. Second, the extent of intracranial disease must be defined. Finally, preoperative imaging is necessary to define specific anatomical criteria that will affect treatment choices.

This first function of preoperative imaging, establishing an accurate diagnosis, depends on both imaging characteristics and patient history. The imaging modality of choice in the evaluation of patients with suspected brain metastases is contrast-enhanced magnetic resonance imaging (MRI) because of its superior tissue detail and its ability to define multiple characteristics of both lesions within the brain and the brain surrounding these lesions. There are several roles for computed tomography (CT), however, in the evaluation of the patient with suspected metastatic disease. There are a small number of patients who cannot undergo MRI scanning due to the presence of paramagnetic implants (e.g., pacemaker) or metallic fragments in their bodies. CT is not just reserved for patients who cannot undergo MRI scanning. CT scans provide better bony detail than MRI, which is sometimes helpful in evaluating metastatic lesions, especially when there is extensive involvement of the calvarium or the skull base.[23]

The MRI characteristics of parenchymal brain metastases are as follows: hypointensity compared with brain on unenhanced T1-weighted images and hyperintensity on T2-weighted images. Metastases usually enhance intensely with contrast administration. In metastases smaller than 3 cm, the enhancement pattern is frequently dense and homogeneous. For larger lesions, the enhancement is more often heterogeneous and frequently is ring enhancing. On CT, parenchymal metastases are either hypo- or isointense to brain prior to contrast administration, and either densely enhancing or ring enhancing following contrast administration.[23]

The differential diagnosis for suspected metastatic lesions includes primary, intra-axial brain tumor (astrocytoma), meningioma, abscess, evolving hematoma, thrombosed giant aneurysm, vascular malformation, granuloma, and demyelinating disease (**Fig. 37–1**).[10] The patient's history is a crucial factor in determining the diagnosis. Certainly, in patients with known systemic cancer and lesion(s) consistent in appearance with metastases, the most likely diagnosis is metastatic tumor. However, in patients with a remote history of cancer; in patients with a new, intracranial lesion and a primary cancer that rarely spreads to brain parenchyma (e.g., prostate cancer); or in patients with a risk factor for either acute or chronic infection, careful consideration must be given to other diagnoses. In Patchell et al's series of 54 patients suspected of having intracranial metastases based on history and imaging characteristics, three patients had tumors of astrocytic origin, one patient had an inflammatory lesion, and one patient had an abcess.[15]

The second function of preoperative imaging is to determine the extent of intracranial disease because this will clearly affect the choice of therapy. Again, MRI is the imaging modality of choice, given the superior anatomical detail it provides when compared with CT. It is important to

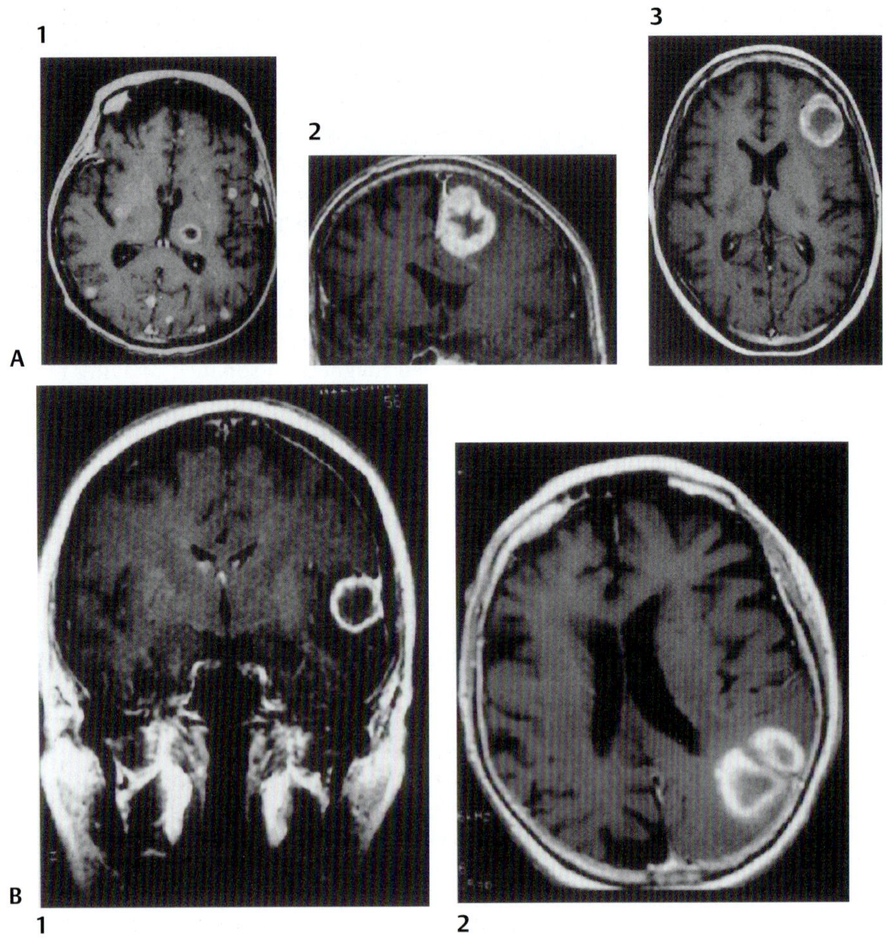

Figure 37–1 **(A)** Typical metastatic lesions. (1) A 68-year-old with disseminated breast cancer. (2) A 67-year-old with thyroid cancer. (3) A 29-year-old with non-small-cell lung cancer. **(B)** (1) A 57-year-old with breast cancer and presumed metastatic lesion. Pathology was meningioma. (2) A 69-year-old with disseminated lung cancer. Resolving hematoma.

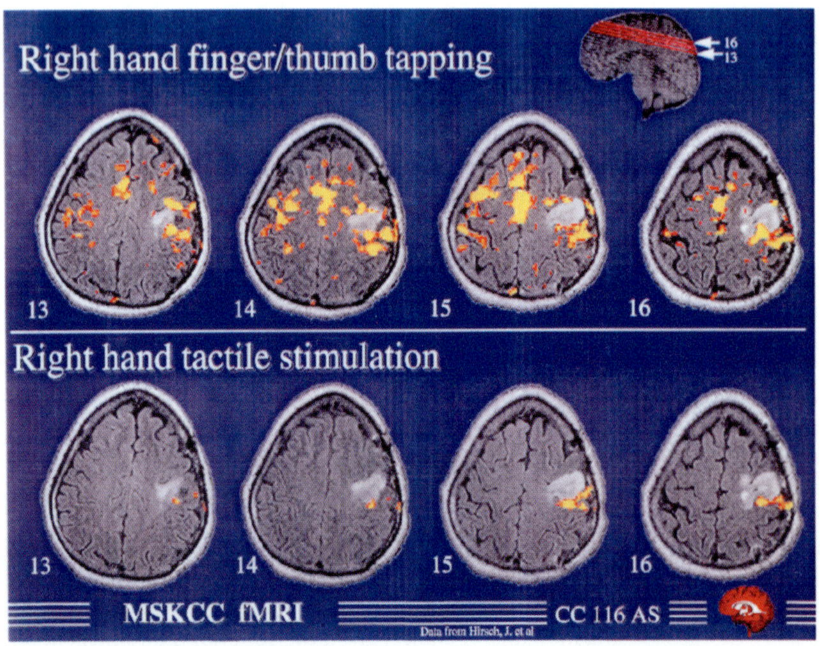

Figure 37–2 Functional magnetic resonance imaging scan in a patient with a left frontal tumor. The top sequence of scans demonstrates motor localization, with the majority of left hemisphere motor function located posterior to the tumor. The bottom sequence of scans demonstrates the sensory cortex.

remember that either high-dose or triple-dose contrast studies should be performed to optimize visualization of small metastases. Currently the resolution of MRI for identifying metastatic lesions is ~5 mm.[23]

The third role of preoperative imaging is to determine certain specific anatomical information. The location of a tumor with respect to surrounding structures within the brain is important for determining (1) if a lesion is safely resected and (2) the best route of approach to a lesion. Also, for those lesions near eloquent cortex, anatomical information may be helpful in determining a tumor's relationship to functional cortex or in planning an approach to a tumor that avoids functional cortex. Although routine MRI may identify eloquent cortex based on anatomical criteria, this is frequently insufficient for surgical planning. Functional imaging, such as magnetoencephalography (MEG) or functional MRI are much more reliable for identifying the location of functional cortex (**Fig. 37–2**). With either functional MRI or MEG, it can often be established that a tumor is outside of adjacent eloquent cortex and is safe to resect. Functional imaging can also be helpful in planning an approach to a tumor to avoid the functional cortex. In some cases, functional imaging may obviate the need for intraoperative localization.

◆ Surgical Technique

Positioning

The positioning of patients for craniotomy for metastatic tumors depends on both the location of the tumor and the desired approach to the tumor. The most common positions used are supine, supine-lateral, full lateral, and prone. Generally, patients with frontal tumors are positioned in either the supine or the supine-lateral position. Patients with temporal or parietal tumors are usually positioned in either supine-lateral or lateral positions. Patients with occipital lesions or posterior fossa lesions are either positioned prone or full lateral with the head turned toward the ground. Although there is usually a choice of positions for any given metastatic lesion, there are often special considerations that favor one position over another. For example, if localizing modalities such as frame-based or frameless stereotaxy are used, the particular system employed may dictate the use of a particular position. Another special situation occurs when multiple lesions are being resected. In such instances, a particular position that is not optimal for some of the tumors may allow for access to all lesions in one position rather than requiring a change of position during surgery. Another consideration involves the limitations imposed by a patient's medical condition. For example, patients who have undergone partial or complete pneumonectomy may not be suitable for the full lateral position with the intact lung in the dependent position.

Incision

The initial exposure for craniotomy for metastatic tumors utilizes standard craniotomy skin incisions (linear, curvilinear, reverse question mark, and U-shaped). Bone flaps are usually circular or rectangular in shape. There are, however, some special considerations for metastatic tumors. When resecting smaller lesions localized with either frame-based or frameless stereotaxy, very small craniotomies utilizing short linear incisions are often used. These miniature craniotomies are most often used when there are several small and superficial lesions being resected.

Approach

Once the initial exposure has been obtained, the next phase of the operation begins. The body of the operation may be divided into two parts: (1) the approach to the tumor and (2) the resection of the tumor. The approach to the tumor is composed of two steps, localization of the tumor followed by the approach to the tumor. There are many methods of tumor localization including manual exploration, localization by anatomical landmarks, CT/MRI localization, intraoperative ultrasound and intraoperative imaging (CT/MRI), frame-based stereotaxy, and frameless stereotaxy (**Table 37–1**).

Table 37–1 Methods of Cranial Localization

Method	Advantages	Disadvantages
Manual localization	Ease of application	Limited accuracy
CT/MRI localization	No special equipment necessary	Requires an additional imaging study No real-time imaging capability
Frame-based stereotaxy	High degree of accuracy Helps with incision and bone flap planning	No real-time imaging capability Frame may limit access to operative site Requires an additional imaging study
Frameless stereotaxy	High degree of accuracy Helps with incision and bone flap planning	No real-time imaging capability Requires special equipment Requires an additional imaging study
Intraoperative ultrasound	Real-time imaging	Requires special equipment Does not help design incision/bone flap
Intraoperative Imaging	Real-time imaging High degree of accuracy	Requires special equipment in the OR Intraoperative MRI requires special surgical instruments

CT, computed tomography; MRI, magnetic resonance imaging; OR, operating room.

Localization by exploration involves either the use of digital palpation of the brain or the insertion of a probe such as a brain needle into the brain to identify changes in the consistency of the brain indicative of the increased density of a tumor relative to the brain. This is the oldest and the least exact localization method. Localization by means of anatomical landmarks involves performing measurements on preoperative imaging to determine the distance of a tumor either from surface landmarks, such as the external auditory canal, or from intracranial landmarks, such as prominent blood vessels. CT/MRI localization involves using imaging to place a marker on the scalp over the region in which a tumor is located, thus indicating the region in which a tumor is located. Frame-based stereotactic localization involves placing the patient in a stereotactic frame and using stereotactic coordinates to guide the approach to a tumor and to design the skin incision and the bone flap. Frameless stereotaxy utilizes specialized computer software and either a robotic arm or a camera-based system to correlate the location of a mobile probe anywhere in or on a patient's head with the MRI scan. This is done by performing a preoperative MRI or CT scan with specialized skin markers, known as fiducials, in place and then registering the position of the fiducials once the patient has been positioned for surgery. The computer then rapidly correlates the position of the probe with the CT or MRI scan (**Fig. 37–3A**). Intraoperative ultrasound involves the use of a specialized ultrasound probe placed on the brain's surface to identify echogenic structures within the brain. Because most metastatic tumors are highly echogenic, they are easily visualized by ultrasound (**Fig. 37–3B,C**).[11]

Each of these localization techniques has distinct advantages and disadvantages, and the reader is referred to **Table 37–1** for a more complete list. The most important considerations when evaluating the advantages and disadvantages of a localization method are the accuracy of the technique, the ability of the technique to help design the incision and the bone flap, and whether the technique allows for real-time imaging. Of the techniques already mentioned, only ultrasound and intraoperative imaging allow for real-time imaging. This is important because the brain frequently undergoes some shifting during intracranial surgery due to

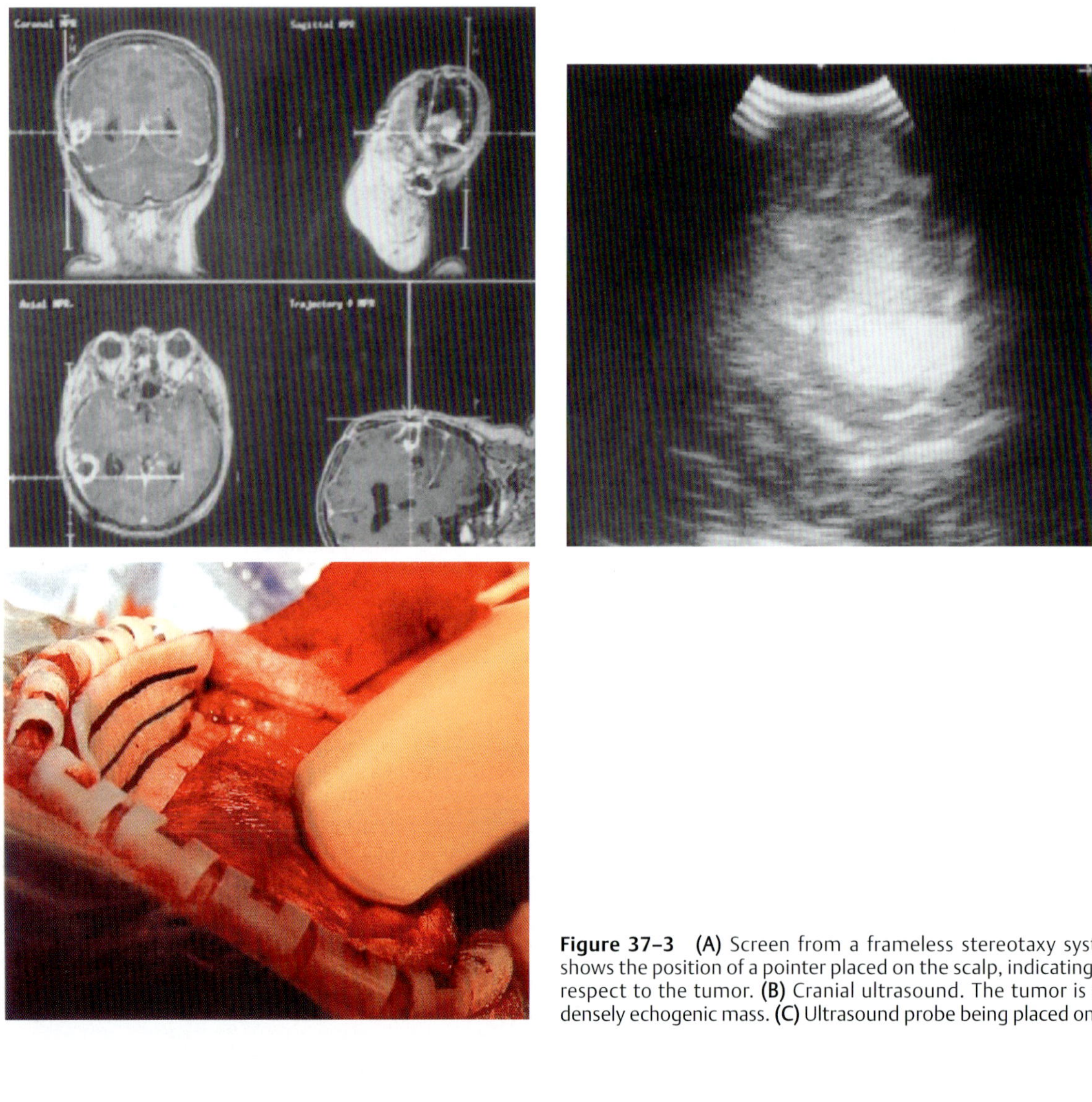

A B C

Figure 37–3 **(A)** Screen from a frameless stereotaxy system. The cursor shows the position of a pointer placed on the scalp, indicating its position with respect to the tumor. **(B)** Cranial ultrasound. The tumor is seen as a white, densely echogenic mass. **(C)** Ultrasound probe being placed on the dura.

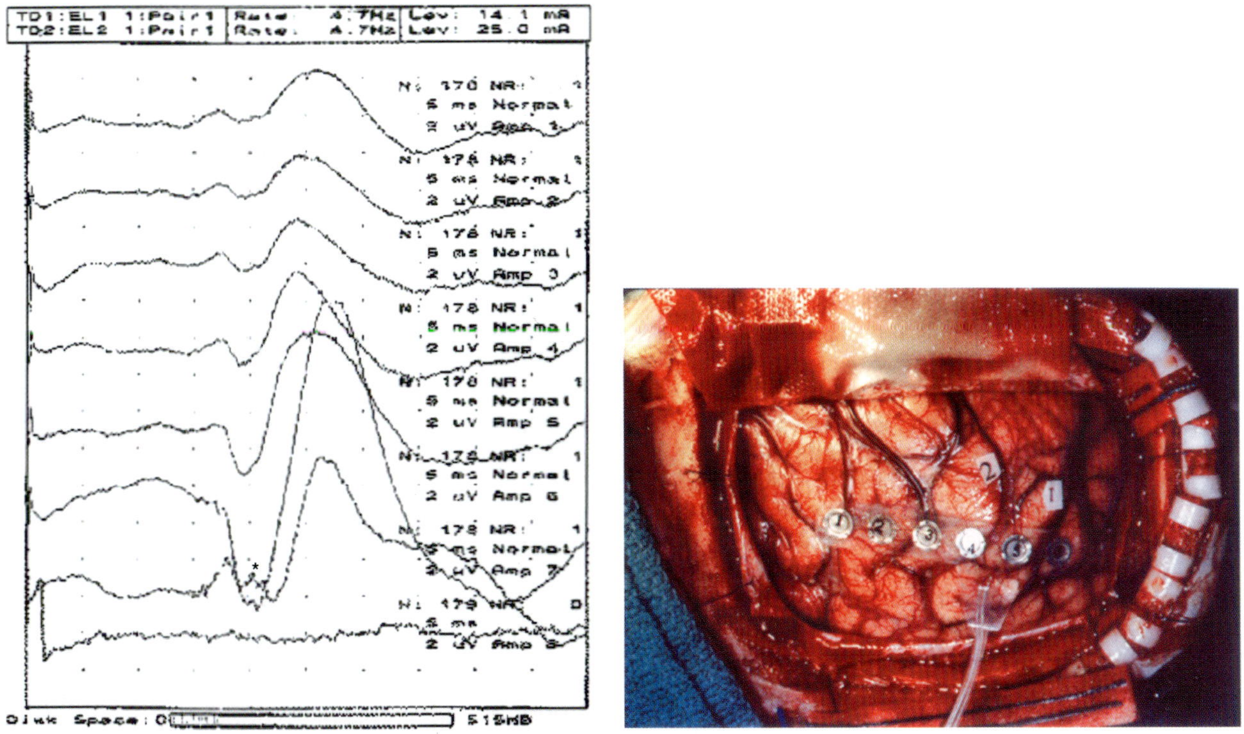

A B

Figure 37–4 **(A)** Phase reversal recording. The polarity changes between the two electrodes are marked by the asterisk, indicating the location of the central sulcus. **(B)** Electrode array for recording evoked potentials positioned on the brain. The central sulcus is located between the white markers no. 1 and no. 2.

manipulations of $PaCO_2$, osmotic diuresis, and the effects of removal of a mass from the brain. This shift can be significant and may cause the brain to shift by a centimeter or more. Because both frame-based and frameless stereotactic techniques are based on preoperative imaging and do not have the capacity to perform real-time imaging, any shift of the brain from its preoperative configuration may lead to inaccuracies in stereotactic systems.

The localization process may also involve cortical mapping. The localization of motor cortex can be performed either by phase reversal techniques or by direct stimulation of the brain.[22] The phase reversal technique involves the use of median nerve sensory evoked potentials.[12] A strip electrode placed on the brain will register this stimulation of the median nerve as positive in the electrode over the motor cortex and negative in the electrode over the adjacent sensory cortex (**Fig. 37–4**). Direct brain stimulation involves stimulating the cortical surface with bipolar current ranging from 1 mA to 16 mA and observing the patient for contralateral motor movement.[12] This technique may also be employed in the subcortical white matter to identify motor pathways through subcortical regions. Phase reversal mapping cannot identify subcortical motor pathways. Speech localization involves direct stimulation of the brain in the awake patient. Speech regions are identified when brief cortical stimulation causes speech errors or arrest during the period of the stimulation.

Once the tumor has been localized and any potential functional cortex has been identified, the optimal approach to the tumor is selected. This is dependent on both the particular region in which the tumor is located as well as the tumor's relation to the surface of the brain. For supratentorial tumors, there are five locations in which tumors can be divided for the purpose of defining the potential approaches to a tumor (**Table 37–2**). These locations are lateral cortical/subcortical, medial cortical/subcortical, deep white matter, intraventricular, and insular. Posterior fossa

Table 37–2 Different Surgical Approaches to Metastatic Tumors According to Their Location

	Tumor Location	Approaches
Supratentorial		
	Lateral cortical/ subcortical	Transcortical Trans-sulcal
	Medial cortical/ subcortical	Interhemispheric
	Deep white matter	Transcortical Trans-sulcal
	Intraventricular	Interhemispheric Transcortical
	Insular	Trans-sylvian Transcortical
Infratentorial		
	Medial parenchymal	Posterior transparenchymal
	Lateral parenchymal	Posterior transparenchymal Lateral (transcisternal)
	Vermian	Transvermian

tumors may be divided into medial parenchymal tumors, lateral parenchymal tumors, and vermian tumors.

The lateral subcortical tumors are those tumors that reside within 2.5 cm of the cortical surface except for those tumors in which the nearest cortical surface is the medial surface of the hemisphere. There are two potential approaches to these superficial supratentorial tumors, either the transcortical or the trans-sulcal route. If the tumor is within 1 to 2 cm of the cortical surface but not does come to the surface, the most direct approach is usually the transcortical approach to the tumor. However, if the tumor underlies functional cortex, the shortest transcortical route may not be the best approach. For tumors that reside more than a centimeter from the surface, a trans-sulcal route usually provides more direct access to the tumor with less disruption of normal tissue. However, the trans-sulcal route has two disadvantages when compared with the trans-sulcal route. First, it involves manipulation and possibly sacrifice of blood vessels within the sulcus. Second, it is limited as to the amount of exposure it may provide. Often, especially with larger tumors, a combination of the transcortical and trans-sulcal approaches is used. Tumors within the deep white matter may be approached with a transcortical, trans-sulcal, or combined approach. Purely trans-sulcal approaches often do not provide sufficient access to deep white matter lesions. Tumors that are located within approximately 1.5 cm of the medial surface of the hemisphere are best approached by an interhemispheric dissection. Intraventricular tumors are approached by either a transcortical or an interhemispheric, transcallosal approach, depending on their location within the ventricular system. Insular tumors may be approached either by a trans-sylvian or a transcortical approach (**Fig. 37–5A**).

There is a more limited choice of approaches for posterior fossa tumors. The majority of these tumors may be approached with a posterior transparenchymal route. Laterally located tumors may be approached by either the posterior transparenchymal route or a lateral, transcisternal approach through the cerebellopontine angle. Vermian tumors may be approached by splitting the vermis, usually with very little disruption of cortical tissue (**Fig. 37–5B**).

Dissection

After the tumor has been exposed, the resection is initiated. There are certain anatomical principles that guide the resection of a metastatic tumor. These tumors tend to displace rather than invade the surrounding brain and these lesions rarely have any brain tissue within the tumor mass. Metastatic tumors do not invade the brain as aggressively as glial

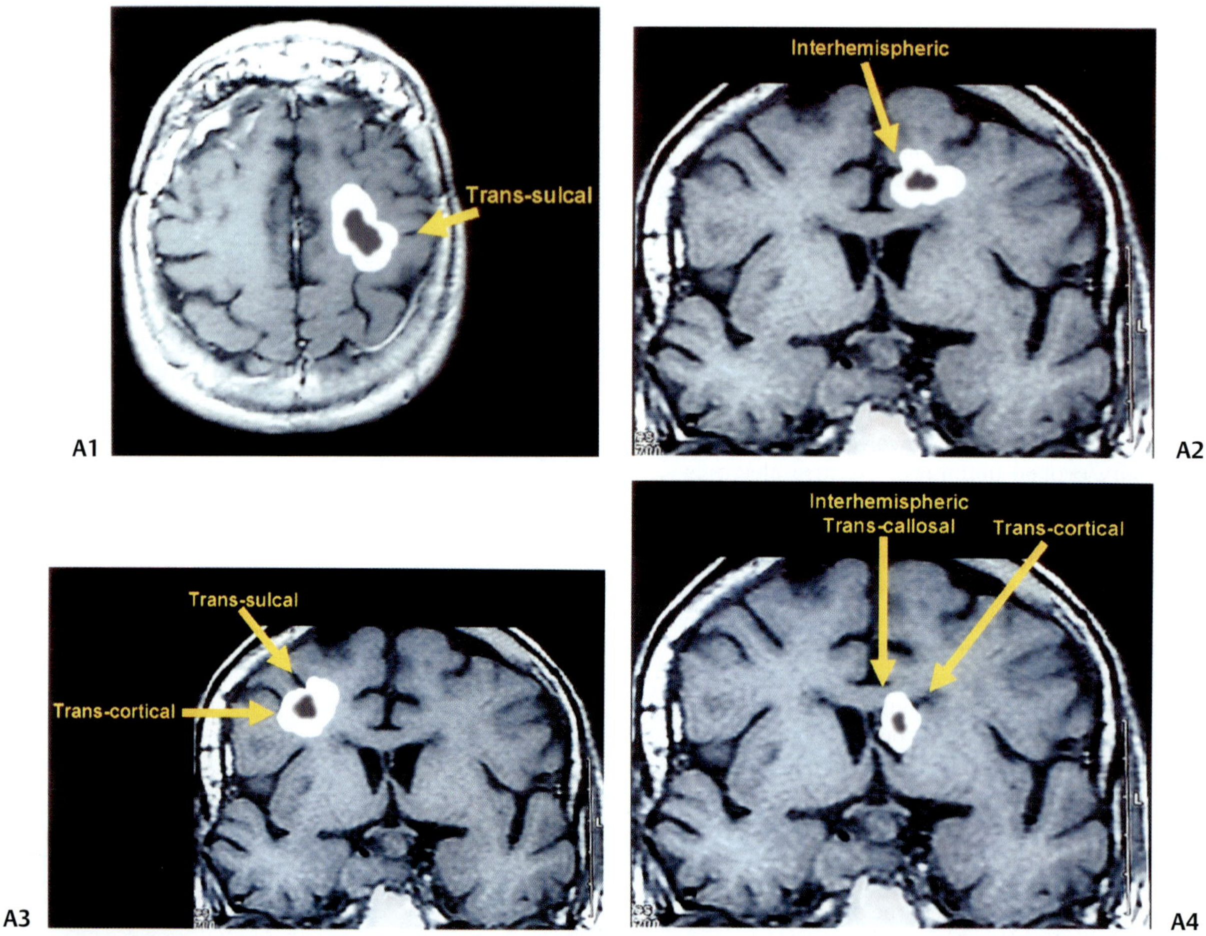

Figure 37–5 **(A)** Approaches to supratentorial lesions: (1) lateral cortical/subcortical tumors, (2) medial cortical/subcortical tumors, (3) deep white matter tumors, (4) intraventricular tumors,

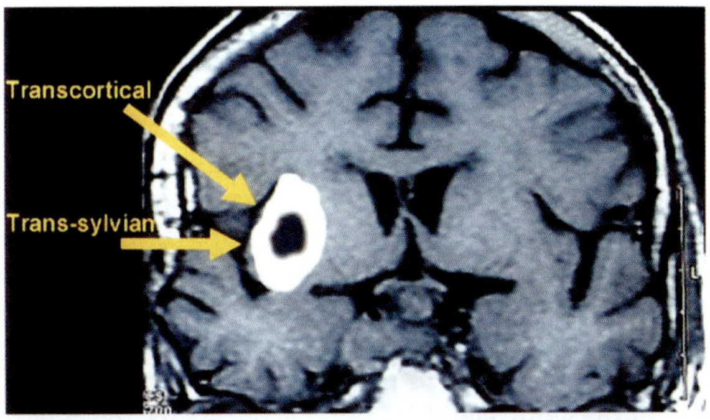

A5

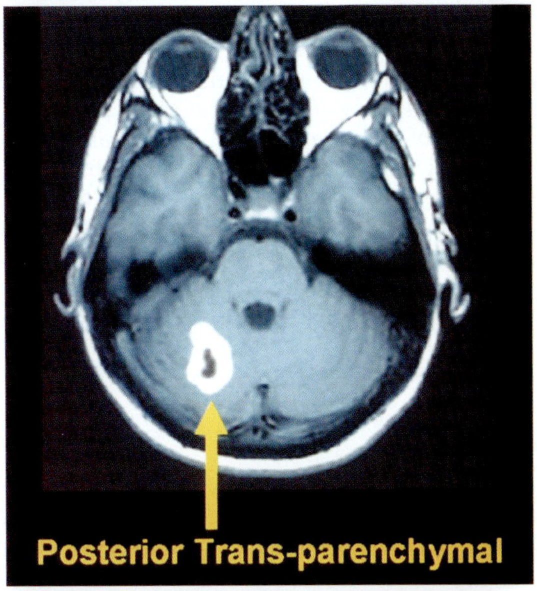

B1

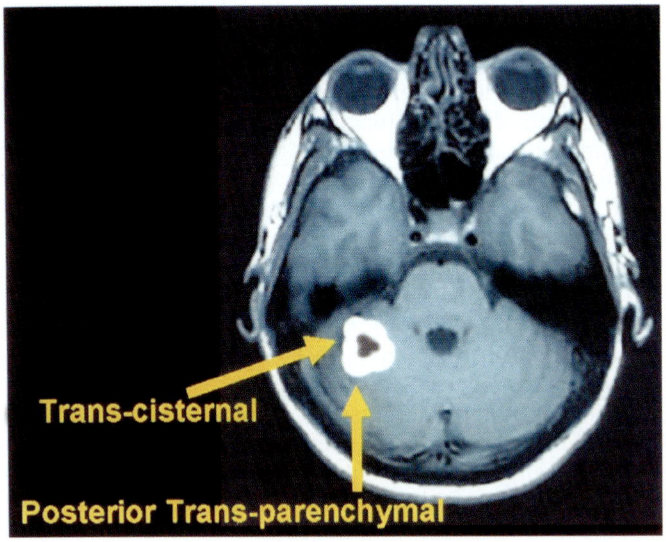

B2

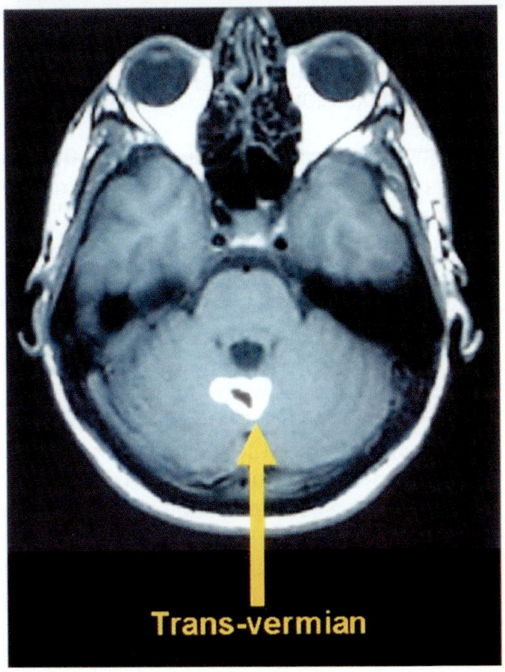

B3

(*Continued*) **Figure 37–5** (5) insular tumors. **(B)** Approaches to infratentorial lesions: (1) medial parenchymal tumors, (2) lateral parenchymal tumors, (3) vermian tumors.

tumors do, although metastatic cells may be found up to 5 to 10 mm from the main mass of tumor cells.[10,12] There is usually a gliotic pseudocapsule surrounding metastatic tumors, and these tumors are usually quite distinct in appearance from the surrounding brain. Whenever possible, a metastatic tumor should be resected by dissection around the tumor, either within or just outside the pseudocapsule, to perform an en bloc resection. This allows the surgeon to control the blood supply to the tumor and gradually devascularize it. Inadvertent entry into the tumor mass may cause significant bleeding, which can be difficult to control until the entire tumor has been removed. Certain types of metastatic tumors, most notably renal cell and medullary thyroid tumors, tend to be very vascular tumors. En bloc resection also prevents spillage of tumor cells. Ideally, a margin of white matter of at least 5 mm in thickness should be obtained around a metastatic lesion. However, this is not always possible when tumors are adjacent to functional cortex. For tumors less than approximately 3 cm in diameter, an en bloc resection is usually feasible. Larger tumors, however, may require excessive brain retraction to be resected in an en bloc fashion. Some of these larger tumors will have a central cyst, and decompression of the cyst allows for the remainder of the tumor to be dissected away from the brain and folded inward to facilitate an en bloc resection. If a large tumor does not contain a central cyst, then it may be necessary to centrally debulk the tumor. The ultrasonic tissue aspirator is often helpful in accomplishing this. When large tumors are resected in this piecemeal fashion, there is often a significant amount of bleeding that is difficult to control. Fortunately, once the tumor has been removed, the bleeding decreases significantly and may be easily controlled.

Following removal of the tumor, the cavity must be carefully inspected for residual tumor. Although smaller metastases tend to be spherical in nature, larger tumors are usually irregular in shape and may have areas that are partially hidden by folds of cortex. Small areas of continued bleeding within the resection cavity are often clues to the presence of residual tumor. If intraoperative ultrasound is used, the resection cavity can be filled with saline and an ultrasound performed. Residual tumor will show up as an area of increased echo at the periphery of the resection cavity. The frameless stereotactic systems may also be used to assess for residual tumor. However, if significant brain shift has occurred, the system may not be accurate enough to assess for small deposits of residual tumor.

Closure

After resection of the tumor, meticulous hemostasis must be obtained. This may be accomplished with a combination of bipolar cautery and any of several hemostatic agents. If there is persistent bleeding from the resection cavity, this may be an indication of some residual tumor, and the cavity should be carefully explored for any remaining tumor. Hemostasis may be assessed by the application of a brief Valsalva maneuver to transiently increase venous pressure and potentially identify any areas of less than optimal hemostasis.

Once hemostasis has been obtained, the dura should be closed in a watertight fashion. This is important to help prevent postoperative cerebrospinal fluid leaks as well as to seal off the intradural space as a barrier to potential infection. Occasionally, the dural flap is insufficient for closure and requires augmentation with either endogenous materials (e.g., pericranium) or dural substitutes. The next step is replacement of the bone flap. There are many methods that may be used to position the bone flap, including suture, wires, miniplates, and pins. There are two important considerations in the choice of a bone fixation system. The system must have sufficient strength to withstand the stresses placed on it, and it needs to adequately reestablish the contours of the skull. On occasion, it is necessary to cover bony defects from the bur holes, and they may be filled with acrylic or covered by a plate. In this population of patients, the scalp is often thinner than normal due to previous radiation or chemotherapy, and many of these patients have poor coverage of their scalp by hair. This means that even relatively small defects may be more visible. After the bone flap has been replaced, the scalp is closed in a routine fashion. Careful attention must be paid to the scalp closure to prevent compromise of blood flow to the scalp given that many of these patients already have diminished blood supply to the scalp because of prior systemic treatments.

◆ Complications

Traditionally, complication rates in patients undergoing craniotomy for metastatic tumor were quite high. Although this complication rate has been substantially reduced in the last 25 years, there is always potential for improvement. When considering potential complications and the goal of minimizing these complications, it is helpful to think of three stages: the preoperative period, the operation, and the postoperative period.

There are many preoperative considerations in the patient about to undergo craniotomy for metastatic tumor. This population of patients tends to have significant medical comorbidity due to factors such as advanced age, diffuse disease, and the effects of prior treatments for their primary disease. A thorough assessment of the patient prior to surgery is critical and particular attention must be directed to the organ system in which the primary disease arises. For example, patients with lung cancer, especially those who have undergone prior lung resections, must undergo pulmonary function testing to ensure that they may be safely ventilated during surgery and after surgery. In addition to optimizing a patient's medical status, the neurological status should be stabilized by minimizing the cerebral edema that is associated with most metastases. This involves the use of high-dose corticosteroids, typically, 12 to 24 mg of dexamethasone per day. Whenever possible, the minimum dose of steroids possible should be used, and the steroids tapered in the postoperative period when the patient is stable. The serum sodium level should not be overlooked because hyponatremia can exacerbate brain edema. In patients who have had a seizure prior to surgery, anticonvulsants should be given. There is no evidence that anticonvulsants will prevent the occurrence of a seizure in a patient with brain metastases.[1] Thus there is not a compelling reason to start anticonvulsants prior to surgery in patients who have not had a preoperative seizure.[1]

There are two categories of complications during surgery in patients undergoing craniotomy for tumor. The first category involves issues of neurosurgical technique. The neurosurgeon must carefully follow standard neurosurgical principles. This implies that the neurosurgeon should minimize brain retraction, prevent unnecessary sacrifice of cerebral veins, minimize the size of cortical incisions, and use proper illumination and magnification. Careful attention to these principles should minimize the risk of postoperative neurological changes and decrease the incidence of postoperative hemorrhage and persistent postoperative cerebral edema.

The second category includes general anesthetic and medical considerations. Cerebral edema is a particularly important issue in these patients because metastatic tumors tend to have a high degree of associated brain edema. Supplemental steroids and osmotic diuresis just prior to the start of surgery are frequently used to decrease brain edema. Also, mild to moderate hyperventilation is often used to decrease cerebral edema and intracranial pressure. Although these are very helpful interventions, they must be used carefully. Overly aggressive diuresis or hyperventilation can lead to decreased cerebral blood flow by means of hypotension or cerebral vasoconstriction, resulting in either a compensatory increase in cerebral edema, or ischemia and possibly neurological deficit. Another consideration with respect to interventions for controlling cerebral edema is the conformational change in the brain induced by diuresis and hyperventilation. The change in the conformation of the brain may introduce inaccuracies for localization aids such as frame-based and frameless stereotaxy, which are not capable of performing real-time imaging and, therefore, cannot compensate for any conformational changes within the brain. Prophylactic antibiotics should be given because these have been shown to reduce the infection rate following craniotomy. It is important to remember that the critical factor in the use of prophylactic antibiotics in surgery is to have adequate tissue levels of antibiotic at the time of the incision. Although many surgeons continue antibiotics for several doses postoperatively, there is no evidence that this provides any additional benefit over intraoperative antibiotics.

One of the most important interventions in the postoperative period is control of cerebral edema. Steroids should be continued in the postoperative period and rapidly tapered as tolerated by the patient. Patients that do not have any remaining intracranial disease following tumor resection will usually tolerate a decrease in the steroid dose by one half every 2 days. Prior to the use of steroids for cerebral edema, fluid restriction was an integral part of the management of cerebral edema. Currently, many neurosurgeons are not using fluid restriction following supratentorial craniotomies for tumor and are administering normal fluid volumes to these patients. This is due to the belief that abnormal fluid restriction may decrease cardiac output and possibly cerebral blood flow. If cerebral blood flow is compromised, this may lead to a paradoxical increase in cerebral edema due to vasodilitation. Although this has been demonstrated in the head-injured patient, it has not been investigated in the postcraniotomy tumor patient whose cerebral edema is mostly vasogenic in nature.

Another important intervention in the postoperative period is prophylaxis against deep venous thrombosis (DVT) and pulmonary embolism (PE). Patients who have undergone a craniotomy for metastatic tumor are at very high risk for developing DVTs due to multiple risk factors, including the presence of systemic cancer; high-dose steroids, which promote vascular stasis and clotting; and the postoperative state, which induces a hypercoagulable state. Antiembolism stockings and compression boots should be applied prior to the surgery and continued until the patient is fully ambulatory. Compression devices help to prevent venous thrombosis by release of systemic factors that promote clot breakdown and not by mechanical assistance of blood flow through large veins. Low-dose heparin or low molecular weight heparin compounds are beneficial in minimizing DVT and PE. There is no increased risk of postoperative hematoma formation when these compounds are begun 48 hours following craniotomy.

There is also the issue of anticonvulsant use for patients undergoing craniotomy. Although anticonvulsants have been shown not to prevent the occurrence of preoperative seizures, there is conflicting evidence regarding the use of anticonvulsants following craniotomy. Many neurosurgeons opt to use prophylactic anticonvulsants in any patient who has had a significant cortical incision, whereas others prefer to use anticonvulsants only when a patient develops recurrent seizures.

◆ Conclusion

At one time neurosurgeons had a pessimistic attitude concerning resection of metastatic tumors due to the high morbidity associated with the procedure. As both neurosurgery and neuroimaging advanced, craniotomies for metastatic tumors became a safe and acceptable treatment option. Several studies, including some randomized trials, demonstrated improved survival for surgery plus radiation therapy when compared with radiation therapy alone in the treatment of patients with a single metastatic brain tumor. This defined a role for surgery in the treatment of metastatic brain tumors.

A successful craniotomy for metastatic tumors requires more than just meticulous surgical technique. Good preoperative imaging is necessary to accurately establish the diagnosis and to develop a surgical plan. Good patient selection, proper positioning of the patient, and the optimal route of tumor exposure are also critical to the success of the procedure. Optimal medical care, both preoperatively and postoperatively, is also a significant factor in minimizing the morbidity of craniotomy for metastatic tumors. When all these factors have been addressed, craniotomy for metastatic brain tumors should be a safe and rewarding procedure.

References

1. Bender L, Posner JB. Current treatment of brain metastases. In: Maciunas RJ, ed. Advanced Techniques in Central Nervous System Metastases. 1998:1–16
2. Bindal AK, Bindal RK, Hess KR, Shiu A, Hassenbusch SJ, Shi WM. Sawaya. Surgery versus radiosurgery in the treatment of brain metastasis [see comments]. J Neurosurg 1996;84:748–754
3. Bindal RK, Sawaya R, Leavens ME, Lee JJ. Surgical treatment of multiple brain metastases. J Neurosurg 1993;79:210–216
4. Cairncross JG, Posner JB. The management of brain metastases. In: Walker MD, ed. Oncology of the Nervous System. Boston, MA: Nijhoff; 1983
5. Coffey RJ, Flickinger JC, Bissonette DJ, Lunsford LD. Radiosurgery for solitary brain metastases using the cobalt-60 gamma unit: methods and results in 24 patients. Int J Radiat Oncol Biol Phys 1991;20: 1287–1295
6. Delattre JY, Krol G, Thaler HT, Posner JB. Distribution of brain metastases. Arch Neurol 1988;45:741–744
7. Flickinger JC, Kondziolka D, Lunsford LD, et al. A multi-institutional experience with stereotactic radiosurgery for solitary brain metastasis [see comments]. Int J Radiat Oncol Biol Phys 1994;28: 797–802
8. Hendrickson FR, Lee MS, Larson M, Gelber RD. The influence of surgery and radiation therapy on patients with brain metastases. Int J Radiat Oncol Biol Phys 1983;9:623–627
9. Kelly PJ, Kall BA, Goerss SJ. Results of computed tomography-based computer-assisted stereotactic resection of metastatic intracranial tumors. Neurosurgery 1988;22:7–17
10. Kondziolka D, Lunsford LD. Brain metastases. In: Apuzzo MLJ, ed. Brain Surgery: Complication Avoidance and Management. New York: Churchill Livingstone; 1993:615–641
11. Landy HJ, Egnor M. Intraoperative ultrasonography and cortical mapping for removal of deep cerebral tumors. South Med J 1991;84: 1323–1326
12. Lang FF, Sawaya R. Surgical management of cerebral metastases. In: Harsh GR, ed. Management of Cerebral Metastases. 1996:459–484
13. Lunsford LD, Kondziolka D, Flickinger JC. Stereotactic radiosurgery: current spectrum and results. [Review] Clin Neurosurg 1992;38: 405–444
14. Mintz AH, Kestle J, Rathbone MP, et al. A randomized trial to assess the efficacy of surgery in addition to radiation therapy in patients with a single cerebral metastasis. Cancer 1996;78:1470–1476
15. Patchell RA, Tibbs PA, Walsh JW, et al. A randomized trial of surgery in the treatment of single metastases to the brain. N Engl J Med 1990;322:494–500
16. Sause WT, Crowley JJ, Morantz R, et al. Solitary brain metastasis: results of an RTOG/SWOG protocol evaluation surgery + RT versus RT alone. Am J Clin Oncol 1990;13:427–432
17. Sawaya R, Hammoud M, Ligon BL. Intraoperative localization of tumor and margins. In: Berger MS, Wilson CB, eds. Textbook of Gliomas. Philadelphia: Saunders; 1999
18. Sundaresan N, Galicich JH. Surgical treatment of brain metastases: clinical and computerized tomography evaluation of the results of treatment. Cancer 1985;55:1382–1388
19. Vecht CJ, Haaxma-Reiche H, Noordijk EM, et al. Treatment of single brain metastasis: radiotherapy alone or combined with neurosurgery? Ann Neurol 1993;33:583–590
20. Weber F, Riedel A, Koning W, Menzel J. The role of adjuvant radiation and multiple resection within the surgical management of brain metastases. Neurosurg Rev 1996;19:23–32
21. White KT, Fleming TR, Laws ER Jr. Single metastasis to the brain: surgical treatment in 122 consecutive patients. Mayo Clin Proc 1981;56: 424–428
22. Wood CC, Spencer DD, Allison T, McCarthy G, Williamson PD, Goff WR. Localization of human sensorimotor cortex during surgery by cortical surface recording of somatosensory evoked potentials. J Neurosurg 1988;68:99–111
23. Young B, Patchell RA. Brain metastases. In: Youmans, ed. Neurological Surgery. Philadelphia: WB Saunders; 1995:2748–2760

38

Tumors in Eloquent Areas

Mitchel S. Berger and G. Evren Keles

The efficacy of cytoreductive surgery to alleviate focal neurological deficits secondary to mass effect and increased intracranial pressure is unquestionable. However, the role of surgery regarding extent of tumor removal and outcome remains controversial, mainly due to the lack of prospective, randomized studies. The recent trend in the literature has been to support the strategy of removing as much tumor as possible in both low- and high-grade glial tumors, and growing evidence suggests that patients will live significantly longer and have an improved functional status.[1–4]

Here we present intraoperative cortical and subcortical stimulation mapping techniques to maximize safe removal of tumors located in eloquent areas. The surgical aim is to achieve adequate tumor removal without causing any additional permanent morbidity. Cortical stimulation mapping techniques were mainly adapted from the pioneering work of Cushing,[5] Forester,[6] and Penfield and Boldrey.[7] Localization of subcortical motor and sensory tracts was first described by Berger et al.[8]

◆ Indications

Motor Function Mapping

Hemispheric tumors located within or adjacent to functional areas (e.g., rolandic cortex, supplementary motor area, corona radiate, internal capsule, and uncinate fasciculus) constitute the major indications for intraoperative motor function mapping. Due to the tendency of infiltrative gliomas to invade underlying white matter tracts, it is important to identify both cortical motor sites and their descending pathways. It should also be noted that regardless of the gross appearance and consistency of the tumor, functional tissues may reside within the wall itself, and must be identified with stimulation mapping prior to definitive resection.[9]

Language Function Mapping

Cortical language localization, in terms of object naming and reading, is variable in each individual and does not follow any reproducible pattern across the population.[10,11]

Dominant temporal lobe resections guided by standard neurosurgical landmarks (i.e., restricting the temporal lobe resections to within 4 cm of the temporal tip and limiting the removal of the superior temporal gyrus) have been associated with permanent postoperative language deficits.[12,13] The traditional concept regarding the cortical representation of language function involves an anterior language site (i.e., Broca's area, the posterior part of the inferior frontal gyrus) and a posterior site (i.e., Wernicke's area, perisylvian in the temporoparietal cortex). This concept was challenged by some early studies using electrical cortical stimulation.[14,15]

More recently, in patients undergoing awake dominant hemisphere surgery, it has been shown that cortical language localization significantly varies and is distributed randomly from within the first few centimeters of the temporal lobe to within 4 cm of the midline in the posterior frontal–anterior parietal lobe.[10] In this study, no specific region of the temporal lobe cortex was found to be essential for language in more than 55% of the patients. In another study evaluating the localization of essential language sites, data obtained from patients with dominant hemisphere temporal lobe tumors was compared with information obtained from epilepsy patients.[16] The authors showed that the superior temporal gyrus contained significantly more language sites than the middle temporal gyrus, both in patients with and in patients without temporal lobe gliomas, and that 12 to 16% of both patient populations had languages sites anterior to the central sulcus in the superior temporal gyrus.

These studies support the fact that cortical stimulation mapping for the identification of essential languages sites in patients with tumors of the dominant hemisphere temporal lobe will maximize the extent of tumor resection while minimizing permanent language deficits. Therefore, an awake craniotomy with cortical stimulation mapping is indicated for any lesion involving the dominant temporal, mid- to posterior frontal, and mid- to anterior parietal lobes to identify language sites prior to tumor removal.

◆ Preparation

Neurological Evaluation

To determine the extent of motor or language function impairment, if any, the patient's neurological status should be assessed preoperatively. Although motor mapping will often not be useful if the patient has severe hemiparesis, it is usually possible to stimulate both cortical and subcortical motor pathways intraoperatively if antigravity movements are present preoperatively. In children younger than 6 years of age, due to cortical electrical inexcitability, somatosensory evoked potentials must be available and used to identify the central sulcus in case the motor pathways are inexcitable.

Besides testing motor and sensory function, it is imperative to assess the patient's language function preoperatively to determine if the baseline naming error rate is < 25%. Patients who will undergo intraoperative mapping for language sites should be preoperatively tested for language errors by being presented a series of slides with common objects to be named. After confirming that the face motor cortex and Broca's area are functional by asking the patient to protrude the tongue and count to 10, slides of common objects are shown. Each slide will start with a phrase such as "This is a . . ." or "These are . . ." to test reading and speech output. Patients must be able to name common objects with less than a 25% baseline error rate, with each slide presented three times.

Language mapping will not be successful in patients who have moderate to severe dysphasia in either comprehension or expression. Therefore, this group of patients may either be operated on asleep, without any attempt to do more than an internal decompression, or challenged with steroids for 7 to 10 days and reevaluated regarding their baseline error rate in naming. An alternative approach may be to biopsy the tumor and then to radiate the lesion following histopathological confirmation to reduce its size to result in functional improvement that will subsequently allow for intraoperative mapping.

The left hemisphere is dominant for language in 85% of the population, whereas language representation is bilateral in 9%, and right side dominance is present in only 6%.[17] For 98 to 99% of right-handed individuals, the dominant hemisphere is on the left. When in doubt, cerebral dominance is verified using Wada's (i.e., intracarotid amytal) test.[18] Its use is limited to entirely or predominantly left-handed patients.

Neuroradiological Evaluation

The functional organization of the brain in relation to the tumor is assessed for motor pathways on a multiplanar magnetic resonance (MR) scan, which is also the current diagnostic study procedure of choice for neuro-oncological follow-up.[19] The most cranial (rostral, superior) cuts of axial T2-weighted MR images are used to identify the central sulcus and the motor strip, which is located within the gyrus directly in front of it. Regardless of mass effect, this landmark is a reliable marker of the motor cortex and is always present and allows one to predict where the functional motor region will be before surgery. The rolandic (i.e., somatosensory-motor cortex) is identified on midsagittal and near midsagittal MR images by following the cingulated sulcus posteriorly and superiorly to its termination point. The rolandic cortex is located directly in front of this sulcus. On far lateral images, the inferior to midportion of the motor cortex is located to a region bisected by a perpendicular line emanating from the posterior corner of the insular triangle. All of these MR landmarks serve as useful guides to preoperatively determine the proximity of the lesion to the motor cortex.

◆ Surgical Technique

Positioning

In the operating room, the patient is placed in the position appropriate for the area to be exposed. The head is placed on a soft donut or secured with a pin fixation device such as a Mayfield if surgical navigation is to be used (**Fig. 38–1**). Special care is given to ensure that all extremities are well padded and protected. A heating blanket is used to avoid the core temperature drifting too low, especially under general anesthesia. An intravenous propofol (Diprivan) drip maintains the sedative-hypnotic anesthesia to keep the patient asleep. Oxygen is administered through a nasal cannula in case of a decrease in the arterial oxygen saturation. Regardless of the need for osmotic diuretics, a Foley catheter is inserted. Prophylactic antibiotics are routinely used and given during the induction phase of anesthesia.

The head is shaved and washed and the incision marked. In general, a wide exposure will be necessary to ensure that enough cortical sites are available for testing. The area of the scalp around the incision is infiltrated with a local anesthetic consisting of lidocaine (0.5%) and Marcaine (0.25%). The craniotomy should be wide enough to expose the tumor and surrounding brain, including areas where language

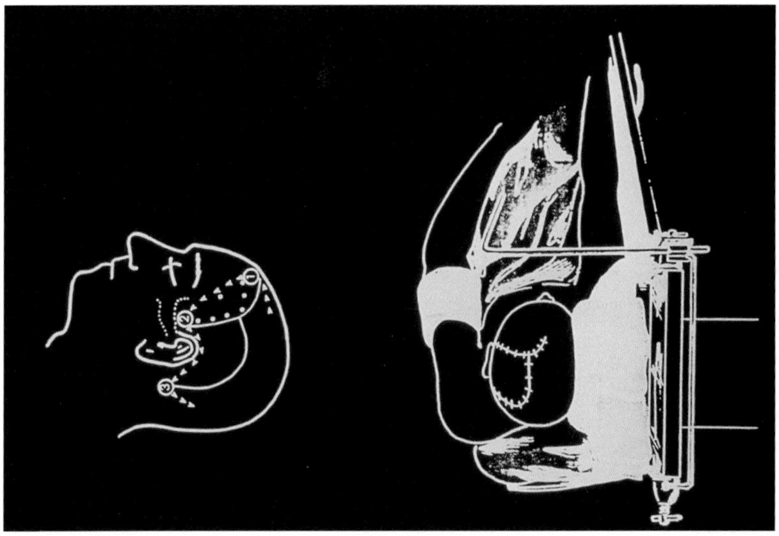

Figure 38–1 The patient is positioned and the scalp incision drawn.

is likely to be located, to provide adequate cortical areas for language mapping. The tumor is localized with intraoperative ultrasound of surgical navigation systems. Because the dura is pain sensitive, the area around the middle meningeal artery should be infiltrated with the lidocaine–Marcaine mixture to alleviate discomfort during wakefulness.

Identification of the Motor Cortex and Subcortical Pathways

Following dural opening, the stimulation mapping should begin by first identifying the motor cortex. A bipolar electrode (5 mm spacing) on the surface for 2 to 3 seconds with a current amplitude between 2 and 16 mA is used. A constant generator is utilized to produce biphasic square wave pulses at 60 Hz and a 1.25 msec single peak (pulse) duration.

Depending on the anesthetic condition of the patient, the current necessary to evoke motor movement will vary, with lower currents used under awake conditions. The motor strip is stimulated in the asleep patient with a starting current of 4 mA and reduced to 2 mA when stimulating the awake patient. The amplitude of the current is adjusted in 1 to 2 mA increments until motor movements are identified. A current above 16 mA has never been necessary to evoke sensory or motor response.[8] At this point cold Ringer's lactate solution should be immediately available for irrigation of the stimulated cortex. If a focal motor seizure occurs, [rapid cortical etc.] rapid cortical irrigation at the stimulation site with ice cold Ringer's solution will abruptly stop the seizure activity originating from the irritated cortex without using short-acting barbiturates.[20]

First, the inferior aspect of the rolandic cortex is identified by eliciting responses in the face and hand. Because the leg motor cortex is tucked away against the falx, a strip electrode may be inserted along the falx, and stimulation using the same current applied to the lateral cortical surface may be delivered through it to evoke leg motor movements. This maneuver is safe due to the lack of bridging veins between the falx and the leg motor cortex. Similarly, a subdural strip electrode may be inserted and stimulated to evoke the desired response if the craniotomy is near but not overlying the rolandic cortex.

Following identification of the motor cortex, the descending tracts may be found using similar stimulation parameters. Descending motor and sensory pathways may be followed into the internal capsule and inferiorly to the brain stem and spinal cord (**Fig. 38–2A–D**). This is especially important during resection of infiltrative glial tumors because functioning motor, sensory, or language tissue can be located within a grossly obvious tumor or surrounding infiltrated brain.[9] A final postresection stimulation of cortical sites should be performed to confirm that pathways are intact. This will also ensure that the underlying functional tracts have been preserved if subcortical status is worse postoperatively. The presence of intact cortical and subcortical motor pathways will imply that the deficit will be transient and resolved in days to weeks.

Although somatosensory evoked potentials (SEPs) may be helpful in identifying the central sulcus, they do not help to localize descending subcortical motor and sensory white matter tracts. Determination of the subcortical pathways is important while removing a deeply located tumor within or adjacent to the corona radiata, internal capsule, insula, supplementary motor area, and thalamus. Because the current spread from the electrode contacts is minimal during bipolar stimulation,[21] resection should be stopped when movement of paresthesia is evoked.

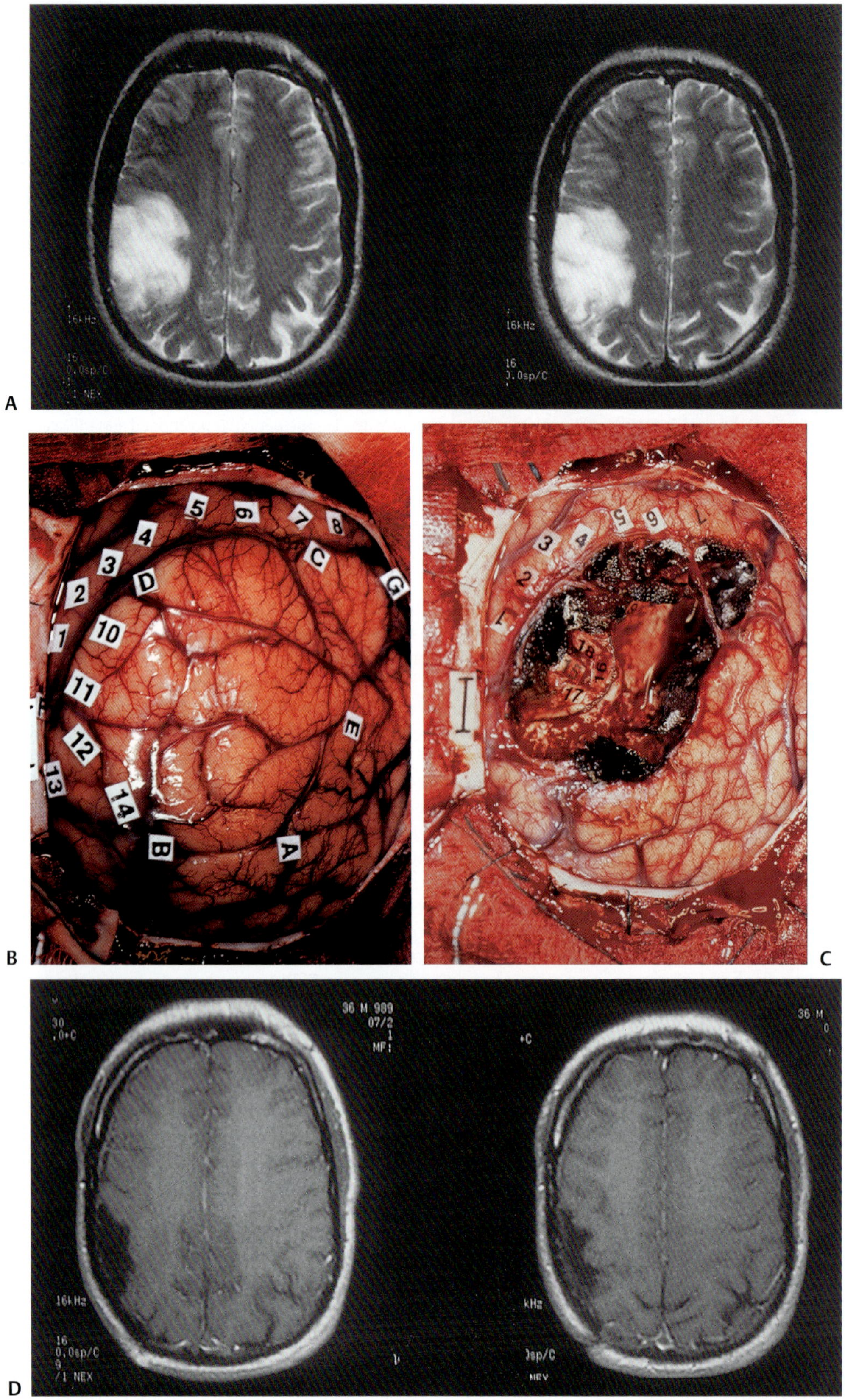

Figure 38–2 **(A)** Preoperative axial magnetic resonance (MR) scan showing a right frontal mass. **(B)** Preresection cortical mapping data, where numbers 1 to 8 depict the motor strip, 10 to 14 the cortical sensory sites. **(C)** Postresection image, with the numbers within the cavity corresponding to subcortical sensory areas. **(D)** Early postoperative axial T1-weighted MR scan.

Identification of Language Sites

Following the scalp opening and bone removal under propofol anesthesia, the patient is kept awake during language mapping. The electrocorticography equipment is placed on the field and attached to the skull after the motor pathways have been identified. With the electrocorticogram in progress, the recording electrode–cortex contact point is stimulated with the bipolar electrode, which may result in afterdischarge potential seen on the monitor (**Fig. 38–3**). The presence of such afterdischarge potentials indicates that the stimulation current is too high and must be decreased by 1 to 2 mA until no after discharge potential is present following stimulation. Using this ideal stimulation current, object-naming slides are presented and changed every 4 seconds, and the patient is expected to correctly name the object during stimulation mapping. The answers are carefully recorded. Each cortical site is checked three times to ensure that there is no stimulation-induced error in the form of anomia and dysnomia. All cortical sites essential for naming are marked on the surface of the brain with sterile numbered tickets. At this point, the patient is asked to count from 1 to 50 while the bipolar stimulation probe is placed near the inferior aspect of the motor strip to identify Broca's area. Interruption of counting (i.e., complete speech arrest without oropharyngeal movement) localizes Broca's area. Speech arrest (e.g., complete interruption of counting) is

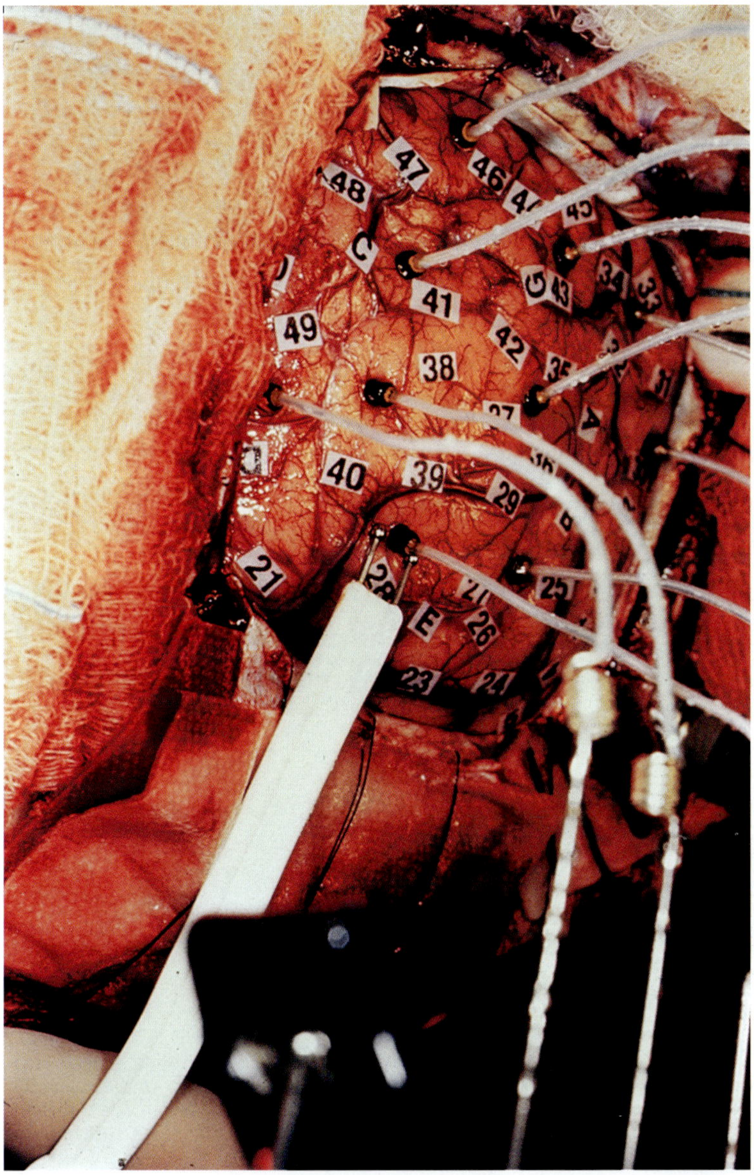

Figure 38–3 Electrocorticography equipment is placed, and the contact point of a recording electrode with the cortex is stimulated with the bipolar electrode.

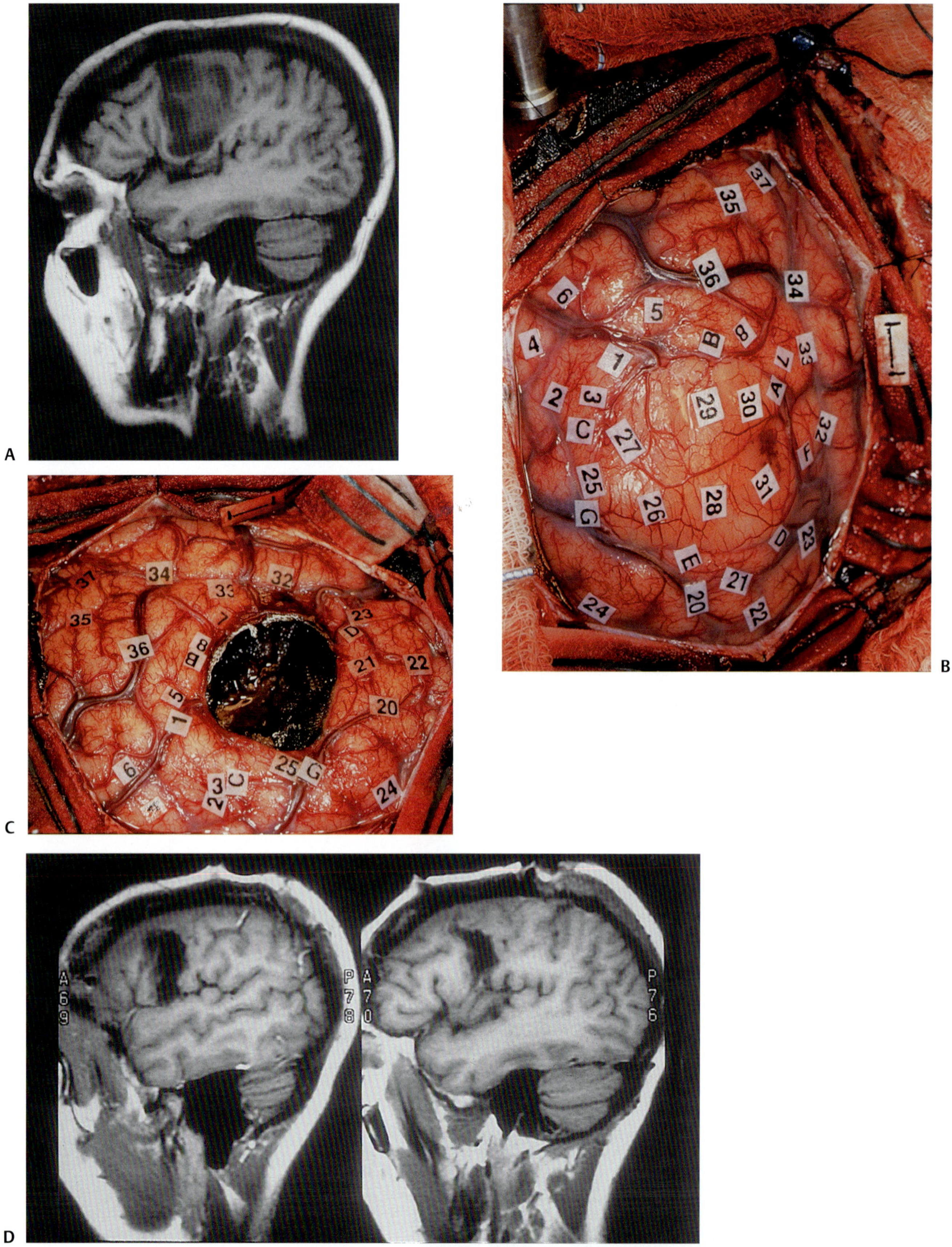

Figure 38–4 **(A)** Preoperative far sagittal T1-weighted magnetic resonance (MR) scan showing the tumor involving the inferior aspect of the face motor cortex. **(B)** Preresection cortical mapping data, where numbers 1 to 3 depict the face motor area, number 4 is finger motor, and numbers 5 and 6 correspond to the sensory areas of the face and finger, respectively. Broca's area could not be identified, and stimulation of no cortical site caused anomia. **(C)** Postresection view. Postoperatively, the patient could not open her mouth, which was transient. **(D)** Early postoperative sagittal T1-weighted MR scan showing the resection cavity.

usually localized to the area directly anterior to the facial motor cortex (**Fig. 38–4A–D**).

The electrocorticogram is continuously monitored throughout language mapping to signal multiple afterdischarge spikes, both to reduce the chances of evoking a seizure by continued stimulation at that current and to reduce the chance that naming errors are caused by the propagated effects of the current.

It is essential to document where language is as well as where it is not located (**Fig. 38–5A–D**). A negative stimulation mapping may not provide the necessary security to proceed confidently with the resection. This is also the

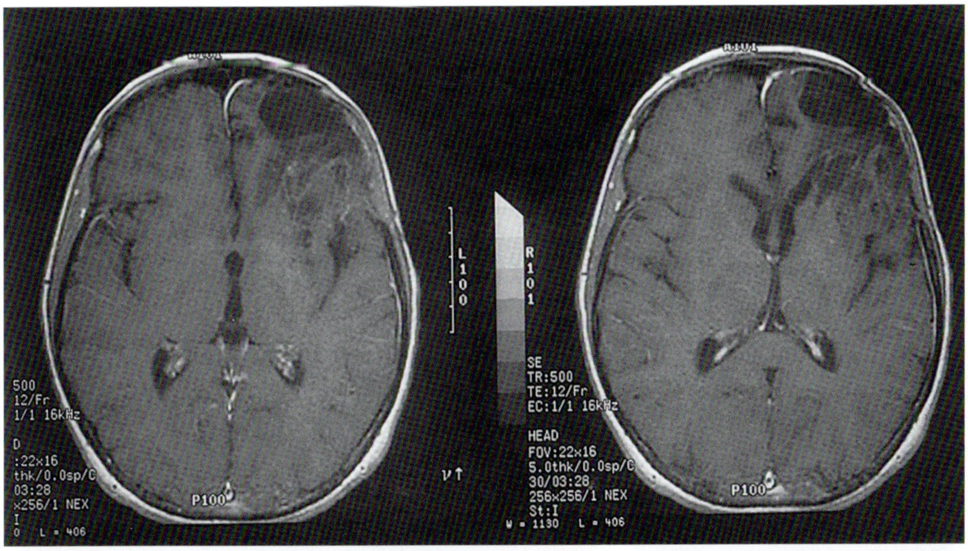

A

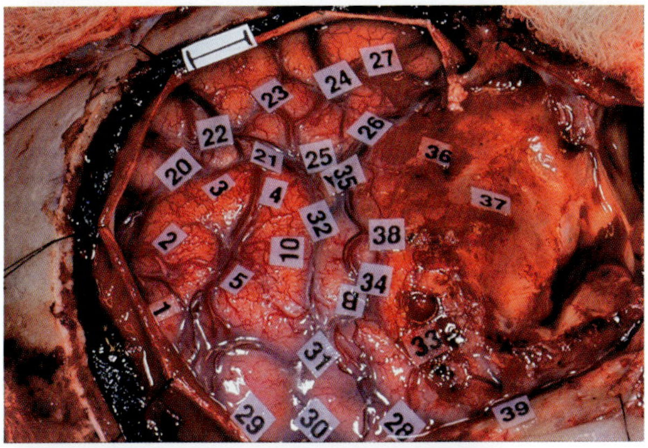

B

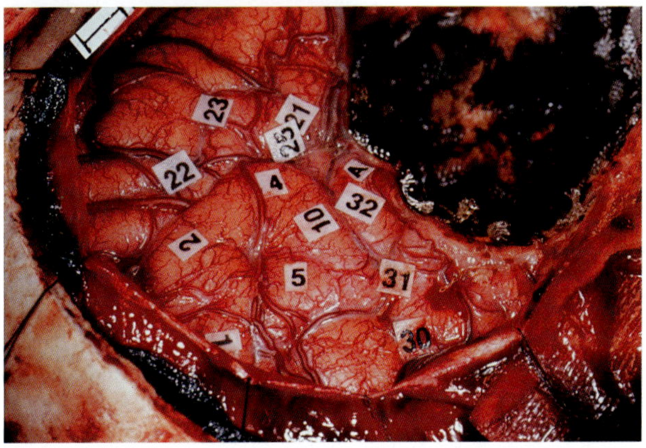

C

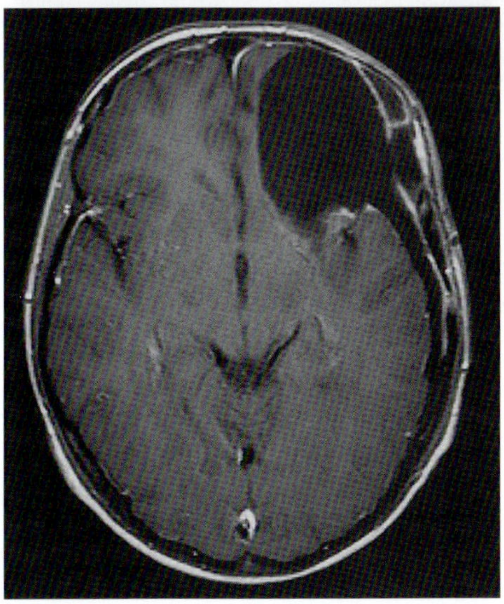

D

Figure 38–5 **(A)** Preoperative axial T1-weighted magnetic resonance (MR) scan showing the left frontal recurrent tumor. **(B)** Preresection cortical mapping data, where numbers 4 and 5 depict the motor strip, 1 and 2 cortical sensory sites. Number 10 is Broca's area, and stimulation of 22 caused anomia. **(C)** Postresection view. **(D)** Early postoperative axial T1-weighted MR scan showing the resection cavity.

reason for having a generous exposure, not only to maximize the extent of resection but to minimize the possibility of obtaining negative data.

The distance of the resection margin from the nearest language site is the most important factor in determining the improvement in preoperative language deficits, the duration of postoperative language deficits, and whether the postoperative language deficits are permanent.[16] Significantly fewer permanent language deficits occur if the distance of the resection margin from the nearest language site is > 1 cm.

◆ Postoperative Care

In the postoperative period, patients are managed in the intensive care unit for up to 48 hours. Because of the relatively long duration of mapping procedures, antibiotics are administered for 48 hours postoperatively. Antiepileptic levels are maintained above the upper limit for 3 to 5 days postoperatively, and then gradually lowered to the therapeutic range. A postoperative scan is obtained within 48 to 72 hours of surgery to avoid postoperative enhancement representing surgical trauma. Dexamethasone is maintained at the dose of 16 mg/d and tapered slowly depending on the remaining mass effect on the postoperative scan. Patients with a transient and resolving paresis or speech deficit may benefit from a short course of inpatient rehabilitation and speech therapy, although not necessary in all.

◆ Conclusion

In the management of cerebral gliomas, an extensive resection has possible advantages, including reduction in the signs and symptoms related to wall effect, lowered risk of tissue sampling error due to small biopsy size, control of seizures, and decreased possibility of malignant differentiation for low-grade gliomas. However, the effect of the extent of resection on outcome remains controversial.

The resection of tumors located in or near functional brain areas may not be safe even if the surgeon remains within the boundaries of the macroscopically obvious tumor. In addition to its use to determine functional cortical sites, stimulation mapping is the only available method that provides reliable identification of descending subcortical motor, sensory, and language tracts.[22,23] Patients with normal preoperative language function bearing dominant hemisphere temporal lobe tumors who undergo cortical stimulation mapping for the identification of language sites will not have a permanent postoperative language deficit if the tumor resection margin is 1 cm or more distant to the essential language site.

In summary, identification of functional tissue by intraoperative stimulation mapping of cortical and subcortical areas in and around a tumor will enable its preservation and thus will minimize the risk of permanent postoperative deficit.

References

1. Berger MS, Deliganis AV, Dobbins J, Kelles GE. The effect of extent of resection on recurrence in patients with low-grade cerebral hemisphere gliomas. Cancer 1994;74:1784–1791
2. Chandler KL, Prados MD, Malec M, et al. Long-term survival in patients with glioblastomas multiforme. Neurosurgery 1993;32:716–720
3. Ammirati M, Vick N, Liao Y, et al. Effect of extent of surgical resection on survival and quality of life in patients with supratentorial glioblastomas and anaplastic astrocytomas. Neurosurgery 1987;21:201–206
4. Ciric I, Ammirati M, Vick N, et al. Supratentorial gliomas: surgical considerations and immediate postoperative results: gross total resection versus partial resection. Neurosurgery 1987;21:21–26
5. Cushing H. A note upon the faradic stimulation of the postcentral gyrus in conscious patients. Brain 1909;32:44–53
6. Forester O. The motor cortex in man in the light of Hughlings Jakson's doctrines. Brain 1936;59:135–159
7. Penfield W, Boldrey E. Somatic motor and sensory representation in the cerebral cortex of man as studied by electrical stimulation. Brain 1937;60:386–443
8. Berger MS, Ojemann GA, Lettich E. Neurophysiological monitoring to facilitate resection during astrocytoma surgery. Neurosurg Clin N Am 1990;1:65–80
9. Skirboll SS, Ojemann GA, Berger MS, et al. Functional cortex and subcortical white matter located within gliomas. Neurosurgery 1996;38: 678–685
10. Ojemann G, Ojemann J, Lettich E, et al. Cortical language localization in left, dominant hemisphere: an electrical stimulation mapping investigation in 117 patients. J Neurosurg 1989;71:316–326
11. Ojemann GA, Creutzfeldt OD. Language in humans and animals: contribution of brain stimulation and recordings. In: Plum F, Geiger S, eds. Handbook of Physiology, Nervous System V. Part 2. Bethesda, MD: American Physiological Society Press; 1987:675–700
12. Heilman K, Wilder B, Malzone W. Anatomic aphasia following anterior temporal lobectomy. Trans Am Neurol Assoc 1972;97:291–293
13. Hermann BP, Wyler AR, Somes G. Language function following anterior temporal lobectomy. J Neurosurg 1991;74:560–566
14. Penfield W, Jasper H. Epilepsy and Functional Anatomy of the Human Brain. Boston: Little, Brown; 1954
15. Penfield W, Rasmussen T. The Cerebral Cortex of Man: A Clinical Study of Localization of Function. New York: Macmillan; 1950
16. Haglund MM, Berger MS, Shamseldin M, et al. Cortical localization of temporal lobe language sites in patients with gliomas. Neurosurgery 1994;34:567–576
17. Woods R, Dodrill C, Ojemann GA. Brain injury, handedness and speech lateralization in a series of amobarbital studies. Ann Neurol 1988;23:510–518
18. Wada J, Rasmussen T. Intracaroid injections of sodium amytal for the lateralization of cerebral speech dominance. J Neurosurg 1960;17: 266–282
19. Berger MS, Cohen WA, Ojemann GA. Correlation of the motor cortex using intraoperative brain mapping data with preoperative magnetic resonance imaging anatomy. J Neurosurg 1990;72:383–387
20. Sartorius CJ, Berger MS. Rapid termination of intraoperative stimulation-evoked seizures with application of cold Ringer's lactate to the cortex. J Neurosurg 1998;88:349–351
21. Haglund MM, Ojemann GA, Blasdel GG. Optical imaging of bipolar cortical stimulation. J Neurosurg 1993;78:785–793
22. Berger MS, Kincaid J, Ojemann GA, et al. Brain mapping techniques to maximize resection, safety and seizure control in children with brain tumors. Neurosurgery 1989;25:786–792
23. Berger MS. Functional mapping guided resection of low grade gliomas. In: Loftus C, ed. Clinical Neurosurgery. Vol 42. Baltimore: Williams & Wilkins; 1995:437–452

39

Convexity Meningiomas

Satish Krishnamurthy and Brian Holmes

Historical Background

Felix Platter is credited with the first description of the tumor we now call a meningioma, and his account appeared in 1614.[1] In the eighteenth and nineteenth centuries, meningiomas were diagnosed during life only if they caused changes in the overlying skull that could be appreciated by inspection or palpation. Few attempts were made to remove these lesions, and only a few of these attempts were beneficial to the patient. Between 1743 and 1896, 13 such operations were performed, and nine patients died.[2] John Cleland, professor of anatomy in Glasgow, suggested that meningiomas arise from arachnoid rather than from dura.[3] In 1915 Cushing and Weed reconfirmed this opinion that meningiomas were derived from arachnoid cell clusters.[4] The sequential nomenclature of meningiomas has included names such as *fungoid tumors, sarcomas, cylindromas, endotheliomas,* and *fibromas.* Harvey Cushing proposed the term *meningothelioma* in an effort to describe these tumors according to a tissue name. Later, he opted for the term *meningioma* in an attempt to rise above the controversy raging at the time concerning the histogenesis of this tumor by simply using the near-constant relationship of this tumor to the meninges to refer to these tumors. In 1938 Cushing and Eisenhardt published a 32-chapter monograph on meningiomas that did much to solidify the understanding of the clinical presentation and surgical treatment of meningiomas for neurosurgeons and remains a classic on the subject today.[5]

Francis C. Grant summarized the state of the art on surgical treatment of meningiomas prior to the advent of microneurosurgery in his article in 1954[6]:

> Removal of the convexity tumor requires a flap to expose the longitudinal sinus, for most of them lie close to it. Once adequate exposure of the tumor is obtained, the dura mater should be cut about the lateral edge of the lesion. . . . [A]fter a line of cleavage is found between dura mater and brain, careful and cautious finger dissection should be used to separate the lesion from the surrounding brain. The tip of the dissecting finger can feel the one or two large vessels running into the mass from below and these can be readily clipped or coagulated.

Advent of the surgical microscope, evolution of techniques in microneurosurgery, availability of a wide variety of microinstruments, ultrasonic surgical aspirator, laser, and improvements in neuroanesthesia and critical care have all been responsible for improved outcomes in the treatment of meningiomas. However, Cushing's statement in 1922,[7] "There is today nothing in the whole realm of surgery more gratifying than the successful removal of a meningioma with subsequent perfect functional recovery," still holds true after more than 80 years.

◆ Surgery, Recurrence, and Incidental Tumors

Meningiomas account for ~30% of incidental tumors found at autopsy. Generally, their incidence increases with age, ranging from a low of 0.3 per 100,000 in childhood to a high of 8.4 per 100,000 in the elderly population.[8] In adults 90% of all intracranial meningiomas occur in the supratentorial compartment. Because meningiomas are presumed to arise from arachnoid or arachnoid cap cells or both, it is not surprising that the majority of supratentorial meningiomas are clustered around the venous sinuses and dural folds where arachnoid granulations are found. Convexity meningiomas are the second most common location for supratentorial meningiomas.

In 1957, Simpson established a classification of surgical resection of meningiomas and its relationship with tumor recurrence.[9] Grade I was described as a microscopically complete removal of tumor, including the dural attachment and any abnormal bone and involved sinus. Grade II was complete removal of tumor with coagulation to the point of charring of its dural attachment. Grade III was macroscopically complete removal but without resection or coagulation of the dural attachment and no removal of involved sinus or hyperostotic bone. Grade IV was a subtotal resection leaving gross macroscopic tumor. Grade V was a simple decompression with or without a biopsy. The recurrence rates for patients with surgical grades I, II, III, IV, and V were 9, 16, 29, 39, and 100%, respectively. Jaaskelainen reviewed 657 patients who had grade I or II resections and found a 9% recurrence after a median of 7.5 years.[10] Multivariate analyses showed that the factors strongly associated with risk of recurrence were coagulation rather than excision of the dura, invasion of bone, and soft tumor consistency at the time of surgery. Most investigators agree that atypical, malignant, and papillary meningiomas, as well as hemangiopericytomas, have a higher rate of recurrence than classic meningiomas and their subtypes.

Borovich and Doron evaluated 14 patients with convexity meningiomas in whom a 3 cm linear strip of dura was removed and pathologically examined.[11] In 64% of the specimens, macroscopic nodules protruded from the inner surface of the dura at 1 to 3 cm from the margin of the original tumor. Fifty-seven percent had microscopic aggregates of cells at a similar distance from the main mass. An additional grade 0 was subsequently proposed as a surgical resection of all gross tumor, including a 4 cm margin of dura around the attachment of tumor. A first recurrence predicted a shorter interval to the second recurrence in a study of 225 patients by Mirimanoff et al.[12] The probability of having a second operation 5, 10, or 15 years after a total excision was 6, 15, and 20%, respectively. In patients who had a second resection, the probability of a third operation was 42% at 5 years and 56% at 10 years, indicating that the chance for surgical cure declines with each successive recurrence, and that the time to a second or a third recurrence tended to be shorter than the time to a first recurrence.

Obviously, the initial operation offers the best chance for a surgical cure. The surgeon should perform as complete a resection as possible, removing a cuff of normal tissue adjacent to the tumor attachment if possible. Hyperostotic bone, which contains meningothelial cells, should be removed.

◆ Alternative and Adjunctive Therapies

External Beam Radiation Therapy

Clinically there seems little question of benefit of irradiating malignant meningiomas, although irradiation of subtotally resected or recurrent meningioma is still controversial because of the risks of acute, early-delayed, and late-delayed radiation toxicity. Irradiation itself has been identified as being responsible for the development of new meningiomas.[8]

Several retrospective studies since 1980 support the use of external beam irradiation therapy for subtotally resected meningiomas. External beam radiation therapy apparently improves tumor control and survival over simple observation alone in subtotally resected nonrecurrent, recurrent, and malignant meningiomas. When meningiomas recur, continued observation and surgery or external beam radiation therapy or both may be considered. Generally speaking, recurrent disease is best managed with the use of both radiation therapy and reoperation.[8]

Radiosurgery

Radiosurgery is a relatively new neurosurgical treatment modality that has been used for meningiomas. Further follow-up is required to compare the results of radiosurgery with those of external beam irradiation or surgery. Early reports do suggest that radiosurgery is effective and that the sharp fall-off in dose that occurs outside the tumor edge should protect the surrounding brain and dura from the risks of late-delayed radiation complications. Whether the treatment is delivered with linear accelerator, gamma knife, or proton beam should not have much influence on the end result.[8] It is to be mentioned that serious complications have been reported with the use of this modality, and more follow-up is needed to assess the durability and maintenance of the responses seen.

Hormonal Therapy

The clinical association of pregnancy with meningioma growth and presence of hormonal receptors in meningiomas has prompted research into hormonal manipulation for treatment. Tamoxifen (an estrogen antagonist), Bromocriptine (a dopamine antagonist), Mifepristone (RU486, a progesterone and cortisol blocking agent), and Trapidil (a platelet-derived growth factor antagonist) have all been found to be effective in vitro and have been tried clinically.[13] Although progress in treating meningiomas has been steady, much detailed and arduous work needs to be done before advocating hormonal antagonist therapy in the management of meningiomas.

◆ Indications

Not all patients with intracranial meningiomas require surgery. The decision to operate involves consideration of many factors related to the patient, the tumor, and the surgical risk:benefit ratio. If diagnostic studies are consistent with a radiological diagnosis of meningioma, the tumor location should correspond with the patient's symptoms and signs. If the clinical history and examination are at odds with imaging studies, then the whole issue of surgical intervention needs to be reexamined. If the patient has no symptoms and the meningioma is discovered incidentally on imaging studies performed for other reasons, then the question must be asked as to whether there is documented growth.

The neurosurgeon should consider the patient's age, expected survival based on life-table analyses, Karnofsky performance status, and neurological condition when deciding to operate. Younger patients (< 60 years) with evidence of a growing tumor that is in a critical location (dominant hemisphere near sylvian fissure or sensorimotor cortex) are more likely to benefit from surgery. Patients in their 70s with an incidental small tumor without accompanying edema or "dural tail" sign are best left alone. Associated medical conditions, such as uncontrolled hypertension and diabetes, increase surgical risk. The patient should understand the aims of the recommended surgery well ahead of time. Patients should also understand how surgery influences their symptoms and future prognosis. If the surgeon decides that immediate surgery is not necessary, the patient should agree with that approach and be available for regular clinical and radiological follow-up.[8]

◆ Imaging

Plain Radiographs

Plain radiographs are no longer used to confirm a clinical diagnosis of meningioma. Radiographs are useful to a surgeon if a patient has already had a craniotomy or if a metallic cranioplasty such as tantalum is in place. In these situations plain radiographs clearly show the extent of previous operations, which can assist the surgeon in planning an extension of an existing bone flap.

Computerized Axial Tomography

Computerized axial tomography can be used to determine the extent of bone involvement, particularly that adjacent to skull base or associated with hyperostosis. It may also help establish the relationship of the tumor to important bony landmarks. Calcification of the tumor is seen more clearly on computed tomography (CT) than on magnetic resonance imaging. Examination of the surrounding bone on bone window settings may reveal new formation of hyperostotic bone that is less homogeneous than cortical bone and usually has irregular margins. The underlying cortical bone may be thickened. Bony erosion may also be seen.

Magnetic Resonance Imaging

Magnetic resonance imaging is the current standard for two-dimensional imaging of the intracranial compartment when a meningioma is suspected. Direct imaging in the coronal, sagittal, and axial planes with and without gadolinium enhancement is preferred. Meningiomas are typically dural-based lesions, with the greatest diameter of the tumor occurring at its dural margin (**Fig. 39–1A,B**). Approximately 60% of the tumors are isointense, and 30% are

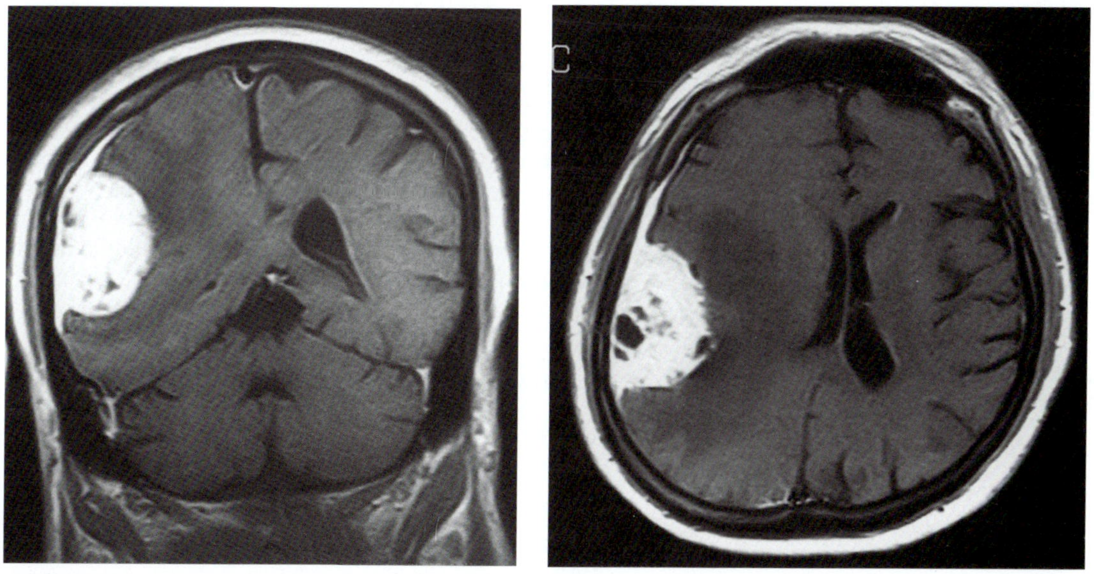

A B

Figure 39–1 Common magnetic resonance imaging characteristics of a convexity meningioma. The coronal view **(A)** demonstrates a wide base, robust enhancement and a "dural tail." On the axial view **(B)**, the dural tail is also evident, along with significant surrounding white matter characteristic of meningioma. The extent of surrounding white matter edema is variable.

hypointense on T1-weighted images. On T2-weighted images, the tumors may be hypointense to hyperintense. An interface is frequently seen between the tumor and the surrounding brain on T1- and T2-weighted images. The tumor typically enhances uniformly with gadolinium administration. The so-called dural tail sign is thought to be relatively specific for meningiomas as opposed to other extra-axial neoplasms. This tail extends a few millimeters from the edge of the base of the tumor, but when it is several millimeters long or is associated with nodularity, it may represent extension of meningioma through the dura. T2-weighted images are much better than CT scans in showing surrounding peritumoral edema.

Cerebral Angiography

Cerebral angiography, although not necessary in every meningioma case, can provide additional information to assist the surgeon in planning surgery and tumor removal, as well as in reducing the vascularity of these tumors with embolization. Angiographic information about the tumor blood supply, displacement of major arteries and their position relative to the tumor, and position and displacement of major draining cortical veins may be useful in operating a large convexity meningioma. Angiography also permits embolization, which may reduce the tumor's blood supply, making resection easier. The surgeon should be aware of the fact that preoperative embolization of external carotid vessels may be associated with ischemic necrosis of the scalp flap if scalp incisions have not been properly planned based on knowledge of the blood supply of the scalp.

Typically, a convexity meningioma derives blood supply from meningeal blood vessels (either or both superficial temporal and middle meningeal arteries) with variable contribution from the adjacent pial vessels. Control of vascular supply to the tumor can be easily done by making a durotomy around the edge of the tumor. Hence preoperative embolization is rarely required for a convexity meningioma.

Octreotide Scan

A high density of high affinity somatostatin receptors is found on meningioma cells both in vitro and in vivo. Octreotide is a somatostatin analogue that has been developed as a stable substitute for somatostatin in the clinical setting. Octreotide has been used in the preoperative radiological evaluation of meningiomas. Radioactive ^{111}indium labeled octreotide (Octreoscan) is being used to confirm a diagnosis of meningiomas preoperatively. Several studies have shown that Octreoscan is 100% sensitive in detecting meningiomas using this method. This can also be used to evaluate completeness of resection and recurrence.[14]

◆ Preparation

Associated medical conditions such as hypertension and diabetes need to be addressed prior to planned surgery. Steroids aggravate diabetes, and this may require insulin infusion. Optimal cardiac functioning should be ascertained, especially in the elderly and in patients with known cardiac history.

The patient is given steroids for at least 48 hours before surgery and longer if there is considerable edema in the adjacent brain tissue. This is important in helping to prevent the problems with cerebral edema that may follow removal of meningioma. Although the use of prophylactic anticonvulsants is controversial, patients with meningiomas are clearly at high risk for perioperative and postoperative seizures. Most physicians would agree that the standard of practice is to administer anticonvulsants until therapeutic serum concentrations are reached before surgery.

The surgeon should review the relevant intracranial anatomy and relationship of arteries and veins to the tumor. Imaging studies should be collected, and the appropriate operating room equipment should be obtained and coordinated. The neurosurgeon should have available an anesthesiologist who is knowledgeable in the field of neurosurgery. The operating room should be dedicated to neurosurgery and include the availability of trained personnel, operating microscope, bipolar coagulator, laser, and ultrasonic surgical aspirator. Contingencies for unexpected intraoperative events, such as intraoperative brain swelling, holes in the venous sinuses, and brisk arterial bleeding, should be planned for. The recovery room and intensive care unit should be staffed with personnel familiar with neurosurgical problems.

◆ Surgical Technique

Anesthesia

When the patient arrives in the operating room, a radial artery catheter is inserted for continuous monitoring of blood pressure and evaluation of blood gases. The $PaCO_2$ is maintained near 30 mm Hg during the operation. Thigh-high alternating pressure boots are placed for thromboembolism prophylaxis. An indwelling Foley catheter is inserted. A central venous line or a pulmonary artery catheter is inserted depending on the cardiovascular status of the patient. If the semisitting position is used, then a central venous line is necessary, as is Doppler monitoring for air embolism.

A smooth induction of anesthesia without the patient straining or coughing and careful control of blood pressure are important factors in getting surgery off to a good start. Prior to making the skin incision, an antibiotic, usually a cephalosporin, is administered and usually continued for 24 hours.

Positioning

In general, the patient is positioned so that the tumor is uppermost in the operative field. The tumor's location therefore determines the operative position of the patient. After careful positioning, the patient's head is held with a three-point skeletal fixation headrest (e.g. Mayfield's clamp) (**Fig. 39–2**). The clamp should be positioned clear of the incision. Care is taken to keep the head above the heart level and to avoid compression of the jugular veins in the neck.

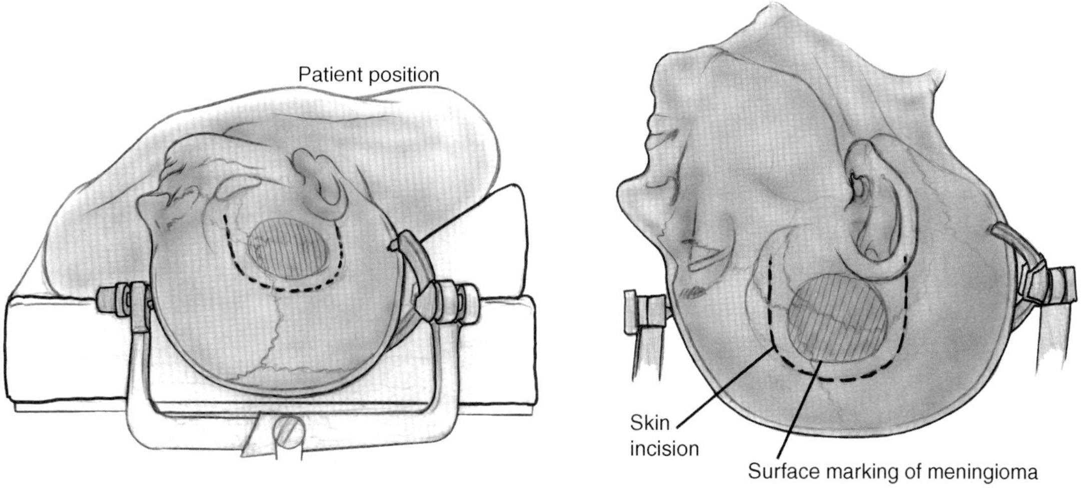

Figure 39–2 Positioning and planning of the surgical incision are of primary importance. The incision may be planned based upon standard surface landmarks such as the pterion. For smaller lesions, preoperative computed tomography or magnetic resonance imaging with placement of a surface marker may help plan an economical incision. Frameless stereotactic technology allows for precise exposure.

The position must take into account the effects of gravity, the need to minimize brain retraction, and the avoidance of compression of the brain against the edge of the dura. Care should be taken to pad all the pressure points in the extremities. The abdomen should be left free when the patient is in the prone position. Some type of magnification (either loupes or operating microscope) is used for the entire operation.

Incision

The skin incision is marked prior to draping and must allow for full exposure of the tumor (**Figs. 39–2** and **39–3**). Blood supply to the scalp flap must be adequate, and a wide enough base must be left to provide good vascularization. The cosmetic result of the scar and bone flap must be considered. The pericranial tissue is left attached to the back of the scalp flap so it can be taken at the end of the operation to repair any dural defects. It is always preferable to slightly oversize the skin and bone flaps in operating meningiomas.[15]

Dissection

A free bone flap will allow for a wide, unimpeded exposure of the tumor and may be enlarged if necessary (**Fig. 39–4**). The bone flap is elevated using a power drill and craniotomes, and adequacy of the bone flap is ensured, if necessary by using ultrasound. As a rule, the dura mater at the attachment of the meningioma appears very bloody as soon as the bone is removed. This is perhaps the trickiest moment in the surgery of a convexity meningioma because the inexperienced surgeon might lift all or part of the meningioma together with the bone, and thus tear the dura and vascular connections between the tumor capsule and the cerebral cortex. In addition to copious bleeding in such an event, there is bound to be cortical damage resulting in intraoperative or postoperative edema and neurological deficits that could have been avoided. It is, therefore, prudent to elevate the flap gently by levering it and detaching the dura bit by bit from the inner table with a periosteal elevator. Bleeding from the dural surface can be controlled by bipolar coagulation of the meningeal vessels and by rapidly opening the dura around the dural attachment. Bleeding from the arachnoid granulations can be controlled by placing pieces of oxidized cellulose or Surgicel over them and exerting slight pressure with cottonoid strips rather than by coagulation, which often widens the bleeding sources and causes dural shrinkage. Twist drill holes are made around the edge of the flap, and duropericranial sutures ("hitch" stitches) are placed and tied to these twist drill holes.

The operating microscope is brought in at this point. The dura is opened circumferentially around the tumor with a 2 to 3 cm margin starting away from the most sensitive cortex, that is, the motor or speech cortex[16] (**Fig. 39–5**). Care should be taken to expose as little cortex as possible so the brain does not bulge around the tumor. While opening the dura near the sagittal sinus or in the region of the vein of Labbé, care should be taken to preserve the draining veins, especially in their transdural course. Unplanned sacrifice of draining veins may result in postoperative cortical venous thrombosis. The dural margins around the tumor are then coagulated with bipolar coagulation, causing shrinkage and enhancing the dissection of the tumor from the underlying brain.

The first step in excision of the tumor is identification of the arachnoidal plane between the meningioma and the adjacent cortex (**Fig. 39–6**). The arachnoid is then incised using an arachnoid knife or a Rhoton disc. The main principle in tumor removal is to debulk and shrink the tumor by enucleating the center, going from the center to the periphery (**Fig. 39–7**). This increases the working space for further manipulation, dissection, and tumor removal, and simultaneously aids in decompressing the brain. This can be done using dissectors, curettes, ultrasonic surgical aspirator, laser, or monopolar or bipolar cautery loops, in a cutting mode.

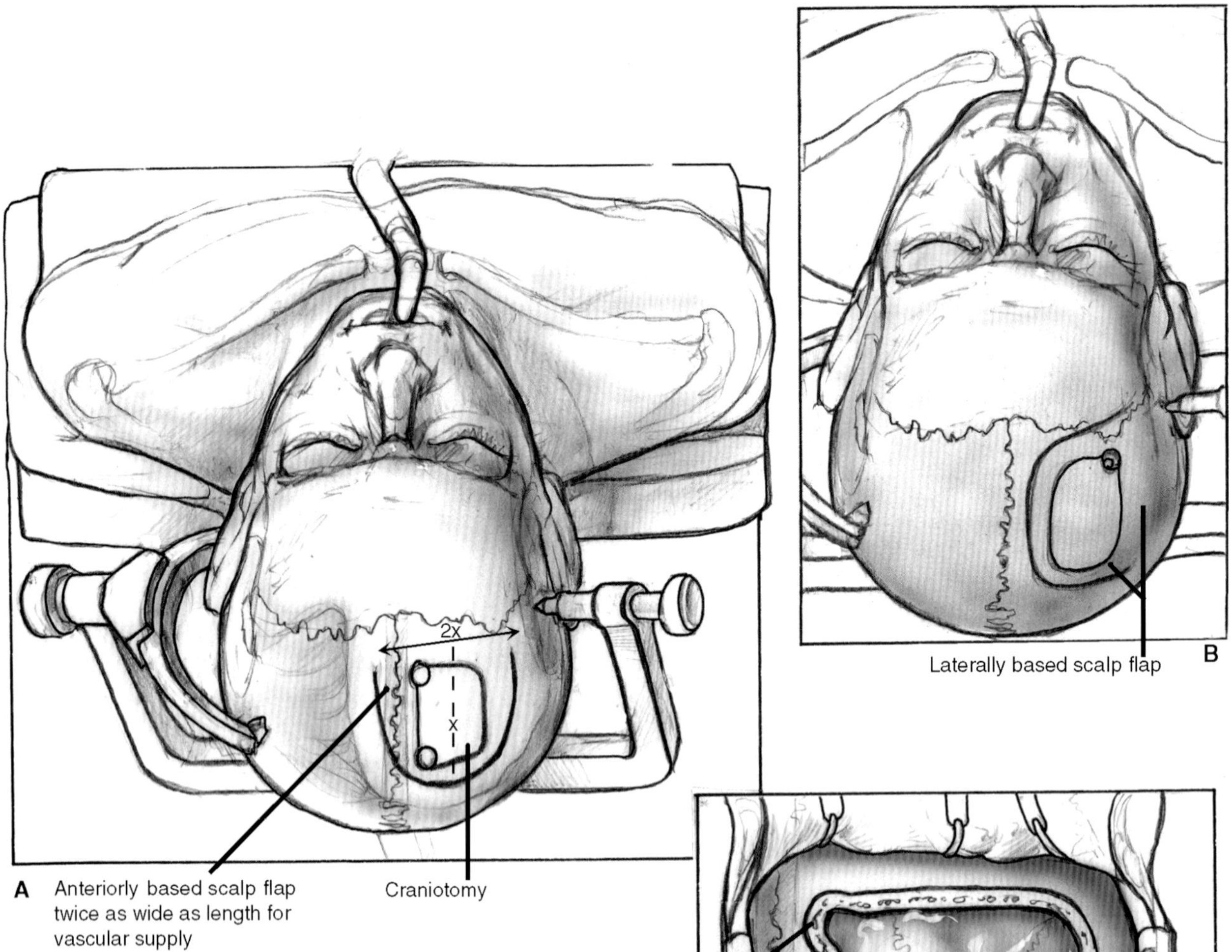

Figure 39–3A,B Initial exposure of the tumor. Use of the free bone flap has supplanted the use of the osteoplastic flap. Bone removal must be adequate to allow for resection of a cuff of surrounding dura.

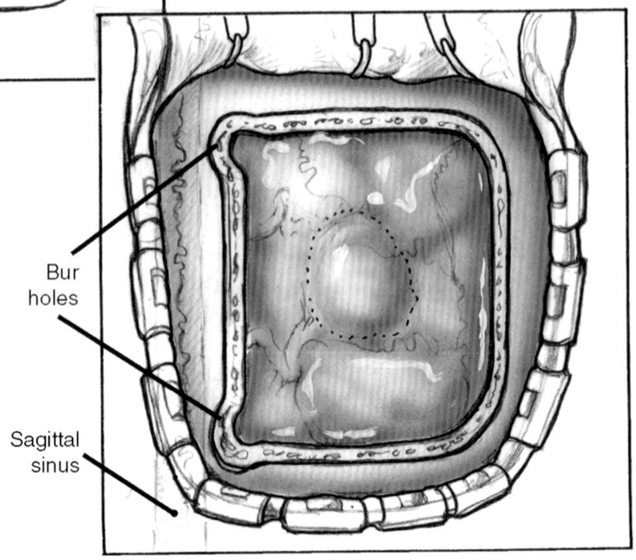

Figure 39–4 A free bone flap allows for wide exposure for tumor dissection, resection of surrounding dura, and dural reconstruction.

Sometimes it is necessary to excise portions of tumor with a knife or scissor. It is imperative that the surgeon remain within the tumor itself, and the capsule of the tumor should not be breached.[14]

Once adequate decompression is achieved, then resection of the capsule is begun (**Fig. 39–8**). The capsule (pseudocapsule) is gently levered circumferentially, and patties (cottonoid strips) or Telfa Strips can be placed in the cleavage between the brain and tumor. The pial supply to the tumor needs to be coagulated during this process and then divided. If a freed portion of the tumor hinders progress, then that part is excised. No new openings are made in the capsule because it is important to maintain the integrity and shape of the capsule to sustain the exact plane of cleavage and prevent hemorrhage. Placing two or three cotton balls into its interior gives the capsule substance and may make it more manageable. The tumor capsule may also be coagulated with bipolar forceps on the internal or external wall, thus

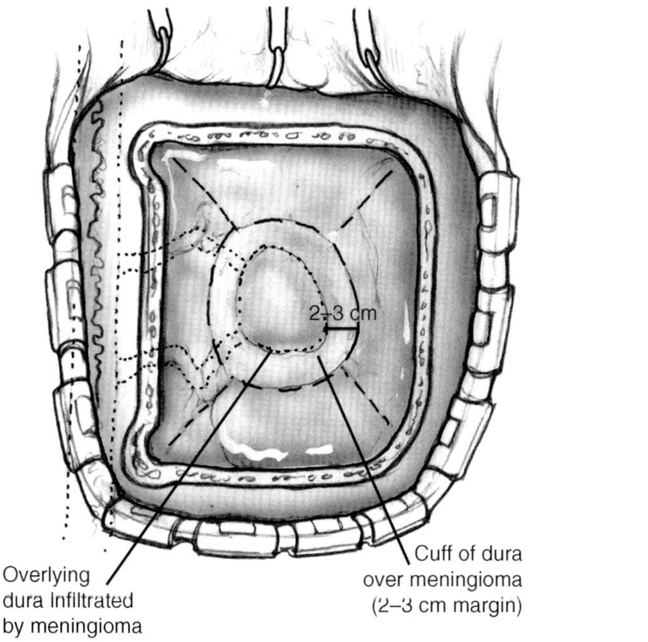

Figure 39–5 Exposing the tumor and surrounding cortex. The cuff of attached dura serves as a "handle" during tumor dissection.

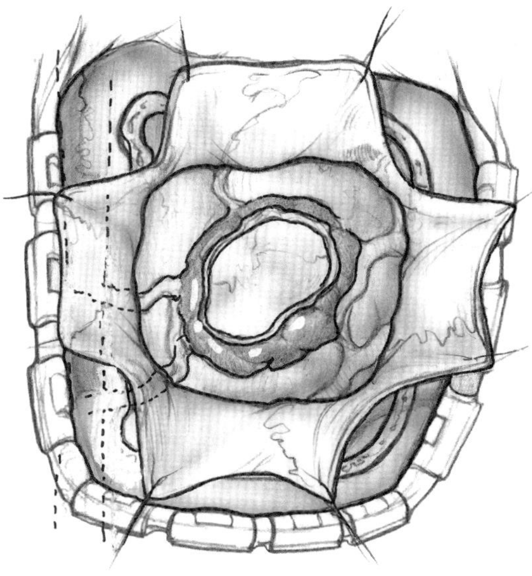

Figure 39–6 The arachnoid plane surrounding the tumor is identified. The plane is developed with careful retraction of the tumor capsule. Judicious directing of irrigating solution from a bulb syringe may help to establish the plane.

shrinking and toughening the capsule or pseudocapsule. Isolation of the capsule from the sylvian vessels can be done by starting at a point where the vessels are not involved by the tumor and then following them to the involved area.

Large tumors usually have destroyed the arachnoidal planes at the depths, leaving denuded cortex in this area. Great care is taken to separate the tumor from important sylvian vessels to avoid unnecessary cortical damage. If there is adherence to the brain, consideration should be given to leaving the capsule attached to the brain. However, every attempt should be made to resect the tumor completely.

Tumor tissue sent for frozen section will help in confirmation of the histological diagnosis. The rest of the tumor tissue can be sent for permanent sections, immunochemical stains, electron microscopy, DNA ploidy, and cell proliferation indices where facilities are available.

Once the tumor is taken out, meticulous hemostasis is achieved by means of bipolar coagulation, and if there are no major bleeders, then irrigation with hydrogen peroxide is useful in controlling bleeding. The cortical surface is then covered with strips of Surgicel after confirming all the bleeding points are coagulated. The surgeon should ensure

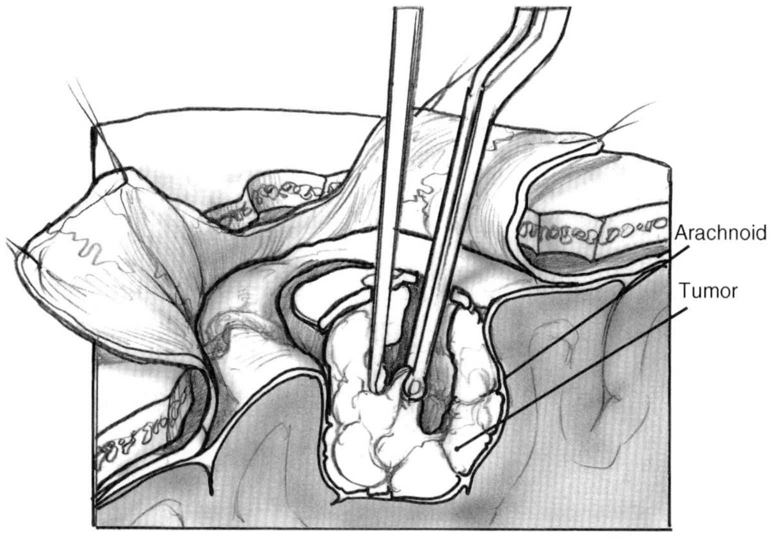

Figure 39–7 The first step in excision of the tumor: debulking and shrinking the tumor by enucleating the center.

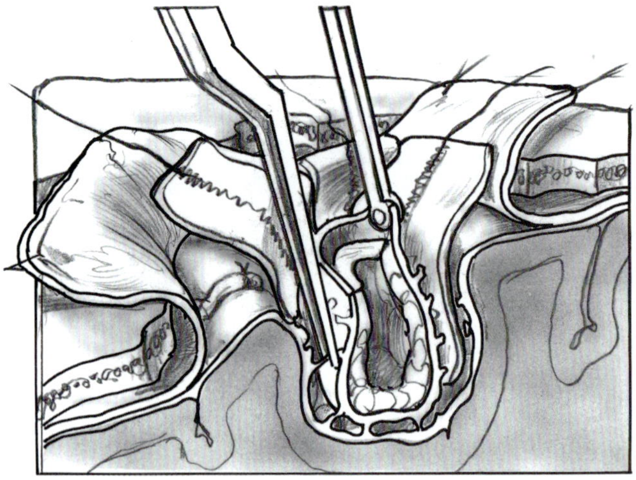

Figure 39–8 The second step in excision of the tumor: removal of the tumor capsule once adequate decompression is achieved.

that the patient has normal blood pressure, and some surgeons use a Valsalva maneuver to check the efficacy of hemostasis.

Once the tumor is removed, the underside of the adjacent dura is examined for evidence of dural invasion and is excised as widely as necessary. Sometimes islets of tumor tissue can be found separate from the main tumor mass. This resected dura should be submitted for histopathological examination.

Closure

The dural defect must always be repaired to prevent cortical adhesions as well as cerebrospinal fluid (CSF) fistulas and infections. Autologous grafts with pericranium or fascia lata are easily available and usually used. Foreign materials, such as lyophilized dura mater, are also used with satisfactory results. A piece of Gelfilm is used to prevent the formation of dural adhesions in addition to a tissue graft.

The bone flap must be examined thoroughly for evidence of invasion by the meningioma. If this has occurred, the invaded part should be generously removed or the whole flap devitalized by autoclaving the bone or boiling it in distilled water for 30 minutes to ensure regrowth from the bone.[15] If there is a substantial volume of hyperostatic bone, the high-speed air drill may be used to thin the bone flap. If there is transdural extension of the tumor, then the bone is resected, and a methacrylate or titanium mesh cranioplasty is performed.

The bone flap is replaced and secured with wire suture, or miniplates and screws (**Fig. 39–9**). The scalp flap is closed in two layers with a galeal closure and skin closure. Unless the flap is very large and hemostasis of the scalp is felt to be inadequate, placement of a subgaleal drain is not advantageous.

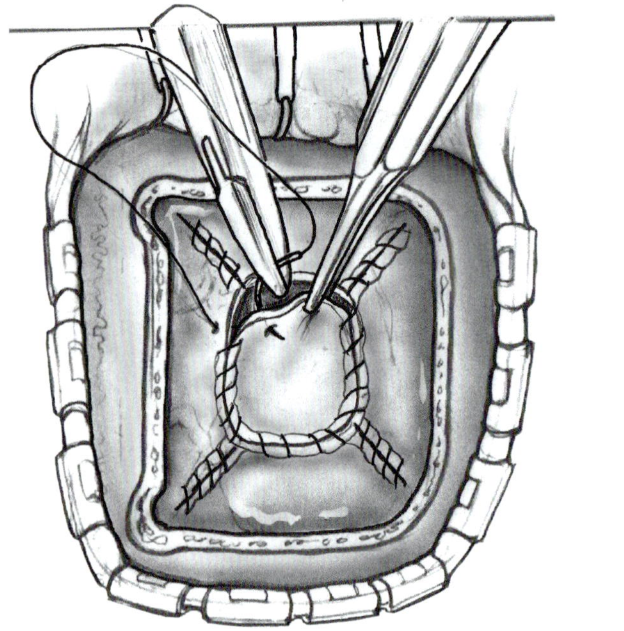

Figure 39–9 Closure, securing of the bone flap with wire/suture.

◆ Postoperative Care

The postoperative course after meningioma removal is usually uneventful, but general principles of supervision and postoperative care apply to these patients, as to all others who undergo intracranial surgery. An unsatisfactory or incomplete recovery from anesthesia, progressive obtundation or focal neurological deficits, or the onset of one or more epileptic seizures calls for a CT scan without contrast enhancement to look for a postoperative hematoma. Persistence of leak despite a lumbar drain is an indication for reexploration and watertight dural closure. If there is evidence of CSF infection, aggressive treatment of infection is essential for the leak to seal over.

A postoperative magnetic resonance imaging scan with gadolinium enhancement is necessary to document complete removal. Histopathological diagnosis is confirmed during this period because a malignant meningioma or hemangiopericytoma will require radiotherapy postoperatively.

◆ Complications

Preoperative

1. **Unnecessary surgery:** This can be prevented by asking the question Why do I need to operate on this tumor? If the reasons are not good enough, then the surgeon should defer surgery or obtain a second opinion to confirm indications for surgery.

Intraoperative

1. **Inadequate exposure:** Typically, large flaps should be used and planned for. Preoperative radiographs are studied carefully to plan the skin and bony flap. Intraoperative ultrasound can be used to localize the tumor after the bone flap has been made to determine if further extension of bony exposure is necessary.
2. **Bleeding during craniotomy:** This complication is serious and is best prevented. Surgical technique to prevent this complication is detailed in the preceding text.
3. **Bleeding during tumor resection:** Bleeding may be minimized by interruption of the tumor blood supply upon initial dural opening and bipolar coagulation of the dural edge. Meticulous hemostasis during internal debulking is mandatory. The arachnoid plane of cleavage must be identified and maintained during surgery to avoid injury to normal cerebral vessels with resultant hemorrhage. Meticulous coagulation of all feeding capsular vessels is imperative during resection of the capsule because these small vessels retract if the capsule is taken out without coagulating these vessels. Uncommonly, diffuse oozing may result from a blood transfusion reaction or iatrogenic thrombocytopenia due to massive blood transfusion. In such an instance, the resection should be suspended until adequate reversal of the coagulopathy is achieved.
4. **Intraoperative brain swelling:** This is prevented by administering preoperative steroids and by careful positioning of the patient. Care should be taken that the head is above the level of the heart, and the neck should not be turned to a degree that jugular venous outflow might be impaired. All of these measures prevent an elevation of intracranial pressure, which might exacerbate cerebral edema. Mannitol is administered at the beginning of craniotomy to reduce cerebral water volume and prevent edema. If substantial brain swelling is identified intraoperatively, the surgical team should verify adequacy of ventilation, endotracheal tube position, and assess for the possibility of air embolism. These conditions are life-threatening and immediate correction is required. Infrequently, there could be a hematoma in the tumor cavity, subdural hematoma, or venous thrombosis of the surrounding brain due to venous occlusion of an important vein that might cause brain swelling. Hematomas can be excluded by using intraoperative ultrasound imaging. These hematomas should be treated prior to tumor resection. If the brain swelling does not subside after all these measures, then hemostasis is obtained, and only the dura is closed using a graft. The bone flap is left out, and the scalp flap is closed. The patient should be transported to the CT scanner while still intubated. The CT findings will dictate the course of treatment.

Postoperative

1. **Progressive neurological deficit or alteration in sensorium:** If a patient exhibits alteration in sensorium or develops progressive neurological deficit, then it is mandatory to exclude a postoperative hematoma by a CT scan. Postoperative hematomas may be prevented by placing duropericranial tacking sutures and meticulous hemostasis prior to the close of the craniotomy. As mentioned earlier, a normal systemic blood pressure at the time of closing and utilizing a Valsalva maneuver is helpful in ensuring adequate hemostasis. A postoperative laboratory assessment should include hematological and coagulation parameters, especially if significant blood loss has occurred. Abnormal values should be addressed promptly.
2. **Seizures:** All patients should receive anticonvulsants preoperatively and intraoperatively. Adequate levels of anticonvulsants should be ensured during the postoperative period and prior to discharge.
3. **CSF leakage:** Any clear discharge from the site of incision is suspicious for a CSF leak. This should be treated aggressively. If there is no intracranial mass (e.g., brain edema, hematoma, significant residual tumor), then a lumbar drain is placed. If the leak does not stop with a lumbar drain, then revision of the wound may be necessary.
4. **Wound infection:** Superficial wound infection is not uncommon. This can be treated with local debridement of skin edges and systemic antibiotics. Osteomyelitis can occasionally result and will necessitate appropriate treatment, which includes resection of infected bone flap and systemic antibiotic therapy. Administration of perioperative antibiotics, meticulous attention to sterile technique, and continuation of antibiotics into the postoperative period in patients who are at a higher risk of infection are helpful in keeping wound infections to a minimum. Excessive coagulation of scalp vessels may result in scalp necrosis and subsequent infection. Careful planning of the scalp flap is also helpful in preventing necrosis.

◆ Conclusion

Meningiomas overlying the cerebral convexities represent the greatest potential for total removal and cure because excision with a wide margin is possible. The initial vital step for resection of any meningioma is the identification of the arachnoidal dissection plane. Defining and staying within this surgical plane minimize the chances of neural or vascular injury.

References

1. Netsky MG, Lapresle J. The first account of a meningioma. Bull Hist Med 1956;30:465–468
2. Al-Rodhan NRF, Laws ER Jr. Meningiomas: a historical study of the tumor and its surgical management. Neurosurgery 1990;26:832–847
3. Cleland J. Description of two tumors adherent to the deep surface of the dura mater. Glasgow Med J 1864;11:148–159
4. Haddad G, Al-Mefty O. Meningiomas: an overview. In: Wilkins RH, Rengachary SS, eds. Neurosurgery. New York:McGraw-Hill;1997:833
5. Cushing H, Eisenhardt L. Meningiomas: Their Classification, Regional Behaviour, Life History, and Surgical End Results. Springfield, IL: Charles C Thomas; 1938:71
6. Grant FC. A clinical experience with meningiomas of the brain. J Neurosurg 1954;11:479–487
7. Cushing H. The meningiomas (dural endotheliomas): their source, and favoured seats of origin. Brain 1922;45:282–316
8. McDermott MW, Wilson CB. Meningiomas. In: Youmans JR, ed. Neurological Surgery. New York: W.B. Saunders; 1997:2782–2825
9. Simpson D. The recurrence of intracranial meningiomas after surgical treatment. J Neurol Neurosurg Psychiatry 1957;20:22–39
10. Jaaskelainen J. Seemingly complete removal of histologically benign intracranial meningioma: late recurrence rate and factors predicting recurrence in 657 patients: a multivariate analysis. Surg Neurol 1986;26:461–469
11. Borovich B, Doron Y. Recurrence of intracranial meningiomas: the role played by regional multicentricity. J Neurosurg 1986;64:58–63
12. Mirimanoff R, Dosoretz DE, Linggood RM, Ojemann RJ, Margwa RL, Meningioma: analysis of recurrence and progression following neurosurgical resection. J Neurosurg 1985;62:18–24
13. Yasargil MG. Meningiomas. In: Yasargil MG. Microneurosurgery of CNS Tumors. Berlin: Georg Thieme Verlag; 1996:134–185
14. Giombini S, Fornari M. Convexity meningiomas. In: Al-Mefty O, ed. Meningiomas. New York: Raven; 1991:321–328
15. Ransohoff J. Removal of convexity, parasagittal, and falcine meningiomas. Neurosurg Clin N Am 1994;5:293–297

40

Torcular and Peritorcular Meningiomas

Fabio Roberti, Carlos Acevedo, and Laligam N. Sekhar

Torcular meningiomas were first described as an individual entity by Cushing and Eisenhardt in 1938. After considering the anatomical relationships between 12 tumors and the torcular, the falx, and the tentorium, Cushing divided the peritorcular area into four corners and thus configured what has been referred to as the four quadrants of possible invasion.[1] Since then, the use of different anatomical classifications (i.e., tentorial, posterior third parasagittal, falcotentorial, posterior fossa)[2–4] has made these uncommon tumors difficult to track in the literature.

Because most torcular meningiomas grow to large sizes before becoming clinically apparent, it is often very difficult to establish whether the tumor originated in the tentorium, falx, sagittal sinus, or adjacent convexity dura mater by the time of diagnosis. It is believed, however, that meningiomas adjacent to or in the confluence of sinuses account for 1 to 4% of the intracranial meningiomas.[5]

Anatomy

The dural sinuses that make up the torcular and the cortical veins that drain into them are the most relevant issues to be considered in planning the surgical strategy.[6] The torcular Herophili is a short and variously shaped intradural sinus lodged in the internal occipital protuberance. Its plexiform structure has its origins in fetal life, which explains the numerous patterns found in adulthood. The torcular Herophili is the confluence of the superior sagittal, straight, occipital, and both transverse sinuses. In addition, minor venous channels in the falx and tentorium form a collateral network around the primary sinuses.[7] These secondary pathways receive blood from the cerebral hemispheres, cerebellum, and brain stem[8] and become important in pathological settings such as neoplastic lesions, arteriovenous malformations, and vascular thrombosis.[9]

According to physiological studies, blood from the superior sagittal sinus empties into the right transverse sinus, whereas the blood from the straight sinus drains to the left transverse sinus. In a study by Woodhall (1978), a partial septation directing these flows was found in 87% of the specimens evaluated.[6] There are also connections from the straight sinus to the transverse sinuses through tentorial veins and venous lakes. These connections take a transdural course and act as collateral channels. Blood flow from the transverse sinuses drains through the respective sigmoid sinuses into the internal jugular veins.

Infratentorially, the occipital sinus connects the torcular with the marginal sinus from which the flow can be directed through emissary veins (i.e., condylar, hypoglossal, or mastoid) to the external jugular vein. These veins and drainage patterns may be prominent in patients with venous obstruction by tumor, or dural arteriovenous malformations. Special attention should be given to the occipital sinus whenever the transverse sinus is not patent because it becomes the main drainage pathway.[10] In some patients, one transverse sinus may be absent, and the occipital sinus may be the main drainage pathway.

◆ Classification

Meningiomas originating in the peritorcular area can be divided as follows:

- Infratentorial: attached to the lower edge of the torcular, inferior surface of the tentorium, and transverse and straight sinuses
- Supratentorial: attached to the upper edge of the torcular, superior surface of the tentorium, and transverse sinuses, and involving the superior sagittal sinuses
- Giant tumors: extending both supra- and infratentorially

◆ Presentation

Torcular meningiomas typically reach large sizes before becoming symptomatic, and signs of intracranial hypertension are the most common early clinical findings. Visual (papilledema, field deficits) and cerebellar (ataxia, dysmetria, nystagmus) signs complete the clinical triad of this pathology.[11] Patients usually complain of instability, visual impairment (the lower quadrants seem to be affected before the upper ones), global headache, occipital/suboccipital pain, neck pain, and stiffness. The later symptoms may result from dural deformation or tonsillar herniation through the foramen magnum and may precede the development of a more complex tumor-related clinical syndrome.

◆ Imaging

Precise location of the origin and extension of these lesions is essential in the selection of the therapeutic strategy and helpful in anticipating potential pitfalls and complications. However, it is only in the rare instance of a small tumor detected early in its development that the dural origin of the tumor can be ascertained by radiological examination. Contemporary techniques in neuroimaging such as magnetic resonance imaging (MRI), magnetic resonance angiography (MRA), magnetic resonance venography (MRV), and digital subtraction angiography (DSA) are used in the evaluation of patients with peritorcular meningiomas.

The single most valuable neurodiagnostic tool is MRI with and without gadolinium. Multiplanar sections give great anatomical detail of the lesion and its relationships with neural and vascular structures. On T1-weighted images, the tumor is isointense with the brain, but after the injection of gadolinium, a marked enhancement is noticed. Intralesional signal voids are associated with either or both patent vessels and calcifications. On T2 images, the tumor appears hyperintense in a varying degree, depending on the fluids contained, and reflects indirectly the consistency of the lesion. This sequence also offers a good opportunity for assessment of the peritumoral cerebrospinal fluid (CSF) spaces and surrounding vessels. Special attention should be paid to long time-relation signal changes, which implies pial invasion. By using spin-echo sequences, the patency of venous sinuses can be evaluated. Partial or complete thrombosis of a sinus is suggested both by its high signal on T1 and low signal on T2 images. However, in the instance of very slow venous flow, the MRI can give equivocal data.

Because the complete evaluation of the venous system is the key to success in surgery, time-of-flight MRV is used along the conventional angiography. MRV provides reliable information concerning the status of major venous sinuses and the architecture of secondary venous pathways. For instance, collateral emissary veins connecting to distended occipital scalp veins have been visualized in cases of transverse sinus occlusion.[12]

The third part of the study is the DSA, the purpose of which is twofold. First, as a diagnostic tool, it defines the vascularity of the neoplasm and identifies its arterial supply. Characteristically these tumors show a dense capillary blush in the late arterial phase. Parasitized blood supply from pial vessels of the posterior cerebral, superior cerebellar, and posteroinferior cerebellar arteries may also be found.[13] The feeding vessels are seen in the early arterial phase and their origins from the external carotid artery (middle meningeal artery, occipital artery), intracavernous carotid artery (meningohypophysial trunk), and vertebral arteries (posterior meningeal artery) are assessed. A careful evaluation of the venous phase after bilateral carotid injection is useful to understand the anatomy of the venous drainage and to assess the presence of collateral flow. Visualization of emissary veins is generally considered abnormal in conventional angiography.[14] Second, as a therapeutic tool, DSA allows embolization of the neoplasm to decrease its vascularity.

◆ Surgical Considerations

Although the ideal objective for surgical therapy of peritorcular meningiomas is the radical resection of the lesion, the surgeon has to balance the risk and the benefits of total tumor resection versus partial tumor resection with observation or radiotherapy of remnants. The choice of treatment must consider the age and clinical condition of the patient, the growth rate of the tumor, the involvement of venous sinuses, and their collateralization.

◆ Surgical Technique

Anesthesia

Anesthesia is induced using intravenous thiopental and a short-acting muscle relaxant. Following hyperoxygenation by mask, the patient is endotracheally intubated and hyperventilated to achieve an arterial $PaCO_2$ of 30 torr. Furosemide or mannitol or both are administered intravenously at the beginning of the operation. A precordial or transesophageal Doppler device is placed to detect air emboli, and a right atrial catheter is inserted to monitor the central venous pressure and to aspirate air in the event of an embolism. The patient is loaded with 1 g of intravenous phenytoin for seizure prophylaxis and administered 2 g of ceftazidime for antibiotic prophylaxis.

The electroencephalogram and somatosensory evoked potentials (SEPs) are monitored continuously during the operation. If the tumor extends bilaterally to involve both calcarine cortexes, visual evoked responses (VERs) may be monitored to reduce the risk of surgically induced cortical blindness. However, VERs are difficult to record and are easily altered by anesthetic agents, and therefore may be difficult to interpret during the operation.

Positioning

Tumors in the torcular area may be operated by placing the patient in prone (Concorde),[15] semiprone, sitting, or semisitting positions, depending on the surgeon's preference. However, we prefer the prone or semiprone positions because it reduces the risk of air emboli and allows the surgeon to sit comfortably at the head of the patient or on the side of the patient, thus facilitating the use of the operative microscope during a long operation. Special attention should be given the brachial plexus and pressure points; gel pads or inflatable beanbags are placed to avoid scars and neuropathies from compression or stretching (**Fig. 40–1**).

Operative Procedure

For unilateral tumors involving a single quadrant, an occipital supratentorial, or occipital paramedian approach may be performed by placing the patient in a three-quarter-prone position.[16] This approach allows the removal of unilateral supratentorial tumors, and, if the borders of the bone flap are extended below the lateral sinus, an infratentorial extension of the neoplasm through the tentorium may be reached and excised.

For supratentorial tumors, the quadrant predominantly involved by the tumor is placed in the superior aspect of the field. A U-shaped incision based just above a line connecting the mastoid tips is performed. The musculocutaneous flap is elevated in a single layer and retracted away from the field, thus exposing the external occipital protuberance, the lambdoid, and the sagittal sutures. After identifying these surgical landmarks, the craniotomy is done in three plates as follows: first, a unilateral occipital craniotomy is placed in proximity to the midline and the transverse sinus. Under tangential vision, the dura mater is dissected free from the calvarium and the second plate elevated from the opposite occipital lobe. This completes the bilateral supratentorial craniotomy while avoiding damage to the superior sagittal sinus. The suboccipital craniotomy is then performed after separating the transverse sinuses under tangential vision.[17] By carrying out the craniotomy in this fashion, the risk of dural or sinus tears is minimized. However, bleeding from sinus surfaces is very

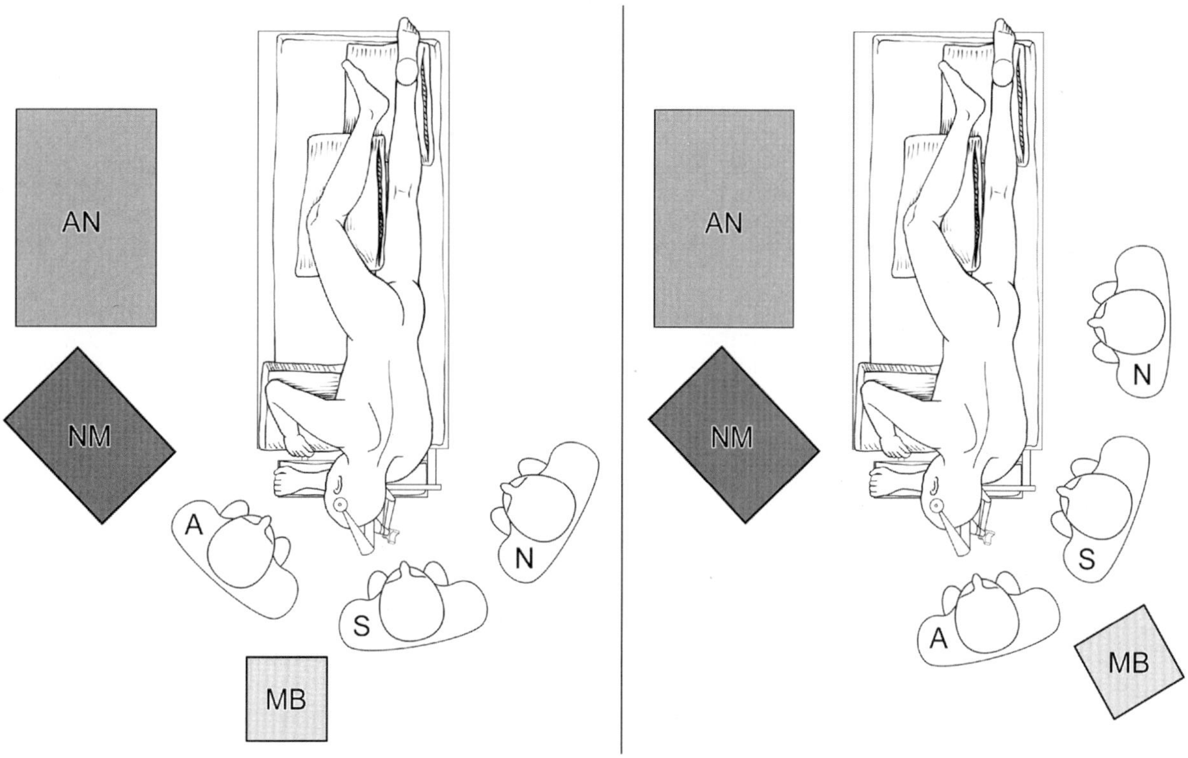

Figure 40–1 Three-quarter-prone position. Surgeon can sit at the head (left in the figure) or on the side (right in the figure) of the patient. S, surgeon; A, assistant; N, nurse; MB, microscope base; AN, anesthesia; NM, neuromonitoring.

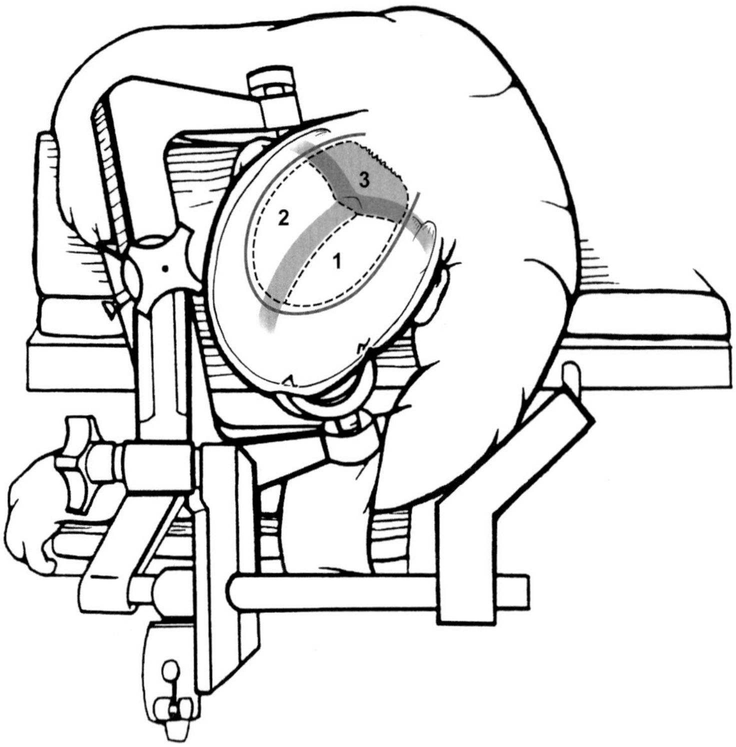

Figure 40–2 Three-quarter-prone position. Musculocutaneous flap (red line), bilateral supratentorial craniotomy (dotted lines), and suboccipital craniectomy (shaded area).

common and may be controlled with dural tack-up sutures, Gelfoam, and bipolar cautery or with Prolene 6–0 stitches in the case of large holes (**Fig. 40–2**).

Frameless stereotaxy may be used in locating the sinuses.

The dura mater is opened in a curvilinear fashion at least 1.5 to 2.0 cm away from the tumor's margin on all three sides, paying special attention to the location of the cortical veins, which must be preserved at any price. If necessary, a small strip of dura may be left attached to the vessels. The dura is then gently elevated from lateral to medial, preserving the large bridging veins. Microsurgical resection of the tumor is then performed. The tumor is debulked with the ultrasonic aspirator or bipolar cautery and scissors. It is then folded into itself and slowly dissected in the arachnoidal plane between the tumor and the brain leading from lateral to medial toward the sinus. No retractors generally need to be placed on the brain, and dissected tumor planes can be protected with a rubber dam and cottonoid. If the tumor invaded the brain, a thin rim should be left on the occipital lobe but may be removed along with the cerebellar cortex. Any involved falx or tentorium are resected, but the venous sinuses are spared. If an involved major venous sinus is still patent, the surgeon's attitude should be conservative, leaving a small piece of tumor firmly adherent to the sinus.[18] Any holes must be repaired by direct suture or by using a small flap of dura mater.

If the sinus is apparently occluded according to the preoperative studies, the surgeon must confirm it intraoperatively. Temporary clips are placed, and the patient is observed for brain swelling or for changes in the SEPs. It is possible that brain swelling due to venous occlusion may not occur for several minutes. For this reason intrasinus pressure is measured by inserting a 20 gauge needle into the proximal part of the clamped sinus, which is connected to a manometer (**Fig. 40–3**). If there is a significant rise of the pressure on test clamping (more than 15 mm Hg after 10 minutes of intraoperative occlusion), the clamp is quickly released, and the sinus cannot be transected. When the intrasinus pressure does not rise above 5 mm Hg, the SEPs do not show changes, and no brain swelling is detected, the sinus is not functional, or it is well collateralized, allowing safe occlusion. If sinus occlusion is elected, an intermediate rise in pressure must be watched for by leaving the needle in place. If the pressure rises progressively, then it should be reconstructed by the use of a short vein or radial artery graft. Any sinus occlusion should be done in a manner that preserves the inflow of the vein of Labbé, and great care should be given to preserve its course.[19] The inner walls of the sinus are evaluated, and any remnant of tumor is resected using angled bipolar forceps, microscissors, or tenotomy scissors. The stumps are then ligated with multiple 4–0 Neurolon or 5–0 Prolene sutures. Tumors partially involving a dominant transverse sinus or the posterior third of the superior sagittal sinus at its junction with the torcular Herophili may be removed along with one wall of the sinus.[20] This can be accomplished by removing the infiltrated edge or lateral wall of the sinus and then replacing the dural defect with a venous patch graft.

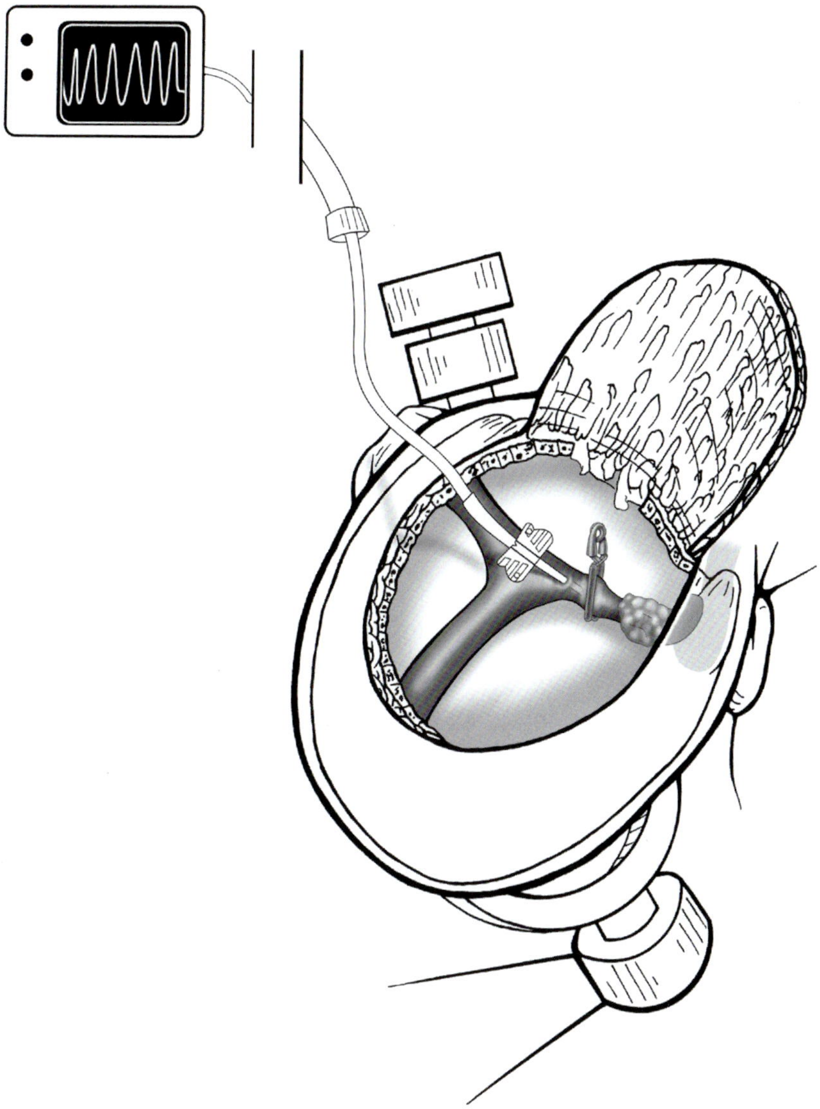

Figure 40–3 A temporary clip has been placed on the sinus, and a 20 gauge needle, connected to a manometer, has been placed to measure intrasinus pressure.

Sinus or Vein Repair

In the event of accidental injury to a patent major sinus or a vein, repair is indicated. The best interposition graft is the radial artery because it is small in diameter as compared with the saphenous vein, and all does not thrombose even when blood flow is of a low volume. The radial artery graft is extracted from the forearm and pressure distended with saline to release vasospasm. The graft is sutured either end to side (when there is size discrepancy) or end to end (when the vessel and graft are evenly matched) using 6–0 or 7–0 Prolene running sutures. When blood flow through the sinus needs to be continued, a balloon shunt should be used, and, in such cases, the patient must be heparinized to prevent thrombosis.

Once the tumor has been resected, a large dural graft is placed. Unless the brain is swollen, the bone plates are repositioned and fixed with titanium microplates. In the case of big defects or large bone gaps, titanium mesh and bone source cement are used for reconstruction.

◆ Postoperative Care

The patients are nursed in the intensive care unit for at least 1 day. Intravenous fluids are replaced to keep the patient euvolemic, and anticonvulsant and steroid medications are continued for at least 1 week. A head CT scan is performed on the first postoperative day before the patient is moved to the regular ward. If brain swelling or hematoma is detected, the patient is kept in the ICU even if clinically asymptomatic.

MRI is performed after 2 to 3 months. If residual tumor is present, consideration should be given to radiosurgery. Subsequent imaging is indicated once a year for 3 to 4 years, and then once every 3 to 4 years thereafter.

◆ Complications

Sinus Opening

If a major venous sinus is accidentally entered or the intrasinus pressure rises above 15 mm Hg after clamping associated with brain swelling and SEP changes, the surgeon must proceed to repair or bypass the segment involved. The anesthesiologist should be prepared for major blood loses. The first step in controlling unexpected sinus bleeding is the application of finger pressure followed by elevation of the head. Once the hole is identified, a Fogarty catheter is introduced, and the sinus is occluded. If brain swelling occurs, a balloon shunt (Pruitt-Inahara shunt)[21] is used, and the patient must be anticoagulated with 2000 U of intravenous heparin.[22] If the opening is a sharp cut, it may be sutured directly using 5–0 Prolene; otherwise a patch is required for closure. Synthetic patches should not be used for repair because of their high risk of thrombosis. Instead, autologous venous grafts (with the endothelial surface facing the lumen of the sinus) or pieces of clean dura mater are used with continuous or interrupted 5–0 Prolene sutures.[20] During the occlusion time it is useful to reduce the blood flow to the brain by inducing controlled hypotension.[23] If the sinus is completely destroyed, reconstruction is performed with a radial artery interposition graft.

Brain Swelling

In case of mild to moderate brain swelling, the patient is kept on mannitol and steroid therapy, and the bone flap is left out and saved for a future cranioplasty. Severe swelling is associated with venous occlusion and may require occipital lobectomies. Swelling should not occur if the procedure has been properly planned and carefully executed.

Air Embolism

The Doppler should be carefully monitored during the procedure. If air emboli are detected, the head should be immediately lowered and the surgical field filled with warm saline solution. The anesthesiologist should increase the inspired fraction of oxygen to 100% and aspirate from the central venous pressure line to recover the air collected in the right atrium.

Venous Infarction

Treatment depends on its size and mass effect. Small infarctions may be treated conservatively with mannitol and serial imaging. In case of a large venous infarct with midline displacements or basal cistern compression, surgical decompression is required. The usual treatment is bone flap removal with a large dural graft.

Seizures

Seizures may be due to brain irritation from either or both the surgical manipulation and venous occlusion. All patients should be treated with anticonvulsants.

◆ Illustrative Cases

Case 1

A 34-year-old previously healthy woman presented with a 1-year history of global headaches, nonspecific visual changes, and inability to work because of difficulties with thought processes. The neurological examination revealed mild impairment of cognitive functions and papilledema. Her visual acuity was normal, as were her visual fields. MRI showed a big (9 × 7 × 7.2 cm) tumor located on and around the torcular (**Fig. 40–4A–C**). Partial arachnoidal plane was visualized as well as some edema in the left occipital lobe. There was no flow signal within the major venous sinuses (**Fig. 40–4C**). The angiographic findings support the occlusion of the sinuses and their collateralization. The tumor was embolized preoperatively.

The patient underwent complete resection of the tumor via the approach herein described. Resection of the venous sinuses was performed along with the tumor after measuring their pressures. Postoperatively, the patient suffered a transient visual deterioration but recovered completely, and at 6-month follow-up, the patient was free of preoperative symptoms. Postoperative MRI imaging showed no evidence of tumor, and she has remained tumor free during a follow-up of 8 years (**Fig. 40–4D,E**).

Case 2

A 65-year-old woman presented with severe headaches located on the vertex associated with memory problems, dizziness, and unsteady gait. On examination, mild ataxia and left upper extremity dysmetria were found. An MRI scan revealed a giant (6 × 4 × 5 cm) meningioma located infratentorially and originating from the inferior aspect of the torcular and tentorium (**Fig. 40–5A,B**). Mild brain stem compression was observed, and a normal arachnoidal plane was seen. The major venous sinuses showed flow signal, and their patency was demonstrated by angiography (**Fig. 40–5C**). The tumor was embolized preoperatively. Using the techniques described previously, a gross total removal of the tumor was performed, preserving the major venous sinuses (**Fig. 40–5D,E**). However, as the tumor was removed from the tentorium, significant bleeding occurred from the inferior aspect of the torcular and the straight sinus, which was controlled by suturing rolls of oxidized cellulose to the dura around the sinus. Postoperatively, edema was observed in the occipital lobe, which was asymptomatic (**Fig. 40–5F**). She has had no tumor recurrence during 9 years of follow-up (**Fig. 40–5G,H**).

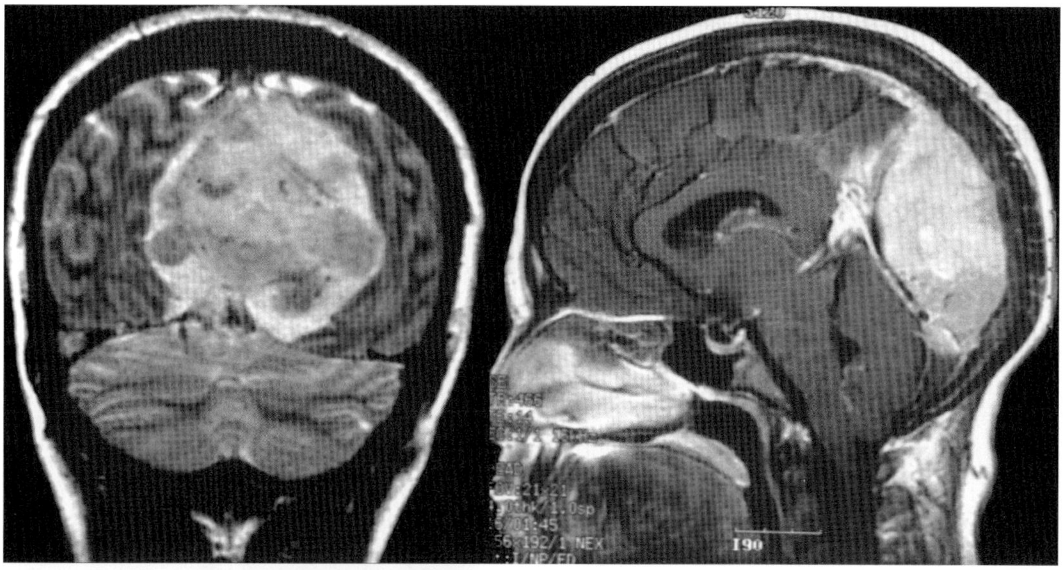

A B

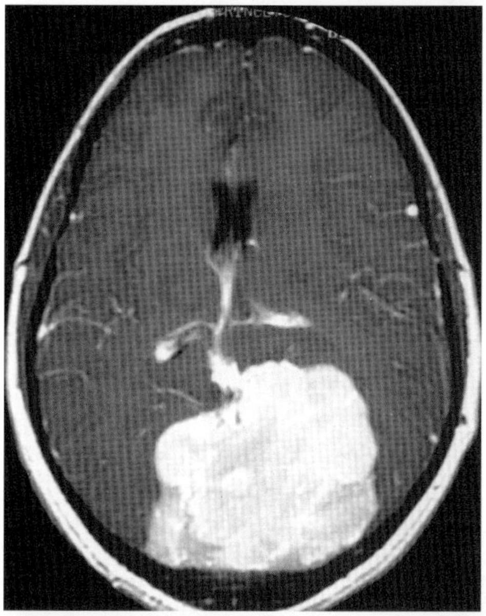

C

Figure 40–4 Preoperative gadolinium-enhanced **(A)** coronal, **(B)** sagittal, and **(C)** axial T1-weighted magnetic resonance imaging (MRI) scans show the tumor involving the torcular. **(D)** Postoperative enhanced MR images confirm gross total resection of the tumor.

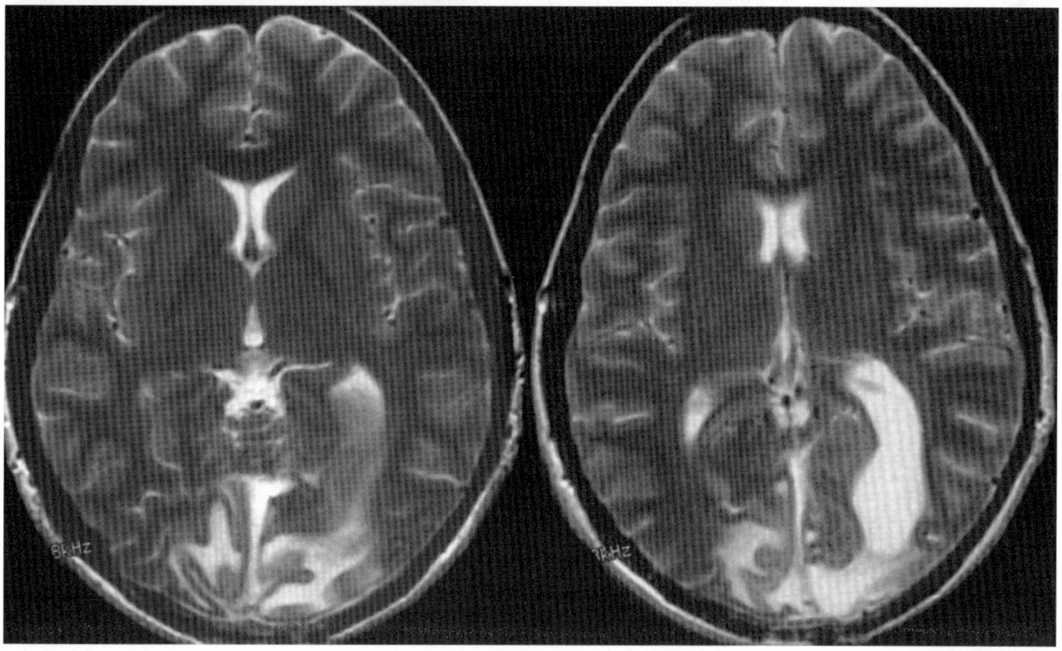

D

(*Continued on page 502*)

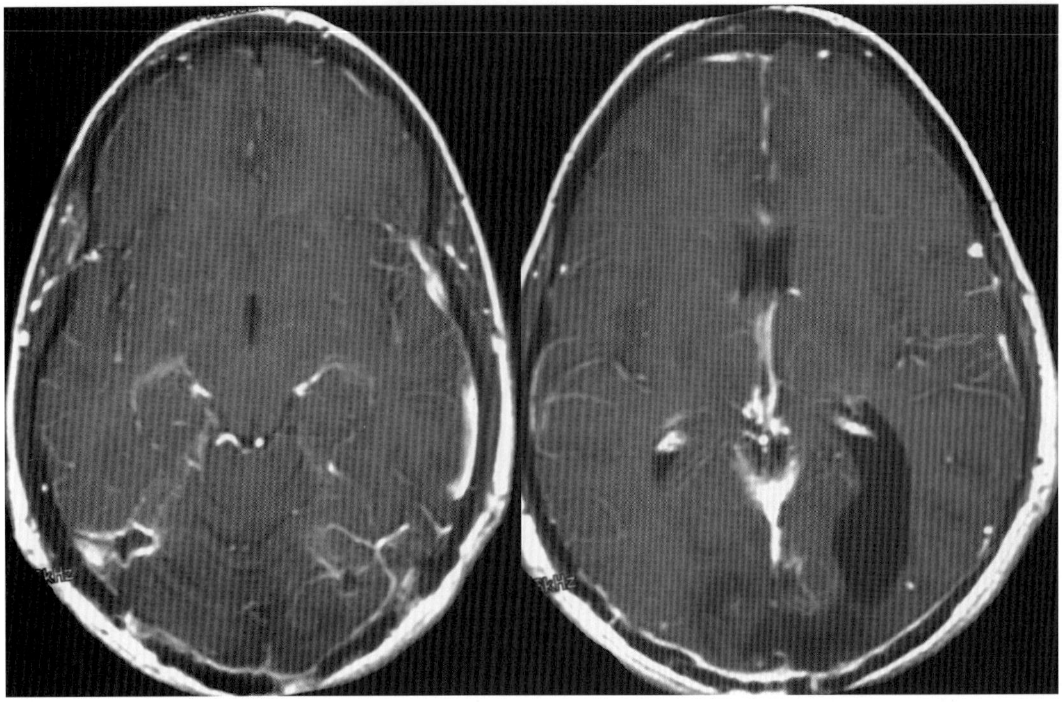

E

(*Continued*) **Figure 40–4 (E)** Postoperative MRI scans show no tumor residue.

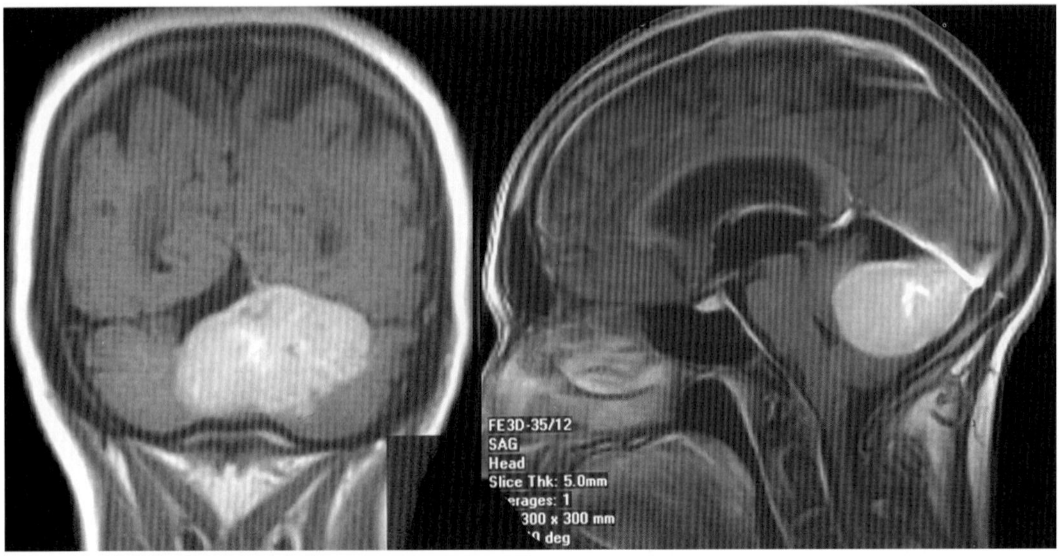

A B

Figure 40–5 (A) Coronal and **(B)** sagittal magnetic resonance imaging (MRI) scans reveal the meningioma involving the inferior aspect of the torcular and tentorium.

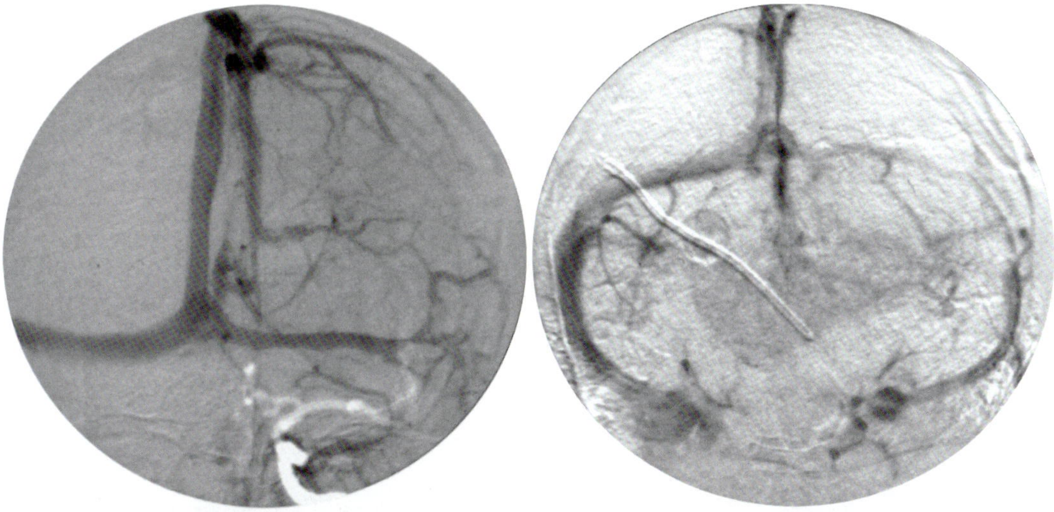

C

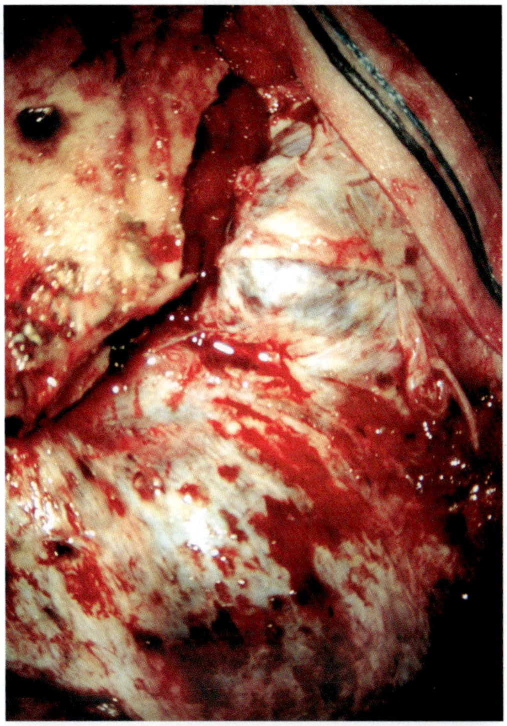

D

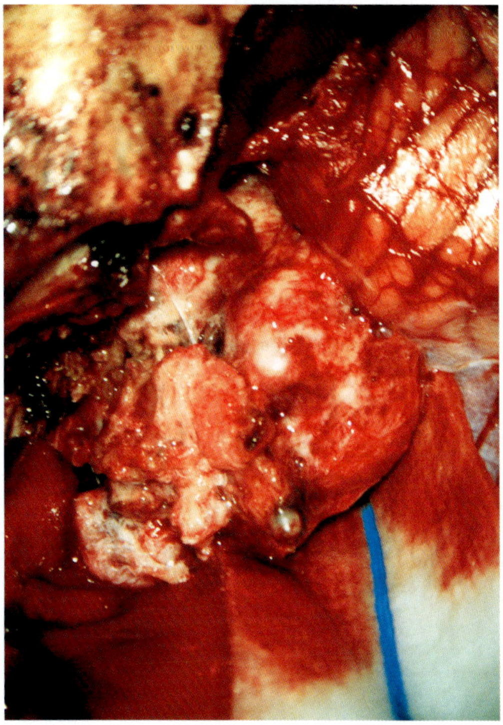

E

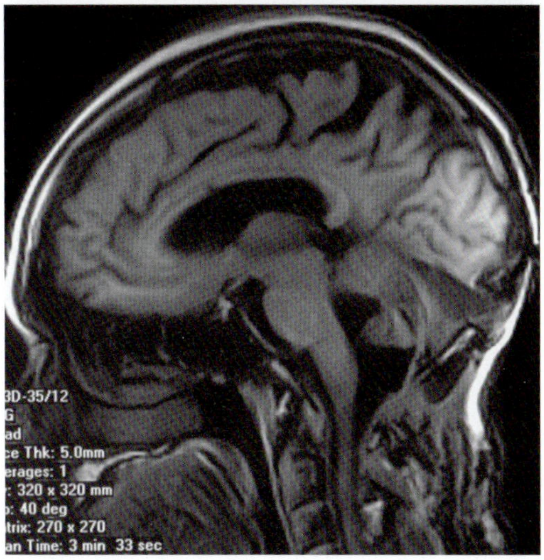

F

(*Continued*) **Figure 40–5 (C)** The preoperative venogram reveals patency of the sinuses. **(D)** The patient has been placed in the semiprone position. An occipital and suboccipital craniotomy has been done, exposing the torcular and both transverse sinuses entirely. **(E)** The tumor has been completely removed. After tumor resection from the inferior aspect of the torcular, venous bleeding occurred from the torcular. This was controlled by suturing on a roll of oxidized cellulose to the surrounding dura mater. **(F)** Postoperative sagittal MRI scan shows some edema of the occipital lobe, which was asymptomatic. Follow-up, enhanced,

(*Continued on page 504*)

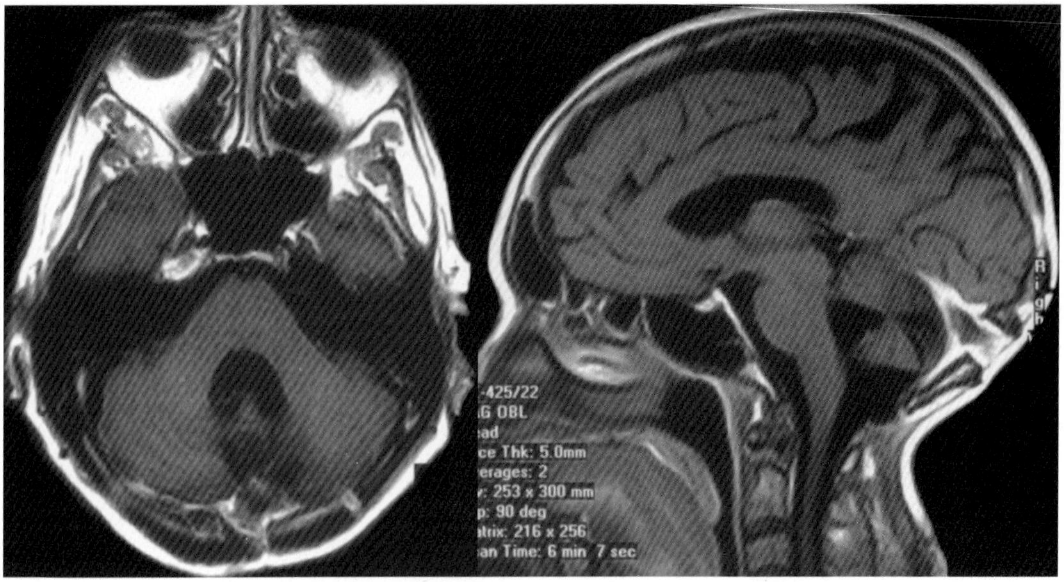

G H

(*Continued*) **Figure 40–5 (G)** axial, and **(H)** sagittal MRI scans show gross total removal of the tumor and resolution of the edema.

References

1. Cushing H, Eisenhardt L. Meningiomas: Their Classification, Regional Behavior, Life History, and Surgical Results. Springfield, IL: Charles C Thomas; 1938
2. Yasargil MG. Microneurosurgery. Vol 4B. Stuttgart: Thieme; 1996: 134–161
3. Castellano F, Ruggiero G. Meningiomas of the posterior fossa. Acta Radiol 1953;104(Suppl):26–69
4. Kondziolka D, Flickinger JC, Perez B, et al. Judicious resection and/or radiosurgery for parasagittal meningiomas: outcomes from a multicenter review. Neurosurgery 1998;43:405–414
5. McDermott MW, Wilson CB. Meningiomas. Vol 4. In: Youmans, JR, ed. Neurological Surgery. Philadelphia: WB Saunders; 1996:2782–2825
6. Lasjaunias P, Raybaud C. Intracranial venous system. In: Lasjaunias P, Bernstein A, eds. Surgical Neuroangiography. Vol 3. New York: Springer-Verlag; 1993:223–245
7. Muthukumar N, Palaniappan P. Tentorial venous sinuses: an anatomical study. Neurosurgery 1998;42:363–371
8. Matsushima T, Suzuki SO, Fukui M, et al. Microsurgical anatomy of the tentorial sinuses. J Neurosurg 1989;71:923–928
9. Oka K, Go Y, Kimura H, et al. Obstruction of the superior sagittal sinus caused by parasagittal meningiomas: the role of collateral venous pathways. J Neurosurg 1994;81:520–524
10. Dora F, Zileli T. Common variations of the lateral and occipital sinuses at the confluens sinuum. Neuroradiology 1980;20:23–27
11. Harsh JR IV, Wilson CB. Peritorcular meningiomas. In: Wilkins RH, Rengachary SS, eds. Neurosurgery. New York: McGraw-Hill; 1996: 891–895
12. Mattle HP, Wentz KU, Edelman RR, et al. Cerebral venography with MR. Radiology 1991;178:453–458
13. Rodesch G, Lasjaunias P. Embolization and meningiomas. In: Al-Mefty O, ed. Meningiomas. New York: Raven; 1991:285–297
14. Anderson CM, Saloner DM, Tsuruda JS, et al. Artifacts in maximum-intensity-projection display of MR angiograms. AJR Am J Roentgenol 1990;154:623–629
15. Kobayashi S, Sugita K, Tanaka Y. Infratentorial approach to the pineal region in the prone position: concorde position: technical note. J Neurosurg 1983;58:141–143
16. Sekhar LN, Goel A. Combined supratentorial and infratentorial approach to large pineal-region meningioma. Surg Neurol 1992;37:197–201
17. Ziyal IM, Sekhar LN, Salas E, et al. Combined supra/infratentorial–transsinus approach to large pineal region tumors. J Neurosurg 1998; 88:1050–1057
18. Sekhar LN, De Oliveira E, Riedel CJ. Parasagittal and falx meningiomas. In: Sekhar LN, De Oliveira E, eds. Cranial Microsurgery: Approaches and Techniques. New York: Thieme; 1999:297–305
19. Morita A, Sekhar LN. Reconstruction of the vein of Labbé by using a short saphenous vein bypass graft: technical note. J Neurosurg 1998;89: 671–675
20. Bonnal J, Brotchi J. Reconstruction of the superior sagittal sinus in parasagittal meningiomas. In: Schmidek HH, ed. Meningiomas and Their Surgical Management. Philadelphia: WB Saunders; 1994:221–229
21. Hakuba A, Huch CW, Tsujikawa S, et al. Total removal of a parasagittal meningioma of the posterior third of the sagittal sinus and its repair by autogenous venous graft. J Neurosurg 1979;51:379
22. Sekhar LN. Radical resection of meningiomas and arteriovenous fistulas involving critical dural sinus segments: experience with intraoperative sinus pressure monitoring and elective sinus reconstruction in 10 patients [Comment]. Neurosurgery 1997;41:1017–1018
23. Schmid-Elsaesser R, Steiger HJ, Yousry T, et al. Radical resection of meningiomas and arteriovenous fistulas involving critical dural sinus segments: experience with intraoperative sinus pressure monitoring and elective sinus reconstruction in 10 patients. Neurosurgery 1997; 41:1005–1018

Section VI

Intraventricular Lesions

41

Surgical Approaches to Lesions Located in the Lateral, Third, and Fourth Ventricles

Hung Tzu Wen, Antônio C. M. Mussi, Albert L. Rhoton Jr., Evandro de Oliveira, and Helder Tedeschi

The cerebral ventricles are cavities encircled by neural structures and are located in the depth of the cerebrum and cerebellum. When the goal is to reach the ventricles, knowledge of the anatomy and the location of each of their components is imperative. As a general rule, any surgical approach directed to the ventricles has to be performed from the surface of either the cerebrum or the cerebellum. Therefore, knowledge of the natural pathways that connect the surface of the cerebrum or the cerebellum to the ventricles is also essential.

These natural pathways are the sulci, fissures, and cisterns. As important as knowledge of the anatomy of the ventricles and the surface of the cerebrum or cerebellum is the correlation between them. This is the so-called x-ray vision concept in which the deep structures can be "seen" through the surface by following some anatomical landmarks located on the surface.

These natural pathways are usually the shortest route to the ventricles. However, they are not necessarily the safest ones because of the risk of trespassing some important fiber systems such as the optic radiation and the pyramidal tract, or some eloquent areas such as the basal ganglia and the thalamus. Therefore, the knowledge of the location of these fiber systems and of the neural structures in relation to the ventricles is also critical. This chapter presents the anatomical aspects of some of the most used surgical approaches to the ventricles, preceded by a brief review of the anatomy of the lateral, third, and fourth ventricles and its correlation with the main sulci, fissures, and cisterns of the brain.

◆ Recommended Surgical Approaches

The general principles that guide surgeons' approach to lesions located in the lateral, third, and fourth ventricles are:

1. The eloquent cortical and subcortical areas, and important fiber tracts that must be avoided (motor, speech areas, optic radiation, motor fibers, memory circuit, thalamus, basal ganglia, etc.), except in those cases where the lesion has already come to the surface of certain eloquent areas. In this case, the lesion can be approached directly.
2. The patients are preferably placed in the usual supine, prone, lateral decubitus, and semisitting positions, and whenever possible with the head preferably in the anatomical position, mostly because a great number of neurosurgeons are more familiar with the anatomy of the head in these positions, making the intraoperative orientation easier.

The surgical approaches recommended by the authors for each part of the lateral, third, and fourth ventricles are:

- Frontal horn: anterior interhemispheric transcallosal approach or superior frontal sulcus approach
- Body: anterior interhemispheric
    - Transcallosal approach
- Temporal horn: transsylvian approach
    - Occipitotemporal sulcus approach
- Atrium: posterior interhemispheric transcingular approach
    - Intraparietal sulcus approach
- Occipital horn: posterior interhemispheric transcingular approach
- Third ventricle: transchoroidea approach
    - Interforniceal approach
    - Subfrontal approach
    - Velum interpositum supracerebellar infratentorial approach
    - Transsylvian approach
- Fourth ventricle: median inferior suboccipital telovelar approach

Surgical Approaches to Lesions Located in the Lateral Ventricle

Lateral Ventricles

The lateral ventricles are two C-shaped cavities that wrap around the mass formed by the basal ganglia and the thalamus (**Fig. 41–1A**). Their morphology resembles two letters *C* obliquely placed with their upper limbs united at the midline. Each ventricle has five components: frontal horn, body, and atrium, and the occipital and temporal horns (**Fig. 41–1B**).[1,2] The frontal horn is located in front of the foramen of Monro, and presents roof, floor, anterior, lateral, medial, and posterior walls. The roof is constituted by the transition between the genu and the body of the corpus callosum, the narrow floor by the rostrum of the corpus callosum, the medial and posterior walls by the septum pellucidum and the thalamus, respectively. The majority of the lateral wall of the frontal horn is represented by the head of the caudate nucleus, except for its most anterior part, constituted by the most anterior part of the anterior limb of the internal capsule. The frontal horn is in close relation to the anterior limiting sulcus of insula (**Fig. 41–1D**).[3] The body of the lateral ventricle is located behind the foramen of Monro and extends to the point where the septum pellucidum disappears and the corpus callosum and fornix meet (**Fig. 41–1C**). The body of the lateral ventricle presents roof, floor, lateral, and medial walls. The roof is formed by the body of the corpus callosum, the medial wall by the septum pellucidum above and the body of the fornix below, the lateral wall by the body of the caudate nucleus, and the floor by the thalamus. The caudate nucleus and the thalamus are separated by the striothalamic sulcus, the groove in which the stria terminalis and thalamostriate vein course (**Fig. 41–1B**). Together, the atrium and occipital horn form a roughly triangular cavity, with the apex posteriorly in the occipital lobe and the base anteriorly on the pulvinar. The atrium has roof, floor, anterior, medial, and lateral walls. The roof is formed by the body, splenium, and tapetum of the corpus callosum, the floor by the collateral trigone, a triangular area that bulges upward over the posterior end of the collateral sulcus (**Fig. 41–1B**). The medial wall is formed by two roughly horizontal prominences; the upper prominence is the bulb of the callosum formed by the large bundle of fibers called the forceps major, which connects the two occipital lobes; the lower prominence is the calcar avis, which overlies the deepest part of the calcarine sulcus (**Fig. 41–1D**). The lateral wall has an anterior part, formed by the tail of the caudate nucleus as it wraps the lateral margin of the pulvinar, and a posterior part, formed by the fibers of the tapetum as they sweep anteroinferiorly along the lateral margin of the ventricle. At the atrium, the optic radiation is separated from the ventricular cavity by the tapetum. The anterior wall has a medial part composed of the crus of the fornix as it wraps around the posterior part of the pulvinar, and a lateral part formed by the pulvinar of the thalamus (**Fig. 41–1E**). The occipital horn extends posteriorly into the occipital lobe from the atrium. It varies in size from being absent to extending far posteriorly in the occipital lobe. The medial wall of the atrium is formed by the bulb of the callosum and the calcar avis. The roof and lateral wall of the atrium are formed by the tapetum, and the floor by the collateral trigone. The fibers of the optic radiation pass laterally and inferiorly to the atrium. These fibers also pass laterally, inferiorly and superiorly in relation to the occipital horn; therefore, the only surface of the occipital horn that is devoid of optic radiation is its medial surface.[4] The temporal horn extends anteriorly, inferiorly, and medially from the atrium into the medial part of the temporal lobe and presents roof, floor, anterior, lateral, and medial walls. The roof is formed by tapetum, the tail of the caudate nucleus, part of the retrolentiform and sublentiform components of the internal capsule, and the amygdaloid nucleus. The retrolentiform component in the roof of the temporal horn is the posterior thalamic radiation that includes the optic radiation; the part of the sublentiform component in the roof of the temporal horn is formed mainly by the acoustic radiation (**Fig. 41–1F**).[5] The amygdaloid nucleus constitutes the anterior wall and the most anterior part of the roof of the temporal horn. The amygdaloid nucleus is located just above the head of the hippocampus[6] anterior to the inferior choroidal point, which is the most anterior site of attachment of the choroid plexus in the temporal horn[3] (**Fig. 41–1G**). The amygdaloid nucleus blends superiorly with the globus pallidus without any sharp demarcation (**Fig. 41–1G**).

The roof of the temporal horn can be considered a lateral extension of the thalamus because all fibers of the optic radiation come from the lateral geniculate body, and there is no clear separation between them[3] (**Fig. 41–1H**). The lateral wall is formed by the tapetum and the optic radiation. The posterior two thirds of the medial wall is constituted by the choroidal fissure, and the anterior third of the medial wall by the head of the hippocampus.[1] The floor is formed medially by the hippocampus and laterally by the collateral eminence, which is the prominence overlying the collateral sulcus (**Fig. 41–1I**).

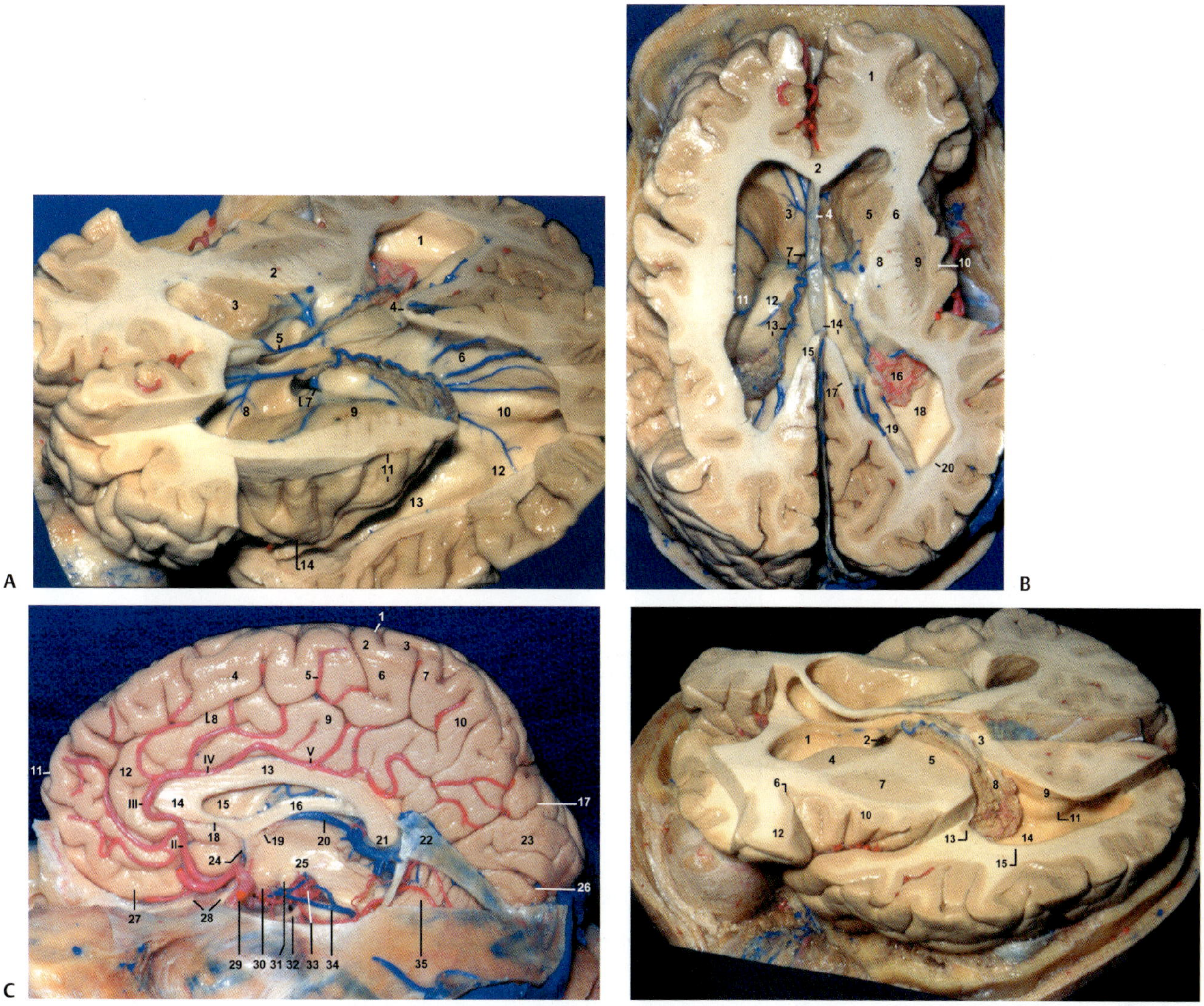

Figure 41–1 **(A)** Superolateral view. **1**, right collateral eminence; **2**, right internal capsule; **3**, right head of the caudate nucleus; **4**, splenium of the corpus callosum; **5**, anterior septal veins; **6**, bulb of the callosum and the medial atrial veins; **7**, foramen of Monro and thalamostriate vein; **8**, left frontal horn; **9**, body of the caudate nucleus; **10**, calcar avis; **11**, insula and its superior circular sulcus; **12**, collateral trigone; **13**, hippocampus; **14**, limen insulae. **(B)** Superior view. **1**, frontal lobe; **2**, genu of the corpus callosum; **3**, rostrum of the corpus callosum; **4**, septum pellucidum; **5**, head of the caudate nucleus; **6**, anterior limb of the internal capsule; **7**, foramen of Monro and thalamostriate vein; **8**, genu of the internal capsule; **9**, lentiform nucleus **10**, insula; **11**, body of the caudate nucleus; **12**, thalamus; **13**, choroid plexus and the superior choroidal vein; **14**, septum pellucidum and the body of the fornix; **15**, splenium of the corpus callosum; **16**, glomus; **17**, bulb of the callosum; **18**, collateral trigone; **19**, calcar avis; **20**, tapetum. **(C)** Medial view of the right hemisphere. **1**, central sulcus; **2**, precentral gyrus; **3**, postcentral gyrus; **4**, medial frontal gyrus; **5**, paracentral ramus of the cingulate sulcus **6**, paracentral lobule; **7**, marginal ramus of the cingulate sulcus; **8**, cingulate sulcus; **9**, cingulate gyrus; **10**, precuneus; **11**, medial frontal gyrus; **12**, cingulate gyrus; **13**, body of the corpus callosum; **14**, genu of the corpus callosum; **15**, head of the caudate nucleus; **16**, fornix; **17**, parieto-occipital sulcus; **18**, rostrum of the corpus callosum; **19**, foramen of Monro and anterior commissure; **20**, internal cerebral vein; **21**, splenium of the corpus callosum; **22**, straight sinus; **23**, cuneus; **24**, lamina terminalis; **25**, hypothalamus; **26**, calcarine sulcus; **27**, rectus gyrus; **28**, olfactory tract and optic nerve; **29**, middle cerebral artery; **30**, tuber cinereum; **31**, mamillary body; **32**, oculomotor nerve; **33**, posterior perforated substance; **34**, basal vein; **35**, cerebellum; **II**, **III**, **IV**, and **(V)**, segments of the anterior cerebral artery. **(D)** Superolateral view. **1**, frontal horn; **2**, fornix and the foramen of Monro; **3**, splenium of the corpus callosum; **4**, head of the caudate nucleus; **5**, thalamus; **6**, anterior limiting sulcus of insula; **7**, lentiform nucleus; **8**, glomus; **9**, bulb of the callosum; **10**, insula, extreme capsule, claustrum, and external capsule; **11**, calcar avis; **12**, pars orbitalis of the inferior frontal gyrus; **13**, tail of the caudate nucleus; **14**, collateral trigone; **15**, tapetum.

(Continued on pages 510 and 511)

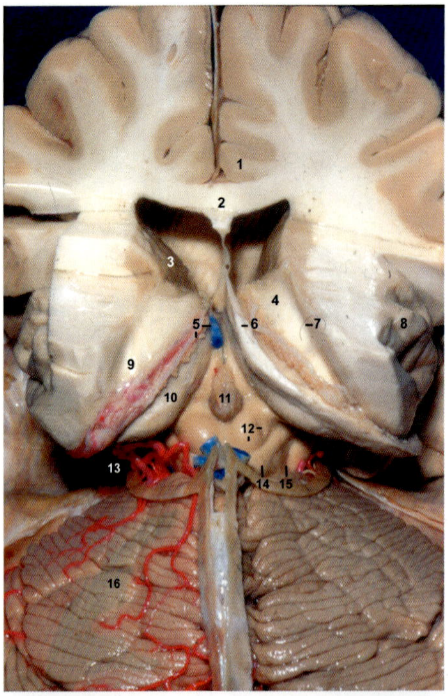
E

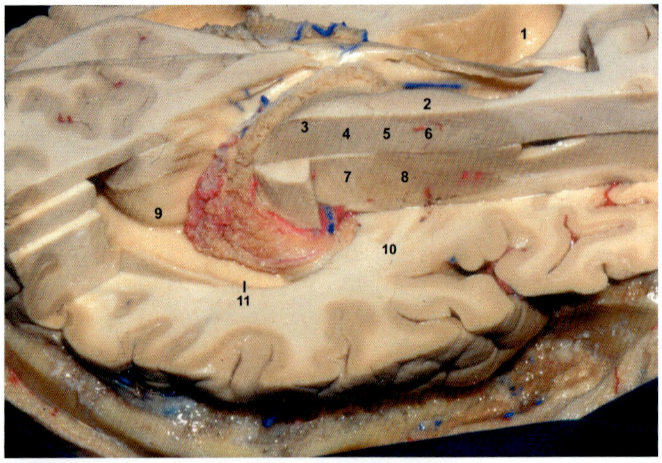
F

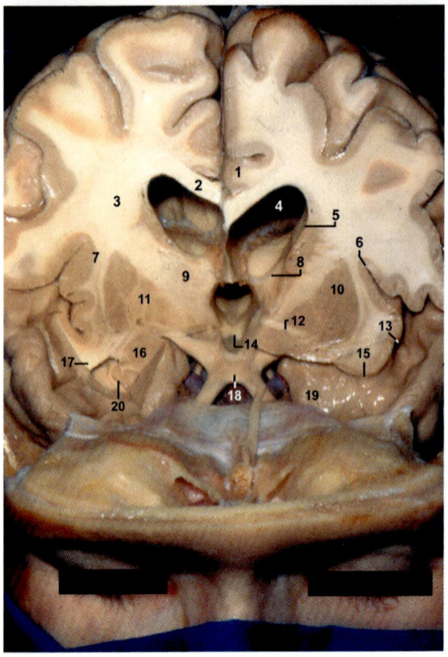
G

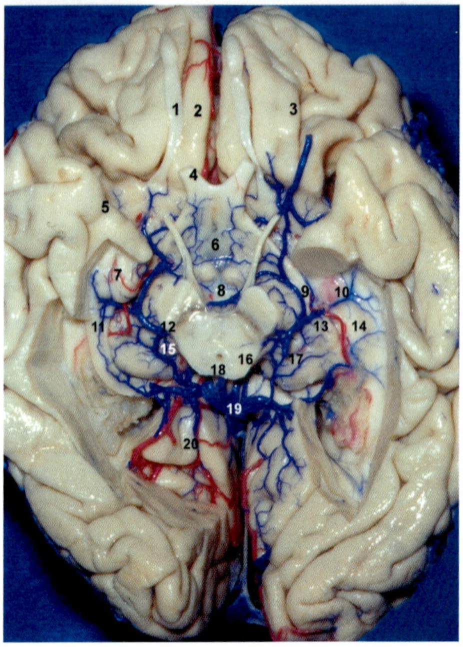
H

(*Continued*) **Figure 41–1** **(E)** Posterior view. **1**, cingulate gyrus; **2**, genu of the corpus callosum; **3**, head of the caudate nucleus; **4**, thalamus; **5**, choroid plexus, thalamus, and the internal cerebral vein; **6**, body of the fornix; **7**, striothalamic sulcus; **8**, insula; **9**, pulvinar of the thalamus (atrial part); **10**, pulvinar of the thalamus (quadrigeminal cistern part); **11**, pineal gland; **12**, superior colliculus and its brachium; **13**, branches of the superior cerebellar artery; **14**, inferior colliculus and its brachium; **15**, crus cerebri and the lateral mesencephalic sulcus; **16**, tentorial surface of the cerebellum and branches of the superior cerebellar artery. **(F)** Superolateral view of the right hemisphere. **1**, left frontal horn; **2**, head of the caudate nucleus; **3**, thalamus; **4**, posterior limb of the internal capsule; **5**, genu of the internal capsule; **6**, anterior limb of the internal capsule; **7**, retrolentiform portion of the internal capsule; **8**, lentiform nucleus; **9**, calcar avis; **10**, sublentiform portion of the internal capsule; **11**, collateral eminence. **(G)** Frontal view. **1**, cingulate gyrus; **2**, genu of the corpus callosum; **3**, pyramidal tract; **4**, body of the lateral ventricle; **5**, body of the caudate nucleus; **6**, superior circular sulcus of the insula; **7**, insula, extreme capsule, claustrum, and external capsule; **8**, thalamostriate vein; **9**, thalamus; **10**, putamen; **11**, globus pallidus; **12**, anterior commissure; **13**, inferior circular sulcus of insula; **14**, mamillary bodies; **15**, limen insulae; **16**, amygdala; **17**, roof of the temporal horn; **18**, optic chiasm; **19**, uncus; **20**, head of the hippocampus. **(H)** Basal view. **1**, olfactory tract; **2**, rectus gyrus; **3**, orbital gyri; **4**, optic nerve; **5**, rhinal sulcus; **6**, tuber cinereum; **7**, inferior surface of the posterior segment of the uncus; **8**, posterior perforated substance, mamillary bodies, and the peduncular vein; **9**, optic tract and the anterior peduncular segment of the basal vein; **10**, inferior ventricular vein; **11**, fornix, dentate gyrus, and anterior longitudinal hippocampal vein; **12**, substantia nigra and lateral mesencephalic sulcus; **13**, lateral geniculate body; **14**, roof of the temporal horn; **15**, medial geniculate body and posterior mesencephalic segment of the basal vein; **16**, tegmentum of the midbrain; **17**, pulvinar of the thalamus (roof of the wing of the ambient cistern); **18**, tectum of the midbrain; **19**, vein of Galen; **20**, precuneus.

(*Continued on page 511*)

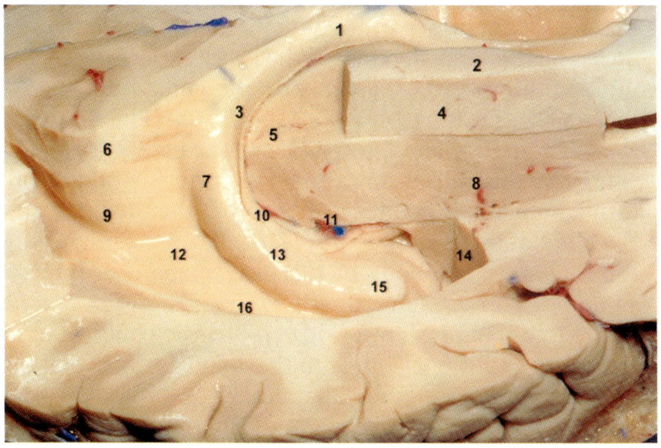

I

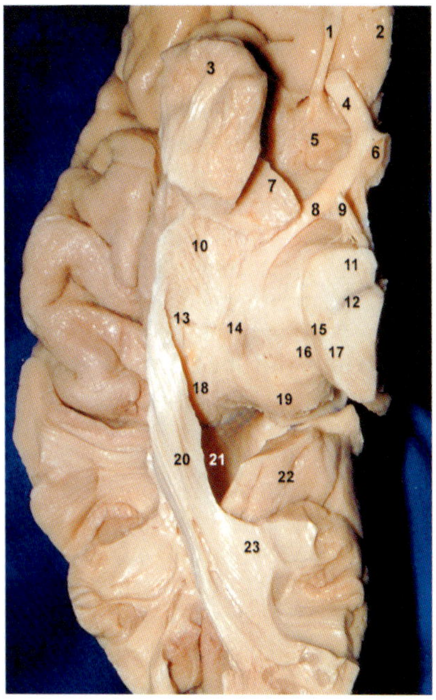

J

(*Continued*) **Figure 41–1** **(I)** Lateral view. The lateral wall of the temporal horn has been removed. **1**, body of the fornix; **2**, head of the caudate nucleus; **3**, crus of the fornix; **4**, internal capsule; **5**, thalamus; **6**, bulb of the callosum; **7**, tail of the hippocampus; **8**, lentiform nucleus; **9**, calcar avis; **10**, fimbria of the fornix; **11**, lateral geniculate body, inferior choroidal vein (in blue), anterior choroidal artery (in red), and inferior choroidal point; **12**, collateral trigone; **13**, body of the hippocampus; **14**, amygdala; **15**, head of the hippocampus; **16**, collateral eminence. **(J)** Basal view of the right hemisphere. **1**, olfactory tract; **2**, rectus gyrus; **3**, temporal pole; **4**, optic nerve; **5**, anterior perforated substance; **6**, optic chiasm; **7**, amygdala; **8**, optic tract; **9**, oculomotor nerve; **10**, anterior part of the optic radiation; **11**, crus cerebri; **12**, substantia nigra; **13**, middle part of the optic radiation; **14**, lateral geniculate body; **15**, lateral mesencephalic sulcus; **16**, medial geniculate body; **17**, tegmentum of the midbrain; **18**, posterior part of the optic radiation; **19**, pulvinar of the thalamus; **20**, optic radiation; **21**, atrium; **22**, isthmus of the cingulate sulcus; **23**, calcarine sulcus.

The neural elements and fiber tracts that are relevant in surgical approaches related to the lateral ventricles are the foramen of Monro, internal capsule, corpus callosum, fornix, thalamus, caudate nucleus, hippocampus, temporal amygdala, choroidal fissure, optic radiation, and pyramidal tract.

Foramen of Monro

The foramen of Monro communicates the lateral ventricle to the third ventricle. It is limited anteriorly and superiorly by the fornix and posteriorly by the thalamus[7] (**Fig. 41–1A**); the elements that run close to the foramen of Monro are the anterior septal vein superior and medially, choroidal plexus posterior and medially, and thalamostriate vein lateral and posteriorly.[1,8]

Internal Capsule

The internal capsule has five parts[5,9]: anterior and posterior limbs, genu, retrolentiform, and sublentiform parts (**Fig. 41–1B,D,F,G**). The anterior limb, located between the head of the caudate nucleus and the anterior part of the lentiform nucleus, contains frontopontine fibers; the posterior limb, located between the thalamus and the posterior part of the lentiform nucleus, contains corticospinal tract, frontopontine fibers, corticorubral fibers, and fibers of the superior thalamic radiation (somaesthetic radiation). The genu comes directly to the ventricular surface and touches the wall of the lateral ventricle immediately lateral to the foramen of Monro in the interval between the caudate nucleus and the thalamus, where the thalamostriate vein usually drains into the internal cerebral vein. The genu contains corticonuclear fibers and anterior fibers of the superior thalamic radiation. The retrolentiform part is located posteriorly to the lentiform nucleus and contains mainly parietopontine, occipitopontine, occipitocollicular, and occipitotectal fibers. The retrolentiform part also contains the posterior thalamic radiation, which includes the optic radiation. The sublentiform part is located below the lentiform nucleus and contains temporopontine and parietopontine fibers, acoustic radiation from the medial geniculate body to the superior temporal, and transverse temporal gyri.

Pyramidal Tract

By definition, the pyramidal tract comprises all fibers that traverse through the pyramids in the medulla. The origin of the fibers of the pyramidal tract includes not only the primary motor area (precentral gyrus), somaesthetic cortex (postcentral gyrus), and paracentral lobule but also a wide area comprising the frontal and parietal lobes.[10]

The motor fibers constitute 40 to 60% of the fibers of the pyramidal tract. The motor fibers arise from the whole precentral gyrus and then converge to the internal capsule. Initially they have a fanlike arrangement. The base of the fan comprises the whole extent of the precentral gyrus from the sylvian fissure laterally to the cingulate sulcus medially. The vertex of the fan is characterized by the convergence of these fibers into the internal capsule, more precisely into the posterior limb of the internal capsule. Because the precentral gyrus possesses a medial to lateral and posterior to anterior orientation, the fibers of the pyramidal tract follow this same orientation throughout the corona radiata. At the internal capsule, between the thalamus medially and the posterior part of the lentiform nucleus laterally, the pyramidal tract begins to twist: the fibers originating close to the sylvian fissure occupy the anterior portion of the posterior limb of the internal capsule, and the fibers corresponding to the leg occupy the posterior portion of the posterior limb of the internal capsule. Therefore, the fibers of the pyramidal tract change its oblique orientation (posterior to anterior and medial to lateral) in the precentral gyrus cortex and the corona radiata, to an anteroposterior orientation in the posterior limb of the internal capsule. At the transition between the corona radiata and the internal capsule, the pyramidal tract is limited medially by the lateral edge of the body of the lateral ventricle (angle formed by the body of the corpus callosum and the body of the caudate nucleus), and laterally by the superior circular sulcus of the insula.

Some conclusions can be drawn from the foregoing information: (1) once inside the body of the lateral ventricle, any further lateral dissection beyond the boundary of the lateral wall can carry a substantial risk of damaging the pyramidal tract. (2) Likewise, any further medial dissection crossing the superior circular sulcus at the posterior half of the insula can also carry the risk of damaging the pyramidal tract. (3) Any further lateral dissection beyond the bottom of the cingulate and the callosal sulci at the level of the paracentral lobule can affect the medial fibers of the pyramidal tract (**Fig. 41–1G**).

Corpus Callosum

The corpus callosum is the largest transverse commissure connecting the cerebral hemispheres. It contributes to the wall of each of the five parts of the lateral ventricle.[2] The corpus callosum has two anterior parts (the rostrum and genu), a central part (the body), and a posterior part (the splenium) (**Fig. 41–1C–E,G**). The rostrum forms the floor of the frontal horn. The genu originates a large fiber tract, the forceps minor, which forms the anterior wall of the frontal horn as it sweeps obliquely forward and laterally to connect the frontal lobes. The genu and the body of the corpus callosum form the roof of both the frontal horn and the body of the lateral ventricle. The splenium originates a large tract, the forceps major, which forms a prominence called the bulb, in the upper part of the medial wall of the atrium and occipital horn as it sweeps posteriorly to connect the occipital lobes. Another fiber tract, the tapetum, which arises in the posterior part of the body and splenium, sweeps laterally and inferiorly to form the roof and lateral wall of the atrium and the temporal and occipital horns. The tapetum separates the fibers of the optic radiations from the temporal horn and the atrium.[2]

Fornix

The fornix is a C-shaped structure that wraps around the thalamus in the wall of the lateral ventricle.[2,3,11,12] The initial portion of the fornix, the fimbria, arises from the alveus, which is the subcortical white matter of the hippocampal allocortex. The fimbria thickens along the medial edge of the body of the hippocampus at the inferior choroidal point, which is the most anterior site of attachment of the choroid plexus in the temporal horn (**Figs. 41–1I, 41–8A, E**). The fimbria is separated from the dentate gyrus by the fimbrodentate sulcus. The fimbria then passes posteriorly to become the crus of the fornix in the atrium, wrapping around the posterior surface of the pulvinar of the thalamus, and arches superomedially toward the lower surface of the splenium of the corpus callosum. The crus constitutes the medial half of the anterior wall of the atrium (**Fig. 41–1E**). At the junction between the atrium and the body of the lateral ventricle, the paired crura meet to form the body of the fornix, which is the inferior portion of the medial wall of the body of the lateral ventricle. At the anterior margin of the thalamus, the body of the fornix separates into two columns that arch along the superior and anterior margins of the foramen of Monro (**Fig. 41–8I**). The columns of the fornix then split unevenly into two bundles: a smaller one, the precommissural fibers that pass anteriorly to the anterior commissure, and a larger, the postcommissural fibers that pass posteriorly to the anterior commissure. The postcommissural fibers are directed inferiorly and posteriorly through the lateral wall of the third ventricle to reach the mamillary bodies at the floor of the third ventricle. In the area below the splenium, the two crura of the fornix are united by the hippocampal commissure (**Fig. 41–8E**).

Thalamus

The thalamus is located in the center of the lateral ventricle. Each lateral ventricle wraps around the superior, inferior, and posterior surfaces of the thalamus. The anterior tubercle of the thalamus is the posterior limit of the foramen of Monro. The posterior part, called the pulvinar (pillow) of the thalamus, is the wall of three different compartments in the cerebrum: the posterolateral part of the pulvinar is the lateral half of the anterior wall of the atrium (**Fig. 41–1E**); the posteromedial part is covered by the crus of the fornix and is part of the superolateral wall of the quadrigeminal cistern (**Fig. 41–1E**); the inferolateral part of the pulvinar is the roof of the wing of the ambient cistern (**Fig. 41–1J**). The medial part of the thalamus is the lateral wall of the third ventricle (**Fig. 41–1C**).[3]

Caudate Nucleus

The caudate nucleus is another C-shaped structure that wraps around the thalamus; it has a head, body, and tail. The head and body are lateral walls of the frontal horn and the body of the lateral ventricle, respectively. The tail extends from the atrium into the roof of the temporal horn and is continuous with the amygdaloid nucleus (**Fig. 41–1B,D**).[2]

Hippocampus

The hippocampus occupies the medial part of the floor of the temporal horn and is divided into three parts: head, body, and tail.[13] The head of the hippocampus, the anterior and the largest part, is directed anterior and inferiorly, and then medially. At the medial end of the tip of the temporal horn, it turns up vertically and bends over laterally forming the medial wall of the tip of the temporal horn ahead of the choroidal fissure; the head of the hippocampus is free of the choroid plexus, and it is characterized by three or four hippocampal digitations; its overall shape resembles that of a feline paw. The head of the hippocampus is directed toward the posterior segment of the uncus[3] and has its posterior limit characterized by the initial segment of the fimbria and the choroidal fissure (**Fig. 41–1J**). Superiorly, the head of the hippocampus is related to the posteroinferior portion of the amygdala, which bulges from the most anterior part of the roof of the temporal horn into the ventricular cavity. Anteriorly, the head of the hippocampus is related to the uncal recess of the temporal horn, the part of the temporal horn located between the anterior wall and the head of the hippocampus, and the uncal recess is also the anterior continuation of the collateral eminence (**Fig. 41–1G**). The emergence of the choroid plexus, the fimbria, and consequently the choroidal fissure mark the beginning of the body of the hippocampus. The body of the hippocampus has an anteroposterior and inferosuperior direction in the medial part of the floor of the temporal horn, and it narrows as it approaches the atrium of the lateral ventricle. Posterior to the head of the hippocampus, the medial wall of the temporal horn is the choroidal fissure, which communicates medially with the ambient cistern. At the atrium of the lateral ventricle, the body of the hippocampus changes its direction and has its longitudinal axis oriented transversely to become the tail of the hippocampus. The tail of the hippocampus is slender and constitutes the medial part of the floor of the atrium; medially the tail of the hippocampus fuses with the calcar avis. Macroscopically, the tail of the hippocampus ends when it meets the medial wall of the atrium (**Fig. 41–1J**), although histologically the terminal segment of the hippocampal tail continues as the subsplenial gyrus, which covers the inferior splenial surface.

Amygdala

The amygdala, along with the hippocampus, constitutes the core of the limbic system. The current concept of the amygdala complex divides it into the temporal or principal amygdala and the extratemporal or extended amygdala, which is located in the primordial floor of the ventricle and is part of the basal forebrain.[6] The temporal amygdala is composed of a series of gray matter nuclei classified into three main groups: basolateral, corticomedial, and central groups. From the neurosurgical viewpoint, the temporal amygdala can be considered as being entirely located within the boundaries of the uncus: superiorly, the amygdala blends with the globus pallidus without any clear demarcation[3]; inferiorly, the posterior portion of the temporal amygdala bulges inferiorly into the most anterior portion of the roof of the temporal horn above the hippocampal head and the uncal recess; medially, it is related to the anterior and posterior segments of the uncus. The temporal amygdala also constitutes the anterior wall of the temporal horn (**Fig. 41–1G,I**).

Choroidal Fissure

The choroidal fissure is a cleft located between the thalamus and the fornix. It is the site of attachment of the choroid plexus in the lateral ventricle. It is a C-shaped arc that extends from the foramen of Monro through the body and atrium to the inferior choroidal point of the temporal horn.[11] The choroidal fissure is divided into three parts: the body part—between the body of the fornix and the thalamus; the atrial part—between the crus of the fornix and the pulvinar of the thalamus; and the temporal part—between the fimbria of the fornix and the stria terminalis of the thalamus. The choroid plexus of the lateral ventricle is attached to the fornix and the thalamus via an ependymal covering called the taenia; in the body and the atrial parts, the taenia fornicis attaches the choroid plexus to the body of the fornix, whereas the taenia choroidea attaches the choroid plexus to the thalamus (**Fig. 41–9B**). In the temporal part, the choroidal plexus is attached to the fimbria via the taenia fimbriae and to the stria terminalis via the taenia choroidea. The choroidal fissure is one of the most important landmarks in microneurosurgeries involving the temporal lobe: it separates those structures located laterally and that can be removed (temporal structures) from those structures located medially that should be preserved (thalamic structures).

Optic Radiation

The optic radiation is a bundle of fibers that extends from the lateral geniculate body to the visual area in the occipital lobe. According to the direction of its fibers, the optic radiation may be divided into anterior, middle, and posterior parts. In the anterior part, the fibers initially take an anterior direction along the roof of the temporal horn, usually reaching as far anteriorly as the tip of the temporal horn and then looping backward in the lateral and inferior aspects of the atrium and occipital horn to end in the lower lip of the calcarine fissure (because of this aspect, the anterior part is also called the lower bundle); the anterior loop is called Meyer's loop, and its anterior extension is variable, ranging from 10 mm in front to 5 mm behind the tip of the temporal horn (average 5 ± 3.9 mm in front).[4] The anterior part of the optic radiation represents the upper quadrants of the visual field. In the middle part, initially the fibers take a lateral direction, coursing along the roof of the temporal horn, and then proceed posteriorly along the lateral wall of the atrium and the occipital horn. The middle part of the optic radiation, also called the central bundle, contains the macular fibers. The fibers of the posterior part of the optic radiation course posteriorly along the lateral wall of the atrium and the occipital horn to end in the upper lip of the calcarine fissure (because of this aspect, the posterior part is also called the upper bundle); these fibers are responsible for the lower quadrants of the visual field[4,7,14,15] (**Fig. 41–1J**).

Cerebral Sulci

The spatial arrangement of the sulci and fissures of the cerebrum follows the pattern of the white matter substance. The white matter substance of the cerebrum is divided into two zones according to Yasargil[16]: the gyral (peripheral) zone and the capsular (central) zone. The central zone is constituted by the external and internal capsules, and the peripheral zone is composed of white matter located between the cortex and the periventricular matrix of the lateral ventricles.

The gyral or peripheral zone is subdivided into many gyral segments. Each gyral segment presents the morphology of a cone or pyramid, with its base occupying a segment of a gyrus and its apex directed perpendicularly toward the underlying periventricular matrix.[17] Because all gyral segments are delineated by the sulci and the fissures, these also converge toward the underlying ventricles.

The main sulci and fissure used to approach the lateral ventricle are the interhemispheric fissure, the superior frontal sulcus, the sylvian fissure, the inferior circular sulcus of the insula, the occipitotemporal sulcus, the intraparietal sulcus, and the parieto-occipital sulcus. Each sulcus will be presented in detail under the specific approach in which that sulcus is involved.

Vascular Relationships

This section emphasizes only the veins located in the ventricular cavity. Other veins or arteries are discussed under each specific approach in which those veins or arteries are involved. The deep venous system is divided in ventricular and cisternal groups.[18,19] The ventricular veins are subependymal veins that drain the basal ganglia, thalamus, internal capsule, corpus callosum, septum pellucidum, fornix, and deep white matter. They converge on the lateral edge of the lateral ventricles, where they split into a forniceal (medial) group or a thalamic (lateral) group, based on whether they course through the thalamic or forniceal side of the choroidal fissure.

The thalamic group drains the lateral wall, floor of the frontal horn, body, atrium, and occipital horn, and roof of the temporal horn. The forniceal group drains the medial wall and the roof of the frontal horn, body, atrium, occipital horn, and floor of the temporal horn. These veins are named mainly according to the location they course: frontal horn: anterior caudate and anterior septal veins (**Figs. 41–1A,B, 41–8E**). Body of the lateral ventricle: thalamostriate, thalamocaudate veins, posterior caudate, and posterior septal veins (**Fig. 41–1B**). Atrium and the occipital horn: medial and lateral atrial veins (**Fig. 41–1A**). Temporal horn: inferior ventricular, amygdala, and transverse hippocampal veins (**Fig. 41–1H.**). Deep thalamic veins: anterior thalamic and superior thalamic veins. Superficial thalamic veins: anterior superficial thalamic, superior superficial thalamic, and posterior superficial thalamic veins; and choroidal veins; superior choroidal and inferior choroidal veins (**Figs. 41–1B, 41–8G**).[2,19]

◆ Surgical Approaches to the Lateral Ventricles

Anterior Transcallosal Interhemispheric Approach

The anterior interhemispheric transcallosal approach can be used to reach the lesions located in the frontal horn, body of the lateral ventricle, and anterior third ventricle (**Fig. 41–2A**). The anatomical aspects involved in this approach are briefly reviewed here.

Anatomical Considerations

The interhemispheric fissure is located in the midline between the medial surfaces of the frontal, parietal, and occipital lobes of the two hemispheres. The interhemispheric fissure contains the falx, a dural fold that is attached anteriorly to the cribriform plate, and arches above the genu, the body, and the splenium of the corpus callosum to fuse posteriorly with the tentorium along the straight sinus. The overall morphology of the falx resembles a sickle, with its posterior part broader than its anterior part. In general, the falx is in contact with the splenium and with the posterior half of the body of the corpus callosum. This information is particularly useful in approaching the corpus callosum through the interhemispheric fissure by following the falx: for the posterior interhemispheric approach, the white neural tissue located immediately ahead of the edge of the falx is the corpus callosum (**Fig. 41–2B**). This landmark is not valid for the anterior interhemispheric approach aiming at the anterior half of the corpus callosum. Because the falx is narrower anteriorly, the edge of the falx usually terminates at the level of the cingulate gyrus or higher and does not reach the corpus callosum. At its superior, anterior, and posterior portions, the two dural sheaths of the falx split to constitute the superior sagittal sinus (**Fig. 41–2A**).

The sulci and gyri involved in the anterior interhemispheric transcallosal approach belong to the medial surface of the frontal lobe. The general organization of the sulci and gyri on this surface can be compared with that of a three-layer roll; the inner layer is represented by the corpus callosum, the intermediate layer by the cingulate gyrus, and the outer layer by the medial frontal gyrus, paracentral lobule, precuneus, cuneus, and lingual gyrus. The cingulate gyrus is separated inferiorly from the corpus callosum by the callosal sulcus, and superiorly from the outer layer by the cingulate sulcus. The cingulate sulcus presents two secondary rami of particular importance: the paracentral ramus, which ascends from the cingulate sulcus at the level of the midpoint of the corpus callosum and separates the medial frontal gyrus anteriorly from the paracentral lobule posteriorly, and the marginal ramus, which ascends from the cingulate sulcus at the level of the splenium of the corpus callosum and separates the paracentral lobule anteriorly from the precuneus posteriorly (**Fig. 41–2B**). The marginal ramus of the cingulate sulcus intercepts the postcentral gyrus in almost 100% of cases.[20,21] The marginal ramus is an important landmark to determine the location of the sensory or motor areas in the lateral convexity through midsagittal magnetic resonance imaging (MRI) because the central sulcus is the one located immediately anterior to the marginal ramus (**Fig. 41–2B**).

The paracentral and the marginal rami determine the paracentral lobule, which is linked with movements of the contralateral lower limb and perineal region and is involved in voluntary control over defecation and micturition.[5,9] The paracentral lobule comprises the anterior part of the postcentral gyrus, the precentral gyrus, and the posterior portion of the superior frontal gyrus. The paracentral lobule is located above the posterior half of the corpus callosum, and it is generally not involved in the anterior interhemispheric transcallosal approaches.

Vascular Relationships

The medial surface of the frontal lobe involved in this approach is drained by the medial frontal veins.[22] They can empty either superiorly into the superior sagittal sinus or inferiorly. Inferiorly, the medial frontal veins can empty either into the inferior sagittal sinus or into the veins that pass around the corpus callosum to drain into the anterior end of the basal vein. The veins that drain into the superior sagittal sinus are the anteromedial frontal, centromedial frontal, posteromedial frontal, and paracentral veins. They drain the majority of the surface of the medial frontal gyrus and the adjoining part of the cingulate gyrus; they commonly curve over the superior margin of the hemisphere onto the upper part of the lateral surface, where they join the terminal end of the veins from the lateral surface before emptying into the superior sagittal sinus (**Fig. 41–2C**). The veins that drain into the inferior sagittal sinus or into the basal vein are the anterior pericallosal, paraterminal, and anterior cerebral veins. The veins that drain the lateral surface of the frontal lobe toward the superior sagittal sinus are the frontopolar; anterior, middle, and posterior frontal; precentral; and central veins (**Fig. 41–2D**).

Involved in this approach are the A3, A4, and A5 segments of the anterior cerebral artery (ACerA). The ACerA is classified according to Fisher in five segments:[23-26] A1 segment: extends from the bifurcation of the internal carotid artery to the anterior communicating artery (ACommA). A2 segment: extends from the ACommA to the junction between the rostrum and the genu of the corpus callosum. A3 segment: extends from the genu of the corpus callosum to the point where the artery turns sharply and posteriorly above the genu of the corpus callosum. The A2 and A3 segments together are also called the ascending segment. The A4 and A5

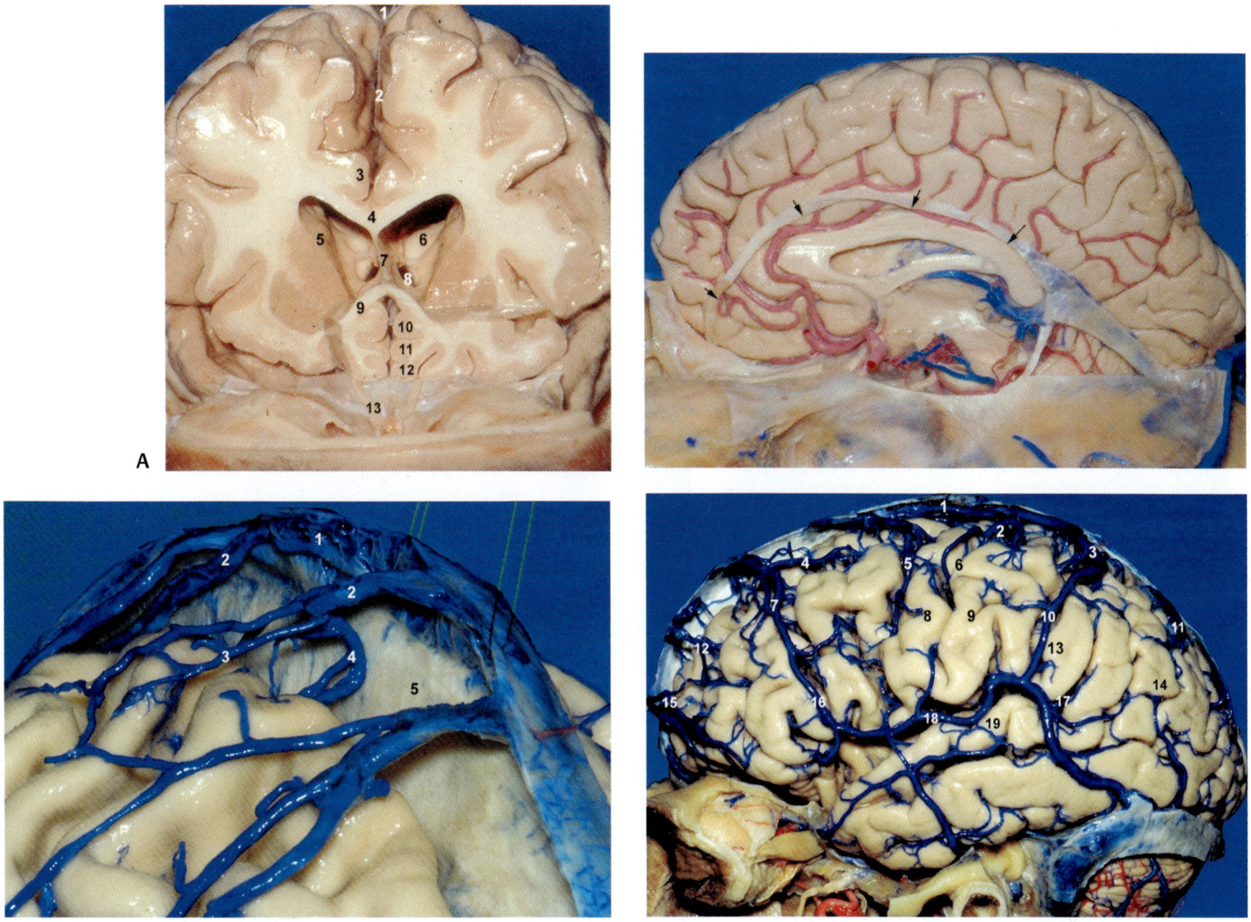

Figure 41–2 **(A)** Frontal view. **1**, superior sagittal sinus; **2**, falx; **3**, cingulate gyrus; **4**, corpus callosum; **5**, head of the caudate nucleus; **6**, thalamus; **7**, septum pellucidum; **8**, foramen of Monro; **9**, rostrum of the corpus callosum; **10**, cingulate gyrus; **11**, medial frontal gyrus; **12**, rectus gyrus; **13**, olfactory tract. **(B)** Midsagittal view. The edge of the falx has been preserved (arrows). For other legends, please refer to **Fig. 41–1C. (C)** Anterolateral view of the parasagittal area of the right hemisphere. **1**, superior sagittal sinus; **2**, veins draining into the superior sagittal sinus; **3**, veins from the lateral surface of the cerebrum; **4**, veins from the medial surface of the cerebrum. **(D)** Lateral view of the left hemisphere. **1**, superior sagittal sinus; **2**, central vein; **3**, vein of Trollard (in this case is also the postcentral vein); **4**, posterior frontal vein; **5**, precentral vein; **6**, central sulcus; **7**, middle frontal vein; **8**, precentral gyrus; **9**, postcentral gyrus; **10**, vein of Trollard; **11**, anterior parietal vein; **12**, anterior frontal vein; **13**, supramarginal gyrus; **14**, angular gyrus; **15**, frontopolar vein; **16**, frontosylvian vein; **17**, anterior ascending ramus of the sylvian fissure; **18**, superficial sylvian vein; **19**, superior temporal gyrus.

(Continued on pages 516,517, and 518)

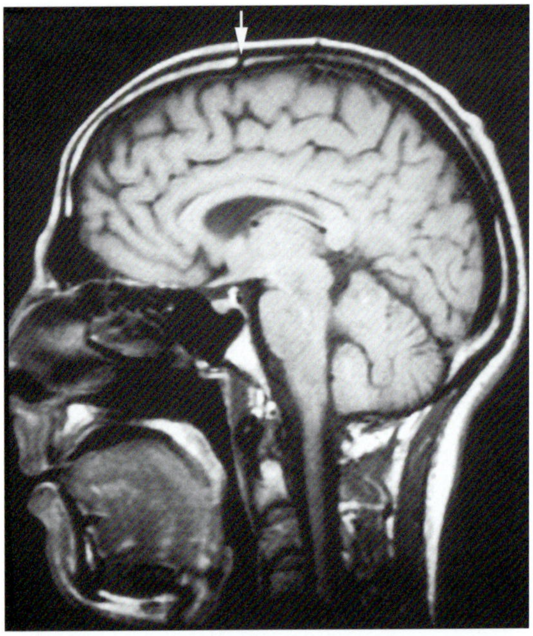

(*Continued*) **Figure 41–2** **(E)** Midsagittal view; coronal suture (arrow). **(F)** A horseshoe skin incision. **(G)** Posterolateral view of **Fig. 41–2F.** **(H)** A bicoronal skin incision. **(I)** The posterolateral view of **Fig. 41–2H.**

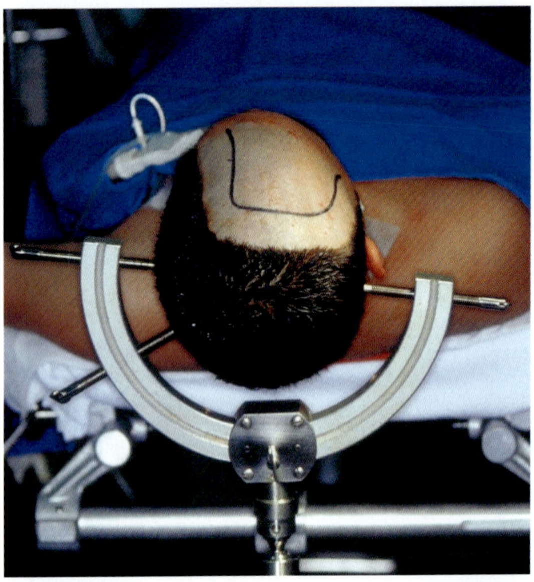

F

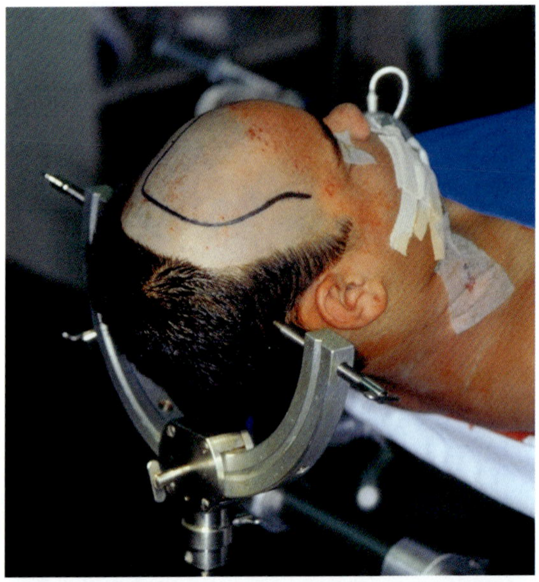

G

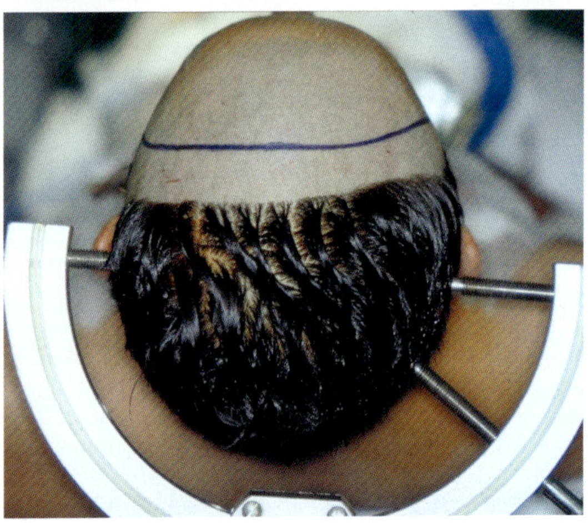

H

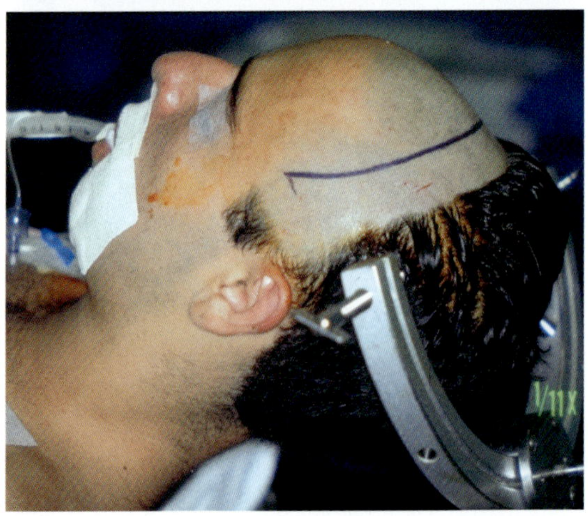

I

(*Continued on pages 517 and 518*)

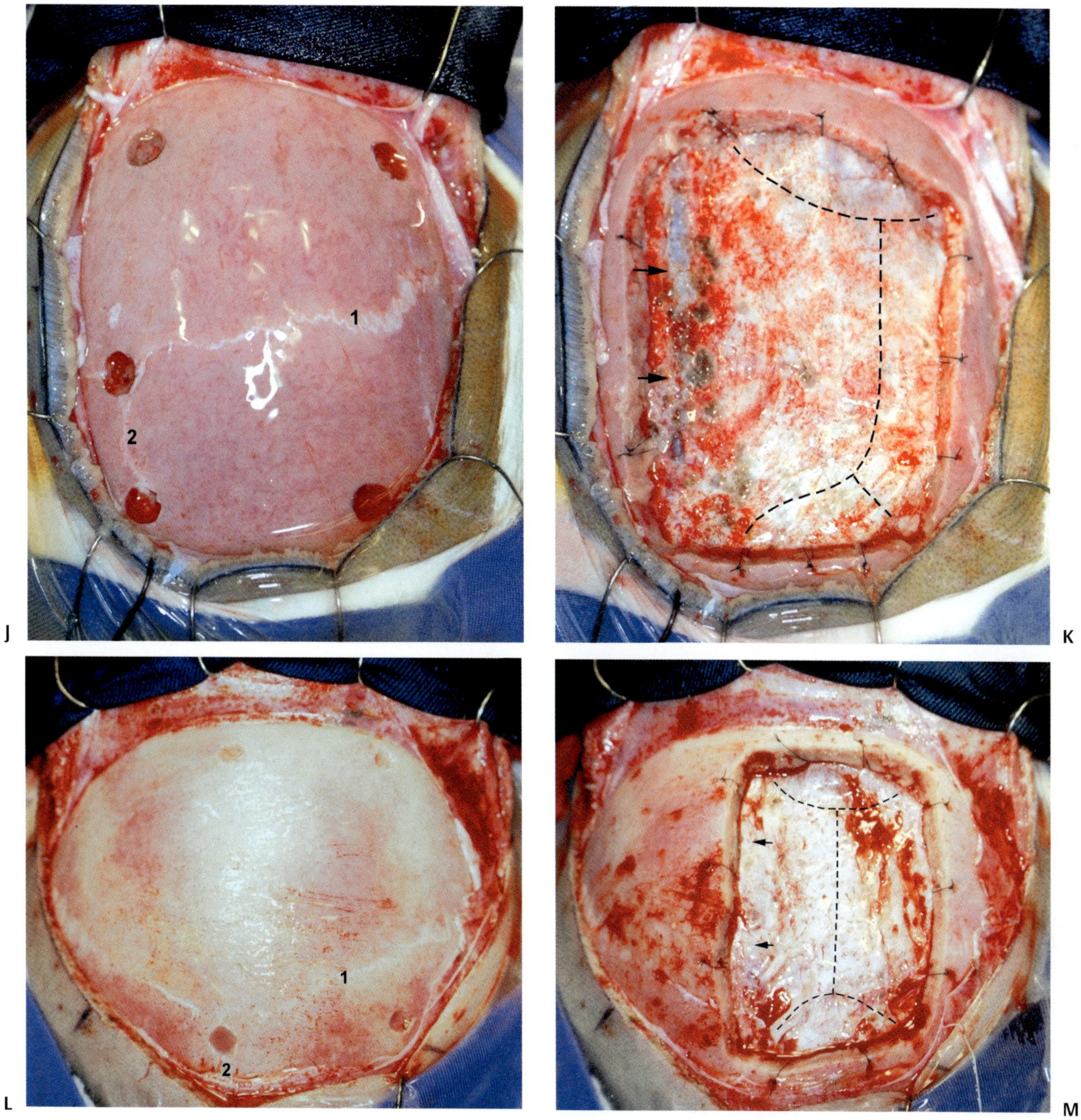

(*Continued*) **Figure 41–2** **(J)** The surgical exposure after the horseshoe skin incision. For the anterior transcallosal approach, it is not necessary to extend the craniotomy as posteriorly to the coronal suture as shown in this figure. **1**, coronal suture; **2**, sagittal suture. **(K)** After the removal of the bone flap, the superior sagittal sinus is exposed. The dotted line shows the dural opening. Superior sagittal sinus (arrows). **(L)** Surgical exposure following the bicoronal incision. **1**, coronal suture; **2**, sagittal suture. **(M)** After the removal of the bone flap, the superior sagittal sinus is exposed. The dotted line indicates an alternative dural opening. Superior sagittal sinus (arrows).

(*Continued on page 518*)

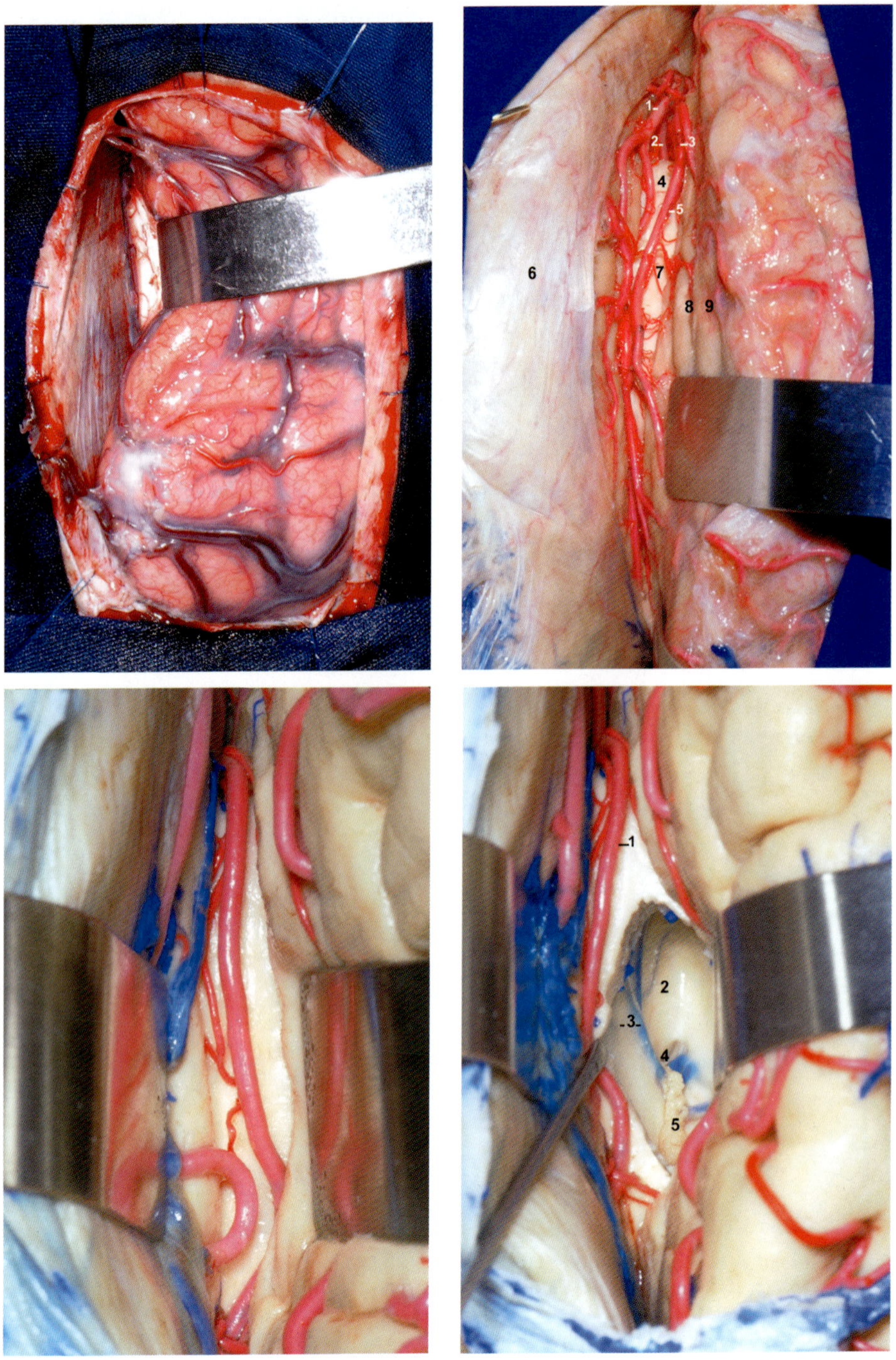

N O P Q

(*Continued*) **Figure 41–2** **(N)** The dura has been opened and the underlying brain tissue exposed. The superior sagittal sinus is further retracted medially, exposing the falx and the interhemispheric fissure. Whenever possible, the veins must be preserved. **(O)** Anatomical dissection of the anterior portion of the interhemispheric fissure. **1**, left pericallosal artery (A3 segment); **2**, left pericallosal artery (A2 segment); **3**, right pericallosal artery; **4**, genu of the corpus callosum; **5**, right pericallosal artery (A4 segment); **6**, falx; **7**, body of the corpus callosum; **8**, cingulate gyrus and sulcus; **9**, medial frontal gyrus. **(P)** Anatomical dissection of the interhemispheric fissure. A magnified view of the body of the corpus callosum after separating both cingulate gyri. **(Q)** Continuation of **Fig. 41–2P.** After the callosotomy, the frontal horn and the body of the lateral ventricle are exposed. **1**, pericallosal artery; **2**, rostrum of the corpus callosum; **3**, septum pellucidum and anterior septal vein; **4**, foramen of Monro; **5**, choroid plexus of the body of the lateral ventricle.

segments extend above the corpus callosum, from the genu to the splenium. These two segments together are also called the horizontal segment. The separation between these two segments is the point bisected in the lateral view behind the coronal suture. The segment of the ACerA distal to the ACommA (A2 to A5) has also been called the pericallosal artery. The two first cortical branches of the ACerA supplying the medial surface, the orbitofrontal and the frontopolar arteries, usually arise from the A2 segment. The segments A3 to A5 give rise to other cortical branches to supply the medial surface of the hemisphere. The A3 segment is a frequent site of origin for the anterior, middle internal frontal, and callosomarginal arteries. The paracentral artery frequently stems from the A4 segment. The A5 segment gives rise to the superior and inferior parietal arteries. All the cortical branches arise more frequently from the pericallosal than from the callosomarginal artery (**Fig. 41–2B**).

For the anterior interhemispheric transcallosal approach, in which the goal is to reach the anterior part or the anterior half of the corpus callosum, the coronal suture can be a very helpful external landmark; the relationship between the coronal suture and the anterior half of the corpus callosum can be visualized in **Fig. 41–2E.** In the anterior transcallosal approach, the patient is in the supine position with the head elevated and slightly flexed (**Fig. 41–2F–I**), without compressing the jugular veins. It is important to have the head flexed in a way that will constitute a comfortable angle for a neurosurgeon sitting on a stool and operating with the microscope. It is obvious but important to emphasize the correct placement of the head holder to avoid limiting the skin incision and obstructing the free movement of the surgeon's hands around the head.

It is helpful, but not mandatory, prior to the insertion of the lumbar drainage, to "relax" the brain and facilitate the exploration through the interhemispheric fissure. The lesions located in the frontal horn and body of the lateral ventricle can be approached through the same side; however, for lesions located in the midline, as in third ventricular lesions, it can be approached from either side depending on the handedness of the surgeon and the hemisphere dominance of the patient. It is more comfortable for a right-handed surgeon to approach the lesion from the right side.

The skin incision can be of several fashions as displayed in **Fig. 41–2F–I,** depending mainly on the hairline of the patient. Care should be taken not to extend into the bare skin. The craniotomy is programmed based on the location of the coronal suture at the midline. The relation between the coronal suture and the corpus callosum can be evaluated preoperatively via MRI (**Fig. 41–2E**). In most cases, the coronal suture is located just before the midway between the splenium and the genu of the corpus callosum. In the anatomical position, the corridor involved for the anterior interhemispheric transcallosal approach can be seen in **Fig. 41–2B.**

An approximate 11 × 7 cm craniotomy is performed (**Fig. 41–2J–M**), exposing the superior sagittal sinus to allow a further medial retraction.

The posterior limit of the craniotomy can be at or slightly behind the coronal suture but does not have to extend too far behind the coronal suture because of the risk of injuring the motor and or supplementary motor areas by retraction. According to Ebeling et al,[27] the central sulcus can be located 2 to 7 cm behind the coronal suture. The dura mater then is anchored to the edge of the craniotomy to avoid the extradural hemorrhage.

The dural opening can be performed in a horseshoe fashion with its base toward the superior sagittal sinus, as demonstrated in **Fig. 41–2K,M.** Whenever possible, all veins draining the lateral surface of the frontal lobe toward the superior sagittal sinus must be dissected and preserved. The dura is reflected toward the midline, and the superior sagittal sinus is retracted medially using sutures (**Fig. 41–2N**) or retractors. This maneuver creates an additional working space and reduces the lateral retraction of the brain. It is important to create an unobstructed pathway from the surface to the corpus callosum (**Fig. 41–2N**).

The dissection is performed through the interhemispheric fissure, separating the arachnoid membrane that covers the medial surface of the brain from the falx. Some small veins that run from the medial surface of the brain to the falx must be coagulated and sectioned. As already mentioned, the anterior portion of the falx is narrower and its edge terminates before reaching the corpus callosum, and then the cingulate gyri appear. Sometimes the two attached cingulate gyri can resemble the corpus callosum, and the callosomarginal artery and the cingulate sulcus can be misinterpreted as pericallosal artery and the callosal sulcus.

Once in the callosal cistern, the pericallosal arteries are identified, and the surface of the corpus callosum is inspected (**Fig. 41–2O,P**). The anterior portion of the corpus callosum is then entered between the two pericallosal arteries, after coagulating its surface. Usually a 1.5 to 2.0 cm callosotomy is sufficient to approach most of the lesions (**Fig. 41–2Q**).

For lesions located more laterally in the frontal horn or the body of the lateral ventricle, the callosal sulcus must be dissected laterally and the callosotomy performed more laterally. Once inside the lateral ventricle, the septum pellucidum can be opened to allow further drainage of the cerebrospinal fluid (CSF) from the contralateral ventricle, allowing further relaxation of the brain. It is advisable to keep in mind that the genu of the internal capsule comes to the surface laterally to the foramen of Monro, usually where the thalamostriate vein turns medially toward the internal cerebral vein.

Sometimes the anatomy is tremendously distorted by the lesion, and it is difficult even to identify which side of the ventricle one is in. In this case the location of the thalamostriate vein in relation to the choroid plexus is helpful: as on the right ventricle, the thalamostriate vein will be located at the right side of the choroid plexus, and vice versa for the left ventricle.[11]

Transsylvian Approach

The transsylvian approach can be used to approach lesions located in the basal cisterns, anterior portion of the temporal horn, and anterior portion of the third ventricle.[17,28–30]

Anatomical Considerations

The sylvian fissure is located on the basal and lateral surfaces of the cerebrum and presents a superficial and a deep part.

The superficial part is constituted by a stem and three rami (**Fig. 41–3A**); the stem extends medially from the semilunar gyrus of the uncus, between the basal surfaces of the frontal and the temporal lobes, to the lateral end of the sphenoid ridge, where the stem divides into anterior horizontal, anterior ascending, and posterior rami on the lateral surface of the cerebrum. The deep (cisternal) part is divided in an anterior part—the sphenoidal compartment, and a posterior part—the operculoinsular compartment.[31] The sphenoidal compartment arises in the region of the limen insulae, at the lateral margin of the anterior perforated substance (**Fig. 41–3B**), and it is a narrow space posterior to the sphenoid ridge between the frontal and temporal lobes that communicates medially with the carotid cistern (sylvian vallecula).[32,33] The operculoinsular compartment is formed by two narrow clefts: the opercular cleft between the opposing

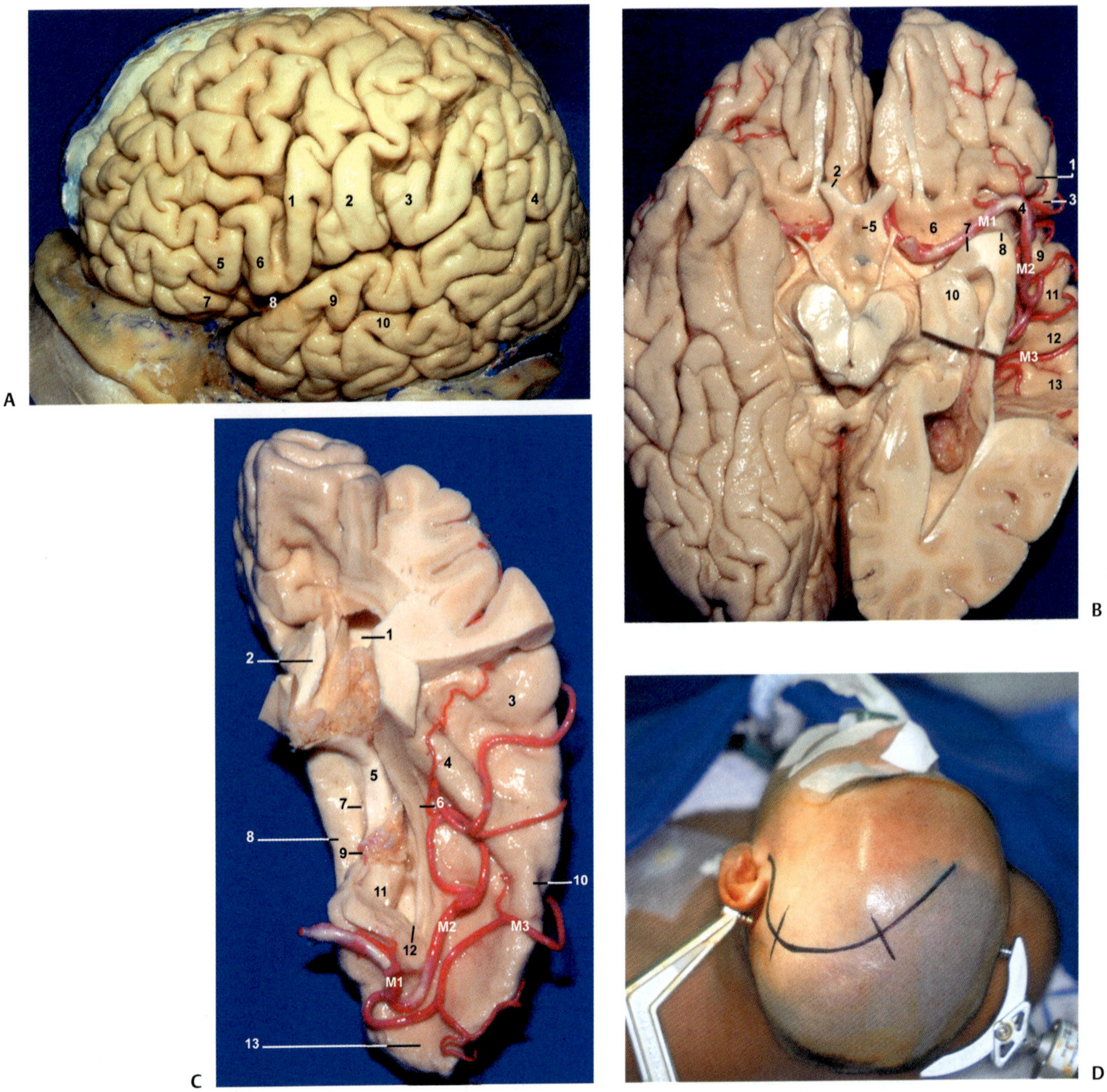

Figure 41–3 **(A)** Lateral view of the left hemisphere. **1**, precentral gyrus; **2**, postcentral gyrus; **3**, supramarginal gyrus; **4**, angular gyrus; **5**, pars triangularis of the inferior frontal gyrus; **6**, pars opercularis of the inferior frontal gyrus; **7**, pars orbitalis of the inferior frontal gyrus; **8**, posterior ramus of the sylvian fissure; **9**, superior temporal gyrus; **10**, middle temporal gyrus. **(B)** Basal view. **1**, pars orbitalis; **2**, optic nerve; **3**, pars triangularis; **4**, genu of the middle cerebral artery; **5**, pituitary stalk; **6**, anterior perforated substance; **7**, amygdala; **8**, limen insulae; **9**, pars opercularis; **10**, head of the hippocampus; **11**, precentral gyrus; **12**, postcentral gyrus; **13**, supramarginal gyrus; **M1**, sphenoidal segment of the middle cerebral artery; **M2**, insular segment of the middle cerebral artery; **M3**, opercular segment of the middle cerebral artery. **(C)** Superior view of the right temporal operculum. **1**, atrium; **2**, bulb of the callosum; **3**, planum temporale; **4**, anterior transverse temporal gyrus (Heschl's gyrus); **5**, fornix; **6**, temporal stem; **7**, dentate gyrus; **8**, parahippocampal gyrus; **9**, inferior choroidal point; **10**, superior temporal gyrus; **11**, head of the hippocampus; **12**, limen insulae; **13**, planum polare; **M1**, sphenoidal segment of the middle cerebral artery; **M2**, insular segment of the middle cerebral artery; **M3**, opercular segment of the middle cerebral artery. **(D)** The patient positioning and the skin incision for the trans-sylvian approach. The incision starts at the superior edge of the zygomatic arch and curves posteriorly to end at the midline behind the hairline. The posterior extension of the incision will vary depending on the extent of the lesion.

(Continued on pages 521and 522)

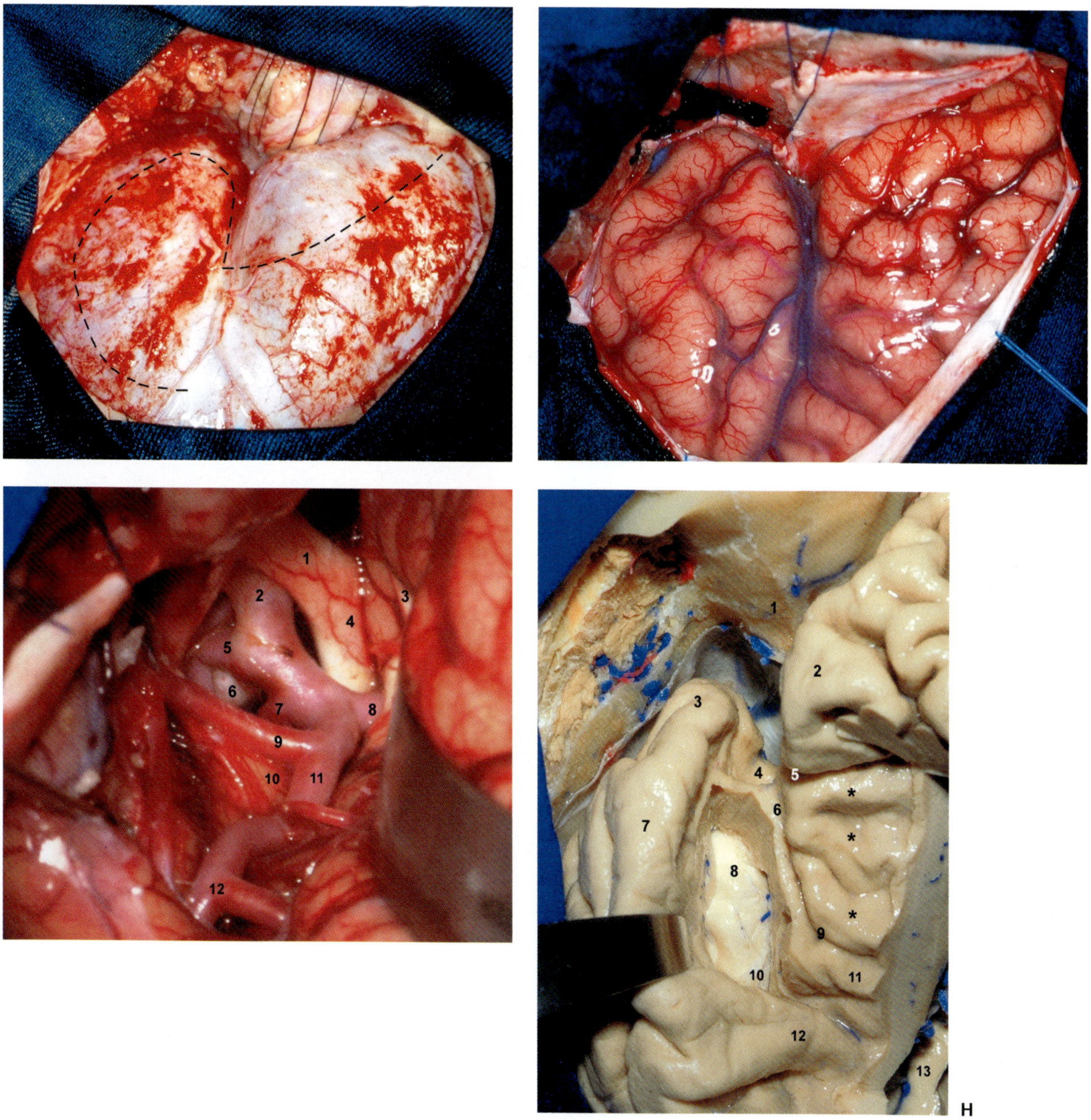

(*Continued*) **Figure 41–3** **(E)** After the craniotomy, the dura is exposed. Sometimes the removal of the orbital ridge (as shown in this case) and/or the removal of the zygomatic arch can increase the exposure. The dotted line shows the dural opening. **(F)** The dura has been opened. The sylvian fissure and the frontal and temporal lobes are exposed. **(G)** After opening the chiasmatic, carotid, and sphenoidal segment of the sylvian fissure, their contents can be identified. **1**, left optic nerve; **2**, carotid artery; **3**, olfactory tract; **4**, chiasm; **5**, posterior communicating artery; **6**, posterior clinoid process; **7**, anterior choroidal artery; **8**, anterior cerebral artery (A1); **9**, early branch of the middle cerebral artery; **10**, anterior segment of the uncus; **11**, middle cerebral artery (M1 segment); **12**, middle cerebral artery (bifurcation). **(H)** Anatomical dissection of the trans-sylvian approach to lesions located in the temporal horn through the inferior circular sulcus of insula. The frontal and parietal opercula have been removed to display the relationship between the insula and the temporal horn. **1**, sphenoid ridge; **2**, pars orbitalis; **3**, temporal pole; **4**, limen insulae; **5**, anterior limiting sulcus of the insula; **6**, inferior circular sulcus of the insula; **7**, superior temporal gyrus; **8**, head of the hippocampus; **9**, central sulcus of the insula; **10**, choroid plexus of the temporal horn; **11**, long gyrus of the insula; **12**, Heschl's gyrus; **13**, atrium; short gyri of the insula.

(*Continued on page 522*)

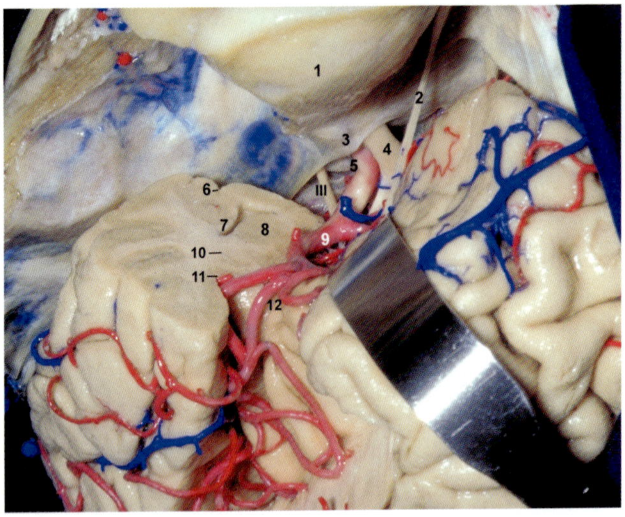

I

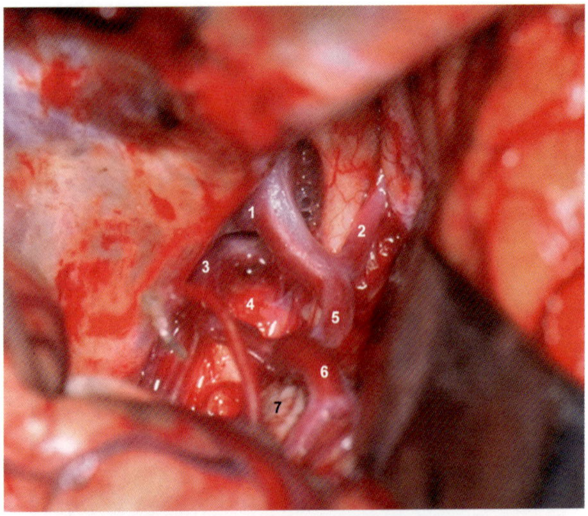

J

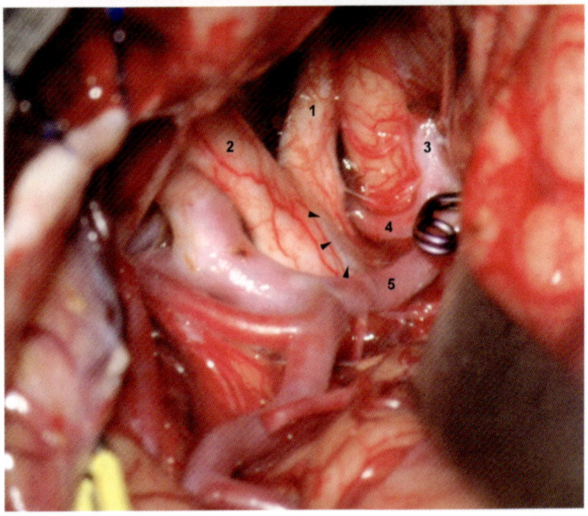

K

(*Continued*) **Figure 41–3** **(I)** Anatomical dissection as in left trans-sylvian approach. A coronal section has been made at the limen insulae to display the normal arrangement of the mesial temporal structures in this approach. **1**, orbit; **2**, olfactory tract; **3**, anterior clinoid process; **4**, optic nerve; **5**, carotid artery and posterior clinoid process; **6**, collateral sulcus; **7**, collateral eminence; **8**, amygdala; **9**, M1 segment; **10**, temporal stem; **11**, inferior circular sulcus of insula; **12**, limen insulae; **III**, oculomotor nerve. **(J)** After removal of the lesion located at the anterior mesial temporal lobe through the trans-sylvian approach, the remaining structures can be seen. **1**, posterior communicating artery; **2**, anterior cerebral artery (A1); **3**, posterior cerebral artery (P2A segment); **4**, crus cerebri (anterior portion); **5**, middle cerebral artery (M1 segment); **6**, genu of the middle cerebral artery; **7**, limen insulae. **(K)** An anterior communicating artery aneurysm case. The anterior portion of the third ventricle can also be accessed through the lamina terminalis, using the trans-sylvian approach. **1**, right optic nerve; **2**, left optic nerve; **3**, right anterior cerebral artery (A2 segment); **4**, right anterior cerebral artery (A1 segment); **5**, left anterior cerebral artery (A1 segment). Lamina terminalis (arrowheads).

lips of the frontoparietal and the temporal opercula; and the insular cleft, which has a superior limb located between the insula and the frontoparietal opercula, and an inferior limb between the insula and the temporal operculum[31] (**Fig. 41–1G**).

The opercular cleft, the gyri that constitute the frontal and parietal opercula of the sylvian fissure, are from posterior to anteriorly the supramarginal, the postcentral, and the precentral gyri, pars opercularis, triangularis, and orbitalis (**Fig. 41–3A**), and the gyri that constitute the temporal operculum of the sylvian fissure, from posterior to anteriorly, are the planum temporale, Heschl's gyrus, and the planum polare[34] (**Fig. 41–3C**). Each gyrus of the frontoparietal opercula is closely related to its counterpart on the temporal side.

The insular cleft is best defined by the anatomy of the insula. The medial wall of the sylvian fissure is the insula or island of Reil, which can be seen only when the lips of the sylvian fissure are widely separated. The insula has the shape of a pyramid with its apex directed inferiorly (**Fig. 41–1A,G**), and it connects the temporal lobe to the posterior orbital gyrus via the limen insulae (**Fig. 41–3B**). The limen insulae is composed of fibers of the uncinate fasciculus covered by a thin layer of gray matter. The word *limen* means threshold, and the term was introduced to indicate that the limen insulae serves as a threshold between the carotid cistern medially and the sylvian fissure laterally.[33] The insula is encircled and separated from the opercula by a deep furrow called the circular or limiting sulcus of the insula, which presents three parts: the superior, anterior, and inferior parts. From the limen insulae the sulci and gyri of the insula are directed superiorly in a radial manner. Anteriorly the insula is formed by three to five short gyri and posteriorly by two long gyri.[35]

From microsurgical and radiological viewpoints, the insula represents the external covering of a mass constituted by the extreme, external, and internal capsules, and the claustrum, basal ganglia, and thalamus. The superior, anterior, inferior, and posterior limits of the insula on the lateral projection correspond to superior, anterior, inferior, and posterior limits of the mass.

The frontal horn, the body, and the temporal horn are related, respectively, to the anterior circular, superior circular, and inferior circular sulcus of the insula; the atrium is related to the junction between the superior and inferior circular sulcus of the insula.

The most important content of the sylvian fissure is the middle cerebral artery,[31,36] which is divided into four segments:

1. The M1 or sphenoidal segment extends from the bifurcation of the internal carotid artery to the limen insulae. The M1 courses first in the carotid cistern then continues in the sphenoidal compartment; it is related superiorly to the anterior perforated substance,[37] inferiorly to the planum polare of the temporal lobe, anteriorly to the lesser wing of the sphenoid; posteriorly, the proximal half of the M1 segment courses in the carotid cistern and is related to the anteromedial surface of the uncus, whereas the distal half courses in the stem of the sylvian fissure and is related posteriorly to the limen insulae (**Fig. 41–3C**). The M1 segment presents two types of branches: the lateral lenticulostriate arteries, which arise mostly from the superior or posterosuperior aspect of the M1 and penetrate the anterior perforated substance, and the early branches that course toward the temporal lobe to supply the temporal pole. The bifurcation of the middle cerebral artery occurs before it reaches the limen of the insulae in 86% of cases.
2. The M2 or insular segment is related to the surface of the insula and extends from the limen insulae to the inferior or superior circular sulcus of the insula; it runs in the insular compartment of the sylvian fissure and is constituted by superior and inferior trunks and their branches. After reaching the superior or inferior circular sulcus of insula, the M2 branches enter the opercular compartment and are called M3 segment.
3. The M3 or opercular segment runs in the opercular compartment and is related to the frontal and parietal opercula superiorly and to the temporal operculum inferiorly, and the M3 depicts exactly the morphology of the opercula to which they are related.
4. The fourth segment, the M4, or cortical, segment, extends from the sylvian fissure to the lateral surface of the cerebrum. The deep middle cerebral vein also travels in the sylvian fissure. It is formed by insular veins that run on the surface of the insula and unite at the limen insulae; the deep middle cerebral vein usually courses in the sphenoid compartment, then proceeds medially into the carotid cistern under the anterior perforated substance to receive the anterior cerebral, olfactory, fronto-orbital, and inferior striate veins to constitute the first segment of the basal vein of Rosenthal.

For the transsylvian approach, the patient is placed in the supine position, and the head is secured with a Mayfield or Sugita head holder. The head, is positioned following four movements: (1) elevation, to facilitate the venous drainage; (2) rotation of ~25 degrees (with exaggerated rotation the temporal lobe will "fall" over the frontal lobe, making the sylvian fissure more difficult to be split); (3) extension of the neck; and (4) "tilt" of the neck (to bring the sylvian fissure parallel to the surgeon)[28,29] (**Fig. 41–3D**).

The skin incision is usually an arch, with a variable posterior temporal extension, depending on how posteriorly the lesion extends. After the interfascial dissection[17] and the reflection of the temporalis muscle, the craniotomy is performed. For lesions located in the temporal horn, it is advisable to have a good exposure of the temporal lobe, having the craniotomy performed down to the floor of the middle fossa, allowing additional working space for the surgeon. For larger lesions with a considerable posterior extension, the removal of the orbital ridge, allowing a greater anteroposterior angulation of the surgeon's view, can sometimes be helpful (**Fig. 41–3E**).

The dura is then opened (**Fig. 41–3F**); the dural opening should take advantage of the craniotomy and allow a full exposure of the underlying brain involved in the surgical approach. The usual dural opening performed by the authors is displayed in **Fig. 41–3E.**

The splitting of the sylvian fissure is then performed, and the basal cisterns are opened. The contents of the sylvian fissure and those of the basal cisterns are identified[38] (**Fig. 41–3G**). The inferior circular sulcus of the insula and the limen insula are important landmarks to enter the temporal horn. Under normal conditions, the temporal horn can be reached by dissecting the bottom of the inferior circular sulcus of the insula following its direction, 1 cm posteriorly to the limen insulae; however, it is interesting to emphasize that the more posteriorly is the dissecting site in the inferior circular sulcus, the easier will be the entry into the temporal horn (**Fig. 41–3H**).

The location of the mesial temporal structures and the temporal horn under normal conditions can be seen in **Fig. 41–3I.** Needless to say, the normal anatomy will most likely be distorted by the presence of a lesion; therefore, each case must be carefully examined, and the spatial relationship between the lesion located in the temporal horn and the sylvian fissure evaluated.

After the resection of the anterior mesial temporal structures, the cerebral peduncle and the posterior cerebral artery (PCA) can be visualized (**Fig. 41–3J**). The transsylvian approach can also be utilized for lesions located adjacent to the lamina terminalis, which is the anterior wall of the third ventricle (**Fig. 41–3K**).

Posterior Interhemispheric Transcingular Approach

This approach is indicated to reach the lesions located in the atrium and in the occipital horn of the lateral ventricle. It consists of opening the posterior portion of the interhemispheric fissure and making a small opening on the precuneus or on the isthmus of the cingulate gyrus, just posteriorly to the splenium of the corpus callosum.[17,30]

Anatomical Considerations

As mentioned earlier for the interhemispheric fissure, the posterior portion of the interhemispheric fissure is limited medially by the falx, closely in contact with the splenium of the corpus callosum, inferiorly by the tentorium, and laterally by the precuneus, cuneus, and lingula gyrus.

The precuneus along with the part of the paracentral lobule behind the central sulcus forms the medial part of the parietal lobe. The parieto-occipital and the calcarine sulci determine the cuneus; the cuneus and the medial part of the lingual gyrus are the medial portion of the occipital

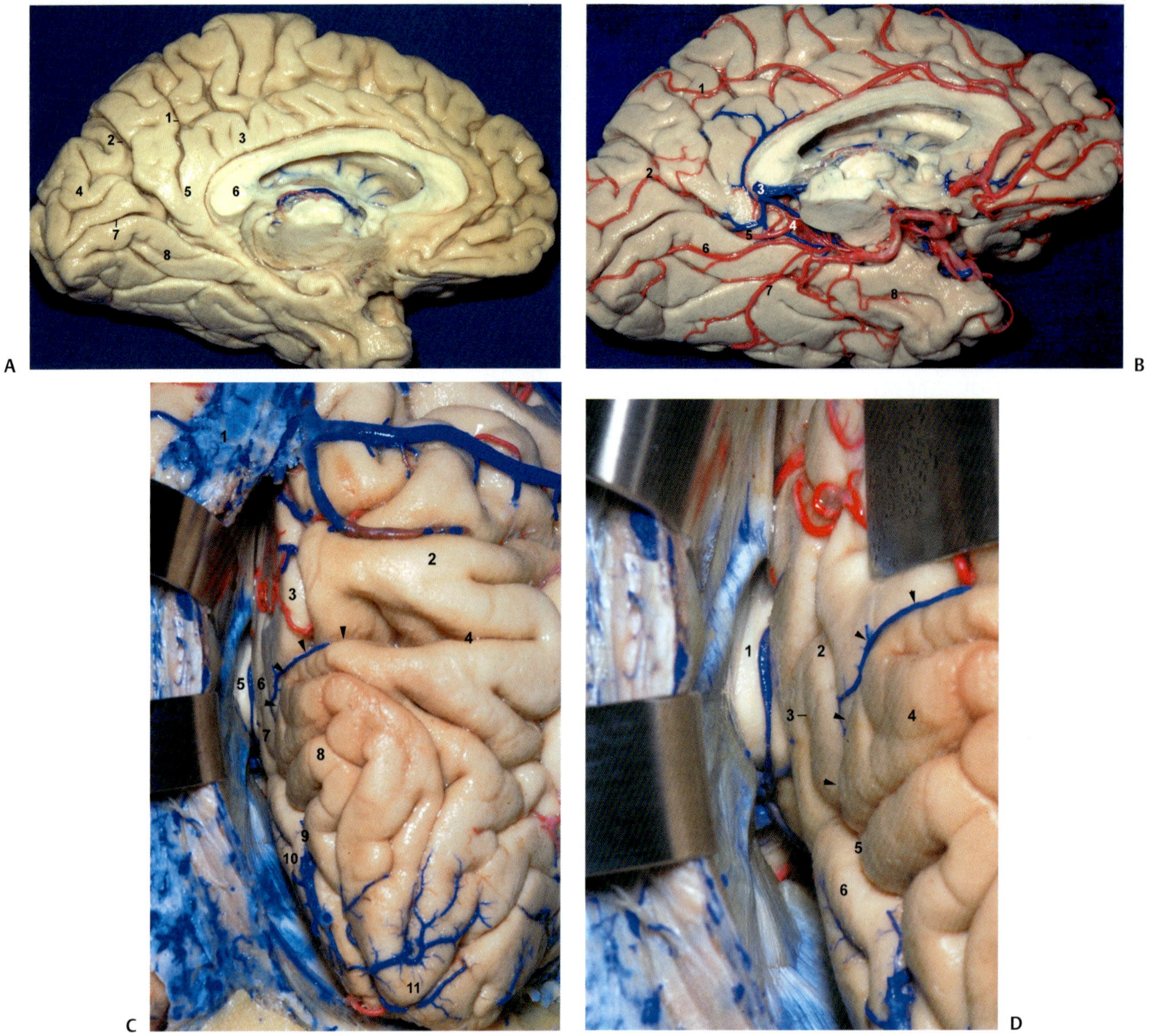

Figure 41–4 **(A)** Midsagittal view of the left hemisphere. **1**, precuneus and subparietal sulcus; **2**, parieto-occipital sulcus; **3**, cingulate gyrus; **4**, cuneus; **5**, isthmus of the cingulate gyrus; **6**, splenium of the corpus callosum; **7**, calcarine sulcus; **8**, lingual gyrus. **(B)** The vascular structures involved in the posterior interhemispheric transcingular approach. **1**, branches from the anterior cerebral artery; **2**, branches from the parieto-occipital artery; **3**, vein of Galen and its tributaries; **4**, P3 segment of the posterior cerebral artery; **5**, P4 segment of the posterior cerebral artery; **6**, inferior temporal artery (posterior group); **7**, inferior temporal artery (intermediate group); **8**, inferior temporal artery (anterior group). **(C)** Posterosuperior view of the right posterior interhemispheric fissure, as in posterior interhemispheric transcingular approach. **1**, superior sagittal sinus; **2**, superior parietal lobule; **3**, precuneus; **4**, parieto-occipital sulcus (on the lateral surface); **5**, splenium of the corpus callosum; **6**, isthmus of the cingulate gyrus; **7**, anterior calcarine sulcus; **8**, cuneus; **9**, calcarine sulcus; **10**, lingual gyrus; **11**, occipital pole. Parieto-occipital sulcus (arrowheads). **(D)** Magnified view of **Fig. 41–4C. 1**, splenium of the corpus callosum; **2**, isthmus of the cingulate gyrus; **3**, anterior calcarine sulcus; **4**, cuneus; **5**, calcarine sulcus; **6**, lingual gyrus. Parieto-occipital sulcus (arrowheads).

lobe. The calcarine sulcus starts at the occipital pole and directs anteriorly, presenting a slightly curved course with its characteristic upward convexity. The calcarine sulcus joins the parieto-occipital sulcus superficially at an acute angle behind the isthmus of the cingulate gyrus, then continues anteriorly to intercept the isthmus of the cingulate gyrus. The portion of the calcarine sulcus anterior to the junction with the parieto-occipital sulcus is called the anterior calcarine sulcus.[39] It is crossed by a buried anterior cuneolingual gyrus and bulges into the medial wall of the atrium of the lateral ventricle as the calcar avis. The part of the calcarine sulcus posterior to the union is called the posterior calcarine sulcus, and it presents the striate (visual) cortex on its upper and lower lips, whereas the anterior calcarine sulcus presents the visual cortex only on its lower lip.[39]

The eloquent areas in this region that must be avoided are the optic radiation and the primary visual cortex; the atrium is devoid of optic radiation on its medial and superior walls, whereas the occipital horn is devoid of optic radiation only on its medial wall (**Fig. 41–4A**).

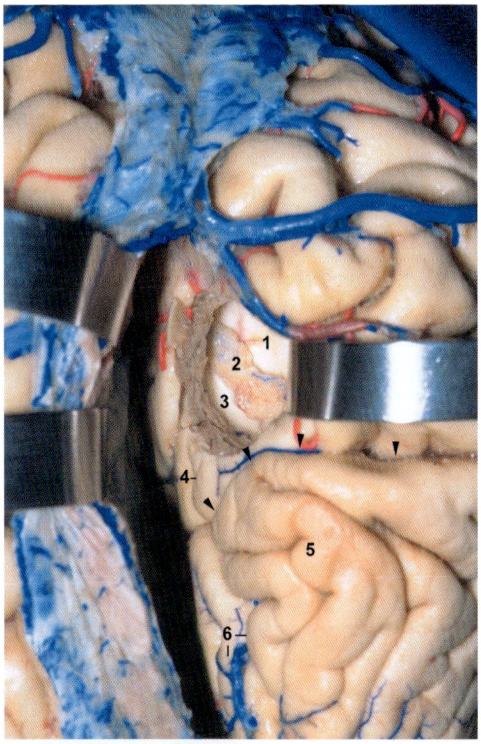

E

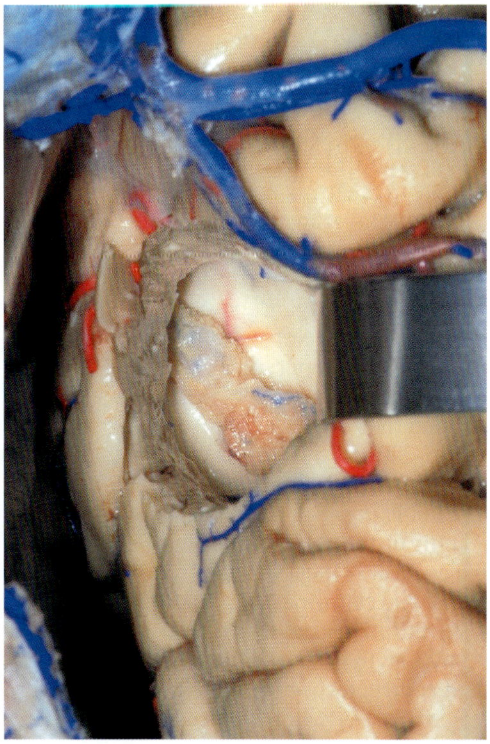

F

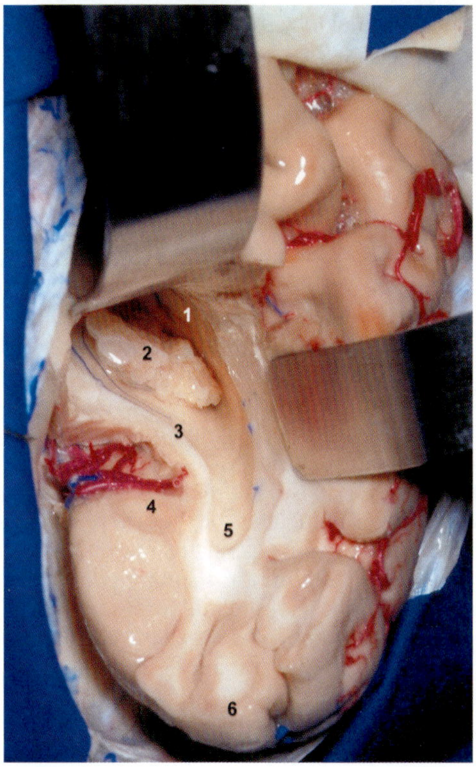

G

(*Continued*) **Figure 41–4 (E)** The isthmus of the cingulate gyrus has been removed to display the atrium of the lateral ventricle. **1**, pulvinar of the thalamus; **2**, choroid plexus; **3**, crus of the fornix; **4**, anterior calcarine sulcus; **5**, cuneus; **6**, calcarine sulcus and the lingual gyrus. Parieto-occipital sulcus (arrowheads). **(F)** Magnified view of **Fig. 41–4E. (G)** The cuneus has been removed to display the arrangement of the intraventricular structures involved in this approach. **1**, thalamus; **2**, glomus; **3**, calcar avis; **4**, lingual gyrus; **5**, occipital horn; **6**, occipital pole.

The surgeon should also be aware of the exact location of the primary visual cortex, when entry is intended into either or both the atrium and the occipital horn from their medial wall. As mentioned earlier, the primary visual cortex is located at the superior and inferior lips of the posterior calcarine sulcus and also at the inferior lip of the anterior calcarine sulcus.

The PCA[40,41] and its terminal branches are the most important vascular elements present in this approach, and it is classified, according to Yasargil and Rhoton, in four segments: P1, P2, P3, and P4. The P1 segment, which extends from the basilar bifurcation to the site where the posterior communicating artery (PCommA) joins the PCA. The P2 segment, which extends from the PCommA to the posterior aspect of the midbrain, is further divided into P2A (anterior) and P2P (posterior) segments. The P2A segment begins at the PCommA and courses around the crus cerebri, inferiorly to the optic tract, AChA[42,43] and basal vein, and medially to the posteromedial surface of the uncus, up to the posterior margin of the crus cerebri. The P2P segment begins at the posterior margin of the crus cerebri and runs laterally to the tegmentum of the midbrain within the ambient cistern, parallel and inferiorly to the basal vein, inferolaterally to the geniculate bodies and pulvinar, and medially to the parahippocampal gyrus to enter the quadrigeminal cistern. The P3 segment begins under the posterior part of the pulvinar in the lateral aspect of the quadrigeminal cistern and ends at the anterior limit of the anterior calcarine sulcus. The P3 is often divided into its major terminal branches, the calcarine and the parieto-occipital arteries, before reaching the anterior limit of the anterior calcarine sulcus. The point where the PCAs from each side are closer to each other is called the collicular or quadrigeminal point. It marks the posterior limit of the midbrain on angiogram. The P4 segment is the cortical branches of the PCA (**Fig. 41–4B**). The parieto-occipital and calcarine arteries are usually terminal branches of the PCA. They arise predominantly from the P3 segment; however, they may sometimes arise from the P2P segment and course, respectively, in the parieto-occipital and the calcarine sulci. As the calcarine sulcus reaches laterally to bulge into the medial wall of the atrium and the occipital horn, the calcarine artery also follows laterally into the depth of the calcarine fissure. The splenial or posterior pericallosal artery supplies the splenium of the corpus callosum, arising from the parieto-occipital artery in 62% of the cases and from the calcarine artery in 12%.

For the surgical approach the patient can be either in the semisitting position or the three-quarter-prone position, with the ipsilateral hemisphere closer to the floor, allowing it to "fall" down by gravity and expose the interhemispheric fissure.

The usual horseshoe skin incision is used by the authors, and a square craniotomy is performed exposing the superior sagittal sinus. This is an important maneuver because it allows a further contralateral retraction of the superior sagittal sinus and the falx, either by sutures or by retractors, increasing the surgeon's working space and visual angle, reducing the unnecessary lateral retraction of the ispilateral hemisphere. The craniotomy does not have to expose either the torcula or the transverse sinus; if necessary a ventricular catheter can be placed to release CSF prior to the dural opening. Then the dura is also opened in a horseshoe fashion with its base toward the superior sagittal sinus; sutures are placed to retract the sinus toward the opposite side, as shown in the anterior interhemispheric approach. The aimed surgical corridor for the parieto-occipital interhemispheric approach is displayed in **Fig. 41–4A,B.**

The bridging veins are dissected and whenever possible preserved. The extension of the parieto-occipital sulcus on the lateral surface of the hemisphere is identified, and the interhemispheric fissure is dissected following the falx and the parieto-occipital sulcus. The splenium of the corpus callosum is identified at the end of the falx (**Fig. 41–4C,D**). If possible, the P3 segment of the PCA is identified as it leaves the quadrigeminal cistern toward the parieto-occipital and the calcarine sulci; the calcarine sulcus is also identified. Direct retraction over the calcarine sulcus should be avoided because it is preferred to retract the cuneus laterally to gain working space. Sometimes significant additional working room can be obtained by dissecting the parieto-occipital sulcus, separating completely the precuneus from the cuneus, to then apply a retractor over the cuneus. At the isthmus of the cingulate gyrus, above the upper edge of the anterior calcarine sulcus, just behind and laterally to the splenium of the corpus callosum, a corticectomy is performed and the dissection proceeds anteriorly and laterally until the atrium is entered (**Figs. 41–4E,F**). The anatomical location of the atrium and the occipital horn for this approach can be seen in **Fig. 41–4G,** after the complete removal of the cuneus.

Occipitotemporal Sulcus Approach

This approach is designed to reach lesions located in the posterior portion of the temporal horn, from the basal surface of the temporal lobe, to avoid the optic radiation that forms part of the roof and mainly the lateral wall of the temporal horn. Any superior or lateral approach to the temporal lobe (e.g., trans-sylvian, via middle temporal gyrus, inferior temporal sulcus) theoretically carries the risk of injuring the optic radiation.

On the basal surface, the temporal lobe is separated posteriorly from the occipital lobe by the basal parietotemporal line, which extends from the preoccipital notch to the junction between the parieto-occipital and calcarine fissures. The basal surface of the temporal lobe presents, from lateral to medially, the inferior temporal gyrus, occipito-temporal sulcus, fusiform gyrus, collateral sulcus, and parahippocampal gyrus (**Fig. 41–3B**). The occipitotemporal sulcus is a lateral to medial, inferior to superiorly oriented sulcus, located medial to the inferior temporal gyrus and pointing toward the collateral eminence (**Fig. 41–5A**). The occipitotemporal sulcus has an anteroposterior orientation and frequently fuses anteriorly and posteriorly with the collateral sulcus, delimiting the fusiform gyrus between them.

For the surgical approach a lumbar catheter is placed before the patient is positioned; the patient is placed in a lateral decubitus position with the head tilted toward the contralateral shoulder as in the subtemporal approach; care should be taken in this maneuver for the risk of impairing the venous drainage. The skin incision can be either horseshoe or question mark fashion, and a square craniotomy is performed down to the base of the middle fossa. Some CSF is drained before the dural opening if this is felt to be tense. The dura is then opened in a horseshoe fashion with its base toward the base of the skull.

The temporal lobe is then inspected, and the inferior temporal gyrus is followed and retracted to expose its continuation on the basal surface. The first sulcus medial to the inferior temporal gyrus on the basal surface is the occipitotemporal sulcus (**Fig. 41–5B**). The occipitotemporal sulcus is continuous in only 36% of cases[39]; therefore, one cannot expect to find it every time on the site intended for entry into the temporal horn. The occipitotemporal sulcus is then dissected beyond its bottom, following its orientation until the temporal horn is reached (**Fig. 41–5C,D**) (the occipitotemporal sulcus points toward the collateral eminence).

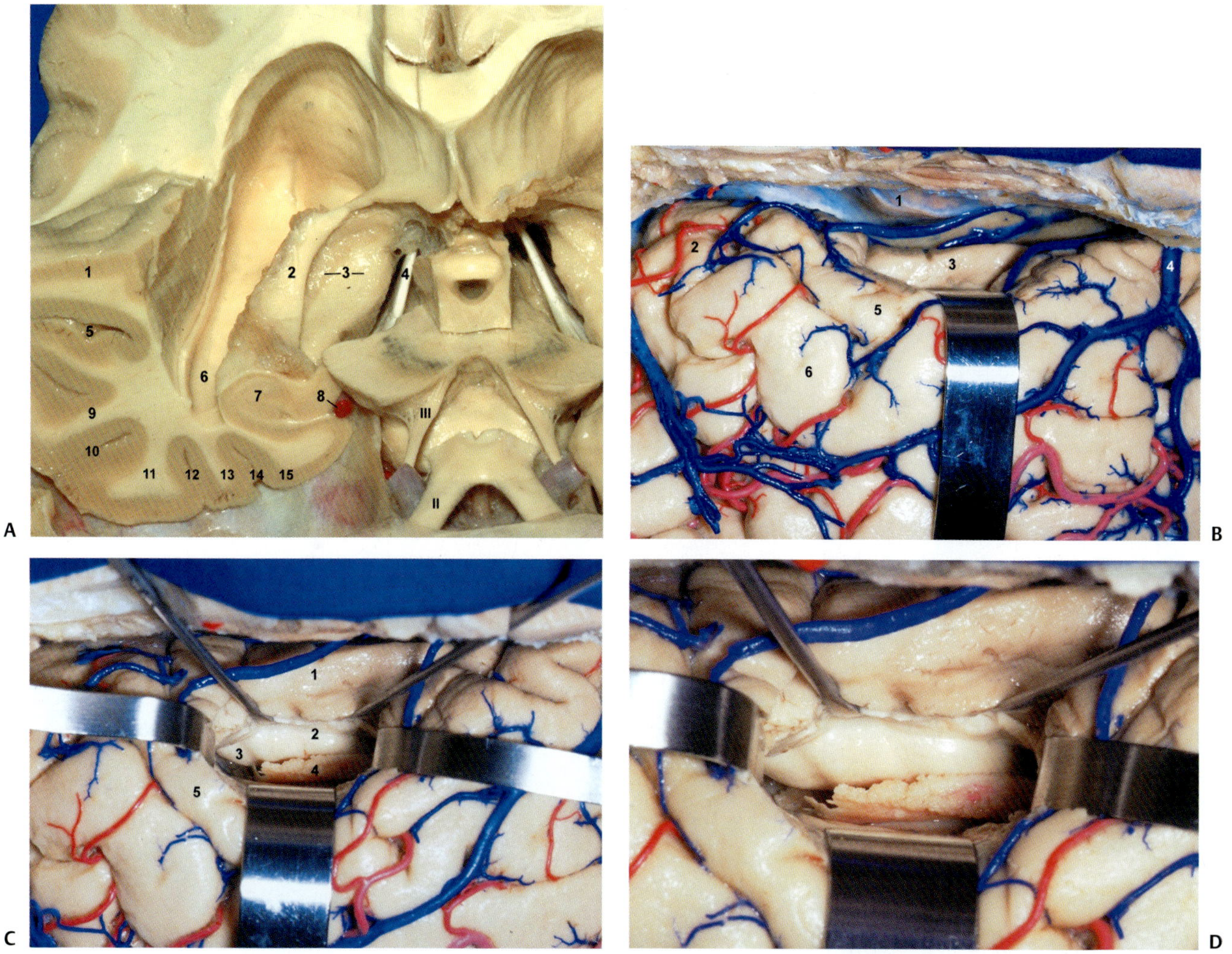

Figure 41–5 **(A)** Frontal view. A coronal section on the right temporal lobe has been performed to display the arrangement of the sulci and gyri of the temporal lobe and their relationships to the temporal horn. **1**, superior temporal gyrus; **2**, fornix; **3**, dentate and parahippocampal gyri; **4**, tentorial edge; **5**, superior temporal sulcus; **6**, collateral eminence; **7**, hippocampus; **8**, posterior cerebral artery; **9**, middle temporal gyrus; **10**, inferior temporal sulcus; **11**, inferior temporal gyrus; **12**, occipitotemporal sulcus; **13**, fusiform gyrus; **14**, collateral sulcus; **15**, parahippocampal gyrus; **II**, optic nerve; **III**, oculomotor nerve. **(B)** Subtemporal view of the right hemisphere. A retractor has been placed in the occipitotemporal sulcus, and the inferior temporal gyrus retracted. **1**, Arcuate eminence; **2**, temporal pole; **3**, fusiform gyrus; **4**, vein of Labbé; **5**, inferior temporal gyrus; **6**, middle temporal gyrus. **(C)** The occipitotemporal sulcus has been dissected and its floor removed down to the temporal horn. **1**, fusiform gyrus; **2**, body of the hippocampus; **3**, head of the hippocampus; **4**, choroid plexus; **5**, inferior temporal gyrus. **(D)** Magnified view of **Fig. 41–5C.**

Superior Frontal Sulcus Approach

This approach is mainly indicated for those lesions located in the frontal horn but extending either or both laterally off the midline and superolaterally toward the surface of the frontal lobe, which makes complete removal difficult via anterior transcallosal interhemispheric approach.

The superior frontal sulcus is an anteroposteriorly oriented sulcus, extending from the frontal pole anteriorly to the precentral sulcus posteriorly (**Fig. 41–3A**). It is continuous in 36% of cases[39] and separates the superior frontal gyrus from the middle frontal gyrus. Its average depth is 14.7 mm,[39] and its bottom points toward the frontal horn (**Fig. 41–1G**). It is frequently used as an alternative route to reach the frontal horn when it is dilated.

The patient is placed in the supine position, with the head elevated above the heart level and slightly flexed; the skin incision can be a semiarc or an arc, depending mostly on the patient's hairline. A paramedian square-shaped craniotomy with its posterior limit at the coronal suture is then performed. There is no need for entirely exposing the superior sagittal sinus; however, the exposure of the lateral edge of the superior sagittal sinus could be helpful as a landmark for intraoperative orientation.

The dura is then opened in a horseshoe fashion following the edges of the craniotomy, leaving the base of the dura toward the superior sagittal sinus. Following the dural opening, the surface of the frontal lobe is inspected and the superior frontal sulcus identified (**Fig. 41–6A, B**) and dissected beyond its bottom until the hydrocephalic frontal horn or the lesion is reached (**Fig. 41–6C**).

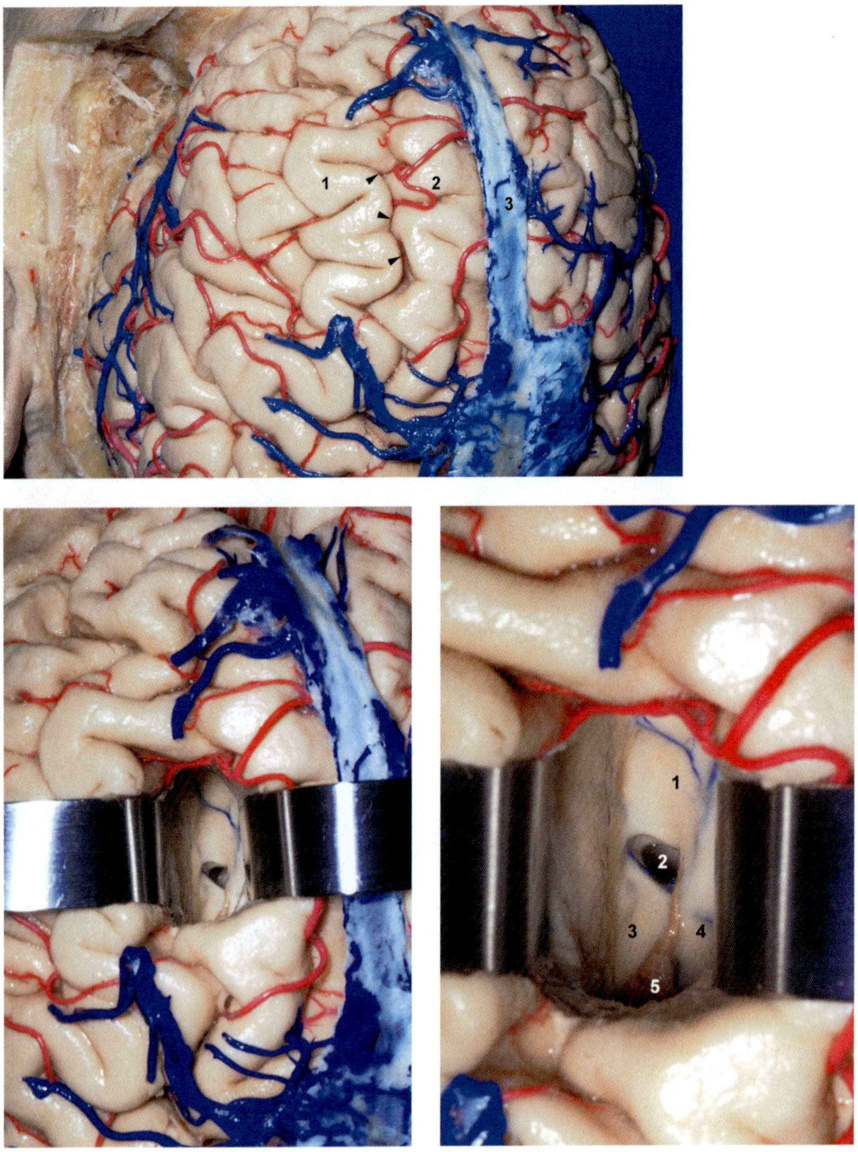

Figure 41–6 **(A)** The left superior frontal sulcus in the surgical position to approach the frontal horn and the body of the left lateral ventricle. **1**, middle frontal gyrus; **2**, superior frontal gyrus. Superior frontal sulcus (arrowheads). **(B)** The left superior frontal sulcus has been dissected and its floor removed to reach the lateral ventricle. **(C)** Magnified view of **Fig. 41–6B**. **1**, rostrum of the corpus callosum (frontal horn); **2**, foramen of Monro; **3**, thalamus; **4**, fornix; **5**, choroid plexus.

Intraparietal Sulcus Approach

This approach is indicated for lesions located in the atrium of the lateral ventricle. As mentioned earlier, the superior and medial walls of the atrium are devoid of the optic radiation; the surgical corridor through the medial wall has been mentioned in the posterior interhemispheric transcingular approach. The surgical corridor to the atrium through its roof is the subject of this section.

The intraparietal sulcus is located in the parietal lobe. It starts at the postcentral sulcus and is directed posteriorly and inferiorly toward the occipital pole; its direction is often parallel and 2 to 3 cm lateral to the midline. The bottom of the intraparietal sulcus is related to both the roof of the atrium and the occipital horn of the lateral ventricle. The intraparietal sulcus divides the lateral surface of the parietal lobe into two parts: the superior parietal lobule, which is the superomedial and smaller part, and the inferior parietal lobule, which is the inferolateral and larger part. The inferior parietal lobule is constituted by the supramarginal and angular gyri (**Fig. 41–7A**). The intraparietal sulcus is continuous in 28% on the right side and 72% on the left, with an average depth of 19.4 mm.[39]

The patient is placed in either the elevated supine or the prone position. In the elevated supine position, the decubitus is ~30 degrees, and the head of the patient is practically in its anatomical position facing forward; in the prone position the head is practically in its anatomical position facing

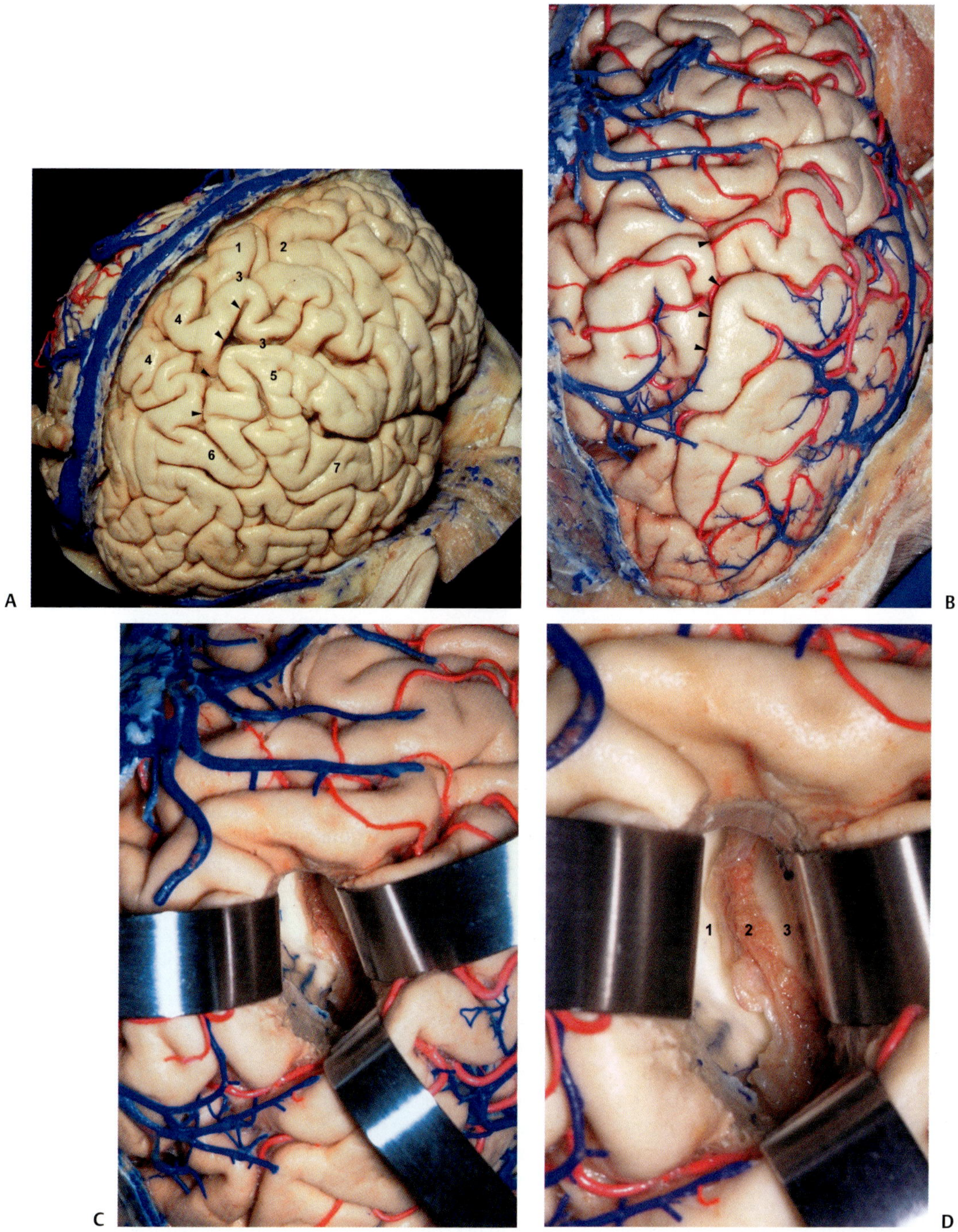

Figure 41–7 **(A)** Posterolateral view of the right hemisphere. **1**, postcentral gyrus; **2**, precentral gyrus; **3**, postcentral sulcus; **4**, superior parietal lobule; **5**, supramarginal gyrus; **6**, angular gyrus; **7**, superior temporal gyrus. Intraparietal sulcus (arrowheads). **(B)** Anatomical dissection displaying the position of the right intraparietal sulcus in surgical position (dorsal decubitus with the head slightly flexed). Intraparietal sulcus (arrowheads). **(C)** The intraparietal sulcus has been dissected and its floor removed to reach the atrium of the lateral ventricle. **(D)** Magnified view of **Fig. 41–7C. 1**, fornix; **2**, choroid plexus of the atrium; **3**, thalamus.

the floor perpendicularly. A horseshoe-shaped incision is used and a paramedian square-shaped craniotomy is performed. Once again, it is not necessary to expose the whole extent of the superior sagittal sinus; however, the exposure of the lateral edge of the superior sagittal sinus can sometimes be useful as a landmark for intraoperative orientation.

A horseshoe-shaped dural opening with its base directed toward the superior sagittal sinus is then performed and the cerebral surface inspected (**Fig. 41–7B**). The intraparietal sulcus is the only sulcus oriented parallel to the midline in this location. It is then dissected beyond its bottom until the atrium is entered (**Fig. 41–7C,D**).

◆ Surgical Approaches to Lesions Located in the Third Ventricle

Third Ventricle

The third ventricle is a narrow, funnel-shaped, unilocular midline cavity located between the two thalami, under the body of the lateral ventricle, in the center of the head (**Fig. 41–8A**). The third ventricle has anterior, lateral, posterior, and superior walls and a floor.[8,44]

The anterior wall of the third ventricle, which extends from the foramen of Monro above to the optic chiasm below, is composed mainly of the lamina terminalis. It is related anteriorly to the longitudinal fissure of the brain. The anterior commissure is found behind the junction between the anterior wall and the roof of the third ventricle (**Fig. 41–1C**). On the lateral wall, the third ventricle presents the hypothalamic sulcus—a sulcus that runs from the foramen of Monro toward the opening of the aqueduct of Sylvius, and it divides the lateral wall of the third ventricle in two parts: the superior part (the thalamus) and the inferior part (the hypothalamus).

The posterior wall of the third ventricle extends from the suprapineal recess above to the aqueduct of Sylvius below when viewed from anteriorly and within the third ventricle. The posterior wall of the third ventricle consists of, from above to below, the suprapineal recess, the pineal gland, the habenular commissure, the pineal recess, the posterior commissure, and the aqueduct of Sylvius (**Fig. 41–8B**). The posterior wall of the third ventricle is related posteriorly to the quadrigeminal cistern.

The floor of the third ventricle extends from the optic chiasm anteriorly to the aqueduct of Sylvius posteriorly. The anterior half of the floor is formed by diencephalic structures: optic and infundibular recesses, related to the chiasmatic cistern; tuber cinereum; mamillary bodies; and posterior perforated substance, related to the interpeduncular cistern. The posterior half is formed by mesencephalic structures (**Fig. 41–8C,D**).

The roof of the third ventricle has five layers[12]: the most superior layer is the fornix. The posterior portion of the third ventricle is covered by the hippocampal commissure, a neural structure that unites the two crura of fornix; the anterior and middle portions of the third ventricle are covered by the body of the fornix (**Fig. 41–8E**). The second layer is the superior membrane of the tela choroidea (**Fig. 41–8F**); the third layer is the vascular layer, which consists basically of the internal cerebral veins and medial posterior choroidal artery and branches, located between the superior and inferior membranes of the tela choroidea, in a space known as the velum interpositum. The fourth layer is therefore the inferior membrane of the tela choroidea; the fifth layer, located beneath the fourth layer, is the choroid plexus (**Fig. 41–8G**). The choroid plexus of the third ventricle, which is the most inferior layer of the roof of this cavity, is continuous with the choroid plexus of the lateral ventricle and runs as two strands from the foramen of Monro to the posterior aspect of the third ventricle, proceeding superior and lateral to the pineal gland (**Fig. 41–8H**).

At the level of the foramen of Monro, the body of the fornix splits into two columns that run anteriorly, inferiorly, and laterally. The columns have their major component running behind the anterior commissure, in the lateral walls of the third ventricle toward the mamillary bodies, located at the floor of the third ventricle (**Fig. 41–8G**). The foramen of Monro therefore is limited anteriorly and superiorly by the columns of the fornix and posteriorly by the thalamus (**Fig. 41–8G**).

Transchoroidal Approach

The transchoroidal approach is designed to approach the lesions located mainly at the anterior two thirds of the third ventricle from its roof through the choroidal fissure in the body of the lateral ventricle.[12] In the body of the lateral ventricle, the choroid plexus is located in the medial part of the floor; medially to the choroid plexus is the body of the fornix, and laterally to it is the thalamus (**Fig. 41–9A**). The choroidal fissure is located between the thalamus inferiorly and the body of the fornix superiorly.

Through the choroidal fissure, the two membranes of the tela choroidea of the third ventricle proceed to the body of the lateral ventricle to originate the choroidal plexus (**Fig. 41–8F**).

Histologically, the choroid plexus has a villous structure with a stroma (leptomeningeal cells, connective tissue, and blood vessels) covered by an epithelium derived from ependyma. The choroid plexus in the body of the lateral ventricle is attached medially to the body of the fornix and laterally to the thalamus; the attachment of the choroid plexus to these two structures is made by ependyma that covers not only the ventricular wall but also the choroid plexus (**Fig. 41–9B**). Consequently, the taenia fornicis and taenia choroidea that attach the choroid plexus, respectively, to the fornix medially and to the thalamus laterally are in fact the continuation of the ependyma from the ventricular cavity to the choroid plexus.[12]

The venous drainage of the body of the lateral ventricle can be divided in two groups: a medial group that drains mainly via posterior septal veins, and a lateral group that drains mainly via thalamostriate, anterior, and posterior caudate veins and superior thalamic veins.

The anterior septal vein, which comes from the septum pellucidum in the frontal horn, runs posteriorly to join the internal cerebral vein along with the thalamostriate and superior choroidal veins, usually at the foramen of Monro. At the body of the lateral ventricle, the main venous drainage is made via the thalamostriate vein, which is subependymal in location (**Fig. 41–9A**).

The thalamostriate vein runs anteriorly in the striothalamic sulcus, between the body of the caudate nucleus and the thalamus in a subependymal location; at the foramen of Monro or behind the foramen of Monro, it enters the choroidal fissure under the taenia choroidea to pierce the inferior membrane of the tela choroidea of the third ventricle and gain the velum interpositum and internal cerebral vein. The thalamostriate vein loses its ependymal cover when the taenia choroidea leaves the upper surface of the thalamus to cover the choroid plexus of the lateral ventricle (**Fig. 41–9B**).

After entering the body of the lateral ventricle through the anterior transcallosal interhemispheric approach,[45] the

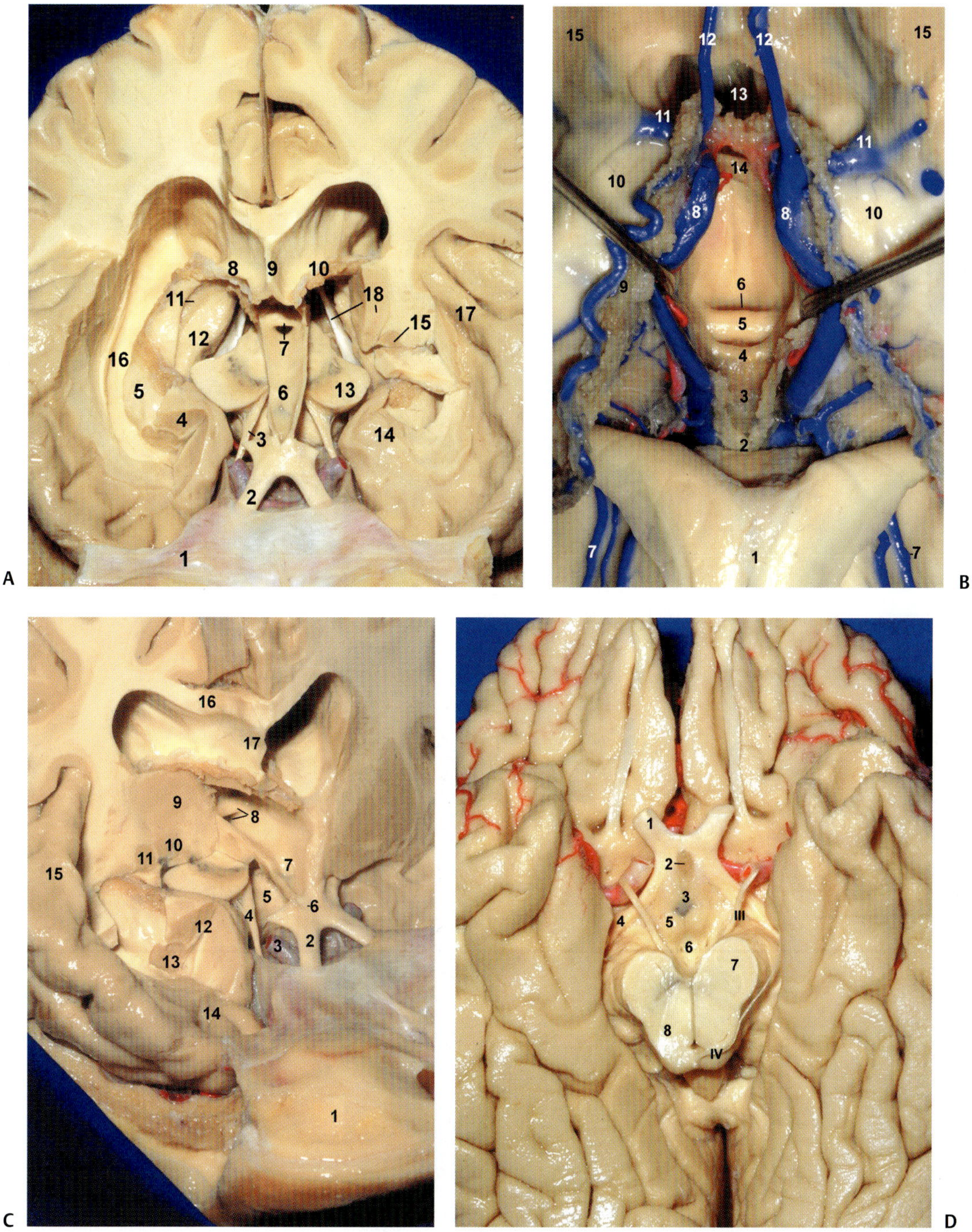

Figure 41–8 **(A)** Frontal view. A coronal section has been performed at the optic chiasm, and both basal ganglia and thalami have been removed via choroidal fissure. The floor of the third ventricle has been kept intact to display the central location of the third ventricle in the head. **1**, right orbit; **2**, optic nerve; **3**, oculomotor nerve; **4**, amygdala; **5**, hippocampus; **6**, floor of the third ventricle; **7**, aqueduct of Sylvius and posterior commissure; **8**, fornix; **9**, septum pellucidum; **10**, choroid plexus; **11**, dentate gyrus; **12**, parahippocampal gyrus; **13**, crus cerebri; **14**, semilunar gyrus; **15**, lateral geniculate body; **16**, collateral eminence; **17**, Heschl's gyri; **18**, thalamus and tentorium. **(B)** Axial view. The columns of the fornix have been cut, and the fornix has been reflected posteriorly. **1**, fornix; **2**, choroid plexus; **3**, pineal gland and suprapineal recess; **4**, habenular commissure; **5**, pineal recess and posterior commissure; **6**, aqueduct of Sylvius; **7**, medial atrial veins; **8**, internal cerebral vein; **9**, superior choroidal vein and choroid plexus of the lateral ventricle; **10**, thalamus; **11**, thalamostriate vein; **12**, anterior septal vein; **13**, foramina of Monro; **14**, massa intermedia; **15**, head of the caudate nucleus. **(C)** Right anterior oblique view. The floor of the third ventricle extends from the optic chiasm anteriorly to the aqueduct of Sylvius posteriorly. **1**, orbital roof; **2**, optic nerve; **3**, carotid artery; **4**, oculomotor nerve; **5**, pons; **6**, optic recess; **7**, mammillary bodies; **8**, aqueduct and posterior commissure; **9**, thalamus; **10**, medial geniculate body; **11**, lateral geniculate body; **12**, amygdala and uncus; **13**, hippocampus; **14**, temporal pole; **15**, Heschl's gyri; **16**, corpus callosum; **17**, septum pellucidum. **(D)** Basal view. **1**, optic nerve; **2**, pituitary stalk; **3**, tuber cinereum; **4**, optic tract; **5**, mammillary bodies; **6**, posterior perforated substance; **7**, crus cerebri; **8**, tegementum; **III**, oculomotor nerve; **IV**, trochlear nerve.

(*Continued on pages 532 and 533*)

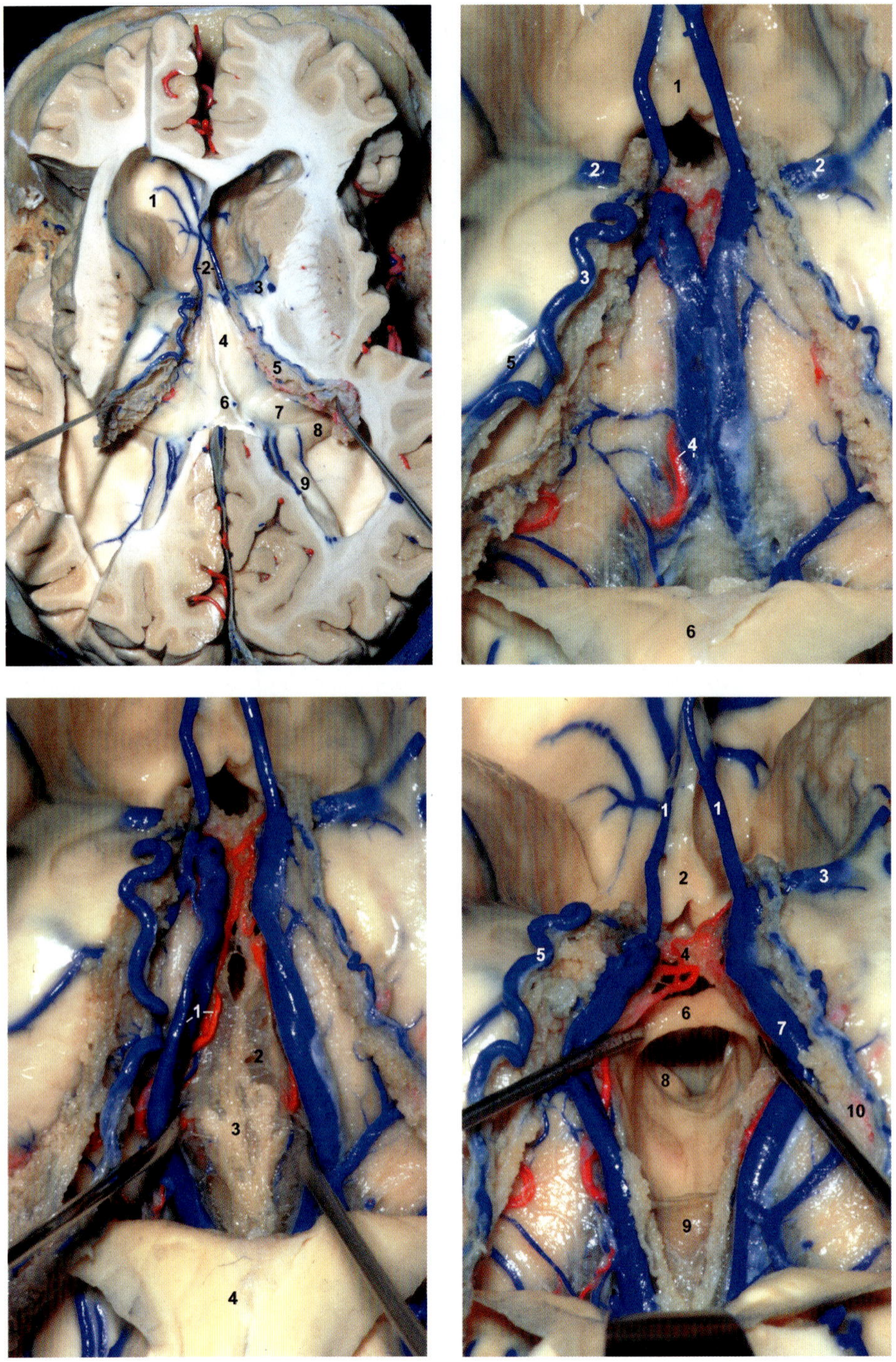

E F G H

(*Continued*) **Figure 41–8** **(E)** Superior view. The septum pellucidum and part of the splenium of the corpus callosum have been removed to display the fornix. **1**, frontal horn; **2**, anterior septal vein; **3**, thalamostriate vein; **4**, body of the fornix; **5**, choroid plexus; **6**, hippocampal commissure; **7**, crus of the fornix; **8**, hippocampus; **9**, calcar avis. **(F)** Superior view. The fornix has been cut and reflected posteriorly to display the tela choroidea. **1**, columns of the fornix (cut) and the anterior septal vein; **2**, thalamostriate vein; **3**, superior choroidal vein; **4**, internal cerebral vein and medial posterior choroidal artery (covered by the superior membrane of the tela choroidea); **5**, superficial superior thalamic vein; **6**, fornix (reflected). **(G)** Superior view. The superior membrane of the tela choroidea has been removed and the vascular elements displaced laterally to show the inferior membrane of tela choroidea. **1**, internal cerebral vein and branches of the medial posterior choroidal artery; **2**, inferior membrane of the tela choroidea; **3**, choroid plexus of the third ventricle; **4**, fornix (reflected). **(H)** Posteroanterior view. The inferior membrane of the tela choroidea has been removed and the two strands of choroid plexus separated. **1**, anterior septal vein; **2**, columns of the fornix (cut); **3**, thalamostriate vein; **4**, choroid plexus and branches of the medial posterior choroidal artery; **5**, superior choroidal vein; **6**, massa intermedia; **7**, internal cerebral vein; **8**, mammillary body; **9**, pineal gland; **10**, choroid plexus of the lateral ventricle.

(*Continued on page 533*)

I 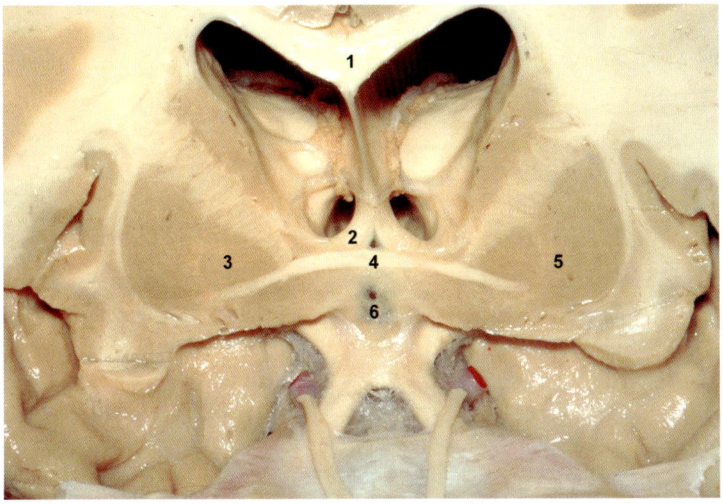

(*Continued*) **Figure 41–8 (I)** Coronal view. A coronal section has been performed at the optic chiasm. **1**, corpus callosum; **2**, column of the fornix; **3**, globus pallidus; **4**, anterior commissure; **5**, putamen; **6**, lamina terminalis.

choroid plexus of the body of the lateral ventricle is identified. The body of the fornix is located medially to the choroid plexus, and the thalamus is located laterally to it (**Fig. 41–9C**). The taenia fornicis is then opened to approach the choroidal fissure. After careful opening of the taenia fornicis, the superior membrane of the tela choroidea and the underlying branches of the medial posterior choroidal artery and the internal cerebral vein, which are the contents of the velum interpositum, can be seen. The internal cerebral vein, the branches of the medial posterior choroidal artery, and the inferior membrane of the tela choroidea can be better visualized after the superior membrane of the tela choroidea is opened (**Fig. 41–9D**).

The dissection is then proceeded medially to the internal cerebral vein (between the two internal cerebral veins), with the opening of the inferior membrane of the tela choroidea. It is important to emphasize that the approach to the third ventricle by going between the two internal cerebral veins is the key step in the transchoroidal approach for two reasons: to avoid the veins that come from the upper surface of the thalamus and run medially toward the internal cerebral vein (e.g., thalamostriate vein), and because there is no bridging vein connecting the two internal cerebral veins.

After the last layer of the roof of the third ventricle has been opened, the cavity of the third ventricle, the massa intermedia (when present), and the floor of the third ventricle can be fully seen (**Fig. 41–9E**). The roof of the third ventricle, therefore, has been completely opened from the foramen of Monro to its posterior part, just above the pineal gland, through the choroidal fissure. Consequently, the posterior limit of the foramen of Monro has been expanded through the choroidal fissure, without sacrificing any neural or vascular structures. If additional space is needed for surgery, the only structure that restricts further expansion of the foramen of Monro is the anterior septal vein, which can be sacrificed if necessary.

The transchoroidal approach can be summarized in **Fig. 41–9B.**

Interforniceal Approach

The interforniceal approach is another alternative for approaching lesions located at the anterior two thirds of the third ventricle from its roof, and it has been popularized by Apuzzo.[46,47] After entering the body of the lateral ventricle through the anterior transcallosal interhemispheric approach, the septum pellucidum is identified. The cavum of the septum pellucidum is then entered, separating the two layers of the septum pellucidum. The reason for this maneuver is to assure that the fornix will be split exactly in the midline because the base of the septum pellucidum is attached exactly in the midline (**Fig. 41–2A**) between the two fornices.

After splitting the fornix and the superior membrane of the tela choroidea, the contents of the velum interpositum come into view (**Fig. 41–10A**). The dissection then proceeds inferiorly between the two internal cerebral veins, splitting the inferior membrane of the tela choroidea and the choroid plexus of the third ventricle to reach the cavity of the third ventricle (**Fig. 41–10B**).

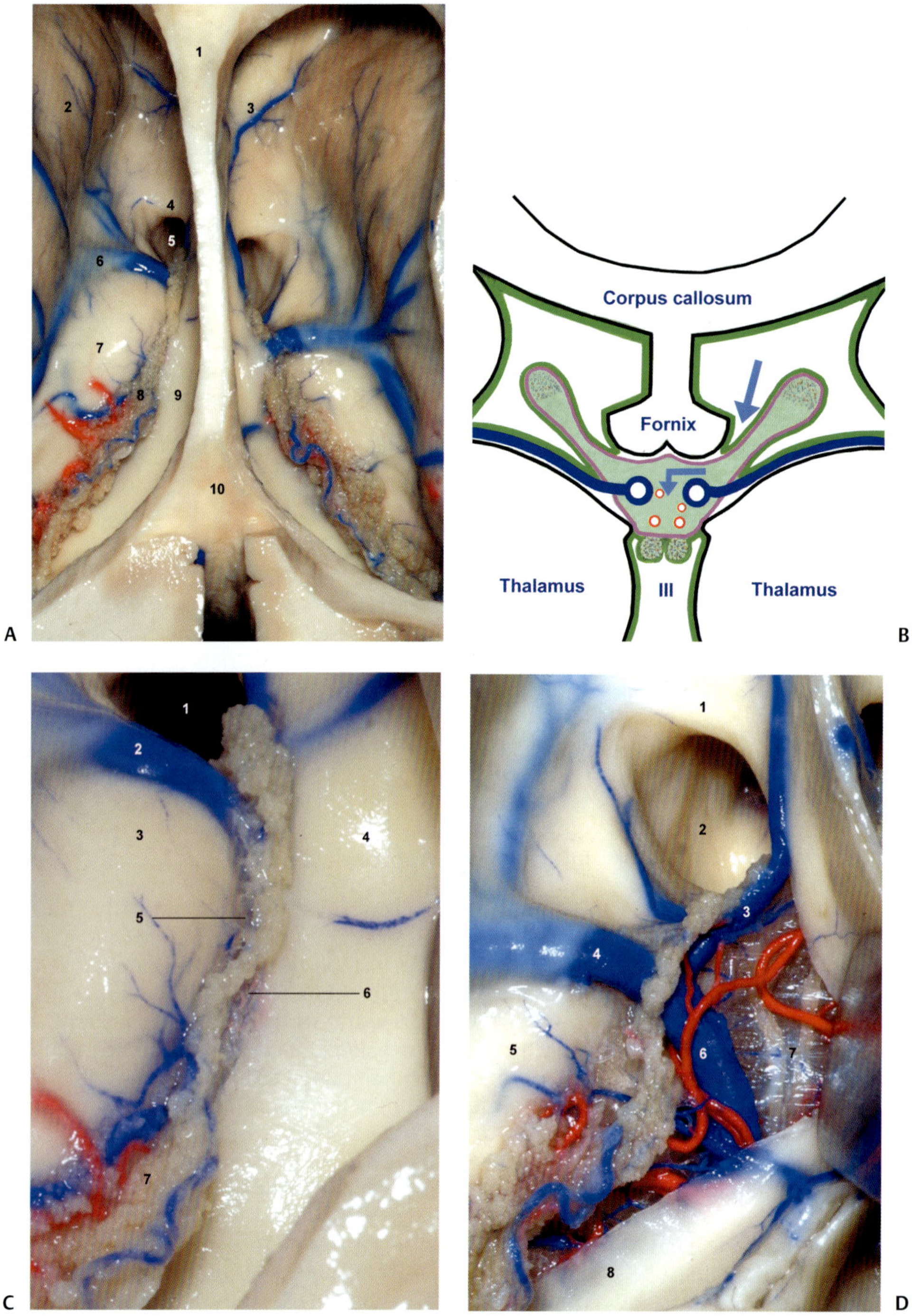

Figure 41–9 **(A)** Superior view. In the body of the lateral ventricle, the choroid plexus is located in the medial part of the floor; the body of the fornix is located medially to the choroid plexus, and the thalamus is located laterally to the choroid plexus. **1**, corpus callosum; **2**, head of the caudate nucleus; **3**, rostrum of the corpus callosum; **4**, left column of the fornix; **5**, foramen of Monro; **6**, thalamostriate vein; **7**, thalamus; **8**, choroid plexus; **9**, body of the fornix; **10**, splenium of the corpus callosum. **(B)** Diagram of a coronal section through the body of the lateral ventricle. The two membranes of the tela choroidea are shown in purple, the ependyma is in green, and the thalamostriate veins are in dark blue. **Left**, the five layers of the roof of the third ventricle are the fornix, the superior membrane of the tela choroidea, the vascular layer (the internal cerebral vein and the medial posterior choroidal artery), the inferior membrane of the tela choroidea, and the choroid plexus. The inferior membrane of the tela choroidea is attached to the taenia thalami, which are small ridges on the free edge of the striae medullaris thalami, on the superomedial border of the thalamus, from the foramen of Monro to the habenular commissure. The choroidal fissure is a natural cleft between the thalamus and the fornix. Through the choroidal fissure, the two membranes of the tela choroidea advance to the body of the lateral ventricle to originate the choroid plexus. The ependyma that covers the ventricular wall also covers the choroid plexus in the lateral ventricle; the choroid plexus of the lateral ventricle is attached medially to the fornix by the taenia fornicis and laterally to the thalamus by the taenia choroidea. Both taenia fornicis and choroidea are extensions of the ependyma, from the ventricular wall to the choroid plexus. The thalamostriate vein and other subependymal veins that run on the upper surface of the thalamus and drain medially into the internal cerebral vein lose their ependymal covering when they pierce the inferior membrane of the tela choroidea and enter the velum interpositum, as the ependyma reflects upward to cover the choroid plexus. **Right**, arrows indicate the route of the transchoroidal approach. After the taenia fornicis is opened, it is better to proceed medially, instead of laterally, to the internal cerebral vein, to avoid the subependymal veins that drain into the internal cerebral vein.

(*Continued on page 535*)

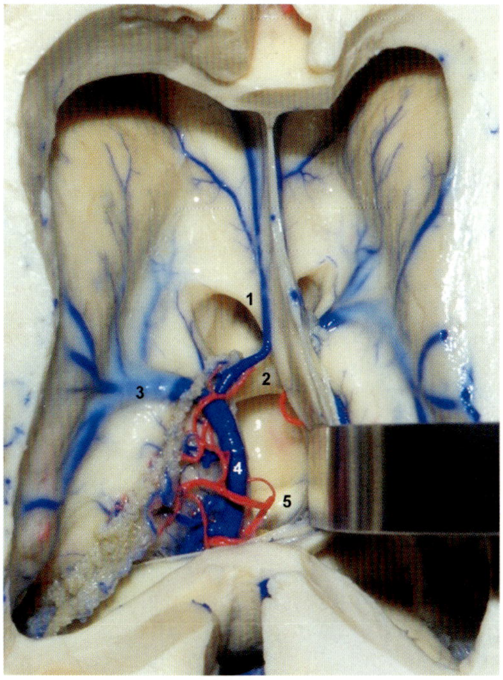

E

(*Continued*) **Figure 41–9** **(C)** Magnified view of the choroid plexus in the body of the left lateral ventricle. The choroid plexus is attached medially to the body of the fornix by the taenia fornicis and laterally to the thalamus by the taenia choroidea. The taenia is actually a continuation of the ependyma that covers the ventricular cavity over the choroid plexus of the lateral ventricle. **1**, foramen of Monro; **2**, thalamostriate vein; **3**, thalamus; **4**, fornix; **5**, taenia choroidea; **6**, taenia fornicis; **7**, choroid plexus and branches of the medial posterior choroidal artery. **(D)** Superior view. After splitting the taenia fornicis and the superior membrane of the tela choroidea, the internal cerebral vein, the branches of the medial posterior choroidal artery, the inferior membrane of the tela choroidea, and the choroid plexus of the third ventricle come into view. **1**, column of the fornix; **2**, foramen of Monro; **3**, anterior septal vein; **4**, thalamostriate vein; **5**, thalamus; **6**, internal cerebral vein; **7**, inferior membrane of the tela choroidea and the choroid plexus of the third ventricle; **8**, crus of the fornix. **(E)** Superior view. After opening the inferior membrane of the tela choroidea, the cavity of the third ventricle, from the foramen of Monro to the posterior commissure is reached. When necessary, the anterior septal vein can be sacrificed to gain additional working space. **1**, anterior septal vein and column of the fornix; **2**, massa intermedia; **3**, thalamostriate vein; **4**, internal cerebral vein; **5**, posterior commissure.

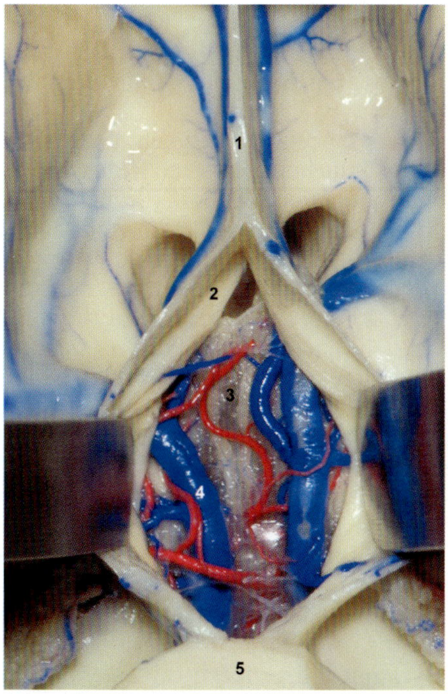

A

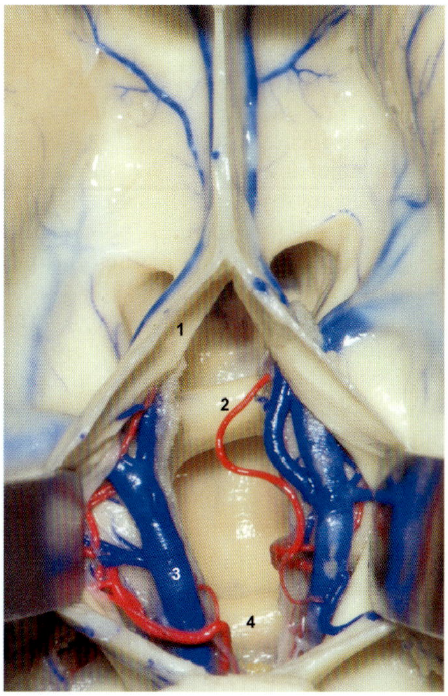

B

Figure 41–10 **(A)** Superior view. After entering the body of the lateral ventricle, the dissection continues between the two leafs of the septum pellucidum down to their attachment at the body of the fornix, then the body of the fornix is divided in the midline. **1**, septum pellucidum; **2**, fornix; **3**, inferior membrane of the tela choroidea; **4**, internal cerebral vein; **5**, splenium of the corpus callosum. **(B)** After the opening of the inferior membrane of the tela choroidea and the choroid plexus of the third ventricle, the cavity of the third ventricle is seen. **1**, fornix; **2**, massa intermedia; **3**, internal cerebral vein; **4**, posterior commissure.

Velum Interpositum Supracerebellar Infratentorial Approach

The space between the tentorium and the tentorial surface of the cerebellum is an excellent natural pathway to access lesions located at the posterior portion of the third ventricle,[48,49] such as those involving the pineal gland or those involving the posterior and posterolateral portions of the midbrain (**Fig. 41–11A**). It is important to emphasize that these lesions do not necessarily have to be accessed through the midline; the lateral part of the space between the tentorial surfaces of the cerebellar hemisphere and the tentorium (under the transverse sinus) can be used as well.

The midbrain is divided by a midline sagittal plane into two halves, called the cerebral peduncles. Each peduncle is further divided into three parts: an anterior part (the crus cerebri or the basis pedunculi), an intermediate part (the tegmentum), and a posterior part located behind the aqueduct (the tectum). The lateral mesencephalic sulcus separates the tegmentum from the crus cerebri. The tectum, which is constituted by the superior and inferior colliculi (quadrigeminal plate), also constitutes the anterior wall of the quadrigeminal cistern.

The midbrain continues superiorly with the diencephalic structures. Just above the quadrigeminal plate, at the midline, is the pineal gland. Nonetheless, internally at the third ventricle, the posterior wall of the third ventricle (posterior commissure, pineal recess, habenular commissure, pineal gland, and suprapineal recess) is also located above the superior colliculi. Externally, the pineal gland is located at the midline above the superior colliculi (**Fig. 41–11A**).

The velum interpositum—the space located between the superior and the inferior membranes of the tela choroidea—is located just above the pineal gland. Therefore, the internal cerebral vein and the vein of Galen are located just above the pineal gland, whereas the terminal portion of the basal vein of Rosenthal is located superolaterally to the pineal gland (**Fig. 41–8H**). The internal cerebral vein and the vein of Galen are expected to be displaced superiorly and the basal vein displaced superolaterally when a pineal tumor is encountered.

Posteriorly, the brain stem is separated from the cerebellum by the cerebellomesencephalic or precentral cerebellar fissure; it presents a posterior wall and an anterior wall. Posteriorly at the midline, the precentral cerebellar fissure is bounded by the anterior part of the culmen above and the central lobule below. Laterally, it is limited by the anterior surface of the quadrangular lobule above and the wing of the central lobule below. Anteriorly, it is limited from the midline to laterally by the lingula and the superior and middle cerebellar peduncles (**Fig. 41–11B**). The interpeduncular or interbrachial sulcus, which separates the superior from the middle cerebellar peduncles, ascends from the bottom of the cerebellomesencephalic fissure toward the lateral aspect of the pons, where it is joined by the pontomesencephalic sulcus to proceed superiorly as the lateral mesencephalic sulcus up to the medial geniculate body[50] (**Fig. 41–11B–D**). The lateral mesencephalic sulcus constitutes an important intraoperative landmark because it separates the crus cerebri anteriorly from the tegmentum mesencephali posteriorly. The lateral mesencephalic sulcus is frequently recognized intraoperatively by the lateral mesencephalic vein, a longitudinal vein that runs on the corresponding sulcus and connects the basal vein superiorly to the brachial veins inferiorly.

Two important veins that are involved in this approach are the precentral cerebellar vein,[51,52] or vein of the cerebellomesencephalic fissure, and the superior vermian vein. Both drain into the vein of Galen (belong to the galenic group).[53,54] The precentral cerebellar vein, formed by the union of two brachial veins, runs superiorly on the anterior surface of the vermis in the cerebellomesencephalic fissure, just anterior to the central lobule (**Fig. 41–11B**). On the angiographic anteroposterior view, the precentral cerebellar vein along with the two brachial veins has an inverted Y configuration.

The superior vermian vein runs posteroanteriorly between the upper surface of the vermis inferiorly and the straight sinus superiorly. Along its way on the superior vermis, the superior vermian vein is joined by supraculminate and intraculminate tributaries.[53,55] Frequently the superior vermian vein joins the precentral cerebellar vein before draining into the vein of Galen (**Fig. 41–11B**).

Also running in the cerebellomesencephalic fissure is the superior cerebellar artery (SCA).[56–58] It is the most rostral of the infratentorial vessels, and it arises near the apex of the basilar artery and encircles the pons and the lower midbrain. The SCA supplies the tentorial surface of the cerebellum, the upper brain stem, the deep cerebellar nuclei, and the inferior colliculi. The SCA is divided into the anterior pontomesencephalic, lateral pontomesencephalic, cerebellomesencephalic, and cortical segments (**Figs. 41–11C,D**). The segments of the SCA directly involved in this approach are the lateral pontomesencephalic, cerebellomesencephalic, and cortical segments.

The lateral pontomesencephalic segment begins at the anterolateral margin of the brain stem and follows caudally onto the lateral side of the upper pons in the infratentorial portion of the ambient cistern to terminate at the anterior margin of the cerebellomesencephalic fissure; this segment is related medially to the brain stem, laterally to the wing of the central lobule, and inferiorly to the middle cerebellar peduncle. The anterior part of this segment is often visible above the free edge of the tentorium, whereas its caudal loop projects toward and often reaches the root entry zone of the trigeminal nerve. The bifurcation of the SCA into its rostral and caudal trunks often occurs in this segment; the rostral trunk supplies the vermis and a variable portion of the adjacent tentorial surface, and the caudal trunk supplies the surface lateral to the area supplied by the rostral trunk.

The cerebellomesencephalic segment courses in the cerebellomesencephalic fissure through a series of hairpin curves, then passes upward to reach the anterosuperior margin of the cerebellum. Inside the cerebellomesencephalic fissure, the cortical branches from the rostral and caudal trunks send off small arterial twig branches called precentral branches. Those precentral branches arising from the rostral trunk supply the inferior colliculi (the superior colliculi are supplied by the PCA) and superior medullary velum, and those arising from the caudal trunk supply the deep cerebellar nuclei.

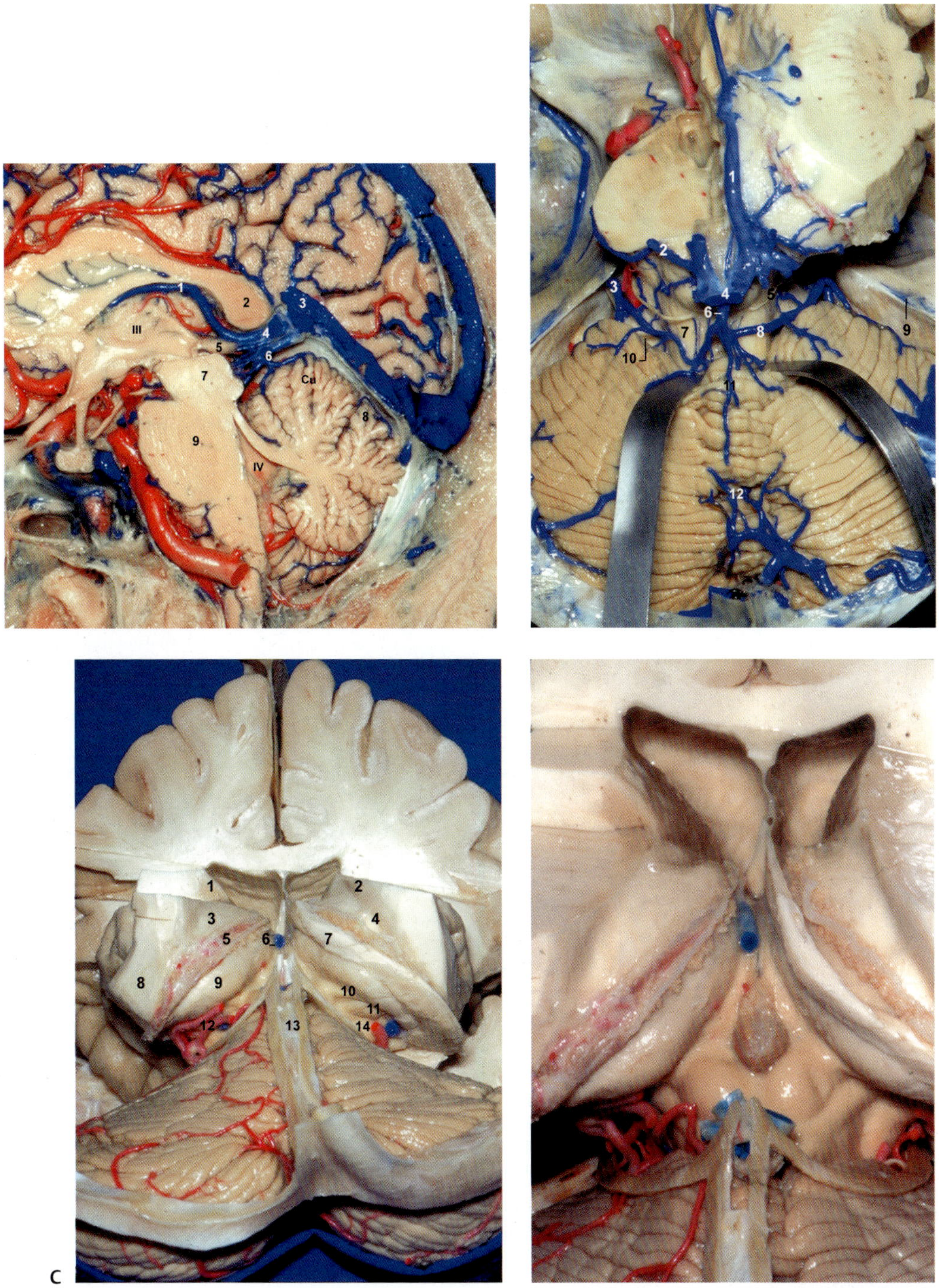

Figure 41–11 **(A)** Midsagittal view to show the route of the infratentorial supracerebellar approach, between the tentorium above and the superior vermis below. It is important to emphasize that the supracerebellar infratentorial approach can be performed above the culmen (in the midline) or lateral to it, above the hemispheric part of the tentorial surface of the cerebellum. **1**, internal cerebral vein; **2**, splenium of the corpus callosum; **3**, straight sinus; **4**, vein of Galen; **5**, pineal gland; **6**, precentral cerebellar vein; **7**, midbrain; **8**, declive; **9**, pons; Cu, culmen; IV, fourth ventricle. **(B)** Posterosuperior view. The posterior wall of the cerebellomesencephalic fissure has been retracted posteriorly to display the related venous structures. **1**, internal cerebral vein; **2**, basal vein; **3**, superior petrosal vein; **4**, vein of Galen; **5**, trochlear nerve; **6**, precentral cerebellar vein; **7**, superior cerebellar peduncle; **8**, brachial vein; **9**, superior petrosal sinus; **10**, middle cerebellar peduncle; **11**, supraculminate vein (on its way to form the superior vermian vein); **12**, declival veins (belong to the tentorial group). In this case the precentral cerebellar vein is formed by the superior vermian vein and the brachial veins. **(C)** Posterior view. Both occipital and temporal lobes have been removed. **1**, head of the caudate nucleus; **2**, body of the caudate nucleus; **3**, thalamus (body of the lateral ventricle); **4**, striothalamic sulcus; **5**, choroid plexus of the atrium; **6**, internal cerebral vein; **7**, crus of the fornix; **8**, pulvinar of the thalamus (anterior wall of the atrium); **9**, pulvinar of the thalamus (roof of the quadrigeminal cistern); **10**, brachium of the superior colliculus; **11**, brachium of the inferior colliculus; **12**, branches of the superior cerebellar artery; **13**, straight sinus; **14**, posterior cerebral artery and basal vein. **(D)** Magnified view of **Fig. 41–11C.**

(Continued on page 538)

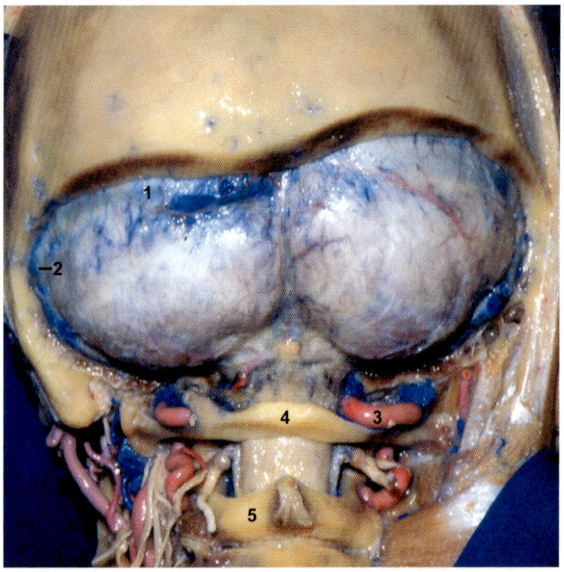

E

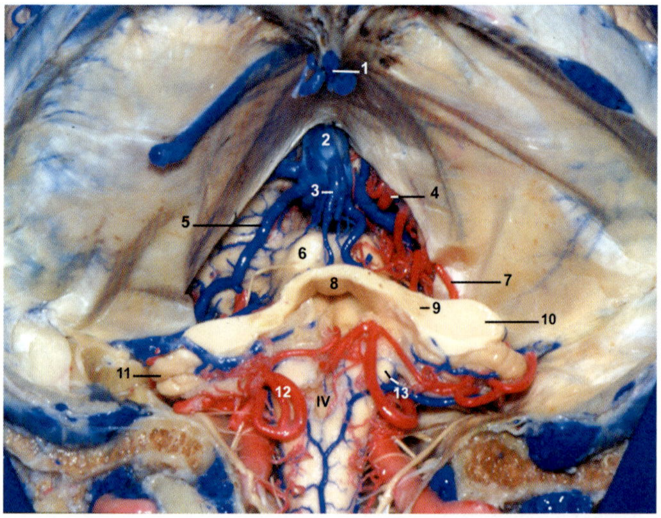

F

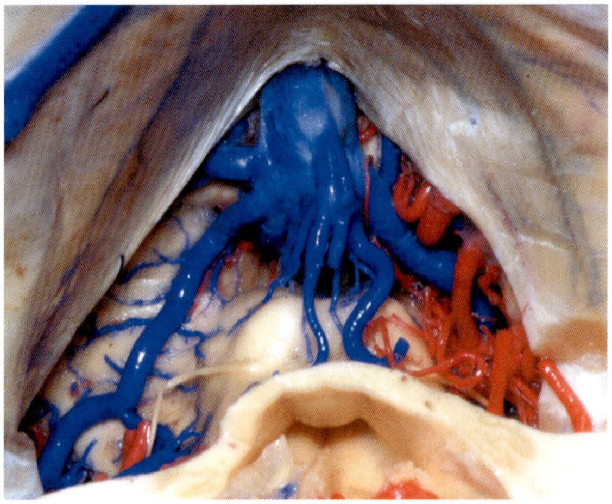

G

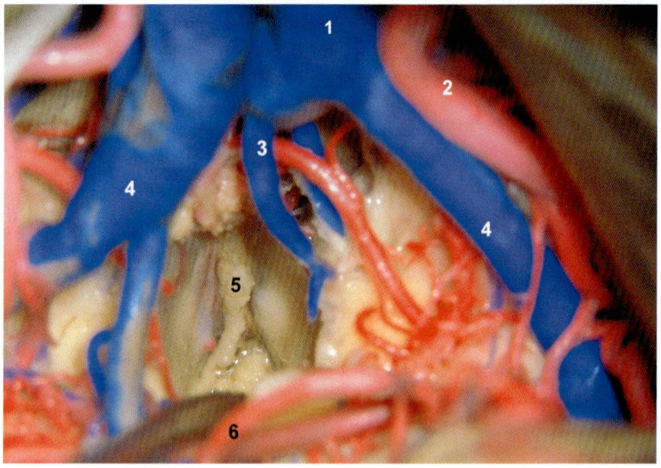

H

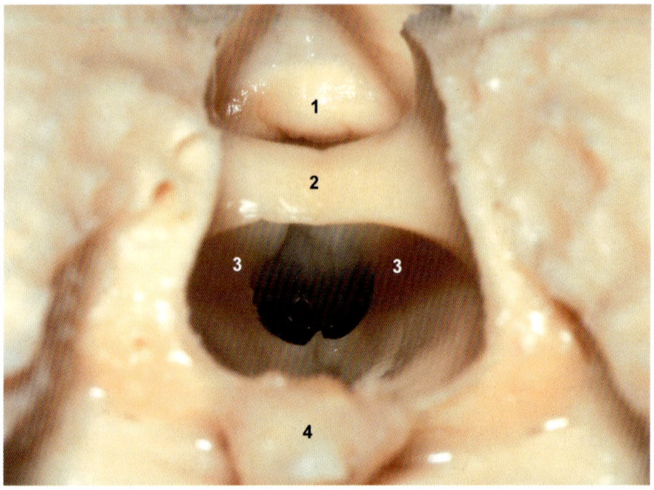

I

(*Continued*) **Figure 41–11** **(E)** Anatomical dissection displaying the craniotomy or craniectomy for the supracerebellar infratentorial approach. It is important to expose the transverse sinus. **1**, transverse sinus; **2**, sigmoid sinus; **3**, vertebral artery; **4**, C1; **5**, C2. **(F)** Anatomical dissection with infratentorial supracerebellar view with the cerebellum removed. **1**, site of drainage for inferior vermian veins; **2**, vein of Galen; **3**, superior vermian vein; **4**, posterior cerebral artery; **5**, basal vein (under the pulvinar of the thalamus); **6**, inferior colliculus; **7**, superior cerebellar artery; **8**, lingula; **9**, dentate nucleus; **10**, middle cerebellar peduncle; **11**, flocculus; **12**, posterior inferior cerebellar artery; **13**, inferior cerebellar peduncle; IV, floor of the fourth ventricle. **(G)** Magnified view of **Fig. 41–11F**. **(H)** Anatomical dissection showing the roof of the third ventricle via infratentorial supracerebellar approach. **1**, internal cerebral vein; **2**, posterior cerebral artery; **3**, precentral cerebellar vein; **4**, basal vein; **5**, choroid plexus of the roof of the third ventricle. **(I)** Anatomical dissection displaying the third ventricle from behind, approximately the view as in infratentorial supracerebellar approach, after the removal of a lesion located at the posterior portion of the third ventricle. **1**, anterior commissure; **2**, massa intermedia; **3**, column of the fornix; **4**, pineal gland.

The cortical segment is represented by the hemispheric and vermian branches to supply the tentorial surface of the cerebellum. In the surgical approach, the patient is placed in the semisitting or sitting position with the neck flexed; excessive flexion of the neck might cause compression of the jugular veins, compromising the venous drainage. Frequently, a tumor arising from the posterior region of the third ventricle is accompanied by an obstructive hydrocephalus. The placement of an external shunt prior to the positioning of the patient may sometimes be helpful. The external shunt can be placed either in the frontal horn or in the occipital horn; because the surgical procedure takes place in the posterior region of the head, the authors prefer to place the external shunt in the frontal horn. After the placement of the shunt, it is kept shut and is opened whenever necessary.

A midline incision is then performed and the suboccipital muscles split through the midline and retracted laterally to expose the suboccipital surface. A craniotomy or a craniectomy is then performed; it is advisable to have the torcula and the transverse sinuses exposed because they can be retracted superiorly using sutures, and precious additional working space can be gained.

In those cases with a shunt placed, the craniotomy or craniectomy does not necessarily include the edge of the foramen magnum. For those without shunt and when the dura mater is felt to be tense after the removal of the bone flap, it is helpful for the surgeon to have access to some subarachnoidal space to drain CSF; the removal of the bone down to the foramen magnum edge will allow access to the cisterna magna. The shunt can be opened if the dura mater is felt to be tense before the dural opening or if a small dural opening at the cisterna magna can be made and the CSF drained.

The dura can be opened in a curved fashion, exposing only the upper portions of the suboccipital surface of the cerebellum (**Fig. 41–11E**). The rest of the intact dura will hold the cerebellum in place, preventing it from "herniating" through the bone opening by gravity. After the drainage of the CSF, and still contained inferiorly by the dura, the cerebellum will fall down from the tentorium, creating the needed working space. The torcula and the transverse sinuses are further retracted superiorly using sutures. The arachnoidal adhesions between the cerebellum and the transverse sinuses and the torcula are cut, and the space between the tentorial surface of the cerebellum and the tentorium is entered. There are veins draining the tentorial surface of the cerebellum toward the sinuses located in the tentorium; most of these veins come from the cerebellum at the level of the postclival fissure. Those veins located in the surgical corridor are sacrificed.

The surgical corridor can be between the tentorium and the vermis or between the tentorium and the cerebellar hemisphere, depending basically on the size of the lesion to be approached. For large lesions located at the posterior part of the third ventricle, it is advisable to perform a larger craniotomy, and both corridors above the two cerebellar hemispheres and the vermis can be used.

The midline corridor between the straight sinus and the superior vermis presents the culmen as the main obstacle. The culmen, due to its morphology (**Fig. 41–11A**), is usually retracted downward during the procedure. As the surgeon advances toward the cerebellomesencephalic fissure and the quadrigeminal cistern, either or both the superior vermian vein and the precentral cerebellar vein commonly have to be sacrificed (**Fig. 41–11A,G**). The quadrigeminal cistern, characterized by the presence of a very thick arachnoid membrane, has to be opened carefully because underlying vessels (branches of the SCA, PCA) can be injured if the dissection and the section of this arachnoid membrane are not adequate.

Usually at this stage, after the removal of the arachnoid membrane, the lesion located at the posterior portion of the third ventricle comes to the surgeon's view before visualization of the vein of Galen, internal cerebral vein, or basal vein because they are usually displaced upward (**Fig. 41–11F,G**). The branches from the PCA can be distinguished from those arising from the SCA because the branches from the PCA are supratentorial; they run and disappear above the tentorium, whereas those branches of the SCA continue below the tentorium to supply the cerebellum (**Fig. 41–11F,G**).

After the removal of the lesion, the anterior and superior aspects of the third ventricle can be inspected from behind (**Fig. 41–11H,I**).

Subfrontal Approach

This approach is indicated for lesions located at the anterior portion of the third ventricle, and it has been popularized by Suzuki.[59,60] The patient is placed in the supine position with the head facing the ceiling and with a slight extension of the neck. A lumbar catheter can be inserted prior to positioning the patient to withdraw CSF whenever necessary (**Fig. 41–12A**).

A bicoronal skin incision and a bifrontal craniotomy down to the orbital ridge are performed exposing the anterior portion of the superior sagittal sinus. The dura is then opened as two horseshoes with their base facing the lateral border of the craniotomy, leaving the anterior portion of the superior sagittal sinus in the midline.

The frontal lobes are then elevated to separate the olfactory tracts from the basal surface of the frontal lobes, therefore allowing additional mobility to the frontal lobes (**Fig. 41–12B**).The anterior portion of the superior sagittal sinus is ligated and removed along with the anterior portion of the falx. The interhemispheric fissure is then completely dissected, and both frontal lobes and the ACerA are retracted laterally, exposing the lamina terminalis (**Fig. 41–12C**). It is interesting to keep in mind that the anterior commissure is located just at the junction between the superior portion of the lamina terminalis and the fornix, and the hypothalamus is located at the lower lateral wall of the third ventricle. The lamina terminalis is then opened (**Figs. 41–12D,E**) to enter the third ventricle.

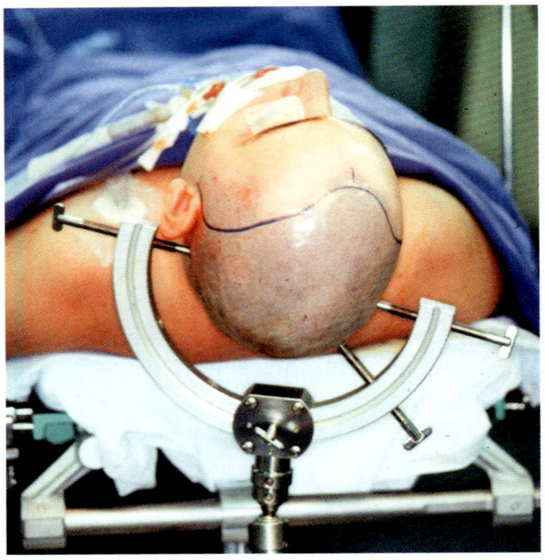

A

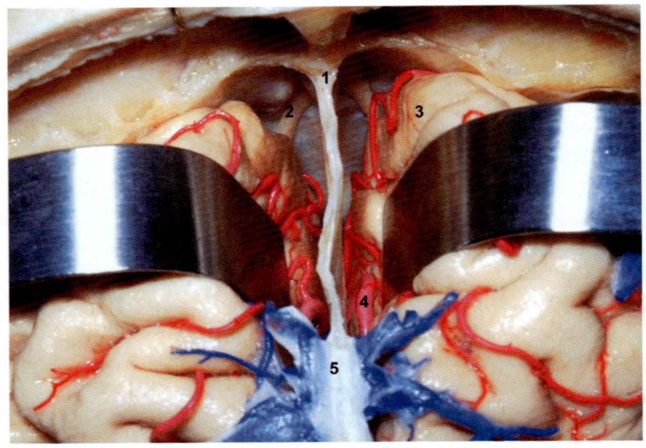

B

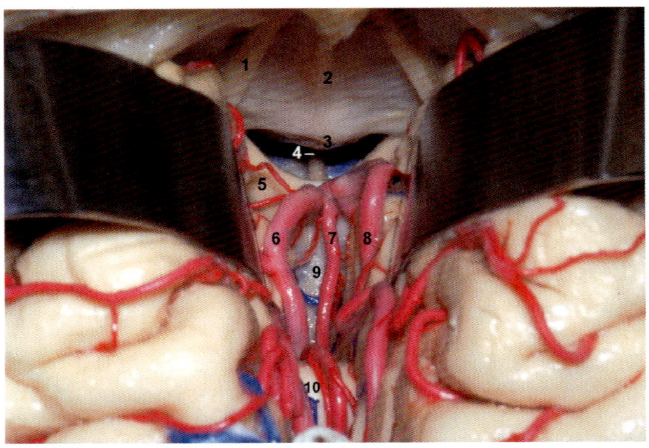

C

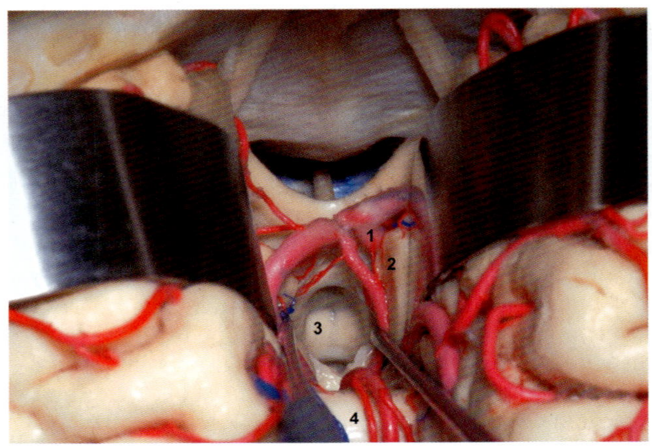

D

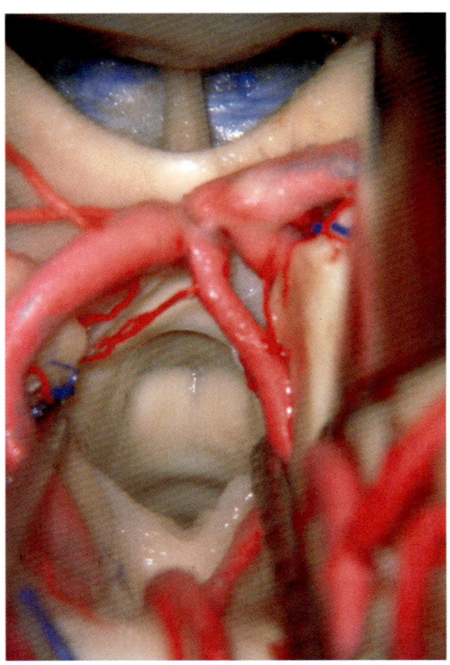

E

Figure 41–12 **(A)** Positioning of the patient and the skin incision for the subfrontal interhemispheric approach to the third ventricle. **(B)** Anatomical dissection of the interhemispheric fissure as in the subfrontal interhemispheric approach to the third ventricle. **1**, falx; **2**, olfactory tract; **3**, medial frontal gyrus; **4**, pericallosal artery; **5**, superior sagittal sinus. **(C)** The anterior portion of the superior sagittal sinus and the falx have been removed. **1**, left olfactory tract; **2**, planum sphenoidale; **3**, tuberculum sellae; **4**, pituitary stalk; **5**, left optic nerve; **6**, left A2; **7**, additional A2; **8**, right A2; **9**, lamina terminalis; **10**, genu of the corpus callosum. **(D)** The anterior cerebral arteries have been retracted laterally and the lamina terminalis opened. **1**, right A1; **2**, right rectus gyrus; **3**, mammillary bodies; **4**, genu of the corpus callosum. **(E)** A magnified view of **Fig. 41–12D.**

◆ Surgical Approach to Lesions Located in the Fourth Ventricle

The Telovelar Approach to the Fourth Ventricle

The fourth ventricle is often described as a tent-shaped midline structure[61,62] surrounded mainly by the vermian components of the cerebellum (**Fig. 41–13A**). A normal tent has a roof that is divided into halves, a floor, and two lateral walls; the actual overall shape of the fourth ventricle resembles that of a tent turned with its base facing forward and two open lateral walls (**Fig. 41–13B**): the floor is represented by the pons and medulla (**Fig. 41–13C,D**); the superior cerebellar peduncles, the superior medullary velum, and the adjacent lingula constitute the superior part of the roof of the fourth ventricle; the inferior part of the roof is composed of the inferior medullary velum, the tela choroidea, the choroid plexus, the uvula, and the nodule (**Figs. 41–13E,F**); the two open lateral walls of the fourth ventricle are open corridors represented by lateral recesses that communicate the fourth ventricle with the cerebellopontine angle.[63,64] When viewed from the front, the two petrosal surfaces of the cerebellum are separated by the brain stem, which comprises the midbrain, the pons, and the medulla (**Fig. 41–13C**).[50]

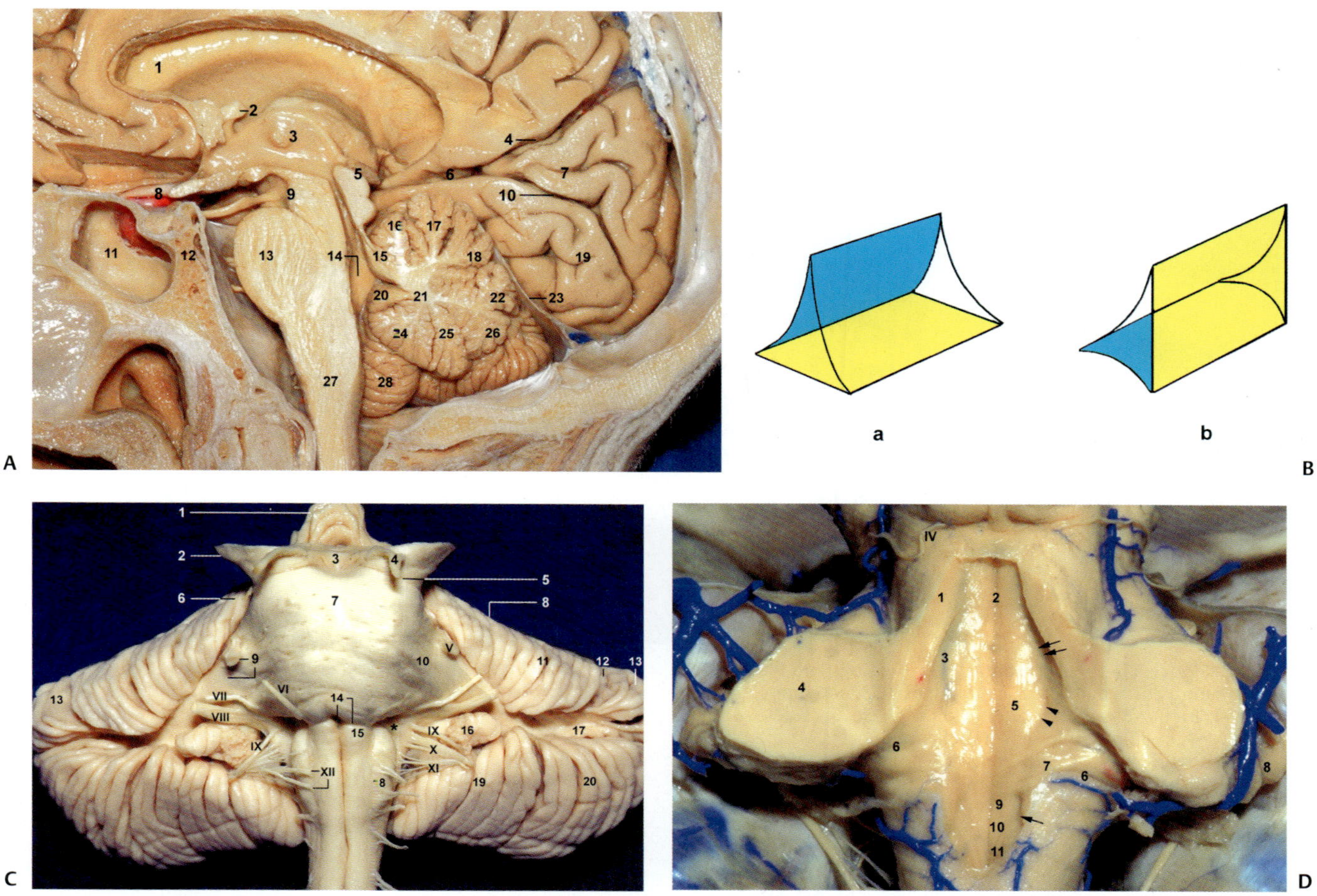

Figure 41–13 **(A)** Midsagittal view. **1**, head of the caudate nucleus; **2**, column of the fornix; **3**, massa intermedia; **4**, parieto-occipital sulcus; **5**, pineal gland and the superior colliculus; **6**, anterior calcarine sulcus; **7**, cuneus; **8**, optic nerve and the carotid artery; **9**, midbrain; **10**, calcarine sulcus; **11**, sphenoid sinus; **12**, clivus; **13**, pons; **14**, fourth ventricle; **15**, lingula; **16**, central lobule; **17**, culmen; **18**, declive; **19**, lingual gyrus; **20**, nodule; **21**, fastigium; **22**, folium; **23**, tentorium; **24**, uvula; **25**, pyramid; **26**, tuber; **27**, medulla; **28**, tonsil. **(B) a**, a regular tent is constituted by a floor (in yellow), a roof that has two parts (one displayed in cyan and another transparent), and two lateral walls (transparent). **b**, the fourth ventricle resembles a turned-over tent, with its floor facing forward (in yellow), and one part of the roof facing upward (transparent) and another part facing downward (cyan); the two lateral walls are an open corridor represented by the lateral recesses. **(C)** Frontal view. **1**, culmen; **2**, crus cerebri; **3**, interpeduncular fossa; **4**, oculomotor nerve; **5**, pontomesencephalic sulcus; **6**, wing of the central lobule; **7**, pons; **8**, quadrangular lobule; **9**, trigeminal nerve and middle cerebellar peduncle; **10**, lateral pontine sulcus; **11**, simple lobule; **12**, postclival sulcus; **13**, superior semilunar lobule; **14**, inferior foramen cecum and pontomedullary sulcus; **15**, pyramid; **16**, flocculus and choroid plexus; **17**, great horizontal fissure or petrosal fissure; **18**, olive; **19**, biventral lobule; **20**, inferior semilunar lobule; *, supraolivary fossette; **V**, trigeminal nerve; **VI**, abducent nerve; **VII**, facial nerve; **VIII**, vestibulocochlear nerve; **IX**, glossopharyngeal nerve; **X**, vagus nerve; **XI**, cranial accessory nerve; **XII**, hypoglossal nerve. **(D)** Posterior view of the floor of the fourth ventricle. **1**, superior cerebellar peduncle; **2**, median sulcus; **3**, vestibular area; **4**, middle cerebellar peduncle; **5**, facial colliculus; **6**, inferior cerebellar peduncle; **7**, stria medullary; **8**, flocculus; **9**, hypoglossal trigone; **10**, vagal trigone; **11**, area postrema. Inferior fovea (double arrow); superior fovea (double arrowhead); sulcus limitans; IV, trochlear nerve.

(Continued on pages 542 and 543)

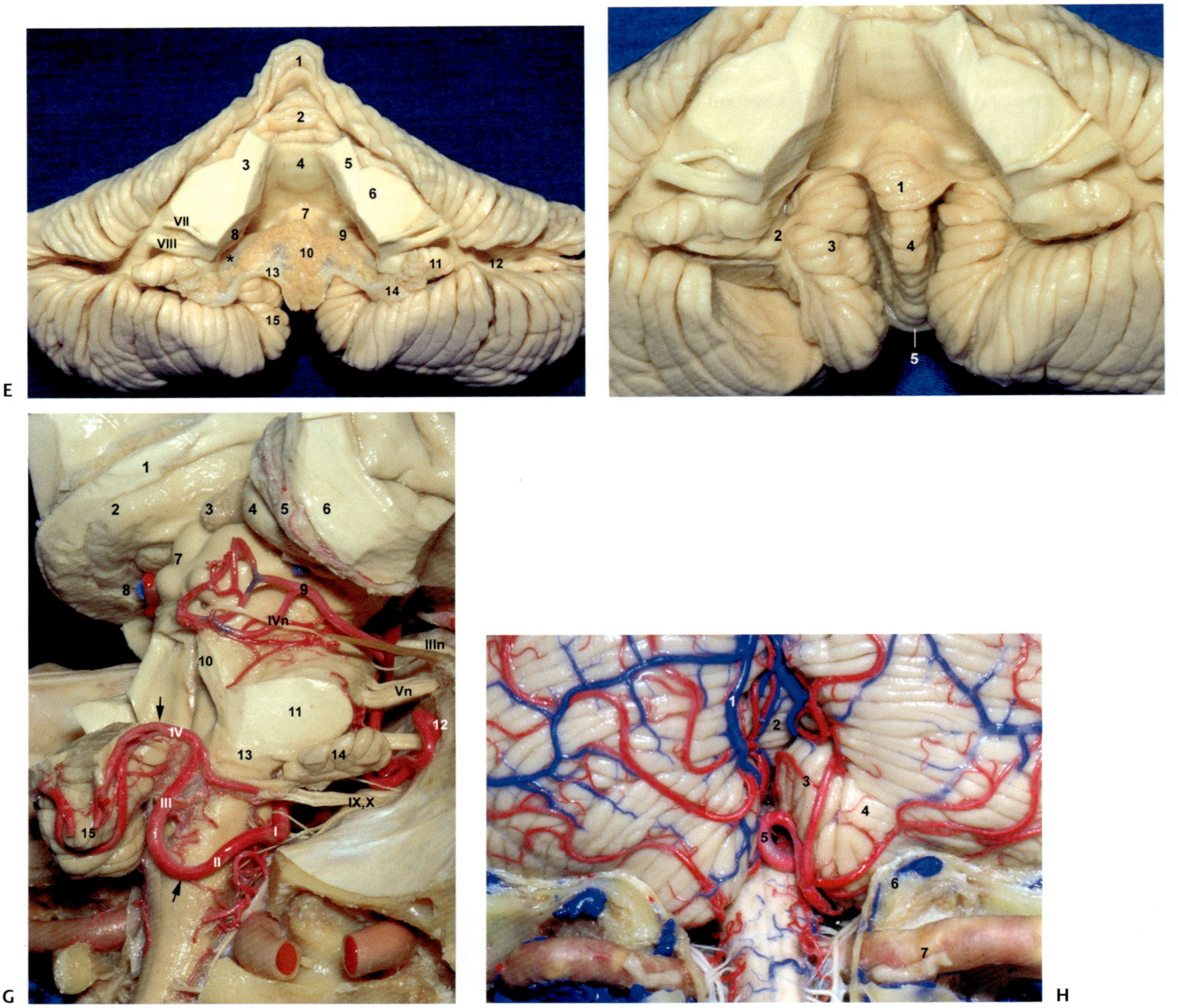

(*Continued*) **Figure 41–13** **(E)** Frontal view. The pons and the medulla have been removed. **1**, culmen; **2**, central lobule; **3**, superior cerebellar peduncle; **4**, lingula; **5**, superior cerebellar peduncle; **6**, middle cerebellar peduncle; **7**, nodule; **8**, inferior cerebellar peduncle; **9**, superolateral recess; **10**, choroid plexus; **11**, flocculus; **12**, petrosal or great horizontal fissure; **13**, tela choroidea; **14**, rhomboid lip; **15**, tonsil; **VII**, facial nerve; **VIII**, vestibulocochlear nerve. **(F)** Magnified view of the roof of the fourth ventricle. The choroid plexus and the tela choroidea have been removed to display the underlying tonsil and inferior vermis. **1**, nodule; **2**, peduncle of the tonsil; **3**, tonsil; **4**, uvula; **5**, pyramid. **(G)** Posterolateral view of the right posterior inferior cerebellar artery (PICA) to display its relationship to the roof of the fourth ventricle. **1**, fornix; **2**, pulvinar of the thalamus (cisternal); **3**, pineal; **4**, pulvinar of the thalamus; **5**, choroidal fissure; **6**, pulvinar of the thalamus (atrial); **7**, quadrigeminal plate; **8**, basal vein and posterior cerebral artery; **9**, superior cerebellar artery; **10**, superior cerebellar peduncle; **11**, middle cerebellar peduncle; **12**, internal acoustic meatus, anterior inferior cerebellar artery, facial and vestibulocochlear nerves; **13**, inferior cerebellar peduncle; **14**, flocculus; **15**, pyramid; **IIIn**, oculomotor nerve; **IVn**, trochlear nerve; **Vn**, trigeminal nerve; **IX**, **X**, glossopharyngeal and vagus nerves; **(I)**, anteromedullary segment of PICA; **II**, lateromedullary segment of PICA; **III**, posteromedullary segment of PICA; **IV**, supratonsillar segment of PICA. Caudal and cranial loops (arrows). **(H)** Anatomical dissection to display the exposure of the suboccipital surface of the cerebellum for the telovelar approach to the fourth ventricle. **1**, inferior vermian vein; **2**, uvula; **3**, tonsil; **4**, biventral lobule; **5**, posterior inferior cerebellar artery; **6**, lateral margin of the foramen magnum; **7**, vertebral artery and C1 nerve.

(*Continued on page 543*)

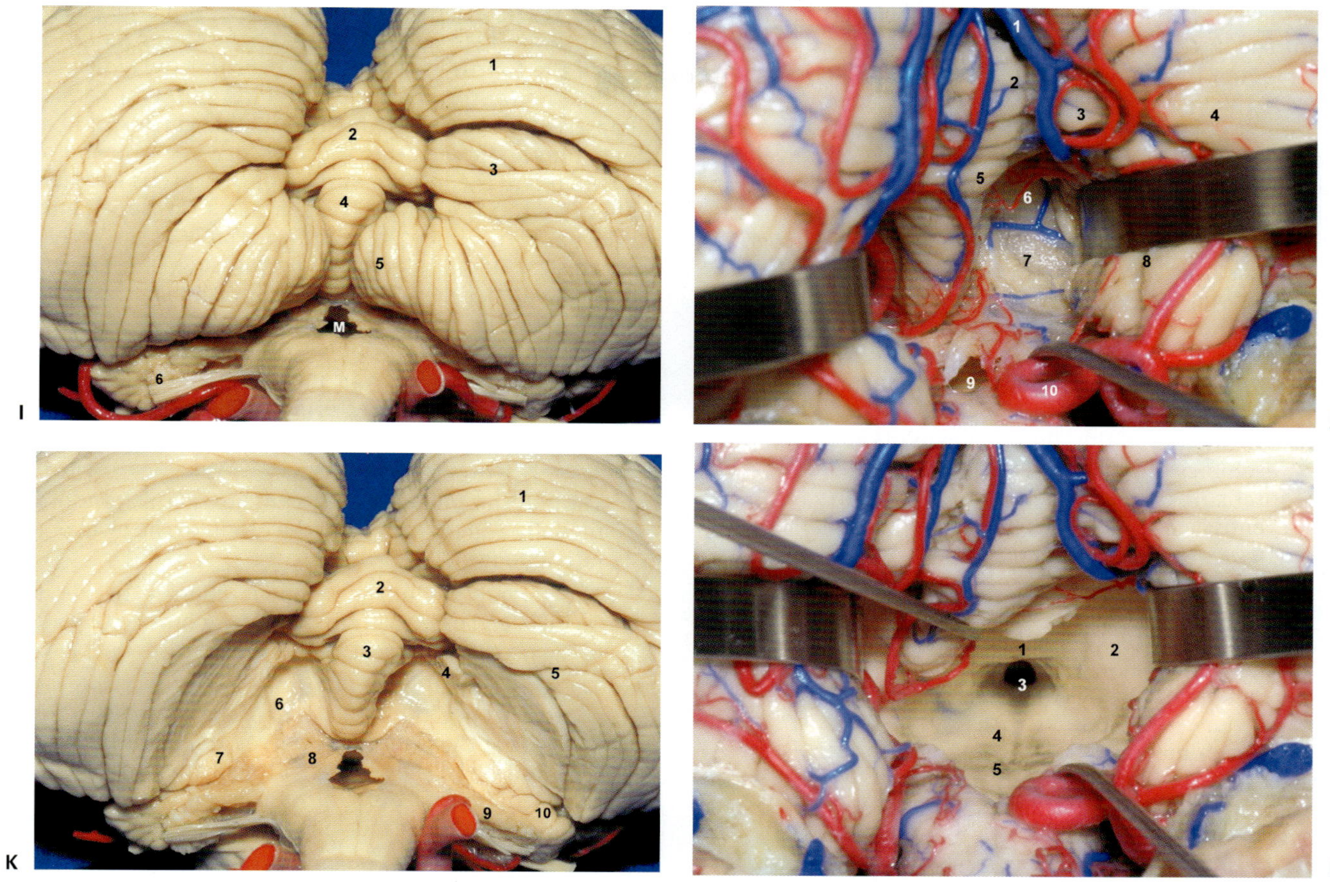

(*Continued*) **Figure 41–13** **(I)** Anatomical dissection displaying the neural structures of the suboccipital surface of the cerebellum. **1**, inferior semilunar lobule; **2**, pyramid; **3**, biventral lobule; **4**, uvula; **5**, tonsil; **6**, flocculus and choroid plexus from the foramen of Luschka; **(J)** Anatomical dissection displaying the telovelar approach to the fourth ventricle. The right tonsil has been "freed" by dissecting the spaces around it (medial, anterior, and superior spaces) and retracted laterally. **1**, inferior vermian vein; **2**, pyramid; **3**, copula pyramidis; **4**, biventral lobule; **5**, uvula; **6**, inferior medullary velum; **7**, tela choroidea; **8**, tonsil; **9**, foramen of Magendie; **10**, posterior inferior cerebellar artery. **(K)** Suboccipital view. Anatomical dissection displaying the inferior portion of the roof of the fourth ventricle, after the removal of both tonsils and part of the biventral lobules. **1**, inferior semilunar lobule; **2**, pyramid; **3**, uvula; **4**, peduncle of the tonsil (cut); **5**, biventral lobule; **6**, inferior medullary velum; **7**, peduncle of the flocculus; **8**, tela choroidea; **9**, rhomboid lip; **10**, flocculus. **(L)** Suboccipital view of the fourth ventricle. The right tonsil has been removed; the uvula has been retracted superiorly and the left tonsil retracted laterally. **1**, superior medullary velum; **2**, superior cerebellar peduncle; **3**, aqueduct; **4**, facial colliculus; **5**, stria medullary of the fourth ventricle.

The lateral recess is the lateral extension of the fourth ventricle and connects the fourth ventricle to the cerebellopontine angle. It is directed from medial to lateral, slightly from superior to inferior, and from posterior to anterior, forming an angle of ~45 degrees with the sagittal plane. The lateral recess presents an anterior, a superior, and a posterior wall and a floor. The anterior and superior walls of the lateral recess are constituted by the inferior cerebellar peduncle as it runs upward and then turns backward toward the white matter of the cerebellum. The floor of the lateral recess is constituted by the tela choroidea anteriorly, the choroid plexus in the middle, and the inferior medullary velum posteriorly; at the foramen of Luschka the inferior medullary velum becomes thicker and is called the peduncle of the flocculus. The peduncle of the flocculus constitutes the posterior wall of the foramen of Luschka **(Fig. 41–13E)**.

The superolateral recess is the space in the fourth ventricle limited medially by the nodule and inferiorly by the lateral extension of the inferior medullary velum, which covers the superior pole of the tonsil laterally. The superolateral recess is also limited superiorly by the superior cerebellar peduncle and anteroinferiorly by the junction between the tela choroidea and the inferior medullary velum (telovelar junction) **(Figs. 41–13E,F)**. After the removal of the pons and the medulla, which is the anterior wall of the cerebellomedullary fissure, the whole extent of the roof of the fourth ventricle is visualized **(Fig. 41–13E)**. The upper half of the roof of the fourth ventricle is constituted by the superior cerebellar peduncles, the superior medullary velum, and the lingula. The lingula can be visualized through transparency behind the superior medullary velum **(Fig. 41–13E,F)**. The lower half of the roof is composed of a horizontal portion and a vertical portion. The horizontal portion is constituted by the inferior medullary velum, which covers the nodule at the midline, and the superior pole of the tonsils laterally. The vertical portion is constituted by the tela choroidea and the choroid plexus, covering the anterior aspect of the nodule, uvula, and partly the tonsils. The two portions of the lower half of the roof of the fourth ventricle unite at the telovelar junction and continue laterally as the floor of the lateral recess. At the midline, the upper and lower halves of the roof of the fourth ventricle converge at the fastigium **(Fig. 41–13E)**.

The morphology of the choroid plexus of the fourth ventricle resembles the letter *T* with two vertical bars.[65–67] The horizontal part of the choroid plexus that starts from the fourth ventricle and protrudes into the cerebellopontine angle resembles the horns of a bull **(Fig. 41–13E)**. The vertical part and the proximal half of the horizontal part of the choroid plexus of the fourth ventricle is usually supplied by the posterior inferior cerebellar artery (PICA); the lateral half of the horizontal part and the choroid plexus located at the cerebellopontine angle is generally supplied by the anterior inferior cerebellar artery (AICA).

The inferior medullary velum separates the tonsil inferiorly from the superolateral recess superiorly. In anatomical position the tonsils are located behind the tela choroidea and under the inferior medullary velum **(Fig. 41–13E,F)**.

The tonsils are two uniform structures that are hemispheric components of the uvula and are attached to the cerebellum through the peduncles of the tonsil located at the superolateral aspect of each tonsil **(Fig. 41–13F)**. The superior, the medial, the anterior, the posterior, and most of the lateral surfaces of the tonsils are free and can be separated easily from the adjacent structures. The tonsils determine, along with surrounding neural structures, important spaces: between its superior pole and the inferior medullary velum is the supratonsillar space; between the medial surfaces of the two tonsils is the vallecula; between the anterior surface of the tonsil and the medulla is the cerebellomedullary fissure; between the posterior surface of the tonsil and the adjacent vermis is the retrotonsillar space, where the inferior vermian veins originate.[68,69]

The superior and inferior portions of the roof of the fourth ventricle are related respectively to the SCA and to the PICA. The inferior portion of the fourth ventricle is the one directly involved in the surgical approach to the lesions of the fourth ventricle.

The PICA arises from the vertebral artery and supplies the medulla, the inferior vermis, the inferior portion of the fourth ventricle, the tonsils, and the inferior aspect of the cerebellum.[70,71] It arises from the vertebral artery, usually at the anterolateral aspect of the brain stem near the inferior olive, and passes posteriorly around the medulla. At the anterolateral margin of the medulla it passes rostral or caudal to or between the rootlets of the hypoglossal nerve. At the posterolateral margin of the medulla the PICA passes rostral to or between the fila of the glossopharyngeal, vagus, and accessory nerves. After passing those latter nerves, it courses around the cerebellar tonsil and passes posteriorly to the lower half of the roof of the fourth ventricle. After turning away from the roof of the fourth ventricle, the PICA enters a series of deep fissures between the tonsil, the vermis, and the hemisphere. Upon exiting these fissures, its branches are distributed to the inferior surface of the vermis and hemisphere and to the tonsil. It often has a tortuous course, and its area of supply is the most variable of the cerebellar arteries. The PICA gives off perforating, choroidal,[67,72] and cortical arteries; when the PICA is absent, the AICA usually supplies this area. The entire inferior cerebellar hemispheres may be supplied by the contralateral PICA. The "normal" PICA has the most complex and variable course of the cerebellar arteries and is divided into five segments **(Fig. 41–13G)**:

1. The anterior medullary segment lies on the front of the medulla and extends from the origin to the level of the inferior olive.
2. The lateral medullary segment courses beside the medulla and extends from the inferior olive to the origin of the glossopharyngeal, vagus, and accessory nerves.
3. The tonsillomedullary or posterior medullary segment courses around the caudal half of the cerebellar tonsil; it begins at the level of the nerves and loops below the inferior pole of the cerebellar tonsil and upward along the medial surface of the tonsil toward the inferior medullary velum (caudal loop).
4. The telovelotonsillar or supratonsillar segment courses in the cleft between the tela choroidea and the inferior medullary velum rostrally, and the superior pole of the cerebellar tonsil caudally. It begins below the fastigium, where the PICA turns posteriorly over the medial side of the superior pole of the tonsil. This segment forms the "cranial loop." It sometimes passes posteriorly before reaching the superior pole of the tonsil, thus giving the cranial loop a variable relationship to the fastigium.
5. The junction of the posterior medullary segment and the supratonsillar segment is called the choroidal point cortical segment. After a short distance distal to the apex of the cranial loop, the PICA continues posteriorly downward in the retrotonsillar fissure, where it usually bifurcates into two terminal trunks, the tonsillohemispheric and the inferior vermian branches. The inferior vermian branch lies on the lower aspect of the inferior vermis and forms a loop convex around the copula pyramidis (pyramidal loop). The most anterior point of the curve of the pyramidal loop is also called the copular point.[73] The terminal portion of the vermian branch curves around the tuber in the posterior cerebellar notch. The tonsillohemispheric branch runs inferiorly near the prepyramidal sulcus and gives off anterior or tonsillar branches and posterior or hemispheric branches, which curve downward and backward around the biventral lobule to the under aspect of the cerebellar hemisphere.

The posterior medullary and supratonsillar segments of the PICA are directly related to the inferior part of the roof of the fourth ventricle **(Fig. 41–13G)**. For the surgical approach,[73] the patient is placed either in the semisitting or the prone position with the neck adequately flexed without compromising the venous drainage. A median linear incision is then performed, and the suboccipital muscles are dissected and retracted laterally. A suboccipital craniotomy or craniectomy is performed. Usually, there is no need to expose any of the sinuses to approach a lesion located in the fourth ventricles. However, adequate opening and drilling of the lateral edge of the foramen magnum has been shown to be very helpful. Sometimes, the removal of the posterior arch of the C1 can enhance the surgical corridor as well, mainly when the fourth ventricle is approached from below as in the semisitting position.

The dura is then anchored to the edge of the craniotomy and opened in a Y fashion. The surgeon should be careful when cutting the falx cerebelli, where the occipital sinus is located, and also when dividing the dura over the foramen magnum, where the marginal sinus is located.

After the dural opening, the suboccipital surface of the cerebellum comes into the surgeon's view (**Fig. 41–13H,I**). The spaces around the tonsil, namely, the vallecula, the supratonsillar space, and the cerebellomedullary fissure, are then dissected and the tonsil freed from the opposite tonsil, uvula, inferior medullary velum, tela choroidea, and posterior medullary segment of the PICA. The tonsil is then retracted laterally, exposing the inferior roof of the fourth ventricle (**Fig. 41–13J**). The inferior part of the roof of the fourth ventricle, from the surgical perspective, can be seen in **Fig. 41–13K**. The tela choroidea or the inferior medullary velum or both can be resected to gain a better view of the fourth ventricle (**Fig. 41–13L**). Removal of the tonsil after freeing it from the surrounding structures has also proven to be very helpful to gain additional space to the fourth ventricle.

These 11 surgical approaches are the ones preferred by the authors to approach the lesions located in the lateral, third, and fourth ventricles. They reflect the experience of the authors accumulated over the years in the anatomy laboratory and in a well-equipped operating room with a well-established team of anesthesiologists and circulating staff as well as adequate intensive care unit support. Because different surgeons have different working backgrounds (operating room, instruments, anesthesiologists, surgical skills, anatomical knowledge, etc.), these factors are absolutely relevant and must be considered and carefully evaluated before any decision on one approach over another is made.

Acknowledgments The authors thank Ronald Smith, M.S., director of the microneuroanatomy laboratory, Department of Neurosurgery, University of Florida, and Toshiro Katsuta, M.D., Department of Neurosurgery, Kyushu University, for their constant support. The authors also thank Cecília Emi Tsukamoto for help in preparing the manuscript.

References

1. Ono M, Ono M, Rhoton AL Jr. Microsurgical anatomy of the region of the tentorial incisura. J Neurosurg 1984;60:365–399
2. Timurkaynak E, Rhoton AL Jr, Barry M. Microsurgical anatomy and operative approaches to the lateral ventricles. Neurosurgery 1986;19:685–723
3. Wen HT, Rhoton AL Jr, de Oliveira E, et al. Microsurgical anatomy of the temporal lobe, I: Mesial temporal lobe and its vascular relationship as applied to amygdalohippocampectomy. Neurosurgery 1999; 45:549–592
4. Ebeling U, Reulen HJ. Neurosurgical topography of the optic radiation in the temporal lobe. Acta Neurochir (Wien) 1988;92:29–36
5. Warwick R, Williams PL. Gray's Anatomy. 35th ed. Philadelphia: WB Saunders; 1973
6. Gloor P. The Temporal Lobe and Limbic System. New York: Oxford University Press; 1997
7. Falconer MA, Wilson JL. Visual field changes following anterior temporal lobectomy: their significance in relation to "Meyer's loop" of the optic radiation. Brain 1958;81:1–14
8. Yamamoto I, Rhoton AL Jr, Peace D. Microsurgery of the third ventricle, I: Microsurgical anatomy. Neurosurgery 1981;8:334–356
9. Williams PL. Gray's Anatomy. 38th ed. London: Churchill Livingstone; 1995
10. Ebeling U, Reulen HJ. Subcortical topography and proportions of the pyramidal tract. Acta Neurochir (Wien) 1992;118:164–171
11. Dunker RO, Harris B. Surgical anatomy of the proximal anterior cerebral artery. J Neurosurg 1976;44:359–367
12. Wen HT, Rhoton AL Jr., de Oliveira E. Transchoroidal approach to the third ventricle: an anatomic study of the choroidal fissure and its clinical application. Neurosurgery 1998;42:1205–1219
13. Duvernoy HM. The Human Hippocampus: An Atlas of Applied Anatomy. Munich: JF Bergmann Verlag; 1988
14. van Buren JM, Baldwin M. The architecture of the optic radiation in the temporal lobe of man. Brain 1958;81:15–4o
15. Rasmussen AT. The extent of recurrent geniculo-calcarine fibers (loop of Archambault and Meyer) as demonstrated by gross brain dissection. Anat Rec 1943;85:277–282
16. Yasargil MG. Microneurosurgery: CNS Tumor: Surgical Anatomy, Neuropathology, Neuroradiology, Neurophysiology, Clinical Considerations, Operability, Treatment Options. Vol 4A. Stuttgart/New York: Georg Thieme Verlag; 1994
17. Yasargil MG. Microneurosurgery: Microneurosurgery of CNS Tumors. Vol 4B. Stuttgart/New York: Georg Thieme Verlag; 1996:29–68
18. Huang YP, Wolf BS. The basal cerebral vein and its tributaries. In: Newton TH, Potts DG, eds. Radiology of the Skull and Brain. Vol 2, book 3. St. Louis: CV Mosby; 1974:2111–2154
19. Ono M, Rhoton AL Jr, Peace D, et al. Microsurgical anatomy of the deep venous system of the brain. Neurosurgery 1984;15:621–657
20. Naidich TP, Brightbill TC. The pars marginalis, I: A "bracket" sign for the central sulcus in axial plane CT and MRI. Int J Neuroradiol 1996;2:3–19
21. Naidich TP, Brightbill TC. The pars marginalis, II: The pars deflection sign: a white matter pattern for identifying the pars marginalis in axial plane CT and MRI. Int J Neuroradiol 1996;2:20–24
22. Oka K, Rhoton AL Jr, Barry M, et al. Microsurgical anatomy of the superficial veins of the cerebrum. Neurosurgery 1985;17:711–748
23. Dunker RO, Harris B. Surgical anatomy of the proximal anterior cerebral artery. J Neurosurg 1976;44:359–367
24. Lin JP, Kricheff II. The anterior cerebral artery complex, I: Normal anterior cerebral artery complex. In: Newton TH, Potts DG, eds. Radiology of the Skull and Brain. Vol 2, book 2. St. Louis: CV Mosby; 1974:1391–1410
25. Perlmutter D, Rhoton AL Jr. Microsurgical anatomy of the distal anterior cerebral artery. J Neurosurg 1978;49:204–228
26. Perlmutter D, Rhoton AL Jr. Microsurgical anatomy of the anterior cerebral-anterior communicating-recurrent artery complex. J Neurosurg 1976;45:259–272
27. Ebeling U, Rikli D, Huber P, Reulen HJ. The coronal suture, a useful bony landmark in neurosurgery? Craniocerebral topography between bony landmarks on the skull and the brain. Acta Neurochir (Wien) 1987;89:130–134
28. de Oliveira E, Tedeschi H, Siqueira MG, Peace DA. The pretemporal approach to the interpeduncular and petroclival regions. Acta Neurochir (Wien) 1995;136:204–211

29. de Oliveira E, Tedeschi H. Pterional and pretemporal approaches. In: Sekhar LN, de Oliveira E, eds. Cranial Microsurgery: Approaches and Techniques. New York/Stuttgart: Georg Thieme Verlag; 1999:124–129
30. Yasargil MG. Microneurosurgery: AVM of the Brain. Vol 3B. Stuttgart New York: Georg Thieme Verlag; 1988
31. Gibo H, Carver CC, Rhoton AL Jr. Microsurgical anatomy of the middle cerebral artery. J Neurosurg 1981;54:151–169
32. Wolf BS, Huang YP, Newman CM. The superficial sylvian venous drainage system. Am J Roentgenol Radium Ther Nucl Med 1963;89: 398–410
33. Wolf BS, Huang YP. The insula and deep middle cerebral venous drainage system: normal anatomy and angiography. Am J Roentgenol Radium Ther Nucl Med 1963;90:472–489
34. Szikla G, Bouvier T, Hori T, Petrov V. Angiography of the Human Brain Cortex. Berlin: Springer; 1977
35. Türe U, Yasargil DCH, Al-Mefty O, et al. Topographic anatomy of the insular region. J Neurosurg 1999;90:720–733
36. Gibo H, Lenkey C, Rhoton AL Jr. Microsurgical anatomy of the supraclinoid portion of the internal carotid artery. J Neurosurg 1981;55: 560–574
37. Rosner SS, Rhoton AL Jr, Ono M, et al. Microsurgical anatomy of the anterior perforating arteries. J Neurosurg 1984;61:468–485
38. Warwick R, Williams PL. Gray's Anatomy. 35th ed. Philadelphia: W.B. Saunders Co. 1973;
39. Ono M, Kubik S, Abernathey CD. Atlas of the Cerebral Sulci. Stuttgart: Georg Thieme Verlag; 1990
40. Margolis MT, Newton TP, Hoyt WF. The posterior cerebral artery, II: Gross and roentgenographic anatomy. In: Newton TH, Potts DG eds. Radiology of the Skull and Brain. Vol 2, book 2. St. Louis: CV Mosby; 1974:1551–1576
41. Zeal AA, Rhoton AL Jr. Microsurgical anatomy of the posterior cerebral artery. J Neurosurg 1978;48:534–559
42. Rhoton AL Jr, Fujii K, Fradd B. Microsurgical anatomy of the anterior choroidal artery. Surg Neurol 1979;12:171–187
43. Theron J, Newton TH. Anterior choroidal artery, I: Anatomic and radiographic study. J Neuroradiol 1976;3:5–30
44. Rhoton AL Jr. Microsurgical anatomy of the third ventricular region. In: Apuzzo MLJ, ed. Surgery of the Third Ventricle Region. Baltimore: Williams & Wilkins; 1987:570–590
45. Stein BM. Transcallosal approach to tumors of the third ventricle. In: Schmidek HH, Sweet WH, eds. Operative Neurosurgical Techniques: Indications, Methods, and Results. Vol 1. Orlando: Grune & Stratton; 1988:381–387
46. Apuzzo MLJ, Giannotta SL. Transcallosal interforniceal approach. In: Apuzzo MLJ, ed. Surgery of the Third Ventricle Region. Baltimore: Williams & Wilkins; 1987:354–380
47. Apuzzo MLJ. Transcallosal interforniceal exposure of lesions of the third ventricle. In: Schmidek HH, Sweet WH, eds. Operative Neurosurgical Techniques. Indications, Methods, and Results. Vol 1. Orlando: Grune & Stratton; 1988:389–395
48. Rhoton AL Jr, Yamamoto I, Peace D. Microsurgery of the third ventricle, II: Operative approaches. Neurosurgery 1981;8:357–372
49. Stein BM. Supracerebellar approach for pineal region neoplasms. In: Schmidek HH, Sweet WH, eds. Operative Neurosurgical Techniques: Indications, Methods, and Results. Vol 1. Orlando: Grune & Stratton; 1988:401–409
50. Huang YP, Wolf BS, Antin SP, et al. The veins of the posterior fossa: anterior or petrosal draining group. Am J Roentgenol Radium Ther Nucl Med 1968;104:36–56
51. Huang YP, Wolf BS. Precentral cerebellar vein in angiography. Acta Radiol Diagn (Stockh) 1966;5:250–262
52. Huang YP, Wolf BS. Veins of the posterior fossa. In: Newton TH, Potts DG, eds. Radiology of the Skull and Brain. Vol 2, book 3. St Louis: CV Mosby; 1974:2155–2216
53. Huang YP, Wolf BS. The veins of the posterior fossa: superior or galenic draining group. AJR Am J Roentgenol 1965;95:808–821
54. Salamon G, Huang YP. Radiologic Anatomy of the Brain. New York: Springer; 1976:332–344
55. Matsushima T, Rhoton AL Jr, de Oliveira E. Microsurgical anatomy of the veins of the posterior fossa. J Neurosurg 1983;59:63–105
56. Hardy DG, Peace D, Rhoton AL Jr. Microsurgical anatomy of the superior cerebellar artery. Neurosurgery 1980;6:10–28
57. Hoffman HB, Margolis MT, Newton TH. The superior cerebellar artery, I: Normal gross and radiographic anatomy. In: Newton TH, Potts DG, eds. Radiology of the Skull and Brain. Vol 2, book 2. St. Louis: CV Mosby; 1974:1809–1830
58. Mani RL, Newton TH, Glickman MG. The superior cerebellar artery: an anatomic-roentgenographic correlation. Radiology 1968;91: 1102–1108
59. Suzuki J, Katakura R, Mori T. Interhemispheric approach through the lamina terminalis to tumors of the anterior part of the third ventricle. Surg Neurol 1984;22:157–163
60. Suzuki J. The bifrontal anterior interhemispheric approach. In: Apuzzo MLJ, ed. Surgery of the Third Ventricle. 2nd ed. Baltimore/Philadelphia: Williams & Wilkins; 1998:489–515
61. Corrales M, Greitz T. Fourth ventricle, I: A morphologic and radiologic investigation of the normal anatomy. Acta Radiol Diagn (Stockh) 1972;12:113–133
62. Matsushima T, Rhoton AL Jr, Lenkey C. Microsurgery of the fourth ventricle: Part 1: microsurgical anatomy. Neurosurgery 1982;11: 631–667
63. Bentson JR, Alberti JB. Lateral recess of the fourth ventricle. Radiology 1972;104:593–599
64. Huang YP, Wolf BS. The basal cerebral vein and its tributaries. In: Newton TH, Potts DG, eds. Radiology of the Skull and Brain. Vol 2, book 3. St. Louis: CV Mosby; 1974:2111–2154
65. Bradac GB, Simon RS, Fiegler W, et al. A radioanatomical study of the choroid plexus of the fourth ventricle. Neuroradiology 1976;11:87–91
66. Fujii K, Lenkey C, Rhoton AL Jr. Microsurgical anatomy of the choroidal arteries: fourth ventricle and cerebellopontine angles. J Neurosurg 1980;52:504–524
67. Takahashi M, Okudera T, Fukui M, et al. The choroidal and nodular branches of the posterior inferior cerebellar artery. Radiology 1972;103:347–351
68. Huang YP, Wolf BS, Okudera T. Angiographic anatomy of the inferior vermian vein of the cerebellum. Acta Radiol Diagn (Stockh) 1969;9:327–344
69. Wolpert SM. Normal angiographic anatomy of posterior fossa (plates I and II). In: Wolpert SM, ed. Angiography of Posterior Fossa Tumors. New York: Grune & Stratton; 1976:31–90
70. Lister JR, Rhoton AL Jr, Matsushima T, et al. Microsurgical anatomy of the posterior inferior cerebellar artery. Neurosurgery 1982;10:170–199
71. Wolf BS, Newman CM, Khilnani MT. The posterior inferior cerebellar artery on vertebral angiography. AJR Am J Roentgenol Radium Ther Nucl Med 1962;87:322–337
72. Belloni G, du Boulay G. The choroidal point and the copular point. Br J Radiol 1974;47:261–264
73. Mussi ACM, Rhoton AL Jr. Telovelar approach to the fourth ventricle: microsurgical anatomy. J Neurosurg 2000;92:812–823

Section VII

Pineal Region Lesions

42

Supracerebellar Approach to Pineal Region Lesions

Jeffrey N. Bruce

The refinement of microsurgical techniques has dramatically improved the surgical outcome for patients with pineal region lesions, leading to improved survival and quality of life. Historically, beginning with Krauses's, first description of the supracerebellar approach in 1926 and Dandy's report of the interhemispheric approach in 1936, attempts at surgical resection of pineal region tumors had been plagued by high mortality and morbidity. The resurgence of surgical favor can be traced back to the early 1970s, when Stein's incorporation of microsurgical techniques in the supracerebellar approach successfully reversed much of the intraoperative complications.

The supracerebellar approach takes advantage of the fact that these tumors are centrally midline and beneath the deep venous system. With the patient in the sitting position, allowing the cerebellum to fall away from the tentorium with minimal retraction, this approach provides a natural corridor with an unobstructed view of the pineal region and without interference of the venous structures. Furthermore, the sitting position minimizes venous bleeding, which can obscure the operative field. Alternate approaches, including the parietal interhemispheric and the occipital transtentorial, may be useful for patients whose tumors extend laterally to the trigone or superiorly above the tentorium. Although these approaches may be useful for large tumors, they have the disadvantage of requiring either or both brain retraction and sacrifice of bridging veins, resulting in hemiparesis with the parietal approach or visual field loss with the occipital approach. Furthermore, by coming from above, these approaches are encumbered by the deep venous system, which lies in the center of the operative field. Overall however, the surgeon should also keep in mind that the choice of approach is dependent on personal preference as well as understanding of the risks and benefits of each approach.

◆ Indications

All patients require surgery because the wide variety of histological subtypes that occur in the pineal region make a tissue diagnosis mandatory for enlightened clinical management. The only exception is for patients whose preoperative evaluation reveals the presence of elevated germ cell markers in the serum or cerebrospinal fluid. These patients have malignant germ cell tumors by definition and are best managed with a combination of radiation therapy and chemotherapy without a histological diagnosis.

Stereotactic biopsy can be a useful alternative for obtaining a tissue diagnosis in certain specific instances. Although less labor intensive and associated with less morbidity, stereotactic approaches have several drawbacks that make them less desirable than open procedures. The limited tissue sampling with a biopsy can result in an erroneous diagnosis, especially in light of the heterogeneity of the tumors and the difficulties that neuropathologists have in characterizing such rare and varied tumors with small sampling sizes. Although generally a safe procedure, stereotactic biopsy carries a risk of hemorrhage related to the adjacent vascular structures and to intratumoral bleeding from the high incidence of vascular tumors that occur in this region. Furthermore, open procedures allow the tumors to be maximally debulked or, in cases of benign tumors, surgically cured. The primary indications for stereotactic biopsy are patients whose medical conditions contraindicate an open procedure or patients who have obvious disseminated tumors. Certain patients whose tumors are obviously invasive within the brain stem or thalamus may have little benefit from an open procedure; however, this characteristic is not always readily apparent on magnetic resonance (MR) scanning, and some tumors that appear invasive actually turn out to have a reasonably well-developed tumor margin.

◆ Preparation

The essential test for all patients is a high-resolution magnetic resonance imaging (MRI) scan with and without gadolinium. Open MRI scans should be avoided if possible because it is important to have the best detail available to delineate the tumor margins and the relationships with the surrounding brain stem and deep venous system. Angiography is not necessary unless a vascular anomaly is suspected or a tentorial meningioma is present and the patency of the deep venous system needs evaluation. All patients should have β-human chorionic gonadotropin (HCG) and α-fetoprotein measured in the serum. If possible, cerebrospinal fluid (CSF) levels should be obtained as well. An elevated β-HCG or α-fetoprotein level is indicative of a malignant germ cell tumor. In these situations, no tissue diagnosis is necessary, and the patient should be treated with radiation or chemotherapy or both.

◆ Surgical Technique

Hydrocephalus

Many patients with pineal region tumors have hydrocephalus from aqueductal obstruction at the time of diagnosis. Optimum management preoperatively consists of an endoscopic third ventriculostomy. Ventriculoperitoneal shunting is a less favorable alternative because of the risk of peritoneal seeding and the risk of shunt malfunction. Patients with mild hydrocephalus can be managed with a ventricular drain placed at the time of surgery in anticipation of sufficient tumor removal to relieve the obstruction.

Anesthesia

There are no special considerations beyond standard anesthetic technique. Although inhalation anesthesia can cause an increase in intracranial pressure, this risk is counterbalanced by hyperventilation, the sitting position, and the relief of hydrocephalus. A Doppler monitoring system is used to detect the presence of air emboli when the sitting position is used. A central venous catheter is useful to remove entrapped air if the situation should arise.

Positioning

The sitting position is generally preferred for the supracerebellar approach because it allows gravity to work in the surgeon's favor by facilitating cerebellar retraction and reducing venous bleeding and pooling in the operative field. The disadvantage involving the risk of air embolus can be minimized by taking proper precautions. As an alternative, the supracerebellar approach can be performed in the three-quarter-prone or Concorde position, which may be desirable for patients under 3 years of age or patients with excessively large ventricles that might be predisposed to ventricular collapse.

For the sitting position, the patient is placed supine, and the table back is maximally inclined (**Fig. 42–1**). The

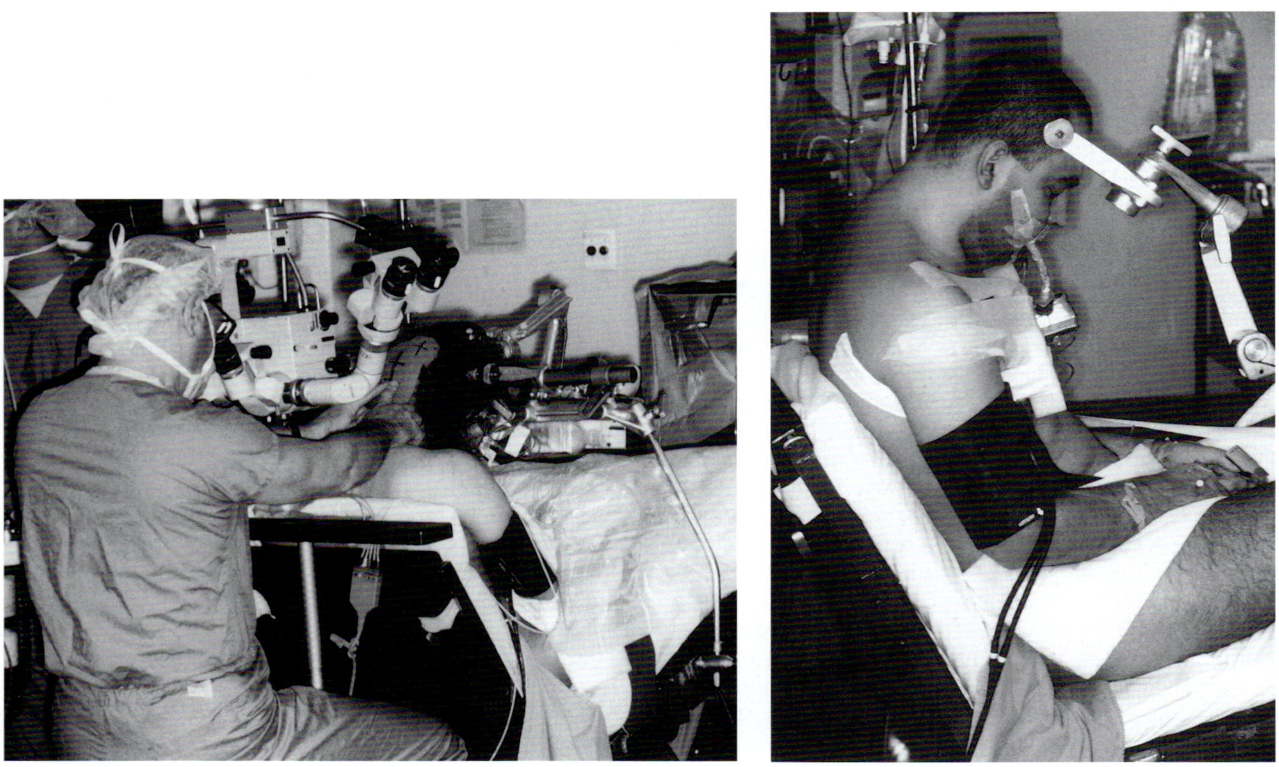

A B

Figure 42–1 **(A)** Operative setup for the supracerebellar approach to the pineal region. **(B)** Lateral view of patient in the sitting position.

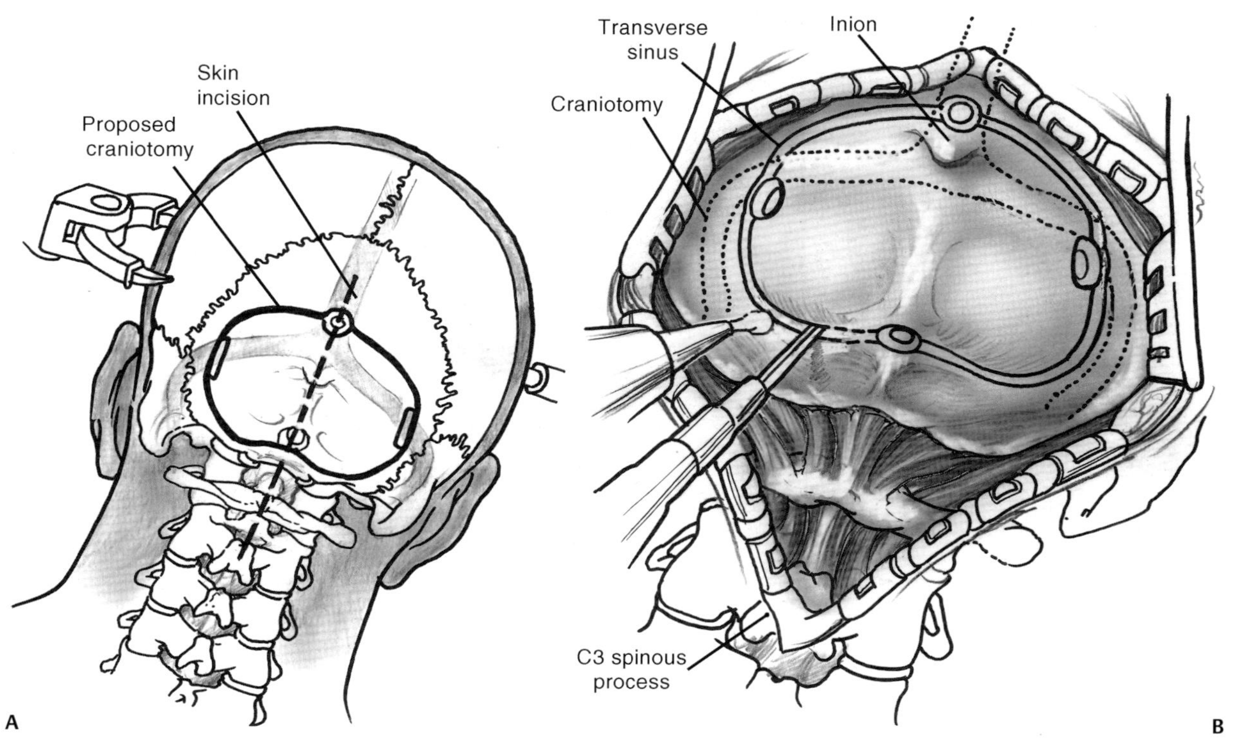

Figure 42–2 **(A)** Midline skin incision for the supracerebellar approach. **(B)** Suboccipital bone flap extending above the transverse sinus.

operating table is usually best used in a reverse position, and a table that goes low to the floor is desirable. A pin-vise head fixation device such as the Mayfield head holder is fixed in front of the patient. The head should be flexed enough so that the tentorium is approximately parallel to the floor without compromising the airway or jugular venous return. The patient is tilted forward so the surgeon is actually working over the back of the patient's shoulders.

A midline incision is used extending from just above the external occipital protuberance and down to approximately the spinous process of C3 (**Fig. 42–2**). A subperiosteal dissection is performed, elevating the muscle and fascia layers and preserving their continuity. The widest part of the exposure should be at the level of the transverse sinus. A craniotomy is preferred over a craniectomy because it is faster and seems to reduce postoperative discomfort. Slotted bur holes are made at the sagittal sinus just above the torcula, at the lateral aspect of the transverse sinus bilaterally and in the suboccipital midline above the foramen magnum. It is not necessary to open the foramen magnum. After elevating the dura, a craniotome is used to complete the craniotomy. Bone edges should be carefully waxed and the sinuses covered with Gelfoam to avoid air emboli.

The dura is opened with a gentle curving incision extending from the lateralmost exposure of the transverse sinus to its contralateral exposure (**Fig. 42–3A**). The incisions should extend from each side down to the midline, where the midline venous sinus can be ligated and the small cerebellar falx can be divided. If the cerebellum appears tense at this point, further relaxation can be facilitated by removal of spinal fluid from the ventricular drain or at the foramen magnum, or with the use of mannitol.

Exposure of the Tumor and Resection

After the dura is opened, the bridging veins will be visible (**Fig. 42–3B**). These should be cauterized and divided, thereby freeing up the cerebellum from the tentorium. The combined effect of gravity, the weight of cottonoids on the dorsal surface of the cerebellum, and some gentle retraction with a copper brain retractor can provide an unobstructed corridor to the pineal region (**Fig. 42–4**).

The operating microscope is brought into place at this time. Ideally a microscope with a variable objective is useful to adjust the focal length for specific parts of the procedure. If one is not available, then a 275 mm objective is utilized. Use of a longer focal distance will allow for easier manipulation of surgical instruments but will leave the surgeon too far from the operative field, resulting in arm fatigue. A freestanding armrest is essential to reduce tremor and arm fatigue.

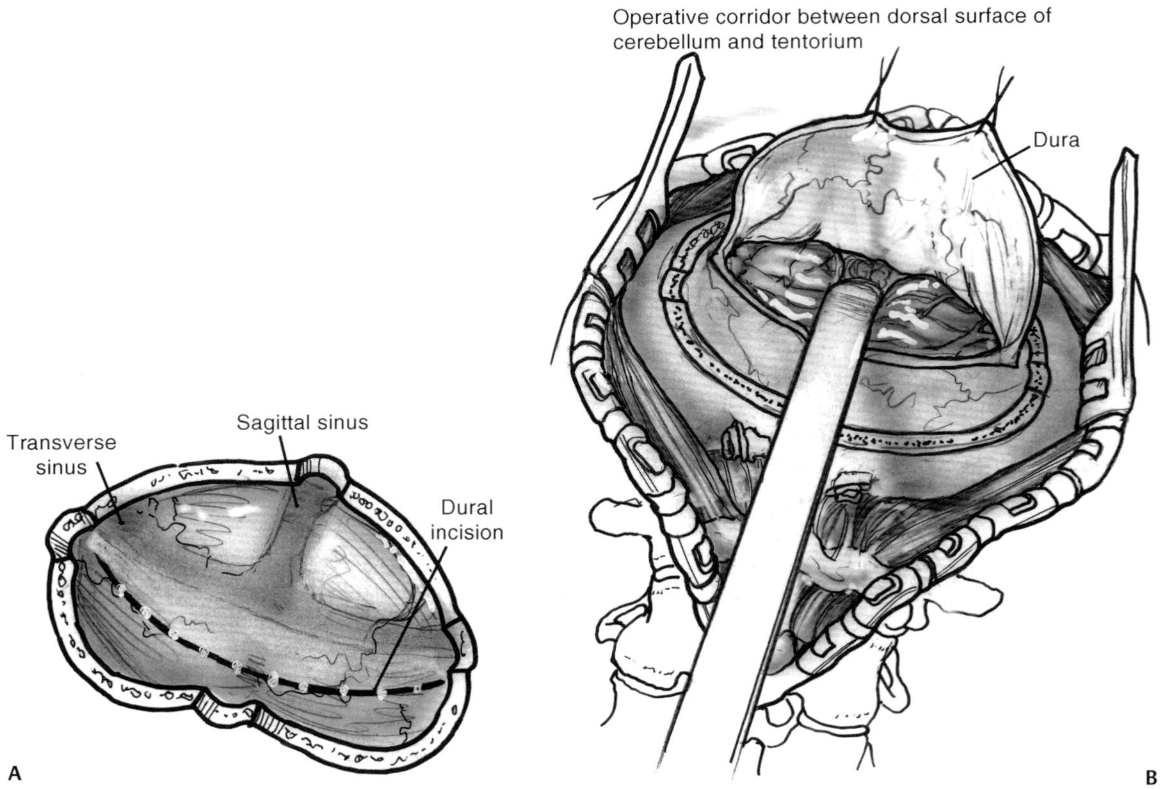

Figure 42–3 **(A)** Semilunar dural incision is reflected toward the transverse sinus. **(B)** Intradural view of the operative corridor.

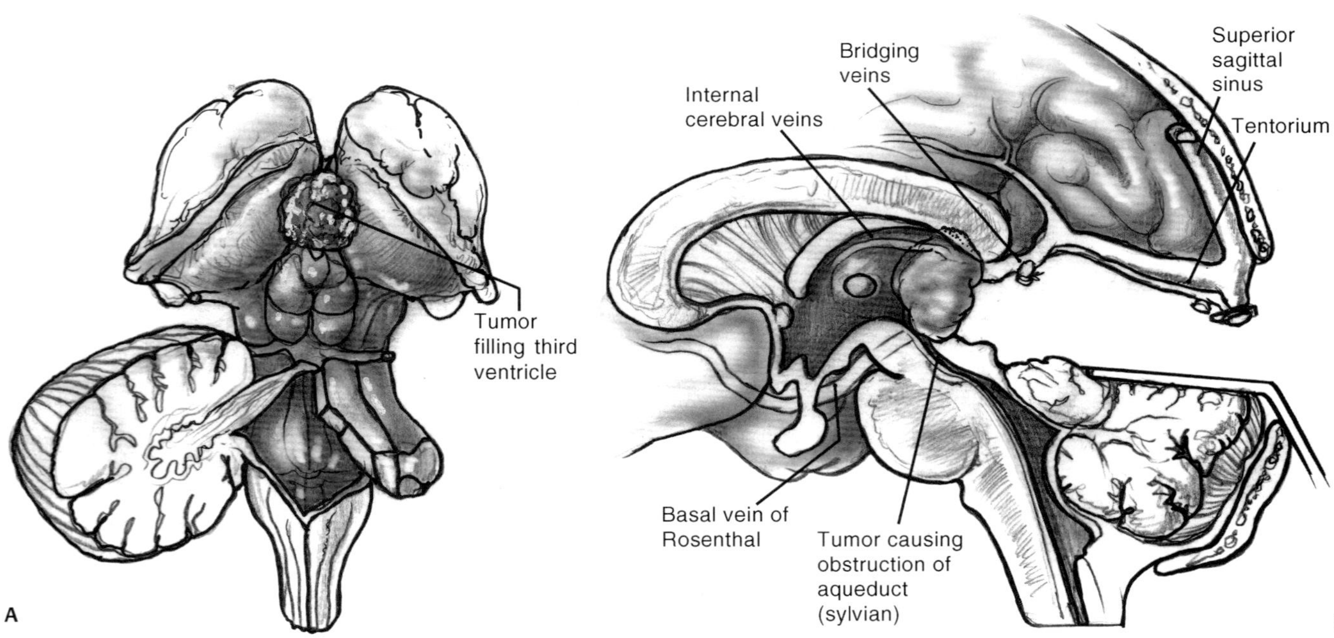

Figure 42–4 **(A)** Anatomy surrounding the pineal region. **(B)** Sagittal view of anatomy surrounding pineal tumor.

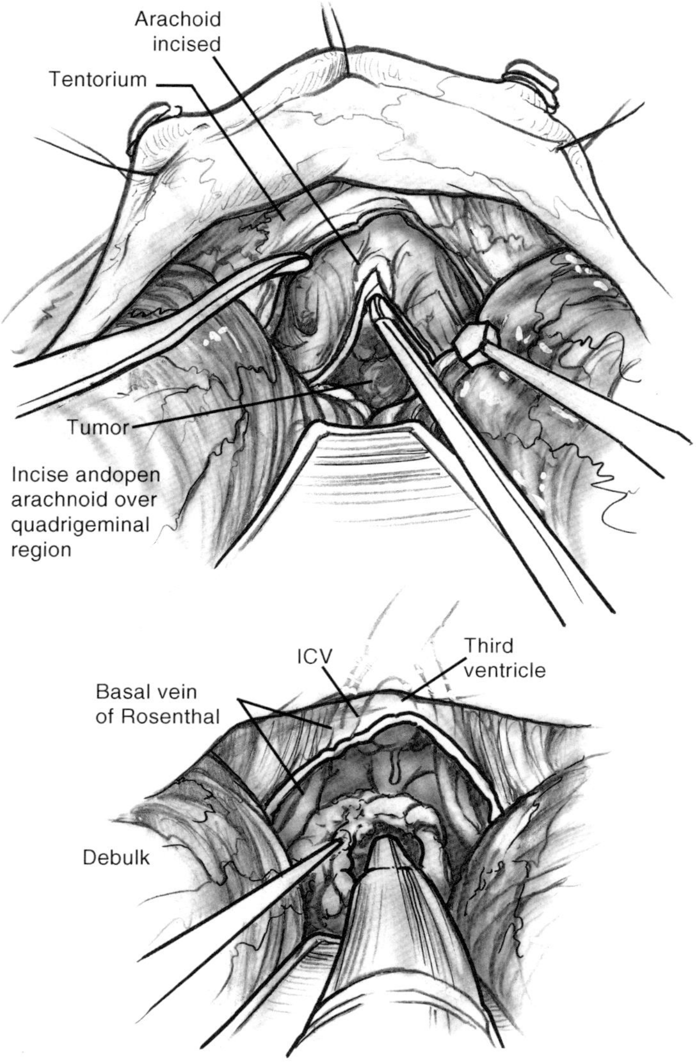

Figure 42–5 **(A)** Microsurgical view of quadrigeminal cistern as arachnoid overlying the pineal tumor is incised. **(B)** Tumor debulking is necessary prior to dissecting the tumor capsule. ICV, internal cerebral vein.

With the microscope in place, the arachnoid overlying the quadrigeminal region is opened sharply (**Fig. 42–5A**). This arachnoid is usually thickened and partially opaque when tumors are present. Advancing the retractor will allow the precentral cerebellar vein to be seen extending from the vermis to the vein of Galen, where it can be cauterized and divided. The vein of Galen and the internal cerebral vein are well above the tumor, and the veins of Rosenthal come from laterally to connect to the vein of Galen. These vessels should be sufficiently outside the tumor field to avoid injury. To avoid injury, it is important to realize that until the arachnoid has been opened and the cerebellum freed of its arachnoid adhesions with the brain stem, the operative trajectory is aimed at the vein of Galen. Once this is accomplished and the cerebellum can be retracted, the trajectory can be lowered so that it is aimed through the central axis of the tumor. The posterior surface of the tumor should be readily visualized and likely is supplied by branches of the choroidal arteries. A small portion of the posterior surface of the tumor is cauterized, then sharply opened to facilitate internal debulking (**Fig. 42–5B**). Depending on the consistency of the tumor, debulking can be performed with suction, cautery, tumor forceps, small curettes, or a Cavitron with a long curved tip. A portion of the tumor is sent for frozen tissue diagnosis, which may be used to guide intraoperative decisions. Many of these tumors are difficult for the neuropathologist to characterize on frozen section, and therefore the inaccuracy must be kept in mind when making decisions.

Once the tumor has been debulked, the capsule can be dissected from the surrounding structures. Tumors can extend anteriorly into the third ventricle for a considerable distance, and extra-long microinstruments are essential for removing those portions. The most difficult and potentially dangerous portion of dissection involves the inferior portion of the tumor, where it may be adherent to the dorsal midbrain. Small dental mirrors and angled instruments can facilitate this dissection. Experienced surgical judgment is important to determine whether the capsule can be completely removed without damage to the brain stem.

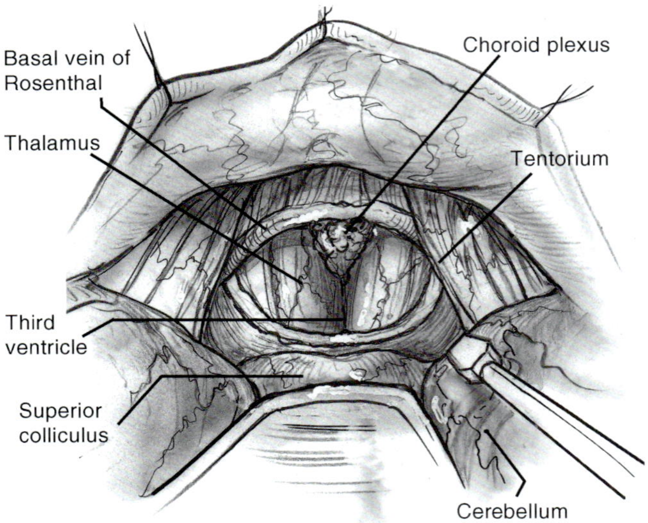

Figure 42–6 View into the third ventricle after the tumor has been removed.

Following tumor resection, the third ventricle can be visualized (**Fig. 42–6**).

When benign tumors are encountered, a gross total resection is desirable. For malignant tumors, an aggressive resection will improve the response to adjuvant therapy, and radical resection is often possible. Obviously, the benefits of resection must be weighed against potential morbidity from dissection at the tumor margin. Additionally, postoperative hemorrhage, one of the most serious complications, can be avoided by complete tumor removal. One exception to an aggressive resection is in the presence of pure germinomas where the exquisite radiosensitivity means that minimal benefit is derived from surgical resection.

Closure

The operative field and the third ventricle should be copiously irrigated with warm saline to ensure meticulous hemostasis and to make sure there are no hidden clots to block the aqueduct. Similarly, excess hemostatic agents should be avoided because they will float in the ventricles and eventually obstruct the aqueduct. The dura should be closed as completely as possible, although getting a watertight closure is often difficult. The bone flap is plated into place, and the soft tissue layers are reapproximated in a standard fashion.

◆ Postoperative Care

Patients should be monitored in an intensive care unit until neurologically stable. It is not unusual for patients to temporarily have mild cognitive impairment, extraocular disabilities, or ataxia. A computed tomographic (CT) scan should be performed on the first postoperative day to monitor ventricular size and the degree of pneumocephalus. If a ventricular drain is placed at the time of surgery, its necessity should be assessed to allow it to be either removed or converted to a ventricular shunt by day 3.

Patients should remain on high-dose steroids for the first several days. Until it has resolved, the subdural air that is present may result in lethargy. Any changes in neurological condition should be vigilantly investigated with a CT scan to rule out hydrocephalus, postoperative hemorrhage, or air. Acute hydrocephalus from debris or an obstructed shunt can resolve in a very rapid deterioration.

As with any surgery, patients should be encouraged to mobilize and ambulate as soon as possible. This may be difficult in the setting of lethargy and ataxia; however, rapid evaluation by a rehabilitation therapist and a physical therapist can facilitate a more expeditious recovery.

◆ Complications

Patients can expect to have some degree of impaired extraocular movements following surgery, particularly with limited upgaze and convergence, which may result in some difficulties focusing. These problems normally last anywhere from a few days to weeks but rarely persist more than several months. Similarly, ataxia from cerebellar retraction is often present for a few days but also resolves spontaneously. Most of these complications are directly related to the structures in the operative field, and their effects can be reduced intraoperatively by careful retraction and minimizing manipulation. In its most extreme form, excess manipulation can cause cognitive impairment or forms of akinetic mutism. The likelihood of these complications can be anticipated because they are more frequent in patients who have either more severe neurological deficits preoperatively, previous radiation, or invasive tumors.

One of the most severe forms of morbidity is postoperative hemorrhage into an incompletely resected tumor. This is most common in the setting of very vascular tumors, particularly of pineal cell origin. Complete resection reduces the risk of hemorrhage; however, this may not always be feasible. Although a small hemorrhage can be managed conservatively, a large hemorrhage requires rapid evacuation.

In the sitting position, subdural hematomas or hygromas or ventricular collapse can occur. These conditions are generally self-limiting and rarely severe. Air embolus is also rarely a problem, but it can be anticipated by a drop in end-tidal carbon dioxide levels or by detection with Doppler monitoring.

◆ Conclusion

Surgery in the pineal region via the supracerebellar approach can be successful and rewarding if careful attention is given to intraoperative technique and judgment. Experience has been a factor with this challenging surgery, resulting in improved operative outcome as experience increases. Much of the outcome is dependent upon rational patient selection and planned operative approach along with intraoperative decisions concerning extent of tumor removal.

Under optimal conditions, mortality and morbidity rates are in the 5 to 10% range. One third of pineal tumors are benign and potentially curable with surgery alone at a rate approaching 100%.

Suggested Reading

Bruce JN. Management of pineal region tumors. Neurosurg Quart 1993;3:103–119

Bruce JN, Fetell MR, Balmaceda CM, Stein BM. Tumors of the pineal region. In: Black PM, Loeffler JS, ed. Cancer of the Nervous System. Malden, MA: Blackwell Science; 1996:576–592

Bruce JN, Stein BM. Infratentorial approach to pineal tumors. In: Wilson CB, ed. Neurosurgical Procedures: Personal Approaches to Classic Operations. Baltimore: Williams & Wilkins; 1992:63–76

Bruce JN, Stein BM. Supracerebellar approaches in the pineal region. In: Apuzzo MLJ, ed. Brain Surgery: Complication Avoidance and Management. New York: Churchill-Livingstone; 1993:511–536

Bruce JN, Stein BM. Surgical management of pineal region tumors. Acta Neurochir (Wien) 1995;134:130–135

Dandy WE. Operative experience of cases of pineal tumor. Arch Surg 1936;33:19–46

Edwards MSB, Hudgins RJ, Wilson CB, et al. Pineal region tumors in children. J Neurosurg 1988;68:689–697

Fetell MR, Bruce JN, Burke AM, et al. Non-neoplastic pineal cysts. Neurology 1991;41:1034–1040

Fetell MR, Stein BM. Neuroendocrine aspects of pineal tumors. Neurol Clin 1986;4:877–905

Goodman R. Magnetic resonance imaging-directed stereotactic endoscopic third ventriculostomy. Neurosurgery 1993;32:1043–1047

Kobayashi S, Sugita K, Tanaka Y, Kyoshima K. Infratentorial approach to the pineal region in the prone position: Concorde position. J Neurosurg 1983;58:141–143

Krause F. Operative Frielegung der Vierhugel, nebst Beobachtungen uber Hirndruck und Dekompression. Zentralbl Chir 1926;53: 2812–2819

Kreth F, Schatz C, Pagenstecher A, Faist M, Volk B, Ostertag C. Stereotactic management of lesions of the pineal region. Neurosurgery 1996;39: 280–291

Page LK. The infratentorial-supracerebellar exposure of tumors in the pineal area. Neurosurgery 1977;1:36–40

Quest DO, Kleriga E. Microsurgical anatomy of the pineal region. Neurosurgery 1980;6:385–390

Reid WS, Clark K. Comparison of the infratentorial and transtentorial approaches to the pineal region. Neurosurgery 1978;3:1–8

Sawamura Y, de Tribolet N, Ishii N, Abe H. Management of primary intracranial germinomas: diagnostic surgery or radical resection? J Neurosurg 1997;87:262–266

Schmidek HH. Pineal Tumors. New York: Masson; 1977

Stein BM. The infratentorial supracerebellar approach to pineal lesions. J Neurosurg 1971;35:197–202

Tien RD, Barkovich AJ, Edwards MS. MR imaging of pineal tumors. AJR Am J Roentgenol 1990;155:143–151

43

Occipital Transtentorial and Parietal Approaches to Pineal Region Lesions

Kazuhiro Hongo, Shigeaki Kobayashi, and Yuichiro Tanaka

Dandy[1] made the first direct surgical approach to the pineal region by splitting the corpus callosum. Van Wagenen[2] used a transventricular approach. The infratentorial supracerebellar approach was first used by Krause[3] and further developed by Stein.[4] Poppen[5] performed a suboccipital approach, and Jamieson[6] modified this approach by mobilizing the occipital pole upward and laterally.

Before the advent of microscopic techniques and modern neuroanesthesia, surgery in the pineal region had a high mortality and morbidity. After introducing these techniques, direct surgery in this region has been performed safely using various surgical approaches, of which the occipital transtentorial and infratentorial supracerebellar approaches are currently used predominantly. A parietal transcortical approach is often indicated for lesions in the thalamus or laterally extending tumors (**Fig. 43–1**),[7] but this procedure is rarely used for the pineal region.

The infratentorial supracerebellar approach allows easy orientation; however, it provides a limited operative field when the lesion extends laterally, anteriorly into the third ventricle and superior to the deep venous plexus. It is usually used for tumors located below the galenic system in the pineal region. On the other hand, the occipital transtentorial approach provides a wide operative field permitting dissection of a tumor extending laterally. For both approaches, great care should be taken not to injure the deep venous system. This chapter describes the occipital transtentorial approach primarily.

◆ Indications

Indications for direct surgery in this area using the occipital transtentorial approach include pineal region tumors such as teratomas, germ cell tumors, and meningiomas, with or without obstructive hydrocephalus. Vascular lesions, such as varices of the vein of Galen, arteriovenous malformations in the pineal region, and aneurysms of the distal portion of P3 to P4 of the posterior cerebral artery are another indication for this approach.

When a germ cell tumor is suspected from preoperative neuroimaging and tumor marker studies, either a stereoscopic or an endoscopic biopsy via the third ventricle is usually performed, followed by radiation or chemotherapy. For typical pineal lesions, the occipital transtentorial approach utilized nowadays[8–10] is preferred by the authors. The parietal approach is mainly indicated for thalamic gliomas or intra-axial tumors extending laterally around the trigone of the lateral ventricle and is rarely used for pure pineal lesions.

◆ Preparation

Magnetic resonance imaging (MRI) with gadolinium enhancement is essential to visualize the tumor and its size and relationship with surrounding structures. A sagittal plane demonstrates especially well the anatomical relationships with the tentorium, third ventricle, splenium, and midbrain. The angle of the straight sinus and the tentorium can also be evaluated. This information is important for selecting the appropriate operative approach. A cerebral angiogram, both carotid and vertebral, is also essential to display the venous anatomy because the position of the torcular Herophili and the course of the transverse sinus can vary. It is important to confirm these venous structures at the time of craniotomy. Usually there are no big cortical veins over the occipital lobe. If the tumor is highly vascular and fed by an arterial branch, preoperative embolization is indicated.

To help make the preoperative diagnosis, it is useful to measure tumor markers, such as α-fetoprotein (AFP) and

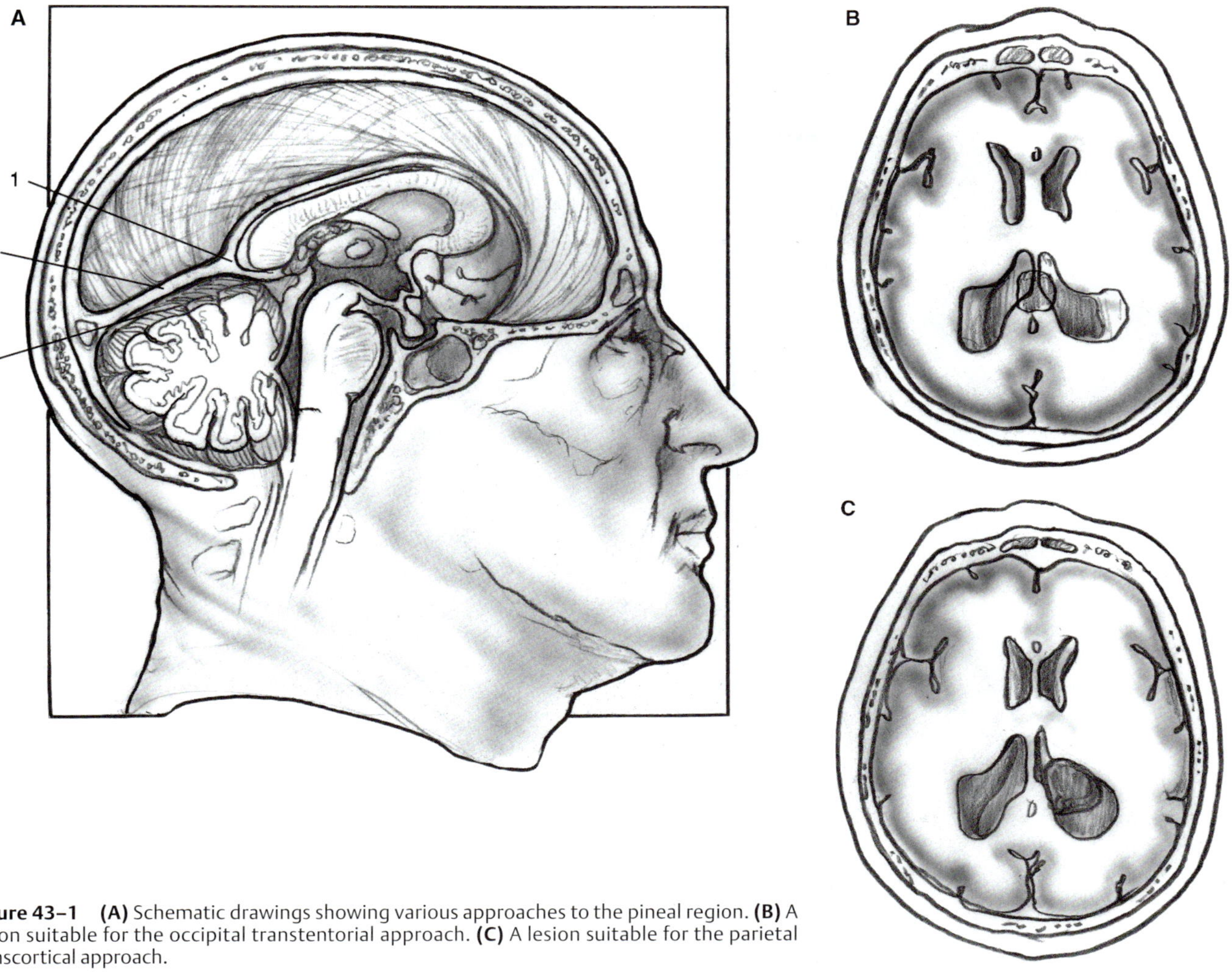

Figure 43–1 **(A)** Schematic drawings showing various approaches to the pineal region. **(B)** A lesion suitable for the occipital transtentorial approach. **(C)** A lesion suitable for the parietal transcortical approach.

human chorionic gonadotropin (HCG). For giant pineal region tumors causing obstructive hydrocephalus, we prefer to perform endoscopic third ventriculostomy first. The tumor is biopsied simultaneously unless the tumor is vascular. We are reluctant to place a ventriculoperitoneal (VP) shunt preoperatively because the hydrocephalus usually disappears once the tumor is removed.

◆ Surgical Technique: Transtentorial Approach

Anesthesia

Standard general anesthesia is used with endotracheal intubation. Mannitol 1 g/kg body weight is administered intravenously for brain relaxation just before surgery.

Neurophysiological Monitoring

No specific neurophysiological monitoring is routinely performed with an occipital transtentorial approach. When the tumor extends downward, pushing the inferior colliculus, the auditory brain stem response (ABR) is helpful.

Positioning

The patient is placed in the semiprone position with the head flexed so that the surgeon can sit behind the patient (**Fig. 43–2**). For typical pineal lesions, the operative approach is from the right side. Therefore, the patient is placed right side down in the semiprone position. It is important to make the craniotomy on the lower side of the skull, usually on the right, to ensure that gravity will help retract the occipital lobe. When the lesion extends right laterally, an approach is made on the contralateral side via a left craniotomy to avoid over-retraction of the occipital lobe.

The patient's hair is shaved where the U-shaped skin incision will be made, and the head is fixed in a Sugita multipurpose head frame with four pins. After the skin is incised, the skin flap and muscles are reflected as a single layer (**Fig. 43–3A**). Next, the craniotomy is performed using six bur holes: two on the left side and two on the right side along the superior sagittal sinus, one just

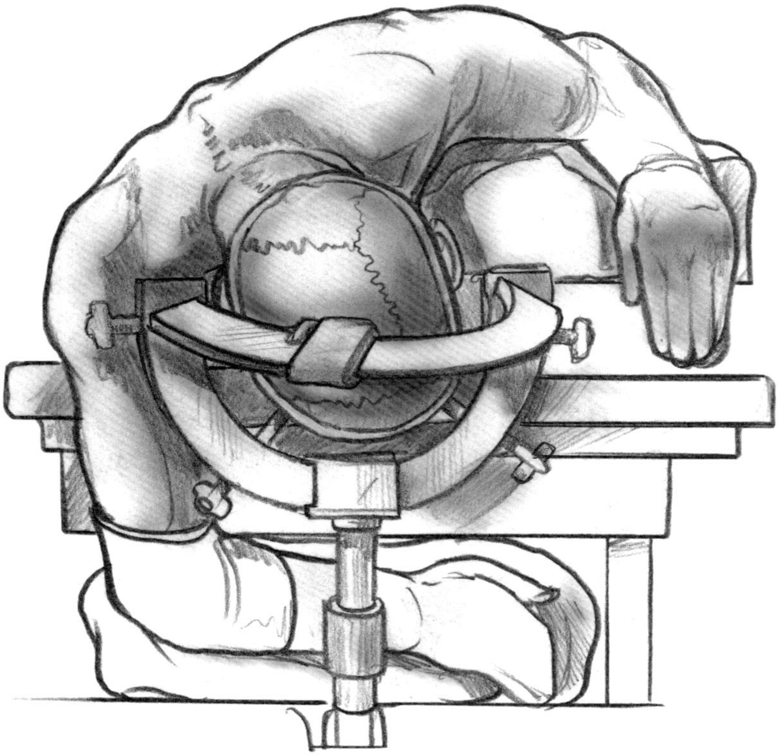

Figure 43–2 Patient's position.

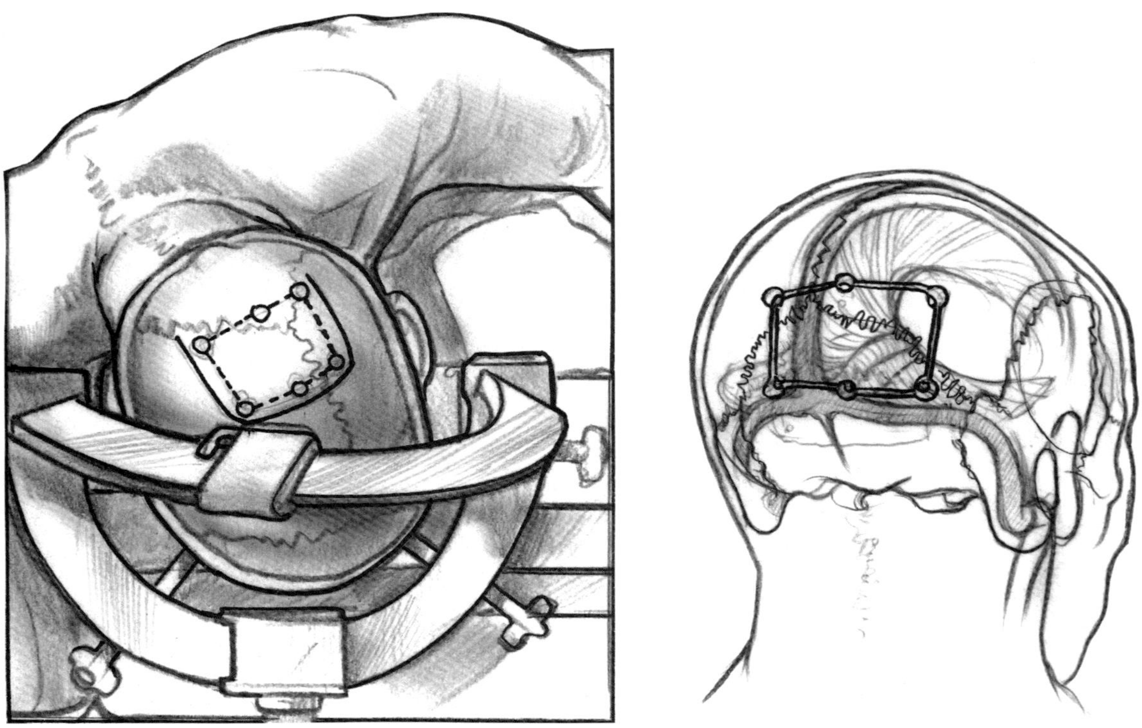

A B

Figure 43–3 **(A)** Skin incision and **(B)** craniotomy.

rostral to the transverse sinus, and the other on the parietal, to fully expose the superior sagittal sinus (**Fig. 43–3B**). The craniotomy is extended caudally to expose the transverse sinus at the torcular portion. The surface of the superior sagittal sinus is covered with Spongel or Gelfoam patties for hemostasis; there is often some bleeding from the pacchionian granulations over or along the sinus.

Procedure

The dura mater is opened with a T-shaped incision and reflected to the side of the sinuses, exposing the occipital lobe. A self-retaining retractor is gently applied to the occipital lobe. Usually there are no big cortical veins. At this point, it is important not to place the brain spatula directly on the calcarine cortex; apply the spatula to the inferior surface of the occipital lobe, rather than deep into the interhemispheric fissure, to avoid visual field deficits postoperatively (**Fig. 43–4**). The falx is also retracted medially with a retractor. A ventricular drain is placed in the occipital horn of the right lateral ventricle in cases with associated obstructive hydrocephalus. Spinal or ventricular drainage is not mandatory when there is no associated obstructive hydrocephalus; the cerebrospinal fluid (CSF) can usually be aspirated from the quadrigeminal cistern before it reaches the lesion after gentle retraction of the right occipital lobe.

The tentorium is then cut open (**Fig. 43–5**). An incision is made parallel to and 1.0 to 1.5 cm from the straight sinus, starting from the edge of the tentorium. Because there are variations in the tentorial sinus, which sometimes forms a vascular lake, adequate coagulation of the cutting edge with a bipolar coagulator is needed. Retention sutures are placed to retract the cut tentorial edge laterally. To widen the operative field, the medial cut end is retracted with a tapered brain spatula.

The arachnoid membrane is usually thick in this area. Great care should be taken not to injure the underlying deep venous system when cutting the arachnoid membrane. It is important to perform sharp dissection with a pair of fine microscissors, without retracting the venous system excessively. CSF gradually drains after the quadrigeminal cistern is opened, and the brain becomes slack. The brain spatula retracting the occipital lobe is repositioned in a stepwise fashion to gradually widen the operative field.

The first vein seen is usually the great vein of Galen, followed by the right basal vein of Rosenthal. Then the internal cerebral and precentral cerebellar veins are visualized (**Fig. 43–6**). These veins are shifted according to the location and extension of the lesion, which is why the preoperative MRI and angiogram evaluation is extremely important.

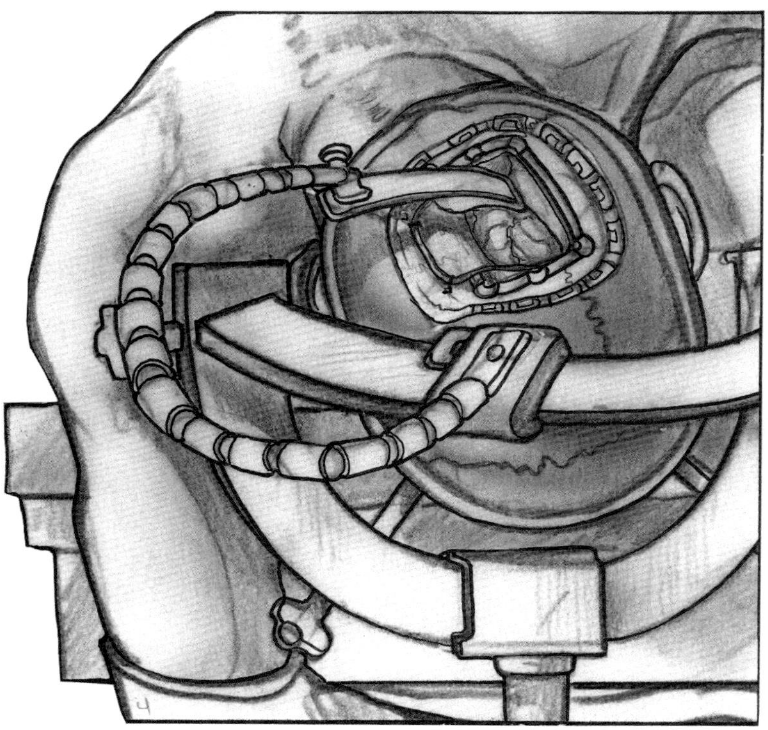

Figure 43–4 Dural incision and retraction of the occipital lobe with a self-retaining retractor.

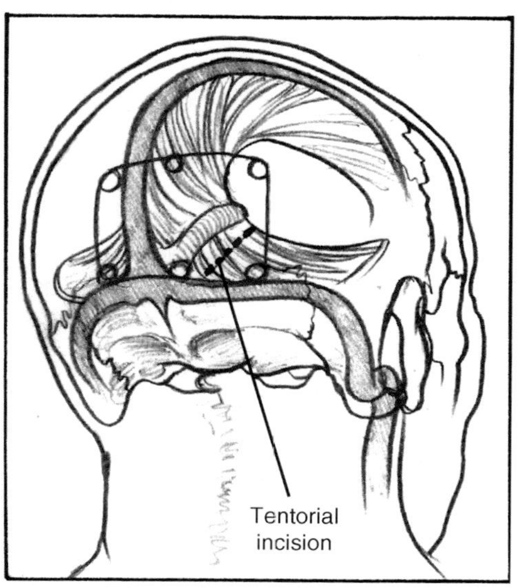

Figure 43–5 Tentorial incision.

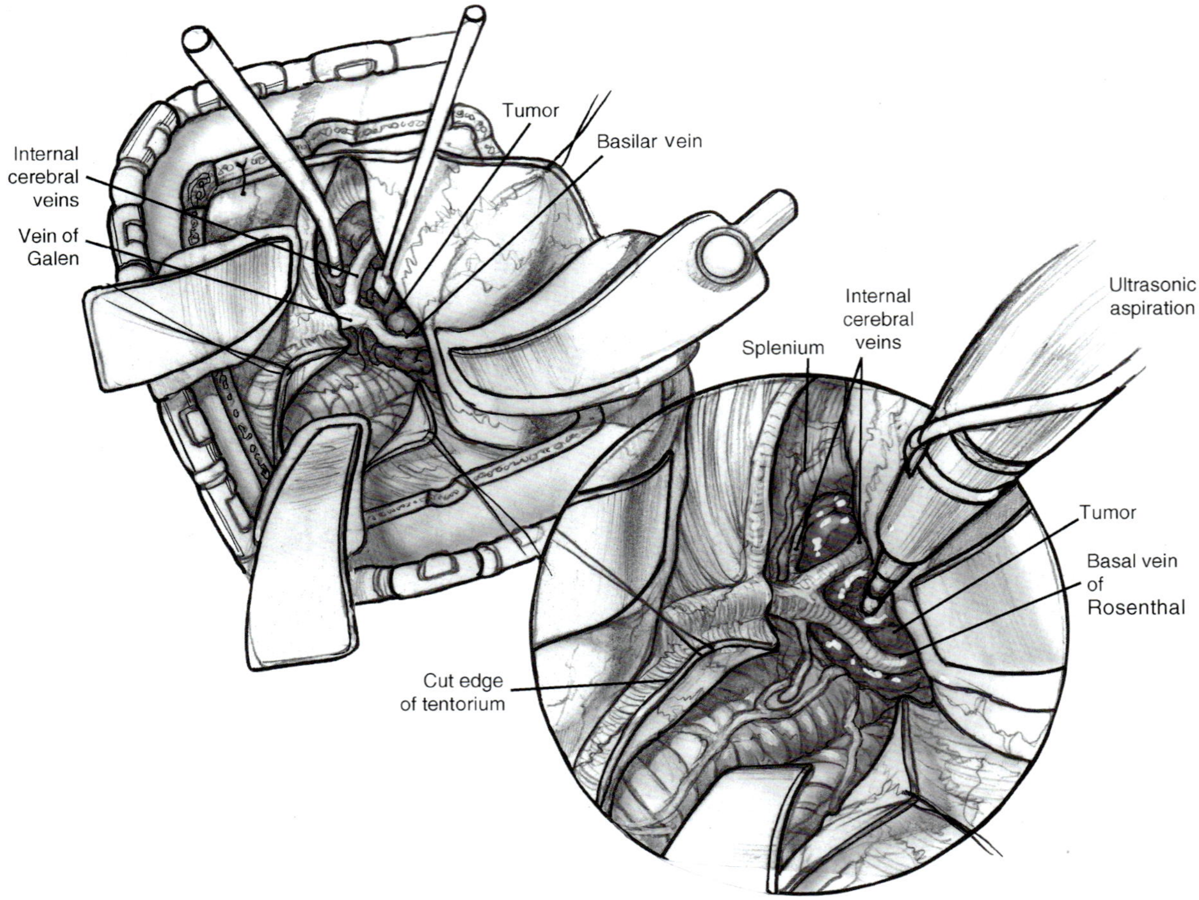

Figure 43–6 Schematic drawing of a tumor in the pineal region.

Once the tumor is reached, its border is found and carefully dissected. If the tumor is small, the dissection proceeds, keeping this cleavage as a surgical plane. On the other hand, when the tumor is large, internal decompression is performed after the border of the shallower part has been dissected. Depending on the tumor consistency, suction or a Cavitron Ultrasound Aspirator (CUSA) is used to debulk the tumor. If the tumor is hypervascular and its feeding arteries are identified, then the arteries are first coagulated and cut as much as possible prior to debulking the tumor. Usually, the medial posterior choroidal arteries supply the tumor. The tumor capsule is then dissected from the surrounding structures. When a clear border is not present or identified, a thin layer of the tumor should be left unresected. Tumors extending into the third ventricle are usually dissected relatively easily anteriorly once the dissection enters the third ventricle.

The extent of the resection depends on the nature of the tumor. To avoid injury of venous and critical neural structures, total resection is not necessary and should not be attempted once the intraoperative histological diagnosis makes it clear that the tumor is sensitive to chemotherapy or radiation.

A navigation system is often helpful for a large tumor in this area. Although it is obvious that intraoperative knowledge of the anatomical relationships is important, a system lets the surgeon know what is being dissected, especially in relation to the deep area in the operative field beyond the tumor margin. If available, an examination with a rigid or flexible neuroendoscope, prior to surgery, is very helpful. A long bipolar coagulator, microscissors, and a microdissector are all essential basic instruments.

Closure

After removing the tumor, hemostasis must be immaculate. Then the wound is thoroughly irrigated. The closure of the dura mater must be as watertight as possible with fibrin glue. The tentorium need not be closed, although a few sutures will prevent the occipital lobe from herniating downward. The bone flap is replaced and fixed with titanium miniplates. The scalp is closed in a two-layer closure of the galea and skin. No special reconstruction is needed in this region. A ventricular drain is left in place. It can be removed when it becomes unnecessary postoperatively.

◆ Postoperative Care

A computed tomographic (CT) scan is taken immediately after surgery to assess postoperative hemorrhage, in the operating room if possible. Patients with large lesions compressing the brain stem should remain in the intensive care unit for at least 1 night and their respiratory function carefully observed. Ventricular drainage is removed after it has been clamped for 1 day, to confirm that there is no increase in the intracranial pressure or no hydrocephalus developing.

Adjunctive therapy, such as chemotherapy or radiotherapy, is started after a definitive histological diagnosis.

◆ Complications

Homonymous hemianopsia is a specific complication of this approach. It is primarily caused by inappropriate and excessive retraction of the occipital lobe. Gentle, gradual retraction of the occipital lobe is necessary to avoid this complication. For cases of hydrocephalus, ventricular drainage is placed beforehand. When there is no ventricular drainage, care should be taken not to retract the brain until adequate CSF has drained after opening the quadrigeminal cistern.

The position of the head is another important issue. The head should be rotated to the side of the approach, which is usually the right side, so that the occipital lobe tends to fall away spontaneously, lessening the need for retraction. Because there is considerable anatomical variation in the tentorial sinus, bleeding sometimes occurs when it is cut. To prevent this, adequate electrocoagulation is needed to cut the tentorium in a stepwise fashion with bipolar coagulating forceps. The preoperative MRI and angiogram must be checked carefully to determine whether there is any deviation in the course of the superior sagittal, transverse, and straight sinuses.

Another important complication is venous injury. This can be caused at any step during dissection and removal of the tumor. The key to avoiding deep venous injury is sharp dissection of the arachnoid membrane and the tumor from the surrounding venous structures, under direct vision at the highest magnification.

◆ Parietal Approach

The parietal transcortical approach is usually indicated for lesions such as posterior thalamic and posterior parathalamic tumors that occur in the posterior paraventricular portion, and arteriovenous malformations around the posterior half of the third ventricle (around the trigone) that are located in the lateral wall of the third ventricle.[7] This approach is not usually used for lesions in the pineal region, but is indicated when the lesion extends laterally.

The patient is placed in the prone position, and the head is fixed in the Sugita multipurpose head frame to enable a perpendicular approach (**Fig. 43–7A**). A-shaped skin incision is made in the medial parietal area, and then the craniotomy is performed. The center of the craniotomy is roughly 4 to 5 cm posterior to the central sulcus and 3 cm lateral to the midline. A cortical incision less than 3 cm long is made coronally on the superior parietal lobule. Coronal sectioning of the cortex and brain helps to minimize damage to the connecting fibers of the corpus callosum. Positioning four tapered spatulas with four self-retaining retractors (**Fig. 43–7B**) facilitates the approach. These retractors are attached to the Sugita multipurpose head frame, so that the spatulas can be placed at any

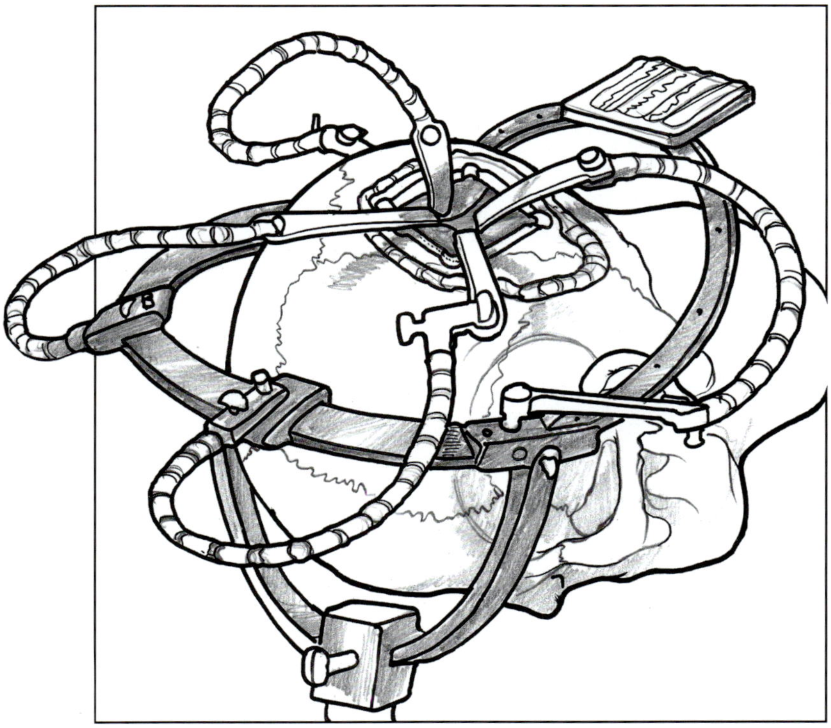

Figure 43–7 Patient's head fixed in a Sugita head frame with four tapered spatulas.

point around the operating field. With this approach, there are two particularly important points regarding the use of tapered spatulas for brain retraction. It is important to use an appropriately sized spatula; three kinds are available with different tip widths: 2, 4, and 6 mm. The use of tapered spatulas permits an ample operating field with less brain retraction. However, it is also important that only one pair of spatulas at a time is used to retract the brain; the other pair is kept loose. Retraction with one pair of spatulas facilitates visualization of a wider operating field than retraction with four spatulas, even through a 3 cm cortical incision.

The procedure for tumor removal is essentially the same as with the transtentorial approach: employ sharp dissection under a high magnification. If the cortical incision is made in the far lateral portion of the parietal lobe, there is a higher possibility of postoperative complications such as homonymous hemianopsia or sensory aphasia. The complication that one must be most careful to avoid is injury of the normal internal capsule. In this area, one must leave a small portion of the tumor when the tumor border is not clear.

◆ Conclusion

For lesions in the pineal region, the occipital transtentorial approach allows a nice operative view and good operative results when performed carefully to avoid complications such as homonymous hemianopsia, venous infarction, and brain swelling due to injury of the deep venous system. Preoperative evaluation with MRI and angiograms and a full understanding of the anatomy of the lesion are essential to accurately and safely perform the surgery.

References

1. Dandy WE. Benign Tumors in the Third Ventricle of the Brain: Diagnosis and Treatment. Springfield: Charles C Thomas; 1933
2. Van Wagenen WP. A surgical approach for the removal of certain pineal tumors: report of a case. Surg Gynecol Obstet 1931;53: 216–220
3. Krause F. Operatiave Freilegung der Vierhugel, nebst Beobachtungen uber Hirndruck und Decompression. Zentralbl Chir 1926;53: 2812–2819
4. Stein BM. The infratentorial supracerebellar approach to pineal lesions. J Neurosurg 1971;35:197–202
5. Poppen JL. The right occipital approach to a pinealoma. J Neurosurg 1966;25:706–710
6. Jamieson KG. Excision of pineal tumors. J Neurosurg 1971;35: 550–553
7. Hongo K, Kobayashi S. The posterior transcortical approach. In: Apuzzo MLJ, ed. Surgery of the Third Ventricle. 2nd ed. 1998: 683–696
8. Clark WK, Batjer HH. The occipital transtentorial approach. In: Apuzzo MLJ, ed. Surgery of the Third Ventricle. 2nd ed. 1998: 721–741
9. de Tribolet N. Surgical approaches to tumours of the pineal region. In: Sawamura Y, Shirato H, de Tribolet N, eds. Intracranial Germ Cell Tumors. New York: Springer; 1998:203–220
10. Ausman JI, Sadasivan B. Occipital transtenStorial approach to pineal region neoplasms. In: Rengachary SS, Wilkins RH, eds. Neurosurgical Operative Atlas. Vol 3. AANS; 23–28

44

Combined Supra- and Infratentorial-Transsinus Approach to Large Pineal Region Tumors

Ibrahim M. Ziyal and Laligam N. Sekhar

The removal of a pineal tumor with the transcallosal approach was first performed by Dandy.[1] This approach required splitting the corpus callosum and resecting 2 to 4 cm of the splenium. Occasionally, an occipital lobectomy was required as well. Cushing noted the difficulty of removing a pineal region tumor and wrote that he personally had never succeeded in exploring a pineal tumor sufficiently enough to justify an attempt at removing it.[2] The transventricular approach, first described by Van Wagenen, was another attempt at removing pineal tumors.[3] He used a 6 to 7 cm, reversed, L-shaped incision in the cortex, extending from the posterior end of the superior temporal gyrus posterosuperiorly to the superior parietal lobule.

The results of previous approaches prompted neurosurgeons to search for safer approaches for removing pineal region tumors. The occipital transtentorial approach was preferred by several surgeons after its initial description.[4] This technique carries no risk of air embolism, and the surgeon has a comfortable position from which to work. In addition, the occipital lobe requires minimal retraction because of gravity. The dissection of laterally extended tumors is even easier. However, the technique is not without difficulty. Occasionally, a small part of the splenium needs to be resected. A tumor located on the contralateral side is also difficult. Furthermore, the retraction of the occipital lobe can be significant, and the exposure of tumor extensions well below the tentorial notch and toward the contralateral side can also be difficult.

Krause's infratentorial supracerebellar approach was modified and improved by Stein,[5] who added microsurgical techniques. This approach allowed easy orientation and did not require destruction of parenchymal tissue. Although the sitting position was preferred, this position allowed the cerebellum to retract by gravity, and there was no accumulation of blood in the operating field. An additional difficulty of this approach is that it provides limited exposure of the tumors that extend laterally, anteriorly into the third ventricle, and superior to the deep venous plexus. It is usually employed for tumors located below the galenic system in the pineal region. In addition to the risk of air embolism, the sitting position is not comfortable for the surgeon, causing discomfort to the arms and neck.

The combined approach for removal of large pineal region tumors with the section of a nondominant transverse sinus was developed by Sekhar.[5,6] The exposure of large pineal tumors with this approach is better than with the other two approaches, and it substantially minimizes the risk of brain retraction. The deep venous structures are well exposed, allowing exposure and resection of lateral, superior, and inferior tumor extensions. A semiprone position can be employed, which is comfortable for the surgeon. The disadvantages with the approach include a longer exposure time and the need to divide the sinus.

Indications

- Large tumors with a diameter of greater than 4.5 cm
- Tumors extending well above and below the planes of the tentorium or tumors arising from the tentorium

- Tumors well below the plane of cerebellar retraction (more than 2 cm below the superior surface of the cerebellum)
- Tumors encasing important venous structures of the region
- Tumors that are very vascular, such that during tumor resection the surgeon has to come around the tumor without the benefit of internal debulking

◆ Preoperative Imaging

A magnetic resonance imaging (MRI) scan is necessary to display the tumor adequately and to determine its relationship to the tentorium, cerebellum, midbrain, third ventricle, and deep venous structures. A cerebral angiogram is necessary, especially to display the venous anatomy. Particular attention must be paid to the size of and communication between the transverse sinuses and the deep venous system.

◆ Advantages

- Less brain retraction
- Deep venous structures well exposed
- Semiprone position more comfortable

◆ Disadvantages

- Longer exposure time
- Need to divide the sinus

◆ Surgical Technique

Anesthesia

A standard endotracheal anesthesia induced with thiopental and a short-acting muscle relaxant is used. Either or both intravenous furosemide 40 mg and mannitol 0.5 to 1.0 g/kg body weight are administered for brain relaxation when the skin incision is made. Precordial Doppler monitoring is used to detect air embolism, and central venous pressure is monitored with a right atrial catheter.

Neurophysiological Monitoring

Somatosensory evoked potentials (SEPs) from the upper and lower extremities and bilateral brain stem auditory evoked responses (BAERs) are monitored during surgery.

Preoperative Shunt or Ventriculostomy

For giant pineal region tumors causing hydrocephalus, some surgeons prefer to insert a ventriculoperitoneal shunt 2 to 4 weeks prior to surgery. Alternatively, a ventriculostomy may be inserted at the beginning of the operation.

Positioning

The semiprone position is preferred for the combined supra- and infratentorial-transsinus approach, so that the surgeon can sit behind the patient (**Fig. 44–1**). If a prone position is used, the surgeon will have to sit at the head of the patient and work with an inverted view. The side of the proposed transverse sinus section is placed inferiorly to allow gravity-aided retraction of the occipital lobe.

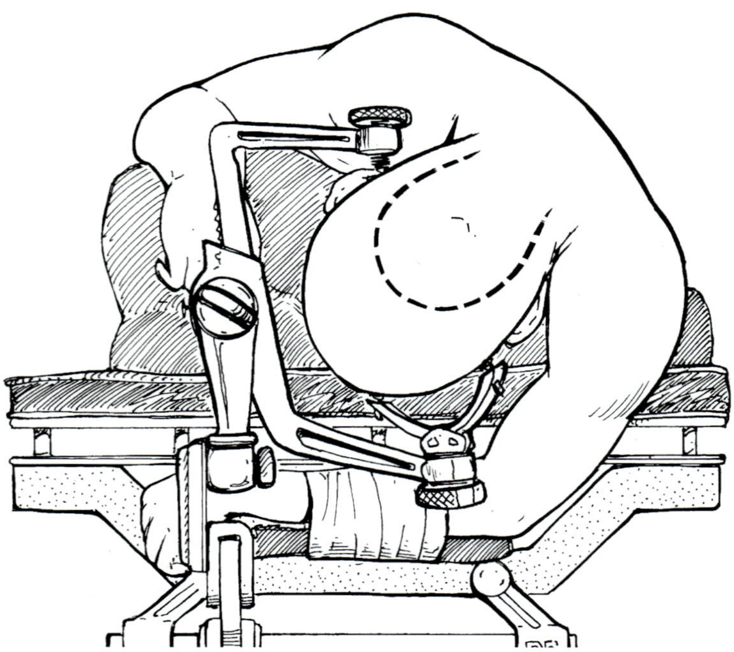

Figure 44–1 The semiprone position is preferred for the combined approach. The position allows the surgeon to sit behind the patient.

Dissection

A U-shaped incision is cut, and the skin flap and muscles are elevated as a single layer. A three-step craniotomy technique, which avoids injury to the venous sinuses, is performed as follows. First, two bur holes are placed inferior to the external landmark of the transverse sinus (a line drawn from the inion to the base of the mastoid), and two additional holes are placed just above the foramen magnum on either side. After separating the dura, a suboccipital craniotomy is performed (**Fig. 44–2A**). The transverse sinus is separated from the dural elevator under tangential vision,

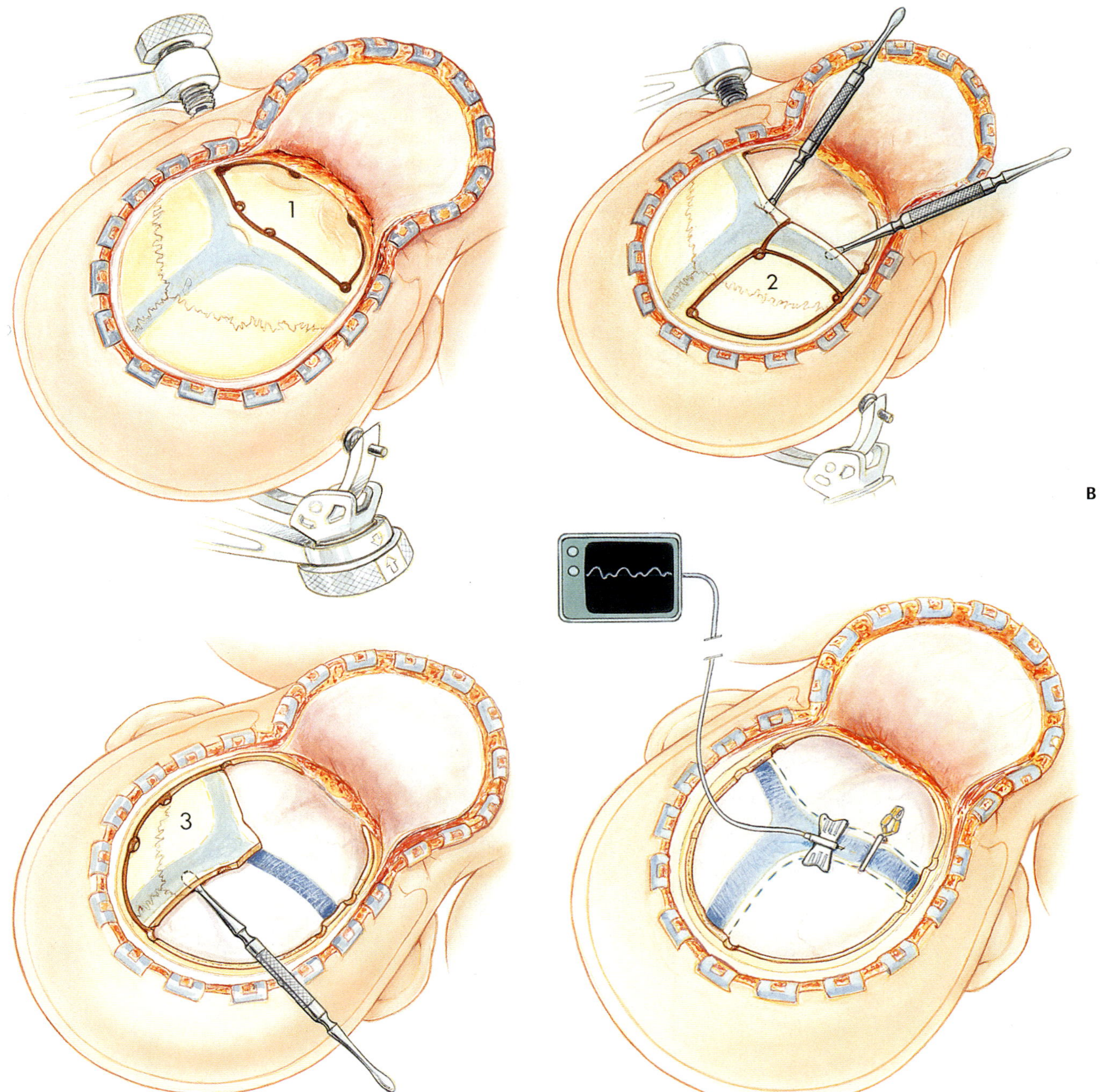

A B C D

Figure 44–2 **(A)** The craniotomy is usually performed in three pieces, with the first plate being suboccipital. **(B)** After separating the transverse sinus under tangential vision, an occipital craniotomy is performed on one side, up to the superior sagittal sinus. **(C)** After separating the superior sagittal sinus from the bone, the occipital craniotomy on the other side is performed. **(D)** The suboccipital dura is opened in a transverse fashion just inferior to the transverse sinus. The occipital dura is then opened parallel to the venous sinuses on the inferior side. A 20 gauge butterfly needle attached to a manometer is placed into the transverse sinus, just lateral to the torcular, and test occlusion of the sinus with a temporary clip lateral to the needle is performed.

and an occipital craniotomy is performed on one side, up to the superior sagittal sinus (**Fig. 44–2B**). After separating the superior sagittal sinus under direct vision, the occipital craniotomy on the other side is performed (**Fig. 44–2C**).

The suboccipital dura is opened horizontally just inferior to the transverse sinus, on either side of the midline, and after ligating the sinus, it is divided completely. If necessary, a small paramedian vertical incision can be made in the suboccipital dura to allow the opening of the cisterna magna, which will relax the brain. The occipital dura on the inferior side is then opened in an L-shaped fashion, medial to the superior sagittal sinus and superior to the transverse sinus. A 20 gauge butterfly needle attached by the anesthesiologist to a pressure transducer is placed into the transverse sinus, just lateral to the torcular, and test occlusion of the sinus lateral to the needle is performed for 5 minutes. If the venous pressure does not increase more than 5 mm Hg, if no brain swelling is observed, and if there are no changes in the evoked potentials, the nondominant transverse sinus can be safely sectioned (**Fig. 44–2D**). The sinus is clipped with two temporary clips and divided (**Fig. 44–3A**). Very rarely, bridging veins may be encountered inferior or medial to the occipital lobe. With gentle retraction of the occipital lobe and cerebellum, the tentorium is exposed, and the straight sinus is identified. The tentorium is then carefully sectioned parallel to, and ~1 cm lateral to, the straight sinus. Venous sinuses or tumor-directed arteries in the tentorium may bleed, requiring bipolar cautery or titanium hemoclips. The occipital lobe and the cerebellum are gently retracted to expose the whole tumor (**Fig. 44–3B**). Some veins draining the cerebellum into the tentorium will have to be divided without adverse effects. Once the tentorium has been divided, the arachnoid overlying the tumor will be exposed. It often appears quite thickened. After the arachnoid membrane is carefully opened, the precentral cerebellar vein and the tumor will be exposed. The basal veins of Rosenthal are usually anterior to the tumor, and the internal cerebral veins and the vein of Galen usually lie superior to the tumor. However, all of these veins may be encased by tumor, and great care must be taken to preserve them. The tumor is initially debulked centrally and then gradually dissected from surrounding structures and removed. While dissecting the tumor from the brain stem and the occipital lobe, the tumor–brain arachnoidal plane must be carefully preserved. When this plane is absent, a thin rim of tumor must be left on the brain to avoid irreversible neural injury.

If the tumor extends forward into the third ventricle, the neuroendoscope can be used to assist in the resection. If the tumor is extraordinarily vascular, the surgeon may need to come around it circumferentially (except anteriorly) and devascularize it as much as possible before removal. If there is inadvertent injury to the deep veins during the surgery, they should be temporarily clipped and reconstructed, if possible, by direct suture using 7–0 Prolene or 8–0 nylon. At

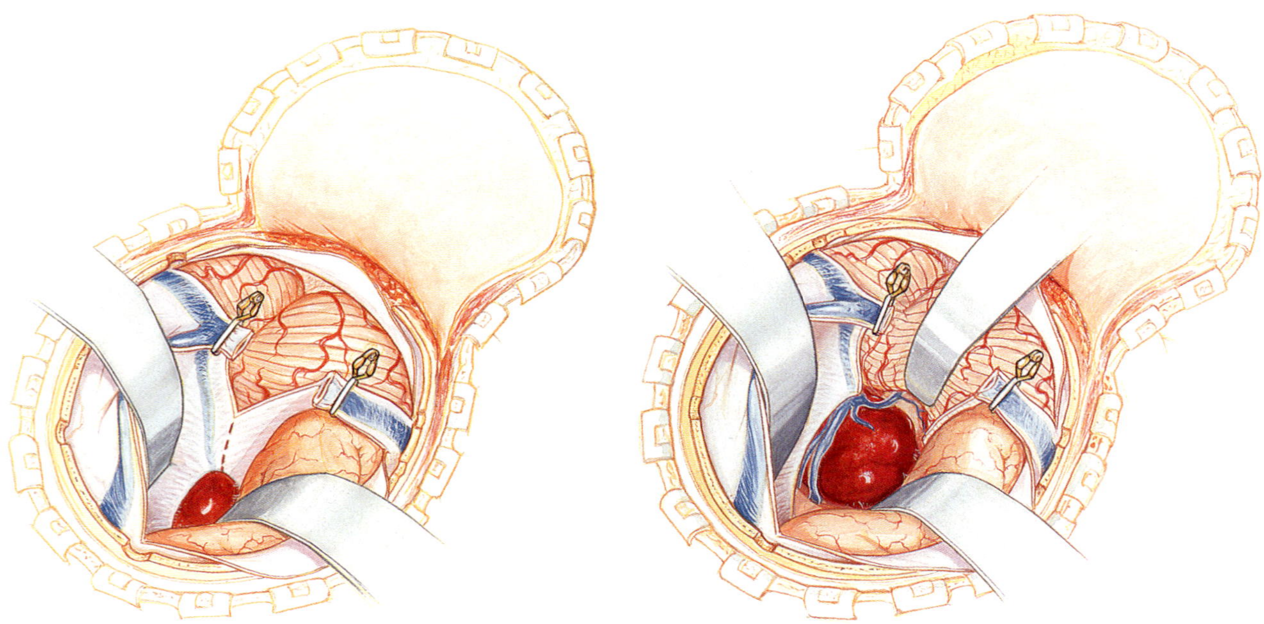

A B

Figure 44–3 **(A)** A combined supra- and infratentorial-transsinus approach to a large pineal region tumor. The nondominant transverse sinus has been clipped with two temporary clips and divided. The occipital lobe and the cerebellum are gently retracted to expose the tentorium. **(B)** The tentorium is then cut just lateral to the straight sinus toward the tentorial notch area. The large exposure of the tumor together with important venous structures is seen.

the end of the procedure, the transverse sinus may be permanently ligated. We prefer to reconstruct by direct suture using 6–0 Prolene or with a short vein graft interposed between the two sinuses.

Closure

Closure of the combined supra- and infratentorial-transsinus approach should be performed meticulously. It is not necessary to suture the tentorium. We usually employ a pericranial or fascia lata dural graft to allow both watertight closure and expansion of the posterior fossa. If no brain swelling exists at surgery, the bone flaps are reapproximated. If brain swelling is observed, the suboccipital bone flap may be left out and a pericranial graft may be used to allow the expansion of the posterior fossa. The remaining muscle and skin layers are closed in the usual manner.

◆ Postoperative Care

Patients who have lesions compressing the brain stem should be monitored carefully for respiratory difficulties in the postoperative period. An apnea monitor is essential if the patient is in a stepdown unit. We usually perform a computed tomographic (CT) scan on the first postoperative day to assess for pneumocephalus or postoperative clots. Significant degrees of nystagmus, ataxia, and oscillopsia may be present. However, these deficits are usually temporary and resolve gradually within 3 months. If a pre- or postoperative ventriculostomy has been placed, ventricular drainage is maintained for 3 to 4 days. At that point, the surgeon must decide whether to remove the ventriculostomy or to place a permanent postoperative shunt by first elevating it to 20 cm above head level for 24 hours and then test clamping it for 24 hours, with intracranial pressure (ICP) monitoring. A postoperative CT scan is performed at this stage. The ventriculostomy can be removed if the ventricles are smaller in size than preoperatively, and if the ICP remains normal after test occlusion.

◆ Complications

The variations of the normal anatomical structures should be kept in mind. Anomalies of the venous sinuses such as duplication of the transverse or superior sagittal sinuses, the presence of an occipital sinus, and different types of the confluence of venous sinuses at the torcular Herophili are common. These must be recognized preoperatively by angiography. Before dividing the tentorium, the straight sinus must be carefully localized to avoid its injury.

The galenic venous system consists of important venous structures. The preoperative angiographic studies or intraoperative inspection may reveal the possible invasion or occlusion of the vascular structures by the tumor. If any of these veins are injured at surgery, the blood pressure must be lowered to reduce the blood flow through them, and repair must be performed with 7–0 Prolene or 8–0 nylon. If these veins are permanently occluded, severe brain swelling or edema may be the end result.

Tumor removal is performed by first debulking the lesion and then removing it piecemeal. This will minimize excessive brain stem compression during tumor removal. Tumors that are vascular and tend to bleed may not allow debulking. In such cases, the surgeon will need to come around it circumferentially as much as possible (except anteriorly) and devascularize it by coagulating feeding arteries before tumor removal. During the tumor resection, the tumor–brain stem arachnoidal plane must be carefully maintained. When it is absent, a small part of the tumor must be left on the brain to avoid irreversible neural injury. If the posterior third ventricle is opened, thorough irrigation of the ventricle to clean any blood clot at the end of the procedure is important to avoid a possible postoperative hydrocephalus. A large opening into the ventricle may be closed with a piece of Gelfoam and fibrin glue, after completion of tumor resection, to avoid the accumulation of cerebrospinal fluid in the subdural space.

When the tumor is giant in size, damage to cranial nerve (CN) IV or V is possible. Knowledge of this risk will usually allow them to be preserved. Although air embolism is more common in the sitting position, it is also possible in the semiprone position, when the head is higher than the heart. Precordial Doppler and end-tidal CO_2 monitoring, aspiration of air through a central venous catheter in the right atrium, and recognition and occlusion of the source of air leak are important steps in its treatment.

The combined approach necessitates less retraction than the occipital transtentorial approach to the occipital lobe and than the infratentorial supracerebellar approach to the cerebellum. However, excessive retraction of the occipital lobe may cause occipital lobe contusion or injury, resulting in transient or permanent vision loss.

Postoperatively, the occurrence of excessive pneumocephalus in the subdural space may require aspiration through a small bur hole and the inhalation of 100% oxygen. If a postoperative hemorrhage is recognized in the tumor bed, a reexploration and removal will be necessary.

◆ Conclusion

The combined supra- and infratentorial-transsinus approach provides the greatest exposure for large pineal region tumors and requires less brain retraction than either the infratentorial supracerebellar approach or the occipital transtentorial approach. It is useful for selected giant-sized and extensive tumors of this region.

Acknowledgments The article "Combined supra/infratentorial-transsinus approach to large pineal region tumors" was published in *Journal of Neurosurgery* (June 1998). The use of all figures in the chapter are with permission from *Journal of Neurosurgery.*

References

1. Dandy WE. An operation for the removal of pineal tumors. Surg. Gynec. Obstet. 1921;33:113–119
2. Cushing H. Intracranial tumors: Notes upon a series of 2000 verified cases with surgical mortality pertaining thereto. Springfield: Charles C Thomas; 1932:64
3. Van Wagenen WP. A surgical approach for the removal of certain pineal tumors: report of a case. Surg. Gynec. Obstet. 1931;53: 216–220
4. Horrax G. Treatment of tumors of the pineal body: experience in a series of 22 cases. Arch Neurol Psychiatry 1950;64:227–242
5. Sekhar LN, Goel A. Combined supratentorial and infratentorial approach to large pineal-region meningioma. Surg Neurol 1992;37: 197–201
6. Ziyal IM, Sekhar LN, Salas E, Olan WJ. Combined supra/infratentorial-transsinus approach to large pineal-region tumors. J Neurosurg 1998; 88:1050–1057

45

Stereotactic Approaches to Pineal Region Lesions

Douglas Kondziolka and L. Dade Lunsford

Management depends on the specific histological nature of the disorder. Some diseases, such as pineal cysts, are indolent and require only intermittent observation by high-resolution imaging. Others, such as astrocytoma, meningioma, and pineocytoma, change slowly over time and require judicious management for effective treatment and to maintain neurological function. Some malignant lesions, for example, teratomas, enlarge in size more rapidly, cause rapid neurological decline, and are curable with microsurgical resection. Other malignant processes, germinomas and pineoblastomas, are not curable with resection and yet may be effectively managed with radiation or chemotherapy. Finally, vascular disorders such as arteriovenous malformations (AVMs) or cavernous malformations can be managed both by resection and by stereotactic radiosurgery. For some patients, imaging alone may allow for a diagnosis suitable for guiding management. An example would be the typical-appearing meningioma at the confluence of the falx and tentorium. However, for most neoplastic processes, histological sampling is required. Stereotactic biopsy provides an effective way to achieve a histological diagnosis with low risk.

As outlined in this book, there exist several sophisticated microsurgical approaches to the pineal region. We believe that such surgery is important when a large tumor (not believed to be radiation responsive) is causing progressive neurological deficits and when curative resection of a tumor can be achieved with minimal if any morbidity.

Indications

- For stereotactic biopsy, to achieve a diagnosis of an intrinsic pineal region neoplasm
- For stereotactic aspiration, to drain cystic masses of the pineal region (cysts and tumors)
- For stereotactic radiosurgery, as definitive management for meningiomas, pineocytomas, and vascular malformations
- As adjuvant management with chemotherapy for germ cell neoplasms and pineoblastomas

Imaging

Multiplanar, contrast-enhanced magnetic resonance imaging (MRI) is necessary to display the lesion adequately and to determine its relationship to the tentorium, deep venous structures, third ventricle, and midbrain. A cerebral angiogram is necessary to diagnose an AVM, although we do not recommend angiography when the MRI characteristics suggest a cavernous malformation.

Surgical Technique

Anesthesia

Stereotactic procedures in adults and adolescents (over 12 years) are performed under local infiltration anesthesia supplemented with intravenous sedation. We apply the Leksell Model G stereotactic frame (Elekta Instruments, Atlanta, GA) using a mixture of lidocaine and bupivacaine in buffered solution. Children undergo stereotactic surgery under general endotracheal anesthesia.

Stereotactic Imaging

For most patients, we use stereotactic, contrast-enhanced computed tomographic (CT) imaging. Axial images spaced by

3 mm or 5 mm are obtained through the level of the lesion and up to the skull surface. Reformatted coronal and sagittal views are used to determine a trajectory from the bone down to the target. In patients where the lesion is poorly identified on CT, stereotactic magnetic resonance (MR) is used with short relaxation time, contrast-enhanced images.

Selection of the Trajectory

Because most patients have midline pineal lesions, biopsy or aspiration is performed via a low-frontal entry point (**Fig. 45–1**). In this manner, we avoid crossing multiple pial and ependymal surfaces. The instrument enters the brain at the hairline (mid- or high-forehead level) and proceeds through the frontal horn of the lateral ventricle or just lateral to it. It traverses the thalamus and occasionally the third ventricle and then enters the tumor. Our goal with this trajectory is threefold:

1. To have the instrument pass below the roof of the third ventricle and internal cerebral veins (usually displaced just superior to the tumor)
2. To remain within less critical brain tissue and within brain parenchyma for as much of the trajectory as possible
3. To allow sampling of cerebrospinal fluid should that be desired

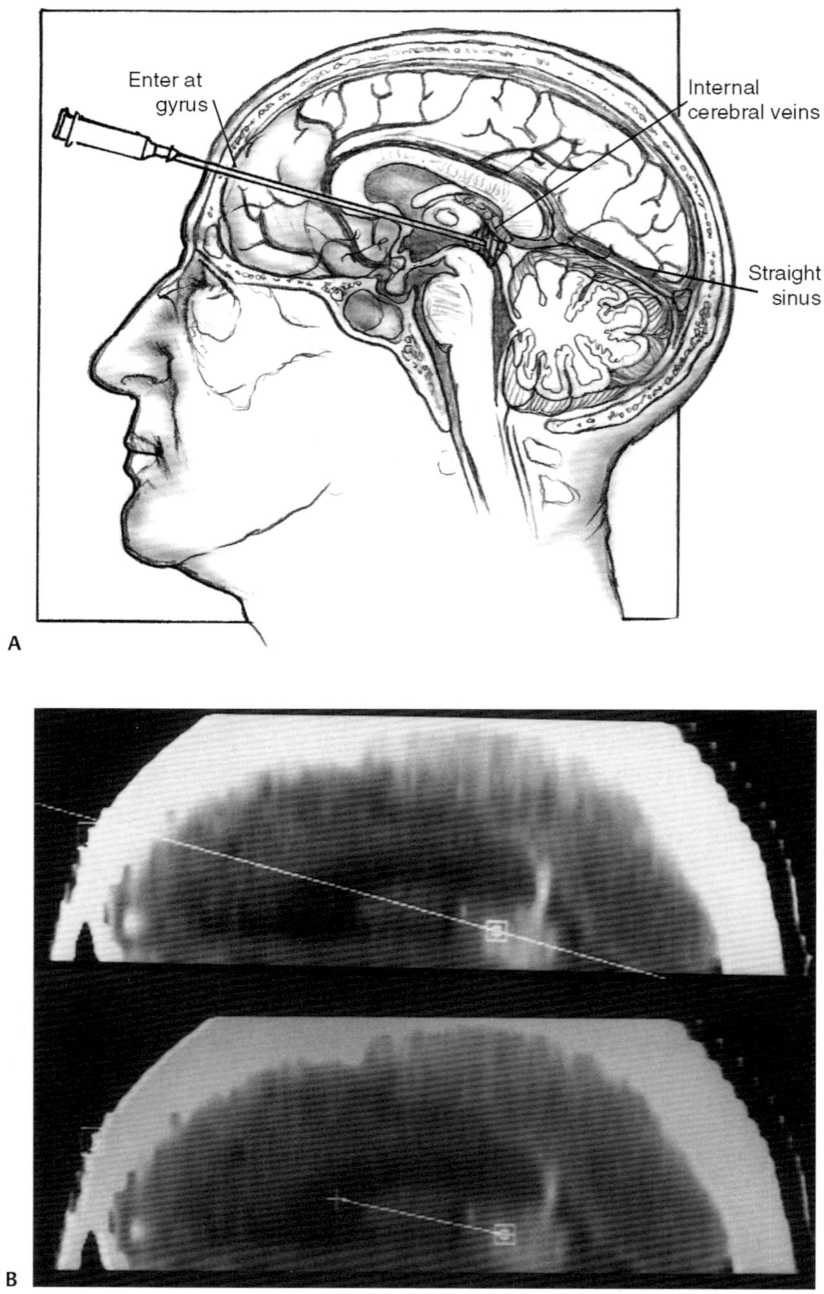

Figure 45–1 The low frontal stereotactic approach to midline pineal region lesions. This trajectory avoids the internal cerebral veins above the tumor and the superior midbrain anterior and inferior to the tumor. **(A)** Artist drawing. **(B)** Imaging photo.

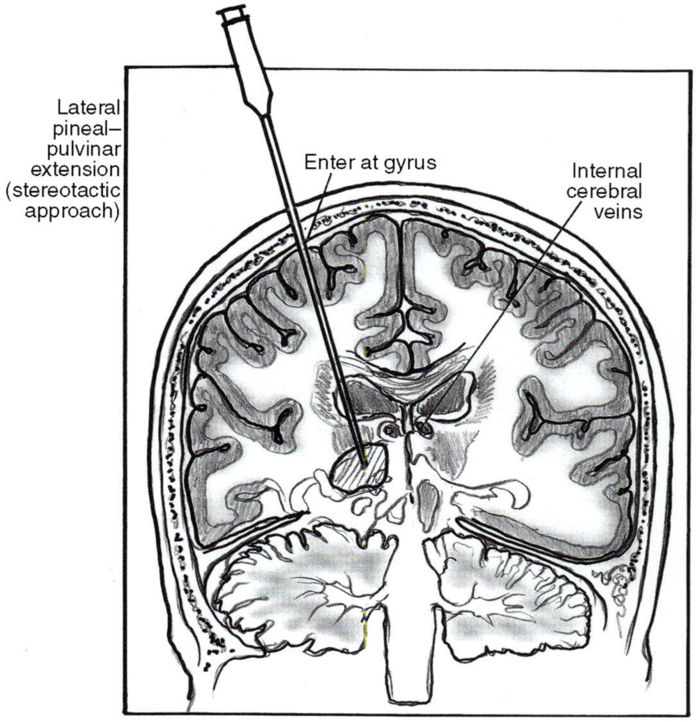

A

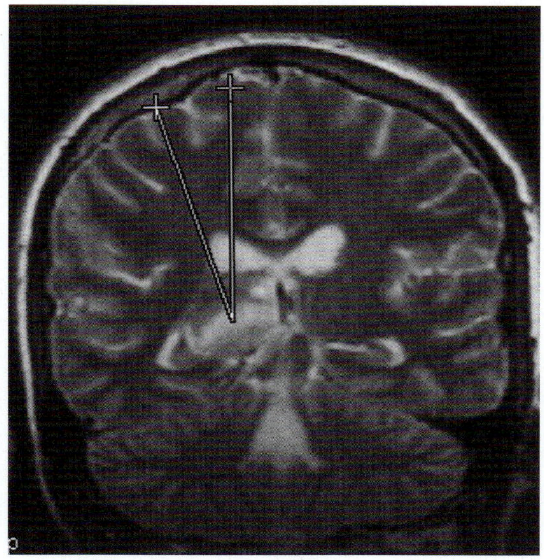

B

Figure 45–2 The parietal stereotactic approach to lateral pineal region lesions. This trajectory stays lateral to the deep veins. A trajectory through the lateral ventricle may be necessary. **(A)** Artist drawing. **(B)** Imaging photo.

For lateral pineal region or pulvinar tumors that might better be approached from the side, we use a parietal trajectory (**Fig. 45–2**). Images are used to define a probe entrance at the crest of a gyrus rather than a sulcus to avoid pial blood vessels that might lead to superficial brain hemorrhage. Utilizing these approaches, we have not sustained a symptomatic hemorrhage in a pineal region stereotactic surgery procedure.

Tissue Sampling

Stereotactic diagnostic biopsy of pineal region tumors must be performed judiciously. Enough tissue must be obtained from within the tumor to make a proper histological diagnosis, but taking too many samples significantly increases the risk for hemorrhage. Usually we obtain two to three samples at different depths within the neoplasm. In most cases, a 1–5 mm side-coring instrument is used for aspiration biopsy. Specimens are given to an experienced neuropathologist, who attends each procedure and performs a touch preparation of the tissue. During the biopsy we identify whether potential diagnostic tissue has been obtained but do not make a specific diagnosis per se. As guided by the clinical situation or by the touch preparation, other samples can be sent for culture or electron microscopy if necessary.

◆ Complications

If bleeding occurs during the stereotactic procedure, a 1.9 mm outer diameter stereotactic needle is left in place at the hemorrhage site. In the vast majority of cases, blood will egress through the instrument and eventually stop if the surgeon remains patient. Injection of peroxide is potentially fatal, and cauterization of the instrument or copious irrigation may be ineffective, dangerous, or both. We keep the instrument open with gentle irrigation. If bleeding continues or neurological deterioration occurs, an immediate CT scan is performed.

Closure

After the biopsy samples are obtained, we withdraw the needle by 5 mm increments to check for hemorrhage at all locations of the trajectory. Once the instrument is removed, the skin puncture is closed with 4–0 suture. An immediate postoperative CT scan is performed to check for hemorrhage and confirm the accuracy of sampling. Usually a dot of air can be seen at the biopsy site. The stereotactic frame is removed, and a local dressing is placed. Patients are observed for 24 hours in the hospital and discharged the next day. We do not place temporary external ventricular drains after biopsy. In some patients with preoperative hydrocephalus, we have performed endoscopic third ventriculostomy 1 or 2 days before stereotactic surgery.

Stereotactic Aspiration

For patients undergoing cyst aspiration, we measure the volume of the cyst using MR or CT axial imaging. The trace and region-of-interest function of the imaging software can be used to define a surface area on each axial slice. The serial surface areas are summed and then multiplied by the image slice separation. This gives an accurate measurement of cyst volume. After instrument placement (usually with a

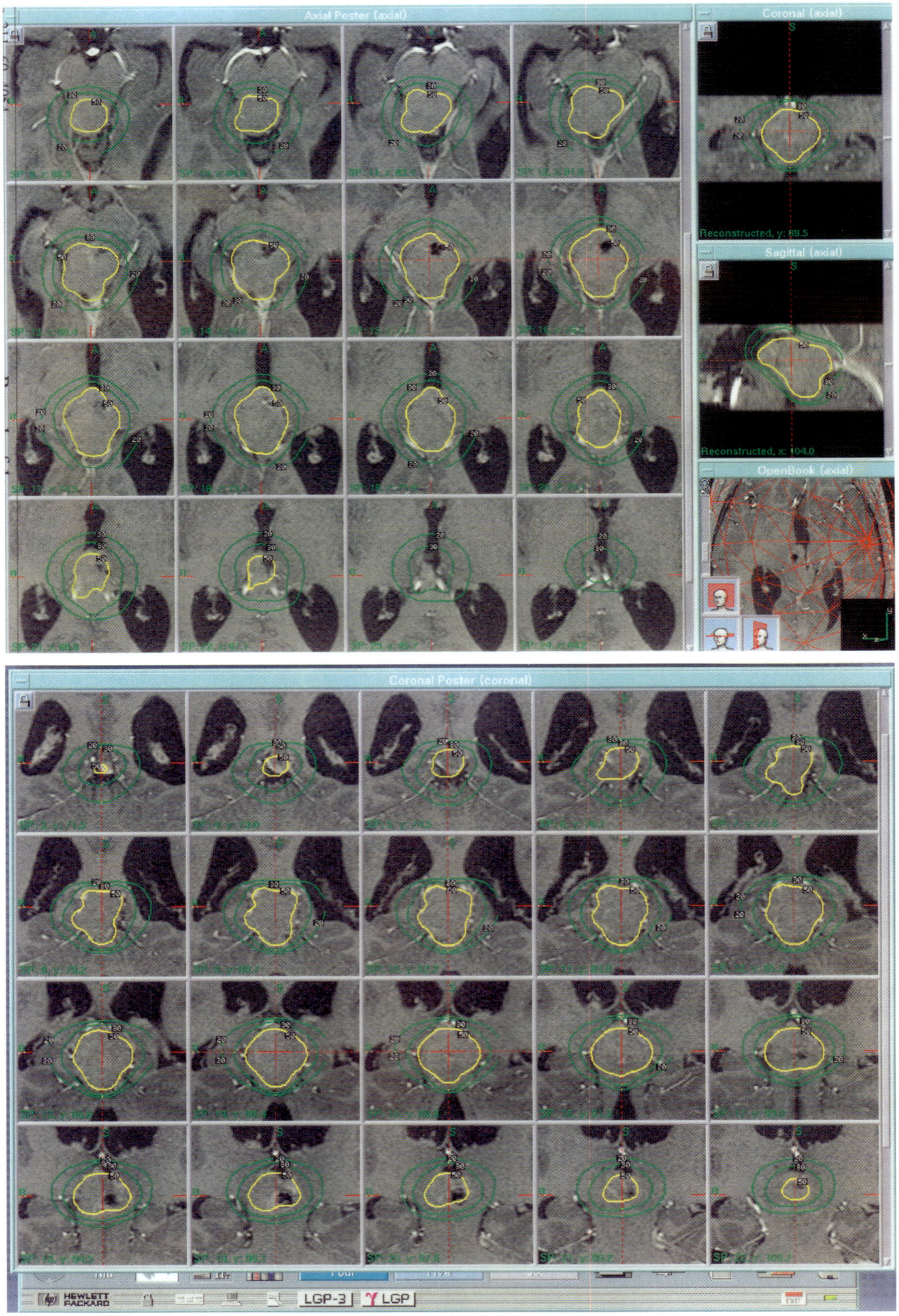

A

B

Figure 45–3 Stereotactic gamma knife radiosurgery dose planning for a pineal region germinoma. Note the conformal peripheral isodose (50% line) targeted to the tumor margin (yellow line). One millimeter magnetic resonance axial (top) and coronal (bottom) images are shown. The plan was created using six 14 mm and four 8 mm isocenters to deliver a 50% margin dose of 13 Gy and a maximum dose of 26 Gy.

1.8 mm blunt puncture needle), we try to gently aspirate 60 to 80% of the cyst volume. Aspiration is performed slowly, and the patient is frequently asked about development of new symptoms, including headache, that might indicate any displacement of regional brain structures.

◆ Stereotactic Radiosurgery for Tumors and Vascular Malformations

Stereotactic surgeries performed on an intraoperative CT scanner table allow immediate intraoperative or postoperative imaging as required. The bony opening is made with a twist-drill craniostomy. We use stereotactic MRI for target definition. An initial sagittal sequence is obtained to localize the lesion, and then an axial volume, contrast-enhanced acquisition (spoiled gradient recalled acquistion [SPGR]) sequence is divided into 1 mm thick slices. Cavernous malformations additionally benefit from long relaxation time images that emphasize the hemosiderin rim surrounding the malformation.

A formal radiosurgery dose plan is achieved using small isocenters of radiation to cover the tumor mass. For most patients we use the 50% isodose line to envelop the lesion margin. The dose is restricted away from regional anatomical structures, with particular concern paid to the midbrain. The radiation dose fall-off into the brain stem is identified using the calculated lower isodoses (**Fig. 45–3**). Dose selection is based upon several factors that include lesion volume, prior radiation exposure, patient age, and regional brain tolerance. Although most patients appear to tolerate 15 Gy to the brain stem surface at the edge of the lesion, this dose might be lowered further depending on tumor volume. We do not limit dose because of the proximity of the deep cerebral veins or the corpus callosum. For patients with pathology such as germinomas, rapid tumor regression is often identified following radiosurgery (in the first month). For patients with benign histologies, follow-up imaging is performed 3 to 6 months later.

Table 45–1

Advantages over Alternative Approaches
Resection may not be necessary, depending on histology
Biopsy may guide effective nonsurgical therapies
Radiosurgery may be an appropriate management alternative for smaller-volume pathologies
Disadvantages Compared with Alternative Approaches
Small biopsy specimens may make the neuropathological diagnosis difficult to achieve
An experienced neuropathology team is critical
There is a small risk for radiation-related neurological deficits after stereotactic radiosurgery

◆ Conclusion

The advanatages and disadvantages of stereotactic approaches are summariged in **Table 45–1.**

Section VIII

Cranial Base Lesions

46

General Principles of Cranial Base Surgery

J. J. van Overbeeke

Skull base surgery has progressed in recent years because of the close cooperation between surgeons from neurosurgical, otolaryngological, maxillofacial, neuroanesthesiological, and neuroradiological disciplines. Modifications to already existing techniques such as a selective resection of the skull base have been developed to reduce the amount of brain retraction and to improve the approach to the tumor to preserve the function of the cranial nerves, brain, and brain stem. Although skull base surgery deals largely with neoplasms, developmental, aneurysmal, and traumatic lesions of the skull should be included in skull base surgery. Skull base surgery requires a multidisciplinary team including an anesthesiologist and neuroradiologist who are familiar with the demands and techniques of skull base surgery. There is no place for occasional skull base surgery. Familiarity with the anatomy by means of extensive practice in an anatomical laboratory of the different approaches is not only desirable but also obligatory.

◆ Preparation

Skull base surgery starts with a careful general and neurological examination. The preoperative neurological deficits should be documented because the neurological deficits are predictive of the postoperative neurological status and because these deficits strongly contribute to the surgical decision-making process. Already existing preoperative neurological deficits may indicate evidence of tumor growth and may be indicative for surgery. Associated visual, auditory, and endocrine abnormalities require preoperative testing. Although hearing should be preserved, a unilateral hearing loss is likely and the hearing function of the contralateral ear should be known. Major diseases will have a major impact on the postoperative outcome and rehabilitation and may even exclude surgery.

Surgical procedures involving the cavernous sinus or petroclival region risk permanent damage of the internal carotid artery (ICA) resulting in a transient or permanent occlusion. Therefore, balloon occlusion test (BOT) of the involved ICA is recommended for the occlusion tolerance of the ICA. Patients who tolerate the BOT without clinical evidence of cerebral ischemia undergo a xenon cerebral blood flow (CBF) study to define a medium or low risk.[1] A BOT is an attempt to imitate the physiology after surgical interruption of the ICA but may fall short in its predictive ability in certain cases. Recently, the occurrence of synchronous filling of the cortical cerebral veins in both hemispheres at angiography during BOT has been described as a reliable predictor of tolerance for ICA occlusion.[2] The BOT has complications in 3.7%, such as intimal dissections of the ICA and transient and permanent ischemic events.[3] However, this technique can be considered safe if performed by an experienced neuroradiologist.

◆ Neuroradiological Evaluation

Contrast-enhanced computed tomography (CT) and magnetic resonance imaging (MRI) are both complementary. CT is focused on bony lesions of the skull base and tumor calcifications and should be performed in thin sections ($\leq$ 3 mm), especially when tumors with skull base erosion and hyperostosis are suspected. MRI demonstrates the relation of the tumor to soft tissue structures, arteries, and venous sinuses, including the jugular vein. The existence of an arachnoidal space between the lesion and the brain, especially the brain stem, is best demonstrated on T2-weighted images in multiple directions and is of paramount importance to the surgeon in determining whether a total removal with minimal neurological changes is possible.

Cerebral angiography is mandatory not only for the vascular anatomy but also to demonstrate the vascularity of the lesion that can be indicative for preoperative embolization. Although embolization may reduce the perioperative blood loss and consequently may improve the postoperative outcome, the risks of embolization such as the skin necrosis, cranial nerve dysfunction, stroke, blindness, and even death should be weighed against the perioperative and postoperative advantages.

◆ Surgical Technique

Anesthesia

The anesthetic management of skull base surgery is focused on general neuroanesthetic principles such as the maintenance of perioperative hemodynamic stability, lower intracranial pressure and an adequate cerebral pressure, oxygenation, and blood volume. Furthermore special brain protection is necessary in case of temporary vascular occlusion, and long-acting muscle relaxation is to be avoided to permit electrophysiological monitoring. Smooth and rapid emergence from anesthesia is indispensable after surgery to examine the postoperative neurological state, especially the function of the cranial nerves such as the lower cranial nerves.

Positioning

The preoperative positioning is of supreme importance and should be discussed with the anesthesiologist. Special care should be given to the shoulders and extremities to prevent stretching and compression of the nerves. Every positioning option should be weighed against anesthesiological and position-related complications. Intermittent compression of the lower limbs should be used to prevent deep vein thrombosis.

A preoperative slow withdrawal of 20 to 50 mL of cerebrospinal fluid (CSF) by means of a lumbar subarachnoid catheter usually results in excellent relaxation of the brain. However, this procedure decreases the visibility of the subarachnoidal spaces.

Electrophysiological Monitoring

Intraoperative monitoring of the cranial nerves is a useful tool allowing for safer and faster identification of the cranial motor nerves in pathological anatomical conditions. It allows the surgeon a degree of comfort by providing immediate information regarding the status of the nerves. It may also improve the postoperative outcome and shorten the operating time. Moreover, it provides some information about the expected postoperative nerve function. Methods have also been developed that allow monitoring of sensory system function such as that of the auditory system, and it has been shown that brain stem auditory evoked potentials can provide important information about the integrity of the auditory nervous system.[4]

The brain function is routinely monitored by means of somatosensory evoked responses (SEPs), brain stem evoked responses (BEARs) and electroencephalography (EEG).

If available, neuromonitoring should be used routinely in skull base surgery.

Instrumentation

The surgeon should use the special equipment that has been designed for the anterior approach to the clivus and craniocervical region. Without the aid of these instruments, no responsible surgery in this region can be performed.

Apart from all the equipment being used in intracranial neurosurgery, skull base surgery also requires long microinstruments for midline approaches. A reciprocating saw and various types of high-speed burs and drills are essential. Bipolar cautery should be irrigating, with various sizes of straight and curved tips used.

Microinstruments for vessel and nerve repair should be available. The use and function of cotton pledgets is numerous: they provide protection of the neural structures and are helpful in the dissection of the arachnoid planes. They should be removed or covered by a spatula before using the high-speed drill.

The use of fibrin glue is recommended for its sealing and hemostatic qualities.

A Cavitron Exel (Ultrasonic Surgical Aspirator, Valley Laboratory, Boulder, CO) ultrasonic aspirator with a microtip is indispensable; however, it should be used only in malleable tumors with a relatively avascular consistency.

The use of laser is not widely advised and does not contribute significantly to ultrasonic aspiration.

Neuronavigation increases efficacy and safety in skull base surgery.[5] The preoperative data preparation for planning and orientation contributes useful information during surgery. Osseous structures are easily identified because there is no problem of shift due to CSF withdrawal. Information regarding soft structures can be obtained from image fusion of the CT and MRI data. By means of subtraction techniques the invasion of the tumor in bony structures and the encasement in the major vessels can be visualized.

Approach

It is important to consider the effects of surgery not only on the normal but also on surgically manipulated tissues to select the optimal approach.

The main principles of approach selection in skull base surgery are (1) avoiding brain retraction, (2) designing the simplest and shortest route to the lesion, (3) obtaining adequate surgical access with optimal visualization of the lesion, and, when feasible, (4) protecting the key anatom-ical structures such as the arteries, venous sinuses, and cranial nerves.

Brain retraction should be avoided by the exposure osteotomies, which enable the surgeon to reach the lesion as safe as possible, and which may create the shortest route to the lesion. Adequate visualization of the lesion aids complete removal and the preservation critical anatomical structures. Each skull base approach has strengths and weaknesses regarding the areas to be exposed and associated morbidities. Every approach needs to be balanced with an acceptable functional and aesthetic morbidity.

The literature regarding the various skull base approaches is somewhat confusing because of the inconsistent nomenclature for essentially the same approaches.

This chapter classifies the approaches based on anatomical characteristics and standard approaches in neurosurgery.[6]

Approaches to the Anterior Clivus and Craniocervical Region

Generally an anterior approach should be used for the surgical treatment of lesions anterior to the skull base. This requires a choice of transfacial or transcranial approaches because of the anteroinferior relationship of the facial structures to the skull base.

Anterior approaches to the skull base are advantageous in that the facial anatomy contains sinuses, which facilitate access to the skull base. Furthermore, the facial and oronasal anatomy develops from the midline, which allows the surgeon to separate the facial structures from the midline with the least traumatic consequences. The vascularization to the facial structures comes from a lateral source such as the external carotid artery, which will be preserved during surgery in the midline. Improvements in maxillofacial surgery facilitate a wide exposure of the skull base with relatively great acceptance of postoperative swelling not affecting the neural structures. The techniques of facial restoration have improved to such a level that there is acceptable functional and aesthetic success.

Disadvantages include contamination of the wound with oropharyngeal bacterial flora, CSF leakage, and the potential for postoperative upper airway obstruction problems.

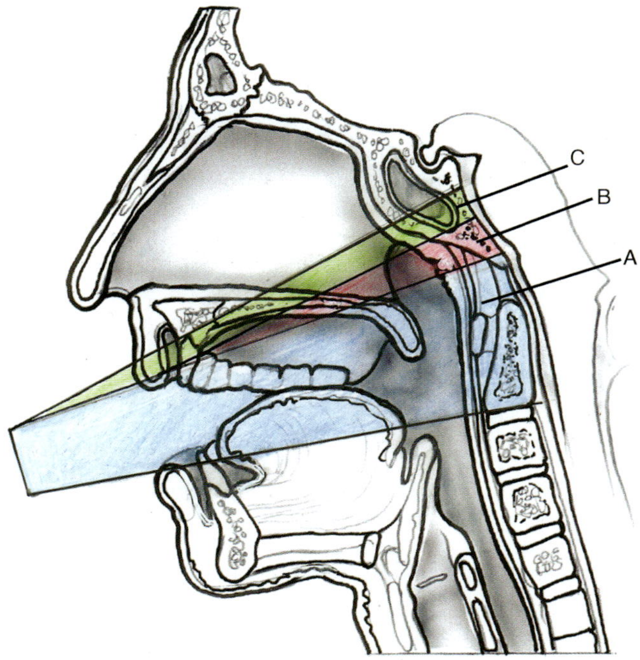

Figure 46–1 Areas of exposure to the clivus by means of transoral approaches. A, transoral approach; B, transpharyngeal approach; C, transpalatal approach.

Transoral Approaches

This approach primarily provides access to the lower midline skull base, craniocervical junction, and upper cervical spine and is mainly used for ventral midline pathology of the craniovertebral junction (**Fig. 46–1** and **Table 46–1**).

Complications of the oral approaches are especially related to the approaches themselves. Prolonged retraction of the tongue may result in ischemic necrosis of the tongue, which can be avoided by intermittent release of the retractor during surgery. Special attention should be paid to the postoperative instability of this region. In all patients stability should be assessed before and after surgery. This is to be repeated until 6 months postsurgery. Patients with rheumatoid disease need by definition a stabilization procedure.[7]

Table 46–1 Anterior Approaches to the Clivus and Anterior Skull Base

		Transpharyngeal approach	Lower anterior third of the clivus and foramen magnum
		Transpalatal approach	Lower anterior half of the clivus
	Transoral approach	Transmandibular approach	Anterior aspect foramen magnum to sphenoid sinus and infratemporal fossa
		Transmaxillary approach	Upper anterior half of the clivus and sphenoid sinus
		Extended maxillectomy	Upper anterior half of the clivus, sphenoid sinus and craniocervical junction
Transfacial approach		Facial translocation	Nasopharynx, anterior clivus and infratemporal fossa
		Facial splitting	Upper half of the anterior clivus and nasal sinuses
	Craniofacial resection	Lateral rhinotomy	Superior and inferior region of the anterior skull base Combined with craniotomy
		Facial degloving	

The transoral approach provides limited access to the midcranial part of the clivus. Therefore the transoral approach can be extended by splitting the soft palate in the midline (the transpharyngeal approach) (**Fig. 46–1**), which gains access to the lower third of the clivus and anterior aspect of the foramen magnum, and by splitting the hard palate (the transpalatal route) (**Fig. 46–1**), which provides access to the lower half of the clivus. The most significant postoperative problem is velopalatine insufficiency and persistent nasal speech. Many of these patients require corrective surgery.[7] In case of CSF leakage a postoperative lumbar drain is mandatory. Closure of the dura is very difficult because of the poor quality of the clival dura and because the dura is often stretched by the tumor. Closure techniques such as a multilayer closure with fat, fascia, and fibrin glue covered with mucosal tissue mobilized from the nasal septum are used to prevent a liquor CSF leakage. The patient should be observed for at least 48 hours on a high-level intensive care unit because a postoperative upper airway obstruction may occur due to swelling of the oropharyngeal soft tissue and the tongue. This should be treated by corticosteroids.

Even combined with splitting the soft and hard palate the transoral approach is not optimal for lesions that have a lateral or an upward extension, and it offers poor control of the internal carotid arteries.

Another variation of the transoral approach is the transmandibular approach (**Fig. 46–2** and **Table 46–1**). This approach provides access to the middle compartment of the skull base from the upper cervical spine and clivus to the sphenoid sinus and infratemporal fossa, inferior surface of the temporal bone, and parapharyngeal space. The mandible is cut in the midline; the floor of the mouth is incised, allowing lateral or transglottal access to the infratemporal fossa. Complications are related to the extent of this approach and include conductive hearing loss due to negative middle ear pressure, dysphagia, and recurrent aspirations.

Lesions that extend beyond the lateral and upper limitations of the transoral approach can be approached by the transmaxillary approach (**Fig. 46–2**). This route is suitable for extradural lesions extending in the upper and middle part of the clivus and sphenoid sinus. The maxilla is saw cut bilaterally through the maxillary buttresses according to a LeFort I osteotomy, and the hard palate is fractured down. The extended maxillectomy (**Fig. 46–2**) also provides access to the craniocervical junction by means of a midline incision of the hard and soft palate. Both approaches require teamwork and have, apart from tongue complications, basically the same complications as the transoral and transpalatine approaches.

Anterolateral skull base procedures such as the facial translocation approach permit greater access to the nasopharynx, clivus, and infratemporal fossa.[8] This approach includes removal of the posterior wall of the maxillary sinus and the pterygoids and osteotomy of the coronoid process. Further steps are isolation of the facial nerve, isolation of the upper and cervical ICA, and opening of the sphenoid

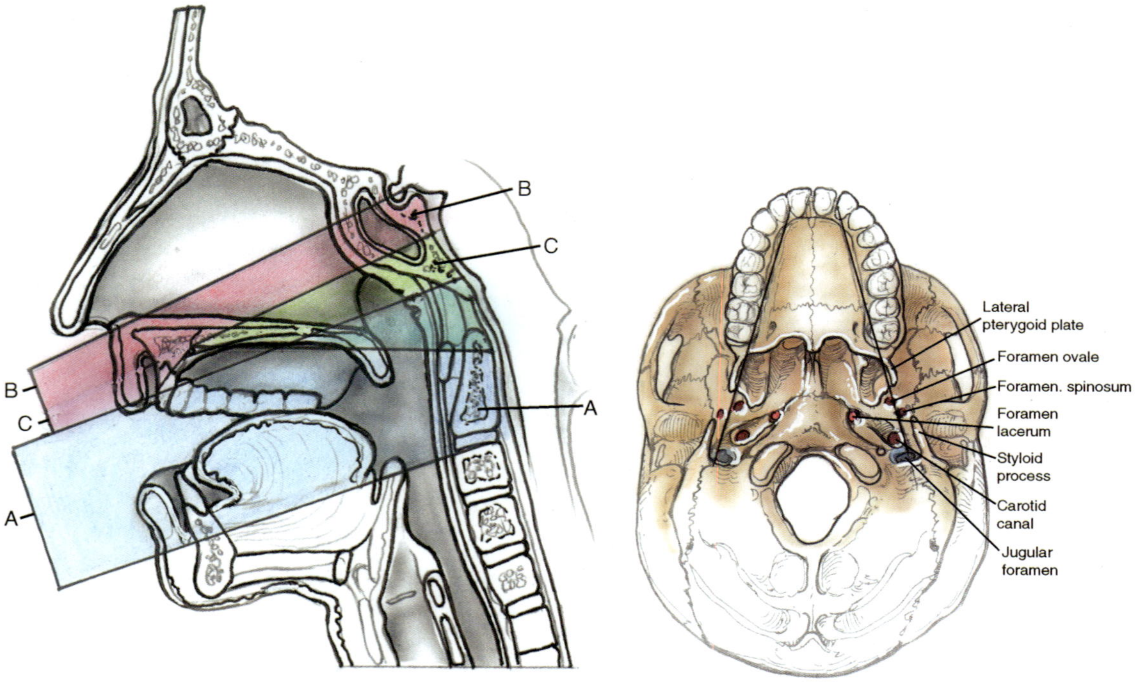

Figure 46–2 Areas of exposure to the clivus and pterygopalatinal regions by means of the transfacial approaches. A, transmandibular approach; B, transmaxillary approach; C, extended maxillectomy; D, extent of the parasagittal extensions of the transfacial approaches.

sinus and orbit. Although this approach involves extensive tissue removal, possible complications are similar to anterior and anterolateral cranial skull base procedures.

The craniofacial resection gives access to lesions of the anterior skull base and facial and oropharyngeal structures. Here the standard uni- or bilateral frontal craniotomy serves as the basis of an extra or intradural approach. A transbasal approach (**Fig. 46–3**) is composed of a standard bicoronal bone flap. This flap should be as low as possible through the frontal sinuses. The anterior skull base and, if necessary, the dura is opened. Dural lacerations in the area of the cribriform plate are almost unavoidable. The orbital roofs and medial walls, optic canals, and ethmoid and sphenoid sinuses can be reached. In the depth the anterior arch of C1 can be reached. The portion behind the sella turcica remains inaccessible. For this reason the extended frontal or basal frontal approach (**Fig. 46–3**) was developed, which combines a bifrontal craniotomy with an orbitofrontoethmoidal (frontal bar) osteotomy. This extension provides more access to the upper clivus. However, the lateral extension of this approach is blocked because of the cavernous sinus and its structures. Wider exposure to the anterior skull base and naso- and oropharynx can be obtained from several facial incisions (**Fig. 46–3**). The facial skin can be incised in the midline from the nasion through the upper lip (facial splitting) or at the paranasal side of the nose either with or without a lip splitting (lateral rhinotomy). These facial incisions can be prevented by incisions of the mucosa through the gingivolabial sulcus and elevation of the soft tissues of the face and nose. This procedure allows enough freedom for osteotomies of the facial bones, and when combined with the craniotomy they provide a wide exposure of the superior and inferior region of the skull base of the anterior fossa. This procedure is known as the facial degloving procedure.

Midline tumors from the dorsum sellae to the foramen magnum can be reached with minimal frontal brain retraction. Because this approach avoids destruction of the nasogastric tract, postoperative upper airway obstruction is less evident. The optic nerves, the cavernous sinus, the ICA, and the hypoglossal nerves at their lowest point limit this approach laterally.

Frontal approaches necessitate the removal of the crista galli and sacrifice of the olfactory nerves with the concomitant risks of anosmia, CSF leakage, and the need for a complex reconstruction of the frontal floor. Therefore a large pericranial flap should be preserved for dural closure. CSF leaks, meningitis, and osteomyelitis of the bone flap are reported as serious complications of the frontal approach procedure. However, considerably fewer complications have been described due to improved surgical techniques and, in particular, more effective treatment of the early postoperative complications.[9] The sense of smell is an important function; its absence is an impairment of the quality of life. Spetzler et al[10] described an en bloc removal of the cribriform plate to preserve the olfactory unit in anterior cranial facial approaches. However, this technique is still a matter of debate regarding its results.

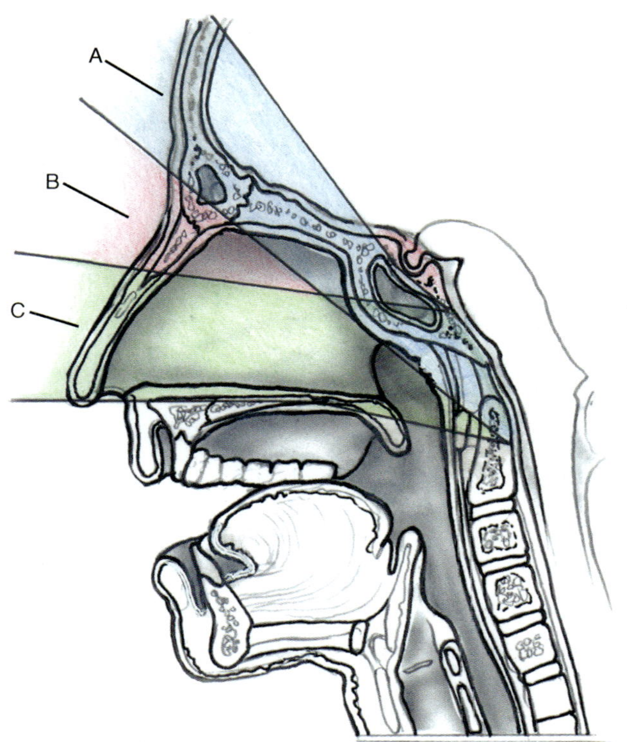

Figure 46–3 Areas of exposure to the clivus by means of the craniofacial resection. A, transbasal approach; B, extended frontal approach; C, transfacial approach.

Approaches to the Anterior Intracranial Fossa

From a surgical point of view it is important to recognize that the anterior cranial skull base is deeper medially than it is laterally. The anterior posterior distance of the anterior cranial fossa is relatively long; the posterior floor region, the planum sphenoidale, is located 4.25 cm behind the foramen caecum, which lies immediately behind the frontal bone in the midline. Furthermore, the orbital roofs are irregular in shape and the vascularization may come from an inferior-medial direction from the posterior and anterior ethmoidal arteries. To deal with these anatomical characteristics, each approach to the intracranial part of the anterior skull base, especially in the midline, should be as low as possible. In this respect the superior and lateral walls of the orbit should be removed. The unavoidable entry into the frontal sinus is not a serious event; large series report an incidence of less than 1% of fatal meningitis.[11] Surgical approaches are the standard bifrontal or unilateral craniotomy. Proponents of the unilateral approach consider that a unilateral approach may avoid bifrontal retraction, thereby avoiding intellectual deterioration with manipulation of both frontal lobes. Also, it may be possible to save one of the olfactory tracts in case of small tumors. Generally the size of the bone flap, either unilateral or bifrontal, depends on the size and location of the lesion.

A unilateral frontotemporal (pterional) osteotomy may be used to gain access to the middle fossa for extensive lesions involving the posterior part of the anterior fossa and the middle fossa. The pterional approach combines the benefit of the subfrontal and the trans-sylvian approach and is the shortest route to the para- and suprasellar region. It allows early identification of the carotid artery and optic nerves soon after the start of the surgery. Compared with the two frontal approaches, there is less compression on the frontal lobes.

The frontal and pterional standard approaches can be extended by removal of the superior and lateral orbital rim to allow a more basal access, allowing an approach under the frontal lobes with less elevation of the brain and a shorter distance to the lesion.

Approaches to the Middle Cranial Fossa, Supra- and Parasellar Region

The frontotemporal (pterional) craniotomy serves as the standard approach to the middle cranial fossa and supra- and parasellar structures. Dependent on the site, nature, and volume of the lesion this approach can be extended by means of the orbitozygomatic osteotomy. Basically this should be a routine procedure in skull base surgery. Sectioning the superior and lateral part of the orbit and zygoma or incorporating these bony structures into the pterional flap enhances the low exposure and increases the access in the anterior middle fossa and parasellar region. It minimizes the brain retraction and provides the shortest approach via either or both an intra- and an extradural route. Furthermore, it offers a multidirectional view of the lesion. The optic canal and superior orbital fissure are exposed and can be unroofed and the vascular supply to the lesion coming from the skull base can be interrupted prior to the tumor removal. By means of this approach the sphenoid sinus and infratemporal and sphenopalatine fossa can be reached. The bony reconstruction is uncomplicated, especially when the orbitozygomatic osteotomy is incorporated in the bone flap and CSF leaks can be easily repaired with the aid of the temporalis muscle.

Avoidable complications related to this approach are sectioning of the frontal branches of the facial nerve and temporal lobe problems because of brain retraction.

Approaches to Intracranial Posterior Middle Fossa and Petrous Bone

The middle fossa approach (**Fig. 46–4** and **Table 46–2**) provides a standard extradural access to the posterior temporal floor. A small subtemporal craniotomy located superior to the external auditory canal is performed, and the middle fossa dura is elevated. This approach provides access to the internal auditory canal (IAC) and the petrous part of the ICA for proximal control of the ICA.[12]

The arcuate eminence and the greater petrosal nerve are landmarks to be identified. The middle fossa approach can be extended to provide access to the posterior fossa. In this respect the petrous bone can be divided into zones.[13] The first zone is defined as the area from the dorsum sellae to the IAC and can be approached by the anterior petrosectomy[14] (**Fig. 46–4**). In this approach the middle fossa approach is extended with a resection of the medial petrous apex, known as Kawase's approach (the petrous tip medial to the carotid artery and anterior to the internal auditory meatus). This approach can be used for lesions in the middle fossa, Meckel's cave, and the upper third of the clivus above the internal auditory meatus. This approach is ideal for dumbbell trigeminal schwannomas located in Meckel's cave and extending into the upper posterior fossa. With this

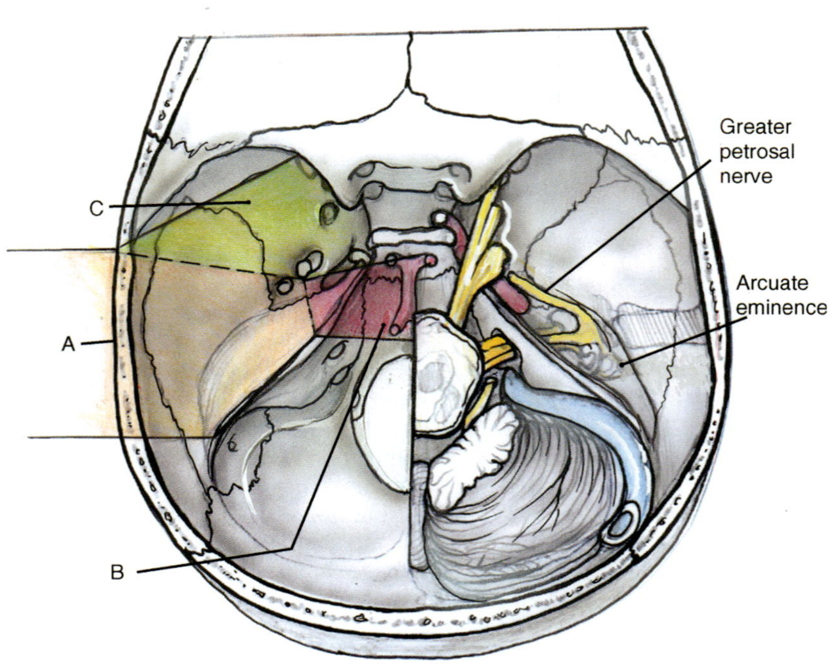

Figure 46–4 Areas of exposure to the posterior middle fossa and petrous bone by means of a middle fossa approach. A, middle fossa approach; B, anterior petrosectomy; C, temperozygomatic approach.

Table 46–2 Approaches to the middle and posterior fossa and petrous bone

	Anterior petrosectomy (posterior extension)	Middle fossa, Meckle's cave and upper posterior aspect of the clivus
Middle fossa approach	Temperozygomatic approach (anterior extension)	Lateral wall of the cavernous sinus and middle fossa
	Preauricular subtemporal-infratemporal approach (inferior extension)	Infratemporal fossa
Transpetrosal approach	Retrolabyrinthine approach	Cerebellopontine angle (exposure limited by labyrinth)
	Translabyrinthine approach	Cerebellopontine angle and IAC
	Transcochlear approach	Ventral aspect of brainstem and posterior clivus (limited by tentorium and jugular bulb)
Suboccipital approach	Lateral suboccipital approach	Ipsilateral posterior aspect clivus, IAC, jugular foramen and foramen magnum
	Transcondylar approach	Craniovertebral junction, anterior space brainstem, upper anterior spinal cord and posterior aspect lower clivus
	Extreme lateral approach	Craniovertebral junction, anterior portion of spinal cord and brainstem, posterior aspect of the lower and middle clivus

approach there is no need for transposition of cranial nerves or vascular structures. The disadvantage is that most surgeons are not familiar with the anatomy of the anterior petrous bone. Furthermore, the surgical field becomes progressively narrow as the field is limited by the IAC, the amount of temporal lobe retraction, and the posterolateral wall of the cavernous sinus. A combination of the anterior petrosectomy with the division of the tentorium, superior petrosal sinus, and a posterolateral dissection of the cavernous sinus may provide additional room.[15]

Enhanced anterior exposure of the middle fossa can be obtained with a temperozygomatic approach (**Fig. 46–4**) that is an inferior-anterior extension of the middle fossa approach. This approach provides access to the lateral wall of the cavernous sinus including Meckel's cave.

The middle fossa approach and the related combined approaches carry a risk of a temporal lobe retraction and obstruction of the venous outflow of the vein of Labbé. Manipulation of the greater petrosal nerve may result in a (temporary) dysfunction of the facial nerve.

The middle fossa approach is part of the preauricular subtemporal-infratemporal fossa approach designed to expose lesions extending in the infratemporal fossa. Bone over the glenoid fossa is removed, and the ICA is isolated from its extracranial portion to the cavernous sinus. The base of the skull can be removed anteriorly up to the foramen ovale. The V3 can be traced from Meckel's cave to the infratemporal fossa and sectioned to reach the foramen rotundum. This approach is derived from the Fisch infratemporal fossa approach for cases in which the middle or inner ear is not affected by the lesion.[16]

Posterolateral Intracranial Approaches to the Petrous Bone and Clivus

Posterior approaches access the skull base mainly via the posterior fossa. These approaches use the suboccipital and transpetrosal routes.

The transpetrosal approaches (**Table 46–2**) are the retrolabyrinthine, partial labyrinthectomy, (partial) translabyrinthectomy, and transcochlear approach. The jugular bulb limits all transpetrosal exposures inferiorly. Therefore, only lesions between the tentorium and cranial nerves IX and X can be reached.

The retrolabyrinthine approach (**Fig. 46–5**) consists of a mastoidectomy exposing the presigmoid dura of the posterior fossa and sigmoid sinus and the dura of the middle fossa with preservation of the structures of the inner ear. This approach requires no extensive cerebellar retraction and offers a short route to the cerebellopontine angle and cranial nerves V, VII, and VIII. The labyrinth limits the anterolateral exposure to the clivus, and the IAC is not accessible. The use of this approach in skull base surgery is limited. However, the combination of this approach with a middle fossa craniotomy is a versatile skull base technique providing access to the lateral aspect of the pons and midbrain. Sectioning of the tentorium is necessary to combine both approaches and to relax the sigmoid sinus to retract this sinus posteriorly.

When sectioning the tentorium and elevating the temporal lobe, the vein of Labbé can be injured. This should be prevented by gentle elevation of the temporal lobe and localization of the vein of Labbé before coagulation and cutting of the superior petrosal vein and tentorium.

The labyrinth limits the exposure of the retrolabyrinthine approach. Therefore, the labyrinth can be removed. The degree of the labyrinthectomy is dependent on several factors. When hearing is absent, the labyrinth can be removed without consequences to improve posterior fossa exposure. Some surgeons advocate a partial labyrinthectomy when hearing is intact. The loops of the superior and posterior semicircular canals can be removed and sealed with bone wax with preservation of hearing.[17] Sacrificing hearing by means of a complete labyrinthectomy should be balanced against the risks of a limited exposure. Also, if the location and the size of the lesion exclude any hope of preservation of cranial nerve VIII, the labyrinth can be sacrificed first.

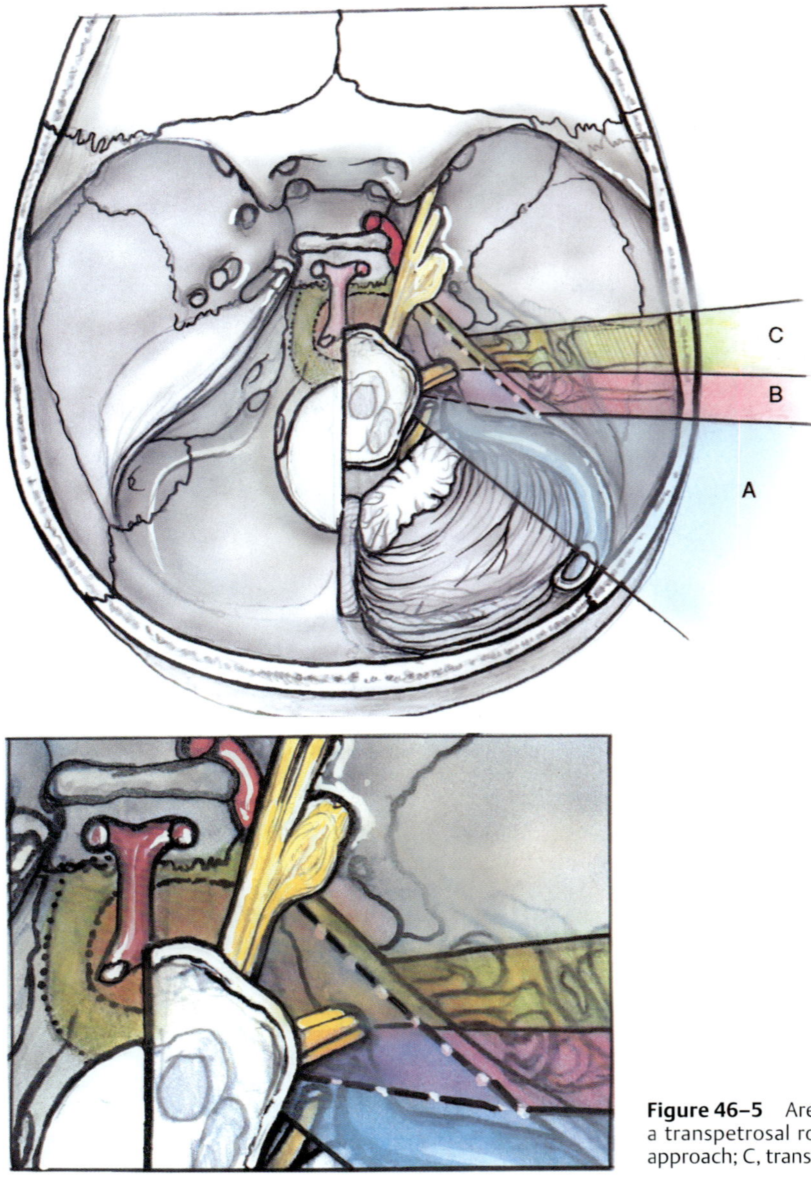

Figure 46–5 Areas of exposure to the petrous bone and clivus by means of a transpetrosal route. A, retrolabyrinthine approach; B, translabyrinthine approach; C, transcochlear approach.

The translabyrinthine approach (**Fig. 46–5**) consists of the retrosigmoid approach and the removal of the labyrinth with anatomical preservation of the facial nerve. The full length of the IAC can be exposed. This approach provides wide access to the cerebellopontine angle and the IAC to its most lateral extent and is mostly used in surgery of acoustic neuromas in patients who do not have useful hearing.

The transcochlear approach (**Fig. 46–5**) is a translabyrinthine approach with an anterior extension. The audiovestibular nerve is cut, and the facial nerve is rerouted posteriorly from the IAC to the stylomastoid foramen. The cochlea is then drilled out to expand the ventral exposure to the posterior fossa. Compared with the translabyrinthine exposure, the transcochlear approach improves the exposure of the ventral brain to provide a wide view of the basilar artery and clivus. The anatomical restrictions are the sigmoid sinus posteriorly, the tentorium and superior petrosal sinus superiorly, the eustachian tube and the vertical portion of the ICA anteriorly, and the jugular bulb inferiorly. A caudal extension of this approach requires additional exposure gained by a retrosigmoid approach and partial condylar resection. An anterior extension can be combined with the approach to the middle fossa such as the temperozygomatic approach. A cranial extension is possible by cutting the tentorium and elevating the temporal lobe.

All transpetrosal craniotomy defects require a meticulous closure of the dura with strips of fat to obliterate the dead space and to prevent CSF leakage. The best method is to plug the dural opening with subsequent strips of fat, harvested from the anterior abdominal wall, and glue. The use of fascia is only recommended in cases of large defects.

The suboccipital approach (**Fig. 46–6** and **Table 46–2**) is the standard neurosurgical exposure to the posterior fossa

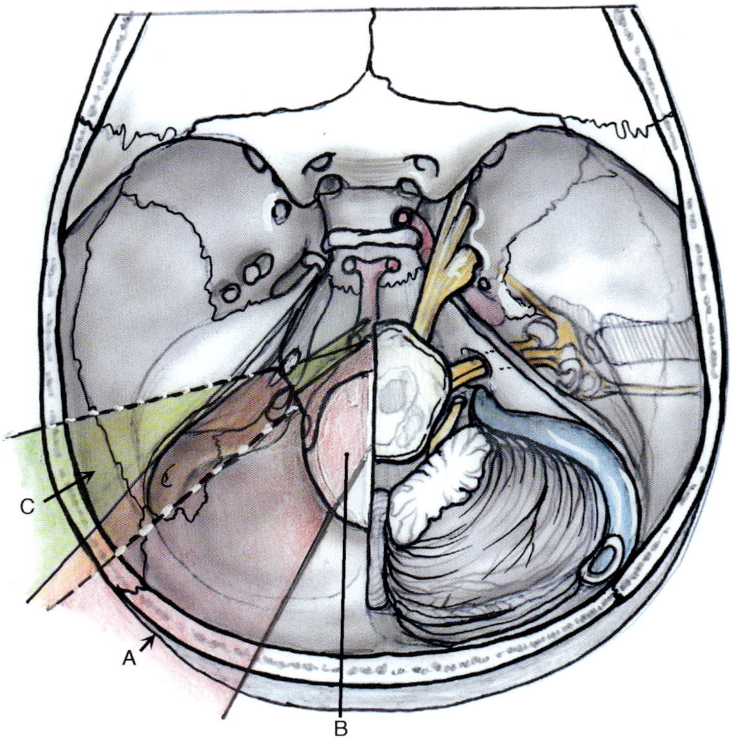

Figure 46–6 Areas of exposure to the petrous bone, clivus, and craniocervical junction. A lateral suboccipital approach; B, far lateral (transcondylar) approach; C, extreme lateral approach.

and can be extended as far lateral as the retrosigmoid (lateral occipital) approach (**Fig. 46–6**). The traditional suboccipital approach entails a craniotomy in the occipital bone and removal of the posterior ring of the foramen magnum. The lateral occipital approach is more lateral and extends just posteriorly to the sigmoid sinus, which may expose the mastoid cells. It provides access to the posterior fossa from the tentorium to the foramen magnum. By drilling its posterior wall, the IAC can be exposed. This approach is well suited for removal of lesions in the cerebellopontine angle such as acoustic neuromas and meningiomas. Lesions of the jugular foramen and ipsilateral lower clivus can be reached. However, because cranial nerves VII, VIII, and IX through XII run through the cerebellopontine angle, lesions ventral to these nerves, such as lesions located on the clivus, are less accessible by this approach, and the approach is purely intradural. Cerebellar retraction is a disadvantage of the retro approach, which can be avoided as much as possible by thorough drainage of the CSF from the cerebellomedullary cisterns immediately after opening the dura. Modern microsurgical techniques have considerably reduced the morbidity of this approach.

Based on the suboccipital approach, the far lateral approach (transcondylar approach) (**Fig. 46–6**) provides access to the craniovertebral junction for lesions anterior to the foramen magnum, on the lower clivus, and the space anterior to the spinal cord at the C1–C2 level. A standard suboccipital or low retrosigmoid craniotomy including the rim of the foramen magnum and a laminectomy of at least half the arch of C1 is performed. To improve the viewing angle across the front of the brain stem, the lateral exposure of the foramen magnum can be extended by means of the removal of the posterior portion of the occipital condyle. More ventrally located tumors require more extensive drilling of the condyle and a transposition of the vertebral artery. The vertebral artery is dissected from the transverse foramen of C1 and mobilized inferomedially. Approximately the posterior half of the condyle can be removed, leaving sufficient bony structure for stability of the craniovertebral junction. More aggressive condylar removal may necessitate occipitocervical fusion.[18] The advantage of the condylar removal is based on the fact that the jugular tubercle can be removed, providing a view to the space anterior to the brain stem.[19]

In the extreme lateral approach the vertebral artery is exposed. The mastoid process until the vertical segment of the facial nerve is skeletonized, and the sigmoid sinus and jugular bulb are fully unroofed. Depending on the site and volume of the tumor, a retrosigmoid craniotomy can be performed, and the condyle can be (partially) removed. Because of its true lateral direction, this approach offers a good view along the anterior portion of the brain stem and spinal cord. Furthermore, this approach can be extended and combined with the subtemporal and infratemporal approach, allowing the resection of the majority of extradural tumors in the region of the middle and lower clivus. An extra risk of this approach compared with the transcondylar approach is injury of the vertebral artery from cauterization of the venous plexus and due to manipulation of the vertebral artery. If dysfunction of cranial nerves IX to XII preexisted or was caused during surgery, a tracheostoma and feeding gastrostomy should be considered during or immediately after operation because dysfunction of these nerves is the greatest cause of postoperative morbidity and mortality.

CSF leaks may occur due to insufficient dural closure due to bipolar manipulation or to extensive removal of the dura in the case of meningiomas in this region.[20]

◆ Complications

Complications are closely related to the histology of the lesion, its involvement with neural and vascular structures, and the feasibility of dissection of these structures from the tumor.

Well-encapsulated neuromas are more easily dissected than meningiomas, and not all meningiomas are easily removable because of their different consistencies.

Despite the number of different approaches in skull base surgery complications from long-term brain retraction and venous outflow obstruction still occur. Therefore, a combination of approaches should be carefully chosen. In this respect skull base surgery is not keyhole surgery; temporary or permanent removal of bony structures in addition to standard craniotomy procedures should provide a low, wide, and close exposure to the lesion. If possible the cisterns should be opened first to drain the CSF before approaching and removing the lesion. Also, especially in extradural approaches, drainage of CSF by a lumbar catheter may provide considerable brain relaxation. However, supra- and infratentorial pressure differences should be kept in mind. Despite the aforementioned measures, some amount of brain retraction is inevitable. Brain retraction must be done intermittently during long-lasting surgical procedures, and the brain surface should be covered with moistened spongy strips under the blades of the retractor. Sometimes it is better to perform a well-judged brain resection of no eloquent areas, such as the anterior tip of the temporal lobe. Although it is not clear which vein is allocated for drainage of blood to a particular area of the brain, the venous drainage should be preserved during the operation.[21] Much attention is focused on the preservation of the vein of Labbé along the posterior temporal lobe, but other temporal bridging veins should also be preserved in lateral cranial base approaches.[22]

Tumor resection should be done by preserving the arachnoidal planes. If the arachnoidal planes are missing, efforts should be made to preserve the pial plane. When no dissection planes can be found, the tumor removal should be considered incomplete.

The surgical team should be prepared to occlude vessels temporarily and to repair by direct suture or reconstruct with a vein graft.[23]

Because of the lack of an epineurium and firm perineurium, cranial nerves are much more prone to damage during surgery than are the peripheral nerves.[24] As a consequence of their histological characteristics, these nerves are easily damaged during prolonged retraction and repeated contact with surgical instruments, such as the suction device, and dehydration. Retraction should be avoided by sharp dissection, and a continuous drip with saline in the operating field is advised. The use of wet cottons pledgets to protect the cranial nerves is strongly discouraged, especially if the high-speed drill is used. After dissection of a cranial nerve, the nerve can be coated with a drop of fibrin glue to protect the nerve from inadvertent injury during further surgery and to prevent the nerve from dehydration.[25] If cranial nerves are definitely injured, reconstruction is performed by suture or with a graft.[26,27]

Manipulation of the lower cranial nerves leads to a temporary or permanent loss of function. Depending on the age of the patient and the function of the contralateral lower cranial nerves, serious postoperative problems of uncoordinated swallowing, aspiration, and speech problems may occur.

A tracheotomy and gastrostomy should be performed at the time of the definite skull base surgery or be considered soon after surgery. Usually these measures are temporary until swallowing function returns or are compensated by the opposite side.

References

1. Sekhar LN, Pomeranz S, Sen CN. Management of tumors involving the cavernous sinus. Acta Neurochir Suppl (Wien) 1991;53:101–112
2. Van Rooij WJ, Sluzewski M, Metz MH, et al. Carotid balloon occlusion for large and giant aneurysms: evaluation of a new test occlusion protocol. Neurosurgery 2000;47:116–121
3. Tarr RW, Jungreis CA, Horton JA. Complications of preoperative balloon test occlusion of the internal carotid arteries: experience in 300 cases. Skull Base Surg 1991;1:240–244
4. Moller AR. Neuromonitoring of operations in skull base surgery. Keio J Med 1991;40:151–159
5. Sure U, Alberti O, Petermeyer E, et al. Advanced image-guided skull base surgery. Surg Neurol 2000;53:563–572
6. van Overbeeke JJ. Neurosurgical approaches to the skull base. Riv. Neuroradiologica 1994;7:515–520
7. Bhangoo RV, Crockard HA. Transoral exposures. In: Kaye AH, Black PM, eds. Operative Neurosurgery. Vol 2. New York: Churchill Livingstone; 2000:1399–1415
8. Janecka IP. Anterior skull-base tumors: general considerations. In: Kaye AH, Black PM, eds. Operative Neurosurgery. Vol 2. New York: Churchill Livingstone; 2000:1373–1383
9. Solero CL, DiMeco F, Sampath P, et al. Combined anterior craniofacial resection for tumors involving the cribriform plate: early and postoperative complications and considerations. Neurosurgery 2000;47:1296–1305
10. Spetzler RF, Herman JM, Beals S, et al. Preservation of olfaction in anterior craniofacial approaches. J Neurosurg 1993;79:48–52
11. Al Mefty O, Smith RR. Combined app in the management of brain lesions. In: Apuzo MLJ, ed. Brain Surgery: Complications, Avoidance and Management. New York: Churchill Livingstone; 1993:2283–2327
12. von Overbeeke JJ, Dujovny M, Dragovic L, Ausman JI. Anatomy of the sympathetic pathways in the carotid canal. Neurosurgery 1991;29:838–844
13. Abdel Aziz KM, Sanan A, van Loveren HR, et al. Petroclival meningiomas: predictive parameters for transpetrosal approaches. Neurosurgery 2000;47:139–150
14. Miller CG, van Loveren HR, Keller JT, et al. Transpetrosal approach: surgical anatomy and technique. Neurosurgery 1993;33:461–469
15. Harsh GR, Sekhar LN. The subtemporal, transcavernous, anterior transpetrosal approach to the upper brainstem and clivus. J Neurosurg 1992;77:709–717
16. Chang CY, O'Rourke DK, Cass SP. Update on skull base surgery. Otolaryngol. Clin North Am 1996;29:467–501
17. Hirsch BE, Cass SP, Sekhar LN, et al. Translabyrinthine approach to skull base tumors with hearing preservation. Am J Otol 1993;14: 533–543

18. Jackler RK. Far lateral approach to foramen magnum. In: Jackler RK, ed. Atlas of Neurotology and Skull Base Surgery. St. Louis: Mosby; 1996:185–196

19. Diaz Day J, Tschabitscher M. The lateral suboccipital transtubercular approach. In: Diaz Day J, Tschabitscher M, eds. Microsurgical Dissection of the Cranial Base. New York: Churchill Livingstone; 1996: 118–128

20. Sen CN, Sekhar LN. An extreme lateral approach to intradural lesions of the cervical spine and foramen magnum. Neurosurgery 1990;27: 197–204

21. Bartels RH, van Overbeeke JJ, Wesseling P. A new technique for the assessment of the draining area of a cerebral vein. Surg Neurol 1999;52: 78–80

22. Sakata K, Al-Mefthy O, Yamamoto Y. Venous consideration in petrosal approach: microsurgical anatomy of the temporal bridging vein. Neurosurgery 2000;47:153–161

23. Linskey ME, Sekhar LN, Sen C. Cerebral revascularisation in cranial base surgery. In: Sekhar LN, Janecka IP, eds. Surgery of Cranial Base Tumors. New York: Raven Press; 1993:45–69

24. Menovsky T, van Overbeeke JJ. On the mechanism of transient postoperative deficit of cranial nerves. Surg Neurol 1999;51:223–226

25. de Vries J, Menovsky T, Grotenhuis JA, et al. Protective coating of cranial nerves with fibrin glue (Tissucol) during cranial base surgery: technical note. Neurosurgery 1998;43:1242–1246

26. van Overbeeke JJ, Cruysberg JR, Menovsky T. Intracranial repair of a divided trochlear nerve. J Neurosurg 1998;88:336–339

27. Menovsky T, van Overbeeke JJ. Repair of intracranial nerves during intracranial neurosurgery: theoretical and practical considerations. Neurosurgery Quarterly 1998;8:48–54

47

Malignant Tumors of the Anterior Cranial Base

Ehab Hanna, Mark Linskey, and Daniel Pieper

Malignant neoplasms involving the anterior cranial base most commonly represent extension of malignant tumors of the nasal cavity and paranasal sinuses.[1] The mucosal lining of the nose—the schneiderian membrane—is derived from ectoderm. This is uniquely different from the rest of the upper respiratory tract mucosa, which is derived from endoderm. Olfactory neuroepithelium lines the superior portion of the nasal cavity and the nasal roof. The sinonasal epithelium also has mucinous and minor salivary glands. The unique histology of this region is reflected in the histogenesis of a complex variety of epithelial and nonepithelial tumors (**Table 47–1**). These tumors have a wide range of

Table 47–1 Tumors of the Sinonasal Tract

Benign	Angiofibroma	Sinonasal undifferentiated carcinoma (SNUC)
Epithelial	Ameloblastoma	**Nonepithelial**
Papilloma	Fibrous dysplasia	Chordoma
Adenoma	Ossifying fibroma	Chondrosarcoma
Dermoid	Giant cell tumor	Osteogenic sarcoma
Nonepithelial	**Malignant**	Soft tissue sarcoma
Fibroma	**Epithelial**	Fibrosarcoma
Chondroma	Squamous cell carcinoma	Malignant fibrous histiocytoma
Osteoma	Differentiated (well, moderately, poorly)	Hemangiopericytoma
Neurofibroma	Basaloid squamous	Angiosarcoma
Hemangioma	Adenosquamous	Kaposi's sarcoma
Lymphangioma	Nonsquamous cell carcinoma	Rhabdomyosarcoma
Nasal glioma	Adenoid cystic carcinoma	Lymphoproliferative
Intermediate	Mucoepidermoid carcinoma	Lymphoma
Schneiderian papilloma	Adenocarcinoma	Polymorphic reticulosis
Inverted	Neuroendocrine carcinoma	Plasmacytoma
Papillary	Hyalinizing clear cell carcinoma	Metastatic
Cylindrical	Melanoma	
	Olfactory neuroblastoma	

(With permission from Stern SJ, Hanna E. Cancer of the nasal cavity and paranasal sinuses. In: Myers EN, Suen JY, eds. Cancer of the Head and Neck. 3rd ed. Philadelphia: WB Saunders; 1996:205–233.)

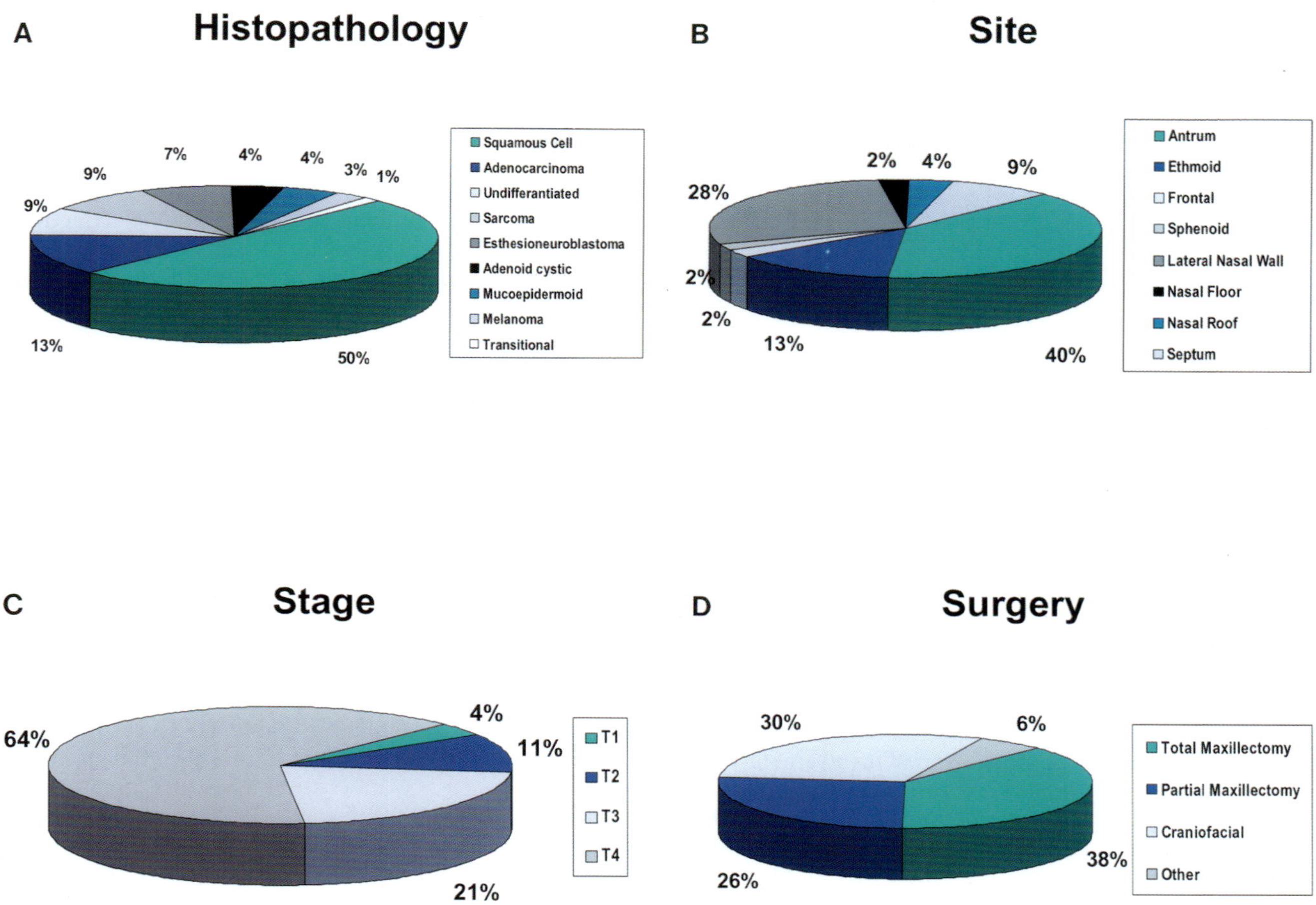

Figure 47–1 Data of 86 consecutive patients with sinonasal malignancy treated at the University of Arkansas for Medical Sciences between 1988 and 1998. Patients are classified according to **(A)** histopathologic diagnosis, **(B)** site of tumor origin, **(C)** stage of disease, and **(D)** type of surgical resection. (With permission from Hanna E, Vural E, Teo C, Farris P, Breau R, Suen JY. Sinonasal tumors: the Arkansas experience. Skull Base Surg 1998;8(Suppl):15.)

biological behavior and, therefore, various propensities for invasion of the anterior cranial base.[1–6]

The most common malignancy of the sinonasal tract is squamous cell carcinoma (**Fig. 47–1A**). Although the maxillary antrum is the most commonly involved sinus (**Fig. 47–1B**), anterior skull base invasion is most frequently encountered with malignant neoplasms of the nasal cavity and ethmoid sinus. Upward extension of these neoplasms toward the cribriform plate or fovea ethmoidalis is not uncommon and heralds intracranial extension. Unfortunately, despite significant improvement in diagnostic techniques such as nasal endoscopy and high-resolution imaging,[7] most patients present with advanced stage disease (**Fig. 47–1C**).

Although recent advances have allowed more accurate delivery of radiation therapy and have offered more effective chemotherapeutic agents, surgical resection is the mainstay of treatment for patients with sinonasal cancer.[1,5] Involvement of the anterior skull base frequently requires combined intracranial and extracranial approaches for achieving optimal surgical exposure and adequate tumor resection. In our experience, approximately one third of patients with sinonasal cancer required a combined approach and resection of the anterior cranial base[3] (**Fig. 47–1D**).

◆ Indications

En bloc resection of the anterior cranial base is indicated for malignant neoplasms involving the cribriform plate or fovea ethmoidalis. This is done, by definition, for most cases of esthesioneuroblastoma[2] as well as carcinomas of the ethmoid sinuses or the nasal cavity approaching or involving the anterior cranial base.[8,9] Tumors transgress the cribriform plate either by direct bony invasion or by perineural spread along the filaments of the olfactory nerves. The dura of the anterior cranial fossa forms a barrier that delays, to a certain extent, brain invasion. Dural resection in patients with intracranial but extradural disease or patients with limited dural involvement often provides an adequate oncological margin. Tumors that transgress the dural barrier and involve the underlying brain parenchyma are usually associated with poor prognosis.[10–13] However, even in some cases with limited frontal lobe involvement, anterior craniofacial resection may still be indicated for local control of the disease.

◆ Contraindications

In the presence of distant metastasis, extensive intracranial involvement, bilateral cavernous sinus extension, or disease involving both orbits, surgery is probably contraindicated.[1] However, in selected cases, surgery may offer the most effective palliation, even in the presence of extensive disease.

◆ Preparation

A thorough preoperative assessment should determine the patient's candidacy for surgical management of a neoplasm. This involves careful "mapping" of the tumor extent, as well as evaluating the general medical condition and functional status of the patient. A detailed history and physical examination including endoscopy of the sinonasal region, cranial nerve examination, as well as neuro-ophthalmologic evaluation should be done. High-resolution imaging should be obtained using computed tomography (CT) or magnetic resonance imaging (MRI) or both to accurately assess the tumor extent.[7] In certain cases, angiography will be needed to determine the extent of carotid arterial involvement. The balloon occlusion test should be performed if carotid artery resection or reconstruction is contemplated. Preoperative embolization may be indicated in certain vascular tumors. The plan for the surgical approach, the extent of resection, and reconstructive options should then be formulated. This plan should be communicated clearly among the various members of the surgical team, particularly the neurosurgeons and otolaryngologists–head and neck surgeons. If free vascularized flaps will be utilized for reconstruction, expertise with microvascular surgery is needed, and appropriate consultation should be obtained. Patients requiring maxillary osteotomies should be evaluated by a maxillofacial prosthodontist to obtain preoperative dental impressions and design surgical obturators or splints for maintenance of proper dental occlusion and oral rehabilitation. A metastatic workup is required for complete oncological staging of the patient.

Careful assessment of the patient's general medical condition should be done. Preoperative chest radiograph, blood counts, liver and renal function tests, blood sugar, electrolytes, coagulation studies, and an electrocardiogram (ECG) should be done routinely. Appropriate consultations from medical colleagues should be obtained to optimize the patient's medical status before surgery and help in management postoperatively. The patient's nutritional status should be evaluated, and if indicated, enteral or parenteral feeding may be considered.

Finally, the surgical team should discuss with the patient and family the nature of the disease, the workup procedures, and the indications, risks, possible complications, sequelae, and alternatives of therapy. The expected postoperative course, including length of stay in the hospital, feeding, rehabilitation, and need for adjunctive therapy, should be described. This ongoing communication should be done in a clear, honest, and sympathetic fashion throughout the course of patient care.

◆ Surgical Technique

Approach

A variety of surgical approaches for resection of malignant tumors of the anterior cranial base have been described. Generally, these approaches may be classified as (1) intracranial, (2) extracranial, and (3) combined. Selection of the optimal surgical approach depends on several factors, including tumor location, extent of disease, and expertise of the surgical team. Whatever approach is used, certain surgical principles should be followed to achieve the best possible outcome (**Table 47–2**).

Intracranial approaches to the anterior cranial base usually involve a frontal craniotomy. Subfrontal approaches involve the addition of osteotomies that allow incorporation of either or both the superior orbit and the nasal skeleton to the craniotomy.[14–16] These skeletal elements may be removed in several subunits or as a single bone flap. The advantage of subfrontal approaches is that they allow wider exposure of the anterior skull base while minimizing brain retraction. This is especially helpful in more posteriorly located lesions, such as those involving the planum sphenoidale, clivus, orbital apex, and optic chiasm.

Several extracranial approaches have been described to access the anterior skull base (**Table 47–3**). The most commonly used extracranial approaches utilize the nasomaxillary route because it offers several advantages. First, most tumors involving the anterior skull base originate from the sinonasal tract, and nasomaxillary approaches allow direct exposure of this region. Second, the air-filled spaces of the nose and paranasal sinuses offer a wide exposure of the anterior cranial base without the need for dissection or retraction of major neurovascular structures.[17] Finally, bony and soft tissue reconstruction of the nasomaxillary region is

Table 47–2 Surgical Principles of Resection of Malignant Tumors of the Anterior Skull Base

Adequate oncological resection
Minimal brain retraction
Protection of critical neurovascular structures
Meticulous reconstruction of the anterior skull base
Optimal aesthetic outcome

Table 47–3 Extracranial Approaches to the Anterior Skull Base

Transmandibular
Transoral
Transpalatal
Transnasal
Transmaxillary
Transethmoid
Transfrontal

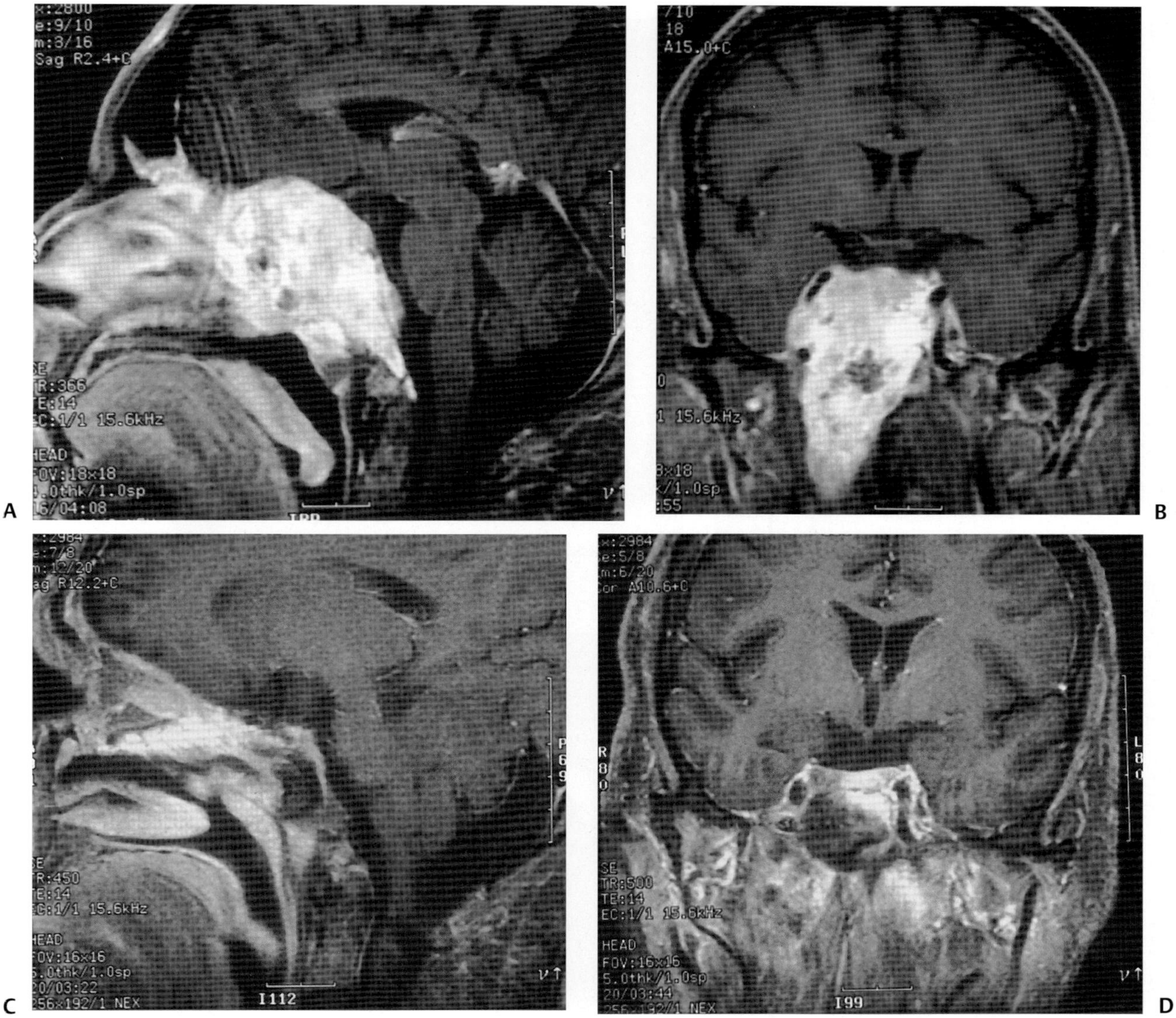

Figure 47–2 Magnetic resonance imaging (MRI) of a patient with large sphenoclival chordoma involving the anterior cranial base superiorly and extending to the level of the foramen magnum inferiorly. The tumor was completely removed through the cranio-nasal-orbital approach. Preoperative **(A)** sagittal and **(B)** coronal and postoperative **(C)** sagittal and **(D)** coronal T1-weighted MRI with gadolinium.

relatively simple and results in excellent functional and aesthetic outcome. Soft tissue access to the nasomaxillary region can be achieved with either transfacial incisions (e.g., lateral rhinotomy) or sublabial incisions (e.g., facial degloving). The advantage of facial degloving is the lack of any facial scars. However, well-executed facial incisions heal with excellent cosmetic result.

We describe a modified subfrontal approach, the cranio-orbital-nasal approach, for resection of tumors of the anterior cranial base. This approach offers wide exposure of the cribriform plate, fovea ethmoidalis, planum sphenoidale, orbital roof, orbital apex, optic chiasm, cavernous sinus, and clivus to the level of the foramen magnum and occipital condyles (**Fig. 47–2**). In addition to the excellent exposure, this provides a shorter working distance to the central skull base. The single cranio-orbital-nasal bone flap allows for simple, effective, and aesthetic bone reconstruction (**Fig. 47–3**).

Incision and Soft Tissue Dissection

The patient is placed supine on the operating room table. The incision is started at the level of the zygoma, in a preauricular crease anterior to the tragus. The main trunk of the superficial temporal artery (STA) should be preserved. The incision is extended in the coronal plane, staying behind the hairline along its entire course, to the contralateral zygoma. We prefer to gently curve the incision anteriorly at the midline (**Fig. 47–4A**). Using sharp dissection, the scalp incision proceeds anteriorly until the prominence of the superior orbital rims is appreciated, staying superficial to the pericranium and temporalis fascia. The scalp flap is reflected anteriorly, while carefully preserving the STA. The anterior branch of the STA can be cut distally and reflected with the scalp flap, whereas the posterior branch should remain adherent to the temporalis fascia. The dissection of the scalp

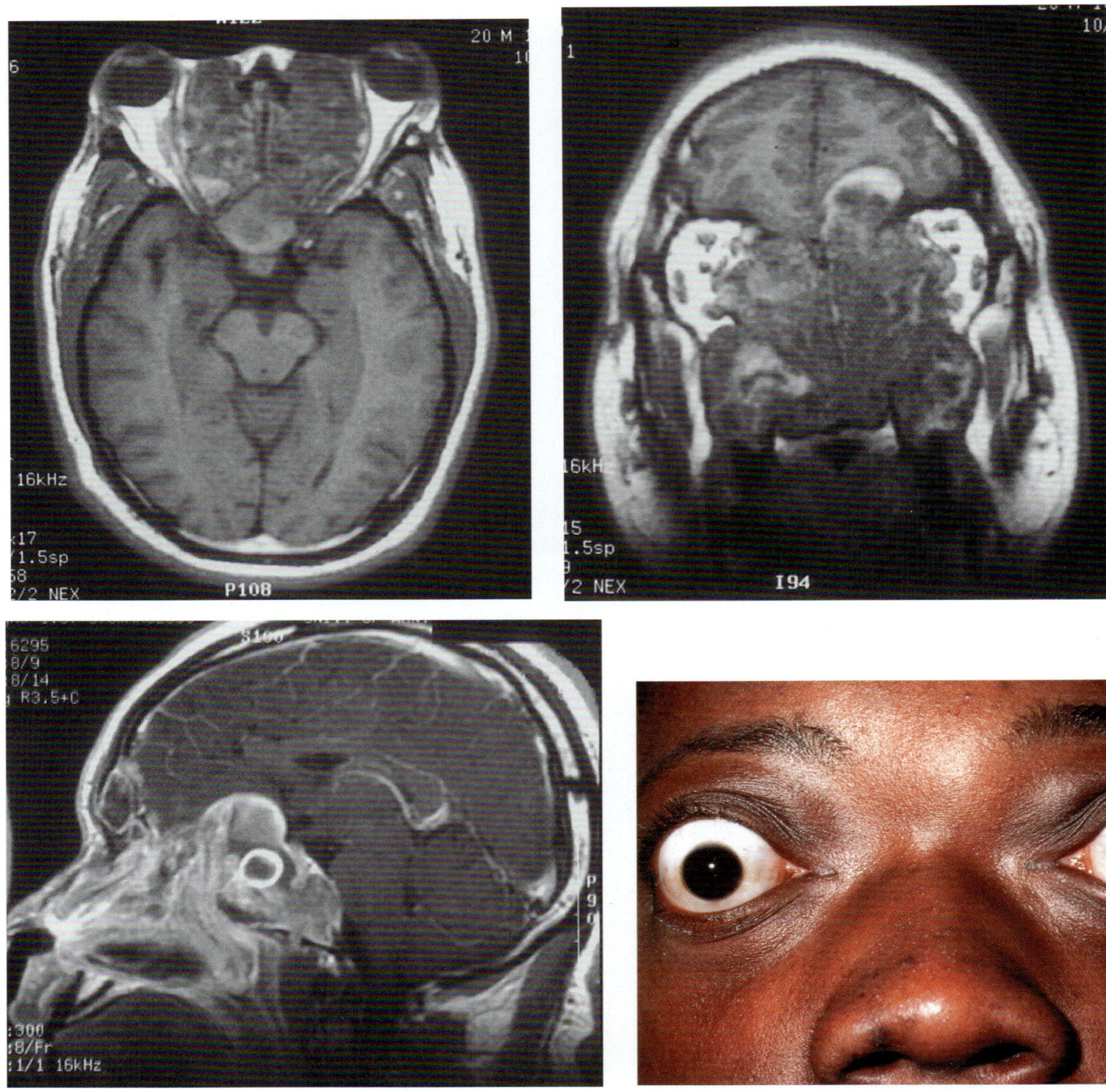

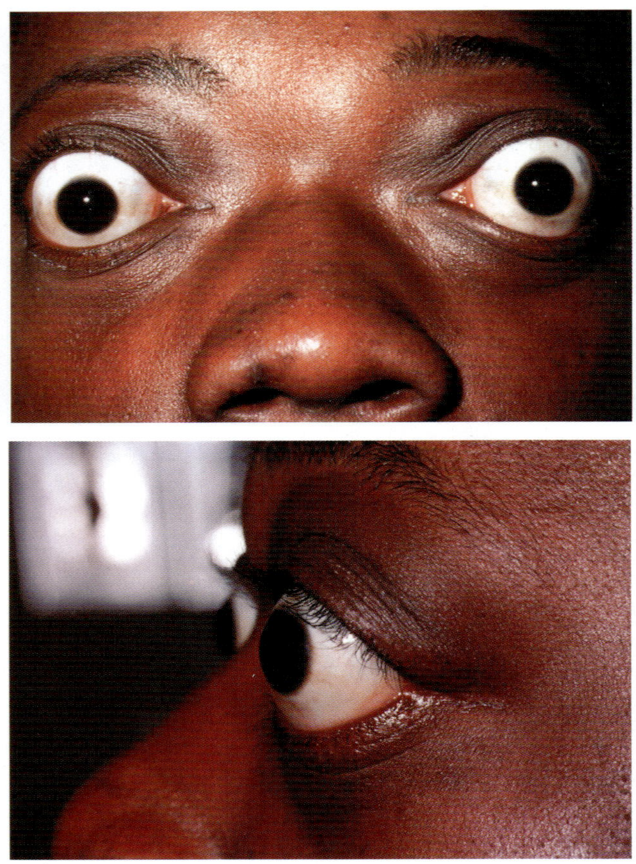

Figure 47–3 T1-weighted magnetic resonance imaging (MRI) **(A)** axial, **(B)** coronal, **(C)** sagittal with gadolinium showing a large enhancing lesion involving the nasal cavity, paranasal sinuses (maxillary, ethmoid, sphenoid), central skull base, and orbits compressing the optic nerve bilaterally. **(D,E)** The patient presented with progressive visual loss and significant proptosis.

from the pericranium is then continued posterior to the vertex, and a pericranial incision is made at the posterior border of the exposed pericranium. The pericranium is dissected free from the bone and reflected anteriorly along the superior temporal line bilaterally, providing a well-vascularized pericranial flap for reconstruction. At the level of the superior orbital rim, care must be taken to identify the supraorbital nerve, typically located along the medial one third of the superior orbital rim. This nerve may exit the skull either through a notch or through a true foramen. Should the former be

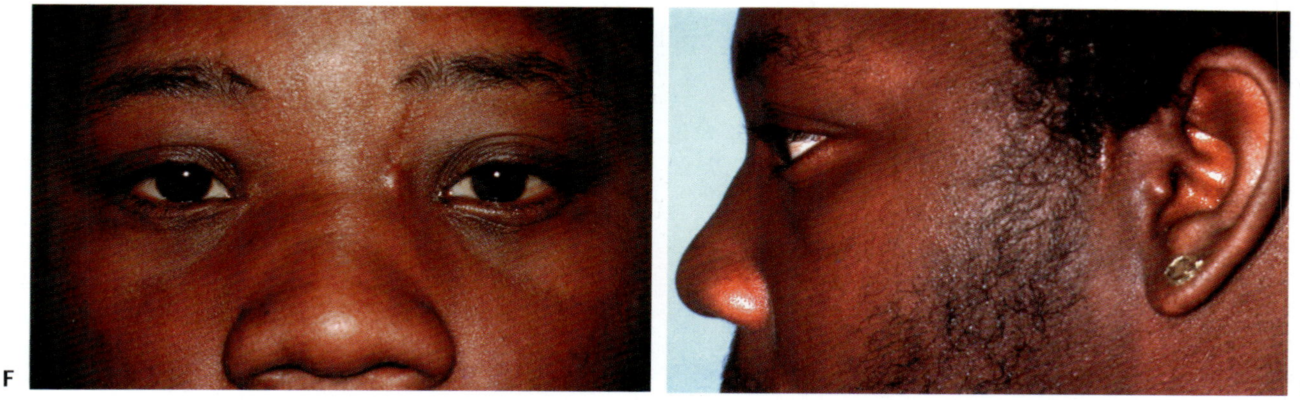

(*Continued*) **Figure 47–3** **(F,G)** Postoperative appearance after removal of this lesion through a cranio-orbital-nasal approach.

present, the nerve can be dissected free without injury; however, if the latter presentation exists, the nerve must be dissected free to avoid injury. Using the Midas Rex B1 attachment (Midas Rex Pneumatic Tools, Inc., Fort Worth, TX) a small osteotomy is performed around the supraorbital foramen and the nerve dissected free with its bony attachment and reflected anteriorly with the scalp and pericranium (**Fig. 47–4A**). The dissection continues anteriorly along the nasion to the level of the lower border of the nasal bones (**Fig. 47–4A**). The medial periorbita is dissected until the anterior and posterior ethmoidal arteries are exposed. These should be coagulated and transected sharply.

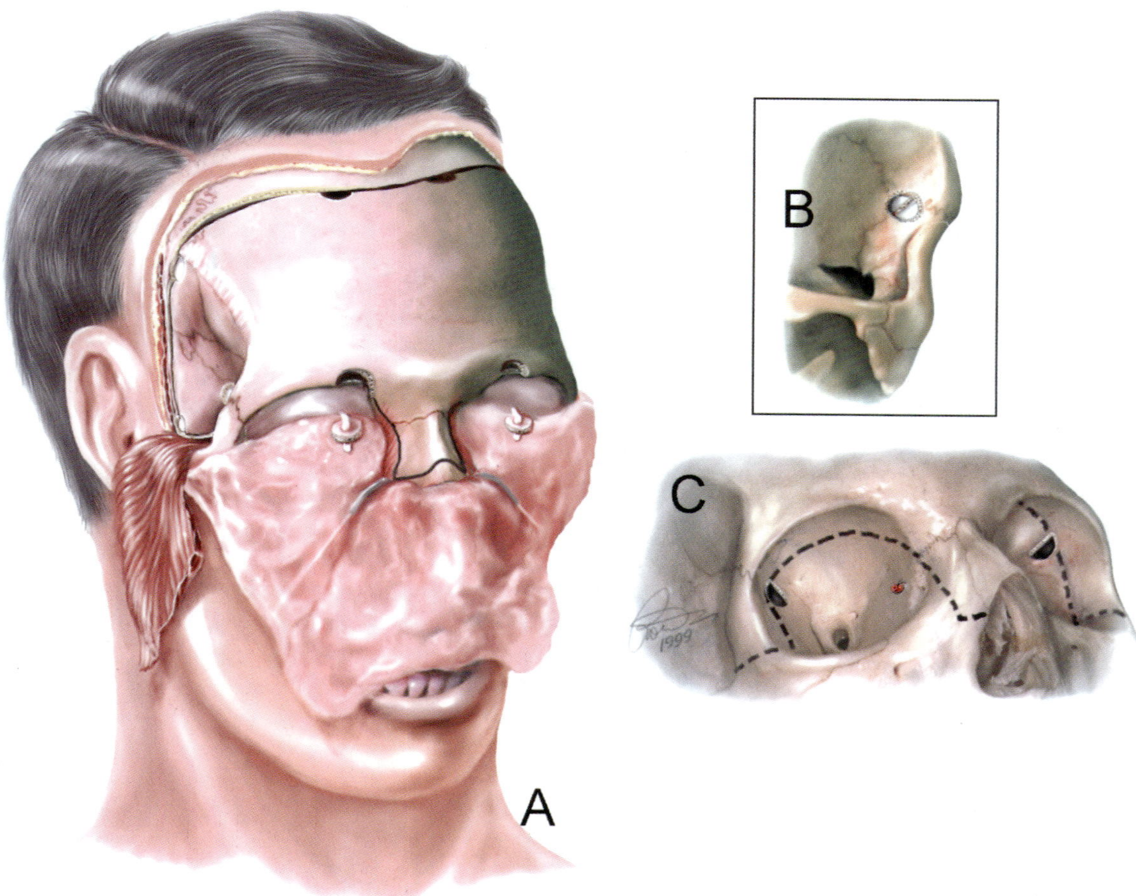

Figure 47–4 **(A)** Bicoronal incision and soft tissue dissection. Note the scalp flap is reflected anteriorly down to the level of the nasal bones. The supraorbital nerves were surrounded by complete foramina rather than a notch. Osteotomies around the foramina allow downward reflection of the nerves with the soft tissue flap. Bur holes are placed on either side of the superior sagittal sinus, anterior to the coronal suture. **(B)** Bilateral bur holes are placed posterior to the frontal-zygomatic sutures. These anatomical keyholes provide access to the anterior fossa dura and periorbita, separated by the bony orbital roof. **(C)** Orbital and nasal osteotomies.

Laterally, an incision is made through the superficial layer of the temporalis fascia 1 to 1.5 cm posterior to the superior orbital rim and extends posteriorly parallel to the course of the zygomatic arch. The temporalis fascia is then dissected along the lateral orbital rim in a subperiosteal fashion and reflected with the skin flap. This maneuver preserves the frontal branch of the facial nerve, which is superficial to the fascia. The temporalis muscle is then cut at its attachment along the superior temporal line and reflected inferiorly to expose the frontozygomatic suture line. We prefer to leave a cuff of fascia adherent to the bone to reattach the muscle at the conclusion of the case.

Craniotomy

Bilateral bur holes are then placed in the depression posterior to the frontal-zygomatic sutures (**Fig. 47–4B**). These anatomical keyholes provide access to the anterior fossa dura and periorbita, separated by the bony orbital roof. Bur holes are then placed on either side of the superior sagittal sinus (SSS), well anterior to the coronal suture (**Fig. 47–4A**). Using a high-speed cutting bit (Midas Rex B1) a cut is made through the inferior aspect of the lateral orbital rim flush with the malar eminence, then directed, under direct vision, superiorly to the anatomical keyhole, carefully avoiding lacerations to the periorbita. The bifrontal craniotomy is performed between the bur holes, with the bur holes straddling the SSS connected last. The dura of the anterior fossa is dissected from the orbital roofs. Under direct vision orbital roof osteotomies are performed using a small osteotome.

Nasal Osteotomies

Bilateral nasal osteotomies are done along the lower border of the nasal bones and then along the suture line between the nasal and lacrimal bones (**Fig. 47–4C**). The osteotomies are connected across the midline below the fronto-ethmoid suture line and in front of the anterior ethmoidal vessels. This avoids injury to the cribriform plate and olfactory nerves.

Orbital Osteotomies

After the dura and periorbita have been carefully dissected from the bone, the lateral wall and roof of each orbit are removed in separate osteotomies (**Fig. 47–4C**). Under direct visualization, taking care to protect the periorbita and dura, an anteroposterior cut is made at the medial aspect of the orbital roof staying lateral to the ethmoid sinus. A second anteroposterior cut is made at the inferior aspect of the lateral orbital wall. These cuts are connected posteriorly taking care to avoid the superior orbital fissure (SOF). The bone flap, consisting of the frontal bone, orbital roof, superolateral orbital rims, and nasal bones can be removed for wide exposure (**Fig. 47–5A,B**).

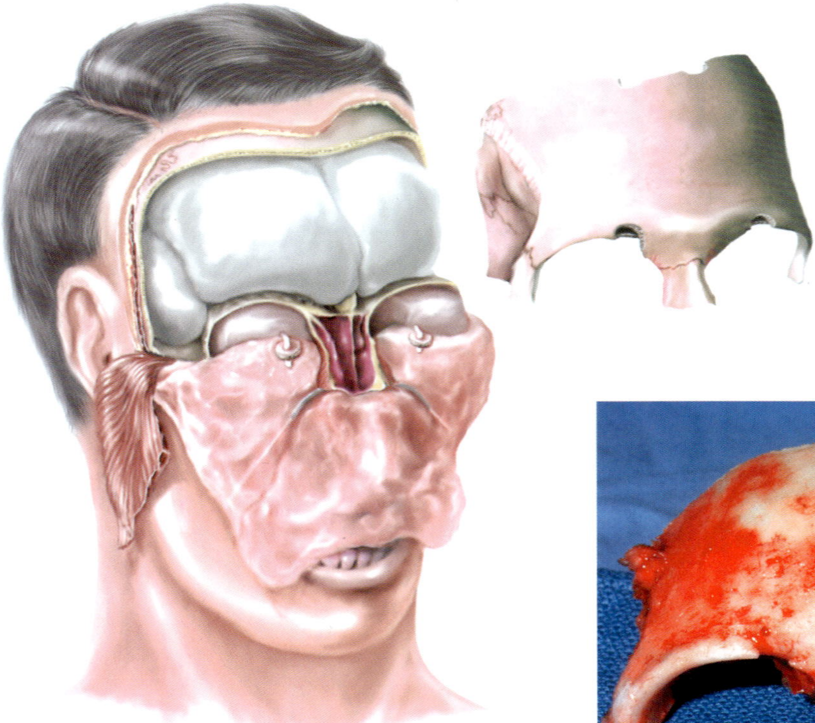

A

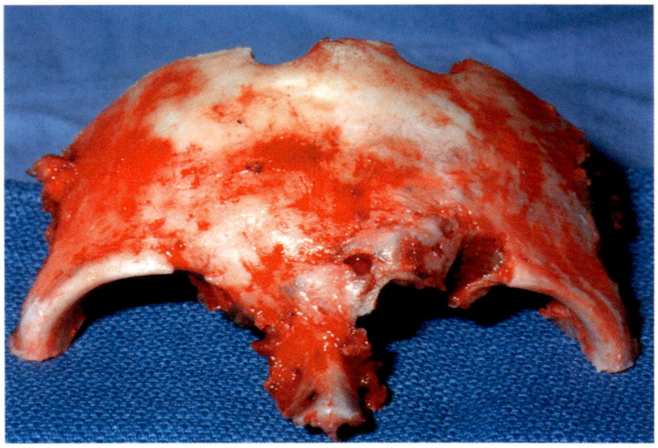

B

Figure 47–5 **(A)** The cranio-orbital-nasal bone flap is removed as a single unit. **(B)** Intraoperative photograph.

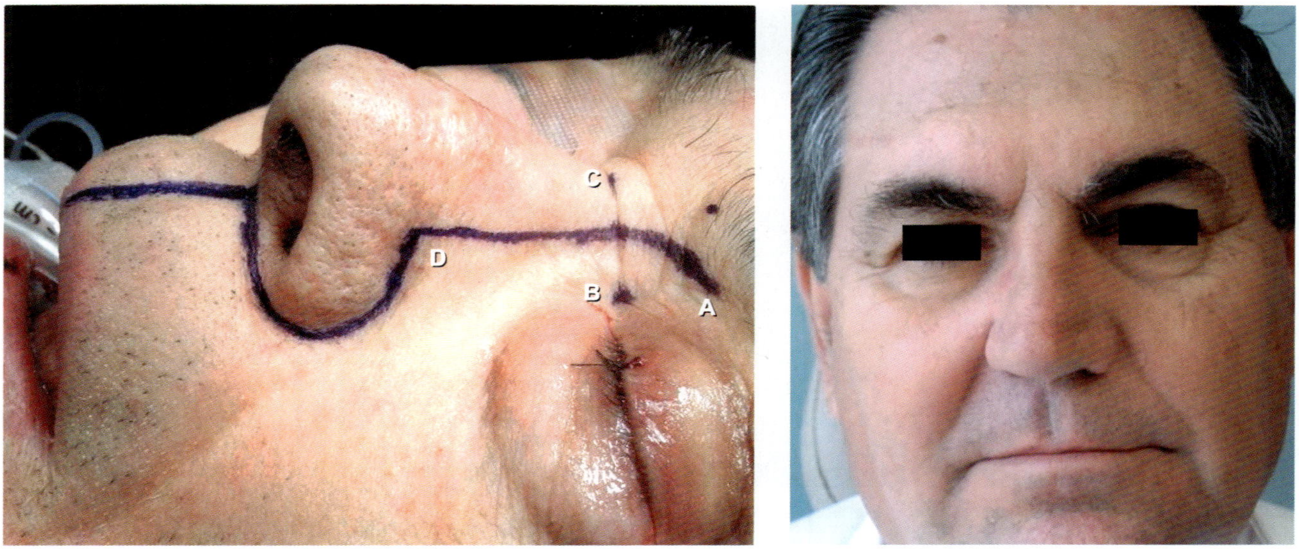

A B

Figure 47–6 **(A)** The extended lateral rhinotomy incision. The incision is outlined using three surface points. The first point (A) is marked at the inferior hairline of the medial eyebrow ~1 cm lateral to its medial end. The second point is marked halfway between the medial canthus (B) and the midline (C). The last point (D) is the medial end of the alar crease where the crease blends with the skin of the nasal tip. The incision starts with connecting the first two points with a gentle curve at the medial canthal area, corresponding to the concavity of this region. The second and the third reference points are then connected with a straight line. The incision then follows the alar crease, turns toward the midline, makes a right angle inferiorly at the columellar base, and continues as a lip-splitting incision at the midline. **(B)** Postoperative photograph showing excellent healing and good aesthetic outcome of the lateral rhinotomy incision.

Transfacial Approach

Removing the nasal bones with the bone flap allows exposure of the superior aspect of the nasal cavity including the nasal septum, cribriform plate, superior and middle turbinates, and ethmoid and sphenoid sinuses. If more exposure of the nasal cavity or paranasal sinuses is needed, a transfacial approach can be added. One of the most commonly used incisions for transfacial approaches is the lateral rhinotomy incision. Vural and Hanna described a modification of this incision, which enhances surgical exposure while improving the functional and aesthetic outcome[18] (**Fig. 47–6A,B**). Intraorally, either or both gingivobuccal and palatal incisions are made according to the location and extent of maxillary osteotomies necessary for exposure or tumor resection. The cheek flap is then elevated subperiosteally, and the periorbita is separated from the inferior and medial orbital walls. Slight retraction of the cheek flap laterally and the orbital content superiorly exposes the nasomaxillary region from the pyriform aperture and nasal cavity medially, to the zygomaticomaxillary suture line laterally. Maxillary and palatal osteotomies can then be done to either resect (maxillectomy) or temporarily displace (maxillotomy or maxillary translocation) various segments of the nasomaxillary facial skeleton, as dictated by the location and extent of the tumor.

Surgical Resection

With simultaneous exposure both intra- and extracranially, the central portion of the anterior cranial base consisting of the cribriform plate, fovea ethmoidalis, and planum sphenoidale can be safely removed. If more lateral resection is needed, the remaining bone around the SOF, located at the intersection of the lateral wall and roof of the orbit, is removed using a small rongeur or high-speed drill. The optic canal, located at the apex of the orbit, medial to the SOF, is then opened extradurally and the optic strut drilled to allow the removal of the anterior clinoid process exposing the subclinoid portion of the internal carotid artery (ICA). Decompression of the optic canals, if needed, can be completed under magnification. During the drilling of the optic canals, copious irrigation is necessary to avoid thermal injury to the optic nerves. During the drilling of the petrous bone, the horizontal portion of the ICA can be identified. If necessary, the cavernous sinus can be entered and the remainder of the cavernous portion of the ICA can be exposed. Drilling along the inferior third of the clivus will expose the lower cranial nerves (IX–XII). Copious irrigation during exposure of these cranial nerves is necessary to avoid thermal injury. Further drilling at this level will expose the vertebral artery at its entrance into the dura.

Surgical Reconstruction

During the reconstruction any dural tears are carefully repaired by direct suture or dural grafts. The vascularized pericranial flap (**Fig. 47–7**) is interposed between the dura and sinonasal cavity to reconstruct the anterior skull base and provide watertight cranionasal separation. This step is crucial to minimize postoperative cerebrospinal fluid (CSF) leakage or pneumocephalus.[19]

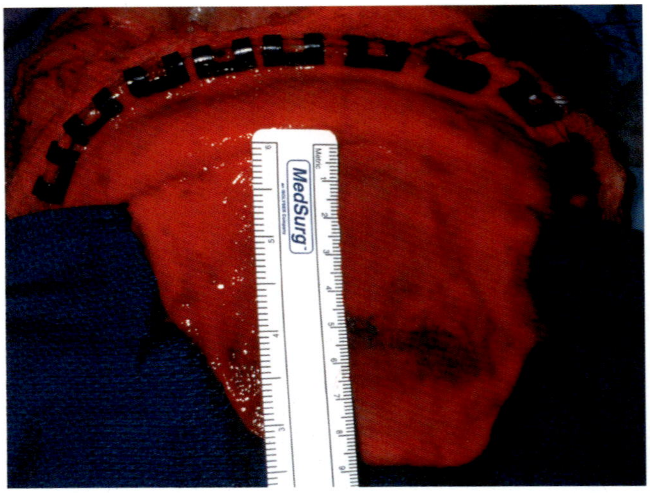

Figure 47–7 A well-vascularized pericranial flap is used for reconstruction of the anterior skull base defect.

If the carotid artery is exposed to the nasopharynx, it should be covered with well-vascularized flaps such as a pedicled temporalis muscle flap or a microvascular free flap. This is done to prevent desiccation of the arterial wall and carotid artery blowout. This is particularly important if the patient received prior radiation therapy or will receive postoperative adjuvant radiation.

The medial canthal ligaments are carefully reattached using a figure-of-eight stitch, to avoid telecanthus. If the nasolacrimal duct has been transected, the lacrimal sac should be marsupialized into the nasal cavity and lacrimal tubes or stents placed to prevent epiphora. The orbital wall osteotomies are reattached to the bone flap.

To prevent future development of frontal sinus mucocele, cranialization of the frontal sinus should be done by drilling out the posterior wall and meticulously stripping the mucosa off the anterior wall. The cranio-orbital-nasal bone flap is reattached using craniofacial plates.

Accurate repositioning and rigid fixation of the nasomaxillary segments and meticulous closure of facial incisions should be done to achieve optimal functional and aesthetic facial reconstruction. Dental splints may be needed for maintenance of proper occlusion, and obturators may be needed for rehabilitation of palatal defects.

◆ Outcome

Any critical assessment of the outcome of a surgical approach should evaluate both the safety and the efficacy of the procedure. Safety is usually measured by the incidence of complications, morbidity, and mortality associated with the surgical procedure. Efficacy of oncological surgery is traditionally measured by disease control and survival rates.

◆ Complications

Combined craniofacial resection has become the standard approach for malignant tumors involving the anterior cranial fossa. Despite its widespread application, however, many surgeons agree that the procedure carries a risk of significant morbidity and even mortality (**Table 47–4**). The rate of major complications correlates with the type of surgical approach,[15] extent of resection,[20] and experience of the surgical team.[21]

Complications can be divided as those related to the intracranial or to the extracranial approach (**Table 47–5**). CSF leakage, pneumocephalus, and transient alteration in mental status were the most common complications associated with the intracranial approach[9,21]. Transient mental status changes were mostly attributed to brain edema, contusion, or hematoma. These complications are less likely to occur when brain retraction is minimized, which is one of the main advantages of subfrontal approaches.[15] Invasion of the dura and the type of reconstruction of the anterior skull base were the most important factors related to CSF leakage and meningitis.[20] Overall, infectious complications were the most devastating[21] and bacterial contamination leading to septic complications was the principal cause of morbidity, accounting for over half of the major complications.[20] The risk of pneumocephalus following craniofacial procedures is significant and may be increased by the use of lumbar

Table 47–4 Morbidity and Mortality of Anterior Craniofacial Resection

Study	No. of Patients	Mortality (%)	Morbidity (%)
Catalano et al 1994[21]	73	2.7	63.0
Kraus et al 1994[27]	85	2.0	39.0
Shah et al 1997[12]	115	3.5	35.0
Dias et al 1999[20]	104	7.6	48.6
Solero et al 2000[9]	168	4.7	30.0

Table 47–5 Complications of Anterior Craniofacial Resection

Intracranial Approach	Extracranial Approach
Brain contusion/hematoma	Epiphora
Cerebrospinal fluid leakage	Telecanthus
Pneumocephalus	Ectropion
Meningitis/abscess	Enophthalmos
Cranial nerve deficits	Dystopia
Cerebrovascular accidents	Palatal fistula
Frontal sinus mucocele	Malocclusion
Osteomyelitis of the frontal bone	Facial deformity

drainage of CSF intraoperatively. In one series, the use of lumbar CSF drainage during the operation correlated most strongly with the development of pneumocephalus.[22] Tension pneumocephalus is a potentially devastating complication that may occur after craniofacial resection. It usually presents with rapid neurological deterioration and requires prompt recognition and treatment to minimize permanent neurological deficits.

Ocular complications are frequent after anterior craniofacial resection. In one series of 58 patients, ocular complications occurred in over 40% of patients and consisted of epiphora in 21 patients, diplopia in eight, vision loss in six, and pain and enophthalmos in two.[23] Twelve patients required revision surgery consisting of dacryocystorhinostomy in eight, ectropion repair in three, drainage of orbital mucocele in one, and corneal transplant in one. Ocular complications, particularly vision loss, are more common in patients treated with postoperative radiation therapy. During surgery, delicate handling of the orbital contents, adequate corneal protection, accurate reconstruction of the bony orbit, and meticulous repair of the medial canthal ligament and lacrimal system can minimize ocular complications, and functional vision can be preserved in most patients.

◆ Disease Control and Survival

Although the literature is replete with reports describing the oncological outcome of combined craniofacial resection of anterior skull base tumors, several confounding factors make meaningful interpretation of the results extremely difficult. Such factors include the diversity of histological diagnoses, site of origin, extent of tumor invasion, prior therapy, extent of surgical resection, status of surgical margins, postoperative adjuvant therapy, and length of follow-up. Despite these limitations, several recent reports demonstrated that combined craniofacial approaches for resection of malignant tumors of the anterior skull base offer good local control of disease and acceptable survival rates (**Table 47–6**). These survival rates are not significantly different from those of patients with sinonasal cancer in general[3] (**Fig. 47–8**).

Tumor grade and histology have a significant impact on disease-control and survival in patients treated with craniofacial resection of anterior skull base malignancy. Sekhar and others have found that 64% of patients with low-grade malignancies and 44% of patients with high-grade lesions were alive with no evidence of disease at an average follow-up of 26 months.[16] Eibling and others performed a meta-analysis of the outcome of anterior skull base resection and reported a 2-year or greater survival of 64% for patients with squamous cell carcinoma, but only 45% for those with undifferentiated carcinoma.[24] The lowest survival rate was observed in patients with mucosal melanoma and highest in those with esthesioneuroblastoma.[12,13] In one study, there was a statistically significant difference between the 5-year disease-free survival for the esthesioneuroblastoma patients and the nonesthesioneuroblastoma patients (90% vs 59.1%; $p = .028$), and aggressive salvage therapy appeared to be a more successful option in the esthesioneuroblastoma group of patients.[25]

Table 47–6 Disease-Specific Survival of Patients Treated with Anterior Craniofacial Resection of Malignant Sinonasal Tumors Involving the Anterior Cranial Base

Study	No. of Patients	5-year (%)	10-year (%)
Shah et al 1997[12]	115	58	48
Lund et al 1998[11]	167	44	32
Bridger et al 2000[26]	73	69	69

Tumor stage and the extent of surgical resection also have a significant influence on tumor control and survival. Dural invasion, brain involvement, and positive resection margins were significantly correlated with poorer prognosis.[10,13] Survival was significantly better for those whose tumors could be excised with a limited resection in comparison with those requiring an extended procedure.[12] Most local recurrences occurred within 6 months of surgery, with the exception of adenocarcinoma of the ethmoids, in which recurrence occurred up to 36 months postoperatively.[10] Patients without prior treatment have a better prognosis than those with recurrent cancer.[8]

Survival of patients undergoing craniofacial resection also depends on their functional status and the presence or absence of comorbidity. For example, in a study of 73 patients treated with craniofacial resection Bridger and colleagues[26] found that the 5-year *cancer-specific* survival was 69%, which was unchanged at 10 years. By contrast, the actuarial *overall* survival at 5 and 10 years was 61% and 48%, respectively. This highlights the fact that a significant number of patients die of cancer-unrelated comorbidities.

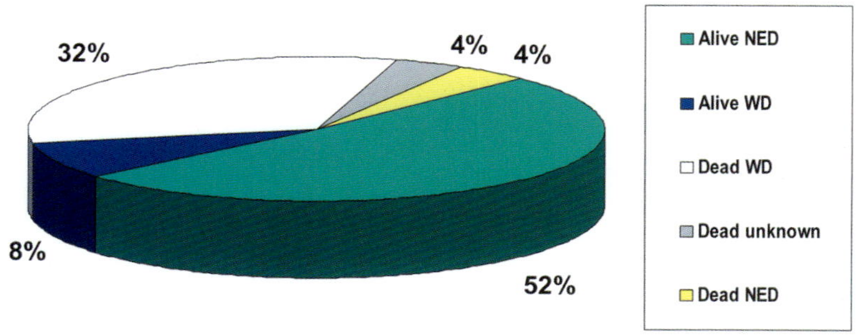

Figure 47–8 Overall outcome of 86 consecutive patients with sinonasal malignancy treated at the University of Arkansas for Medical Sciences between 1988 and 1998. Minimum follow-up of 2 years. NED, no evidence of disease; WD, with disease. (With permission from Hanna E, Vural E, Teo C, Farris P, Breau R, Suen JY. Sinonasal tumors: the Arkansas experience. Skull Base Surg 1998;8(Suppl):15.)

◆ Conclusion

Craniofacial resection is feasible and effective in controlling malignant tumors of the anterior cranial base in well-selected patients. This careful selection should consider tumor grade, histology, extent of disease, and the patient's general condition. It is hoped that earlier diagnosis and more effective adjuvant therapy will improve the outcome of patients with malignant tumors involving the skull base.

References

1. Stern SJ, Hanna E. Cancer of the nasal cavity and paranasal sinuses. In: Myers EN, Suen JY, eds. Cancer of the Head and Neck. 3rd ed. Philadelphia: WB Saunders; 1996:205–233
2. Girod D, Hanna E, Marentette L. Esthesioneuroblastoma. Head Neck 2001;23:500–505
3. Hanna E, Vural E, Teo C, Farris P, Breau R, Suen JY. Sinonasal tumors: the Arkansas experience. Skull Base Surg 1998;8:15
4. Vural E, Suen JY, Hanna E. Intracranial extension of inverted papilloma: an unusual and potentially fatal complication. Head Neck 1999;21:703–706
5. Pitman KT, Prokopakis EP, Aydogan B, et al. [PM7]The role of skull base surgery for the treatment of adenoid cystic carcinoma of the sinonasal tract. Head Neck 1999;21:402–407
6. Teo C, Dornhoffer J, Hanna E, Bower C. Application of skull base techniques to pediatric neurosurgery. Childs Nerv Syst 1999;15:103–109
7. Lund VJ, Howard DJ, Lloyd GA, Cheesman AD. Magnetic resonance imaging of paranasal sinus tumors for craniofacial resection. Head Neck 1989;11:279–283
8. Cantu G, Solero CL, Mariani L, et al. Anterior craniofacial resection for malignant ethmoid tumors: a series of 91 patients. Head Neck 1999;21:185–191
9. Solero CL, DiMeco F, Sampath P, et al. Combined anterior craniofacial resection for tumors involving the cribriform plate: early postoperative complications and technical considerations. Neurosurgery 2000;47:1296–1304
10. Rutter MJ, Furneaux CE, Morton RP. Craniofacial resection of anterior skull base tumours: factors contributing to success. Aust N Z J Surg 1998;68:350–353
11. Lund VJ, Howard DJ, Wei WI, Cheesman AD. Craniofacial resection for tumors of the nasal cavity and paranasal sinuses: a 17-year experience. Head Neck 1998;20:97–105
12. Shah JP, Kraus DH, Bilsky MH, Gutin PH, Harrison LH, Strong EW. Craniofacial resection for malignant tumors involving the anterior skull base. Arch Otolaryngol Head Neck Surg 1997;123:1312–1317
13. Bilsky MH, Kraus DH, Strong EW, Harrison LB, Gutin PH, Shah JP. Extended anterior craniofacial resection for intracranial extension of malignant tumors. Am J Surg 1997;174:565–568
14. Derome P. Spheno-ethmoidal tumors: possibilities for exeresis and surgical repair [in French]. Neurochirurgie 1972;18(Supp 1):1–164
15. Raveh J, Laedrach K, Speiser M, et al. The subcranial approach for fronto-orbital and anteroposterior skull-base tumors. Arch Otolaryngol Head Neck Surg 1993;119:385–393
16. Sekhar LN, Nanda A, Sen CN, Snyderman CN, Janecka IP. The extended frontal approach to tumors of the anterior, middle, and posterior skull base. J Neurosurg 1992;76:198–206
17. Janecka IP, Sen CN, Sekhar LN, Arriaga M. Facial translocation: a new approach to the cranial base. Otolaryngol Head Neck Surg 1990;103:413–419
18. Vural E, Hanna E. Extended lateral rhinotomy incision for total maxillectomy. Otolaryngol Head Neck Surg 2000;123:512–513
19. Snyderman CH, Janecka IP, Sekhar LN, Sen CN, Eibling DE. Anterior cranial base reconstruction: role of galeal and pericranial flaps. Laryngoscope 1990;100:607–614
20. Dias FL, Sa GM, Kligerman J, et al. Complications of anterior craniofacial resection. Head Neck 1999;21:12–20
21. Catalano PJ, Hecht CS, Biller HF, et al. Craniofacial resection: an analysis of 73 cases. Arch Otolaryngol Head Neck Surg 1994;120:1203–1208
22. Yates H, Hamill M, Borel CO, Toung TJ. Incidence and perioperative management of tension pneumocephalus following craniofacial resection. J Neurosurg Anesthesiol 1994;6:15–20
23. Andersen PE, Kraus DH, Arbit E, Shah JP. Management of the orbit during anterior fossa craniofacial resection. Arch Otolaryngol Head Neck Surg 1996;122:1305–1307
24. Eibling DE, Janecka IP, Snyderman CH, Cass SP. Meta-analysis of outcome in anterior skull base resection for squamous cell and undifferentiated carcinoma. Skull Base Surg 1993;3:123–129
25. Levine PA, Debo RF, Meredith SD, Jane JA, Constable WC, Cantrell RW. Craniofacial resection at the University of Virginia (1976–1992): survival analysis. Head Neck 1994;16:574–577
26. Bridger GP, Kwok B, Baldwin M, Williams JR, Smee RI. Craniofacial resection for paranasal sinus cancers. Head Neck 2000;22:772–780
27. Kraus DH, Shah JP, Arbit E, Galicich JH, Strong EW. Complications of craniofacial resection for tumors involving the anterior skull base. Head Neck 1994;16:307–312

48

Orbital Tumors

Jack Rootman and Felix A. Durity

The last quarter century has witnessed the emergence of orbital disease management as an ophthalmic subspecialty, requiring specific training in the pathogenesis, epidemiology, and management of both medical and surgical disorders of the orbit. For the most part, the surgical component of this discipline has culled from skills in the areas of ophthalmology, neurosurgery, oculoplastic and general plastic surgery, and sinonasal and endoscopic surgery. The practice at the Orbital Clinic at the University of British Columbia/Vancouver General Hospital spans the past 30 years of this century and reflects the development of this subspecialty[1–6]. Having managed over 4000 cases of orbital disease, it is worthwhile to contextualize orbital tumors within the spectrum of processes affecting these structures. Approximately 50% of these cases represent the clinical management of thyroid orbitopathy, with neoplasia representing 18.1%, structural lesions, 12.5%, inflammatory lesions 8.6%, vascular disorders 4.6%, functional disease 2.9%, and atrophy and degeneration 1.7%.[7] In terms types of tumors encountered in the orbit, 27.0% were neurogenic, 22.5% lymphoproliferative, 13.2% vascular, 13.0% secondary from adjacent structures, 8.9% mesenchymal, 8.5% metastatic, and 6.8% lacrimal.

In addition to the broad range of medical disorders that dominate the discipline of orbital disease, there has been a significant paradigm shift in the surgical management of tumors of the orbit and adjacent structures. For the most part, the development of new techniques and sophisticated interventions has led to more frequent use of anterior and lateral orbitotomies with a reduction in the number of cranial incursions into the orbit. These influences have led to a significant advance in our ability to deal with a broader range of surgical disorders of the orbit using a wider variety of techniques, often with increasingly minimalistic approaches. The role of the neurosurgical discipline in managing orbital tumors has shifted from being a primary operator to more multidisciplinary surgery that involves orbital surgeons who have more knowledge of the physiological, pathological, and surgical aspects of orbital disease. In our institution, we have formed a very strong multidisciplinary team that extends the armamentarium to the real benefit of the patient. This chapter focuses on the cross-disciplinary area of neurosurgery and orbital surgery.

Indications

The major neoplastic indications for orbitocranial surgery are tumors of the optic nerve or orbital apex, lesions of the sphenoid wing, and lesions of the nasopharynx and sinus that have extended into the orbit and cranial cavities.[4]

Tumors of the Optic Nerve

Increased understanding of the natural history and pathogenesis of optic nerve tumors has led to a shift from surgical management to either observation or surgical debulking in combination with external beam radiotherapy or stereotactic fractionated radiotherapy.[8] In the case of optic nerve gliomas, the indication for excision of the optic nerve remains profound proptosis with deteriorated visual function in an isolated optic nerve glioma that is anterior to the chiasm. In patients who suffer from neurofibromatosis type 1 (NF1) with optic nerve glioma, it has become clear that these tumors have a much better prognosis for vision than the isolated optic nerve glioma and are best managed with a conservative nonsurgical approach. In our clinic, we have seen several patients with NF1 who have shown fluctuations of vision between 20/400 and 20/20 with ultimate stabilization at very acceptable levels of vision. In addition, these patients are prone to the development of secondary gliomas within the nervous system, which appear to be a much more serious issue than the optic nerve glioma.

Optic nerve meningiomas have also been increasingly treated conservatively. The general consensus is that, unless the patient is blind with significant proptosis, orbital optic nerve meningiomas can be observed with serial imaging. We have also seen success both visually and in terms of arresting progress with direct radiotherapy of optic nerve meningiomas that had deteriorating vision.[9,10] Meningiomas that extend to the chiasm, however, with a significant intracranial component require excision with or without adjuvant radiotherapy.

◆ Tumors of the Orbital Apex[4,11]

Heretofore, it has been the axiom that apical orbital tumors require a combined panoramic orbitotomy, but the newer techniques have allowed safer apical approaches from anterior, extended lateral, and medial orbitotomies. Lesions in the posterior third of the orbit require special considerations and are best approached on an individualized basis depending on the location of the tumor. Lesions in the medial posterior third of the orbit can be approached, depending on their type and nature, via semilunar fold or caruncular incision with or without disinsertion of the medial rectus muscle, direct cutaneous incision, combined lateral orbitotomy and medial conjunctival incision, or via a craniotomy with a coronal incision. Direct approaches can also be utilized more easily by recognizing that they are potentially expandable by virtue of removal of either the medial or lateral apical orbital bony structures. Lesions in the superior orbital fissure can be very adequately approached by an extended lateral orbitotomy with removal of the whole of the lateral and posterolateral walls of the orbit up to the superior orbital fissure (**Fig. 48–1**).[12,13] In particular, this method avoids the potential for damage from a superior approach for tumors that are inferolateral to the nerve. These are best approached by customized lateral marginotomies, including the zygoma, allowing direct en face excision without having to dissect through the superior orbital fissure. On the other hand, lesions that are in the superolateral and superior locations, particularly those that have transgressed beyond the orbital space to include the intracranial cavity, obviously may need a panoramic orbitotomy and craniotomy.

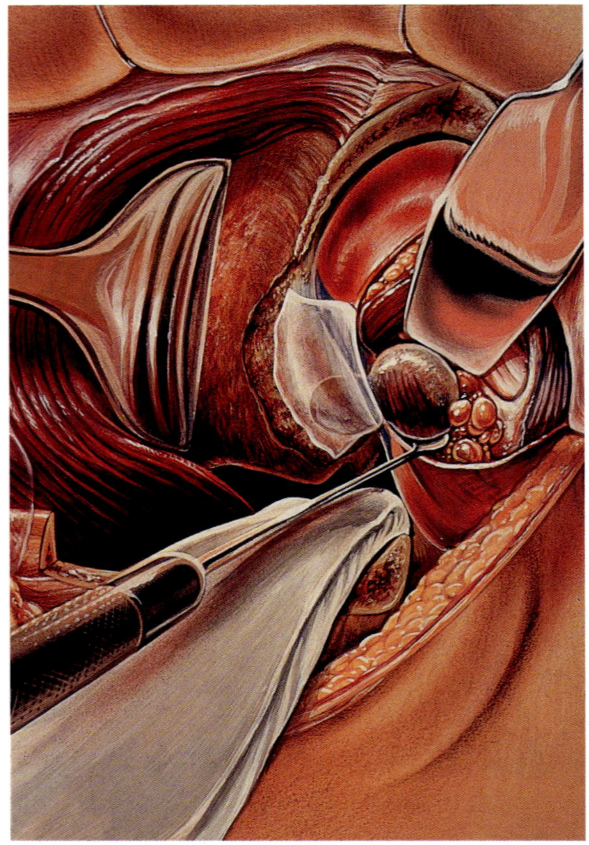

Figure 48–1 This diagram illustrates an extended lateral orbitotomy with removal of the posterolateral wall and part of the zygoma to access a tumor of the apex, inferolateral to the optic nerve. This en face view allows for a safer approach than a superior craniotomy by virtue of avoiding the structures in the superior orbital fissure above it, thereby minimizing ptosis and cranial nerve palsies. (With permission from Rootman J, Stewart B, Goldberg R. Orbital Surgery: A Conceptual Approach. Philadelphia: Lippincott-Raven; 1995:283; Fig. 8–70b.)

◆ Tumors of the Sphenoid Wing

Sphenoid wing meningiomas have been successfully treated by combined orbitocranial and skull base procedures over the last 2 decades.[14,15] Our experience includes 16 out of 34 tumors in this location that had surgery without any requiring repeat surgery so far. The approach we favor is to debulk the overwhelming majority of the gross tumor and add radiotherapy when a significant or functionally disabling component is left as a residuum, or regrowth is demonstrated.

Complex lesions that involve the triple fossa of the orbit, middle cranial, temporalis, and pterygopalatine areas require combined techniques that include removal of the zygomatic arch, roof, and lateral wall of the orbit. We have used these techniques for the management of triple fossa meningiomas, extensive combined venous-lymphatic malformations (so-called lymphangiomas), orbital reconstruction, and complex neurofibromas (**Fig. 48–2**).

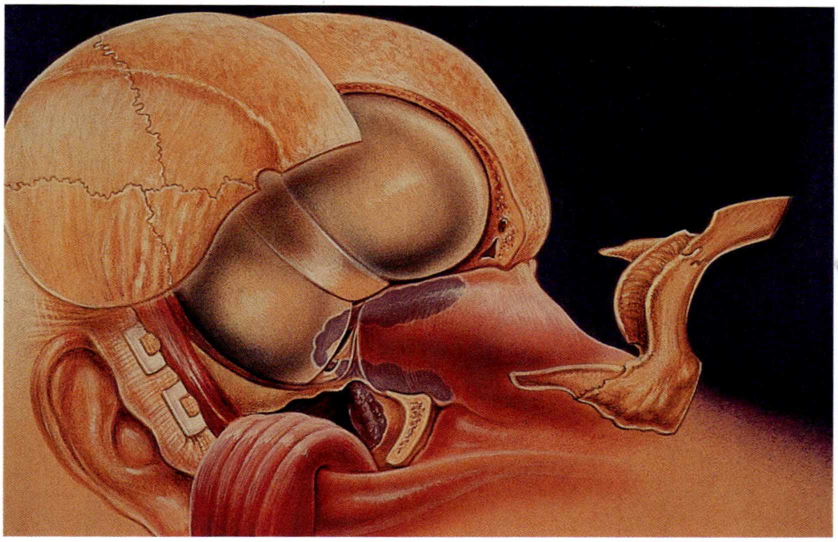

Figure 48–2 A disarticulated view of access to a triple fossa lesion. It may be necessary to remove the arch of the zygoma to gain access to this space. (With permission from Rootman J, Stewart B, Goldberg R. Orbital Surgery: A Conceptual Approach. Philadelphia: Lippincott-Raven; 1995:319; Fig. 9–19b3.)

◆ Lesions of the Nasopharynx and Sinus Extending into the Orbit and Cranial Cavities

Lesions that transgress these three cavities can be handled by combined intracranial, orbital, and ear-nose-throat (ENT) approaches that may include removal of involved dura, periorbita, and sinus/nasopharyngeal structures.

◆ Preparation

The most valuable techniques for the study of cranio-orbital neoplasia are high-resolution computed tomography (CT) and magnetic resonance imaging (MRI), with or without the use of vascular techniques. Vascular studies are sometimes necessary to determine the need for preoperative embolization. In addition, the orbital veins may be used as an access site for the retrograde management of some dural cavernous fistulae. Generally, imaging studies allow us to assess orbital masses as to contour, presence or absence of infiltrative features, vascularity, and effect on adjacent structures. In our opinion, high-resolution CT scans are the best method for studying the effect of disease on bone, and MRI is particularly useful for studying soft tissue disease, especially those of the optic nerve or meninges. CT identifies calcification easily but MRI, especially postgadolinium contrast with fat suppression, allows for clear delineation of the extent of optic nerve tumors, particularly meningiomas.

◆ Surgical Technique

Anesthesia

For procedures requiring noncranio-orbital approaches, routine anesthetic methods are adequate. In some instances, particularly vascular lesions, mild hypotensive anesthesia may be necessary. For combined procedures, patients are premedicated with dexamethasone 10 mg PO or IM 10 hours and repeated IV on call to the operating room (OR) preoperatively. A lumbar subarachnoid drain is inserted and furosemide 1 mg/kg and mannitol 1 g IV are administered before the incision. Postoperatively the clamped lumbar drain is removed in 48 hours if there is no cerebrospinal fluid (CSF) rhinorrhea. With the patient supine, the head is placed in three-point pin fixation and rotated 30 degrees to the opposite side.

Neurophysiological Monitoring

In the unlikely and rare instances where these tumors may extend through the tentorium and into the posterior fossa, making contact with the brain stem structures and cranial nerves, somatosensory evoked potentials (SEPs), brain stem auditory evoked responses (BAERs), and motor evoked potentials (MEPs) as well as compound motor action potentials of motor V and VII cranial nerves would be indicated. In our experience to date, we have not encountered this pattern of growth. Tumors that involved the cavernous sinus may benefit from monitoring of cranial nerve III, with bipolar stimulating electrodes inserted into the appropriately supplied muscles. We do not favor monitoring cranial nerves IV or VI, and actually believe that even monitoring of cranial nerve III is of limited value.

Dissection Procedures for Cranio-orbital Lesions

Tumors of the Sphenoid Wing[10]

Sphenoid wing meningiomas may be primarily en plaque dural lesions with associated hyperostotic bone, or they may involve the periorbita and intraorbital tissues, and occasionally may have a globoid intradural component. More rarely, a sphenoid wing meningioma (particularly those of the inner third) may extend down the sheath of the optic nerve. In most instances, a standard coronal flap is adequate but if the intention is to operate on the cavernous sinus, the carotid bifurcation is exposed to ensure proximal control of the blood supply. Vascular meningiomas may be embolized preoperatively. Our experience has led us to the surgical goal of major debulking as opposed to aggressive attempts to remove all visible tumor, particularly at the risk of significant damage to important neural structures. We then add adjuvant radiotherapy if there is evidence of significant residuum, progressive functional deficit, or significant growth postoperatively.

With the patient supine, the head is placed in three-point pin fixation and rotated 30 degrees to the opposite side. Fine silk sutures are placed under the tendons of the lateral and superior recti and levator complex for later identification during orbital dissection. A coronal scalp incision is made and may be extended to just below the tragus for tumors extending into the pterygopalatine or infratemporal fossa. In most instances, we have moved to a more minimalist approach, aiming for smaller incisions and gross total removal as described.

Injury to the superior division of the seventh nerve is avoided by dissection beneath the interfascial superficial temporalis fat pad from the body of zygoma to just anterior to the pterion ("key" point) to avoid damage to the nerve superficial to it. This dissection is carried over the edge of the lateral orbital margin in a subperiosteal plane.

The superficial temporalis fascia is incised along the frontozygomatic process to the body of the zygoma and along the zygomatic arch. The temporalis muscle is cut and disinserted 1 cm below the superior temporal line, dissected from the temporal fossa, and retracted inferiorly. If we intend to remove the zygomatic arch, the origin of the masseter muscle is removed from the undersurface of the arch up to the body of the zygoma. The pericranium is reflected over the supraorbital margin and the supraorbital nerve is dissected free of its notch or foramen. The periorbita is then dissected off the superior and lateral walls of the orbit to the superior orbital fissure and lateral aspect of the inferior orbital fissure, or to the anterior limit of bone and soft tissue invaded by the tumor. This allows one surgeon to protect the periorbita during the creation of the second bone flap, avoiding troublesome herniation of orbital fat. The superomedial and medial periorbita can be stripped, including the trochlear region up to and including the apex of the orbit, thereby giving broad access to the orbital space and protection from incision above. This also provides access to the anterior and posterior ethmoid arteries, which can be clipped or cauterized as adjunctive procedures to reduce the vascularity of some frontal base or olfactory groove meningiomas.[16]

The extradural component begins with creation of two bone flaps, frontal (-temporal as bony disease dictates) and orbital, or in more limited procedures, only the orbital rim is removed. Only a single bur hole at the pterion is required for the bone flap (**Fig. 48–3**). The frontal (-temporal) dura is reflected off the orbit while the orbital surgeon protects the periorbita as the roof, as far posteriorly as possible, and lateral orbital walls are cut. The lateral end of the inferior orbital fissure marks the medial and inferior limit of the lateral bony wall incision. The body of the zygoma is then cut through its midportion on a line directed outward from the inferior orbital fissure, thereby avoiding the maxillary sinus. The zygomatic arch is cut posteriorly when needed just anterior to the temporomandibular joint, allowing the superior and lateral orbital margins, with zygomatic arch, to be removed en bloc and thus gaining wider access to the pterygopalatine and middle cranial fossae when needed. This also allows for further retraction of the temporalis muscle and good exposure to the remaining orbital bone, orbital contents, apex, pterygopalatine, and infratemporal fossae. If more limited access to the orbital apex is required for a tumor in this location, only the roof and lateral wall down to the zygoma are removed. The remaining roof of the orbit when involved with tumor can be removed with rongeurs

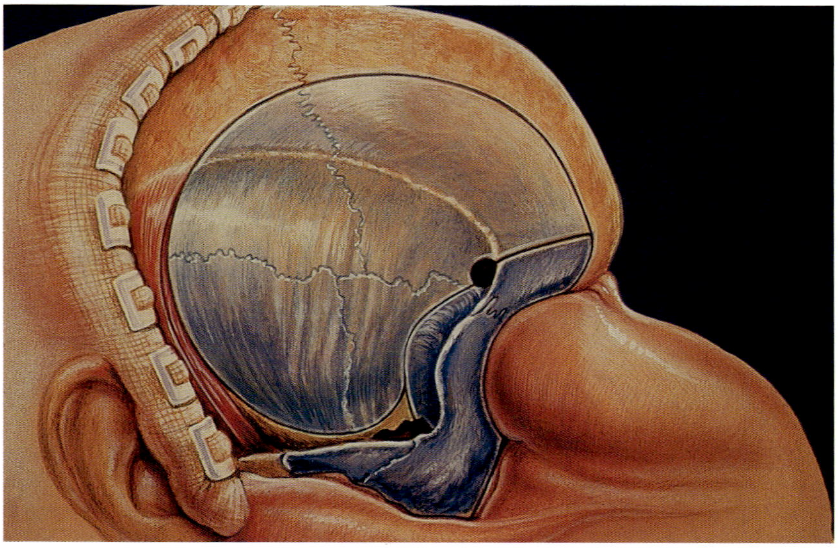

Figure 48–3 Demarcation of the scope of bony cuts necessary for access to lesions that extend intracranially and into the pterygopalatine and temporalis fossa. The temporalis muscle has not been shown for better visualization. (With permission from Rootman J, Stewart B, Goldberg R. Orbital Surgery: A Conceptual Approach. Philadelphia: Lippincott-Raven; 1995:335; Fig. 9–19b2.)

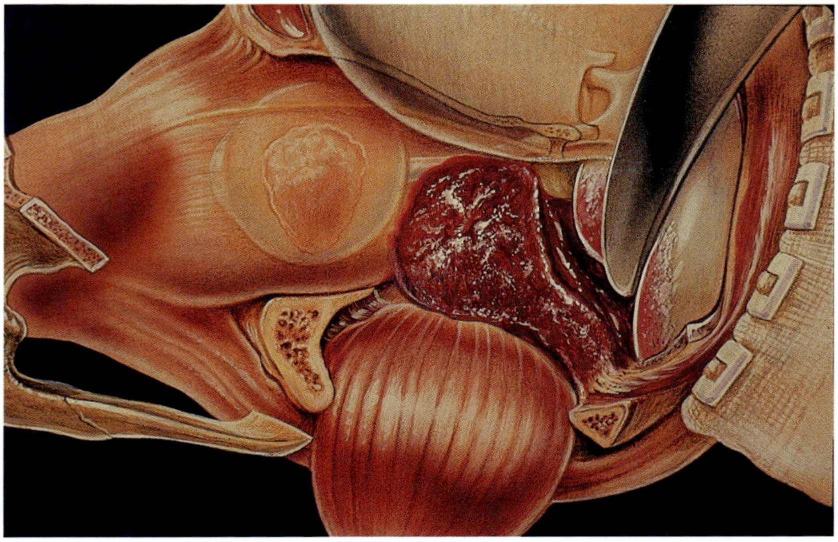

Figure 48–4 Exposure of meningioma involving the orbital cranial junction. The bone, periorbita, and temporal lobe dura are involved and have been exposed for excision by this approach. (With permission from Rootman J, Stewart B, Goldberg R. Orbital Surgery: A Conceptual Approach. Philadelphia: Lippincott-Raven; 1995:313; Fig. 9–16.)

and high-speed drills, exposing the superior orbital fissure and ultimately the optic canal in those cases in which the optic nerve is to be removed or when the apical periorbita or anulus of Zinn is involved. Tumor invading the greater wing of the sphenoid along the floor of the middle cranial fossa can be removed medially to the foramina rotundum and ovale, posteriorly to the foramen spinosum, and laterally to the squamous temporal bone anterior to the temporomandibular joint (**Fig. 48–4**). The sphenoid sinus and the outer wall of the cavernous sinus can be reached if necessary. At this point, depending on the extent, removal of all extradural tumor in bone, pterygopalatine, and infratemporal fossae proceeds. Thereafter, the intradural and intraorbital removal is performed. If the intradural tumor is bulky and retraction of this mass would increase pressure on the surrounding brain, the intradural component is removed as a first step.

The periorbita when involved is excised by the orbital surgeon after delimiting the amount involved. This dissection extends into the orbital soft tissues using microdissectors to lift the en plaque lesion from the orbit. The superior rectus, levator, and lateral rectus are manipulated with previously placed external sutures to dissect or remove the tumor. If the tumor has invaded the deeper orbit in an infiltrative manner and it is not possible to remove it without doing damage, a gross total removal is attempted and postoperative radiation is offered. The excised periorbita or dura is replaced with pericranium, fascia, or cadaver dura (Tutoplast [10P Inc., Costa Mesa, CA]) as necessary.

After replacement of the superior and lateral orbital margins and zygomatic arch, the roof and lateral wall of the orbit are reconstructed with autologous inner table split-thickness frontal bone graft (**Fig. 48–5**). Two triangular pieces of bone are wired, sutured, or secured with microfixation osteosynthesis plates. In some instances, we have harvested bone from the scalp posterior to the bony incision or

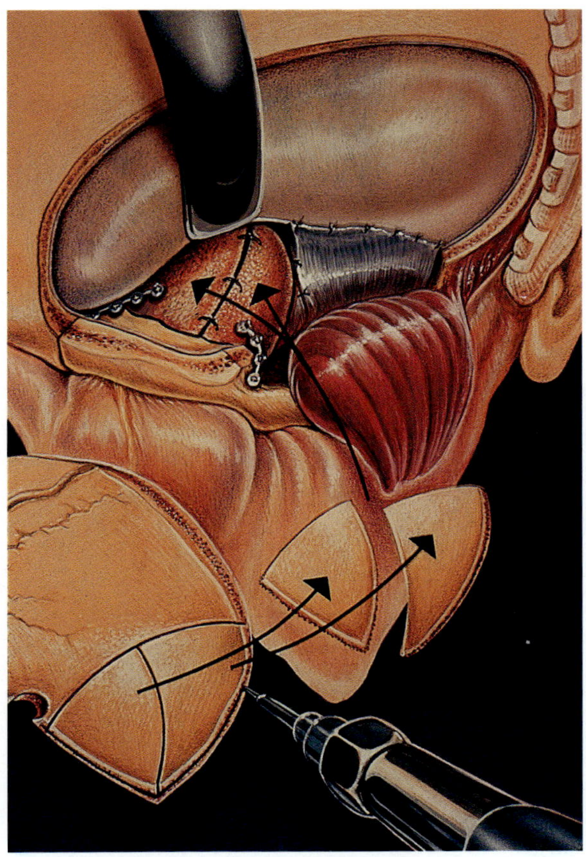

Figure 48–5 Reconstruction of the roof and lateral wall of the orbit using autologous inner-table split-thickness frontal bone graft. The two triangular pieces of bone are wired or sutured together at their apices and then secured to the orbital rim segment. (With permission from Rootman J, Stewart B, Goldberg R. Orbital Surgery: A Conceptual Approach. Philadelphia: Lippincott-Raven; 1995:348; Fig. 10–21.)

have used sculpted alloplastic material to reconstruct the orbit to avoid enophthalmos and pulsation. Reconstruction also provides a useful plane of dissection if repeat surgery becomes necessary. The floor of the middle cranial fossa, however, is not usually reconstructed. The freed pterional flap is repositioned and if no sinus has been opened, acrylic or metallic screen is used to fill the bony defect at the pterion prior to resuturing the temporalis muscle. A subgaleal hemovac (Zimmer, Inc., Warsaw, IN) drain is placed, and the skin is closed in the standard fashion.

Utilizing these techniques, we have been able to obtain gross total or aggressive subtotal removal of the overwhelming majority of our sphenoid wing meningiomas with relief of proptosis in all and a complication of enophthalmos in only 12% of our patients. Surgical limits have been governed by involvement of the cavernous sinus, subarachnoid seeding, and extensive bony disease. There have been no deaths. Twelve of our patients experienced diplopia in extreme gaze, 25% had temporalis fossa excavation, 12% experienced V1 or V2 dysesthesia, and 12% had ptosis of up to 3 mm. Half of our patients received postoperative radiotherapy, and in the whole series only 12% had evidence of regrowth, none of which have required surgery to date (average follow-up = 4 years). Of the patients with visual involvement, 60% have improved visual outcome and 40% have had either persistent field loss or moderate optic pallor. Adjunctive radiotherapy has been 5000 to 6000 cGy in 25 fractions over 5 weeks. We conclude that for sphenoid wing meningiomas, this technique allows for aggressive but limited surgery with low morbidity and mortality, preservation of vision, good cosmetic results, and very slow evidence of recurrence.

◆ Intraorbital Optic Nerve Tumors with or without Intracranial Extension

Excision of Dural Optic Nerve Tumor

Some localized optic nerve tumors that are noninfiltrative can be removed but it should be noted in the literature that the majority of optic nerve meningiomas have recurred following local excision. The best case scenario is removal of an anterior superior localized meningioma. As an example, using a panoramic orbitotomy-craniotomy to obtain complete access to the superior portion of the optic nerve from both a superomedial and a superolateral viewpoint, we have been able to remove a superior, anterior optic nerve tumor. This was achieved by raising a superior periorbital flap and distracting the superior muscle group medially and the lateral muscle group laterally. The orbital soft tissues are dissected using blunt microdissectors and dry neuropatties. The anterior optic nerve is exposed and the posterior ciliary nerves and arteries dissected off the tumor. The tumor can then be excised along with adjacent and involved dura (**Fig. 48–6**).

Removal of the Optic Nerve

For removal of the optic nerve, the periorbita is incised in a U-shaped flap between the lateral and superior rectus muscles and between the superior rectus/levator complex and the superior oblique medially. It is then reflected and by blunt microdissection, the orbital contents are distracted to identify the optic nerve and tumor, posterior emissarial vessels, and ciliary nerves, which are dissected free of the sheath

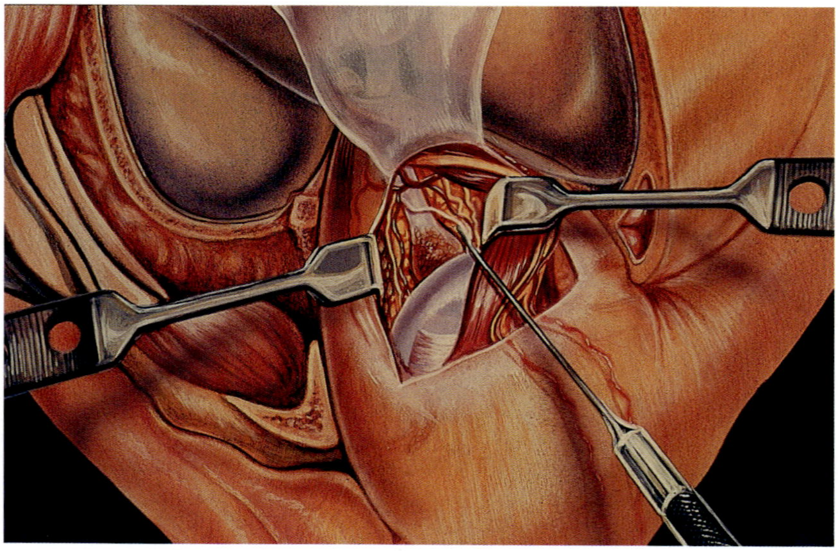

Figure 48–6 This demonstrates an orbitocranial access to a localized anterior optic nerve meningioma. The periorbita had been incised and the superior muscle complex distracted to allow a clear view of the optic nerve. (With permission from Rootman J, Stewart B, Goldberg R. Orbital Surgery: A Conceptual Approach. Philadelphia: Lippincott-Raven; 1995:319; Fig. 9–13b.)

of the nerve and tumor. The fourth cranial nerve is mobilized apically using blunt microdissectors. The optic nerve is resected at the globe with serial placement of sutures to close the distal end and prevent spillage of tumor (**Fig. 48–7**). The nerve is identified, distracted, and dissected free to the apex either superomedially or superolaterally. The anulus of Zinn is incised apically to mobilize that portion of the nerve. This incision is best made medially to avoid damage to structures in the superior orbital fissure. The nerve is then freed from the anulus by sharp dissection intimate to the dura. The proximal nerve is cut intracranially prechiasmally, and the ophthalmic artery identified and either dissected free or clipped. The roof of the optic canal has been removed so the nerve can be freed from the floor where it is frequently relatively firmly attached. The entire optic nerve and tumor is now free and can be removed by distracting it anteriorly, or, using the previously placed distal sutures, it can be pulled superiorly behind the dissected fourth nerve. Closure of the anulus is optional as long as the dura is repaired or patched.

A modification of this procedure can be used for removal of tumors of the inner third of the sphenoid wing that have extended down the optic nerve by adding removal of the affected bone and dura.

Triple Fossa Lesions

Removal of triple fossa lesions involves increasingly complex procedures. Some of these can be removed by a direct anterior approach with a modified lateral orbitotomy that includes excision of part of the wing of the zygoma to expose the pterygopalatine fossa. We have removed several tumors of the sphenoid wing, such as hemangiomas of bone, in an essentially extradural approach anteriorly (**Fig. 48–8**). On the other hand, complex lesions involving the intracranial, orbital, and pterygopalatine structures require a more extensive orbitotomy-craniotomy with

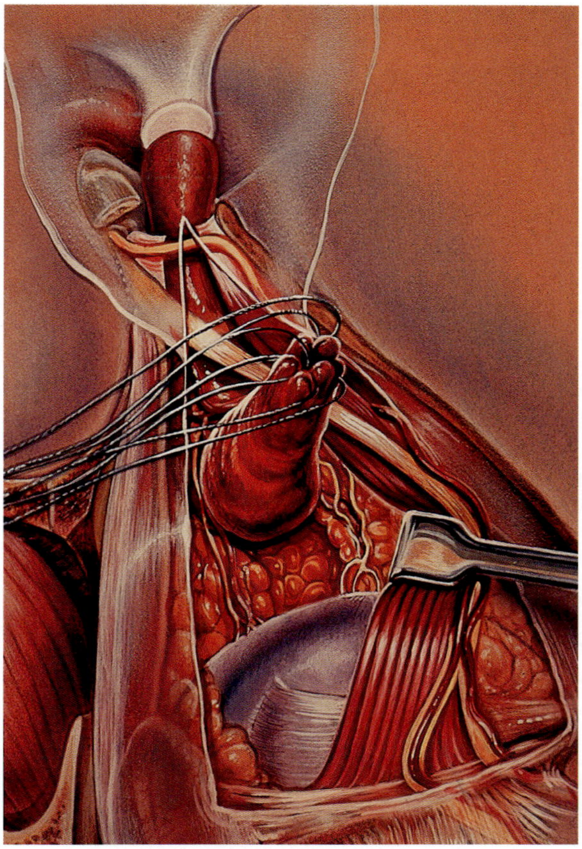

Figure 48–7 This demonstrates removal of an intrinsic optic nerve tumor. Intracranially, the nerve is transected anterior to the chiasm. The fourth nerve has been dissected apically and the anulus opened. The nerve and tumor have been excised from the globe and are held by sutures. (With permission from Rootman J, Stewart B, Goldberg R. Orbital Surgery: A Conceptual Approach. Philadelphia: Lippincott-Raven; 1995:325; Fig. 9–14 part B10)

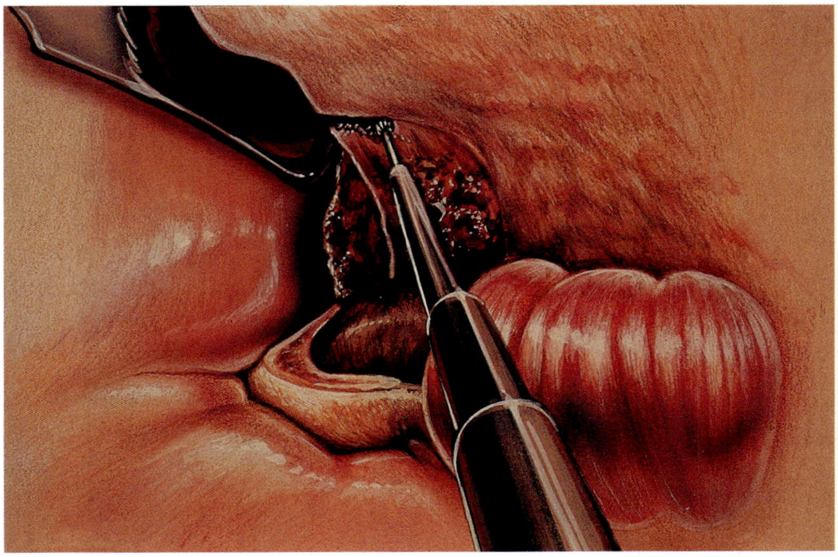

Figure 48–8 Access to and excision of a previously embolized cavernous hemangioma of bone involving the greater wing of sphenoid and posterolateral orbital wall by an extracranial orbital approach. (With permission from Rootman J, Stewart B, Goldberg R. Orbital Surgery: A Conceptual Approach. Lippincott-Raven; 1995:333; Fig. 9–12 part B2.)

removal of the zygomatic arch as described, allowing for exposure of the pterygopalatine fossa, orbit, and middle cranial fossa for excision. This can be shown in a complex tumor of the gasserian ganglion, orbital roof, and pterygopalatine fossa wherein the structures were unlocked allowing access to these fossae and excision of a painful neurofibroma (**Fig. 48–2**). This approach can also be used to reconstruct the orbital walls in cases of trauma or complex malformations.

En Bloc Orbitectomy

Lesions that may require en bloc orbitectomy include malignancies of the lacrimal gland, orbit, and adjacent bony structures. If the procedure is essentially extradural, it can be managed with a modified exenteration incision of the periorbital skin with or without inclusion of the brow. The walls of the orbit can then be removed en bloc without necessarily having to resort to a frontal bony cut. However, in more extensive lesions, a frontal flap is also included (**Fig. 48–9**).

A coronal skin flap is then prepared and brought down. A frontotemporal sphenoidal craniotomy is performed, the subfrontal dura is mobilized and retracted extradurally to just behind the lesser wing of the sphenoid and the tip of

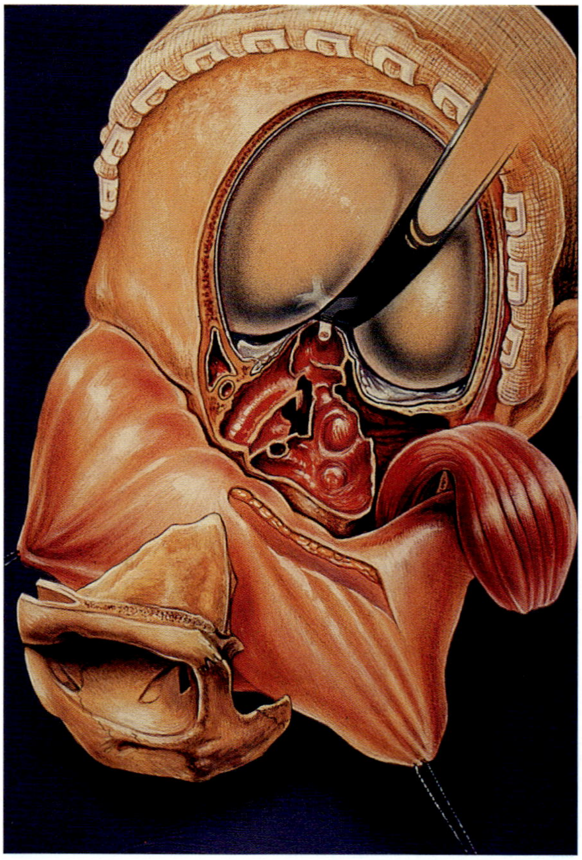

Figure 48–9 Bone and soft tissue excision for a complete en bloc orbitectomy including the medial wall. (With permission from Rootman J, Stewart B, Goldberg R. Orbital Surgery: A Conceptual Approach. Philadelphia: Lippincott-Raven; 1995:316; Fig. 9–19.)

the anterior clinoid and adjacent tuberculum sellae, and the anterior temporal dura is mobilized posterior to the greater wing of sphenoid so that the superior orbital fissure and its contents are well exposed intracranially. Only the medial portion of the extraperiosteal space is entered in the case of lacrimal gland tumors where the periorbita is elevated to guide the bony incision superomedially. The bone is then incised from above and below the superomedial orbit.

For malignant tumors involving the medial or central orbit requiring en bloc orbitectomy, the medial incision includes the medial wall and thus is through the cribriform plate superiorly. The inferomedial orbit is then dissected free of the periorbita, and en bloc bony excision is performed, including the floor of the orbit through the upper portion of the zygomatic arch. The posterior roof of the orbit is incised to the region of the superior orbital fissure and connected to a bony cut deep through the temporalis fossa into the middle cranial fossa beyond the most posterior reaches of the lateral wall of the orbit, just anterior to the foramen rotundum. The incision is carried superiorly just anterior to the posterior tip of the anterior clinoids and infralaterally into the temporalis fossa to avoid entering the orbit or damaging the carotid artery. The orbit is then completely free for en bloc excision as shown (**Fig. 48–9**).

After replacement of the frontal bone, there are several reconstructive options for repairing the defect. We usually use bone from the inner table of the frontal craniotomy or, occasionally, a rib graft to perform primary bone reconstruction of the orbit, and more recently alloplastic materials. The orbitectomy cavity can be either filled with a deltopectoral myocutaneous vascularized flap or an extended trapezius musculocutaneous flap. If the superficial temporal artery has been preserved, it can be anastomosed to a free latissimus dorsi myocutaneous vascular flap or one from another site, such as the radial forearm.

Combined Orbito-cranial-otorhinolaryngologic Lesions

Modifications of the various techniques that have already been described can be utilized in the management of lesions that transgress these cavities. The involved dura, periorbita, and sinus structures can be approached from both above and below, thereby allowing for en bloc resection of midline tumor masses.

◆ Complications

There are three major potential complications of this surgery. CSF leaks are a possible consequence, and a meticulous dural repair and retention of the lumbar drain for potential postoperative use deal effectively with this problem. Cranial neuropathies may also be encountered. To avoid this possibility, gentle handling and aggressive but limited tumor removal is useful, avoiding undue manipulation within the cavernous sinus. Pulsating enophthalmos, which occurred significantly in only one of our patients, is best avoided by a two-wall reconstruction of the superior and lateral bony orbit with bone or prosthetic material.

◆ Conclusions

We have attempted to describe the expanded pantheon of techniques that can be used for more minimal approaches to tumors of the orbit. In addition, we have described the value of multidisciplinary surgical approaches to these often very complex and difficult lesions. The multidisciplinary approach allows for creative and ever-changing technical advancement and for sharing the burden of heretofore very difficult and complex surgery.

References

1. Jones BR. Surgical approaches to the orbit. Trans Ophthalmol Soc U K 1970;90:269–281
2. McCord CD Jr. Surgical approaches to orbital disease. In: McCord CD, Jr, Tanenbaum M, eds. Oculoplastic Surgery. 2nd ed. New York: Raven; 1987:257–278
3. Rootman J, Durity FA. Orbital surgery. In: Sekhar LN, Janecka IF, eds. Surgery of Cranial Base Tumors: A Color Atlas. New York: Raven; 1992:769–786
4. Rootman J, Stewart B, Goldberg R. Orbital Surgery: A Conceptual Approach. Philadelphia: Lippincott-Raven; 1995
5. Wright JE. Orbital surgery. In: Silver B, ed. Ophthalmic Plastic Surgery. 34th ed. San Francisco: American Academy of Ophthalmology' 1977:213
6. Wright JE. Surgical exploration of the orbit. Trans Ophthalmol Soc U K 1979;99:238–240
7. Rootman J. Diseases of the Orbit: A Multidisciplinary Approach. 2nd ed. Philadelphia: Lippincott Williams and Wilkins, 2003
8. Eng TY, Albright NW, Kuwahara G, et al. Precision radiation therapy for optic nerve sheath meningiomas. Int J Radiat Oncol Biol Phys 1992;22:1093–1098
9. Saeed P, Rootman J, Nugent RA, White VA, MacKenzie IR, Koorneef L. Optic nerve sheath meningiomas. Ophthalmology 2003;110:2019–30
10. Kennerdell JS, Maroon JC, Malton M, Warren FA. The management of optic nerve meningiomas. Am J Ophthalmol 1988;106:450–457
11. Maroon JC, Kennerdell JS. Microsurgical approach to orbital tumors. Clin Neurosurg 1979;26:479–489
12. Goldberg RA, Shorr N, Arnold AC, Garcia GH. Deep transorbital approach to the apex and cavernous sinus. Ophthal Plast Reconstr Surg 1998;14:336–341
13. Kennerdell JS, Maroon JC. Microsurgical approach to intraorbital tumors. Technique and instrumentation. Arch Ophthalmol 1976;94: 1333–1336
14. Maroon JC, Kennerdell JS. Surgical approaches to the orbit: indications and techniques. J Neurosurg 1984;60:1226–1235
15. McDermott MW, Durity FA, Rootman J, Woodhurest WB. Combined frontotemporal-orbitozygomatic approach for tumors of the sphenoid wing and orbit. J Neurosurg 1990;26:107–116
16. McDermott MW, Rootman J, Durity FA. Subperiosteal, subperiorbital dissection and division of the anterior and posterior ethmoid arteries for meningiomas of the cribriform plate and planum sphenoidale: technical note. Neurosurgery 1995;36:1215–1218

49

Olfactory Groove and Planum Sphenoidale Meningiomas

Christopher A. Bogaev and Laligam N. Sekhar

Resection of basal frontal tumors has undergone a steady evolution that has paralleled the evolution of cranial base techniques. The goal of these more specialized cranial base methods is to remove more bone to access and resect a tumor with minimal brain retraction.

Prior to the development of contemporary skull base techniques, the cosmetic problems, morbidity, high incidence of cerebrospinal fluid (CSF) leakage, and longer exposure time precluded the more extensive exposures needed to fully minimize brain retraction. The techniques listed give some insight into the evolution of anterior cranial base procedures in providing acceptable cosmetic results with low morbidity.

Evolution of Anterior Fossa Approaches

- **Bifrontal craniotomy**—with inferior bone cut across basal frontal bone avoiding the orbital roofs[1,2]
- **Extended pterional craniotomy**—to optimally view the optic apparatus and cerebral vasculature[1]
- **Orbital osteotomy techniques**—to enhance exposure and reduce brain retraction
  - **Supraorbital approach**—for exposure of the frontal fossa floor[3,4]
  - **Supraorbital-pterional approach**—for a more anterolateral exposure of anterior cranial fossa lesions[5]
- **Frontal sinus approach**—for a cosmetically acceptable method of exposing the floor of the anterior cranial fossa in the midline.[6]

Currently, the most common approaches to olfactory groove and planum sphenoidale meningiomas fall into two main categories: anterior and lateral approaches. Each has its own set of possible modifications as well as its own set of strengths and weaknesses.

◆ Lateral (Pterional) Approach (with or without Orbital Osteotomy)

Advantages

- Early exposure of supraclinoid carotid artery, anterior cerebral arteries, and optic nerve such that they can be dissected free of the tumor and protected

Disadvantages

- With large skull base defect, more difficult to repair with pedicled pericranial graft with this approach
- Inadequate visualization of the contralateral side of the tumor, particularly if it extends across the midline

◆ Anterior (Subfrontal) Approach (with or without Orbital Osteotomy)

Advantages

- Provides an excellent view of both sides of the tumor
- Easier cranial base reconstruction with pedicled pericranial flap

Disadvantages

- More frontal lobe retraction may be necessary for adequate tumor exposure
- Optic nerves, supraclinoid carotid artery, and anterior cerebral arteries are not seen until the end of the tumor resection.

The optimal approach, particularly for tumors of moderate to large size, would provide the advantages of both by combining a pterional with a subfrontal approach. The one-and-a-half fronto-orbital approach accomplishes this, along with the advantages of an orbital osteotomy as described by Jane[3] and Al-Mefty.[1] Using this approach, the surgeon is able[1] to begin working laterally to split the root of the sylvian fissure and find and dissect free the supraclinoid carotid, optic nerve, and anterior cerebral arteries. The subfrontal exposure can then be used to visualize both sides of the tumor to facilitate resection while providing excellent exposure of the cranial base for reconstruction once the resection is complete.

An additional advantage of this approach is the opportunity for sparing contralateral olfaction by not performing bilateral orbital osteotomies and removing the cribriform plate. Instead, a unilateral orbital osteotomy is performed and the contralateral olfactory tract is dissected free from the frontal lobe to prevent its avulsion during the resection.

◆ One-and-a-Half Fronto-orbital Approach

Advantages

- Early exposure of the optic nerve, supraclinoid carotid, and anterior cerebral arteries
- Excellent view of both sides of the tumor
- Potential preservation of the contralateral olfactory tract with olfactory groove meningiomas
- Excellent exposure of the anterior cranial base to facilitate reconstruction
- Minimizes brain retraction

Disadvantages

- Longer exposure time
- Possible increased risk of postoperative pneumocranium due to exposure of such a large area of dura

Indications

- Moderate to large-sized olfactory groove meningiomas
- Olfaction present preoperatively
- Anterior cranial fossa tumors that involve the anterior cerebral arteries, supraclinoid carotid artery, optic nerves, or chiasm
- Tumors of the anterior fossa floor with significant posterior and contralateral extension
- For large planum sphenoidale meningiomas, a large predominantly frontal frontotemporal craniotomy extending near the midline combined with a large orbital osteotomy is usually adequate for the tumor resection and subsequent reconstruction

◆ Preparation

Head Computed Tomography

- Bone windows useful to determine extent of bony destruction by the tumor as well as hyperostosis. Also useful to assess for tumor calcification

Brain Magnetic Resonance Imaging

- Contrasted study in multiple planes best shows the relationship of the tumor to surrounding structures including frontal lobes, optic chiasm, and optic nerves.
- Flow voids can reveal locations of critical vascular structures such as the supraclinoid carotid artery and anterior cerebral arteries and can show degree of displacement or encasement of these vessels. Irregular appearance of a flow void could represent vascular invasion by tumor.

- T2-weighted images are most useful for assessing the integrity of the arachnoid plane around the tumor as well as the extent of surrounding brain edema present.

Cerebral Angiography

- Determines vascularity of tumor as well as its blood supply
- Can allow for embolization if needed
- Can definitively determine the course and configuration of the anterior cerebral arteries and supraclinoid carotid
- Irregularity of vessel walls more sensitive indicator of vessel wall invasion than magnetic resonance imaging (MRI) appearance.

For the reasons already listed, computed tomographic (CT) and MRI scanning are useful in every case of olfactory groove or planum sphenoidale meningioma. Due to the fairly predictable pattern of blood supply to these tumors, cerebral angiography is most useful for cases with vascular encasement on MRI or for cases needing embolization. Carotid artery temporary balloon occlusion is reserved for cases of carotid encasement or invasion by tumor.

◆ Surgical Technique

Anesthesia

Standard general endotracheal tube anesthesia with muscle relaxation is usually given as for most intracranial procedures. Commonly used agents for intracranial surgery include isoflurane, fentanyl, pancuronium, midazolam, and nitrous oxide in combinations customized by the neuroanesthesiologist for the needs of a given patient. Mild to moderate hyperventilation ($PaCO_2 = 30–35$) is often used during the exposure and resection portions of the procedure to facilitate brain relaxation. Mannitol (0.5–1.0 g/kg) is usually administered just prior to initiation of the bone work, also for brain relaxation. If an adequate response is not obtained, IV furosemide (20–40 mg) can potentiate the effects of the mannitol.

For changes on intraoperative monitoring possibly indicating ischemia, usually temporary release or removal of brain retractors or a mild increase in blood pressure will reverse these abnormalities. More extensive cerebral protective measures are usually not needed unless there is vascular encasement or invasion by tumor requiring prolonged temporary clipping or vascular bypass. These additional measures include elevation of the blood pressure 20% above its normal range, mild to moderate hypothermia to ~34°C, mild hemodilution, and finally burst suppression on electroencephalogam (EEG) (usually by the use of thiopental, etomidate, or propofol).[7]

A lumbar drain is used unless there is a mass in the tentorial notch. The drain is opened as soon as anesthesia is induced, and 50 mL of CSF are slowly drained to relax the brain prior to craniotomy. Rapid CSF drainage may induce the formation of an acute subdural hematoma. Postoperative drainage of CSF is rarely needed, but the drain may be left in place for about 3 days to drain small amounts of CSF (~20 mL every 6 to 8 hours).

Intraoperative Monitoring

The most useful neurophysiological intraoperative monitoring for olfactory groove and planum sphenoidale meningiomas includes multimodality monitoring common to other cranial base tumor operations:

Somatosensory Evoked Potentials

- Able to detect changes in cortical function due to ischemia or from temporal lobe or brain stem retraction[8]
- Upper and lower extremity somatosensory evoked potentials (SEPs) are usually monitored.
- Changes in SEP waveforms can be conveyed to the operative team to allow the surgeon to reduce brain retraction or the anesthesiologist to elevate the blood pressure.

Brain Stem Auditory Evoked Responses

- Used as an index of brain stem function
- Contralateral brain stem auditory evoked responses (BAERs) monitoring most common
- Waveform changes can also indicate ischemia or overly aggressive brain retraction and can be conveyed to the operative team so that appropriate measures can be taken.

Electroencephalogram

- Slowing is a sensitive indicator of ischemia.[9]
- Most useful in cases where induction of burst suppression is needed such as during the performance of vascular bypasses

Specific cranial nerve monitoring is usually not indicated for olfactory groove or planum sphenoidale meningiomas. As with other cranial base operations, the use of monitoring should be customized according to the individual needs of the patient.

Positioning

The patient is placed in the supine position with the head placed in pins. The patient is firmly secured (taped) to the table with profuse padding to allow significant table rotation during the operation. The skull pinning is performed for a planned bicoronal incision. The head is turned 20 degrees to the opposite side to facilitate dissection of the root of the sylvian fissure, optic nerve, and anterior cerebral arteries without compromising the bilateral view needed for the subfrontal aspect of the procedure (**Fig. 49–1**). The head is placed in slight extension to aid exposure of the basal frontal lobes with minimal retraction, but only slightly so the view of the anterior cranial base, which is optimal with the head in neutral (horizontal) position, is not compromised.[10]

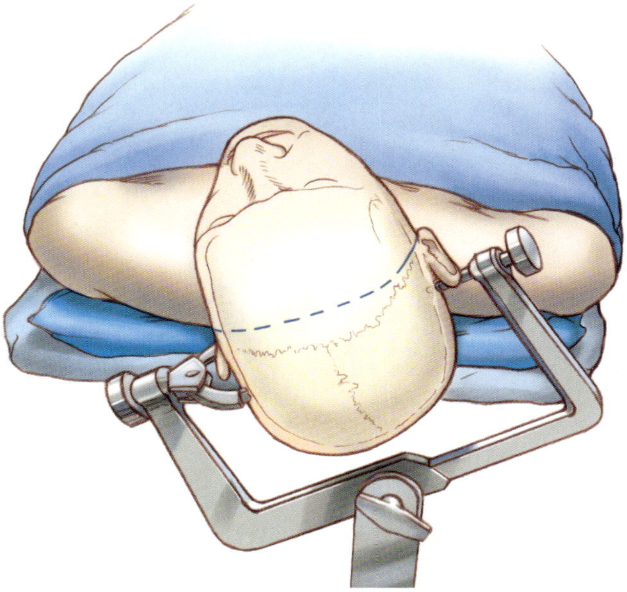

Figure 49–1 Head positioning for one-and-a-half fronto-orbital approach.

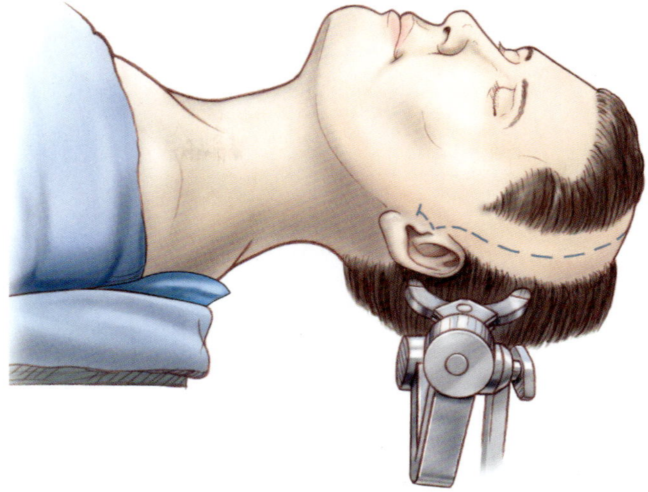

Figure 49–2 Bicoronal skin incision in the skin crease anterior to the tragus.

Head depression and elevation during the course of the procedure are usually performed with Trendelenburg or reverse Trendelenburg maneuvers. Flexion at the patient's hip can also be done, but this is usually avoided because flexion at the hip in a patient in pins can change the relationship of the head to the table resulting in unwanted cervical traction.[10] Careful positioning with the patient firmly secured to the operating table with adequate tape and padding can allow for a significant amount of rotational mobility about the patient's long axis during the procedure.

When the patient is prepped and draped, the lateral thigh or lower abdomen should be included for possible autologous fat or fascial grafts needed during the reconstruction phase of the procedure.

Incision

A bicoronal skin incision is used, but it is kept well behind the hairline. This not only allows a larger pericranial flap to be harvested but it is more cosmetic, leaving hair anterior to the incision when only a strip of hair is shaved. The lower end of the incision is made in the skin crease just anterior to the tragus, which is more cosmetic and also avoids injury to the frontotemporal branch of the facial nerve and the superficial temporal artery (**Fig. 49–2**).

Dissection

The pericranium is elevated with the scalp to protect it and prevent its desiccation during a potentially lengthy procedure. The pericranium is incised separately from the scalp so that the scalp posterior to the incision can be undermined for a larger pericranial flap if needed. Elevation of the scalp and pericranium is continued anteriorly until the superficial temporal fat pad is encountered, at which time an interfascial dissection of the frontotemporal branch of the facial nerve is performed ipsilateral to the tumor. Because this nerve lies superficial to the superficial fascia of the temporalis muscle, this fascia is sharply incised, usually ~2 cm posterior to the zygomatic process of the frontal bone[11] and extended from the keyhole anteriorly to the root of the zygoma inferiorly (**Fig. 49–3**). More blunt dissection

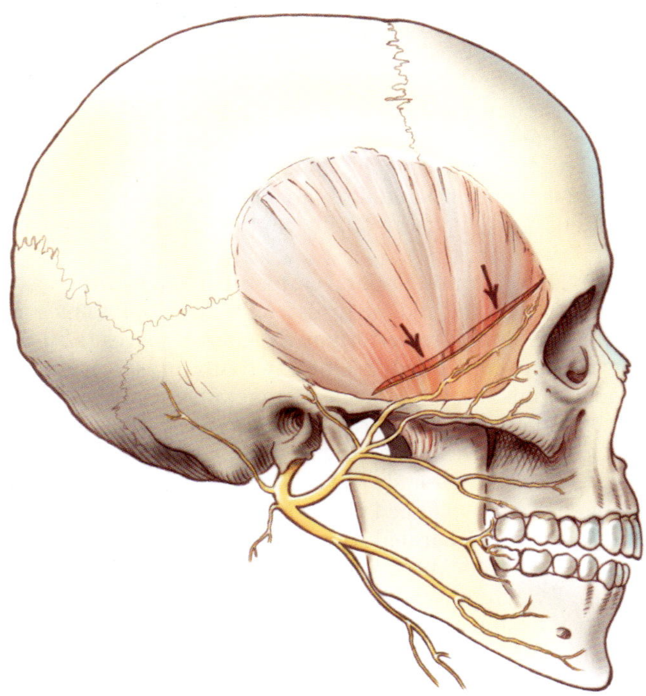

Figure 49–3 Interfascial dissection of the frontotemporal branch of the facial nerve.

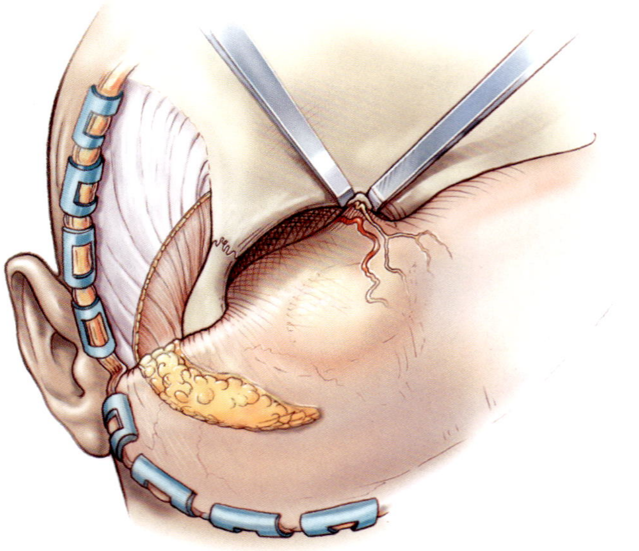

Figure 49–4 Freeing the neurovascular bundle from the supraorbital foramen.

is then used to elevate this fascia and fat pad together from the deep temporalis fascia until the lateral orbital rim and superior zygomatic arch are exposed.

The elevation of the pericranium and scalp is continued down to the orbital rims bilaterally, with exposure of only the medial orbital rim needed contralaterally. If the ipsilateral supraorbital nerve and artery are in a complete foramen instead of a notch, the foramen is opened with a small osteotome on either side of these structures to free them without injury[4] (**Fig. 49–4**).

The ipsilateral temporalis muscle is then carefully elevated completely with periosteal elevators with care being taken to preserve the thin fascial layer on the underside of the muscle. The posterior edge of the incision is undermined to avoid cutting the temporalis muscle to preserve its innervation and blood supply. The temporalis muscle is then retracted laterally and inferiorly providing excellent bony exposure of the frontotemporal region and orbital rim.

A unilateral frontotemporal craniotomy flap is turned extending just off the midline ipsilaterally. The craniotomy and orbital osteotomy are performed as separate pieces to allow for a more controlled osteotomy with preservation of enough orbital roof to prevent postoperative enophthalmos. The craniotomy can be started with bur holes at the keyhole and just above the zygomatic root. An additional bur hole can be placed ipsilaterally just off the midline along the posterior edge of the planned craniotomy flap for separating the dura. A slot is then drilled connecting the first two bur holes using a Midas Rex M8 (Midas Rex Pneumatic Tools, Inc., Fort Worth, TX) or equivalent drill bit that proceeds around the temporal tip and across the root of the sphenoid wing. An alternative and preferred method is to perform no bur holes but drill the slot along the same route with the ends at the keyhole and zygomatic root just being large enough to accommodate the Midas Rex B1 footplate or its equivalent.

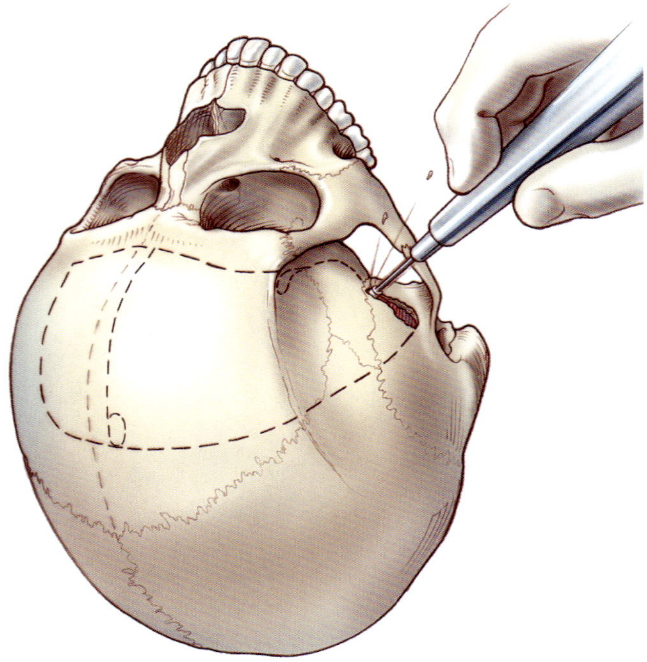

Figure 49–5 Craniotomy flaps for one-and-a-half fronto-orbital approach with optional bur holes.

Dural stripping can then be performed with a Woodson elevator prior to turning the craniotomy flap.

With the initial craniotomy flap turned by either method, the superior sagittal sinus can be stripped from the overlying bone under direct vision. A second craniotomy flap is then turned 2 to 3 cm across the midline, exposing the contralateral frontal dura while minimizing the risk of superior sagittal sinus injury (**Fig. 49–5**).

Prior to performing the orbital osteotomy, the periorbita must be stripped from the orbital roof and walls. The periorbita is most densely adherent to the orbital rim, so care must be taken to prevent holes. A small periosteal elevator, a freer, or the sharp end of a Penfield no. 1 are often used for this dissection. Once the orbital rim is free, the periorbita of the orbital roof and walls must be separated. Because it is less adherent here, more blunt dissection is performed with such instruments as the blunt end of a Penfield no. 1 along with the use of cottonoids for added blunt dissection and protection. Along the superomedial orbital wall, a very adherent area is noted, which represents the trochlea of the superior oblique muscle. This area is separated as well and will eventually heal to its original position with replacement of the orbital osteotomy.[11]

To prevent postoperative pulsatile enophthalmos, at least 2.5 cm or two thirds of the orbital roof must be preserved.[11] For this reason, the periorbita is usually stripped ~3 cm from the orbital rim to ensure adequate protection of the periorbita and orbital contents.

The frontal dura is separated from the orbital roof back to the superior orbital fissure. The contralateral frontal dura is stripped from anterior to the cribriform plate to the edge of the craniotomy defect to facilitate the osteotomy. The dural sleeves of the olfactory nerves and the cribriform plate itself are not disturbed. This is a major point of differentiation with the standard subfrontal approach in that the one-and-a-half fronto-orbital approach is designed to provide the necessary expose yet spare olfaction.

The orbital osteotomy cuts are begun with a reciprocating saw. Malleable brain retractors are placed over the frontal dura and the orbital contents for protection, and the saw cuts are generally made away from the brain for additional safety. The medial saw cut is made along a line extending from the contralateral edge of the craniotomy defect to the superomedial ipsilateral orbital rim. The lateral cut is made at the junction of the orbital rim with the zygomatic arch. The reciprocating saw is always used for the cosmetically important cuts on the face and through the thick areas of the orbital rim. The cuts along the orbital roof and lateral orbital wall where the bone is thin can then be done with either the reciprocating saw, the Midas Rex M8 or equivalent drill bit, or small osteotomes. These posterior cuts are made to preserve at least 2.5 cm (two thirds) of the orbital roof and lateral orbital wall while staying out of the superior orbital fissure and orbital apex, which are opened later. This preserves adequate bone while minimizing the risk of optic nerve injury or injury to the nerves of the superior orbital fissure (**Fig. 49–6**).

In the one-and-a-half fronto-orbital approach, the medial orbital osteotomy cut is designed to spare the contralateral orbit yet remove the contralateral basal frontal bone, circumventing the cribriform plate while providing excellent basal exposure (**Fig. 49–7**). Large tumors that have completely destroyed olfaction and eroded through the cribriform plate may require a more extensive osteotomy, perhaps including the contralateral orbit. Once the osteotomy cuts have been made, the entire block of bone is loosened with a mallet and chisel and removed. Care must be taken to check for any residual adherence of the periorbita to the osteotomy when removing it to avoid producing or extending tears. Openings in the frontal sinus are dealt with during the reconstruction phase of the procedure.

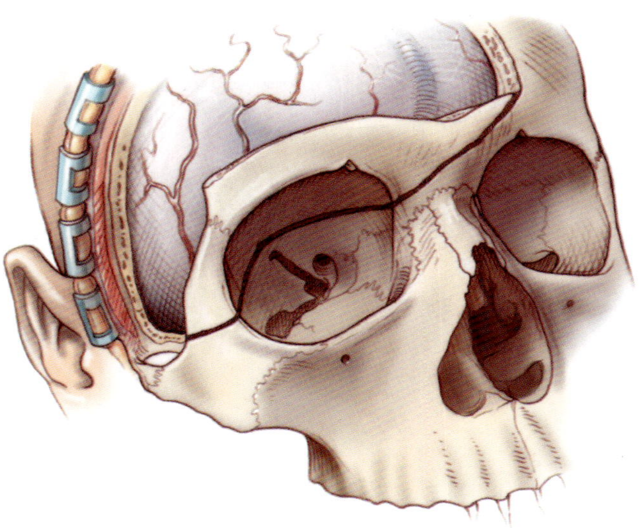

Figure 49–6 Orbital osteotomy for one-and-a-half fronto-orbital approach.

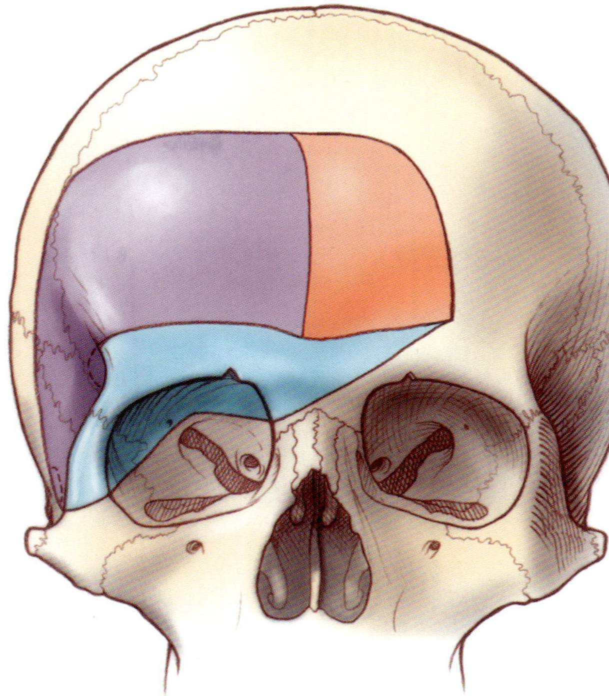

Figure 49–7 External view of bone removal for one-and-a-half fronto-orbital approach. Purple, first bone flap; orange, second bone flap; blue, orbital osteotomy.

The operating microscope is then brought into the field. The remaining orbital roof and lateral orbital wall are then carefully removed with a small rongeur (Lempert or Sekhar; Codman Johnson & Johnson Professional Products Ltd., Berkshire, UK)) after their associated dura and periorbita have been separated. The superior orbital fissure is widely decompressed to take full advantage of the exposure gained by the orbital osteotomy. The anterior clinoid process can then be removed, and the optic canal widely opened extradurally providing an extensive decompression of the ipsilateral optic nerve prior to opening the dura. Early decompression of the optic nerve aids in protecting it in cases where there is tumor extending into the optic canal or abutting or surrounding the optic nerve and significant optic nerve manipulation will be required during the tumor resection.

If an extradural anterior clinoidectomy is needed, sectioning the orbital meningeal artery and stripping temporal dura away from the orbital apex and anterior cavernous sinus provides the necessary exposure.[12] The anterior clinoid process is then cored using a Midas Rex K2 or K3 or equivalent drill bits until only a fine shell of cortical bone remains. This remaining bone can be removed with fine rongeurs. The optic canal can be opened further by removing the optic strut, which should be well visualized at this time. Any cavernous sinus bleeding elicited by these maneuvers can usually be controlled with Surgicel or Gelfoam.[12]

With all of the bone work completed, the intradural portion of the procedure begins. A curvilinear dural incision is made circumventing the sylvian fissure and extending over the low anterior frontal dura where it is continued to a

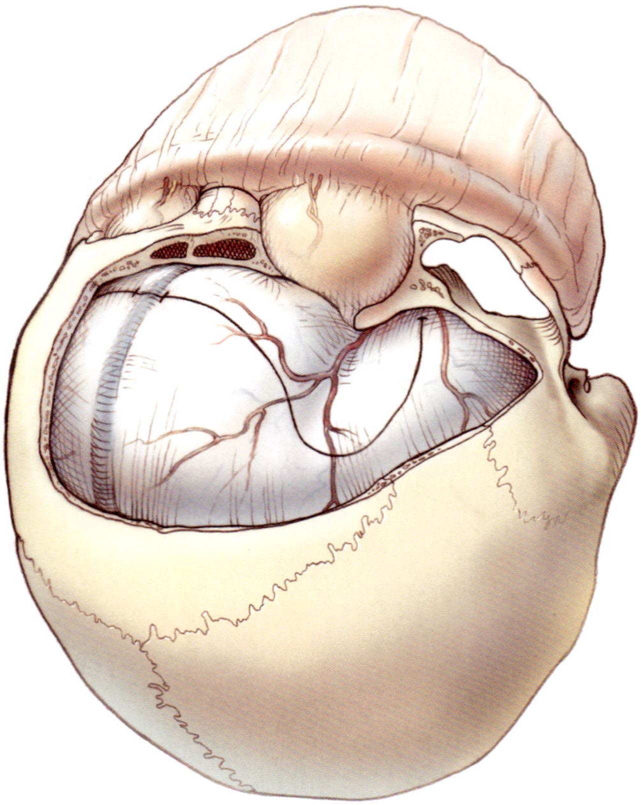

Figure 49–8 Dural incision for one-and-a-half fronto-orbital approach.

point just off the midline. A low anterior frontal dural incision is then made contralaterally, which is also extended near midline. The superior sagittal sinus is then ligated and sectioned near its base, and the falx cerebri is then completely cut along the anterior fossa floor (**Fig. 49–8**). The flap of dura obtained laterally by posteriorly circumventing the sylvian fissure is then retracted anteriorly over the orbital osteotomy site, effectively retracting the orbital contents inferiorly, thereby maximizing exposure.

Tumor Exposure and Resection

The surgeon is now able to open the sylvian fissure to identify the optic nerve intradurally, the supraclinoid carotid, and one or both anterior cerebral arteries. These structures can then be dissected as free from the tumor as possible and protected (**Fig. 49–9**). An additional advantage is that the basal cisterns can be drained of CSF during this dissection, providing significantly more overall brain relaxation. Attention is then directed subfrontally for the tumor resection.

Due to the bilateral dural incision, CSF removal and extensive bone work performed by this point, the basal frontal lobes should be well exposed with minimal brain retraction, particularly ipsilaterally. Early during the subfrontal dissection, the contralateral olfactory tract should be dissected from the inferior frontal lobe to protect it and

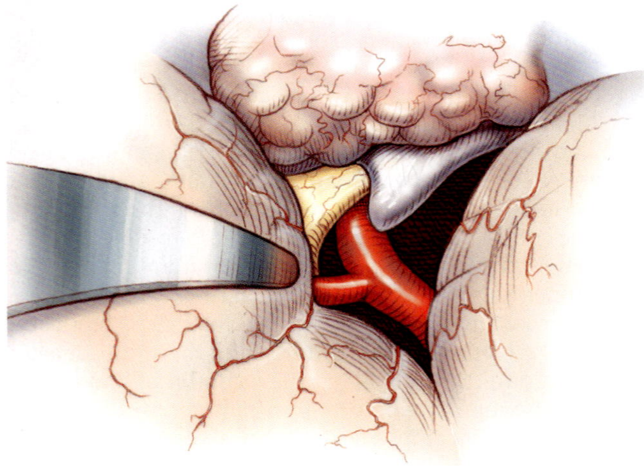

Figure 49–9 The sylvian fissure is split to identify and protect the optic nerve, the carotid artery, and its branches.

prevent it from being avulsed during the tumor resection. The anterior margin of the tumor is then exposed, and the tumor is internally debulked using sharp dissection, spituitary forceps, ultrasonic surgical aspirator, or any combination of these techniques (**Fig. 49–10**). The debulking is focused toward the base of the tumor in an attempt to devascularize it and disconnect it from the skull base as much as possible. Internal debulking is continued until only a rind of tumor

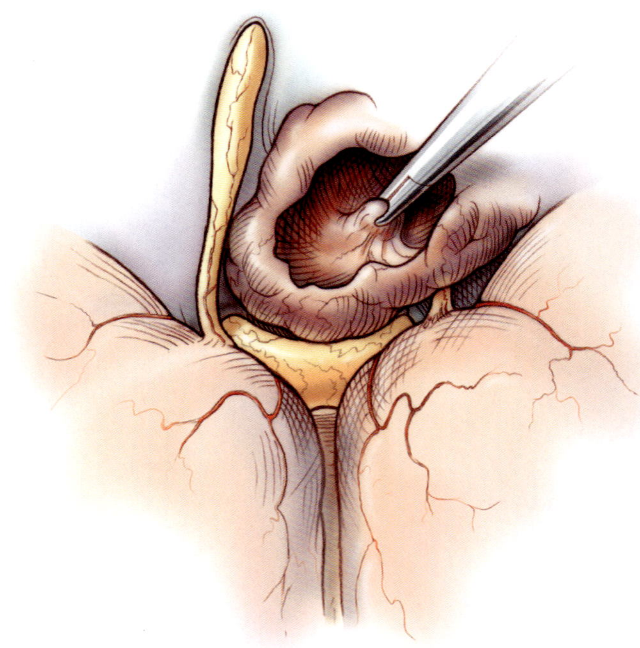

Figure 49–10 Internal debulking of a typical tumor.

remains attached to surrounding structures. The tumor is then microsurgically dissected from the pial surface of the brain and the dissection of the tumor from the optic nerves and cerebral vasculature is completed.

Olfactory Groove versus Planum Sphenoidale Meningiomas

Although the operative techniques discussed to this point are essentially the same for both olfactory groove and planum sphenoidale meningiomas, there are several important differences. For planum tumors, both olfactory tracts are dissected from the inferior frontal lobes initially so that if it is necessary to divide one during the tumor resection, the other is left intact.[13] The ipsilateral olfactory tract is usually the one divided. Also, for large planum tumors, the frontal portion of a frontotemporal craniotomy is extended near the midline and combined with a large orbital osteotomy. This exposure is usually adequate for the resection and subsequent repair, avoiding the need for a full one-and-a-half fronto-orbital approach.

Another important difference is that planum tumors often extend into the optic canals, requiring the optic nerves to be decompressed both extradurally and intradurally. The extensive extradural bone work, including anterior clinoidectomy and optic canal decompression, facilitates the tracing of tumor from intra- to extradurally by opening the dura propria of the optic nerve along the tumor extension (**Fig. 49–11**). Additional intradural bone work, including more anterior clinoid process, tuberculum sellae, or planum sphenoidale removal can be performed at this stage if necessary to supplement the extradural work performed earlier

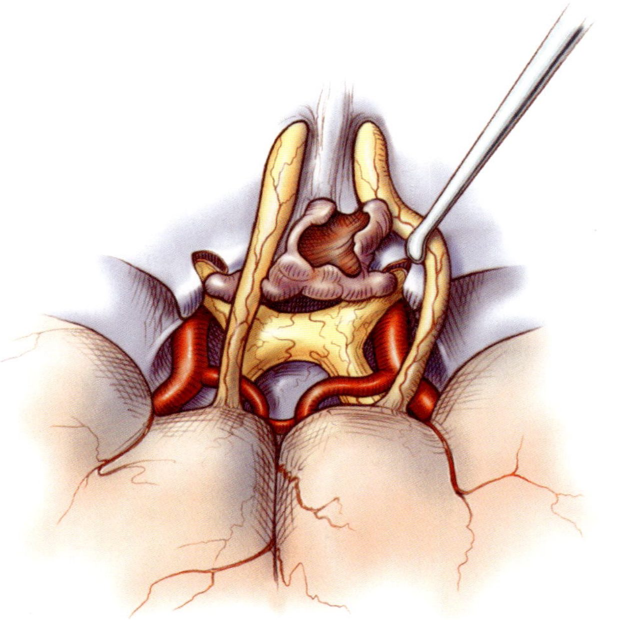

Figure 49–11 Opening of the dura propria of the optic nerves to remove a planum sphenoidale meningioma extending into the optic canals.

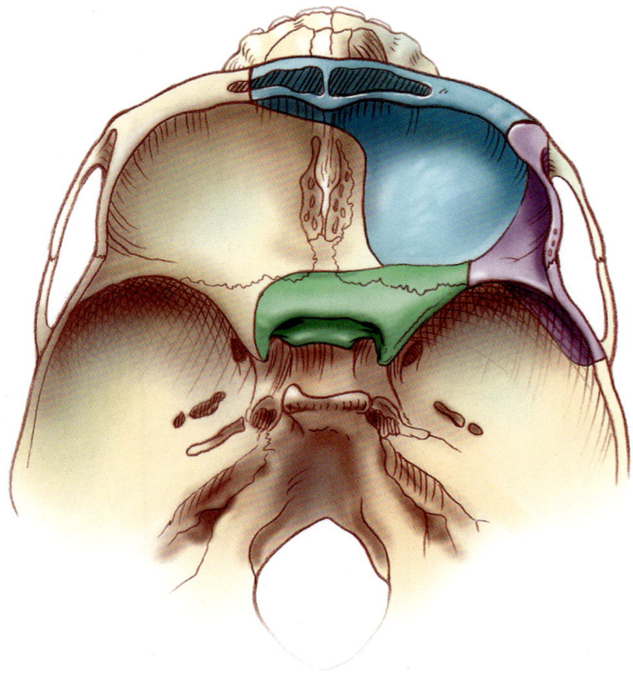

Figure 49–12 Total bone removal possible through the one-and-a-half fronto-orbital approach. Purple, craniotomy flap; blue, orbital osteotomy; green, drilled and rongeured bone.

in the procedure. Alternatively, the dural flap can be retracted posterosuperiorly to allow for additional extradural bone removal to avoid the additional dural incisions needed for intradural bone work. The combined bone removal possible through the one-and-a-half fronto-orbital approach is illustrated in **Fig. 49–12.**

Tumor extension into the cavernous sinuses or sella turcica can occur with either type of tumor but is much more likely with planum sphenoidale meningiomas. For total removal, all of the abnormal dura associated with the tumor and its various extensions is also excised.

Closure

Attempts are made to obtain a watertight primary closure of the main dural incision. Dural defects are generally repaired with autologous tissue. Free pericranial grafts are used for smaller defects. For large defects, abdominal fascia can be used. These grafts are sewn to the dural edges in a circumferential fashion using the operating microscope. Although watertight closure is not possible, when combined with fibrin glue and sinus repair, this closure is usually adequate. The fibrin glue is usually placed after the pericranial flap is secured over the frontal sinus or skull base defect to reinforce the entire construct.

Once the dura is closed, the frontonasal ducts are packed with rolls of Surgicel after the frontal sinus is exenterated. The remainder of the frontal sinus is then packed with autologous abdominal fat to obliterate the sinus and provide proper support for a pericranial flap. To close sphenoid and

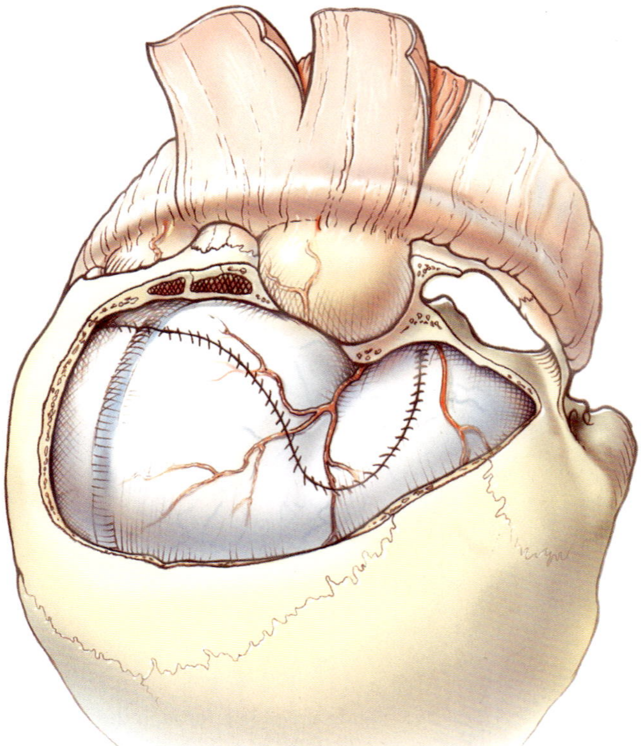

Figure 49–13 Primary dural closure and harvesting of the pericranial flap on its vascular pedicle. The slit in the pericranial graft is to allow it to surround the region of the cribriform plate.

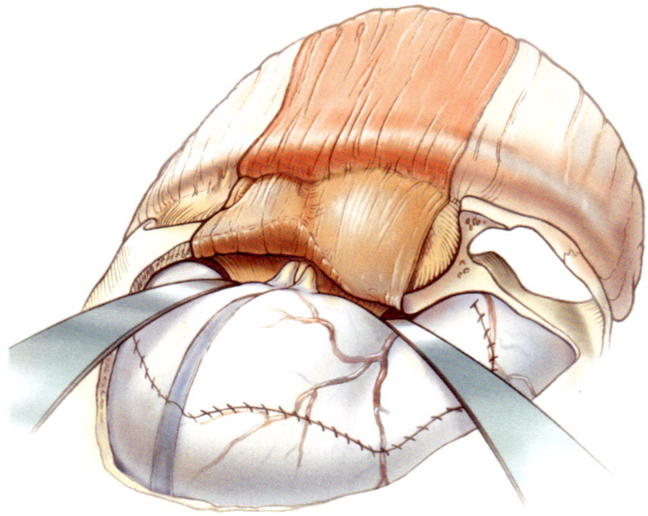

Figure 49–14 The pericranial graft is sutured in position over fat grafts placed in the open paranasal sinuses. The entire reconstruction is then augmented with fibrin glue.

ethmoid sinus defects, a pericranial flap is elevated and secured to the clival bone with titanium mesh and screws. Autologous fat is then packed between to fill the dead space, along with fascial graft and pericranium. Care is taken not to overpack this dead space to prevent optic nerve compression. Muscle is not used to pack the sinus because its high metabolic rate makes it less likely to remain viable.[11]

The pericranial flap is harvested on its vascular pedicle (**Fig. 49–13**). The best method to separate the pericranium from the remainder of the scalp without putting holes in the graft is to use a combination of sharp and scissor dissection in a direction parallel to the coronal suture. The flap is then gradually elevated from posterior to anterior until the anterior origin of the pericranium at the orbital rims is reached. The dissection is continued this far inferiorly to prevent puckering of the skin of the forehead when the graft is placed, which can produce a significant cosmetic defect. A large flap is harvested if the ethmoid or sphenoid sinuses have been entered or if there is a large anterior fossa floor defect. A smaller flap can be used if only the frontal sinus is involved. The pericranial flap is then placed in its final position over the fat grafts and secured to the surrounding dura with 4–0 braided nylon sutures (**Fig. 49–14**).

After the dura has been closed, the pericranial flap has been secured in its final position, and the entire construct is reinforced with fibrin glue, the orbital osteotomy is placed over the pericranial graft into its original position and secured with titanium miniplates. Care is taken not to replace the bone so tightly that it occludes the vascular supply of the pericranial flap. The craniotomy flaps are replaced with titanium miniplates as well. Any residual defects in the bone that are potentially cosmetically significant can be repaired with hydroxyapatite cement. The temporalis muscle is then replaced in its original position and secured with multiple sutures to the miniplates of the bone flaps and to multiple small holes in the bone along the superior temporal line. These holes in the bone are made at oblique angles with a Midas Rex C1 or equivalent drill bit so the suture needle can pass through easily. With the temporalis muscle secured at multiple places along its entire superior margin, it is firmly fixed in its original position with minimal disruption of its anatomical or functional integrity. The scalp is then closed in two layers in the usual fashion.

◆ Complications

Ischemic Complications

Internal carotid and anterior cerebral artery (ICA and ACerA) injury may occur during tumor resection resulting in associated ischemic complications. One of the advantages of the one-and-a-half fronto-orbital approach for resection of large olfactory groove meningiomas affecting these vessels is the ability to open the sylvian fissure early in the intradural stage of the procedure so that these structures can be dissected free from surrounding tumor and protected. If a normal ICA or ACerA is injured, it can usually be repaired by trapping the damaged segment with temporary clips and direct microsurgical suturing.

Previously irradiated tumors or prior surgery substantially increase the chances of vascular injuries because the arachnoid plane around the ICA or ACerA may be absent. In these patients, great care must be taken in dissecting these vessels because they may be thin-walled and may rupture with little provocation. If these vessels are injured beyond repair, revascularization of the affected area of the brain is recommended. A detailed discussion of microsurgical cerebral revascularization is beyond the scope of this chapter.

Cerebrospinal Fluid Leakage

The best way to prevent postoperative CSF leakage is to perform a meticulous reconstruction of the surgical defect at the end of the tumor resection as described earlier in this chapter. If a postoperative leak does occur despite adequate reconstruction, it can often be managed with a lumbar drain. Transsphenoidal packing with fascia and fat can close leaks from a sphenoid sinus defect refractory to lumbar drainage. Other leaks refractory to lumbar drainage may require reexploration and revision of the reconstruction along with simultaneous lumbar drainage continuing for 3 to 5 days after the revision.

Cranial Nerve Injuries

Cranial nerves I and II are most frequently at risk during these cases. Preservation of olfaction is another advantage of the one-and-a-half fronto-orbital approach. Despite preservation of the cribriform plate during the approach, the olfactory tracts may be easily avulsed during the tumor resection or from frontal lobe retraction. To avoid this, the contralateral olfactory tract is dissected from the inferior frontal lobe early during the resection of olfactory groove meningiomas. For planum meningiomas, both olfactory tracts are dissected from the inferior frontal lobes early in the resection. Occasionally, it may be necessary to divide one of the olfactory tracts during the tumor resection. Early dissection of the olfactory tracts can accommodate for this and maximize the chances of useful postoperative olfaction.

During the resection of large olfactory groove meningiomas, visualizing and protecting the optic nerves and chiasm early by opening the sylvian fissure prior to tumor resection best prevents optic nerve injury. Also, the optic nerves and chiasm are manipulated as little as possible, and high doses of dexamethasone are given preoperatively and intraoperatively to increase their tolerance to what manipulation is necessary.

For the removal of planum sphenoidale meningiomas, the optic nerves are decompressed both extradurally and intradurally due to their frequent extension into the optic canals. Early decompression of the optic nerves, particularly ipsilaterally, allows for more manipulation of the optic nerve without damaging it.

Brain Injury

Using contemporary cranial base approaches along with good brain relaxation and CSF drainage, brain injury from retraction should be minimal. If contusion does occur, it is most often present in the frontal lobe. Such contusions should be monitored closely with postoperative CT to insure that an intracerebral hemorrhage does not develop. Rarely, reoperation to evacuate a parenchymal hemorrhage may be needed.

◆ Conclusion

The one-and-a-half fronto-orbital approach combines the advantages of both the pterional and subfrontal approaches while eliminating their limitations. This approach is ideally suited for moderate- to large-sized olfactory groove meningiomas with olfaction present preoperatively, contralateral extension, and involvement of the optic nerves, chiasm, supraclinoid carotid, or ACerAs. For planum sphenoidale meningiomas, a medially extended frontotemporal craniotomy, a wide orbital osteotomy, extradural optic nerve decompression, and planum sphenoidale removal facilitate tumor resection. In either case, complete removal is the goal to prevent recurrence. Also, reconstruction must be meticulous to prevent postoperative CSF leakage. Presented here is only a set of general guidelines intended to illustrate the principles and techniques involved in this approach, which should be modified according to the pathology encountered.

References

1. Al-Mefty O. Supraorbital-pterional approach to skull base lesions. Neurosurgery 1987;21:474–477
2. Jane JA, Newman SA. Transcranial orbital surgery. Clin Neurosurg 1996;43:53–71
3. Jane JA, Park TS, Pobereskin LH, Winn HR, Butler AB. The supraorbital approach: technical note. Neurosurgery 1982;11:537–542
4. Lee DS, Peck M. Anesthetic considerations for cranial microsurgery. In: Sekhar LN, Oliveira Ed, eds. Cranial Microsurgery: Approaches and Techniques. New York: Thieme; 1999:19–22
5. Ojemann RG. Surgical management of anterior basal meningiomas: olfactory groove. In: Schmidek HH, Sweet WH, eds. Operative Neurosurgical Techniques. Philadelphia: WB Saunders; 1995:393–402
6. Persing JA, Jane JA, Levine PA, et al. The versatile frontal sinus approach to the floor of the anterior cranial fossa. J Neurosurg 1990;72: 513–516
7. Ransohoff J, Nockels RP. Olfactory groove and planum meningioma. In: Apuzzo MLJ, ed. Brain Surgery: Complication Avoidance and Management. New York: Churchill Livingstone; 1993:203–218
8. Sclabassi RJ, Krieger DN, Weisz DJ, et al. Methods of neurophysiological monitoring during cranial base tumor resection. In: Sekhar LN, Janecka IP, eds. Surgery of Cranial Base Tumors. New York: Raven; 1993:83–98
9. Sekhar LN, Raso J. Orbitozygomatic frontotemporal approach. In: Sekhar LN, Oliveira ED, eds. Cranial Microsurgery: Approaches and Techniques. New York: Thieme; 1999:130–133
10. Sekhar LN, Tzortzidis F. Resection of tumors by the fronto-orbital approach. In: Sekhar LN, Oliveira ED, eds. Cranial Microsurgery: Approaches and Techniques. New York: Thieme; 1999:61–75
11. Sekhar LN, Tzortzidis F, Bucur SD. Patient positioning for cranial microsurgery. In: Sekhar LN, Oliveira ED, eds. Cranial Microsurgery: Approaches and Techniques. New York: Thieme; 1999:12–18
12. Sekhar LN, Tzortzidis F, Raso J. Fronto-orbital approach In: Sekhar LN, Oliveira ED, eds. Cranial Microsurgery: Approaches and Techniques. New York: Thieme; 1999:54–60
13. Vera PL. Intraoperative neurophysiological monitoring. In: Sekhar LN, Oliveira ED, eds. Cranial Microsurgery: Approaches and Techniques. New York: Thieme; 1999:23–30

50

Fibrous Dysplasias, Osteopetrosis, and Ossifying Fibromas

Sunil J. Patel

Osseous lesions of the skull are a rare group of heterogeneous disorders that are either a manifestation of a systemic skeletal disorder or a localized solitary process. Neurological manifestation of these disorders often results from compression of the cranial nerves in the exiting foramina at the skull base, and the optic nerve is most commonly affected. Osteopetrosis is a diffuse disease in which skeletal sclerosis is formed by thickening of both the cortical and the spongy bone due to osteoclast deficiency. Albers-Schonberg first described this as "marble bone disease," which was later identified as osteopetrosis by Karshner.[1,2] This disorder is a subtype of a broad category of congenital abnormalities of bone formation known as craniotubular bone modeling disorders. There is a proclivity for involvement of the skull base, and as a result patients most often present with deficits of cranial nerve (CN) II, VII, and VIII.[3] Blindness from optic nerve compression is almost exclusively associated with the juvenile autosomal recessive form of this disease.

Fibrous dysplasia is also a rare skull disorder, accounting for only 2.5% of all bone tumors.[4] Involvement of the skull occurs in up to 10% of patients with the monostotic form of the disease, rising up to 100% involvement in the rarer polyostotic form.[5] The etiology of fibrous dysplasia is unknown, with the bone in localized areas being replaced by fibrous tissue resulting in expanded, softened, and fragile bone. The monostotic form most often affects the fronto-orbital region, presenting with equal frequency in both sexes; the polyostotic form affects multiple bones, including the facial and orbital areas, and occurs more often in females. Progressive visual loss, proptosis, and cosmetic deformity are the usual manifestations of the skull involvement. There is a 0.5% incidence of malignant transformation.[6]

Ossifying fibroma is a neoplastic process affecting the bones of the skull. There is still confusion as to the distinctiveness of this disease, and these lesions have often been mislabeled as fibrous dysplasia, cementifying fibroma, fibrous osteoma, and ivory osteoma.[7] The distinct histological finding is the presence of osteoblasts and lamellar bone (fibrous dysplasia has woven bone with dysplastic bony spicules without osteoblasts). Head and neck lesions are most often in the mandible and maxilla, with rare occurrences reported in the paranasal and sphenoid bones and occasionally in the orbit. They tend to occur in the third and fourth decades, with the younger patients noted to have a more aggressive (faster growing) lesion.

◆ Indications

Progressive cranial nerve deficit is the main indication to decompress the affected nerve. Because neurosurgeons are more often called upon to manage optic nerve compression, the latter will be the focus of this chapter. Deficits of CN VII and VIII may require transmastoid decompression, usually the domain of neuro-otologists. Occasionally proptosis from direct orbital compression (ossifying fibroma and fibrous dysplasia) alone may be an indication for orbital decompression. Bilateral procedures are often required in patients with osteopetrosis.

◆ Preparation

Once the primary disease is confirmed, frequent monitoring (every 3–6 months) of cranial nerve functions is important in these patients. Periodic objective visual testing (acuity and visual field testing) is especially important in osteopetrosis, although in infants, this may be difficult, and behavioral manifestations of visual compromise may be the only indication of visual dysfunction. Patients with proptosis from orbital or periorbital involvement in both fibrous dysplasia and ossifying fibroma should also have objective visual testing to evaluate for any optic nerve dysfunction. Radiographic confirmation of optic canal narrowing is essential for the diagnosis and surgical planning. Optic atrophy, as noted on funduscopy, and abnormalities in visual evoked potentials (VEPs) are additional tests of confirmation of optic nerve compression, especially in the younger population. It is important to realize that optic atrophy can also be caused by either or both chronic increased intracranial pressure and hydrocephalus in patients with osteopetrosis. There is still controversy that the failure of decompression to improve visual loss in the latter disease may be due to a primary retinal degeneration. For the latter reason preoperative evaluation with electroretinography is recommended to rule out retinopathy as the primary cause of the visual loss. Preoperative evaluation in patients with osteopetrosis must include making certain that the bone marrow is not suppressed so that both anemia and leukopenia have to be ruled out before the operation. Patients with the McCune-Albright form of polyostotic fibrous dysplasia (associated with hyperpigmentation and endocrinopathy) should also have adequate preoperative endocrinological evaluation.

◆ Surgical Technique

Neurophysiological Monitoring

Intraoperative VEPs have not proven useful in this procedure. Early enough changes are not usually seen in the potentials to evaluate the adequacy of the decompression during the procedure. However, VEPs are essential and often the only objective measure of the efficacy of the decompression in infants.

Anesthesia

The anesthesiologist should make every effort to help with brain relaxation. Often the intracranial pressure is high, especially in cases with advanced osteopetrosis. Some important maneuvers to achieve this include hyperventilation, intravenous mannitol infusion, barbiturates, elevation of the head above the level of the chest, and uncompromised venous drainage (avoid internal jugular lines when possible).

Positioning

With the patient in a supine position, the head is turned 30 to 45 degrees to the opposite side and very slightly extended. This should be done with caution in patients with osteopetrosis to avoid injury to the craniovertebral junction, which is often involved.

Approach

A curvilinear incision is made in the frontotemporal area as would be required for a pterional exposure. Include with the scalp the superficial fatty later of the temporalis muscle fascia to avoid injury to the frontalis branch of the facial nerve. The temporalis muscle is then separately reflected posteroinferiorly. Bur holes are then placed in the temporal squama behind, and the frontal area just behind the superior temporal line and orbital rim. Often multiple bur holes may be necessary in cases where the calvarium is quite thick. The pterional craniotomy alone is adequate in cases where the orbital roof is not very thick (**Fig. 50–1**). When the orbital roof is quite thick, removing the lateral and superior orbital rim (orbital osteotomy) can provide more room and helps to minimize frontal lobe retraction (**Fig. 50–2**). In addition, extradurally drilling down the orbital roof and lateral sphenoid wing is helpful. The latter is also done in cases where the intent of the operation is to treat proptosis from a lesion involving the superior or lateral walls of the orbit. In infants with bilateral disease, it is not unreasonable to stage the operation and perform separate operations on either side. In infants blood loss should be replaced.

Procedure

It is essential to bear in mind that the objective of the operation is to decompress the optic nerve or orbit or both, and not necessarily to excise the entire lesion. For orbital decompression alone, the extradural approach alone usually suffices. Decompression of the optic nerve, however, is best done intradurally from above. It is much less cumbersome to identify the intradural portion of the nerve and follow it

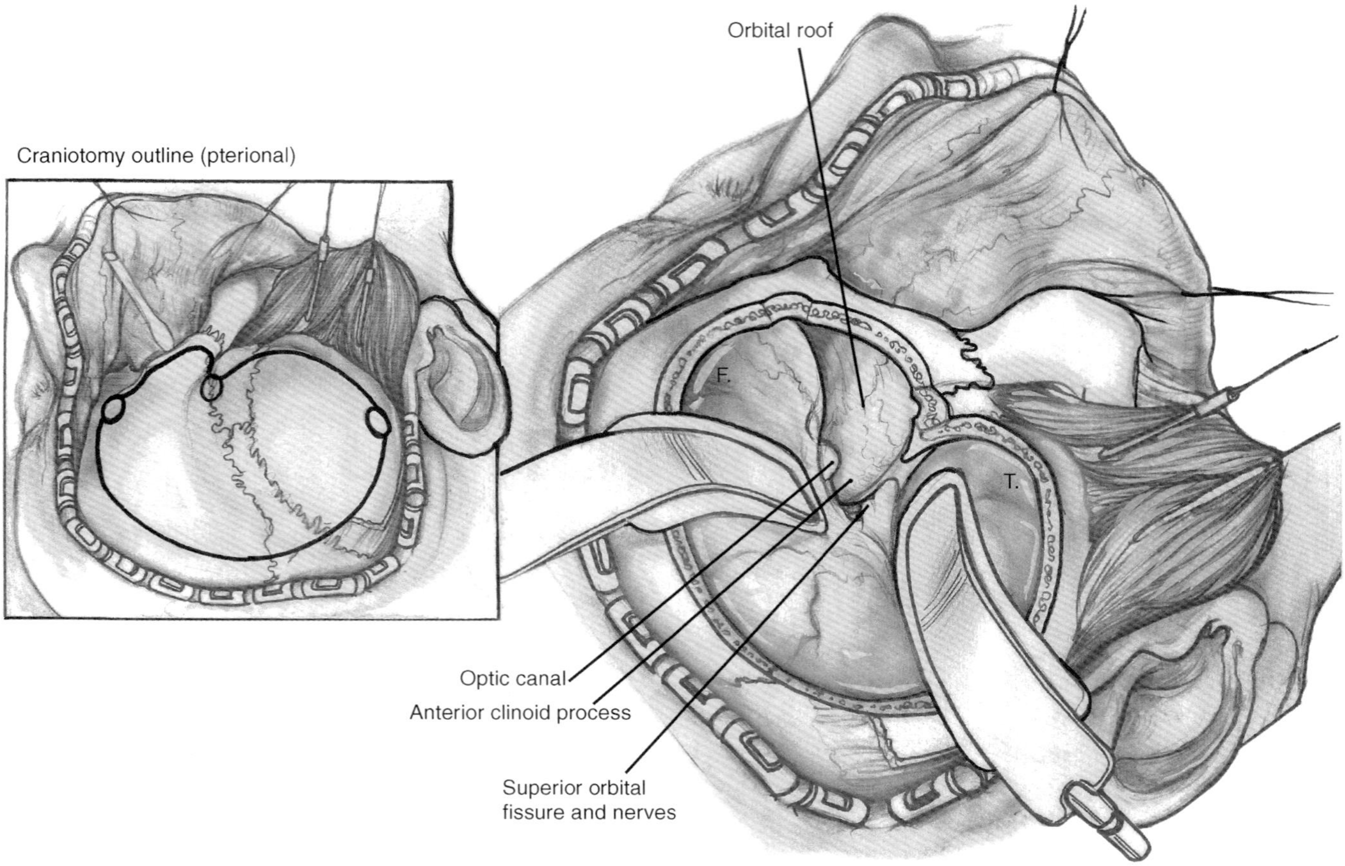

Figure 50–1 Initial pterional craniotomy illustrating orbital rim osteotomy cuts when this is necessary.

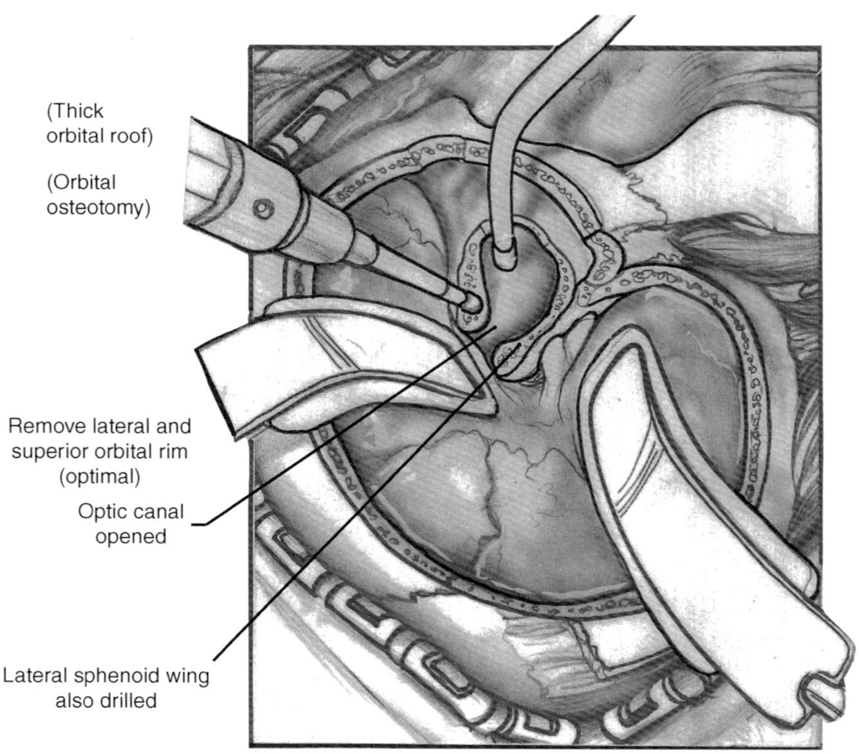

Figure 50–2 Extradural drilling of the enlarged orbital roof to minimize frontal lobe retraction.

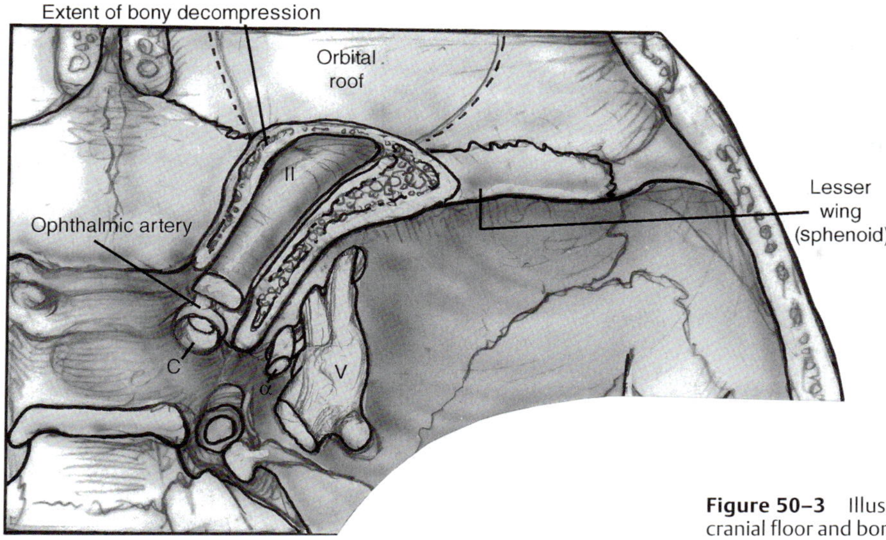

Figure 50–3 Illustration of the final drilled surface of the anterior cranial floor and bony decompression of the optic canal.

outward into the canal than to do the entire nerve decompression extradurally. The dura is opened curvilinearly around the remaining sphenoid wing from the frontal lobe to the temporal lobe. Immediate access to the perioptic subarachnoid cistern is important to release cerebrospinal fluid (CSF) and provide more relaxation of the frontal lobe. Occasionally CSF ventricular drainage with a catheter can be done to facilitate any retraction of the frontal lobe. With the brain adequately relaxed, the rest of the operation is done under the magnification of an operating microscope. The dura overlying the roof of the optic canal is then dissected away, and a high-speed air drill is used to unroof the optic canal from side to side (180 degrees). The last layer of bone is drilled with a diamond bit, with adequate irrigation to avoid heat injury to the nerve. Bone punching instruments (Kerisson rongeurs) should be avoided because the canal is quite compromised. Often, with the bone thinned enough, a flattened microdissector can be used to gently crack off the last bit of it. The bony decompression is illustrated in **Fig. 50–3.** The benefit of opening the optic sheath is controversial, and this should be done with the utmost care because it can sometimes be quite thinned from the chronic compression.

Closure

Closure is standard, with watertight closure of the pterional dura. Prophylaxis with an antibiotic is necessary. In cases where the orbital rim is also involved (fibrous dysplasia and ossifying osteoma), the older patient may desire cosmetic reconstruction of this. A prefabricated, computer-generated mesh or acrylic cranioplasty may be used to replace the rim.

◆ Postoperative Care

Immediate postoperative care is similar to routine craniotomy. Serial postoperative VEPs are essential in following infants, and changes in VEPs have been seen as early as 4 days postop. The older patients should have visual acuity and fields tested to document the efficacy of the procedure. Children who have had significant blood loss may need to have transfusion.

◆ Complications

Frontal contusion and retraction injury from inadequate relaxation of the brain can occur, especially in patients with osteopetrosis and untreated hydrocephalus. Any hydrocephalus should be shunted first, and then if the vision does not improve, consider nerve decompression. It is also useful to remember that the goal of the operation is to decompress the nerve and not to eradicate all diseased bone. Through the intradural approach the nerve is decompressed from the top 180 degrees, avoiding unnecessary penetration of posterior ethmoid or sphenoid sinus air spaces. If these sinuses are penetrated, then they should be packed from above with fat graft, and external drainage of CSF should be done for a few days.

◆ Conclusion

Patients with these rare bone diseases should have frequent objective surveillance of their vision, so that they may benefit from early decompression if deficits occur. Nerve decompression is the primary goal. The surgeon should be familiar with performing orbital osteotomies when needed.

References

1. Albers-Schonberg H. Rontgenbilder einer seltenen Knochenerkrankung. Munch Med Wochenschr 1904;51:365–368
2. Karshner RG. Ostoepetrosis. AJR 1926;16:405–419
3. Johnston CC Jr, Lavy N, Lord T, Vellios F, Merritt AD, Deiss WP Jr, Osteopetrosis: a clinical, genetic, metabolic, and morphologic study of the dominantly inherited, benign form. Medicine 1968;47:149–167
4. Derome PS, Visot A, Akerman M, Oddou B, Mazabraud A, Tessier P. La dysplasia fibreuse cranienne. Neurochirurgie 1983;29:1–117 Akerman M, Oddou B, Mazabraud A, Tessier P.
5. Nager GT, Kennedy DW, Kopstein E. Fibrous dysplasia: a review of the disease and its manifestations in the temporal bone. Ann Otol Rhinol Laryngol Suppl 1982;92:1–52
6. Beuerlein ME, Schuller DE, DeYoung BR. Maxillary malignant mesenchymoma and massive fibrous dysplasia. Arch Otolaryngol Head Neck Surg 1997;123:106–109
7. Levine PA, Wiggins R, Archibald RWR, et al. Ossifying fibroma of the head and neck: involvement of the temporal bone: an unusual and challenging site. Laryngoscope 1981;91:720–725

51

Sphenoid Wing Meningiomas

Jacques Brotchi and Benoit Pirotte

◆ Definition

Sphenoid wing meningiomas account for about 20% of intracranial meningiomas and represent a real surgical challenge due to their invasion of the bone and their being in proximity to the main arteries and cranial nerves.

Anatomically, the sphenoid wing extends from the anterior clinoid process to the pterion, with the greater wing constituting the outer third and the lesser wing the inner two thirds.

◆ Classification

Cushing and Eisenhardt[1] in 1938 were the first to describe sphenoid wing meningiomas, which they classified into three groups: (1) deep, inner, or clinoidal; (2) middle or alar; and (3) outer or pterional. Later, Bonnal et al[2,3] and Brotchi and Bonnal[4] divided sphenoid wing meningiomas into five groups that raised specific surgical problems: group A, deep or clinoidal or sphenocavernous; group B, invading en plaque of the sphenoid wings; group C, invading en masse of the sphenoid wings, which combines the features of groups A and B; group D, middle ridge meningiomas; and group E, pterional or sylvian point meningiomas **(Fig. 51–1).** Al-Mefty[5] subdivided clinoidal meningiomas into three groups. All these classifications are based on surgical considerations and related to operative strategy and challenge. The details may be found in the cited references.

◆ Treatment Options

Surgery is the gold standard treatment of sphenoid wing meningiomas. The chance of total removal during a second operation is much smaller than during the first one, and the complications are greater. Thus, complete removal at first surgery is the best choice. However, one should keep in mind that complete removal signifies total removal of the tumor and of the invaded dura and bone (hyperostotic bone is tumoral bone!), which is not easy when the tumor extends far down in the face and encases the carotid artery and its branches or the cranial nerves. Neurological deficits can occur, even in experienced hands, but everything should be done to avoid them. Quality of life must always be kept in mind, and that is why some alternative treatments have been considered, such as radiotherapy, radiosurgery, hormonal therapy, and chemotherapy, all of which remain controversial because we have no long-term follow-up for some of them (such as stereotactic radiosurgery) or not enough patients treated for others (chemotherapy and hormonal therapy) and no randomized prospective study for any of them.

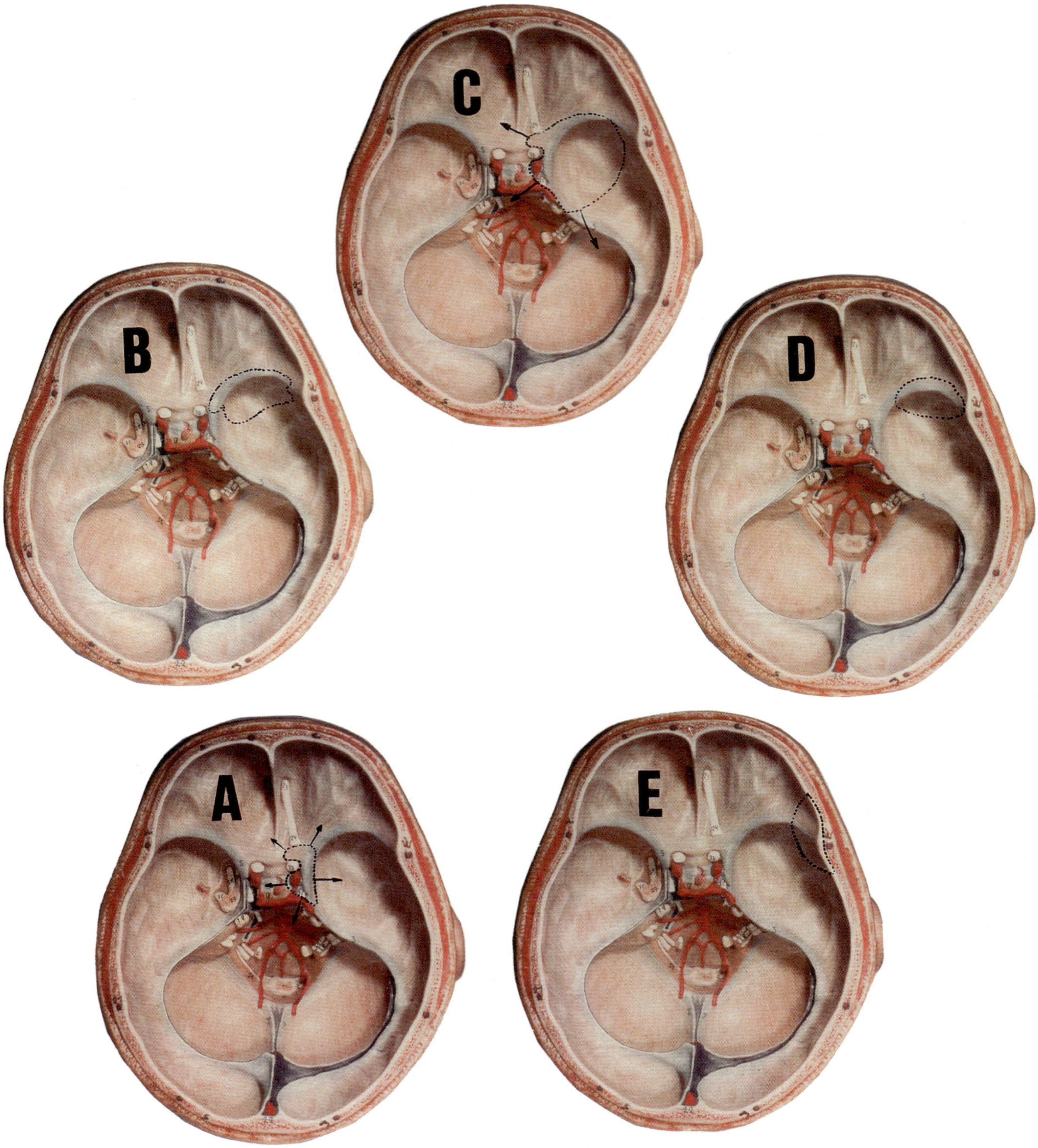

Figure 51–1 Sphenoid wing meningiomas, types A to E.

◆ Indications

Indications for Surgery

Sphenoid wing meningiomas should be operated after diagnosis when they are symptomatic, even when symptoms are limited to an isolated exophthalmia, pterional pain, or diplopia. In patients older than 70 or if the diagnosis is done by chance without any peritumoral edema, a growth in tumoral size should be demonstrated on repeated magnetic resonance imaging (MRI) before considering surgery. However, when the tumor is adjacent to the optical canal, surgery is always indicated to avoid extension toward the optic tract and midline. Finally, the use of Simpson's[6] grading for the extent of tumor removal should be standardized in every surgical protocol.

Indications for Alternative Therapies

The cavernous sinus is for us an important landmark. We consider postoperative diplopia a major deficit; thus we recommend stopping surgery when it is obviously impossible to achieve a total removal without injuring the internal carotid artery or the cranial nerves. In that situation, we advise stereotactic radiosurgery on the small tumoral remnant. Few patients have a long follow-up after radiosurgery, but until now we haven't observed any progression of the disease after more than 5 years' follow-up in several cases monitored annually by MRI. In recurrent meningiomas, we are testing new chemotherapy protocols when a new surgery seems hazardous. It is too early to draw any conclusion or make any suggestions in this area, but this technique should be kept in mind for the future.

Indications for Specific Approaches

Neuronavigation techniques are promising in sphenoid wing meningiomas as in other skull base tumors because of the fixed bony landmarks and the technique's safety in localizing the carotid artery and its major branches, especially when they are encased by the tumor. Image-guided neurosurgery has become routinely used in the treatment of these tumors, allowing the introduction of precise anatomical landmarks in the preoperative three-dimensional (3D) planning.

◆ Preparation

What Must We Know before Surgery and What Workup Do We Use?

Decisions regarding treatment of sphenoid wing meningiomas are often difficult to make.[7]

Several questions should be raised and answered before planning surgery[8]:

- *Is it a meningioma?* Special attention should be paid to bony structures on computed tomography (CT) or MRI. If the anterior clinoid process in particular is missing, a lytic malignant tumor such as a metastasis or a chordoma may be suspected. A preoperative CT scan with bony windows is therefore useful to check whether the bone is hyperostotic or eroded.
- *What blood supply exists for the tumor?* The tumor may be vascularized by external carotid artery branches only, by the internal carotid artery only, or by both. Angiography remains necessary to depict the tumor's vascularity and blood supply and to determine the accuracy of preoperative embolization.
- *What are the meningioma/arteries and veins relationships?* The internal carotid artery and its branches may be displaced, stretched, or encased. The precise anatomy of arteries and veins (including the dominant and collateral veins) is important to know to reduce the risk of perioperative injury. Today, the best tools showing the vessels inside and around the meningioma are MRI and MR angiography (MRA), which provide great safety for surgical dissection **(Figs. 51–2** and **51–3).**
- *What are the tumor limits and dural invasion?* The dural invasion may be very extensive in en plaque meningiomas (our B and C groups[2–4]). Gadolinium-enhanced MRI is the best way to see the tumor limits and dural invasion. However, dural enhancement doesn't necessarily mean invasion but is highly suggestive. Nevertheless, resection of enhanced dura is mandatory to lessen the risk of recurrence.
- *What is the extent of skull base and craniofacial cavities invasion?* It is very important to know whether the tumor invades the pterygomaxillary fossa, parapharyngeal space, and eustachian tube. Indeed, the long-term prognosis of meningiomas in terms of recurrence is closely correlated to the degree of tumor removal. One therefore should aim to achieve gross total removal of Simpson grade I or II. These types of resection include resection of the involved dura by a wide margin and bone. It is also important to assess the extent of bone invasion because hyperostotic bone means invaded bone. Coronal sections (CT scan and MRI) are the best tools to study the extent of the meningioma into the skull base and through craniofacial cavities. Furthermore, one should pay attention to the risk of cerebrospinal fluid (CSF) leakage when ethmoidal or sphenoidal sinuses must be opened during surgery. Finally, penetration downward must be observed by the surgeon to avoid catastrophic situations.
- *Are the optic nerves and tract concerned?* It is of great benefit to know before surgery the potential contact between the meningioma and the optic nerves to avoid visual postoperative sequelae. In clinoidal meningiomas (group A), as in groups B and C, a neuro-ophthalmological examination is mandatory before surgery. A tumoral extension to the optic canal, however, may exist without any clinical deficit. One should be able to see it on coronal MRI views and then make the appropriate intraoperative decisions.
- *Is the pituitary stalk involved?* It may be encountered in juxtasellar meningiomas. Therefore, an endocrinological workup is also mandatory. However, normal endocrine parameters do not exclude a surgical adherence of the pituitary stalk to the tumor.

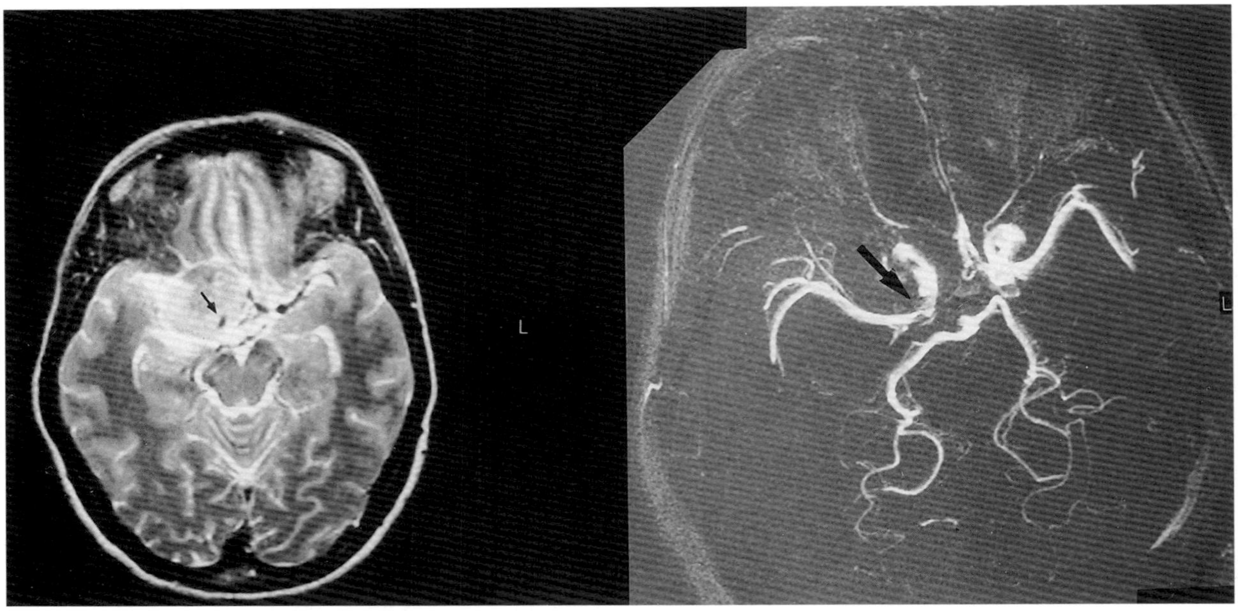

Figure 51–2 Type C sphenoid wing meningioma. Axial magnetic resonance imaging shows internal carotid and sylvian arteries encased in and around the tumor (arrows).

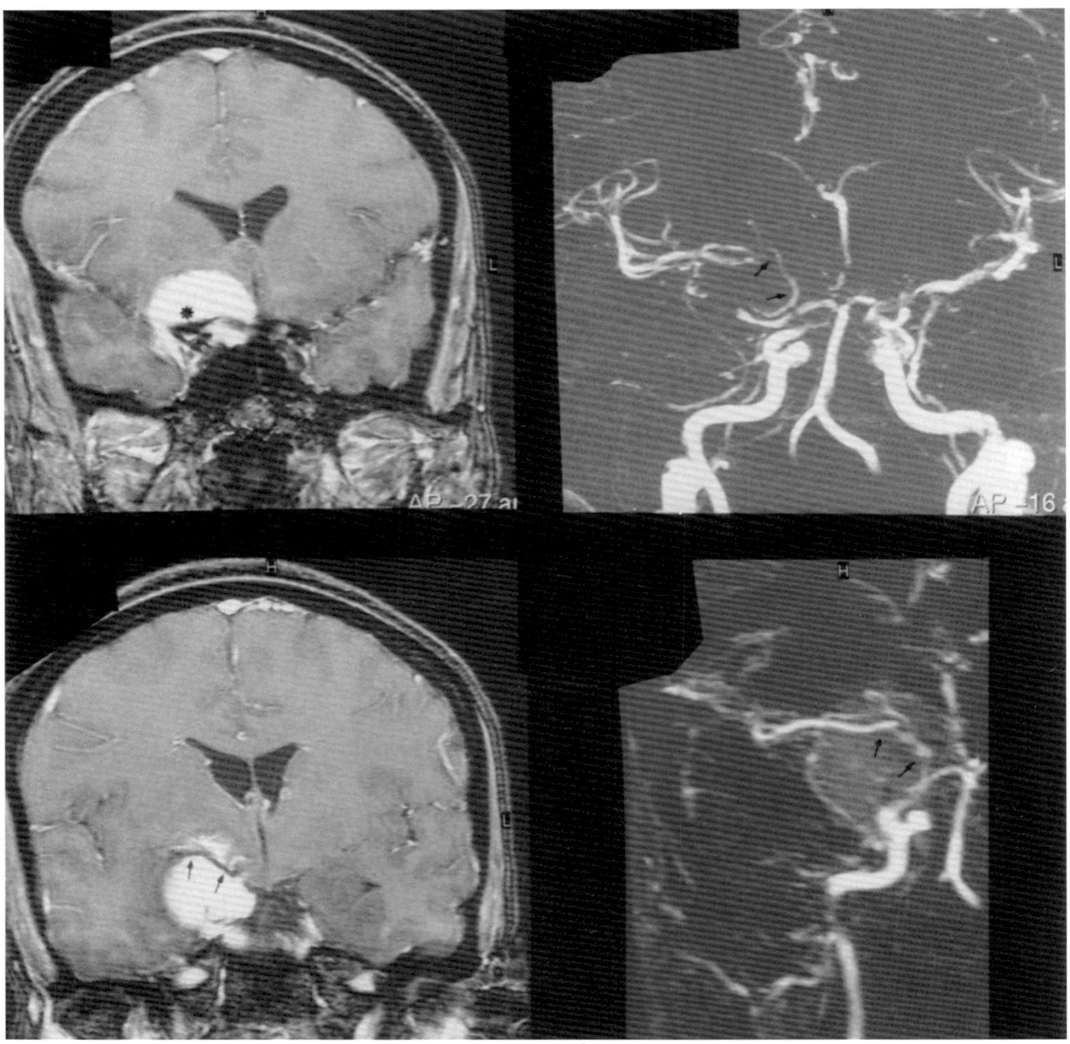

Figure 51–3 Type C sphenoid wing meningioma. Coronal magnetic resonance imaging and magnetic resonance angiography views showing bone structures and sylvian artery encased in and around the tumor (arrows).

- *Why is exophthalmia present?* Exophthalmia may be due to bony hyperostosis, orbital invasion by the meningioma, or cavernous sinus involvement. It is very important to determine if the cavernous sinus is involved and to remember that its tumoral invasion may be encountered without any cranial nerve deficit. One must determine before surgery the cause of the exophthalmia. Coronal MRI views are essential.
- *Why is diplopia present?* The two major causes of diplopia are orbital and cavernous sinus invasion. But sometimes diplopia may be due to a herniated tumoral bud into the posterior fossa between the upper brain stem and the tentorial free edge. In such a situation, the third and the fourth cranial nerves may be sticking to the tumor. Frontal, axial, and coronal MRI views are essential in the preoperative planning. Careful dissection must avoid nerve rupture, which can happen if the tumor is strongly mobilized.

In summary, in all cases of sphenoid wing meningiomas, the preoperative planning requires a CT scan with bony windows, a three-plane gadolinium-enhanced MRI, an MRA, and internal/external carotid artery angiography. In juxtasellar insertion, we like to perform a neuro-ophthalmological and endocrinological workup. The question of a preoperative embolization should be raised in all cases and performed when branches feeding the tumor arise from the external carotid system.

◆ Surgical Technique

Anesthesia

Patients are anesthetized using intravenous pentothal, sufentanil, and cis-atracurium. After endotracheal intubation anesthesia is maintained followed by Isoflurane. Venous and arterial pressures are monitored with a central venous jugular or subclavicular catheter and a radial artery catheter.

When starting the anesthesia, patients receive intravenously an antiepileptic cover (diphenylhydantoin 1 g), antibiotics (cefazolin 2 g), and glucocorticoids (Solu-Medrol 40 mg) to reduce postoperative risk of seizure, meningitis, and brain edema. Two doses of Solu-Medrol 40 mg are administered further during the duration of surgery. Perioperative mannitol delivery and lumbar CSF drainage are performed only after dural opening.

Neurophysiological Monitoring

Perioperative neurophysiological monitoring is not mandatory for sphenoid wing meningioma surgery. However, electromyographic (EMG) monitoring with electrodes directly inserted into the lateral rectus, superior rectus, and superior oblique muscles may be helpful when the meningioma invades the orbit or has some connection with the third and fourth cranial nerves or the cavernous sinus.

Positioning

The patient lies in the supine position with the head fixed in a Mayfield clamp to secure it from any movement. Except for groups D and E, which are close to convexity, we like to insert a controlled lumbar CSF drainage to help the brain in retraction. In groups A, B, and C, the head is turned ~30 degrees to the opposite side (45 degrees in groups D and E), moderately hyperextended, and elevated from heart level by giving a 20 degree angle to the table. When neuronavigation is used, reference points are registered and the microscope is calibrated at that stage.

The choice of the opening is made according to careful preoperative neuroradiological study.

We prefer a simple, large, pterional flap for most sphenoid wing meningiomas, keeping the frontal sinus intact and allowing us to enter the orbit whose lateral roof and wall are removed, keeping intact the periorbita **(Fig. 51–4)**. When the tumor invades the orbit and the periorbita, we use a pteriono-orbital approach, which can be extended to the zygoma when the meningioma is extending backward to the tentorium **(Fig. 51–5)**.

In the pterional approach, we deflect the skin, galea, pericranium, and muscle in one layer to avoid injury to the frontal branches of the facial nerve **(Fig. 51–6)**. In a pteriono-orbital flap, great care is taken to preserve the supraorbital nerve. When the zygoma has to be sectioned, the superficial and deep layers of the temporalis fascia are incised along the zygomatic arch 10 mm posterior and parallel to the course of the frontal branches of the facial nerve. The arch is then dissected subperiostally and cut. The muscle can be detached from the temporal fossa and retracted downward or kept on the bone flap when we want to keep them both together.

A technical detail concerning the keyhole: it is essential that it opens both the orbit and the cranium. One must see through it the orbital roof separating the periorbita from the frontal dura.

Exposure of the Tumor and Resection

The dura is opened under the microscope in a semicircular fashion centered on the pterion, and CSF is drained by the anesthesiologist on the request of the surgeon only **(Fig. 51–7)**. In groups A to C, the sylvian fissure is opened. Frontal and temporal lobes are separated and gently kept away with a self-retaining retractor. Great care is taken to protect the sylvian veins **(Fig. 51–8)**. We always search for the distal branches of the middle cerebral artery first, which we follow from distal to medial. This is a safe maneuver to find the middle and anterior cerebral arteries and then the internal carotid artery itself. By going straight on the clinoid process, one can injure the carotid artery and the optic nerve. Neuronavigation will perhaps modify this risk, but in the meantime we find it safer to go distally first. The tumor is debulked either with the ultrasonic aspirator or with bipolar cutting or coagulation and scissors when the tumor consistency is hard. Great care must be taken in the vicinity of arteries and nerves when using the ultrasonic aspirator. This instrument doesn't distinguish tumoral, arterial, or neural tissues, contrary to what the surgeon might believe!

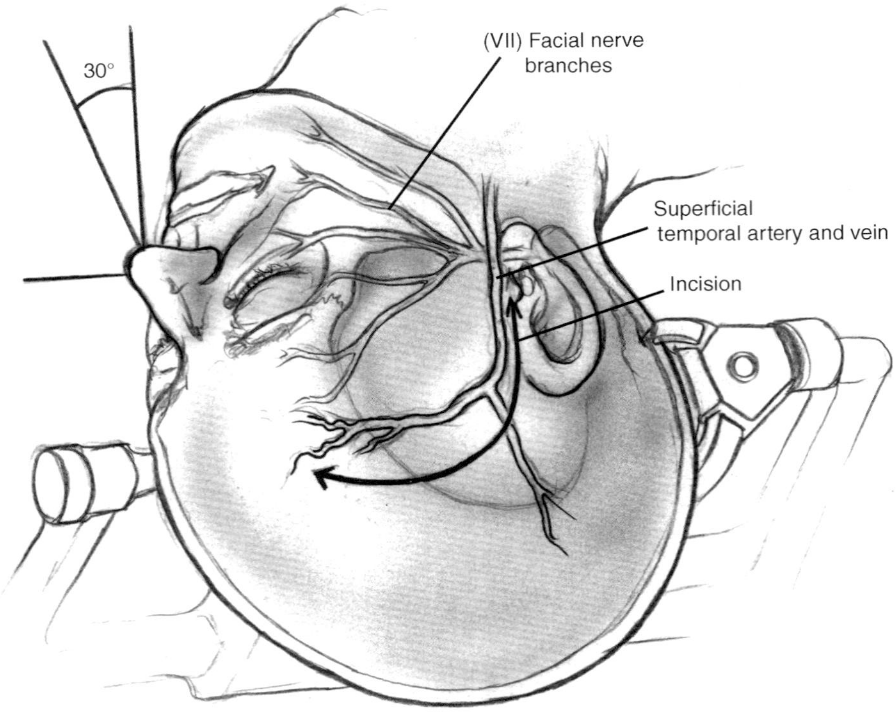

Figure 51–4 The head is slightly hyperextended and turned by 30 degrees from the midline for a right sphenoid wing meningioma. Note the skin incision and the usual location of the supraorbital branch of the facial nerve (VII).

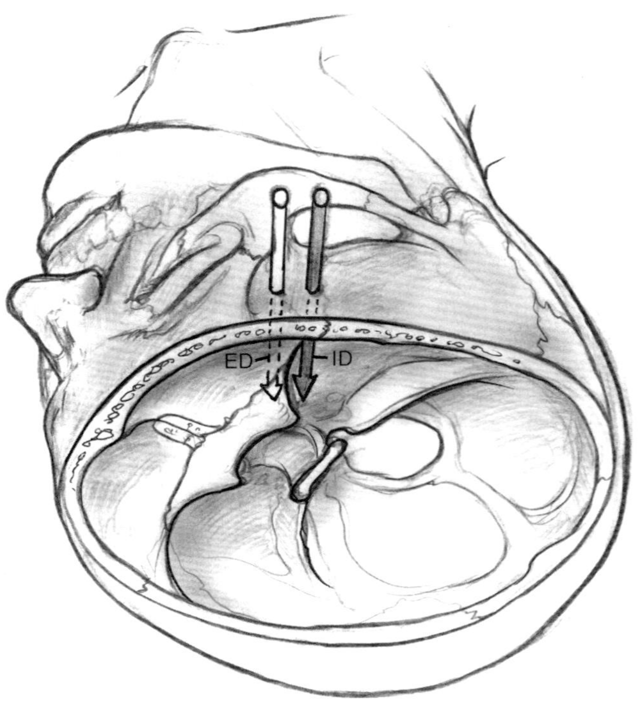

Figure 51–5 Pterional intradural (ID) and extradural (ED) routes for right sphenoid wing meningiomas.

Every small artery must be preserved in that area and dissected. Lenticulostriate arteries may be stretched or encased and are very fragile **(Fig. 51–8).** By following the arteries, the brain is progressively separated from the meningioma, giving access to the optic nerves and tract, which are dissected as the pituitary stalk in medial tumors. We never lose the arachnoidal membranes during dissection. They represent the best natural protection for arteries and cranial nerves and are very useful for separating the third cranial nerve, the posterior communicating artery, and anterior thalamic or lenticulostriate perforators.

When the tumor mass has been removed, the invaded dura and bone are resected **(Fig. 51–9).** We stop close to the cavernous sinus whose lateral and superior walls are often superficially involved. It is possible to peel these walls and to achieve complete tumor removal with cautious bipolar coagulation. The last problem is bone and orbital invasion.

The whole hyperostotic bone should be removed from the pterion to the sphenoid body by opening the foramen rotundum, the foramen ovale, and the sphenoid fissure whenever necessary. The use of high-speed drills with diamond burs and irrigation is recommended. One should be very cautious with Zinn's common tendinous ring, whose removal compromises the ocular mobility and stability. The supraorbital rim and orbital roof may be removed, and the optic canal opened. In clinoidal (group A) and in large invading (group C) meningiomas, the anterior clinoidal process

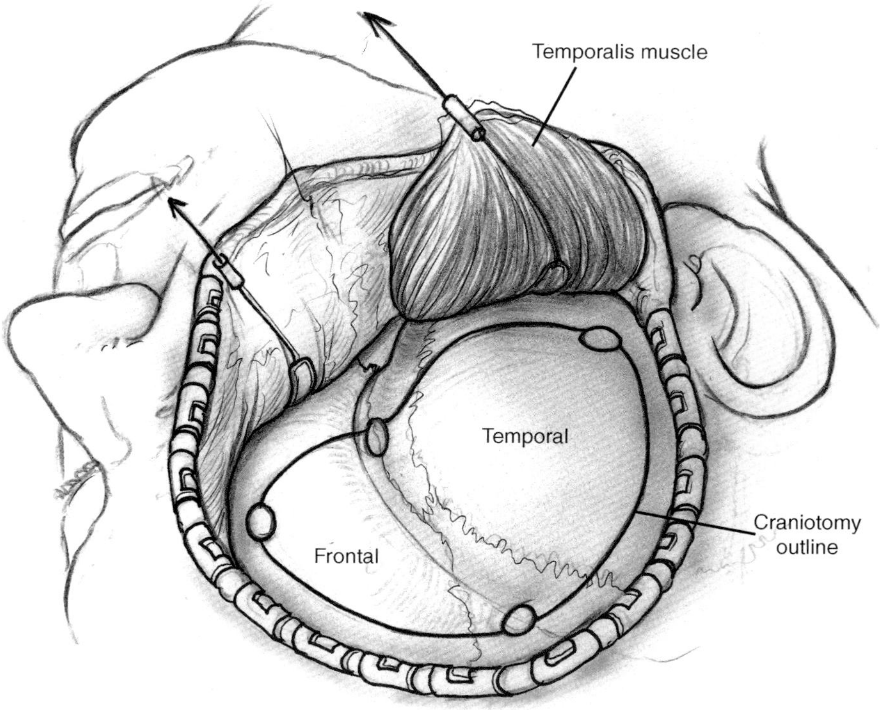

Figure 51–6 Bone opening for right pterional approach.

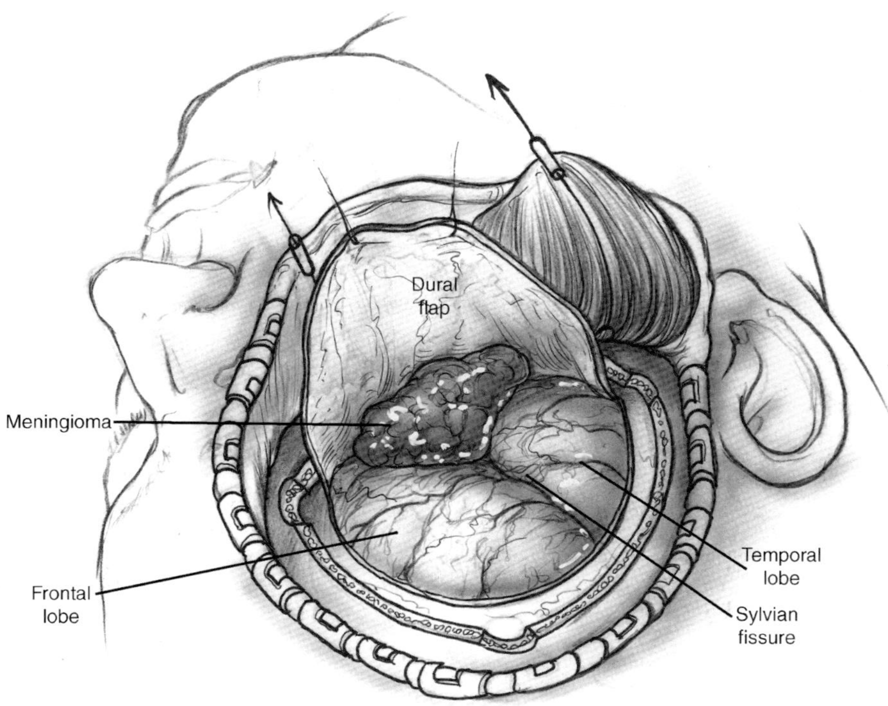

Figure 51–7 After extradural drilling of the right sphenoid wing (not shown), the U-shaped opening of the dura shows the lateral portion of the meningioma.

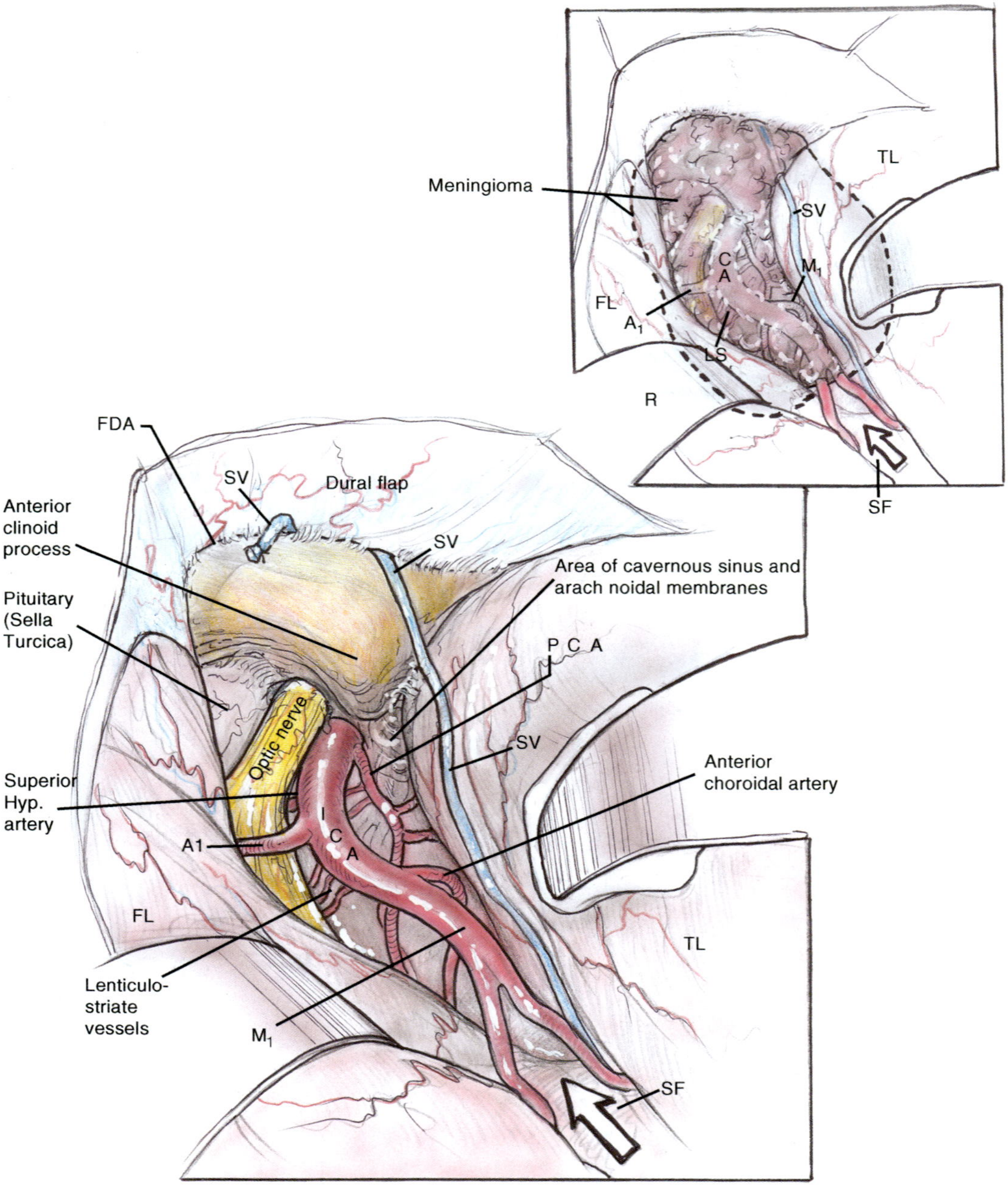

Figure 51–8 Starting dissection of a type C meningioma: retraction (R) of the frontal and temporal lobes (FL, TL), conservation of the sylvian veins (SV), opening the sylvian fissures (SF) from distal to proximal (arrow), following the distal sylvian arterial branches to the M1 segment, lenticulostriates (LS), internal carotid artery (ICA), anterior cerebral artery (A1). FDA, feeding dural arteries.

must be removed because it is very often the starting point of recurrence. When the tumor spreads into the lower part of the orbit and the nasoethmoidal cells, a second operation through an anterior approach[9] is a possibility. An alternative is a combined frontotemporal and lateral infratemporal fossa approach to the skull base,[10] or a transmalar or transzygomatic approach through a subciliary incision.[11]

Group D meningiomas are easier to remove. No lumbar CSF drainage is necessary. Indeed, keeping CSF in place makes the subarachnoidal dissection easier. The sylvian fissure is superficially opened. The only difficulty may come from the dural entry point of the sylvian veins into the sphenoparietal sinus. Either preoperative MRA has shown other collateral veins, allowing division of the sylvian vein, or the sylvian vein must be preserved with a

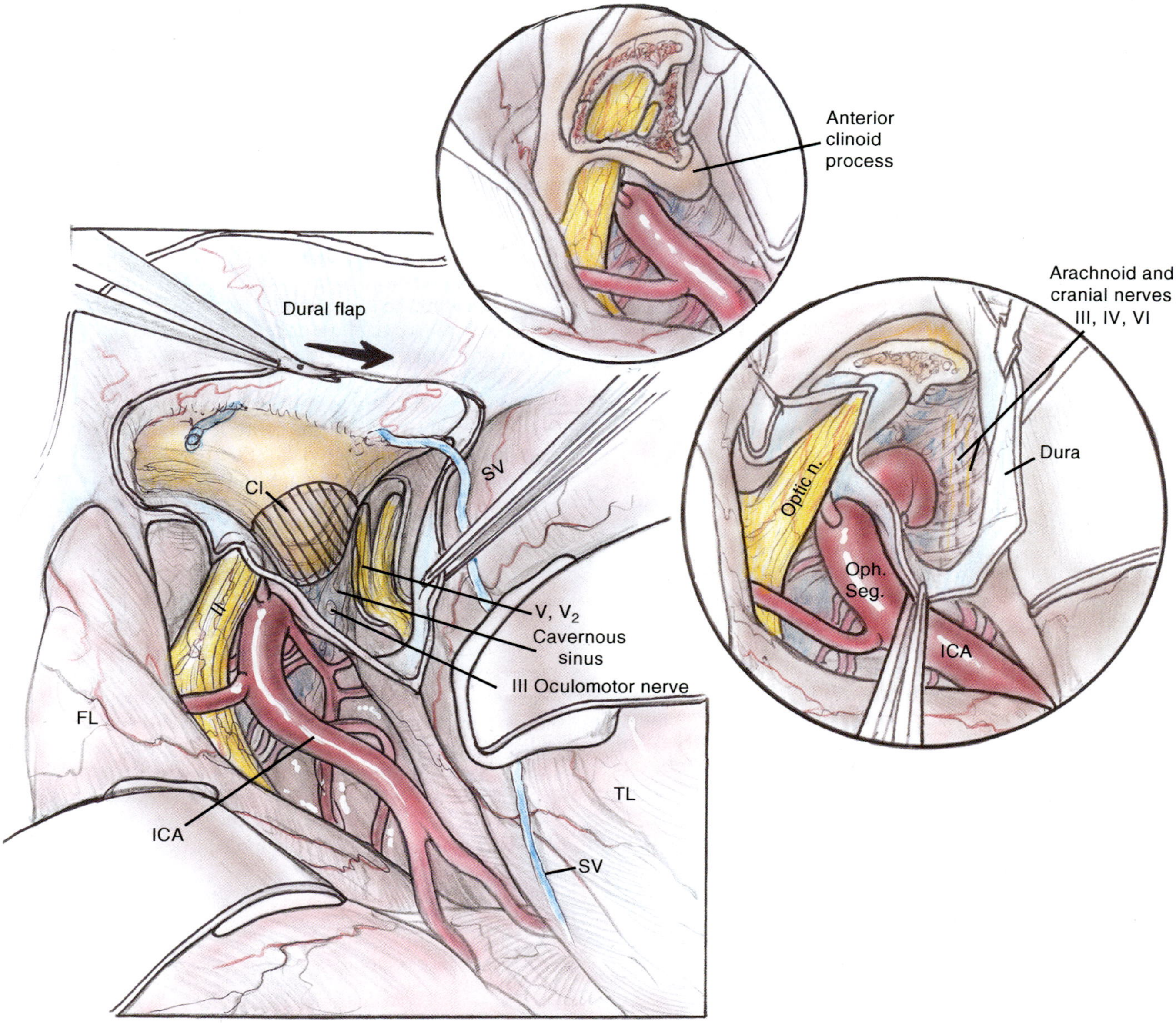

Figure 51–9 After tumor removal, the dural implantation of a type C meningioma including the anterior clinoid process (CL), needs to be resected. The use of dissectors, curettes, drills (for the CL), and scissors is required, alternating with an extradural view (arrow) by mobilizing the dural flap. The insertion of the sylvian vein (SV) is conserved. The common oculomotor nerve (III) and cavernous sinus are neighboring this area. FL, frontal lobe; ICA, internal carotid artery; TL, temporal lobe.

piece of dura around it, sometimes with a small nub of tumor with it.

In group E, the operation essentially concerns bone, dura, and periorbita. A very wide opening of the roof and lateral wall of the orbit must be made, taking care to keep the periorbita intact. After removal of as much hyperostotic bone as possible with the help of drills, it is possible to open the periorbita. If done earlier, orbital fat will herniate and obscure the surgical space. When involved, the periorbita must be removed, with care taken not to injure the extraocular muscles and Zinn's annulus. Finally, these tumors may sometimes invade maxillary and malar bones and require complex surgery.

Closure and Reconstruction

Closure must be planned before the surgery. But before closing, one should have a very clean operative field, without any bleeding from the skull base. Hemostasis should be meticulous. The dura is sutured in a watertight manner either primarily or with pericranial or fascia lata graft. If the sinus cavities have been opened and if the opening is wide and covered with a sutured dural graft, the cavities should be plugged with muscle or fat. Any potential CSF leakage should be avoided. Bone flap is cosmetically replaced using either nonresorbable sutures or microplates whose location has been planned before opening the bone. When cut, the zygomatic arch is reattached with microplates. The orbital rim can be nicely reconstructed with either a rib or a piece of split bone flap from the convexity. The temporal muscle is sutured to the fascia at the orbital rim and along the temporal bone when separated from the skin. Otherwise, it is sutured at its posterior margin only and the skin is closed in two layers.

◆ Postoperative Care

The patient should be monitored in the intensive care unit for a minimum of 24 hours. During the first postoperative day, we usually perform a CT scan to look for postoperative clots or pneumocephalus. When the main arteries have been dissected, ultrasonic Doppler is performed daily during the first week for prediction of vasospasm. Corticosteroids are prescribed for 8 to 10 days.

◆ Complications

One of the main risks is overlooking some important preoperative information regarding the extension of the tumor and its connection with cranial nerves and vessels. That can be avoided by a meticulous clinical and radiological preoperative evaluation. If the opening is not adapted to the type of meningioma, removal will be hazardous.

Every detail is important, starting with the skin opening, which must preserve the branches of the facial nerve. Bad cosmetic results may happen with bone removal without repair. However, it is mandatory to remove all the hyperostotic bone to protect against recurrence. So frontal, pterional, facial, and orbital repair is often necessary. Don't hesitate to collaborate with surgeons who specialize in cosmetic correction. A CSF fistula may lead to meningitis and may compromise a superb surgery. Be meticulous in sinus plugging and dural repair.

Accessing the sphenoid wings requires some surgical space, which can be achieved by making a sufficient basal bone opening, by putting the patient's head in the right position, by CSF drainage, and by opening the sylvian fissure. The greatest enemy of the neurosurgeon is the brain retractor, which may cause extended neurological deficits. A postoperative diplopia is a major handicap. To avoid it, great care must be taken with third and fourth cranial nerve dissection, as with the cavernous sinus. A postoperative loss of vision is highly disabling. Don't place a retractor on the optic nerve. Place it slightly on the carotid artery. Pay attention when drilling the optic canal. Use copious irrigation to prevent thermal injury to the nerve.

A motor deficit may occur if anterior thalamic or lenticulostriate arteries are injured. Be sure that the vessel is going to the meningioma only before coagulating and dividing it. This is not easy with stretched or encased vessels. Patience is our best ally.

◆ Conclusion

The best treatment of sphenoid wing meningiomas is radical surgery, with meticulous dissection of shifted, stretched, or encased vessels, as of cranial nerves. Total removal (meningioma, dura, and bone) should be the aim of the first surgery. Indeed, if several surgical procedures are considered, one should be aware that the dissection of vessels, nerves, and orbital content becomes more difficult with every new operation. Thus it is important to plan the surgery carefully with a very complete preoperative workup.

References

1. Cushing H, Eisenhardt L. Meningiomas: Their Classification, Regional Behaviour, Life History and Surgical Results. Springfield, IL: Charles C Thomas; 1938
2. Bonnal J, Thibaut A, Brotchi J, Born J. Invading meningiomas of the sphenoid ridge[CR5]. J Neurosurg 1980;53:587–599
3. Bonnal J, Brotchi J, Born J. Meningiomas of the sphenoid wings. In: Sekhar LN, Schramm VL Jr, eds. Tumors of the Cranial Base: Diagnosis and Treatment. Mount Kisco, NY: Futura; 1987:373–392
4. Brotchi J, Bonnal J. Lateral and middle sphenoid wing meningiomas. In: Al-Mefty O, ed. Meningiomas. New York: Raven; 1991: 413–425
5. Al-Mefty O. Clinoidal meningiomas. J Neurosurg 1990;73:840–849
6. Simpson D. The recurrence of intracranial meningiomas after surgical treatment. J Neurol Neurosurg Psychiatry 1957;20:22–39
7. Ojemann RG. Meningiomas: clinical features and surgical management. In: Wilkins RH, Rengachary SS, eds. Neurosurgery. New York: McGraw-Hill; 1985:635–654
8. Brotchi J, Levivier M, Raftopoulos C, Noteran J. Invading meningiomas of sphenoid wings: what must we know before surgery? Acta Neurochir Suppl (Wien) 1991;98–100
9. Derome PJ, Guiot G. Bone problems in meningiomas invading the base of the skull. Clin Neurosurg 1978;25:435–451
10. Mickey B, Close L, Schaffer S, Sanson D. A combined fronto-temporal and lateral infratemporal fossa approach to the skull base. J Neurosurg 1988;68:678–684
11. Basso AJ, Carrizo A. Sphenoid ridge meningiomas. In: Schmiedek HH, ed. Meningiomas and Their Surgical Management. Philadelphia: WB Saunders; 1991:233–241

52

Cavernous Sinus Tumors

Christopher Bogaev and Laligam N. Sekhar

The cavernous sinus remains one of the most challenging anatomical regions of the cranial base. For many years, lesions in the cavernous sinus were considered inoperable because of the risk of injury to the cavernous carotid artery and cranial nerves traversing this small but complex space. Advances in neuroanatomy, neuroimaging, and microsurgical techniques have only recently made surgery of these lesions possible with acceptable morbidity. Cavernous sinus tumor surgery requires the surgeon to be an expert in microsurgical techniques and to have a detailed and practical knowledge of the relevant anatomy. The advent of radiosurgery has caused a reevaluation of surgical indications and strategies, which remain controversial. This chapter focuses on the surgical aspects of treating cavernous sinus tumors.

◆ Anatomy

The term *cavernous sinus* is commonly used, but this entity has been more accurately termed the lateral sellar compartment in that the veins are neither cavernous nor a true dural sinus, but are complex and multiple and are a segment of the extradural neural axis compartment.[1] The term *cavernous sinus* is used in this chapter because of its common usage. The overall schema of the cavernous sinus is a truncated pyramid whose base faces the posterior fossa (petrous apex) and whose apex faces the orbital apex (superior orbital fissure). This results in a lateral, superior, medial, anterior, posterior, and inferior surface, with all of the surgical approaches to the cavernous sinus being through one of these surfaces **(Fig. 52–1)**.

Dural Layers

The lateral wall of the cavernous sinus consists of two layers of dura. The inner dural layer is continuous with the periosteum of the temporal, clival, and sphenoid bones and is partially formed by the epineurium of cranial nerves (CN) III, IV, and V. The thicker outer layer is continuous with the dura of the middle fossa, the tentorium, and the outer layer of the clival dura. Proximal and distal dural rings demarcate the clinoidal segment of the internal carotid artery (ICA). These rings fuse medially and are separated by the anterior clinoid process (ACP) laterally. The distal dural ring is continuous with the outer layer of the lateral wall of the cavernous sinus, and the proximal ring (carotico-oculomotor membrane) is continuous with the inner layer of the lateral wall.[1] The proximal dural ring forms the roof of the cavernous sinus.[3] The cavernous venous plexus can variably extend around the clinoidal ICA, making the clinoidal ICA variably intra- or extracavernous.[4] In addition, there is a third fibrous ring around the cavernous ICA that consists of a periosteal ring at the entrance of the petrous ICA into the cavernous sinus.

The medial wall of the cavernous sinus is continuous with the dura of the floor of the sella and the inner layer of the dura of the clivus. The medial aspect of the cavernous sinus is covered by a thin rim of bone formed by the lateral wall of the sphenoid sinus. The anterior loop of the cavernous ICA produces an impression in the bone of the sphenoid sinus that is known as the carotid prominence.[3]

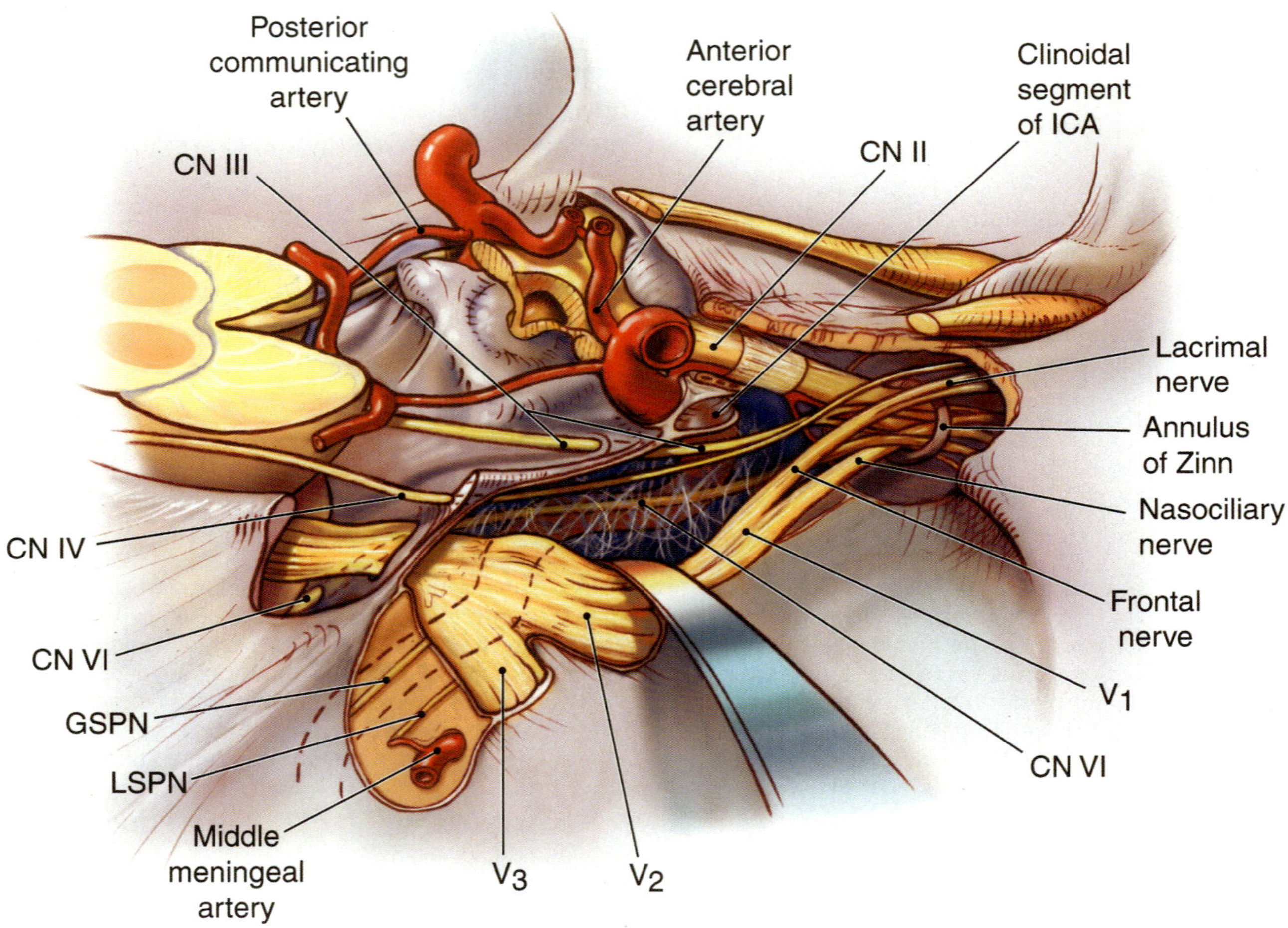

Figure 52–1 Anatomy of the right parasellar region including the cavernous sinus. CN, cranial nerve; GSPN, greater superficial petrosal nerve; ICA, internal carotid artery; LSPN, lesser superficial petrosal nerve.

Cavernous Internal Carotid Artery

Various nomenclatures have been used to describe the segments of the cavernous ICA. For the purposes of this chapter, the following descriptive terms are used to describe the segments of the cavernous ICA beginning with the periosteal fibrous ring at the junction with the petrous ICA and continuing distally:

- Trigeminal segment (junctional segment with petrous ICA covered by trigeminal ganglion and root)
  - Posterior vertical segment
  - Posterior bend
  - Horizontal segment
  - Anterior bend
  - Anterior vertical segment
  - Clinoidal segment (delineated by the proximal and distal dural rings)

The cavernous ICA has two consistent branches (the meningohypophyseal trunk and the inferolateral trunk), as well as other more variable branches:

- Meningohypophyseal trunk—usually arises between the posterior vertical and horizontal segments of the ICA.[3] Divides into:
  - Tentorial artery (Bernasconi-Cassinari)
  - Dorsal meningeal artery (supplying the clival dura)
  - Inferior hypophyseal artery
- Inferolateral trunk (lateral main stem artery[2])—arises from the inferolateral aspect of the horizontal segment of the ICA and passes over CN VI.[3] Divides into[9]:
  - Anterolateral branch following V2
  - Anteromedial branch supplying CN III, IV, V1, and VI near the superior orbital fissure
  - Posterior branch following V3 through the foramen ovale
  - Superior branch usually anastomosing with the tentorial artery
- Capsular arteries of McConnell—usually arise from the distal horizontal segment of the ICA. Present on only ~30% of anatomical dissections.[5]
- Ophthalmic artery—approximately 3% to 8% of cases have an intracavernous origin or originate from the clinoidal segment of the ICA.[2,3]

Cranial Nerves of the Cavernous Sinus

Cranial nerves III, IV, V1, and V2 course between the two dural leaves of the lateral wall of the cavernous sinus. Only CN VI and the sympathetic nerve fibers run within the cavernous sinus.

CN III: enters the roof of the cavernous sinus lateral to the posterior clinoid process and acquires a sheath of dura in the lateral part of the anterior petroclinoid fold.[2] It continues in the lateral wall of the cavernous sinus and exits through the superior orbital fissure (SOF).

CN IV: enters the tentorial edge lateral to the cerebral peduncle and courses in a groove on the undersurface of the tentorium before entering its dural canal in the tentorium.[1] The trochlear nerve then runs in the lateral wall of the cavernous sinus inferior to CN III until it crosses over CN III about 5 to 7 mm posterior to the bony margin of the SOF to assume a medial position in the apex of the orbit.

Ophthalmic division of CN V: travels in the lateral wall of the cavernous sinus to the SOF. The triangular space formed by CN IV, V1, and the fold of dura between them is Parkinson's triangle.[2]

Maxillary division of CN V: courses in the lateral wall of the cavernous sinus inferior to V1 to the foramen rotundum.

CN VI: has a cisternal segment, a clival segment, a cavernous segment, and an orbital segment. It pierces the dura of the clivus and courses several millimeters inside the basilar venous plexus before passing through Dorello's canal into the cavernous sinus.[3] The roof of Dorello's canal is mainly formed by the petroclinoid ligament, which extends from the petrous apex to the posterior clinoid process and dorsum sellae.[3] Once the abducens nerve has entered the cavernous sinus, it runs lateral to the posterior vertical segment of the ICA and then inferolateral to the horizontal segment prior to its exit through the SOF. The posterior part of CN VI travels medial to the trigeminal root and Meckel's cave, but in the anterior cavernous sinus CN VI lies inferior and medial to V1 near the orbital apex, eventually becoming the most lateral nerve inside the annulus of Zinn.[3]

Cavernous Sinus Venous Spaces

The sizes and shapes of the cavernous sinus venous spaces vary depending on the exact course of the cavernous ICA. They are generally divided into four main areas:

Lateral venous space: between the cavernous ICA and the lateral wall of the cavernous sinus.[3]

Medial venous space: between the cavernous ICA and the sella.[3]

Posterior venous space: below the roof of the cavernous sinus, but superior to the posterior vertical and horizontal segments of the ICA.[3]

Anterior venous space: a narrow space located posterior to the SOF and anterior to the anterior bend and anterior vertical segments of the cavernous ICA.[3]

The cavernous sinuses communicate via the anterior and posterior intercavernous sinuses within the sella. The largest anastomosis between the two cavernous sinuses is the basilar venous plexus, which lies between the two leaves of the clival dura. Other venous connections to the cavernous sinus include the superior and inferior ophthalmic veins, the pterygoid plexus, and the superior and inferior petrosal sinuses.

◆ Classification of Cavernous Sinus Tumors

Tumors involving the cavernous sinus can be classified according to tumor pathology, biological behavior, tumor extension and size, or extent of involvement of the cavernous sinus and cavernous ICA. The following classification schemes are listed in order of increasing complexity, but are all useful, particularly when applied together:

Tumor Extension and Size[6]

Confined tumors: those < 2.5 cm in diameter and predominantly confined to the cavernous sinus and surrounding areas (such as petrous apex, tentorial notch, sella, or middle cranial fossa).

Extensive tumors: those ≥ 2.5 cm in diameter that extend into multiple regions (e.g., petroclival meningioma extending into the cavernous sinus).

Biological Behavior

- Benign: meningioma
- Nonmeningioma: trigeminal schwannoma
  - Pituitary adenoma
  - Cavernous hemangioma (although vascular malformations, they behave as tumors)
- Slow-growing malignant: chondrosarcoma
  - Chordoma
  - Hemangiopericytoma
  - Adenoid cystic carcinoma (which can be fast growing)
- Fast-growing malignant: squamous cell carcinoma
  - Adenocarcinoma

Extent of Cavernous Sinus and Internal Carotid Artery Involvement[6]

Grade	Cavernous Sinus Involvement	Cavernous ICA
I	One area only (anterior, posterior, lateral, or medial cavernous sinus)	Not involved
II	More than one area	Displaced, not encased
III	Entire cavernous sinus	Totally encased (at least a short segment)
IV	Entire cavernous sinus	Encased with narrowing, pseudoaneurysm, or occlusion
V	Bilateral cavernous sinuses	Encased

◆ Indications for Surgery

Meningiomas

- Progressive growth on serial imaging
- Progression of cranial nerve deficits
- Possibility of total resection or subtotal resection followed by stereotactic radiosurgery of a small remnant
- Higher threshold for surgery for grades III, IV, and V tumors[7]
- Meningioma originating outside the cavernous sinus and secondarily involving it (e.g., petroclival, Meckel's cave, or clinoidal meningiomas) are easier to resect completely than those originating from within the cavernous sinus.[7]
- Meningiomas that completely infiltrate the cavernous sinus are impossible to completely resect without resection of the cavernous ICA.[7]

Other Benign Tumors

- Trigeminal schwannomas, epidermoids, pituitary adenomas, cavernous hemangiomas, and other benign tumors involving the cavernous sinus are easier to resect than meningiomas, and removal of the cavernous sinus extension should be performed at the time of primary resection in order to obtain a possible cure.[7]

The carotid is more often displaced than encased in these cases and can usually be dissected free from the tumor.

Chordoma and Chondrosarcoma

- Usually fairly straightforward to remove from the cavernous sinus, and extension into the cavernous sinus should not prevent their total excision if it is otherwise possible (even if bilateral cavernous sinuses are involved).[7]
- Because cavernous sinus involvement in these cases represents secondary extensions, it is usually straightforward to dissect the cranial nerves and ICA from tumor.

Other Malignant Tumors

- Because these tumors are usually removed en bloc for an oncologic resection, all other parts of the tumor must be resectable in order to justify radical surgery.[7]
- The cavernous ICA may need to be resected and replaced with a vein graft in selected cases.[6]

- Surgery remains controversial for high-grade lesions.
- Bilateral cavernous sinus involvement is a contraindication to surgery.

Preoperative Studies

Head Computed Tomography

- Bone windows are useful to determine extent of bony destruction by the tumor as well as hyperostosis (axial and coronal images helpful).
- Bone windows are helpful for normal bony anatomy for surgical planning (e.g., degree of pneumatization of the anterior clinoid process).
- Bone windows are useful to assess for tumor calcification.

Brain Magnetic Resonance Imaging

- Best screening procedure for cavernous sinus tumors (particularly the axial and coronal planes); significantly more sensitive than computed tomography (CT)
- The magnetic resonance imaging (MRI) signal characteristics are very helpful in determining the tumor type (e.g., chondrosarcoma and schwannoma have intermediate T1 signal and high T2 signal; hemangioma brightly enhances with gadolinium). The signal characteristics coupled with the location and pattern of tumor extension can often determine the diagnosis preoperatively.
- Contrasted study in multiple planes best shows the relationship of the tumor to surrounding structures, including intradural extension or the presence of a dural tail.
- Flow voids can reveal locations of critical vascular structures such as the cavernous carotid artery or supraclinoid carotid artery and can show displacement or encasement of these vessels. Irregular appearance of a flow void could represent vascular invasion by tumor.
- T2-weighted images are most useful for assessing the integrity of the arachnoid plane around the tumor as well as the extent of surrounding brain edema present.

Cerebral Angiography

- Determines vascularity of tumor as well as its blood supply
- Can allow for embolization if needed
- Defines exact nature and origin of vascular lesions
- Defines degree of involvement of ICA with accurate demonstration of ICA stenosis or occlusion; irregularity of vessel walls more sensitive indicator of vessel wall invasion than MRI appearance
- Can reveal coexisting vascular pathology that can affect operative decision making
- Allows for balloon test occlusion (BTO) (particularly important for tumor grades III, IV, and V):
  - 15-minute occlusion—the contralateral ICA, ipsilateral common carotid, and bilateral vertebral arteries are injected to evaluate collateral blood flow.
  - Value of the test is mainly for temporary occlusion tolerance—carotid reconstruction is preferred for all younger patients with benign or low-grade malignant tumors who undergo carotid resection.[6] Tolerance to temporary occlusion may influence the revascularization technique (see cerebral revascularization chapter).
- Reasons for carotid bypass after carotid resection include delayed ischemic complications, de novo contralateral aneurysm formation, growth or rupture of existing contralateral aneurysms, and the possibility of cavernous sinus tumors eventually involving the contralateral cavernous sinus.[7]

Xenon Computed Tomography/Single Photon Emission Computed Tomography

- Balloon occlusion test (BOT) alone may not detect patients at risk for delayed ischemia.
- BOT combined with xenon CT or SPECT can help screen for these patients. A cerebral blood flow (CBF) study is performed during and after ICA balloon occlusion:
- No change in exam or CBF during occlusion (CBF > 35 mL/100 g/min)(~75% of patients) = low risk[7]
- No change in exam but decreased blood flow (CBF 10–35 mL/100 g/min)(~15% of patients) = intermediate risk[7]
- Neurological deficits during test occlusion (~10% of patients) = high riskal[7]
- CBF studies not performed as commonly due to universal surgical revascularization after carotid resection in young patients with benign or low-grade malignant tumors

Overview of Cavernous Sinus Approaches

Extradural Approaches

Inferior approach: A frontotemporal-infratemporal exposure is followed by exposure of the petrous ICA, which is traced superiorly into the cavernous sinus.[8] The inferior surface can also be exposed by the transmaxillary approach.[8]

Anterolateral approach: A frontotemporal craniotomy with an orbitozygomatic osteotomy is followed by extradural exposure of the superior orbital fissure and V2. The medial temporal dura is dissected from the dura of the lateral wall of the cavernous sinus, and the tumor is followed into the cavernous sinus.[8]

Medial approach: This approach is performed through the sphenoid sinus by either a transsphenoidal or an extended transbasal approach.

Intradural Approaches

Superior approach: This approach provides good exposure of the region superior and medial to the horizontal portion of the cavernous ICA. It provides good exposure of the anterior bend, anterior vertical and clinoidal segments of the ICA, as well as the sella.[7] This approach is usually performed via a frontotemporal craniotomy with an orbitozygomatic osteotomy, anterior clinoidectomy, unroofing of the optic canal, opening of the dura propria of the optic nerve, and opening of the proximal and distal dural rings of the clinoidal ICA.

Lateral approach: For chordomas, chondrosarcomas, or schwannomas extending into the cavernous sinus, a longitudinal incision is made in the lateral wall over the most prominent part of the tumor,[8] so the lateral wall is opened in a limited area. For meningiomas lateral and inferior to the cavernous ICA, the lateral approach is also used. For extensive meningiomas, a complete dissection of the cavernous sinus is often necessary, sometimes combining the superior and lateral approaches. The initial steps of this approach are the same as for a superior approach, but the outer dural layer of the lateral wall is removed, and the dissection is continued between the cranial nerves of the lateral wall.

◆ Surgical Technique

Anesthesia

Standard general endotracheal tube anesthesia with muscle relaxation is usually given as for most intracranial procedures. Commonly used agents for intracranial surgery include isoflurane, fentanyl, pancuronium, midazolam, and nitrous oxide in combinations customized by the neuroanesthesiologist for the needs of a given patient. Mild to moderate hyperventilation ($PaCO_2 = 30–35$) is often used during the exposure and resection portions of the procedure to facilitate brain relaxation. Mannitol (0.5–1.0 g/kg) is usually administered just prior to initiation of the bone work, also for brain relaxation. If an adequate response is not obtained, intravenous (IV) furosemide (20–40 mg) can potentiate the effects of the mannitol.

For changes on intraoperative monitoring possibly indicating ischemia, usually temporary release or removal of brain retractors or a mild increase in blood pressure will reverse these abnormalities. More extensive cerebral protective measures are usually not needed unless there is vascular encasement or invasion by tumor requiring prolonged temporary clipping or vascular bypass. These additional measures include elevation of the blood pressure 20% above its normal range, mild to moderate hypothermia to ~34°C, mild hemodilution, and finally burst suppression on electroencephalogram (EEG) (usually by the use of thiopental, etomidate, or propofol).[9]

A lumbar drain may be placed when there is not a significant tumor mass in the tentorial notch. Slow drainage of ~50 mL of cerebrospinal fluid (CSF) relaxes the brain and reduces the incidence of dural tears and brain injury during performance of the craniotomy and orbitozygomatic osteotomy. However, rapid drainage of CSF during the initial opening may result in the formation of an acute subdural hematoma.

Intraoperative Monitoring

The most useful neurophysiological intraoperative monitoring for cavernous sinus tumors includes multimodality monitoring common to other cranial base tumor operations:

Somatosensory Evoked Potentials (SEPs)

- Used in virtually all cavernous sinus tumor cases
- Able to detect changes in hemispheric function due to ischemia or from temporal lobe or brain stem retraction[22]
- Upper and lower extremity SEPs are usually monitored.
- Changes in SEP waveforms can be conveyed to the operative team to allow the surgeon to reduce brain retraction or the anesthesiologist to elevate the blood pressure.

Brain Stem Auditory Evoked Responses (BASERs)

- Used as an index of brain stem function
- Usually reserved for larger, more complex cavernous sinus tumors with brain stem or posterior circulation involvement
- Contralateral BASER monitoring most common
- Waveform changes can also indicate ischemia or overly aggressive brain retraction and can be conveyed to the operative team so that appropriate measures can be taken.

Electroencephalogram (EEG)

- Used in virtually all cavernous sinus tumor cases
- Slowing is a sensitive indicator of cortical ischemia.[10]
- Most useful in cases where induction of burst suppression is needed such as during the performance of vascular bypasses

Specific cranial nerve monitoring (e.g., CN III and VI) has been found to be less helpful and is generally not used.[6] As with other cranial base operations, the use of monitoring should be customized according to the individual needs of the patient.

Positioning

The patient is placed in the supine position with the head placed in pins. The patient is firmly secured (taped) to the table with profuse padding to allow significant table

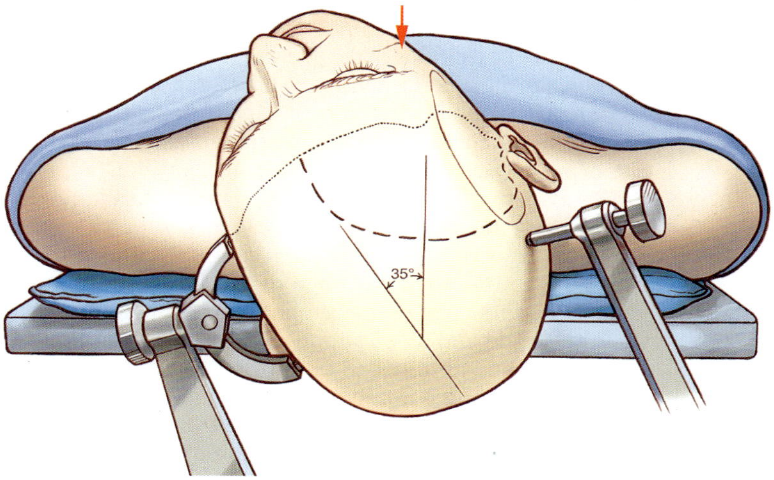

Figure 52–2 Optimum head position for most cavernous sinus tumors: head 35 degrees to the contralateral side with the malar eminence being the highest point.

rotation during the operation. Sequential compression stockings are used to prevent venous stasis. The head is turned ~35 degrees to the opposite side with the head positioned so that the malar eminence is the highest point[1] **(Fig. 52–2).** This maximizes the exposure of the region of the cavernous sinus without compromising venous drainage.

Head depression and elevation during the course of the procedure are usually performed with Trendelenburg or reverse Trendelenburg maneuvers. Flexion at the patient's hip can also be done, but this is usually avoided because flexion at the hip in a patient in pins can change the relationship of the head to the table, resulting in unwanted cervical traction.[11] Careful positioning with the patient firmly secured to the operating table with adequate tape and padding can allow for a significant amount of rotational mobility about the patient's long axis during the procedure.

When the patient is prepped and draped, the lateral thigh or lower abdomen should be included for possible autologous fat or fascial grafts needed during the reconstruction phase of the procedure.

Approach

The operative approach depends on the expected tumor type. The most common approach to the cavernous sinus is a frontotemporal craniotomy with an orbitozygomatic osteotomy. Tumor extensions beyond the cavernous sinus will need modifications of the standard approaches.

Meningiomas

Meningiomas are the most complex and difficult of cavernous sinus tumors. Those that begin outside of the cavernous sinus and secondarily extend into it are much easier to completely resect than primary cavernous sinus meningiomas.

There are three main types of resection of cavernous sinus meningiomas depending on the involvement of the cavernous ICA:

- Non–ICA-encasing
- ICA-encasing with vein graft reconstruction
- ICA-encasing with tailored resection

(Except for selected cases of the third type, cervical ICA exposure is needed. The cervical ICA is used more commonly for proximal control than the petrous carotid for reasons discussed later in the chapter.)

Non–ICA-Encasing Meningiomas

The most common exposure for tumors of this type is a frontotemporal craniotomy with an orbitozygomatic osteotomy (OZO). Extensions beyond the cavernous sinus require modifications, such as possible extension of the frontotemporal craniotomy with an OZO to a one-and-a-half fronto-orbital approach, extension of the OZO to include the condylar fossa, or the addition of a petrosal approach. Most non–ICA-encasing meningiomas are sphenocavernous or medial sphenoid wing tumors originating outside of the cavernous sinus and secondarily extending into it.

Frontotemporal Craniotomy with Orbitozygomatic Osteotomy

A question-mark skin incision is usually made beginning in the skin crease just anterior to the tragus and inferior to the root of the zygoma and extending to the hairline in the midline anteriorly **(Fig. 52–3).** The incision is question-mark–shaped to circumvent the bulk of the temporalis muscle to facilitate its elevation during the next step of the procedure. The incision in the pretragal skin crease is not only more cosmetic but avoids injury to the frontotemporal branch of the facial nerve or the superficial temporal artery.

The pericranium is elevated with the scalp to prevent its desiccation or injury until it is needed for the reconstruction phase of the procedure. Elevation of the scalp and pericranium is continued anteriorly until the superficial temporal fat pad is encountered, at which time an interfascial dissection of the frontotemporal branch of the facial nerve is performed. Because this nerve lies superficial to the superficial fascia of the temporalis muscle, this fascia is

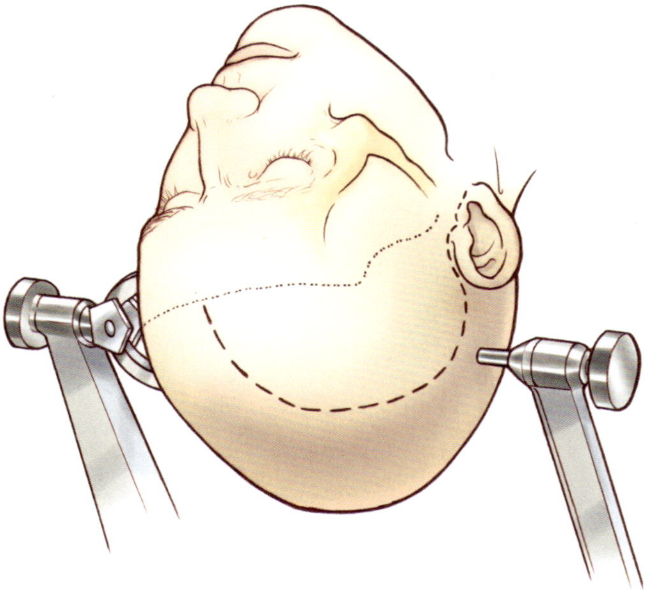

Figure 52–3 Skin incision for a frontotemporal craniotomy with an orbitozygomatic osteotomy.

sharply incised usually ~2 cm posterior to the zygomatic process of the frontal bone[20] and extended from the keyhole anteriorly to the root of the zygoma inferiorly **(Fig. 52–4).** More blunt dissection (usually with a periosteal elevator) is then used to elevate this fascia and fat pad together from the deep temporalis fascia until the lateral orbital rim and superior zygomatic arch are exposed. A periosteal elevator is then used to expose the entire zygomatic arch from its root posteriorly to just inferior to the zygomaticofacial foramen anteriorly. The inferior aspect of the zygomatic arch is freed by sharply incising the masseter muscle along its insertion on the arch. The elevation of the pericranium and scalp is continued down to the superior and lateral orbital rim. If the ipsilateral supraorbital nerve and artery are in a complete foramen instead of a notch, the foramen is opened with a small osteotome on either side of these structures to free them without injury.[13]

The ipsilateral temporalis muscle is then carefully elevated completely with periosteal elevators, with care being taken to preserve the thin fascial layer on the underside of the muscle. The posterior edge of the incision is undermined to avoid cutting the temporalis muscle to preserve its innervation and blood supply. The temporalis muscle is then retracted laterally and inferiorly, providing excellent bony exposure of the frontotemporal region.

The craniotomy and OZO are performed as separate pieces. This allows for a more controlled osteotomy, preserving the necessary two thirds or 2.5 cm of orbital roof to prevent postoperative enophthalmos. In addition, the OZO is sufficiently vascularized by surrounding tissue that it can be left in situ if the craniotomy flap has to be discarded in the event of postoperative epidural abscess.

The craniotomy can be started with bur holes at the keyhole and just above the zygomatic root. A slot is then drilled connecting the first two bur holes using a Midas Rex (Pneomatie Tools, Inc., Fort Worth, TX) M8 or equivalent drill bit that proceeds around the temporal tip and across the root of the sphenoid wing. Dural stripping can then be performed with a Woodson elevator prior to turning the craniotomy flap. The ends of the slot can be made larger if the dura is adherent and difficult to strip. A standard frontotemporal craniotomy flap is then turned with its medial extent approximating the level of the supraorbital notch **(Fig. 52–5).** The residual bone in the

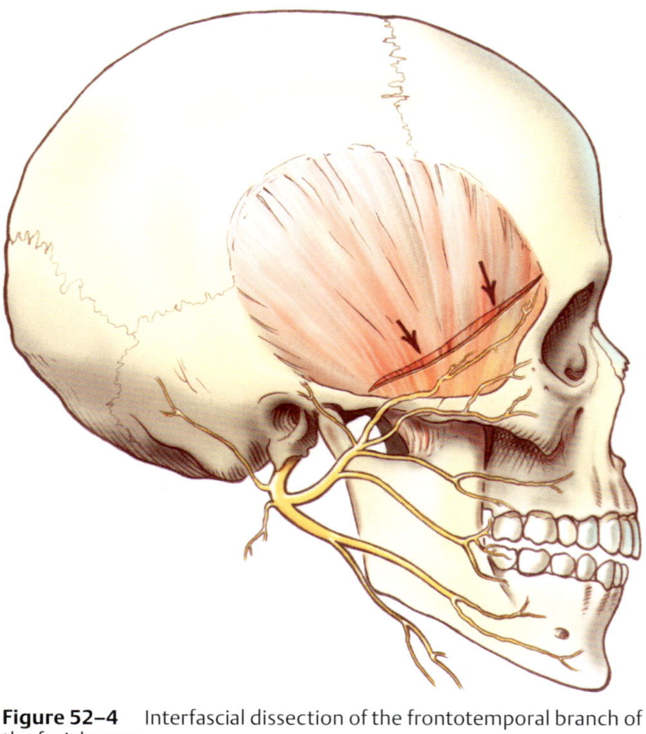

Figure 52–4 Interfascial dissection of the frontotemporal branch of the facial nerve.

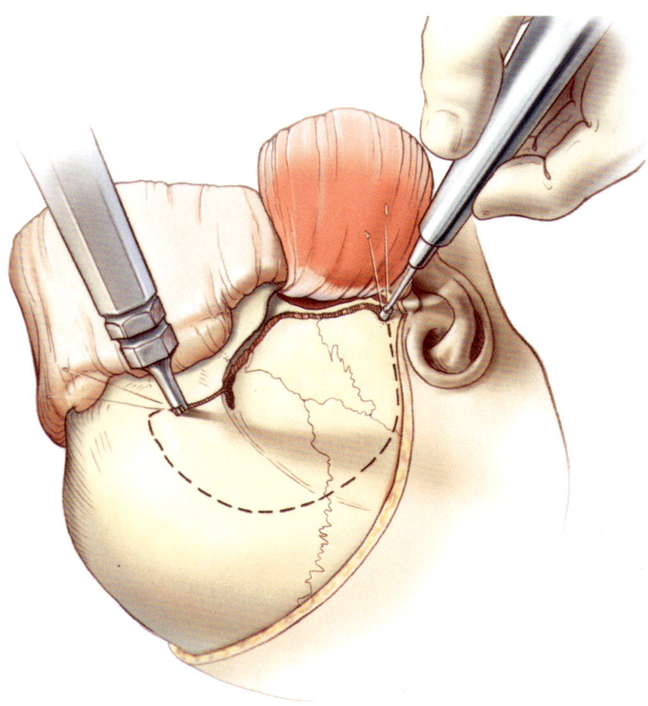

Figure 52–5 Frontotemporal craniotomy flap.

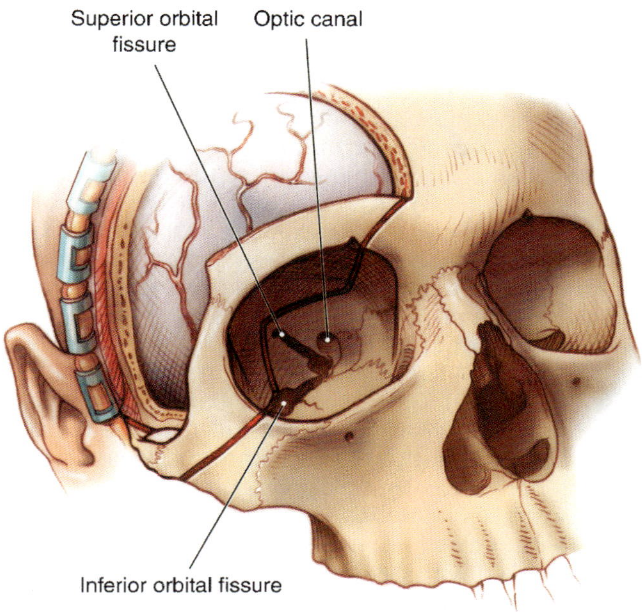

Figure 52–6 Reciprocating saw cuts for an orbitozygomatic osteotomy.

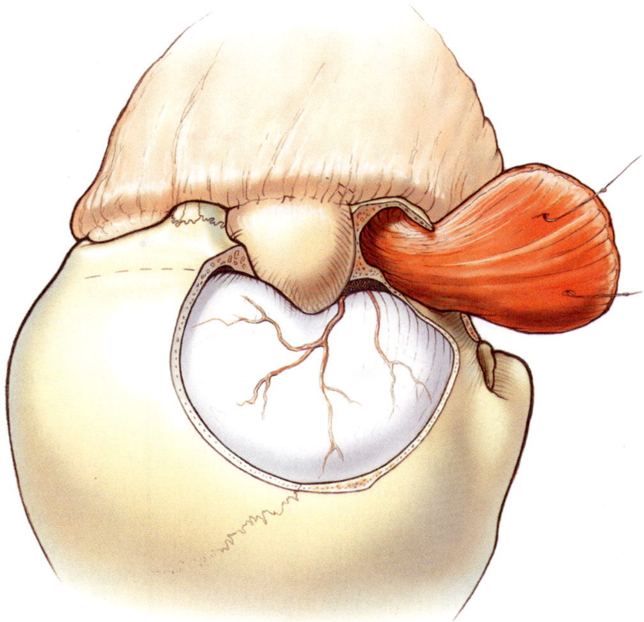

Figure 52–7 Exposure obtained from a frontotemporal craniotomy with an orbitozygomatic osteotomy.

temporal region can then be drilled down to be flush with the floor of the middle fossa.

The temporal and frontal dura are then stripped from the orbital roof and lateral orbital wall, and the periorbita is stripped from these same areas to at least 3 cm from the orbital rim. The periorbita is stripped medially to the supraorbital notch and inferolaterally to the inferior orbital fissure (IOF).

The OZO cuts are begun with a reciprocating saw. Malleable brain retractors are placed over the frontal dura and orbital contents for protection, with the saw cuts being made away from the brain. The reciprocating saw is always used for the cosmetically important cuts on the face or through the thick areas of the orbital rim. The cuts through the thin bone of the orbital roof or lateral wall can be made with the reciprocating saw, the Midas Rex M8 or equivalent drill bit, or small osteotomes. The medial reciprocating saw cut is made at approximately the supraorbital notch. The lateral cut is made beginning at the IOF and continuing posteroinferiorly to the level of the zygomaticofacial foramen. Staying at or above this landmark avoids entrance into the maxillary sinus. A third cut is made from the anterior, inferior edge of the zygomatic arch to connect with the posterior aspect of the second cut (making a "V" on the malar eminence centered on the zygomaticofacial foramen). Finally, a fourth reciprocating saw cut is made (in nearly the sagittal plane) across the root of the zygoma at its junction with the squamosal temporal bone **(Fig. 52–6).** The posterior (coronal) cut is made across the roof of the orbit and down the lateral orbital wall to the posterior aspect of the IOF. This cut is generally made 2.5 to 3.0 cm from the orbital rim preserving enough orbital roof and wall (about two thirds) to prevent postoperative enophthalmos.[14] The superior orbital fissure (SOF) and orbital apex are deliberately circumvented with these cuts to prevent injury to the optic nerve or the nerves of the SOF. Once all of the OZO cuts have been made, the entire block of bone is loosened with a mallet and chisel and removed **(Fig. 52–7).** Openings in the frontal sinus are managed during the reconstruction phase of the procedure.

Condylar Fossa Osteotomy

The condylar fossa can be included in the OZO if extensive exposure of the petrous carotid artery is needed. The temporomandibular joint capsule is opened and the meniscus is depressed inferiorly to protect it.[15] The middle fossa dura is then elevated with a Penfield no. 1 until the foramen spinosum, foramen ovale, and middle meningeal artery (MMA) are identified. The MMA is then cauterized and cut, and the foramen spinosum is packed with bone wax. A V-shaped cut is planned that spans the condylar fossa and encompasses the zygomatic root. The junction of the two cuts should be no further medial than the foramen spinosum to avoid petrous carotid injury. Using a fiberoptic light source or endoscope to transilluminate the condylar fossa from below is helpful to more precisely delineate the condylar fossa for optimal cuts.[15] Cuts made too far posteriorly may result in entry into the middle ear. Once the landmarks are well visualized and the osteotomy is planned precisely, the two cuts around the condylar fossa are made with the reciprocating saw directed inferiorly.

Exposure of the Petrous Carotid Artery

Further temporal dura is elevated medially until the arcuate eminence is seen superior to the external ear canal and perpendicular to the long axis of the petrous bone. More medial dissection exposes the hiatus of the greater superficial petrosal nerve (GSPN). The GSPN runs at about a 60 degree angle anteromedially from the arcuate eminence.[15] To avoid confusion with the lesser superficial petrosal nerve (LSPN), the GSPN can be stimulated with 1 to 2 mA delivered through a direct current electrode near the facial hiatus, resulting in facial muscle contractions.[15] The petrous ICA is then identified just posterior and medial to V3 and directly inferior to the GSPN. The horizontal petrous ICA is usually only partially covered with bone, and a hiatus in the floor of the middle fossa can often be seen with the underlying periosteal sheath of the petrous ICA visible. If a hiatus is not present, the bone covering the horizontal petrous carotid is very thin.

Usually, the GSPN is divided when there is extensive work around the petrous carotid to avoid traction injury to the facial nerve. For this reason, for routine cavernous sinus tumors, proximal control of the ICA is obtained through a small incision in a skinfold of the neck instead of at the petrous carotid artery. It is quicker, does not require temporal lobe retraction, and avoids sectioning of the GSPN with the resultant dry cornea. If tumor involves the petrous ICA, this technique of petrous carotid exposure is used for proximal control.[6]

Drilling with a diamond bur is used to expose more of the petrous carotid artery. The lateral aspect is exposed first to determine the exact course and angle of the artery, which is followed to the genu of the artery **(Fig. 52–8).** To avoid the eustachian tube, the artery is generally not followed proximal to its genu. The tensor tympani muscle lies superior to the eustachian tube, making it an excellent landmark to avoid drilling into the eustachian tube. The periosteal sheath of the petrous ICA is left intact to protect the arterial wall, and this periosteum is dissected free from the walls of the carotid canal to mobilize the artery. Drilling posterior to the petrous carotid genu is avoided to prevent drilling into the basal turn of the cochlea. For exposure of the vertical segment of the petrous carotid, the condylar fossa osteotomy is performed as described above, and the horizontal petrous carotid is exposed. The mandibular condyle is then depressed with firm retraction. Drilling is continued beyond the tensor tympani muscle until the eustachian tube is exposed **(Fig. 52–9).** The tensor tympani muscle is divided. The osseous eustachian tube is then drilled to trace the tube anteriorly, where it is sectioned in its cartilaginous portion. The anterior eustachian tube mucosa is then packed with fat or Surgicel and closed with a hemoclip or by oversewing to prevent CSF leak. The posterior portion of the eustachian tube is packed with fat or Surgicel as well.[15] Progressive drilling of the tympanic bone is then continued, following the vertical petrous carotid inferiorly until the dense fibrocartilaginous ring at the entrance of the carotid canal is encountered. This ring is detached from the periosteal sheath, opened, and excised.[15] The cervical carotid can then be traced further proximally if needed.

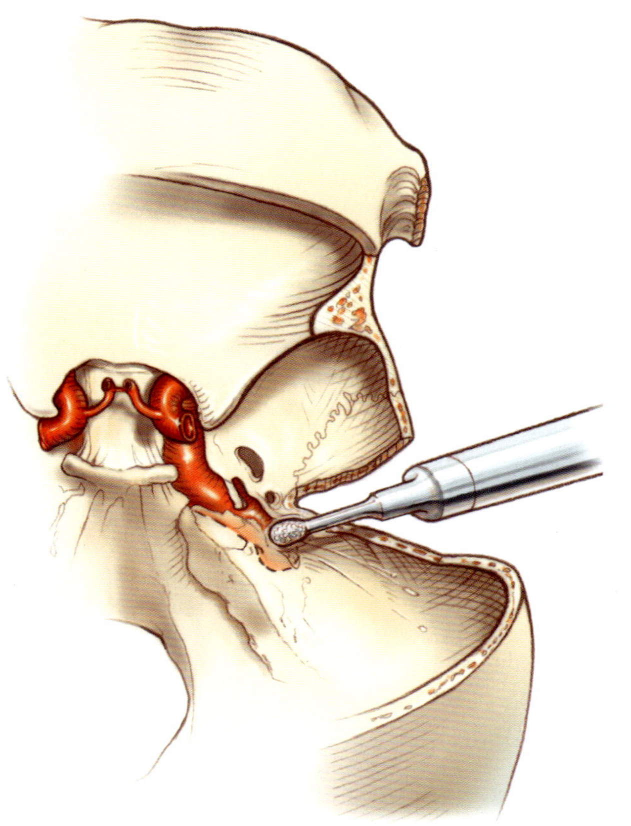

Figure 52–8 Drilling of the horizontal petrous internal carotid artery. Note the location of the condylar fossa osteotomy.

The need for this much proximal exposure depends on the extent of the tumor. Removal of the condylar fossa with the orbitozygomatic osteotomy is generally reserved for cases where exposure of the vertical segment of the petrous ICA is needed.

Anterior Clinoidectomy

After the OZO has been performed, the bone around the SOF is removed. The greater wing of the sphenoid is removed first to expose the dura of the inferolateral SOF, followed by removal of the lesser wing. The lesser wing is removed from lateral to medial until the anterior clinoid process (ACP) is exposed. Wide decompression of the SOF allows the surgeon to take full advantage of the exposure gained by the OZO. Under the guidance of the operating microscope, the ACP can then be removed and the optic canal widely opened extradurally.

Extradural Anterior Clinoidectomy If the ACP is short, it can be resected extradurally. If the ACP is long or complex or a middle clinoid process is present, extradural anterior clinoidectomy may be difficult or impossible. If an extradural anterior clinoidectomy is needed, coagulation and sectioning of the orbital meningeal artery (division of the lateral aspect of the SOF) and stripping temporal dura away from the orbital apex and anterolateral cavernous sinus provide the necessary exposure.[14] A fine diamond drill bit is then used to core the ACP until only a thin rim of cortical bone remains **(Fig. 52–10).** This remaining bone can be removed with fine rongeurs. Cavernous sinus bleeding can be controlled with Surgicel or Gelfoam. The optic strut (inferior wall of the optic canal) can now be well visualized and removed with a fine rongeur or Kerri-

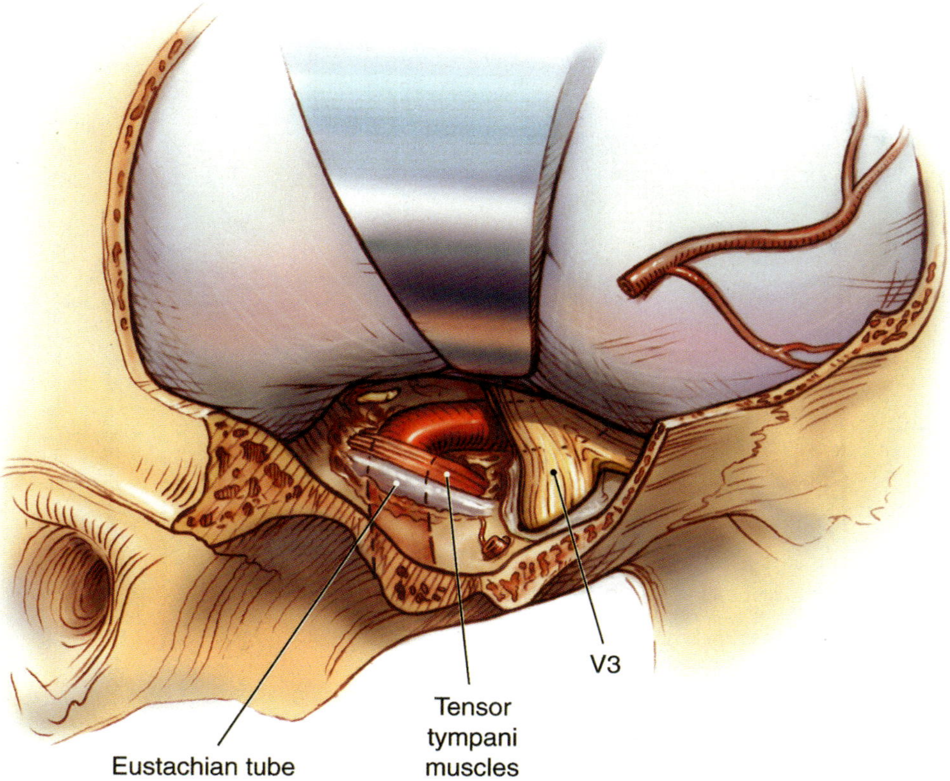

Figure 52–9 Drilling inferiorly from the petrous internal carotid artery genu exposes the tensor tympani muscle followed by the eustachian tube. Note that a condylar fossa osteotomy has been performed.

son punch. The optic nerve is unroofed superiorly, laterally, inferiorly, and as much as indicated medially. If the bone of the optic canal and optic strut are removed prior to the removal of the ACP, the ACP will become disconnected and unstable, making it very difficult or impossible to drill safely.[14]

Pneumatized Anterior Clinoid Process The ACP, optic strut, and lesser sphenoid wing may be pneumatized with extensions of the sphenoid sinus. Some indication of this can be seen on the preoperative CT bone windows. Removal of the ACP or optic strut can then result in a defect in the sphenoid sinus **(Fig. 52–11).** This area should always be inspected for

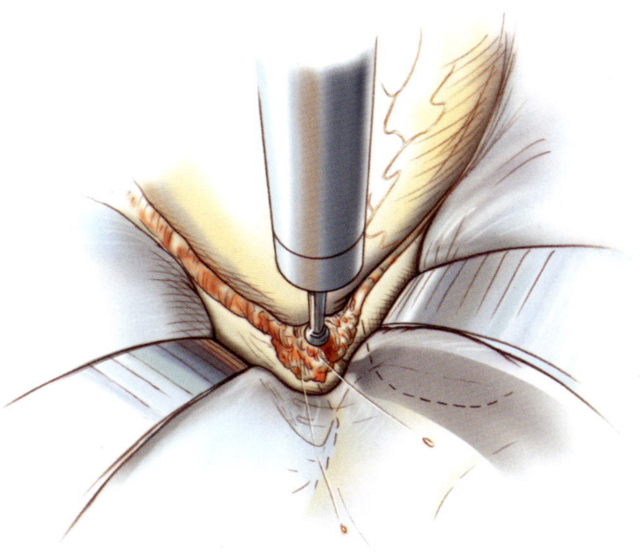

Figure 52–10 Extradural drilling of the anterior clinoid process.

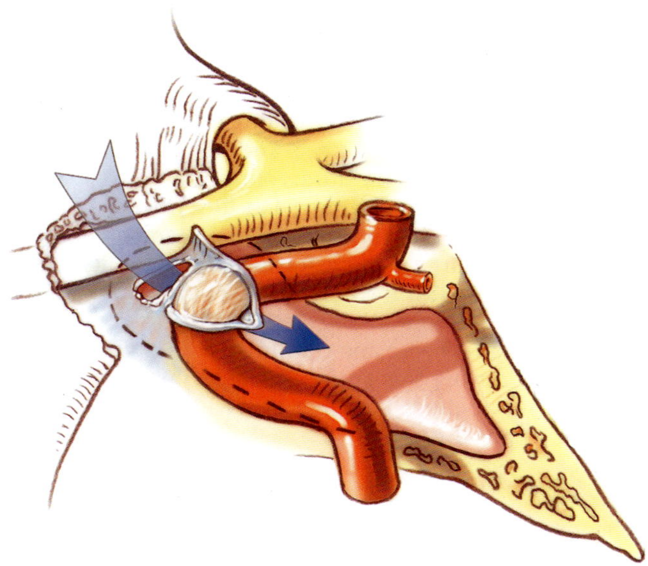

Figure 52–11 A pneumatized anterior clinoid process or optic strut can result in a sphenoid sinus defect after an anterior clinoidectomy.

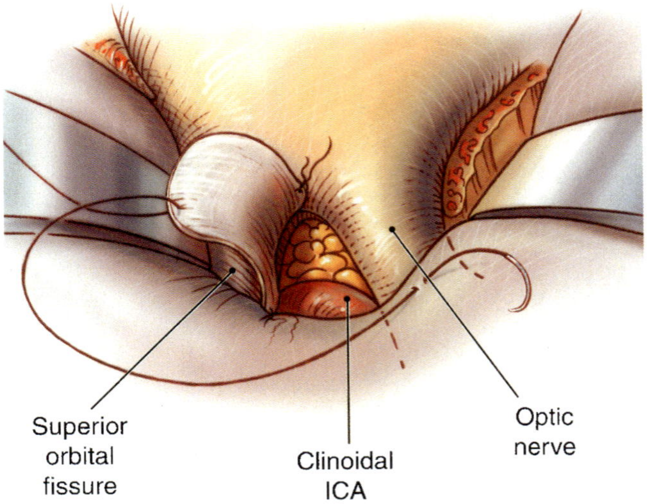

Figure 52–12 Repair of a sphenoid sinus defect after anterior clinoidectomy with the placement of fat and pericranial grafts. ICA, internal carotid artery.

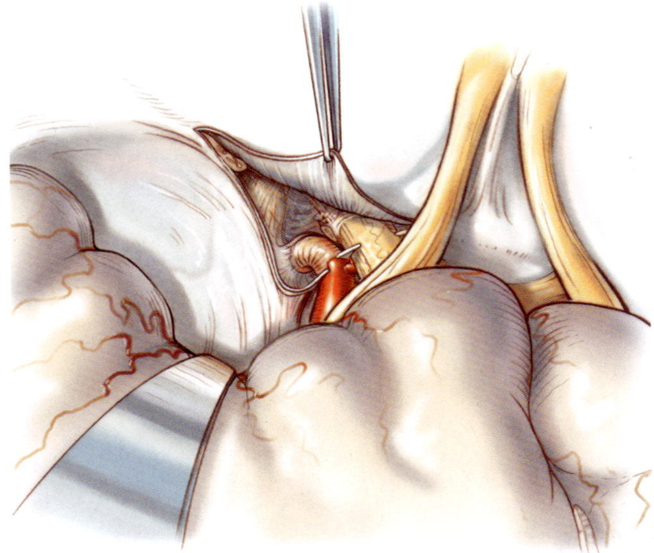

Figure 52–13 Completion of an intradural anterior clinoidectomy. Note the visible roof of the cavernous sinus.

defects to prevent a postoperative CSF leak. If a defect is present, the sinus mucosa is removed as much as possible, and the sinus is packed with autologous fat and covered with a dural graft or a pericranial flap[14] **(Fig. 52–12).** The graft is sutured over the hole circumferentially, using the dura propria of the optic nerve to hold sutures if necessary.[16] Any coexisting dural defect, particularly a clinoidal dural defect from an extradural anterior clinoidectomy, is closed with a dural graft (usually pericranium or fascia lata). The entire reconstruction is supplemented with fibrin sealant.

Intradural Anterior Clinoidectomy The initial steps are the same as for an extradural resection. The SOF is unroofed and the orbital meningeal artery is divided. The orbital roof is removed until the base of the ACP is well visualized. The dura is opened, and the sylvian fissure is dissected from a lateral to medial direction. A flap of dura is then made over the optic canal and ACP that is reflected or excised to expose the underlying bone of the ACP, which is then cored and removed as described for an extradural resection. The optic strut removal and optic canal decompression are also performed as previously described **(Fig. 52–13).** Intradural resection of the ACP is technically easier and allows better visualization of the neighboring optic nerve and carotid artery. Copious irrigation is used during this entire process to prevent excess heat generation during drilling as well as to remove the associated bone dust.

Superior Approach to the Cavernous Sinus

The superior approach provides exposure of the area superior and medial to the horizontal portion of the cavernous ICA. It provides good exposure of the anterior bend, anterior vertical and clinoidal segments of the cavernous ICA, as well as the sella.[7] The posterior vertical segment and posterior bend of the cavernous sinus are generally not well seen by this approach. Although CN III and its intracavernous course are well exposed, and CN VI is sometimes exposed, the remaining cranial nerves of the cavernous sinus are not well seen by this route.[7] When combined with a lateral approach, all cranial nerves and the majority of the cavernous ICA are well visualized.

Initial steps in this approach involve a frontotemporal craniotomy with an OZO. V2 and V3 are exposed further distally with careful extradural drilling if they are affected or involved by tumor **(Fig. 52–14).** The frontotemporal dural opening is made, and the dural flap is retracted over the orbital contents, resulting in maximal exposure with the additional inferior retraction of the orbital contents.[5] An anterior clinoidectomy, optic canal decompression, and opening of the clinoidal dura and dura propria of the optic nerve are performed.

The dural rings around the clinoidal segment of the ICA are opened, and the ICA is followed proximally into the cavernous sinus, mobilizing the distal cavernous carotid. The dural incision is made in the superior cavernous sinus beginning in the clinoidal space and extending toward the posterior clinoid process. This dura must be opened with care to avoid damaging the underlying cavernous ICA because it can sometimes be adherent to the superior wall of the cavernous sinus.[7] A suture can be placed in the tentorial edge for retraction to maximize this exposure. In addition, the dura can be incised following the intracavernous course of the oculomotor nerve to mobilize it completely **(Fig. 52–15).** It can then be retracted laterally along with the tentorium, maximizing the working space of the superior approach. The mobilized distal cavernous ICA can also be displaced laterally

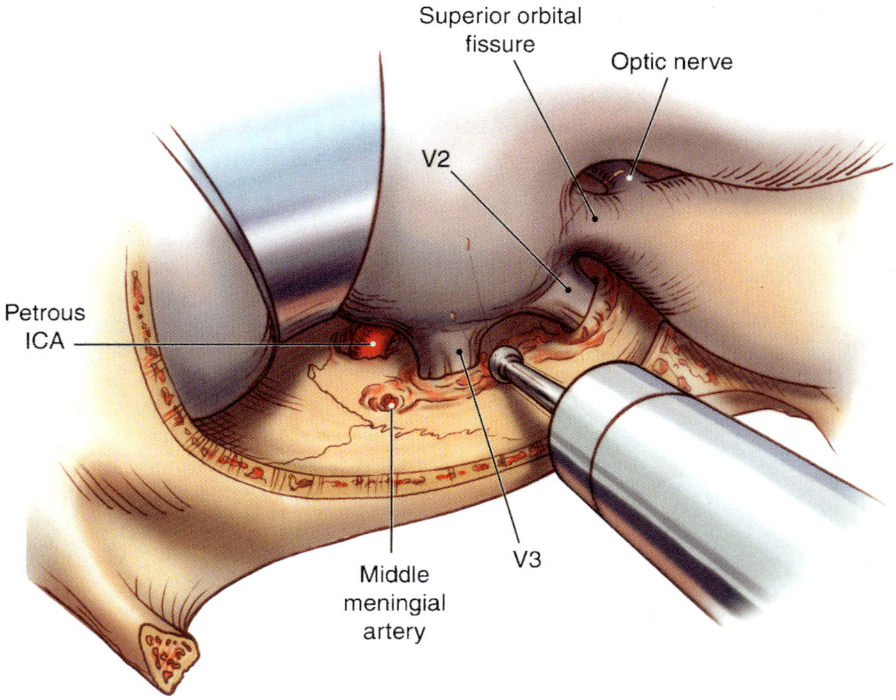

Figure 52–14 Potential extradural exposure provided by a frontotemporal craniotomy with an orbitozygomatic osteotomy. The anterior clinoid process has been removed, and the superior orbital fissure has been decompressed. The horizontal petrous internal carotid artery (ICA) has been exposed, and further exposure of V2 and V3 is provided by drilling the middle fossa floor distally along their dural sleeves.

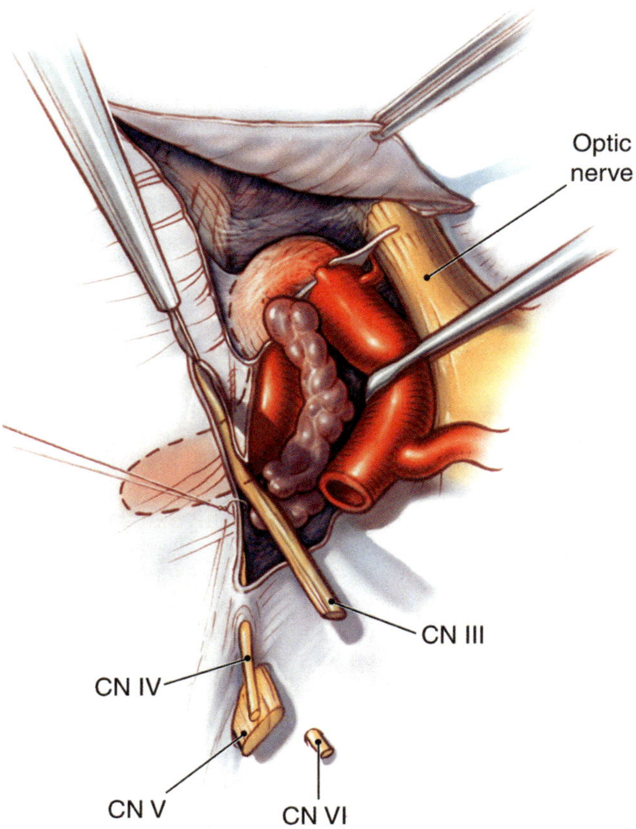

Figure 52–15 Superior approach to the cavernous sinus. The superior wall has been opened, and the dura is incised along cranial nerve (CN) III to maximize exposure. The dural rings of the clinoidal internal carotid artery (ICA) will be opened to mobilize the distal cavernous ICA.

to allow removal of tumor extending into the sella. Dissection can continue around the pituitary gland to reach small extensions of tumor in the opposite cavernous sinus.[17]

Cavernous sinus venous bleeding is controlled with thrombin-soaked Gelfoam or Surgicel. Gelfoam is generally preferred because it is less compressive on surrounding structures. The reverse Trendelenburg position can also be used to reduce venous bleeding, but it may increase the risk of air embolism.

Lateral Approach to the Cavernous Sinus

For extensive meningiomas, a complete dissection of the cavernous sinus is often necessary.[6] Initial steps again include a frontotemporal craniotomy with an OZO. V2 and V3 are further exposed extradurally if they are involved by tumor. A subtemporal/infratemporal approach is occasionally needed to pursue tumor into the infratemporal fossa. The frontotemporal dura is opened and retracted over the orbital contents, and the sylvian fissure is widely dissected. The anterior clinoidectomy, optic canal decompression, and opening or resection of the clinoidal dura and dura propria of the optic nerve are performed as described above. The dural rings of the clinoidal segment of the ICA are opened, and the ICA is followed proximally into the cavernous sinus. The superior wall of the cavernous sinus can be opened for additional exposure of extensive tumors **(Fig. 52–16).**

The lateral wall of the cavernous sinus is then removed by peeling it away from the area of the sphenoparietal sinus anteriorly, V2 and V3 inferolaterally, the region of the superior petrosal sinus posteriorly, and the tentorial edge

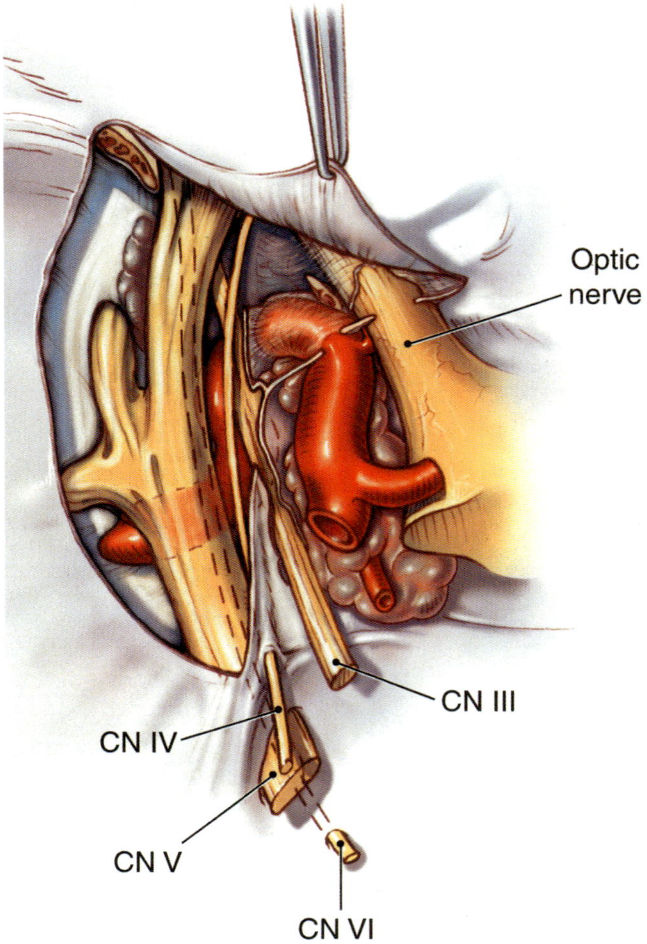

Figure 52–16 The lateral and superior approaches can be combined for extensive tumors.

superomedially[7] **(Fig. 52–17).** If possible, some dura is left attached to cranial nerves III and IV to preserve their vascular supply.[6] Frequently, the dura around the third and fourth cranial nerves may be invaded by tumor requiring resection of this dura to obtain complete tumor removal. This exposure is then extended to open Meckel's cave, and the tentorium is opened widely posterior to the entrance point of the fourth nerve into the cavernous sinus.[21] The inner layer of dura of the lateral wall may be thin or incomplete, requiring Gelfoam or Surgicel to stop venous bleeding.

Cranial nerves III through V are identified in the lateral wall of the cavernous sinus, which is then entered through Parkinson's triangle (between CN IV and V1), between cranial nerves III and IV, between V1 and V2, or posterior to V3.[7] CN V is the most difficult nerve to preserve completely due to its frequent infiltration by tumor and because it covers the majority of the cavernous sinus.[6] The cavernous ICA and the abducens nerve must then be definitively located for safe tumor resection. The sixth nerve is the most difficult structure to locate in the cavernous sinus and for this reason is the most likely cranial nerve to be inadvertently transected during the tumor resection. The abducens nerve can be found either at the anterior end of the cavernous sinus just superior and medial to V1 as it enters the SOF,[6] or at the posterior end of the cavernous sinus as it passes through Dorello's canal medial to Meckel's cave and usually medial to the trigeminal root.[6,7] If the sixth nerve is not found by either of these methods, the petrous apex may be removed subtemporally to expose the clival dura, which is then opened to find the subarachnoid segment of the nerve.[7] An alternative to this last method is to find the nerve between the extraocular muscles in the orbital apex. A difficulty sometimes encountered in locating and protecting the sixth nerve is that it may divide into multiple fascicles within the cavernous sinus.[2,7] The sympathetic nerve can sometimes be identified as well, and attempts should be made to preserve it when identified.

Dissecting the cavernous ICA from non–ICA-encasing tumors is usually straightforward. With the dural rings opened, the cavernous ICA is traced proximally, dissecting tumor away with Rhoton 2 or 3 dissectors **(Fig. 52–18).** Alternatively, the ICA may be traced distally from an exposed petrous segment. At all times, the surgeon must be ready to place temporary clips should carotid injury occur.

Tumor is easily left behind in the blind area medial to Meckel's cave if this area is not explored. If additional exposure is needed to explore this region, the gasserian ganglion can be split between V1 and V2 or between V2 and V3.[7]

Closure and Reconstruction

A detailed description of cranial nerve and cranial base reconstruction can be found in the chapter by that title in this book. Reconstruction of sphenoid sinus defects from anterior clinoidectomy is discussed earlier in this chapter. In some cases, the sphenoid sinus may be opened by the tumor resection along the medial aspect of the cavernous sinus. When this occurs, reconstruction is performed by packing the sinus with fascia and fat, followed by fascial repair of the bony defect. This third layer of fascia may be secured to any surrounding dura with sutures. If surrounding dura is not available, the third fascial layer can be anchored to surrounding bone with titanium screws.

Exenterating the affected sinus, packing with autologous fat, and suturing a pedicled pericranial flap over the defect is generally the method employed to repair defects in other paranasal sinuses including the frontal or ethmoid sinuses. With frontal sinus defects, rolls of Surgicel are placed in the frontonasal ducts prior to packing with fat. Muscle is not used to pack the sinuses because its high metabolic rate makes it less likely to remain viable.[12]

These reconstructions are reinforced with fibrin glue, and the osteotomy pieces and bone flaps are replaced with titanium miniplates. Any residual bone defects can be repaired with hydroxyapatite cement. The temporalis muscle is secured with multiple sutures to an oblique hole in the bone along the superior temporal line made with the Midas Rex C1 or equivalent drill bit. The scalp is closed in the usual two layers.

With tumors having large extracranial extensions, the resection is often done in two stages. The extradural tumor is generally removed first with a local temporalis muscle or free flap reconstruction, followed by a second intradural stage. This is done to minimize the chances of a CSF leak.[6]

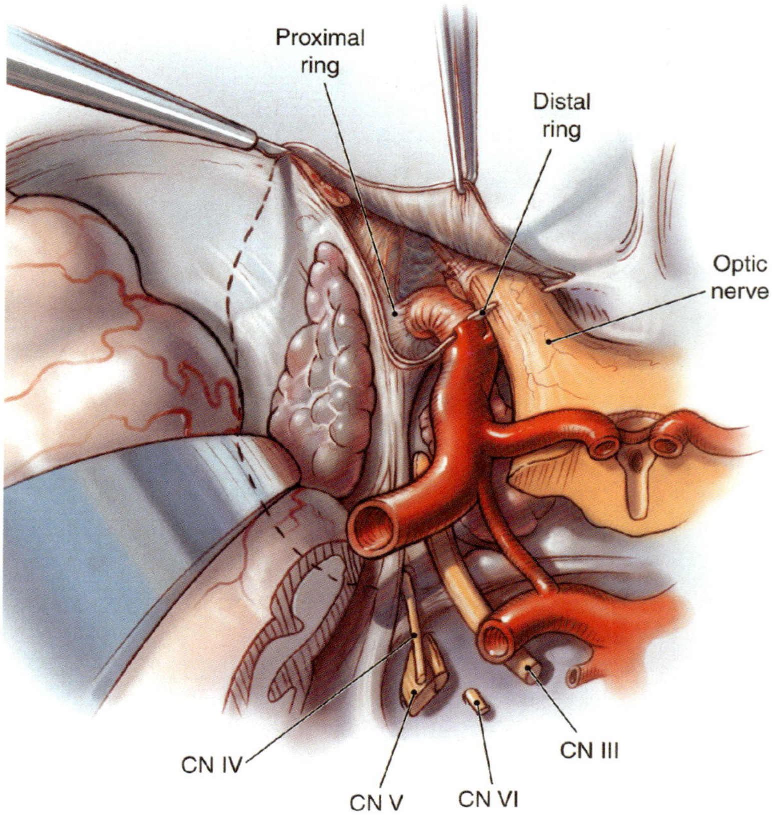

Figure 52–17 Lateral approach to the cavernous sinus. An intradural anterior clinoidectomy has been completed, and the outer layer of the lateral wall is incised and removed.

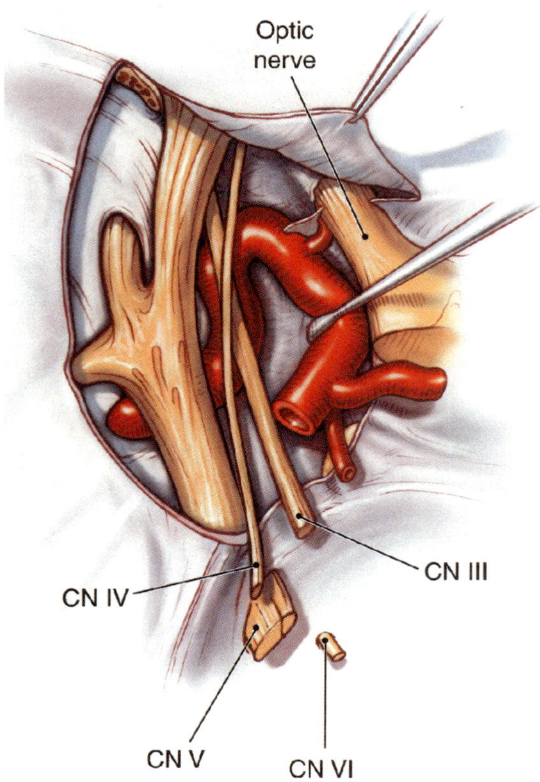

Figure 52–18 Possible exposure from the completion of a combined superior and lateral approach.

ICA-Encasing Meningiomas with Vein Graft Reconstruction

In patients whose tumors encase or narrow the cavernous ICA, carotid artery resection with vein grafting may be needed for gross total resection of the tumor. The exposure and operative techniques for ICA-encasing meningiomas are the same as for non–ICA-encasing tumors except for some important distinctions. During exposure of the cavernous ICA, the tumor is dissected from the carotid with Rhoton 2 or 3 dissectors, or sometimes with sharp dissection using microscissors. The surgeon must be prepared for temporary clipping of the ICA at all times during the dissection. If ICA injury occurs, the injured segment is trapped with temporary aneurysm clips and the carotid is repaired, if the tumor can be dissected from the arterial wall. If the tumor will not peel away from the arterial wall without significant risk of carotid rupture, a bypass with resection of the diseased ICA segment will have to be performed.

The decision to perform a bypass is usually made after the tumor has been explored and it has been determined that the arterial wall has been invaded by tumor, and dissection of tumor from the carotid is not possible. The bypass is then performed, and the tumor resection is completed approximately 2 weeks later. The bypass is usually made with autologous saphenous vein from the thigh and is placed from the cervical ICA or external carotid artery to the

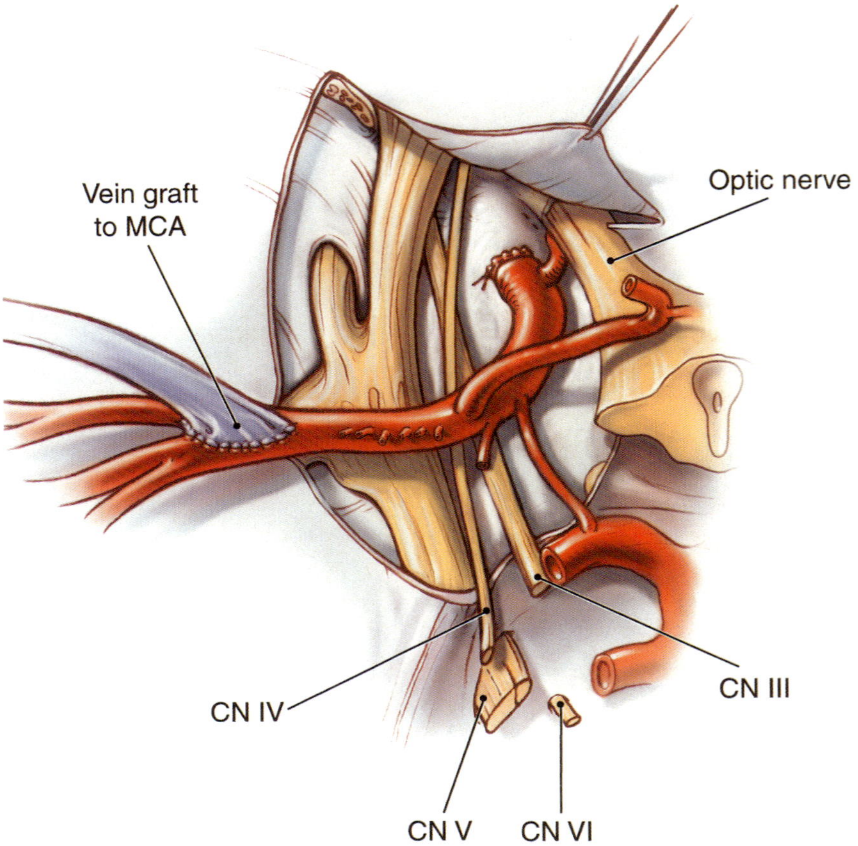

Figure 52–19 Carotid resection proximal to the ophthalmic artery with a saphenous vein bypass from the cervical internal carotid artery to the middle cerebral artery (MCA).

M2 segment of the middle cerebral artery (MCA). The ideal recipient site is the MCA bifurcation **(Fig. 52–19).** If the MCA branches are small, the supraclinoid ICA can be used for the distal anastomosis. Petrous ICA to supraclinoid ICA bypasses are performed less frequently because both anastomoses are performed in a deep working space requiring longer ICA clamping time.[6] Details of these revascularization techniques are beyond the scope of this chapter and are discussed in detail elsewhere in this book.

ICA-Encasing Meningiomas with Tailored Resection

For some larger tumors, resection of tumor from critical areas can be followed by radiosurgical treatment of the remaining tumor. Although this approach is well suited for higher-grade tumors in elderly patients, patients with multiple medical problems, and patients with contralateral cranial nerve deficits, this treatment remains controversial in younger patients with lower-grade tumors. Despite the controversy, tailored resection followed by radiosurgical treatment of the residual tumor remains a viable option to ICA bypass for some ICA-encasing meningiomas.

Many of the techniques are the same as described earlier in this chapter. The optic nerve is decompressed in the same fashion, including anterior clinoidectomy when needed, and tumor is removed from the optic nerve and chiasm to reduce the chances of radiation injury to these structures from subsequent radiosurgery. All of the subdural tumor is removed, and tumor is followed into Meckel's cave, which is also opened. The tentorium is divided posterior to CN IV, and the petroclinoid and tentorial notch extensions of the tumor are resected. The intracavernous tumor is not resected and the cavernous carotid is left alone. Radiosurgical treatment follows once the patient has sufficiently recovered from the craniotomy. The exact timing of the radiosurgery is a matter of judgment related to the amount of residual tumor, rapidity of tumor growth, and postoperative neurological status.

◆ Nonmeningiomatous Tumors

Trigeminal Schwannoma

In general, trigeminal schwannomas are easier to resect than meningiomas. Smaller tumors not extending above the level of the ACP can sometimes be excised extradurally. This can be done with a frontotemporal craniotomy and either a simple zygomatic osteotomy or an OZO. Meckel's cave is then opened extradurally, and the tumor is dissected away from the fascicles of the trigeminal nerve. Because smaller tumors generally arise from only one or two fascicles, the remaining fascicles can often be preserved.[6] The cavernous sinus is usually not involved by small tumors confined to Meckel's cave.

Small tumors can alternatively be resected intradurally, but an intradural resection is always necessary for large tumors extending above the ACP or having posterior fossa extension. For these intradural approaches, the techniques are the same as for meningiomas (including frontotemporal craniotomy with OZO) until the opening of the sylvian fissure is completed. The lesion is then internally debulked, and the tumor capsule is completely removed. The tentorium must be opened so that all of the posterior fossa extension of the tumor can be well visualized and resected. Cavernous sinus involvement usually occurs with larger tumors by extension of the tumor through the medial wall of Meckel's cave.[6] The intracavernous structures are usually displaced by these tumors, which can be removed through a cruciate extension of the defect in the cavernous sinus wall that was the route of tumor entry into the cavernous sinus, or through a linear or cruciate incision in the lateral cavernous sinus wall over the most prominent part of the tumor. A formal cavernous sinus dissection is usually not required. Cavernous sinus bleeding occurs when the margins of the tumor are reached, which is controlled with Gelfoam or Surgicel.

Giant trigeminal schwannomas may extend into the brain stem and may invade the entire trigeminal root. If there is a large posterior fossa extension of tumor, a petrosal approach may be needed. If necessary, a petrosal approach can be combined with a frontotemporal zygomatic or orbitozygomatic approach for complex tumors with extensive cavernous sinus and posterior fossa involvement.

Petrosal Approach

The incision for a standard petrosal approach is illustrated in **Fig. 52–20.** This C-shaped incision extends along the superior temporal line into the retroauricular region to join an upper cervical skin crease. The scalp including the pericranium is elevated, and the temporalis muscle is elevated and reflected anteriorly. A muscle-sparing exposure is performed with the sternocleidomastoid muscle reflected anteriorly with the skin, and the semispinalis capitus and splenius capitus muscles elevated and reflected posteriorly. The mastoidectomy and a small retrosigmoid craniectomy are performed prior to the temporal craniotomy. This allows the surgeon to capitalize on the subtemporal dural and sigmoid sinus exposures from the mastoidectomy, making the craniotomy safer and easier. Once the craniotomy is completed, the temporal bone work is continued with skeletonization of the facial nerve, exposure of the semicircular canals, and exposure of the jugular bulb. A retrolabyrinthine, partial labyrinthectomy/petrous apicectomy, translabyrinthine, or transcochlear approach can then be completed depending on the exposure needed, and any preoperative cranial nerve deficits. The details of these exposures are discussed in a separate chapter.

If a combined frontotemporal/orbitozygomatic/petrosal approach is needed, the incision is made in a curved fashion from the midline hairline to the zygomatic root and is bisected posteriorly by an incision following the posterior aspect of the superior temporal line that ends in an anterior cervical skin crease **(Fig. 52–21).** The soft tissues are elevated as above including an interfascial dissection of the frontotemporal branch of the facial nerve as well as complete mobilization of the temporalis muscle. The mastoidectomy can be performed once the soft tissue work is completed, and then the frontotemporal craniotomy with an OZO (usually incorporating the condylar fossa) is done along with a retrosigmoid craniotomy, if needed. The temporal bone work is completed as above.

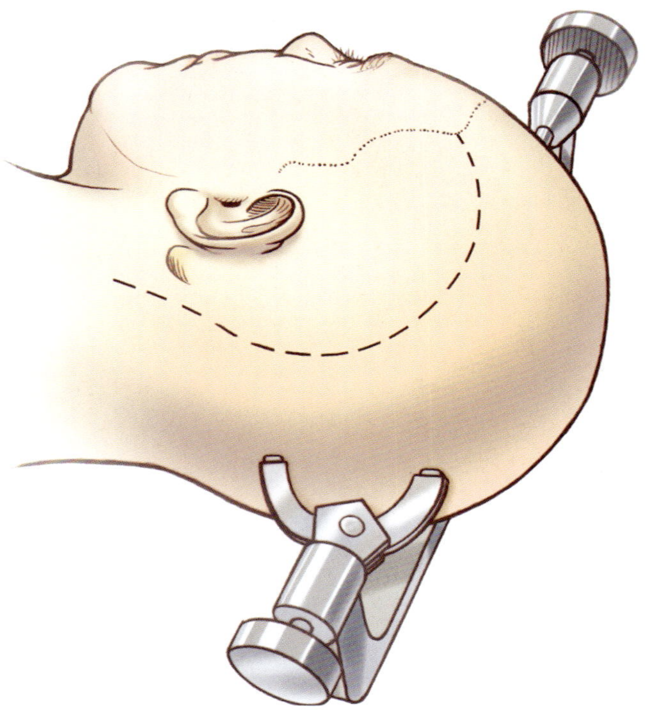

Figure 52–20 Skin incision for a standard presigmoid petrosal approach.

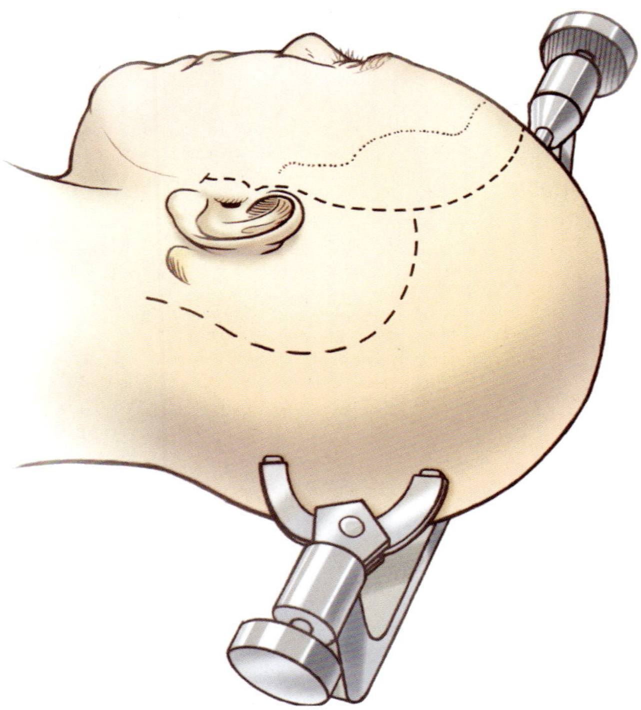

Figure 52–21 Skin incision for a combined frontotemporal/orbitozygomatic/petrosal approach.

The presigmoid dura is opened nearly vertically very close to the sigmoid sinus, and the basal cisterns in the region are opened for the drainage of CSF. This provides significantly more brain relaxation.[18] The presigmoid dural incision is continued up to the superior petrosal sinus (SPS). The temporal dura is opened horizontally over the inferior temporal gyrus and continued to the SPS to nearly intersect the presigmoid dural incision. The SPS is then ligated and cut, and the tentorium is divided from this point to a point just posterior to the entrance of the fourth nerve into the tentorium. Care must be taken to see the trochlear nerve to prevent its injury, and the superior cerebellar artery must be visualized as well because it can sometimes be adherent to the tentorium[18] **(Fig. 52–22).** Of great importance is watching for the vein of Labbé whose proximity can alter the dural incisions, the approach chosen, and the amount of retraction possible. Its visualization on preoperative imaging is extremely helpful for operative planning.

Sutures are placed in the dural edges for purposes of retraction, and the temporal dura is retracted inferiorly with the presigmoid dural edge retracted anteriorly over the residual temporal bone to maximize the exposure obtained from the extensive bone work. The tumor is internally debulked, and the capsule is dissected away from surrounding structures. The petrosal veins are often cauterized and divided, and Meckel's cave is opened widely to mobilize and visualize the trigeminal root. The SPS along the roof of Meckel's cave can be ligated with titanium hemoclips and divided for a wider opening of Meckel's cave.[18]

Once the resection is completed, a primary dural closure is extremely difficult. A dural graft of autologous pericranium or fascia lata can be used. The presigmoid dura and residual temporal bone are covered with an autologous fat graft after the eustachian tube and middle ear are packed with rolls of Surgicel. The entire construct is reinforced with fibrin sealant. The bone flaps are split to perform a split calvarial reconstruction of the mastoid (see the cranial nerve and cranial base reconstruction chapter). All of the bone flaps, including the split calvarial grafts, are secured with

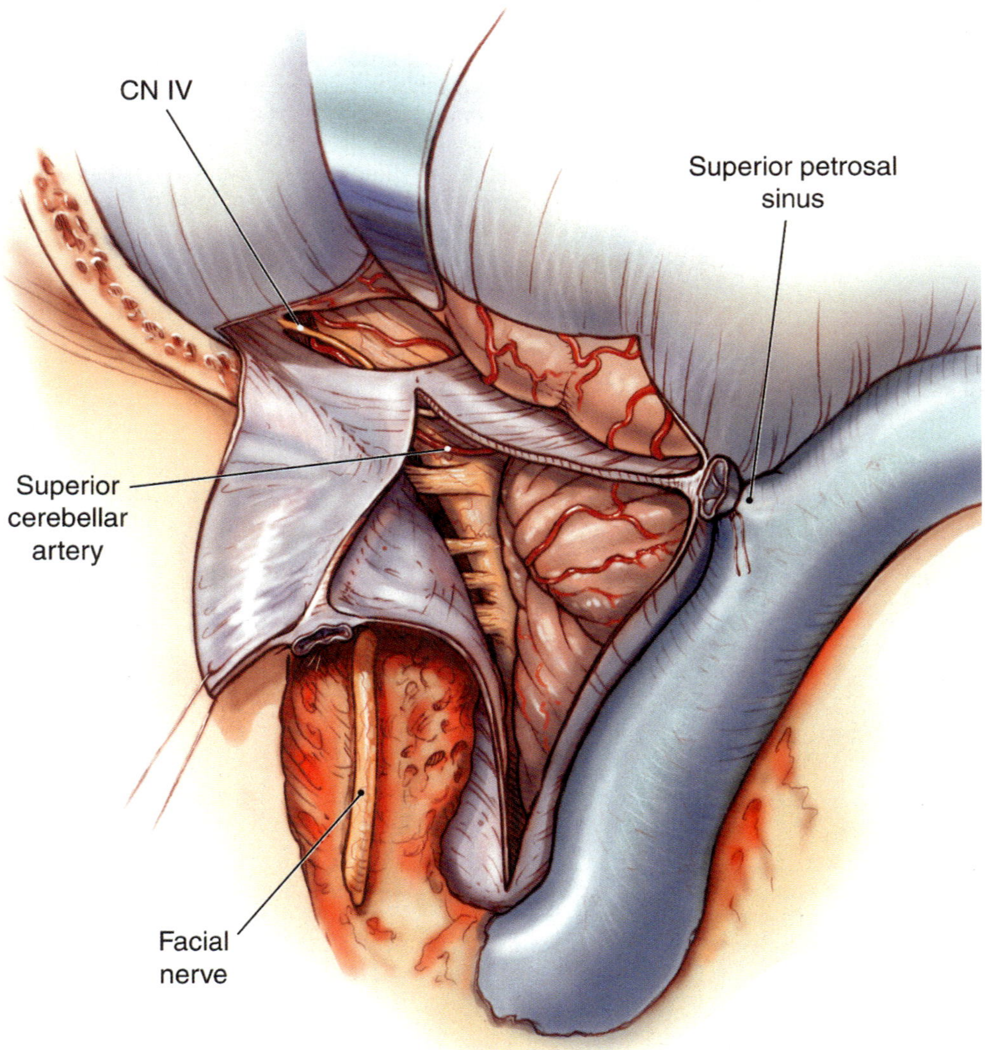

Figure 52–22 Incision in the superior petrosal sinus and tentorium. Care is taken to protect the fourth nerve and the superior cerebellar artery.

titanium miniplates. Alternatively, reconstruction can be performed with titanium mesh and hydroxyapatite cement in addition to autologous fat graft. The temporalis muscle and retroauricular musculature are sutured to small holes in the bone along their lines of insertion. The usual two-layer scalp closure is then performed.

Cavernous Hemangiomas

Cavernous hemangiomas of the cavernous sinus are very rare. Although representing a type of vascular malformation, they are resected in a fashion similar to some tumors. They usually present with signs and symptoms of mass effect like other neoplasms.[19,20] These lesions typically receive their blood supply from multiple small branches of the cavernous ICA. Due to the small size of these branches, these lesions can be angiographically occult,[19] and preoperative embolization is usually not possible.

Surgical Resection

Depending on the size of the lesion, the cavernous sinus is opened by a lateral approach between cranial nerves IV and V1 (Parkinson's triangle), V1 and V2, and V2 and V3. Larger lesions may require a superior approach combined with a lateral approach. Due to the high vascularity of these lesions, piecemeal resection is usually not done.[19] However, when the lesion is very large, it may be removed in two or three pieces. These lesions are usually spongy and are dissected from surrounding structures with a combination of bipolar cautery, Cottle elevator, and Rhoton 2 or 3 microdissectors. The lesion is separated from the cavernous ICA as quickly as possible, with the small arterial feeders being cauterized and divided. Larger lesions may require dissection from the pituitary gland or the opposite cavernous sinus. For larger lesions, temporary trapping of the ICA is beneficial in reducing the bleeding. After total excision of the lesion, the open cavernous sinus is packed with Gelfoam or Surgicel. A few sutures may be required in the dura of the lateral wall to hold the Gelfoam or Surgicel in place.

Pituitary Adenoma with Cavernous Sinus Extension

Pituitary macroadenomas usually penetrate the cavernous sinus through the medial wall. Transsphenoidal resection of these lesions is discussed in a separate chapter. For resection of these tumors with a craniotomy, the cavernous sinus is usually opened through the superior wall, with the sellar diaphragm also being opened to facilitate resection of the intrasellar portion. If tumor has extended lateral to the cavernous ICA, a combined lateral and superior approach to the cavernous sinus must be performed. When the cavernous carotid artery is encased by pituitary tumors, the tumor usually dissects fairly easily from the arterial wall. Carotid resection and bypass are rarely needed.

Chordoma and Chondrosarcoma

Chordomas and chondrosarcomas are usually less adherent to intracavernous structures than meningiomas, making their resection from the cavernous sinus somewhat easier.[16] These tumors may have areas of soft tumor as well as extremely hard areas consisting of invaded or partially eroded bone. This heterogeneity in consistency combined with the expected cavernous sinus bleeding may make structures such as the sixth nerve difficult to visualize and may also obscure residual tumor making it easy to overlook.

Chordomas and chondrosarcomas often require an extradural and an intradural approach.[21] Some of these tumors have minimal cavernous sinus invasion and can be removed extradurally. Because these tumors arise extradurally, dural invasion and intradural extension may not have occurred at the time of surgery. An extradural approach is needed to remove the involved petrous apex and sphenoid bone and to dissect the ICA prior to its entrance into the cavernous sinus. Extradural approaches used include the inferior, anterolateral, and medial approaches described earlier. The medial approach can be done transsphenoidally for small tumors or for a limited resection in older patients, or it can be done for larger tumors via an extended transbasal approach (bifrontal craniotomy and biorbitoethmoidal osteotomy) for a more radical resection.[8] Inferior and anterolateral approaches are often combined for an aggressive extradural resection. Some extensive tumors require a combination of all three extradural approaches.

An intradural approach is needed for tumors with more extensive cavernous sinus involvement or intradural extension. An intradural approach is also needed to resect involved bone of the dorsum sellae because this area is poorly visualized by the extended transbasal approach. From intradurally, the cavernous sinus is usually opened along the lateral wall for chordomas and chondrosarcomas. A vertical or horizontal incision is usually made over the prominent part of the tumor, and the outer layer of the lateral wall is dissected free in an attempt to displace the surrounding cranial nerves.[16,21] Further incisions can be made in the lateral wall if necessary to expose the remaining tumor. Extensive cavernous sinus involvement by tumor may require a combined superior and lateral approach.

Because the extensive extradural component of these tumors often requires combined intradural and extradural resection, the cavernous sinus is packed with fascia and fat and the wall of the cavernous sinus is carefully closed in a watertight fashion to prevent CSF leak.[6] For this reason, it is necessary to consider the closure of the lateral wall when the incision is made. A fascia lata or pericranial graft is sometimes needed, and the entire cavernous sinus wall closure is reinforced with fibrin sealant.

Adenoid Cystic Carcinoma

Adenoid cystic carcinomas generally extend into the cavernous sinus by tracking along the cranial nerves. When the cavernous sinus is involved by these tumors, it is usually the inferior cavernous sinus, so they can sometimes be removed along with cranial nerves V and VI, preserving cranial nerves III and IV. The trigeminal root and tumor are dissected away from the cavernous sinus structures to be preserved back to the entrance point of the trigeminal root into the brain stem.[6] Cases of extensive cavernous sinus involvement or cavernous sinus recurrence may require resection of the entire cavernous sinus.[6]

Another important consideration with adenoid cystic carcinoma is that ICA bypass with a vein graft followed by resection of the tumor with the ICA as a second stage may be the safest option for a younger patient with cavernous ICA encasement to obtain a radical resection. An alternative is resection of the extracavernous tumor followed by radiotherapy, particularly in older patients. Because of these options, the goals of surgery need to be defined beforehand.

Fast-Growing Malignant Tumors

Cavernous sinus surgery is generally not worthwhile for fast-growing malignancies such as squamous cell carcinoma. Occasionally, resection of a metastatic tumor to the cavernous sinus may be beneficial, if it is a solitary lesion.

◆ Complications

Ischemic Complications

Ischemic stroke may occur either from injury to perforating arteries outside the cavernous sinus or from ICA occlusion. Stroke is most commonly due to the presence of extracavernous tumor, with damage occurring intraoperatively to the anterior choroidal artery or lenticulostriate perforators. Previously irradiated tumors or prior surgery substantially increases the chances of such injuries because the arachnoid plane may be absent. In these patients, the ICA or middle cerebral artery (MCA) may be thin-walled and may rupture with little provocation.

Despite a favorable preoperative BTO or xenon-CT scan, injury or sacrifice of the cavernous ICA may result in infarction due to thromboembolic complications. For this reason, revascularization of the brain is recommended whenever the ICA is occluded. Small defects in the cavernous ICA wall can be sutured primarily. In these cases, intraoperative angiography is recommended to assess carotid patency.

If the ICA is exposed to the nasopharynx after resection of a malignant nasopharyngeal tumor, then a carotid pseudoaneurysm and subsequent rupture may result. To prevent this complication, a bypass graft from the cervical ICA to the MCA followed by ICA occlusion and free flap reconstruction is recommended.

Cerebrospinal Fluid Leak

The most common cause of postoperative CSF leak from cavernous sinus surgery is from defects in the sphenoid sinus. Detection and prevention of this problem are discussed in detail earlier in this chapter. If a postoperative leak occurs despite an adequate reconstruction, it can often be managed with a lumbar drain. Most leaks refractory to lumbar drainage can be closed by transsphenoidal packing with fascia and fat. These grafts are usually obtained from the abdomen or thigh.

Cranial Nerve Injuries

The best way to avoid cranial nerve injury is to recognize the anatomy and preserve the nerves' vascularity as much as possible. If a nerve is damaged, repair by primary reanastomosis or interposition graft is recommended. A detailed description of cranial nerve reconstruction can be found in the cranial nerve and cranial base reconstruction chapter of this book.

Postoperative diplopia can be managed with temporary eye patching or botulinum toxin injections, or with strabismus surgery if the deficit persists longer than a year or is expected to be permanent.[6] Close ophthalmologic follow-up is recommended for these patients.

Injury to V1 can result in corneal abrasions from loss of corneal sensation. This is usually temporary if V1 is anatomically intact, but the cornea should be protected and the patient instructed not to scratch the eye until the sensation returns. Ophthalmologic evaluation is recommended should any redness of the eye occur. Sectioning the GSPN complicates corneal anesthesia by causing eye dryness. This can be prevented by sectioning the GSPN only when necessary and gaining proximal control of the ICA in the neck. If petrous ICA exposure is necessary and the GSPN is sectioned, the eye dryness can be managed by punctal plugging by an ophthalmologist and the frequent use of lubricants.[6]

Brain Injury

Using contemporary cranial base approaches along with good brain relaxation and CSF drainage, brain injury from retraction should be minimal. If contusion does occur, it is most often present in the frontal or temporal lobes. These contusions should be monitored closely with postoperative imaging to ensure that an intracerebral hemorrhage does not develop. Rarely, reoperation to evacuate a parenchymal hemorrhage may be needed.

◆ Conclusion

With detailed neuroanatomical knowledge, contemporary neuroimaging, and modern microsurgical techniques, direct surgery in the cavernous sinus is now possible. With an armamentarium of approaches to different areas of the cavernous sinus along with an awareness of the expected morbidity, complications and complication management associated with cavernous sinus surgery, cavernous sinus tumors can be systematically approached with good results. The standard approaches to these lesions used alone or in combination must be modified depending on the patient's age, condition, existing deficits, tumor type, precise location, areas of extension, and available alternative or adjunctive treatments such as radiosurgery. Detailed surgical planning is essential and must be individualized for every case.

References

1. Goel A, Nadkarni TD. Cavernous hemangioma in the cavernous sinus. Br J Neurosurg 1995;9:77–80
2. Sekhar LN, Tzortzidis F, Bucor SD. Patient positioning for cranial microsurgery. In: Sekhar LN, Oliveira ED, eds. Cranial Microsurgery: Approaches and Techniques. New York: Thieme; 1999:12–18
3. Sekhar LN, Linskey ME, Sen C, Altschuler EM. Surgical management of lesions within the cavernous sinus. Clin Neurosurg 1991;37:440–489
4. Kim JM, Romano A, Sanan A, et al. Microsurgical anatomic features and nomenclature of the paraclinoid region. Neurosurgery 2000;46:670–682
5. Sekhar LN, Wright DC. Tumors involving the cavernous sinus. In: Sekhar LN, Oliveira ED, eds. Cranial Microsurgery: Approaches and Techniques. New York: Thieme; 1999:207–230
6. Raso J, Sekhar LN, Tzortzidis F. Anatomy of the cavernous sinus. In: Sekhar LN, Oliveira ED, eds. Cranial Microsurgery: Approaches and Techniques. New York: Thieme; 1999:176–181
7. Lanzino G, Sekhar LN, Hirsch WL, et al. Chordomas and chondrosarcomas involving the cavernous sinus: review of surgical treatment and outcome in 31 patients. Surg Neurol 1993;40:359–371
8. Dolenc VV. Anatomy and Surgery of the Cavernous Sinus. New York: Springer-Verlag; 1989:4–7
9. Jane JA, Park TS, Pobereskin LH, Winn HR, Butler AB. The supraorbital approach: technical note. Neurosurgery 1982;11:537–542
10. Sekhar LN, Tzortzidis F, Raso J. Fronto-orbital approach. In: Sekhar LN, Oliveira ED, eds. Cranial Microsurgery: Approaches and Techniques. New York: Thieme; 1999:54–60
11. Sawamura Y, Tribolet ND. Cavernous hemangioma in the cavernous sinus: case report. Neurosurgery 1990;26:126–128
12. Sekhar LN, Ross DA, Sen C. Cavernous sinus and sphenocavernous neoplasms. In: Sekhar LN, Janecka IP, eds. Surgery of Cranial Base Tumors. New York: Raven; 1993:521–604
13. Sekhar LN, Salas EL. The subtemporal transzygomatic approach and the subtemporal infratemporal approach. In: Sekhar LN, Oliveira ED, eds. Cranial Microsurgery: Approaches and Techniques. New York: Thieme; 1999:413–431
14. Sekhar LN, Raso J. Orbitozygomatic frontotemporal approach. In: Sekhar LN, Oliveira ED, eds. Cranial Microsurgery: Approaches and Techniques. New York: Thieme; 1999:130–133
15. Sekhar LN, Sen C, Jho HD, et al. Surgical treatment of intracavernous neoplasms: a four-year experience. Neurosurgery 1989;24:18–30
16. Osborn AG. The internal carotid artery: cavernous and supraclinoid segments. In: Osborn AG, ed. Introduction to Cerebral Angiography. Philadelphia: Harper & Row; 1980:109–141
17. Sekhar LN, Raso J, Schessel DA. The presigmoid petrosal approach. In: Sekhar LN, Oliveira ED, eds. Cranial Microsurgery: Approaches and Techniques. New York: Thieme, 1999:432–463
18. Parkinson D. Extradural neural axis compartment. J Neurosurg 2000; 92:585–588
19. Sclabassi RJ, Krieger DN, Weisz D, et al. Methods of neurophysiological monitoring during cranial base tumor resection. In: Sekhar LN, Janecka IP, eds. Surgery of Cranial Base Tumors. New York: Raven; 1993: 83–98
20. Sekhar LN, De Jesus O. Clinoid and paraclinoid aneurysms. In: Sekhar LN, Oliveira ED, eds. Cranial Microsurgery: Approaches and Techniques. New York: Thieme; 1999:151–175
21. Lee DS, Peck M. Anesthetic considerations for cranial microsurgery. In: Sekhar LN, Oliveira ED, eds. Cranial Microsurgery: Approaches and Techniques. New York: Thieme; 1999:19–22

53

Transsphenoidal Approach and Its Variants

Ali F. Krisht

◆ Indications

The most common indication for the transsphenoidal approach is the resection of pituitary adenomas. The approach can be safely used in the resection of pituitary microadenomas. It can also be used for the resection of large, broad-based pituitary macroadenomas. The approach is contraindicated in tumors that have a smaller central component compared with a larger parasellar and cavernous sinus component. It is also not the best approach in sellar tumors, which do not have the typical sellar changes and consistency that are similar to a pituitary adenoma. An intrasellar meningioma is an example. Meningiomas are usually firm and can be recognized by a plane separating the tumor from the normal gland with no significant enlargement of the sella. Craniopharyngioma is another tumor that is best operated through a cranial approach in the majority of cases. The transsphenoidal approach is also used in the repair of spontaneous or traumatic cerebrospinal fluid (CSF) leaks from the sphenoid sinus region.

◆ Preoperative Studies

Magnetic resonance imaging (MRI) is the study of choice for the evaluation of intrasellar pathology and the anatomical features of the sella and the parasellar region. It is important to assess the midsagittal and coronal cuts as well as the axial scans to verify the relationship of the floor of the sella to the floor of the sinus, the relationship to the clivus, as well as the location of the sphenoid septum. MRI helps delineate the borders of the tumor and its suprasellar extension. It also helps compare and match the radiological dimensions of the sella with findings during surgery, and it guides the extent of tumor resection. It is also important in recognizing the relationship of the carotid arteries to the tumor any anomalous displacement that may put them at risk of injury during tumor resection. The anatomical aspects of the sphenoid sinus are carefully studied preoperatively using MRI scans. Occasionally there may be more than one septum and more than one or two air cells, the recognition of which will make the surgical findings more familiar and well correlated with the radiological details on the MRI.

◆ Surgical Technique

Anesthesia

After induction of anesthesia and standard endotracheal intubation of the patient, the endotracheal tube is mobilized to the left side of the mouth, which is best suited with the position of the head for a right-handed surgeon. The anesthetic technique involves normotension, normocarbia, and normovolemia. An arterial line is inserted to help monitor the systemic pressure, which can become elevated as a result of surgical stimulation, especially the step of positioning and opening the transsphenoidal retractors. A central venous pressure monitor is not usually used unless otherwise indicated.

Positioning

The head is positioned using the Mayfield three-point headholder. The head of the patient is mildly flexed and rotated toward the surgeon's side (to the right side of the patient for a right-handed surgeon) and it is then tilted in the opposite direction as if the patient is looking face to face at the surgeon. The left lower quadrant of the abdomen is also draped for harvesting a fat graft. The nose is washed at its entry with Betadine solution. Even though intraoperative lumbar drains are commonly used during resection of macroadenomas, we stopped their use without losing any significant surgical advantage and we replaced this with repeated Valsalva maneuvers when needed.

Exposure

There are several ways to achieve the transsphenoidal approach to the sella. The classic way is the sublabial approach, which we rarely use nowadays. The two main approaches we commonly use are either the transseptal transsphenoidal approach or the endonasal transsphenoidal approach, and they are described here. The endoscopic approach uses the same route of the endonasal transsphenoidal approach and they are also described.

Transseptal Transsphenoidal Approach

In the transseptal transsphenoidal approach the cartilaginous septum is approached through the right nostril but the submucosal dissection is done under the mucosa of the left side of the septum **(Fig. 53–1)**. The mucosa at the most anterior portion of the septum is usually most adherent. For this reason, the initial submucosal dissection is carried very slowly and very carefully until the glistening white cartilage of the septum is well visualized. The field should be avascular and the plane should dissect easily. The mucosal dissection is carried posteriorly with enlargement of the submucosal window along the superoinferior plane until the bony septum is reached. Submucosal dissection on the left side of the septum is carried posteriorly until the left side of the anterior face of the sphenoid is reached.

A lot of surgeons obtain intraoperative fluoroscopic evaluation of the dissection plane at this stage, which is a perfectly acceptable step. We have avoided the use of intraoperative fluoroscopy by using the following important anatomical landmarks irrespective of whether fluoroscopy is used or not:

1. During dissection the direction of the nasal speculum should not be at more than a 20 degree angle above the floor of the maxilla **(Fig. 53–2)**.
2. The bony septum at the level of the anterior face of the sphenoid is usually soft and feels malleable or eggshell thin in the majority of cases. When the bony septum is harder than expected, it suggests that the speculum either is too close to the bony spine of the maxilla, which means the direction of the speculum is too low or is against the perpendicular plate of the ethmoid, which means the direction of the speculum is too high.
3. The deepest 130 to 150 mm nasal speculum is enough to reach the anterior face of the sphenoid. If the end of the speculum is too far from what is thought to be the anterior face of the sphenoid, then it is either too low along the roof of the nasopharynx or it is too high and pointing toward the ethmoid air cells and/or anterior frontal fossa **(Fig. 53–3)**.

Using these landmarks we managed to avoid the use of intraoperative fluoroscopy in the last 250 transsphenoidal operations. However, when in doubt take an x-ray. All through this dissection process the midline is kept on the left side of the speculum. Once the location of the anterior face of the sphenoid is identified, the speculum is further opened and rotated to fracture the thin portion of the septum using the left arm of the nasal speculum and followed by advancing it in the submucosal plane on the right side of the patient. The transsphenoidal suction is used to further dissect this submucosal plane superiorly and inferiorly on both sides of the septum. A self-retaining transsphenoidal retractor is then applied in place. This step is done by notifying the anesthesiologist because it is a stimulating step that can cause intraoperative hypertension.

The application of the self-retaining transsphenoidal retractor results in some submucosal oozing, which can easily be controlled by applying cotton balls. The anterior face of the sphenoid has the characteristic look resembling the "keel of a boat" **(Fig. 53–4)**. The anterior face of the sphenoid is then removed by identifying the sphenoid ostium and using the up-biting and down-biting Kerrison rongeurs. We routinely remove the mucosa of the sphenoid sinus. This is a controversial step. We prefer its removal to avoid the possible occurrence of a sphenoid sinus mucocele.

At this stage the dimensions and features of the sella are evaluated and the lateral walls of the anterior face of the sphenoid are further removed until both lateral aspects of the sella are well visualized, especially the infrasellar prominences of the internal carotid arteries. We routinely check the MRI at this stage to correlate what we see in the surgical field with what is shown on the MRI scans. This helps correlate the three-dimensional aspect of the suprasellar portion of the tumor and guides our choice of instruments.

In the majority of pituitary adenomas, the floor of the sella is thin enough to where it can easily be cracked by gently pushing against it with a curet or a dissector. It is then removed using Kerrison rongeurs. The removal of the bone is done without extension into the frontal skull base to avoid bleeding from the anterior intercavernous sinus **(Fig. 53–5)**. In case bleeding is encountered, the use of avetine with gentle pressure is the fastest way to stop the bleeding. After hemostasis is established the dura is opened for tumor removal. It is very important to cut the dura without the insertion of the knife deep into the sellar space. This is a word of caution because in some cases the carotid artery could be displaced both medially and anteriorly and it can easily be injured while opening the dura. We usually open the dura in a cruciate fashion and centered over the expected location of the tumor. The exposed sellar floor is gradually widened as the tumor resection proceeds. The steps of the tumor resection are discussed later.

Endonasal Transsphenoidal Approach

In the endonasal approach the anterior portion of the septum is bypassed and the sphenoid sinus is directly approached through its anterior wall. The landmarks to the location of the sphenoid sinus level are the different anatomical structures of the nasal cavity. The sphenoid ostium is usually located at the level of the middle turbinate. It can also be traced by

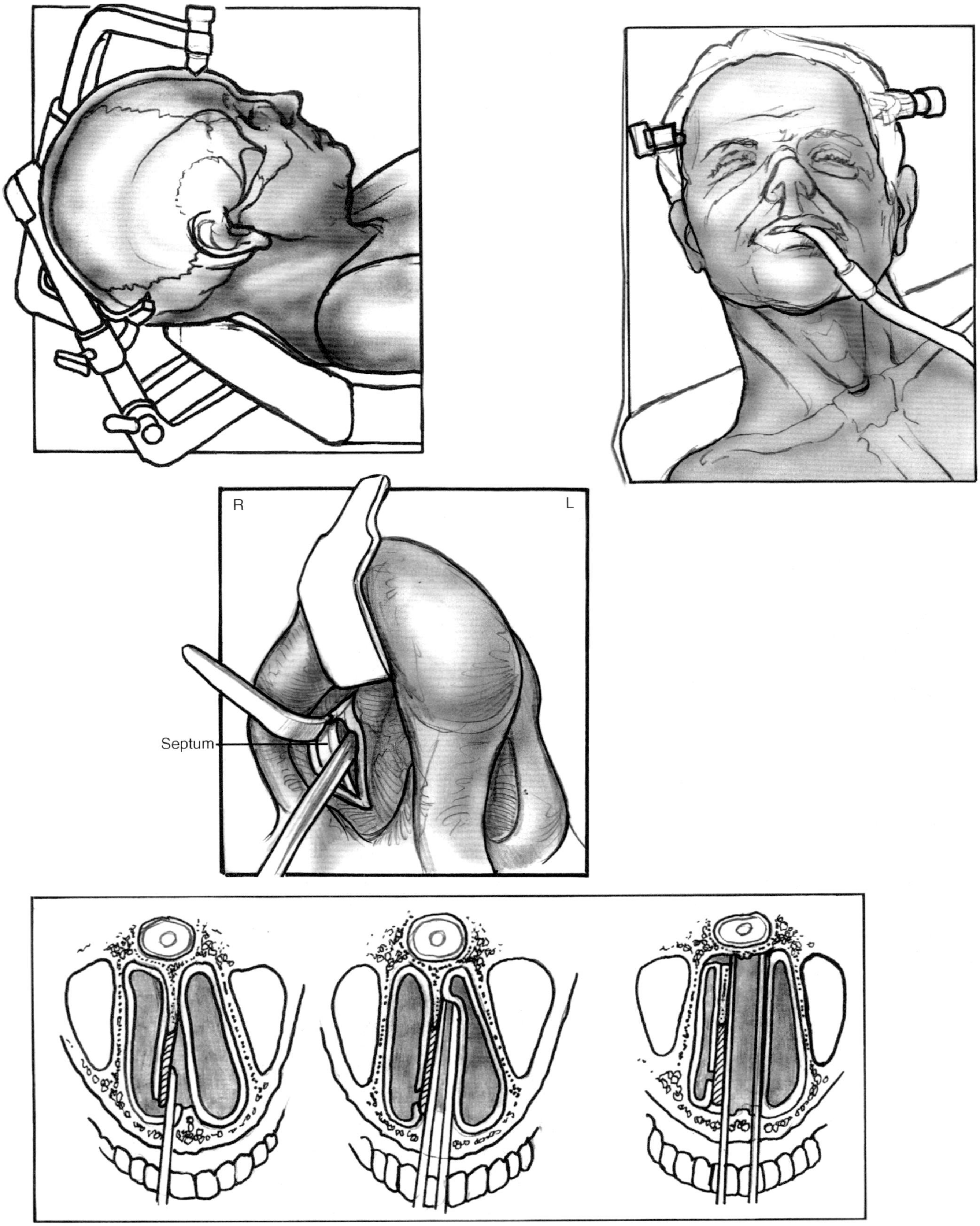

Figure 53–1 **(A)** Schematic diagram showing the transseptal transnasal transsphenoidal approach through the right nostril with left submucosal dissection. **(B)** Intraoperative picture of the approach. M, mucosal; CS, cartilaginous septum.

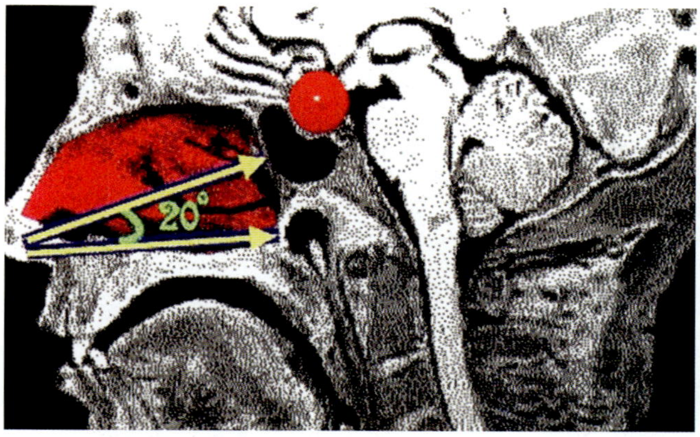

Figure 53–2 The relationship of the direction of transsphenoidal approach to the direction of the floor of the maxilla (about a 20 degree angle).

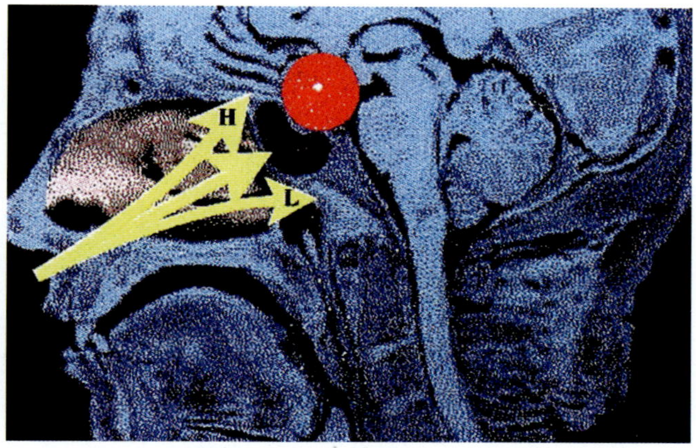

Figure 53–3 The longer the depth of the nasal cavity, the submucosal dissection should go too high (longer arrow H), or too low (longer arrow L).

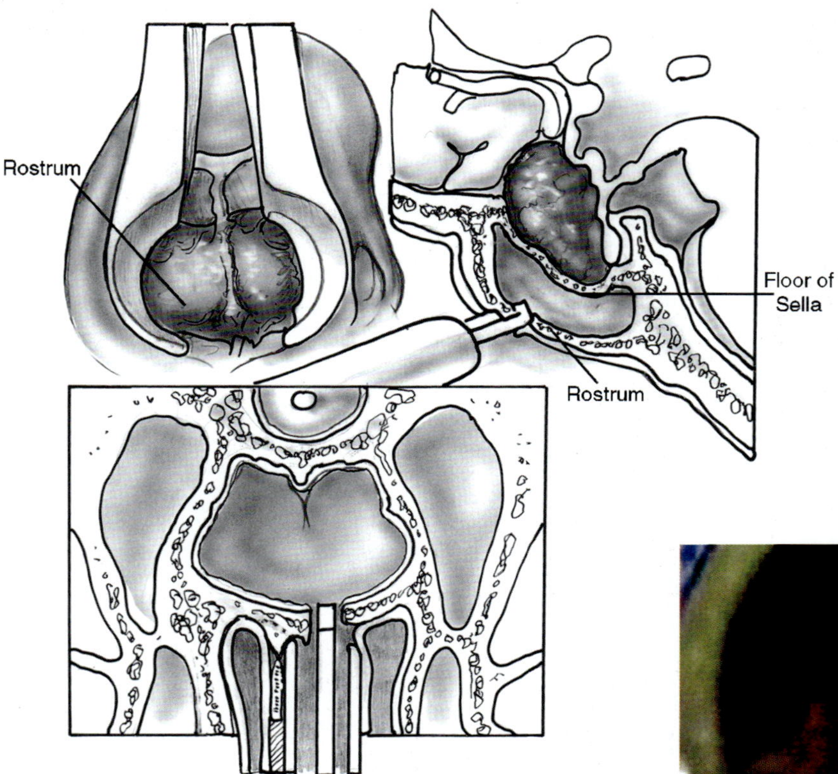

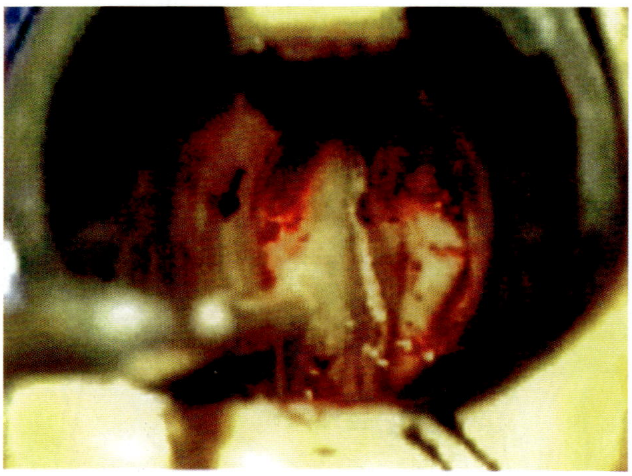

Figure 53–4 An intraoperative picture of the anterior face of the sphenoid, which looks like the keel of a boat.

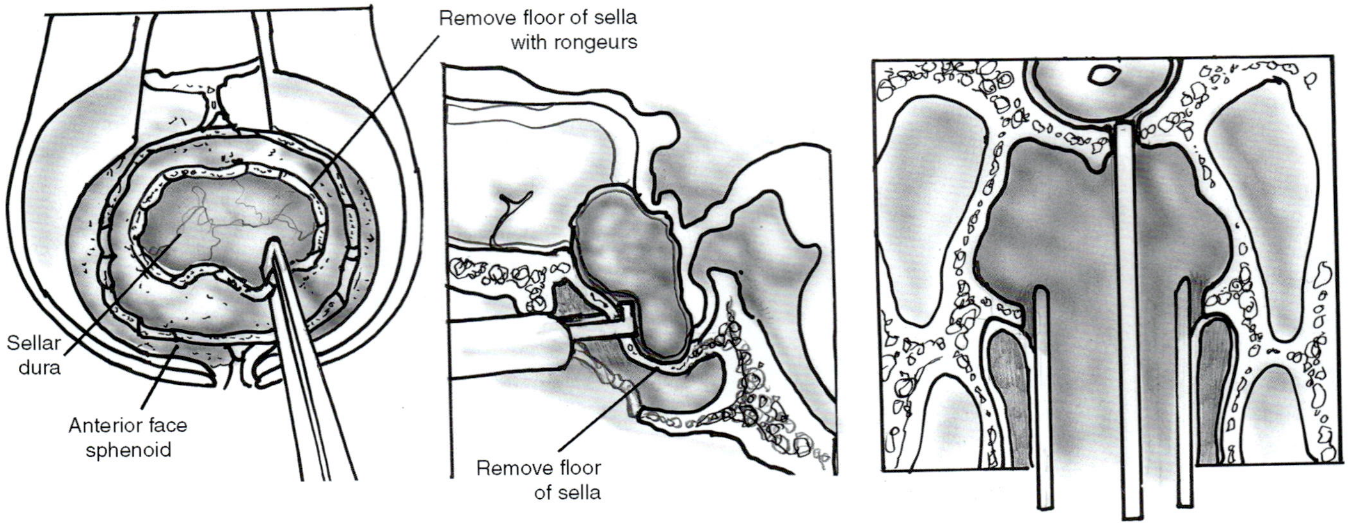

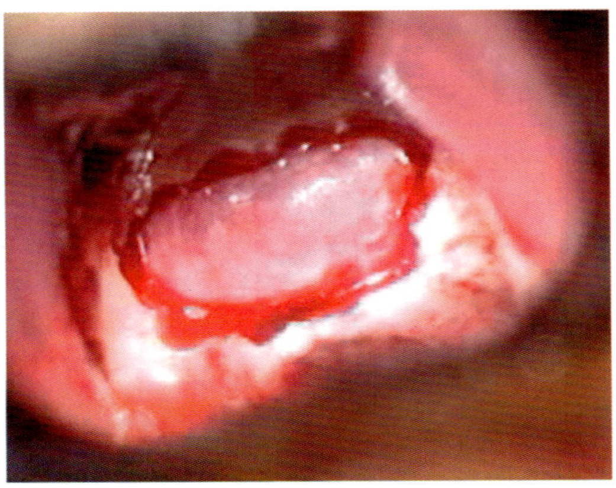

Figure 53–5 An intraoperative picture of the exposed sellar floor in a patient with a pituitary microadenoma.

following the roof of the nasopharynx as it curves anteriorly and superiorly. The meeting point of this course with the middle turbinate is a good entry point to the sphenoid sinus, which leads to the floor of the sella **(Fig. 53–6)**. When the endonasal transsphenoidal approach is used, the mucosa is cut on the side of the nostril through which the approach is made, and then the thin bony septum is mobilized with gentle pressure using the bade of the nasal speculum. The septum is then positioned between the two blades of the speculum, which is positioned in the submucosal plane. Further dissection with the tip of a suction instrument is made until adequate exposure of the anterior face of the

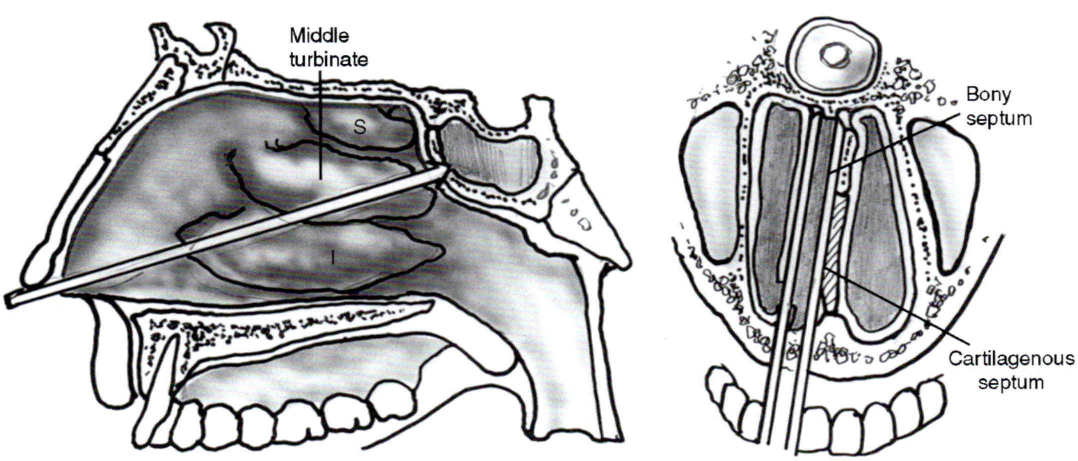

Figure 53–6 The endonasal approach level at the superior aspect of the middle turbinate.

sphenoid is achieved, similar to what is seen in the transseptal transsphenoidal approach. The transsphenoidal self-retaining retractor is then applied and the procedure is continued, very similar to what was described above for the transsphenoidal transseptal approach.

When the endoscope is used the mucosal opening is made at the same entry level, and the sphenoid ostium can be used as the initial entry point. The mucosa is cut and the anterior face of the sphenoid is widened with the Kerrison rongeurs until a window large enough to allow the introduction of the endoscope and two other instruments is achieved. In the majority of cases the site of the opening in the anterior face of the sphenoid is not significantly different or smaller than what is needed in the endonasal approach. The advantage achieved in the endonasal approach is best appreciated in pituitary macroadenomas when the suprasellar component of the tumor and the diaphragma sellae do not fall down into the surgical field. The endoscope can help inspect whether there is residual suprasellar tumor that needs further excision.

Tumor Resection

Excision of Microadenomas

Excision of pituitary microadenomas should be carried as meticulously as possible to avoid the risk of complications related to injury of the normal gland or the pituitary stalk. The proximity of the microadenoma to the stalk makes it more demanding to dissect the tumor without injury to the stalk. We recommend sharp dissection without the use of the bipolar cautery, which can injure the normal gland or the pituitary stalk. When the tumor is located in the lateral aspect of the gland, we find it necessary in the majority of cases to chase the tumor until venous bleeding from the cavernous sinus is encountered. This is a good indication that total resection was achieved.

Excision of Macroadenoma

The majority of pituitary adenomas are soft and suckable. The use of blunt curets is usually enough to scrape and remove the tumor in its majority. The use of a swiveling curet allows for tumor dissection in different directions. We start by resecting the tumor in its most inferior portion, causing the superior part to fall into the surgical field. This stepwise resection plan eventually leads the diaphragma sellae to fall into the field, an indication of adequate removal of the suprasellar component of a macroadenoma. The carotid itself can be felt. With experience the lateral gutters of the sella, especially around the carotid arteries, can be cleaned well. The tumor is then scraped from below and above the carotid arteries. This step is safer using the blunt transsphenoidal ring currette. The normal pituitary gland is usually flattened along the walls of the tumor bed. It is usually more orange to red in appearance, and it is not as suckable as the tumor. Very occasionally the tumor is hard to where it can be difficult to distinguish from the normal gland. In these cases the tumor needs to be carefully dissected off the carotid and the lateral wall of the sella, as well as from its attachment to the diaphragma sellae. These tumors need dissection with sharper curettes and a gentle pull with micropituitary rongeurs with further dissection using the suction tips. The resection of such tumors needs good experience by the surgeon to achieve a total resection without injury to the normal gland and the stalk.

Careful dissection and removal of the tumor can be achieved without significant injury to the diaphragma sellae and the risk of postoperative spinal fluid leak. When we encounter CSF leakage through the diaphragma sellae a small piece of fat harvested from the abdomen is put in the sella and followed by another piece in the sphenoid sinus. This simple step helped us avoid postoperative spinal fluid leakage, which was encountered in only two patients out of our last 250 transsphenoidal operations. When the endonasal approach is used it is important to position the fat well within the sphenoid sinus to avoid its displacement into the nasal cavity. After the fat application we introduce a nasal airway tube through each nostril and into the nasopharynx. They will splint the nasal septum and apply gentle pressure from both sides of the septum to help tamponade any blood oozing from the mucosa. Those tubes are removed the next morning. We rarely if ever use nasal packings.

◆ Postoperative Care

The patients are watched for any signs of diabetes insipidus in the first 24 hours and to see that the drainage from their nose stops by the time they get to the recovery room. The nasal airway tubes are removed the next morning as well as the Foley catheter. The majority of patients leave the hospital by the evening of the first postoperative day. Patients from out of town are advised to stay in a local hotel for another 24 hours. We routinely give patients 100 mg of hydrocortisone every 8 hours in the perioperative period, but they are discharged on 20 mg in the morning and 10 mg in the afternoon. Depending on their preoperative pituitary hormonal functions, a decision is made on how long to keep patients on steroid replacement. When the preoperative hormonal functions are normal the majority of patients undergo a morning fasting cortisol level a week after discharge, and if their cortisol level is adequate, discontinuing the hydrocortisone is tried. Patients are asked to call about any fatigue, decreased appetite, or lethargy in the 48 hours to follow. Our neuroendocrine clinic nurse usually calls the patients 2 days after discontinuing the hydrocortisone to confirm their well-being. The patients are seen on follow-up in 4 to 6 weeks from the time of the surgery at which time their wounds are evaluated and a baseline postoperative MRI is obtained for follow-up. During that visit the other hormonal functions are evaluated and further replacement is decided accordingly.

◆ Complications

The best way to avoid complications is to assume they will happen. This is true in every surgery including transsphenoidal surgery. The most dreaded complication is injury to the carotid artery. Even though it is a rare complication, it is a potentially devastating one and very difficult to manage.

The best way to avoid such a complication is to have good knowledge of the normal anatomy of the pituitary gland and the potential variations as a result of tumor occurrence. The proximity of the carotid artery is not something that most surgeons appreciate. It is also important to know that in pituitary tumors the carotid artery can get in direct contact with the sellar space. The avoidance of scraping along the carotid wall with sharp objects and the assumption that the carotid wall could be very thin in some patients will help avoid its injury.

Cerebrospinal fluid leakage is reported in the literature more often than it should occur. As mentioned above, gentle tumor dissection and attention to the preservation of the diaphragma sellae is a key step. Removal of the tumor starting with its inferior component and followed by the suprasellar component avoids the early protrusion of the diaphragma sellae into the surgical field and thus decreases the chances of its injury. In general, when surgery is done with the plan to preserve the normal pituitary gland, the chance of preserving the diaphragma sellae and avoiding the spinal fluid is increased. This is because in the majority of patients the diaphragma sellae is covered by a thin layer of compressed gland, which does not need to be removed. When residual tumor is suspected we recommend a microbiopsy of the tissue with an intraoperative frozen section evaluation to avoid unnecessary removal of the compressed normal gland and thus avoid the risk of a spinal fluid leak. If spinal fluid is encountered, fat harvested from the abdomen is positioned within the sella and the sphenoid sinus. We rarely use any other agents. Good packing of the sphenoid sinus is usually enough to prevent a CSF leak.

Infection and the risk of meningitis are other rare complications. They are less likely to occur if the diaphragma sellae is preserved. Chronic postoperative sphenoid sinusitis is not infrequent and it usually presents with patients complaining of a foul odor in their nose or excessive sinus drainage and headaches. Patients also develop a nasal voice very similar to the changes that occur after a common cold. These patients are treated with a 2-week course of antibiotics using 500 mg of ampicillin every 6 hours.

◆ Conclusion

The transsphenoidal approach to the pituitary area is a versatile and important approach which should be learned by all neurosurgeons.

54

Pituitary Macroadenomas: Transcranial Approach

Gerardo Guinto, Fabrizio Cohn, Ramiro Perez–de la Torre, and Mauricio Gallardo

Nowadays, most sellar tumors are surgically treated using the transsphenoidal approach because of its very low morbidity and mortality. However, there are several lesions that for some specific reason cannot be treated with this approach, so a transcranial route becomes necessary.[1] This option represents a higher complication risk, but in experienced hands it is possible to obtain more radical resections with preservation of the surrounding neurovascular structures. One of the most important advantages of the craniotomy is that it affords the surgeon a complete view of the effect of the pituitary tumor on the optic system, vessels, and oculomotor nerves, allowing their preservation even in highly aggressive lesions.[2] The main limitation of this approach, however, is that the intrasellar portion of the tumor may be very difficult to remove, especially when a prefixed chiasm also exists.

Throughout the years there have been different surgical alternatives available when choosing an intracranial approach, and the final choice depends on the surgeon's preference and personal experience. The critical point is to select the approach that allows the widest and safest exposure to ensure maximum resection of the tumor. Over the last 2 decades, development of skull base techniques has proved that it is possible to obtain ample exposure of the lesion without increasing morbidity. With this rationale, modern surgeons should be open to and familiar with all these procedures to select the ideal one, according to the circumstances.

◆ Indications

Considering that more than 96% of pituitary adenomas can be treated through a transsphenoidal approach, the main reason for choosing a craniotomy is for those cases where a transsphenoidal route cannot be used or has failed. The following factors have to be considered.

Tumor Size

There still exists some controversy on using the word *giant* or *massive* in referring to a pituitary adenoma.[3] Jefferson was the first to use the word *giant* for certain macroadenomas, but he did not specify the required dimensions. Symon et al[4] defined giant pituitary adenomas as lesions that extend more than 40 mm from the jugum sphenoidale in any direction, or within 6 mm of the foramen of Monro. Wilson[5] and Mohr et al[6] used the word *giant* for tumors that displace the third ventricle, which would imply an extension of 30 mm or higher from the tuberculum sellae. For dealing with all these types of adenomas, the transcranial approach is the preferred method.

Tumor Growth

The transcranial approach is the selected route when the tumor invades the anterior floor or middle cranial fossa, especially the cavernous sinus. Suprasellar extension is not a contraindication to the transsphenoidal approach because the upper part of the tumor usually descends into the sella as the intrasellar portion is being removed. Most dumbbell-shaped tumors can also be removed using the transsphenoidal approach because the aperture in the sellar diaphragm is rarely so narrow as to prevent the descent and removal of the suprasellar portion of the tumor. Considering this, craniotomy is the method of choice for all those cases when the tumor could not be removed by an experienced surgeon using the transsphenoidal approach.

Tumor Consistency

The vast majority of pituitary adenomas are soft and friable, which makes them feasible for removal with gentle dissection and suction. However 5% of all tumors show a higher connective tissue content, which complicates their resection. In these cases, a transcranial approach should be considered.

Sellar Tumors Other Than Pituitary Adenomas

Even though there are some small intrasellar lesions such as craniopharyngiomas, meningiomas, or chordomas that could be removed with a transsphenoidal approach, a transcranial route is safer in the majority of cases. As a general concept, when there is uncertainty about the diagnosis of a sellar lesion, craniotomy should be the preferred approach.

◆ Preoperative Management

A complete endocrine evaluation is mandatory for every patient to be operated on, for several reasons. First, a hormonal deficiency mandates an immediate preoperative replacement therapy, especially because the transcranial approach is clinically correlated with higher postoperative hormonal deficiencies, more than the transsphenoidal route. Second, it is very important to know if the tumor produces some specific hormone, especially prolactin, because in cases of highly invasive functioning tumors, the surgeon may not be so aggressive with portions invading critical areas like the cavernous sinus; these residual fragments could be medically treated thereafter. Finally, preoperative hormone levels, including dynamic tests, can be compared with postoperative ones to determine if the patient could be cured with surgery.

Except for Cushing's disease, stress doses of hydrocortisone are given in divided dosages of 300 mg on the day of surgery and gradually reduced by 50 to 100 mg each day thereafter until they can be discontinued. On the same day of the procedure, antibiotics and anticonvulsants are started. Once the general anesthesia is under way, an arterial line, a peripherally inserted central catheter, and a urinary catheter are placed.

◆ Choosing the Approach

There are some goals that need to be considered when choosing all possible surgical options for the transcranial route:[7] (1) choosing the shortest trajectory from the skin to the lesion, but avoiding critical neurovascular structures; (2) using the anatomical surgical corridors rather than free dissection; (3) retracting the brain as minimally as possible; (4) planning the incisions so as to preserve the va-scular supply of the flaps, taking into account prior scars; (5) respecting cosmesis; (6) ensuring early surgical control over feeding tumor vessels; (7) considering opportunities for reconstruction; and (8) considering the possibility of a redo operation. The most frequent transcranial approaches used for the resection of pituitary macroadenomas are described in the following sections.

Pterional

Popularized by Yasargil and Fox,[8] the pterional surgery is probably the most versatile and frequent approach used not only in sellar lesions but also in neurosurgical procedures in general.[9] This is particularly recommended for tumors with lateral extension that can be removed through the optico-carotid space. The name of the approach comes from the anatomical point called the pterion, which is a small circular area where the frontal bone, parietal bone, greater wing of the sphenoid, and the squamous part of the temporal bone meet. The patient is placed in a supine position, with the head secured with a head holder. The position is obtained after four basic movements: elevation of the head, 20 to 30 degree contralateral rotation, extension, and lateral tilt of the neck **(Fig. 54–1)**.

The surgical incision starts at the upper edge of the zygomatic arch (less than 1 cm in front of the tragus) and extends superiorly to the superior temporal line, where it turns anteriorly to end at the midline behind the hairline. The superficial temporal artery can be dissected and preserved in most of the cases, and the fascia of the temporalis muscle is kept intact. Interfascial dissection of the temporal muscle follows to avoid damage to the frontal branch of the facial nerve. This can be accomplished by making an oblique incision in the superficial temporal fascia behind and superior to the zygomatic arch.[10] The temporal fat pad is separated from the deep layer of the deep temporal fascia and reflected over the zygomatic arch. The temporal muscle is detached entirely from the superior temporal line and reflected anteroinferiorly. The craniotomy is usually initiated with only a single bur hole, placed at the most anterior extension of the superior temporal line, just above the frontozygomatic suture (keyhole). The size of the craniotomy depends on the growth pattern of the tumor. When there is a big suprasellar component, the craniotomy has to be extended toward the frontal bone. If the tumor grows toward the middle or posterior fossa, the craniotomy has to be extended backward. The next step is drilling along the sphenoid ridge. This drilling has to be continued medially up to the superior orbital fissure, and, during this maneuver, the meningo-orbital artery is coagulated and cut. The dura is then opened in a C-shaped fashion, parallel to the posterior edge of the craniotomy and reflected over the orbital roof. It is sometimes necessary to perform some relaxing incisions on its posterior aspect. Now a surgical microscope is brought in the field to start with the sylvian fissure dissection. This is a critical point in this approach because it allows the disengagement of the temporal lobe from the frontal lobe and allows the

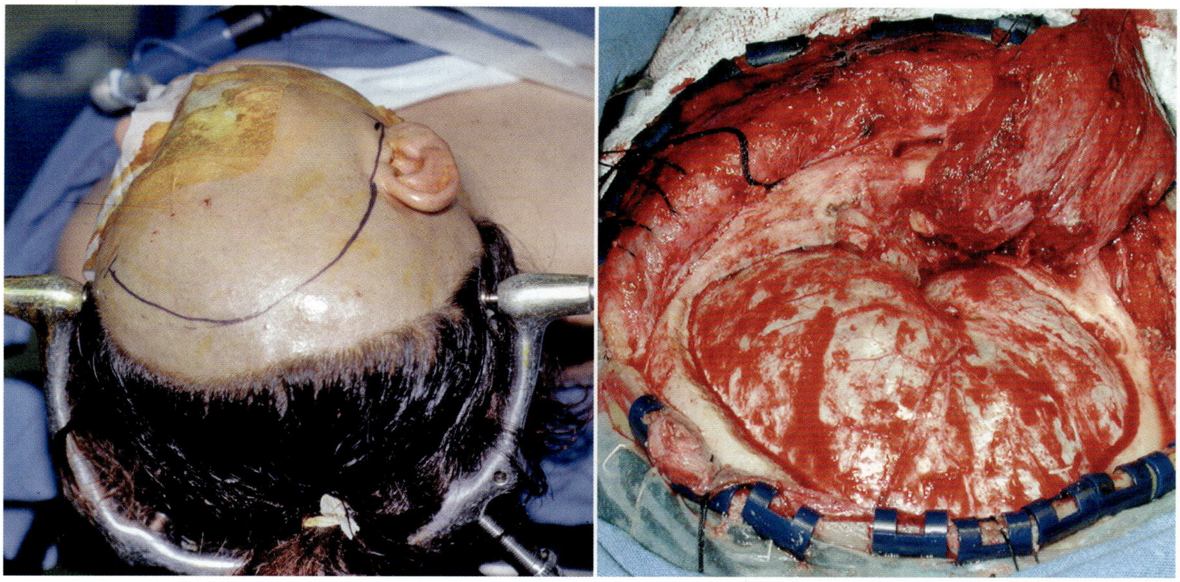

Figure 54–1 Pterional approach. Left: Positioning. Right: Details of the craniotomy.

frontal lobe to fall backward and the temporal lobe to fall downward through the force of gravity, almost without the need for a retractor. It also helps in the early visualization of the middle cerebral artery, the anterior cerebral artery, and the carotid bifurcation. The splitting process of the sylvian fissure usually initiates (using a no. 11 blade and microscissors) at the level of the pars triangularis, where the space between the frontal and temporal lobes is wider. Dissection is usually performed on the frontal side of the superficial sylvian vein, leaving this vein to the temporal side, preserving its drainage to the sphenoparietal sinus. The dissection is then continued to the chiasmatic and carotid cisterns, allowing the cerebrospinal fluid (CSF) to leak out freely.

Once the tumor has been identified, the resection process begins with an intratumoral debulking. Cystic components are also drained first to decrease tumor size. In cases of solid tumors, with the optic nerve stretched, it is recommended to drill the optic canal first and to cut the overlying fibrous dural band. This will decompress and relax the nerve so it can be more tolerant of manipulation during tumor removal. Then the tumor can be reached using several windows (**Fig. 54–2**). Moving toward the frontal extension of the approach, it is possible to access the lesion through the interoptic space, bearing in mind that this window is reduced or absent in cases of prefixed chiasm. The space between the optic nerves allows for good exposure of the intrasellar tumor, and through dissection of the lamina terminalis it is possible to have access to the third ventricle. Another window provided by the pterional approach is the opticocarotid space, which can be widened when removing the anterior clinoid process. When the tumor is reached through this window, extreme care should be taken with the perforating arteries that originate in the medial wall of the internal carotid artery and that become the superior hypophyseal artery complex, which supplies the optic chiasm, the pituitary stalk, and the optic nerves. The last window offered by this approach is the space between the internal carotid artery and the oculomotor nerve. However, this is the narrowest space to reach the tumor, and there is a high risk of oculomotor deficit. Other important structures that can be identified in this space include the choroidal artery and the posterior communicating artery. Finally, with the drilling of the posterior clinoid process, access to the posterior fossa can also be obtained.

The initial debulking can be done with the aspirator, bipolar, biopsy forceps, and curets. In pituitary adenomas it is almost never necessary to use another surgical tool like an ultrasonic aspirator or laser. Once the tumor has been decompressed, it is now possible to remove the pseudocapsule, dissecting it from

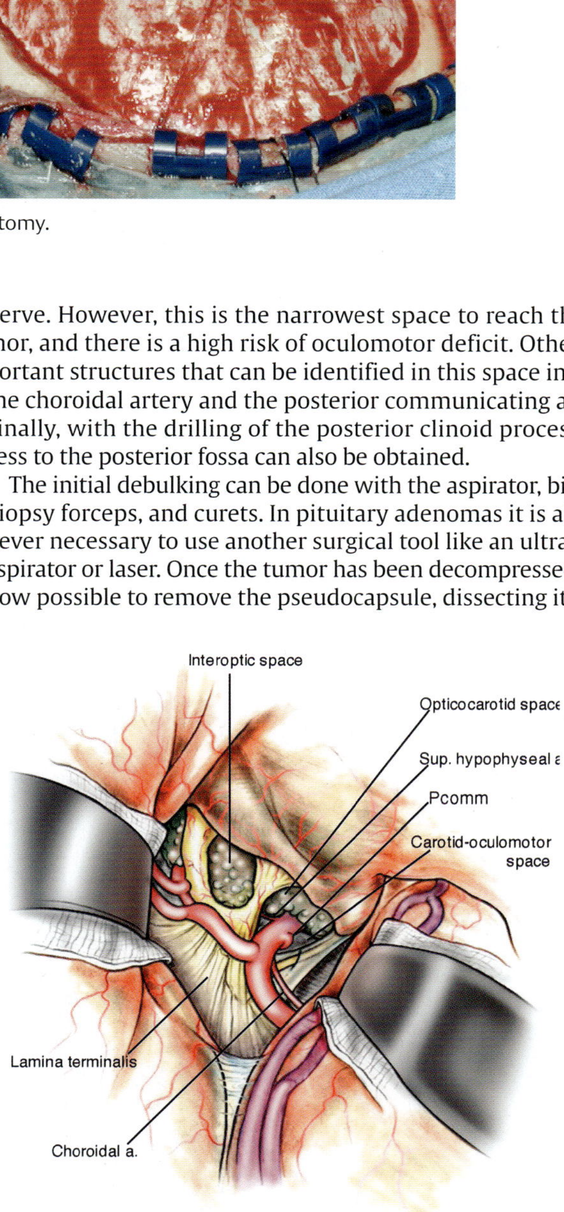

Figure 54–2 Schematic representation of exposure in the pterional approach. The tumor can be removed through the following spaces: interoptic, opticocarotid, and carotid-oculomotor. Lamina terminalis could also be opened to gain access to the third ventricle.

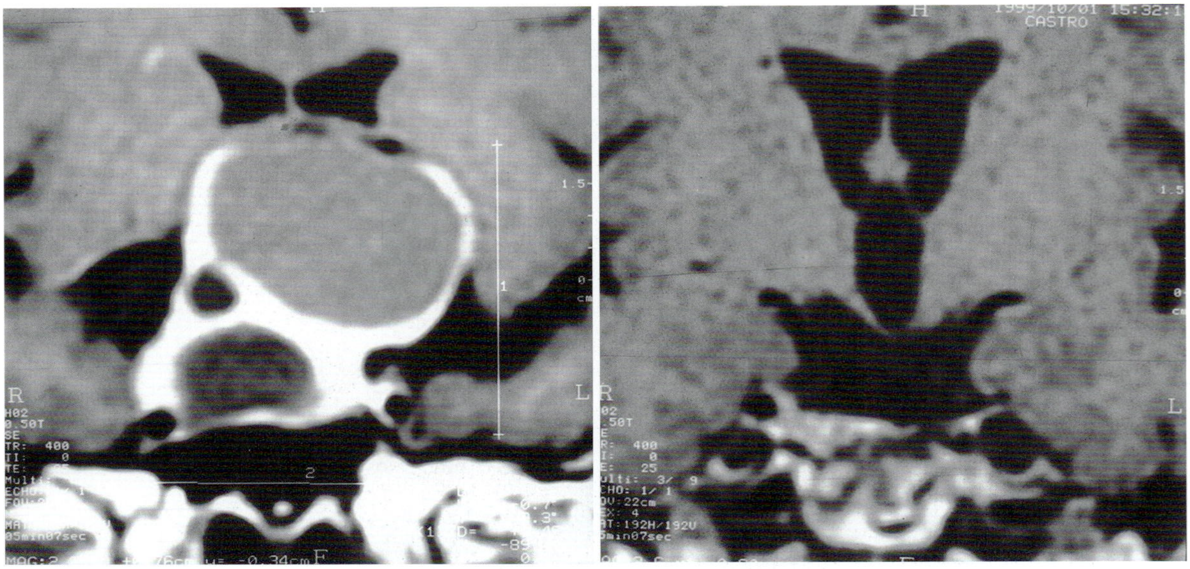

Figure 54–3 Case no. 1. A 37-year-old woman with a severe visual deficit, mainly in the left eye. Left: Preoperative magnetic resonance imaging showing a multicystic pituitary adenoma with lateral extension. Right: Tumor was totally removed through a left pterional approach.

the surrounding structures. In some special situations where there has been a history of prior surgery or radiotherapy, there are firm adherences between the tumor, arteries, and nerves, which make the dissection process difficult.

Fig. 54–3 shows a large tumor that was removed through the pterional approach.

Orbitozygomatic

This approach is especially appropriate for tumors with extension into the paranasal sinuses, orbit, cavernous sinus, and petroclival region.[11] Patient positioning and the craniotomy process are similar to those for the pterional approach. Once this step has been completed, an osteotomy is performed, which includes the orbital rim, the roof and lateral wall of the orbit, and the zygomatic arch **(Fig. 54–4).**

When access to the cavernous sinus is required, it becomes necessary to expose the petrous portion of the internal carotid artery. Then the major part of the condylar fossa of the temporal bone has to be included in the zygomatic osteotomy. The extradural stage of the approach must also include the complete resection of the anterior clinoid process and the drilling of the middle cranial fossa until exposing the second and third divisions of the trigeminal nerve. The

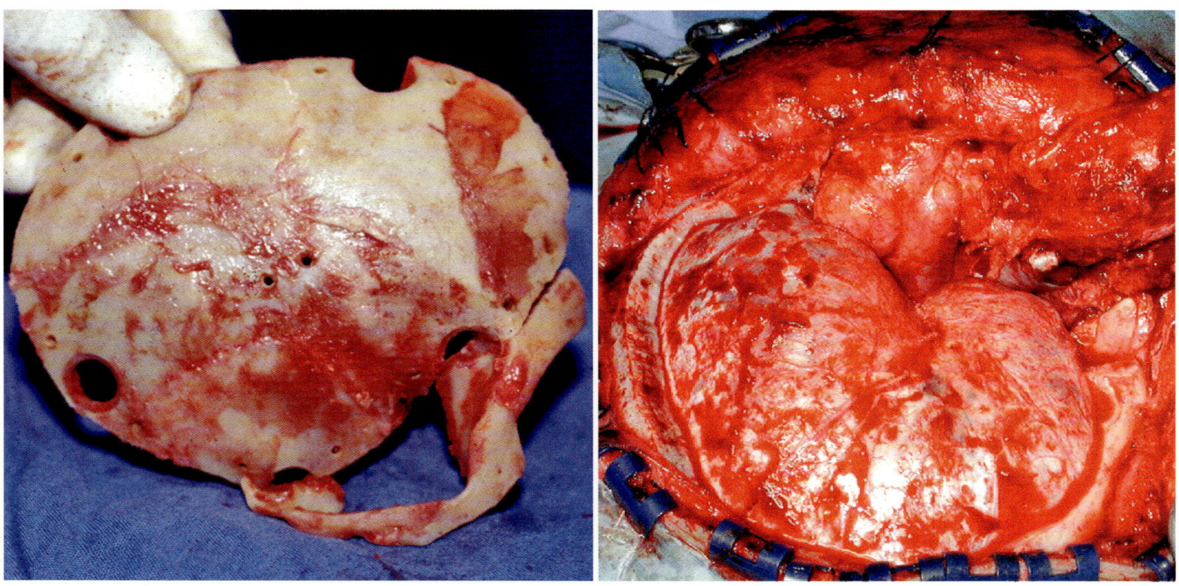

Figure 54–4 Orbitozygomatic approach. Left: Details of the frontotemporal craniotomy and the orbitozygomatic osteotomy. Right: Surgical exposure. Note how the complete displacement of the temporalis muscle allows for wide exposure of the middle cranial fossa, orbit contents, and base of the infratemporal fossa.

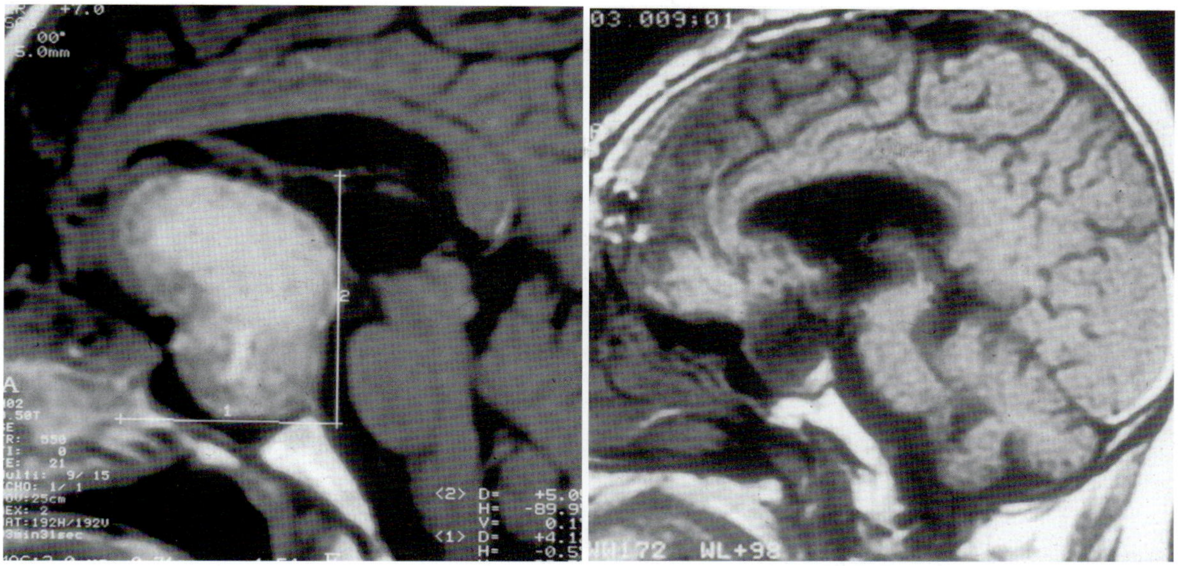

Figure 54–5 Case no. 2. A 43-year-old man with headache, bitemporal hemianopsia, and frontal syndrome. Left: A giant sellar tumor with an evident extension to the anterior floor is shown. Right: Postoperative result. A bifrontal interhemispheric approach was used, and there is no evidence of residual tumor. Intrasellar hyperintensity corresponds to the neurohypophyseal tissue.

middle meningeal artery and the greater superficial petrosal nerve have to be sectioned.

With this approach, exposure of the orbit, middle fossa, and base of the infratemporal fossa is wide and safe. Finally, if the petrous apex is drilled, access to the petroclival region and the upper third of the clivus is also obtained.

Bifrontal Interhemispheric

Although this approach was originally described for clipping anterior communicating aneurysms,[12] it allows excellent exposure of the sellar region with bilateral control of the optic nerves and internal carotid arteries. It also provides preservation of the olfactory nerves. This approach is particularly suitable when anterior midline extension of a sellar tumor is observed **(Fig. 54–5).**

The patient is placed in a supine position with the head slightly extended. A bicoronal skin incision is performed, running from one root of the zygomatic arch to the other. The myocutaneous flap is anteriorly reflected until both orbital rims can be seen; it is not necessary to detach the periorbita or to expose the supraorbital nerves **(Fig. 54–6).** A

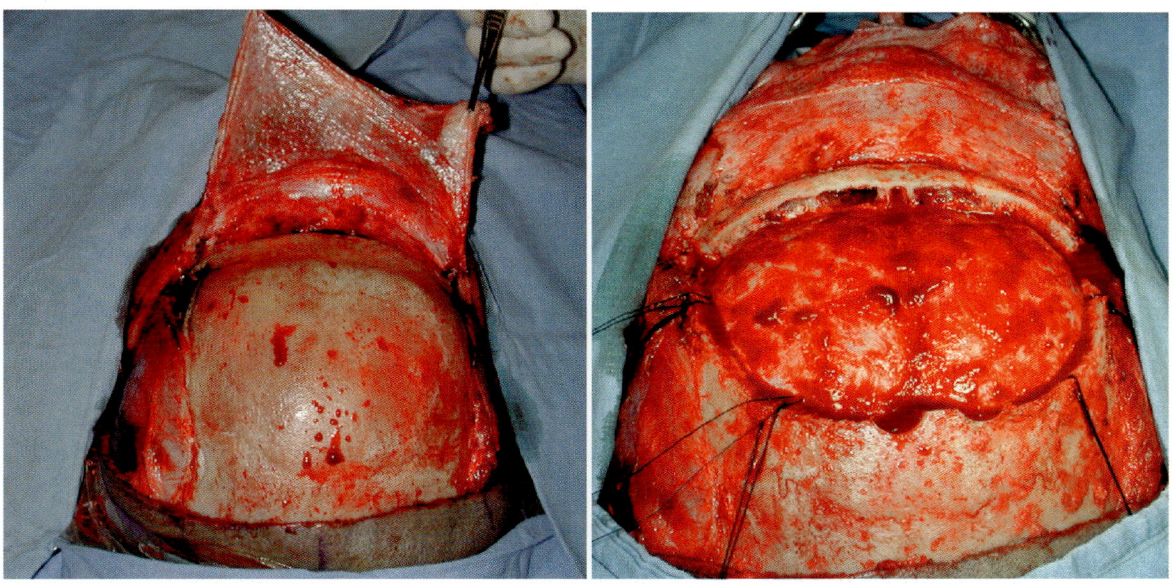

Figure 54–6 Bifrontal interhemispheric approach. Left: Exposure of the frontal squama. Note the preservation of the pericranial flap. Right: Details of the craniotomy.

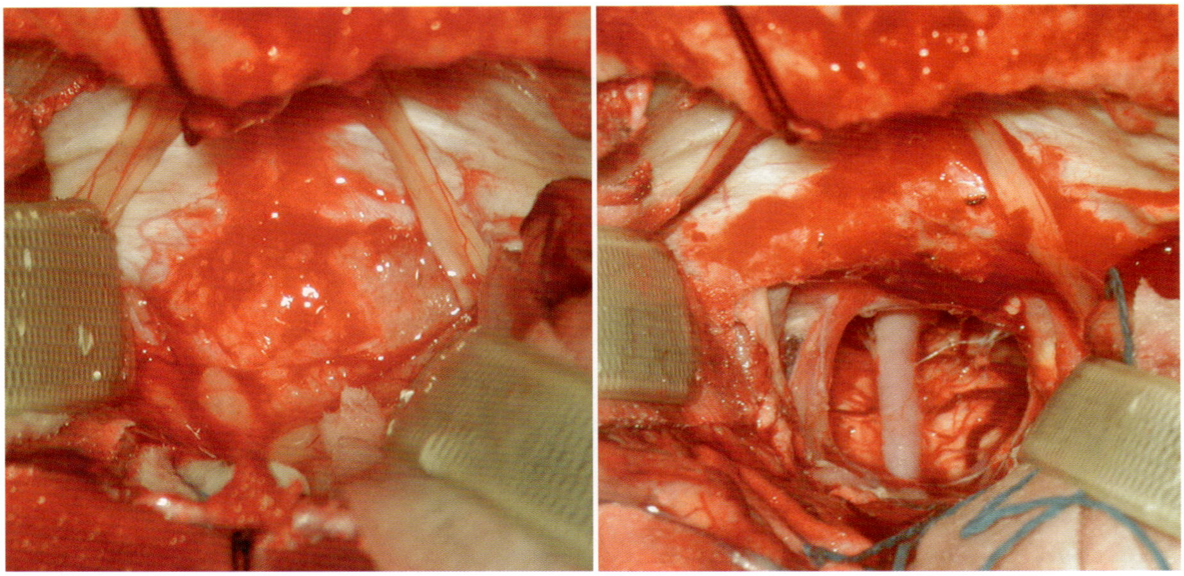

Figure 54–7 Exposure of a sellar tumor through the bifrontal interhemispheric approach. Left: the frontal lobes are retracted laterally and the sellar tumor is clearly seen. Note the preservation of both olfactory nerves. Right: tumor has been completely removed with preservation of the olfactory nerves. The basilar artery and the anterior surface of the brain stem is exposed.

craniotomy is performed, centered in the frontal bone, 2 cm in front of the coronal suture, 1 cm above the superior insertion of the temporalis muscles, and 1.5 cm above the orbital rims. The dural incision is performed in a U-shaped fashion with its arms opened backward. The sagittal sinus is sutured and cut as far anterior as possible, and the falx cerebri is also sectioned. The dural flap is reflected backward, identifying and preserving the superficial frontal veins that directly drain into the sagittal sinus. Working under the microscope, the interhemispheric frontal fissure is divided while gentle lateral retraction on the frontal lobes is maintained. The dissection is continued toward the anterior floor of the skull base up to the identification of the *crista galli* and both olfactory nerves. Every nerve is carefully detached from the orbital surface of the frontal lobe. It is advisable to invest as much time as needed until both olfactory nerves are totally free. Sometimes dissection of the olfactory nerves is time-consuming, but surgeons must be conscientious about ensuring that olfaction can be preserved in the majority of cases. Next, the *jugum sphenoidale* and *tuberculum sellae* are identified; however, quite often these structures are hidden by the tumor, and thus initial internal debulking has to begin at this point. In cases of a prefixed chiasm, access to the intrasellar component of the tumor is very difficult. Drilling of the *tuberculum sellae* could help, being careful not to open the sphenoid sinus to avoid risk of CSF leakage.

Once tumor decompression has been performed, the pseudocapsule can be freed from the surrounding neurovascular structures. Every small perforating artery in this area has to be preserved because they represent the main vascular supply to the chiasm, pituitary stalk, and hypothalamus. The lamina terminalis can also be opened to obtain access to the third ventricle. Traction on the pituitary stalk should be avoided; however, in very large tumors, identification of this anatomical structure is almost impossible. Finally, when the tumor is completely removed, it is possible to see the basilar artery and the ventral surface of the brain stem **(Fig. 54–7).**

Extended Subfrontal

This approach is selected when lesions invade the sphenoid sinus, ethmoid sinus, orbits, and inferior two thirds of the clivus up to the anterior surface of C1.[13] The main limitation of this approach is lateral exposure, toward the cavernous sinus, petrous bone, and internal carotid arteries, and the need to cut the olfactory nerves. Even though this access is more frequently used in other lesions such as chordomas, sometimes pituitary adenomas have such a growth pattern that its use is justified **(Fig. 54–8).**

The patient is placed in the supine position, with the head slightly extended. A bicoronal skin incision is made behind the hairline, starting right in front of the ear and extending vertically up to the opposite side. The incision is taken down to the pericranium, which is dissected from the skin flap posteriorly and divided about 3 to 4 cm behind the line of the skin incision. Then the skin flap (with the pericranium) is reflected forward and dissection is performed to expose the superior orbital rims bilaterally and the frontonasal suture in the midline. The supraorbital nerves and vessels are freed from their corresponding notches; the periorbita is dissected from the superior, lateral, and medial walls of the orbit, at least 3 cm posterior to the supraorbital ridges.

A similar craniotomy to the one described in the previous approach is performed, but a little wider and as anterior as possible, sometimes including the superior wall of the frontal sinus. Care should be taken in the dissection of the sagittal sinus. In elderly patients this sinus is usually firmly adhered to the bone, so the craniotomy may be done in two pieces, allowing sinus detachment under direct vision. The frontal sinus

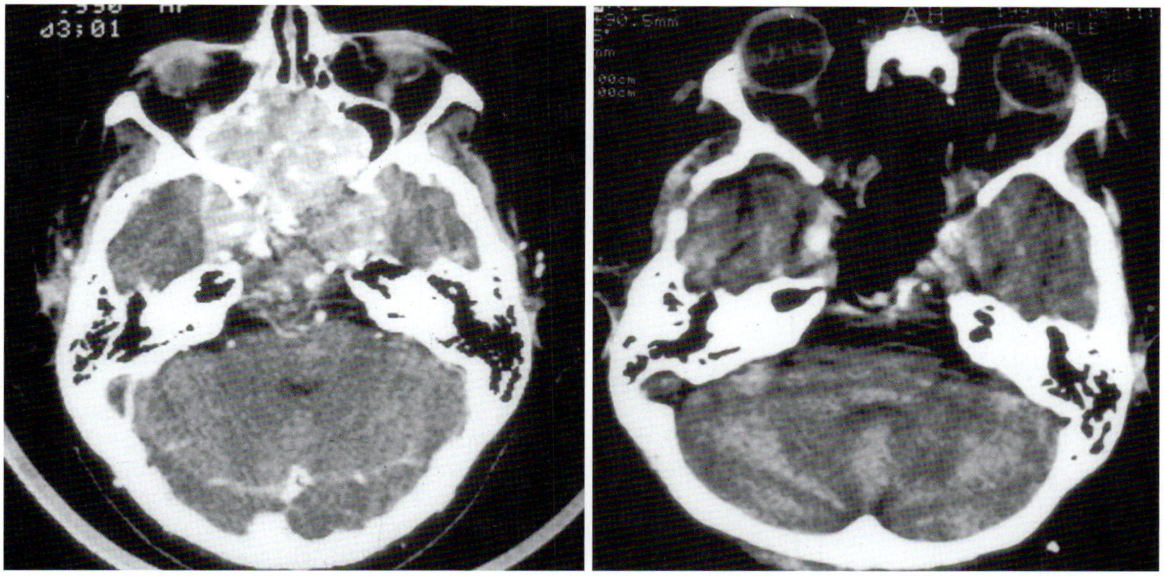

Figure 54–8 Case no. 3. A 45-year-old woman with amenorrhea and galactorrhea and a very high prolactin level. She was treated with bromocriptine but with no response. Left: A giant tumor with invasion to the sphenoid, ethmoid sinus, and orbits. Right: Tumor was completely removed using an extended frontal approach.

mucosa is then exenterated and the dura is separated from the *crista galli*; the dural sleeves of the olfactory nerves (with the nerves inside) are then bilaterally divided; detachment of the dura is continued on the roofs of the orbits, going back to the *planum sphenoidale*. Suturing of the dural olfactory sleeves can be done at this point or at the end of the procedure.

A bilateral orbital osteotomy is performed by doing two particular cuts: a coronal cut is initially made, at least 2.5 cm back from the supraorbital rim, running through the roof of both orbits, and passing behind the cribriform plate of the ethmoid. The other cut is horizontal or axial and is made at or just below the frontonasal suture and extended posteriorly ~3 cm to meet the coronal cut, which will extend to the anterior ethmoidal foramen, where some bleeding may be seen because of the laceration of the ethmoidal arteries. Both cuts also meet at the lateral walls of the orbits. Once this is complete, the orbito-fronto-ethmoidal osteotomy piece can be removed **(Fig. 54–9).** Working under the microscope, the remaining ethmoid cells and *planum sphenoidale* are removed with rongeurs or drilling. The optic nerves are unroofed and

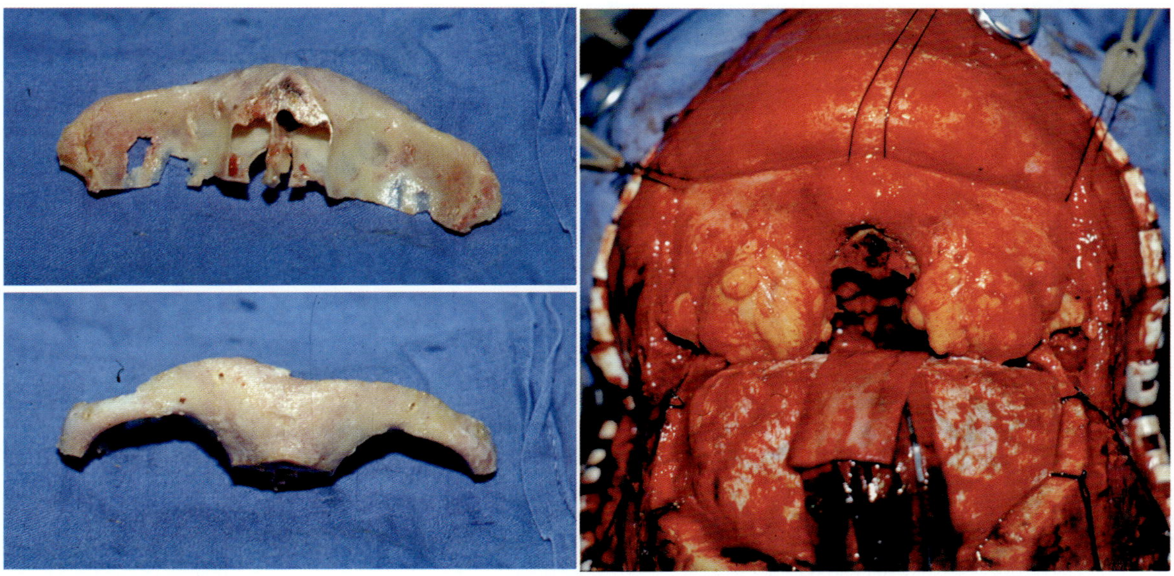

Figure 54–9 Extended frontal approach. Left: Details of the orbito-fronto-ethmoidal osteotomy piece. Right: Tumor exposure is obtained working between both orbits and optic nerves.

the anterior wall of the sphenoid sinus is also drilled, entering the sphenoid sinus, where the contour of the sella and the base of the clivus can be identified.

Tumor removal technique is the same as has already been mentioned. Reconstruction starts by filling the dead space with fat, usually taken from the lateral surface of the thigh. Then the pericranial flap is rotated and brought into the surgical bed, passing underneath the orbital osteotomy piece, and the bone flap is replaced as usual.

Anterior Transcallosal

Some pituitary adenomas grow upward into the third ventricle, and they cannot be reached using a basal access. The anterior transcallosal approach is specially designed for these cases.[14]

The patient is placed in a supine position, with the head fixed and slightly flexed. The incision can be either bicoronal, horseshoe-shaped, or in the shape of a question mark, centered in the nondominant hemisphere over the frontal squama, trying to expose the coronal suture and the midline when retracting the skin flap. A standard craniotomy is performed 2 cm behind the coronal suture, 5 cm in front of it, 5 cm from the midline on the ipsilateral side, and 2 cm from the midline to the contralateral side. The sagittal sinus must be exposed to reduce midline slot retraction and optimize deep view lines. The dural flap is opened to the lateral component of the bone flap and reflected medially to the sagittal sinus. A surgical microscope should be used for this step, because venous structures and pacchionian granulations have to be carefully dissected and preserved. The frontal lobe is then dissected from the falx cerebri and separated laterally with the self-retractor. At this point the callosal marginal and pericallosal arteries, on both sides, should be identified and also separated to expose the *corpus callosum*. A 2.5 cm anterior callosotomy is made, and at this point the lateral ventricle falls into view and the self-retractor is gradually advanced. Once the ventricle has been entered, the choroid plexus should be identified to have a proper orientation because it is not uncommon to penetrate the contralateral ventricle. The plexus can be followed in a forward direction until the foramen of Monro is visualized, from which the third ventricle can be reached to proceed with the tumor resection. In pituitary adenomas this transforaminal approach is usually sufficient to afford tumor resection; however, sometimes it is necessary to increase exposure, which can be obtained using the interforniceal or subchoroidal access.

Once the tumor has been removed, strict hemostasis is mandatory because a minimum residual bleeding in the ventricular cavity represents a high risk of hydrocephalus. However, the placement of a transient ventriculostomy catheter is recommended in most cases.

With this approach only the uppermost part of the tumor can be safely removed; the sellar component should be resected using another access **(Fig. 54–10).**

Subfrontal

This approach can be performed through two possible accesses: midline or lateral. The first is similar to the bifrontal interhemispheric, but here the frontal lobe is retracted upward instead of laterally. The second approach allows access to the sellar region in an oblique direction, entering through a frontolateral or transciliary craniotomy.[15] The main disadvantage of subfrontal approaches is that the cavity of the sella is less accessible because the surgeon must work over the ipsilateral optic nerve.

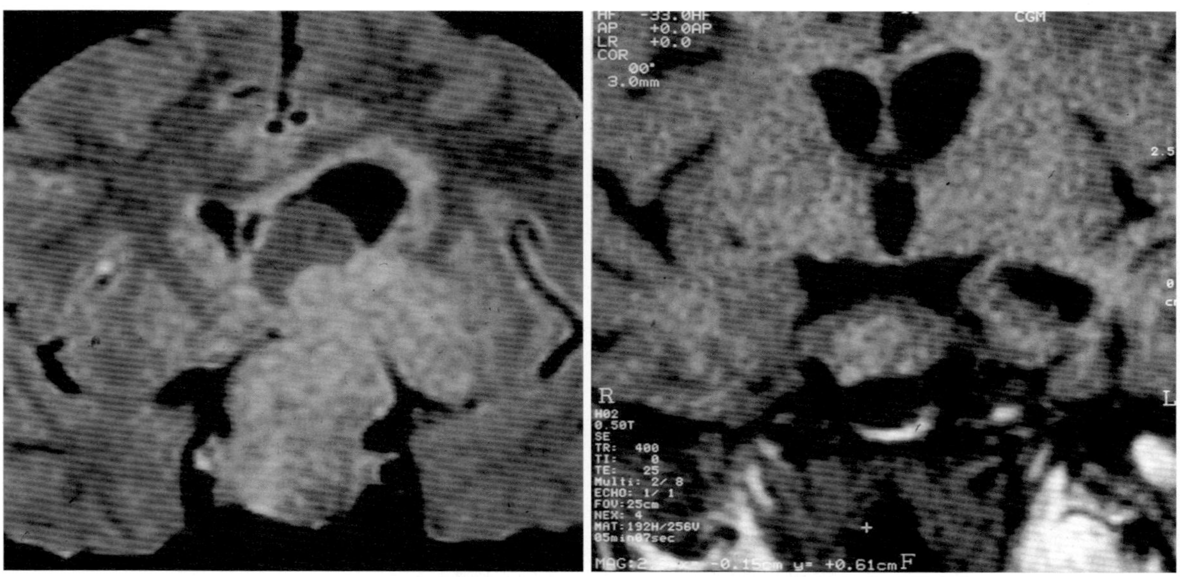

Figure 54–10 Case no. 4. A 47-year-old man with headache and visual deficit. Left: A giant tumor is shown growing upward, invading the third and left lateral ventricles. Right: An anterior transcallosal approach was used; note how the whole intraventricular component of the tumor was removed. There is a small piece of residual tumor located in the sella that was operated on through a transsphenoidal approach 4 months later.

Combined Approaches

In huge tumors with a peculiar growth pattern, a simultaneous combination of two or more approaches can be used; one of these is the supra-infrasellar.[16] This approach is especially recommended for sellar tumors with extension to the middle cranial fossa and consists of the tumor resection using pterional and transsphenoidal routes in the same surgical stage. It has to be performed by two complete surgical teams. The procedure begins with the pterional approach to expose the tumor, dissecting from the surrounding neurovascular structures; then the transsphenoidal team approaches the tumor from below. At this moment, the pterional team gently pushes the tumor down, which is mainly removed by the transsphenoidal team.

Another combination that is also used in this kind of tumor is the pterional with the transcallosal approach.[17] This is particularly indicated for lesions with a huge suprasellar component and invasion into the third ventricle. Both routes do not strictly need to be performed simultaneously, so two surgical teams are not necessary. Because of the high aggressiveness of combined approaches, they would only be preferred for young people without major risk factors.

◆ Postoperative Care

In general, every patient operated on through a transcranial route needs more intensive postoperative care than do patients operated on with the transsphenoidal approach. Thus they have to be routinely transferred to the intensive care unit at the end of the procedure.

The patient is extubated as soon as possible, a strict hydroelectrolyte balance is started, and an early simple computed tomography is performed within the first 48 hours. The patients are usually discharged from the unit within 48 to 72 hours and sent home 4 to 6 days later. Control radiological studies are performed 2 months after surgery.

◆ Complications

General complications are basically the same as in other neurosurgical procedures; they include infection, hematoma, seizures, and CSF leakage. Among them, CSF leakage warrants special mention. This complication occurs mostly when a previous transsphenoidal operation has been done and an inadequate obliteration of the sphenoid sinus was performed. It can also occur because of an inadvertent opening in the sphenoid or ethmoid sinus not properly repaired during surgery.

There are other groups of postoperative complications that are seen more frequently in sellar lesions than in other standard neurosurgical procedures: hypothalamic damage and visual deficit. To avoid hypothalamic damage, preservation of all the perforating arteries is mandatory, as is the gentle manipulation of the upper part of the tumor. Most of the time a visual deficit is secondary to damage in the vascular supply of the optic nerve or chiasm. Comprehensive anatomical knowledge of the microvascular anatomy and a meticulous refined technique are the most important factors to avoid this complication.

References

1. Patterson RH. The role of transcranial surgery in the management of pituitary adenoma. Acta Neurochir Suppl 1996;65:16–17
2. Thapar K, Laws ER. Pituitary tumors. In: Kaye AH, Laws ER, eds. Brain Tumors. New York: Churchill Livingstone; 2001:803–854
3. Wilson CB. A decade of pituitary microsurgery: the Herbert Olivecrona Lecture. J Neurosurg 1984;61:814–833
4. Symon L, Jakubowski J, Kendall B. Surgical treatment of giant pituitary adenomas. J Neurol Neurosurg Psychiatry 1979;42:973–982
5. Wilson CB. Neurosurgical management of large and invasive pituitary tumors. In: Tindall GT, Collins WF, eds. Clinical Management of Pituitary Disorders. New York: Raven; 1979:335–342
6. Mohr G, Hardy J, Comtois R, Beauregard H. Surgical management of giant pituitary adenomas. Can J Neurol Sci 1990;17:62–66
7. Torrens M. Factors influencing the choice of approach. In: Al-Mefty O, ed. Operative Skull Base Surgery. New York: Churchill Livingstone; 1997:1–19
8. Yasargil MG, Fox JL. The microsurgical approach to intracranial aneurysms. Surg Neurol 1975;3:7–14
9. Wen HT, De Oliveira E, Tedeschi H, Andrade FC, Rhoton AL. The pterional approach: surgical anatomy, operative technique, and rationale. Oper Techn Neurosurg 2001;4:60–72
10. Yasargil MG, Reichman MV, Kubik S. Preservation of the frontotemporal branch of the facial nerve using the interfascial temporalis flap for pterional craniotomy: technical article. J Neurosurg 1987;67:463–466
11. Sekhar LN, Schramm VL, Jones NF. Subtemporal-preauricular infratemporal fossa approach to large lateral and posterior cranial base neoplasms. J Neurosurg 1987;67:488–499
12. Suzuki J, Mizoi K, Yoshimoto T. Bifrontal interhemispheric approach to aneurysms of the anterior communicating artery. J Neurosurg 1986;64:183–190
13. Sekhar LN, Wright DC, Sen CN. Extended frontal approach to tumors and aneurysms of the cranial base. In: Wilkins RH, Rengachary SS, eds. Neurosurgery. New York: McGraw-Hill; 1996: 1611–1621
14. Apuzzo ML, Litofsky NS. Surgery in and around the anterior third ventricle. In: Apuzzo ML, ed. Brain Surgery: Complication Avoidance and Management. New York: Churchil Livingstone; 1993:541–579
15. Sanchez-Vazquez MA, Barrera-Calatayud P, Mejia-Villela M, Palma-Silva JF, Juan-Carachure I, Gomez-Aguilar JM, et al. Transciliary subfrontal craniotomy for anterior skull base lesions. Technical note. J Neurosurg 1999;91:892–896
16. Loyo M, Kleriga E, Mateos H, de Leo R, Delgado A. Combined supra- infrasellar approach for large pituitary tumors. Neurosurgery 1984;14:485–488
17. Yasargil MG, Curcic M, Kis M, Seigenthaler G, Teddy PJ, Roth P. Total removal of craniopharyngiomas: approaches and long-term results in 144 patients. J Neurosurg 1990;73:3–11

55

Pituitary Macroadenomas: Transsphenoidal Approach

Gerardo Guinto, Fabrizio Cohn, Ramiro Perez–de la Torre, and Mauricio Gallardo

The transsphenoidal approach represents the most frequent surgical procedure for treating intrasellar lesions, particularly pituitary adenomas. It was initially described by Schloffer in 1907 using a superolateral, nasoethmoidal access, and modified later by Harvey Cushing, who designed the sublabial route.[1] He used this approach extensively and with relatively good results but later abandoned it in favor of the transcranial procedure. In the 1960s, Gerald Guiot and Jules Hardy refined the operation using a surgical microscope and intraoperative fluoroscopic guidance, greatly improving the results. The procedure today stands as one of the most effective operative techniques performed by neurosurgeons, with a morbidity of less than 2% and a mortality rate of less than 0.5%.

◆ Indications

The transsphenoidal approach is indicated for the majority of tumors located in the sellar region, such as pituitary adenomas, craniopharyngiomas, and meningiomas. However, there are other nontumoral lesions, including arachnoid cysts and special cases of empty sella syndrome, for which this approach is used as well. In the case of tumors, there are several factors, described in the following sections, that have to be considered in selecting this approach.

Tumor Size

For small lesions confined to the sella, there is no doubt about the greater benefits of the transsphenoidal approach compared with any other transcranial route; however, discussion arises when dealing with larger lesions, but this approach is being used more frequently nowadays[2] because of the dramatic impact in the development of surgical instruments, endoscopically-assisted procedures, and stereotactic guidance.

Growth Pattern

Almost every intrasellar and suprasellar tumor that grows homogeneously can be resected through the transsphenoidal approach, but in cases of a dumbbell-shaped tumor the chances of total resection are reduced. Other conditions that limit the potential resection of these lesions include cavernous sinus involvement and posterior fossa or anterior fossa extension.[3]

Tumor Consistency

Through careful analysis of the preoperative magnetic resonance imaging (MRI), it is possible to predict tumor consistency. In general, lesions that show a bright hyperintensity in the T1-weighted phase tend to be softer and easier to remove and thus can be treated through the transsphenoidal route.

Factors Related to the Approach Itself

It is very critical to consider factors such as the sellar size, the type of sphenoid sinus, the position and tortuosity of the carotid arteries, and the presence of an inflammatory process or infection in the paranasal sinuses.[4]

Patient Conditions

Given its low morbidity and mortality rate, the transsphenoidal approach is the preferred surgical procedure for elder patients or those with severe systemic disease.

◆ Preparation

Once all imaging studies and blood tests have been properly done, it is very important to have a complete endocrinologic study to identify any hormonal deficiency that has to be corrected before surgery. The day of the surgery, an antibiotic and a stress dose steroid (300 mg hydrocortisone) are given intravenously.[5] This regimen applies in all cases, except for patients with Cushing's disease, because of their excessive endogenous steroid production and the alterations in the postoperative hormone evaluation that this dose could cause.

◆ Surgical Technique

Positioning

After anesthetic induction and oral intubation, the oropharynx is packed with moist gauze to avoid swallowing or fluid aspiration. The patient is placed in a comfortable semirecumbent position, with 15 degrees of head flexion and lateral inclination such that the left ear is cocked toward the left shoulder. The head holder application is optional because a horseshoe headrest can also be used to allow minimal head movement during the procedure. The surgical site for donor tissue is prepared; the authors prefer the lower right quadrant of the abdomen given the better cosmetic results. A urinary catheter is placed only in the case of macroadenomas, where active manipulation of the pituitary stalk is expected. Insertion of an arterial line or a subarachnoid lumbar drain is not routinely performed. The portable image intensifier is placed, making sure that the position of the beam is such that it is not obstructed by the head holder. The microscope is prepared, and the monitor is positioned facing the surgeon. The surgical table should be placed in an oblique direction allowing for a shorter distance between the patient's feet and the anesthesia cart, keeping a good alignment of the mouth and nose with the surgeon's position **(Fig. 55–1)**.

Approach

There are two approach options to access the sellar region: the endonasal and the sublabial. Over the past few years there has been a general consensus on using the endonasal route given the lower complication rate,[6] but for larger tumors and small nostrils the sublabial route is preferred.

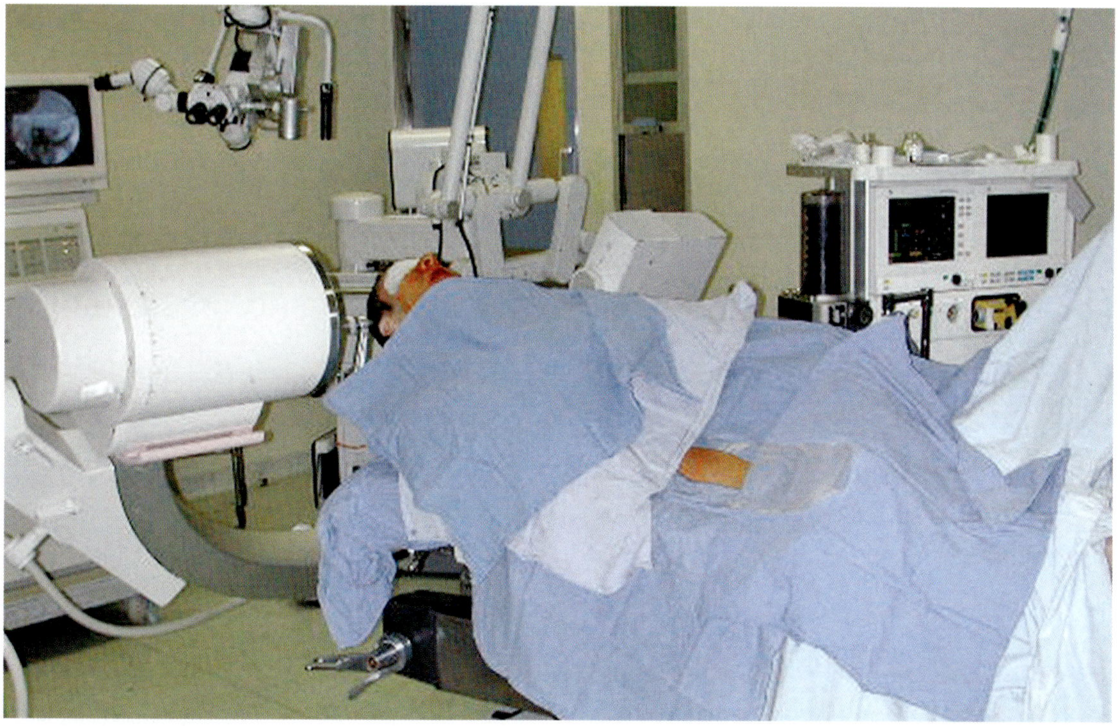

Figure 55–1 Positioning.

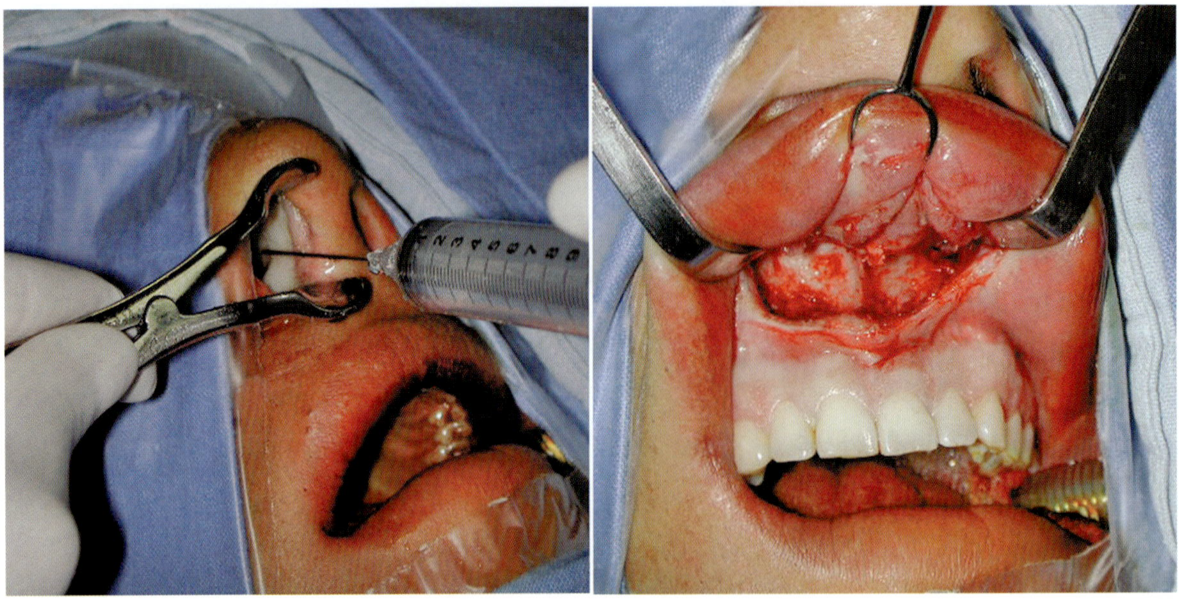

Figure 55–2 Left: Submucosal infiltration of the nasal septum. Note how the mucosa becomes white during the injection, which is a sign of a correct infiltration. Right: Sublabial incision and subperiosteal dissection.

Endonasal Approach

The initial part of the procedure is done with a headlight and surgical loupes. The nasal preparation is immediately done after intubation, using a nasal spray decongestant. A submucosal infiltration of the nasal septum is next, using 0.5% Xylocaine in 1:200,000 epinephrine solution. Proper infiltration greatly facilitates the dissection process **(Fig. 55–2).** Right-handed surgeons prefer a right-sided approach. The procedure begins with the contralateral displacement of the columella, and then a 1 to 2 cm incision is made at the junction of the skin and nasal mucosa. Initially the Cottle knife is used to dissect the mucosa from the cartilage, thus creating the anterior right tunnel **(Fig. 55–3).** At this site, firm adhesions between the mucosa and the nasal spine are frequently encountered, and sharp separation with the scalpel is required. Once this tunnel has been made, a posterior blunt subperichondrial dissection follows, using the Cottle dissector, thus creating the posterior right tunnel. The inferior right tunnel is now made by dissecting the mucosa from the palatine process of the maxilla, and immediately after, both the anterior and inferior right tunnels are connected. The

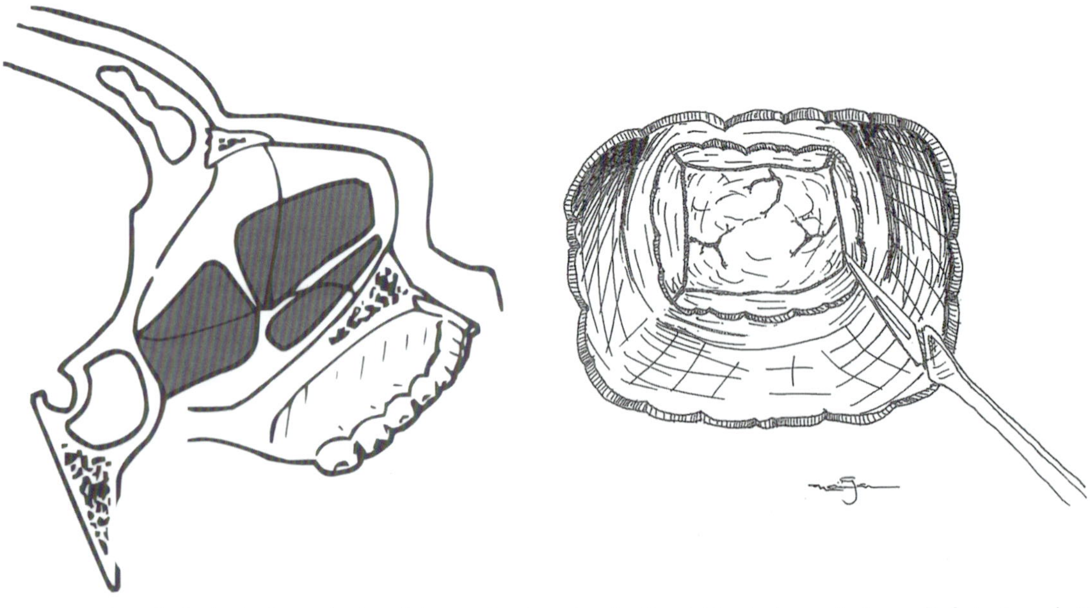

Figure 55–3 Left: Sagittal schematic view of the nasal septum showing the right anterior, posterior, and inferior tunnels. Right: Details of the dural opening.

cartilage septum is then incised at the junction with the perpendicular plate of the ethmoid bone, and the left posterior submucosal tunnel is created, detaching the mucosa from the left surface of the bony septum. The articulation of the cartilaginous septum with the maxilla is then dissected free and an attempt is made to raise the inferior mucosal tunnel on the opposite side so that the cartilaginous septum can be completely displaced toward the left nostril. A nasal speculum is applied, leaving the perpendicular plate, free of its mucosa, at the center, between the blades.

Sublabial Approach

The upper lip is retracted and a transverse incision is made at the buccogingival junction, extending from one canine fossa to the other. Subperiosteal dissection elevates the mucosa to the pyriform aperture. The two inferior nasal tunnels are created by detaching the mucosa away from the superior surface of the hard palate. The inferior border of the cartilaginous septum is exposed by using the scalpel, and then, with sharp dissection, the anterior right tunnel is created. With blunt dissection, the detachment is continued toward the right side of the bony septum to create the right posterior tunnel. Using the Cottle knife again, the right anterior and posterior tunnels are connected with the right inferior one. The cartilaginous septum is detached from the anterior border of the bony septum and the palatine process of the maxilla. By using firm blunt dissection along the right side of the base of the cartilage, this septum is dislocated and reflected to the left; then the left posterior mucosal tunnel is developed along the left side of the perpendicular plate of the ethmoid bone. It is now possible to introduce the nasal speculum, leaving the bony septum at the center. From this point on, the rest of the approach is the same in both routes.

Bony Septum

Once the mucosal dissection is complete, the nasal speculum is changed for the transsphenoidal speculum (Hardy) and care should be taken to place all mucosal tears laterally to the retractor blades. The retractor is gradually opened; this maneuver sometimes fractures the turbinates, but it is not advisable to apply a great deal of force in opening the retractor because the maxilla may also be fractured. Using angled scissors, two cuts are performed in the bony septum, one at the junction with the hard palate and the other 3 cm above it. Using vomer forceps, the fragment of the septum is taken and gentle alternating lateral movements are then applied, trying to fracture the base of this fragment, to obtain a free bony plate. In some cases, however, this fracture may be difficult, and in these cases it is necessary to use a curved chisel. The free bony fragment will be used to reconstruct the sellar floor. The anterior nasal spine has to be left in place to get better cosmetic results, but sometimes, particularly in acromegalic patients, this structure is very prominent; an experienced surgeon has to be prepared to work with this spine in the visual field. Once the nasal septum is removed, the sphenoid rostrum will reveal the so-called keel of the boat. The rest of the procedure has to be done under the microscope.

Sphenoid Sinus and Sellar Access

Toward the rostral end of the surgical field, the paired sphenoid ostia become evident. Entrance to the sphenoid sinus can be gained beginning with a caudal enlargement of the sphenoid ostia with microrongeurs or with a chisel; then the complete sphenoid rostrum is removed. Fluoroscopic guidance is used to confirm the right position of the nasal speculum. Once the anterior wall of the sinus is opened, the sphenoid mucosa is completely exenterated and the sphenoid septa are removed. At this point the sellar floor with its rounded contour can be visualized. It is critical to keep the anatomical orientation in all surgical steps; the most important point is to maintain the appropriate midline trajectory at all times. Using a microchisel, a quadrangular window is opened in the sellar floor, which is then enlarged with a Kerrison rongeur. It is very important to make a wide opening in the floor to gain sufficient control of the sellar structures. The bluish color of the dura identifies the cavernous sinuses and the superior intercavernous or circular sinus. Inferiorly, bone removal should continue until the edge of the sellar floor merges into the clivus. It is better to avoid extensive superior removal of bone because there is usually dense attachment of the dura at the junction with the anterior floor of the skull base, and it could produce cerebrospinal fluid (CSF) leakage at this point. In cases of conchal varieties of the sphenoid sinus, the use of a high-speed drill is mandatory.

Dural Opening and Tumor Resection

Before performing the opening itself, a bipolar coagulation of the dural surface should be made to avoid excessive bleeding from venous sinuses and capillary vessels. The authors prefer to make a quadrangular opening of the dura mater, resecting a square fragment of this membrane. Relaxing incisions can be made in every corner of the opening to improve exposure (**Fig. 55–3**). The dural edges are then coagulated again to avoid bleeding and to ensure even more retraction.

In the case of microadenomas, initial exploration has to be made at the precise location of the tumor, based on preoperative imaging studies; however, sometimes, even with high-resolution MRI, it is not possible to know the exact location of the lesion. In these cases exploration begins with a cruciate X-shaped incision in the pituitary gland. Then, using the 3 mm right-angled curette, slight pressure is applied in every quadrant of the gland. The microadenoma tends to herniate into the surgical field. In the case of macroadenomas, once the dura mater has been opened, it is possible to identify the grayish and friable typical aspect of the tumor. The initial resection is quite simple and is normally made using blunt-tipped curets, a surgical aspirator, and biopsy forceps. It is worth bearing in mind a tridimensional image of the pituitary fossa to fully explore all its regions. The resection process initiates with the intrasellar portion, leaving the suprasellar component for the end of the procedure, because an early descent of the sellar diaphragm would impede the proper exploration of the surgical area. Resection is easier and safer if an anterograde movement of the curet is applied in the interface between the tumor and the sellar

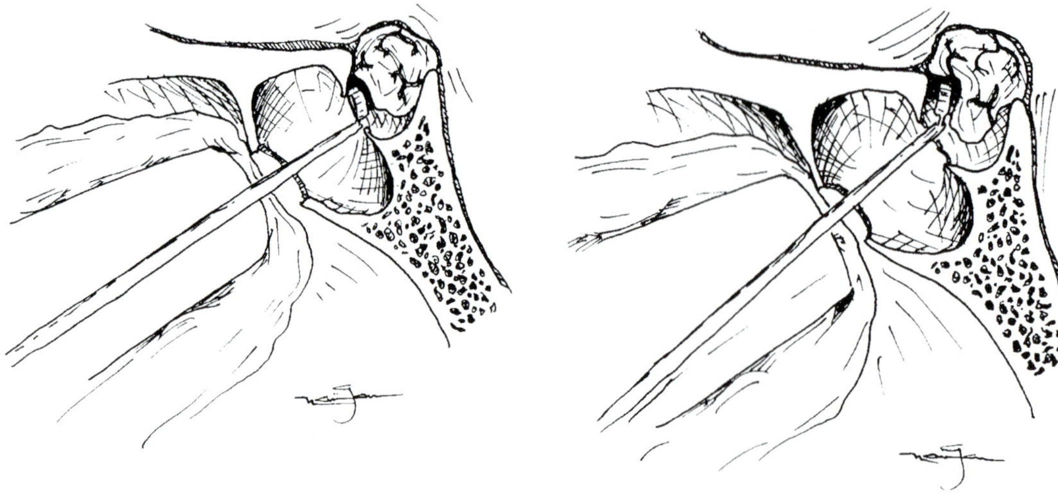

Figure 55–4 Tumor resection. A safer form to achieve the removal is by placing the angled curets at the interface between the tumor and the sellar walls, and then gently pushing it, following the sellar contour, trying to move the lesion toward the sella.

walls, pushing the lesion toward the sella, instead of pulling it toward the surgeon (**Fig. 55–4**). With this maneuver, there is less surgical trauma to the surrounding tissue. For the resection of the suprasellar portion, several surgical strategies have been reported,[7] such as bilateral jugular vein compression, and air or saline solution application through a subarachnoid lumbar catheter. All these methods are not strictly necessary because, by using a series of Valsalva maneuvers and with gentle manipulation of the sellar diaphragm, maximal descent can be obtained in the majority of cases (**Fig. 55–5**). Sometimes this suprasellar portion does not descend into the sella; in these cases, the patients can be reoperated on 2 or 3 months later, waiting for the spontaneous descent of this portion during that time.[8] The surgeon must avoid any brusque movement in the diaphragm because of the risk of subarachnoid hemorrhage due to rupture of the suprasellar arteries. On the other hand, the complete descent of the diaphragm is not an unequivocal sign of total tumor removal, so every corner of the surgical field has to be explored under direct vision. One of the most difficult areas to explore is toward the medial wall of the cavernous sinus. This is because quite often the dura mater shows several venous plexus in the proximity of the cavernous sinus and it cannot be widely opened. In that

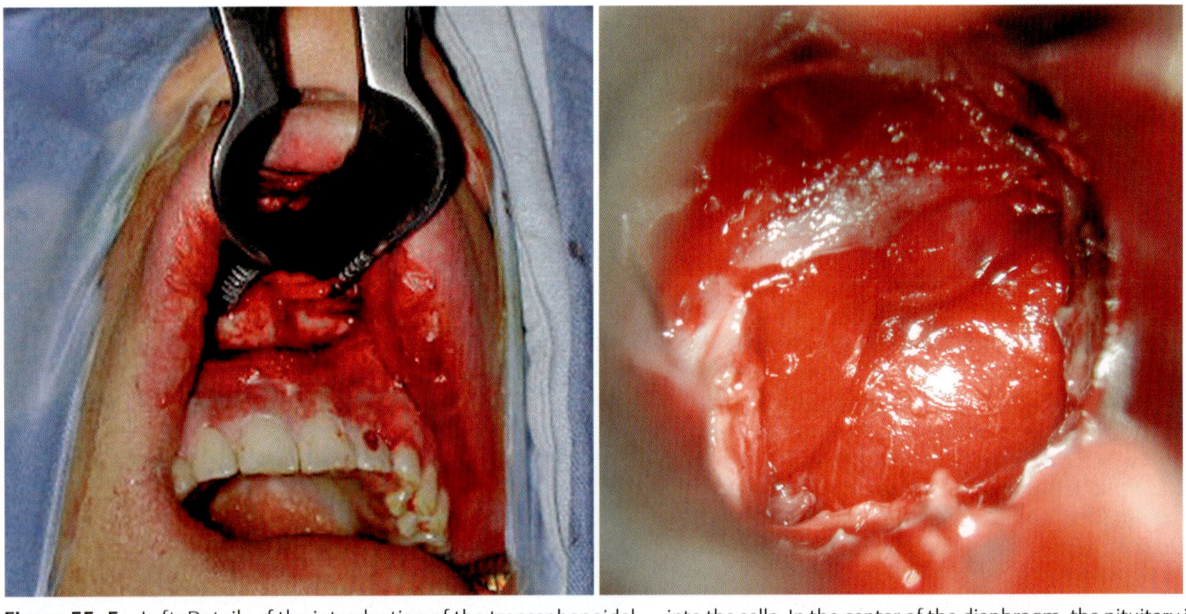

Figure 55–5 Left: Details of the introduction of the transsphenoidal speculum in a sublabial access. Right: Microscopic view after a complete tumor removal; observe how the diaphragm has completely descended into the sella. In the center of the diaphragm, the pituitary infundibulum can be observed.

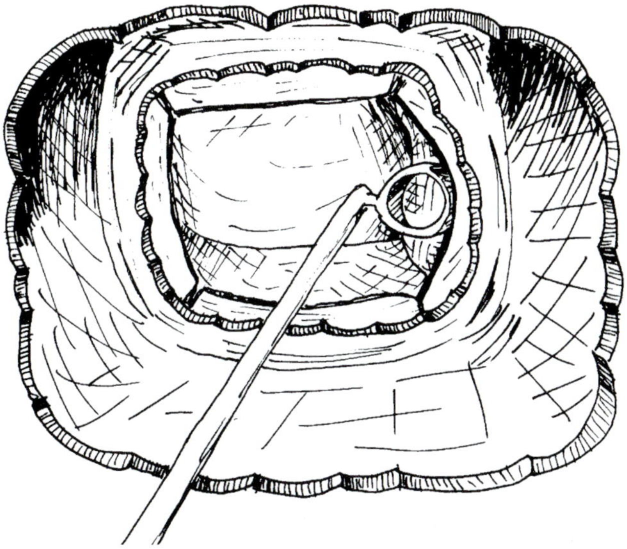

Figure 55–6 To explore the lateral parts of the sella, the dural edge can be pushed with a blunt right-angled curet to check for the medial wall of the cavernous sinus under direct vision.

case, a blunt right-angled curet can be used to push the dural edge, exposing the reddish dark color of the medial wall of the cavernous sinus and the transmitted pulsations of the internal carotid artery **(Fig. 55–6)**. Another area that it is difficult to explore is toward the tuberculum sellae, mostly when the diaphragm has descended. In this situation, the diaphragm can be lifted up with the surgical aspirator, together with the simultaneous introduction of the right-angled curet using fluoroscopic guidance; also, a cottonoid can be used to maintain the diaphragm elevation to free both hands for the resection of this anterior portion of the tumor. The endoscopic enhanced vision greatly facilitates this removal by allowing us to "see around the corner."[9,10]

In all cases, efforts are made to preserve normal pituitary tissue, which usually appears as a thin membrane adhered to the diaphragm, or superolaterally against the sellar wall. Experienced surgeons do not have any difficulty in differentiating the orange-yellow color of the gland and its firm consistency from the grayish color and granular texture of the tumor. Identification of the pituitary stalk is also mandatory because firm traction on it can cause hypothalamic damage with permanent endocrine deficiencies.

Reconstruction and Closure

Once the tumor has been removed and hemostasis achieved, reconstruction begins with the exploration of the sellar diaphragm, looking for small tears that could inadvertently have occurred during the procedure. Minor tears can be managed with surgical reposition of the arachnoid edges and the placement of a small fragment of aponeurosis. In the case of major tears, a larger aponeurotic patch is placed to substitute the lost diaphragm, but it is also necessary to put some fat tissue in the sellar cavity to maintain the aponeurosis in place. Fibrin glue can also be applied to keep the surgical area hermetically closed. Subarachnoid drainage is not routinely used because meticulous repair of the tears in this manner is sufficient to avoid the risks of CSF leakage.

For microadenomas, it is not necessary to put any graft in the surgical dead space created by tumor removal; on the other hand, in the majority of cases of macroadenomas, a fragment of hemostatic material is left in the sella. Only in particular cases with huge tumors do we place a fat graft in the surgical bed. Reconstruction of the sellar floor is made using the fragment of the bony septum obtained during the approach. The ideal placement location of this fragment is in the epidural space.[11] Sometimes, due to the wide opening on the sellar floor, a single fragment is not enough to perform this reconstruction, so small fragments of the cartilaginous septum can also be used. In most cases, it is not necessary to introduce any graft tissue in the sphenoid sinus; however, when there is a high risk of CSF leakage, the sinus can also be completely occluded with fat tissue.

During the closing procedure, careful attention should be paid to achieving anatomical and physiological restoration of the nasal portion of the procedure. Crushed nasal bone and cartilage can be put in the posterior septal space; then the septal flaps are reapproximated and the cartilaginous septum is returned to its midline insertion; at this time all mucosal tears can be identified and sutured with absorbable material. The incision in the columella is closed with the same absorbable suture, and bilateral nasal packing is placed. In the sublabial approach, nasal packing is applied first, followed by suture of the sublabial mucosa and application of a gauze moustache dressing.

◆ Postoperative Care

Most patients can be extubated in the operating room, and only those with very large tumors and a large suprasellar component are transferred to the intensive care unit. Steroid support is tapered from 100 mg twice a day on the first postoperative day to 20 mg every morning and 10 mg every night for the next 3 days. This dosage is stopped according to the results of postoperative hormonal levels. Antibiotic treatment is ordinarily given for a maximum of three doses using a third-generation cephalosporine. Topical nasal decongestants (pseudoephedrine) are prescribed to alleviate the feeling of nasal fullness. Additional postoperative orders include a nasal humidifier for alleviating oral breathing discomfort. For all patients postoperative monitoring of water and electrolyte balance is mandatory. Postoperative images are usually made 2 to 3 months after the surgical procedure,[12] and their hormonal profile is monitored on a regular basis to determine suitable replacement therapy strategies.

◆ Clinical Examples

The following cases were operated on using the transsphenoidal approach.

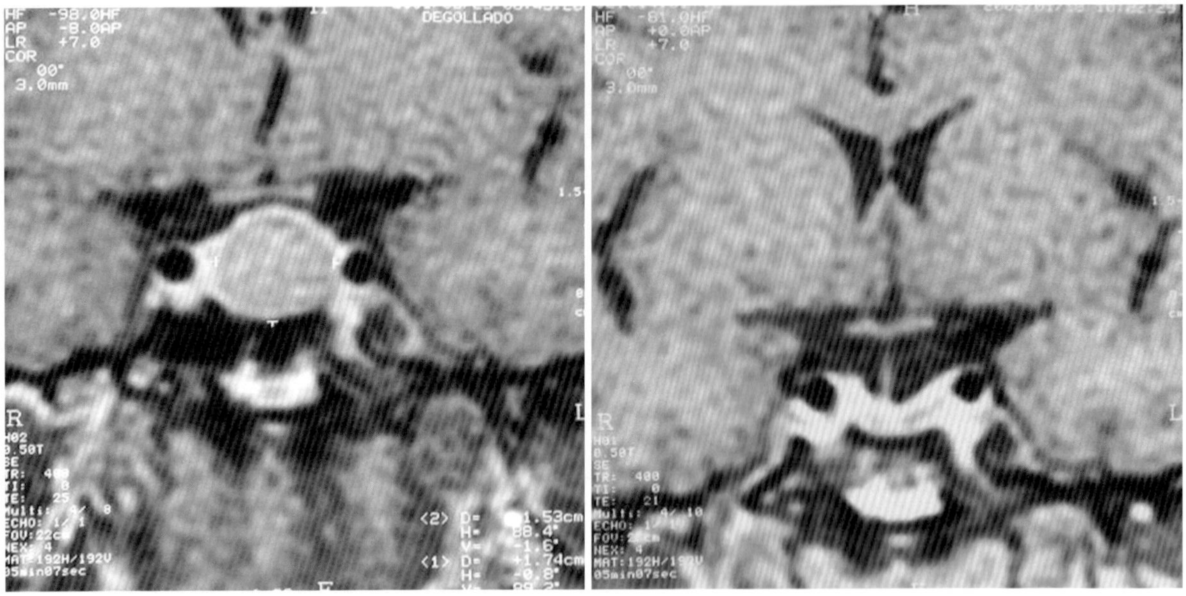

Figure 55–7 Case no. 1. Left: Preoperative magnetic resonance imaging (MRI). An intrasellar macroadenoma (1.7 cm) can be observed. Note the hyperintensity of the pituitary gland displaced superolaterally, in close contact with the diaphragm and the right carotid artery. Right: Postoperative MRI. A complete removal of the tumor was possible, with preservation of the pituitary gland.

Case No. 1

A 34-year-old man presented with clinical manifestations of acromegaly and left temporal hemianopsia. An MRI showed an intrasellar macroadenoma that was completely removed. The hormonal postoperative analysis showed remission of the disease, with complete preservation of his endocrine function and visual recovery (**Fig. 55–7**).

Case No. 2

A 36-year-old woman presented with a chronic history of headache. Six months before her admission to the hospital she presented with an evident and progressive bitemporal hemianopsia. The tumor was removed and the visual deficit improved (**Fig. 55–8**).

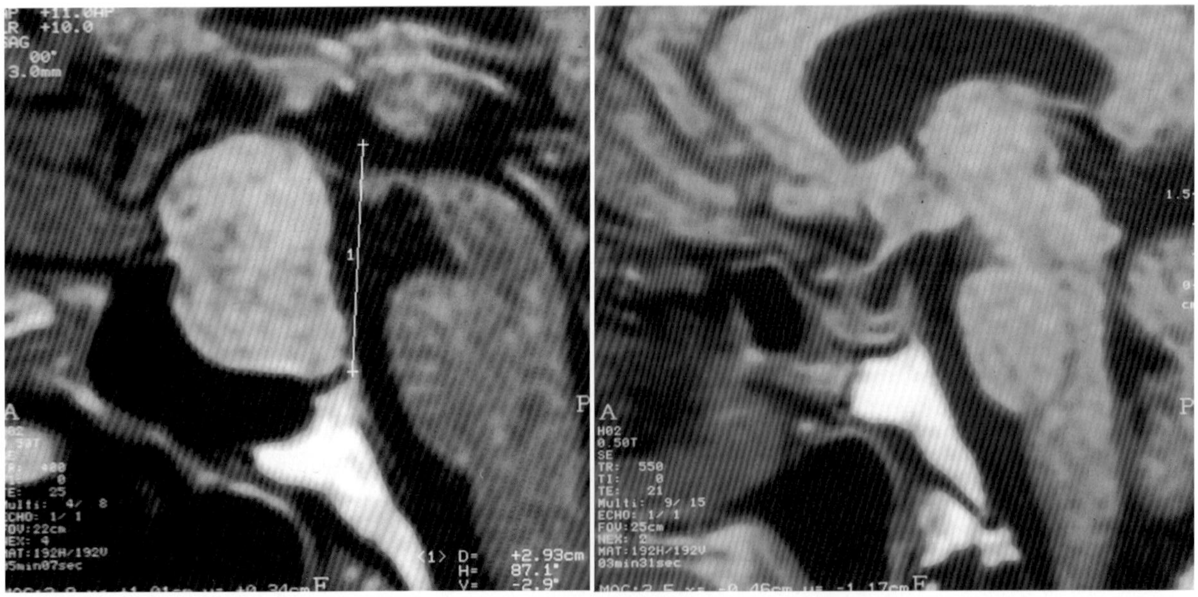

Figure 55–8 Case no. 2. Left: Preoperative magnetic resonance imaging (MRI). A large intrasellar and suprasellar tumor is shown. Right: Postoperative MRI. There is no residual tumor and the preservation of the pituitary tissue and the stalk can be observed.

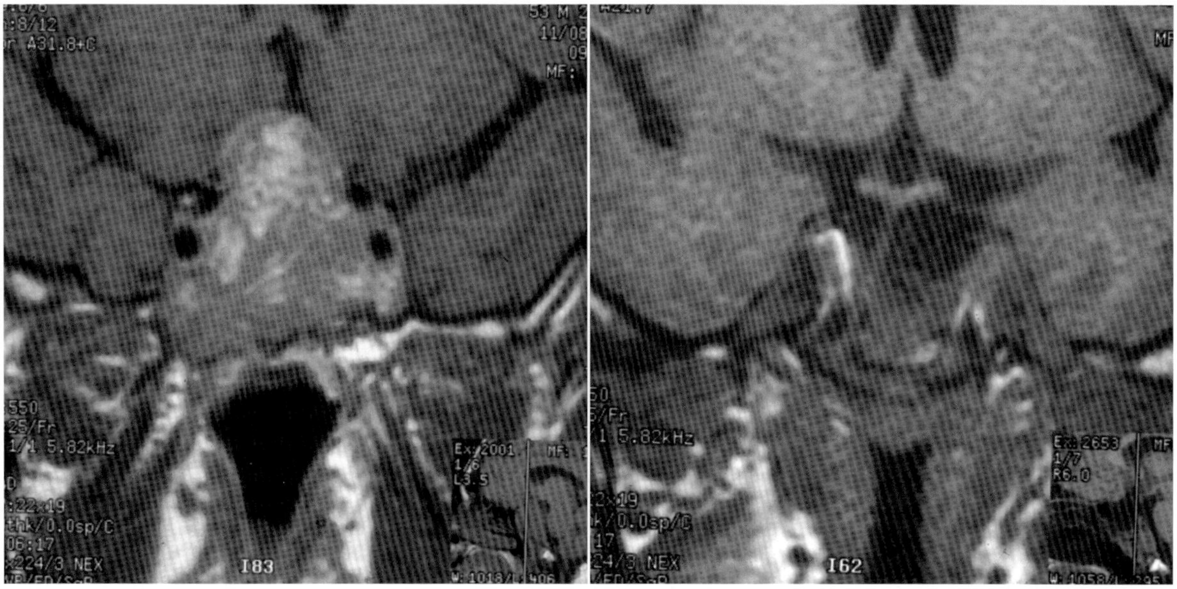

Figure 55–9 Case no. 3. Left: Preoperative magnetic resonance imaging (MRI). The tumor is pushing the optic chiasm from below; note the portion of the tumor growing under the right cavernous sinus. Right: Postoperative result that shows total removal. The optic chiasm was freed of its compression and the pituitary stalk could be preserved.

Case No. 3

A 46-year-old man with a rapidly progressive reduction in his visual field and clinical signs of hypothyroidism. The tumor was totally removed, preserving his endocrine function, except for the thyroid hormone, for which he is now under hormone substitution (**Fig. 55–9**).

Case No. 4

A 47-year-old woman presented with left blindness and right temporal hemianopsia. The tumor was removed, and she recovered her right eye vision (**Fig. 55–10**).

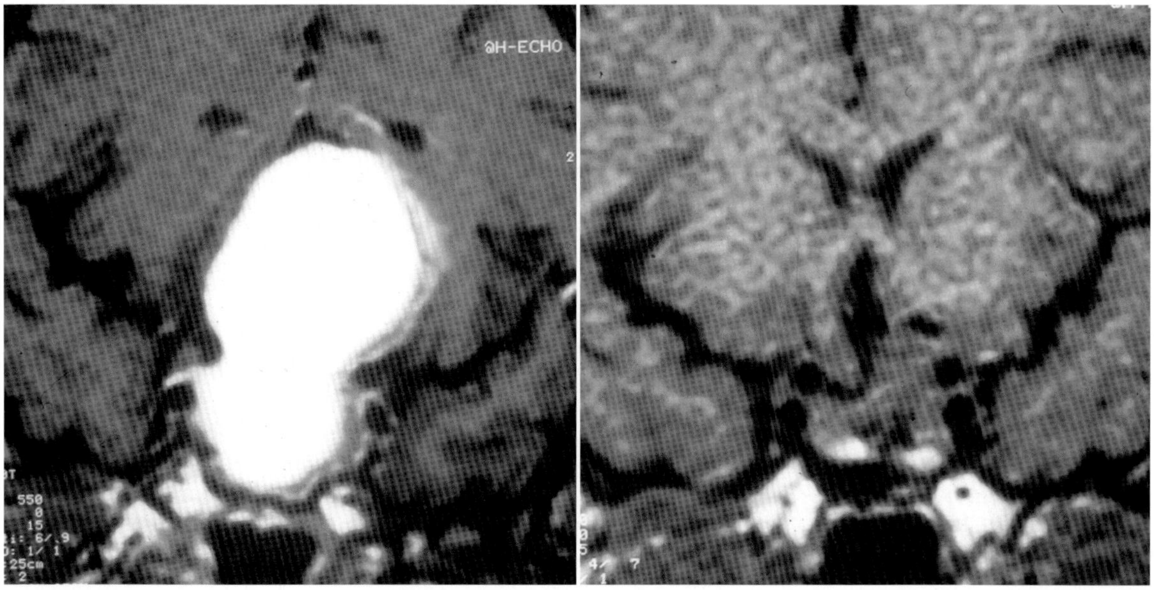

Figure 55–10 Case no. 4. Left: Preoperative magnetic resonance imaging. A huge tumor with an extensive suprasellar growth. The tumor shows a bright hyperintensity, which is why the transsphenoidal approach was the right one for this particular case. Right: Postoperative result. Only the pseudocapsule of the tumor can be seen within the sella.

◆ Complications

Vascular Injury

Although rare, this is the main source of operative mortality following this procedure.[13] The intracavernous segment of the internal carotid artery is the most frequent vessel injured in this approach. There are two critical steps during which this vessel can be damaged. One is during the sellar floor opening when chiseling; to avoid this, it is very important to begin the opening right along the midline. When there are doubts about the midline location or when the bone is thick, it is preferable to use a high-speed drill instead of a chisel. If additional lateral bone removal is needed, it is safer to do this once the dura mater is opened and the precise location of the medial wall of the cavernous sinus is identified. The second time when the carotid artery can be injured involves tumor resection at the lateral portions of the sella. To avoid this complication, preoperative radiological studies have to be carefully evaluated, attempting to define if there is only a displacement of the artery or if there is a real invasion of the cavernous sinus. In the first case, it is possible to try to remove this part of the tumor using blunt curets with gentle movements, but in the second case it is safer to consider different treatment options, like a transcranial approach or radiosurgery, to manage this portion.

Laceration of the carotid artery or any of its branches is a very difficult situation to deal with critically. Direct repair of the vessel is very difficult to obtain through this procedure, so a tamponade should be used to control hemorrhage. Fibrin glue can be added to enhance better adhesion of the hemostatic material to the injured vessel. Even when the vascular defect has been successfully repaired, there is still a risk of spontaneous detachment of the packing several weeks after the procedure. This is why it becomes necessary to maintain the patient in absolute rest for about 6 to 8 weeks after surgery, with close monitoring and frequent visits. When an arterial injury has occurred, a postoperative angiography must be performed to search for carotid-cavernous fistula or a pseudoaneurysm.[14] The cavernous sinus is another structure that also can be injured during this approach, but in this case the repair work is easier and does not require any special postoperative radiological study.

Visual Problems

Damage to the optic nerve or chiasm may occur after this type of surgery; the main causes of this damage are direct surgical trauma, hemorrhage, and ischemia.[15] There are several causes of visual system damage in this procedure; for example, fractures of bony structures of the skull base when opening the sellar floor; aggressive opening of the transsphenoidal retractors; brusque maneuvers during tumor resection, particularly when pulling down the anterosuperior portion of the tumor; and finally, overpacking the sellar floor during reconstruction.

When an immediate postoperative visual deficit is present, the patient should be critically evaluated. Computed tomography (CT), including a bone window algorithm, is ordered, searching for fractures or free bone fragments compressing the nerves. Also an MRI should be performed to identify a hematoma or ischemic insult in the visual pathways. The surgeon has to bear in mind that almost every patient who shows immediate postoperative visual deficit has to be surgically reexplored as soon as possible.

Endocrine Complications

Diabetes insipidus is a common problem in 30% of patients during the postoperative period, but it is generally transient, being permanent in only 3% of patients.[16] The specific management includes adequate hydroelectrolyte replacement, and in only a very few cases the use of antidiuretic hormone substitutes. In some patients with huge tumors, severe hypothalamic damage could be observed following this procedure. This clinical state can cause alterations in the vegetative system, deep coma, or even death. To avoid this complication, the upper portions of tumor have to be managed very gently, avoiding brusque traction.

Permanent postoperative endocrine alterations are more frequently seen if the patient has already had a preoperative hormonal deficiency or if radiotherapy was applied.

Cerebrospinal Fluid Leakage

Fortunately, the frequency of this complication and associated meningitis has been reduced over the past few years. This is due to better surgical control of arachnoid tears, the use of fibrin sealants, which greatly enhances the watertight closure, and the use of a new generation of antibiotics.[17]

Cerebrospinal fluid rhinorrhea has to be immediately identified. Leakage is not always present at the time the nasal packing is removed, so the patient and relatives have to be well instructed about this possibility at the time of discharge from the hospital, to call for care as soon as it appears. Initial management includes strict bed rest, the use of diuretics, and, in some cases, the placement of a subarachnoid lumbar drain. Very few patients have to be reoperated on to seal the defect.

Complications Related to the Approach

There are a whole series of clinical situations that can arise after a transsphenoidal approach and that in general are not life threatening, but they are uncomfortable. Mucoceles, sinusitis, epistaxis, septal perforation, nasal bridge deformity, hoarseness, olfactory function loss, and dental anesthesia are the most frequent problems reported.[18,19] Careful and meticulous surgical techniques during exposure and anatomical reconstruction at the time of closure are the best options to avoid them.

References

1. Rosegay H. Cushing's legacy to transsphenoidal surgery. J Neurosurg 1981;54:448–454
2. Romano A, Zuccarello M, van Loveren HR, Keller JT. Expanding the boundaries of the transsphenoidal approach: a microanatomic study. Clin Anat 2001;14:1–9
3. Fraioli B, Esposito V, Santoro A, Iannetti G, Giuffre R, Cantore G. Transmaxillosphenoidal approach to tumors invading the medial compartment of the cavernous sinus. J Neurosurg 1995;82:63–69
4. Saeki N, Yamaura A, Numata T, Hoshi S. Bone window CT evaluation of the nasal cavity for the transsphenoidal approach. Br J Neurosurg 1999;13:285–289
5. Cawley CM, Tindall GT. Transsphenoidal surgery. operative techniques. In: Krisht AF, Tindall GT, eds. Pituitary Disorders. Baltimore: Lippincott Williams & Wilkins; 1999:349–359
6. Das K, Spencer W, Nwagwu CI, Schaeffer S, Weuk E, Weiss MH, et al. Approaches to the sellar and parasellar region: anatomic comparison of endonasal-transsphenoidal, sublabial-transsphenoidal, and transethmoidal approaches. Neurol Res 2001;23:51–54
7. Elias WJ, Laws ER. Transsphenoidal approaches to lesions of the sella. In: Schmidek HH, Sweet WH, eds. Operative Neurosurgical Techniques. Orlando, FL: Grune & Stratton; 1988:373–384
8. Saito K, Kuwayama A, Yamamoto N, Sugita K. The transsphenoidal removal of non-functioning pituitary adenomas with suprasellar extensions: the open sella method and intentionally staged operation. Neurosurgery 1995;36:668–675
9. Jarrahy R, Berci G, Shahinian HK. Assessment of the efficacy of endoscopy in pituitary adenoma resection. Arch Otolaryngol Head Neck Surg 2000;126:1487–1490
10. Jho HD. Endoscopic transsphenoidal surgery. In: Schmidek HH, Sweet WH, eds. Operative Neurosurgical Techniques. Orlando, FL: Grune & Stratton; 1988:385–397
11. Spaziante R, de Divitiis E, Cappabianca P. Reconstruction of the pituitary fossa in transsphenoidal surgery: an experience of 140 cases. Neurosurgery 1985;17:453–458
12. Rajaraman V, Schulder M. Postoperative MRI appearance after transsphenoidal pituitary tumor resection. Surg Neurol 1999;52: 592–598
13. Laws ER. Vascular complications of transsphenoidal surgery. Pituitary 1999;2:163–170
14. Cappabianca P, Briganti F, Cavallo LM, de Divitiis E. Pseudoaneurysm of the intracavernous carotid artery following endoscopic endonasal transsphenoidal surgery, treated by endovascular approach. Acta Neurochir (Wien) 2001;143:95–96
15. Trautmann JC, Laws ER. Visual status after transsphenoidal surgery at the Mayo Clinic, 1971–1982. Am J Ophthalmol 1983;96:200–208
16. Laws ER, Kern EB. Complications of transsphenoidal surgery. In: Tindall GT, Collins WF, eds. Clinical Management of Pituitary Disorders. New York: Raven; 1979:435–445
17. Van Velthoven V, Clarici G, Auer LM. Fibrin tissue adhesive sealant for the prevention of CSF leakage following transsphenoidal microsurgery. Acta Neurochir (Wien) 1991;109:26–29
18. Koren I, Hadar T, Rappaport ZH, Yaniv E. Endoscopic transnasal transsphenoidal microsurgery versus the sublabial approach for the treatment of pituitary tumors: endonasal complications. Laryngoscope 1999;109: 1838–1840
19. Sharma K, Tyagi I, Banerjee D, Chhabra DK, Kaur A, Taneja HK. Rhinological complications of sublabial transseptal transsphenoidal surgery for sellar and suprasellar lesions: prevention and management. Neurosurg Rev 1996;19:163–167

56

Craniopharyngiomas

J. J. van Overbeeke

Cushing described the removal of a craniopharyngioma as a "baffling problem to neurosurgeons." Although slow-growing and histologically benign, craniopharyngiomas' intimate adherence to the infundibular stalk, hypothalamus, and optic system predisposes to several endocrinological, neurobehavioral, and visual postoperative problems.

Despite advances in radiosurgery,[1] total removal is still the most important treatment with the best long-term prognosis.[2]

The success of a total removal with minor deficits is dependent on the volume and the site of the tumor, the neurosurgeon's knowledge of the pathological growth and surgical anatomy, and, most importantly, the neurosurgeon's experience and approach to the tumor.

◆ Incidence

Craniopharyngiomas account for about 1.2 to 4% of all intracranial tumors, and for 13% of the sellar and suprasellar tumors in all age groups. In children they represent 56% of all sellar and suprasellar tumors.[3]

◆ Pathology

Craniopharyngiomas are histologically benign. From a surgical point of view it is important to realize that they are thought to arise from embryonic ectodermal rests in the pituitary stalk. This means that there are varying primary sites resulting in various origins of growth in or near the stalk.[4] Infradiaphragmatic growth results in an intrasellar tumor that is separated from the brain by the dura and arachnoidal tissue. In the suprasellar region the tumor is always surrounded by the arachnoid. However, closely to the tuber cinereum, tumor nests are surrounded by a firm glial tissue instead of the arachnoid.

Because the origin of craniopharyngiomas is from the anterior diencephalon, they share the same blood supply, meaning that craniopharyngiomas are vascularized by the perforators of the internal carotid artery, the posterior communicating artery, the anterior cerebral arteries, and the anterior communicating artery. The basilar and posterior cerebral arteries are normally not involved in the vascularization of the diencephalon, and therefore they play no part in the vascularization of these tumors.

◆ Surgical Anatomy

Because craniopharyngiomas originate in the suprasellar region they are closely related to the pre- and postchiasmatic cisterns, the cistern of the lamina terminalis, and the interpeduncular cistern. They distort and obliterate this area depending on their size and direction of growth. Most craniopharyngiomas contain a solid part, sometimes with calcifications, and a cystic part. They grow by expansion, which comes mostly from the cystic part.

The suprasellar craniopharyngiomas may start to grow in a vertical direction toward the arachnoid layers of the chiasmatic cisterns and the cisterns of the lamina terminalis. In the cranial direction they expand against the floor of the third ventricle and may elevate the floor to the level of the foramen of Monro. The ventricular floor becomes paper-thin. Because of the slow growth, the hypothalamic structures become gradually adapted so that hypothalamic functions remain mostly normal. Because of the arachnoid layer between the dome of the craniopharyngioma and the floor of the ventricle, the tumor does not infiltrate into the third ventricle. This is often in contrast with the magnetic resonance imaging (MRI) study, which does not show a clear line between the tumor and the ventricle. This also may be an argument for not approaching a craniopharyngioma transcallosally.

Craniopharyngiomas may grow in the direction of the optic chiasm either retrochiasmatically or against the chiasm. In the first case the pituitary stalk is displaced forward and the chiasm is displaced forward and upward. In the latter case the pituitary stalk is pushed backward and the chiasm upward. Here the optic nerves become severely stretched laterally on the tumor capsule and the tumor can even infiltrate into the frontal lobes. In the case of a lateral growth the temporal lobes become compressed and the lower poles of the craniopharyngioma may become firmly attached to the dura of the sellar diaphragm and lateral wall of the cavernous sinus.

Several transcranial approaches have been described. The choice mostly depends on the experience of the surgeon. Every approach should meet the criterion that the craniopharyngioma is exposed by routes to essential spaces, such as the subchiasmatic route to the space between the optic nerves and the chiasm; the opticocarotid route to the space between the optic nerve and carotid artery (the opticocarotid triangle), which contains the superior hypophyseal arteries and their small perforating arteries and the feeding arteries to the capsule of the tumor from the internal carotid artery, posterior communicating artery, and anterior cerebral arteries; the route to the space between the carotid artery and sylvian fissure (caroticosylvian space); and the route to the lamina terminalis, which should be chosen if the tumor pushes the chiasm into a prefixed position and if the tumor extends into the third ventricle.

The transsphenoidal approach is preferred if the tumor is situated in or extends upward out of an enlarged sella turcica.

◆ Preoperative Studies

Radiology

An MRI provides, especially by means of its multiplane displays, the necessary insight into the relation of the tumor to adjacent soft structures such as the diencephalon. On the T2-weighted images a possible arachnoidal plane between the capsule and neural structures can be noted, which may be predictive for radical removal. A computed tomographic (CT) scan can be used for the demonstration of intratumoral calcifications and the bony anatomy of the skull base. If available, MR angiography demonstrates the displacement of the major vessels; otherwise, four-vessel angiography is necessary.

Before an osteotomy of the superolateral rim of the orbit and zygoma is considered in children, the development of the dental elements should have a radiological evaluation.

Endocrinological Evaluation

Endocrinological evaluation is done routinely before any treatment of a craniopharyngioma. Because the patient is expected to have a transient or permanent postoperative panhypopituitarism, the preoperative endocrine status is of importance to guide selective intraoperative and postoperative replacements of the hormones because adequate endocrine replacements reduce the postoperative morbidity.

Hypoadrenalism should be treated with high doses of corticosteroids pre- and intraoperatively. Hypothyroidism should already be supplemented by thyroxine some days before the surgery, and diabetes insipidus needs to be treated by adequate fluid and electrolyte replacement and antidiuretic hormone.

Neuro-ophthalmic Evaluation

The ophthalmologic status is obtained in the preoperative phase, and particular attention must be paid to the extent of damage to the visual system by the tumor itself, to follow the patient's postoperative status.

Neurobehavioral Evaluation

In children a preoperative neuropsychological examination may be of interest because of the existence of pre- and postoperative neurobehavioral syndromes. These tests are of importance because of the evaluation and estimation of the further expected progress of the intellectual development of children after the surgery.

◆ Surgical Techniques

Anesthesia

Unless the preoperative endocrinological evaluation prescribes a different regime, 5 mg of dexamethasone three times a day combined with a protecting agent against gastric ulcers should be taken 1 day prior to the operation, and after induction mannitol 1 g/kg is administered for further brain relaxation.

Preoperative Shunt

Especially in children the craniopharyngioma becomes manifest by an obstructive hydrocephalus. Depending on the preoperative clinical condition of the patient, an external ventricular drain (EVD) prior to the surgery may be placed, especially if brain retraction is required, such as in patients with large craniopharyngiomas. Here an external lumbar drain before and during surgery is highly recommended.

Approach

The approach is dependent on the volume and site of the tumor.

The pterional approach provides the shortest distance to the suprasellar region. The sylvian fissure can be opened as far as possible, and the craniopharyngioma can be approached via the already-mentioned routes (see Surgical Anatomy, earlier in chapter). Furthermore, this approach provides an easy opening to the basal cisterns so that cerebrospinal fluid (CSF) can be removed first. Due to the location and volume of the craniopharyngioma, the hypothalamus and optic chiasm have been elevated upward, creating a large space for dissecting the neurovascular structures also on the contralateral side. However, it is essential that the approach is as basal as possible. Therefore, an orbital or orbitozygomatic osteotomy should be performed. In cases that require primary visualization of both optic nerves, the approach should be extended more frontally (the frontolateral approach).

In contrast to the bifrontal approach, the frontolateral approach preserves one of the olfactory nerves, and only one (usually right) frontal lobe has to be retracted. Additionally, the bifrontal approach gives no primary access to the basal cisterns.

Therefore, for most craniopharyngiomas a pterional approach with an anterior subfrontal extension (the frontolateral approach) is the recommended approach.

Frontolateral Approach

Position and Initial Exposure

Unless there is a significant parasellar extension of the craniopharyngioma into the left sylvian fissure, a right-sided approach is used by the right-handed surgeon.

The patient is placed in the supine position, and the head is fixed in a pin-type headholder. The trunk is slightly elevated and the head is turned about 20 degrees to the contralateral side. The body is fixed to the table to allow a rotation of the head of 20 to 30 degrees more to either side.

The skin incision starts as a routine "pterional" skin incision with an inferior extension in an orbitozygomatic approach and a variable extension beyond the frontal midline, in the hairline, in a more frontolateral approach **(Fig. 56–1)**.

The skin and external fascia temporalis are reflected in one layer anteriorly until the fascia covering the supraorbital and lateral-orbital rim is exposed. The pericranial flap is elevated from the skull and dissected from the superior and lateral wall of the orbit. The flap should be preserved for the repair of skull-base defects. The supraorbital nerve is preserved; the temporalis muscle is dissected from the skull starting at the level of the zygoma in an upward direction **(Fig. 56–2)**.

A craniotomy is performed beginning at the root of the zygoma moving upward anterosuperiorly to end medial or lateral to the supraorbital foramen. The latter is dependent

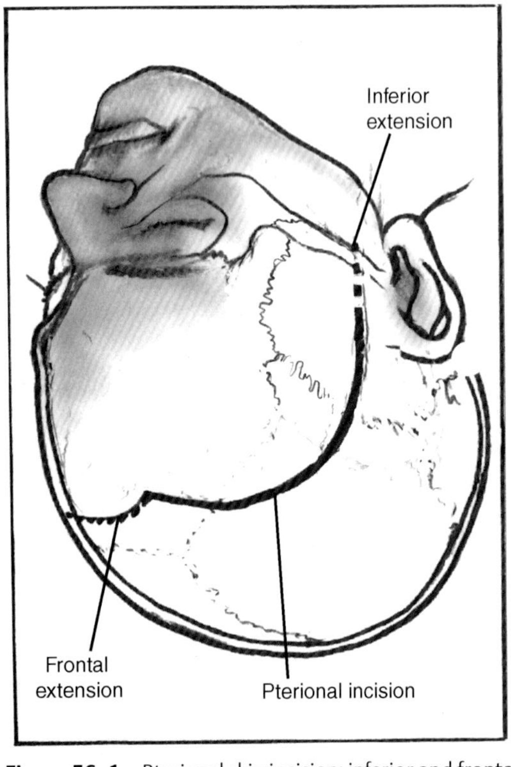

Figure 56–1 Pterional skin incision: inferior and frontal extension.

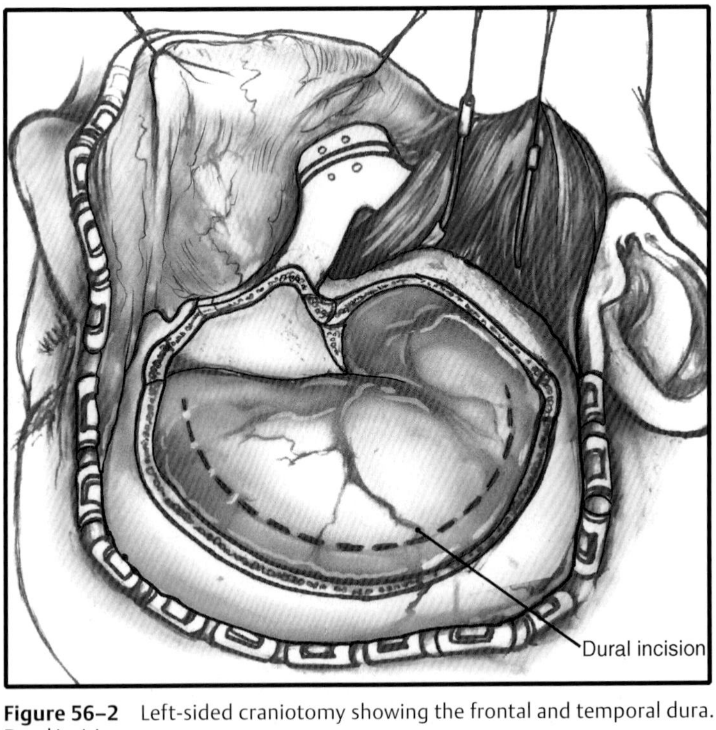

Figure 56–2 Left-sided craniotomy showing the frontal and temporal dura. Dural incision.

on the extent of the frontal-basal approach. The craniotomy is continued at the level of the frontal base to the sphenoid ridge downward to the base of the squama temporalis.

The craniotomy is extended by an osteotomy of the superolateral rim of the orbit and zygoma (**Figs. 56–2** and **56–3**). By means of the high-speed drill the sphenoid rim is removed until a smooth contour is obtained from the frontal floor to the middle fossa. If the frontal sinus has been opened, it should be packed with the cranial flap and surgical glue before opening the dura.

The dura is opened by means of a frontotemporal incision (**Fig. 56–2**). The optic nerve is approached by opening of the arachnoid cisterns and slight elevation of the frontal lobe. The sylvian fissure is opened as much as necessary. It is essential to remove the CSF as much as possible to retract the frontal lobe and to expose the optic nerves. The basal cisterns are opened and more CSF can be removed.

Exposure of the Tumor and Resection

The anterosuperior part of the craniopharyngioma becomes visible. A recommended sequence of resection is advised (**Fig. 56–4A**).

If possible, a dissection is done of the arachnoidea from the capsule and from the optic nerves and superior hypophyseal arteries. As long as the capsule is expanded, this dissection is easier than after the puncture or debulking of the tumor.

After this dissection, an interoptic debulking or puncture of the cystic component should be performed.

In contrast to the arteries, the adherence of the craniopharyngioma to the nervous tissue is less dense, so that in the intraoptic space the tumor can be debulked and mobilized by means of a gentle retraction on the capsula (**Fig. 56–4B**). Once the tumor has been partially mobilized, the pituitary stalk may come into view. This structure can be recognized because of its striated appearance caused by the portal veins on the surface of the stalk. Because of the different places of the onset of growth of the craniopharyngioma, the stalk can be found on all parts of the capsule. The stalk can most easily be found on its fixed entrance through the diaphragma sellae. If there is no infiltration of the tumor, the pituitary stalk can be dissected by gently pulling the capsule from the lower part of the pituitary stalk. Otherwise a part of the stalk or complete stalk should be sacrificed. The stalk should be cut as distal as possible because of its ability to restore the production of antidiuretic hormone (ADH).

Because the superior hypophyseal arteries mainly enter the optic nerve on the lateral inferior side and the pituitary stalk, they are not always visible in this stage of surgery. Therefore, cauterization should be avoided here, and the arachnoid membranes should be respected as much as possible. In the case of a prefixed chiasm or a pseudoprefixed chiasm caused by the tumor itself, the small preoptic space can be enlarged by drilling away the bone of the planum sphenoidale as much as possible, avoiding an opening and disruption of the mucosa of the sphenoid sinus.

The next step is the dissection and removal of the craniopharyngioma through the opticocarotid triangle (**Fig. 56–4C**).

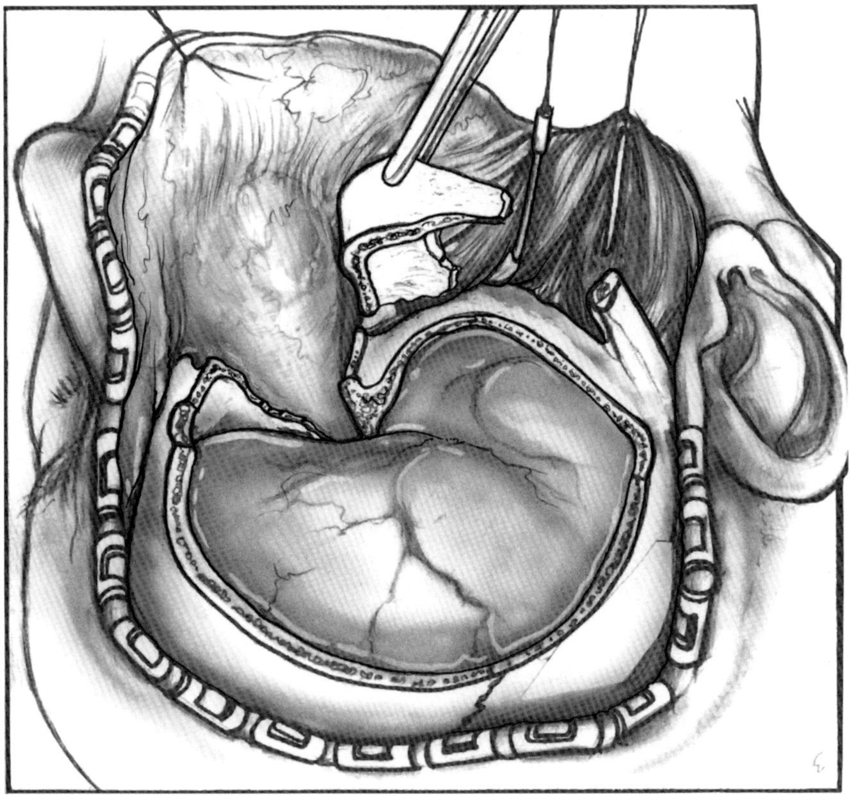

Figure 56–3 Frontal side of the craniotomy showing the osteotomy of the superolateral rim of the orbit and zygoma.

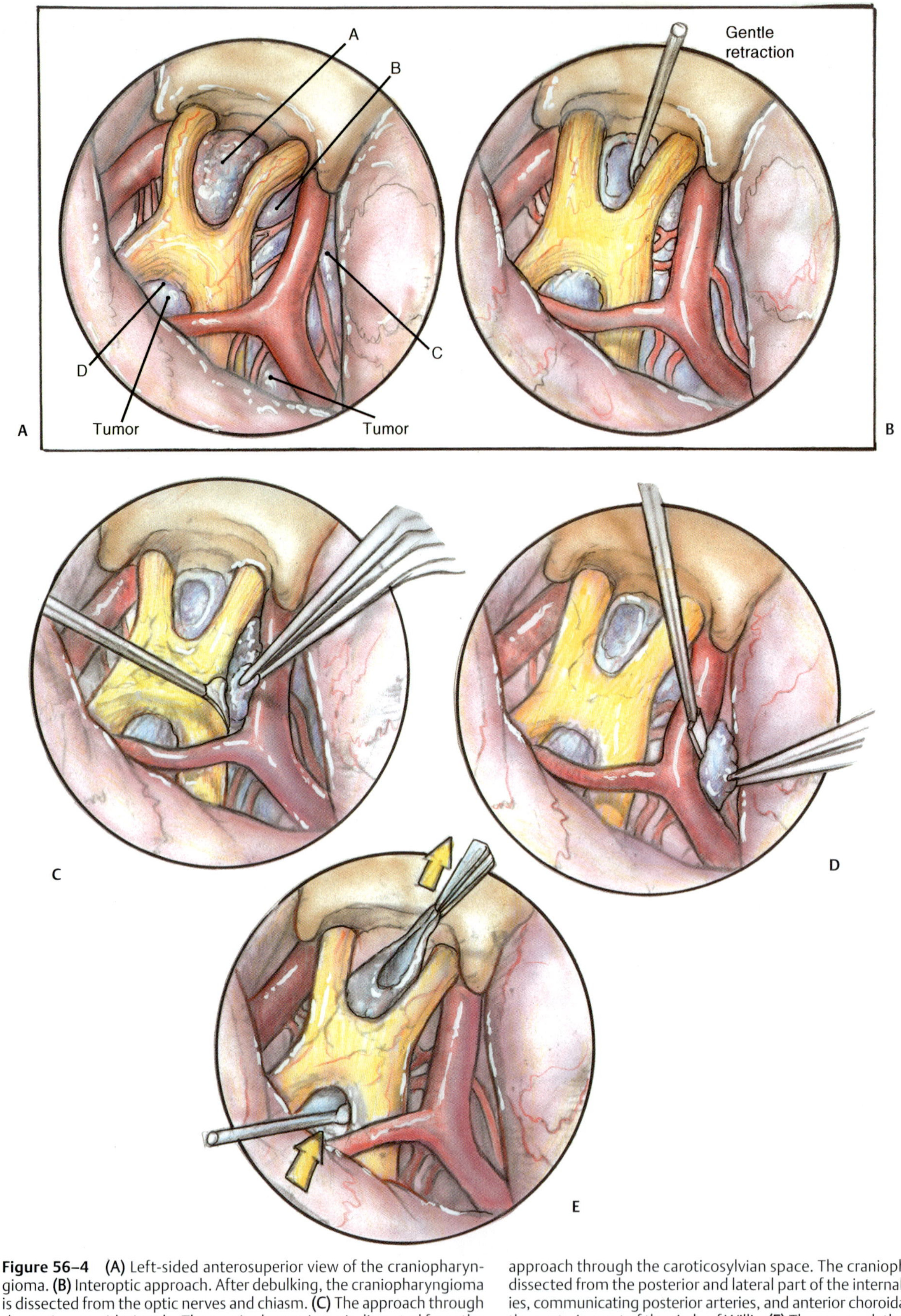

Figure 56–4 **(A)** Left-sided anterosuperior view of the craniopharyngioma. **(B)** Interoptic approach. After debulking, the craniopharyngioma is dissected from the optic nerves and chiasm. **(C)** The approach through the opticocarotid triangle. The craniopharyngioma is dissected from the lateral parts of the optic nerves, the internal carotid arteries, and the superior hypophyseal arteries and anterior part of the circle of Willis. **(D)** The approach through the caroticosylvian space. The craniopharyngioma is dissected from the posterior and lateral part of the internal carotid arteries, communicating posterior arteries, and anterior choroidal arteries, and the posterior part of the circle of Willis. **(E)** The approach through the lamina terminalis. The craniopharyngioma is dissected from the hypothalamic area and posterior part of the circle of Willis.

The most common obstacle here is the identification and dissection of the superior hypophyseal arteries and the dense adhesions of the tumor to these arteries. The lateral capsule is manipulated medially toward the collapsed central cavity. The arterial feeders of the tumor from the internal carotid artery, the posterior communicating artery, and the anterior part of the circle of Willis become stretched and can be recognized. Parts, especially calcified parts, of the tumor adherent to the circle of Willis without a dissection plane should be left behind to prevent a disruption or weakening of the adventitia of the arteries.

The lateral capsula is further exposed through the caroticosylvian space. The brain and inferolateral surface of the internal carotid artery is dissected; the posterior communicating and anterior choroidal arteries can be recognized. The posterior communicating artery can be followed until the posterior part of the circle of Willis, which can be dissected from the capsula together with the oculomotor nerve (**Fig. 56–4D**). Also, the contralateral wall can be pulled medially as far as possible and dissected from the feeding arteries and adjacent structures.

After removal of the two lateral portions, the upper pole of the tumor is dissected from the optic chiasm and hypothalamus through the lamina terminalis (**Fig. 56–4E**). The lamina terminalis should be opened in the midline behind the crossing of the macular fibers of the optic chiasm, which is the most transparent area of the optic chiasm. Opening of this membrane offers an excellent view on the dome of the craniopharyngioma and if performed in the midline will not produce hypothalamic deficiencies. In the tuber cinereum the layer of glial tissue may help in separating the capsule from the hypothalamus. Only gentle pulling is allowed to prevent hypothalamic dysfunctions. The posterior pole of the tumor can now pull anteriorly (**Fig. 56–4E**). This procedure is relatively safe because there are no feeding arteries from the posterior part of the circle of Willis and the firm membrane of Lillequist separates the tumor from the brain stem and basilar artery.

After the dissection of all the parts of the capsule, the tumor can be debulked as much as possible and removed.

Closure

If the frontal and sphenoid sinus were opened, the skull base defects are closed by suturing the pericranial flap to the basal dura and by the use of surgical glue.The dura is sutured watertight, and the bone flap and the orbital–zygoma complex are fixed by miniplates.

The temporal muscle and fascia temporalis and skin layers are closed in the usual manner.

◆ Postoperative Care

Endocrinological disturbances are always present after surgery. Cutting or damaging the stalk results in both early and late postoperative endocrine disorders. The earliest endocrine disorder is diabetes insipidus, which usually becomes manifest in three stages. An excessive diuresis begins within 24 hours after the damage of the stalk and can sometimes be noted during the surgery. This first stage is determined by the sudden cessation of the normal intraaxonal transport of ADH, whereas the second stage is due to the degeneration of the hypothalamo-hypophyseal tract and neurohypophysis. In this stage there is an uncontrolled release of ADH 1 to 4 days after surgery, resulting in paradoxical water retention. In the third stage the stored ADH disappears and massive diuresis returns. Daily fluid balance and electrolyte control are essential, especially to prevent water intoxication during the second stage, which can aggravate the postoperative brain edema.

Hypoadrenalism may be suspected; therefore, high doses of corticosteroids, which are usually given in the preoperative phase, should be continued. The hypothyroidism is considered to occur and L-thyroxine is usually supplemented in the second postoperative week. Further endocrinological disturbances are treated in the late postoperative phase according to the physiological requirements. The visual acuity and fields should be tested in the postoperative phase, and the tests should be repeated in cases of known residual tumor. Especially in children neurobehavioral tests should be repeated to identify and treat social and psychological problems.

◆ Complications

Perioperative Surgical Complications

Between the craniopharyngioma and neuroendocrine and neurovascular structures an arachnoid membrane is present. The loss of this membrane may result in inadequate tumor removal and more risk of peri- and postoperative complications. The initial debulking of the craniopharyngioma should be restricted to prevent a redundant and folding capsule and arachnoid, which then become more difficult to separate.

To mobilize the tumor and to dissect the arachnoid, the surgeon needs a perfect overview of all margins of the tumor. Therefore, the choice of the craniotomy is essential and should be as wide as possible. Depending on the volume of the tumor an orbitozygomatic osteotomy and frontolateral extension of the pterional approach should be performed. This is also advised if a prefixed chiasm is expected and the craniopharyngioma extends into the third ventricle. The intraoperative use of the endoscope offers great value in the visualization of the capsule, especially of the capsule of the opposite site of the tumor.

Injury of the Optic Nerve and Chiasm

The optic nerve and chiasm are very sensitive to surgical manipulations, which may result in infarctions of the optic nerves and decreased vision. Therefore, only small amounts of extra space can be obtained by gentle retraction of the optic nerve. In this respect the removal of the dural pouch at the entrance of the optic canal allows the optic nerve to be retracted more. The opticocarotid triangle should be enlarged only by a gentle retraction of the internal carotid artery. As the superior hypophyseal arteries have a tortuous course to the optic nerve, these arteries can be stretched.[5]

Injury of the Pituitary Stalk

The fixed entrance of the pituitary stalk through the diaphragma sellae is the main point to be recognized as early as possible. From here the stalk can be dissected, preserving the arachnoid membrane. In case the stalk should be sacrificed, the stalk should be cut as distal as possible to reestablish the production of ADH.

Hypothalamic Injury

Because craniopharyngiomas are slow growing and histologically benign and hypothalamic injury may cause tremendous neurological, neurobehavioral, and neuroendocrinological complications, hypothalamic injury should be avoided in all cases. Only a very gentle pulling of the tumor is allowed in this region. If the tumor capsule cannot be separated from the hypothalamic structures, it should be left behind. In this respect the transcallosal approach is very prone to hypothalamic injury, especially because the tumor is approached through the hypothalamic structures. The tumor, not the neural structures, should be dissected free from the arachnoid layers.

Vascular Injury

The anterior part of the circle of Willis and perforating arteries are displaced by the tumor. As long as there is an arachnoid plane between the vascular structures and the tumor capsule, removal of the tumor from the vascular structures remains possible. Special attention should be paid to the perforating arteries, because they could be firmly attached to the tumor capsule. Small vessels become more visible after stretching the capsule, and the vessels can be dissected sharply off the capsule.

Aseptic Meningitis

Great care must be taken to avoid spilling tumor material and leakage of the cyst content to prevent aseptic meningitis. During surgery continuous irrigation by means of a drip into the surgical field may dilute the cystic content, and tumor material can be sucked easily. Furthermore, continuous irrigation helps the surgeon in dissecting the arachnoid membrane from the tumor capsule.

A postoperative communicating hydrocephalus may be another sequela of aseptic meningitis. A routine postoperative CT scan should be performed to exclude hydrocephalus.

Tumor Recurrence

Although a radical removal is the first choice of treatment, residual or recurrent tumors are not uncommon features. A second attempt of surgery may not be advised because of the existence of scar tissue, resulting in a very high postoperative complication rate.

Fractionated external-beam radiation therapy is advised; however, it carries the risk of damaging the hypothalamus and optic pathways. Recently, the results of gamma knife radiosurgery proved to be superior to conventional radiation therapy. It is suggested that gamma knife radiosurgery should be used as an alternative in the treatment of recurrent and residual craniopharyngiomas if further microsurgical excision cannot be performed.[6]

References

1. Scott RM, Pomeroy LS, Tarbell NJ. Craniopharyngioma. In: Black PMcL, Loeffler JS, eds. Cancer of the Nervous System. Cambridge: Blackwell Science; 1997:414–422
2. Hoffman HJ, De Silva M, Humphreys RP, Drake JM, Smith ML, Blaser SL. Aggressive surgical management of craniopharyngiomas in children. J Neurosurg 1992;76:47–52
3. Samii M, Tatagiba M. Craniopharyngioma. In: Kaye AH, Laws ED Jr, eds. Brain Tumors: An Encyclopedic Approach. New York: Churchill Livingstone; 1995:873–894
4. Russel DS, Rubinstein LJ. Pathology of Tumors of the Nervous System. 4th ed. Baltimore: Williams & Wilkins; 1977:35
5. van Overbeeke JJ, Sekhar LN. The microanatomy of the blood supply to the optic nerve. Orbit 2003;22:81–88
6. Chung WY, Pan DH, Shiau C-Y, Guo W-Y, Wang L-W. Gamma knife radiosurgery for craniopharyngiomas. J Neurosurg 2001;93(Suppl):47–56

57

Tumors of the Tentorium

Saleem I. Abdulrauf and Ossama Al-Mefty

Surgical excision of tumors involving the tentorium can be challenging, mainly due to access, especially for medially located lesions, as well as their relationship to the brain stem, cranial nerves, temporal lobe, blood vessels, and venous sinuses. The downward sloping of the tentorium, from its apex anteriorly to the petrous bones laterally, and the occipital bones posteriorly add an extra geometric complicating factor to accessing these lesions. More recent advances in microsurgical techniques and skull-base approaches have made access and resection of some of these larger and medially located tumors less difficult.

Although medial tentorial ring meningiomas may appear very similar to petroclival and sphenopetroclival meningiomas on radiographic examination, they differ significantly in their local anatomical relationships, and ultimately this is reflected in the operative difficulty and outcome.[1] Petroclival meningiomas originate medial to cranial nerve V, and, based on the senior author's (SIA) observations, usually have only one layer of arachnoid separating them from the brain stem, to which they are usually adherent, thus making total resection technically difficult. Tentorial meningiomas, on the other hand, arise from the tentorial edge, where there is a convergence of the interpeduncular, crural, and ambient cisterns, and as they grow, they push multiple layers of arachnoid ahead of them. This provides a clear demarcation between the tumor, brain stem, and cranial nerves, thus making total resection relatively less risky.

◆ Surgical Planning

Detailed radiological studies are crucial for surgical planning. Computed tomography (CT) and magnetic resonance imaging (MRI) are complementary. They should be obtained in coronal, sagittal, and axial planes to specifically identify the location of the tumor and any extensions as well as the tumor's relationship to the brain stem, and to delineate any encasement of vessels and involvement of the cavernous sinus and the temporal bone.

Delineation of the vascular anatomy, especially the venous system, is crucial for planning surgery. This should include bilateral demonstration of the transverse and sigmoid sinuses and their connection at the torcular Herophili for lateral and posterior approaches. Venous drainage of the temporal lobe must be thoroughly studied. This system includes the vein of Labbé and basal temporal veins, and it is important to identify their relationship to the superior petrosal sinus, tentorium, and sigmoid sinus. The jugular bulb and its location must also be delineated. These structures are best seen during the venous stage of angiography; however, magnetic resonance venography (MRV) may be sufficient to obtain this information.[2]

◆ Surgical Approaches

This chapter systematically reviews varying approaches to the tentorium based on the anatomical location of the tumor **(Fig. 57–1).** Meningioma is the most common tumor to involve the tentorium, and much of the dissection in this chapter is based on the management of this lesion. The classification system for tumors of the inner ring of the tentorium utilized in this chapter is modified after Yasargil's[3] classification system.

We advocate the use of neurophysiological monitoring, including cranial nerve, somatosensory, and brain stem evoked potentials.

The Zygomatic Extended Middle Fossa Approach

Tumors involving the anterior to mid-medial incisural ring and the petrous apex with extension into the perimesencephalic area **(Fig. 57–2)** can be resected using the extended middle fossa (EMF) approach. We prefer this transzygomatic approach to the standard subtemporal approach because it allows for a larger inferior window and thus less

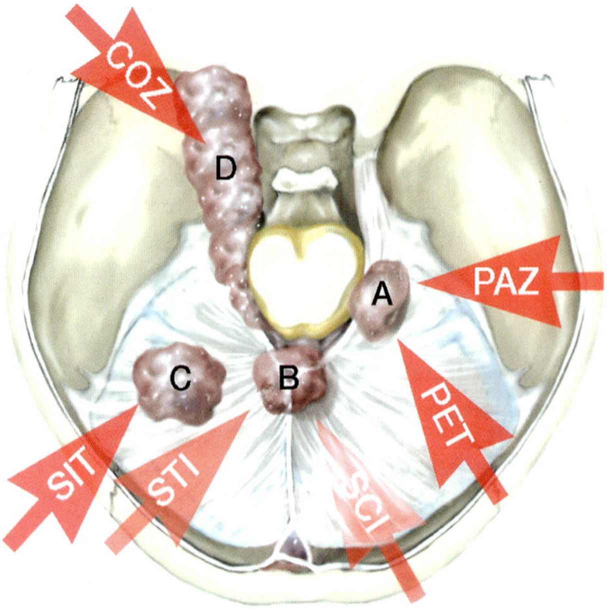

Figure 57–1 Surgical trajectories for lesions of the tentorium. A, petrosal (PET) approach; B, supratentorial interhemispheric (STI) approach; C, suprainfratentorial (SIT) approach; D, cranio-orbital zygomatic (COZ) approach.

temporal lobe retraction. This approach can be combined with an anterior petrosectomy for lesions extending posteriorly into the lateral pontine area.

Positioning

The patient's head is rotated to the contralateral side ~30 degrees, tilted slightly contralaterally, combined with elevation of the ipsilateral shoulder. The head is fixed in this position using the Mayfield head holder. Spinal drainage is placed.

Surgical Technique

A reverse question-mark–shaped incision is made starting at the inferior margin of the root of the zygoma, anterior to the tragus, encircling posteriorly just above the external auditory meatus, and then curved anteriorly and medially toward the midline just behind the hairline. The skin flap is separated from the underlying temporalis fascia. The superficial and deep temporalis fascia layers are cut sharply anteriorly, preserving the frontal branches of the facial nerve. The zygoma root and arch are dissected in the subperiosteal plane and cut obliquely anteriorly and posteriorly. The zygoma with its masseter muscle attachment is reflected inferiorly. The temporalis muscle is sharply separated from the underlying bone and is retracted inferiorly. Two bur holes are placed low in the middle fossa. One or two additional bur holes can be placed at the superficial temporal line. The bur holes are all connected using a high-speed drill. Additional craniectomy is done to ensure maximal middle fossa inferior access **(Fig. 57–3).**

For sphenopetroclival meningiomas with extension along the tentorium, the anterior petrosal approach may be needed. The dura of the middle fossa is separated under the operative microscope magnification. Spinal drainage is useful during this portion of the procedure. The second and third divisions

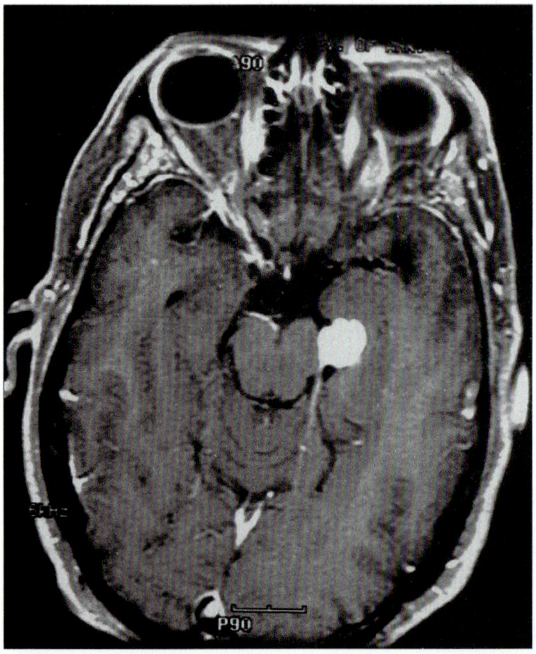

Figure 57–2 Postgadolinium contrast axial T1-weighted magnetic resonance imaging showing a meningioma involving midincisural ring.

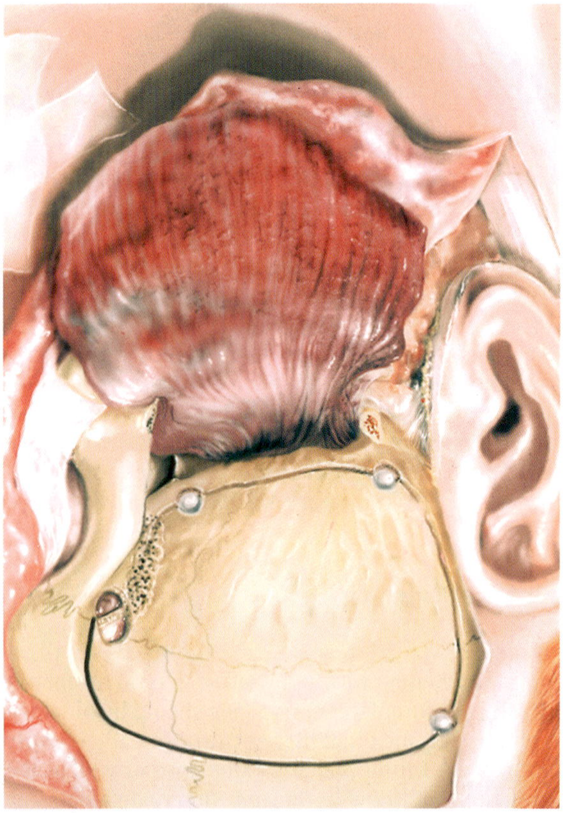

Figure 57–3 Artist's depiction of a right-sided craniotomy for a zygomatic middle fossa approach.

of the fifth cranial nerve are identified. The middle meningeal artery is identified at its entrance from the foramen spinosum and is coagulated and cut. The greater petrosal nerve is identified posteriorly. Inferior and medial to the greater petrosal nerve lies the petrous internal carotid artery (ICA). In the majority of cases, the petrous ICA is separated from the middle fossa by only a thin fibrous layer of tissue. Exposure of the petrous internal carotid artery is done in cases where lateral entry into the cavernous sinus is anticipated. Detailed understanding of the anatomy of the temporal bone is required for performing an anterior petrosectomy.[4]

The dural opening for the standard EMF approach, can be performed more medially to avoid excessive direct manipulation of the temporal lobe and its underlying veins.

Petrosal Approach

Tumors of the middle to posterior part of the inner ring of the tentorium with involvement of the petroclival area and extension into perimesencephalic/peripontine structures can be approached using the petrosal approach **(Figs. 57–1 and 57–4).** To access these regions, the petrosal approach offers several advantages: (1) the surgeon's operative distance to these regions is shorter than in the retrosigmoid approaches; (2) there is minimal retraction of the cerebellum and temporal lobe; (3) the neural structures (seventh and eighth nerves) are preserved; (4) the otologic structures (cochlea, labyrinth, semicircular canals) are preserved; (5) and the major venous sinuses (transverse and sigmoid) along with the vein of Labbé and other temporal and basal veins are preserved.[5]

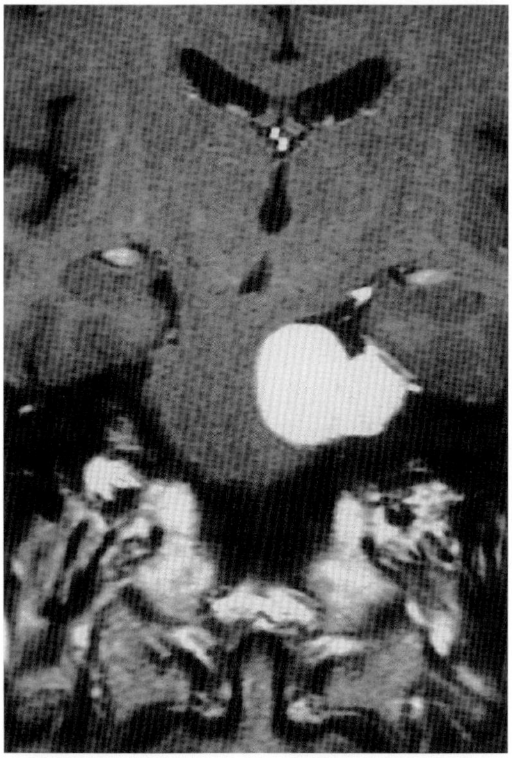

Figure 57–4 Postgadolinium coronal T1-weighted magnetic resonance imaging demonstrating a meningioma attached to inferior surface of the tentorium.

Positioning

The patient is placed in the supine position on the operating table. The table is flexed ~30 degrees to allow head and trunk elevation. The patient's ipsilateral shoulder is slightly elevated using a shoulder roll. The head is rotated away from the side of the tumor (~50 degrees) and is flexed slightly toward the floor. The head is fixed in a three-point Mayfield headrest.

Surgical Technique

A reverse question-mark–shaped incision is made starting at the zygoma anterior to the tragus, and carried about 2 to 3 cm above and encircling the ear, and descending 1 cm medial to the mastoid process. The skin flap is sharply dissected from the underlying pericranium and fascia. The temporalis fascia is reflected sharply and is kept in continuity with the sternocleidomastoid muscle, which is subsequently sharply dissected off the bone and reflected inferiorly. The surgeon must take special care during the dissection at the mastoid process to avoid injury to the seventh nerve. The temporalis muscle is then reflected anteriorly in a similar fashion.

Four bur holes, two on each side of the transverse sinus, are made. The first bur hole is placed just medial and inferior to the asterion, which is located at the inferior junction of the transverse and sigmoid sinuses. The second bur hole is placed at the squamous and mastoid junction of the temporal bone, along the projection of the superior temporal line, which would open into the supratentorial compartment. The final two holes are placed about 2 to 3 cm more medially and closer together on either side of the transverse sinus. A temporoparietal craniotomy as well as a lateral occipital craniotomy are performed without connecting the bur holes across the sinus **(Fig. 57–5)**. The holes across the sinus are then connected using the B-1 attachment (without a footplate) of the Midas-Rex drill (Midas-Rex, Fort Worth, TX). Following meticulous separation of the wall of the sinus from the flap, the bone plate is elevated.

This stage of the operation requires that the surgeon be familiar with the anatomy of the temporal bone and its surrounding structures. The operating microscope, mounted on a Contraves stand, is used. A complete mastoidectomy is performed using a high-speed air drill. The diamond bit should be used when drilling near vital neural and otologic structures. The sigmoid sinus is drilled down to the jugular bulb. The sinodural angle, Citelli's angle, which identifies the location of the superior petrosal sinus, is exposed. The surgeon next drills the superficial mastoid air cells as well as the deep (retrofacial) air cells. The facial canal and the lateral and posterior semicircular canals are identified. The petrous bone is thinned by drilling along the pyramid toward the apex.

The posterior fossa dura just anterior to the sigmoid sinus is opened. The dura at the floor of temporal fossa is also opened to the drainage point of the superior petrosal sinus. Depending on the specific anatomy of the vein of Labbé, it may need to be dissected along its course to avoid injury during temporal lobe retraction. The superior petrosal sinus is coagulated or ligated and then transected. The dural

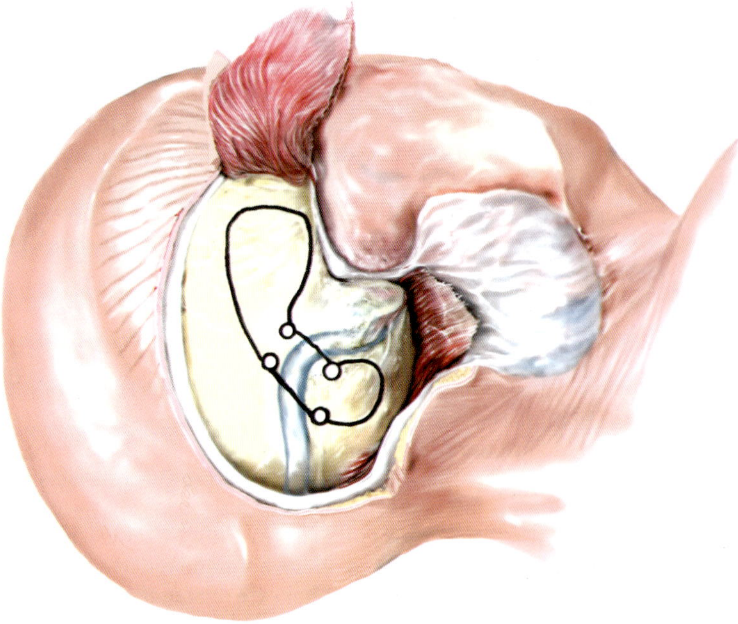

Figure 57–5 Skin incision and bur hole demarcations for a posterior petrosal approach.

incision is now extended, parallel to the pyramid toward the incisura. Care must be taken to avoid injury to the fourth nerve, by cutting the tentorial edge posterior to the insertion of the fourth nerve **(Fig. 57–6).** Additionally, for larger tumors with great extension into the posterior fossa and cerebello-pontine angli (CPA), the dura posterior to the sigmoid sinus can also be opened allowing wider and more inferiorly directed access **(Fig. 57–7).**

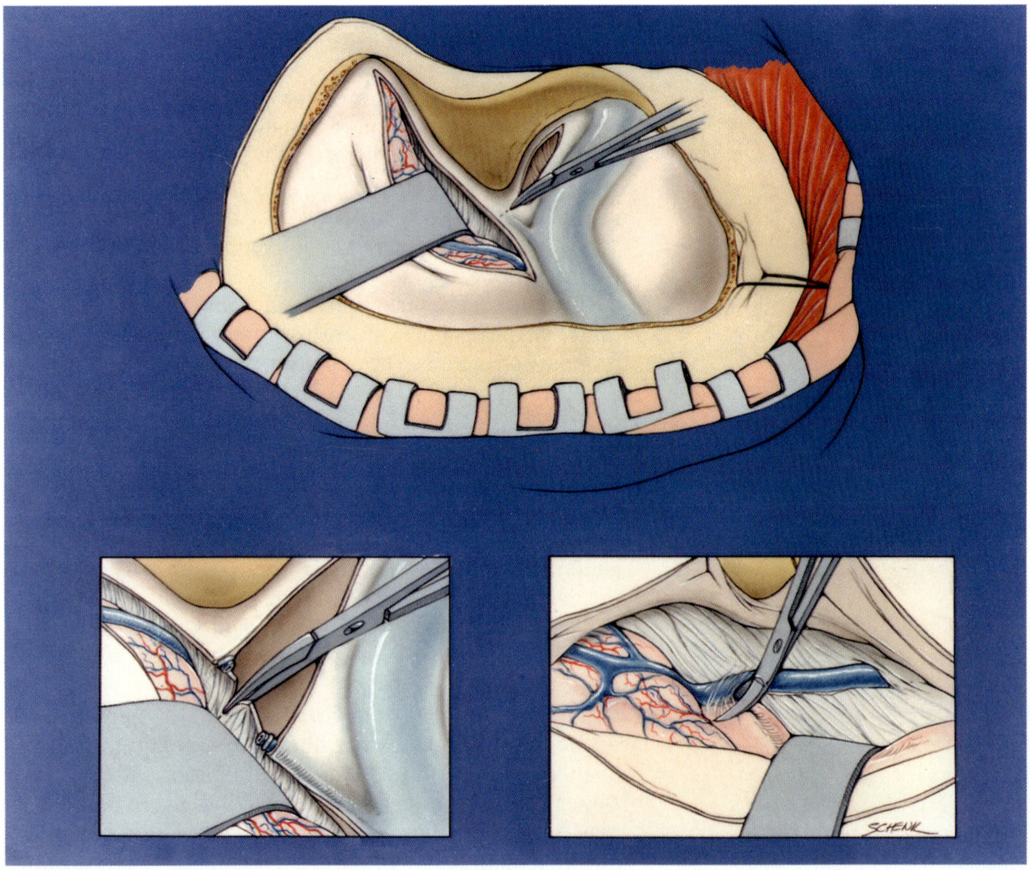

Figure 57–6 Ligation of the superior petrosal sinus and cutting of the tentorium steps.

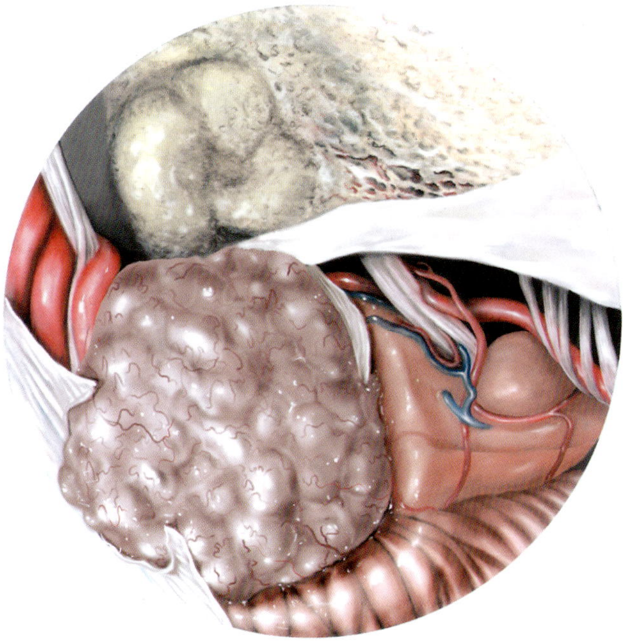

Figure 57–7 Artist's depiction of a tumor of the upper clivus through the posterior petrosal trajectory.

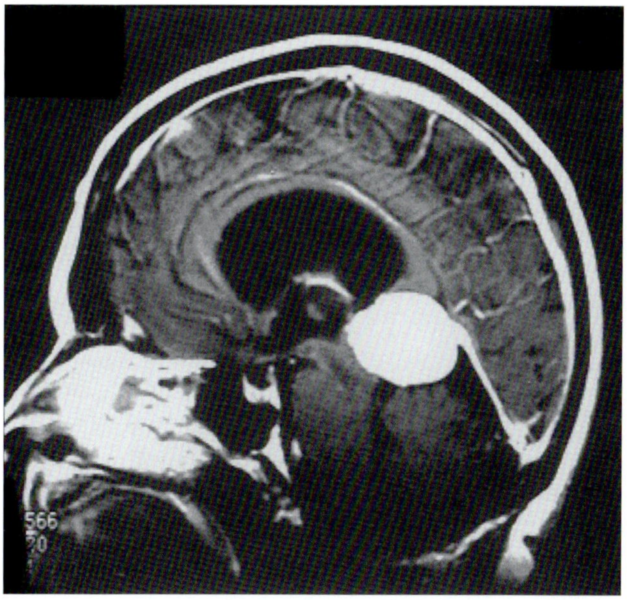

Figure 57–8 Postgadolinium contrast-enhanced midsagittal magnetic resonance imaging of a falcotentorial meningioma projecting infratentorially.

The Supratentorial Interhemispheric and the Supracerebellar Infratentorial Approaches

Falcotentorial lesions (**Figs. 57–1** and **57–8**) are accessed using a posterior interhemispheric transtentorial approach. Tumors at the falcotentorial junction, which are mainly infratentorial, can be accessed via the supracerebellar infratentorial (SCI) approach **(Fig. 57–9).**

The posterior supratentorial interhemispheric (STI) approach, combined with tentorial splitting if needed, is achieved using a low occipital craniotomy that is fashioned to expose the superior sagittal sinus, the torcula, and the transverse sinus. We prefer to approach the tumor from the nondominant side. The patient is placed in a three-quarter prone position, allowing gravity to "retract" the occipital lobe.

The SCI approach is performed with the patient in the sitting position, with the head slightly flexed. A suboccipital craniotomy exposing the torcula and the transverse sinus is made. Microsurgical dissection above the cerebellum in the

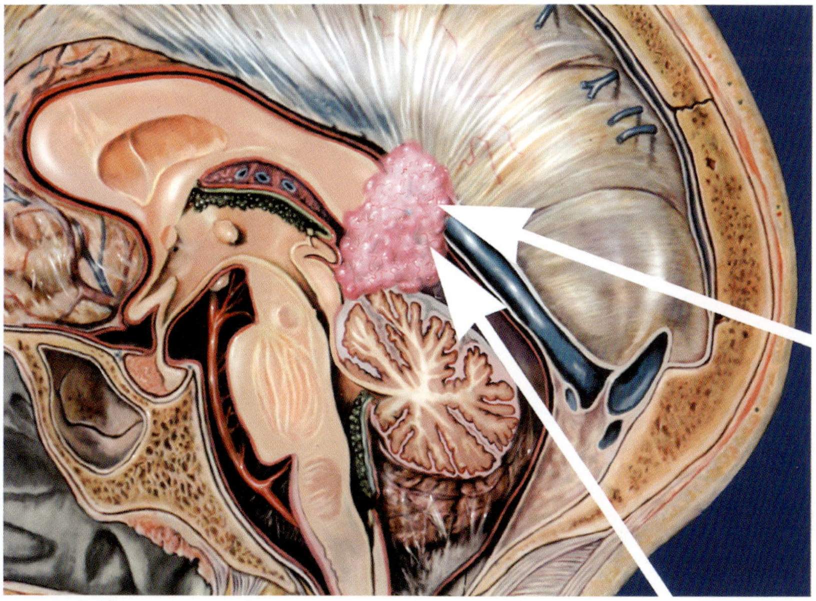

Figure 57–9 Artist's depiction of a falcotentorial junction meningioma with arrows delineating the supratentorial interhemispheric (upper arrow) and the supracerebellar infratentorial (lower arrow) trajectories.

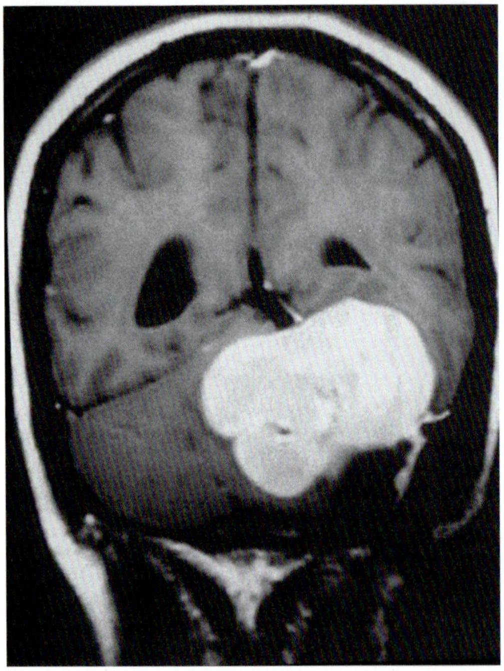

Figure 57–10 Postgadolinium contrast-enhanced coronal T1-weighted magnetic resonance imaging showing a posterior tentorial meningioma projecting both above and below the tentorium.

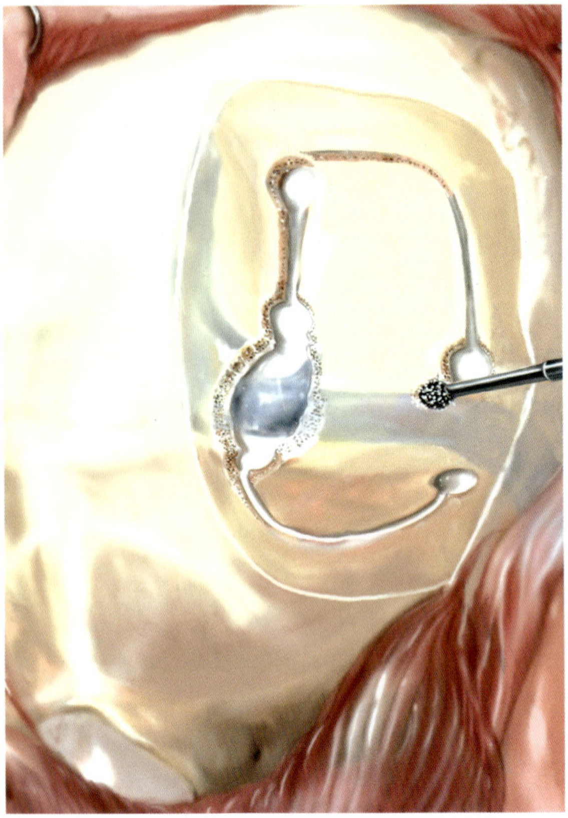

Figure 57–11 Bur holes straddling the lateral sinus for the suprainfratentorial approach.

midline, or laterally when large vermian veins are present, is performed. Preservation of the veins draining into the vein of Galen is crucial.

Suprainfratentorial Approach

Larger tentorial leaf tumors with superior extension into the occipital lobe and inferior extension into the cerebellum can be approached using the suprainfratentorial approach (SIT) **(Figs. 57–1** and **57–10).**

In this approach, a single occipital suboccipital bone flap is made in a similar fashion to the one described for the petrosal approach above **(Fig. 57–11).** Wide exposure of the transverse sinus is achieved above and below the sinus **(Fig. 57–12).** We advocate the avoidance of sinus sacrifice in this and all other approaches.

The Cranio-orbital Zygomatic Approach

For skull-base meningiomas that involve the parasellar region and secondarily involve the tentorium, the cranio-orbital zygomatic (COZ) approach should be considered **(Figs. 57-1** and **57–13).** This approach allows the surgeon wide access to the anterior clinoid process (extradurally and intradurally), the posterior clinoid process, and the middle fossa. For larger lesions in this location, this approach allows the surgeon early identification of decompression of the optic nerve(s) and chiasm.

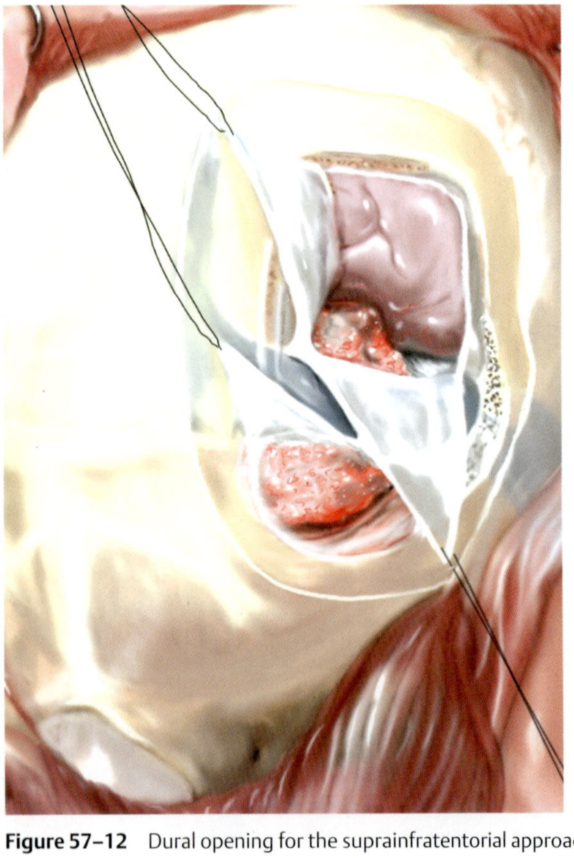

Figure 57–12 Dural opening for the suprainfratentorial approach.

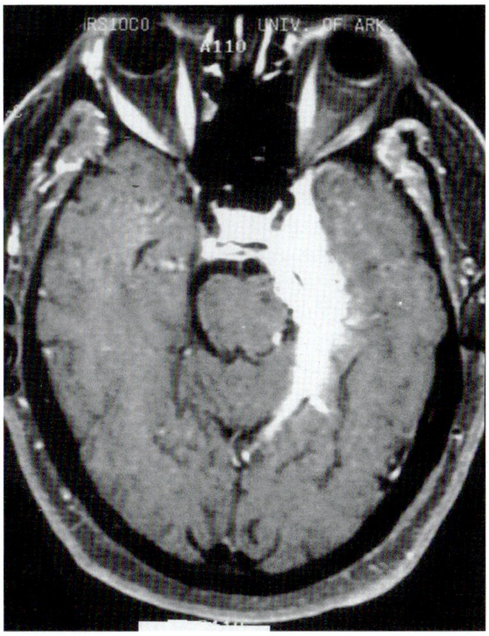

Figure 57–13 Axial magnetic resonance imaging demonstrating meningioma involving the tentorial incisura.

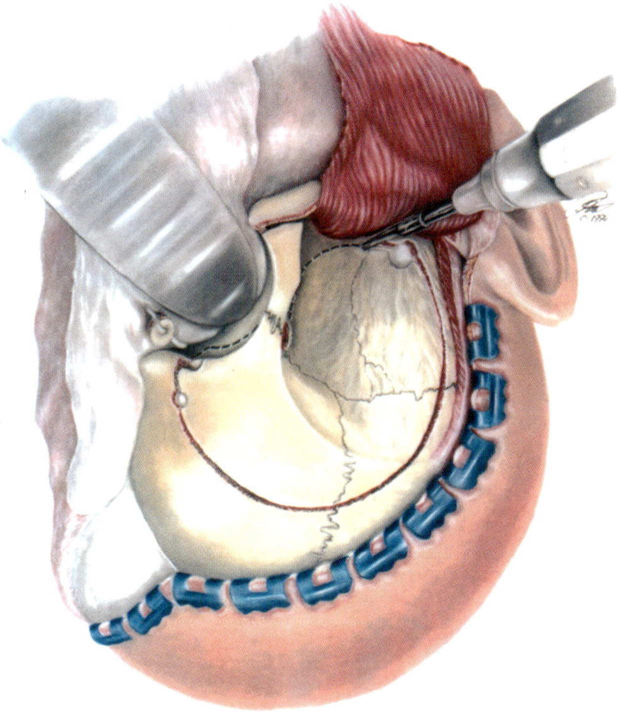

Figure 57–14 Bur hole locations and osteotomies for a single-piece cranial-orbital-zygomatic approach.

Positioning

The patient is placed in the supine position. The head is rotated 30 to 40 degrees to the opposite side and is slightly tilted toward the floor. The head is fixed in position using the Mayfield head holder.

Surgical Technique

A bicoronal incision is made behind the hairline extending from the zygomatic arch on the ipsilateral side to the superior temporal line of the opposite side. The superficial and deep fascia of the temporalis muscle are cut parallel to the zygomatic arch, preserving the frontal branches of the facial nerve. A large vascularized pericranial flap is reflected. The zygomatic arch is incised obliquely anteriorly and posteriorly. The zygoma is then reflected inferiorly. The temporalis muscle is detached from its insertions and retracted inferiorly. A bur hole is placed in the anatomical keyhole. This allows access to both the anterior cranial fossa as well as the periorbita. Bur holes are then placed on the floor of one middle fossa. Using a high-speed drill, the bur holes are connected **(Fig. 57–14)**. The orbital roof is cut using a small osteotome. The bone flap is reflected as one piece. The lateral wall and roof of the orbit are removed in a separate osteotomy.

Further steps are dependent on the size and extent of the lesion **(Fig. 57–15)**. Extradural removal of the anterior clinoid process, exposure of the subclinoid internal carotid artery, and exposure of the petrous internal carotid artery are key steps to unlocking the cavernous sinus. The approach and site of entering into the cavernous sinus depend on the anatomy of the tumor within it.

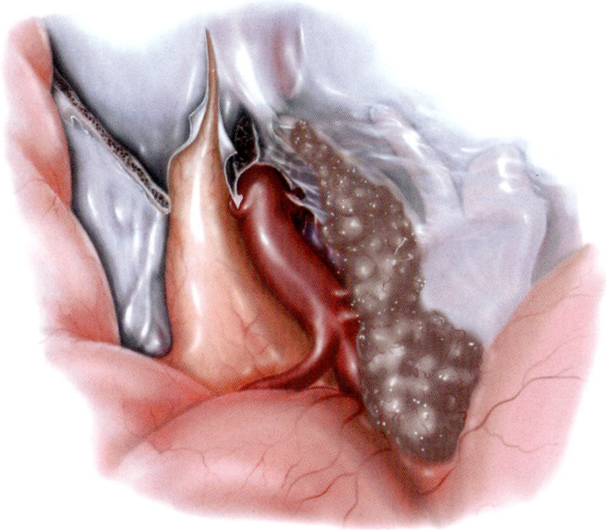

Figure 57–15 Carotid cistern and cavernous sinus regions as accessed via a single-piece cranial-orbital-zygomatic approach combined with an anterior sylvian fissure opening (artist's depiction).

◆ Closure and Reconstruction

Skull-base approaches require especially meticulous closure. Cerebrospinal fluid leakage needs to be avoided by achieving a watertight dural closure. The dura may be expanded using an autologous fascia lata graft. Vascularized pericranial graft provides the principal protective layer for skull-base reconstruction. Vascularized temporalis muscle graft can also provide an additional strong reconstructive element for the larger temporally based approaches. Microplating systems have enhanced the cosmetic results, especially in the zygomatic and maxillary areas.

◆ Conclusion

The resection of tentorial tumors (i.e., meningiomas) has traditionally been associated with significant morbidity and mortality. Advanced microsurgical techniques and skull-base approaches in combination have significantly improved surgical outcome and facilitated achieving total lesion resection. Intraoperative neurophysiological monitoring, minimal brain retraction, preservation of vascular (arterial and venous) connections, preservation of cranial nerves, watertight dural closure, and the use of vascularized pericranial and temporalis muscle flaps to reconstruct the skull base are the principal elements of successful resection of lesions in these locations.

References

1. Harrison MJ, Al-Mefty O. Tentorial meningiomas. In: Congress of Neurological Surgeons, eds. Clinical Neurosurgery: Proceedings of the Congress of Neurological Surgeons, Montreal, Quebec, Canada, vol 26. Baltimore: Williams & Wilkins; 1996:451–466
2. Al-Mefty O. Operative Atlas of Meningiomas. Philadelphia: Lippincott-Raven; 1998:209–286
3. Yasargil MG. Microsurgery. Vol 1. Stuttgart: Thieme; 1996:134–161
4. Kawase T, Shiobara R, Toya S. Anterior transpetrosal-transtentorial approach for sphenopetroclival meningiomas: surgical method and results in 10 patients. Neurosurgery 1991;28:869–876
5. Al-Mefty O, Fox JL, Smith RR. Petrosal approach for petroclival meningiomas. Neurosurgery 1988;22:510–517

58

Petroclival Meningiomas

Christopher Bogaev and Laligam N. Sekhar

Petroclival meningiomas remain a surgical challenge despite their usually benign pathology. The complex anatomy and difficult exposure of this region have led to the development of multiple techniques designed to minimize morbidity but potentially obtain a surgical cure with a complete resection. Sometimes a complete resection is not possible, such as with very large tumors involving multiple regions, adherence or invasion of the brain stem, or encasement of the vertebrobasilar circulation. A systematic approach to these tumors based on their size, location, brain stem involvement, preoperative deficits, and radiographic appearance optimizes the extent of resection and minimizes perioperative morbidity. There is no substitute for proper preoperative planning, including detailed imaging and multidisciplinary involvement. Equally essential is a detailed knowledge of the anatomy of the region and of the surgical techniques involved, including their indications, strengths, and limitations. This chapter provides a systematic approach to these difficult lesions.

◆ Preoperative Evaluation

Head Computed Tomography

- Bone windows are useful in evaluating bone destruction or hyperostosis as well as the bony anatomy of the skull base.
- Computed tomography (CT) is useful in assessing tumor calcification.
- Fine cuts through the temporal bone on the side of the approach are useful for surgical planning by defining temporal bone anatomy and the degree of pneumatization, which can facilitate the surgical exposure.

Brain Magnetic Resonance Imaging

- Contrasted study in multiple planes best shows the relationship of the tumor to the surrounding structures.

- Flow voids can reveal locations of important regional vascular structures such as the basilar or internal carotid arteries and their larger branches. It can show the degree of encasement or displacement of these vessels (best seen on T2-weighted images). Irregularity in the appearance of a flow void could represent vascular invasion by tumor.
- T2-weighted images are useful for assessing the integrity of the arachnoid plane of the tumor as well as associated brain edema.
- Edema of the brain stem on T2-weighted images can indicate pial invasion, particularly if a well-defined arachnoid plane is not seen.
- Higher T2 signal of the tumor can sometimes correlate with the softer tumor consistency.

Cerebral Angiography

- For small tumors, magnetic resonance (MR) angiography is preferred instead of a conventional angiogram to evaluate the size and collateral flow of the transverse and sigmoid sinuses. Visualization of the location, size, and configuration of the superficial venous anatomy, particularly the vein of Labbé, is extremely useful but is not always possible with this study.
- For large and giant tumors, cerebral angiography is performed to evaluate the venous anatomy precisely, as well as the vertebrobasilar circulation and the blood supply and vascularity of the tumor.
- Clival branches of the meningohypophyseal trunk are the most common arterial supply to these tumors.
- Additional blood supply may come from external carotid branches or from the vertebrobasilar circulation if pial invasion is present.[1]
- Angiography allows for embolization, which can greatly facilitate tumor removal by decreasing the blood supply, but some necrosis may occur that can soften the tumor. Aggressive small particle embolization should be used carefully because some tumor edema may occur that can acutely exacerbate brain stem compression in patients with larger or giant tumors with severe preexisting mass effect on the brain stem.
- Detailed angiographic delineation of the venous anatomy is crucial in planning the surgical strategy of large and giant tumors.
- Size and dominance of the transverse of sigmoid sinuses and collateralization through the torcular can affect the surgical approach by revealing a very large sigmoid or high-riding jugular bulb, either of which significantly affects the amount of exposure. Similarly, a small sigmoid with excellent collaterals affords more exposure with lesser consequences should sigmoid sinus occlusion occur.
- The configuration, relative sizes, and anastomotic relationships of the veins draining the temporal lobe are extremely important. In most patients, the veins of Labbé and Trolard and the superficial middle cerebral vein form an anastomotic relationship, with these veins being relatively equal in size.[1] In some patients, one or more of these veins may predominate and be correspondingly larger in size. The consequences of occluding a large or dominant vein must be factored into the surgical planning to protect them and avoid venous infarction.

Audiogram

- A baseline audiogram to evaluate preoperative hearing function is essential for surgical planning. Lack of useful hearing on the side of the tumor may simplify the approach.

Neurological Function

- Facial function and function of the lower cranial nerves (IX, X, XII) should be evaluated very carefully preoperatively because as this also influences choice of operative approach (e.g., facial weakness from complete mobilization of the facial nerve from a total petrosectomy is not a concern if there is no facial function on that side preoperatively).
- Patients with chronic paresis of cranial nerves IX and X are likely to have compensated for these deficits and will better tolerate complete paralysis of these nerves postoperatively.[1]

◆ Selection of Operative Approach

For the purposes of surgical planning, the clivus can be divided into three regions[1]:

Upper clivus: above the crossing point of the trigeminal nerve root over the clivus, including the dorsum sellae

Midclivus: from the trigeminal root inferiorly to the level of the glossopharyngeal nerve root

Lower clivus: from cranial nerve IX to the foramen magnum

Also for more detailed surgical planning, the petrous ridge is divided into two areas:

Medial area: area medial to the internal auditory canal (IAC)

Lateral area: area lateral or posterior to the IAC

The presigmoid petrosal approach is the one used for the majority of these tumors, but there are several important variations to this approach. The location, size, extension, vascular encasement, and prior surgery or radiation are major considerations in designing the optimal approach to be used.

◆ Variations of the Presigmoid Petrosal and Related Approaches

Retrolabyrinthine Petrosal (Presigmoid Petrosal without Labyrinthectomy)

This variation is indicated for small or medium-size laterally located tumors of the petrous ridge or midclivus **(Fig. 58–1)**. It is also useful for larger tumors of the lateral petrous ridge or cerebellopontine angle.

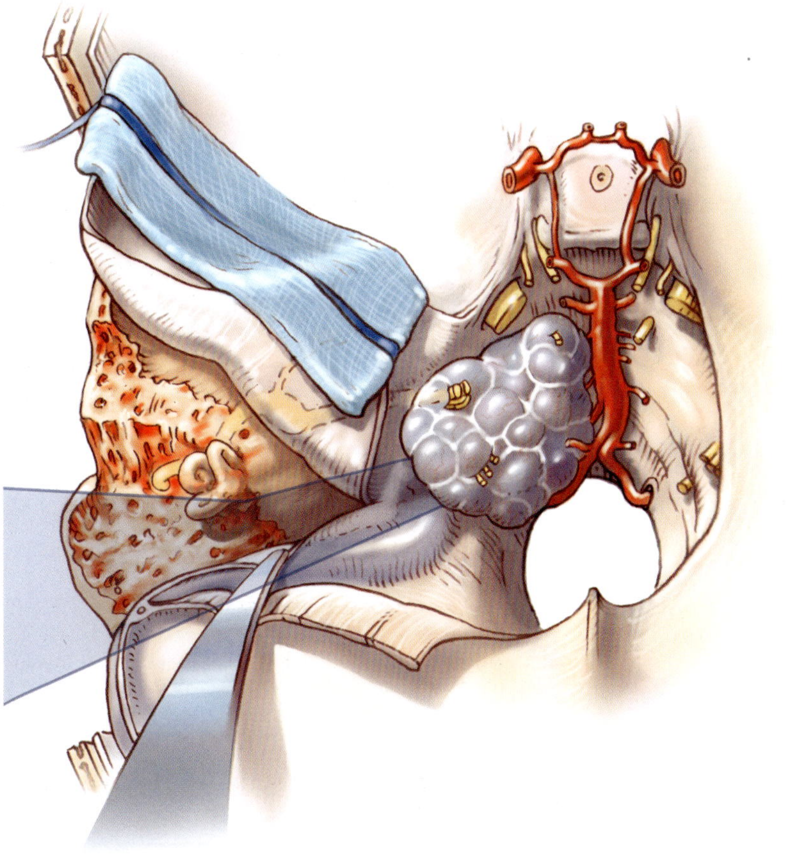

Figure 58–1 Superior view of a petroclival meningioma appropriate for a retrolabyrinthine petrosal approach. The shaded region represents the corridor of exposure provided by this approach.

Partial Labyrinthectomy Petrous Apicectomy Petrosal Approach

- Indicated for small or medium-size centrally placed tumors of the petrous ridge or midclivus in patients with useful ipsilateral hearing **(Fig. 58–2)**
- Especially useful for small centrally placed tumors that have not displaced the brain stem significantly because less room laterally en route to the mass has been created by the mass
- Also useful for some patients with previously untreated giant tumors encasing the vertebrobasilar complex. For large tumors such as those extending to the lower clivus, this approach can be combined with a retrosigmoid craniotomy.

Translabyrinthine Petrosal Approach

- Similar indications as for the partial labyrinthectomy petrous apicectomy but best used in patients with no hearing ipsilateral to the side of the approach
- Advantages are that it is simpler and quicker than the Partial labyrinthectomy petrous apicectomy (PLPA) approach and provides additional exposure, particularly to the IAC **(Fig. 58–3).**

Total Petrosectomy Petrosal Approach

- Indicated for giant-size tumors with prior surgery or radiation, bilateral extension, extensive vascular encasement, and/or if the brain stem is tilted away from the side with no useful hearing, and when more exposure is needed than with a translabyrinthine petrosal approach **(Fig. 58–4)**

Frontotemporal Orbitozygomatic Approach

- Indicated for tumor extension superior to the dorsum sellae toward the thalamic region or where there is encasement of the posterior communicating or posterior cerebral arteries **(Fig. 58–5).** For extension into these areas as well as below the upper clivus, a frontotemporal orbitozygometic (OZO) approach can be combined with a petrosal approach.

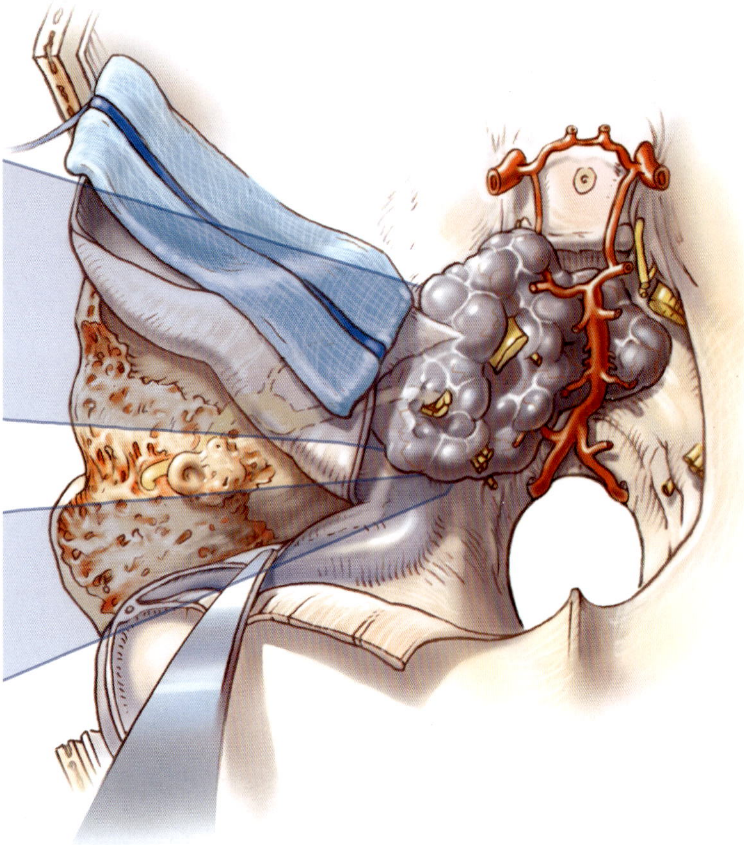

Figure 58–2 Superior view of a petroclival meningioma appropriate for a partial labyrinthectomy petrous apicectomy petrosal approach. The shaded region represents the corridor of exposure provided by this approach.

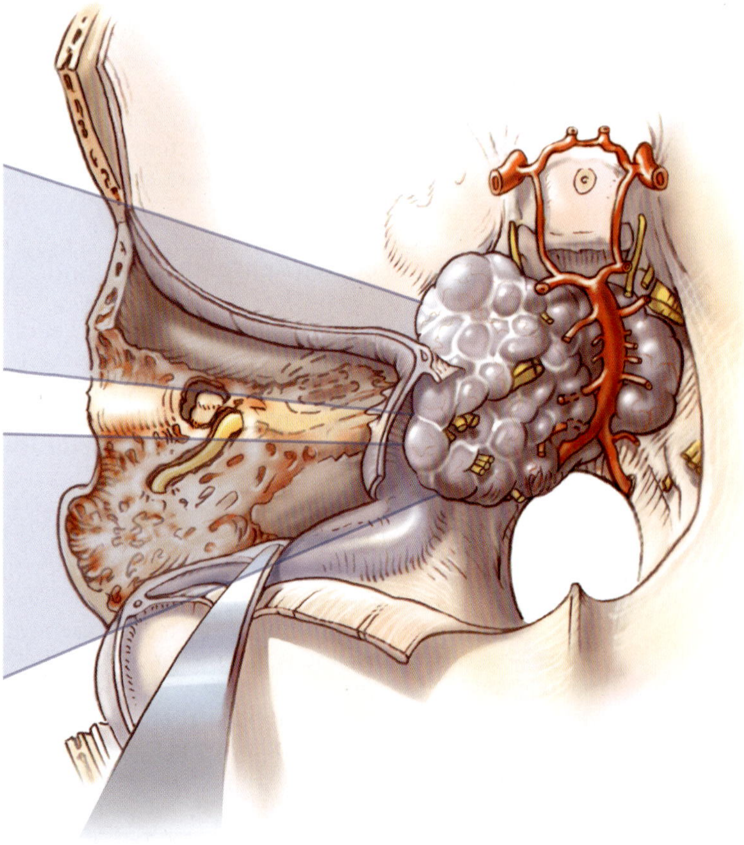

Figure 58–3 Superior view of a petroclival meningioma appropriate for a translabyrinthine petrosal approach. The shaded region represents the corridor of exposure provided by this approach.

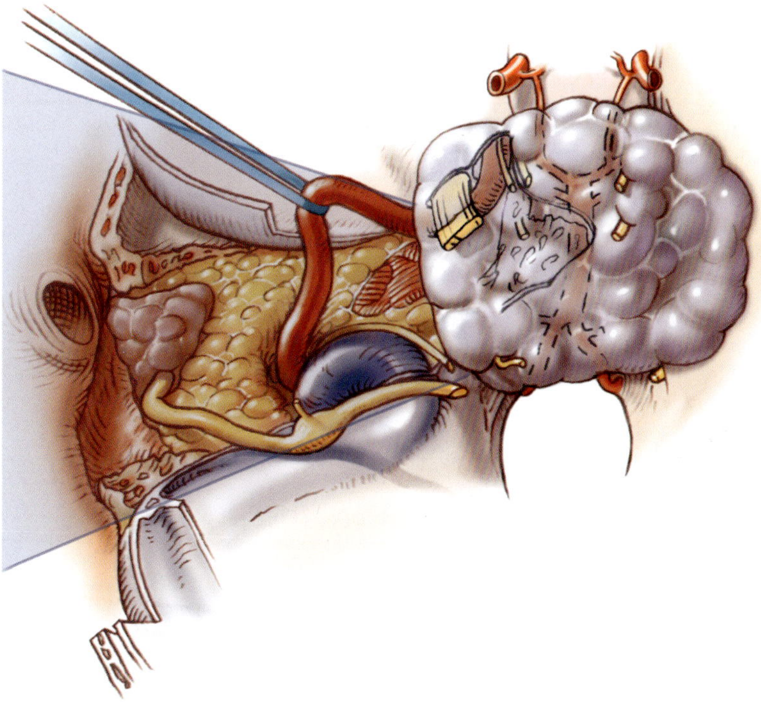

Figure 58–4 Superior view of a petroclival meningioma appropriate for a total petrosectomy approach. The shaded region represents the corridor of exposure provided by this approach.

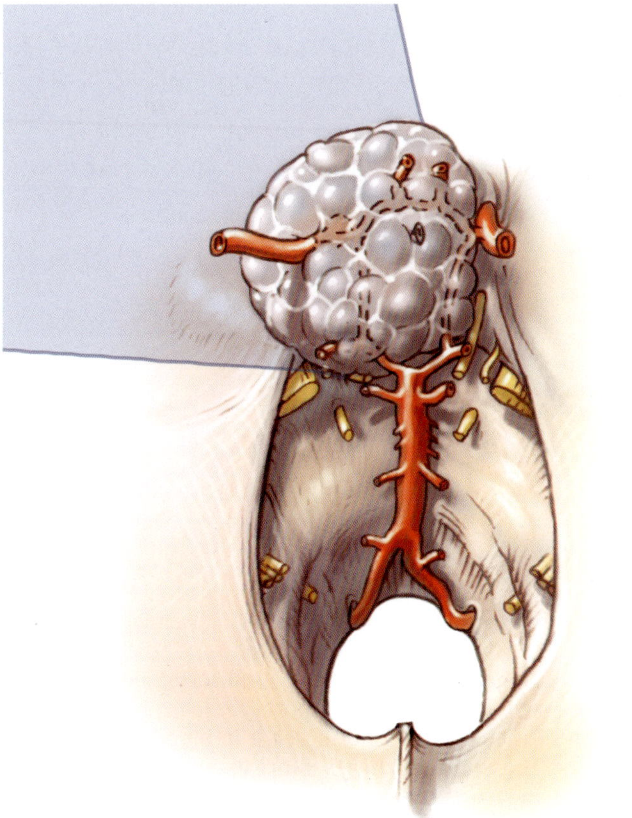

Figure 58–5 An upper clival meningioma appropriate for a frontotemporalorbiztoygomatic approach. The shaded region represents the corridor of exposure provided by this approach.

- In general, progressive dissection superior to the dorsum sellae requires progressively more temporal lobe retraction for a petrosal approach.
- The frontotemporal OZO transsylvian approach provides a much better view of this region with less temporal lobe retraction.

Extreme Lateral Transcondylar Approach

- Indicated for centrally located tumors of the lower clivus
- More laterally placed tumors of the lower clivus can be reached via an extreme lateral retrocondylar approach[2]
- For centrally located lower clival tumors extending to the midclivus or higher, an extreme lateral approach can be combined with a presigmoid petrosal approach.

Retrosigmoid Approach

- Can be used for laterally placed tumors of the petrous ridge or tumors predominantly in the cerebellopontine angle
- For tumors with some central extension, a retrolabyrinthine petrosal approach may be required. For giant tumors in this region, these two exposures can be combined. In general, large tumors extending inferior to cranial nerve IX, indicated for a petrosal approach, would require the addition of a retrosigmoid approach.
- If a patient has a very large sigmoid sinus or a high jugular bulb, a retrosigmoid or extreme lateral approach can also be added to provide the necessary exposure **(Table 58–1).**

Table 58–1 Selection of Approaches to Clival and Posterior Fossa Meningiomas

Tumor Location	Tumor Size	Special Features	Recommended Approach
Upper clivus	Small or medium	With or without middle fossa extension	Frontotemporal, OZO
Upper and midclivus (midline and paramedian)	Large	Extends ≤ 2 cm above dorsum sellae with useful ipsilateral hearing	PLPA petrosal translabyrinthine
		Extends 2 cm above dorsum sellae without useful ipsilateral hearing	Petrosal PLPA petrosal + frontotemporal, OZO
		Extends > 2 cm above dorsum sellae with useful ipsilateral hearing	Translabyrinthine
		Extends > 2 cm above dorsum sellae without useful ipsilateral hearing	Petrosal + frontotemporal, OZO
	Large or giant	Prior surgery or radiation Extensive vascular encasement No deviation of brain stem to opposite side	Total petrosectomy
Midclivus (midline and paramedian)	Small or medium	With useful ipsilateral hearing Without useful ipsilateral hearing	PLPA petrosal Translabyrinthine petrosal
Medial petrous ridge	Small or medium	With useful ipsilateral hearing Without useful ipsilateral hearing	PLPA petrosal Translabyrinthine petrosal
Lateral petrous ridge or cerebellopontine angle	Small or medium	Without useful ipsilateral hearing; with extensive IAC involvement	Retrosigmoid
	Large	Prior surgery or radiation	Retrosigmoid or retrolabyrinthine petrosal
	Giant	Extensive vascular encasement	Translabyrinthine petrosal; total petrosectomy
Mid- and lower clivus	Large	With useful ipsilateral hearing	PLPA petrosal + retrosigmoid
		Without useful ipsilateral hearing	Translabyrinthine petrosal + retrosigmoid
	Giant	Prior surgery or radiation Extensive vascular encasement No deviation of brain stem to opposite side	Total petrosectomy + retrosigmoid or extreme lateral Retrocondylar or transcondylar
Lower clivus (midline and paramedian	Small or medium		Extreme lateral transcondylar
Lower clivus (lateral)	Small or medium		Extreme lateral retrocondylar

IAC, internal auditory canal; OZO, orbitozygometic; PLPA, partial labyrinthectomy petrous apicecfomy.

◆ Surgical Technique

Anesthesia

Standard general endotracheal tube anesthesia is used but with the absence of muscular paralysis to allow for reliable cranial nerve monitoring. Mild to moderate hyperventilation ($PaCO_2$ = 30–35) is often used during the exposure and resection portions of the procedure to facilitate brain relaxation. Mannitol (0.5–1.0 g/kg) is usually administered just prior to the bone work and for optimal brain relaxation. If an adequate response is not obtained, IV furosemide (20–40 mg) can potentiate the effects of the mannitol.

For changes on intraoperative monitoring possibly indicating ischemia, usually temporary release or removal of brain retractors or a mild increase in blood pressure will reverse these abnormalities. More extensive cerebral protective measures are usually not needed unless there is vascular encasement or invasion by tumor requiring prolonged temporary clipping or vascular bypass. These additional measures include elevation of the blood pressure 20% above its normal range, mild to moderate hypothermia to

~34°C, mild hemodilution, and finally burst suppression on electroencephalogram (EEG), usually by the use of thiopental, etomidate, or propofol.[3]

Intraoperative Monitoring

Multimodality neurophysiological intraoperative monitoring including somatosensory evoked potentials, contralateral brain stem evoked responses, and ipsilateral facial nerve function are routinely utilized for these procedures.

Somatosensory Evoked Potentials

- Able to detect changes in cortical function due to ischemia or from temporal lobe or brain stem retraction[4]
- Upper and lower extremity somatosensory evoked potentials (SEPs) are usually monitored.
- Changes in SEP waveforms can be conveyed to the operative team to allow the surgeon to reduce brain retraction or the anesthesiologist to elevate the blood pressure.

Brain Stem Auditory Evoked Responses

- Used as an index of brain stem function
- Contralateral brain stem auditory evoked response (BAER) monitoring is most common.
- Waveform changes can also indicate ischemia or overly aggressive brain retraction and can be conveyed to the operative team so that appropriate measures can be taken.

Electroencephalogram

- Slowing is a sensitive indicator of ischemia.[5]
- Most useful in cases where induction of burst suppression is needed, such as during the performance of vascular bypasses or prolonged vascular temporary clipping.

Cranial Nerve Monitoring

- Ipsilateral facial nerve is routinely monitored for a petrosal approach.
- Lower cranial nerves (IX through XII) are monitored for very large tumors where involvement of these nerves is suspected.
- Cranial nerve V can be easily monitored as well, should trigeminal involvement be anticipated.
- Cranial nerves III, IV, and VI can be monitored by recording the electromyogram (EMG) from the extraocular muscles. These are found to be less helpful and electrode placement can be difficult, so these are generally not monitored.

Positioning

The patient is placed in the supine position with the head in pins. A large ipsilateral shoulder roll is used, and the head is turned ~70 degrees to the contralateral side with the neck laterally flexed to lower the vertex.[6] A component of the preoperative planning should include a check of neck mobility and potential head position. Preoperatively, the patient's head is turned 70 degrees away from the surgeon with a pillow under the ipsilateral shoulder. If the patient is comfortable with no headache, excessive venous compression or kinking of the arteries is unlikely to occur with this position intraoperatively. If the patient experiences significant discomfort in this position preoperatively, less head rotation may be required with an increased need for table rotation to compensate for this.

The patient is positioned with the shoulder approximately 2 inches off the superior end of the operating table. This enables the surgeon to sit under the patient's head with adequate room for the surgeon's knees. The surgeon sits posterior to the patient's ear for the majority of the procedure, but sitting at the head of the table may be needed to view the inferior and posterior medial structures.[1]

Head depression and elevation during the course of the procedure are usually performed with Trendelenburg or reverse Trendelenburg maneuvers. Flexion at the patient's hip can also be done, but this is usually avoided because flexion at the hip in a patient in pins can change the relationship of the head to the table, resulting in unwanted cervical traction.[7] Careful positioning with the patient firmly secured to the operating table with adequate tape and padding can allow for a significant about of rotational mobility about the patient's long access during the procedure.

When the patient is prepped and draped, the lateral thigh or lower abdomen should be included for possible autologous fat or fascial grafts needed during the reconstruction phase of the procedure.

Approach

The operative techniques discussed here focus on the petrosal approach and its variations. Detailed description of the frontotemporal approach with orbitozygomatic osteotomy is provided in the chapter on cavernous sinus tumors.

Incision and Initial Exposure

The skin incision and initial exposure differ depending on whether a presigmoid petrosal approach is performed alone or combined with a frontotemporal/orbitozygomatic approach. The incision for a standard petrosal approach is illustrated in **Fig. 58–6.** This C-shaped incision extends along the superior temporal line into the retroauricular region to join an upper cervical skin crease. The scalp including the pericranium is elevated, and the temporalis muscle is elevated and reflected anteriorly. A muscle-sparing exposure is performed with the sternocleidomastoid muscle reflected anteriorly with the skin, and the semispinalis capitis and splenius capitis muscles elevated and reflected posteriorly. This exposes the temporal, retrosigmoid, and mastoid areas, and the root of the zygoma **(Fig. 58–7).** The mastoidectomy and a very small retrosigmoid craniectomy are performed prior to the temporal craniotomy. This allows the surgeon to capitalize on the subtemporal dural and sigmoid sinus exposures from the mastoidectomy,

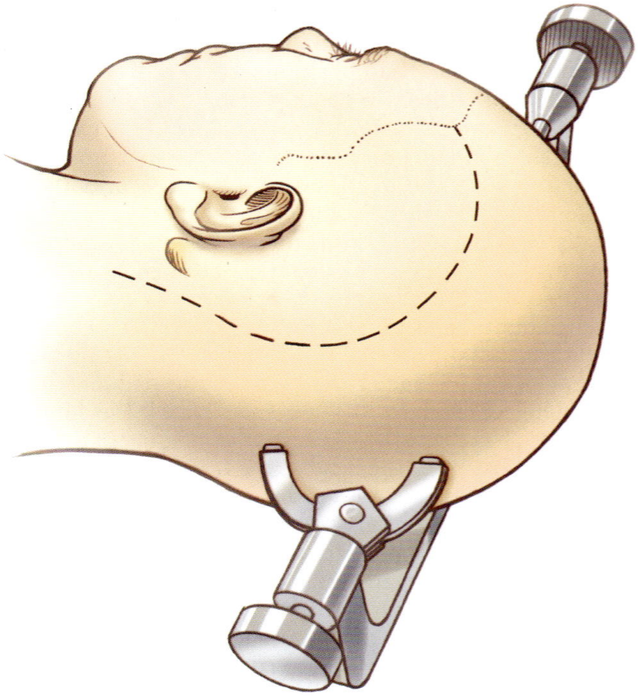

Figure 58–6 Incision for standard presigmoid petrosal approach.

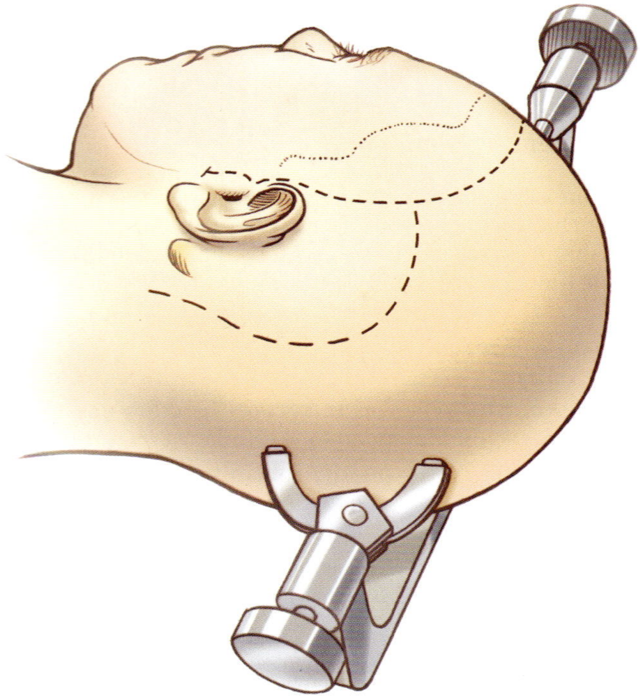

Figure 58–8 Incision for combined frontotemporal/orbitozygomatic/presigmoid petrosal approach.

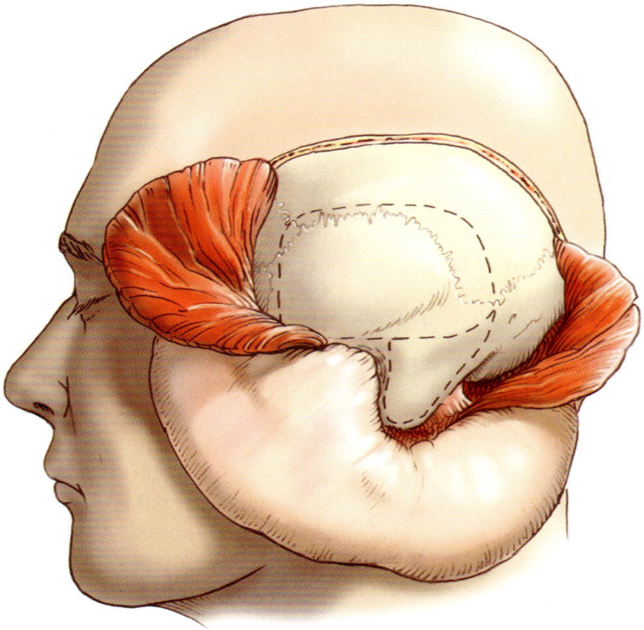

Figure 58–7 Location of planned temporal craniotomy and mastoidectomy with completed soft tissue dissection.

making the craniotomy safer and easier. The extent of the temporal craniotomy should be at least 1 cm anterior and posterior to the extent of the tumor, with the posterior extent extending at least 2 cm posterior to the sigmoid transverse junction to avoid obstruction of the view of the deep areas by bone.[1] The sigmoid sinus can be separated from the overlying bone under direct vision, and a small retrosigmoid craniotomy can be performed if needed. Once the craniotomy is completed, the temporal bone work is continued as a retrolabyrinthine, partial labyrinthectomy/petrous apicectomy, translabyrinthine, or total petrosectomy approach, depending on the exposure needed and any preoperative cranial nerve deficits.

If a combined frontotemporal/orbitozygomatic/petrosal approach is needed, the incision is made in a curved fashion from the midline hairline to the zygomatic root, and is bisected posteriorly by an incision following the posterior aspect of the superior temporal line that ends in an anterior cervical skin crease **(Fig. 58–8).** The soft tissues are elevated as above, including an interfascial dissection of the frontotemporal branch of the facial nerve as well as complete mobilization of the temporalis muscle. The mastoidectomy can be performed once the soft tissue work is completed, and then the frontotemporal craniotomy with an orbitozygomatic osteotomy (usually incorporating the condylar fossa) is done along with a retrosigmoid craniotomy, if needed. The temporal bone work is then completed depending on which variation of the petrosal approach is to be used.

Retrolabyrinthine Approach

A radical mastoidectomy is performed by the neuro-otologist, unroofing the sigmoid sinus, the superior, lateral, and posterior semicircular canals, the vestibular aqueduct, the jugular bulb, and the mastoid segment of the facial nerve. The facial nerve is left inside a thin shell of bone to prevent

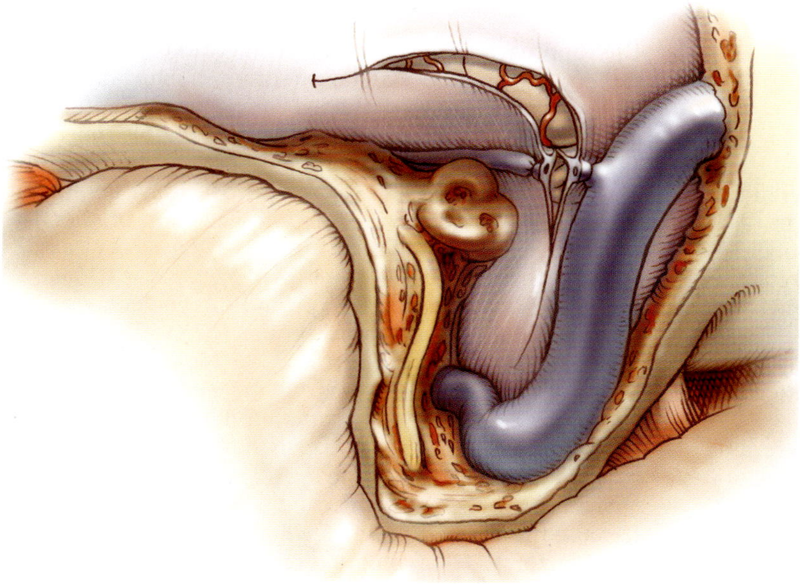

Figure 58–9 Lateral view of a retrolabyrinthine petrosal approach with bone work and initial dural incisions completed. The superior petrosal sinus has been ligated and divided, and the tentorium is being divided.

unnecessary facial nerve trauma. All of the bone of the sinodural angle is removed. Skeletonization of all of these structures maximizes the exposure of the presigmoid dura without removing or manipulating any normal structures within the temporal bone **(Fig. 58–9).** This exposure provides minimal risk of hearing loss or facial weakness but provides fairly limited presigmoid exposure.

Partial Labyrinthectomy/Petrous Apicectomy

The addition of a PLPA to a retrolabyrinthine petrosal approach preserves hearing in most patients while providing better exposure. A radical mastoidectomy is performed as described for the retrolabyrinthine approach. The bone of the superior and posterior semicircular canals is thinned until nearly transparent, and four fenestrations is made: two adjacent to the ampullae, and two adjacent to the common crus.[6] Once open, the semicircular canals are rapidly occluded with bone wax to prevent the loss of endolymphatic fluid and subsequent hearing loss. The remaining bony and membranous portions of the semicircular canals are then removed **(Fig. 58–10).**

The partial labyrinthectomy facilitates the petrous apicectomy, which is the next step. The bone resected by the petrous apicectomy is superior to a line drawn between the ampulla of the superior semicircular canal and the

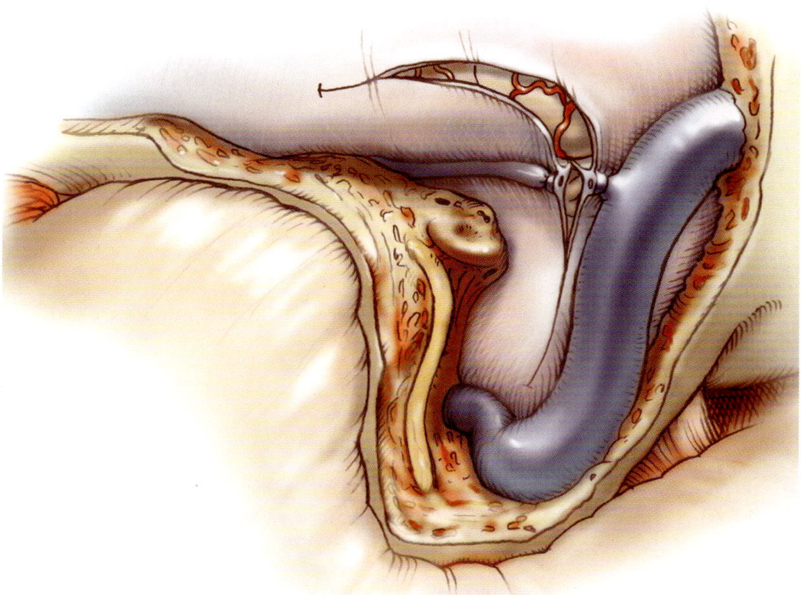

Figure 58–10 Lateral view of a partial labyrinthectomy petrous apicectomy petrosal approach with bone work and initial dural incisions completed. The superior petrosal sinus has been ligated and divided, and the tentorium is being divided.

entrance of the vestibular aqueduct into the petrous dura.[6] The superior wall of the internal auditory canal is skeletonized during the removal of the petrous apex.

Translabyrinthine Approach

When hearing preservation is not an issue, a translabyrinthine petrosal approach can provide additional exposure in cases where a total petrosectomy is not needed. If the patient has no useful hearing on the side of the approach preoperatively, a translabyrinthine approach is easier and quicker to perform than a PLPA approach. If the petrous apex is removed after the labyrinthectomy, a translabyrinthine approach provides more exposure than a PLPA approach, particularly to the IAC.

A radical mastoidectomy is performed as described above, with complete removal of the bone in the sinodural angle. The lateral, posterior, and superior semicircular canals are removed and the vestibule is opened. The facial nerve is skeletonized from the genu inferiorly to near the stylomastoid foramen, leaving a thin shell of bone protecting it. After the labyrinthine bone has been removed to the level of the vestibule, the bone of the IAC is dissected and removed **(Fig. 58–11).** The petrous apicectomy can be performed as described above. When completed, the translabyrinthine exposure is limited posteriorly by the sigmoid sinus, superiorly by the tegmen dura, anteriorly by the facial nerve, and inferiorly by the jugular bulb. When combined with the temporal craniotomy and opening of the tentorium, the full translabyrinthine petrosal approach provides excellent exposure to the petroclival region and can be efficiently performed with low facial nerve morbidity.

Total Petrosectomy

This approach is reserved for giant tumors with prior surgery or radiation, bilateral extension, or extensive vascular encasement due to the added complexity and associated morbidity of this exposure. Due to the lengthy, time-consuming dissection involved in this approach, the operation is usually staged with the total petrosectomy being performed on one day, and the tumor resection on another. The time between the stages varies from 1 day to 1 week depending on the needs of the patient.

The incision and initial exposure are the same as the other petrosal approaches, except that the external auditory canal is transected and oversewn.[8] The temporomandibular joint capsule is dissected free from the glenoid fossa. A radical mastoidectomy and a complete labyrinthectomy are performed, and the facial nerve is exposed from the stylomastoid foramen through the IAC.

The temporal craniotomy can be performed at this time because the added exposure facilitates the remainder of the petrosectomy. The temporal craniotomy is similar to the other petrosal approaches except that it extends further anteriorly to near the sphenoid wing. A zygomatic osteotomy including the condylar fossa is performed to facilitate the exposure of the vertical portion of the petrous carotid artery. For additional exposure, the condyle and neck of the mandible are occasionally resected.[8] The greater superficial petrosal nerve and middle meningeal artery are identified and sectioned. The cartilaginous eustachian tube is exposed, packed with autologous fat, and sutured closed.[8] The petrous carotid artery is completely unroofed from the proximal cavernous portion to the upper cervical segment, elevating the periosteal sheath of the carotid canal with the carotid artery.[8] The fibrocartilaginous ring surrounding the

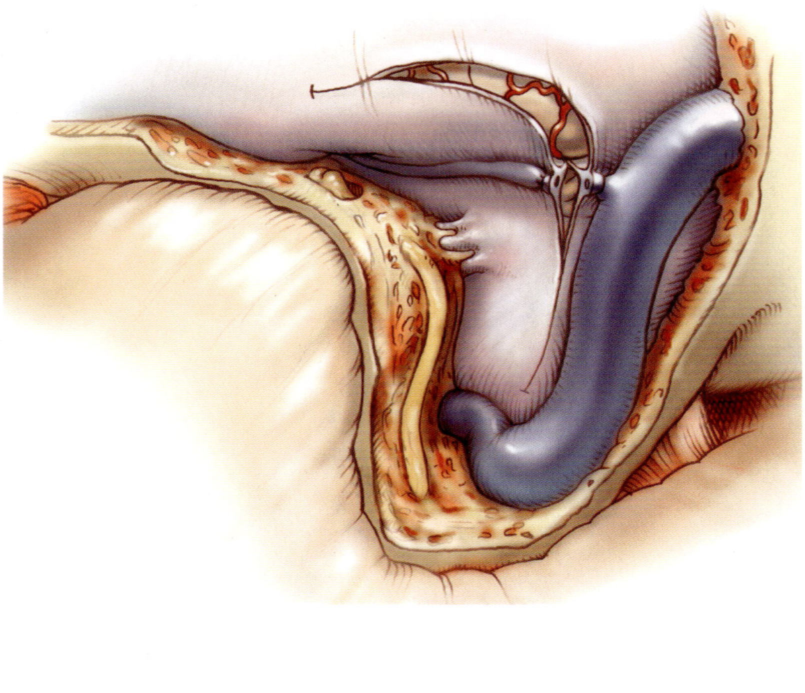

Figure 58–11 Lateral view of a translabyrinthine petrosal approach with bone work and initial dural incisions completed. The superior petrosal sinus has been ligated and divided, and the tentorium is being divided.

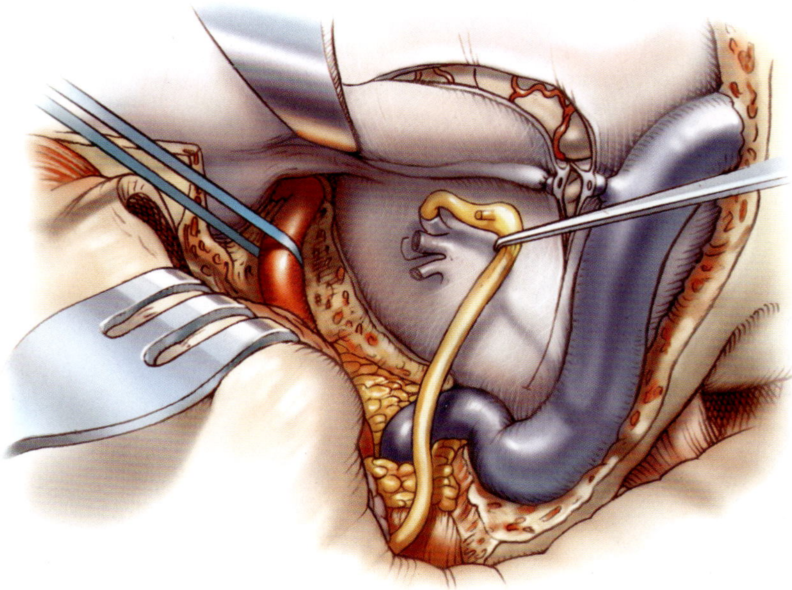

Figure 58–12 Lateral view of a total petrosectomy approach with bone work and initial dural incisions completed. The superior petrosal sinus has been ligated and divided, and the tentorium is being divided.

cervical carotid at its entrance into the skull base is divided, and the internal carotid artery (ICA) is mobilized anteriorly.[5] A detailed discussion of the condylar fossa osteotomy and exposure of the petrous carotid artery is in the chapter on cavernous sinus tumors.

The neuro-otologist is now able to work subtemporally to remove the cochlea and bone medial to the mastoid segment of the facial nerve.[8] The jugular foramen and its associated structures are skeletonized, all bone remaining in contact with the facial nerve is removed, and the facial nerve is mobilized posteriorly.[1,8]

The facial nerve has three important sources of blood supply: the anterior inferior cerebellar artery (AICA) provides branches to the proximal segment, the midsegment is supplied by the petrosal artery that accompanies the greater superficial petrosal nerve (GSPN), and the distal segment is supplied by the stylomastoid artery.[1] The petrosal artery is cut along with the GSPN, but careful preservation of the remaining blood supply to the facial nerve with minimal mechanical trauma during the exposure and tumor resection can result in minimal loss of facial function.[1,8] For this reason, exposure and mobilization of the facial nerve constitute one of the most important, meticulous, and time-consuming aspects of the procedure.

Once the petrous carotid artery and facial nerve have been mobilized, the medial petrous apex and lateral clivus can be resected **(Fig. 58–12).** For a staged procedure, the first stage is usually ended here because the next step is the dural opening followed by the tumor resection. If the procedure is to be staged, the facial nerve is usually covered with Gelfilm, autologous fat is placed over the petrosectomy defect, and the incision is closed in layers after the craniotomy flaps are plated into their original positions. The Gelfilm prevents scar or adhesion formation over the facial nerve or dura in the event the second stage is delayed for any reason.

Dural Opening and Division of the Tentorium

Once the extradural exposure has been completed for any of the presigmoid petrosal approaches, the dura is opened first in the presigmoid region. The incision is begun caudally just anterior and parallel to the sigmoid sinus and superior to the jugular bulb. After only a small dural incision in this region, the basal cisterns are opened and large amounts of cerebrospinal fluid (CSF) are drained to provide considerable brain relaxation and facilitate the remainder of the dural opening. This presigmoid dural incision is then continued just anterior and parallel to the sigmoid sinus until the edge of the posterior aspect of the superior petrosal sinus is reached. The temporal dura is then opened horizontally and low over the inferior temporal gyrus to end at the edge of the superior petrosal sinus just across from the presigmoid dural incision. Care must be taken to avoid damaging the vein of Labbé when opening the posterior temporal dura. Relaxing the brain with CSF drainage and beginning the temporal dural incision anteriorly allows for direct visualization of the vein. Noting its size and location on preoperative angiography is extremely helpful in avoiding vein of Labbé injury. For an anteriorly placed vein of Labbé, the tentorium may need to be divided more anteriorly so that the tentorium can be retracted along with the temporal lobe to avoid excessive stretch on the vein of Labbé.

Once the two dural incisions meet at the edges of the superior petrosal sinus (SPS), the SPS is suture ligated anterior and posterior to this point and subsequently divided, joining the presigmoid and temporal dural incisions. The tentorium is then carefully divided toward its midpoint. The fourth nerve and the superior cerebellar artery are identified and separated from the tentorium for their protection **(Figs. 58–13** and **58–14).** If the tentorium is divided too far anteriorly, these structures, particularly the fourth nerve, may be cut because it may have entered the tentorial edge by this point en route to the cavernous sinus.

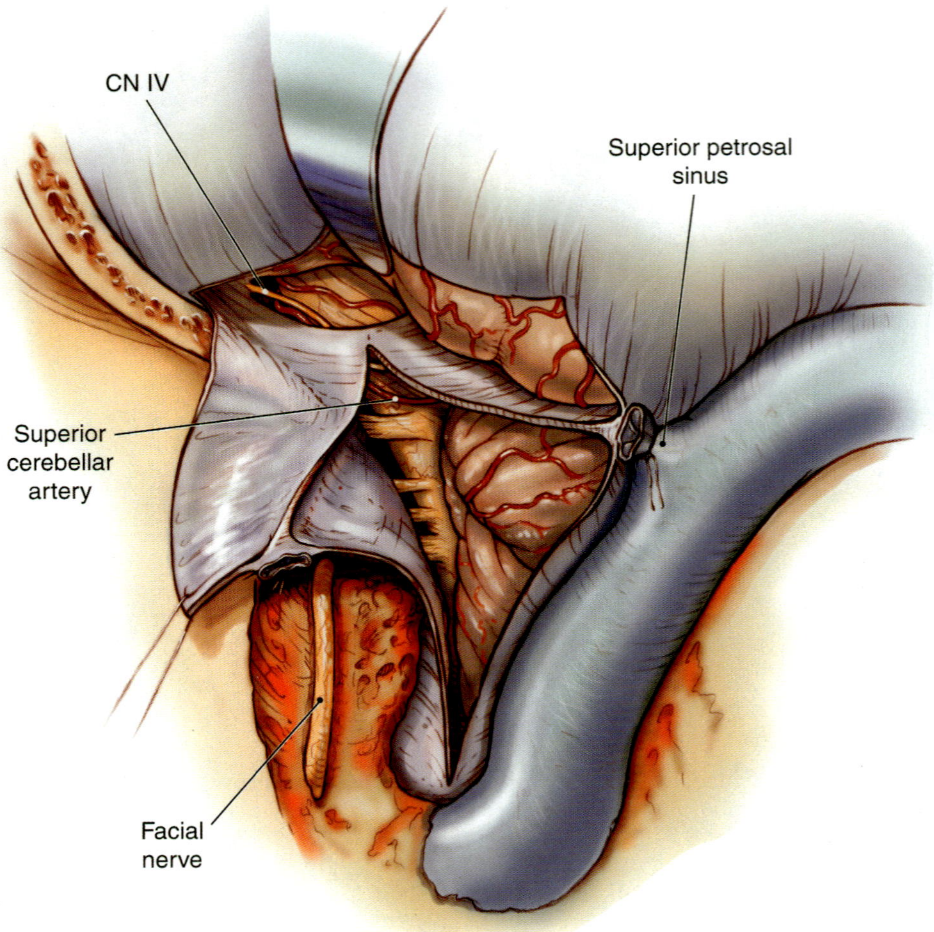

Figure 58–13 Surgical view of the tentorial incision during a presigmoid petrosal approach. The superior petrosal sinus has been ligated and divided. Care is taken to protect the fourth nerve and the superior cerebellar artery.

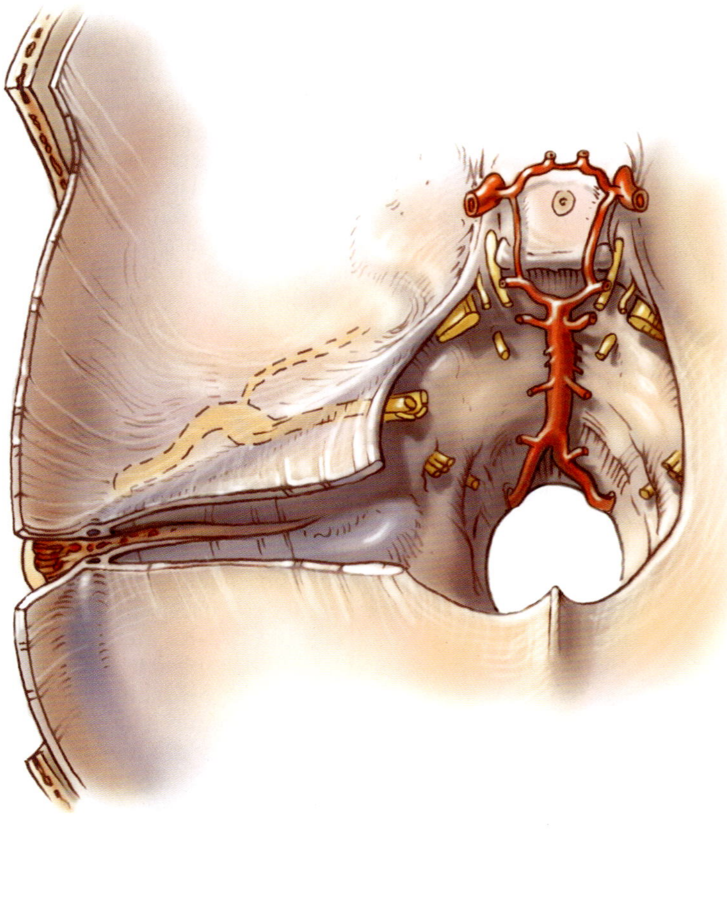

Figure 58–14 Superior view of the dural and tentorial incisions for a presigmoid petrosal approach.

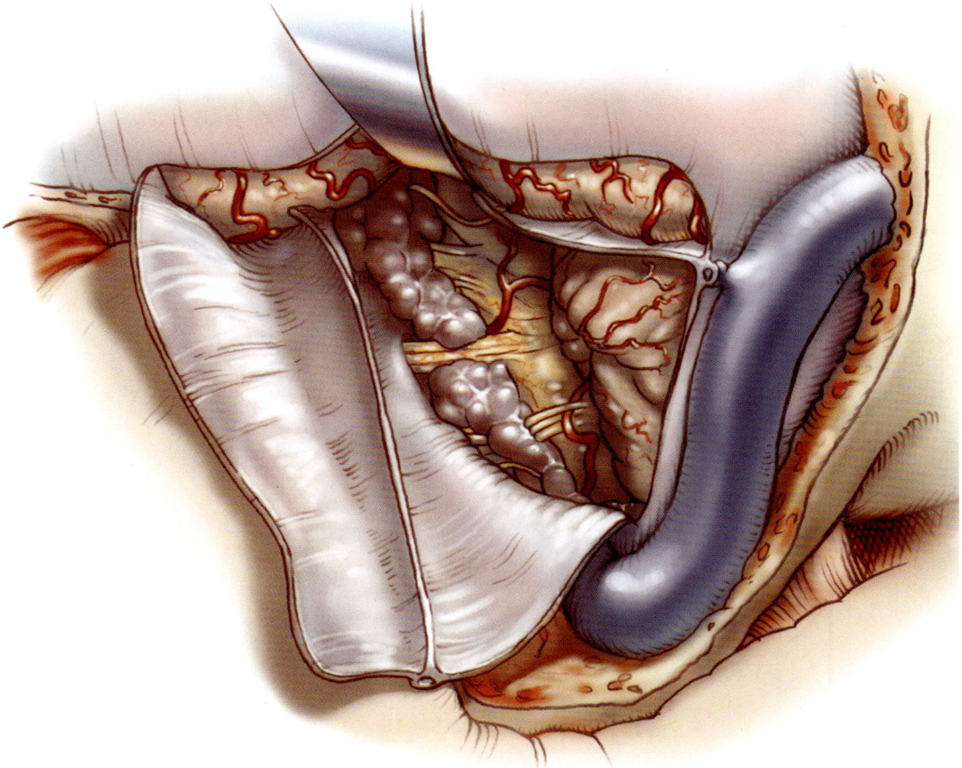

Figure 58–15 Surgical view afforded to a petroclival meningioma and the brain stem by a presigmoid petrosal approach.

Sutures are placed in the dural edges for purposes of retraction, and the temporal dura is retracted inferiorly with the presigmoid dural edge retracted anteriorly over the residual temporal bone to maximize the exposure obtained from the extensive bone work **(Fig. 58–15).**

Tumor Resection

The complex intradural steps involved in the resection of petroclival meningiomas should be followed systematically to minimize cranial nerve, vascular, or brain stem injury:

- The petrosal veins are cauterized and divided.
- Meckel's cave is opened widely to mobilize and visualize the trigeminal root. The entrance to Meckel's cave can be delineated by passing a blunt nerve hook along the trigeminal root.[1] The superior petrosal sinus along the roof of Meckel's cave can be ligated with titanium hemoclips and divided for a wider opening of Meckel's cave.[1]
- The arachnoid is opened between cranial nerves III and IV, IV and V, and V and VIII.[1]
- Tumor debulking begins between cranial nerves IV and V and between cranial nerves V and VIII to minimize manipulation of the VII–VIII nerve complex.[1]
- Tumor debulking then proceeds toward the base and inferior pole of the tumor to identify the sixth nerve proximal to its encasement by tumor.[1] The sixth nerve is then dissected free from tumor from proximally to distally. During this process, the tumor is progressively disconnected from the petroclival dura using bipolar electrocautery and microscissors. This devascularizes the tumor facilitating the remainder of the resection.
- The remainder of cranial nerves III through XII are dissected free as the tumor is intermittently further debulked.
- The basilar artery is dissected free from tumor by following it from a normal to an abnormal area and from the branches to the main trunk. When the basilar artery is totally encased, the anterior surface is dissected first because it is free of branches.[8] If the basilar artery, its branches, or its perforators are invaded or are unable to be dissected free from tumor, some tumor remnants may have to be left behind.
- Tumor dissection from the brain stem is the last and most important step. The arachnoid plane and the brain stem veins must be preserved as much as possible. If there is tumor invasion of the arachnoid plane, some tumor capsule may have to be left adherent to the brain stem to prevent postoperative hemiparesis or other significant brain stem morbidity.[1]
- Resection of the intradural portion of the tumor is completed prior to any extradural tumor extensions. The cavernous sinus can be opened from a posterolateral direction by following the course of the tumor into the cavernous sinus. Extensive cavernous sinus invasion or

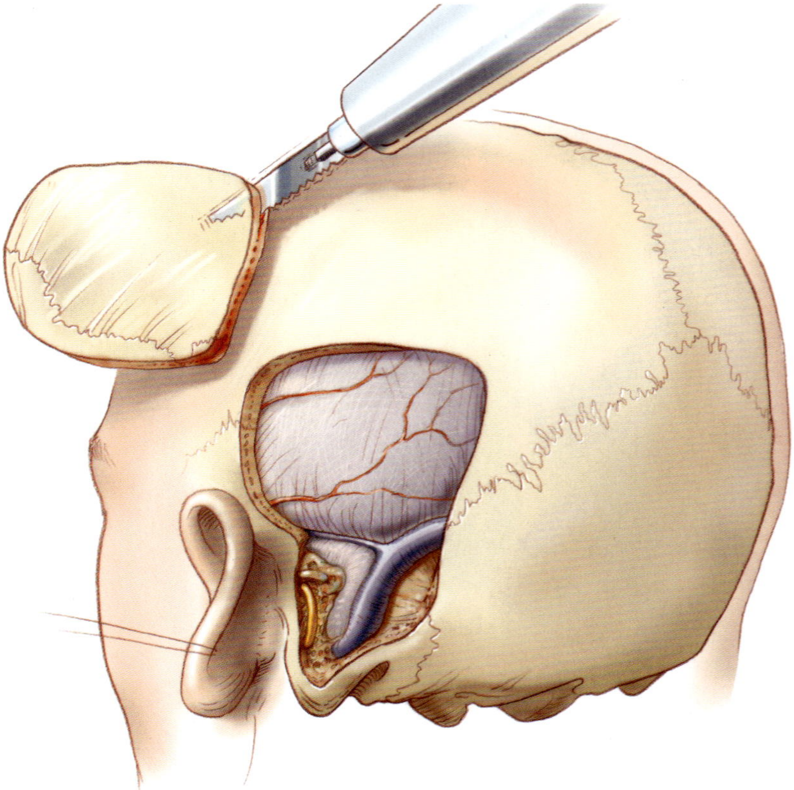

Figure 58–16 The temporal craniotomy flap is split with a reciprocating saw to provide a split calvarial reconstruction of the mastoidectomy defect.

extension of tumor high into the tentorial notch may require a frontotemporal OZO approach combined with this procedure or as an additional stage. Details of tumor resection from the cavernous sinus are present in the chapter on cavernous sinus tumors.

Closure and Reconstruction

Once the resection is completed, a primary dural closure is extremely difficult. A dural graft of autologous pericranium or fascia lata can be used to close the dural defect with circumferential suturing around the defect. The presigmoid dura and residual temporal bone are covered with an autologous fat graft after the eustachian tube and middle ear are packed with rolls of Surgicel. For a total petrosectomy, the large defect is also obliterated with a large autologous fat graft. The entire construct is reinforced with fibrin sealant. The bone flaps are split to perform a split calvarial reconstruction of the mastoid **(Fig. 58–16).** Details of this reconstruction are provided in the cranial nerve and cranial base reconstruction chapter. All of the bone flaps including the split calvarial grafts are secured with titanium miniplates **(Fig. 58–17).** Alternatively, reconstruction can be performed with titanium mesh and hydroxyapatite cement in addition to autologous fat graft. The temporalis muscle and retroauricular musculature are sutured to

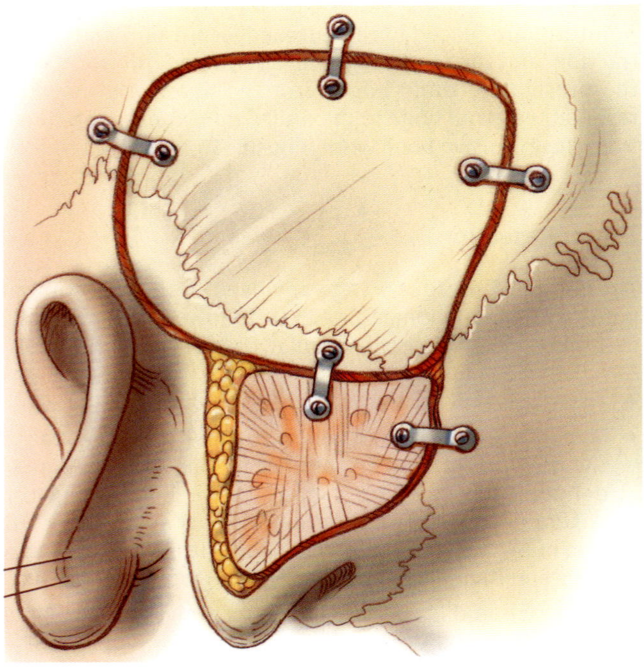

Figure 58–17 Completed bony reconstruction after a presigmoid petrosal approach. Note the split calvarial graft covering the mastoidectomy defect.

small holes in the bone along their lines of insertion. The usual two-layer scalp closure is then performed.

◆ Complications

Ischemic strokes may occur either from injury to the basilar artery, its branches, or its perforators, or from damage to the posterior communicating arteries or their perforators. Temporal lobe venous infarction may occur from damage to the vein of Labbé whose size, location, and configuration must be considered in all stages of the procedure. Injury to the brain stem with its associated morbidity can occur if a sufficient number of the veins of the brain stem are not preserved when the tumor capsule is dissected from the pial surface of the brain stem.

Any arterial injuries should be repaired with temporary clipping and microsutures. In patients with prior surgery, radiation, or invasion of tumor into vessel walls, developing a plane between the tumor capsule and adjacent arteries may be impossible. In these cases, some tumor may have to be left adherent to these structures to avoid major ischemic complications.

Cerebrospinal Fluid Leak

Meticulous reconstruction is the best prevention for postoperative CSF leak. This involves a multilayered closure including autologous fat graft and fibrin sealant as described above. Packing the middle ear and eustachian tube with Surgicel in a PLPA or translabyrinthine petrosal approach, or packing the eustachian tube with fat and oversewing it in a total petrosectomy, is the best method of preventing CSF rhinorrhea.

Should postoperative CSF rhinorrhea occur, it is initially treated with 3 to 5 days of lumbar drainage. If the leak is refractory to adequate lumbar drainage, the wound is reexplored and the reconstruction is augmented. A free flap reconstruction is sometimes required for a large defect with a refractory leak.

Cranial Nerve Injuries

The best way to avoid cranial nerve injuries is to recognize the anatomy and preserve the vascularity as much as possible. If a nerve is damaged, repair by primary reanastomosis or interposition graft is recommended. A detailed description of cranial nerve reconstruction can be found in the cranial nerve and cranial base reconstruction chapter. Postoperative diplopia can be managed with temporary eye patching, botulinum toxin injection, or with strabismus surgery if the deficit persists longer than a year or if it is expected to be permanent.[9] Close ophthalmologic follow-up is recommended for these patients.

Facial nerve weakness is expected with a total petrosectomy due to its complete mobilization. Facial nerve weakness is also seen when there is significant IAC involvement with tumor or when significant dissection is required to free the facial nerve from tumor. If eye closure is a problem postoperatively, placement of a gold weight in the upper eyelid or lateral tarsorrhaphy can be performed to prevent ocular complications. If corneal anesthesia from fifth nerve dysfunction and facial weakness are present simultaneously, tarsorrhaphy is almost always performed to prevent corneal ulceration. Ophthalmologic consultation should be obtained should any redness of the eye occur.

Swallowing is carefully evaluated postoperatively prior to initiation of oral feeding. An ear, nose, and throat consultation is obtained early in cases of significant swallowing dysfunction to prevent aspiration problems. A low threshold is used for thyroplasty to improve coughing and swallowing early and obviate the need for tracheostomy.[1]

Brain Injury

Using contemporary cranial base approaches along with good brain relaxation and CSF drainage, brain injury from retraction should be minimal. If contusion does occur, it is most often present in the temporal lobe. These contusions should be monitored closely with postoperative imaging to ensure that an intracerebral hemorrhage does not develop. Rarely, reoperation to evacuate a parenchymal hemorrhage may be needed.

Brain stem injury may occur from ischemic injury or from violation of the pial surface of the brain stem during tumor resection. If the tumor has violated the pial surface, some tumor capsule is left adherent to the brain stem to prevent hemiparesis or coma that may result from brain stem injury.

◆ Conclusion

Petroclival meningiomas are surgical challenges even under the best of circumstances. A systematic, multidisciplinary approach to these tumors along with a thorough understanding of the operative approaches and their indications are essential for successful treatment with acceptable morbidity. Currently, the presigmoid petrosal approach and its variations provide the cornerstone for surgical management of these lesions. This chapter has presented only a framework of guidelines for this approach and its variations, and specific steps may have to be modified, added, or omitted depending on the specific pathology of each case.

References

1. Sekhar LN, Raso J, Schessel DA. The presigmoid petrosal approach. In: Sekhar LN, Oliveira ED, eds. Cranial Microsurgery: Approaches and Techniques. New York: Thieme; 1999:432–463
2. Salas E, Sekhar LN, Ziyal IM, Caputy AJ, Wright DC. Variations of the extreme-lateral craniocervical approach: anatomical study and clinical analysis of 69 patients. J Neurosurg 1999;90(Suppl 2):206–219
3. Lee DS, Peck M. Anesthetic considerations for cranial microsurgery. In: Sekhar LN, Oliveira ED, eds. Cranial Microsurgery: Approaches and Techniques. New York: Thieme; 1999:19–22
4. Vera PL. Intraoperative neurophysiological monitoring. In: Sekhar LN, Oliveira ED, eds. Cranial Microsurgery: Approaches and Techniques. New York: Thieme; 1999:23–30

5. Sclabassi RJ, Krieger DN, Weisz D, et al. Methods of neurophysiological monitoring during cranial base tumor resection. In: Sekhar LN, Janecka IP, eds. Surgery of Cranial Base Tumors. New York: Raven; 1993:83–98
6. Sekhar LN, Schessel DA, Bucor SD, Rasso JL, Wright DC. Partial labyrinthine petrous apicectomy approach to neoplastic and vascular lesions of the petroclival area. Neurosurgery 1999;44:537–552
7. Sekhar LN, Tzortzidis F, Bucor SD. Patient positioning for cranial microsurgery. In: Sekhar LN, Oliveira ED, eds. Cranial Microsurgery: Approaches and Techniques. New York: Thieme; 1999: 12–18
8. Cass SP, Sekhar LN, Pomeranz S, Hirsh BE, Snyderman CH. Excision of petroclival tumors by a total petrosectomy approach. Am J Otol 1994; 15:474–484
9. Sekhar LN, Wright DC. Tumors involving the cavernous sinus. In: Sekhar LN, Oliveira ED, eds. Cranial Microsurgery: Approaches and Techniques. New York: Thieme; 1999:207–230

59

Epidermoid and Dermoid Cysts

Albino Bricolo

Epidermoid and dermoid cysts are rare nonneoplastic congenital lesions, accounting for about 1% and 0.4% of all intracranial tumors, respectively. Compared with their minor epidemiological relevance, the disproportionate interest they receive is perhaps due to their aesthetic beauty, exemplified in Dandy's description of epidermoids as "the most beautiful tumor of the body." Epidermoids and dermoids are considered together due to their similar natural histories and their macroscopic appearance; thus differentiation often depends entirely on the microscopical findings of the cyst wall and its content. Both are derived from skin-forming epiblastic cells that have detached from their neighbors and have been included in the mesenchyme during the early stage of fetal life. The various locations (midline versus lateral, intradural versus extradural) may be explained by the inclusion at different stages of embryogenesis. The clinical presentation is typically late with respect to the tumors' volume, and their function is variable in the multiple sites they occupy. Prior to the advent of computed tomography (CT) and magnetic resonance imaging (MRI), these lesions were difficult to diagnose preoperatively, whereas today the diffusion of these imaging techniques has facilitated identification and diagnosis of asymptomatic or incidental epidermoids. Most of these surgical lesions may now be completely and safely removed using microsurgical techniques thus reducing morbidity and the possibility of recurrence.[1–3]

◆ Pathology

Epidermoid cysts, also described as cholesteatomas, have an irregular nodular capsular surface that has a striking mother-of-pearl sheen; thus the term *pearly tumor*[4] **(Fig. 59–1)**. Their thin and nearly transparent wall transmits the characteristic appearance of its content, which is creamy-white and glistening, the latter resulting from cholesterol crystals. Epidermoids consist of an inner lining of heavily keratinized, stratified, well-differentiated squamous epithelium supported by an outer collagenous layer.[5] The overwhelming bulk of its content consists of layered anucleate squames resulting from progressive desquamation and breakdown of keratin from the epithelium lining the cyst. The content, comprising also a variable amount of cholesterol crystals, may be described as waxy, crumbly, or flaky, with a greasy texture, sometimes forming concentric lamellae in an onion-like manner. The escape of cyst content into surrounding tissue may lead to a localized granulomatous inflammation in which foreign-body giant cells are prominent; a glial reaction may be produced when the cyst is adjacent to brain tissue.

Epidermoids are typically intradural in nature yet may also arise from the diploë or the petrous apex. They tend to occupy a lateral position in the neuraxis, and the sites of predilection are the cerebellopontine angle, where epidermoids represent the third most common tumor following acoustic neuroma and meningioma, the parasellar region, the petrous bone, the diploë, and the spinal canal.

Dermoid cysts are oval or round multilobular masses, well demarcated by a wall, usually thicker than epidermoids, and are essentially dermis with adnexal structures such as hair follicles, sebaceous glands, and fibroadipose tissue. Also the cyst content, more greasy than flaky, is usually thicker and buttery-yellow due to secretion of sebaceous material and epithelial desquamations. Hairs may be found mixed within the content.[5] Dermoids may be related externally to a dermal sinus overlying the lesion, especially in the spinal cord or the posterior fossa, and may be the pathway of pyogenic infections of the cysts.

Dermoid cysts have a greater tendency than epidermoids to occupy midline positions: the cerebellar vermis, cauda equina, scalp, orbit, and paranasal region.[6,7] Rupture often leads to the spread of inflammation into the neighboring tissues, the nature of which depends on the content. Dermoid cysts may also be associated with skeletal or cutaneous abnormalities.[8] These pealike subcutaneous swellings are usually noticed in childhood, lying in a depression in the skull and occurring along the lines of fusion of the facial processes and in the sagittal plane of the scalp.

Epidermoids and dermoids are so rare that their percentage of incidence cannot reasonably be assessed and their division into two distinct entities appears somewhat arbitrary. **Table 59–1** summarizes some differences between the two types of cysts. Although epidermoids and dermoids are benign lesions, rare transformation to squamous carcinoma has been reported for both.[9]

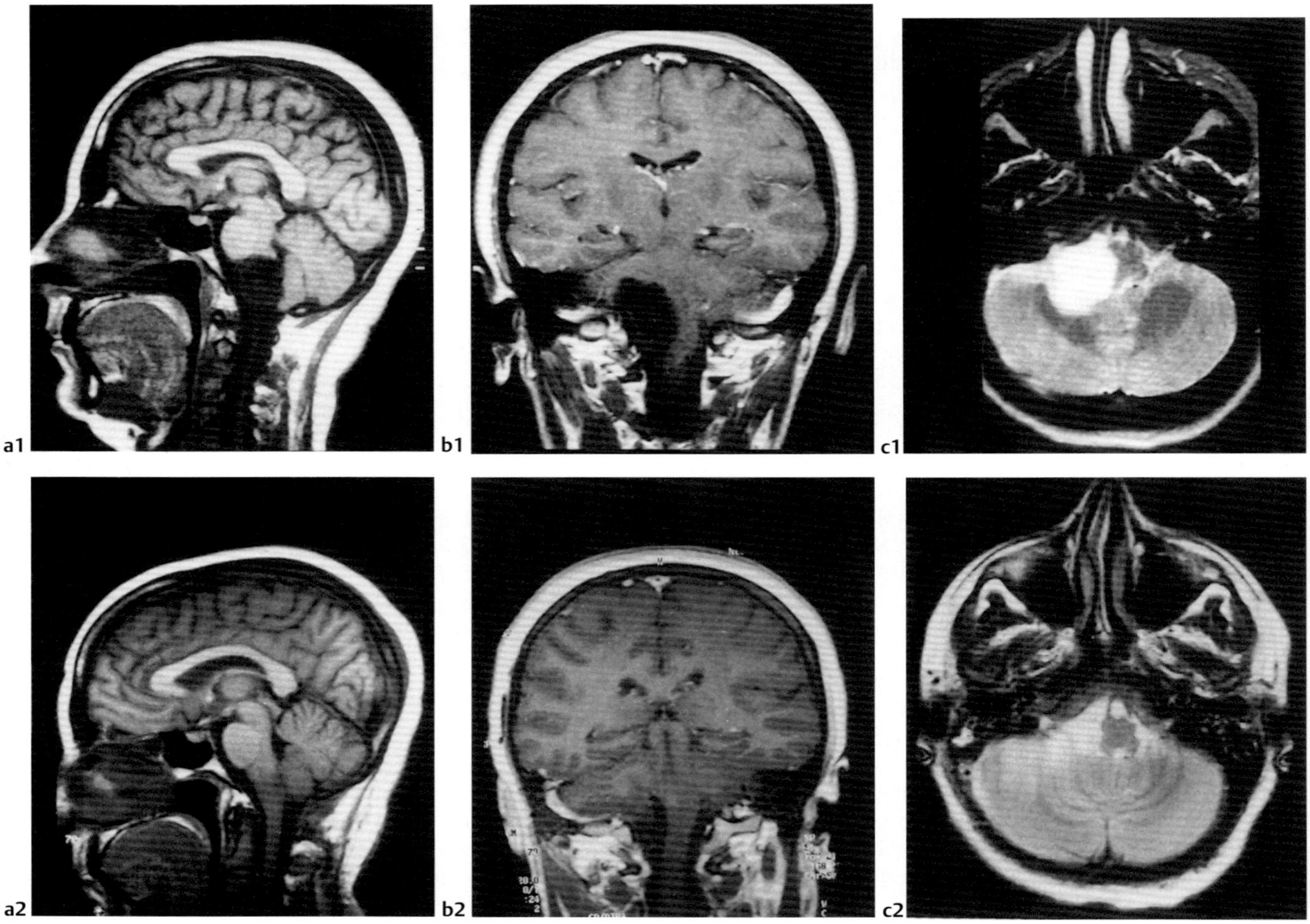

Figure 59–1 A 38-year-old woman presented long-standing swallowing disturbances associated with diplopia and positional vertigo. *Imaging:* (**a$_1$**) MR, magnetic resonance(1) unenhanced T1-weighted sagittal, (**b$_1$**) contrast-enhanced coronal, and (**c$_1$**) T2-weighted axial images showing a large epidermoid cyst at the level of the right cranial cervical junction. Comparable MR images (**a$_2$**, **b$_2$**, **c$_2$**) obtained 4 days after surgery demonstrating unexpected early reexpansion of the brain.

(Continued on page 713)

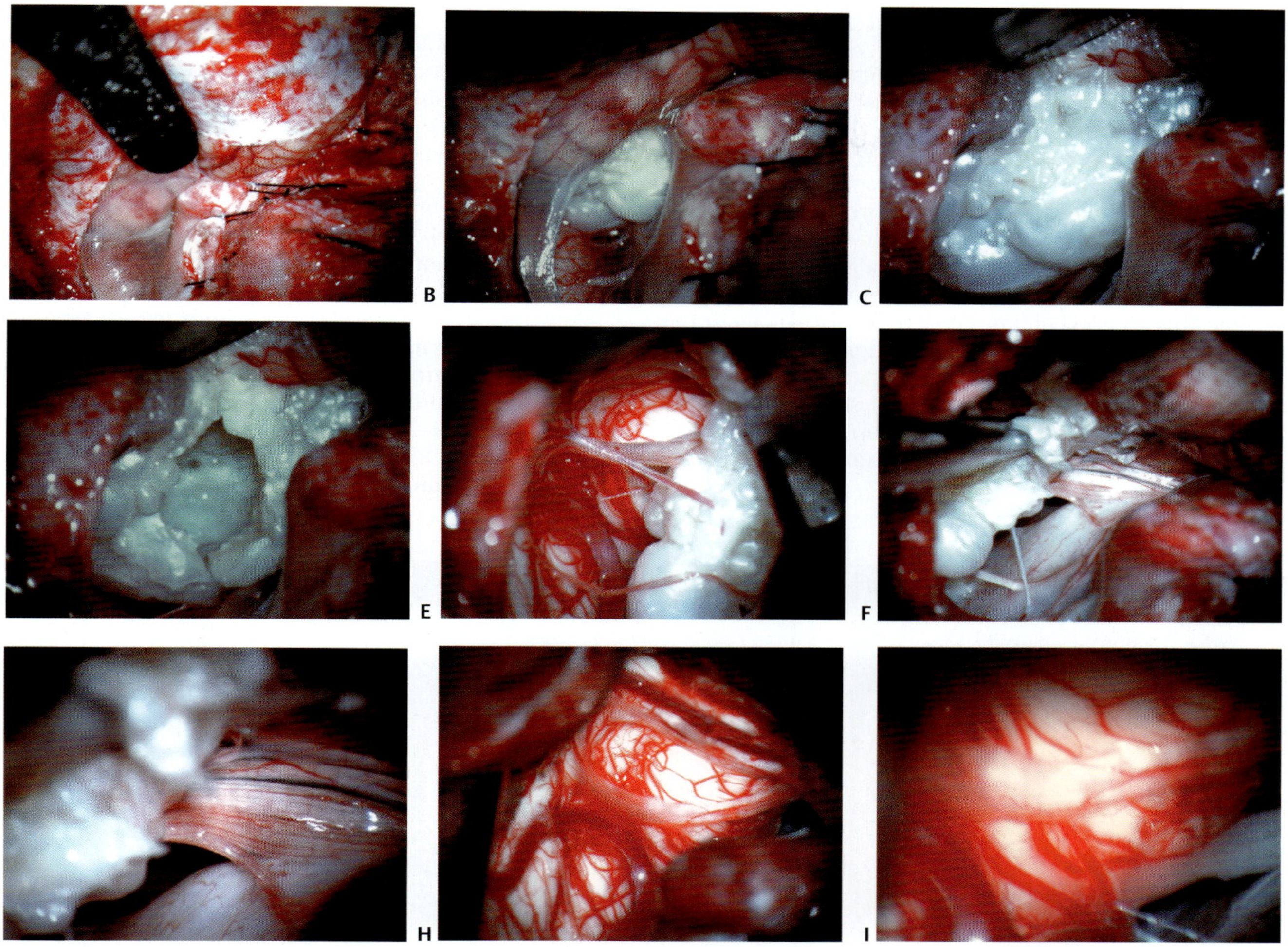

(*Continued*) **Figure 59–1** *Intraoperative views*: **(A)** Using a right dorsolateral approach with the patient in a semisitting position, the cranial cervical junction is exposed **(B,C)** at the opening of the cisterna magna, the pearly tumor protrudes under the cerebellar tonsil in the foramen magnum, **(D)** the tumor capsule is entered, and the flaky contents are removed by aspiration; **(E)** the capsule is gently detached from the cervicomedullary junction, posteroinferior cerebellar artery, and involved cranial nerves; **(F,G)** the firm adhesion of the capsule to cranial nerves IX and X entering the jugular foramen is noted; **(H,I)** at the end of tumor removal, the brain stem, the lower cranial nerves, VI, VII, and VIII, appear to be untouched. The postoperative course was uneventful, and the patient is well.

Table 59–1 Features of Epidermoid and Dermoid Cysts

	Epidermoid	Dermoid
Incidence	1%	0.4%
Sex	None	Male
Age	Third to fifth decades	Childhood
Lining	Keratinized squamous epithelium	Cutaneous-type epithelium with adnexal structure
Content	Keratinous debris, cholesterol	+ Hair and sebum
Preferred compartment	Cranium	Spinal canal
Location	Lateral	Midline
Connection	None	Dermal sinus tract
Meningitis	Chemical	Chemical and/or bacterial

◆ Rate and Pattern of Growth

Epidermoid growth occurs by the desquamation of normal cells in a cystic cavity, whereas in dermoids, enlargement is caused also by the secretion of dermal elements. Differing from true neoplasms, which grow by progressive cell division, the growth rate of these lesions is a linear progression comparable to the turnover time of normal skin.[10] Consequently, it has been calculated that a patient with a small fragment of residual tumor is at risk for a symptomatic recurrence due to the production of a lesion with the same volume after a period of time equal to the patient age at the time of resection plus 9 months,[10] suggesting that even near-total removal may result in cure for middle age or elderly patients.[3] Applying statistical analysis in a clinical setting, an increasing time-dependent recurrence-free survival rate was observed in patients with subtotal removal up to 65% at 13 years.[11]

In a landmark review, Lepoire and Pertuiset[12] offered an ingenious explanation regarding the seemingly haphazard anatomical distribution of the intradural tumors, considering that the epiblastic inclusions are carried to their final destinations by the developing network of cerebral arteries. Based on this hypothesis, the authors classified the location according to the major arterial territories: carotid (chiasmal and parasellar, frontal, supracallosal, and sylvian), vertebrobasilar (cerebellopontine angle, prepontine, cerebellar), and choroidal (intraventricular). These slow-growing histologically benign lesions present a unique capacity to flow across the basal surface of the brain into any available space dissecting along natural occurring planes,[13] and only in later stages of their growth do they behave as expanding lesions and surround and embed rather than displace the cranial nerves **(Fig. 59–2)**. Furthermore, due to their irregular shape, it is difficult to determine their exact size by measuring the maximum diameter; as a consequence, published

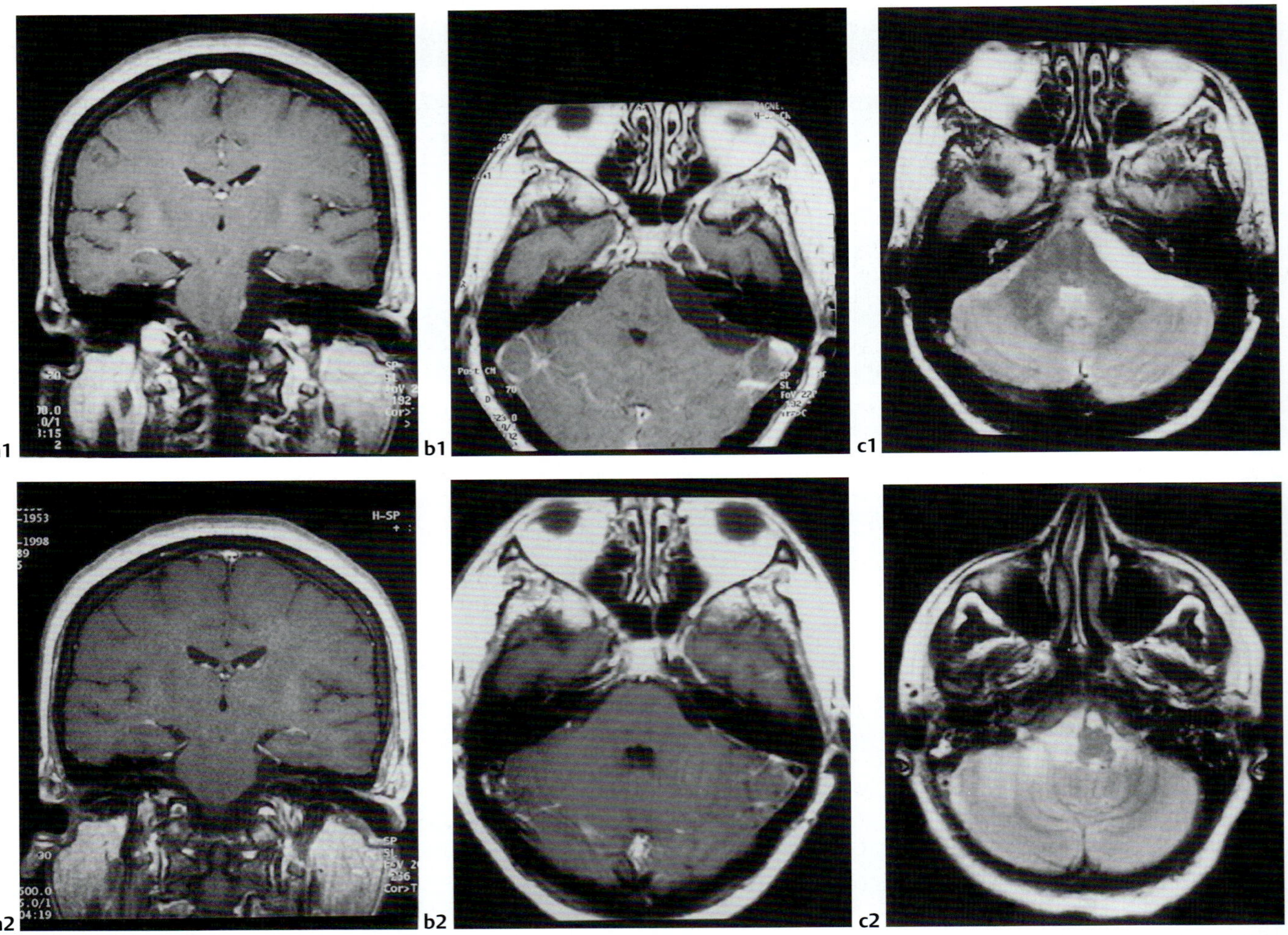

a1 b1 c1 a2 b2 c2

Figure 59–2 A 44-year-old woman presented with facial numbness and left-sided tinnitus. *Imaging:* **(a_1,b_1)** The coronal and axial T1-weighted contrast-enhanced and **(c_1)** axial T2-weighted scans show a left cerebellopontine angle (CPA) epidermoid cyst with transtentorial-subtemporal extension. Comparable magnetic resonance images **(a_2, b_2, c_2)** obtained 8 months after surgery demonstrate apparent complete removal of the tumor.

(Continued on page 715)

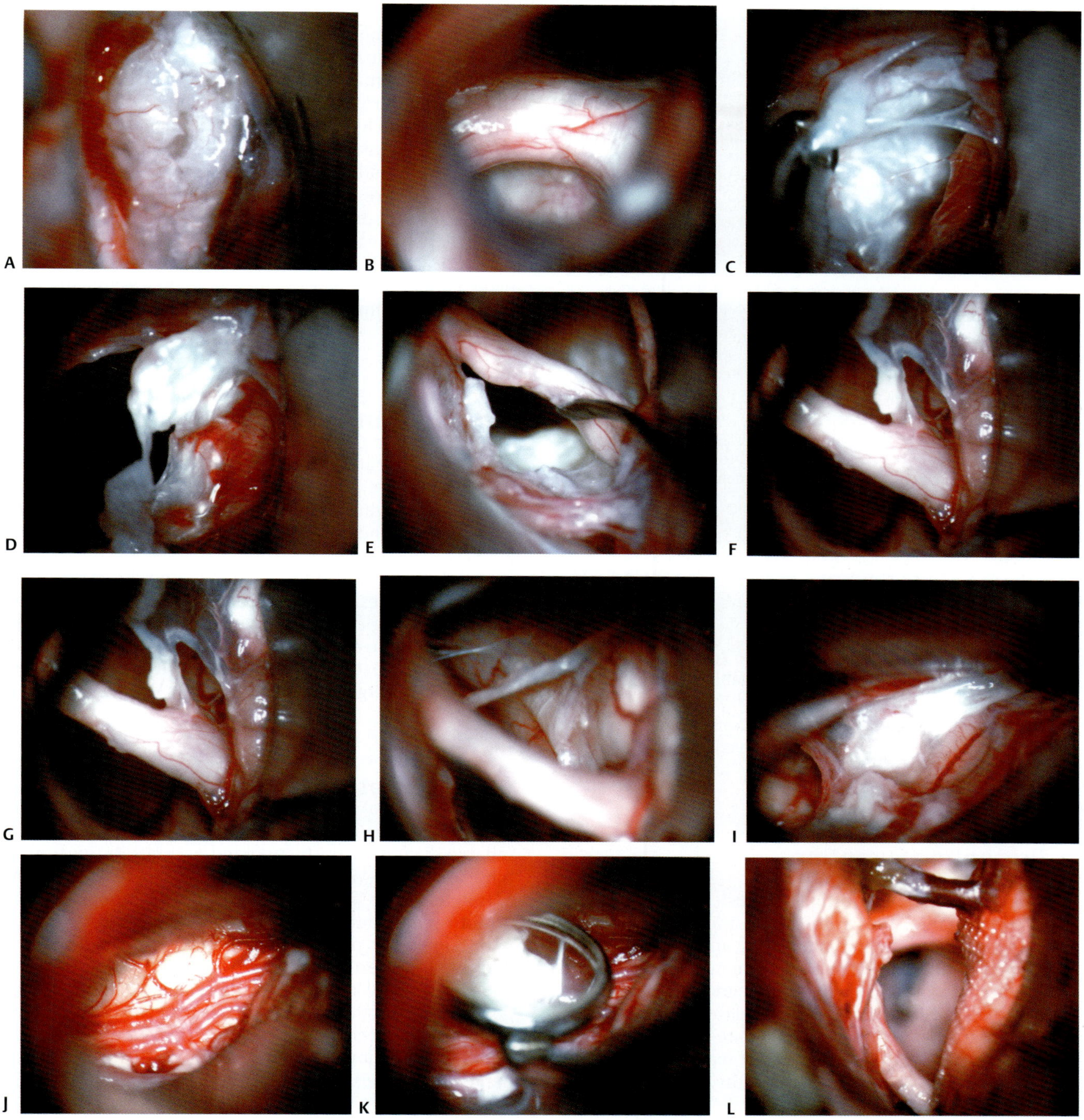

(*Continued*) **Figure 59–2** *Intraoperative views:* **(A)** Using a retrosigmoid approach with the patient in a semisitting position, the left CPA-situated tumor covering all the neurovascular structures is carefully debulked, exposing **(B)** the trigeminal nerve, which was completely engulfed as the other cranial nerves and arteries. **(C,D)** The capsule of the superior expansion of the tumor detached from the brain stem; **(E,F)** the VII and VIII cranial nerves and the lower cranial nerves are exposed and freed from the tumor; **(G,H)** a capsule remnant is detached from the pons; **(I)** the cerebellomesencephalic fissure at the tentorial incisure is filled by the tumor, and **(J)** cleaned; **(K)** the supratentorial extension of the tumor is removed with the help of a mirror; **(L)** the surgical field is seen at the end of removal. The postoperative course presented severe trigeminal and facial nerves dysfunction associated with ataxia. The patient is now neurologically well 1 year after surgery.

Table 59–2 Subgrouping Epidermoid Cysts by Primary Location and Extension

Primary Location	Extension
Cerebellopontine angle	None Foramen magnum Temporobasal/parasellar Mesencephalic/pineal
Petroclival	Cerebellopontine angle Suprasellar/chiasmatic Mesencephalic/pineal
Fourth ventricle	None Cerebellopontine angle Foramen magnum
Mesencephalic/pineal	Third ventricle Temporobasal Infratentorial
Parasellar/temporobasal	None Sylvian fissure Suprasellar/chiasmatic Anterosellar/frontobasal Cerebellopontine angle
Cerebral hemispheres	None Lateral ventricles

series are not comparable; thus these tumors are better classified by their primary site, presumably the largest, and their eventual secondary extension(s).[11,14] **Table 59–2** summarizes the various possible combinations of location and extension, which assists the surgeon in choosing the surgical strategy.

◆ Presenting Symptoms

Symptoms are often long-lasting and misleading; irritations rather than cranial nerve deficits, remittent symptoms including recurrent aseptic meningitis, and seizures unaccompanied by intracranial hypertension may mimic neurological disease and delay accurate diagnosis, resulting in one of the primary problems in effective treatment.

The slow growth of these lesions due to gradual accumulation of normal dividing cells and their tendency to insinuate along the subarachnoid cisterns at the base of the brain around the neurovascular structures, rather than compressing them, explain their clinical silence or indolence for many years.[15] These lesions often attain a large size prior to the onset of symptoms and signs typically regarded as the presenting symptoms of the disease, and as a result, the clinical findings may remain trivial for several years because they are rarely associated with intracranial hypertension. Furthermore, once the epidermoid has proliferated widely, the neurological picture may appear bizarre, thus making the clinical diagnosis obscure and even making the clinician suspect disseminated sclerosis or brain stem tumor; yet at diagnosis, they may present as any mass lesion in the same site. Suprasellar/chiasmatic lesions present visual acuity impairment and hemianoptic defects, sometimes associated with diabetes insipidus. Parasellar lesions are associated with seizures and trigeminal sensory loss, whereas retrosellar lesions are associated with trigeminal neuralgia or hemifacial spasm, ataxia, nystagmus, and hemiparesis. Cerebellopontine angle and petroclival cysts usually present trigeminal, facial, and auditory disturbances associated with lower cranial nerve palsies and ataxia. Hydrocephalus, even with tumors filling the aqueduct, curiously enough, is uncommon.

◆ Indications for Surgery

Surgery is indicated for symptomatic tumors and tumors with evidence of progressive growth. The optimal surgical treatment is radical removal of the tumor capsule at first operation, for the reason that leaving the capsule in place appears to guarantee recurrence.[14,16] However, the peculiar growth features along with the wide extension of the tumor and its firm adhesion to important neurovascular structures make total surgical removal not always possible or advisable.[2] There is no considered alternative therapy to surgery. Conservative treatment including a "wait and see" strategy and palliative surgery may be adopted in select cases.

◆ Preoperative Neuroimaging Studies

The investigative method of choice is MRI, which assists in reliable diagnostic evaluation and accurate surgical planning. T1- and T2-weighted images show *epidermoids* as hypoisointense and hyperintense, respectively, compared with cerebrospinal fluid (CSF) and brain tissue as seen in the figures. Some cysts may exhibit a higher intensity signal, reflecting the difference in the amount of low-density lipids and high-density keratin in the desquamated debris. Proton density (PD) weighting is the sequence of choice for CSF differentiation, whereas T2-weighted images provide additional information on the position of distorted cranial nerves and vessels **(Fig. 59–3).** CT shows epidermoids to be isodense with respect to the CSF and hypodense with the brain tissue, and due to their low absorption values they do not increase after intravenous contrast. Calcifications and capsule-like enhancement occur in a minority of cases. Differential diagnosis is posed with arachnoid cysts and craniopharyngioma. When adopting a combined supra-infratentorial approach, angiography is necessary to assess venous drainage, the depth venous system, the dominant transverse sinus, and the position and site of drainage of the vein of Labbé into the transverse sinus.[1]

In the *petrous* lesion, the signal is the same as that of its intradural counterpart. CT with a bone window algorithm provides additional information on the extent of petrous erosion, pneumatization, and the relationship with the cochlea and labyrinth. Differential diagnosis is posed with cholesterol granuloma.

Diploic epidermoids, on x-ray, typically appear as osteolytic lesions with well-defined, sometimes sclerotic, margins. CT demonstrates a diploë thickness, which may be described as surrounding the lesion, thin, or absent. MRI is rarely described. Differential diagnosis is posed with metastasis or eosinophil granuloma.

In *dermoids*, MRI demonstrates variable relaxation times based on the fat content, typically showing high-signal intensity on T1- and T2-weighted images. Also on CT, variable relaxation times show hypodense images yet with greater inhomogeneity. Calcifications and enhancement are uncommon, similar to epidermoids, and the lipid content are peculiar features of these tumors. Differential diagnosis is posed for epidermoids, teratoma, and other germ-cell tumors.

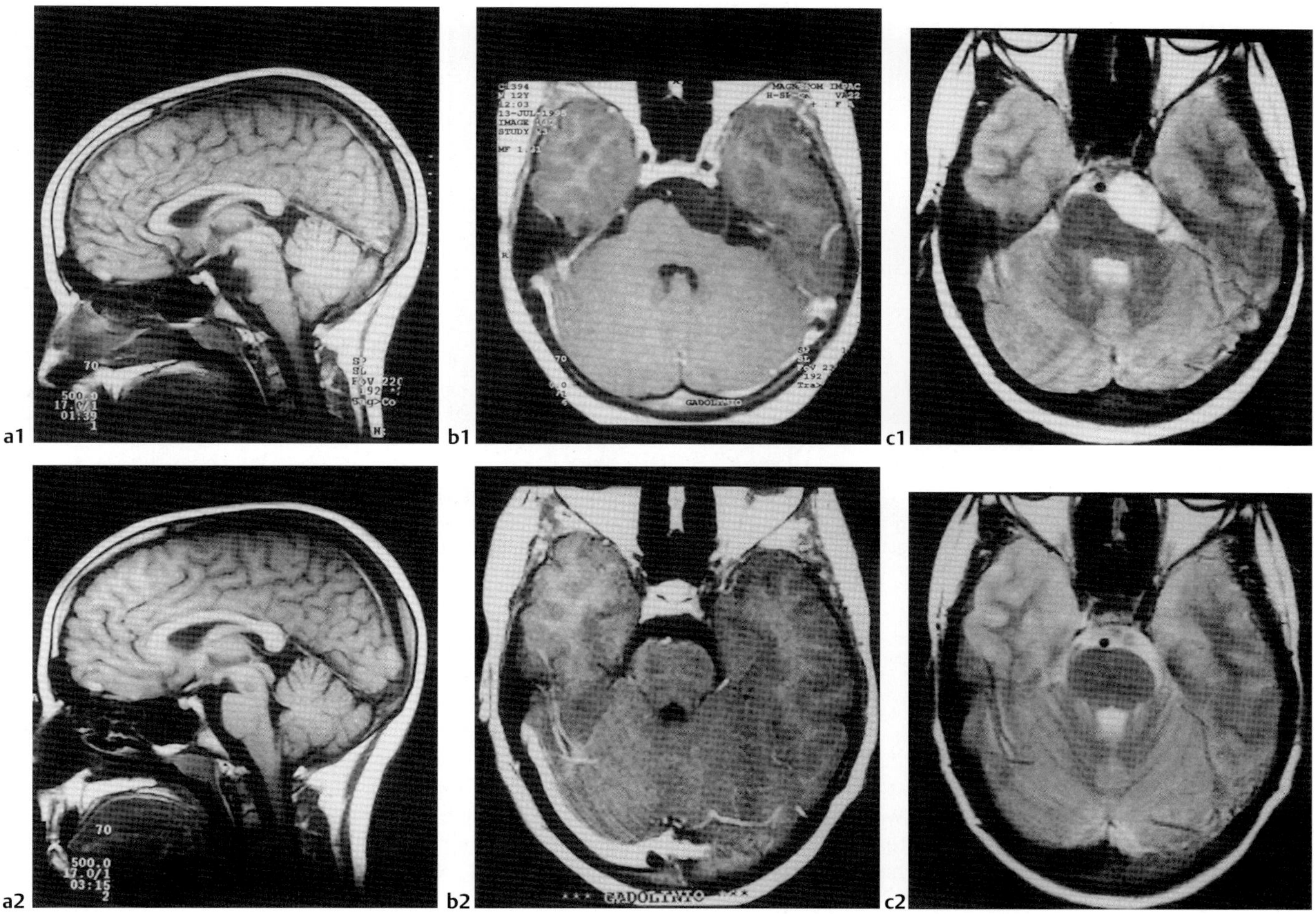

Figure 59–3 An 11-year-old boy presented with headache, neck pain, and visual disturbances. *Imaging:* (a_1) MR unenhanced sagittal, (b_1) contrast-enhanced axial, and (c_1) T2-weighted images clearly delineate a petroclival epidermoid lying medial to the trigeminal nerve. Comparable MR images (a_2, b_2, c_2) obtained 2 years after surgery demonstrate no signs of residual tumor.

(*Continued on page 718*)

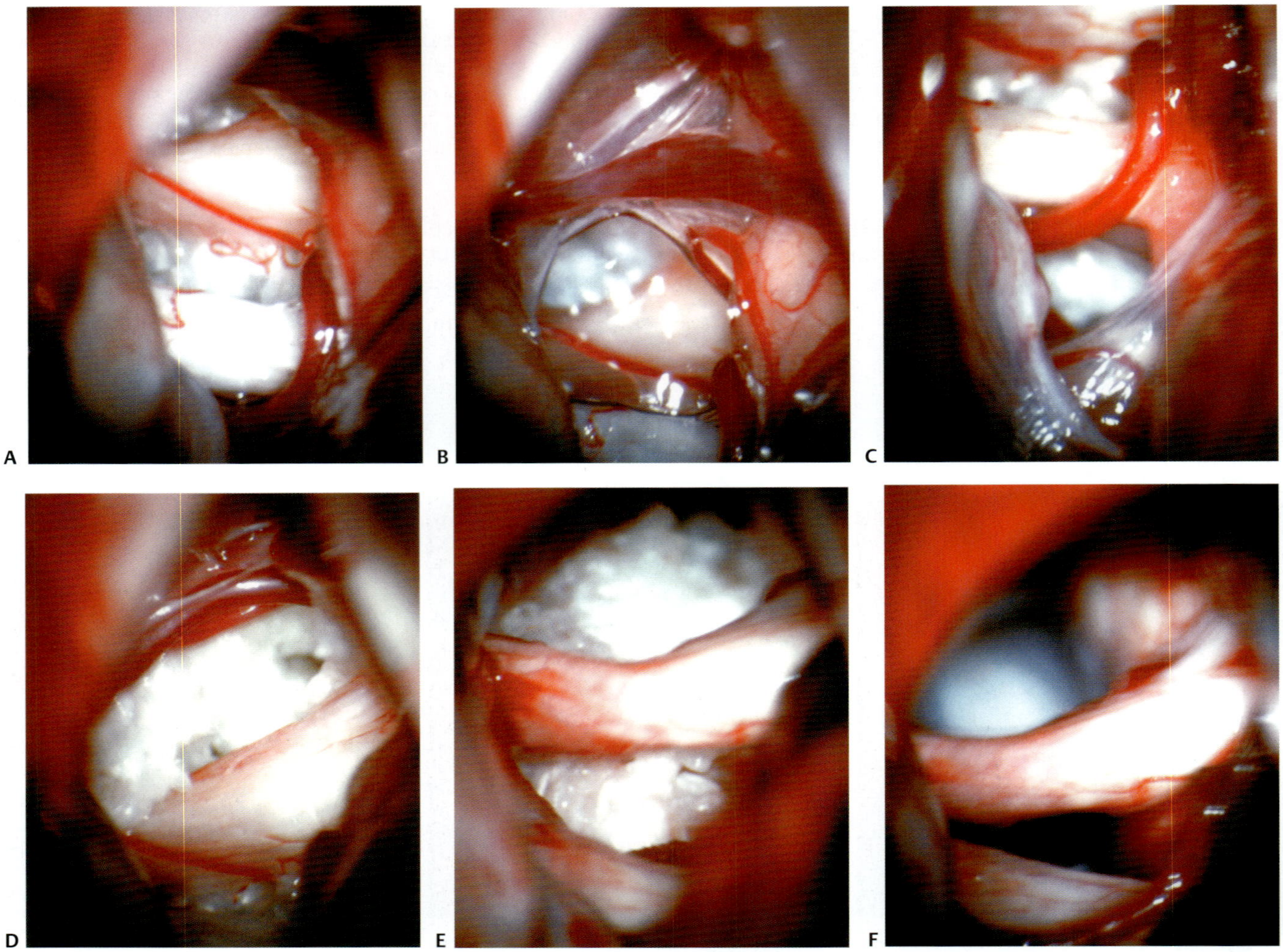

(*Continued*) **Figure 59–3** *Intraoperative views:* **(A–C)** After exposing the cerebellopontine angle through a retrosigmoid approach, the epidermoid appears completely ventral to the trigeminal, superior petrosal vein, and cranial nerves VII and VIII. **(D,E)** Working between the tentorium and trigeminal and the trigeminal and VII–VIII nerves, the tumor is debulked and removed. **(F)** The brain stem, trigeminal, and VII–VIII nerves are shown before dura closure. The child is neurologically intact 3 years after surgery.

◆ Surgical Technique

Approach

Simple standard surgical approaches may be used for epidermoid and dermoid cysts. The primary location, usually the largest when the tumor occupies two or more regions, determines the choice. The classical pterional and the laterosuboccipital retrosigmoid approaches are valid in the majority of cases. A favorable aspect of these approaches is that as tumor debulking progresses, the brain does not collapse, thus avoiding the need for retraction and permitting further removal (**Figs. 59–1** to **59–3**).

Suprasellar/chiasmatic and parasellar lesions are best accessed by pterional craniotomy, and the lesions in the cerebellopontine angle and petroclival region are approached via retromastoid craniectomy (**Figs. 59–2** to **59–4**). A midline suboccipital craniectomy associated with a C1 laminectomy is suitable to approach and remove fourth ventricle center tumors. A high suboccipital midline craniotomy permits opening of the supracerebellar infratentorial corridor to access a pineal-mesencephalic lesion expanding in the quadrigeminal cistern (**Fig. 59–5**). A dorsolateral extension of the lateral suboccipital retrosigmoid approach is indicated for tumors extending from the cerebellopontine angle into the foramen magnum (**Fig. 59–1**). Hourglass epidermoids involving both the middle fossa and the cerebellopontine angle may also be removed by the pterional approach with division of the medial tentorium.

More extensive approaches are indicated only in cases where greater superficial exposure is necessary to perform multiple trajectories or to be closer to an otherwise inaccessible location. Midline-located tumors of uniform size and tumors growing above and below the tentorium, insinuating into contralateral spaces, present particular difficulty. For these tumors, a combined supra- and infratentorial approach, tailored in its variants; namely, the presigmoid retrolabyrinthine, translabyrinthine, and transcochlear, may be adopted.[17] The transsigmoid variant of the retromastoid approach enhances downward exposure.

Petrous apex cholesteatomas are best approached via extradural routes (**Table 59–3**). Residual hearing and facial function dictate the choice of a conservative approach (middle fossa transpetrous apex and infratemporal) or a more aggressive approach (transcochlear) to the tumor. Supra- and infralabyrinthine approaches are typically adopted for incomplete total removal.

Anesthesia

The standard anesthesia is induced by thiopental and a short-acting muscle relaxant (succinylcholine), whereas other agents are selected for anesthetic maintenance. Isoflurane, N_2O, opioid analgesics, and muscle relaxants may be used based on the general condition of the patient, surgical position, and need of electromyography, or cranial nerve motor function testing.

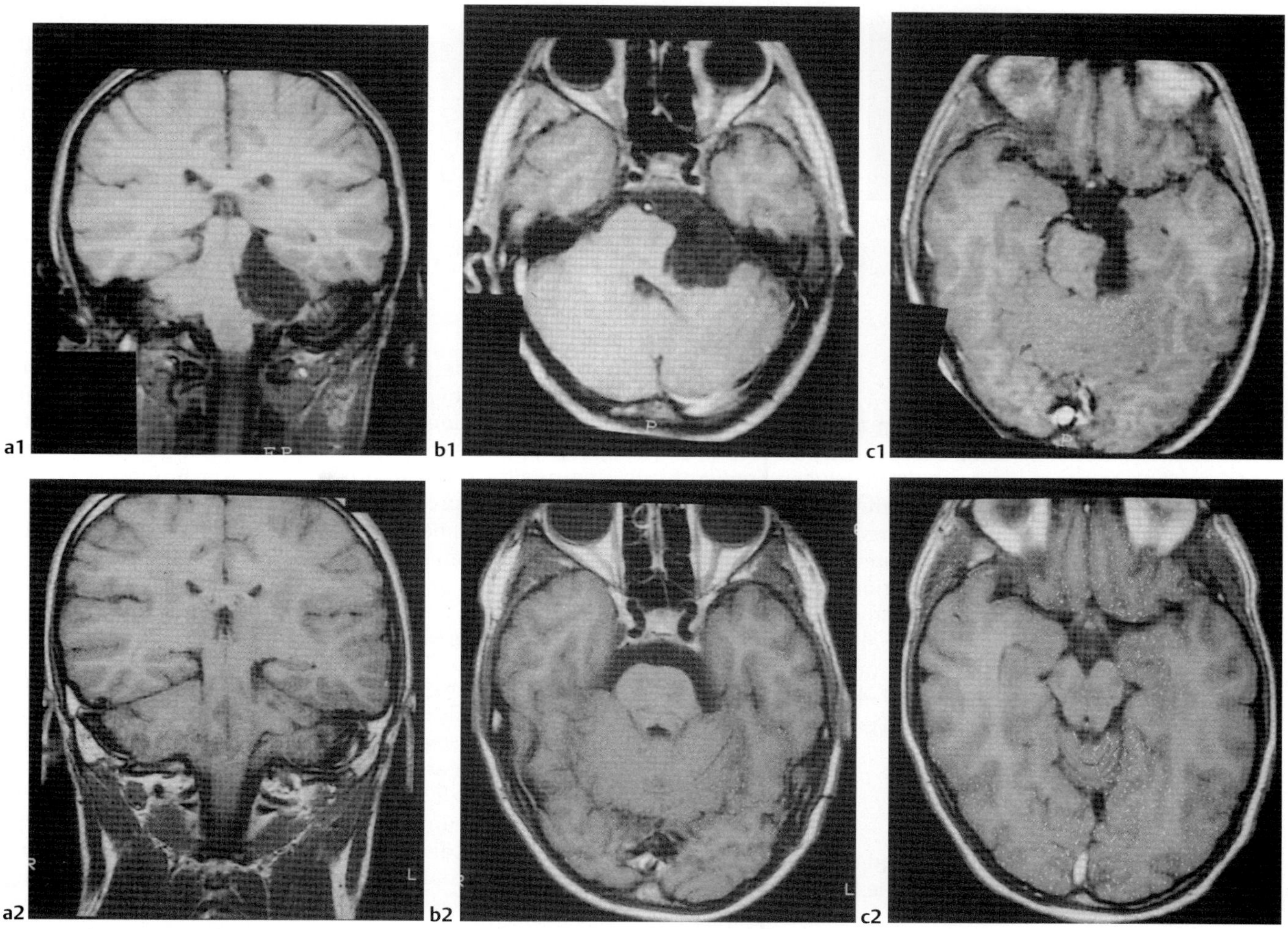

Figure 59–4 A 15-year-old boy presented with worsening positional vertigo, torticollis, diplopia, and gait ataxia. *Imaging:* (**a**$_1$, **b**$_1$, **c**$_1$) Magnetic resonance (MR) unenhanced T1-weighted coronal and axial images showing a huge cerebellopontine and upper clival epidermoid. Comparable MR images (**a**$_2$, **b**$_2$, **c**$_2$) obtained 6 years after surgery demonstrate total removal using a simple retrosigmoid approach.

(Continued on page 720)

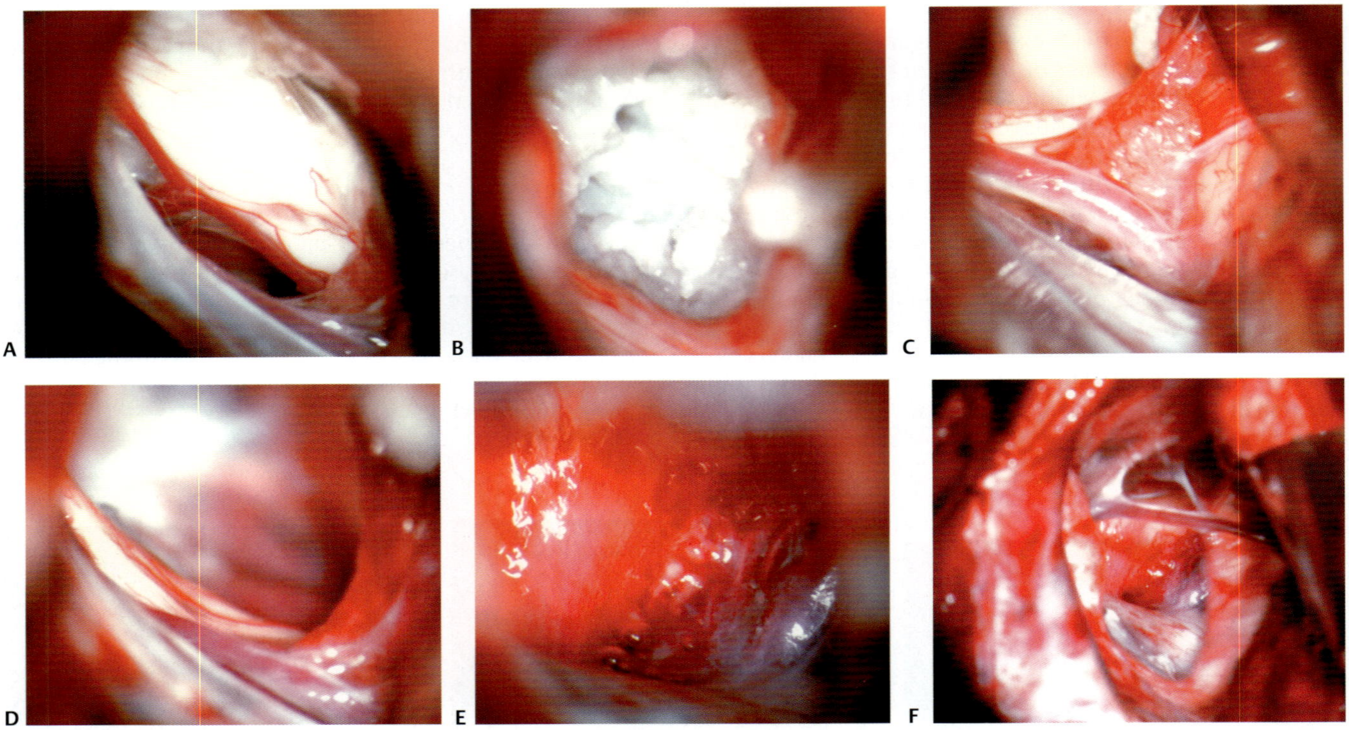

(*Continued*) **Figure 59–4** *Intraoperative views:* **(A)** The epidermoid pushing downward and stretching the VII–VIII nerves and the internal carotid artery is **(B)** debulked and removed without injury to **(C,D)** the cranial nerves and arteries. **(E)** At the end of removal, the pituitary stalk is visible from below, and **(F)** the panoramic view of the operative field before closure is shown. The patient is now neurologically normal.

Positioning

The three common positions for surgery are the supine, lateral decubitus, and semisitting. There is considerable concern regarding the semisitting position, yet the potential risks (air embolism and hypotension) are nearly eliminated by prevention, early detection, and treatment. Some approaches may be performed in alternate positions and tailored accordingly. In surgery of posterior fossa-based epidermoids, the semisitting position is advocated because it provides greater exposure from below, allowing removal of higher portions of tumors up to the mesencephalic and suprasellar regions (**Figs. 59–2** and **59–4**). Differently, lateral decubitus provides a wider lateral exposure to allow a contralateral view.

Monitoring

Hemodynamic monitoring is performed to provide the following information: compromise of the brain stem (variations of heart pulse and arterial pressure); trigeminal sensory function (hypertension, bradycardia); and vagal function (hypotension, bradycardia). Additional warning signs are helpful due to frequent brain stem involvement. Brain stem auditory evoked responses and somatosensory evoked potentials can provide early detection of local injury. Electromyography and direct electrical stimulation assist safe dissection of cranial nerves.

Table 59–3 Petrous Apex Epidermoids: Surgical Approaches

Middle fossa transpetrous apex:
Petrosal transcochlear
Infratemporal
Supralabyrinthine
Infralabyrinthine

Operative Procedure

After opening the dura, the arachnoid is divided and the tumor capsule is exposed: its unmistakable white and lucent appearance provides immediate histological confirmation of epidermoid (**Fig. 59–1**). After coagulation of the small vessels seldom covering the capsule, the cyst is entered and tumor debulking begins (**Figs. 59–2** and **59–3**). Due to the soft and totally avascular content composed of keratin lamellae, this stage is performed using suction, curet, and cuplike forceps. The surgical strategy adopted is to follow the path created by the tumor via a single simple route. The dissector assists the surgeon to mobilize parts of the tumor allowing the surgeon to enter the visual field. An important concept to bear in mind during debulking is that epidermoid tumors, rather than displacing cranial nerves and vessels, more often engulf them. Cranial nerves and arteries, encountered inside the tumor may be distorted in an abnormal position; thus the removal of cyst content must be performed with particular attention and an understanding of the involved anatomy until the nerves and arteries are identified (**Fig. 59–2**). Because cranial nerves have fixed entry and exit points at the brain stem and cranial foramina, a useful trick is to start by identifying the cranial nerve at these points and then following the path of the nerve into the tumor. During debulking, the tumor capsule is simultaneously dissected (**Figs. 59–1** and **59–2**). Externally, the tumor has a nodular surface, and although clearly demarcated, its capsule is often firmly adherent to blood vessels, cranial nerves, arachnoid, pia, and choroid plexus (**Figs. 59–1** and **59–4**).

Limiting factors for radical removal include the tenuous nature of the wall; its tenacious adhesion to vessels, nerves, and/or brain matter; and the impossibility of reaching distant and hidden tumor remnants (**Fig. 59–2**). In the latter case, an angled mirror or a neuroendoscope assists in decreasing the amount of tumor remnant, which is critical to recurrence. Firm portions of capsule left in situ are more often the result of the strategy of an experienced surgeon rather than an inappropriate approach.[2] It is still uncertain whether diagnosis delay or tumor extension influences capsule adhesion to important neurovascular structures. In the literature, heterogeneous results concerning the extent of tumor removal are partially due to subjective evaluation of total removal. It is not clear if leaving thin portions of capsule is overlooked by some authors.

A good view of the entire cyst wall is difficult to obtain regardless of the technique in removal of petrous apex

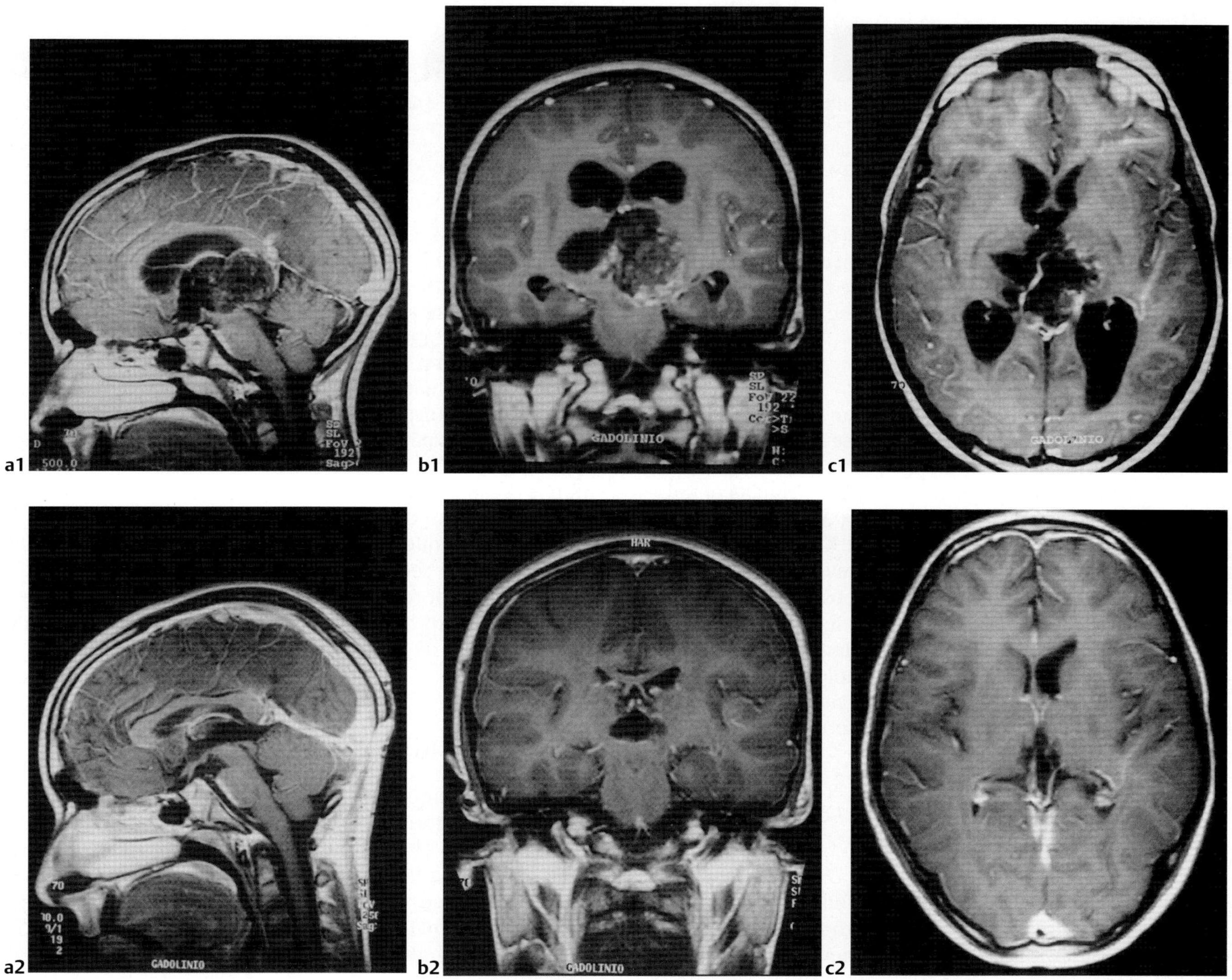

Figure 59–5 A 12-year-old boy presented with signs of intracranial hypertension due to a rapid onset of hydrocephalus that required ventriculoperitoneal shunting. *Imaging:* Magnetic resonance (MR) contrast-enhanced (**a_1**) T1-sagittal, (**b_1**) coronal, and (**c_1**) axial scans demonstrating a large dermoid cyst invading the quadrigeminal cistern and invaginating into the third ventricle with a huge mass effect on the mesencephalon. The postoperative comparable MR scans (**a_2, b_2, c_2**) suggest a complete surgical removal.

(*Continued on page 722*)

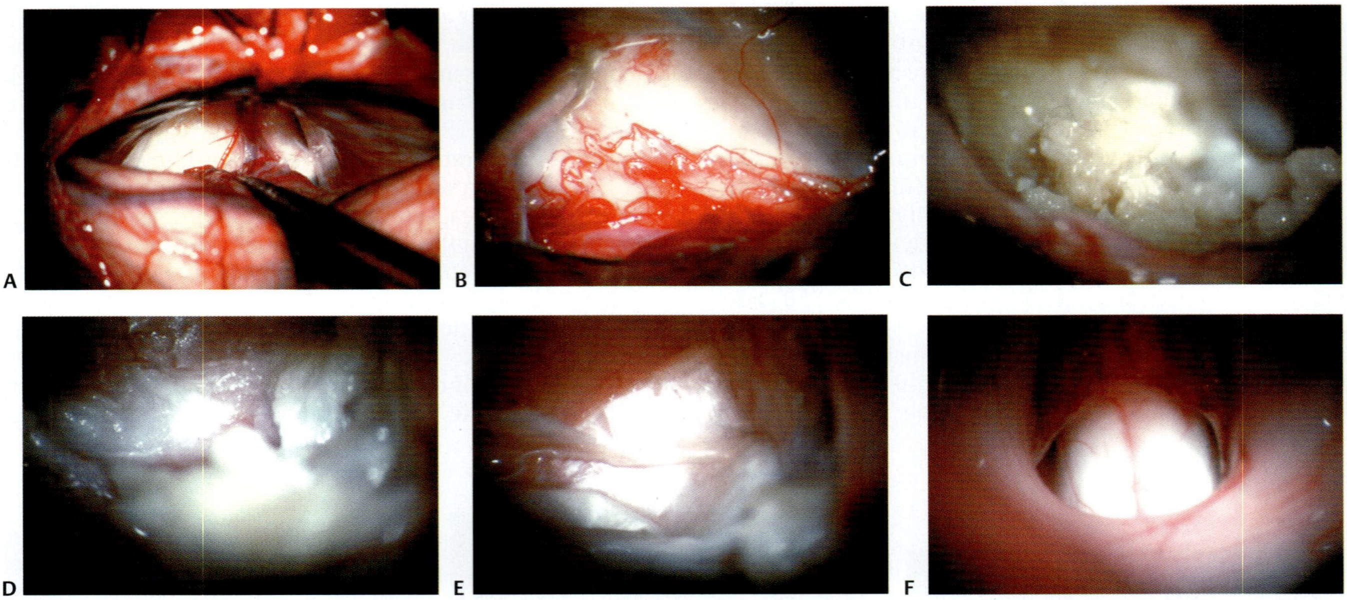

(*Continued*) **Figure 59–5** *Intraoperative views:* **(A)** The epidermoid is exposed at the quadrigeminal cistern through a suboccipital-infratentorial supracerebellar approach. **(B)** The quadrigeminal plate is slid down, and the tumor entered. **(C,D)** The cyst contents, consisting of a creamy, greasy texture and strands of hair, are removed. **(E)** The ventral chitin-like lining is detached and resected enabling entry into the **(F)** third ventricle chamber. The postoperative course was uneventful, and the patient is well except for slight upward gaze disturbance.

epidermoids, yet adjacent structures (bone and dura) facilitate safe dissection of adherent capsule. This is similar also for diploic tumors. In cases where the tumor capsule cannot be removed, dural plastic may be performed.

Closure and Reconstruction

Care should be taken during dural closure, particularly following temporal bone drilling, because of the risk of CSF leakage. The middle ear and eustachian tube are the final pathways that lead to rhinorrhea. Fixing the couche of muscle between the edges of dural opening with a few stitches and fibrin glue, possibly combined with autologous fat in the petrous cavity, is a very useful preventive procedure. Fascia lata may be used to pack the eustachian tube, the antrum, and the cells of the middle ear. In petrous apex epidermoids, the cavity should be obliterated if such complication is considered. In diploic epidermoids with extensive bone excision, skull repair with acrylic cement may be necessary in the same procedure or some months following surgery.

◆ Postoperative Care

During the early postoperative period, functional neurological impairment remains unchanged, although nearly half of the patients suffer mild transient deterioration typically related to cranial nerve dysfunction. Trigeminal, VII, and IX to X cranial nerve deficits require particular care to prevent cheratitis and aspiration pneumonia, respectively.

Because epidermoids are benign in nature, assessment is required not only to determine the extent of surgical removal but also to monitor tumor recurrences. During the initial follow-up period, the surgeon's assessment of the extent of removal is more reliable than neuroimaging information due to the immediate shrinkage of the hypodense and hypointense area on CT and T1-weighted MRI, respectively; yet the surgeon's intraoperative judgment may prove inaccurate in later follow-up.

To better evaluate the rate of recurrence, longer follow-up periods are required for patients with total or near-total removal than for patients with subtotal removal. Follow-up serial MRI studies at 2-year intervals after the initial operation is recommended to monitor any eventual regrowth of the tumor before the recurrence becomes symptomatic. The timing of subsequent surgery is controversial. Surgeons still debate whether second surgery should be performed at first MRI evidence of recurrence, or at the time the tumor presumably extends beyond the original operative field, or after the renewal of symptoms.

◆ Complications

The operative mortality for intracranial epidermoid and dermoid cysts decreased dramatically from 70% before 1936 to 10% by 1977[13,18]; more recent series have reported zero mortality and a very low surgical morbidity of less than 10%.[3,14,19] At surgery, meticulous care must be taken to avoid spilling tumor material to prevent distant seeding or aseptic meningitis. Although distant seeding remains a theoretical concern, aseptic meningitis and hydrocephalus have demonstrated the most dangerous complications, occurring in 40% of reported cases.[20] Basal arachnoiditis, ependymitis, or aqueduct stenosis may lead to dense cranial nerve deficits and hydrocephalus. Satisfactory results have been obtained by irrigating the surgical field and the adjacent cisterns with hydrocortisone (2 g) before dural closure, and postoperatively maintaining the patient on a high-dosage steroid (parenteral dexamethasone) regimen. Carcinomatous degeneration is not a complication but a possible consequence of incomplete removal.

◆ Conclusion

Epidermoid and dermoid cysts are histologically benign lesions of maldevelopmental origin. They are extraaxially located in the subarachnoid and cisternal spaces and tend to grow, insinuating into the natural extensions of these virtual channels. Surgery is the only effective treatment, with the gold standard being radical removal of the cyst content and lining wall at the first operation. In cases when the cyst wall is too firmly adherent to important neurovascular structures to allow extirpation, the priority remains the preservation of neurological function due to the fact that the linear slow growth of these tumors renders the symptomatic recurrence a distance event.

The primary concerns in the management of epidermoid and dermoid cysts remain misdiagnosis, incomplete removal at the first operation, and delayed detection of recurrences. Contemporary microsurgical techniques with a more extensive exposure increase the possibility of obtaining safe total or near-total cyst removal with near-zero mortality, acceptable morbidity, and definite cure.

References

1. Sabin HI, Bordi LT, Symon L. Epidermoid cysts and cholesterol granulomas centered on the posterior fossa: twenty years of diagnosis and management. Neurosurgery 1987;21:798–805
2. Samii M, Tatagiba M, Piquer J, Carualha CA. Surgical treatment of epidermoid cysts of the cerebellopontine angle. J Neurosurg 1996;84: 14–19
3. Yasargil MG, Abernathy CD, Sarioglu AC. Microneurosurgical treatment of intracranial dermoid and epidermoid tumors. Neurosurgery 1989;24:561–567
4. Cruveilhier J. Anatomie Pathologique du Corps Humain. Vol 1, book 2. Paris: J.B. Bailliere; 1829–1835:341
5. Russell DS, Rubenstein LJ. Pathology of Tumors of the Nervous System. 5th ed. Baltimore: Williams & Wilkins; 1989:663–695
6. Baxter JW, Netsky MG. Epidermoid and dermoid tumors: pathology. In: Wilkins RH, Rengachary SS, eds. Neurosurgery. New York: McGraw-Hill; 1985:655–661
7. Ulrich J. Intracranial epidermoids: a study on their distribution and spread. J Neurosurg 1964;21:1051–1057
8. Lunardi P, Missori P, Innocenzi G, et al. Long term results of surgical treatment of cerebello-pontine angle epidermoids. Acta Neurochir (Wien) 1990;103:105–108
9. Lewis AJ, Cooper PW, Kassel EE, et al. Squamous cell carcinoma arising from a suprasellar epidermoid cyst. J Neurosurg 1983;59: 538–341
10. Alvord ED Jr. Birthrates of epidermoid tumors. Ann Surg 1977;2: 367–370
11. Talacchi A, Sala F, Alessandrini F, et al. Assessment and surgical management of posterior fossa epidermoid tumors: report of 28 cases. Neurosurgery 1998;42:242–252
12. Lepoire DM, Pertuiset B. Les Kistes Epidermoides Cranioencephaliques. Paris: Masson; 1957:20–25
13. Johnston FG, Crockard HA. Dermoid, epidermoid and neuroenteric cysts. In: Kaye AH, Laws ER, eds. Brain Tumors. Edinburgh: Churchill Livingstone; 1995:895–902
14. Altschuler EM, Jungreis CA, Sekhar LN, Jannekka PJ, Skptak PE. Objective treatment of intracranial epidermoid cysts and cholesterol granulomas: report of 21 cases. Neurosurgery 1990;26:606–614
15. De Micheli E, Bricolo A. The long history of a cerebello-pontine angle epidermoid tumour: a case report and lessons learned. Acta Neurochir (Wien) 1996;138:350–354
16. Long DM. Intracranial epidermoid tumours. In: Apuzzo MLJ, ed. Brain Surgery. Vol 1. New York: Churchill Livingstone; 1993:669–688
17. Spetzler RF, Daspit CP, Pappas CT. The combined supra- and infratentorial approach for lesions of the petrous and clival regions: experience with 46 cases. J Neurosurg 1992;76:588–599
18. Guidetti B, Gagliardi F. Epidermoid and dermoid cysts: clinical evaluation and late surgical results. J Neurosurg 1977;47:12–18
19. Yamakawa K, Shitara N, Genka S, Monaka S, Takakura Ka Clinical course and surgical prognosis of 33 cases of intracranial epidermoid tumors. Neurosurgery 1989;24:568–573
20. Conley FK. Epidermoid and dermoid tumors: clinical features and surgical management. Neurosurgery 1985;1:668–673

60

Craniovertebral Junction: An Extreme Lateral Approach

Chandranath Sen and Chun Siang Chen

Surgical lesions at the anterior aspect of the craniocervical junction include a variety of benign and malignant neoplasms, aneurysms, and skeletal anomalies. This region, which includes the lower clivus, foramen magnum,[1] and the upper two cervical vertebrae, contains the lower brain stem, the cervicomedullary junction, the caudal cranial nerves, and the vertebral arteries. The jugular bulbs and the occipitocervical articulation are in the vicinity and can be involved by the tumor or in the way of the surgical approach. Traditionally, the lateral suboccipital approach that has been used is limited by the fact that it provides a long, narrow exposure of the field, and it is necessary to work in between the cranial nerves, which may limit the access.[2] This approach is inadequate in dealing with tumors that extend extradurally. The extreme lateral approach is designed to provide relatively wide and shallow access to this area along with complete control of the ipsilateral vertebral artery with minimal brain stem or cerebellar retraction. It provides excellent access to both intradural and extradural lesions as well as vertebral and vertebrobasilar junction aneurysms.[3–9]

Indications

- Anterior and anterolaterally placed intradural tumors of the lower clivus, C1, C2
- Extradural tumors of the lower clivus, C1, C2
- Aneurysms of the vertebral artery and the vertebrobasilar junction

Salient Features of the Approach

1. The skin incision is placed on the side of the neck and suboccipital region and the muscles are dissected in layers, allowing the soft tissues to be away from the area of the surgical access.
2. The vertebral artery is identified and exposed at an early stage, allowing the approach to be carried as laterally as needed with proximal control of the vessel.
3. The bony opening is behind the sigmoid sinus and below the jugular bulb. Drilling of the occipital condyle and jugular tubercle is needed in lesions that are situated entirely along the anterior surface of the foramen magnum. The extent of this drilling is determined according to the particular case.
4. If the vertebral artery is intimately involved by the lesion, it is freed from the dura circumferentially at its entry into the posterior fossa so that it can be followed into the tumor and adequately freed from the tumor under total control.
5. It is important to note that the direction of visualization is from the upper cervical area, looking up into the foramen magnum and the posterior fossa. This allows the surgeon to minimize the manipulation of the lower cranial nerves to access the anterior surface of the lower clivus.

Preoperative Studies

Preoperative assessment of the caudal cranial nerve function is an important part of the neurological examination. A long-standing insidious paralysis of any of these nerves can go unnoticed by the patient. It indicates that such a patient would tolerate manipulation of these nerves without much adverse problems. However, an acute lower cranial nerve palsy is quite disabling. Detailed imaging studies include magnetic resonance imaging (MRI) and computed tomographic (CT) scans. MRI provides an accurate assessment of the soft tissue, neural, and arterial relations of the lesion. CT is important for the bony anatomy of the foramen magnum region and for depicting the nature and location of the bony changes. An MR angiogram gives sufficient information about the vertebral arteries (VAs). An arteriogram is used specifically for aneurysms and for tumors that encase the artery where the specific details about the artery and its branches and the collateral vessels need to be studied. The extent of the tumor blood supply from the VAs is also noted. If the jugular bulb is involved by tumor, the venous anatomy is evaluated.

◆ Surgical Technique

Anesthesia and Intraoperative Monitoring

The operations are always performed under general endotracheal anesthesia. Somatosensory evoked potentials (SEPs) are monitored routinely. The monitoring is usually started prior to the surgical positioning so that any alterations during positioning can be detected and remedied before starting the operation. Anterior flexion of the head on the neck must be avoided because it causes further compromise of the cervicomedullary junction. Motor evoked potentials monitoring if available is also helpful. Although the vocal cords, the trapezius, and the tongue muscles can be directly monitored with electromyography (EMG) electrodes, cranial nerve monitoring of the lower nerves has not been found to be particularly useful in locating the nerves or facilitating their dissection. An intraarterial and a central venous catheter are always used. Meticulous blood pressure control is exercised to avoid hypotension, which may produce an ischemic insult on a compromised cord. Sequential compression stockings are used for prophylaxis against deep venous thrombosis during such lengthy operations.

Positioning

We prefer placing the patient in a full lateral decubitus position with the involved side up in a three-point pin head holder (**Fig. 60–1**). We find that in this position it is easier to manage the hemodynamic status of the patient, and it is more comfortable for the surgeon than the sitting position. The sitting position has the main advantage of reduced venous bleeding, and the blood drains away from the surgical field. The head is maintained in a neutral position, slightly flexed on the side of the dependent shoulder to open up the space between the mastoid and the side of the neck, but without rotation or ventral flexion. The torso of the patient is secured to the operating table with several bands of adhesive tape because the table may be rotated in several directions during the operation. The contact surfaces must be well padded. A soft roll is placed against the dependent chest wall to prevent a brachial plexus injury, and excessive traction on the superior shoulder should be avoided. More recently, the park-bench position has been used with the dependent shoulder hanging off the table, but the rest of the positioning remains unchanged. This prevents a pressure sore from the axillary roll on the chest wall that is necessary in the true lateral position.

Incision and Muscle Dissection

An inverted L-shaped incision is usually preferred unless the tumor extends higher up in the clivus. Then a C-shaped incision is made centered on the ear. The short horizontal limb of the L is made at the level of the top of the ear, whereas the vertical limb is made behind the ear on the side of the neck, just posterior to the mastoid process and brought down to the middle of the neck below C2 (**Fig. 60–2**). The muscles of the posterior cervical triangle (behind the sternomastoid) are identified and taken down in individual layers (**Fig. 60–3**).

These muscles are detached from their occipital attachments and attachments on the transverse process of C1 and reflected inferiorly, and can be resutured at the end of the operation (**Fig. 60–4**). This type of dissection is anatomical and is helpful in providing a wide unimpeded viewing angle, and there is no hindrance from a bulk of soft tissues on either side of the retractor. These points are important to follow, so that one does not end up working in a deep, narrow hole during the tumor resection. The tip of the mastoid process and the transverse process of C1 are used as the bony landmarks. These steps are useful in identifying and isolating the vertebral artery extracranially. The deepest

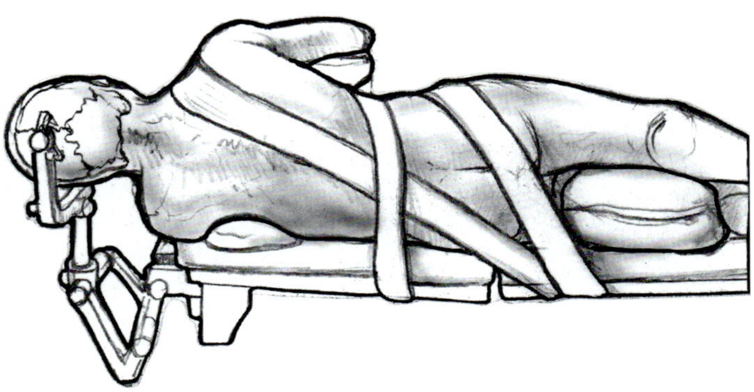

Figure 60–1 The lateral decubitus position is shown with a cushion below the dependent axilla. The head is tilted toward the dependent shoulder but otherwise neutral.

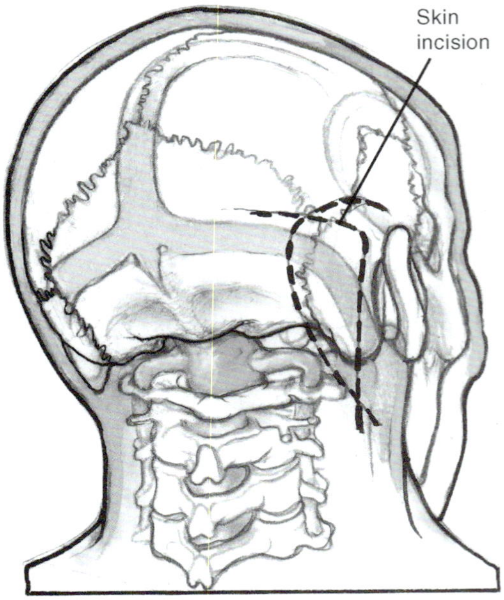

Figure 60–2 The inverted L- or C-shaped incision is positioned behind the mastoid process.

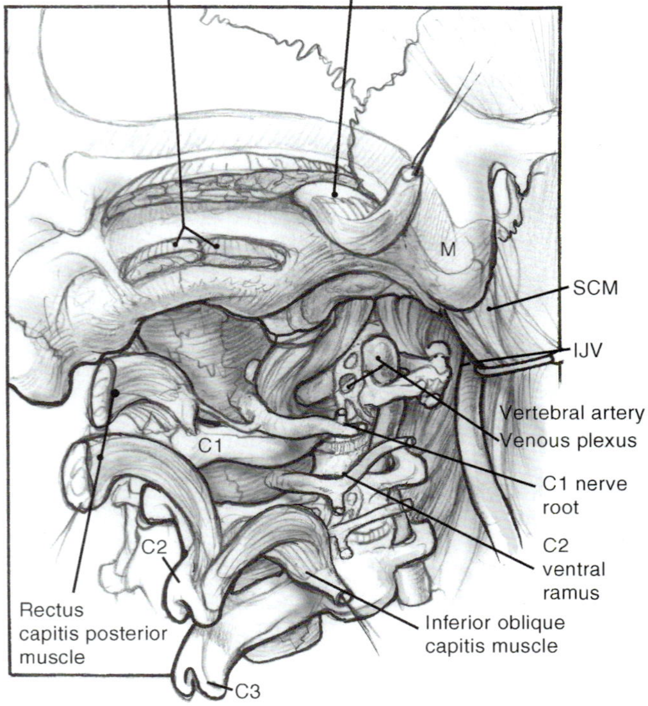

Figure 60–4 Diagram illustrating the muscles being detached and reflected inferiorly.

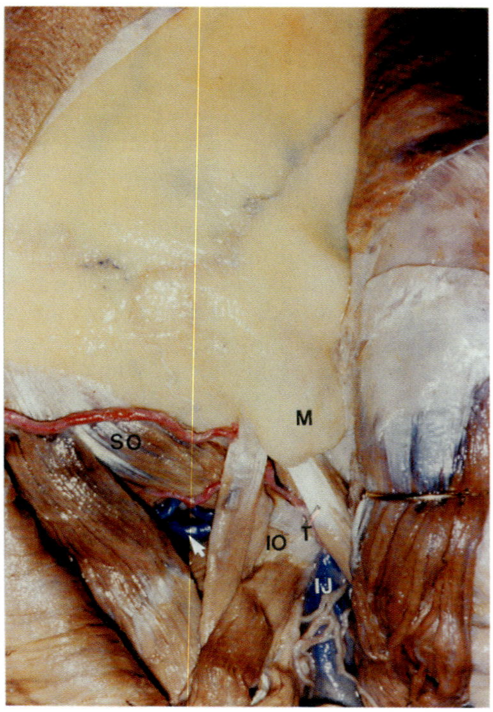

Figure 60–3 The right side posterior cervical triangle is dissected in the cadaver specimen. M, mastoid process; IJ, internal jugular vein; SO, superior oblique muscle; IO, inferior oblique muscle; T, transverse process of C1; arrow, venous plexus around the vertebral artery (VA) above C1.

layer of muscles is composed of the superior and inferior obliqui and the levator scapulae. These muscles are used as a guide to finding the VA, which is just deep to this layer.

Identification and Isolation of the Vertebral Artery

Proximal control of the VA is obtained early in the operation, either above C1 or below C1 as dictated by the location of the lesion.[10] The muscles are detached from the transverse process and arch of C1 as well as the occipital bone, and the VA covered by the venous plexus is identified. The VA identification and isolation is done under magnification because the arterial pulse is not always a reliable guide due to the surrounding soft tissues.

The extent to which the artery is isolated and manipulated varies with the pathology and location of the tumor. Tumors that intimately involve the artery usually require that the vessel be isolated from the venous sheath before it enters the dura. This allows complete control of the artery, which can then be released circumferentially from the dura, facilitating its dissection from the tumor. The venous sheath is coagulated and opened longitudinally along the course of

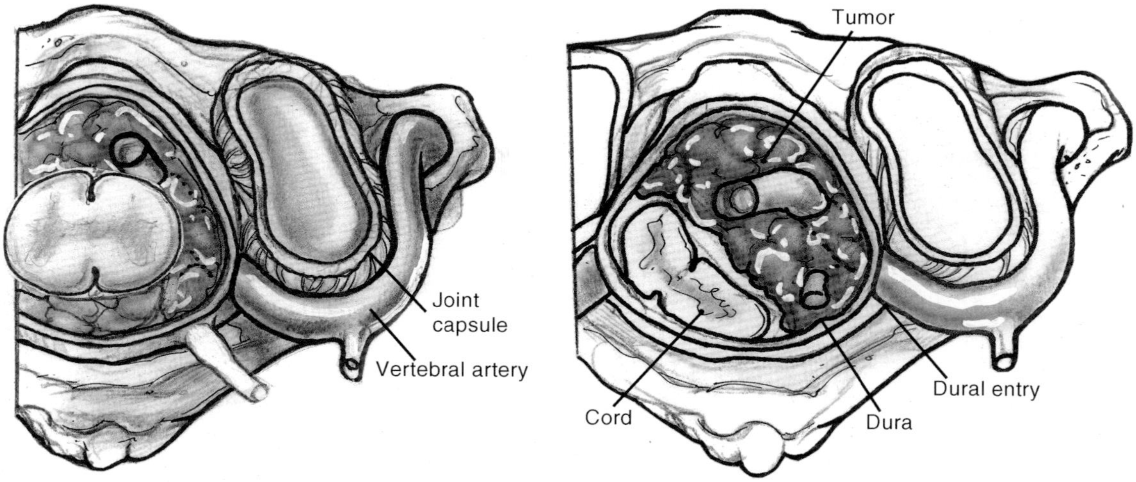

Figure 60–5 **(A)** The vertebral artery at C1 is closely adherent to the joint capsule. **(B)** Mobilization of this segment of the artery is needed when the tumor involves the vessel at its dural entry.

the artery. The artery is then completely taken out of the sheath. There is usually a lot of venous bleeding during this maneuver, but once the artery is removed from the sheath, the venous bleeding is easily controlled with the bipolar cautery or Surgicel packing. The condylar emissary vein is also handled in a similar manner. A rubber vessel loop is placed around the VA, which is followed to the dural entry. The joint capsule of the articulation between the occipital condyle and C1 lateral mass is adherent to the venous sheath around the VA and needs to be carefully separated under the microscope during mobilization of the artery for proximal control **(Fig. 60–5)**. It is also necessary to be aware that the posterior inferior cerebellar artery may arise from the VA outside the dura.[11] Such extensive degree of mobilization of the extradural artery may not be necessary if there is sufficient room to obtain proximal control intradurally.

Bony Exposure

The posterior portion of the mastoid process, occipital bone, and ipsilateral C1 posterior arch are exposed, including the occiput–C1 articulation. A suboccipital craniectomy is made to include the foramen magnum **(Fig. 60–6)**. The posterior border of the sigmoid sinus is exposed but the entire sinus need not be unroofed. Inferior to the jugular bulb, the bone removal is taken up to the occipital condyle. The ipsilateral C1 posterior arch is also removed up to the lateral mass. The additional bony dissection is tailored to the lesion at hand.

For lesions that are located anterolaterally at the foramen magnum, the retrocondylar bony opening as described is sufficient **(Fig. 60–7)**. Tumors that are entirely anterior in location require further bone in an anterior direction below the jugular bulb. Using a high-speed drill the posterior one third of the occipital condyle is resected. Superiorly, the jugular tubercle is drilled away below the jugular bulb. This additional bone removal allows the vertebral artery to be circumferentially released at its dural entry point and allows a better exposure of the base of the tumor **(Fig. 60–8)**. The partial condylar resection is used in meningiomas, glomus jugulare tumors, and vertebral and vertebrobasilar aneurysms.

Resection of the entire occipital condyle is performed in bony tumors that involve the condyle **(Fig. 60–9)**. These are usually chordomas, chondrosarcomas, and osteomas that infiltrate the bone, which need to be aggressively drilled

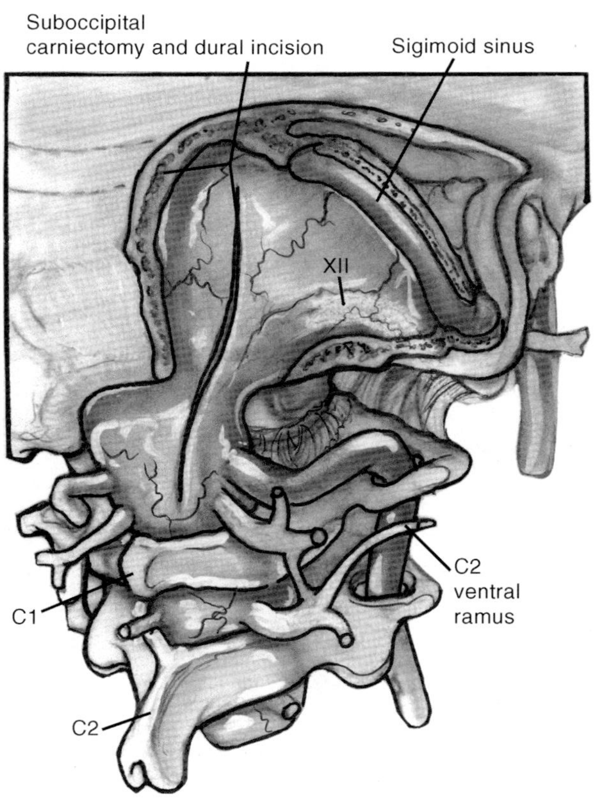

Figure 60–6 The retrocondylar bony opening exposes only the posterior edge of the sigmoid sinus and the occipital condyle.

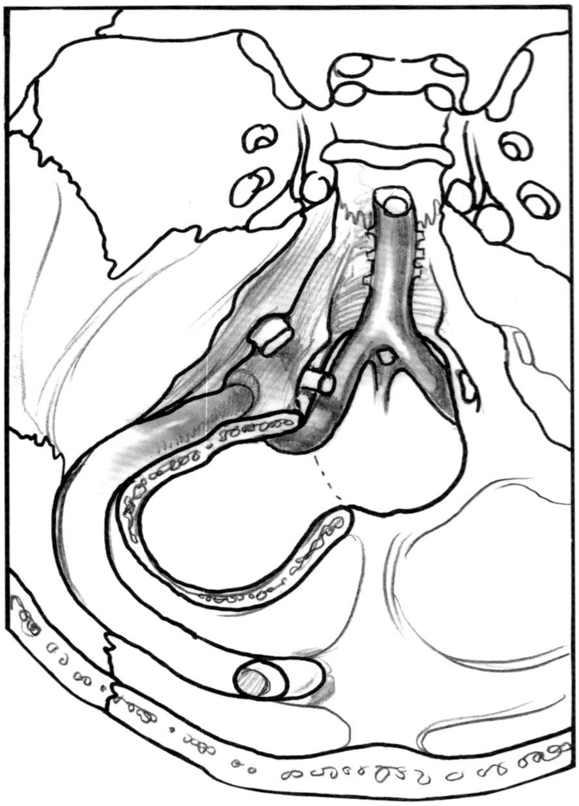

Figure 60–7 Intracranial view of the retrocondylar exposure.

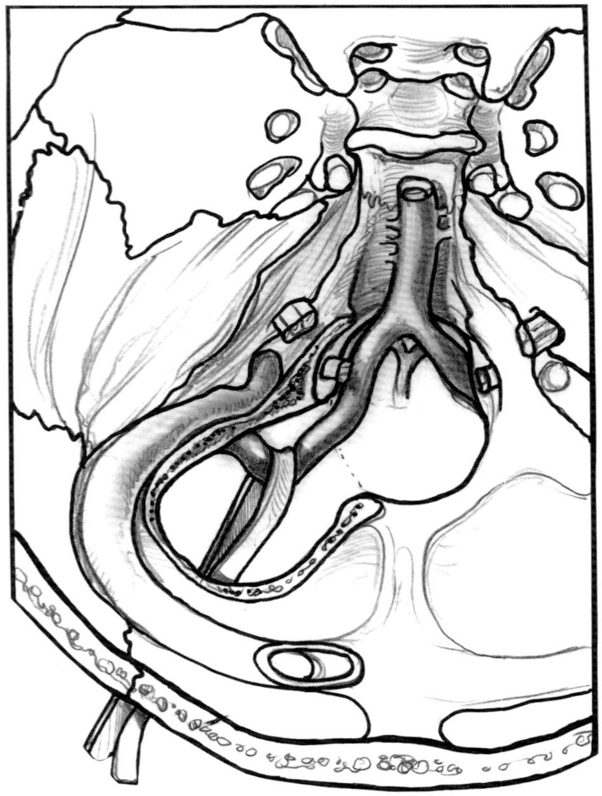

Figure 60–8 Partial resection of the occipital condyle and resection of the jugular tubercle provide better exposure of the anterior surface of the foramen magnum and posterior displacement of the vertebral artery.

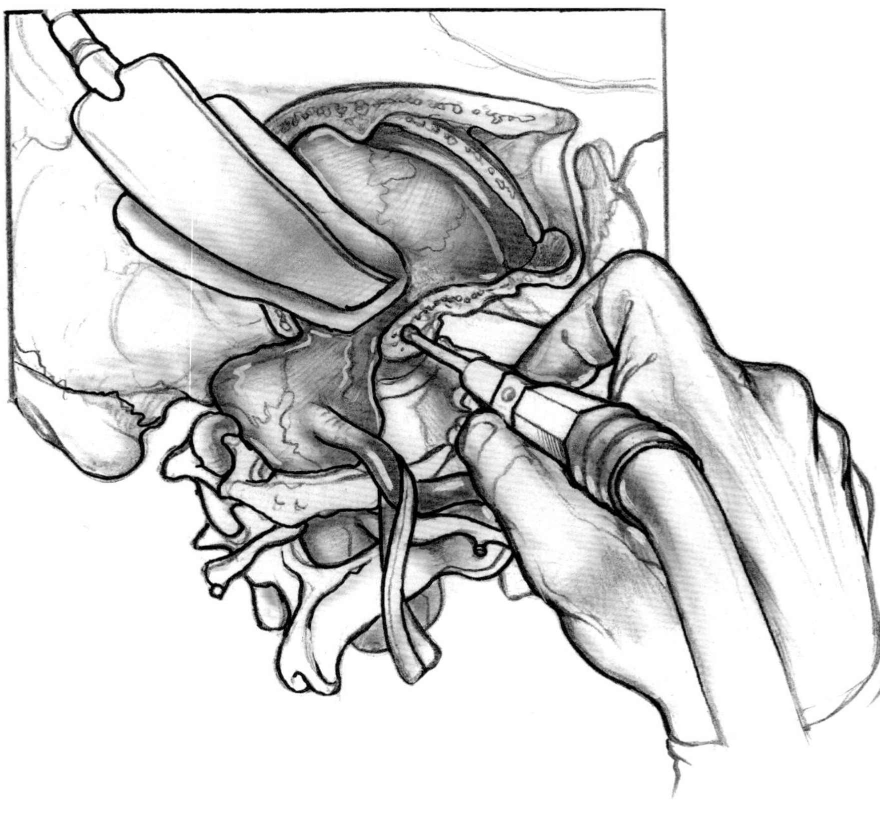

Figure 60–9 Complete resection of the occipital condyle exposes the hypoglossal canal and destabilizes the craniocervical articulation.

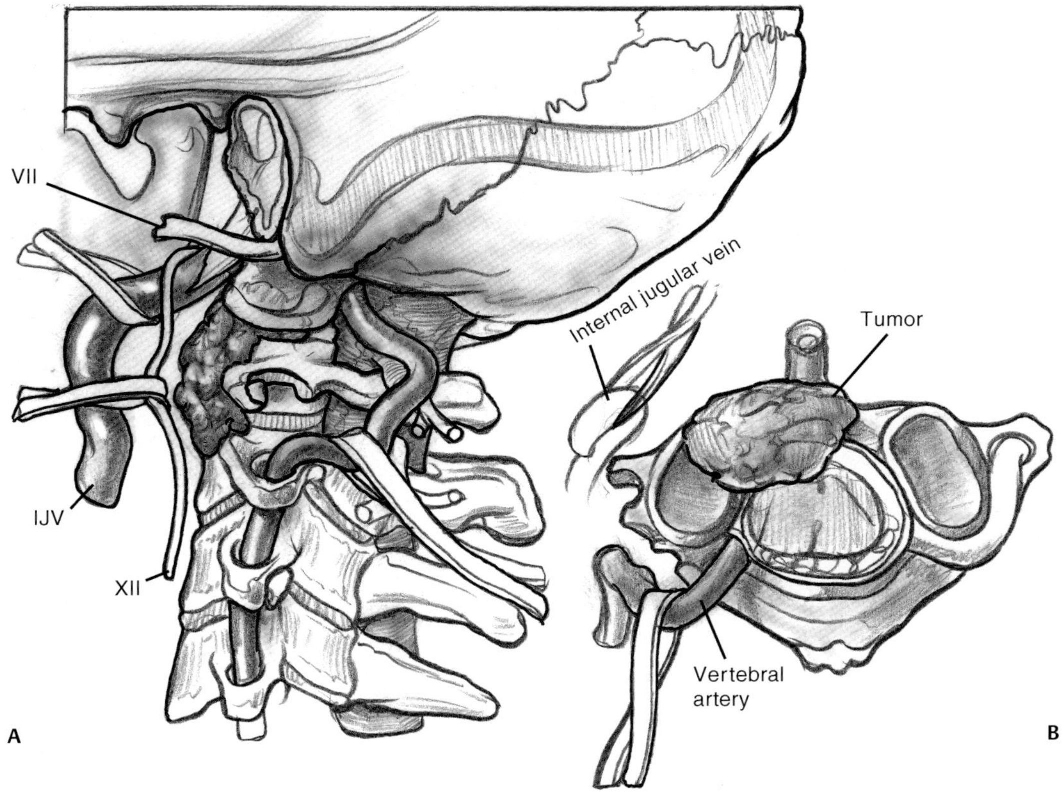

Figure 60–10 **(A)** Exposure of the anterior aspect of C1 and C2 between the vertebral artery posteriorly and the internal jugular vein anteriorly. **(B)** Axial diagram illustrating the same.

away to achieve a radical resection. Partial condylar resection does not render the occiput–C1 articulation unstable, but if the entire condyle is resected, an occipitocervical fusion is necessary for stabilization.

Exposure of the Anterior Aspect of C1-C2

Exposure of the Vertebral Artery

The attachment of the superior and inferior oblique muscles and the levator scapulae to the transverse process of C1 are taken down, and the ipsilateral posterior arch of C1 and the lamina of C2 are uncovered. The internal jugular vein, which is located immediately anterior to the C1 transverse process, is identified. The accessory nerve curves around the vein and passes by the transverse process of C1 to enter the sternomastoid muscle and is carefully protected. The C2 ganglion and the ventral and dorsal roots are fully exposed. The ventral root of C2 crosses the lateral aspect of the VA, between C2 and C1. The transverse process of C1 is freed of the muscle attachments and the transverse foramen for the VA is defined. The VA is completely uncovered by removing the transverse process with rongeurs while protecting the artery and the venous plexus around it. Developing a subperiosteal plane in the bony canal, the artery is displaced out of the canal. The artery is dissected out of the venous sheath beginning at the C2 transverse foramen until where it enters the dura behind the lateral mass of C1. The artery can now be reflected posteriorly with a vessel loop while the internal jugular vein and the accessory nerve are pushed anteriorly, creating access to the anterior aspect of C1 and C2 **(Fig. 60–10)**.

Exposure of the Tumor

The posterior arch of C1 is removed from the lateral mass to the posterior tubercle to expose the lateral surface of the spinal dura from the foramen magnum to C2. If there is higher extension of the tumor, a portion of the occipital bone is also removed at the foramen magnum. Similarly, for a caudal extension, the C2 hemilamina is removed. The dura is opened along the lateral surface of the thecal sac, just posterior to the C2 ganglion. The intradural tumor, a meningioma, or a schwannoma is easily visualized at this point. The dentate ligaments over two or more segments are cut so that the spinal cord can be rotated to some degree, and tumor resection is performed using standard microsurgical techniques.

For extradural neoplasms or removal of the odontoid process,[9] the lateral mass of C1 is completely drilled down from the occipital condyle to the articulation of C2, and the bone removal is continued anteriorly until healthy bone is reached. The prevertebral soft tissues, especially the pharynx, must be carefully dissected from the tumor. The extent of bony removal that is required in resecting extradural lesions usually renders the craniovertebral junction unstable. An occipitocervical stabilization and fusion is necessary and is performed at the same sitting as described elsewhere in this book.

Closure

The dura is closed with a fascial graft, but a watertight closure is usually not possible. The mastoid air cells are thoroughly obliterated with bone wax. The muscles are reapproximated in layers. The subcutaneous and skin layers are approximated with closely applied sutures. A drain is not usually necessary.

References

1. de Oliveira E, Rhoton AL Jr, Peace D. Microsurgical anatomy of the region of the foramen magnum. Surg Neurol 1985;24:293–352
2. Heros RC. Lateral suboccipital approach for vertebral and vertebrobasilar artery lesions. J Neurosurg 1986;64:559–562
3. Bertalanffy H, Seeger W. The dorsolateral suboccipital, transcondylar approach to the lower clivus and anterior portion of the craniocervical junction. Neurosurgery 1991;29:815–821
4. George B, Dematons C, Cophignon J. Lateral approach to the anterior portion of the foramen magnum. Surg Neurol 1988;29:484–490
5. Patel SJ, Sekhar LN, Cass SP, Hirsch BE. Combined approaches for resection of extensive glomus jugulare tumors. J Neurosurg 1994;80:1026–1038
6. Sen C, Sekhar LN. An extreme lateral approach to intradural lesions of the cervical spine and foramen magnum. Neurosurgery 1990;27:197–204
7. Sen C, Sekhar LN. Surgical management of anteriorly placed lesions of the craniocervical junction:—an alternative approach. Acta Neurochir (Wien) 1991;108:70–77
8. Spetzler RF, Grahm TW. The far lateral approach to the inferior clivus and the upper cervical region: technical note. BNI Q 1990;6:35–38
9. Al-Mefty O, Borba LAB, Aoki N, Angtuaco E, Glenn Pait T. The transcondylar approach to nonneoplastic lesions of the craniocervical junction. J Neurosurg 1996;84:1–6
10. Lang J, Kessler B. About the suboccipital part of the vertebral artery and the neighbouring bone, joint and nerve relationships. Skull Base Surg 1991;1:64–72
11. Salas E, Ziyal IM, Bank WO, Santi MR, Sekhar LN. Extradural origin of the posteroinferior cerebellar artery: an anatomic study with histological and radiographic correlation. Neurosurgery 1998;42:1326–1331

61

Foramen Magnum Meningiomas: An Extreme Lateral Approach

Chandranath Sen and Chun Siang Chen

Meningiomas constitute the majority of benign intradural extramedullary neoplasms found at the foramen magnum. There is a female preponderance, as there is elsewhere with meningiomas, and they are commonly found between the fourth and sixth decades of life. They were initially classified as craniospinal and spinocranial, depending on their primary site of attachment. The craniospinal type is anterior and anterolateral in location, whereas the spinocranial type is posterior and posterolateral. However, from a practical standpoint, it is more useful to classify meningiomas as anterior, anterolateral, and posterior. This classification influences the surgical approach and predicts the potential technical difficulties and complications.[1,2] The extreme lateral approach is very well suited for anteriorly as well as anterolaterally situated meningiomas at the foramen magnum region.[3–5]

◆ Considerations in Planning the Surgical Approach

The preoperative magnetic resonance imaging (MRI) and computed tomographic (CT) scans as well as vertebral arteriogram are carefully reviewed for the following findings to formulate the surgical approach:

1. Location of the tumor: anterior, anterolateral, or posterior
2. Craniocaudal extent of the tumor: whether the tumor extends above the jugular foramen
3. The dominance of the vertebral artery and its relation to the tumor, especially where it enters the dura of the posterior fossa
4. The origin of the posterior inferior cerebellar artery in relation to the tumor
5. If the tumor extends above the jugular foramen or into it, the sigmoid sinus, the jugular bulb, and the jugular veins on both sides should be evaluated with an arteriogram or magnetic resonance (MR) venogram.

The operation that is described here pertains to the following situation: the tumor is anteriorly situated at the foramen magnum and is surrounding the vertebral artery (VA) where it enters the dura. The origin of the posterior inferior cerebellar artery (PICA) is also surrounded by the tumor. There are variations in these findings, and the operation needs to be tailored to the particular patient and to the surgical goals. This is especially true in terms of the need for exposure and drilling of the condyle and the amount of exposure and isolation of the VA that may be required.

◆ Operative Procedure

The patient positioning, anesthesia, and intraoperative monitoring are performed as described in Chapter 60 (see Fig. 60–1).

◆ Surgical Technique

Incision, Soft Tissue Dissection, and Exposure of the Vertebral Artery

An inverted-L–shaped incision is used with the horizontal limb directed posteriorly from the mastoid process at the level of the pinna while the vertical limb is directed straight

Figure 61–1 Diagram of the inside view of the posterior fossa showing the relation of the bone drilling carried into the jugular tubercle and the posterior part of the occipital condyle, to allow direct access to the anterior portion of the tumor.

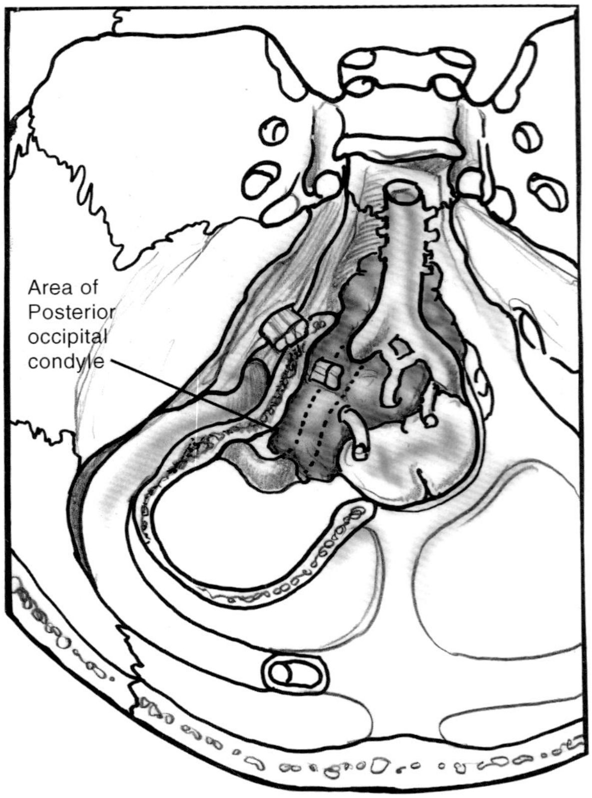

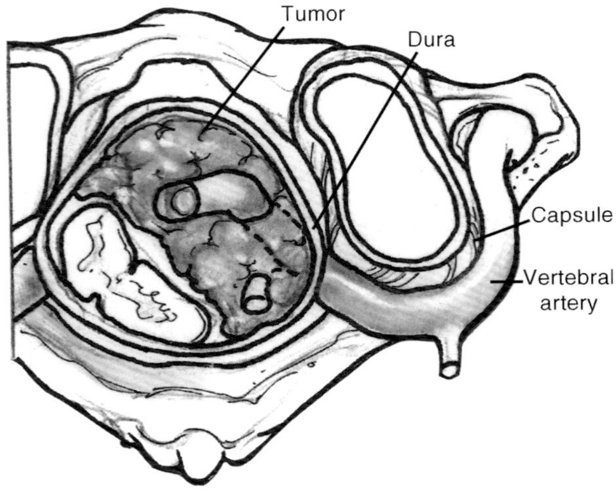

Figure 61–2 Diagram showing the intradural course of the vertebral artery through the tumor and its relation to the occiput–C1 articulation. It can be easily followed that in a situation like this, to expose a small amount of the dura in front of the entry point of the artery, the posterior part of the occipital condyle needs to be drilled away.

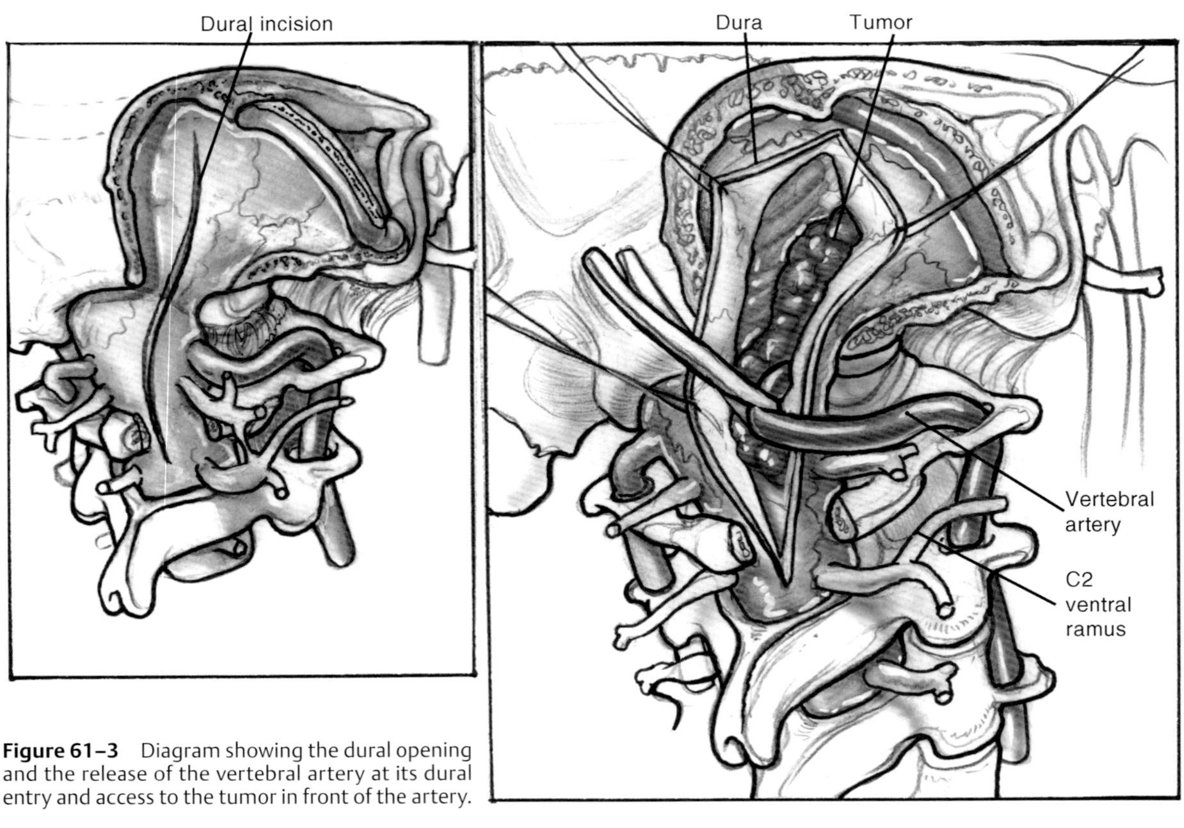

Figure 61–3 Diagram showing the dural opening and the release of the vertebral artery at its dural entry and access to the tumor in front of the artery.

downward into the neck behind the sternomastoid muscle (see Chapter 60, Fig. 60–2). The muscles in the posterior cervical triangle are dissected in layers as described in the Chapter 60, and the suboccipital area of the skull as well as the ipsilateral lamina of C1 and C2 are exposed (see Chapter 60, Figs. 60–3 and 60–4). The VA is identified above the C1 arch and the venous sheath around it is removed to expose the artery itself. The artery is separated from the joint capsule of the occiput–C1 articulation, and a vessel loop is placed around the artery to control it (see Chapter 60, Fig. 60–5). The site where the artery enters the dura of the posterior fossa is identified. Venous bleeding from the area of the condylar emissary vein is controlled with Surgicel packing.

Bony Opening

A craniectomy is made with a high-speed drill in the retrosigmoid area to include the foramen magnum. The posterior edge of the sigmoid sinus and jugular bulb are exposed (**Fig. 61–1**; also see Chapter 60, Fig. 60–6). While protecting the VA, the C1 hemilamina is removed up to the transverse process. Inferior to the jugular bulb, the bone is carefully drilled away, thus removing the jugular tubercle. The bone is drilled down to a thin cortical shell, which is then removed with a small Kerrison punch. In a similar manner, a small amount of the posterior part of the occipital condyle is drilled away to expose some dura anterior to the entry site of the VA (**Fig. 61–2**; also see Chapter 60, Figs. 60–7 to 60–9). This drilling does not extend up to the hypoglossal canal, which traverses the middle of the condyle.

Dural Opening and Tumor Resection

The dura is opened vertically in a linear fashion behind the sigmoid sinus and the VA. The tumor is removed in a piecemeal manner looking for the accessory nerve ascending to the jugular foramen and also the PICA. The dural opening is extended anteriorly, to the VA entry point and then carefully carried around the artery so that the vessel is completely freed from the dura (**Fig. 61–3**; also see Chapter 60, Fig. 60–6). The artery is then followed into the posterior fossa and the tumor is resected around it. In this manner the surgeon is looking up into the foramen magnum, along the course of the artery. The artery is moved posteriorly with the aid of the vessel loop and the tumor at the anterior aspect of the lower clivus is removed. By working initially at the base of the tumor, the remaining tumor is devascularized, making the resection relatively easy and facilitating preservation of the cranial nerves and important vessels that are intimately involved by the tumor. Proceeding superiorly, the caudal cranial nerves are carefully sought out. If these nerves are intimately involved by the tumor, the pros and cons of their manipulation must be carefully considered because impairment of their function can be quite disabling. Because the dural base of the tumor is easily accessible, it can be excised if so desired. Venous bleeding encountered while excising the dural base is also controlled by packing with Surgicel.

Dural Closure

The dura is closed with a dural graft using a fascia or dural substitute, but a watertight closure is seldom possible. A piece of autologous fat is placed on the dura and the VA. The bone is thoroughly sealed with bone wax, especially if the mastoid air cells have been entered. The muscles are reapproximated in a layer-by-layer manner. A local tissue drain is usually not left. The skin and subcutaneous tissues are closed well because a subcutaneous cerebrospinal fluid collection is not uncommon.

◆ Postoperative Care

A cervical collar is not necessary. If a substantial subcutaneous fluid collection forms, a lumbar spinal drain may be inserted for 3 or 4 days to prevent jeopardizing the suture line. Steroid medications are rapidly tapered off. Oral feedings are resumed early unless there is reason to expect impairment of the caudal cranial nerves. In such a situation a swallowing study is undertaken prior to oral alimentation. Dysphagia is an indication for a temporary gastrostomy, especially in the elderly or a frail patient because proper nutrition is essential for recovery and avoidance of complications.

References

1. George B, Lot G, Velut S, Gelbert F, Mourier KL. Tumors of the foramen magnum. [in French] Society of Neurosurgery. 44th Annual Congress. Brussels, June 8–12, 1993. Neurochirurgie 1993;39(Suppl 1):1–89
2. Samii M, Klekamp J, Carvalho G. Surgical results for meningiomas of the craniocervical junction. Neurosurgery 1996;39:1086–1095
3. Babu RP, Sekhar LN, Wright DC. Extreme lateral transcondylar approach: technical improvements and lessons learned. J Neurosurg 1994;81:49–59
4. Kratimenos G, Crockard HA. The far lateral approach for ventrally placed foramen magnum and upper cervical spine tumours. Br J Neurosurg 1993;7:129–140
5. Sen C, Sekhar LN. An extreme lateral approach to intradural lesions of the cervical spine and foramen magnum. Neurosurgery 1990;27: 197–204

62

Acoustic Neuroma: Retrosigmoid and Transpetrosal Approaches

Laligam N. Sekhar, Sajjan Sarma, and Amitabha Chanda

Acoustic neuromas are a commonly encountered neurosurgical problem, but their optimal treatment with excellent outcome requires considerable skill, experience, and judgment, especially important now with the availability of radiosurgery for the treatment of these tumors. This chapter discusses the treatment of these lesions by retrosigmoid and transpetrosal approaches.

Preoperative Diagnosis

The diagnosis of an acoustic neuroma (also termed vestibular schwannoma) is usually made by an audiogram, and a computed tomographic (CT) or magnetic resonance imaging (MRI) scan. If an audiogram has not been performed, it is important to obtain one with pure tones and speech discrimination scores in a reputable audiology laboratory. Magnetic resonance scanning is important, with contrast administration, and T2-weighted images. Coronal images are important to see if the tumor has grown superiorly into the tentorial notch or inferiorly toward the jugular foramen. On T2-weighted images, the surgeon can assess whether the tumor extends all the way into the fundus of the internal auditory canal (IAC), which is of prognostic importance when hearing preservation is a goal of the surgery. We measure the tumor diameters (D_1, D_2, D_3) in three planes in the cerebellopontine angle—axial, sagittal, and coronal—and derive the tumor equivalent diameter (TED = $\sqrt[3]{D1 \times D2 \times D3}$).

A bone window CT scan is usually performed to look for air cells in the petrous bone, and the location of the posterior semicircular canal in relation to the origin of the IAC. A cerebral angiogram is performed in giant-sized tumors ($\geq$ 4.0 cm) in which the transpetrosal approach is being considered—primarily to view the arterial supply to the tumor and the anatomy of the veins and sinus pertinent to the approach. The arterial supply to the acoustic neuromas is usually derived from branches of the anterior inferior cerebellar artery (AICA) and some meningeal branches of the external and internal carotid arteries. Venous information that may be important includes the anatomy of the petrosal vein and the vein of Labbé, and of the sigmoid and transverse sinus and the superior petrosal sinus.

Surgical Treatment Options and Approaches

When the patient is diagnosed as having an acoustic neuroma, several treatment options exist: no treatment with observation, radiosurgery, and microsurgery **(Table 62–1).** When microsurgery is elected, the most common approach is the retrosigmoid. The translabyrinthine approach is used by the senior author (LNS) only for tumors smaller than 2.5 cm in patients with no hearing. Even for intracanalicular tumors reaching into the fundus of the internal acoustic canal, with the use of endoscope-assisted microsurgery, the middle fossa approach is unnecessary.

For tumors larger than 4.0 cm, and particularly those that extend superiorly into the tentorial notch (rather than toward the jugular foramen), the transpetrosal approach is preferred, which allows better dissection of the upper portion of the tumor and better tumor dissection from the brain stem.

Table 62–1 Acoustic Neuroma

Microsurgery	Radiosurgery	No Treatment, Observation
Retrosigmoid approach; most tumors ≤ 4.0 cm	Tumor size ≤ 2.5 cm Physiological problems Patents' preference	Tumor size ≤ 1.0 cm Elderly patient Physiological problems
Translabyrinthine approach; tumor size ≤ 2.5 cm; poor hearing		
Transpetrosal approach; tumor size > 4.0 cm; tumor extends into the tentorial notch and small posterior fossa		

◆ Retrosigmoid Approach

Surgical Technique

Anesthesia

The anesthesia is similar to that for other brain tumors, with control of the airway and intracranial pressure. Of major importance is that the patient cannot be relaxed, to allow the monitoring of facial nerve function. The patient is given 2 g of ceftazidime and 10 mg of dexamethasone at the beginning of the operation. Half a gram per kilogram body weight of mannitol is also administered intravenously at the time of the skin incision.

In a young patient with a small or a medium-size tumor, a lumbar drain can be inserted at the beginning of the operation to relax the brain. In the majority of the patients, steroids, hyperventilation, and cisternal drainage can provide adequate relaxation.

After the facial nerve dissection is completed the patient may be relaxed to facilitate the administration of different anesthetic agents and to allow a smooth and rapid emergence from the anesthesia.

Neuromonitoring

In patients undergoing acoustic neuroma surgery, it is important to monitor the brain stem and cranial nerve (CN) VII and VIII function **(Table 62–2).**

When hearing preservation is the goal of surgery, CN VIII monitoring is performed. Unless the eighth nerve can be seen near the brain stem as a nearly normal nerve, direct electronic monitoring of CN VIII is not possible.

Table 62–2 Neuromonitoring for Acoustic Neuroma Operation

Brain stem function	Somatosensory evoked potential (SEP) Contralateral auditory brain response (ABR)
Facial nerve function	Facial electromyography in frontalis, orbicularis oculi, and mentalis muscles Intraoperative stimulation of cranial nerve (CN) VII
Cochlear nerve function	Ipsilateral ABR Direct electronic monitoring of CN VIII

Retrosigmoid Approach for Small- and Medium-Size Tumors

When the tumor has grown more toward the brain stem, the patient's head is turned slightly toward the surgeon. When it has grown more toward the fundus of the internal acoustic canal, the head is turned slightly toward the floor, from the neutral position. Before making the incision, some landmarks should be marked: the tip of the mastoid process, the bass of the mastoid process, the inion, and the zygomatic arch. A line drawn from the inion to the zygomatic arch represents the approximate course of the transverse sinus, and a second line along the posterior border of the mastoid process represents the sigmoid sinus **(Fig. 62–1).** It must be

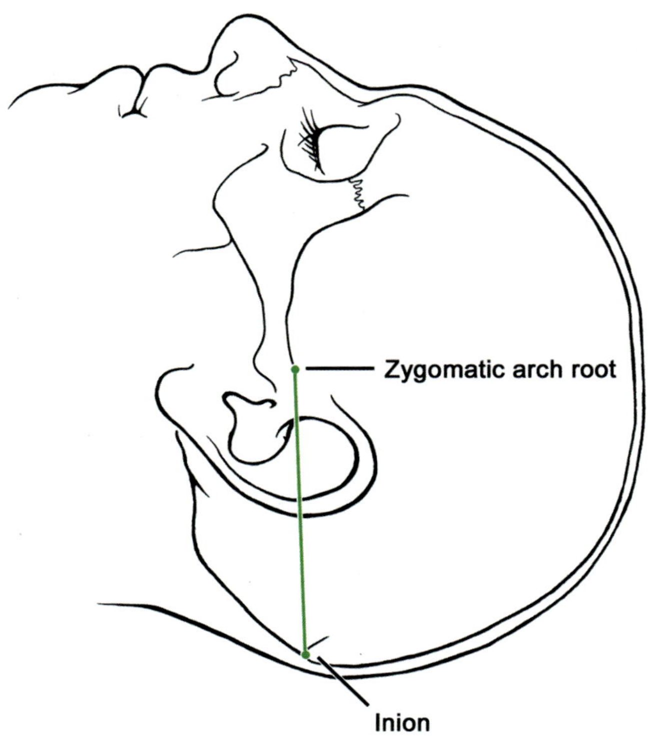

Figure 62–1 The line drawn from the inion to the zygomatic arch represents the approximate position of the lateral sinus, and the line drawn along the posterior border of the mastoid process represents the approximate position of the sigmoid sinus.

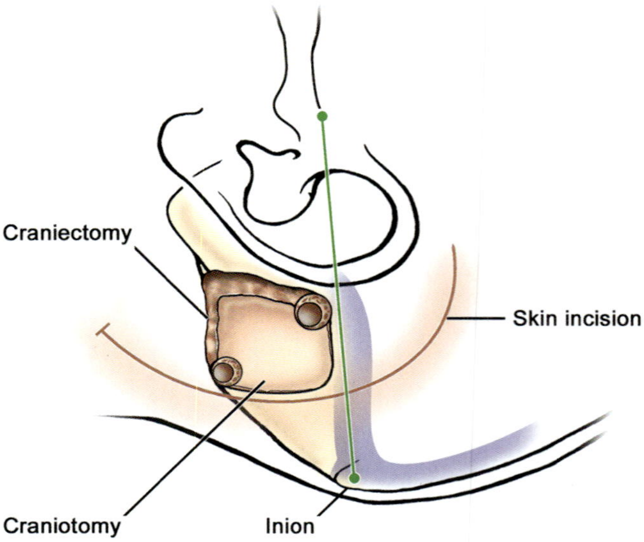

Figure 62–2 Two bur hole sites and the proposed area of craniotomy/craniectomy. The site of the first bur hole in relation to the transverse–sigmoid sinus junction is noted.

recognized that on the right side the sigmoid sinus is usually dominant and large as compared with that on the left, and many variations are possible. The surgeon should observe the anatomy of the sinus on a gadolinium-enhanced MRI scan preoperatively. The outer wall of the sigmoid sinus is curved and may be adherent to the mastoid bone, especially in older patients. Because of this, the position of the bur holes for a craniotomy and craniectomy is very important.

The skin incision is C-shaped, and its apex should be ~4 cm posterior to the posterior edge of the mastoid process **(Fig. 62–2).** It is difficult to retract the skin posteriorly; therefore, the incision should extend as far back as the planned posterior edge of the craniotomy. The skin incision and the suboccipital muscles are infiltrated with 0.5% Xylocaine with epinephrine, which reduces bleeding. The skin flap is raised along with the sternomastoid muscle and fascia. The lesser occipital nerve is frequently divided along the line of the incision. It is tagged with 4–0 neurolon stitch, and reanastomosed at the end of the operation with a 7–0 Prolene stitch. The remaining suboccipital muscles (splenius capitis, semispinalis capitis, longissimus capitis, and recti capitis muscles) are split along the direction of the fibers, at the anterior and the posterior limits of the incision, divided at their cranial attachment, and reflected inferiorly. This technique minimizes the muscle-related pain. The occipital artery is divided deep to the digastric groove and must be ligated or cauterized carefully with bipolar forceps to prevent later reopening of the vessel.

Two bur holes are then made, one just posteroinferior to the presumed location of the sigmoid–transverse sinus junction, and the other at the inferomedial corner of the exposure. The first bur hole is generally just away from the venous sinuses. If it is, the dura mater is separated with a bent Cottle elevator or a Penfield no. 1 instrument, and a craniotomy is performed with the Midas Rex (Medronics Co., Fort Worth, TX) instrumentation. If there is any difficulty with the separation of the dura mater, it is best to limit the craniotomy to the separated region and then perform an additional craniotomy or craniectomy as needed. It may be necessary to drill away some of the mastoid bone to expose the edge of the sigmoid sinus. If the mastoid emissary vein is bleeding, it may be controlled with a small piece of bone wax and Surgicel if still encased by bone, or by bipolar cautery if completely free of bone. All exposed air cells must be closed by bone wax.

Small tears in the sigmoid sinus may be controlled by packing Surgicel. However, if the sinus is a dominant one, it is best to control the bleeding with a cottonoid, then expose the sinus further by drilling away bone, and repair it with 6–0 or 7–0 Prolene sutures. A small dural patch may be needed to repair a large laceration.

Additional craniectomy is usually performed inferiorly to expose the "floor" of the posterior fossa. This refers to the point where the dura mater turns from a vertical to a horizontal direction. Because the sigmoid sinus moves more laterally inferiorly, the craniectomy also extends more laterally in the inferior area. When completed, the dural exposure extends from the edge of the transverse sinus to the floor of the posterior fossa, and laterally from beyond the sigmoid sinus.

The intradural portion of the operation is performed under the surgical microscope, with the surgeon seated comfortably behind the patient. The first step is to make a small dural incision at the anteroinferior portion of the exposure **(Fig. 62–3).** The cerebellum may be full at this time but should not herniate out of the dural opening. If it does, additional measures to reduce the intracranial pressure may need to be instituted, such as additional intravenous mannitol, furosemide, or further hyperventilation, to lower the $PaCO_2$.

The surgeon's objective at this time is to open the arachnoid membrane of the lateral cerebellomedullary cistern to drain cerebrospinal fluid (CSF) and relax the brain. A rubber dam/cottonoid is placed on the cerebellum that is exposed, and with gentle retraction it is advanced to the cistern. If an endoscope is available, a 0 degree, 2.5 mm rigid endoscope

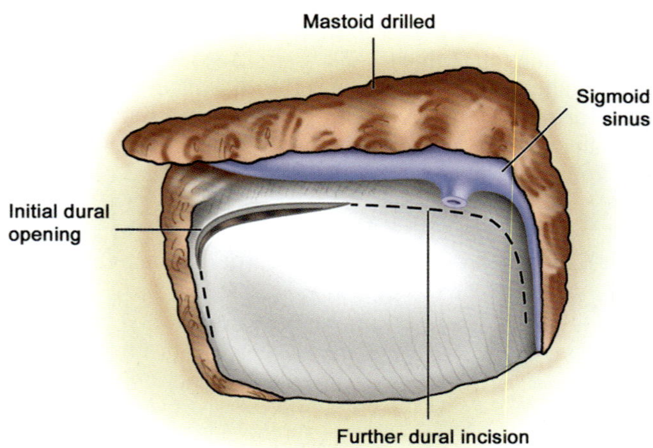

Figure 62–3 The initial dural opening and the line of further dural opening. The proposed craniotomy/craniectomy has been done, and the margin of the sigmoid sinus is seen at the edge of the craniotomy.

can be used instead. The arachnoid is incised with an arachnoid knife with CSF draining out for a few minutes to relax the cerebellum.

In some patients, a small vein may be present in this area, and it may be torn. It should be directly visualized and avoided or cauterized and divided.

The remainder of the dura mater is then opened in a C-shaped fashion, T-ed laterally in one or two places, and tacked up to the tissues laterally, retracting the sigmoid sinus in the process.

The technique for the removal of a medium-size to large tumor (1.0 to 2.5 cm in the cerebellopontine angle) with intact hearing is described first. After the dural opening, the retractor is moved over the midportion of the cerebellum. The cerebellum is never retracted more than 2.0 cm from the petrous dura, and most of the operation can be performed with no retraction at all. The acoustic neuroma is enclosed by two layers of arachnoid, the first being the peripheral layer of the posterior fossa, and the second being the layer that envelops the tumor itself **(Fig. 62–4).** The dissection of the tumor is usually performed between the two layers, or between the tumor and the deep arachnoidal layer. The initial view reveals the tumor (grayish or yellowish in color), the anterior inferior cerebellar artery (AICA) with its subarcuate, the tumoral branches, the petrosal vein, and frequently the eighth cranial nerve **(Fig. 62–4),** with its fibers splayed over the surface of the tumor. The arachnoid membrane is opened, and the subarcuate artery (which goes into the subarcuate fossa superior to the porus acusticus), is cauterized and divided. A rare variant of the AICA is the *subarcuate type* of the artery, in which the main artery itself loops into and out of the dura mater posterior to the internal acoustic canal. In such cases, the dura mater must be incised around the artery and reflected medially along with the vessel. The petrosal vein can generally be preserved in small and medium-size tumors, but may need to be cauterized and divided with large and giant-size tumors, to facilitate the dissection of the upper pole.

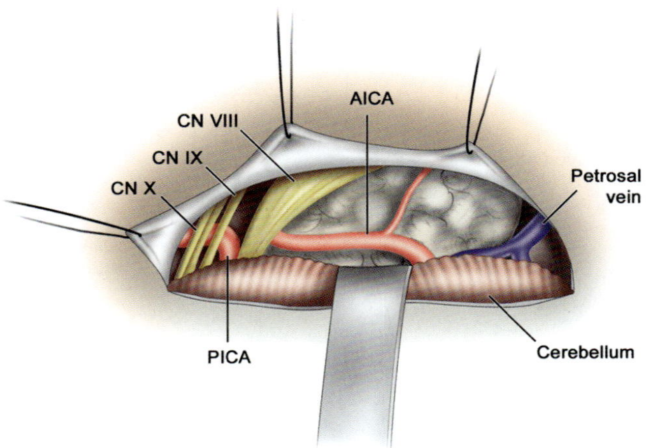

Figure 62–4 The initial view after gentle retraction of the cerebellum and drainage of some cerebrospinal fluid (CSF). The lower cranial nerves, posterior inferior cerebellar artery (PICA), part of cranial nerve VIII, anterior inferior cerebellar artery (AICA), and petrosal vein are seen along with the tumor.

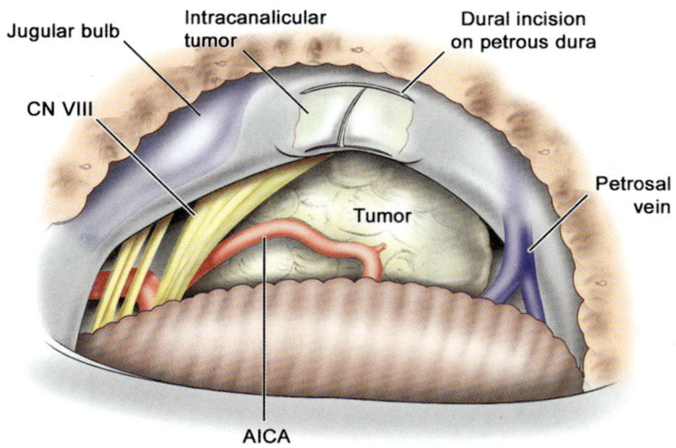

Figure 62–5 The dural incision on the petrous dura before drilling of the internal auditory canal.

The posterior tumor capsule is stimulated at this point to look for the facial nerve. Only with recurrent tumors and in patients with Neurofibromatosis Type 2 may the facial nerve be in this rare location. The petrous bone is usually drilled away at this stage to expose the tumor inside the IAC. The entrance of the IAC is generally apparent, but if it is not, it can be confirmed by placing a small blunt microhook (Rhoton no. 9, V. Mueller, Chicago, IL) into it. There may be adhesions between the tumor capsule and the dura of the petrous bone through which blood vessels enter the tumor, and these are cauterized and divided. Incisions are made into the dura along the axis of the IAC and perpendicular to it **(Fig. 62–5),** extending no more than 1 cm lateral to the porus acusticus. Using a high- or low-speed drill, with frequent irrigation and breaks, the bone is drilled away 180 degrees around the dural envelope of the tumor. It is important to drill the bone more extensively than just a trough to facilitate tumor dissection. In the superior aspect of the drilling, care must be exercised with the facial nerve, which lies in the anteroinferior aspect of the envelope. In the inferior aspect of the bone exposure, a dominant jugular bulb may be found. If this is suspected from the preoperative MR venogram or MRI scan, then this aspect of the drilling must be done with a diamond drill and frequent irrigation to avoid damage to the bulb. The lateral extent of the drilling can be judged from the preoperative CT scans; however, it is unnecessary to drill more than 1 cm laterally because of the use of the neuroendoscope as an adjunct to remove the tumor from this area.

After the drilling is completed, the dural envelope of the tumor in the IAC is opened **(Fig. 62–6).** The next step is to convert a solid tumor into a hollow one because the surgical field is smaller than the tumor. A segment of the posterior tumor capsule is removed, and the interior of the tumor is

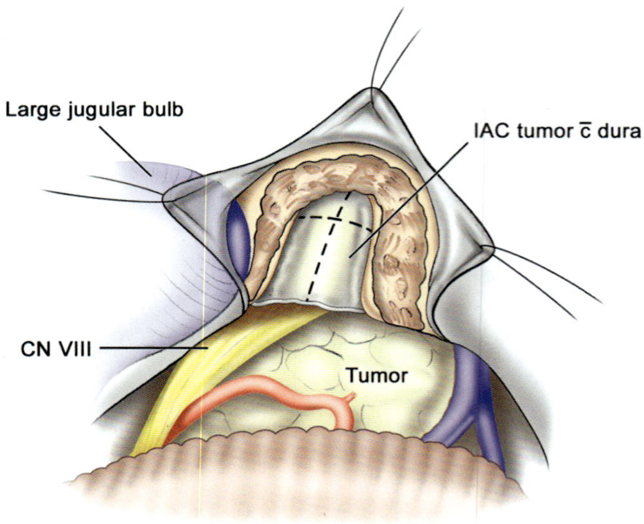

Figure 62–6 The line of incision of the dura of the internal auditory canal (IAC). The roof of the IAC has been drilled off and the tumor is seen going into the IAC.

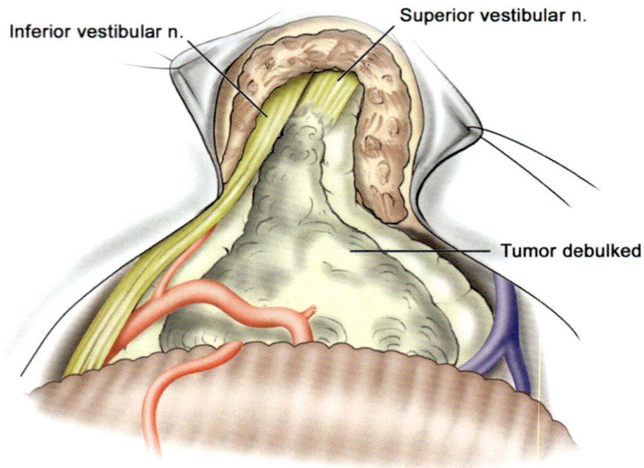

Figure 62–8 The usual position of the vestibular nerve in relation to the tumor. Good tumor debulking has already been done.

debulked by using bipolar cautery, an ultrasonic aspirator, pituitary forceps (used to crush the tumor rather than pull it), or a curved cutting instrument such as a Cottle elevator **(Fig. 62–7).**

Once the tumor is debulked, it is dissected away from the AICA and the eighth cranial nerve. This dissection is best performed sharply by pulling the tumor capsule away from the nerve and creating a cleavage plane using a microscissors or a Rhoton no. 3 dissector. The brain stem evoked responses (or the direct nerve action potentials if an electrode has been placed on the eighth nerve) are carefully watched during the tumor dissection **(Fig. 62–8).** The internal auditory branch of the AICA frequently accompanies the eighth cranial nerve and must be preserved. Vascular dissection is best performed by placing traction on the vessel with a suction tip and dissecting away the adhesions with microscissors **(Fig. 62–9).** Any small branches going to the tumor are coagulated away from the main vessel using low current on an angulated tip irrigating bipolar forceps. Such a forceps is also very useful while working on the tumor capsule in the vicinity of the nerve to avoid damage to it.

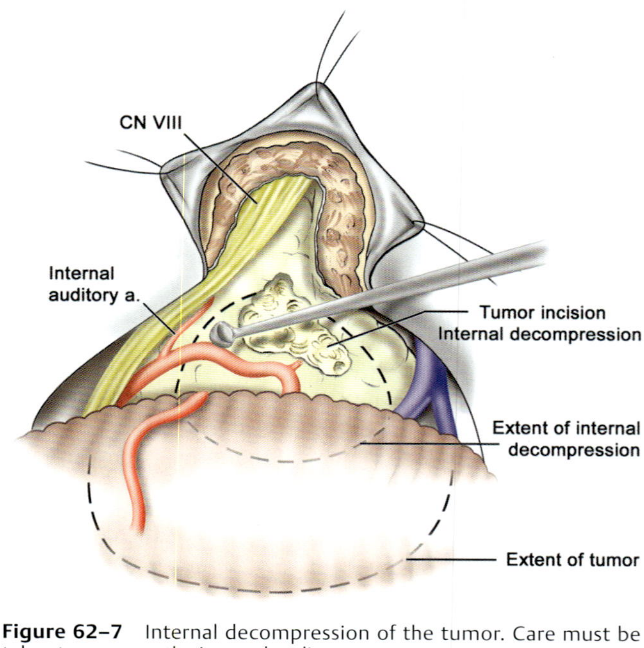

Figure 62–7 Internal decompression of the tumor. Care must be taken to preserve the internal auditory artery.

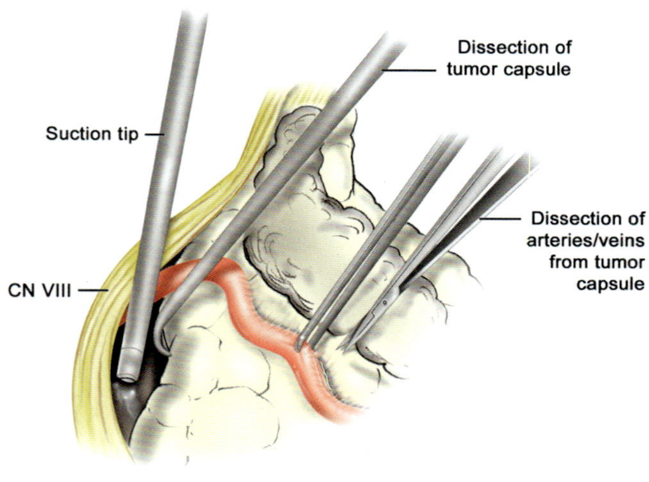

Figure 62–9 The method of separation of the tumor from the cerebellum/brain stem. The tumor is gently lifted from the surface, and with suction or microinstruments, fine adhesions are broken up.

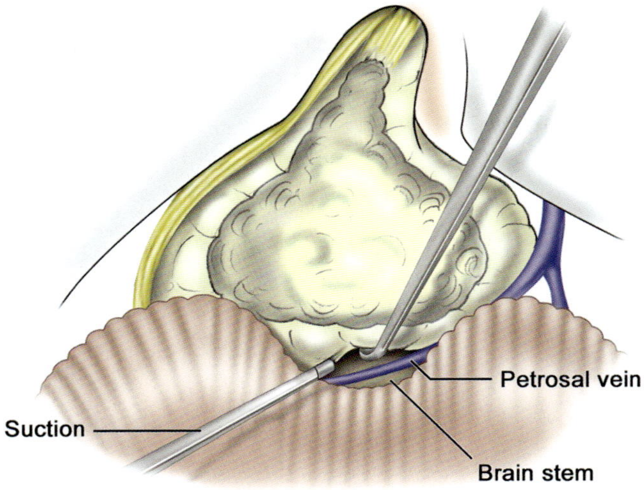

Figure 62–10 The method of dissection of an artery or a vein and CN VIII, from the tumor capsule. The structure is lifted up gently by a forceps or a suction tip, and adhesions are cut by microscissors.

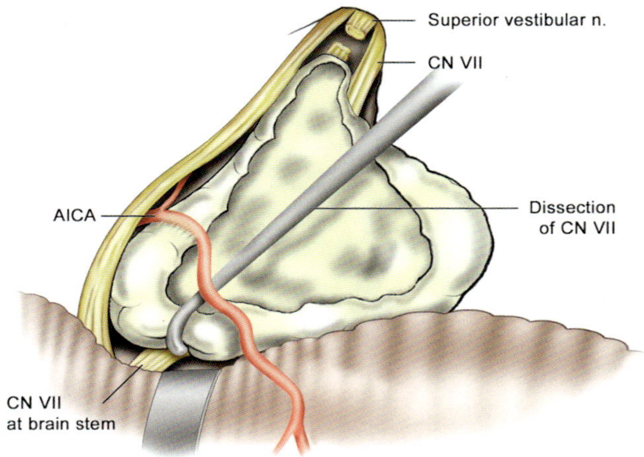

Figure 62–11 Dissection of CN VII at the brain stem from the tumor. Note the usual relation of the nerve to the anteroinferior surface of the tumor.

The next step is to dissect the tumor capsule from the brain stem and cerebellum **(Fig. 62–10).** The dissection is usually started near the upper pole of the tumor where it may be rapidly dissected from the trigeminal root. The upper and the medial pole of the tumor is then pulled away from the brain stem and cerebellum using a *two-hands technique* (suction in left hand to push the capsule away, with the dissector or bipolar forceps in the right hand to develop the plane or achieve hemostasis) or a *three-hands technique* (grasping the capsule with the forceps in the surgeon's left hand, and dissecting with the right, while the assistant provides the suction). This dissection is slowly extended along the middle and then the inferomedial pole of the tumor. This dissection must be strictly maintained in the arachnoid plane between the tumor and the brain stem. Some acoustic neuroma may be very vascular and associated with arterialized veins, which may be very troublesome. Such veins must be carefully cauterized to keep the field bloodless.

As tumor is dissected away, intermittent debulking is performed to reduce its mass. As the surgeon dissects away the inferomedial pole, the brain stem surface is frequently stimulated to look for the facial nerve root exit zone. The facial nerve exits the brain stem quite close to the entrance of the eighth cranial nerve but may be separated from it because of the distortion of the brain stem. The facial nerve is usually seen as a distinct nerve bundle, slightly grayer than the eighth nerve at its exit. With intermittent tumor debulking, the tumor is separated from the facial nerve toward the porus acusticus using a Rhoton no. 3 dissector, a sharp needle dissector, or microscissors. However, the dissection stops when the facial nerve becomes splayed or when it turns up into the porus acusticus **(Fig. 62–11).**

The lateral pole of the tumor is then dissected. It must be first debulked internally, and its capsule dissected away from the facial nerve superiorly and the cochlear nerve inferiorly **(Fig. 62–12).** Approximately 70% of tumors arise from the superior vestibular nerve, whereas 20% of tumors arise from the inferior vestibular nerve. The fascicles of the vestibular nerve that lead into the tumor are divided, whereas normal vestibular nerve fascicles are preserved. The inferior vestibular nerve and the cochlear nerve are usually adherent to each other, and the surgeon should not try to separate them. The auditory

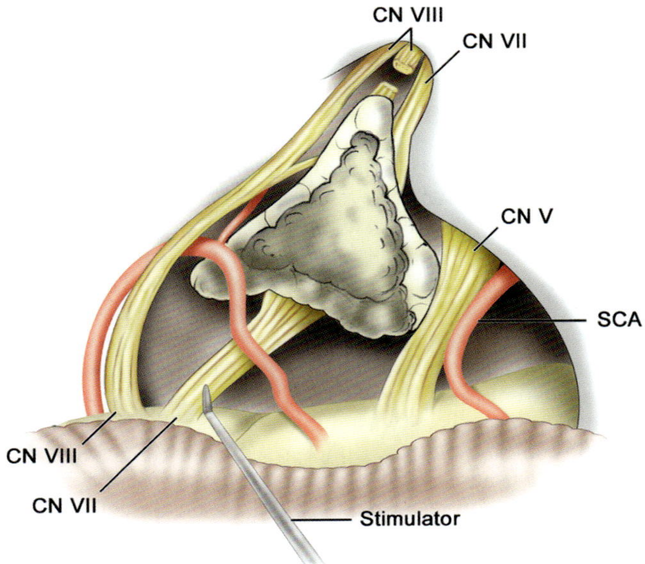

Figure 62–12 The tumor has been separated from the brain stem. The functional integrity of CN VII has been checked by stimulating with the nerve stimulator. A good electromyographic response with low-current stimulation indicates normal functioning of the nerve.

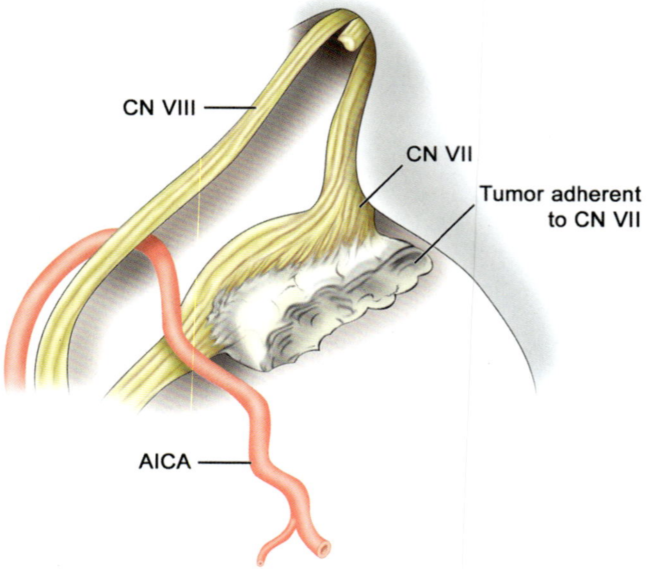

Figure 62–13 A small piece of tumor adherent to the CN VII. This is the most difficult part of the tumor dissection from the nerve. AICA, anterior inferior carebellar artery.

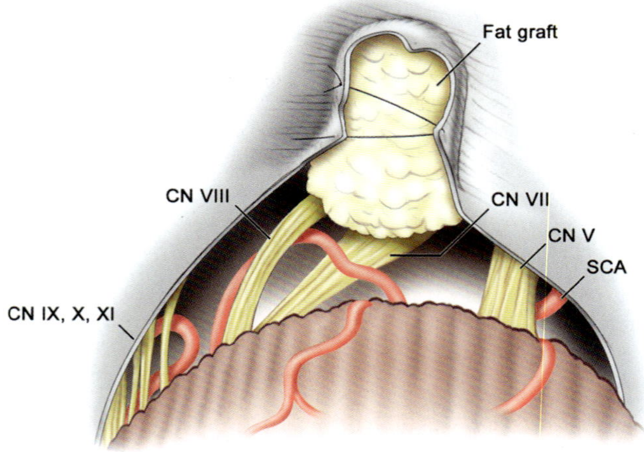

Figure 62–14 After complete tumor excision, the internal auditory canal (IAC) has been filled with fat graft, which has been secured by putting a few stitches through the petrosal dura. The IAC must not be overpacked to avoid compression of CNs VII and VIII.

brain stem response (ABR) must be carefully observed while dissecting tumor in any location. If it changes, the surgeon must pause and allow it to recover. If it does not, the surgeon must try to find the cause, which may require further tumor debulking, moving the tumor away from the eighth nerve, or applying of papaverine to eliminate vasospasm.

The tumor is now dissected away from the facial nerve proceeding in both directions (mediolateral and lateromedial) toward the most difficult area, which lies just proximal to the porus acusticus **(Fig. 62–13).** The facial nerve monitor must be audible at this stage, and intermittent stimulation is used to verify the position of the nerve. Both parallel dissection along the fiber of the nerve and dissection perpendicular to the nerve fascicles may be necessary. Sometimes it is hard to judge whether a filament is facial nerve, arachnoid membrane, or a fascicle of the eighth nerve (vestibular fascicle). Stimulation with low-intensity current (0.1 to 0.2 mA) can distinguish the facial nerve fascicle as long as the nerve is physiologically intact. Rarely, especially in an older person or in a patient with a cystic tumor, the surgeon may need to leave behind a small piece of tumor that is directly adherent to the nerve.

The endoscope is now used to check for tumor in the lateral ends of the IAC. If any tumor is seen, it is removed using angled instruments while looking at the endoscope monitor. The endoscope is also useful to look for air cells in the drilled bone. Small air cells are closed with bone wax, whereas large areas are closed with a piece of Surgicel and bone wax. Additional closure of the IAC is effected with a fat graft. A small piece of fat graft is extracted from the abdomen or thigh and placed so as to fill the opening in the IAC but not compress CN VII and VIII. It is held in place with a few sutures to the dura on the petrous ridge, and reinforced with fibrin glue **(Fig. 62–14).**

For larger tumors in which hearing preservation is not a goal, the dissection steps are very similar. The major difference is that the lower pole of the tumor may have to be elevated away from the lower cranial nerves after initial tumor debulking, which may aid in the identification of the facial nerve. The eighth nerve is divided as it enters the brain stem. The facial nerve exit zone lies just anterior to the entrance of the ninth nerve and the choroid plexus. In addition, the AICA may also be used as a landmark because it usually passes between the seventh and eighth nerves. In rare cases, facial nerve dissection may need to be done entirely from the IAC lateromedially.

The facial nerve must be stimulated at the end of the operation, at the brain stem. If it can be stimulated at an intensity 0.2 mA, near-normal function can be expected postoperatively. If it is stimulated but at a higher threshold, facial nerve weakness may be expected postoperatively. If the facial nerve cannot be stimulated at the brain stem up to a stimulus intensity of 2 mA, the nerve must be carefully inspected along its entire length to determine if it is anatomically intact. The loss of a short segment can be repaired by direct nerve suture. A longer segmental loss requires a nerve graft. The sural nerve or the greater auricular nerve is used to interpose the two ends, and one suture of 10–0 or 9–0 nylon supplemented with fibrin glue is adequate. If the facial nerve stump cannot be found at the brain stem, there is no alternative other than to perform a hypoglossal-facial anastomosis about 1 to 2 months later.

At the conclusion of the operation, the cerebellum must be carefully inspected for contusions, and if any are found, they are resected and covered with Surgicel (Ethicon, Johnson

& Johnson, Somerville, NJ). The dura mater is usually shrunken, and usually a graft of pericranium or Dura-guard (Biovascular Inc., St. Paul, MN) is used to close the posterior fossa with some space allowance for cerebellum swelling. A watertight closure with suture is supplemented with fibrin glue (Haemacure Corp., Sarasota, FL).

The bone flap is reapproximated with titanium microplates. Any small bone defects are covered with Bonesource cement (Stryker Liebinger, Kalamazoo, MI). If the bone defect is large, a titanium mesh (Stryker Liebinger) is used as a scaffolding, and bone-source cement is used for cranioplasty. The muscles and the skin are closed in layers, and if the lesser occipital nerve was divided, it is reattached with 7–0 Prolene sutures.

Transpetrosal Approach

For giant-size acoustic neuromas, larger than 4.0 cm, and especially those that have grown to the tentorial notch area, the transpetrosal approach is used. This approach can be translabyrinthine, or with partial labyrinthectomy, with a presigmoid and retrosigmoid craniotomy and a small temporal craniotomy. Most of the operation is performed through the presigmoid and subtemporal space, although if the tumor extends very low, the retrosigmoid space can also be used. Because the surgeon can view the tentorial notch area and the tumor–brain stem interface directly, this approach is better for giant-size tumors. Additionally, the facial nerve results are better than with the retrosigmoid approach because the tumor can be lifted up and away from the nerve early in the operation.

The major details of this approach are similar to those of the transpetrosal approach for petroclival meningiomas.

◆ Complications

Cerebellar Contusion

Cerebellar contusions and hematomas may occur because of the craniotomy, during the dural opening in the face of a tight brain, or because of severe and prolonged retraction. Cerebellar swelling may also occur because of a venous sinus injury (see later). The best strategy for the surgeon is to avoid this problem altogether. When it does occur, the treatment depends on the severity and the location of the contusion or hematoma. If recognized during the operation, the contused area should be resected, proper hemostasis achieved, and the area covered with Surgicel. Up to a third of the lateral cerebellar hemisphere may be removed without producing a permanent cerebellar deficit. If the swelling is diffused, then it may be best to decompress the posterior fossa widely (including the foramen magnum) and close it with a dural graft. In severe cases, it may be necessary to leave the dura open. This is a very rare situation with modern surgical techniques.

Venous Sinus Injury

Injuries to the sigmoid sinus may occur during the bony opening in the retrosigmoid approach or during a transpetrosal approach. If the nondominant, or equidominant, well-collateralized sinus is impaired, it can be managed by occlusion with Surgicel or suture. However, any injury to a dominant sinus is very dangerous. The bleeding should be stopped by pressure with cottonoids or by finger pressure, and the rest of the sinus unroofed by drilling away the bone. The injury is then repaired with a patch of autologous dura if available. If the venous bleeding cannot be controlled adequately to visualize the injured area, a balloon-carotid shunt is passed inside the sinus and inflated at either end to occlude the sinuses while maintaining venous flow. The patient should be heparinized during the repair.

Cerebrospinal Fluid Leakage

SF leakage may occur through the mastoid bone or the petrous bone (near the IAC) or through the wound. When such a leak occurs, three factors may be present: (1) an opening in the dura and an air cell in the bone; (2) poor wound closure; and (3) elevated spinal fluid pressure, which is quite common after acoustic neuroma operation (due to blood spilled at surgery in the basal cisterns). When the CSF leak does occur, a CT head scan is performed to ensure the absence of pneumocephalus (due to excessive fluid leakage), and to attempt to determine the pathway of the leak. Fluid in the middle ear, seen in the CT scan or on otoscopy, confirms the leakage. If bone window thin sections show fluid in the mastoid air cells, or in a large open air cell in the petrous bone, these findings give indications about the route of the fluid.

Small leaks may be stopped by a pressure dressing on the incision (if a CSF effusion is present), repeated spinal tap and fluid drainage, or by prescribing acetazolamide 250 mg by mouth three times daily. Larger leaks require the institution of spinal fluid drainage by lumbar catheter, ~30 mL every 6 to 8 hours. If the leak does not stop with spinal fluid drainage, or if pneumocephalus is detected by CT scans, then surgical repair is often needed. Such repair may consist of carefully opening and waxing air cells, additional fat grafting, and dural closure with graft. If the patient has no hearing and the leakage is through the middle ear, the leak can be stopped easily by packing the middle ear with autologous fat. When communicating hydrocephalus is present, it may be necessary to perform a shunt procedure as well.

Trigeminal and Facial Paralysis

The combination of trigeminal and facial paralysis, even if temporary, can be devastating because of the possible exposure keratopathy. Although the immediate treatment may consist of a moisture bubble around the eye and lubricants, a lateral tarsorrhaphy will be necessary to prevent an exposure keratitis until recovery of function occurs.

Lower Cranial Nerve Paralysis

The paralysis of the lower cranial nerves (IX, X, and XII) after the excision of giant-size tumors may cause dysphagia and aspiration pneumonia. Unilateral vocal cord paralysis can be managed by laryngeal surgery (arytenoid adduction and thyroplasty). Although this may prevent pneumonia, the swallowing should be carefully evaluated before feeding the patient. Nasogastric tube feeding or a feeding jejunostomy may rarely be necessary.

◆ Surgical Outcomes

From July 1985 to December 1999, 219 patients were consecutively operated by the senior author and another neurosurgeon at the University of Pittsburgh and later at George Washington University and Fairfax Hospital. A neuro-otologist also took part in most of these operations. Fifteen patients (7%) had undergone previous treatment for their tumors, 13 having undergone microsurgery alone and two having undergone both microsurgery and radiosurgery. The patients' ages ranged from 14 to 88 years, with a mean of 48 years. Eight patients had fulfilled the criteria of neurofibromatosis type 2 (NF2).

Tumor size was measured as tumor equivalent diameter (TED). The tumors were classified as small (< 2 cm), medium (2.0 to 3.9 cm), and large (≥ 4 cm); 44% of the tumors were classified as small, 43% as medium, and 13% as large **(Table 62–3).**

The different surgical approaches used are shown in **Table 62–4.** Eight patients were treated in planned two-stage operations. One patient underwent subsequent surgery for tumor recurrence 1 year after initial operation. Thus a total of 228 operations were performed.

Of the 219 patients, 217 underwent total tumor resection evidenced by MRI studies. One patient with NF2 underwent partial tumor resection to preserve hearing in the only functional ear. The tumor regrew after 1 year. The patient underwent subsequent surgery, and the tumor was resected subtotally with excellent facial nerve outcome (House grade I) and functional hearing preservation. The patient has not shown any evidence of further growth. Another patient had subarachnoid hemorrhage during surgery from an undiagnosed internal carotid–posterior communicating artery aneurysm, and the surgery was aborted. This patient expired. Patient follow-up has a mean duration of 59 months (range, 3 to 171 months). Three patients died during follow-up due to reasons unrelated to acoustic neuroma or surgery.

Facial nerve results were classified according to the House-Brackmann facial nerve grading system, with grade I or II function considered to be an excellent result.[3] Tumor size proved to be the most important variable with respect to functional results. Ninety-six percent of the patients with small tumors recovered to postoperative grade I or II function within 3 months, and 4% achieved grade III or IV function. Of the 87 patients with medium-size tumors, 74% had grade I or II function and 25% had grade II or IV functions. One patient died 3 days after surgery due to a ruptured aneurysm. In her case the facial nerve function cannot be commented upon. Of the 26 patients with large tumors, 38% had grade I or II function, 58% had grade III or IV function, and 4% had grade V or VI results **(Table 62–5).** The patients who had facial nerve function of grade III or worse (all due to previous treatment) are not included for assessment of facial nerve function. In four patients (2%) the anatomical continuity of the facial nerve was lost during the operation. In one patient the nerve was directly resutured and a House grade III recovery was achieved. Another patient underwent sural nerve grafting and improved to grade III. The third patient underwent surgery to achieve a partial hypoglossal (CN XII) to facial nerve anastamosis and improved to House-Brackmann grade III.[1] The fourth patient refused the proposed surgery for hypoglossal nerve–facial nerve communication. In two patients who had NF2, the facial nerve was resected because it was severely invaded by tumor, and sural nerve grafting was done. They improved to grade II and III. For three additional patients in whom the facial nerve had been severed during previous operations by other

Table 62–3 Acoustic Neuroma Tumor Size Distribution

Tumor Size (tumor equivalent diameter, TED)	Number	Percentage
Small (< 2.0 cm)	96	44
Medium (2.0–3.9 cm)	94	43
Large (≥ 4.0 cm)	29	13
Total	219	100

Table 62–4 Operative Procedures for Acoustic Neuroma*

Approach	Number	Percentage
Retrosigmoid, transmeatal	191	84
Transpetrosal, retrosigmoid	21	9
Translabyrinthine	11	5
Transmastoid, transpetrosal, partial labyrinthectomy	5	2
Total	228	100

*Two hundred and twenty-eight operations were performed on 219 patients. One patient underwent a second operation for tumor recurrence. Eight patients underwent planned two-staged procedures (four underwent initial retrosigmoid approaches and then second-stage retrosigmoid approaches, two underwent initial retrosigmoid and then second-stage petrosal approaches, and two underwent initial retrosigmoid and then second-stage translabyrinthine approaches.

Table 62–5 Facial Nerve Function According to Tumor Size

Tumor size (TED)	Preoperative Grade* I or II	Postoperative Grade I or II	Postoperative Grade III or IV	Postoperative Grade V or VI
Small (< 2.0 cm)	96	92 (96%)	4 (4%)	0 (0%)
Medium (2.0–3.9 cm)	87	64 (74%)	23 (26%)	0 (0%)
Large (≥ 4.0 cm)	26	10 (38%)	15 (58%)	1 (4%)
Total	209	166 (79%)	42 (20%)	1 (1%)

* House-Brackmann grading system.

surgeons, surgery to achieve hypoglossal nerve–facial nerve anastosis communication was performed to minimize tongue atrophy. One patient improved to grade III and two improved to grade IV. Two patients had delayed facial nerve palsy, which recovered to grade I.

Functional hearing results were also analyzed with respect to tumor size, which again proved to be the most important outcome-related variable. The Gardner-Robertson classification was used to score hearing results.[2] Patients with class I or II results [i.e., speech reception threshold (SRT) ≤ 50 dB combined with speech discrimination score (SDS) ≥ 50%] were considered to have functional hearing. All patients were tested preoperatively and postoperatively. Hearing preservation was not attempted in patients with preoperative hearing function worse than class II. Based on these criteria, only 90 of the 219 patients were considered to have preoperative functional hearing **(Table 62–6).** The rate of hearing preservation was better in smaller tumors. The overall hearing preservation rate was 42%.

The most frequent postoperative complication was CSF leakage, which occurred in 32 patients (14%). Twenty-three of these leaks were transient and resolved with lumbar spinal fluid drainage. Nine patients required subsequent surgery (six middle ear packing, two wound revision, and one lumboperitoneal shunt). CSF leakage occurred after 26 (14%) of the 191 retrosigmoid procedures, two (18%) of the 11 translabyrinthine procedures, two (40%) of the five transmastoid partial labyrinthectomy procedures, and two (10%) of the 21 transpetrosal retrosigmoid procedures. One patient suffered cerebellar and sigmoid sinus injury during craniotomy and brain stem injury during operation to remove the tumor. This patient is partially disabled, with gait ataxia and hemisensory loss. The injury occurred before we modified our operative technique to expose the medial aspect of the sigmoid sinus before the craniotomy. One more patient had sigmoid sinus injury during surgery. However, the sinus was repaired by direct suturing and the patient did very well after surgery. A postoperative MR venogram showed a patent sinus. The most common complaint of the patients after surgery was headache, which was temporary in most cases. Six patients had communicating hydrocephalus, for which a ventriculoperitoneal shunt was done in five patients and a lumboperitoneal shunt was done in one. The other complications are listed in **Table 62–7.**

There were three deaths in our series. One patient with a medium-size tumor died suddenly on the sixth postoperative day as a result of a myocardial infarction. Another patient with a small tumor and chronic obstructive lung disease died as a result of pulmonary complications and systemic sepsis 1 month after his operation. Both of them

Table 62–6 Functional Hearing Preservation According to Tumor Size

Tumor Size (TED)	Preoperative Class* I or II	Postoperative Class I or II
Small (< 2.0 cm)	60	32 (53%)
Medium (2.0–3.9 cm)	27	6 (22%)
Large (≥ 4 cm)	3	0 (0%)
Total	90	38 (42%)

*Gardner-Robertson classification.

Table 62–7 Complications after Acoustic Neuroma Surgery

Complications	Number	Percentage
CSF leak	32	14*
Aseptic meningitis	5	2
Hydrocephalus/VP or LP shunt	6	3
Wound infection	3	1
Lower cranial nerve palsy	3	1
Cerebellar/brain stem injury	1	0.4
Death	3	1.4

CSF, cerebrospinal fluid; VP, ventriculoperitoneal; LP, lumboperitoneal.

*Nine patients (4%) of the total required some sort of surgery for CSF leak.

had undergone uncomplicated tumor resections. The third patient had a medium-size tumor. During surgery there was sudden brain swelling. Surgery was aborted and a CT scan was done. The patient had suffered a subarachnoid hemorrhage due to a ruptured internal carotid–posterior communicating artery aneurysm, which was unknown before surgery. She died after 3 days in the hospital.

◆ Conclusion

The retrosigmoid approach is very important for the removal of acoustic neuromas, especially when hearing preservation is attempted. Many nuances of the approach need to be learned so that the surgeon can perform it safely and effectively.

Suggested Readings

Cusimano MD, Sekhar LN. Partial hypoglossal to facial nerve anastomosis for reinnervation of paralyzed face in patients with lower cranial nerve palsies: technical note. Neurosurgery 1994;35:532–533

Gardner G, Robertson JH. Hearing preservation in unilateral acoustic neuroma surgery. Ann Otol Rhinol Laryngol 1988;97:55–66

House WF, Brackmann DE. Facial nerve grading system. Otolaryngol Head Neck Surg 1985;93:184–193.

63

Cranial Base Lesions: Translabyrinthine and Middle Fossa Approaches

Derald E. Brackmann, Jose N. Fayad, and Robert M. Owens

Modern neurosurgery began in the early 1960s when William F. House and others began employing the microscope in their approach to neurotological disease. House promoted the concept of teams of neurotologists and neurosurgeons approaching lesions in the cerebellopontine angle (CPA). The lateral transtemporal approaches, using this combined expertise, resulted in the development of multiple approaches to the CPA. Now neurotologists and neurosurgeons have an armamentarium of operative techniques to approach different areas and pathologies of the CPA and skull base. The use of the operating microscope and the development of these approaches have significantly reduced the mortality and morbidity for treatment of CPA lesions. The translabyrinthine and middle fossa approaches are discussed in this chapter.

House[1,2] was the first to use the translabyrinthine approach to remove acoustic tumors in 1960. More than 4000 acoustic tumors have been resected using this approach by the doctors of the House Clinic. The translabyrinthine approach allows wide access to the CPA with little cerebellar retraction and permits exposure of the entire facial nerve from the brain stem to the stylomastoid foramen.[3,4] The exposure is mostly extradural, minimizing possible injuries to the brain and the cerebellum. In addition, it provides a more direct and anterior perspective. A shorter distance separates the surgeon from the contents of the CPA[5–9]. The translabyrinthine approach allows for identification of the facial nerve at the lateral end of the internal auditory canal (IAC) before tumor dissection. The main disadvantages of the translabyrinthine approach are the need to sacrifice hearing in the operated ear, the limited exposure of the lower part of the CPA, and the limited access to the neural contents of the foramen magnum and foramen jugulare.

House[5] refined the middle fossa approach in 1961. Initially he used this approach to decompress the IAC in cases of extensive otosclerosis with sensorineural hearing loss. Although not beneficial for that condition, it quickly became evident that this approach was suitable for small acoustic tumors with good hearing.[6,7] The middle fossa procedure is a hearing preservation approach.[8–10] For tumors, it allows complete exposure of the lateral end of the IAC, so no blind dissection is necessary at the fundus. This is a definite advantage over the retrosigmoid approach, which does not allow exposure of the lateral third of the IAC without loss of hearing. When used for facial nerve tumors or facial nerve injuries, the areas of the geniculate ganglion, the site of multiple pathologies, can be exposed very adequately to allow decompression and repair of the nerve, if needed. Disadvantages include the fact that this is a technically difficult approach. Because of the superior location of the facial nerve in the canal, dissection of the tumor may subject the facial nerve to more manipulation than in other approaches. But with the advent of facial nerve monitoring, problems of the facial nerve are kept to a minimum and facial nerve outcome is no different than when using the translabyrinthine approach.[11] Retraction of the temporal lobe is required for the duration of the drilling and tumor removal, which usually does not exceed 1 to 1 $^{1}/_{2}$ hours.

In the treatment of acoustic neuromas, the translabyrinthine and middle fossa approaches are often compared with the retrosigmoid approach. The retrosigmoid approach provides a panoramic view of the posterior fossa from the tentorium to the foramen magnum. Access is provided to the cerebellar hemisphere, the lateral aspect of the pons and medulla, and the root entry zone and cisternal course of cranial nerves V to XI. Although exposure superiorly is limited by the tentorium, this approach represents a modification of the classical suboccipital approach. Krause[12] and others first employed the suboccipital route during the latter portion of the 19th century. In this procedure, a large bone flap is removed from the suboccipital area, with the anterior limit of the dissection being the first mastoid cell. Superiorly, bone is removed up to the inferior margin of the transverse sinus. The retrosigmoid approach offers a more favorable angle of view into the CPA and a markedly reduced need for cerebellar retraction than the classical suboccipital approach. It does not pose a risk of air embolism or quadriplegia as does the classical suboccipital approach, which has the patient in the sitting position. Advantages are wide access of the CPA and the potential for hearing preservation. The retrosigmoid approach is capable of addressing most lesions of the CPA.[13] Disadvantages include a higher incidence of postoperative headaches and cerebrospinal fluid (CSF) leaks.[14,15] When compared with the retrosigmoid approach, the translabyrinthine approach has somewhat lower morbidity. The incidence of postcraniotomy headaches is lower than in the retrosigmoid approach, perhaps due to lesser cerebellar retraction, reduced dissection of the suboccipital musculature, and completion of all the bony work before dural opening. The CSF leak is also less following the translabyrinthine approach than the retrosigmoid craniotomy.[16,17] The higher incidence of CSF leaks is explained by the difficulty in sealing all the cells in the petrous apex, especially when it is extensively pneumatized. Another disadvantage is poor exposure of the ventral aspect of the pons and medulla due to the relatively posterior angle of view. The posterior aspect of the clivus is obstructed by the course of cranial nerves V to XI. The retrosigmoid approach is discussed elsewhere in this book.

◆ Indications

Translabyrinthine Approach

The translabyrinthine approach is ideal for many lesions of the CPA in patients with poor or no hearing. Such lesions include acoustic neuromas, meningiomas, facial nerve tumors, cholesteatomas of the petrous bone extending to the posterior fossa, cholesterol granulomas, paragangliomas and adenomas of the temporal bone, traumatic facial nerve injuries, and aneurysms of the midportion of the basilar artery. Cochleovestibular neurectomy may also be accomplished through this route. The translabyrinthine approach can be combined with a middle fossa craniotomy for transtentorial lesions.

The translabyrinthine approach is used most commonly in acoustic neuroma surgery and is indicated for any size tumor when the hearing is nonserviceable. It is also indicated in tumors larger than 2.5 cm regardless of the status of the hearing.[18] Our definition of serviceable hearing is a pure-tone average threshold better than 50 dB, a speech discrimination score of greater than 50%, or both. This definition is referred to as the 50/50 rule. Exceptions to this rule do exist, as in the case of poor hearing in the contralateral ear or in bilateral tumors. In those cases, a middle fossa craniotomy or a retrosigmoid approach may be pursued depending on the size and the exact location of the tumor.

Middle Fossa Approach

A major indication for the middle fossa approach is removal of small ($\leq$ 2 cm) acoustic neuromas with serviceable hearing,defined as just noted.[19]

Other lesions approached through the middle fossa include facial nerve neuromas, hemangiomas, and meningiomas. Other indications include repair of the facial nerve after injury by temporal bone fractures; decompression of the fallopian canal in Bell's palsy and herpes zoster oticus; and vestibular neurectomy and bony decompression of the IAC in neurofibromatosis type 2 in an effort to retard progressive hearing loss.

◆ Preoperative Studies

Magnetic resonance imaging (MRI) is necessary to show the exact location and size of the tumor. It determines the relationship of the tumor to the brain stem, cerebellum, and IAC. Particular attention should be paid to a major vessel loop crossing within the tumor. The nature of the tumor and its consistency, cystic versus solid, can also be evaluated.

◆ Surgical Technique

Anesthesia

A standard endotracheal anesthesia induced with thiopental and a short-acting muscle relaxant is used. Intravenous furosemide 40 mg and mannitol 1 g/kg body weight are administered for brain relaxation when the skin incision is made. Preoperative antibiotics are also administered. The blood pressure is monitored using an arterial line.

Neurophysiological Monitoring

Facial nerve monitoring is used for the whole length of the operation. When hearing preservation is attempted, cochlear nerve function is monitored using auditory brain stem responses; once the tumor is exposed, direct cochlear nerve potentials are obtained just prior to tumor removal.

Patient Positioning and Initial Exposure

For both the translabyrinthine and middle fossa approaches, the patient is placed in the supine position, with the head rotated away from the surgeon. A head holder may be used if greater posterior exposure is required. The operating room table is reversed so that the patient's head is located at the foot of the bed; this allows the surgeon to sit and work comfortably during the procedure without any obstruction under the table. A long anesthesia circuit permits the anesthesiologist to stay at the other end of the surgical site. An electrically controlled table allows the frequent turning from side to side needed during neurotologic procedures.

Translabyrinthine Approach

The translabyrinthine approach allows exposure of the CPA anterior to the sigmoid sinus. Exposure includes the lateral aspect of the pons, the ventral aspect of the lateral cerebellar hemisphere, and cranial nerves V, VI, VII, and VIII. The root entry zone of the lower cranial nerves IX, X, and XI is also seen to a variable degree, depending on the location and the anatomy of the jugular bulb.

Hair is shaved from the postauricular area, and the skin is prepped using povidone-iodine (Betadine). A plastic Vi-Drape (Medical Concepts Development; Woodbury, MN) is used to cover the surgical site. The lower abdomen is also prepared and draped in the usual fashion to allow harvesting of fat.

The postauricular skin is injected with 1% lidocaine (Xylocaine) with epinephrine 1:100,000. The incision is performed 4 cm posterior to the postauricular sulcus in a C-shaped fashion. This allows the pinna to be retracted anteriorly. This incision is carried through the soft tissue covering the mastoid process. A Lempert elevator is used to elevate the periosteum off the mastoid bone. The spine of Henle and the mastoid bone are uncovered.

A complete mastoidectomy is performed with a high-speed drill, using different sizes of cutting, diamond, and rough diamond burs **(Fig. 63–1A).** The antrum and the incus are identified. Bone overlying the sigmoid sinus is removed, and the sigmoid is skeletonized. Removal of bone is carried posteriorly over the suboccipital dura to allow for retraction of the sigmoid and for wider exposure. Some surgeons prefer to leave an island of bone (Bill's island) over the sigmoid sinus to protect this structure from the shaft of the bur. The dissection continues with bone removal over the middle fossa dura and the sinodural angle as well as over the posterior fossa dura medial to the sigmoid sinus. Once all of the bony work has been completed (i.e., the dura posterior to the sigmoid is uncovered, the sigmoid sinus is skeletonized, and the middle fossa dura and the posterior fossa dura anterior to the sigmoid sinus are uncovered), the labyrinthectomy is started.

The labyrinthectomy is accomplished with a cutting bur **(Fig. 63–1B).** It starts with removal of the lateral semicircular canal and is extended toward the posterior semicircular canal. The bone removal is continued inferior and anterior toward the ampullated end of this canal. The posterior semicircular canal is opened inferiorly to the vestibule and superiorly to the crus commune and the vestibule. The facial nerve is identified in its descending segment, and care is taken not to injure the nerve while working on the lateral end of the vestibule. Now that the facial nerve is identified, the remainder of the bone of the inferior IAC is removed to the vestibule. Then we proceed to remove the superior portion of the posterior canal to the common crus, which is formed by the nonampulated ends of the superior and posterior semicircular canal. The superior canal is then followed and removed to its ampullated end in the vestibule. This ampullated end identifies the area where the superior vestibular nerve exits the lateral end of the IAC. The saccule, the utricle, and the posterior semicircular canal ampulla are identified; they represent the areas where the inferior vestibular and singular nerves exit the lateral end of the IAC. Removing the bone posterior to the IAC uncovers the vestibular aqueduct and the endolymphatic sac. By now, the superior and inferior ends of the IAC are outlined.

To properly expose the IAC and the contents of the CPA, bone needs to be removed from around the canal superiorly and inferiorly up to 270 degrees of the circumference of the canal **(Fig. 63–1C).**

The inferior limit of the dissection is represented by the jugular bulb and the cochlear aqueduct. By staying superior to the cochlear aqueduct, injury to cranial nerves IX, X, and XI is avoided. Bone located between the middle fossa dura and the IAC is removed. At the lateral end of the canal, Bill's bar, or the vertical crest, is identified. It separates the facial nerve from the superior vestibular nerve. Because the facial nerve is located in the anterior and superior part of the IAC, care must be taken not to injure the nerve while removing the bone of the superior lip. Pressure should not be applied over the canal. The dissection in this area is done with the side of the bur.

Once the bony removal is completed, attention is turned to the antrostomy and the middle ear cleft. The incus is removed from the fossa incudis; the area of the facial recess is widened to obtain a good view of the eustachian tube and the tensor tympani muscle. The tensor tympani is sectioned to allow for better packing of the middle ear space.

The dura of the canal and the posterior fossa is not opened until all bone removal has been accomplished. During the drilling, the wound is irrigated periodically with bacitracin solution. The craniotomy defect is again irrigated prior to dural opening.

Middle Fossa Approach[21]

The middle fossa approach allows the unroofing of the IAC and the exposure of the fundus of the canal **(Fig. 63–2A).** The facial nerve is located at the lateral end of the canal, where it enters the temporal bone and becomes the labyrinthine segment between the cochlea and the superior semicircular canal. This approach makes possible the removal of laterally placed tumors in the IAC without the need for blind dissection. When used for facial nerve lesions, the floor of the middle fossa can be removed lateral to the otic capsule, exposing the middle ear and the upper tympanic portion of the facial nerve above the cochleariform process.

The incision starts in the pretragal area, curves initially posteriorly above the ear, and then runs vertical for 4 cm before curving at a right angle anteriorly in the temporal area. The shape of the incision resembles a question mark. Once the skin is elevated, an incision is made in the temporalis muscle and fascia, and the muscle is reflected anterior inferiorly.

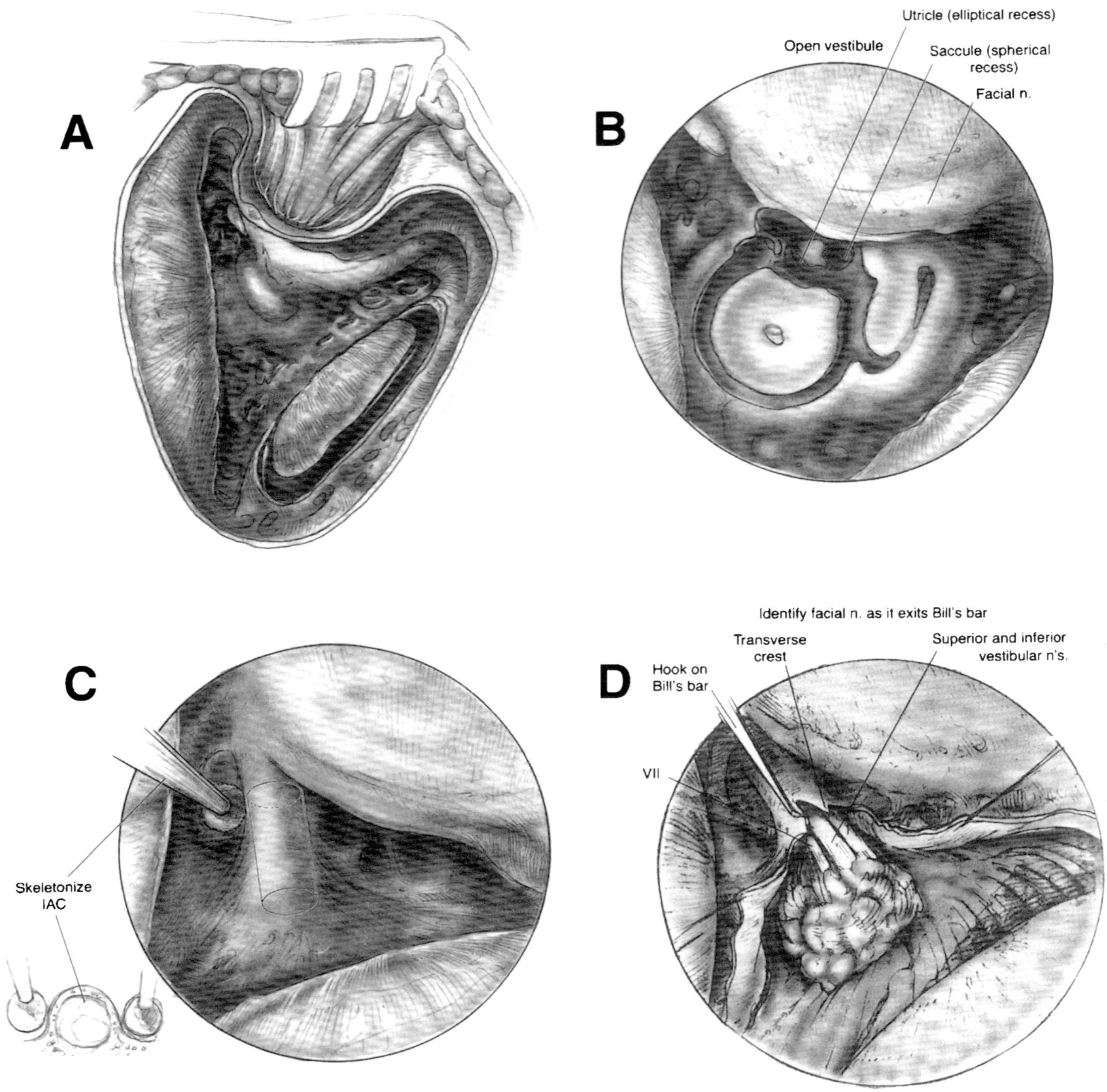

Figure 63–1 **(A)** Cortical mastoidectomy, and sigmoid decompression. **(B)** Opening of the lateral, superior, and posterior semicircular canals. **(C)** Skeletonizing of the internal auditory canal. **(D)** Opening of the dura and removal of the tumor.

Using a cutting bur, an opening is made in the squamous portion of the temporal bone. The craniotomy measures 5 × 5 cm and is located two thirds anterior and one third posterior in relation to the external auditory canal. The bone flap is kept in antibiotic solution and is placed back at the conclusion of the case. The dura is now elevated from posteriorly to anteriorly from the floor of the middle fossa, and any remaining bone over the root of the zygoma is drilled away as close as possible to the floor of the middle fossa. The anterior extent of dural elevation is marked by the initial landmark, the middle meningeal artery. Frequently, bleeding is encountered in this area and is controlled by packing Surgicel in the foramen spinosum. Dissection of the dura continues until the petrous ridge is identified. Once the dura is completely elevated, the House-Urban retractor is placed into position over the porus acusticus. At this time, the arcuate eminence and the greater superficial petrosal nerve have been identified **(Fig. 63–2B).** In a small proportion of patients, the geniculate ganglion is dehiscent, and care is taken not to injure it while elevating the dura. Posterior to anterior

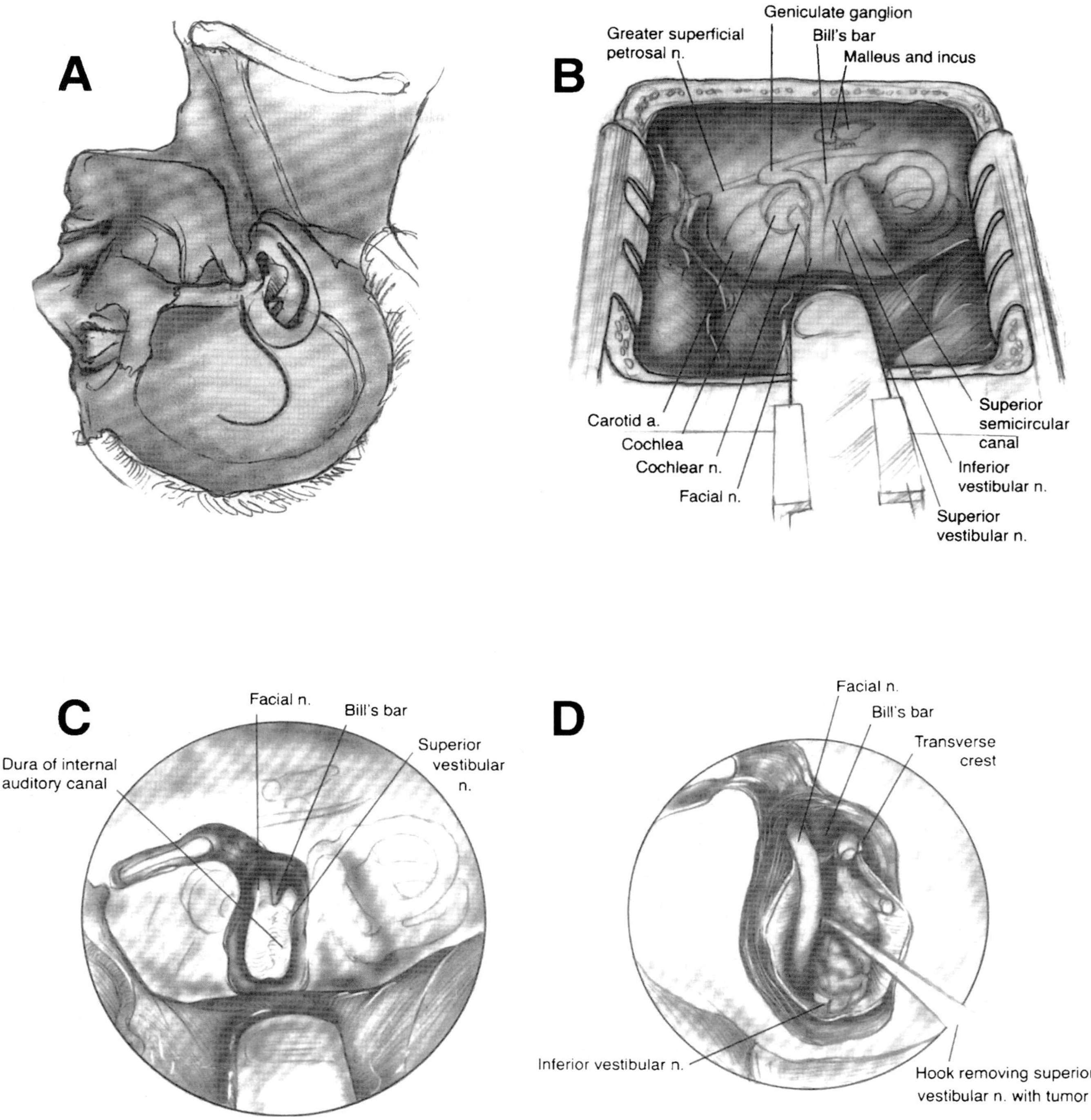

Figure 63–2 **(A)** Incision. **(B)** Surgical anatomy of the temporal bone from above. **(C)** The internal auditory canal is identified medially, the labyrinthine segment of the facial nerve is followed to the geniculate ganglion, and the internal auditory canal is exposed completely. **(D)** The dura is opened and dissection of the tumor proceeds.

elevation avoids elevating the ganglion. Using suction irrigation and diamond burs, dissection of the IAC is started medially. The IAC bisects the angle formed by the greater superficial petrosal nerve and the arcuate eminence as described by Garcia-Ibanez. Identifying the IAC medially and anteriorly is safest because medially there are no important anatomical structures. Once the IAC is identified, bone surrounding it in the area of the porus is removed. Bone removal extends posteriorly to the level of the arcuate eminence and the common crus, anteriorly to Kawase's triangle. Bone is removed 270 degrees around the canal, including the entire posterior lip. Lateral dissection of the IAC then proceeds. The exposure narrows laterally because of the presence of the cochlea anteriorly and the ampullated end of the superior semicircular canal posteriorly. At the lateral end of the canal, Bill's bar is identified. The facial nerve is followed into its labyrinthine portion. The ligament surrounding it at the beginning of the labyrinthine segment is cut to allow for decompression of the nerve in this portion **(Fig. 63–2C).**

Tumor Resection and Closure

Translabyrinthine Approach

A 3 mm hook is used to elevate the dura over the superior vestibular nerve and to palpate the vertical crest. The superior vestibular nerve is then dissected away from the facial nerve. Scissors are used to complete the dural opening and obtain wide access to the CPA **(Fig. 63–1D).** After division of the facial-vestibular anastomosis, the plane between the superior vestibular nerve and the facial nerve leads the surgeon into the plane between the facial nerve and the tumor. Cottonoids are placed between the tumor and the cerebellum posteriorly. Partial tumor removal then proceeds by incising the tumor capsule and debulking the tumor by using the House-Urban dissector. Once enough gutting of tumor has been accomplished, the tumor is separated from the brain stem by cottonoids. Inferiorly the ninth nerve is identified and protected using small cottonoids. Often large vessels are located at the inferior pole of the tumor. Care is taken to gently separate the tumor from those vessels. Further debulking of the tumor, at this point, is achieved. Now the lateral end of the IAC is dissected. The facial nerve has been identified and separated from the tumor. A hook is used to remove the inferior vestibular nerve, and the dura is opened along the inferior aspect of the tumor. Along the superior aspect of the tumor, dissection proceeds, keeping in mind the position of the facial nerve in relation to the tumor. The tumor is now gently retracted posteriorly. The plane along the facial nerve is further developed. Dissection of the tumor at the level of the porus can be difficult. If it is, the tumor is rotated posteriorly in order to identify the facial nerve medially at the brain stem. The facial nerve is then followed from medial to lateral. Developing the facial nerve plane from medial to lateral leads to the medial extent of the tumor. The continuing plane of the facial nerve is then developed back to the porus. Once the facial nerve is cleared, the tumor is easily delivered.

After tumor removal, the wound is copiously irrigated with Ringer's solution to remove all the blood clots. Careful hemostasis is achieved. The dura is reapproximated with 4–0 silk. The eustachian tube is packed with Surgicel and the middle ear cleft is filled with muscle. The craniotomy defect is filled with fat obtained from the lower part of the abdomen. Strips of fat are packed tightly to prevent leakage of CSF. A titanium mesh is used to recontour the skull and reconstruct the lateral wall of the mastoid. The wound is closed in layers with 0-chromic and 3–0 Vicryl sutures. Steri-Strips are applied to the postauricular incision, and a head pressure dressing is applied.

Middle Fossa Approach

The dura of the IAC is opened along the posterior aspect. The facial nerve is identified clearly and stimulated **(Fig. 63–2D).** The superior vestibular nerve is cut at the end of the IAC. Following this, the vestibulofacial anastomotic fibers are cut. The tumor is then separated from the end of the IAC and from the facial nerve. The goal is to free the tumor from the facial nerve and to deliver it from under the nerve. Dissection of the lateral end of the inferior compartment of the IAC can be very difficult. It is best to cut both superior and inferior vestibular nerves to avoid postoperative unsteadiness. Once the lateral end of the tumor has been delivered, the plane between the cochlear and facial nerves and tumor becomes apparent. This plane is developed using fine hooks. Tumor dissection proceeds from lateral to medial. At this point, a search for the anterior inferior cerebellar artery is begun. Great care is taken to identify and not injure this important artery. At this time, the tumor is separated gently from this vessel. Debulking of the tumor begins using small cup forceps. At all times, care is taken not to injure the facial nerve with the suction or by stretching it. Finally, the medial end of the tumor is freed with small hooks. Once tumor removal is completed, hemostasis is obtained. The tumor bed is irrigated copiously. Abdominal fat is obtained and is used to close the dural defect. The temporal lobe retractor is removed. The dura is suspended on either side of the craniotomy to limit the dead space. A Penrose drain is placed into the wound. The bone flap is repositioned and secured by microplates. The wound is closed in layers and a mastoid-type pressure dressing is applied.

◆ Postoperative Care

The patient is observed in the intensive care unit for a period of 36 hours. Steroids and antibiotics are not routinely used. Steroids are used in patients who exhibit signs of cerebellar swelling after removal of large tumors. For the middle fossa approach, the Penrose drain is removed from the wound on the first postoperative day. A new pressure dressing is applied. The wound is inspected every day thereafter. The mastoid dressing remains in place for 4 days, and the patient is instructed not to lift or strain during the early postoperative period.

◆ Complications

Translabyrinthine Approach

Although rare, the most common early postoperative complication is a hematoma in the CPA. This is manifested by signs of increased CPA pressure. This complication is managed by immediate opening of the wound in the intensive care unit and removal of the fat. The patient is then taken to surgery to secure hemostasis and repack the wound.

Meningitis is an uncommon complication and is managed with appropriate antibiotics following culture and identification of the offending organisms.

CSF leak occurs in a small percentage of patients. Most leaks can be stopped with a pressure head dressing and bed rest with the patient's head elevated. If the leak continues despite the dressing in place, a lumbar spinal drain is inserted and kept in place for 3 to 4 days. Reexploration of the wound and repacking of the wound with additional fat is done if the leak persists despite the above steps. If facial weakness occurs, the eye is protected by using conservative measures first. These include artificial tears, moisture chambers, and soft contact lens. In certain situations, the insertion of a gold weight or a palpebral spring may be necessary.

Middle Fossa Approach

An epidural hematoma is an uncommon early postoperative complication. The incidence of this complication is lowered by leaving a Penrose drain in the wound for the first 24 hours, and by obtaining meticulous hemostasis prior to closure of the wound. Patients with this complication exhibit increased intracranial pressure. Treatment is immediate evacuation of the hematoma in the intensive care unit. Further hemostasis is secured in the operating room. Other complications are those that are common to any intracranial procedure, such as meningitis. Possible problems related to temporal lobe retraction include memory loss, auditory hallucinations, and speech disturbances. These are rarely significant clinical problems. Seizures are often cited as a possible complication of the middle fossa approach, but in reality this problem is seldom encountered. Older patients do not tolerate the middle fossa approach as well as younger patients due to the fragility of the dura and retraction of the temporal lobe. Fortunately, all of the above complications have been very rare in our experience.[10]

References

1. House WF. Acoustic neuroma (monograph). Arch Otolaryngol Head Neck Surg 1964;80:598–757
2. House WF. Translabyrinthine approach. In: House WF, Luetje CM, eds. Acoustic Tumors. Vol 2: Management. Baltimore: University Park Press; 1979:43–87
3. Brackmann DE. Translabyrinthine removal of acoustic neurinomas. In: Brackmann DE, ed. Neurological Surgery of the Ear and Skull Base. New York: Raven; 1982:235–241
4. House WF, Luetje CM, eds. Acoustic Tumors. Vol 1: Diagnosis. Baltimore: University Park Press; 1979
5. House WF. Surgical exposure of the internal auditory canal and its contents through the middle cranial fossa. Laryngoscope 1961;71: 1363–1385
6. House WF. Middle cranial fossa approach to the petrous pyramid: report of 50 cases. Arch Otolaryngol 1963;78:460–469
7. House F, Hitselberger WE. The middle fossa approach for removal of small acoustic tumors. Acta Otolaryngol 1969;67:413–427
8. Shelton C, Brackmann DE, House WF, Hitselberger WE. Acoustic tumor surgery: prognostic factors in hearing conversation. Arch Otolaryngol Head Neck Surg 1989;115:1213–1216
9. Gantz BJ, Parnes LS, Harker LA, McCabe BF. Middle cranial fossa acoustic neuroma excision: results and complications. Ann Otol Rhinol Laryngol 1986;95(5 pt 1):454–459
10. Slattery WH III, Brackmann DE, Hitselberger W. Middle fossa approach for hearing preservation with acoustic neuromas. Am J Otol 1997;18:596–601
11. Arriage MA, Luxford WM, Berliner KI. Facial nerve function following middle fossa and translabyrinthine acoustic tumor surgery: a comparison. Am J Otol 1994:15:620–624.
12. Krause F. Zur Freilegung der hinteren Felsenbeinflache und des Kleinhirns. Beitr Klin Chir 1903;37:728–764
13. Shelton C, Alavi S, Li JC, Hitselberger WE. Modified retrosigmoid approach: use for selected acoustic tumor removal. Am J Otol 1995;16: 664–668
14. Smith PG, Leonetti JP, Grubb RL. Management of cerebrospinal fluid otorhinorrhea complicating the retrosigmoid approach to the cerebellopontine angle. Am J Otol 1990;11:178–180
15. Schessel DA, Nedzelski JM, Rowed W, Feghali JG. Headache and local discomfort following surgery of the cerebellopontine angle. In: Tos M, Thomsen J, eds. Acoustic Neuroma. Proceedings of the First International Conference on Acoustic Neuroma. Amsterdam: Kugler Publications; 1991:899–904
16. House JL, Hitselberger WE, House WF. Wound closure and cerebrospinal fluid leak after translabyrinthine surgery. Am J Otol 1982;4:126–128
17. Tos M, Thomsen J. Cerebrospinal fluid leak after translabyrinthine surgery for acoustic neuroma. Laryngoscope 1985;95:351–354
18. Briggs RJ, Luxford WM, Atkins JS Jr, Hitselberger WE. Translabyrinthine removal of large acoustic neuromas. Neurosurgery 1994;34:785–790 discussion 790–791
19. Shelton C, Brackmann DE, House WF, Hitselberger WE. Middle fossa acoustic tumor surgery: results in 106 cases. Laryngoscope 1989;99: 405–408
20. Slattery WH 3rd, Francis S, House KC. Peciooperative morbidity of acoustic neuroma surgery. Otol Neurotol 2001;22:895–902

64

Paragangliomas and Schwannomas of the Jugular Foramen

Derald E. Brackmann, Jose N. Fayad, and Robert M. Owens

Jugular foramen tumors are rare. Due to their deep location, the diagnosis and management of these tumors remain very challenging. Interdisciplinary cooperation among neuroradiologists, neurosurgeons, otologists, and head and neck surgeons is needed to achieve an optimal therapeutic outcome.[1]

Frequently, jugular foramen tumors have intracranial and extracranial extensions. The surgical approach adopted should be able to address both components of the tumor if complete surgical excision of these generally benign tumors is to be achieved. New advances in diagnostic imaging techniques, improvements in anesthetic agents, and new surgical techniques make this goal achievable.[2]

Paragangliomas, schwannomas, and meningiomas are the most common benign tumors that involve the jugular foramen. The differential diagnosis also includes malignant neoplasms such as squamous cell carcinomas, chondrosarcomas, and chordomas. Aneurysms of the vertebral or posterior inferior cerebellar artery should be considered. This chapter focuses on paragangliomas and schwannomas of the jugular foramen.

◆ Paragangliomas

This is the most common benign tumor of the jugular foramen. Paragangliomas are benign neoplasms arising from the extraadrenal neural-crest–derived paraganglia. In 1941, Guild described glomus tissue formation along the jugular system, which he termed glomus jugulare. In 1945, Rosenwasser described the first carotid-body–like tumor occurring in the temporal bone. Glomus jugulare tumors occur in the adventitia of the jugular vein, as opposed to glomus tympanicum tumors, which are associated with Arnold's and Jacobson's nerves. These tumors affect more females than males. The incidence of multiple glomus tumors is 7 to 10%. The most common symptom is a conductive hearing loss. Other symptoms include pulsatile tinnitus, ear pain, bleeding, vertigo, and facial nerve problems. Paragangliomas are locally invasive neoplasms, with extension into and destruction of adjacent structures, including the temporal bone and mastoid. Typically, paragangliomas bleed profusely on manipulation. They are polypoid, red, friable masses, identified behind an intact tympanic membrane or within the external auditory canal. Histologically, the cell nest or "zellballen" pattern is characteristic of paragangliomas. The neoplasm is composed predominantly of chief cells, which are round or oval with uniform nuclei, dispersed chromatin pattern, and abundant eosinophilic, granular, or vacuolated cytoplasm. Sustentacular cells may be seen; these cells represent modified Schwann cells and are seen at the periphery of the cell nests as spindle-shaped, basophilic-appearing cells. The immunohistochemical profile for the chief cells is chromogranin, synaptophysin, neuron-specific enolase, and neurofilament positive; for the sustentacular cells, S-100 protein is positive. Neurosecretory granules are present on electron microscopy.[3] Endocrinologically active tumors occur in 1 to 3% of glomus tumors. These tumors have been found to secrete epinephrine, norepinephrine, and dopamine. These active tumors are screened preoperatively by testing urinary vanillylmandelic acid (VMA) and metanephrine. Paragangliomas of the temporal bone have been classified by many authors. In the classification system of Jenkins and Fisch, later modified by Fisch and Mattox, tumors are divided into four categories:

1. Tumors limited to the middle ear and promontory
2. Tumors involving the hypotympanum
3. Tumors originating in the jugular bulb
   a. There is erosion of the carotid foramen but no involvement of the internal carotid artery (ICA).
   b. There is involvement of the vertical carotid canal.
   c. There is invasion of the vertical and horizontal carotid.
   d. There is invasion of the ICA from the carotid foramen to the foramen lacerum.
4. Tumors with intracranial extension

Although these are slow-growing neoplasms, prognosis is guarded because they often infiltrate and invade adjacent structures. Preoperative embolization is useful to decrease the vascularity of the tumor and allow for safer surgery. Complete surgical excision is the treatment of choice; however, the location and invasive nature of these lesions sometimes preclude complete surgical eradication. In such cases, radiotherapy can be a useful adjunct to surgery, resulting in decreased vascularity and promoting fibrosis.[4] Malignant paragangliomas do occur and can metastasize to the cervical lymph nodes, lungs, and liver (3%).

◆ Schwannomas

Although schwannoma of the jugular foramen is an unusual skull base tumor, it is the second most common benign tumor of that region. It may take origin from any cranial nerve at the skull base, but most jugular foramen schwannomas are thought to originate from the tenth cranial nerve, and this incidence has been reported to be as high as 50%. When the tumor enlarges, it can compress adjacent cranial nerves and adjacent extracranial and intracranial structures. The patient usually presents with a unilateral lesion of cranial nerve IX, X, or XI or a combination of these. Occasionally, a retrocochlear finding is the initial presentation.[5] These tumors were categorized by Kaye et al[6] into three categories: types A, B, and C. The position of the tumor depends on its point of origin from the nerve as it passes through the pars nervosa of the jugular foramen.

Pathological examination of schwannomas shows a circumscribed, tan-white, rubbery to firm mass that may appear yellow and have cystic changes. Tumors contain alternating regions that are composed of compact spindle cells called Antoni A areas, and loose, hypocellular zones called Antoni B areas. Nuclei are vestibular to hyperchromatic, elongated and twisted, with indistinct cytoplasmic borders. Cells are arranged in short, interlacing fascicles. Whorling or palisading of nuclei may be seen. Retrogressive changes, including cystic degeneration, necrosis, hyalinization, calcification, and hemorrhage may be seen. Immunohistochemistry of these tumors shows a uniform and intense positive reaction with S-100 protein.[7] Complete surgical excision is the treatment of choice and is curative. Malignant degeneration of a benign schwannoma rarely occurs.[8]

◆ Indications for Surgery

Paragangliomas

For small tumors limited to the jugular bulb, we use the transjugular approach. For tumors eroding the carotid foramen but not invading the carotid artery (Fisch type C1 tumors), we use a mastoid-neck approach with limited transposition of the facial nerve. For bigger tumors involving the internal carotid artery (types C2, C3, and C4) an infratemporal approach type A is indicated.

Schwannomas

The decision to recommend surgery is similar to that made with other benign lesions of this region. Little is known about the natural history. Usually these are slow-growing tumors. One would anticipate progressive loss of cranial nerve function and mass effect within the posterior cranial fossa. The patient's age and general medical condition are taken into consideration when the surgical option is contemplated.

Usually, schwannomas of the jugular foramen can be removed using the transjugular approach. Sometimes a mastoid-neck approach with limited transposition of the facial nerve may be indicated. For possible intracranial extension, the dura is usually opened anteriorly to the sigmoid sinus (presigmoid).

◆ Preoperative Studies

The preoperative evaluation includes a history and complete physical examination, with full neurological exam assessing all preexisting nerve deficits of the lower cranial nerves, facial nerve, and hearing nerve; high-resolution computed tomography (CT) (1.5 mm thin sections) with and without intravenous contrast medium in axial and coronal projections; and a magnetic resonance imaging (MRI) study with gadolinium, and dynamic studies if a highly vascularized lesion is suspected.

An area extending from the craniocervical junction up to the tentorial notch is examined using 1.5 mm overlapping CT cuts. Bone windows of the skull base look for destruction or erosion of the jugular foramen, carotid, hypoglossal, and facial canals, the petrous bone, and the clivus areas. CT is helpful in differentiating a jugular foramen schwannoma from glomus jugulare tumor. CT shows a smooth tumor capsule and smooth bony erosion of the jugular foramen in the case of a schwannoma. In the case of a paraganglioma, there are irregular tumor margins and irregular bony destruction of the jugular foramen.

An MRI with gadolinium, with sagittal and coronal projections, helps define the tumor and its relationship to the carotid artery, the brain stem, the medulla oblongata, as well as the intracranial and extracranial extensions. MRI demonstrates a smooth-contoured, soft tissue mass nearly isointense with the brain stem on T1-weighted images. Gadolinium enhancement is similar to that seen in glomus tumors, but the flow voids noted in glomus tumors are absent. MR angiography is helpful in evaluating blood vessel involvement.

If a highly vascular lesion is suspected from previous studies, a four-vessel angiogram is obtained. It is essential for the evaluation of feeding vessels, the vascular composition of the tumor, the venous return, and the circulation time through the vascular bed. Collateral circulation as well as the position of the jugular bulb and venous sinuses are also evaluated. The blood supply to the tumor could be coming from the external carotid artery, internal carotid artery, or intracranial or extracranial branches of the vertebrobasilar artery.

Collateral circulation should be evaluated by balloon test occlusion if the petrous ICA is involved by the tumor. If the vertebral artery is involved, balloon test occlusion is not usually done; the size of the arteries as well as the size of the posterior communicating arteries provide the necessary information about the patient's tolerance to vascular occlusion.

Usually, all vascular tumors are embolized preoperatively by an interventional radiologist.[9] Embolization procedures are not without a risk, especially when the feeding vessels are coming from the internal carotid system or the vertebrobasilar system.

All patients with paragangliomas should be screened for the presence of vasoactively secreting substances to avoid severe hypertensive episodes intraoperatively.

◆ Surgical Technique

Anesthesia

Anesthesia requirements include maintaining adequate cerebral blood flow, sedation, and analgesia, with the avoidance of paralytic agents. Although dissection of the lower cranial nerves while removing a jugular foramen tumor can compromise the function of these nerves, care must be taken to save those nerves when dealing with benign pathology. Patients with cranial nerve deficits preoperatively have already somewhat compensated, and the need for tracheostomy may be obviated initially and the patient reassessed postoperatively.

Neurophysiological Monitoring

Cranial nerve monitoring usually includes the facial nerve and the lower cranial nerves IX, X, XI, and XII.

Positioning

The patient lies in the supine position. The head is turned away from the surgeon and flexed. We do not use head pins or a Mayfield headrest. Usually, the abdomen is prepared and draped in the usual fashion for later harvesting of an abdominal fat graft or, more rarely, for a rectus abdominis muscle free flap if this type of reconstruction is needed. If facial nerve reconstruction is anticipated, the greater auricular nerve will be harvested for nerve grafting. All patients get elastic and pneumatic compression stockings.

Approach

The choice of a surgical approach depends on the exact location of the tumor and the presence of vascular encasement. For benign tumors of the jugular foramen, a transtemporal or an infratemporal approach is needed to remove these tumors.[10]

For tumors involving only the jugular bulb, the transmastoid approach combined with an upper cervical approach with or without anterior translocation of the nerve is recommended (transjugular approach or mastoid-neck approach with limited facial nerve translocation). For limited involvement of the clivus, we recommend the transmastoid approach with facial nerve translocation (mastoid-neck approach with limited facial nerve translocation). For extensive involvement of the clivus, the subtemporal and infratemporal approaches with dissection and displacement of the petrous ICA are needed. We describe here the transjugular approach, the mastoid-neck approach with limited transposition of the facial nerve, and the infratemporal type A approach.

Transjugular Approach or Mastoid and Neck Approach

This approach (**Fig. 64–1**) is used for tumors limited to the jugular bulb without extension into the neck, the carotid artery, or the posterior fossa.

A postauricular incision is made 2 cm posterior to the postauricular fold. A complete mastoidectomy is performed. The facial nerve is identified and skeletonized anteriorly, the tegmen is identified superiorly, and the sigmoid sinus and the jugular bulb are identified posteriorly and inferiorly. Then the mastoid tip is amputated lateral to the digastric muscle. The skin incision is carried down to the neck following the anterior border of the sternocleidomastoid muscle. This muscle is freed from its insertion to the mastoid tip and reflected posteriorly. The digastric muscle is removed from its groove and reflected anteriorly. At this point, the major neurovascular structures are identified. The spinal accessory nerve is identified lateral to the internal jugular vein. The ninth and tenth cranial nerves are also identified and preserved. The internal jugular vein is doubly ligated in the neck. Attention is now directed to the area of the sigmoid sinus and the jugular bulb. These structures are completely decompressed using diamond burs. Bone is preserved over the proximal portion of the sigmoid to allow for extraluminal packing of the sigmoid with Surgicel. The lumen of the sinus is opened. Further bleeding coming from the inferior petrosal sinus is controlled using Surgicel. Avoiding tightly packing the sinus can help preserve the function of the lower cranial nerves. The tumor is now ready for resection. It is usually removed with the dome of the jugular bulb. Hemostasis is secured after tumor removal. Usually, minimal morbidity is associated with this approach.

Mastoid and Neck Approach with Limited Facial Nerve Rerouting

If more room is needed superiorly, the facial nerve can be rerouted anteriorly (**Fig. 64–2**). Further exposure can be obtained by removing bone in the area of the vertical portion of the facial canal and retrofacial air cells along the infralabyrinthine air cell tract.

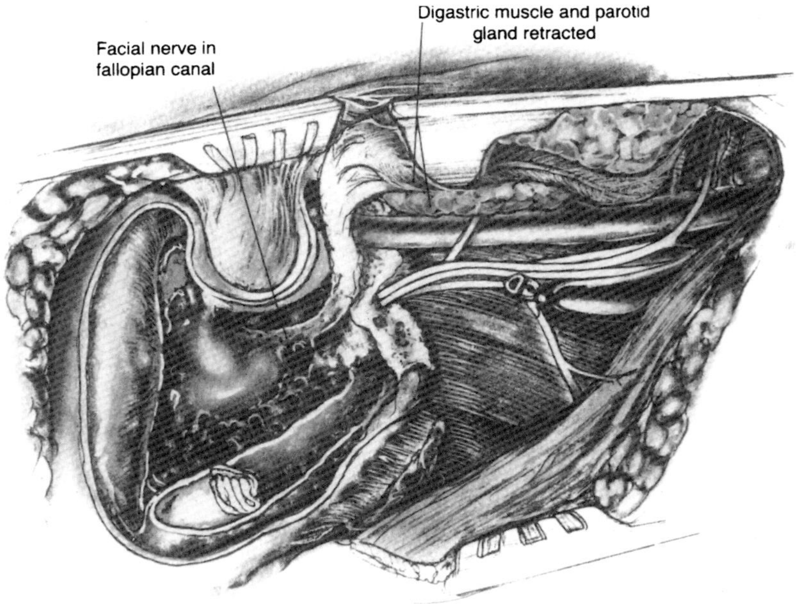

Figure 64–1 Transjugular approach.

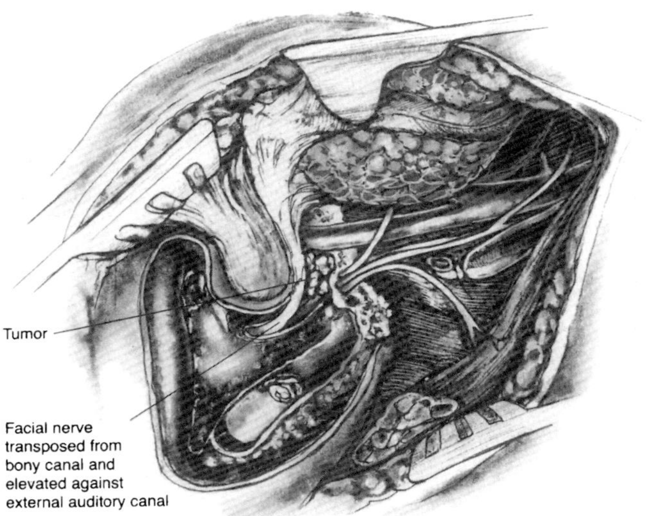

Figure 64–2 Mastoid-neck approach with limited transposition of the facial nerve.

The facial nerve is totally decompressed from the second genu to the stylomastoid foramen. The periosteum of the facial nerve at the stylomastoid foramen is preserved but the fibrous attachments to the nerve in its vertical portion are sharply transected. The completely mobilized nerve is now transposed anteriorly and laterally.[11]

This modification of the mastoid and neck approach with limited rerouting of the facial nerve is ideal for neuromas of the jugular foramen because they are not as intimately involved with the internal carotid artery as are paragangliomas. This approach is also suitable for paragangliomas limited to the jugular bulb (C1 type in the Fisch classification). For tumors involving the vertical portion of the carotid, the infratemporal approach is indicated.

Infratemporal Approach

For paragangliomas intimately involving the carotid artery, further exposure is needed to obtain control of the carotid artery and achieve complete resection of the tumor (**Fig. 64–3**). The infratemporal approach type A is indicated in these cases.[12]

The skin incision is C-shaped and is placed 4 cm behind the postauricular crease. The superior limb extends to the frontotemporal hairline and extends inferiorly to the neck following the anterior border of the sternomastoid muscle up to the level of the thyroid cartilage.

Superiorly, the incision is deepened to the deep layer of temporalis fascia, and the dissection is pursued between the two layers of fascia. In the postauricular area, dissection is performed superficial to the fibroperiosteal layer of the mastoid cortex. The posterior wall of the external auditory canal is identified at this point. Dissection of the cervical skin flap is done deep to the platysma muscle. The greater auricular nerve is identified and prepared for later use if needed. The infratemporal approach consists of the following steps:

1. *Transection of the ear canal.* Transection of the ear canal is performed medial to the bony cartilaginous junction. The cartilage is removed from the ear canal, and the skin is fashioned as a cuff ready to be everted and sutured with 4–0 nylon. Periosteum from the postauricular area is elevated and turned as a flap to buttress the previous suture line.
2. *Mastoidectomy, extended facial recess, and decompression of the facial nerve.* A complete mastoidectomy is accomplished. The facial recess is opened widely. The chorda tympani is sacrificed to extend the facial recess. Next, the posterior wall of the external auditory canal is removed. The tympanic membrane, malleus, incus, and the remaining skin of the external auditory canal are then removed. The facial nerve is decompressed from the area of the geniculate ganglion to the stylomastoid foramen. The tympanic ring is then removed, exposing the jugular bulb

posteriorly. Bone is removed from the area of the temporomandibular joint, exposing the petrous carotid artery.

3. *Vascular control in the neck.* The incision is extended inferiorly along the anterior border of the sternocleidomastoid muscle, which is dissected away from the mastoid tip. The mastoid tip is removed. Vascular control of the internal, common carotid, and internal jugular vein is obtained.

4. *Facial nerve rerouting.* The facial nerve is transposed anteriorly and laterally as described previously **(Fig. 64–3A).** The use of continuous facial nerve monitoring during this maneuver has significantly improved postoperative facial nerve function.

5. *Proximal and distal control of the neurovasculature.* The entire mandible is retracted forward. The remaining bone over the sigmoid sinus, jugular bulb, and vertical portion of the petrous carotid artery is removed. The internal carotid is followed from the neck through the skull base and into the temporal bone. The lower cranial nerves are identified and followed to the jugular foramen. The internal jugular vein is doubly ligated and transected **(Fig. 64–3B).** The external carotid artery is ligated. The sigmoid sinus is doubly ligated and divided if the tumor has an intracranial extension; otherwise, it is packed extraluminally.

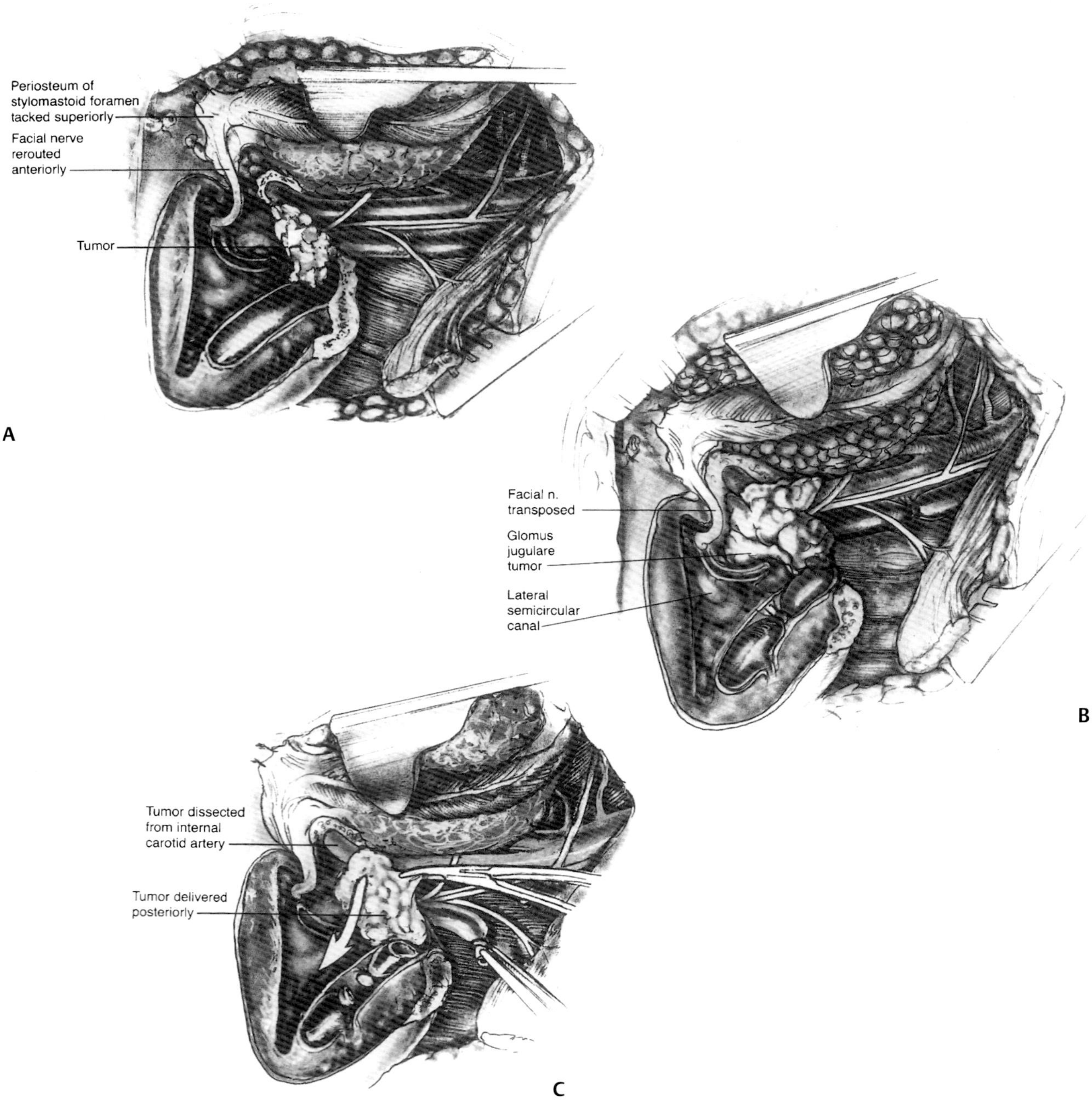

Figure 64–3 Infratemporal fossa approach. **(A)** Exposure. **(B)** Jugular vein and sigmoid sinus ligations. **(C)** Tumor dissection in the area of the internal carotid artery.

(*Continued on page 757*)

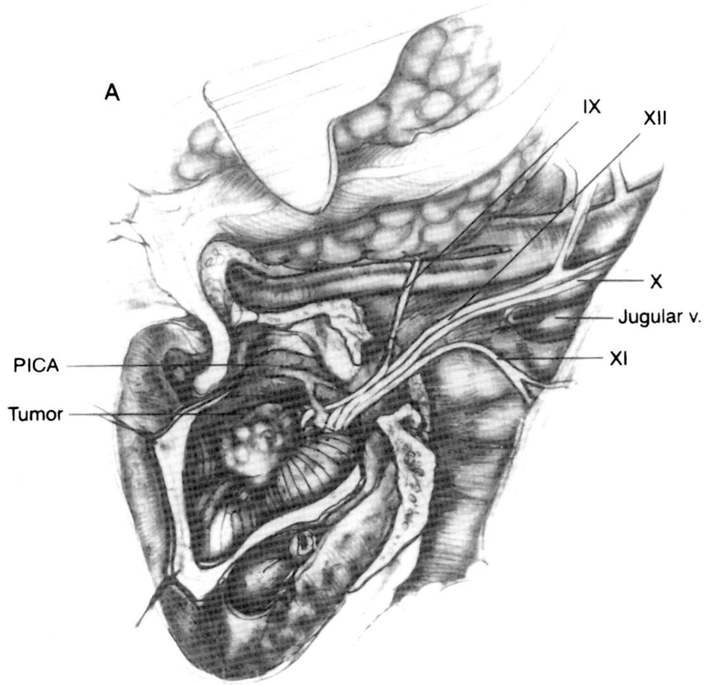

D

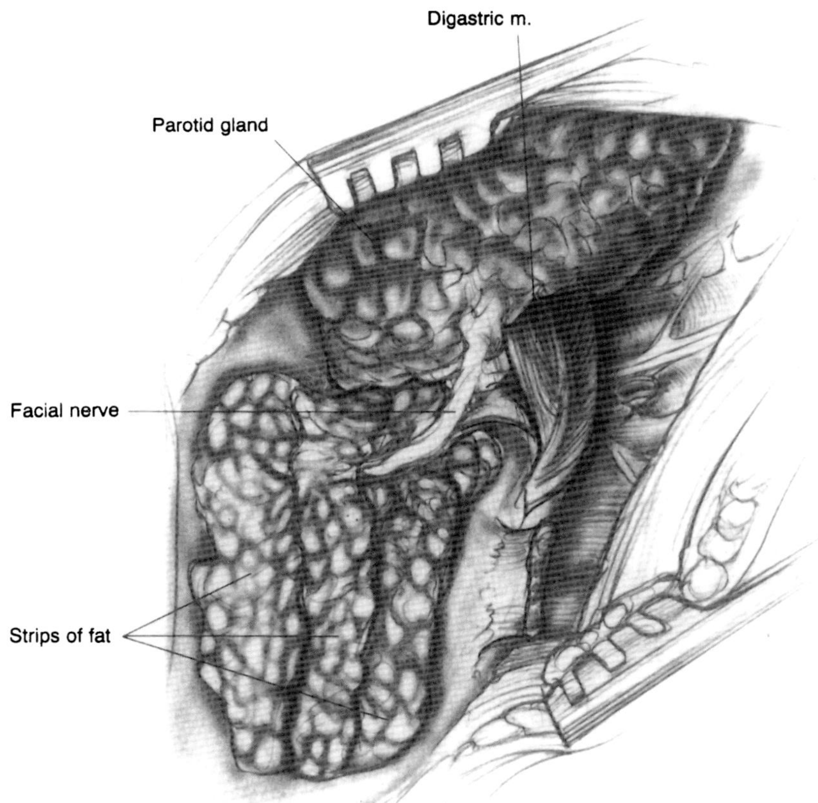

E

(Continued) **Figure 64–3** **(D)** Removal of the intracranial extension. **(E)** Closure. PICA, posterior inferior carotid artery.

6. *Tumor dissection.* Dissection of the tumor proceeds from inferiorly to superiorly following the internal jugular vein into the area of the jugular bulb. The tumor is then freed from the carotid artery anteriorly **(Fig. 64–3C).** Attention is then focused on removing the intracranial part of the tumor **(Fig. 64–3D).** Once this is done, hemostasis is secured.
7. *Wound closure* **(Fig. 64–3E).** Wound closure starts with eustachian tube closure using Surgicel and muscle. Abdominal fat is used to pack the surgical defect. The wound is then closed in layers. A Penrose drain is left in the neck and removed the following morning.

◆ Postoperative Care

The patient stays in the intensive care unit for 2 days. The Penrose drain is removed from the neck the following morning. The lumbar drain is left in place for 5 days until the wound is sealed. The pressure dressing is left in place for 4 days.

◆ Complications

Possible complications include facial nerve injury, lower cranial nerve dysfunction, carotid artery injury, hemorrhage, and intracranial complications.

Facial Nerve Injury

The advent of facial nerve monitoring has significantly improved postoperative nerve function in temporal bone surgery.[13] Transection of the facial nerve and reanastomosis using nerve graft may be needed if the tumor has invaded the facial nerve.

Lower Cranial Nerves Injury

In our experience, the need for tracheostomy or gastrostomy has been infrequent (<4%). In patients where the tumor has already weakened the lower cranial nerves, we recommend early intervention: thyroplasty or vocal cord augmentation for vagal paralysis.

Internal Carotid Artery Injury

Careful preoperative imaging, including CT, MRI, and angiography helps define the anatomical relationship of the tumor to the ICA. Balloon occlusion testing helps predict if the patient will be able to tolerate total occlusion of the ICA.

Hemorrhage

The possibility of severe blood loss when approaching the jugular foramen and a resecting glomus jugulare tumor should be anticipated. Autologous blood donation has been helpful in avoiding transfusion of banked blood. Similarly, the use of cell saver may reduce the requirement for banked blood transfusions.

Intracranial Complications

These include intracranial hemorrhage, cerebrospinal fluid (CSF) leakage, and wound infections. Intracranial tumor resection is done cooperatively with a neurosurgeon. Careful hemostasis is achieved in the posterior fossa by the neurosurgeon before closure. Most CSF leaks are managed conservatively using pressure dressing and lumbar drainage. Meningitis and wound infections are treated with the appropriate antibiotics.

References

1. Samii M, Bini W. Surgical strategy for jugular foramen tumors. In: Sekhar LN, Janecka IP, eds. Surgery of Cranial Base Tumors. New York: Raven; 1993:379–387
2. Horn KL, Hankinson H. Tumors of the jugular foramen. In: Jackler RK, Brackmann DE, eds. Neurotology. St. Louis: Mosby; 1994:1059–1068
3. Wenig BM. Neoplasms of the ear. In: Weing BM, ed. Atlas of Head and Neck Pathology. Philadelphia: WB Saunders; 1993:368–371
4. Brackmann DE, House WF, Terry R, Scanlan RL, Hardij RW Jr., Bay JW Parker JC Jr. Glomus jugulare tumors: effect of irradiation. Trans Am Acad Ophthalmol Otolaryngol 1972;76:1423–1431
5. Kinney SE. Jugular foramen neurilemmoma. In: Sekhar LN, Janecka IP, eds. Surgery of Cranial Base Tumors. New York: Raven; 1993:731–735
6. Kaye AH, Hahn JF, Kinney SE, et al. Jugular foramen schwannomas. J Neurosurg 1984;60:1045–1053
7. Weing BM. Neoplasms of the ear. In: Weing BM, ed. Atlas of Head and Neck Pathology. Philadelphia: WB Saunders; 1993:371–373
8. Maniglia AJ, Chandler JR, Goodwin WJ Jr, et al. Schwannomas of the parapharyngeal space and jugular foramen. Laryngoscope 1979;89:1405–1414
9. Murphy TP, Brackmann DE. Effects of preoperative embolization on glomus jugulare tumors. Laryngoscope 1989;99:1244–1247
10. Hirsch BE, Sekhar LN, Kamerer DB. Transtemporal and infratemporal approach for benign tumors of the jugular foramen and temporal bone. In: Sekhar LN, Janecka IP, eds. Surgery of Cranial Base Tumors. New York: Raven; 1993:267–289
11. Brackmann DE. The facial nerve in the infratemporal approach. Otolaryngol Head Neck Surg 1987;97:15–17
12. Fisch U, Fagan P, Valvanis A. The infratemporal fossa approach for glomus tumors of the temporal bone. Ann Otol Rhinol Laryngol 1982;91:474–479
13. Leonetti JP, Brackmann DE, Prass RC. Improved preservation of facial function in the infratemporal fossa approach to the skull base. Otolaryngol Head Neck Surg 1989;101:74–78

65

Nonvestibular Schwannomas of the Brain

Laligam N. Sekhar, Sajjan Sarma, David A. Schessel, and Foad Elahi

Schwannomas are slow-growing benign tumors, arising from Schwann cells of the covering membrane of the nerves. Sixty percent of all symptomatic schwannomas arise from cranial nerves. Vestibular schwannomas are the most frequently occurring schwannoma of the brain. Among nonvestibular schwannomas, trigeminal schwannomas are the commonest; they represent 0.8 to 8% of intracranial schwannomas.[1-4] Other nonvestibular schwannomas are uncommon and usually arise from the glossopharyngeal, vagal, facial, accessory, hypoglossal, oculomotor, trochlear, and abducens nerves, in descending order of frequency[5-7] Complete excision of these tumors usually results in long-term recurrence-free survival, whereas subtotal excision usually results in recurrence.[8] Application of various skull-base approaches is useful for complete and safe excision of these tumors. This chapter describes the operative techniques for removal of different varieties of nonvestibular schwannomas.

◆ Preoperative Studies

A thorough clinical examination is important. Magnetic resonance imaging (MRI) with and without contrast is the primary investigation necessary to define the tumor size, its various extensions, and its relationship with major blood vessels. T2-weighted images define any invasion into the surrounding brain, including the brain stem. Coronal and sagittal images are important to assess the superior and inferior extent of the tumor and to determine if there is any infratemporal extension of the tumor. Magnetic resonance venogram (MRV) should be performed to study the venous drainage and dominance of the sinuses pertinent to the approach to be used. A computed tomographic (CT) scan is important to define any bone erosion by the tumor. When the tumor encases a major artery such as the internal carotid artery (ICA) or the vertebral artery (VA), a preoperative angiogram is needed to define the anatomy and to assess the adequacy of cross-circulation. When the ICA is encased, an arteriogram with cross-compression can give the surgeon a good idea of the collateral circulation. Note should be made of the source of collateral arterial supply, such as the anterior communicating artery or the posterior communicating artery, because if the artery is damaged in addition to the ICA, then a bypass is required. A balloon occlusion test is usually not necessary because most encased arteries can be dissected free of tumor. However, if a major artery is damaged, a bypass graft is always performed. An audiogram is done whenever the tumor extends near cranial nerve (CN) VIII, or if the patient complains of hearing loss.

◆ Anesthesia and Intraoperative Monitoring

Standard neuroanesthetic techniques, without muscle relaxation, are used. Placement of a lumbar drain prior to surgery and controlled release of cerebrospinal fluid (CSF) will help in adequate brain relaxation. When there is significant hydrocephalus preoperatively or if there is significant mass in the tentorial notch, a ventricular catheter is placed instead of a lumbar drain. Continuous monitoring of somatosensory evoked potentials (SEPs) and electroencephalography (EEG) are performed routinely. When the tumor extends near CN VIII and VII, electromyographic (EMG) monitoring of the facial nerve, intraoperative direct stimulation of the nerve, and ipsilateral monitoring of the brain stem auditory evoked responses (BAERs) are performed. If there is significant brain stem compression, bilateral monitoring of the BAER is recommended. Monitoring of the function of the CNs X (vocal cord EMG monitoring), IX, and XII is performed when these CNs are involved.

◆ Trigeminal Schwannoma

Trigeminal schwannomas are the most commonly occurring nonvestibular schwannomas of the brain. They may arise from one of the roots of the nerve, from the ganglionic segment of the nerve, or from the cisternal segment. Accordingly they may be localized to the infratemporal region, the orbit, the middle fossa, the posterior fossa, or their combinations. A large or giant trigeminal schwannoma may extend to all three regions.[9] The tumor generally arises from one of the fascicles of the nerve and expands, compressing the remaining healthy fascicles. The goal of surgery is to preserve all uninvolved fascicles, so that near-normal function of the nerve can be preserved or nerve function can be improved.[10,11]

We classify these tumors into (1) precavernous and cavernous type, (2) cavernous type, and (3) cavernous and postcavernous type, depending on the location of the tumor in relation to the cavernous sinus (CS). Surgical strategies change according to the location of the tumor. For example, to remove a precavernous and cavernous type of trigeminal schwannoma, when the tumor extends to the orbital apex, an orbital osteotomy is performed, whereas for a tumor limited to the CS and infratemporal fossa, a zygomatic osteotomy is performed to remove the tumor (**Table 65–1**; also see cases 1 to 4, later in chapter.)

Table 65–1 Different Surgical Strategies According to Trigeminal Schwannoma Location

Location of the Tumor	Approach Used
CS	Temporal craniotomy + zygomatic osteotomy
CS + orbit	FT + orbital osteotomy
CS + infratemporal fossa	FT + zygomatic osteotomy
CS + small posterior fossa	Temporal craniotomy + zygomatic osteotomy
Large posterior fossa + CS	Transpetrosal PLPA approach

CS, cavernous sinus; FT, frontotemporal; PLPA, partial labyrinthectomy and petrous apicectomy.

Anterior-Lateral Approaches

These approaches are used to remove a trigeminal schwannoma localized to the precavernous, cavernous, and small postcavernous areas. The patient is placed in the supine position with the head in a three-pin head holder. The head is rotated 45 degrees away from the surgeon, and a roll is placed under the ipsilateral shoulder to minimize excessive stretching of the neck. A frontotemporal craniotomy[11] and an orbital or orbitozygomatic osteotomy are performed[12] **(Fig. 65–1A,B).** Subsequent steps of the operation depend on where the major portion of the tumor is located. When the tumor involves only a small portion of the CS anteriorly or inferiorly, an extradural approach is adequate. When a large mass of the tumor is located in the CS, especially in the superior and posterior portion, then an intradural approach is required.

Extradural Approach

The temporal dura is gradually elevated from the floor of the middle cranial fossa from the posterior to anterior direction after coagulating and dividing the middle meningeal vessels. Bone is removed from the floor of the middle cranial fossa with the help of rongeur and high-speed drill and the superior orbital fissure (SOF) or the CN V branches are decompressed under surgical microscope as needed. CSF is drained through the lumbar drain to relax the brain before retracting the temporal lobe. The bulging of the tumor is seen in the lateral wall of the CS at this time. An incision is made in the lateral wall of the CS at its attachment at the SOF, V2, and V3, and the dura is peeled away to expose the tumor **(Fig. 65–1C).** The tumor is debulked internally with the help of a Cottle dissector, pituitary forceps, and the Cavitron ultrasonic surgical aspirator (CUSA [Valley Lab, Boulder, CO]). After sufficient internal debulking has been achieved, the capsule of the tumor is then dissected from the other fascicle of the nerve using a no. 3 Rhoton dissector (V. Mueller, Chicago, IL), microscissors, and bipolar forceps. The surgeon should gently grasp and pull the tumor capsule and separate it from the other fascicles with fine instruments, while the assistant provides the suction. One should be careful to find the petrous

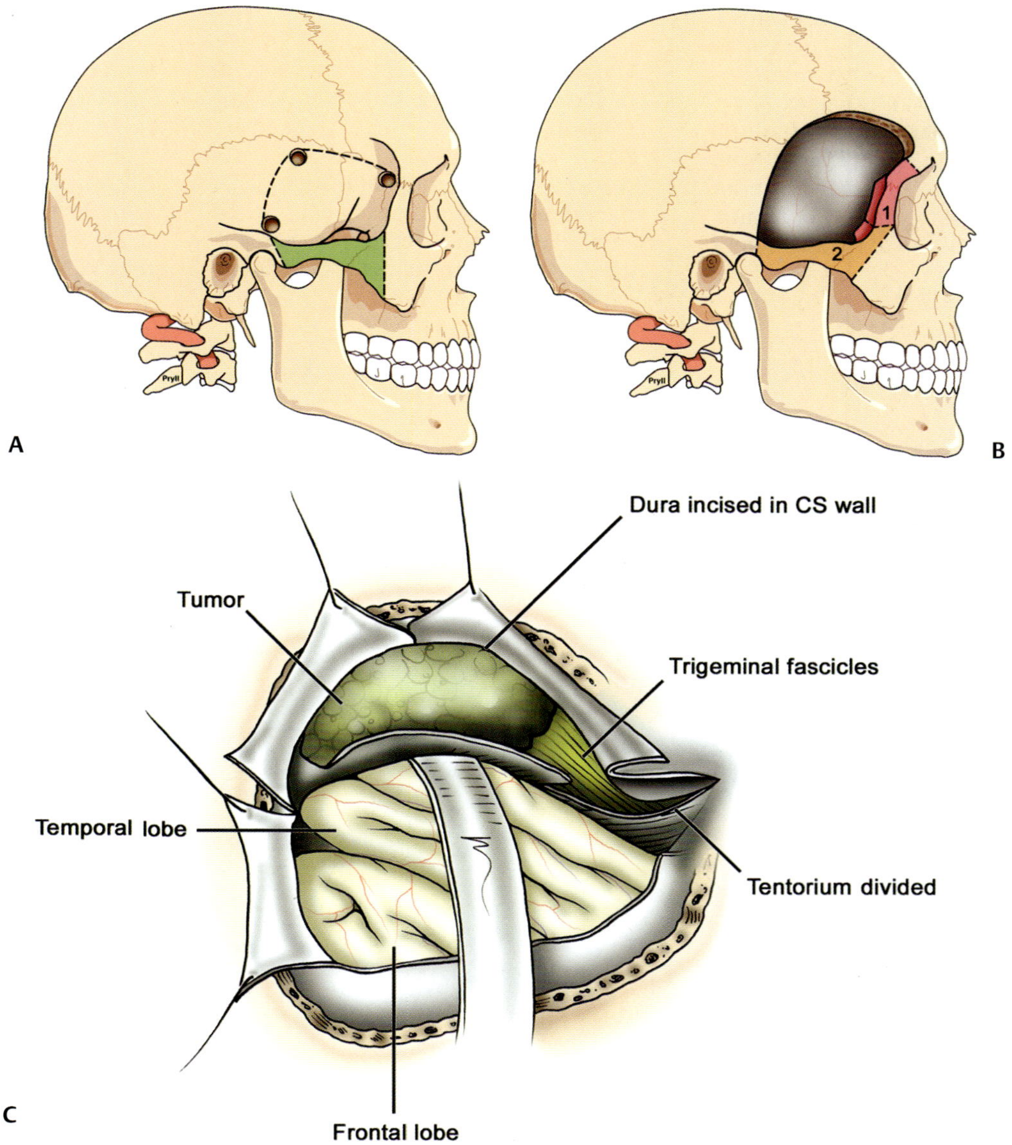

Figure 65–1 Anterolateral approach for a trigeminal schwannoma. **(A)** Temporal craniotomy and zygomatic osteotomy. **(B)** Frontotemporal craniotomy and orbitozygomatic osteotomy. **(C)** Tumor exposure by the subtemporal approach. CS, cavernous sinus.

carotid artery at this stage. The surrounding bone may be eroded by the tumor, and the artery may be displaced from its normal position. A Doppler probe may be helpful to find a displaced artery. Rarely, the artery may be completely surrounded by the tumor, and in this situation the artery should be identified in the relatively normal area and traced up to the pathological area. Usually one can find a good dissection plane between the tumor capsule and the adventitia of the artery unless the tumor has been previously operated or irradiated. In this situation, it is advisable to have the proximal control of the artery in the neck, and the patient may require a bypass procedure if the artery cannot be preserved. Although small and medium-size schwannomas do not invade the CS, large tumors frequently invade the CS. During removal of the tumor from inside the CS, CNs III, IV, VI, and the cavernous carotid artery should be carefully preserved. The capsule of the tumor should be carefully followed during the whole dissection, which is important for complete removal of the tumor. At the final stage of removal of the tumor from the cavernous sinus, there may be brisk bleeding from the sinus, which can be easily controlled by packing the sinus with Surgicel (Ethicon, division of Johnson & Johnson, Somerville, NJ) or thrombin-soaked Gelfoam (Upjohn, Kalamazoo, MI). If a small portion of the tumor extends into the posterior fossa, it can be easily removed after drilling away the petrous apex and opening the Meckel's cave.

Intradural Approach

After opening the dura of the frontotemporal area, the sylvian fissure is opened, and the temporal lobe is mobilized as needed, to pursue the anterior subtemporal or transsylvian approaches. When the tumor is visualized in the lateral wall of the CS, a cruciate incision is made over the maximum tumor bulge and the dura of the lateral wall is peeled away. The steps of tumor removal are similar to the extradural approach. Generally, the surgeon should stay away from CNs III and IV as much as possible. If there is small posterior fossa extension of the tumor, the tentorium is cut behind the CN IV and the Meckel's cave is opened to remove tumor from the posterior fossa.

Lateral Approach

Whenever there is large postcavernous location of the tumor, it is removed by a lateral approach. A partial labyrinthectomy and petrous apicectomy (PLPA) and transpetrosal approach (**Fig. 65–2**) is performed for this approach.[13] We do not recommend the retrosigmoid approach for posterior fossa trigeminal schwannomas because with that approach the tentorial notch and Meckel's cave are difficult to access, and there is greater stretching of the already stretched CNs VII

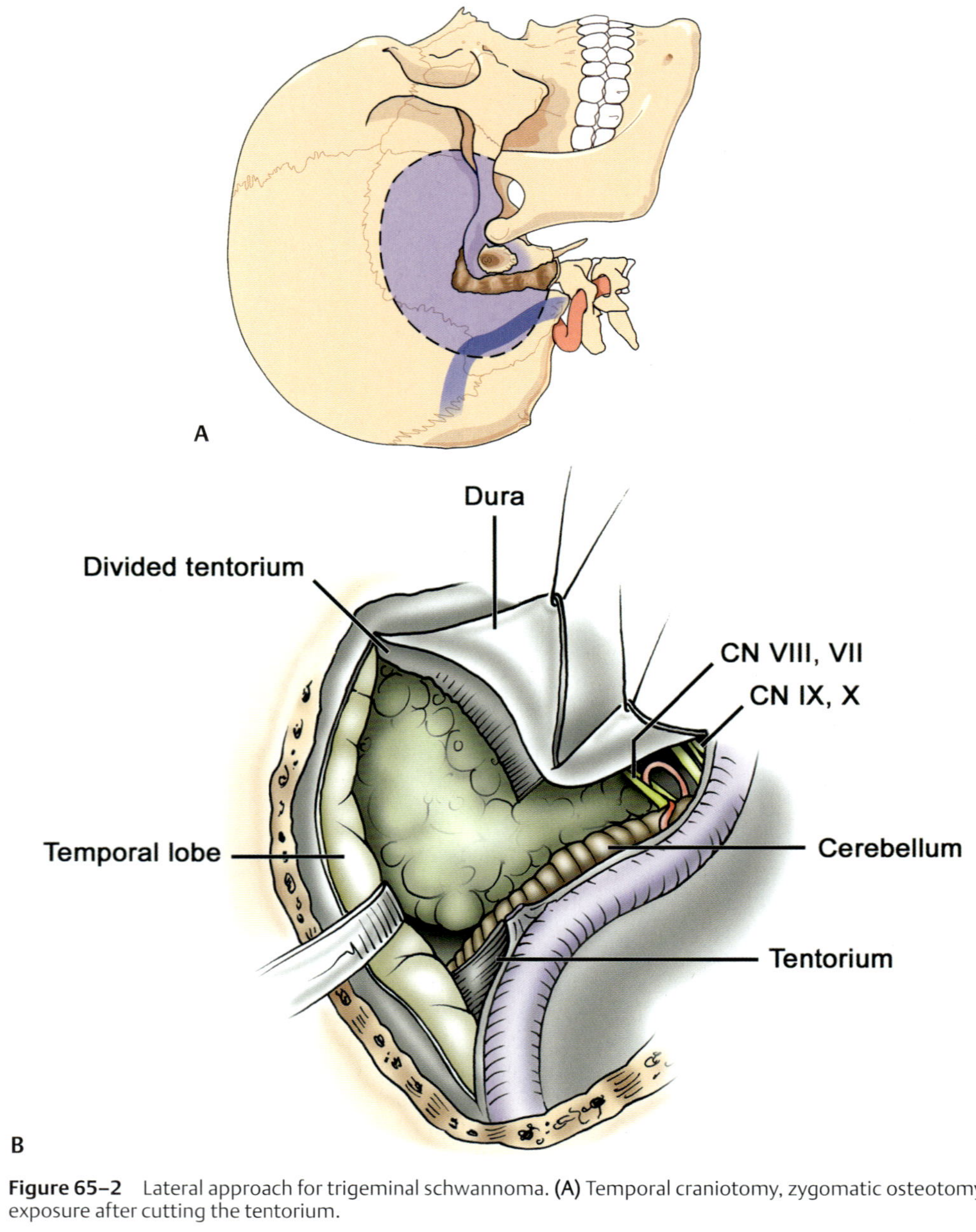

Figure 65–2 Lateral approach for trigeminal schwannoma. **(A)** Temporal craniotomy, zygomatic osteotomy, and transpetrosal approach. **(B)** Tumor exposure after cutting the tentorium.

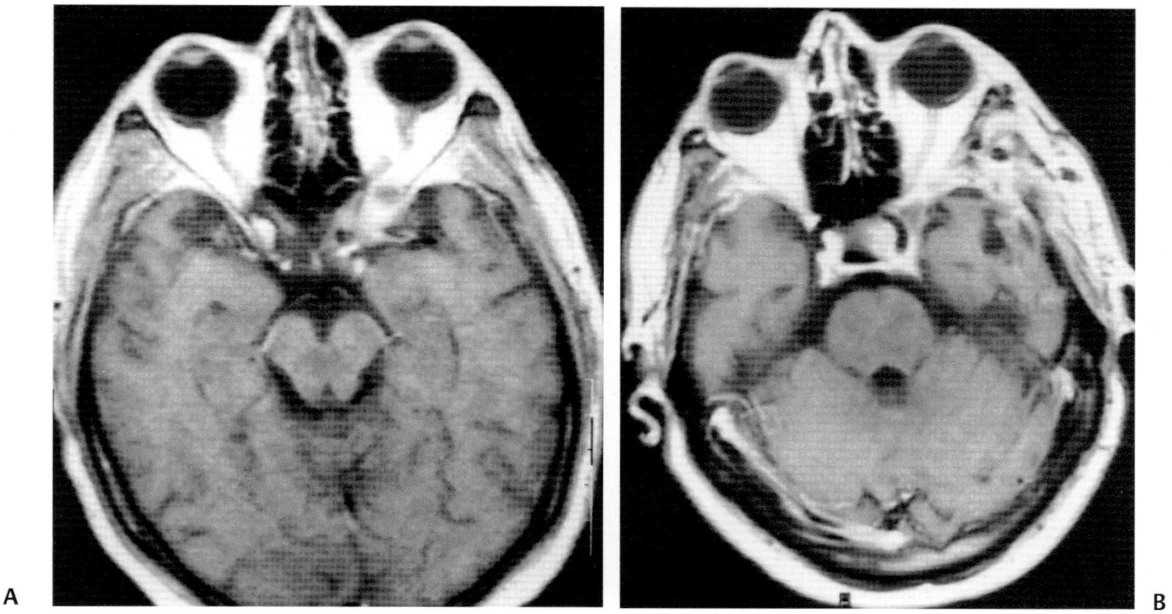

Figure 65–3 (A) This 69-year-old man presented with severe visual impairment of the left eye, and on magnetic resonance imaging (MRI) examination a trigeminal schwannoma extending from the cavernous sinus into the orbital apex was detected. The tumor was excised completely after a frontotemporal craniotomy and an extradural subtemporal approach. (B) Postoperative MRI showing complete excision of the tumor.

and VIII during cerebellar retraction. With the transpetrosal approach, the entire tumor can be exposed easily, and there is less stretching of CNs VII and VIII. The details of the lateral approaches are described in the chapter on petroclival meningiomas. The steps of tumor removal are the same as with the anterolateral approach.

Illustrative Cases

Case 1: **Fig. 65–3**

Case 2: **Fig. 65–4**

Case 3: **Fig. 65–5**

Case 4: **Fig. 65–6**

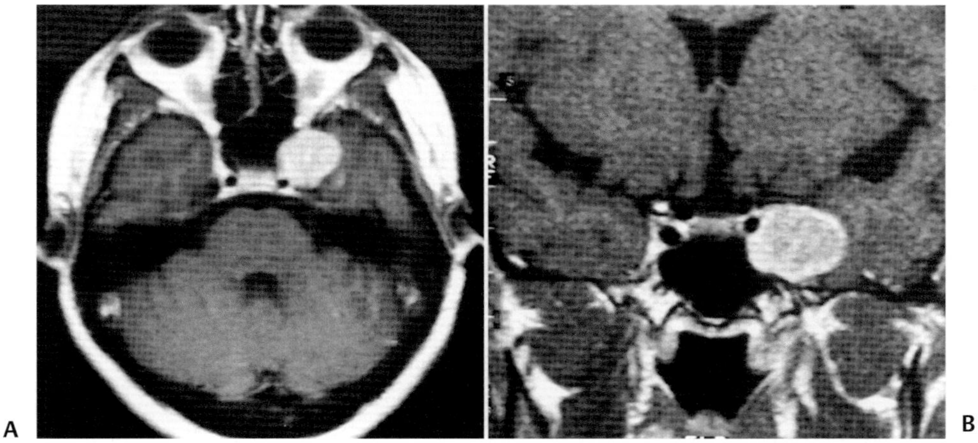

Figure 65–4 (A,B) A case of trigeminal schwannoma where the tumor was localized to the lateral wall of the anterior and inferior cavernous sinus.

(*Continued on page 764*)

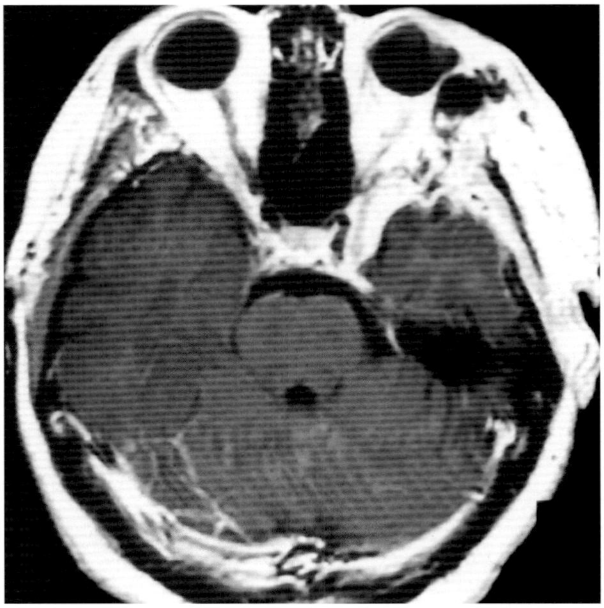

C

(*Continued*) **Figure 65–4** **(C)** The tumor was excised completely after a frontotemporal craniotomy and an orbital osteotomy and a subtemporal extradural approach.

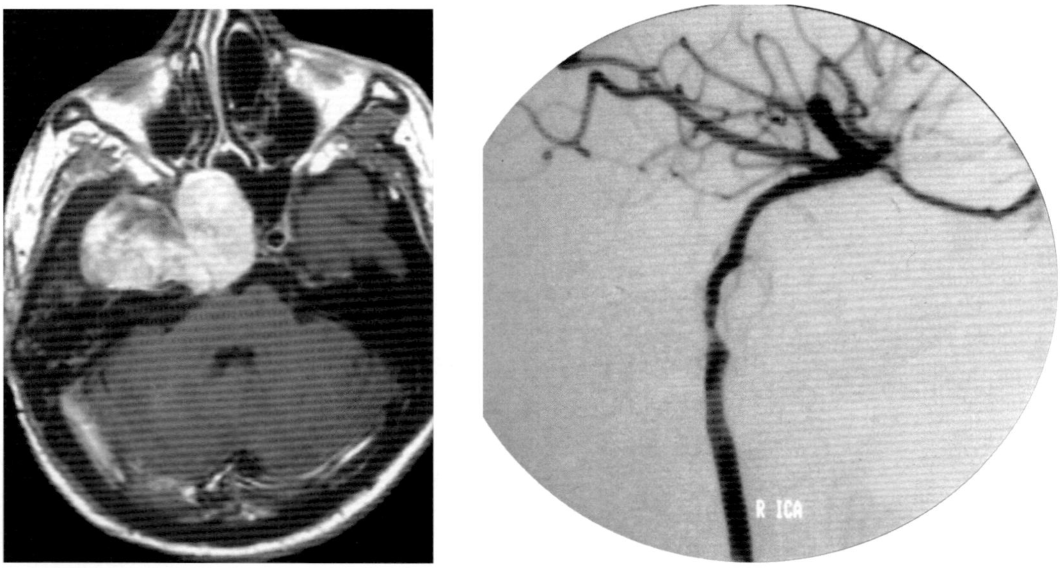

A

B

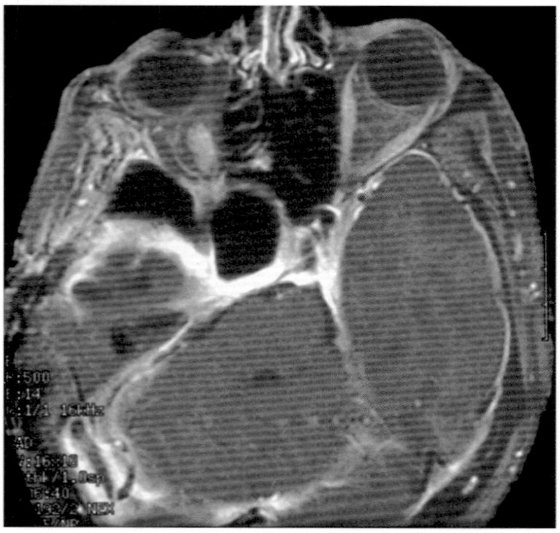

C

Figure 65–5 **(A)** This 33-year-old man had a partial resection of the trigeminal schwannoma elsewhere and presented with a large recurrence extending to the cavernous sinus and infratemporal area. **(B)** The preoperative angiogram showed severe narrowing and displacement of the internal carotid artery. **(C)** The patient underwent a first-stage cervical internal carotid artery to middle cerebral artery bypass procedure followed by complete excision of the tumor in a second stage by a frontotemporal craniotomy, an orbitozygomatic osteotomy, and subtemporal/infratemporal approach.

(*Continued on page765*)

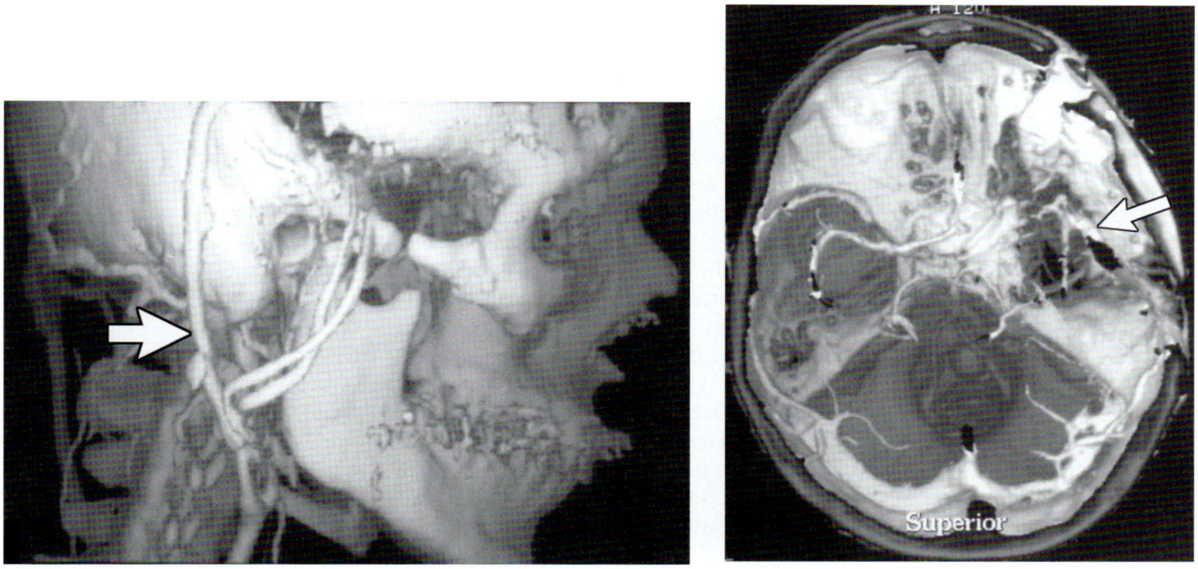

D E

(*Continued*) **Figure 65–5** **(D,E)** The follow-up CT angiogram shows good filling of the bypass graft (arrow).

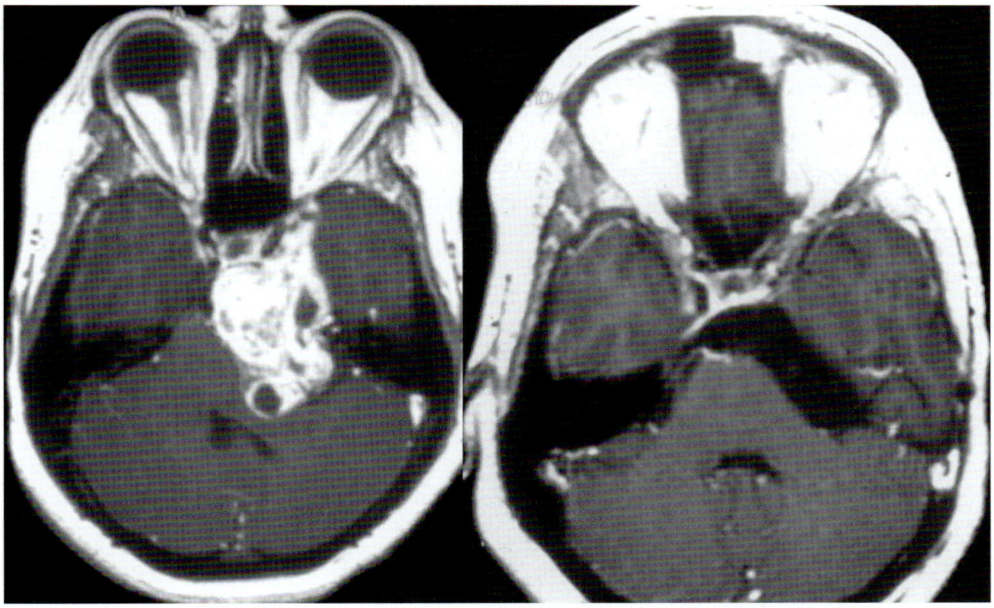

A B

Figure 65–6 **(A)** This woman with trigeminal schwannoma had a large postcavernous extension into the posterior fossa. The tumor was excised by a partial labyrinthectomy and petrous apicectomy and the transpetrosal approach. **(B)** Postoperative magnetic resonance imaging shows complete excision of the tumor. The patient suffered delayed postoperative cerebrospinal fluid rhinorrhea due to communicating hydrocephalus, which was relieved after a ventriculoperitoneal shunt.

◆ Facial Nerve Schwannoma

Facial nerve schwannomas can arise from anywhere from the cisternal segment of the nerve up to its extracranial branches. Depending on the location of these tumors, they can be categorized as (1) cerebellopontine angle, (2) geniculate (most common variety), and (3) tympanomastoid type. Medium-size and large schwannomas may extend into more than one segment of the nerve, making it difficult to ascertain the precise site of origin of the tumor. There are some controversies regarding the timing of surgery of these tumors because facial palsy is frequent after surgery. King and Morrison[7] and Lipkin et al[14] discourage early surgery in young patients with intact facial nerve function. But our philosophy is to perform early surgery because there is a better chance of hearing preservation and a better result of facial reconstruction when the tumor is small. In some patients with small tumors, it may be possible to preserve the uninvolved fascicles of CN VII and peel the tumor away, even improving the function of the nerve. The selection of the approach to tumor removal is based on the extent of the lesion. Due to the circuitous course of the facial nerve, and thus the tumor, access to these lesions may involve the middle fossa or suboccipital approach alone, but more commonly includes combinations of the above approaches, as well as some degree of removal of the intervening temporal bone. In many cases, the surgeon must be prepared to uncover all parts of the nerve, both to ensure complete removal of the lesion and to expose sufficient uninvolved nerve to enable grafting, if necessary.

Preoperative determination of the degree of nerve involvement is not always possible. Although the extent of enhancement of the nerve on gadolinium-enhanced MRI may reflect the location of the lesion, the authors have encountered tumors that overreach these imaging boundaries, and others that demonstrated extensive enhancement of the uninvolved nerve, but the tumor was confined to a small segment. It has been our practice that unless the tumor can be resected with preservation of the nerve, intraoperative biopsy is used to define the margins of the tumor. This not only ensures complete tumor excision but also avoids dissection and resection of uninvolved nerve.

Purely cerebellopontine tumors can be removed by a retrosigmoid approach. The steps of removal of such a tumor are very similar to the removal of an acoustic neuroma, but nerve reconstruction with graft is usually necessary.

Schwannomas arising from the geniculate segment of the facial nerve may grow superiorly through the roof of the temporal bone into the middle fossa or through the fallopian canal into the posterior fossa or in both directions. For tumors extending into the middle fossa alone, a standard middle fossa approach can be used. In such cases, localization of the nerve is facilitated by the presence of the tumor already extending through the tegmen tympani. It is often necessary to remove a portion of the ossicular chain to gain adequate access to the entire lesion.

In the case of more extensive lesions, a combined transmastoid and middle fossa approach is used. In this case, access is gained through a C-shaped incision starting posterior to the mastoid tip, curving behind the ear, and extending over the ear as far forward as the tragus. Bone dissection begins with a cortical mastoidectomy with definition of both the involved and distal uninvolved nerve. Removal of some elements of the ossicular chain is necessary for this dissection. These elements are replaced after tumor excision. A small middle fossa craniotomy allows exposure of the roof of the temporal bone. In this instance, localization of the lesion and the facial nerve in the middle fossa floor is facilitated by removal of the overlying tegmen during the mastoidectomy.

After defining the complete extent of the tumor as well as the surrounding uninvolved nerve, the tumor is removed with preservation or resection of the uninvolved nerve as needed. If nerve resection is necessary, repair is accomplished with a sural nerve interposition graft **(Fig. 65–7C,D)**. Anastomosis is made with one or two 10–0 nylon suture proximally and two to three 9–0 sutures for the distal connection.[15,16] The anastomosis is reinforced with fibrin glue (Haemacure Corp., Sarasota, FL). Reconstruction of the craniotomy is done with fat graft, titanium mesh, and bone source cement.

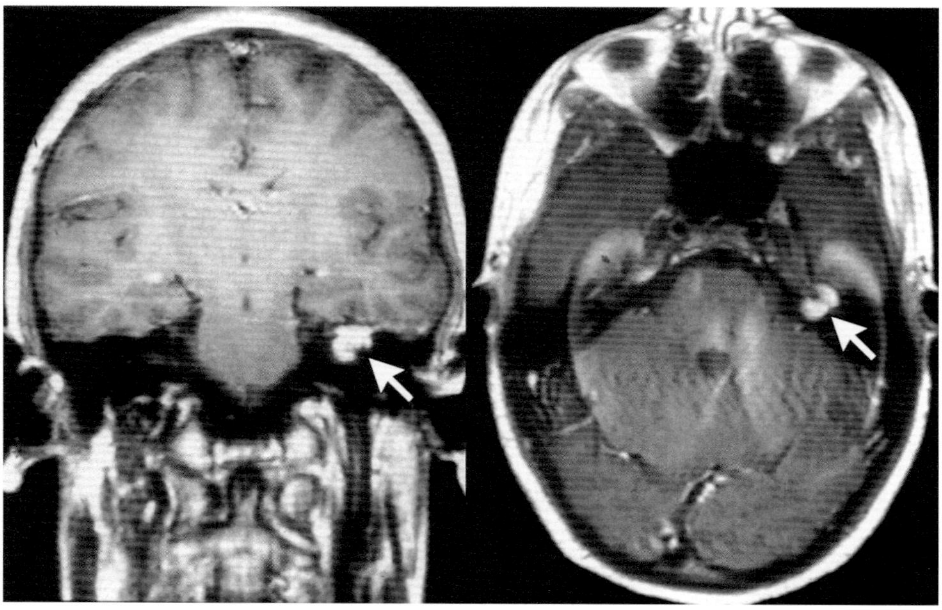

A B

Figure 65–7 This 15-year-old girl presented with a sudden-onset persistent facial weakness, not improved with steroids. **(A,B)** Magnatic resonance imaging (MRI) examination showed a facial nerve schwannoma arising from the geniculate segment (arrows). The tumor was excised by a middle fossa and transmastoid approach and the tumor was excised with transection of the facial nerve and facial nerve repair by a sural nerve graft. **(C,D)** The artist's diagram shows the technique of tumor excision and facial nerve repair by a nerve graft.

(Continued on page 767)

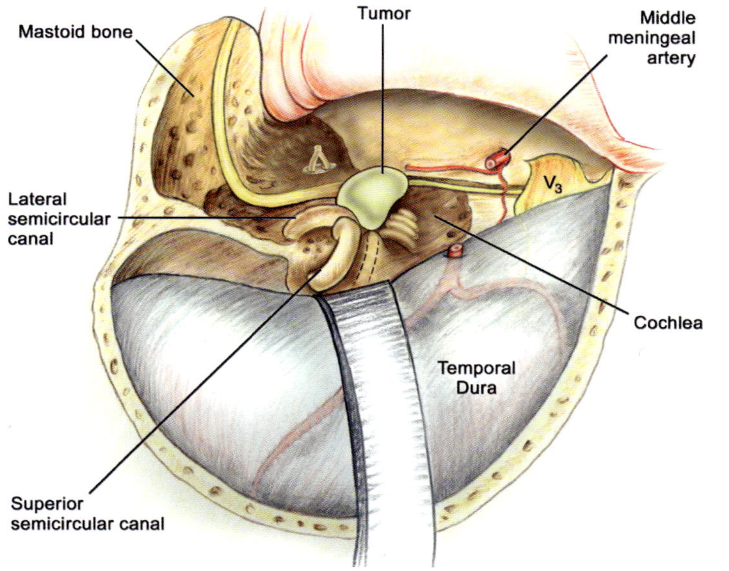

C

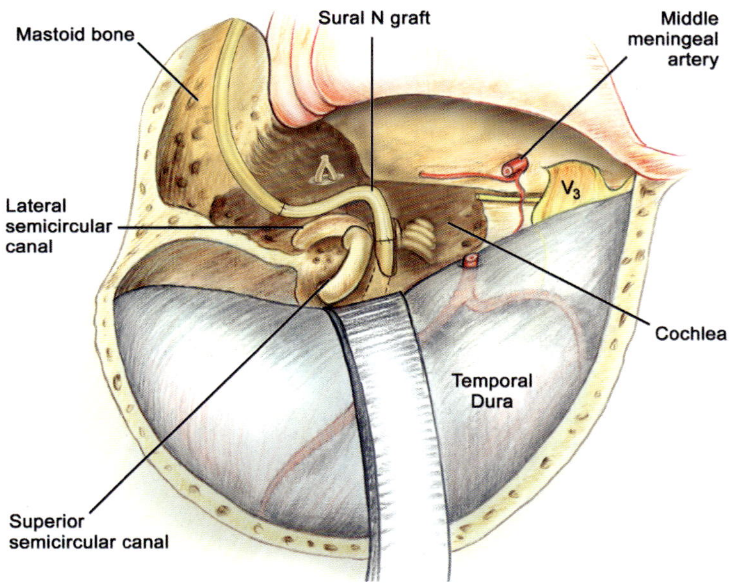

D

(*Continued*) **Figure 65–7** **(E)** Follow-up MRI shows complete excision of the tumor, and **(F)** the patient's photograph taken 2 years after surgery shows House-Brackmann grade III recovery of the facial nerve function.

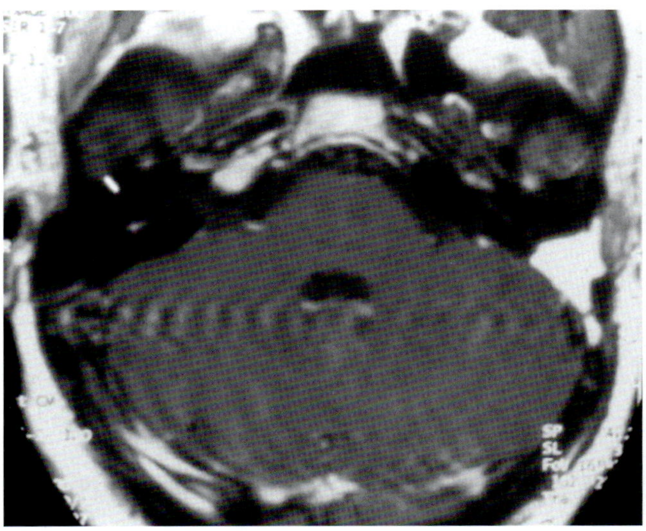

E

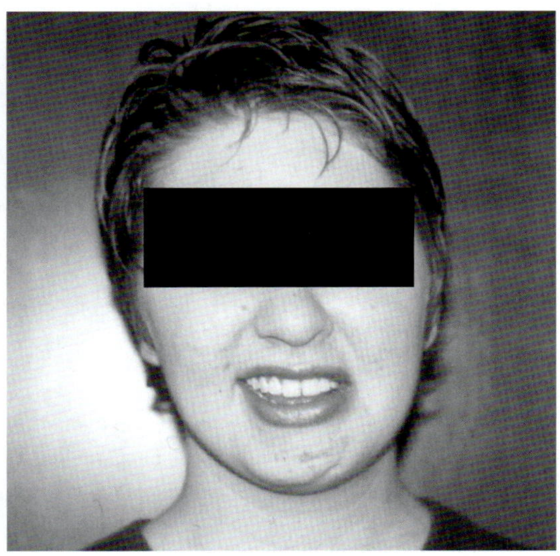

F

When the tumor is in the mastoid or extracranial segment, the nerve should be exposed proximal and distal to the tumor location. Exposure of the extracranial segment of the facial nerve may be difficult. The nerve can be exposed at the stylomastoid foramen by following the digastric muscle, the styloid process, and the cartilage of the external ear canal. When followed out distally, the nerve divides into two branches in the parotid gland. This anatomical fact helps in confirming the identity of the nerve, which can also be stimulated by a nerve stimulator.

Illustrative Case 5: Fig. 65–7

◆ Schwannomas of Cranial Nerves IX, X, and XI

Schwannomas arising from CNs IX, X, and XI occur in the jugular foramen area. CN IX schwannomas are the commonest among these three. In addition, because CN XII crosses through the jugular foramen, schwannomas of this nerve may also involve the jugular foramen. There are three types of growth pattern of these tumors, depending on the origin of the tumor from the nerve: (1) The tumor may be localized entirely to the posterior fossa if it arises from the proximal segment of the nerve. (2) The tumor may originate in the pars nervosa of jugular foramen and extend both intradurally and extradurally in a dumbbell-shaped manner. (3) The tumor may be in the jugular foramen extradurally and extracranially. Extradural tumors may also extend into the petroclival and cavernous area (see case 7, later in chapter). The approaches used to excise these tumors vary according to their location. If the tumor is intradural in the posterior fossa, it can be removed by a retrosigmoid approach. For the dumbbell-shaped tumors, with intracranial and extracranial extension, a combined retrosigmoid and transjugular approach is chosen **(Fig. 65–8).** A long skin incision is made starting just above the ear and curving behind the ear and extending down along a skin crease in the neck to enable exposure of the mastoid and retrosigmoid bone as well as the jugular vein in the neck. A complete mastoidectomy is performed with exposure of the sigmoid and distal transverse sinuses, which facilitates the subsequent retrosigmoid craniotomy as well as proximal control of the vessels. The facial nerve is identified and retrofacial bone removed until the jugular bulb and tumor are exposed. Smaller lesions confined to the region of the jugular bulb can be removed in this way. In the case of large lesions with greater extracranial extension under the skull base toward the upper cervical and petrous carotid artery, the facial nerve will be in the way and requires mobilization. Only the vertical segment of the nerve below the otic capsule bone is mobilized along with its soft tissue attachments to the stylomastoid foramen and digastric muscle. It has been found that if the inferior tympanic bone is removed in front of the facial nerve, then the nerve can be lifted laterally and pushed forward to enable complete access to the extracranial tumor as far anterior as the carotid

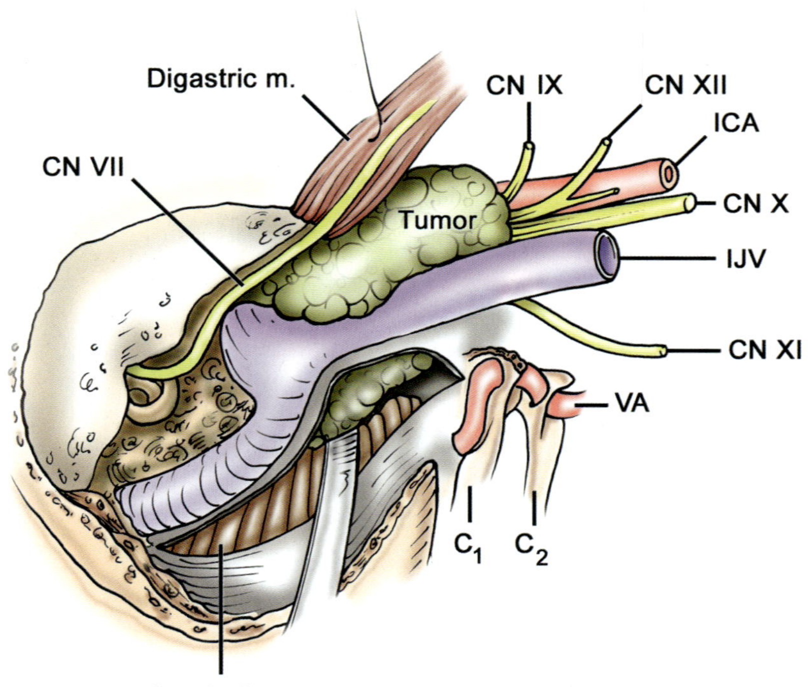

Figure 65–8 Artist's diagram of the retrosigmoid-transjugular approach for an intra- and extradural jugular foramen schwannoma.

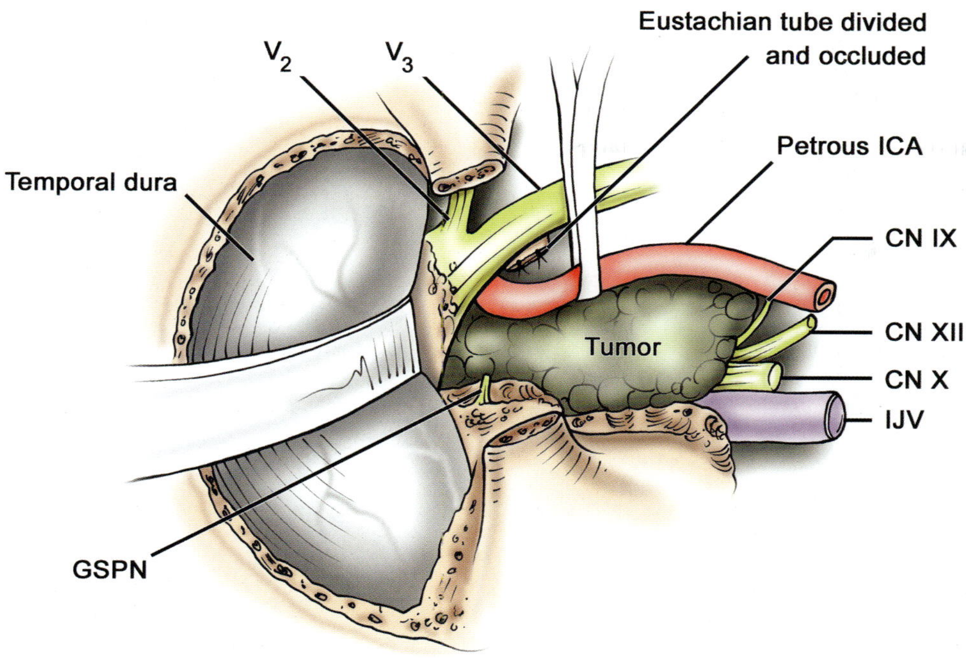

Figure 65–9 Diagram of the subtemporal-infratemporal approach for an extradural petroclival and cavernous sinus extension of a jugular foramen/hypoglossal schwannoma. ICA, internal carotid artery; IJV, inernal jugular vein.

artery. Furthermore, this partial mobilization of the nerve is not usually followed by significant permanent facial nerve dysfunction. Auditory function is disturbed with this approach.

The extradural tumor is removed first. Although the lesion can usually be dissected off the jugular bulb or the vessel repaired after removal of the invading tumor, the sigmoid sinus and the jugular bulb must occasionally be transected to allow complete tumor excision. The decision to sacrifice the vessel is made only if the vessel is clearly completely occluded by the lesion, if it is proven to be nondominant by angiography, or upon temporary occlusion, the proximal intravascular pressure does not rise by more than 5 mm Hg (pressure measured both before and after temporary clipping by cannulating the vessel with a needle connected to a pressure transducer). When the jugular vein is sacrificed, it is usually necessary to occlude the inferior petrosal sinus. There may be multiple venous connections present, each of which should be controlled with packing. Care must be taken in doing this to avoid injury to the intact lower cranial nerve fibers that run near this sinus.

Once exposed, the steps of tumor excision include (1) initial debulking of the tumor, (2) careful separation of the capsule from the surrounding structures while maintaining the cleavage plane of the tumor, and (3) preservation of all uninvolved nerve fascicles.

If the jugular foramen Schwannoma is primarily localized extradurally, an extreme lateral and transmastoid approach is used to remove the tumor from the jugular foramen area, whereas a preauricular subtemporal-infratemporal approach is used if the tumor is localized to the petroclival and CS area (**Fig. 65–9**).[17] These approaches have to be tailored according to the extension of the tumor. Postoperatively, the swallowing function of the patient is tested carefully before allowing the patient to eat. If the patient fails the swallowing test, an arytenoid adduction and thyroplasty procedure are performed first. If the patient still has trouble with swallowing, a temporary percutaneous endoscopic jejunostomy (PEJ) may be needed until the swallowing function recovers (usually 2 to 3 months). A tracheostomy is rarely needed.

Illustrative Cases

Case 6: **Fig. 65–10**
Case 7: **Fig. 65–11**
Case 8: **Fig. 65–12**

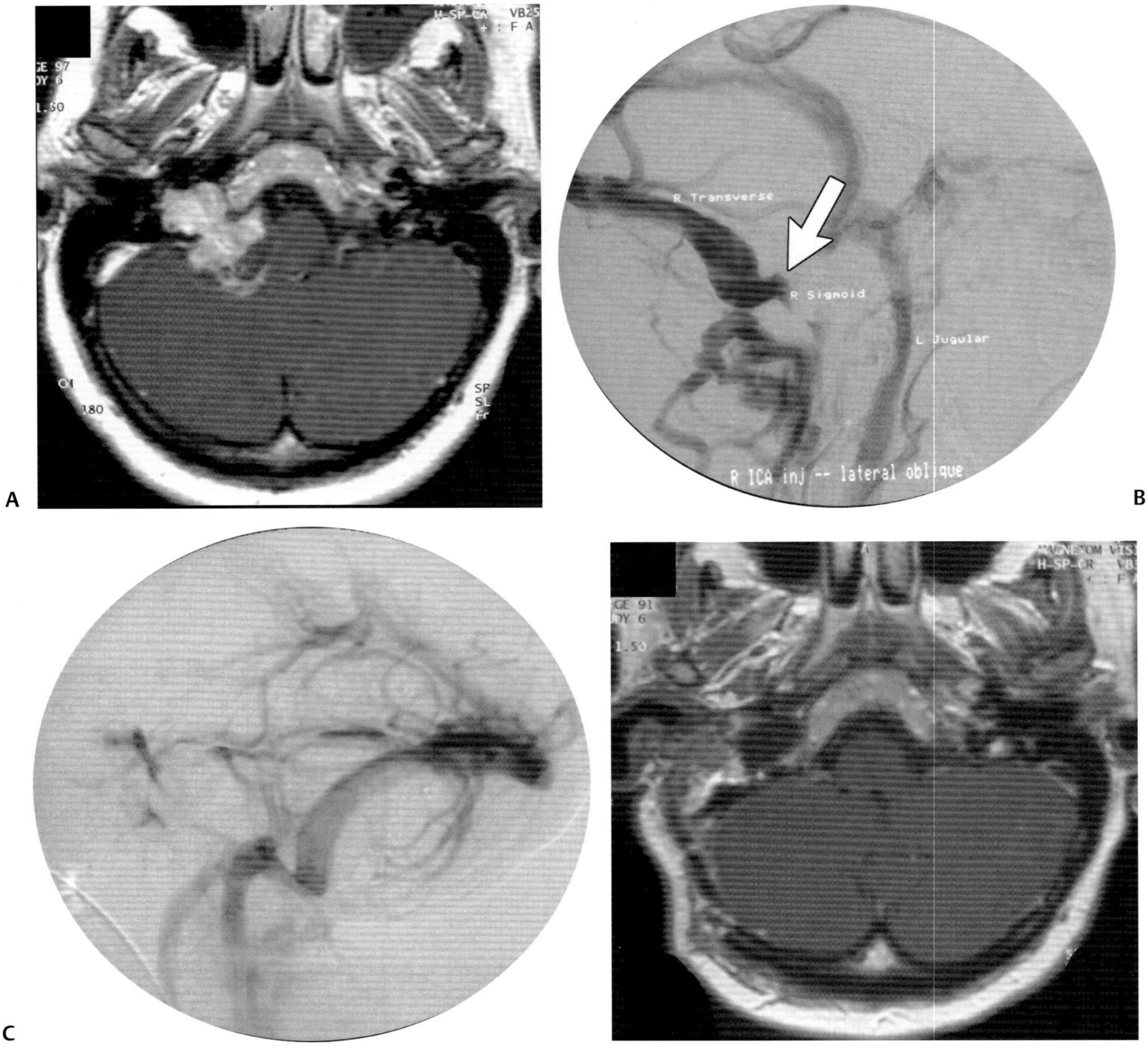

Figure 65–10 **(A)** This patient presented with a sudden loss of hearing, severe vertigo, and impairment of balance due to a dumbbell-shaped jugular foramen schwannoma arising from CN IX. **(B)** The sigmoid sinus and jugular bulb were severely narrowed by tumor invasion (arrow). The tumor was excised by a retrosigmoid transjugular approach. The sigmoid sinus was opened for tumor extraction from inside the sinus, and the sinus was reconstructed at the end of the tumor resection. **(C)** Postoperative angiogram shows good flow across the sinus, and **(D)** postoperative magnetic resonance imaging shows complete resection of the tumor.

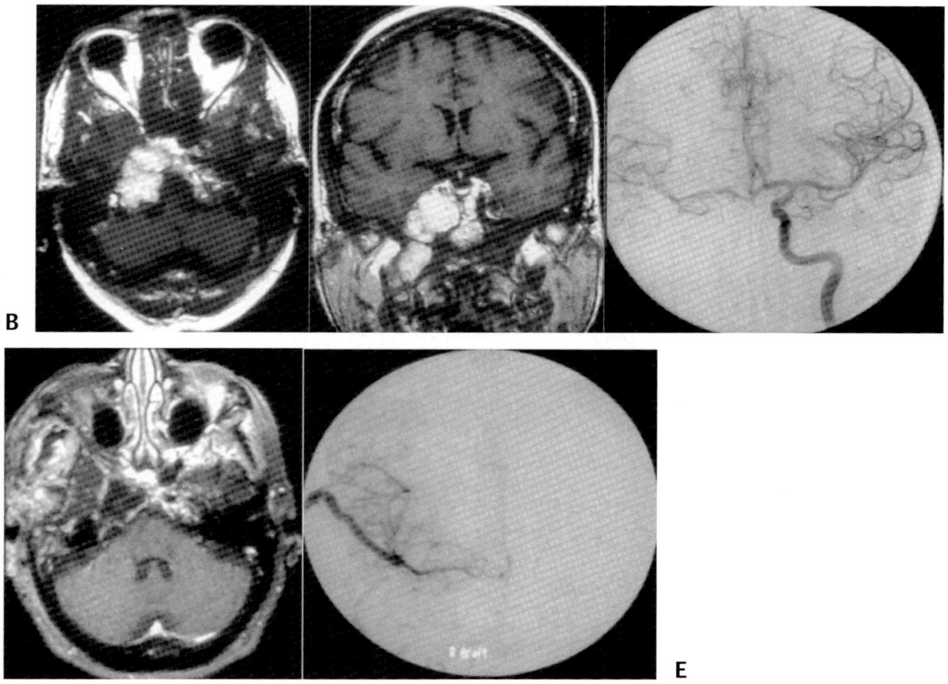

A – B C

D E

Figure 65–11 **(A,B)** A case of jugular foramen schwannoma, where the tumor extends extradurally to the petroclival and cavernous sinus area. **(C)** The preoperative angiogram shows severe narrowing of the carotid artery without adequate cross-circulation, and the evoked potentials became very attenuated during transient hypotension during surgery. The patient underwent a carotid artery bypass procedure in the first stage and complete tumor excision by a subtemporal-infratemporal approach in the second stage. **(D)** Postoperative magnetic resonance imaging shows complete tumor resection, and **(E)** the postoperative angiogram shows good filling of the graft.

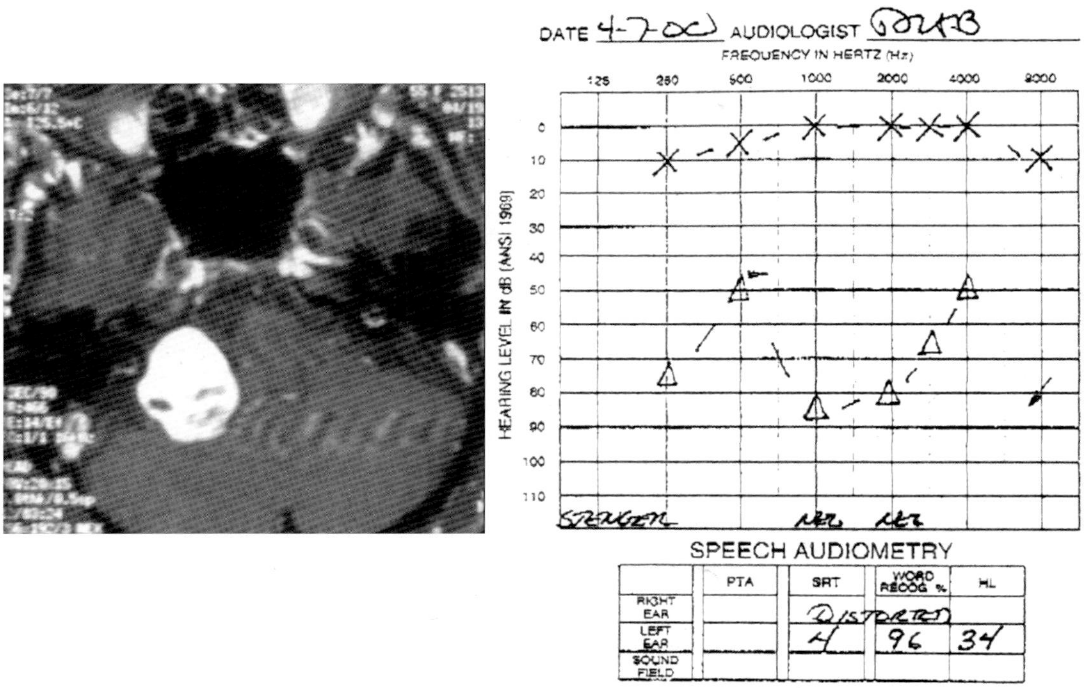

A B

Figure 65–12 **(A)** This patient with vagal nerve schwannoma presented with severe loss of hearing of the right ear with mild impairment of balance. **(B)** Preoperative audiogram of the patient shows significant loss of hearing of that ear.

(*Continued on page 772*)

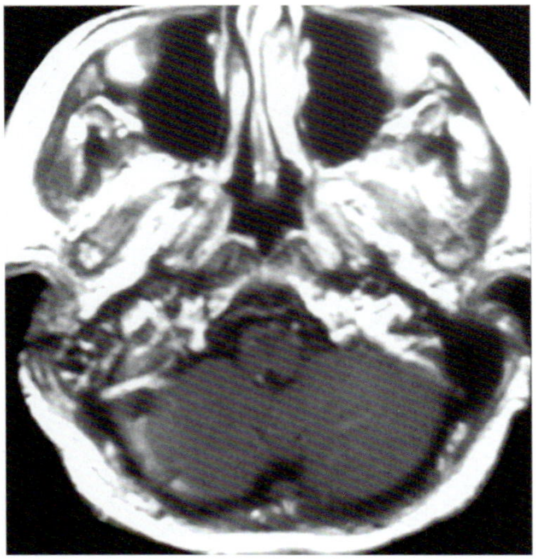

C

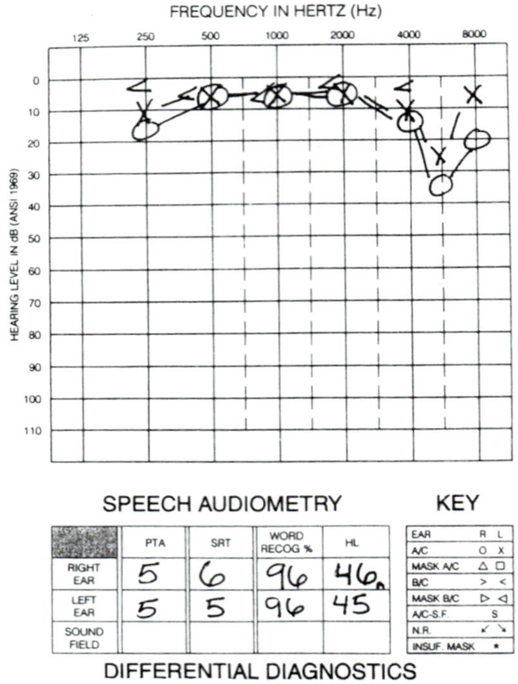

D

(*Continued*) **Figure 65–12** **(C)** The tumor was excised by a retrosigmoid approach, and follow-up magnetic resonance imaging shows complete resection of the tumor. **(D)** Complete recovery of the hearing of that ear was noted 3 months after surgery.

◆ Hypoglossal Schwannoma

These tumors may be completely intradural, intra- and extradural, or completely extradural. When they are localized extradurally, they occupy the jugular foramen area and have to be differentiated from schwannomas arising from CNs IX, X, and XI. The only way to distinguish them may be by seeing the nerve of origin of the tumor proximally at surgery (see case 9, later in chapter). Associated tongue wasting and enlargement of the hypoglossal foramen in bone window CT scans are clues to the diagnosis. A cerebral angiogram with injection of both vertebral arteries is important to see the dominance of the vertebral artery and its position in relation to the tumor and the size and dominance of the jugular bulb and vein.

A hypoglossal schwannoma is generally removed by an extreme lateral partial transcondylar approach **(Fig. 65–13)**. The patient is positioned in lateral position with slight lateral flexion of the neck to the opposite side, to open up the angle between the head and shoulder. A C-shaped incision is made in the retroauricular and upper cervical area extending along a skin crease. The sternomastoid muscle may be reflected along with the skin flap or it may be separated from the skin flap and reflected inferiorly after stripping off from its mastoid attachment, if the tumor extends below the C2 level.

The splenius capitis, longissimus capitis and cervicalis, the superior and inferior oblique muscles, and the rectus capitis major muscles are reflected from lateral to medially and the vertebral artery is identified in the suboccipital triangle. The vertebral artery is mobilized from the foramen transversarium of the C1 and reflected medially and held by a stitch taken through the adventitia of the artery. It is important to guard that the artery does not get kinked when it is reflected medially. A low retrosigmoid craniotomy is performed extending up to the foramen magnum. A portion of the lateral mass of C1, a portion of the occipital condyle, and the mastoid bone are drilled away, depending on the extension of the tumor. The tumor can be removed both extradurally and intradurally as shown in **Fig. 65–6.** If the tumor extends extradurally to the petroclival area, it is removed by a subtemporal-infratemporal approach **(Fig. 65–4).**[18] Basic steps of tumor removal are the same as for other schwannomas.

Illustrative Cases

Case 9: **Fig. 65–14**

Case 10: **Fig. 65–15**

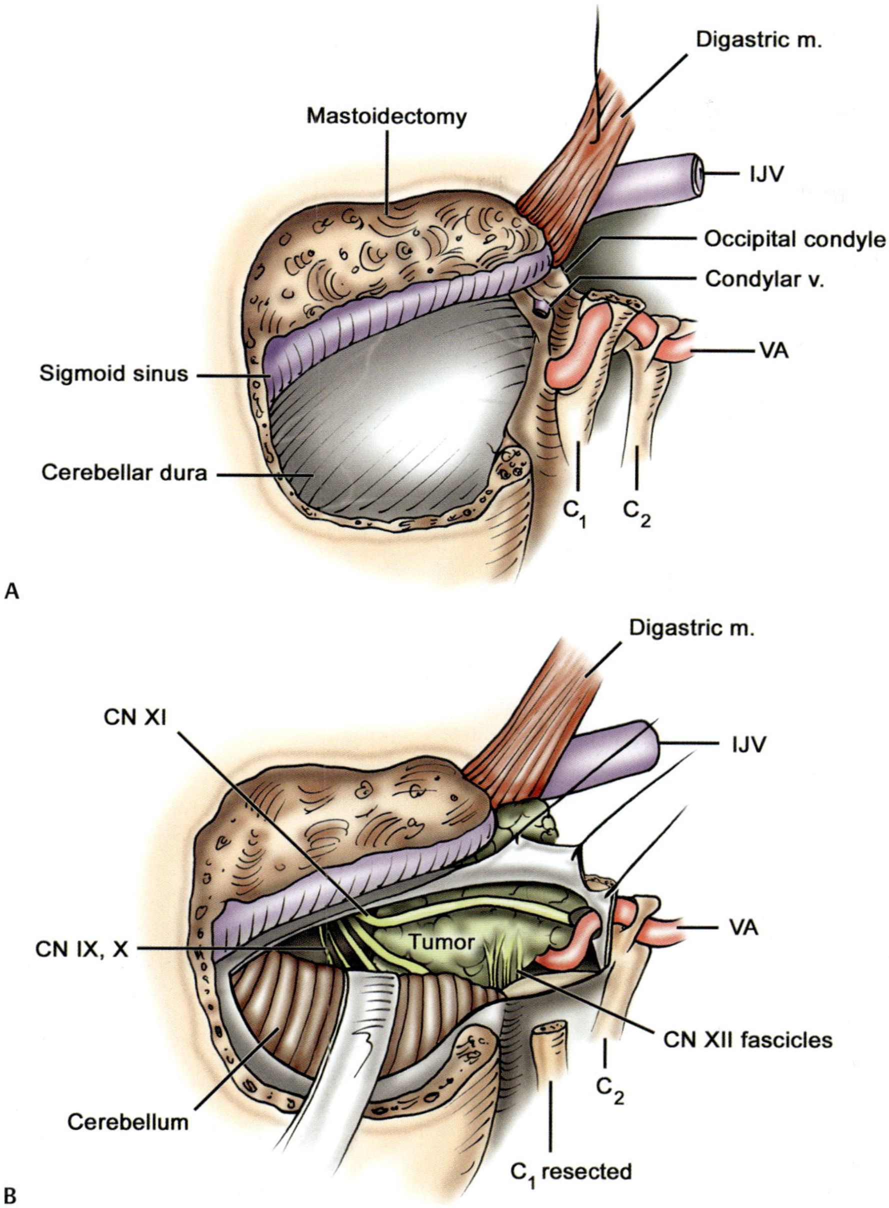

Figure 65–13 Artist's diagram of the extreme lateral partial transcondylar approach for a hypoglossal schwannoma. **(A)** Extradural exposure. **(B)** Intradural exposure shows the location of a hypoglossal schwannoma. IJV, internal jugular vein.

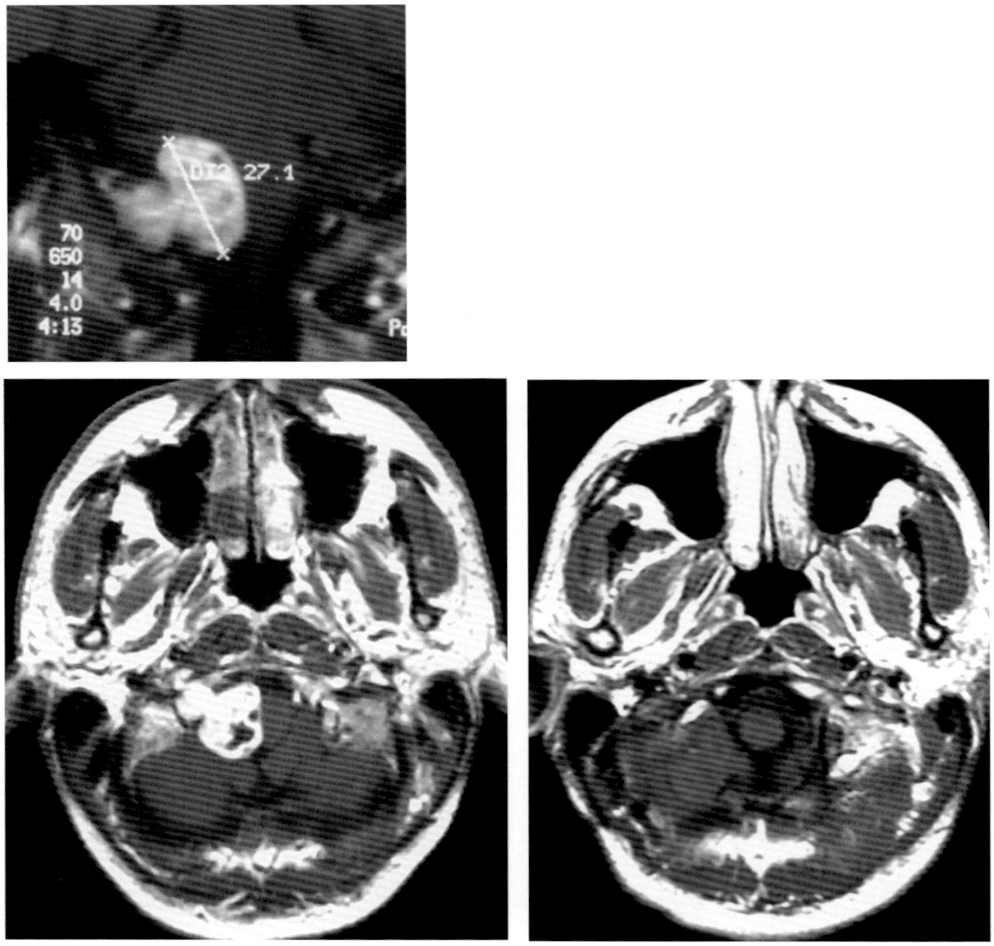

A

B

C

Figure 65–14 **(A,B)** This 42-year-old man was found to have a hypoglossal nerve schwannoma when he was being investigated for cervical spondylosis. The tumor was excised by an extreme lateral partial transcondylar approach. **(C)** Postoperative magnatic resonance imaging shows complete resection of the tumor.

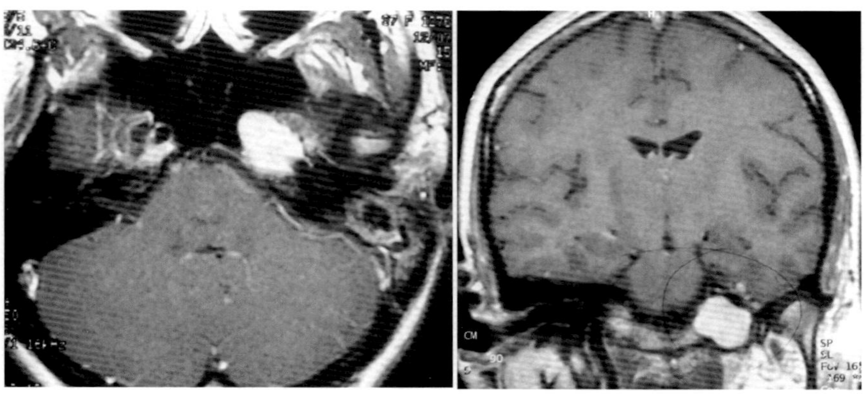

A

B

Figure 65–15 This patient presented with wasting of the tongue and was subsequently found to have a hypoglossal schwannoma. **(A,B)** The tumor extends extradurally to the petroclival and cavernous sinus area. It was excised by a subtemporal-infratemporal approach.

(*Continued on page 775*)

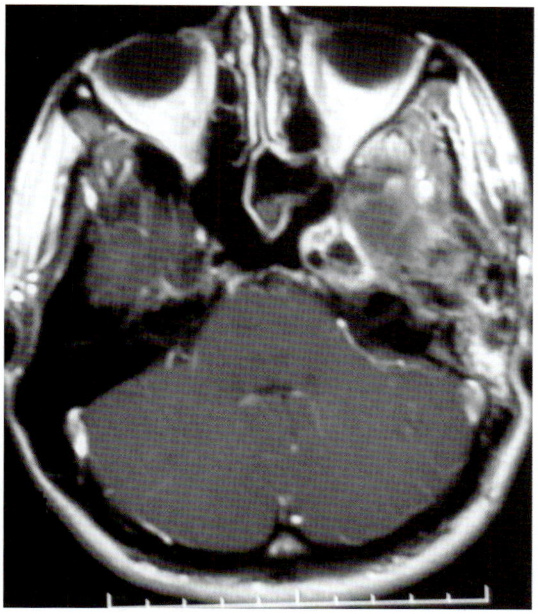

C

(*Continued*) **Figure 65–15** **(C)** Postoperative magnatic resonance imaging shows complete resection of the tumor.

◆ Schwannomas Arising from Cranial Nerves III, IV, and VI

Schwannomas arising from CNs III, IV, and VI are very uncommon unless associated with neurofibromatosis.[6] Celli et al[1] divided these tumors into three types: (1) cisternal, (2) cisternocavernous, and (3) cavernous, of which the cisternocavernous type is the most common. Approaches to be used for these tumors depend on their location. If the tumor is localized to the prepontine or the ambient cistern, it can be excised by a transpetrosal approach.[10] If it is localized to the interpeduncular cistern and cavernous sinus, a transsylvian approach is used after an orbitozygomatic osteotomy. After excision of the tumor, total or near-total paralysis of the involved nerve is the usual consequence. Nerve reconstruction by a nerve graft may result in partial (CN III) or nearly complete (CNs IV and VI) recovery of the nerve function. However, oculomotor nerve reconstruction is important for cosmetic reasons (ptosis avoidance) and in case of blindness of the other eye.

Illustrative Case 11: Fig. 65–16

A

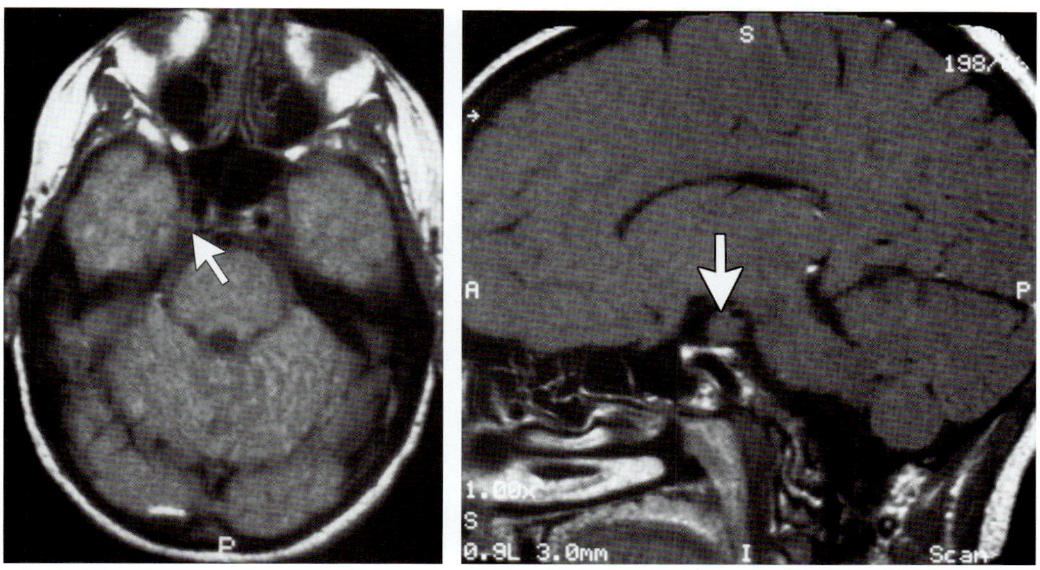

B

Figure 65–16 This patient with an oculomotor schwannoma presented with diplopia due to CN III paresis. **(A,B)** The tumor was localized to the cisternocavernous location (arrows). The tumor was excised after a frontotemporal craniotomy, an orbital osteotomy, and a transsylvian intradural approach. The tumor was completely excised along with totally invaded oculomotor nerve, and the nerve was repaired with a sural nerve graft.

(*Continued on page 776*)

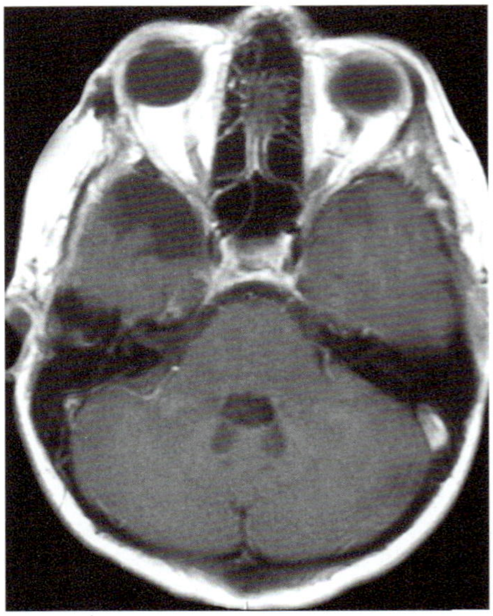

C

(*Continued*) **Figure 65–16** **(C)** Postoperative magnetic resonance imaging shows complete resection of the tumor. **(D)** Photographs of the patient's ocular movements show partial recovery of the oculomotor nerve function.

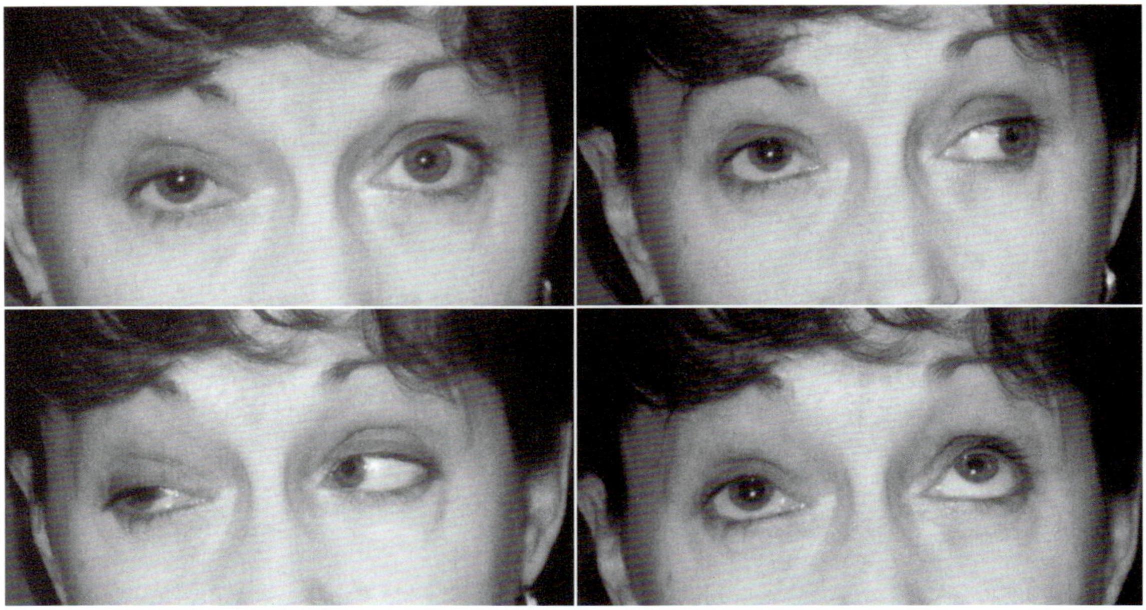

D

◆ Complications

Brain Contusion

This complication usually results from retraction injury of the brain. The use of various skull-base approaches has greatly decreased the incidence of such injuries. They are easier to prevent than treat. One should remember that brain should never be retracted for more than 2 cm from the base of the skull. A better guideline is not to retract the brain more than what can be achieved with gravity. Adequate measures should be taken to reduce the intracranial pressure (ICP) by the use of mannitol, furosemide, hyperventilation, CSF drainage, and the like, before brain retraction is started. If brain contusion has occurred, the contusion should be removed and the raw area of the brain covered with pieces of oxidized cellulose. The overlying dura should be closed with a piece of pericranial graft to accommodate brain swelling. If the brain still remains very tight, the bone flap may be left out, to be replaced at a later time.

Injury to the Draining Veins and Venous Sinuses

Injury to the draining veins can occur while performing a transpetrosal approach. Preoperative study of the venous anatomy before contemplating such an approach is very important. If the preoperative study shows a very anterior drainage of a dominant vein of Labbé, the PLPA petrosal approach may still be used because it moves the surgery well anterior to the sigmoid–transverse sinus junction. In rare patients, because of a markedly dominant jugular bulb and sigmoid sinus, the surgeon may have to use a different approach, such as a subtemporal-transzygomatic[15] or retrosigmoid approach. When the venous injury is detected intraoperatively and the vein is considered to be a dominant vein, it should be reconstructed with a segment of short saphenous vein. If the venous infarction is detected postoperatively, the only option left is evacuating the contused brain and providing space to accommodate brain swelling. The management of injury to the sigmoid sinus is described in the acoustic neuroma chapter.

Cerebrospinal Fluid Leakage

CSF leakage may occur through the mastoid bone, petrous bone, or sphenoid sinus, or through the wound. A CT scan should be done to rule out pneumocephalus/hydrocephalus and to determine the route of fluid leakage. If the leak is through the mastoid or petrous bone, fluid in the middle ear may be seen on otoscopy. Incisional leakage may be stopped by a pressure dressing over the incision (in case of CSF effusion) and institution of repeated spinal taps or temporary lumbar spinal drainage of CSF, ~30 mL every 6 to 8 hours. If pneumocephalus is detected in the CT scan or if the leak persists despite CSF drainage, surgical exploration of the wound may be needed, which consists of carefully waxing all opened air cells, additional fat graft, dural closure with graft, and so forth. If the leak is through the sphenoid sinus, it can be stopped by transnasal packing of the sphenoid sinus with fascia and autologous fat. After a transpetrosal approach,[13] the eustachian tube is always temporarily occluded via a facial recess approach after tumor excision. In the case of postoperative CSF leakage via the eustachian tube, conservative treatment with CSF diversion is usually effective. If not, surgical closure of the eustachian tube can be performed as noted above, combined with several days of CSF drainage. If hearing preservation is not important, the ear canal can be obliterated and the eustachian tube permanently occluded. CSF leak may be due to communicating hydrocephalus, which occurs after some of these operations, and in those instances a CSF shunt procedure is needed in addition to repair of the leakage.

Injury to Other Cranial Nerves

Temporary paresis of CNs III, IV, and VI is very common after excision of tumor from the cavernous sinus. These deficits usually resolve completely within 2 to 3 months.[18] If mild weakness of the ocular muscles persists after 2 to 3 months of the surgery, the correction of the diplopia can be tried using prism lenses. If there is complete paralysis of CN VI, the medial rectus muscle of the same eye may be made temporarily weak by injecting botulinum toxin into the muscle, which will help in the correction of diplopia, and also help in early recovery of the lateral muscle function. If moderate to severe diplopia persists even after 1 year postoperatively, diplopia can be corrected partially by a corrective ocular muscle surgery.

Paralysis of the lower cranial nerves (CNs IX, X, and XII) can occur after excision of a jugular foramen schwannoma, which can produce dysphagia and aspiration pneumonia. After excision of a jugular foramen schwannoma, a swallowing study should always be done before allowing the patient to eat. Unilateral vocal cord paralysis can be managed by laryngeal surgery (arytenoid adduction and thyroplasty). If the swallowing study still indicates aspiration, a temporary feeding jejunostomy should be done. If bilateral lower cranial nerve weakness exists, then a tracheoesophageal separation procedure may be necessary.

References

1. Konovalov AN, Spallone A, Mukhamedjanov DJ, Tcherekajev VA, Makhmudov UB. Trigeminal neurinomas: a series of 111 surgical cases from a single institution. Acta Neurochir (Wien) 1996;138: 1027–1035
2. Samii M, Migliori MM, Tatagiba M, Babu R. Surgical treatment of trigeminal schwannomas. J Neurosurg 1995;82:711–718
3. Tancioni F, Paolo G, Laura V, Federica Z, Baena RRY. Neuroma of the trigeminal root and atypical trigeminal neuralgia: case report and review of literature. Surg Neurol 1995;44:36–42
4. Yamada K, Ohta T, Miyamoto T. Bilateral trigeminal schwannomas associated with von Recklinghausen's disease. AJNR Am J Neuroradiol 1992;13:299–300
5. Celli P, Ferrante L, Acqui M, Mastronardi L, Fortuna A, Palma L. Neurinoma of the third, fourth and sixth cranial nerves: a survey and report of a new fourth nerve case. Surg Neurol 1992;38:216–224
6. Kachhara R, Nair S, Radhakrishnan VV. Oculomotor nerve neurinoma: report of two cases. Acta Neurochir (Wien) 1998;140:1147–1151
7. King TT, Morrison AW. Primary facial nerve tumors within the skull. J Neurosurg 1990;72:1–8
8. Huang CF, Kondziolka D, Flickinger JC, Lunsford LD. Stereotactic radiosurgery for trigeminal schwannomas. Neurosurgery 1999;45: 11–16
9. Yoshida K, Kawase T. Trigeminal neurinomas extending into multiple fossae: surgical methods and review of literature. J Neurosurg 1999; 91:202–211
10. Day JD, Fukushima T. The surgical management of trigeminal neuromas. Neurosurgery 1998;42:233–241
11. Dolenc VV. Frontotemporal epidural approach to trigeminal neurinomas. Acta Neurochir (Wien) 1994;130:55–65
12. Sekhar LN, Raso JL. Orbitozygomatic frontotemporal approach. In: Sekhar LN, Oliveira ED, eds. Cranial Microsurgery: Approaches and Techniques. New York: Thieme; 1999:130–133
13. Sekhar LN, Raso JL, Schessel DA. The presigmoid petrosal approach. In: Sekhar LN, Oliveira ED, eds. Cranial Microsurgery: Approaches and Techniques. New York: Thieme; 1999:432–463
14. Lipkin AF, Coker NJ, Jenkins HA, Alford BR. Intracranial and intratemporal facial neuroma. Otolaryngol Head Neck Surg 1987;96:71–79
15. Dott NM. Facial nerve reconstruction by graft bypassing the petrous bone. Arch Otolaryngol 1963;78:426–428
16. Drake CG. Acoustic neuroma: repair of facial nerve with autogenous graft. J Neurosurg 1960;17:836–842
17. Sekhar LN, Salas EL. The subtemporal transzygomatic approach and the subtemporal infratemporal approach. In: Sekhar LN, Oliveira ED, eds. Cranial Microsurgery: Approaches and Techniques. New York: Thieme; 1999:413–431
18. Pollock BE, Kondziolka D, Flickinger JC, Maitz A, Lunsford LD. Preservation of cranial nerve function after radiosurgery for nonacoustic schwannomas. Neurosurgery 1993;33:597–601

66

Chordomas and Chondrosarcomas

Robert C. Rostomily, Laligam N. Sekhar, and Foad Elahi

Skull-base chordomas and chondrosarcomas are histopathologically and histogenetically distinct neoplasms that are often grouped together because of their similar biologia, radiologia, anatomical, and surgical features. Although they are rare, with each representing ~0.15% of all intracranial tumors, they are nonetheless important because of the difficulties inherent in their management. This chapter focuses on surgical approaches and strategies used in their management. Some background is given as it relates to specific surgical considerations. For a more extensive discussion of clinical and biological features of these tumors, the reader should refer to several available reviews and articles[1–3] (**Table 66–1**).

◆ Origins and Pathology

Chordomas develop from notochordal remnants that exist in normal adults as the nucleus pulposus of the intervertebral disks. However, other remnants may be found in the clival bone marrow, accounting for the extradural location

Table 66–1 Characteristics of Chordomas and Chondrosarcomas

	Chordoma	Chondrosarcoma
Percent of brain tumors	0.15%	0.15%
Skull-base location	Midline paramedian	Paramedian
Age range (years)	6–78	25–57
Median age (years)	45	40
Male : female ratio	1.5:1	3.7:1
Pathological types	Chondroid Nonchondroid Dedifferentiated	Classical (grade I, II, III) Mesenchymal Dedifferentiated
Histopathologic markers	Positive for EMA and cytokeratin	EMA* and cytokeratin negative

EMA, epithelial membrane antigen.

of most chordomas. Primary intradural chordomas have been reported, but they are rare.[4] Although the main bulk and epicenter of tumor growth is extradural, intradural extension can occur with aggressive tumors, recurrent tumors, or previously irradiated tumors. A rare variant of chordoma, called the chondroid chordoma, has been described, which appears to confer a better prognosis, but many pathologists believe this variant is actually a low-grade chondrosarcoma.[5] Although chordomas can metastasize, the vast majority of patients succumb to the effects of local recurrence. Rarely, chordomas demonstrate anaplastic histologic features and the clinical picture of a tissue sarcoma, and are referred to as "dedifferentiated" chordomas.[6]

Chondrosarcomas probably arise from embryonal mesenchymal remnants in the petrosphenoclival region.[2] Three histopathological types are recognized—classic, mesenchymal, and dedifferentiated—with the latter two types conferring a worse prognosis. The majority of skull-base chondrosarcomas are of the classic type and are graded from I to III, according to the degree of malignancy. The majority of skull-base chondrosarcomas are of the grade I variety. Unlike chordomas, which arise primarily in the midline clival region, most chondrosarcomas arise in a paramedian location, with the most common site of origin being the petrosphenoclival junction.

◆ Imaging Characteristics

Imaging studies cannot definitively distinguish between chordoma and chondrosarcoma, other than their location. Both lesions can enhance to varying degrees, cause local bone destruction, have similar signal intensities on magnetic resonance imaging (MRI) (isointense or hypointense to brain on T1- and hyperintense to brain on T2-weighted images). Intralesional calcification and a paramedian location are two characteristics that are thought to be more prevalent in chondrosarcomas. Histologically, the two types of tumors are distinguished by epithelial membrane antigen (EMA) and cytokeratin staining. Chordomas stain positively, whereas chondrosarcomas do not show positivity. However, in some patients, the distinction between the two tumors may still be difficult to make.

◆ Prognostic Factors

The reported average survivals for *untreated* chordoma and chondrosarcoma of 0.6 to 2.0 years are derived mainly from series that predate the computed tomography (CT) and MRI.[7–9] The value of these data in assessing the effects of contemporary treatments on outcome is questionable because patients today are probably diagnosed earlier in the course of their disease, and few patients with a chordoma or chondrosarcoma go untreated.

Prognostic factors associated with poorer outcomes include higher histologic grades and certain pathological subtypes (mesenchymal or dedifferentiated chondrosarcoma and anaplastic chordoma). For example, grade I, II, and III classic chondrosarcomas have reported 5-year survival rates of 90%, 81%, and 43%, respectively.[10] Chordomas, as a whole, have shorter survivals than classic chondrosarcomas. One study has reported a bimodal survival pattern for patients with skull-base chordomas, with one group having an aggressive course and high 5-year mortality, whereas the other group has a very indolent course with nearly normal life expectancy.

◆ Treatment Options

Surgery

Surgery is the mainstay of treatment for chordoma and chondrosarcoma. The association between a larger extent of resection and a better outcome underscores the importance of surgery. Large tumor volumes, irregular geometry, slow growth, and inherent resistance all limit the effectiveness of radiation, and no chemotherapy regimen has yet to show significant activity against these lesions. In a series of patients treated primarily by surgery alone (20% received postoperative radiation), the 5-year recurrence-free survival rate was 80% for all patients, 90% for chondrosarcoma, and 65% for chordoma.[1] In this same study, those patients with total, or near-total resection (questionable remnants), had an 84% 5-year recurrence-free survival compared with 64% for patients with known residual disease. Prior surgery reduced the 5-year recurrence-free survival rates from 93 to 64%. In a series of patients receiving proton-beam radiation after surgery, smaller residual tumor volumes were independently associated with prolonged survival.[11] Thus the extent of resection appears to have a strong association with outcomes in these patients.

The surgical risks reported by Gay et al[1] in 1995 included nonsurgical mortality (pulmonary embolism, myocardial infarction) in three of 60 patients (5%), hemiparesis in three (5%), and gait ataxia in three (5%). There were 92 new cranial nerve deficits in 48 patients, with 57 deficits being permanent. The single most common complication was a cerebrospinal fluid (CSF) leak. Eighteen patients had CSF leaks (30%), of which 10 required operation (17%) and six developed meningitis (10%). This risk profile must be interpreted in light of the patient population. In this series, 39(65%) of patients had had either previous surgery ($n = 29$) or radiation ($n = 10$), and the tumors were either large (volume between 15 and 85 cm^3) or giant (volume > 85 cm^3) in 69% and 16% of patients, respectively.

Radiation Therapy

Chordomas are radiosensitive only in the 70 to 80 Gy dose range,[12] whereas chondrosarcomas are probably more radiosensitive. Multiple delivery methods have been used to treat chordomas and chondrosarcomas. The most common approaches include external-beam photon radiation, charged particle (protons and helium or neon ions) radiation (with or without photons), and stereotactic radiosurgery.

Proton Beam

In 1989, Austin-Seymour et al[2] reported an 82% 5-year local control rate in 68 patients with chordoma and chondrosarcoma treated with proton-beam supplemented with photons. An update from these authors in 1995 reported 5-year control rates of 53% and survival rates of 50% for chordoma, whereas six patients with chondrosarcoma were alive without disease progression.[13] A report of helium and neon ion-charged particle therapy augmented with photons reported 5-year local control rates of 78% for chondrosarcoma and 63% for chordoma with 5-year survival of 83% and 75%, respectively.[14] The report utilizing proton beam with a mean follow-up of only 33 months reported local control rates of 76% for chordoma and 92% for chondrosarcoma and actuarial 5-year survival rates of 76% for chordoma and 100% for chondrosarcoma.[13] Better local control was related to tumor size ($< 25\ cm^3$) and absence of brain stem involvement.

Stereotactic Radiosurgery

Stereotactic radiosurgery (SRS) is emerging as a means to provide local control to small tumor volumes. In a recent small series of 15 patients, 10 of 11 surviving patients followed for an average of 4 years had either reduction or stabilization of their tumor after SRS, but the mean tumor volume treated was only 4.6 cm^3.[15] In contrast the mean volume in a surgical series was 58 cm^3.[1]

Complications

An analysis of a combined high-dose photon and proton beam irradiation protocol for chordoma and chondrosarcoma revealed a 13.2% 5-year incidence of temporal lobe damage with 80% of those affected suffering severe to moderate symptoms.[16] In another study, the use of helium/neon ions produced a 20% rate of serious complications ranging from cranial nerve injury to death over a mean follow-up period of 45 months.[14]

Chemotherapy

Chemotherapy has not been used extensively as a front-line treatment of chordoma and chondrosarcoma. The vast majority of these tumors are low grade and relatively slow growing. In rare instances of a highly malignant lesion with a high mitotic rate, or in the equally rare instance of tumor dissemination, chemotherapy regimens have been used that show efficacy for the treatment of sarcoma and other malignant bone tumors.

◆ Indications for Treatment

The majority of newly diagnosed chondromas and chondrosarcomas are candidates for microsurgical removal. However, very small tumors and some elderly patients may be followed for several months or even years to see if there is tumor growth. Radiotherapy is reserved for small tumor remnants not excised by surgery. Patients who have been operated previously are at slightly higher risk for surgery. However, previously irradiated patients are at high risk and are more amenable to palliative surgery.

◆ Preoperative Studies and Patient Preparation

All patients must have a preoperative MRI. In most cases an angiogram or high-quality CT angiogram or MR angiogram (MRA) is needed to assess the anatomy of the large venous sinuses, draining veins, the extent of any arterial involvement, and the pattern of potential collateral circulation. Carotid occlusion testing (COT) is reserved for those lesions encasing the internal carotid artery (ICA) where a gross total resection is planned. Various means are used to determine the adequacy of collateral blood flow, but of those patients who pass such a test, there is still a significant 10 to 25% risk of stroke when the ICA is occluded at surgery. For this reason, we do not plan permanent carotid occlusion at surgery, and we use the COT only to assess tolerance to temporary occlusion. If the artery is occluded at surgery, reconstruction must be performed by direct repair or by bypass grafting.

Embolization is not used because these lesions are relatively avascular. For lesions involving the sellar and parasellar regions, preoperative endocrine testing and neuroophthalmological testing are mandatory. Lesions involving the cerebellopontine angle or petrous bone should have preoperative audiology studies. CT scans are obtained to view the details of the bony anatomy and extent of bone involvement or destruction.

◆ Surgical Technique

Anesthesia

The appropriate anesthesia management of a cranial base patient requires good communication among the anesthesiologist, neurophysiologist, surgeon, and nursing team. Like any patient undergoing general anesthesia, the patient with a cranial base chordoma or chondrosarcoma must have a thorough preoperative evaluation of general health, a thorough clinical examination of cranial nerve function, and in certain cases neuroendocrine testing. All patients have two large-bore intravenous lines (and a central venous catheter if needed), a radial artery catheter, a Foley catheter with temperature probe, and sequential compression stockings placed before final patient positioning. If a vascular graft is planned, a femoral sheath is placed by the radiologist, and the thigh is prepared in a sterile fashion. Lumbar drains are placed only for extradural exposures where brain retraction is required or where a significant dural opening and reconstruction are anticipated.

Positioning

Patient positioning must be closely coordinated between the surgeon and anesthesiologist. At the start of the operation, every patient is given steroids (10 mg dexamethasone) and antibiotics. Mannitol is also given before the bone work has started (0.5 to 1.0 g/kg). If an intradural supratentorial approach is planned, the patient is loaded with 1 g of intravenous phenytoin as well.

The anesthetic regimen should allow for reliable neurophysiological monitoring. A common plan includes the use of short-acting narcotic with a sub-minimal alveolar concentration (MAC) of Forane, an amnesic dose of midazolam, fentanyl, pancuronium infusion, and nitrous oxide (no more than 60%). The infusion of a small amount of muscle relaxant that can be reversed as needed will not affect cranial nerve monitoring. Fluid management is designed to maintain cerebral perfusion but avoid cerebral edema. Urine output and blood loss are carefully monitored. Hematocrits are kept in the 30 to 35% range to maximize rheology and microvascular perfusion. With ongoing large blood losses, coagulation parameters (prothrombin time, partial thromboplastin time, and platelet count) must be closely monitored and corrections made while communicating abnormalities to the surgeon. Burst suppression is employed during vascular occlusion in bypass procedures (see chapter on cerebral revascularization).

Neurophysiological Monitoring

Intraoperative neurophysiological monitoring includes brain stem auditory evoked responses (BAERs), bilateral upper and lower extremity somatosensory evoked potentials (SEPs), facial nerve electromyogram (EMG) and stimulation, and electroencephalogram (EEG) (to evaluate burst suppression during vascular bypass). The BAER provides reliable trends that can guide the use of retraction on the cerebellum. In the event of significant changes, the surgeon may alter retraction or work elsewhere until the potentials recover or stabilize. SEPs monitor dorsal column impulses that are recorded at the cortical level, and can help gauge retraction effects on the cerebral cortex. Significant SEP changes thus alert the surgeon to release or reposition retractors, search for other causes of vascular compromise or cerebral edema, or assess the potential risk of deliberate vessel interruption. When working in the cerebellopontine angle, facial nerve EMGs and direct stimulation are invaluable for anatomical identification of the nerve and for guiding the surgical technique, based on spontaneous EMG activity.

Resection

Grossly, these lesions have a soft cartilaginous or gelatinous core that can be removed easily. However, some heavily calcified chondrosarcomas must be removed piecemeal or by light drilling if they are heavily ossified. The scarring present in previously irradiated or operated tumors also makes resection more difficult. The key to complete resection is to drill off all adjacent tumor-infiltrated bone until normal marrow and cortical bone is encountered. Dural invasion by tumor is common, especially in recurrent lesions. Resection of a wide dural margin is recommended if adequate dural reconstruction is possible. The need to resect bone at the margins of the tumor to achieve a gross total resection should be factored into planning the surgical approach. In general, extradural approaches are preferred for these predominantly extradural tumors. Intradural approaches are reserved for intradural invasion and extensive upper clivus or cavernous sinus tumor.

◆ Surgical Approaches

Overview

The surgical approach for treating chordomas and chondrosarcomas is dictated by the tumor location, surgical goals, and results of preoperative studies. Unless there are extenuating medical factors, the surgical goal should be a gross total resection with minimal morbidity. Combined approaches or staged operations are often necessary because of the growth patterns of these lesions. In a surgical series of 60 patients, only eight tumors were confined to one anatomical region. In total, 93% of tumors invaded the clivus, 75% invaded the cavernous sinus, and 63% invaded the petrous bone.[1]

The predilection for these tumors to involve the clivus has spawned a wide variety of anterior surgical approaches that can be roughly categorized as either cranial or transfacial. The transfacial approaches involve access through the face, palate, or respiratory sinuses, and include the transsphenoidal, extended transsphenoidal, transethmoidal, various maxillotomies, and transoral approaches. Although these approaches provide a direct route to the clivus, they have restricted lateral access, and dural reconstruction and management of CSF fistulae are difficult. Although many surgeons advocate the use of such approaches, the senior author (RCR) prefers the use of the alternative cranial approaches outlined below because they provide the best chance for a definitive resection. For instance, the extended transfrontal cranial approaches provide access to the entire clivus, anterior cranial fossa, and medial cavernous sinus (CS) in one approach, and dural reconstruction, if needed, is not technically as challenging. Nevertheless, the anterior transfacial approaches are valuable for cases where palliation or diagnosis alone is the surgical goal, in the rare instance of a localized midline tumor, or in combination with other approaches for attempted radical resection.

The following four cranial approaches are the most frequently used, alone or in combination, for resection of cranial base chordoma or chondrosarcoma: (1) extended subfrontal; (2) frontotemporal transcavernous; (3) subtemporal (transpetrous apex or subtemporal-infratemporal); and (4) extreme lateral transcondylar. We describe these approaches separately, but they are often combined to provide individualized access for a particular tumor. The surgical anatomy of the clivus is shown in **Fig. 66–1.**

Extended Frontal Transbasal Approach

Indications

This approach is useful for midline tumors of the upper to lower clivus and with extension into the sphenoethmoidal region, medial CS, petrous apex, occipital condyles, or foramen magnum.[17] The lateral limits for resection are the optic nerves, carotid arteries, abducens nerves (petrous apex), and hypoglossal nerves. The dorsum sella cannot be reached directly by this approach, and tumors with extensive lateral components are also not totally resectable by this approach using conventional microsurgical techniques. However, the use of the endoscope can augment lateral or superior visualization and the ability to resect additional tumor.

Operative Procedure

A spinal drain is inserted for brain relaxation and the patient is positioned supine, secured in pins with the head neutral or slightly extended to allow the frontal lobes to fall away

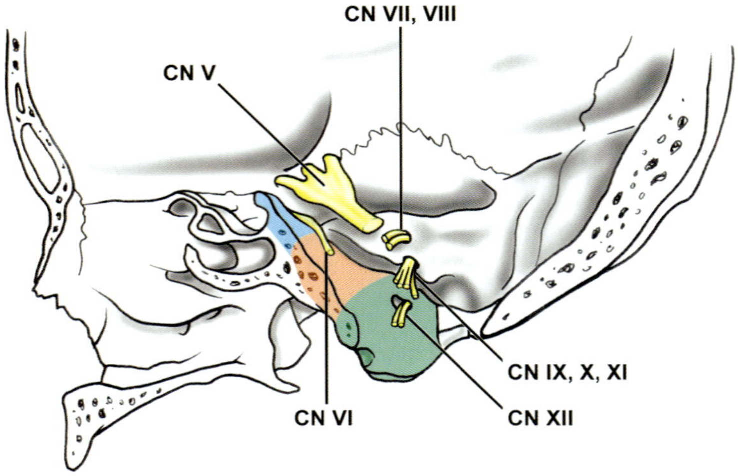

Figure 66–1 Surgical anatomy of the clival region in a sagittal section showing the delineation of the upper, middle, and lower clivus.

from the frontal base. A bicoronal skin incision is made from zygoma to zygoma. An additional 2 to 4 cm of pericranium is harvested from under the posterior edge of the incision for use in the repair of the frontal base. The scalp flap is reflected to the orbital rims and the frontonasal suture (**Fig. 66–2A**). If the supraorbital nerve and vessels are tethered in their bony foramen, they are released by chiseling out the foramen. The temporalis muscle is reflected laterally from over the keyhole, and bilateral bur holes are drilled. A low unilateral frontal craniotomy up to the sagittal sinus is performed and then completed across the sinus on the contralateral side (**Fig. 66–2B**). In a younger patient, wherein the dura mater is not very adherent to the sagittal sinus, the bifrontal craniotomy may be performed in a single piece. A bilateral orbitofrontal or fronto-orbital-ethmoidal osteotomy is then performed. The orbitofrontal osteotomy is used for lesions confined to the anterior fossa region, whereas the more extensive orbitofrontoethmoidal osteotomy provides access to the sphenoclival region (**Fig. 66–2C,D**).

For the bilateral fronto-orbital osteotomy, bone cuts are made at the nasofrontal suture and then laterally across the medial orbital wall to the anterior ethmoidal foramen, and then superolaterally to the orbital rim just medial to the orbitozygomatic suture. Cuts are then made in the medial orbital roof encircling the ethmoid bone. The bone is then released with an osteotome as needed. The olfactory dura is gradually drilled free of bone, the nasal septum and olfactory mucosa are divided and retracted up with the frontal dura; at the end of the operation, the dura is attached to a hole in the pericranial flap. This preserves olfaction in many but not all patients. To perform the orbitofrontoethmoidal osteotomy, the bone cuts are the same except that the ethmoid bone is not encircled but included in the osteotomy by cutting across the back of the cribriform plate and then laterally and anteriorly across the orbital roof. The dural invagination into the cribriform plate must be detached to allow exposure behind the cribriform plate. This step then allows the ethmoids to be included in the bone flap. Olfaction is thus sacrificed. This approach provides a better exposure and a lower risk of CSF leakage. This is the preferred exposure in older or irradiated patients whose dura is very thin and adherent.

For the extradural resection, the nasal mucosa is identified and dissected intact anteriorly into the nasal cavity. The ethmoidal mucosa is vascular and is coagulated along with the feeding anterior and posterior ethmoidal arteries. The optic foramina lie approximately 1 cm posterior to the posterior ethmoidal arteries. The medial and superior portions of the bony optic canal are drilled off using a high-speed drill to expose the optic nerves. The anterior clinoid processes do not need to be resected with this approach.

The middle and posterior ethmoidal cells are removed to increase working room and expose the sphenoid sinus (**Fig. 66–2E**). The planum sphenoidale is then resected. The superior and lateral walls of the sphenoid sinus are then removed by drilling to expose the sella and medial wall of the CS (**Fig. 66–2F**). The sella obscures the region of the dorsum sella, which generally cannot be reached by this approach (**Fig. 66–2G**). The anterior bend of the ICA is then identified in the medial wall of the CS. By following the medial surface of the cavernous ICA posteriorly along the horizontal and vertical segments, the junction of the petrous bone and CS is encountered. This exposure allows resection of tumor in part of the petrous apex, medial CS, and anterior wall of the sphenoid (**Fig. 66–2H**). Venous bleeding from the medial CS is controlled with Surgicel or Gelfoam packing. The mucosa of the nasopharynx lies just anterior to the anterior wall of the sphenoid and must not be violated.

The clival bone is then removed by drilling in a superior to inferior direction to expose the dura. The foramen magnum can be reached inferiorly. The lateral limits of exposure in the midclivus are in line with the intradural course of the abducens nerve, whereas in the lower clivus the dural sleeve of the hypoglossal nerve and part of the condyle can be accessed (**Fig. 66–2H**). The dura should be left intact if possible. It is usually thick in young patients but can be extremely thin in the elderly. Bleeding from the basilar venous plexus can be substantial and is controlled by packing with Surgicel or Gelfoam. If the dura has to be opened and excised due to tumor invasion, a watertight repair is not possible. However, a small piece of intradural tumor in the middle of lower clivus can be safely removed.

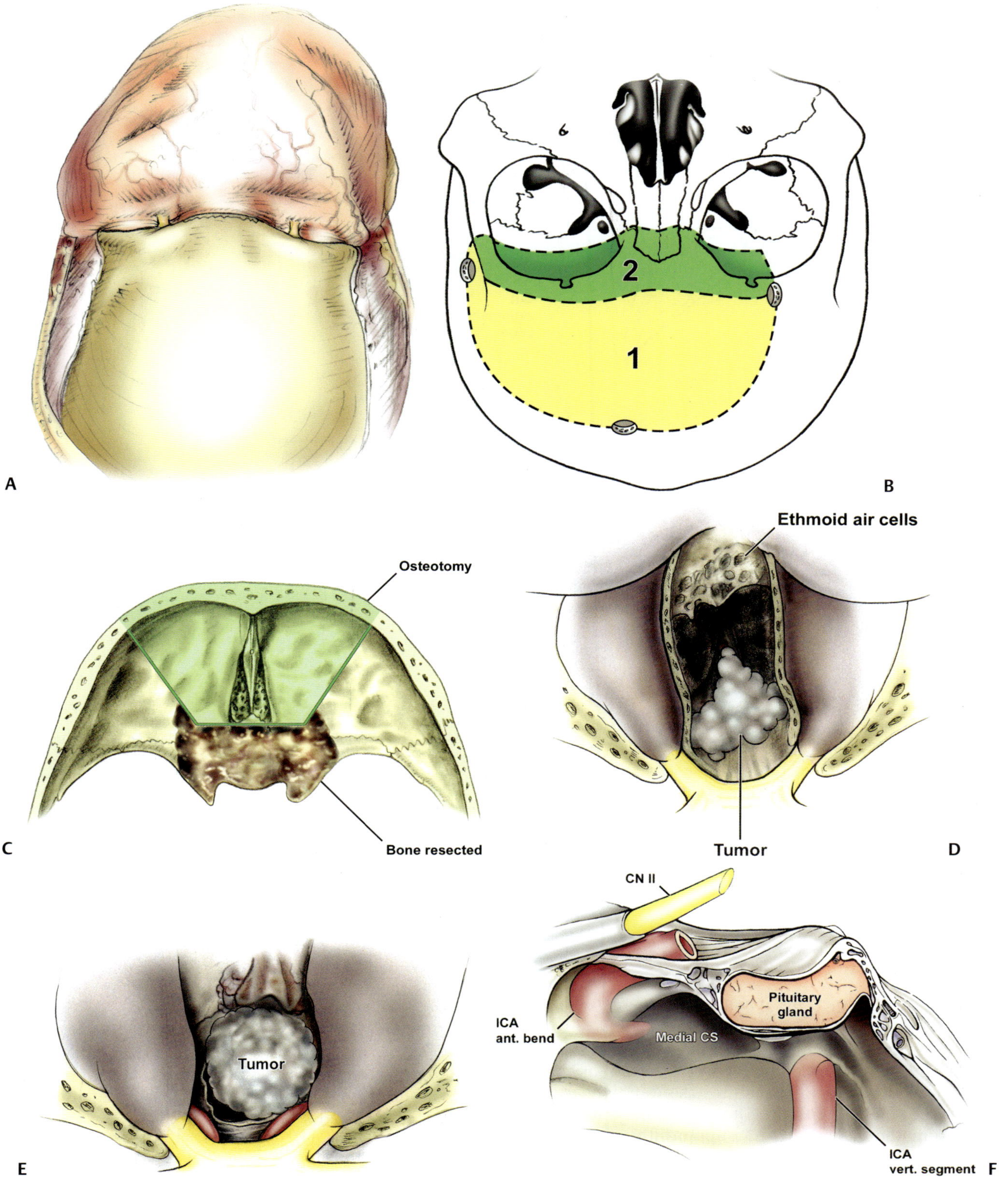

Figure 66–2 **(A)** After a bicoronal incision, the pericranium is reflected with the scalp flap. **(B)** The craniotomy (1) and osteotomy (2) are shown. **(C)** The frontoorbitoethmoidal osteotomy is shown. This is most common for use in resection of clival chordomas. **(D)** The middle and posterior ethmoid air cells have been removed to provide more working space. The orbit and optic nerves have been unroofed. **(E)** The optic nerves have been unroofed and the planum sphenoidale removed. The cavernous carotid arteries have been unroofed and tumor resection begins. **(F)** A lateral view of the wall of the sphenoid sinus in a normal person shows the relationship between the anterior bend and vertical segment of the internal carotid artery (ICA) and the medial wall of the cavernous sinus (CS).

(*Continued on page 784*)

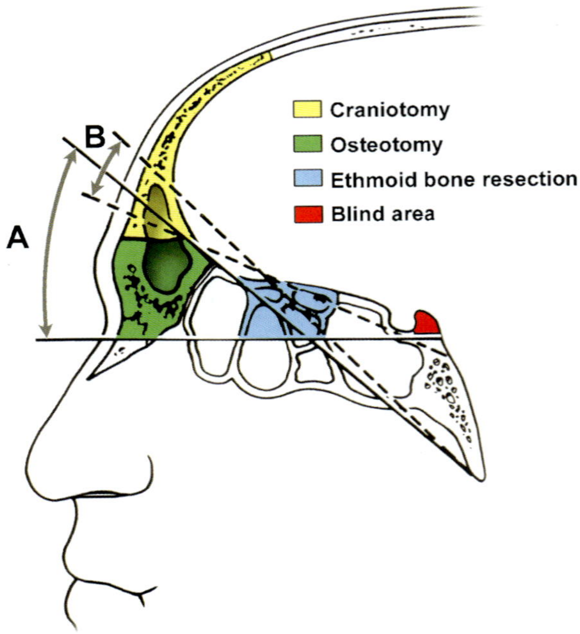

G

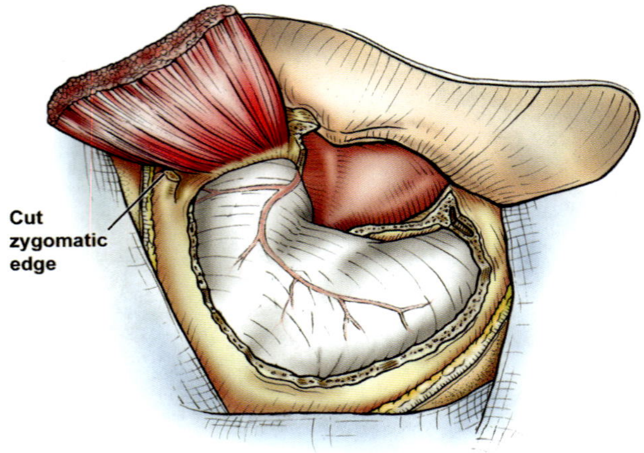

H

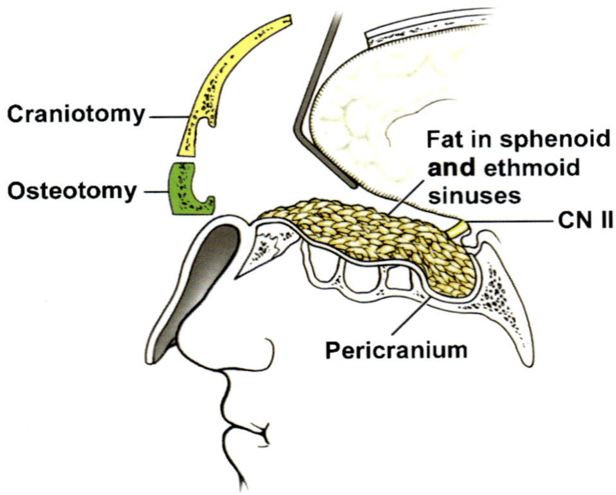

I

(*Continued*) **Figure 66–2** **(G)** Schematic view showing the advantages of the extended transfrontal approach (A) over craniotomy alone (B). The limitations of the approach in viewing the dorsum sella are also shown. **(H)** A parasagittal section in a normal person showing the anatomy of the abducens and hypoglossal nerves, the lateral limits of the resection with the extended frontal approach. **(I)** Reconstruction of the cranial base with free fat grafts and a pericranial graft.

Closure and Reconstruction

Primary suture repair of dural defects is difficult, so a fascia lata or pericranial patch is approximated and secured with suture and augmented with autologous fat and tissue adhesives. The remaining mucosa of the frontal or sphenoid sinuses is exenterated, and the nasofrontal ducts and sinuses are plugged with fat. The pericranial flap is elevated from the scalp with its supraorbital and supratrochlear vascular pedicles. The flap is incised just at the junction of the frontoorbitoethmoidal bone flap with the nasal bone to allow direct bone contact. The pericranial flap is tucked into the tumor cavity along the anterior-inferior margin to separate the subsequent autologous fat graft from the nasopharynx. Free fat grafts are then used to obliterate dead space from the resection cavity above the pericranial flap. Provided enough pericranium is available, the flap can also be brought up over the fat and secured to the planum with suture, thus providing a three-layered closure **(Fig. 66–2I)**. The closure is also augmented with fibrin glue. Orbital reconstruction is necessary only if the medial orbital wall or an extensive portion of the orbital roof has been resected. This is best performed with a titanium mesh that is attached to the orbital bone.

Postoperative Management

The appropriate time for extubation depends on many factors that must be determined by both the surgeon and anesthesiologist. In cases of difficult intubations, long burst suppression, large fluid loads, extended operative time,

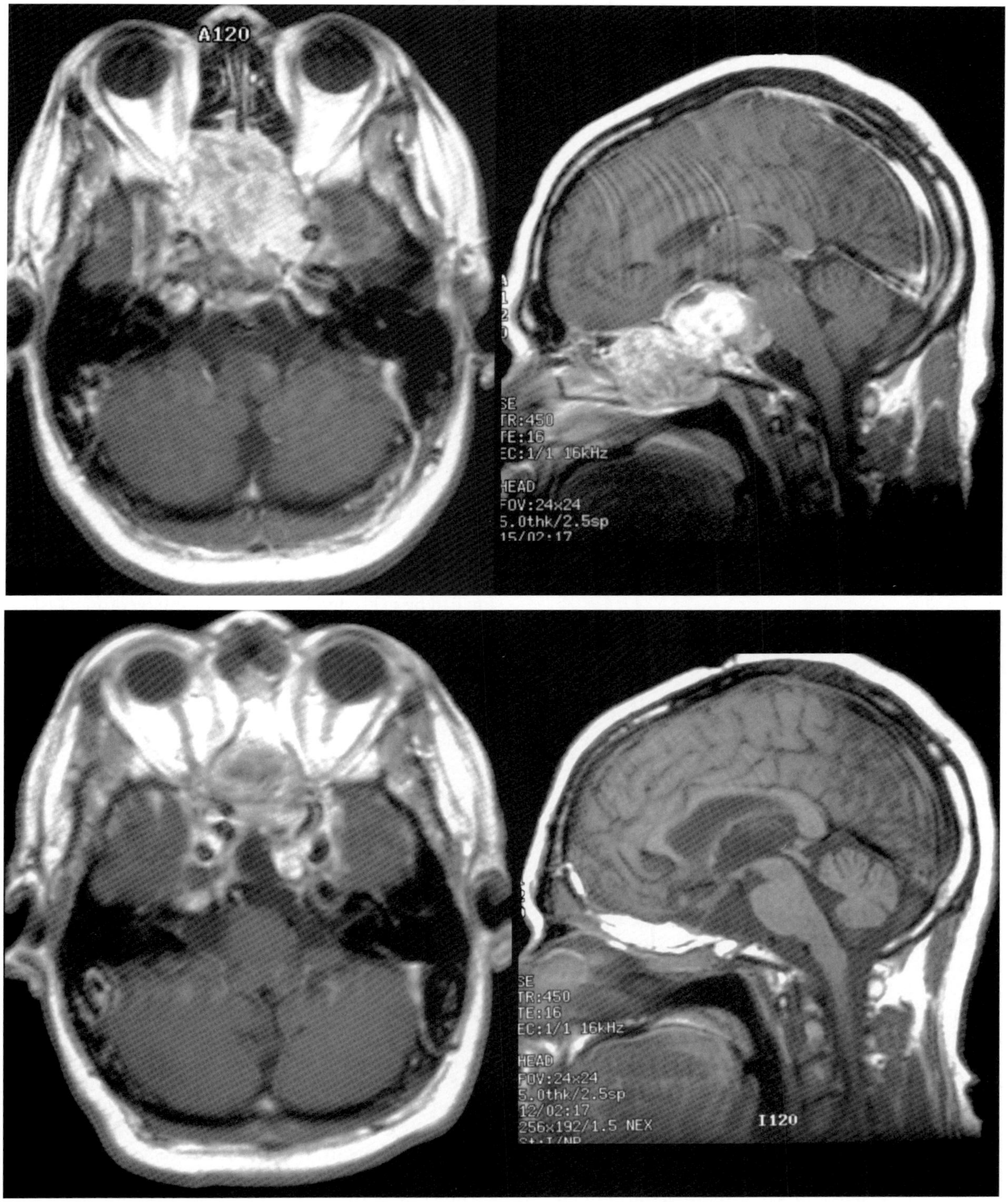

A B C D

Figure 66–3 **(A,B)** Illustrative case 1. A 50-year-old man with an extreme midline chordoma extending into both cavernous sinuses. The tumor was resected nearly completely by an extended subfrontal approach. **(C,D)** A small remnant was treated by radiosurgery. He has a tumor recurrence in the nasal septum 6 years after the original surgery, and after resection, remains free of tumor, 10 years after the original resection.

facial or pharyngeal edema, depressed level of consciousness, or possible lower cranial nerve dysfunction, it is often best to monitor the patient intubated in the recovery room or overnight in the intensive care unit (ICU). Postoperative recovery room and ICU management includes monitoring of neurological status, arterial blood pressure, urine output, O_2 saturations, arterial blood gases, coagulation profiles, anticonvulsant levels, serum electrolytes, and urine specific gravity (in cases with sellar involvement). Patients with significant brain swelling, or who are difficult to follow clinically, may require intracranial pressure (ICP) monitoring. Any patient with an unexpected neurological deficit postoperatively or who is slow to awaken should have an immediate CT scan to rule out a mass lesion. Otherwise, a CT scan with and without contrast, and with fine bone window cuts, is obtained on the first postoperative day to document the extent of tumor resection and unexpected complications. Intraoperative angiograms are obtained to evaluate vascular grafts, and CT angiograms or MR angiograms are used to follow the grafts postoperatively. Patients can be transferred in 24 to 48 hours to the step-down units, if close neurological or general systemic assessment and monitoring without intubation are still needed, or to the general ward if only routine evaluations are required.

Pitfalls and Complications

The critical structures that are at highest risk of injury in this approach are the optic nerves, cavernous ICA, and sixth nerve. The position of the optic nerves must be anticipated as bone is removed along the planum. A helpful landmark is the posterior ethmoidal artery and foramen. These are found ~1.0 cm anterior to the optic foramen in the posteromedial wall of the orbit. Bone removal in this area should be performed only with drills. During the procedure care is taken not to retract the optic nerves. The cavernous ICA is identified along the medial CS wall and should not be exposed unless tumor infiltrates this area. Inadvertent opening of the medial dural wall can occur especially in the elderly in whom the dura is often attenuated. Injuries to the ICA are more likely to occur during reoperation and may require either direct suture repair or saphenous vein bypass grafting if the laceration is irregular or large. The abducens nerve is at risk, particularly in the posterolateral corner, because no landmark marks its course from its entrance point in the leaves of the clival dura to the CS. Careful bone removal helps prevent injury. All the structures of the anterior brain stem are at theoretical risk, particularly if there is dural invasion of tumor.

The use of mannitol and lumbar CSF drainage reduces the risks of frontal lobe retraction. CSF leak can be a problem if inadequate primary repair or reconstruction is performed. In the event of a CSF leak, lumbar drainage is instituted and a lumboperitoneal (LP) or ventriculoperitoneal (VP) shunt is placed as needed. Large leaks may require additional repair, and in previously operated or radiated patients a free-tissue vascularized graft may be necessary.

Illustrative Case 1: ***Fig. 66–3A–D***

Frontotemporal Transcavernous Approach

Indications

This approach allows excellent intradural access to the CS, and, in combination with the subtemporal approach (described later), the upper clivus and petrous apex. It provides excellent direct vision of any intradural tumor that compresses the upper brain stem or extensively involves the CS. It does not address any associated major bony involvement, and so an auxiliary second approach may be needed to achieve a total resection.

Operative Procedure

The patient is placed supine with a roll under the ipsilateral shoulder and the head turned between 30 and 60 degrees with the head extended. The degree of rotation is increased for posterior fossa lesions and decreased for middle fossa lesions. An incision is made starting at the level of the zygomatic process of the temporal bone and less than 1 cm from the tragus (to avoid the facial nerve) and curved up and then forward behind the hairline to the midline. The incision can be extended in a partial or full bicoronal fashion, if the hairline is not favorable, to get adequate inferior mobilization of the scalp flap, or if a possible subsequent contralateral approach is being considered. The skin, galea, and pericranium are elevated as a layer, preserving the superficial layer of the deep temporalis fascia. The flap is advanced forward until the superficial fat pad is visualized and an interfascial approach is used to protect the frontotemporal branch of the facial nerve while completing the mobilization of the flap.[18,19] The temporalis fascia attached to the zygomatic arch is dissected in a subperiosteal fashion. The temporalis muscle is then elevated from its attachments along the superior temporal line and inferiorly in the temporal fossa under the zygoma.

Orbitozygomatic Osteotomy

The bone removal is accomplished in two steps with a separate frontotemporal craniotomy and orbitozygomatic osteotomy (OZO). Although this can be accomplished in a single step, the use of two steps is technically easier, and in the event of a bone flap infection the orbitozygomatic bone can usually be left in situ. A frontotemporal craniotomy is performed taking the anterior temporal bone cut low under the reflected temporalis muscle and inferomedially along the junction of the lateral orbital wall and the medial sphenoid wing **(Fig. 66–4A).** The frontal bone cut is taken just medial to the supraorbital notch. The temporalis muscle is returned to its normal anatomical position for the completion of the OZO **(Fig. 66–4B).** The OZO can be performed with or without an osteotomy involving the condylar fossa, depending on the need for additional middle fossa exposure. The orbital part of the osteotomy should include at least two thirds of the orbital roof and half of the lateral wall to prevent enophthalmos postoperatively. Additional exposure is gained from

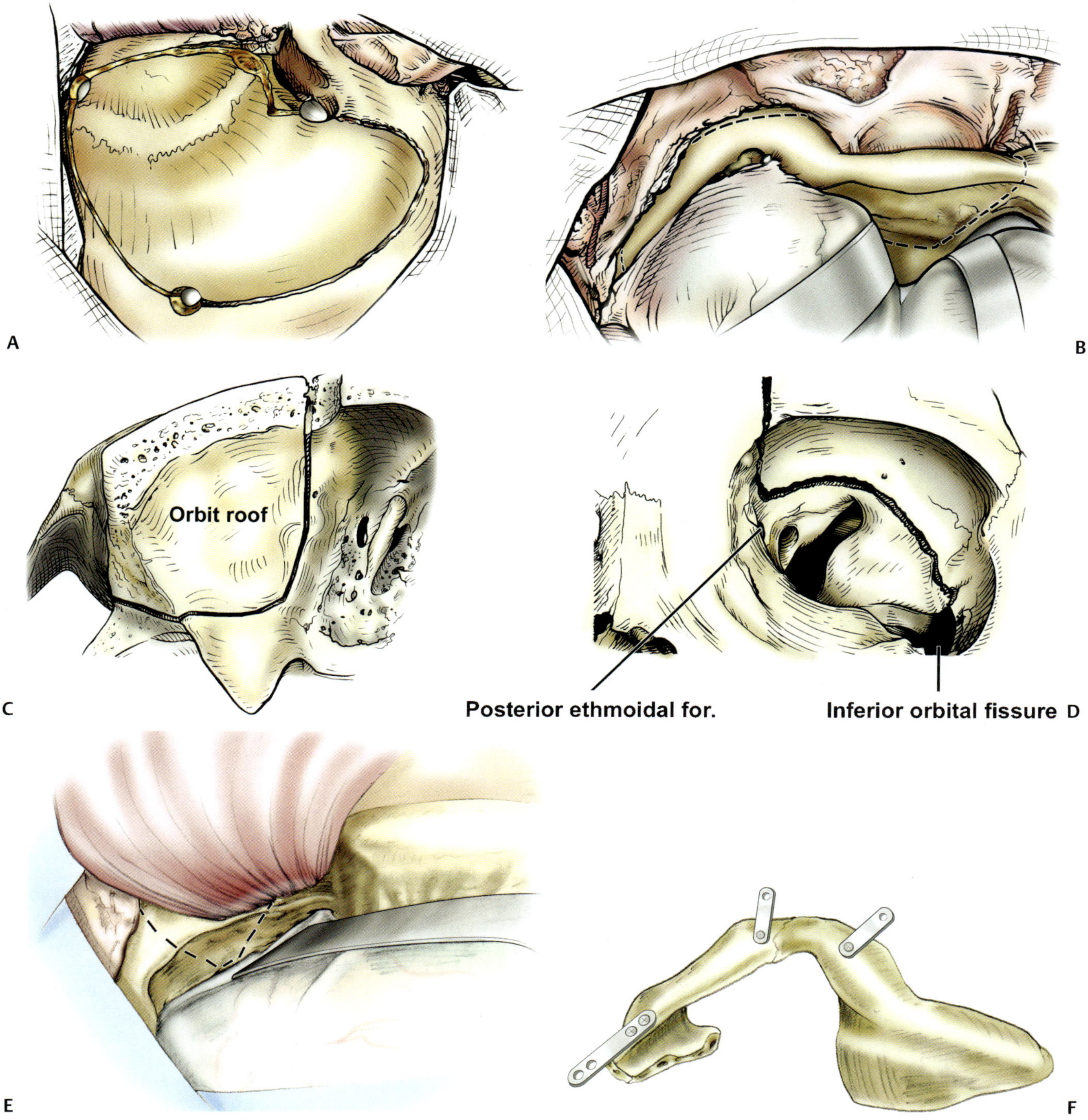

Figure 66–4 **(A)** The frontotemporal craniotomy. **(B)** The osteotomy cuts for a standard orbitozygomatic osteotomy (OZO) without a condylar osteotomy. **(C)** The osteotomy cuts in the orbit roof. **(D)** The orbital osteotomy from an anterior perspective, showing the lateral and inferior extension to the inferior orbital fissure. **(E)** The V-shaped condylar osteotomy cuts originating at the foramen spinosum. **(F)** The final appearance of a completed OZO including a condylar osteotomy.

(*Continued on page 788*)

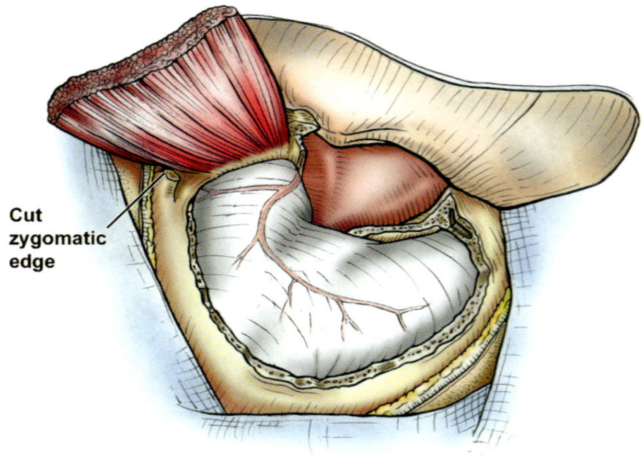

G

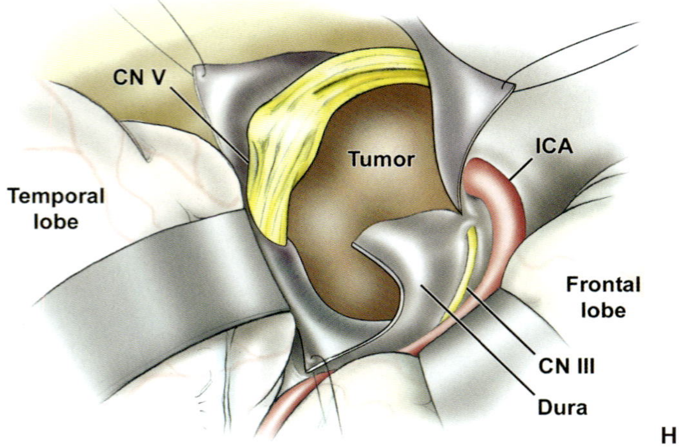

H

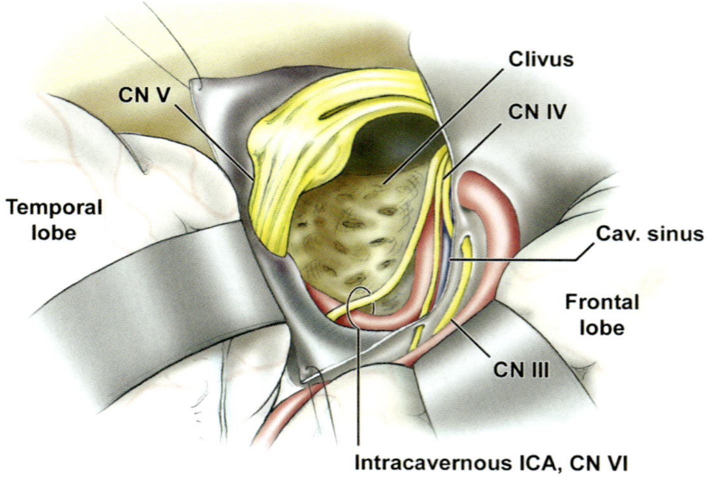

I

(*Continued*) **Figure 66–4** **(G)** The final appearance after the craniotomy and OZO for the frontotemporal transcavernous approach. **(H)** The intradural exposure of tumor in the cavernous sinus. The sylvian fissure is split and the lateral dural wall over the tumor has been incised. The distortion of cranial nerves by the tumor is shown. **(I)** After removal of intracavernous tumor. The uninvolved cavernous sinus and the clivus that has been exposed after resection are shown. ICA, internal carotid artery.

extradural or combined extra- and intradural resection of the clinoid.

The tightly adherent periorbita is dissected off the orbital rim using a sharp dissector, and then a cottonoid patty is used to protect the periorbita. The frontal and temporal dura are elevated from the orbital roof and the remaining sphenoid wing is rongeured or drilled. The orbital meningeal artery is identified, coagulated, and divided. This artery is a landmark for the superior aspect of the superior orbital fissure.

The osteotomies are then made with a reciprocating sagittal saw. The medial orbital rim is cut in line with the medial margin of the craniotomy while the periorbita and dura are protected with retractors. This is carried through the thin bone of the orbital roof toward the apex in line with the clinoid process just over the prominence of the orbital roof (3 to 3.5 cm). Then the anterolateral part of the inferior orbital fissure (IOF) is identified in the orbit and a cut is made across the zygomatic bone just above the zygomaticofacial foramen. The medial orbital cut is continued laterally across the orbital roof and then the lateral wall to connect to the IOF **(Fig. 66–4C,D).** The OZO is completed with either a simple zygomatic osteotomy by making an oblique forward-angled cut at the root of the zygoma or a condylar osteotomy that provides additional middle fossa exposure.

The condylar osteotomy is performed only for the subtemporal-infratemporal approach (see below) but is described here because it is a modification of the standard OZO. The condylar osteotomy requires incision of the superficial temporomandibular capsule and then dissection above the meniscus of the condylar joint. This allows the mandible to be retracted inferiorly if needed. The temporal lobe dura is retracted to expose the middle meningeal artery (MMA), which is coagulated and divided. A V-shaped osteotomy is made with the anterior limb connecting the MMA to a point at the anteriormost aspect of the root of the zygoma. The posterior cut must angle posteriorly behind the mandibular fossa without entering the external ear canal **(Fig. 66–4E).** After completion of these steps a bur and chisels are used to ensure complete bony disarticulation. The appearance of the final OZO with condylar osteotomy is shown in **Fig. 66–4F.** The remaining soft tissue attachments such as the temporalis muscle fascia and masseter muscle are divided. The final bone removal involves drilling away the remainder of the posterior orbital roof to the optic foramen and over the optic canal to the clinoid. The clinoid can be removed extradurally by drilling and disarticulating the remaining bone from the optic strut with fine rongeurs. Alternatively, the clinoid can be removed intradurally under direct vision. The appearance of the exposure after completion of the craniotomy and OZO is shown in **Fig. 66–4G.**

Resection of Cavernous Sinus Tumor

The CS is involved in up to 75% of patients with chordoma and chondrosarcoma. Therefore, understanding the surgical approaches and techniques in this area is mandatory in most cases for attempts at total resection. The CS can be approached from either extradural (discussed in later sections) or intradural approaches, or both. The frontotemporal approach is designed for intradural resection of tumor in the CS. The principles of resection of tumor in the CS include the need for adequate exposure and proximal and distal ICA control.

Proximal ICA control is achieved in the neck via a small skin crease incision. Exposure of the petrous ICA is avoided because it requires division of the greater superficial petrosal nerve (GSPN), which leads to a dry eye. After splitting the sylvian fissure, the CS is entered through a *lateral approach* at the most prominent part of tumor involvement using a horizontal or vertical incision in the outer dural layer that is dissected from the inner dural layer. In most cases this access is through the lateral wall. Cranial nerves are dissected and displaced gently to increase exposure and allow tumor removal **(Fig. 66–4H,I).** Multiple incisions can be made, but to preserve their vascularity and function, the dura overlying cranial nerves III and IV must be preserved. Chordomas and chondrosarcomas are generally not firmly adherent to the nerves or ICA. A *superior approach* can also be used. The optic canal is unroofed, the anterior clinoid process is resected, and the dural rings around the optic nerve and ICA are divided and dissected free. This allows access to the superior and medial CS between the optic and third nerves.

Occasionally, the cavernous ICA may be invaded by the tumor, or it may be lacerated by tumor removal. This requires resection and graft reconstruction.

Closure and Reconstruction

The resection of the anterior clinoid process can lead to CSF leak by communication with the air sinuses through a pneumatized clinoid or inadvertent entry into the sphenoid sinus. CSF leakage may also occur through dural openings into the CS or dorsum sellae. The dura must be closed as carefully as possible, using a fascial graft if necessary. The sphenoid sinus must be packed with fat and sealed with a pericranial or fascial graft and tissue glue. Pneumatized air cells must be waxed or packed with fat and sealed with tissue glue. The dura is closed in a watertight fashion, and the OZO osteotomy is secured with titanium miniplates. A miniplate can be placed across the site of the mandibular fossa cut and drilled before removing the bone to ensure good occlusion.

Pitfalls and Complications

The frontotemporal branch of the facial nerve must be avoided in the exposure by using the interfascial approach. Preservation of the supraorbital nerve and vessel prevents forehead numbness and ensures maximal blood supply to the pericranium should it be needed for reconstruction. Large lacerations of the periorbita that expose muscle should be repaired with suture or a patch to prevent entrapment syndromes. Care must be taken in resecting the clinoid to avoid injury to the optic nerve or cranial nerves III and IV, which traverse the superior orbital fissure (SOF) just under the clinoid. The ICA can be injured with resection of the clinoid or tumor resection in the sinus, but this is rare because chordomas and chondrosarcomas are generally not extremely adherent. However, in patients with recurrent tumors, ICA injury must be anticipated, and preparations made for possible bypass grafting. Excessive packing of the cavernous sinus with Surgicel may create a stenosis of the ICA. At the end of the procedure, excess Surgicel must be removed and may be replaced with Gelfoam. Entry into the sphenoid sinus or air cells must be dealt with by a two-layered closure (pericranium and graft) as discussed above, to prevent postoperative CSF leaks and infection.

Illustrative Case 2: ***Fig. 66–5***

Subtemporal (Transpetrous Apex Transcavernous) and Subtemporal-Infratemporal Approaches

Indications

The subtemporal-infratemporal approach (ST-ITA) is an inferior extension of the transzygomatic approach and is used when the petroclival bone is involved inferior to the level of the horizontal segment of the petrous ICA.[23] Tumor extension inferior to the level of the hypoglossal canal or across the midline may be difficult to remove by this approach. The subtemporal approach (STA) provides access to the middle fossa, petrous apex, upper clivus, horizontal petrous ICA, and posterior CS. The ST-ITA provides additional exposure of the clivus to the level of the foramen magnum; the CS; the sphenoid, maxillary, and ethmoid sinuses; the infratemporal fossa; and the retro- and parapharyngeal space and the orbit. If the tumor has both intra- and extradural involvement, the extradural portion is performed first unless there is significant mass effect from the intradural portion. Involvement of the nasopharynx is important to recognize because it precludes a one-stage intra- and extradural procedure due to the risk of infection and the integrity of the vascular grafts (see below).

Operative Procedure

A lumbar drain is placed before positioning for these approaches to aid in brain relaxation and reduce retraction injury. The patient is positioned supine with the head turned 70 degrees, and the neck in slight extension, in pins. Fat grafts and fascia lata are needed for reconstruction, so the head, face, neck, abdomen, and ipsilateral thigh are all prepped and draped. The medial thigh and anterior aspect of the forearm are also prepped in the event that a vascular graft is needed. The preauricular limb of the incision extends

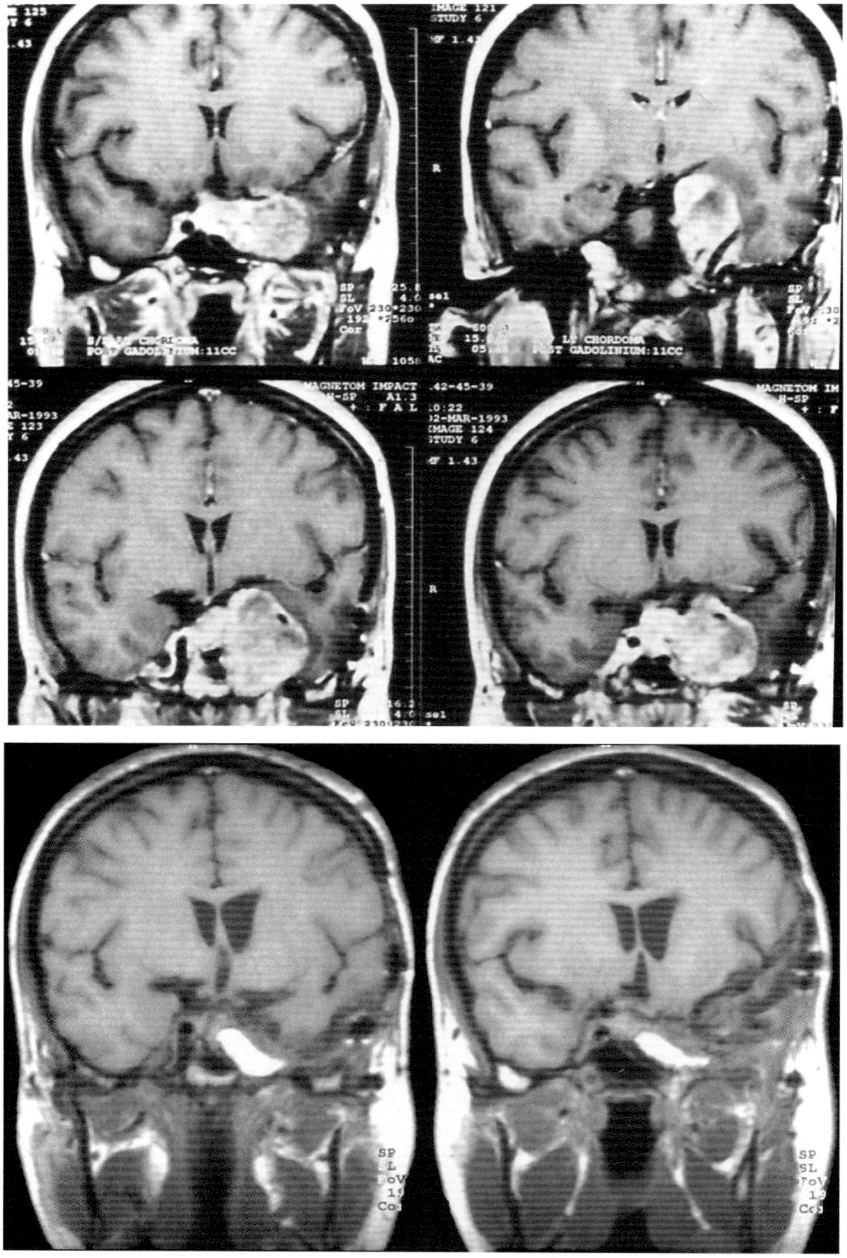

A B C D E F

Figure 66–5 Illustrative case 2. This 30-year-old women presented with a recurrent chondrosarcoma including the left cavernous sinus. **(A–D)** The intracavernous internal carotid artery (ICA) is encased and narrowed. Tumor resection required a saphenous vein graft replacement of the ICA. **(E,F)** Postoperative MRI scan and

(*Continued on page 791*)

G

H

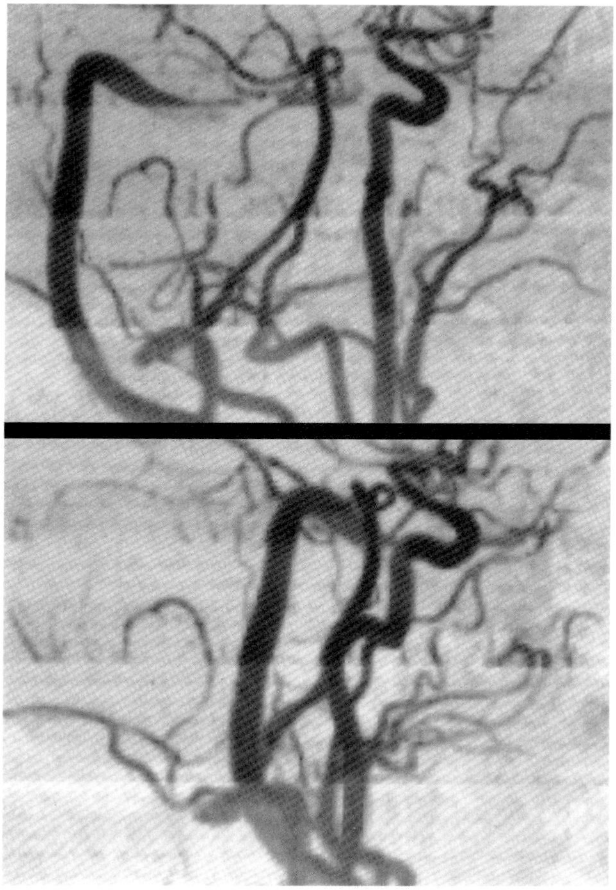

(*Continued*) **Figure 66–5** **(G,H)** magnetic resonance angiography show the absence of tumor and the patent grafts. This patient had a small recurrence 8 years later, treated successfully by radiosurgery.

from the inferior border of the ear lobule for the ST-ITA and just below the zygomatic process for the STA **(Fig. 66–6A).** At the junction of the tragus and helix the incision is angled around the tragus of the ear to form a 90 degree indentation. This provides a better cosmetic result. The incision then can be either extended slightly behind the ear and then brought forward along the superior temporal line or taken bicoronally. These options provide the necessary anterior skin exposure. The mobilization of the skin flap and temporalis muscle is the same as described for the OZO (see earlier); however, for the ST-ITA, the superficial temporal artery and vein, the upper branches of the facial nerve, and the parotid gland tissues are elevated from the masseteric fascia ("reverse degloving procedure") **(Fig. 66–6A).** Soft tissues below the zygoma are mobilized anteriorly with the scalp flap along the plane of the masseteric fascia. This provides adequate additional inferior exposure in the infratemporal region and avoids direct dissection of the facial nerve. The cervical ICA is exposed only if the ICA is encased by tumor and a bypass is planned.

A free temporal bone flap is elevated with one bur hole at the pterion and another just above the base of the mastoid process **(Fig. 66–6B).** No frontal exposure is needed. The capsule of the temporomandibular joint is opened and a zygomatic (or orbitozygomatic) osteotomy is performed including the condylar fossa. The temporalis muscle is reflected inferiorly, and for the ST-ITA the meniscus of the condyle is dissected, and the condyle is depressed with a retractor to provide additional exposure. Under magnification, the middle fossa dura is elevated to expose the MMA, the GSPN, the mandibular nerve (V3), and the arcuate eminence of the petrous bone. The MMA is cauterized and divided and the GSPN is divided to avoid injury to the geniculate ganglion. The greater wing of the sphenoid is rongeured to expose the foramen ovale laterally, the foramen rotundum anteriorly, and the inferior edge of the SOF **(Fig. 66–6C).**

To allow for continued medial dural retraction, an incision is made in the dural reflections over V2 and V3, which allows the middle fossa dura (including the outer layer of cavernous sinus dura) to be peeled away from V2, V3, the semilunar ganglion, and the trigeminal rootlets. This maneuver improves access to the petrous apex and the intracavernous and dorsum sellae portions of the tumor, if present. Bleeding from entry into the margins of the cavernous sinus is controlled with Surgicel.

The petrous ICA is now identified at the junction of the GSPN and V3 **(Fig. 66–6C).** The petrous ICA lies inferior to V3 and medial to its exit at the foramen ovale and immediately beneath the GSPN. If the ICA requires dissection, the GSPN should be divided near the geniculate ganglion to avoid facial nerve injury. At this point the tensor tympani muscles overlie the bony eustachian tube lateral to the ICA and GSPN. If the eustachian tube is divided and excised to gain better access to the ICA and petrous apex, the posterior end in the petrous bone is packed with fat and the anterior cartilaginous end is sealed with suture or a hemoclip. The genu of the petrous ICA lies medial to the eustachian tube covered by a thin layer of bone or no bone at all. The ICA is unroofed with small punches inferiorly and superiorly. The vertical segment of the petrous ICA is exposed inferiorly. A dense cartilaginous ring adheres to the periosteum of the carotid canal at the entrance point of the ICA **(Fig. 66–6D).** This ring is divided to mobilize the ICA at the cervical-petrous junction. The cervical ICA is dissected free to the level of the styloid process in the neck **(Fig. 66–6E).**

The horizontal segment of the ICA is then traced forward. The petrous bone posterosuperior to the ICA genu is carefully avoided to prevent injury to the geniculate ganglion and cochlea. To trace the ICA to the CS one must remove bone posterior, anterior, and medial to V3, or resect it if it is invaded by tumor. Once the upper cervical and petrous ICA have been fully mobilized, the entire ICA segment is rotated forward and held with vessel loops.

With the ICA out of its canal, the bone medial to the carotid canal and the petrous apex posterosuperior to the horizontal segment of the petrous ICA can be drilled away to expose the petroclival synchondrosis and clivus. The clivus can now be drilled away from the level of the petrous apex to foramen magnum. Posterior to the tympanic bone, care is taken to avoid injury to cranial nerves IX to XII and the jugular bulb. The hypoglossal nerve can be unroofed and traced into the posterior fossa. The anterior arch of the atlas and tip of the odontoid can also be removed by this approach. Exposure below this level can be achieved by working below the facial nerve and in front of the ICA and external carotid

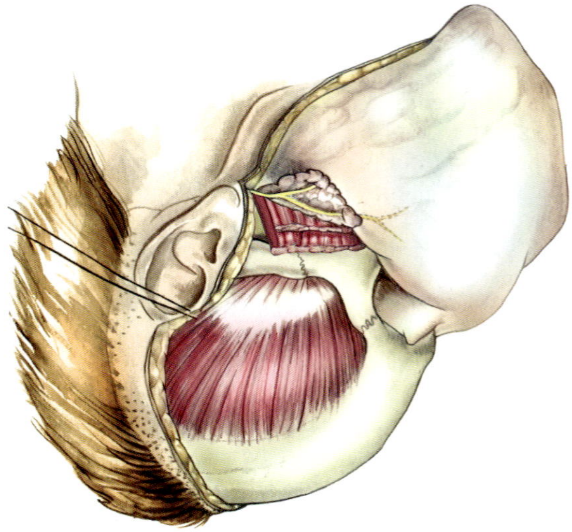

A

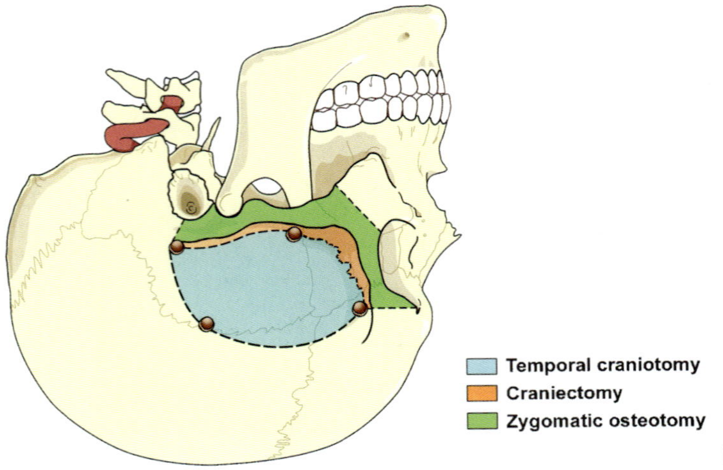

B

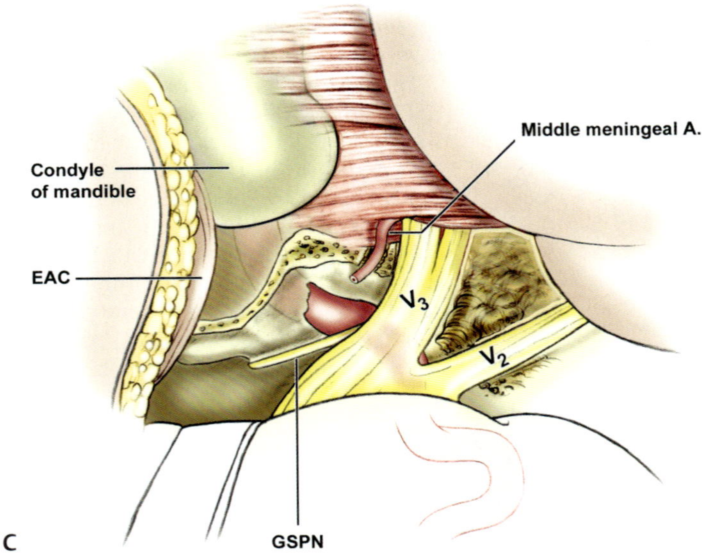

C

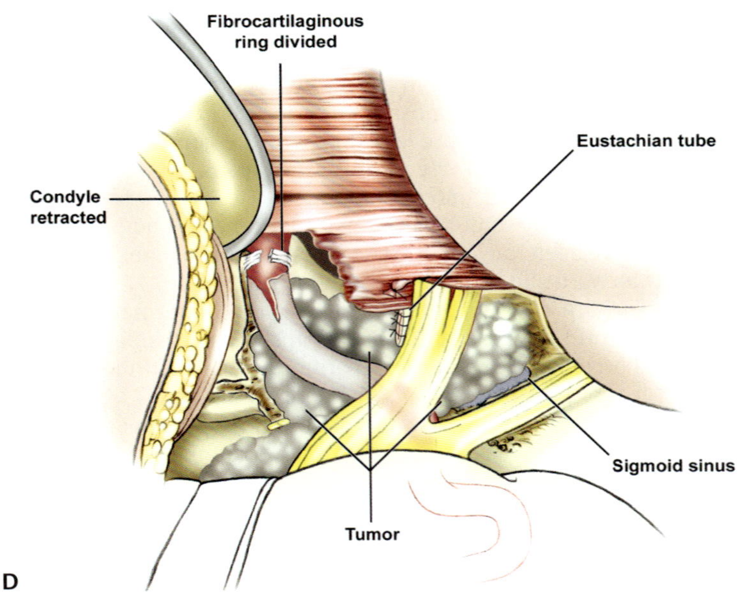

D

Figure 66–6 **(A)** The incision for the subtemporal-infratemporal approach and "reverse-degloving" of the parotid and facial nerve from the masseteric fascia. **(B)** The craniotomy and osteotomies for the subtemporal-infratemporal approach. Depending on the planned access, either an orbitozygomatic osteotomy or a simple zygomatic osteotomy is performed. **(C)** After elevation of the temporal lobe dura and division of the middle meningeal artery, the greater superficial petrosal nerve (GSPN) and the partially exposed horizontal portion of the internal carotid artery (ICA) are seen. V3 and V2 have been unroofed. EAC, external auditory canal. **(D)** After incising the dura propria over the semilunar ganglion and V2 and V3, the temporal lobe dura is further retracted for additional exposure. Note the relationships among the GSPN, ICA, and V3. Also note the access to the sphenoid sinus between V2 and V3, and the retraction of the mandibular condyle.

(*Continued on page 793*)

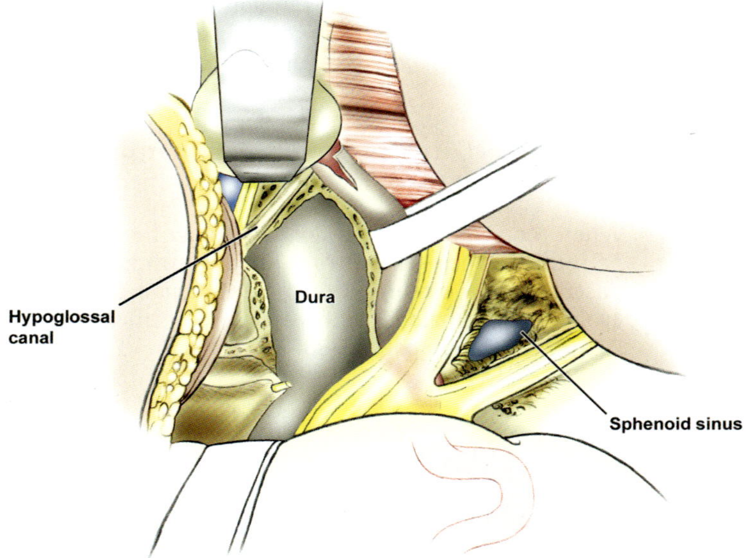

E

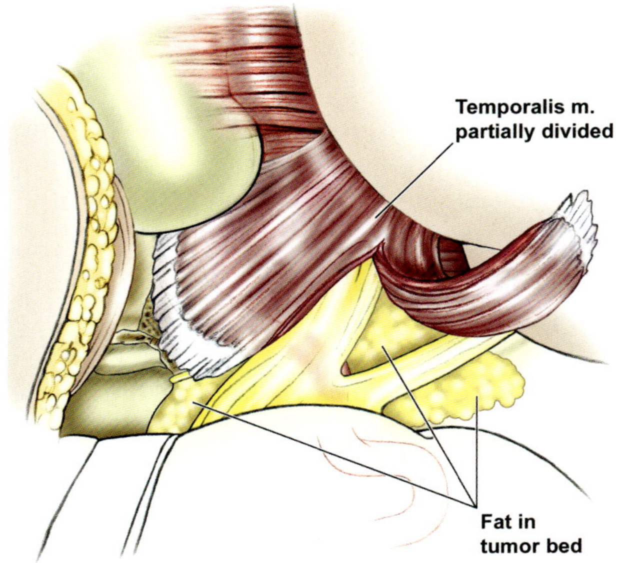

F

(*Continued*) **Figure 66–6** **(E)** Mobilization of the petrous ICA from the carotid canal. Note the exposed jugular bulb and lower cranial nerves. **(F)** Tumor has been resected, and reconstruction is done using temporalis muscle and fat.

artery.[21] Significant bleeding, which can occur from the basilar venous plexus, is controlled with packing and head elevation. If the clival dura is opened, a direct repair or fascia lata patch must be fashioned to prevent CSF leak.

The lateral wall of the sphenoid bone medial to the maxillary division of the trigeminal nerve (V2) can be removed to provide access to the sphenoid sinus. However, V2 may have to be divided to gain adequate access. It can be resutured at the end of the procedure. The inferior and medial portion of the cavernous ICA will also be exposed in this dissection. The posterior inferior aspect of the CS can be entered by following the ICA. Alternatively, the anterior portion of the sinus can be entered between the ophthalmic division of the trigeminal nerve (V1) and V2 between the leaves of the dura. The growth plane of tumor can also be followed as it extends into the CS to provide good access for resection. Extension of tumor into the orbit, maxillary sinus, ethmoid sinus, infratemporal fossa, and retro- and parapharyngeal space can easily be removed.

Management of the Internal Carotid Artery and Indications for Bypass

When tumor encases the ICA in patients who have been previously operated and irradiated, bypass may be necessary for attempted radical resection. Depending on the caliber of the M2 recipient vessel, either a saphenous vein or radial artery graft is used and is tunneled behind the ear and away from the main operative field. Regardless of the nature of the collateral circulation, if the ICA is damaged, it must be reconstructed to avoid a stroke. Greater caution must be exercised in patients with a poor collateral circulation, either by a more conservative resection or by a prophylactic radial artery ICA to MCA bypass, before aggressive dissection of the intracavernous ICA.

Closure and Reconstruction

Dural defects must be closed with a free fascial graft and circumferentially tacked in place. This graft is fortified with autologous fat and tissue glue. When the nasopharynx, paranasal air sinuses, or external surface communicates with the resection cavity, it must be reconstructed with vascularized tissue. Small defects are closed with a temporalis flap (**Fig. 66–6F**), whereas for larger defects, or in patients who have had prior surgery, a vascularized free tissue flap may be required. The rectus abdominis muscle free microvascular flap is a good choice because it is easily accessible and provides generous coverage to large defects.

Subtemporal, Transcavernous, Transpetrous Apex Approach

When the tumor does not extend below the genu of the petrous ICA, the entire petrous ICA does not have to be exposed, and the occlusion of the eustachian tube may be avoided. The remainder of this exposure is similar to the ST-ITA and is illustrated in **Fig. 66–7.**

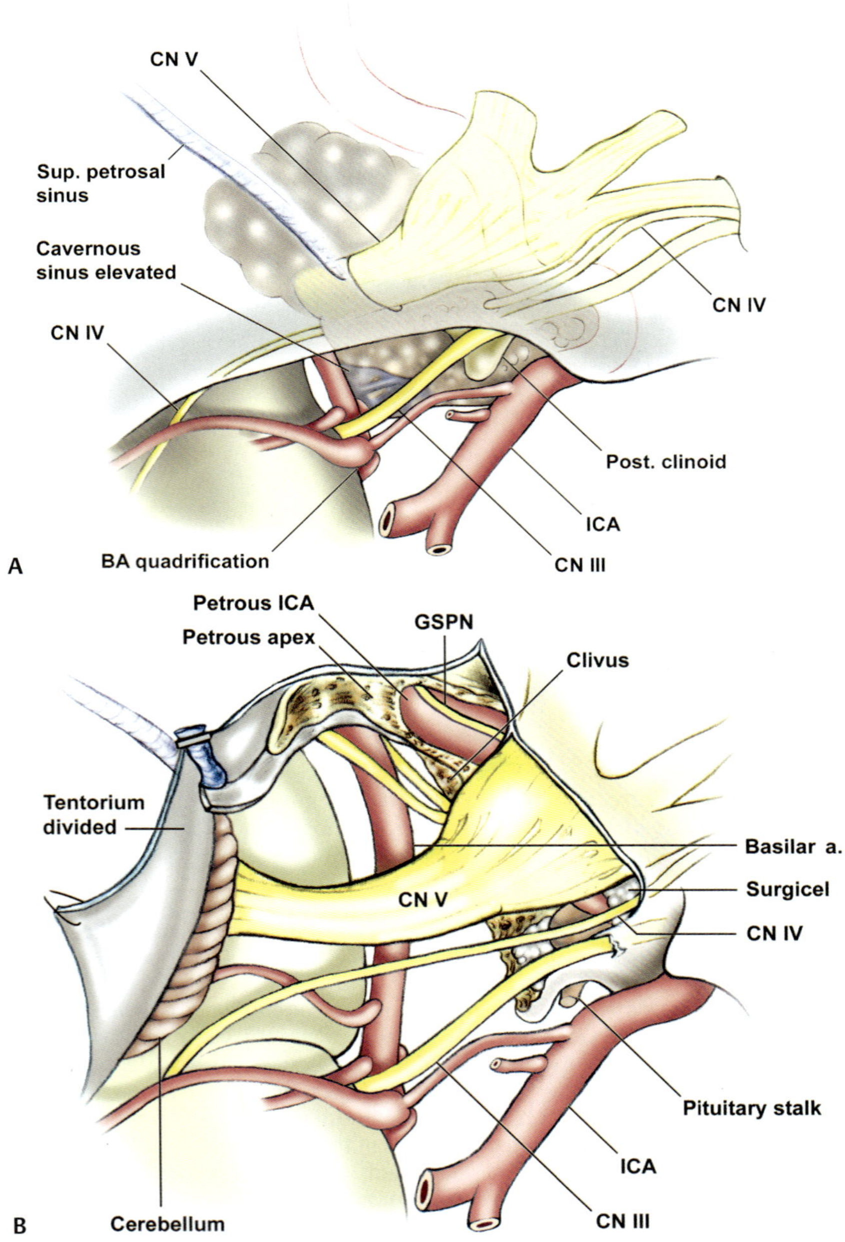

Figure 66–7 **(A)** Subtemporal-transzygomatic and transpetrous apex approach, with tumor in place. It lies in the cavernous sinus, and extends to the level of the horizontal petrous internal carotid artery (ICA). **(B)** The exposed anatomy after tumor resection using this approach. BA, basilar artery; GSPN, greater suprfrcial petrosal nerve.

Pitfalls and Complications

A CSF leak is the most common complication and is best avoided by careful reconstruction with the use of a vascularized tissue flap if the repair is tenuous and by prophylactic postoperative lumbar drainage. If a CSF leak develops, it usually resolves with a short course of intermittent lumbar drainage. Infection is also avoided by the same measures that ensure adequate reconstruction. The eustachian tube must be identified, packed with fat, and then sutured or clipped shut anteriorly to prevent CSF leaks.

Almost all of the cranial nerves can be exposed and injured in the more extensive subtemporal-infratemporal approaches. The use of good microsurgical techniques prevents most permanent injuries, but if tumor is adherent or the patient has previously been operated or irradiated, then it may not be possible to spare a nerve without leaving adherent tumor behind. The facial nerve must be dissected into the parotid to the point of its major branching to reduce traction when the mandible is distracted. Petrous bone resection must respect the position of the cochlea and geniculate ganglion, which are located posterior and superior to the genu of the petrous ICA. In addition, the GSPN should be divided as it is exposed, to prevent facial nerve palsy from traction injuries or bleeding into the geniculate ganglion. The ICA can be injured during drilling or from retraction and may also be compromised when tumor is invading it. Mild trismus and malocclusion may be present after the distraction or resection of the condyle, but resolves over time and with jaw exercises.

Illustrative Case 3: **Fig. 66–8**

Illustrative Case 4: **Fig. 66–9**

Illustrative Case 5: **Fig. 66–10**

Illustrative Case 6: **Fig. 66–11**

Extreme Lateral Transcondylar Approach

Indications

The extreme lateral approach includes a variety of posterolateral approaches useful for tumors involving the ventral upper cervical spine, lower clivus, foramen magnum, and occipital condyles.[21] The specific subtypes of the extreme lateral approach vary in the degree of bony resection to facilitate exposure to specific regions.[22] For extradural resection of chordomas and chondrosarcomas, the complete transcondylar approach (CTCA) is most commonly employed and is described below.

Operative Procedure

When only this approach is planned, the patient is placed in the lateral position with the lower arm hanging away from the top of the table, supported by gel padding, a cloth sling made from the bed sheet under the patient, and an arm

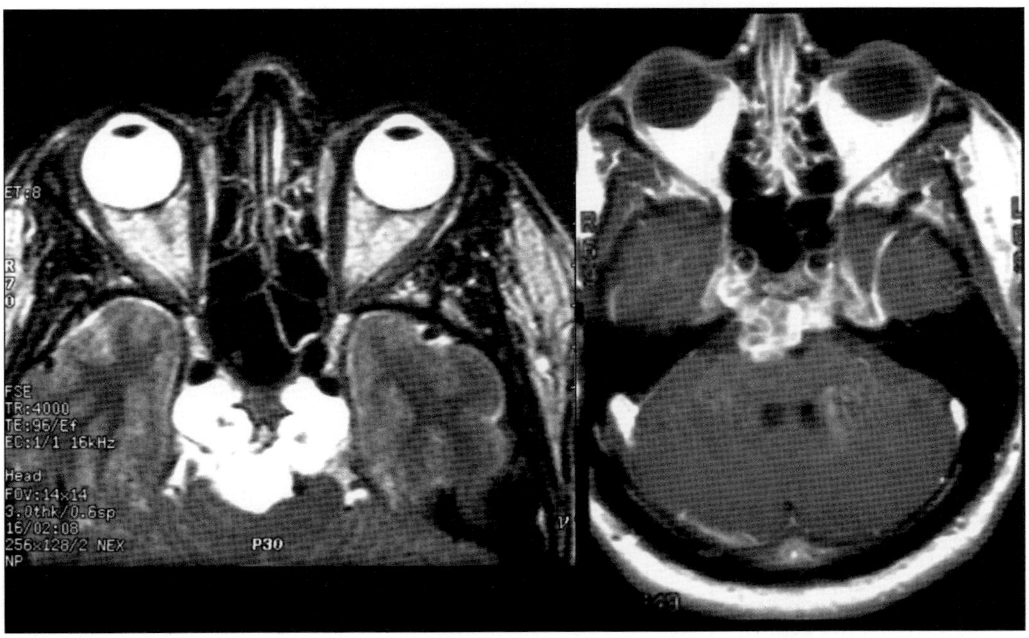

A B

Figure 66–8 Illustrative case 3. **(A,B)** This patient presented with a chondroma involving the posterior aspect of both cavernous sinuses and the clivus. A total resection was performed with a subtemporal-transzygomatic, transpetrous apex approach.

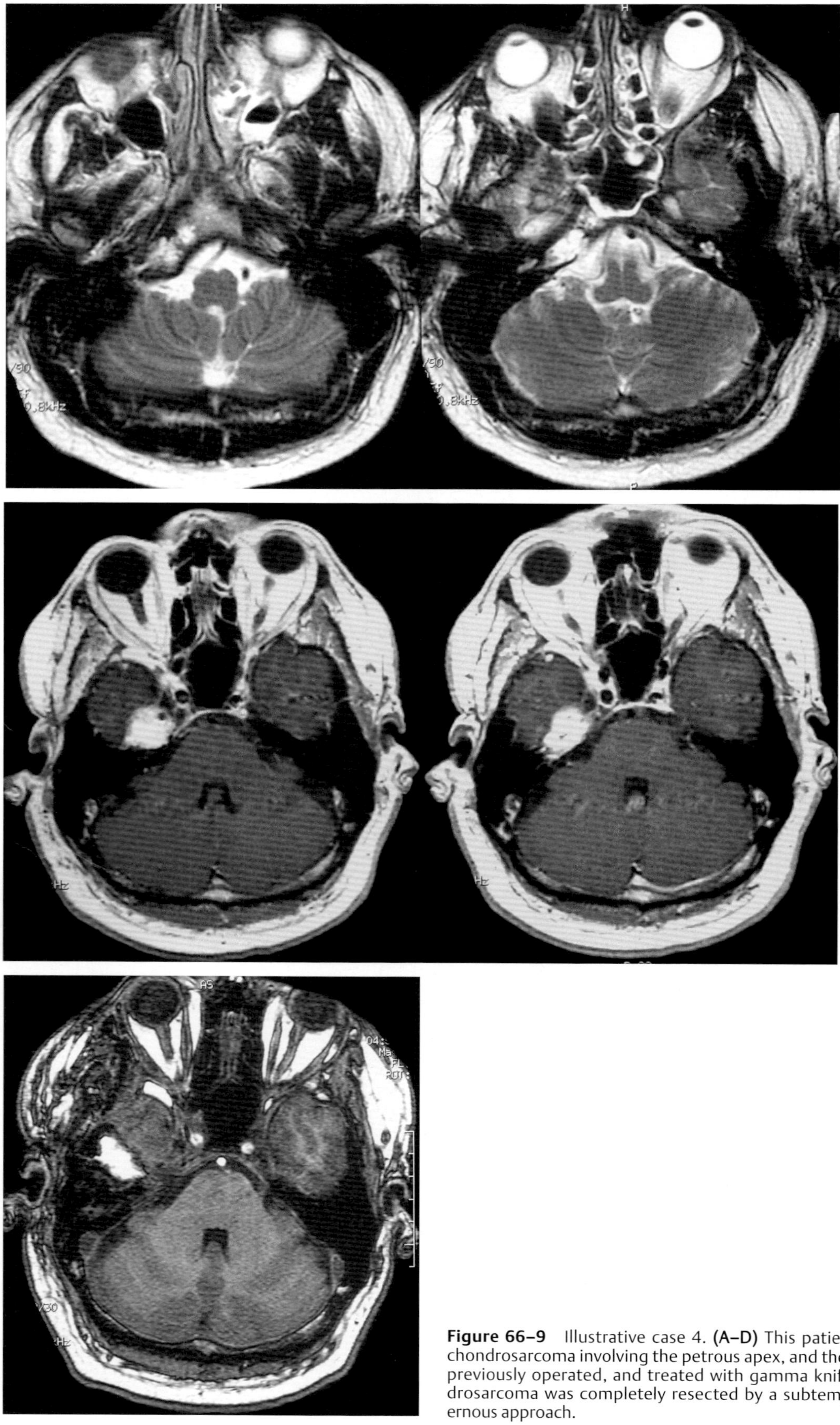

A B C D E

Figure 66–9 Illustrative case 4. **(A–D)** This patient presented with a recurrent chondrosarcoma involving the petrous apex, and the cavernous sinus. He had been previously operated, and treated with gamma knife radiosurgery. **(E)** This chondrosarcoma was completely resected by a subtemporal, transpetrous, transcavernous approach.

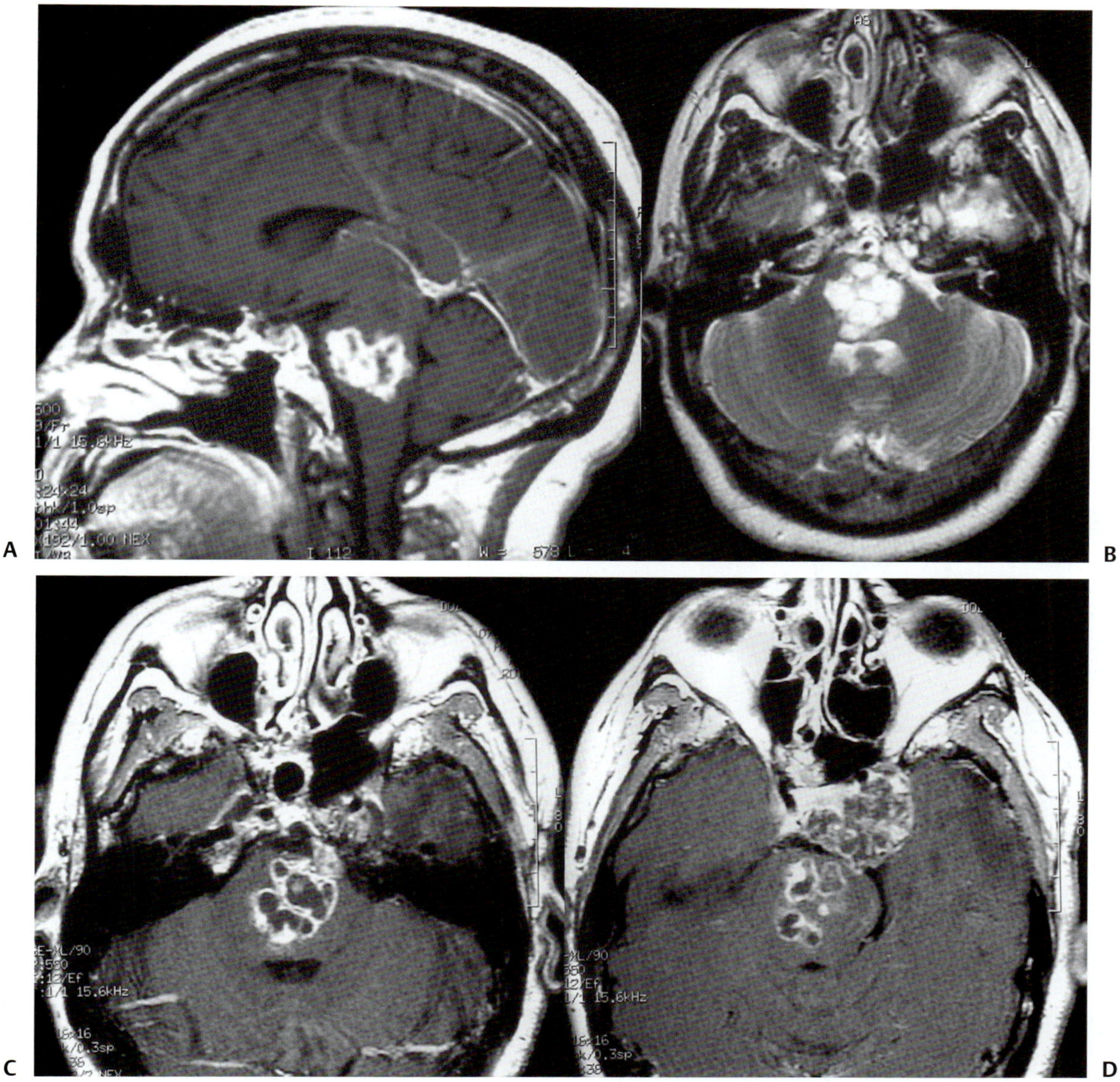

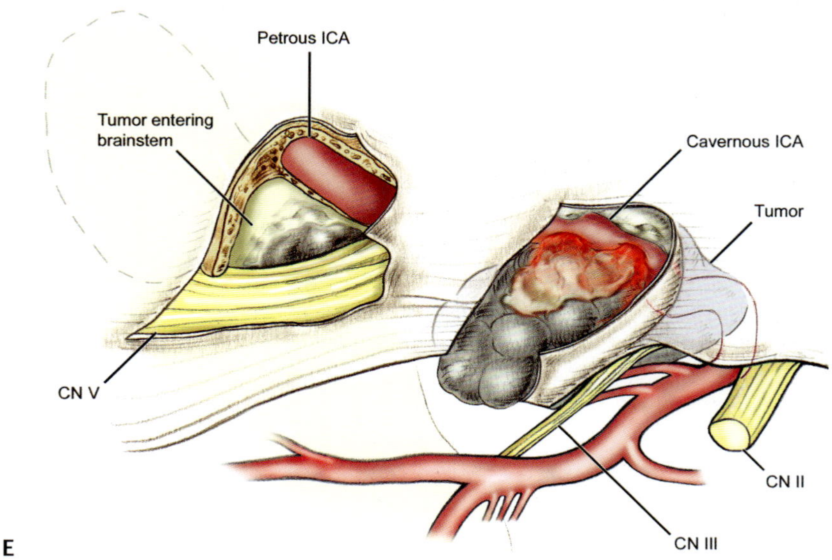

(*Continued on page 798*)

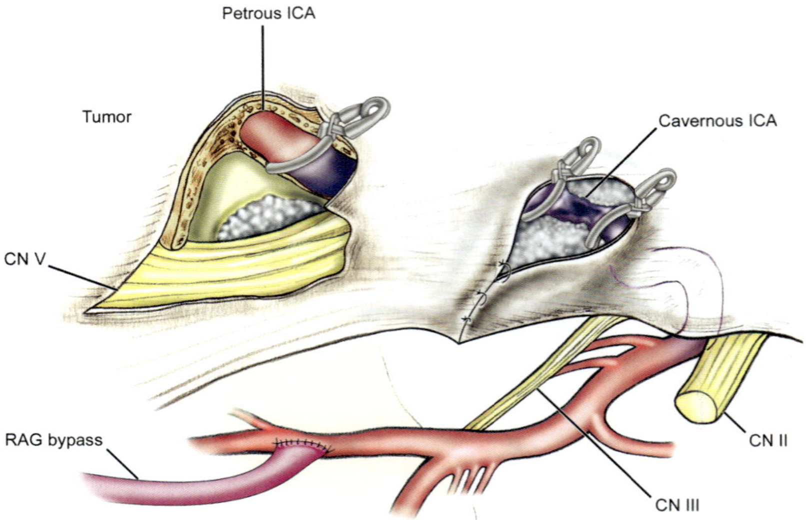

F

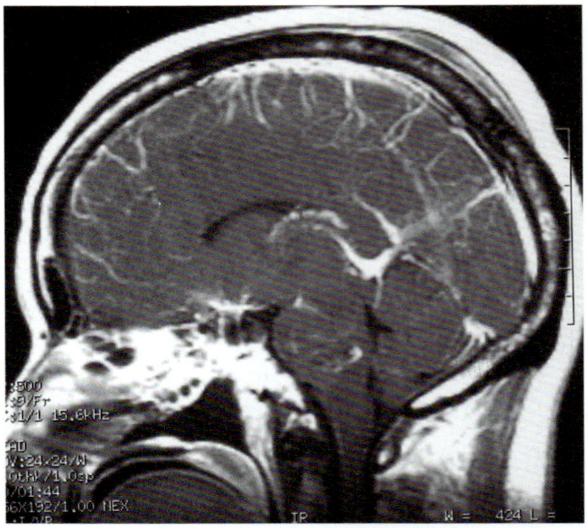

G

Figure 66–10 Illustrative case 5. (A–D) This 59-year-old woman presented with a large chondrosarcoma of the cavernous sinus, petroclival area, and the brain stem. (E) During the first operation for tumor removal, the intracavernous was damaged. (F) A radial artery graft was placed from the cranial internal carotidartery (ICA) to the middle cerebral artery (MCA), and tumor was removed from the brain stem. (G–I) The patient underwent a second operation to remove residual cavernous and clival tumor Postoperative MRI scans do not show residual tumor. She remains well, but with residual paralysis of CNs II and III.

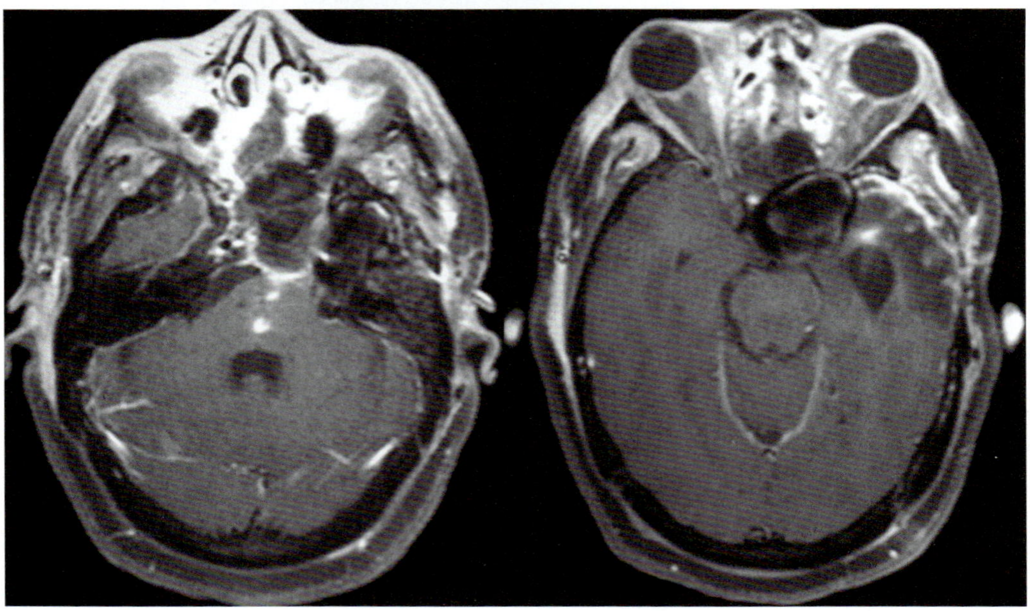

H I

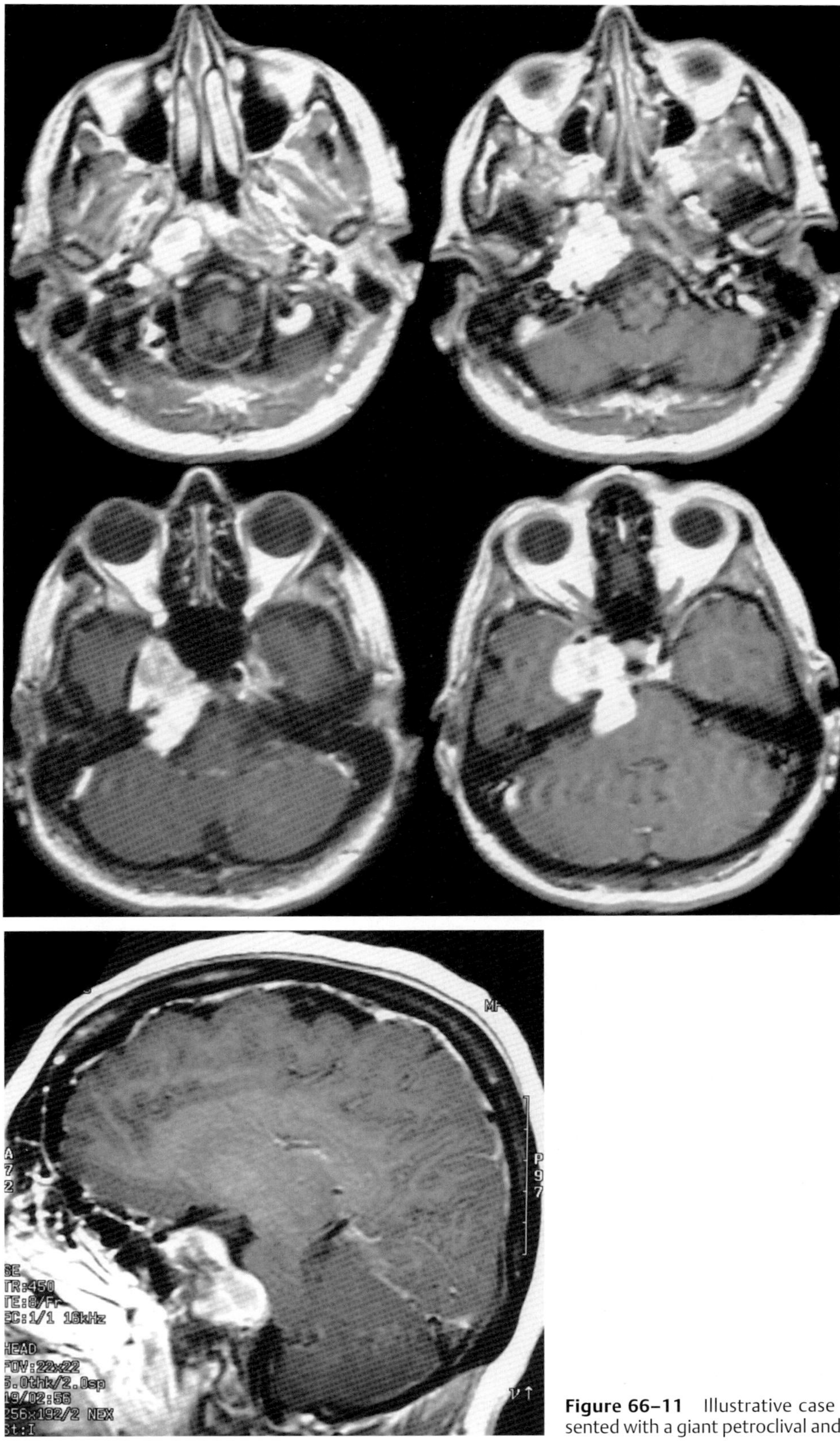

Figure 66–11 Illustrative case 6. **(A–E)** This 43-year-old woman presented with a giant petroclival and cavernous sinus chordoma.

(*Continued on page 800*)

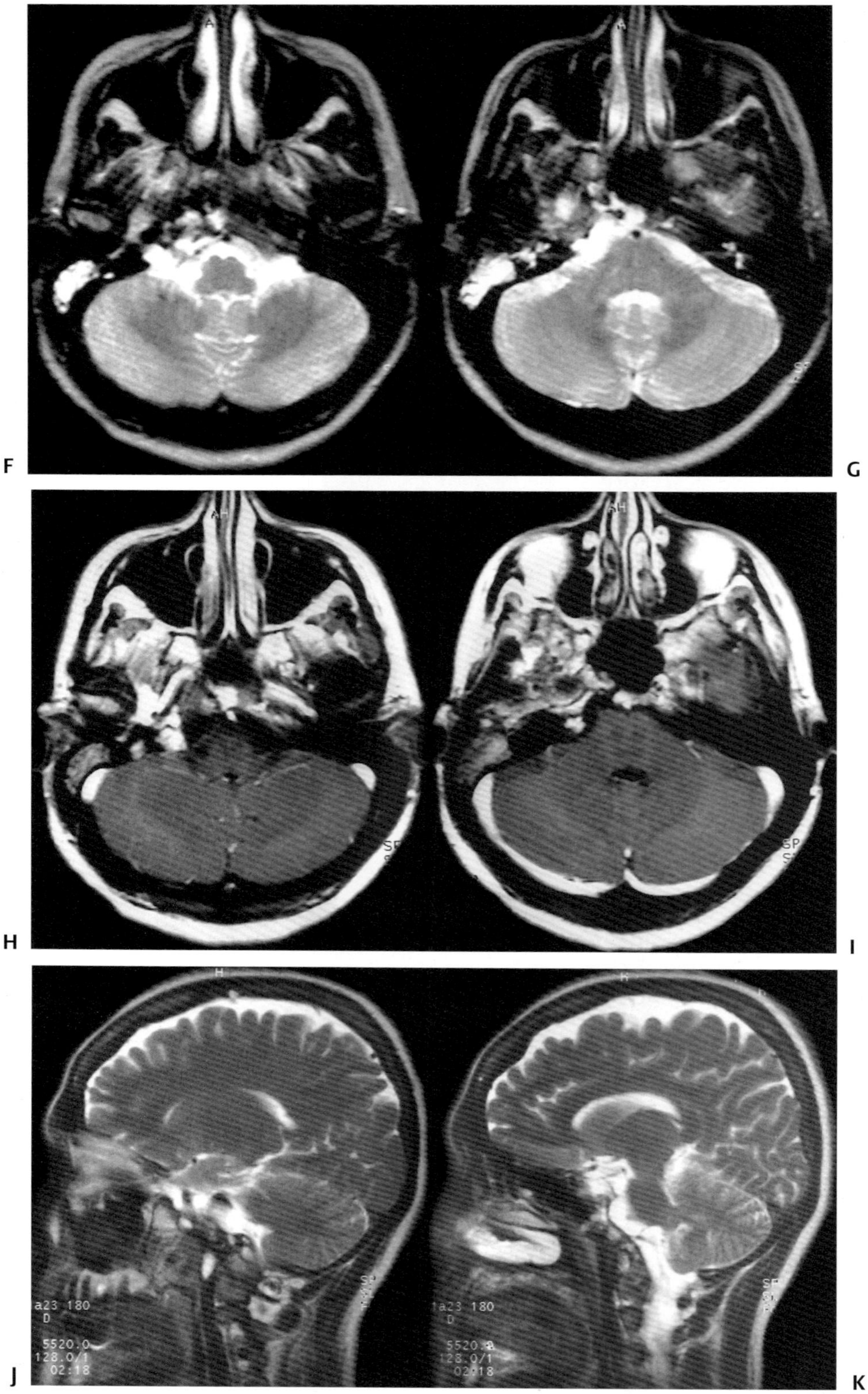

(*Continued*) **Figure 66–11** **(F–K)** Microsurgical total resection was performed in two stages, first by a subtemporal-infratemporal and later by a frontotemporal-transcavernous approach. Patient remains tumor free 1 year postoperatively, without any deficit.

board. The upper arm is supported on an overarm board. If this approach is combined with a petrosal approach, the patient is placed supine with a large ipsilateral shoulder roll and the head rotated 45 degrees away from vertical. One must be aware that the lateral position makes any vein graft harvest more difficult. However, a radial artery graft can be extracted from the inferior forearm. Excessive head turning ($>$ 60 degrees) is avoided because it moves the transverse process and foramen of C1 medial and inferior to the mastoid tip, stretching the vertebral artery (VA) between C2 and C1. If there is extensive involvement of the condyle and complete resection is planned, the lateral position with the head in neutral alignment is preferred. An occipital-cervical fusion is generally necessary but is performed in a second-stage operative procedure.

There are several options for skin incisions for the extreme lateral approaches, but for the CTCA we prefer a C-shaped incision just posterior to the mastoid process. A subsequent occiput to C2–C3 fusion is performed through a midline occipitocervical incision. The C-shaped retroauricular incision and patient postioning are shown in **Fig. 66–12A.**

In elevating the flap of a C-shaped incision, four layers of muscles are sequentially encountered. The sternomastoid constitutes the first layer **(Fig. 66–12B)**. The sternomastoid muscle and fascia are reflected forward with the scalp flap to improve its vascularity. If exposure at or below C2 is required, then the sternomastoid muscle must be separated and reflected inferiorly. Care should be taken to identify and preserve the spinal accessory nerve that exits the posterior border of the sternomastoid. Underlying the sternomastoid muscle is the splenius capitis muscle, which forms the second layer **(Fig. 66–12B,C)**. The occipital artery is identified running horizontally between the second and third muscle layers **(Fig. 66–12C)**. Just deep to the splenius is the third layer of muscles, the semispinalis and longissimus capitis **(Fig. 66–12C)**. All three of these layers are reflected inferomedially with the skin flap to expose the deepest layer of muscles formed by the superior and inferior oblique muscle, the rectus capitis major and minor, and the levator scapulae **(Fig. 66–12D)**. The transverse process of C1 can now be palpated. The superior and inferior oblique muscles (which attach to the transverse process of C1) and the rectus capitis major form an important landmark called the suboccipital triangle **(Fig. 66–12D)**. The VA courses along the superolateral aspect of the C1 arch, and, along with the suboccipital nerves (terminal branches of C1), lies within this space. An extensive venous plexus surrounds the VA and connects with the epidural venous plexus and condylar emissary vein. The condylar emissary vein is the most prominent emissary vein in the region and connects to the sigmoid sinus or jugular bulb.

The suboccipital muscles are reflected as well as the muscular attachments to the C1 transverse process. Between C1 and C2, injury to the VA can be avoided by recognizing that it often takes a tortuous course in this location, and that the dorsal ramus of C2 courses dorsal to the artery **(Fig. 66–12E)**. The fatty fibrous tissue that lies between the occiput and C1 is resected. The VA with its venous plexus is then mobilized from the C1 arch laterally to its foramen. The lateral third of the C1 lamina and the lateral mass (and sometimes C2) is resected and the VA can then be dissected free from its foramen and sutured through the adventitia to provide medial mobilization **(Fig. 66–12F)**.

To gain access to the condyle, a low mastoidectomy is first performed, which can extend laterally to the facial nerve. The inferior sigmoid sinus and jugular bulb are then unroofed and a small suboccipital craniotomy is performed to provide access to the foramen magnum **(Fig. 66–12G)**. Preoperative assessment of the venous sinus anatomy and dominance is mandatory so that complications can be managed appropriately, including the need for ligation or reconstruction of the sinus. If the sinus has to be divided, the intrasinus pressure is measured with temporary clipping. If there is a significant rise in pressure ($>$ 5 cm Hg), then the sinus should be reconstructed either by direct suture of a patch or end-to-end graft with reversed saphenous vein.

Initially the posterior half of the condyle is drilled off to expose the hypoglossal canal. Additional bone removal superior and inferior to the canal completes the condylectomy and partial resection of the jugular tubercle to provide exposure to the midclivus. The removal of the lateral mass of C1 provides access to the lower clivus and odontoid process **(Fig. 66–12H)**. The extradural resection includes all grayish gelatinous bulk tumor and adjacent bone margins infiltrated by small tumor islands until normal marrow bleeding is encountered. The full access afforded by the CTCA is shown schematically in **Fig. 66–12I.**

Closure and Reconstruction

The resection bed is gently packed with autologous fat. If the dura has been violated, it must be primarily sutured, or if this is impossible, a fascial or pericranial graft should be placed and then bolstered with fat and sealed with tissue glue. The stability of the occipitocervical (OC) junction depends on the preservation of the condyle and C1 transverse process and the attachments of the alar and transverse ligaments to the anterior one third of these structures. If more than a half of the condyle has been resected or if the anterior soft tissues have been disrupted, then an OC fusion is indicated. Fusion is usually performed 2 to 3 days postoperatively. When there is evidence of a CSF effusion, the OC fusion is delayed for ~4 weeks to reduce the risk of CSF leaks and infection.

Postoperative Care

Patients must be carefully evaluated for lower cranial dysfunction, aspiration, respiratory difficulty, and CSF leak. Unilateral dysfunction of CNS IX and X may require arytenoid adduction and thyroplasty procedures and temporary feeding tube placement. Bilateral involvement requires tracheostomy and feeding gastrostomy or jejunostomy. CSF leaks are managed with lumbar drainage and rarely may require reexploration.

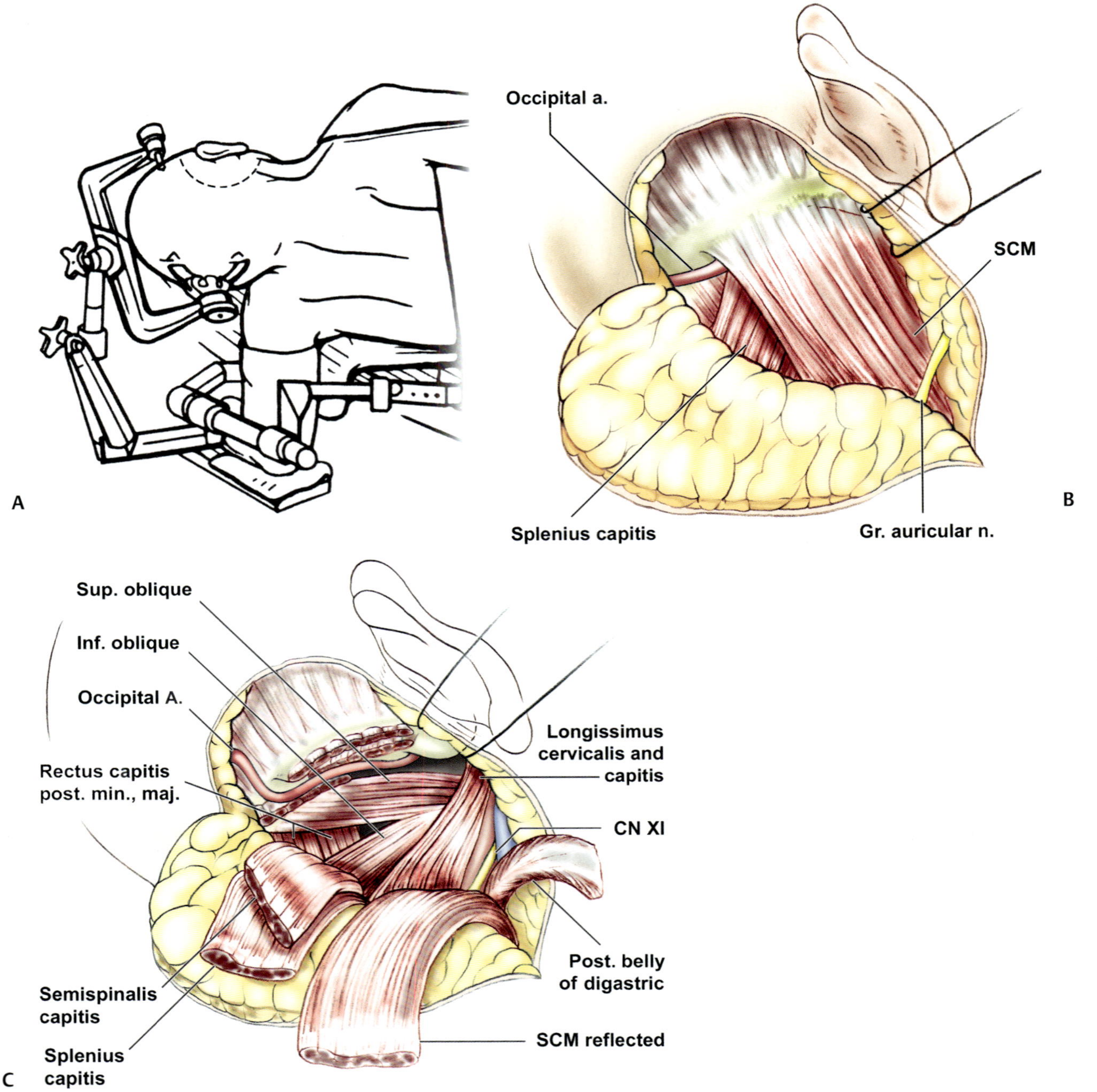

Figure 66–12 **(A)** Patient positioning and incision for a complete transcondylar extreme lateral approach. If this approach is combined with a petrosal approach then the patient is placed supine with the head turned to 45 degrees. **(B)** The initial exposure of the muscle layers. The sternomastoid is either taken forward with the skin flap or detached and retracted inferiorly (for cases where access below C1–C2 is necessary). The occipital artery is demonstrated emerging below the splenius muscle. **(C)** The first, second, and third muscle layers have been reflected, exposing the fourth, and deepest, muscle layer. These three muscles shown here define the suboccipital triangle, an important landmark for the vertebral artery (VA).

(*Continued on pages 803 and 804*)

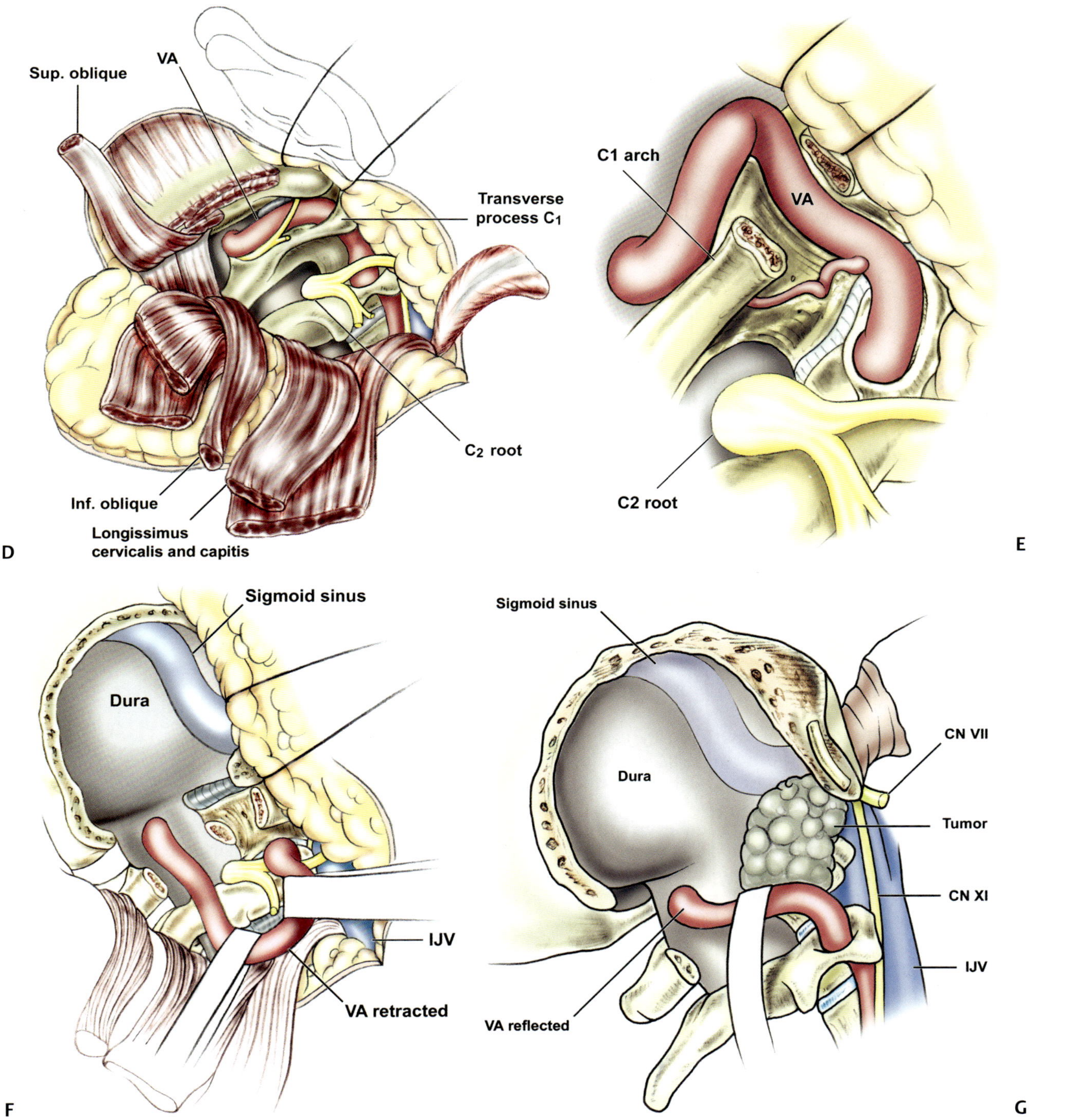

(*Continued*) **Figure 66–12** **(D)** The relationship among the VA, C2 dorsal root, C1 lamina, and occipital condyle. **(E)** After removal of the transverse foramen, the VA is completely exposed. **(F)** A retrosigmoid craniotomy and C1 laminectomy have been performed. The VA has been mobilized medially. The occipital condyle can now be resected as needed for complete tumor removal. **(G)** Tumor resection has commenced.

(*Continued on page 804*)

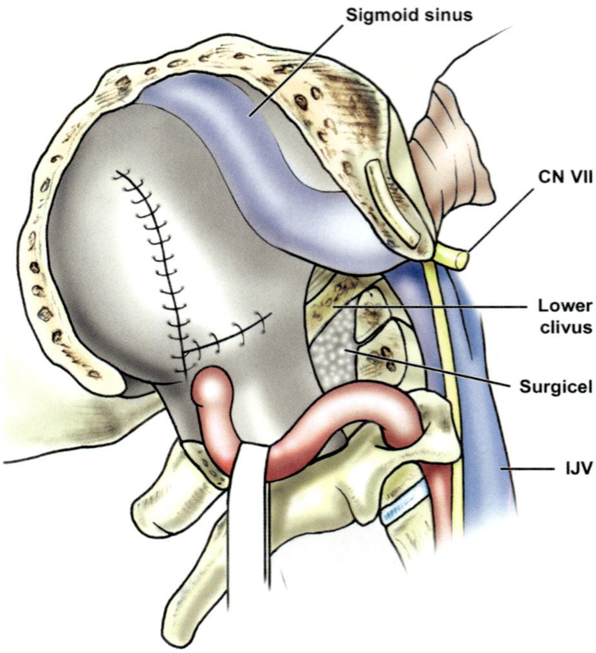

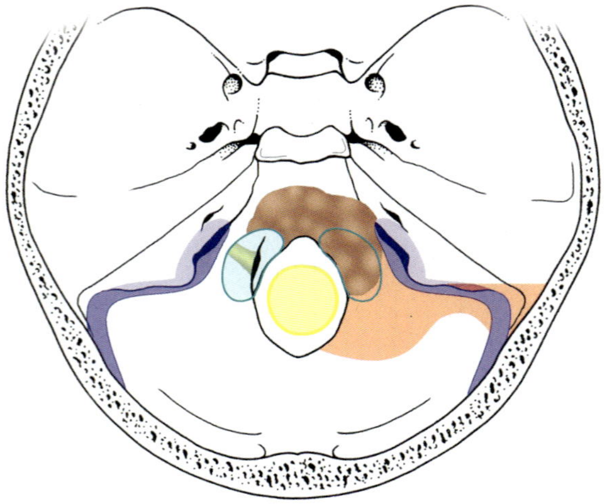

(*Continued*) **Figure 66–12** **(H)** Tumor resection has been completed. **(I)** The extent of exposure provided by the complete transcondylar extreme lateral approach. IJV, internal jugular vein.

Pitfalls and Complications

A CSF leak can be avoided in most patients by careful dural repair, waxing exposed mastoid air cells, and augmentation with fascial grafts and tissue glue as indicated. Cranial nerve dysfunction is generally unilateral and is managed as outlined above. The consequences of unrecognized lower cranial nerve dysfunction can be avoided by careful postoperative evaluation of swallowing and vocal cord function. Vascular injury to the vertebral artery is rare but can occur in recurrent tumors. Injury to branches of the vertebral artery, posterior inferior cerebellar artery (PICA), or basilar perforators can occur during intradural tumor resection causing brain stem or cerebellar infarction. Any damaged arteries must be reconstructed by direct suture or by graft. Excessive retraction of the cerebellum can cause postoperative edema, delay recovery, and cause transient hydrocephalus requiring ventriculostomy. Retraction injury can be recognized by use of intraoperative BAER monitoring and avoided by repositioning or retractor removal until signals return to baseline values.

Occipitocervical instability must be recognized and treated with fusion. Fusion is required when more than 50% of a single condyle is resected or there is bilateral involvement. The potential for fusion should be anticipated based on preoperative imaging studies and factored into the choice of skin incision and staging of the surgeries. Finally, accessory nerve injury can occur during resection of the sternocleidomastoid muscle as it exits from its posterior border.

*Illustrative Case 7: **Fig. 66–13***

Transpetrosal Approach

For tumors with extensive brain stem compression and basilar artery encasement, a transpetrosal intradural approach may be necessary.[4] The details of this approach are similar to petroclival meningiomas (see petroclival meningiomas chapter).

The Use of Combined or Alternative Approaches

Because of the extensive nature of this tumor it is often necessary to employ more than one approach in a staged fashion. The operations are separated by a few days, or rarely by several weeks.[1,3,24]

When the tumor has extensive brain stem compression or intradural invasion, then an intradural transpetrosal[23] or subtemporal-transzygomatic approach is utilized.[25] Dural repair of the excised clival dura must be meticulous to avoid postoperative CSF leakage or subsequent intradural tumor invasion.

The use of single and combined approaches is illustrated in **Fig. 66–14.**

The transsphenoidal or extended transphenoidal approaches are used either as an adjunct to other approaches or in cases where the surgical goal is biopsy or palliation alone because of the limited exposure. Only in rare cases of focal small tumors can these approaches be considered in attempts at definitive surgical resection. The transsphenoidal approach can be augmented by the use of frameless stereotaxy and neuroendoscopy to assist in localization of vital

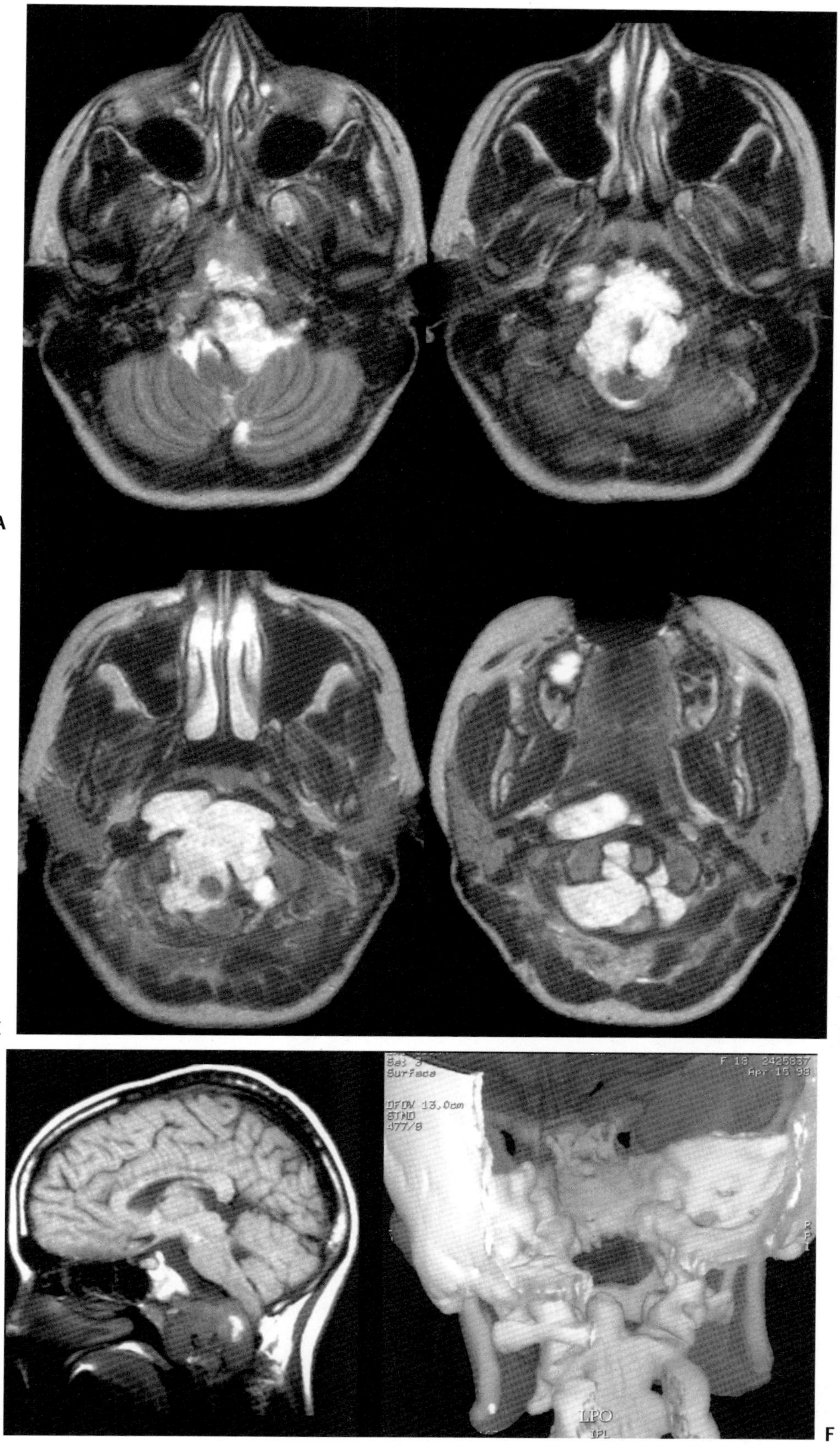

Figure 66–13 Illustrative case 7. **(A–F)** This 19-year-old woman presented with a giant chordoma of the foramen magnum area. A complete resection was performed by an extreme lateral, complete transcondylar approach, and subsequently she underwent an occipitocervical fusion. **(G–I)** She remains free of tumor recurrence, 7 years later.

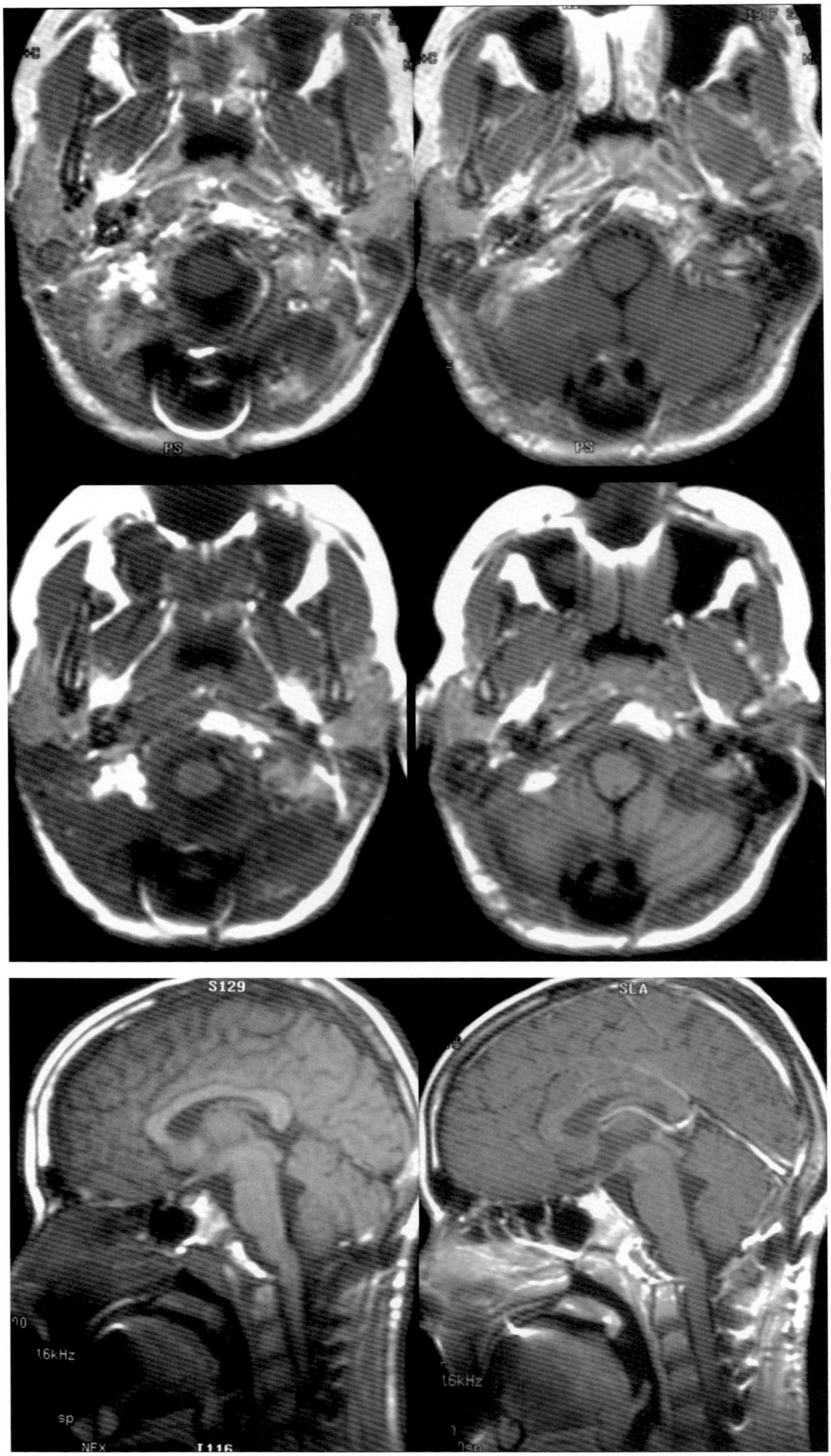

G H I J K L

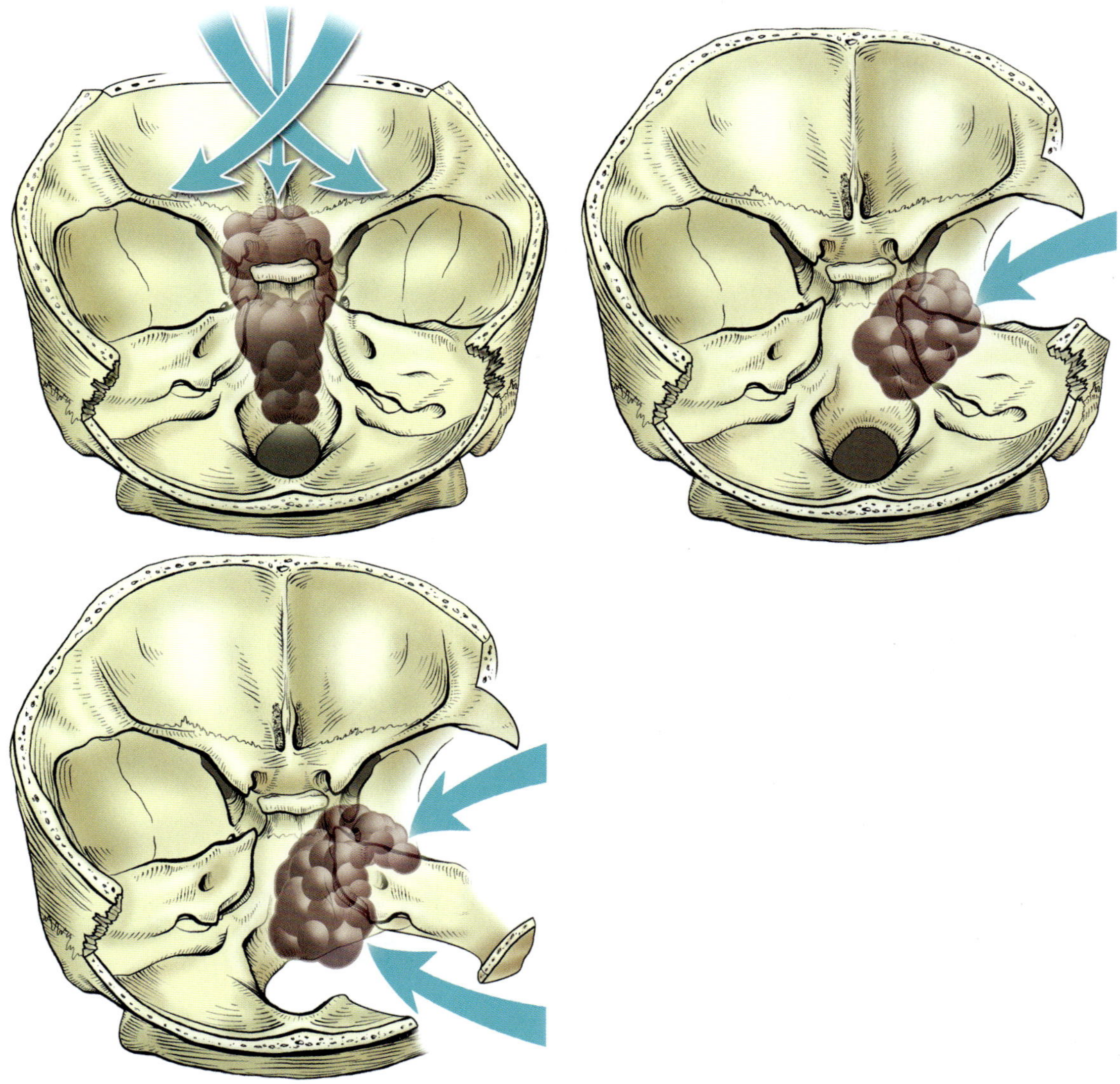

A B C

Figure 66–14 The location of various tumors and the approaches of choice for resection, including **(A)** the extended subfrontal approach **(B)** the subtemporal-infratemporal approach and **(C)** a combined subtemporal-infratemporal approach and extreme lateral approach.

structures and expand the surgical field of view, respectively **(Fig. 66–15)**.

The use of anterior ethmoidal approaches or unilateral maxillotomies must be considered in this same fashion. Transoral approaches provide limited midline exposure to the lower clivus and foramen magnum. The use of the Le Fort I procedure provides extensive rostral-caudal exposure (middle ethmoids to anterior arch C1) but has limitations with lateral access and potential hazards with dural repair and CSF fistulae. Although others have reported success with this approach,[26] the extended frontal approach provides the same rostral-caudal access with a shallower field and more ease in performing dural reconstruction if necessary. Lastly, advances in the use of endoscopy raise the possibility of significantly extending the exposure afforded by various approaches and thus increasing their utility. Ultimately, this technology may allow for less morbid approaches and more extensive tumor resection.

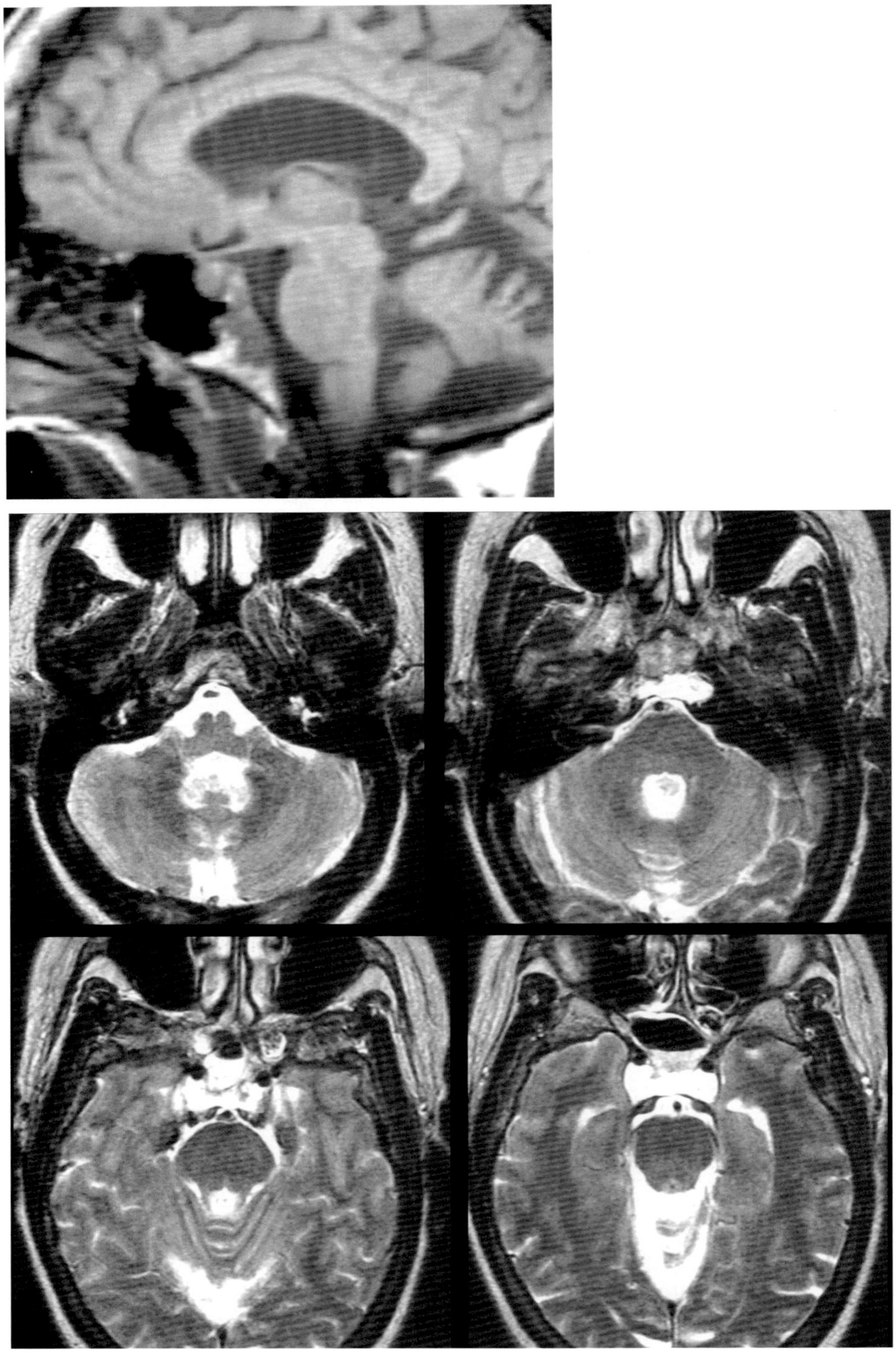

A B C D E

Figure 66–15 Illustrative case 8. **(A–E)** This 67-year-old woman presented with a tumor recurrence after transsphenoidal resection.

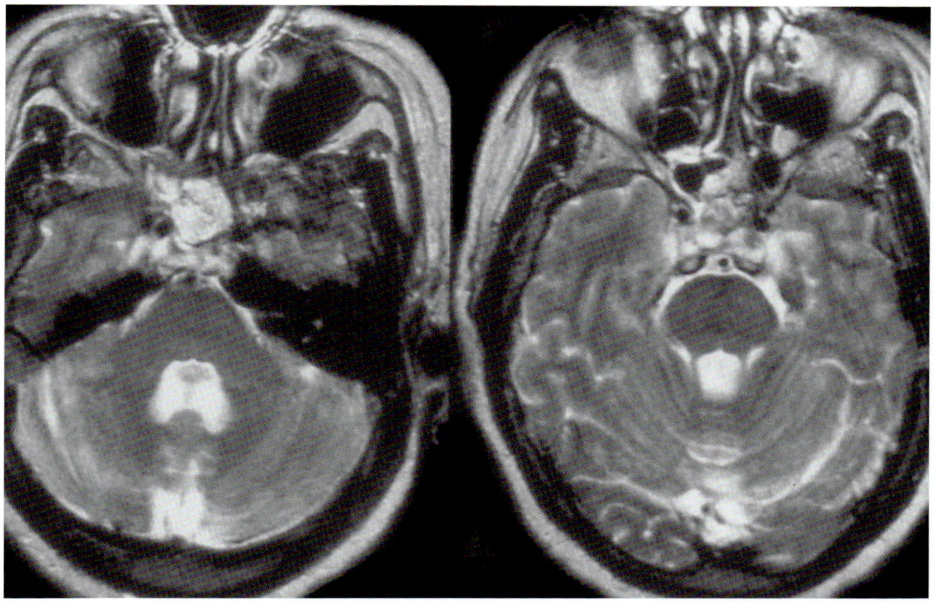

F G

(*Continued*) **Figure 66–15** **(F,G)** An endoscopically and stereotactically assisted microsurgical removal was performed. The patient remained free of tumor until her death from cardiac causes 5 years later.

Illustrative Case 8: ***Fig. 66–15***

◆ Conclusion

Chordomas and chondrosarcomas pose unique challenges to cranial base surgeons. They arise in bone, grow to involve multiple areas of the cranial base, and frequently erode into the intradural space to encompass neurovascular structures and compress the brain stem. Multiple staged approaches are often required to achieve total resection. In most patients, complete resection should be the surgical goal at the time of the initial operation, not only because the only alternative treatment is radiation but also because subsequent operations, particularly after radiation, have a much higher rate of complications. In addition, most of these tumors are large at the time of presentation, and radiation of large tumor volumes is associated with a significant rate of complications and poorer response to the treatment. With the advent of stereotactic radiosurgery, small residual tumor volumes can be left in critical areas to avoid morbidity and be treated with focused radiation. Although initial studies on small numbers of patients report good local control with acceptable complication rates (equal to or less than with microsurgery in similar areas), longer-term follow-up is needed in more patients to evaluate whether a theoretical reduction in immediate morbidity is justified by the longer-term patient outcome.

References

1. Gay E, Sekhar LN, Rubinstein E, et al. Chordomas and chondrosarcomas of the cranial base: results and follow-up of 60 patients. Neurosurgery 1995;36:887–897
2. Korten AG, Berg HJ, Spincemaille GH, van der Laan RT, Van de Wel AM. Intracranial chondrosarcoma: review of the literature and report of 15 cases. J Neurol Neurosurg Psychiatry 1998;65:88–92
3. Sekhar LN, Gay E, Wright DC. Chordomas and chondrosarcomas of the cranial base. In: Wilkins RH, Rengachary SS, eds. Neurosurgery. New York: McGraw-Hill; 1996:1529–1543
4. Nishigaya K, Kaneko M, Ohashi Y, Nukui H. Intradural retroclival chordoma without bone involvement: no tumor regrowth 5 years after operation: case report. J Neurosurg 1998;88:764–768
5. Brooks JJ, LiVolsi VA, Trojanowski JQ. Does chondroid chordoma exist? Acta Neuropathol (Berl) 1987;72:229–235
6. Forsyth PA, Cascino TL, Shae EG, et al. Intracranial chordomas: a clinicopathological and prognostic study of 51 cases. J Neurosurg 1993;78: 741–747
7. Eriksson B, Gunterberg B, Kindblom LG. Chordoma: a clinicopathologic and prognostic study of a Swedish national series. Acta Othop Scand 1981;52:49–58
8. Heffelfinger MJ, Dahlin DC, MacCarty CS, Beabout JW. Chordomas and cartilaginous tumors at the skull base. Cancer 1973;32:410–420
9. Kamrin RP, Potanos JN, Pool JL. An evaluation of the diagnosis and treatment of chordoma. J Neurol Neurosurg Psychiatry 1964;27: 157–165
10. Evans HL, Ayala AG, Romsdahl MM. Prognostic factors in chondrosarcoma of bone: a clinicopathologic analysis with emphasis on histologic grading. Cancer 1977;40:818–831
11. OíConnell JX, Renard LG, Liebsch NJ, Efird JT, Munzenrider JE, Rosenberg AE. Base of skull chordoma: a correlative study and clinical features of 62 cases. Cancer 1994;74:2261–2267
12. Pearlman AW, Friedman M. Radical radiation therapy of chordoma. Am J Roentgenol Radium Ther Nucl Med 1970;108:332–341
13. Hug EB, Fitzek MM, Liebsch NJ, et al. Locally challenging osteo- and chondrogenic tumors of the axial skeleton: results of combined proton and photon radiation therapy using three-dimensional treatment planning. Int J Radiat Oncol Biol Phys 1995;31: 467–476
14. Castro JR, Linstadt DE, Bahary JP, et al. Experience in charged particle irradiation of tumors of the skull base: 1977–1992. Int J Radiat Oncol Biol Phys 1994;29:647–655

15. Muthukumar N, Kondziolka D, Lunsford LD, Flickinger JC. Stereotactic radiosurgery for chordoma and chondrosarcoma: further experiences. Int J Radiat Oncol Biol Phys 1998;41:387–392
16. Santoni R, Liebsch N, Finkelstein DM, et al. Temporal lobe (TL) damage following surgery and high-dose photon and proton irradiation in 96 patients affected by chordomas and chondrosarcomas of the base of the skull. Int J Radiat Oncol Biol Phys 1998;41:59–68
17. Sekhar LN, Nanda A, Sen C, Snyderman CN, Janecka IP. The extended frontal approach to tumors of the anterior, middle, and posterior skull base. J Neurosurg 1992;76:198–206
18. Salas E, Ziyal IM, Bejjani GK, Sekhar LN. Anatomy of the frontotemporal branch of the facial nerve and indications for interfascial dissection. Neurosurgery 1998;43:563–569
19. Yasargil MG, Reichman MV, Kubik S. Preservation of the frontotemporal branch of the facial nerve using the interfascial temporalis flap for pterional craniotomy: technical note. J Neurosurg 1987;67: 463–466
20. Sekhar LN, Schramm VL, Jones NF. Subtemporal-preauricular infratemporal fossa approach to large lateral and posterior cranial base neoplasms. J Neurosurg 1987;67:488–499
21. Sen CN, Sekhar LN. An extreme lateral approach to intradural lesions of the cervical spine and foramen magnum. Neurosurgery 1990; 27:197–204
22. Salas E, Sekhar LN, Ziyal IM, Caputy AJ, Wright DC. Variations of the extreme-lateral craniocervical approach: anatomical study and clinical analysis of 69 patients. J Neurosurg 1999;90(Suppl 2):206–219
23. Cass SP, Sekhar LN, Pomeranz S, Hirsch BE, Snyderman CH. Excision of petroclival tumors by a total petrosectomy approach. Am J Otol 1994;15:474–484
24. Al-Mefty O, Borba LA. Skull base chordomas: a management challenge. J Neurosurg 1997;86:182–189
25. Sen CN, Sekhar LN. The subtemporal and preauricular infratemporal approach to intradural structures ventral to the brain stem. J Neurosurg 1990;73:345–354
26. Uttley D, Moore A, Archer D. Surgical management of midline skull-base tumors: a new approach. J Neurosurg 1989;71:705–710

67

Cranial Nerve and Cranial Base Reconstruction

Christopher A. Bogaev and Laligam N. Sekhar

In cranial base surgery, there are three stages to every procedure: exposure of the lesion, resection of the tumor, and reconstruction of the cerebral vasculature, cranial nerves, cranial base, and related soft tissues.[1] Each phase is crucial, with the exposure and reconstruction phases often being longer than the tumor resection. The primary goals of the reconstruction phase are to reestablish the watertight integrity of the neurocranium and reestablish the continuity of the cranial base by protecting the exposed internal carotid artery and sealing off the pharynx, nasal cavity, and paranasal sinuses. Another goal of this phase is to reestablish the normal bony contour of the craniofacial skeleton for functional and aesthetic purposes.[2]

Because of its importance in cranial base surgery, the reconstruction is planned preoperatively as well as during the exposure and resection phases to optimize the quality of this important third stage. Equal emphasis must be placed on vascular, cranial nerve, bony, as well as soft tissue reconstruction. This chapter discusses some of the more common soft tissue, bone, and cranial nerve reconstructive techniques. Vascular and complex soft tissue reconstruction involving microvascular free flaps are described elsewhere in this book.

◆ Cranial-Base Reconstruction

General Concepts

Vascularized autologous tissue is the primary and preferred material used in cranial base reconstruction. This maximizes the rapidity of primary healing while minimizing the risk of infection or cerebrospinal fluid (CSF) leak. If vascularized grafts are not available, the second choice is free autologous grafts such as pericranium, fascia lata, split calvarium, or sural nerve. Allografts or synthetic materials are used only if autologous tissue is unavailable, due to their lower rate of incorporation, lack of vascularity, and higher potential for infection, particularly in cranial base procedures where contaminated areas are involved such as the paranasal sinuses, middle ear, external ear canal, and nasopharynx.

Soft Tissue Reconstruction

Pericranial Grafts

Pericranial grafts are used in nearly every skull base case. Due to the frequency of orbital or orbitozygomatic osteotomies in anterior and middle fossa procedures, the paranasal sinuses are commonly entered. Incisions are made with the pericranium in mind. The most common incisions for cranial-base surgery are bicoronal incisions or question-mark incisions beginning at the tragus and extending to the midline. This spares cutting the temporalis muscle, which can be elevated intact, and exposes a large area of pericranium, particularly with a bicoronal incision.

Bicoronal incisions are made well behind the hairline to maximize the amount of graft that can be obtained. The pericranium is incised separately from the skin so that the posterior edge of the incision can be undermined to obtain the largest sized graft. This is especially important for anterior cranial fossa procedures, craniofacial resections, or extended frontal transbasal approaches where a large defect is present in the anterior fossa floor, and the frontal sinus, ethmoids, sphenoid sinus, or nasal cavity has been entered.

The pericranial flap is initially taken down with the scalp and is harvested during the reconstruction phase to prevent desiccation or shrinkage of the graft. The supraorbital and supratrochlear neurovascular pedicles are left intact **(Fig. 67–1)**. A smaller flap can be obtained and rotated locally if only a frontal sinus defect exists. The pericranium

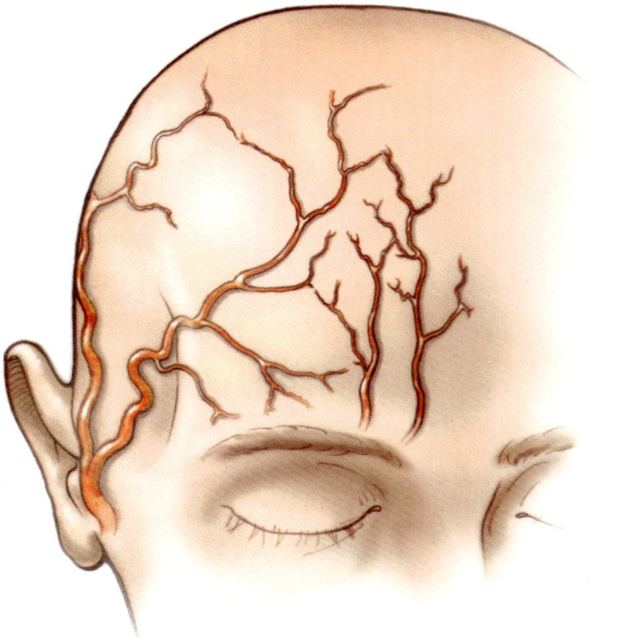

Figure 67–1 The vascular supply of the pericranium must be considered in designing a pedicled pericranial flap.

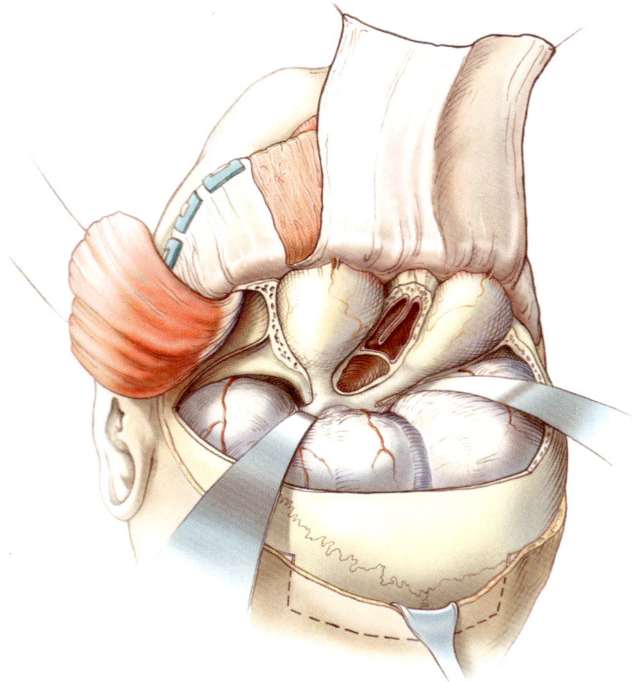

Figure 67–2 The largest possible pericranial flap is needed for large defects, such as for the repair following an extended frontal transbasal approach.

is harvested down to the level of the orbital rims to prevent puckering of the overlying scalp of the forehead, which may result in a cosmetic defect.

In the case of a large defect such as an extended frontal transbasal approach or craniofacial resection, the largest possible pericranial flap is needed **(Fig. 67–2)**. In this way, a double layer of pericranium can be stretched across the defect in addition to a watertight dural closure, resulting in a triple-layer vascularized autologous closure. If a large dead space is present, such as with the resection of a large tumor with local bone destruction, a large fat graft can be placed between the layers of the pericranium to fill the void **(Figs. 67–3** and **67–4)**. This maneuver not only minimizes the amount of intracranial air but also provides apposition of the pericranial flap to dura or adjacent tissue to maximize healing and prevent CSF leak.

For patients who have undergone a previous unilateral craniotomy and have inadequate ipsilateral pericranium, a bicoronal conversion of the scalp flap is made and the contralateral pericranium is mobilized, left attached to its vascular pedicle, and rotated to the opposite side. Maximum mobility of the contralateral pericranium is obtained by incising its base all the way to the vascular pedicle (supratrochlear and supraorbital arteries).[3]

It is important that pericranial flaps used to cover cranial base defects or paranasal sinuses are sewn to surrounding native dura to ensure that they maintain their optimal position and provide the necessary coverage to effect a seal. When osteotomies are involved, the pericranial graft is usually placed first and secured properly, and then the osteotomy

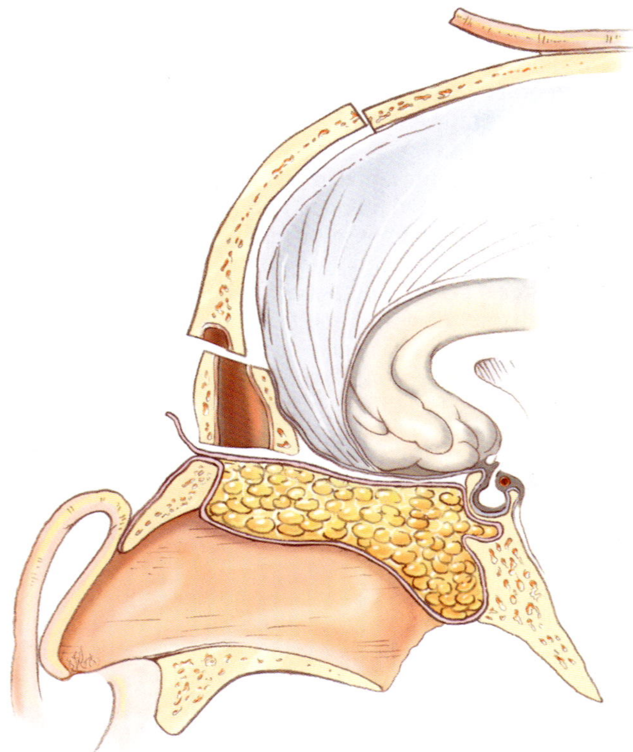

Figure 67–3 Cross-sectional view of a double-layer pericranial graft with autologous fat between the layers.

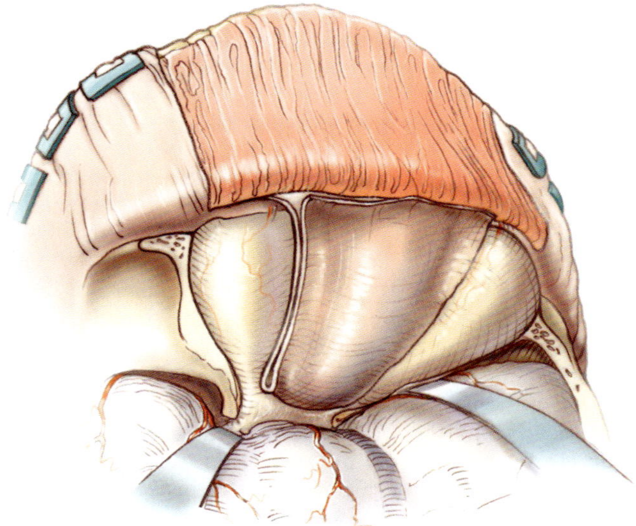

Figure 67–4 A different view of the type of reconstruction depicted in **Figure 67–3.**

is placed in its original position superior to the pericranial flap with care being taken to avoid occlusion of the graft's vascular supply by overly aggressive reapproximation of the bone edges.

Another excellent and frequent use of pericranium is as free pericranial grafts to repair dural defects. The pericranium is easily harvested from neighboring areas of a craniotomy site and is of an excellent thickness and consistency for sewing to native dura. The posterior aspect of a scalp incision is often undermined to provide adequate material for grafting, particularly if the anterior pericranium is needed to cover other defects that are dependent on the vascular pedicle.

Temporalis Fascia and Fascia Lata Grafts

For large dural defects, it is sometimes difficult to obtain a large enough free pericranial graft, particularly if a complex reconstruction requires a large vascularized pericranial flap for an extradural repair of a skull base defect. Two other options for autologous tissue are temporalis fascia, which can be harvested locally **(Fig. 67–5)**, and abdominal fascia and fascia lata, which are obtained through a linear incision on the lateral thigh **(Fig. 67–6)**. Abdominal fascia is especially attractive because it as well as fat can be extracted from near the groin with minimal morbidity. If a large piece of abdominal fascia is removed, reconstruction of the defect is performed with synthetic mesh.

These tissues provide sturdy autologous grafting material that can be obtained in large enough sizes to cover most dural defects. To prevent adhesion formation to the underlying brain, the smooth surface of the respective graft is chosen as the intradural surface. Bovine pericardium or other allografts or synthetic materials are used only when autologous material is not available.

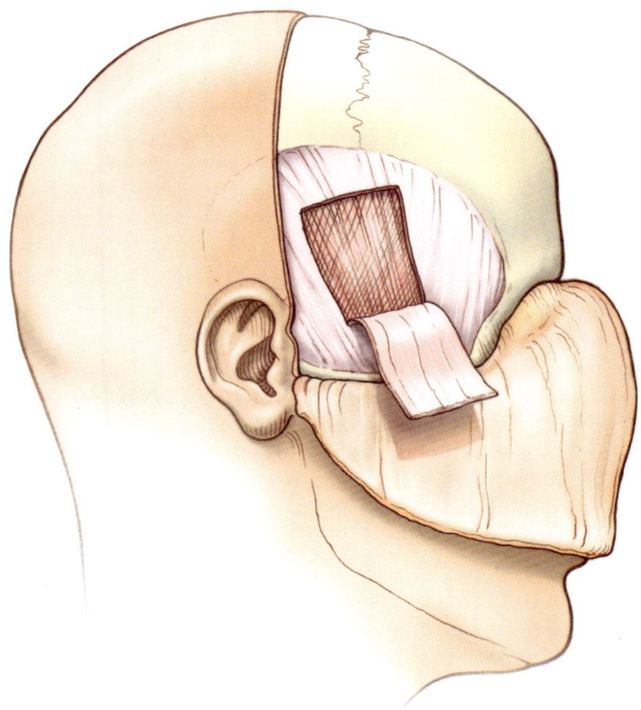

Figure 67–5 Harvesting autologous temporalis fascia.

Fibrin Sealant

With repair of any dural defect in cranial-base surgery, a watertight dural closure is attempted with meticulous suturing using the operating microscope. Given more complex or difficult-to-reach defects, a watertight closure may be difficult or impossible. For this reason, fibrin glue is routinely used to supplement dural closure particularly in cases where there is a high probability of CSF leak. This would include cases with paranasal sinus involvement, mastoidectomy defects, or involvement of the nasopharynx.

Fibrin sealant is generally placed once the dura is closed and any pericranial flaps have been secured in their final

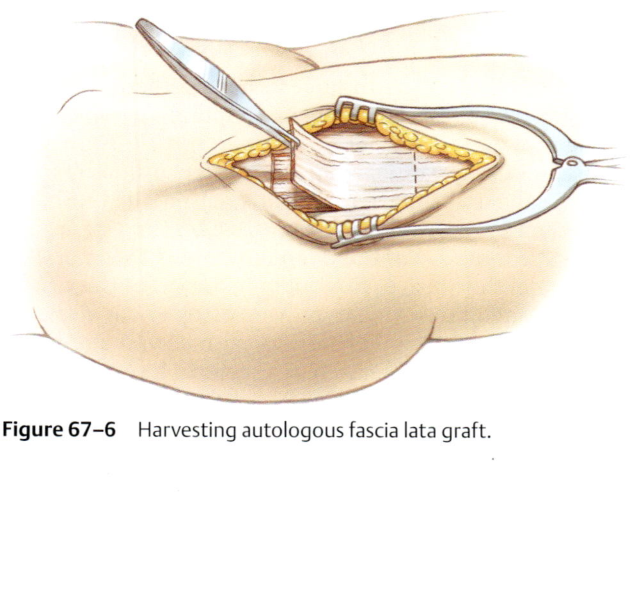

Figure 67–6 Harvesting autologous fascia lata graft.

positions. The entire construct is reinforced with fibrin glue prior to replacement of the osteotomy pieces. Careful observation is necessary during the postoperative period because the fibrin sealant is gradually absorbed, producing an increased incidence of CSF leaks around postoperative day 5.

Autologous Fat Grafts

For filling paranasal sinuses or extracranial dead space, autologous fat taken from the abdomen or thigh is used. Abdominal fat is usually harvested from below the waistline to minimize cosmetic deformity. Fat is used instead of muscle for free grafts because the high metabolic rate of muscle allows it to be absorbed too quickly without preservation of its vascular supply. In the closing of paranasal sinus defects, the mucosa is stripped, and in the case of the frontal sinus, the frontonasal duct is packed with Surgicel rolls prior to obliteration of the sinus with fat to provide additional protection against CSF leak.

Fat can also be used to obliterate the dead space present after the resection of large destructive neoplasms. In the case of anterior fossa tumors of this nature, the fat can be placed between the two layers of a large redundant pedicled pericranial graft. The fat is gradually revascularized by the well-vascularized pericranium.

Additional indications for fat grafts are packing of the sphenoid sinus after transsphenoidal surgery, filling mastoidectomy defects, and sewing a small graft over the internal acoustic meatus after a retrosigmoid approach for a vestibular schwannoma resection to prevent postoperative CSF leak.

Temporalis Flaps

Another useful pedicled soft tissue grafting material for local reconstruction is the temporalis muscle itself. Supplementation of a watertight dural closure and overlying vascularized pericranial flap with this regional muscle transfer provides a three-layer reconstruction with vascularized autologous tissue for protection of the intracranial contents. For smaller cranial base defects, pericranium along with a good dural closure is often enough. For medium-size defects, the three-layer construct with the added bulk of the temporalis muscle provides an excellent reconstruction, often without the need for a bone graft. Large defects, however, often need bone grafts or a microvascular free flap reconstruction.

Controversy exists as to how to handle the temporalis muscle in cranial cases to prevent temporalis atrophy. The most logical way to prevent this is to preserve the innervation as well as the vascular supply, which is primarily from the internal maxillary artery. For this reason, the muscle is elevated en bloc without cutting it, cauterizing it, or disrupting the integrity of the deep temporalis fascia on the underside of the muscle. This not only preserves the vascular supply and innervation to prevent atrophy but also acts to harvest the muscle in its entirety with its vascular pedicle intact so that it can be used as a regional muscle flap for reconstruction if needed. This is the rationale for the technique of elevating the temporalis muscle described here. Even if the flap is not used for reconstructive purposes, this technique mobilizes it extremely well to provide the maximum exposure for the subsequent bone work.

Technique for Handling the Temporalis Muscle

The scalp incision, whether bicoronal or question mark, is made far enough posteriorly that nearly the entire temporalis muscle can be exposed with some undermining of the neighboring scalp so that the muscle can be elevated entirely with no incisions through it. After the scalp has been elevated with the pericranium to expose the keyhole region and the zygomatic root, an interfascial dissection of the frontotemporal branch of the facial nerve is performed. This is accomplished by incising the superficial temporalis fascia from the zygomatic root to the keyhole and elevating the temporal fat pad with blunt dissection to the zygomatic arch. A broad, sharp periosteal elevator is used to elevate the muscle beginning at the superior temporal line and working inferiorly using careful side-to-side motion to preserve the fascia on the deep surface of the temporalis muscle and not leave any muscle fragments remaining on the underlying bone **(Fig. 67–7)**. This not only reduces muscle bleeding and subsequent cauterization, but preserving this plane is also more likely to preserve the innervation and blood supply. The muscle can be elevated below the level of the zygomatic arch into the infratemporal fossa. Cauterization in the region of the foramen ovale is avoided to prevent inadvertent injury to the vascular pedicle of the muscle **(Fig. 67–8)**. In cases requiring extensive head and neck dissection, the internal maxillary artery must be protected more proximally, specifically with care being taken to avoid injury at the point where it curves around the neck of the mandible, which is an area of particular vulnerability.[2]

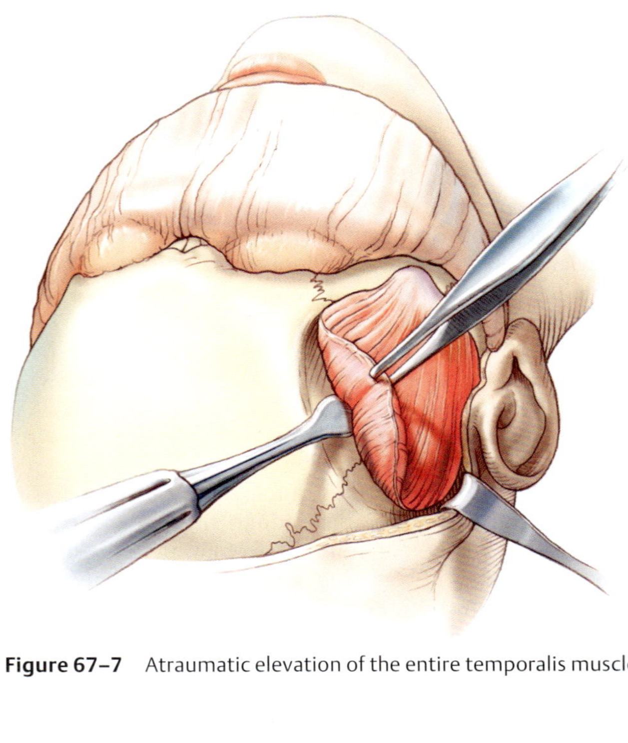

Figure 67–7 Atraumatic elevation of the entire temporalis muscle.

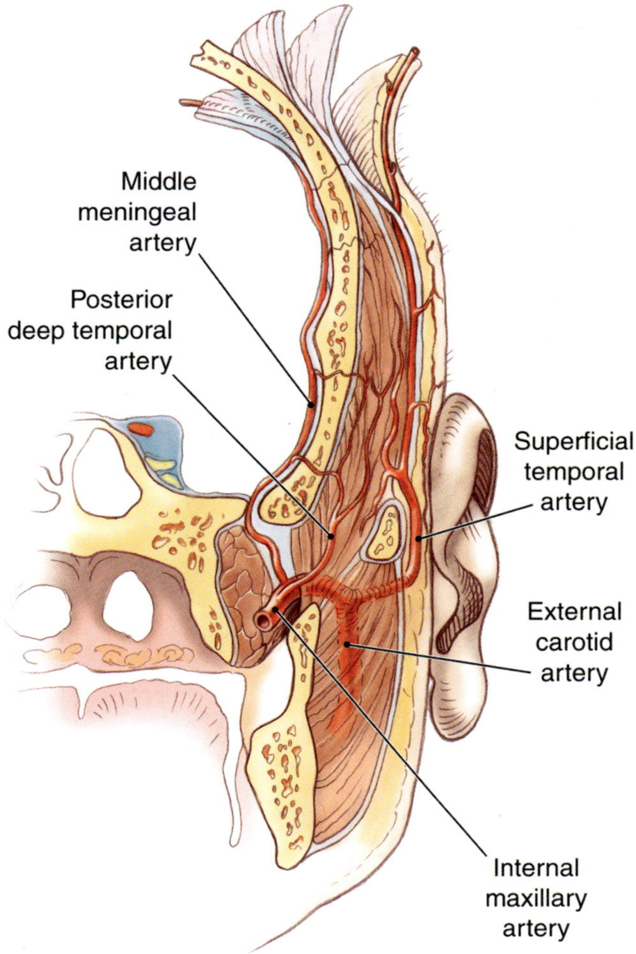

Figure 67–8 Vascular supply of the temporalis muscle.

Temporalis Flap Placement

A temporalis flap provides excellent coverage for anterolateral skull-base defects, particularly to the ipsilateral orbit, nasopharynx, or anterior and middle cranial fossae **(Fig. 67–9).** The muscle can also be doubled back on itself to provide coverage and bulk to the ipsilateral infratemporal fossa, which is particularly important when the petrous carotid artery is exposed to sinus or nasopharyngeal mucosa.[2] Removal of the zygomatic arch maximizes the arc of rotation of the temporalis muscle to allow it to reach medially to the midline or posteriorly to cover the mastoid region.[2]

The temporalis flap is held in position by tacking it to holes made in the surrounding bone or to surrounding soft tissue such as a pericranial flap, periorbita, or dura. If the temporalis flap is used, autologous fat can be harvested from the abdomen or thigh and placed in the temporal fossa to replace bulk and establish symmetry for cosmetic reasons. If the temporalis muscle is not used for reconstruction, it can be tacked up in its original position to multiple oblique holes along the superior temporal line made with the Midas Rex (Medtronics, Fort Worth, TX) C1 or equivalent drill bit. Replacing the muscle in this fashion reestablishes its anatomical as well as functional integrity.

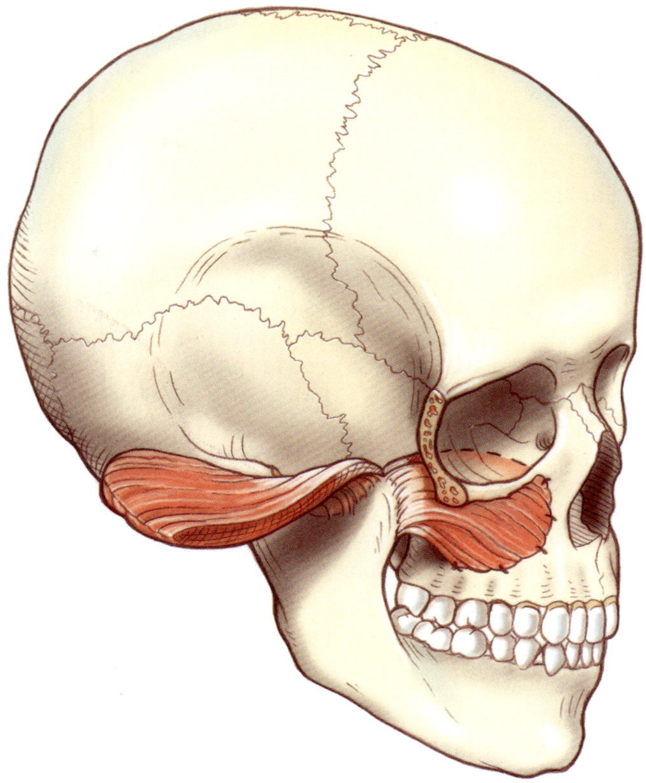

Figure 67–9 An example of a local temporalis flap placement.

Microvascular Free Flaps

For more extensive soft tissue reconstruction where the above methods would provide inadequate coverage, microvascular free flaps can be used. Specific circumstances where microvascular free flaps are needed include cases with inadequate soft tissue for reconstruction due to prior operations, large oncologic resections with their associated margins, and devascularized tissue from prior radiation therapy. Because these free flaps are generally performed by plastic surgeons, a thorough discussion is beyond the scope of this chapter and is described elsewhere in this book.

◆ Bony Reconstruction

General Concepts

Consideration and planning for the bony reconstruction, like the soft tissue reconstruction, usually begins with the approach. Exposures performed with the reconstruction in mind allow preserving important vascular pedicles of soft tissues as well as minimizing bone loss from the craniotomies and osteotomies to simplify and facilitate the bony reconstruction. The craniotomies and osteotomies used in cranial base surgery are designed to provide maximal tumor exposure with minimal brain retraction.

Facial Osteotomies

Osteotomies of the facial skeleton such as orbital or orbitozygomatic osteotomies are made as separate pieces from craniotomy flaps for two major reasons:

1. More controlled bone cuts can be made allowing bony anatomy to be preserved, which facilitates the bony reconstruction. This is especially true with the orbital roof. Two thirds or ~2.5 cm of the orbital roof is removed with orbital osteotomies, preserving enough orbital roof to prevent pulsatile enophthalmos postoperatively.[4] At the end of the procedure, the osteotomy can be replaced with no need for further reconstruction of the orbital roof.
2. Should epidural infection occur at some time postoperatively requiring removal of the craniotomy flap, the osteotomy is a separate piece and is usually sufficiently well vascularized that it can be left in place. This minimizes the cosmetic deformity as well as facilitates the eventual reconstruction.

Craniotomy Flaps

Great care is taken in turning the craniotomy flap to minimize bone loss and facilitate the bony reconstruction. Instead of the standard large 14 mm bur holes being made, small slots in the bone can be made with the Midas Rex M8 or equivalent drill bit. This is especially true with frontotemporal craniotomy flaps where the slot can be made from the keyhole region to the root of the zygoma in a curvilinear fashion following the anterior temporal tip and the root of the sphenoid wing. The dura is exposed all along this line except at the root of the sphenoid wing, which is deeply scored. The ends of this long slot are made just large enough to accommodate the Midas Rex B1 footplate or its equivalent, and the underlying dura is separated with a Woodson elevator. The craniotomy flap is then turned with the B1 footplate, and the root of the sphenoid wing is either fractured along the scoring or is cut with a small osteotome **(Fig. 67–10)**.

When the craniotomy is performed in this way, the temporal tip and the floor of the middle fossa are exposed completely by turning the bone flap with minimal or no further bone removal needed. The same is true of the sphenoid wing because it is scored and fractured at its base. Similar slots or small holes can be made elsewhere in place of bur holes to minimize bone loss and cosmetic deformity. With these techniques, an excellent cosmetic bony reconstruction is as simple as replacing the bone flap with miniplates in the usual fashion.

An alternative method of performing a craniotomy is to make smaller bur holes using the Midas Rex. The bur holes can be placed in the standard locations but are more controlled with regard to size and shape than with a standard 14 mm perforator bit. Some prefer the presence of bur holes to enable more aggressive dural stripping from the overlying bone. If this technique is used, titanium bur hole covers or hydroxyapatite cement can be used in cosmetically significant locations.

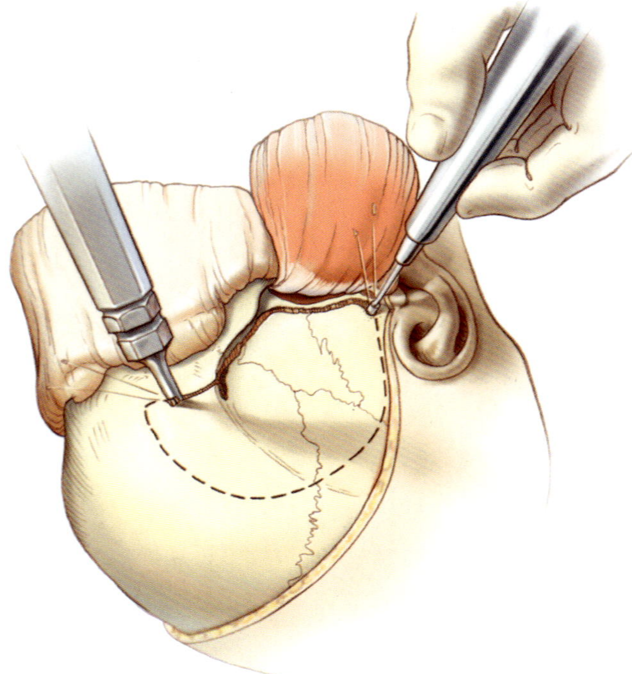

Figure 67–10 Technique of turning a frontotemporal craniotomy flap with minimal bone loss.

Hydroxyapatite Cements

For small cosmetic defects, such as an irregularity in the forehead or other cosmetically significant area, small gaps between the bone flap and craniotomy edge, or covering bur holes or other small defects less than ~1.5 cm in diameter, hydroxyapatite bone cement or similar bone reconstructive materials can be used. Its advantages are its soft, pasty consistency, making it easy to contour; its osteoconductive properties; and its lower relative risk of infection when compared with other alloplastic materials.

A major limitation to the use of hydroxyapatite cement is its fragile, brittle consistency while it is hardening. If this material is setting in the presence of dural pulsations, small fractures may appear within it that may affect the integrity of the final construct. Protecting the cement from these pulsations until it has fully set usually results in a more stable reconstruction with less chance of fracturing or subsidence of the cement.

Split Calvarial Grafts

For larger cranial defects, autologous split-thickness calvarial grafts are often used. This is consistent with the overall preference for autologous tissue for cranial base reconstruction. In general, a reciprocating saw is used to split a calvarial bone flap through the diploë. The Midas Rex C1 or equivalent drill bit can be used to cut through the diploë of smaller flaps, but the cut is generally not as smooth. Potentially any site where a craniotomy can be turned can be used as a donor site, but thicker bone usually has a more developed diploë, making it easier to split. The inner table is then used as the graft, whereas

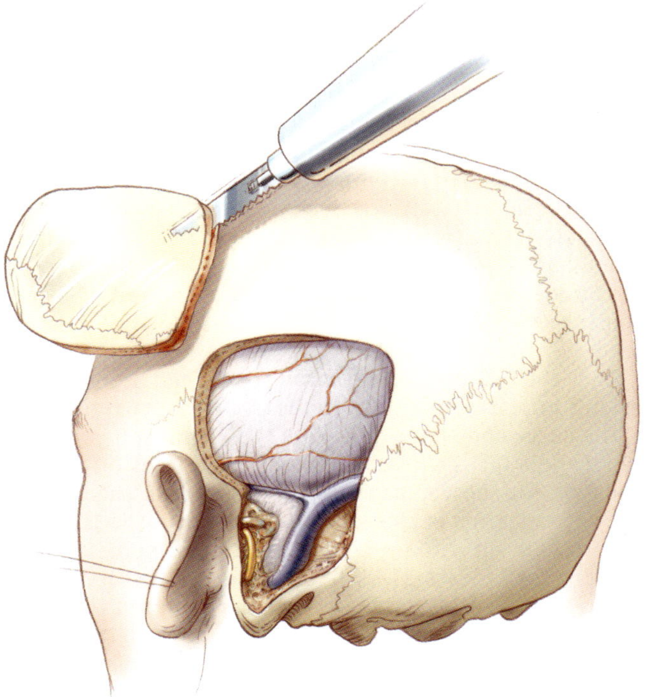

Figure 67–11 Initial stages of a split calvarial reconstruction of the defect following a petrosal approach.

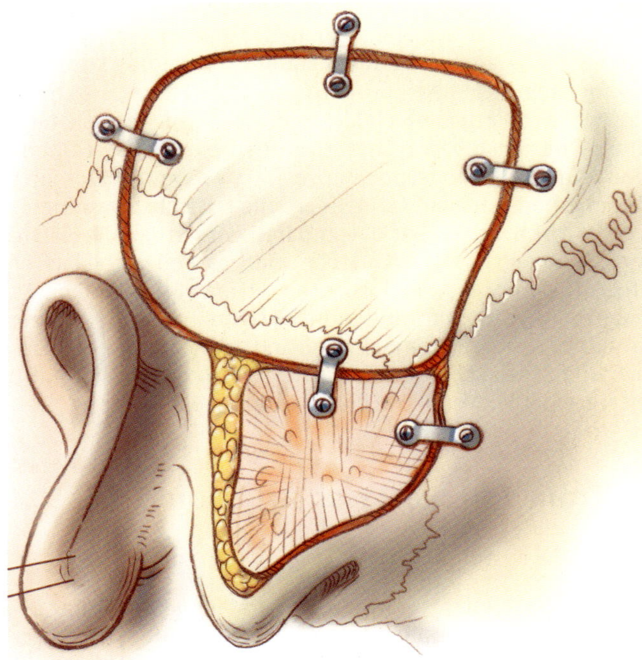

Figure 67–12 Completion of the split calvarial reconstruction following a petrosal approach.

the outer table is secured to its original position using miniplates. Generally, the bone graft is shaped and trimmed to fit as closely as possible the size and contour of the defect to be covered. However, there is often not a perfect fit. A small cutting bur can be used for contouring, and the small gaps and irregularities remaining can be repaired with hydroxyapatite cement. Miniplates are most often used to secure calvarial grafts because of their versatility and rigid fixation.

One of the more routine examples of the use of split calvarial bone is for the reconstruction after a presigmoid petrosal approach. When the mastoidectomy is performed prior to the posterior temporal craniotomy, a standard mastoidectomy defect is present at the end of the operation **(Fig. 67–11)**. The posterior temporal craniotomy flap is then split with the inner table shaped to fit the mastoidectomy defect and plated there to reconstruct the normal surface contour of the mastoid portion of the temporal bone. The outer table of the craniotomy flap is then plated back into its original position **(Fig. 67–12)**.

Another consideration with large anterior or middle fossa defects is the effects of gravity on the frontal or temporal lobes. However, pedicled muscle flaps in combination with meticulous dural repair and pericranial flap placement is usually sufficient.[3] If this repair appears tenuous, split calvarial bone can supplement the reconstruction with the graft secured to the edges of the bony defect. For large oncologic resections, a microvascular free flap may be needed as well.

Split calvarial bone can also be used for functional reconstruction, such as in the repair of the medial orbital walls after an extended transbasal resection of a destructive lesion. Fortunately, meticulous technique in performing osteotomies obviates the need for this in most cases.

An alternative to split calvarial grafts is other forms of autologous bone encountered during the exposure. Perhaps the best example of this is harvesting a piece of vomer during the exposure in an open transsphenoidal procedure. This small piece of autologous bone is then used to reconstruct the floor of the sella at the end of the procedure with no need for allograft or further incisions to harvest autograft.

Alloplastic Reconstruction

In cases where split calvarial graft is not available or not possible, titanium mesh can be used to cover defects that are too large for hydroxyapatite cement alone. The mesh is usually held in position with screws from an available plating system. The advantages of titanium mesh are that it is quick and easy to contour and is of uniform thickness, which is often not true of methacrylate. In addition, titanium mesh can be used as a skeleton for a hydroxyapatite cement overlay, which could allow for some incorporation and replacement by natural bone.

If the mesh with hydroxyapatite overlay is used, the contour of the mesh should be slightly depressed in relation to surrounding bone so that the cement overlay does not produce a cosmetically significant prominence. The mesh provides several advantages over hydroxyapatite alone. The first is that it adds much more stability, providing scaffolding for the brittle hydroxyapatite cement. This strengthens the entire construct, much like reinforced concrete. Furthermore, the mesh can insulate the hydroxyapatite cement from dural pulsations, preventing fractures in the overlying cement. Additional advantages are the possible lower infection risk of hydroxyapatite compared with other alloplastic materials such as methyl methacrylate, as well as the lack of an exothermic reaction during the setting of the cement. As progressively more formulations of hydroxyapatite become available, the ease of preparation and application is increasing. All of these characteristics have resulted in a dramatic increase in the overall use of this technique.

◆ Cranial Nerve Reconstruction

Concepts

The success of microsurgical peripheral nerve repair has led neurosurgeons to apply these techniques to the reconstruction of cranial nerves. Due to the increased incidence of complex procedures involving the cranial base, there has been an increase in problems associated with cranial nerves III, IV, V, VI, and VII because they are often displaced or encased by tumors in this area. These nerves can be invaded by tumor requiring partial nerve resection for complete resection of a tumor, or these nerves can be damaged or cut during the dissection of a tumor from an encased nerve. Fibrous tumors, prior surgery, and prior radiation treatment make the preservation of cranial nerves more difficult. Reconstruction of these nerves by primary repair or interposition graft is performed for functional (binocular vision, facial function, or corneal protection) as well as cosmetic reasons.

General Techniques

Reanastomosis or grafting is begun in all cases by excising the abnormal or damaged segment of the nerve. Due to the small size of cranial nerves and relatively thin epineurium, epineural repair is often the technique of choice. Group fascicular repair is generally not possible here and is reserved for larger somatic peripheral nerves. A notable exception is a primary anastomosis of the facial nerve distal to the stylomastoid foramen where it becomes polyfascicular. It is monofascicular more proximally.[5]

Epineural Repair

For epineural repair, the nerve is inspected for longitudinal blood vessels that can serve as a guide to align the epineurium. Fascicular arrangement is noted if possible, but this can be difficult in cranial nerves due to their small size and sometimes simple organization (for example, cranial nerves IV and VI). With most intracranial segments of cranial nerves, the epineurium is very thin. The sutures in these anastomoses simply approximate the nerve endings free of tension. In general, the smallest number of sutures and the smallest suture type are used to avoid interference with neural regeneration. The 9–0 or 10–0 monofilament nylon sutures are most often used for cranial nerves due to their small size. A tensionless anastomosis is required. If it cannot be approximated easily with 9–0 nylon, then too much tension is present. In cadaveric studies, if the gap between the two ends of cranial nerves III or VI in the region of the cavernous sinus exceeded 0.3 cm, the ends of the nerves could not be adequately approximated by direct suture.[6] If direct anastomosis is not possible, an interposition graft must be used.

Once the two ends of the nerve are aligned properly, the nylon suture is passed through the epineurium of both ends of the nerve and is tied **(Fig. 67–13)**. Care must be taken to avoid knots that are overly tight such that they distort the ends of the nerve, producing a fascicular mismatch.[7] The second stitch is placed 180 degrees opposite the first. One to four sutures are needed for cranial nerve anastomoses depending on the size of the nerve. The number of sutures used is the minimum number required that provides good approximation of the nerve stumps. If the size of the nerve requires it, a third or fourth suture is placed, each halfway between the first two. The anastomosis is then reinforced with fibrin glue.

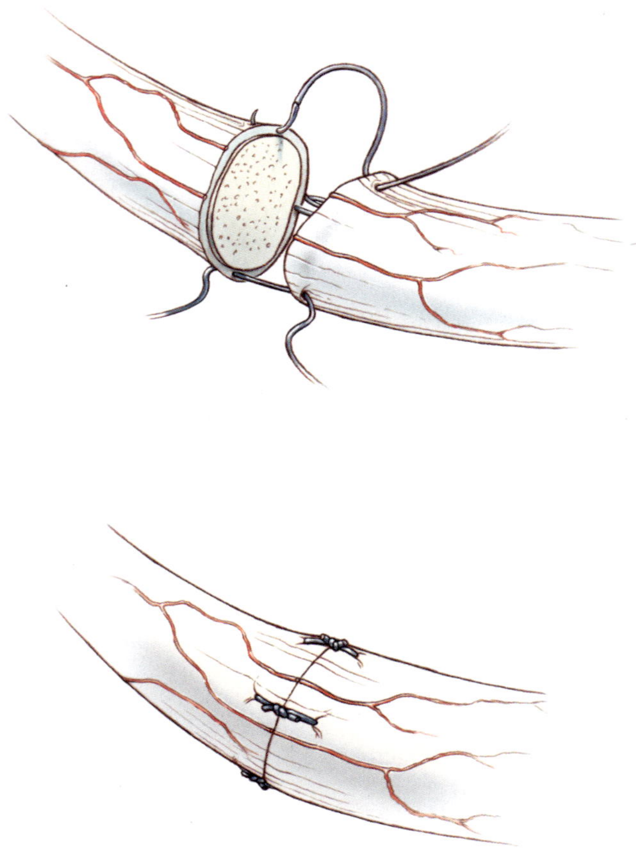

Figure 67–13 Technique of epineural repair using longitudinal blood vessels as a guide for proper alignment of the ends.

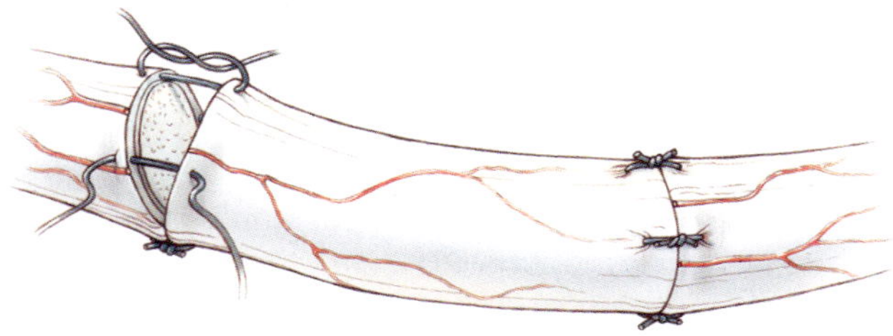

Figure 67–14 Technique of interposition nerve grafting.

Interposition Nerve Grafts

If a tension-free anastomosis is not possible despite maximal freeing of the nerve from surrounding tissue, then an interposition nerve graft is needed. In general, the most common donor site is the sural nerve, followed by the greater auricular nerve, followed by the other sensory branches of the cervical plexus. Interposition nerve graft anastomoses are performed in the same fashion as direct epineural repairs for each end of the graft **(Fig. 67–14)**. The major exception to this type of repair is grafting of the facial nerve distal to the stylomastoid foramen where it becomes polyfascicular. This requires a more complex repair, such as interfascicular and perineural suturing, for best results.[5]

Donor Sites for Nerve Grafts *Sural Nerve* The sural nerve, in ideal circumstances, can provide grafts up to 40 cm long with a diameter comparable to that of the facial nerve.[5] Removal of the nerve results in sensory loss to the lower leg and lateral foot, which is usually not bothersome to patients.

Harvesting Technique Dissection of the sural nerve is much easier if the patient is in the prone or lateral positions, but it can be done in the supine position. A longitudinal incision is made two thirds of the way anteriorly from the Achilles tendon to the lateral malleolus with the lower part being parallel to the posterior curvature of the lateral malleolus. The sural nerve is generally found slightly anterior and deep to the lesser saphenous vein (**Fig. 67–15**). Once it is found, atraumatic dissection is performed with the skin incision gradually lengthened proximally concomitant with the dissection so that the exact proximal course of the nerve is followed. This avoids significant soft tissue flaps. The nerve is cut as sharply as possible to avoid injury to the ends of the graft. The wound is then closed in two layers.

Greater Auricular Nerve During many lateral skull-base operations requiring neck dissections, a greater auricular nerve graft can be obtained through an existing incision, or an incision can be extended inferiorly to expose the posterior border of the sternocleidomastoid muscle to provide a longer segment of nerve. Generally, if the greater auricular nerve is not easily accessible through an existing incision, a sural nerve graft is used, but this requires the prepping and draping of a distant site.

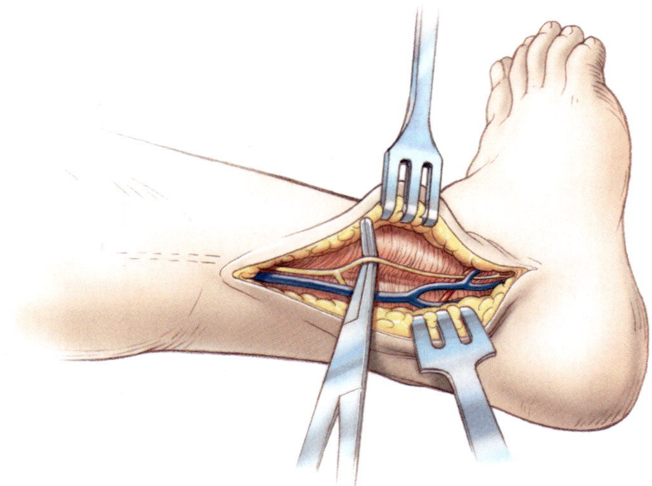

Figure 67–15 Technique of sural nerve graft harvesting. The sural nerve is generally found slightly anterior and deep to the lesser saphenous vein.

The maximum obtainable length of greater auricular or other cervical plexus grafts is generally ~10 cm, and the diameter is often comparable to that of the facial nerve.[5] The sensory disturbance from harvesting cervical plexus grafts is usually well tolerated by patients.

Harvesting Technique for Cervical Plexus Grafts. A postauricular skin incision beginning just above the mastoid tip and extending inferiorly along the posterior border of the sternocleidomastoid muscle usually provides adequate exposure to several possible donor nerves including greater auricular, transverse cervical, and supraclavicular nerves in descending order **(Fig. 67–16)**. Once a given nerve is located as it crosses the sternocleidomastoid muscle, it can be

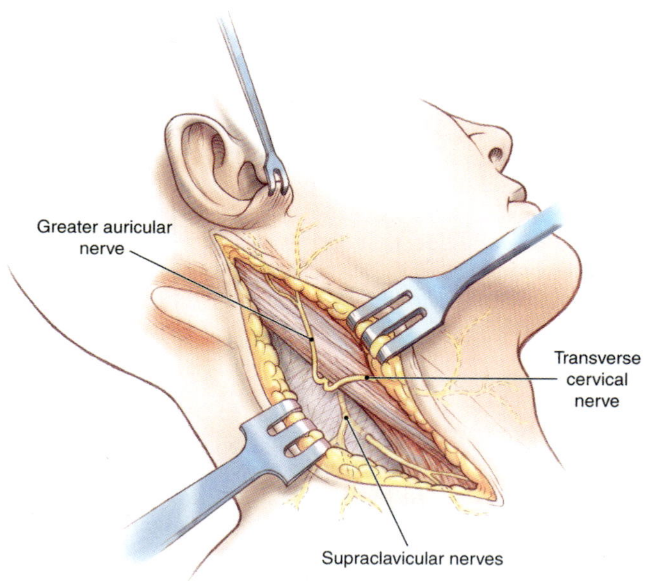

Figure 67–16 Technique of harvesting cervical plexus nerve grafts.

traced proximally and distally until adequate length is obtained. The nerve is cut as sharply as possible and the wound is closed in two layers.

Repair of Specific Cranial Nerves

Oculomotor Nerve

Cranial nerve III injury most likely occurs during cavernous sinus surgery or during surgery in the region of the interpeduncular fossa. Due to its short intracavernous course, its anatomical continuity can often be preserved. However, it is very fragile, and temporary functional impairment can occur with minimal manipulation.

Success of third nerve regeneration after operative repair appears to be limited due to its highly differentiated functions. There are difficulties achieving coordinated motion of the extraocular muscles, which has been attributed to "aberrant neural regeneration."[8] Because only partial functional recovery usually occurs, complete return of binocular vision is rare. For this reason, the primary goals of operative repair of cranial nerve III anatomical disruption is for cosmetic reasons, unless the ipsilateral eye is the only one with useful vision or there is potential for loss of vision in the contralateral eye. Alleviation of ptosis appears to be one of the more successful aspects of oculomotor nerve repair.[8] As with other cranial nerves, the results of reconstruction are significantly better in patients with good preoperative function.

The technique of repair is usually a direct end-to-end epineural anastomosis. If a tension-free anastomosis is not possible, an interposition graft is used.

Trochlear Nerve

Because of its simple organization, its being a motor nerve only, and its innervation of only a single muscle, cranial nerve IV is well suited for operative repair. The fourth nerve is commonly injured in cranial base procedures because of its small size and long length.

Because of its suitability for reconstruction, trochlear nerve operative repair should be attempted despite the fact that fourth nerve injuries can have spontaneous return of binocular vision or can be alleviated with fairly simple measures such as prism glasses. With its low chance of aberrant regeneration, operative repair is attempted to maximize the chance for a full recovery of binocular vision.[8] If there is no recovery, eye muscle surgery can be performed to correct the rotational diplopia that occurs.

The technique used is a direct end-to-end epineural anastomosis. Due to its small size, one 10–0 nylon suture is usually adequate.

Trigeminal Nerve

In the majority of patients, the ophthalmic division innervates the entire cornea, with occasional patients having the lower half innervated by the maxillary division.[8] Corneal anesthesia with its associated keratitis is a significant problem that can result in loss of vision. This is the rationale behind operative repair of loss of V1 or V2 anatomical continuity because even partial return of corneal sensation can have profound functional implications. Reconstruction of the trigeminal root can also be attempted.

The most frequent cause of cranial nerve V (V1 or V2) injury is the resection of cavernous sinus tumors or trigeminal schwannomas. The technique of repair is also by direct epineural anastomosis, or an interposition graft is used if sufficient length is not available.

Abducens Nerve

Similar to cranial nerve IV, cranial nerve VI is well suited to operative repair because of its simple organization with only motor fibers innervating a single muscle, making the chances of aberrant regeneration very low. The sixth nerve is the most likely to be injured because of its long intracranial course and location within the cavernous sinus itself. Functional aspects of the sixth nerve are important, and because of its suitability for reconstruction, a good operative repair could potentially result in a return of binocular vision.

The technique of repair is by direct epineural reanastomosis, as is done for the intracranial segments of the other cranial nerves discussed. If resection of a segment of the sixth nerve is required, an interposition graft may be needed.

Facial Nerve

Of all the cranial nerve injuries requiring operative repair, the seventh nerve warrants special attention due to its profound functional and cosmetic implications. A multitude of reconstructive techniques for reanimation of the denervated face have been developed, but this discussion focuses on facial nerve repair from injuries to the intracranial segment, which is most relevant to neurosurgery.

Primary Reanastomosis Primary nerve repair is superior to all other reconstructive procedures for a transected facial nerve,[5] providing the maximum opportunity for functional recovery. The most common circumstances in which this occurs is in the suboccipital approach to vestibular schwannomas where a large tumor has sufficiently thinned the nerve that it is easy to transect during the tumor resection. The elongated condition of the nerve makes end-to-end anastomosis possible provided the proximal and distal stumps can be located. The elongated nerve usually allows enough overlap that the ends can be properly trimmed of abnormal tissue and still allow a tension-free anastomosis.

Due to the monofascicular arrangement and scant epineurium of the intracranial facial nerve,[5] the technique of repair used is a direct end-to-end epineural anastomosis (**Fig. 67–17**). Precise approximation of the two ends of the nerve and tension-free sutures are essential for a good result. An interposition graft with two tensionless anastomoses is preferable to an end-to-end repair under tension.[5]

Interposition Grafts If the two stumps of the facial nerve can be found but a tension-free primary reanastomosis is not possible due to a gap between the ends, an interposition graft is needed. Sural nerve or greater auricular nerve are most commonly used as donor nerves due to their well-tolerated sensory deficits as well as their sizes (the sural

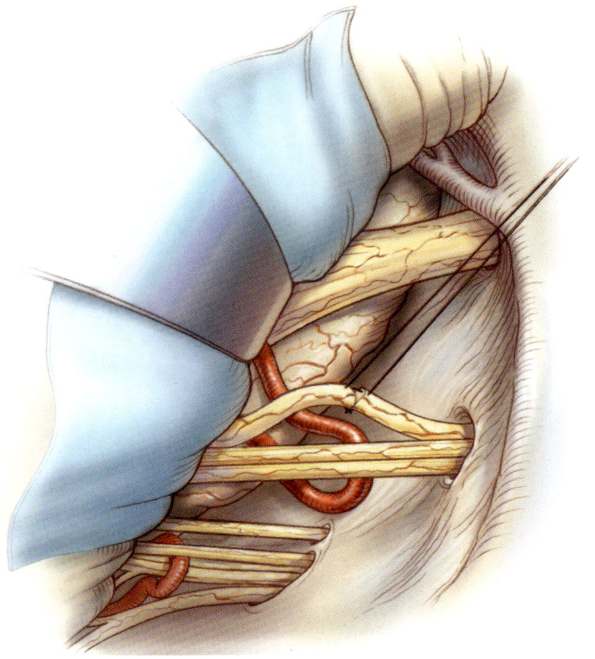

Figure 67–17 Technique of primary repair of a transected facial nerve from a retrosigmoid approach.

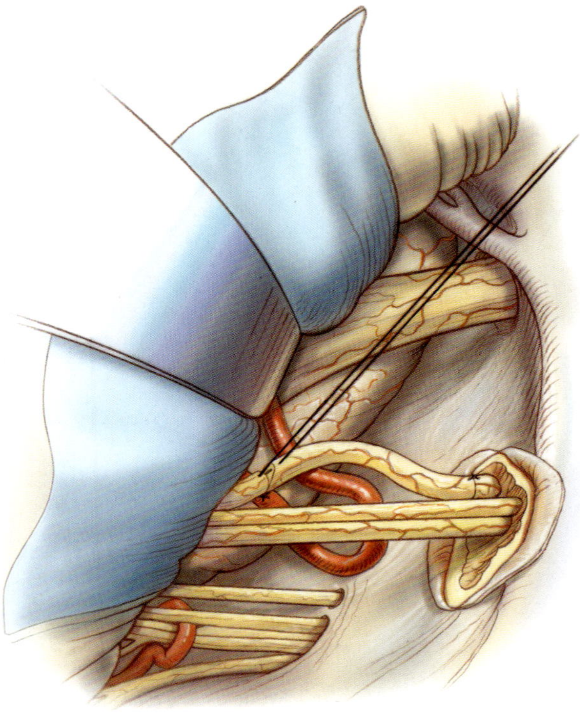

Figure 67–18 Repair of a transected facial nerve using an interposition nerve graft from a retrosigmoid approach.

nerve usually has twice the diameter of the facial nerve, whereas the greater auricular nerve is usually of a comparable diameter to the facial nerve). Techniques of harvesting and advantages of each are described earlier in this chapter. The same end-to-end anastomotic technique used for a primary repair is used for the two anastomoses of the interposition graft **(Fig. 67–18).**

Hypoglossal-Facial Anastomosis In cases where the proximal nerve stump is not available, or when there is no return of facial function 1 year after surgery when either anatomical continuity was present or reestablished by primary repair or interposition grafting, the most successful neural repair is a hypoglossal to facial anastomosis. Inferior results have resulted from phrenic or accessory nerve transfers in regard to facial nerve function as well as donor site deficits.[5] With the XII–VII anastomosis, the hemitongue atrophy is not particularly bothersome, and the possible transient dysarthria and other symptoms of unilateral hypoglossal paralysis usually resolve after several weeks. A more recent technical development is the partial hypoglossal–facial anastomosis. Both the traditional as well as the partial XII–VII anastomoses are discussed here.

The XII–VII anastomosis provides very good resting tone and facial symmetry, and good voluntary function around the mouth and midface (less satisfactory around the eye), but often poor reflex or emotional facial movement. Training in a motivated patient can improve voluntary facial movement substantially. Furthermore, mass movements and the synkinesis that is often present can improve. A XII–VII anastomosis provides a powerful graft with a large number of motor axons for maximal input to the distal stump of the facial nerve. Although cross-facial grafting is an excellent technique that restores some emotional facial reanimation, XII–VII anastomosis is preferred because of the numerically superior input to the distal facial nerve.[5]

Operative Technique The skin incision begins slightly superior to the mastoid tip. If additional superior exposure is needed to facilitate location of the facial nerve, the top of the incision can begin just inferior and anterior to the tragus and loop below the auricle and back superiorly to the mastoid tip. The incision then extends inferiorly to approximate the anterior border of the sternocleidomastoid muscle and then anteriorly to end in a skin crease in the anterior neck for cosmetic reasons **(Fig. 67–19).**

Facial Nerve Dissection The next step involves identification of the extracranial facial nerve as it exits the stylomastoid foramen. Deep dissection is continued anterior to the mastoid tip with the triangular process of the conchal cartilage (pointer of cartilaginous meatus), posterior belly of the digastric muscle, styloid process and tympanomastoid fissure acting as important landmarks for the facial nerve.[9] Use of a nerve stimulator to locate the facial nerve is not useful due to the lack of electrical excitability from chronic denervation. If extra length of facial nerve is needed, or if the nerve is difficult to locate, the mastoid tip can be

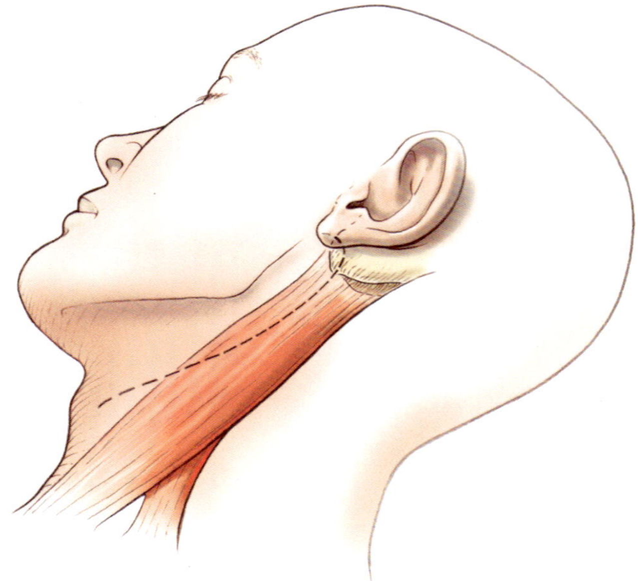

Figure 67–19 Skin incision for a hypoglossal–facial anastomosis.

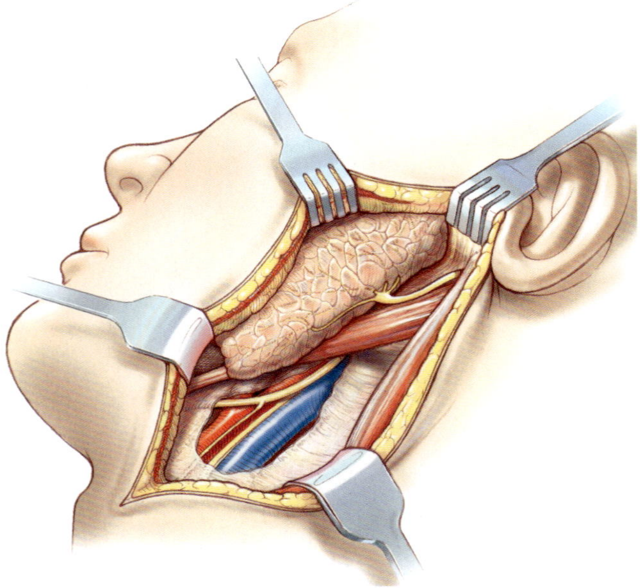

Figure 67–20 The facial nerve is dissected from the stylomastoid foramen to the pes anserinus. The hypoglossal nerve is dissected as far proximally and distally as possible to maximize length and produce a tension-free XII–VII anastomosis.

resected to expose the terminal mastoid segment of the facial nerve. Another potential aid in locating the facial nerve is to trace the branch of the facial nerve innervating the posterior belly of the digastric muscle back to the main trunk of the facial nerve. The facial nerve main trunk is dissected from the stylomastoid foramen to the pes anserinus to maximize length and reduce tension in the anastomosis.

Hypoglossal Nerve Dissection The next step involves dissection of the hypoglossal nerve. The carotid sheath is opened in the angle between the lower border of the posterior belly of the digastric muscle and the anterior border of the sternocleidomastoid muscle. The hypoglossal nerve is identified and followed obliquely down over the carotid bifurcation and as far proximally and distally as possible to maximize length and produce a tension-free anastomosis. The distal dissection should continue well past the descending ramus (ansa cervicalis, descendens hypoglossi), which is also dissected as far peripherally as possible (**Fig. 67–20**).

Performing the Anastomosis The facial nerve is cut proximally as close to the stylomastoid foramen as possible. The hypoglossal nerve and the descending ramus are then sectioned as far distally as possible. The hypoglossal nerve trunk is approximated to the peripheral facial nerve stump and the anastomosis is performed if no tension exists. If there is any tension present, the nerves are further dissected, the hypoglossal nerve is placed medial to the posterior belly of the digastric muscle, or this muscle can be divided. Once a tension-free approximation of the two nerve ends is possible, an epineural repair is performed with the smallest number of 9–0 or 10–0 monofilament nylon sutures required to ensure good approximation of the nerve stumps (usually three or four) (**Fig. 67–21**). The descending ramus can then be anastomosed to the distal hypoglossal stump in a similar fashion to minimize the chances of hemitongue atrophy (**Fig. 67–22**). Greater auricular or sural nerve interposition grafts should only be used in cases where all other measures fail to achieve a tension-free anastomosis.

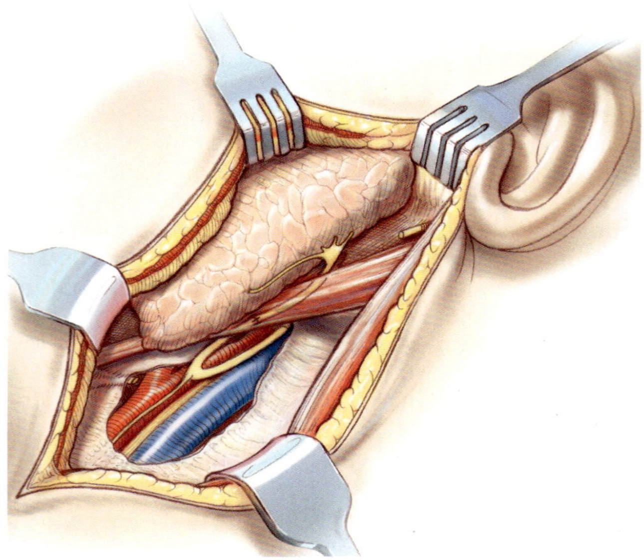

Figure 67–21 The hypoglossal nerve trunk is approximated to the peripheral facial nerve stump and the anastomosis is performed if no tension exists.

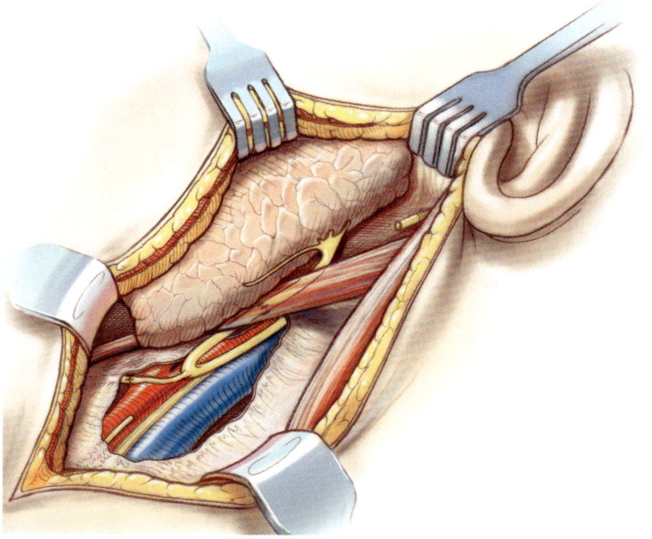

Figure 67–22 The descending ramus (descendens hypoglossi) can be anastomosed to the distal hypoglossal stump to minimize the chances of hemitongue atrophy.

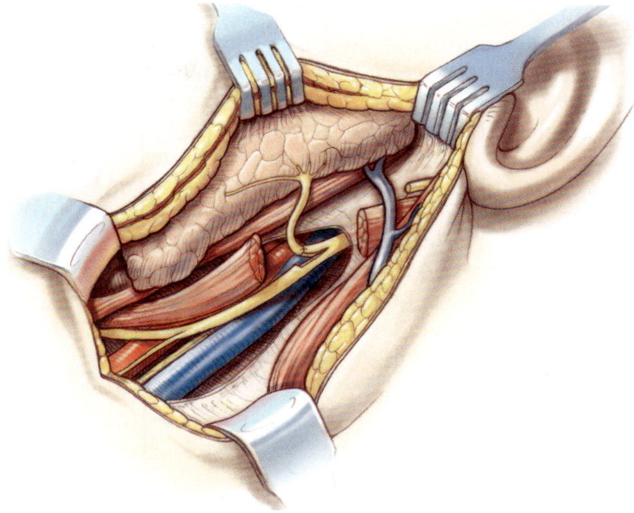

Figure 67–23 Technique of partial hypoglossal–facial anastomosis.

Partial Hypoglossal–Facial Anastomosis The hemitongue paralysis that occurs with a classic XII–VII anastomosis can result in severe deficits related to speech, mastication, and swallowing in patients with unilateral or bilateral CN IX or X deficits, or contralateral CN XII deficits. Also, classic XII–VII anastomoses cannot be performed bilaterally for bilateral facial paralysis. These patients, as well as those whose livelihoods depend on speaking and who would not tolerate loss of CN XII function, could be candidates for a partial hypoglossal to facial anastomosis.[10]

Although the hypoglossal nerve is monofascicular, it is thick enough that half of it can be split under the microscope and be of comparable thickness to the facial nerve. The other half can be left undisturbed to maintain hypoglossal function.[10] Although maximal functional result of the face is obtained with a classic XII–VII anastomosis, the partial XII–VII anastomosis is an alternative for the patient population listed above that is not able to tolerate total ipsilateral CN XII dysfunction.

Operative Technique The hypoglossal and facial nerves are identified and dissected as described for a classic XII–VII anastomosis. Similarly, the facial nerve is sectioned as far proximally as possible. Under the operating microscope, one half to one third of the 12th nerve is split as closely as possible to the skull base and dissected longitudinally proximally for several millimeters.[10]

Proximal to this dissection, CN XII is stimulated at 1 V to check for residual function, which reportedly correlates with postoperative preservation of hypoglossal function.[10] If distal hypoglossal function is not present, the descending ramus (descendens hypoglossi) is anastomosed to the cut end of CN XII. The split segment of CN XII is then anastomosed to the distal cut end of the facial nerve **(Fig. 67–23)**. A tension-free epineural repair is then performed with the smallest number of 9–0 or 10–0 monofilament nylon sutures needed for adequate approximation (usually three or four). An interposition graft is reserved for cases where all other measures fail to produce a tension-free anastomosis.

◆ Conclusion

Every cranial base operation consists of three crucial phases: exposure, resection, and reconstruction. The primary goal of the reconstruction phase is to reestablish the watertight integrity of the neurocranium and reestablish the anatomical integrity of the cranial base to seal off the neurocranial contents from the pharynx, nasal cavity, and paranasal sinuses. Normal bony contours of the craniofacial skeleton are also important for functional and cosmetic reasons.

The simplest way to facilitate a good reconstruction is to plan the reconstruction during the exposure, maintaining vascular pedicles of possible graft tissue and minimizing destruction of normal anatomy with careful soft tissue dissection, craniotomy flap elevation, and osteotomy execution. Meticulous attention to minimizing bone loss in these steps can result in a good functional and cosmetic result simply by replacing the bone flaps and osteotomy pieces. Split calvarial grafts and hydroxyapatite cement can be used to repair residual bony defects.

Vascularized autologous tissue is the tissue of choice for reconstruction to optimize healing and minimize the risks of infection or CSF leak. Commonly used choices include pericranial and temporalis muscle flaps. The next choice would be autologous free tissue grafts such as abdominal or thigh fat grafts, free pericranial grafts, split calvarial bone grafts, or temporalis fascia or fascia lata grafts. Any of these reconstructive materials can be reinforced with fibrin glue.

Autologous free muscle grafts are usually not used due to the high metabolic rate of muscle tissue. Synthetic materials or allografts are used only when autologous material is not available.

Cranial nerve repair is also performed for functional as well as cosmetic reasons. Due to the small size and often monofascicular composition of the intracranial segments of most cranial nerves, the most effective repair is tension-free direct epineural reanastomosis with the fewest number of 9–0 or 10–0 monofilament nylon sutures needed for adequate reapproximation of the two ends. Interposition grafts are reserved for cases where a tension-free anastomosis is not possible. The most common donor sites for interposition grafts are the sural nerve or sensory branches of the cervical plexus such as the greater auricular nerve.

These principles hold for the intracranial course of the facial nerve with direct reanastomosis giving the best chance for functional recovery, and an interposition graft used only when needed. In cases where there has been no return of facial function 1 year after surgical repair or if a facial nerve stump cannot be found, a hypoglossal–facial anastomosis is generally the most successful and well-tolerated neural repair. In cases where the usual CN XII deficits cannot be tolerated, a partial XII–VII anastomosis can be performed.

The use of these techniques and principles in the exposure and reconstruction phases of cranial-base procedures along with careful planning and attention to detail throughout can maximize the chances of a good functional and cosmetic outcome while minimizing the morbidity traditionally associated with cranial-base surgery. Procedures once regarded as prohibitively complicated for routine use are now being integrated into the mainstream neurosurgical armamentarium for this reason.

References

1. Sekhar LN, Goel A, Sen C. General neurosurgical operative techniques and instrumentation in cranial base surgery. In: Sekhar LN, Janecka IP, eds. Surgery of Cranial Base Tumors. New York: Raven; 1993: 1–10
2. Janecka IP, Sekhar LN. Reconstruction of skull base surgical defects. In: Jackson CG, ed. Surgery of Skull Base Tumors. New York: Churchill Livingstone; 1991:251–272
3. Wright DC, Sekhar LN. Management of anterior cranial base tumors. In: Tindall DC, Barrow DC, Cooper PR, eds. The Practice of Neurosurgery. Baltimore: Williams & Wilkins; 1995:949–962
4. Sekhar LN, Tzortzidis F, Raso J. Fronto-orbital approach. In: Sekhar LN, Oliveira ED, eds. Cranial Microsurgery: Approaches and Techniques. New York: Thieme; 1999:54–60
5. Samii M, Draf W. Facial nerve and skull base surgery. In: Samii M, Draf W, eds. Surgery of the Skull Base: An Interdisciplinary Approach. Berlin: Springer-Verlag; 1989:476–499
6. Sekhar LN, Burgess J, Akin O. Anatomical study of the cavernous sinus emphasizing operative approaches and related vascular and neural reconstruction. Neurosurgery 1987;21:806–816
7. Wilgus EFS. Techniques of epineural and group fascicular repair. In: Gelberman RH, ed. Operative Nerve Repair and Reconstruction. Philadelphia: JB Lippincott; 1991:287–293
8. Sekhar LN, Lanzino G, Sen C, et al. Reconstruction of the third through sixth cranial nerves during cavernous sinus surgery. J Neurosurg 1992; 76:935–943
9. Fabian RL. Facial nerve paralysis. In: Gelberman RH, ed. Operative Nerve Repair and Reconstruction. Philadelphia: JB Lippincott; 1991: 461–487
10. Cusimano MD, Sekhar LN. Partial hypoglossal to facial nerve anastomosis for reinnervation of the paralyzed face in patients with lower cranial nerve palsies: technical note. Neurosurgery 1994;35: 532–534

Section IX

Epilepsy and Functional Pain Disorder

68

Surgical Treatment for Intractable Epilepsy

Ghassan K. Bejjani

Epilepsy surgery includes temporal lobectomy for partial complex temporal lobe epilepsy, and corpus callostomy, hemispherectomy, and corticectomy for extratemporal foci. This chapter is limited to temporal lobe surgery for seizure control.[1,2]

◆ Preoperative Workup

Electrophysiological Localization of the Seizure Focus

Once it has been established that a patient's seizure disorder is intractable, an electroencephalographic (EEG) analysis is performed to determine whether or not a discrete seizure focus exists. If a discrete temporal lobe or extratemporal focus is identified, then surgery may be offered as a therapeutic modality.

The workup usually includes complete EEG monitoring with simultaneous video imaging. If necessary, cerebral localization using sphenoidal or foramen ovale electrodes is added. If the scalp EEG has distortion or artifact, then placement of subdural strip electrodes (through a bur hole) or large electrocorticographic grid arrays (via a craniotomy) may be required.

Occasionally, when surface recordings reveal conflicting or inconclusive results, depth electrodes need to be inserted using stereotactic techniques. Intracranial electrodes are indicated if the scalp EEG reveals any of the following:

1. Ictal and interictal foci not localized to the same site
2. Simultaneous bitemporal ictal discharges
3. No discrete seizure focus localized within the same hemisphere
4. Secondary focus or multiple foci for seizure generalization

Radiological Studies

Radiological studies utilized to support the diagnosis and plan the surgical resection of a discrete seizure focus include magnetic resonance imaging (MRI) looking for temporal lobe configuration, single photon emission computed tomography (SPECT), and, if possible, ictal SPECT. Positron emission tomography (PET) and functional MRI localization with MRI spectroscopy may enhance the workup, but these studies are not universally available.

Neuropsychiatric Evaluation

Patients who will be undergoing a temporal lobectomy usually undergo a complete cognitive evaluation with elaborate IQ, memory, and neuropsychological testing. In addition, a Wada test may be performed prior to surgical resection of the temporal lobe. The goal is to document good contralateral memory function prior to hippocampal resection. This test involves selective angiographic catheterization and Amytal injection of the distal cerebral arteries that supply the temporal lobe. Electroencephalography and standardized test questions are then used to determine speech localization as well as memory function in each temporal lobe.

◆ Surgical Anatomy of the Temporal Lobe

The temporal lobe is the only part of the brain where the neocortex **(Fig. 68–1)**, paleocortex **(Fig. 68–2)**, and archicortex **(Fig. 68–3)** coexist yet remain distinct from one another. The temporal lobe can be subdivided into two major subunits: the lateral neocortical subdivision (formed by the superior, middle, and inferior temporal gyri and the

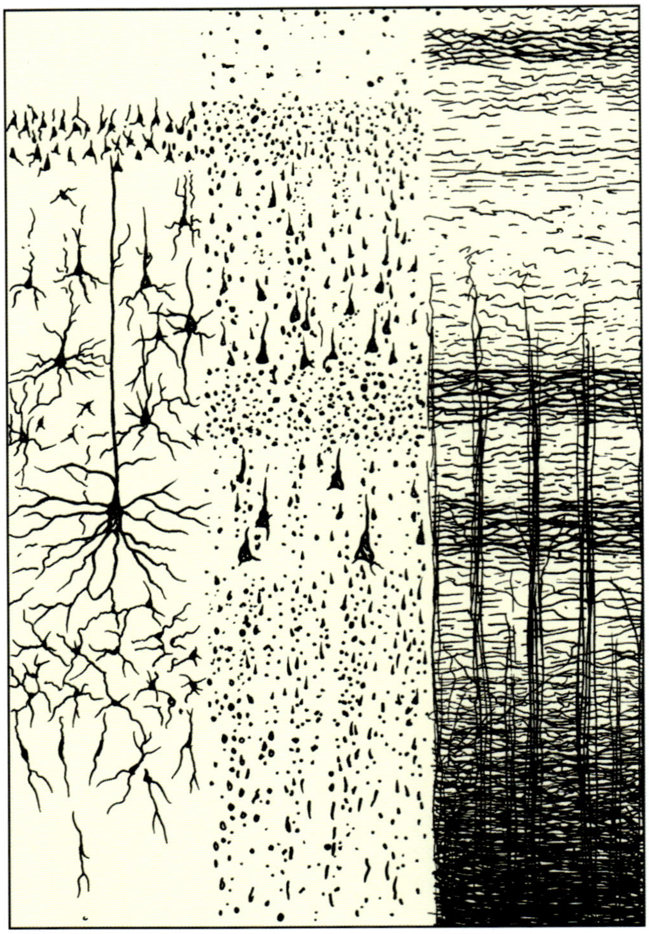

Figure 68–1 The six-layer neocortex forms the majority of the cerebral cortex.

occipitotemporal or fusiform gyrus), and the mediobasal paleocortical and archicortical subdivision [formed by the parahippocampal gyrus (PHG), dentate gyrus, amygdala, hippocampal formation, and fornix].

The medial surface of the temporal lobe (**Fig. 68–4**) has a complex anatomical orientation consisting of three components: opercular, parenchymal, and cisternal (**Fig. 68–5**). The *opercular component* is the enfolded opercular surface of the temporal lobe as it relates to the lateral surface of the insula. The inferior sulcus of the insula is located at the lower border of the inferomedial cleft of the sylvian fissure. The inferior insular vein and the inferior trunk of M2 course over it. The basal ganglia are located medial to the insular cortex. The *parenchymal component* of the medial surface of the temporal lobe corresponds to the white matter tracts connecting the temporal lobe with the remainder of the brain. These fibers, located above the temporal horn, correspond medially to the internal capsule and the thalamus. The *cisternal component* begins anteriorly at the temporal pole, continues posteriorly as the amygdala and uncus, and terminates more posteriorly as the hippocampal formation and associated mediobasal structures.

The *mediobasal structures* of the temporal lobe consist of the amygdala, fimbria, dentate gyrus, hippocampus, and PHG. With the exception of the amygdala, these structures course parallel to each other in an anteroposterior direction. On a coronal cut, they are arranged in a semicircular fashion with a medial convexity (**Fig. 68–5**). Starting from the PHG laterally, the subicular complex is encountered first and the hippocampal sulcus second. The hippocampus is located deep to the hippocampal sulcus. It is seen not at the inferior surface of the temporal lobe but on the floor of the temporal horn, where the white fibers forming the alveus cover its ventricular surface. These fibers converge medially to form the fornix. The enlarged anterior extremity of the hippocampus is called the *pes hippocampi* because of the digitations on its ventricular surface. The dentate gyrus, a very small gyrus also named for its surface digitations, is seen superior to the hippocampal sulcus, on the medial aspect of the temporal lobe. Located above the dentate gyrus is the fimbria, which carries posteriorly the fibers from the alveus and forms the fornix. The choroidal fissure is located above the fimbria. The relationships of the PHG are similar to those of the choroidal fissure. The PHG is related medially to the cerebral peduncle via the ambient cistern. In the ambient cistern, the basal vein of Rosenthal as well as the posterior cerebral artery and trochlear nerve course medial to the PHG.

Arterial Relationships

There are very elegant arterial relationships to the temporal lobe that must be respected by the surgeon during the surgical procedures for temporal lobectomy: the middle cerebral artery branches that course within the sylvian fissure, the dominant temporal lobe vessels that supply the angular gyrus, and Wernicke's region. The *anterior choroidal artery*, which arises from the carotid artery, courses posteriorly between the uncus and cerebral peduncle, inferior and parallel to the optic tract (**Fig. 68–6**). It enters the choroidal fissure near the ambient cistern and then proceeds distally to supply the choroid plexus. The artery's cisternal segment gives off perforating branches that supply the optic tract as well as regions of the basal ganglia, thalamus, and internal capsule. The *posterior cerebral artery* starts in the interpeduncular fossa and curves posteriorly around the cerebral peduncle, traversing the ambient and then the quadrigeminal cisterns. Opening the choroid fissure exposes the posterior cerebral artery in the ambient cistern, where it courses along with the medial posterior choroidal artery, and where it gives off its thalamogeniculate and lateral posterior choroidal branches. The P2 segment of the posterior cerebral artery also gives off important branches (i.e., the hippocampal artery and the anterior, middle, and posterior temporal branches), which supply the hippocampus and the temporal lobe.

Neural Relationships

The neural relationships are with the optic tract, the optic radiation, and the third and fourth cranial nerves. The *optic tract* is in close proximity to the medial portion of the uncus

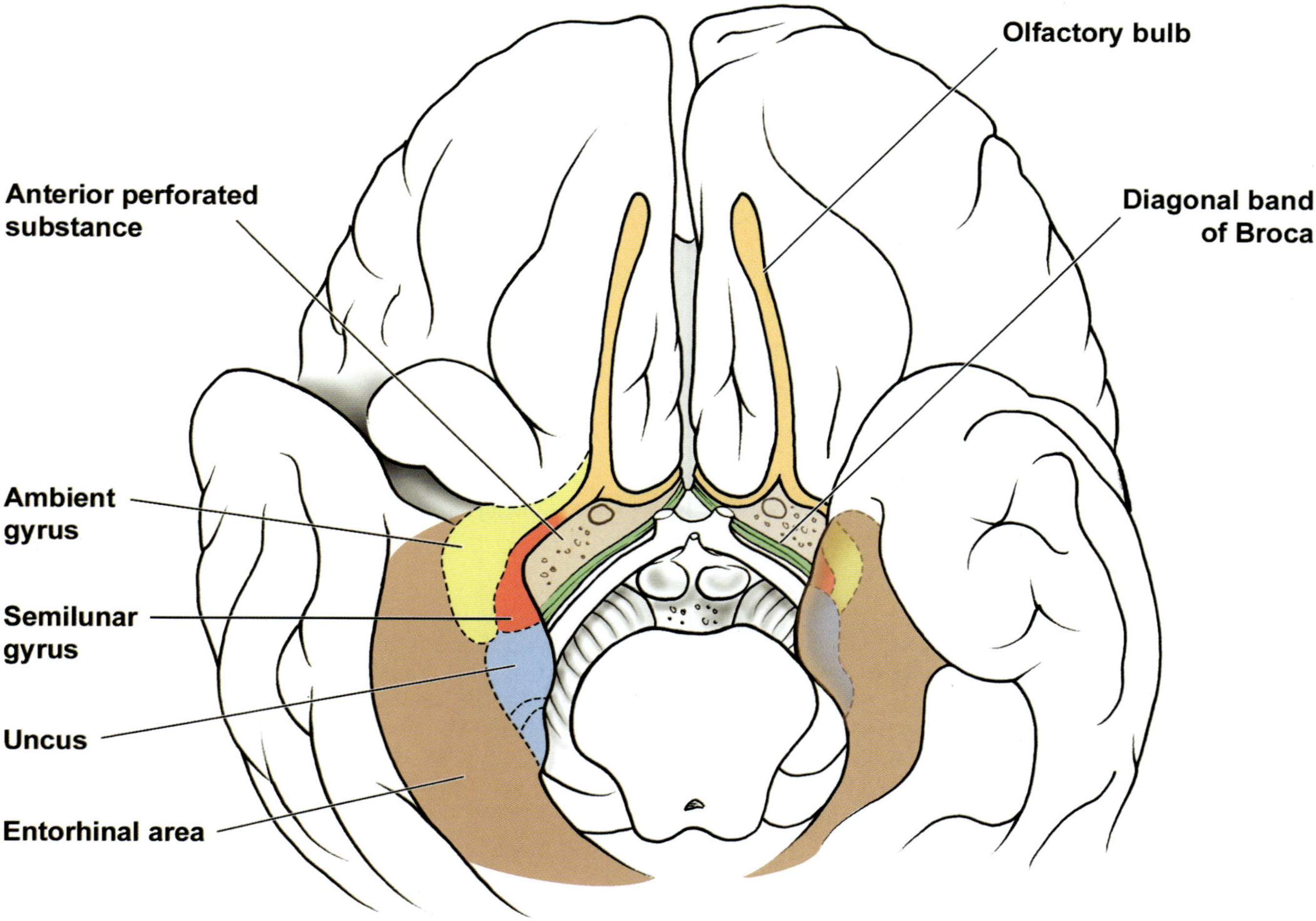

Figure 68–2 The paleocortex is seen along the inferior surface of the brain.

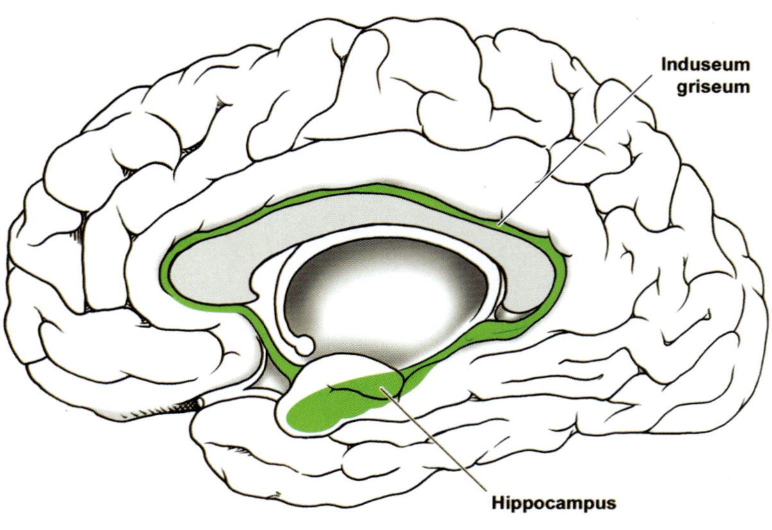

Figure 68–3 The archicortex (in green) is seen along the medial surface of the hemisphere.

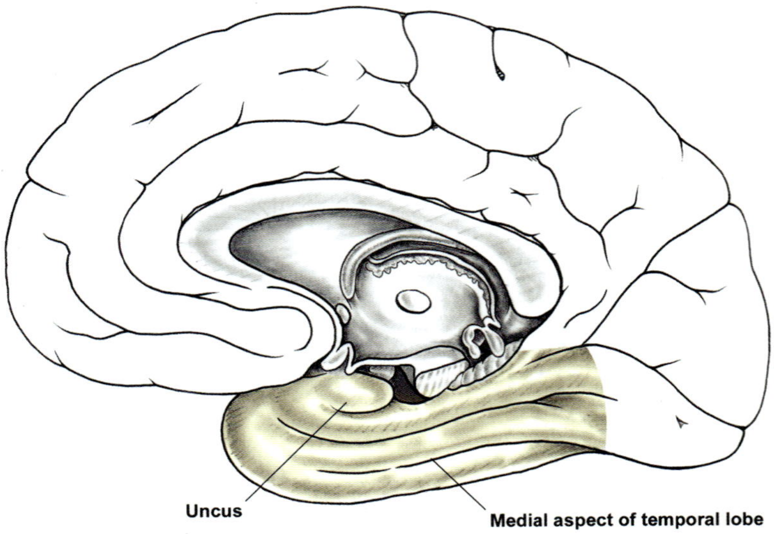

Figure 68–4 Medial view of the temporal lobe illustrates its mesiobasal structures.

as it turns around the cerebral peduncle to reach the lateral geniculate body (LGB). The LGB lies medial to the choroidal point. The *optic radiation* begins at the LGB and projects more posteriorly to the calcarine cortex. The portion of the optic radiation that projects anteriorly, known as Meyer's loop, comes in close proximity to the roof of the temporal horn of the lateral ventricle behind the level of the pes hippocampus and is at risk during temporal lobectomies, leading to a "pie in the sky" visual field defect pattern.

In the interpeduncular cistern, the third cranial nerve is located medial to the uncus. The fourth cranial nerve courses around the midbrain at or below the level of the tentorial incisura and enters the cavernous sinus through the posterolateral angle of the oculomotor triangle.

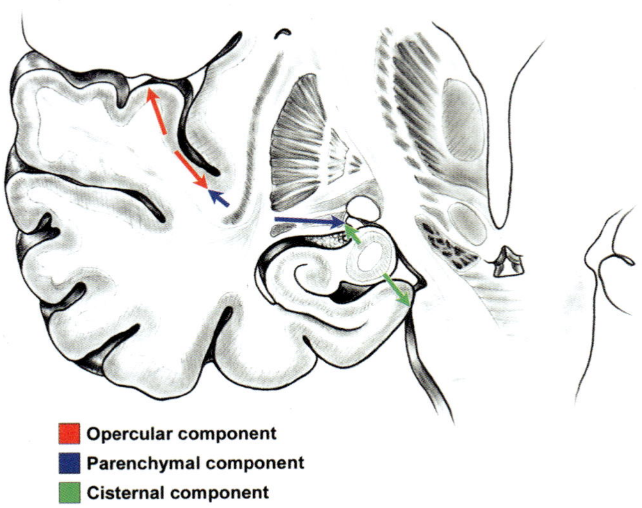

Figure 68–5 Coronal cut through the hemisphere: the opercular, parenchymal, and cisternal components are seen.

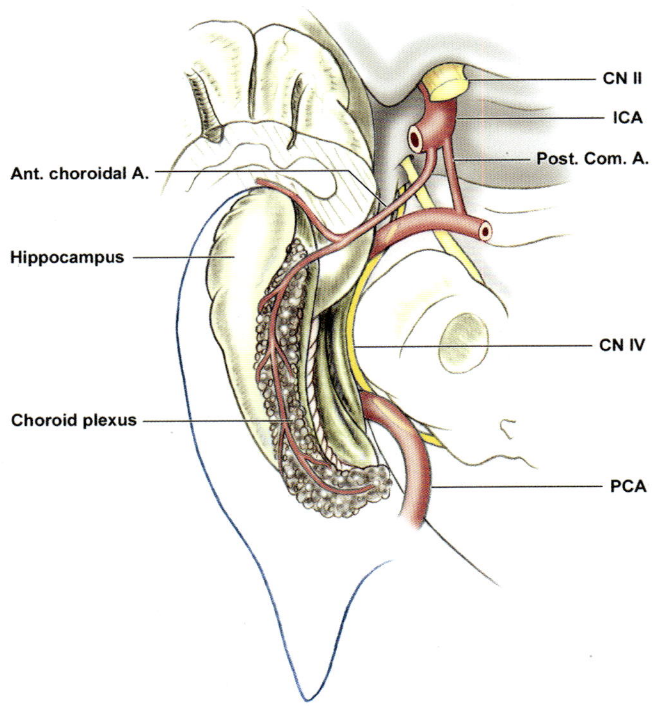

Figure 68–6 Anterior choroidal artery. ICA, internal carotid artery; PCA, posterior cerebral artery.

◆ Surgery for Temporal Lobe Epilepsy

Anatomy of the Temporal Lobe as It Relates to Epilepsy Surgery

The temporal lobe has two main subunits: a lateral neocortical unit and a mesiobasal allocortical unit. The lateral unit is composed of the superior, middle, and inferior temporal gyrus and occipitotemporal or fusiform gyrus, whereas the mesiobasal unit is composed of the amygdala, hippocampus, parahippocampal gyrus, and adjacent allocortical structures. Most temporal resections for seizure control are aimed at resecting the mesiobasal structures. Removing the lateral temporal structures serves as the approach leading to the mesiobasal structures, although some selective resections aim at removing the latter structures without major lateral resection.

The complex medial relationships of the temporal lobe have to be carefully understood. The mesiobasal temporal structures are in close proximity with various neurovascular structures in the basal cisterns: the anterior choroidal artery, the posterior communicating artery, the posterior cerebral artery, the basal vein of Rosenthal, the optic tract, and the third and fourth nerves. Staying subpial during the last stage of the resection helps preserve the integrity of these structures.

General Considerations Regarding Surgery for Temporal Lobe Epilepsy

Two philosophies have developed with respect to surgery for temporal lobe epilepsy: temporal lobectomy and directed temporal lobe resection.

Advocates of temporal lobectomy localize the focus to the temporal lobe via scalp EEG recordings, with long-term seizure monitoring in an epilepsy unit. On occasion, if no precise focus is identified, subdural electrocorticographic grid arrays and depth electrodes are placed surgically. Following localization to either the right or the left temporal lobe, a temporal lobectomy is undertaken, incorporating both the lateral and medial temporal lobe structures including the amygdala and the hippocampus. The amount of lateral resection is variable, with two variants:

- En bloc anterior temporal lobectomy proper, which consists in resecting 6 cm in the nondominant temporal lobe and 4.5 cm in the dominant temporal lobe, as measured from the tip posteriorly, and removing the medial temporal structures along with the lateral structures
- Anteromedial temporal lobectomy, in which 3.5 cm on the nondominant and 3 cm on the dominant side are resected, and the superior temporal gyrus is spared

Advocates of directed temporal lobe resection perform the same standard workup, including scalp electrode EEG and long-term seizure monitoring in an epilepsy unit. In selected cases, they also perform similar subdural electrocorticographic grid array and depth electrode recording. However, the temporal lobe resection is tailored and limited based on very precise mapping of the epileptic focus obtained by intraoperative electrocorticography and stimulation. Selective amygdalohippocampectomy is a variant of the latter approach, in a way such that the resection is limited to the amygdala and hippocampus, sparing the lateral temporal lobe.

Lateral Temporal Lobe Resection (Anteromedial Variant)

A modified frontotemporal craniotomy, contained beneath the confines of the temporalis muscle, and a zygomatic osteotomy are used to provide the surgical approach **(Fig. 68–7).** This approach provides a wide exposure and easy

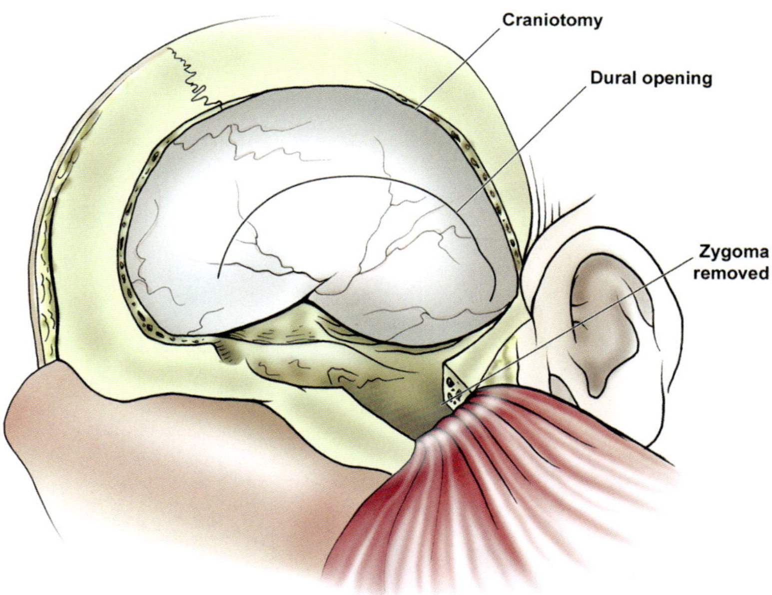

Figure 68–7 Craniotomy and zygomatic osteotomy.

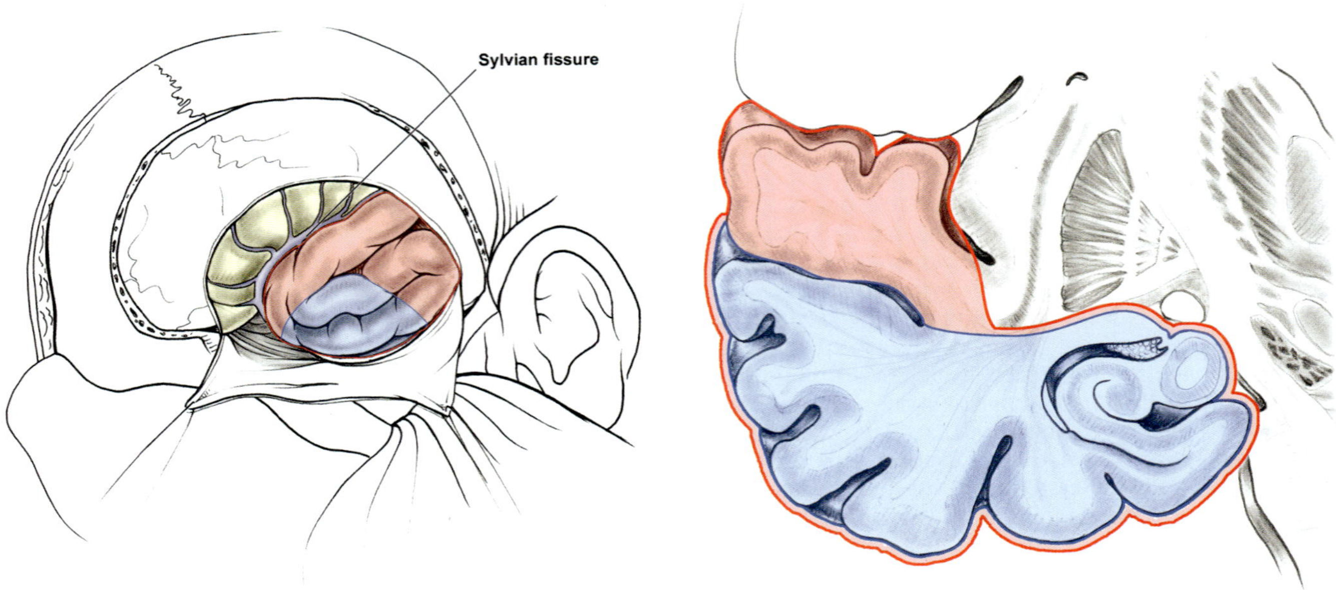

Figure 68–8 Dural opening and outline of an en bloc temporal resection (red) and anteromedial resection (blue).

access to the frontal and temporal lobes, including the medial basal portion of the temporal lobe, and allows for intraoperative electrocorticography and stimulation. The patient is placed in the supine position on the operating table. The head is fixed in the Mayfield three-point head holder, extended ~20 degrees, and rotated to the opposite side 30 degrees off the horizontal. After the craniotomy and zygomatic osteotomy have been completed, a portion of the sphenoid ridge is drilled down as in a standard pterional approach.

The dura is then opened **(Fig. 68–8)**. The lateral cortex is resected. We prefer a limited anteromedial resection. We remove 1.5 to 2 cm of the middle temporal gyrus and 2.5 to 3 cm of the inferior temporal gyrus, in one segment **(Fig. 68–9)**. This lateral cortex is sent as a separate specimen for pathological analysis. The temporal lobe is tagged with respect to anterior, medial, and lateral orientation to allow the pathologist to achieve the proper anatomical configuration. Following the removal of the lateral cortex, the temporal horn of the lateral ventricle is entered **(Fig. 68–10)**. The head of the hippocampus and amygdala are easily identified in the temporal horn.

At this point, the medial portions of the temporal lobe, including the amygdala, hippocampus, and perihippocam-

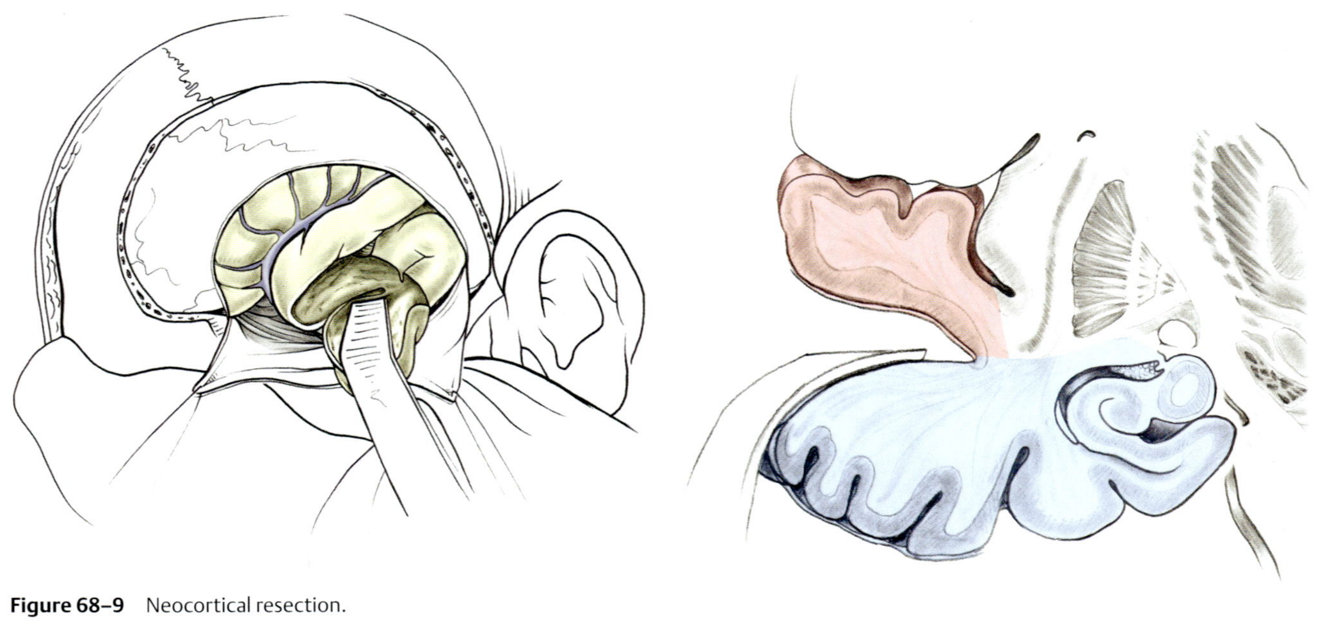

Figure 68–9 Neocortical resection.

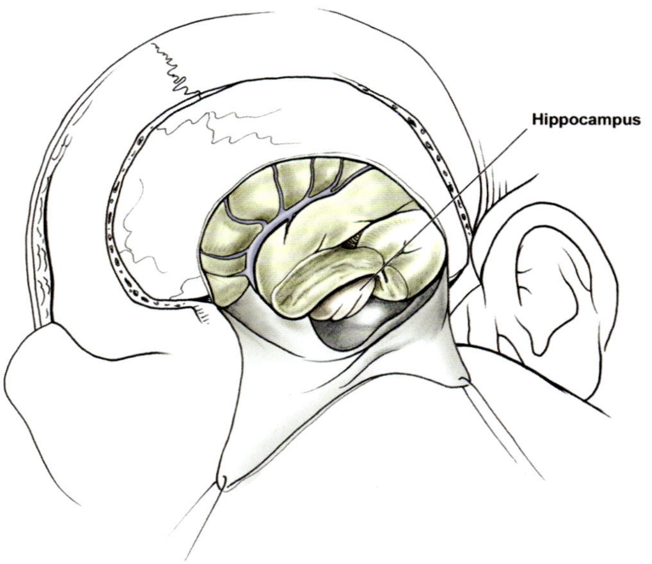

Figure 68–10 Exposure of the mediobasal structures.

pal gyrus, are resected using the operating microscope. The resection is performed in a subpial manner, with care being taken to avoid entry into the subarachnoid space of the sylvian fissure and to maintain a discrete arachnoid barrier medially and posteriorly **(Fig. 68–11).** The optic tract, optic radiation, anterior choroidal artery, posterior cerebral artery, and third and fourth cranial nerves must be respected at all times to avoid injury. Excessive coagulation of the pial arachnoid margin should also be avoided; however, any minor bleeding from this area can be easily controlled with loose placement of Surgicel.

Following the resection of the temporal lobe, the dura is then closed in the usual manner. The craniotomy bone flap and zygomatic arch are reaffixed using miniplates, and the temporalis muscle is closed over the craniotomy site. The remainder of the galea/skin incision is closed in the standard fashion. The use of miniplates and the restriction of the craniotomy bone flap to the area under the temporalis muscle allow for the most aesthetic cosmetic result.

Selective Amygdalohippocampectomy

Selective amygdalohippocampectomy was developed by Yasargil in 1975 for the treatment of temporal lobe epilepsy. A standard pterional approach is used **(Fig. 68–12).** After the dura has been opened, the frontal lobe is lifted and the carotid cistern exposed and opened. The sylvian fissure is then split **(Fig. 68–13),** exposing the internal carotid artery and the middle cerebral artery to the level of the anterior third of the insulae **(Fig. 68–14).** Once the limen insulae is exposed, a 15 mm incision is made along the inferior insular sulcus, lateral to the inferior insular vein and the branch of the middle cerebral artery **(Fig. 68–15).** The amygdala lies a few millimeters deep to this incision, but may be more difficult to see than the temporal horn, which is located behind it. Opening the temporal horn **(Fig. 68–16)** improves the visualization of the amygdala, which can then be partially resected. During this stage of the dissection, the surgeon must take care to avoid injury to the optic tract inferiorly and the basal ganglia medially. The adjacent temporal lobe and PHG are removed subpially. The temporal horn, now well exposed, guides the remainder of the dissection. The hippocampus is exposed over its floor.

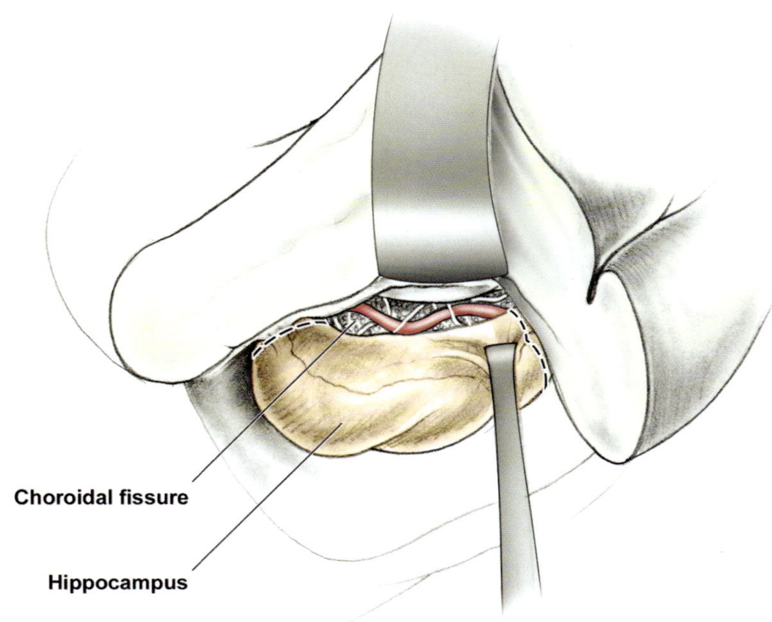

Figure 68–11 **(A)** Resection of the mesiobasal structures, exposing

(*Continued on page 834*)

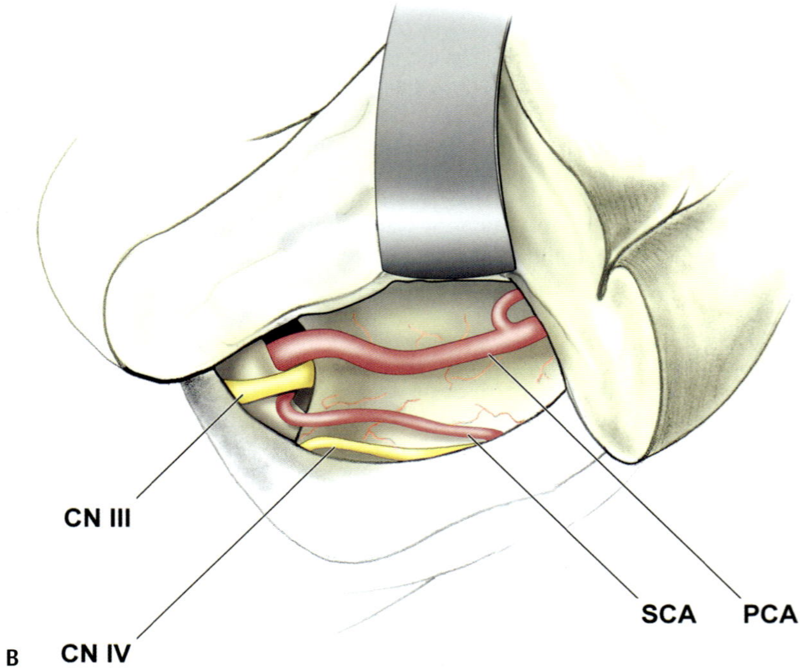

(*Continued*) **Figure 68–11** **(B)** the medial arachnoidal plane. PCA, Posterior cerebellar artery; SCA, superior cerebellar artery.

More posteriorly, the choroidal fissure is opened under the choroid plexus to separate the mediobasal structures from the remainder of the brain. Care must be taken to respect the anterior choroidal artery. Its branches that feed the PHG and uncus are coagulated and sectioned, whereas the feeders to the internal capsule, optic tract, cerebral peduncle, and other structures must be preserved. Posteriorly, the fissure is opened until the level of the posterior border of the cerebral peduncle is reached. A transverse cut is made at that level along the hippocampus and PHG until the collateral eminence is reached. The cut is then carried anteriorly along the collateral eminence, further disconnecting the hippocampus and PHG from the temporal lobe. Once the lateral cut joins the area of the previously resected

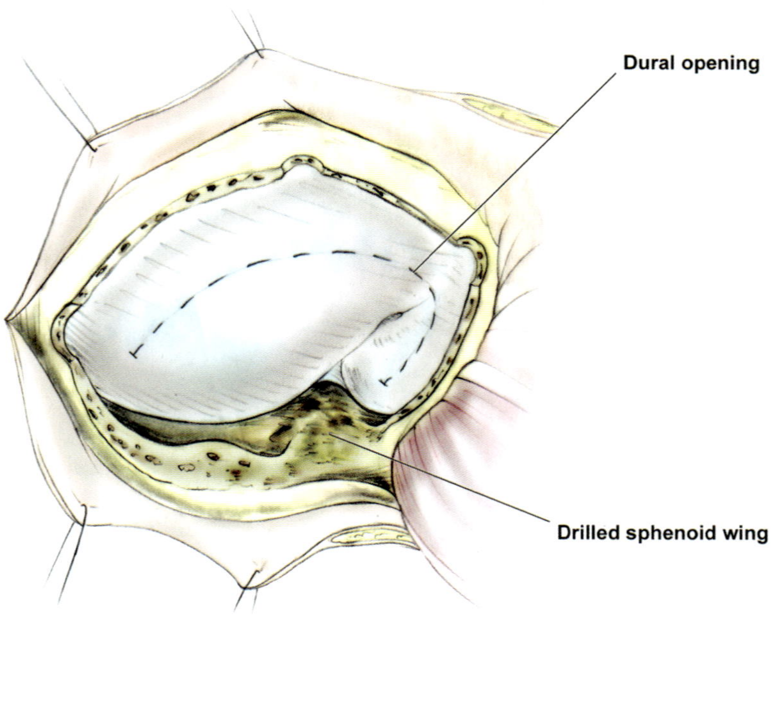

Figure 68–12 Standard pterional approach. (Modified from Yasargil MG. Microneurosurgery of CNS Tumors. Vol 4b: Limbic and Paralimbic Tumors. New York: Thieme; 1995:252–290, with permission of the publisher.)

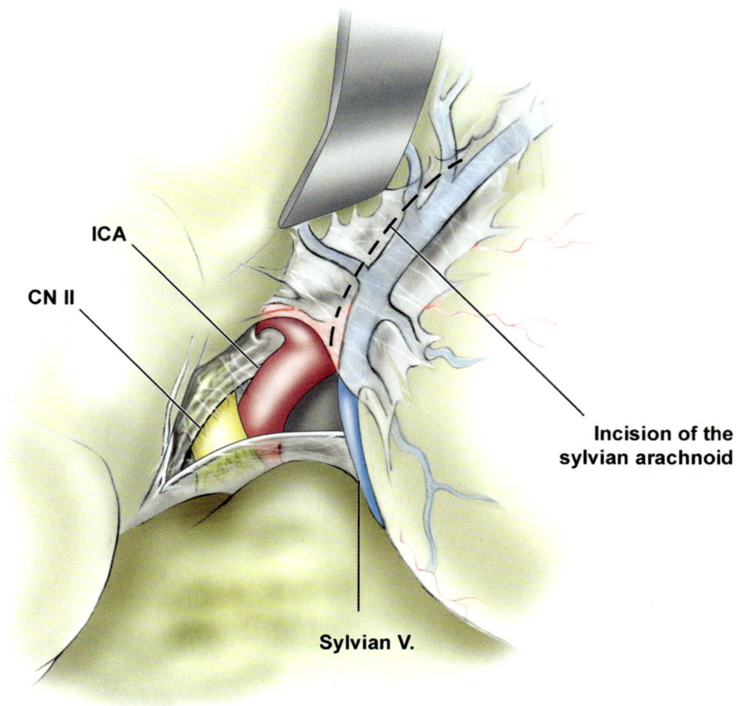

A

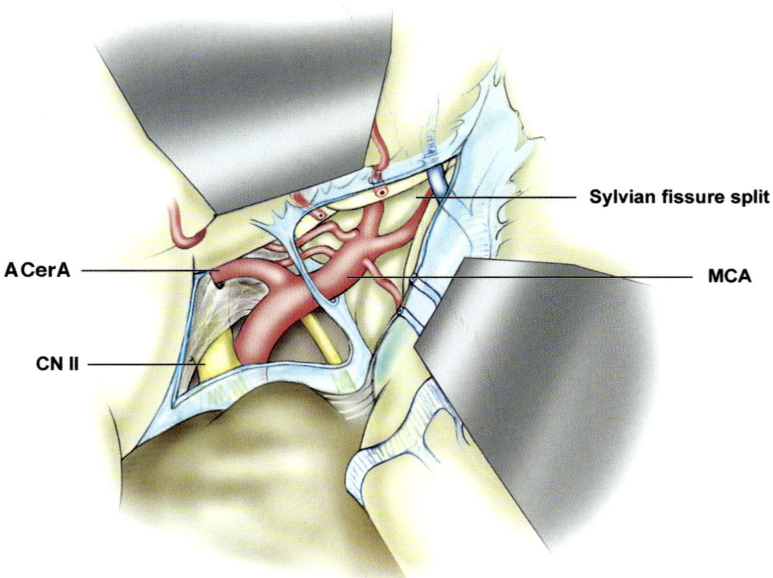

B

Figure 68–13 (A,B) The sylvian fissure is split. AcerA, anterior cerebral artery; MCA, middle cerebral artery. (Modified from Yasargil MG. Microneurosurgery of CNS Tumors. Vol 4b: Limbic and Paralimbic Tumors. New York: Thieme; 1995:252–290, with permission of the publisher.)

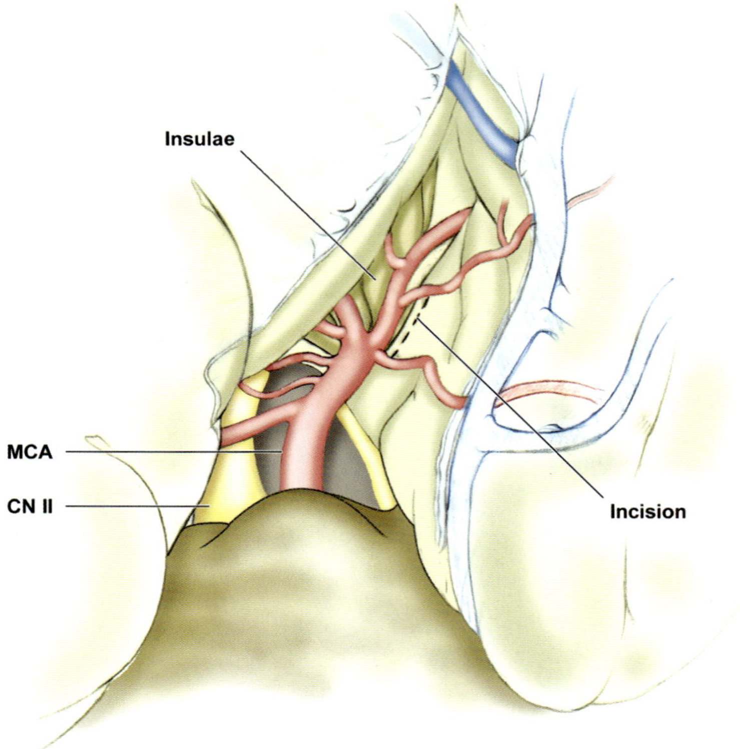

Figure 68–14 The insulae is exposed. The insular incision is marked. MCA, middle cerebral aretery. (Modified from Yasargil MG. Microneurosurgery of CNS Tumors. Vol 4b: Limbic and Paralimbic Tumors. New York: Thieme, 1995: 252–290, with permission of the publisher.)

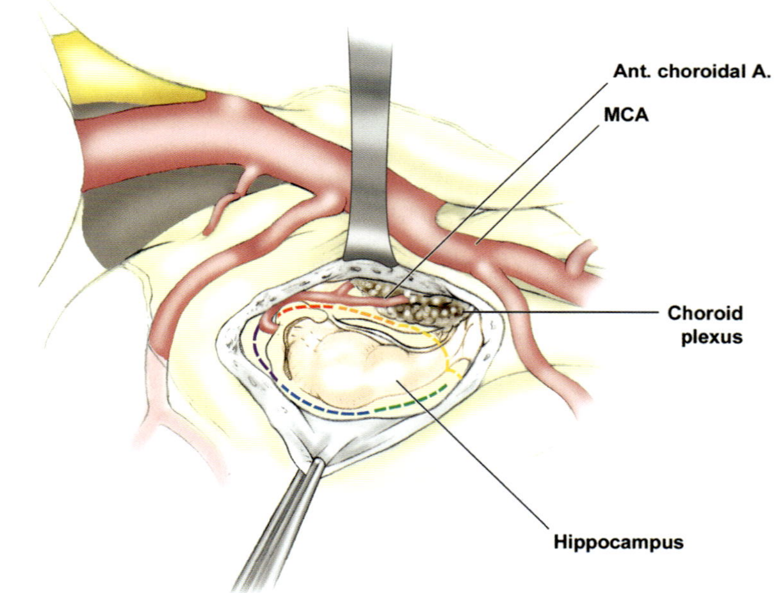

Figure 68–15 The limen insulae is incised. The temporal horn is opened, exposing the hippocampus. The hippocampal incisions are outlined. MCA, middle cerebral artery (Modified from Yasargil MG. Microneurosurgery of CNS Tumors. Vol 4b: Limbic and Paralimbic Tumors. New York: Thieme; 1995:252–290, with permission of the publisher.)

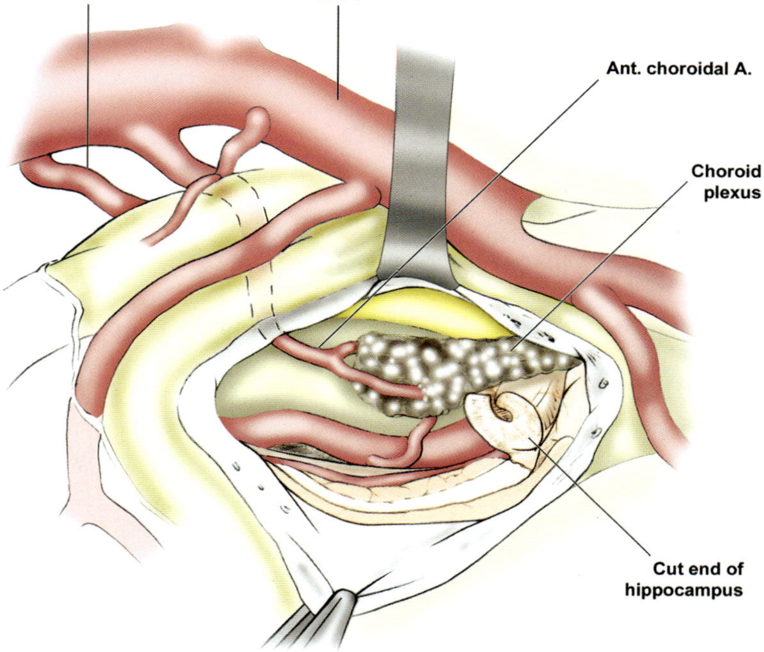

Figure 68–16 The hippocampus is resected. MCA, middle cerebral aretery. (Modified from Yasargil MG. Microneurosurgery of CNS Tumors. Vol 4b: Limbic and Paralimbic Tumors. New York: Thieme; 1995:252–290, with permission of the publisher.)

amygdala anteriorly, the PHG and hippocampus are completely disconnected and removed en bloc. Staying subpial during the resection protects the surrounding structures, especially the third and fourth cranial nerves. Routine closure can be performed after careful hemostasis has been achieved.

◆ Conclusion

Temporal lobe surgery for epilepsy is a useful and relatively safe tool in the armamentarium of the neurosurgeon dealing with patients with intractable epilepsy. In experienced hands and with the correct indications, it is a gratifying procedure.

References

1. Miller JW, Silbergold D. Epilepsy Surgery: Principles and Controversies. New York: Taylor and Francis Group; 2006
2. Yasagil MG. Microsurgery of CNS Tumors. Vol IVb: Limbic and Paralimbic Tumors. New York: Thieme; 1995, 252–290

69

Surgical Treatment for Parkinson's Disease

Prithvi Narayan and Roy A. E. Bakay

Parkinson's disease (PD) is a progressive, degenerative disorder characterized clinically by bradykinesia, rigidity, resting tremor, and postural instability, and pathologically by the loss of dopaminergic cells in the substantia nigra pars compacta (SNc).

Surgical treatment of PD emerged during the early part of the 20th century and involved, for the most part, creating a lesion in the corticospinal system for alleviation of tremor. These interventions resulted in good relief of tremor but were complicated by the development of spasticity and weakness. Establishment of the concept of the extrapyramidal motor system in the 1920s was a turning point for the treatment of movement disorders. Between the 1930s and the 1950s, a large number of surgical procedures lesioning the globus pallidus (GP) and ansa lenticularis for the alleviation of rigidity and tremor were performed. Leksell, by varying the site of the lesion within the pallidum, found that targets in the ventral and posterior portions of the internal segment of the globus pallidus (GPi) were more effective. By the early 1960s, however, empirical observations led to the abandonment of pallidotomy in favor of thalamotomy as the procedure of choice for treating parkinsonian tremor. The advent of L-dopa and its clinical benefit in the treatment of PD marked the decline of all surgical interventions for PD in the mid-1960s. (see Svennilson E. Torvik A, Lowe R. Lekell L)

Resurgence in the surgical treatment of PD in the 1990s was due to multiple factors. Chronic L-dopa therapy is associated with the wearing-off phenomenon as well as motor complications such as on-off fluctuations and dyskinesias. The advancements in stereotactic techniques and instrumentation, improved neuroimaging, better understanding of basal ganglia circuitry, and improved physiological intraoperative localization techniques have led to more consistent improvements in parkinsonian motor symptoms following surgery and to a progressive increase in the use of surgical therapy for the treatment of PD well as other movement disorders.

Surgical treatment for PD involves two basic approaches: ablation and deep brain stimulation (DBS). A third approach, restorative therapy including cell transplantation and growth factor infusion is in the nascent stage and still considered experimental. This chapter discusses the techniques for ablation and DBS.

Targets for ablation and DBS include the sensorimotor portions of the GPi, the motor thalamus [i.e., nucleus ventralis intermedius (Vim), nucleus ventralis oralis posterior and anterior (Vop, Voa)], and the subthalamic nucleus (STN). Pallidotomy is the surgical ablation of portions of the internal segment of the GP and is effective for most parkinsonian motor signs. DBS of GPi or STN also relieves most parkinsonian symptoms and is a viable alternative to pallidotomy. Ablation or DBS of parts of the Vim provide relief from parkinsonian tremor and if extended anteriorly to include the Vop and parts of the Voa, may also improve rigidity and drug-induced dyskinesias, but Gpi and especially STN procedures are equally effective and will affect other parkinsonian motor signs as well, such as bradykinesia and akinesia.

◆ Indications

Patients, with a history of idiopathic PD, who initially benefited but who are no longer adequately controlled by medical therapy, are candidates for pallidotomy. The presence of at least two of the three cardinal signs—tremor, rigidity bradykinesia—and a history of a beneficial response to L-dopa are the criteria for the diagnosis of idiopathic PD. For patients with predominantly disabling tremor, thalamotomy or thalamic DBS is a viable alternative to GPi or STN DBS or ablation. However, most PD patients gradually develop other motor signs over time and require ablation or DBS of either GPi or STN. Thus, rather than perform two operations for these patients, it may be preferable to consider GPi or STN as the preferred surgical target for tremor-predominant PD as well as for akinetic-rigid PD.

◆ Contraindications

Contraindications to DBS or ablation include patients with "Parkinson's plus" syndromes, dementia, extensive brain atrophy, and any systemic medical illness that would significantly increase the surgical risk. For DBS procedures, a stimulator should not be placed in patients who have concurrent infections or demand pacemakers, or who have intolerance to foreign bodies. Diathermy is an absolute contraindication after DBS placement because it can cause severe tissue damage at the lead sites.

◆ Preoperative Studies and Patient Preparation

Preparation for Surgery

To reduce anxiety the patient should be fully informed of the order of events including frame placement, scanning, surgical opening under anesthesia, intraoperative mapping, and lesioning/stimulation. All antiparkinsonian medications should be discontinued at midnight on the day of the procedure to allow manifestation of parkinsonian symptoms in the operating room and prevent the development of drug-induced dyskinesias during frame placement and imaging. No intravenous lines should be placed on the limbs contralateral to the lesion because they are used for neurological assessment.

Frame Placement

Any commercially available stereotactic head frame can be used for localization. The authors use a Leksell series G head frame. The frame must be placed with its axes orthogonal to the standard anatomical planes of the brain to ensure that the preoperative images and the intraoperative microelectrode-derived maps are interpretable in reference to standard brain atlases. The frame is placed on the head, with the aid of earplugs, and aligned with the external auditory meatus (EAM). The earplugs are placed in the middle of three possible holes on the carrier and the carrier is adjusted to a Y position of 95. The earplugs are advanced simultaneously until they fit into the EAM. The *y*-axis of the frame is then angled so that the inferior margin of the anterior bar of the frame aligns with the tip of the nose (**Fig. 69–1,** line a). This places the anteroposterior (AP) axis of the frame parallel to the orbitomeatal line (**Fig. 69–1,** line b), which is itself parallel to the anterior-posterior commissure line (AC-PC line). The pin sites are anesthetized with a local anesthetic such as 1% lidocaine with epinephrine. Short-acting sedatives such as Versed may be necessary to ensure patient comfort. The skull pins are then advanced until all four pins lightly penetrate the skin. The earplugs are then retracted to avoid pain in the EAM, and the pins are then tightened.

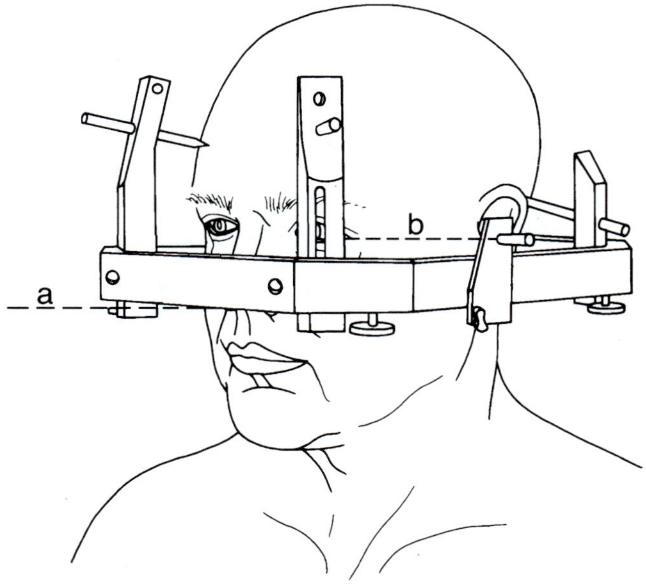

Figure 69–1 Frame placement for ablation or deep brain stimulation.

Target Localization

Three methods are utilized for target localization: image-guided stereotactic localization, microelectrode mapping, and macrostimulation. The latter two are performed intraoperatively and are described later.

Image-guided stereotactic localization is based on location of targets relative to the AC-PC line. The AC and PC can be visualized by computed tomography (CT) or magnetic resonance imaging (MRI). Target selection is based on identification of the AC-PC line and localization of the Vim, GPi, and STN indirectly by measuring fixed distances from the AC-PC line. The inferior border of the GPi target, based on Leksell's coordinates, is 21 to 22 mm lateral, 2 to 3 mm anterior, and 2 to 6 mm below the AC-PC midpoint. The center of Vim is approximately in the same axial plane as AC-PC and approximately 5 mm anterior to the PC. The lateral

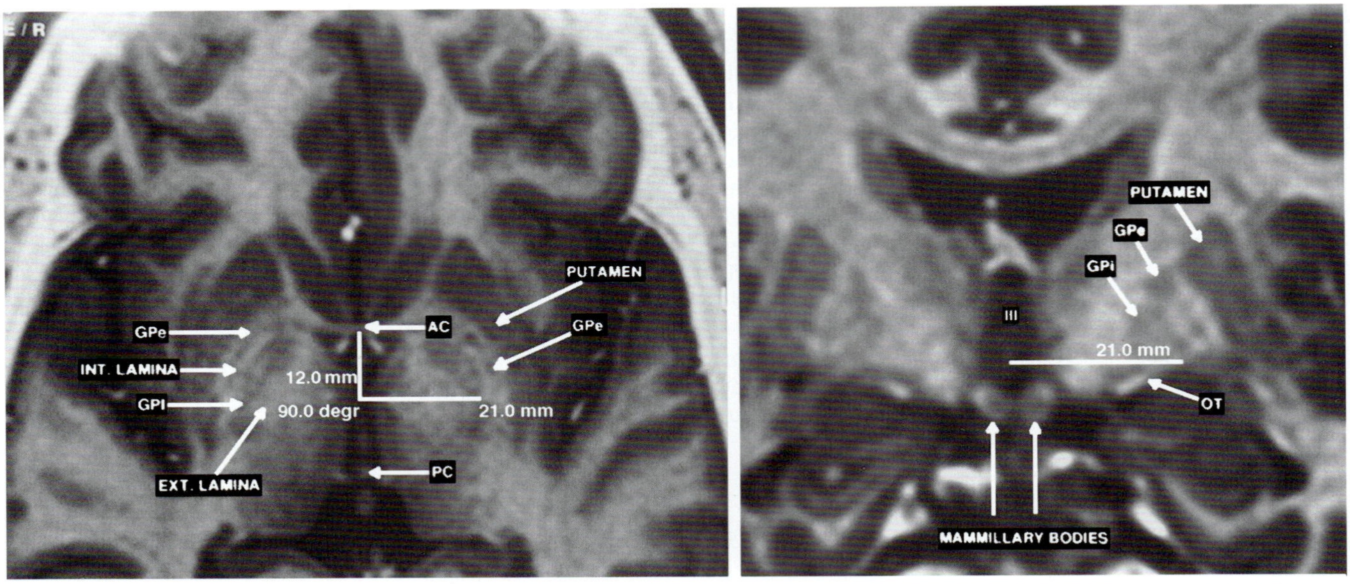

Figure 69–2 Magnetic resonance imaging–based target selection for globus pallidus interna (GPi).

coordinate is 2 mm medial to the border between the thalamus and internal capsule or 11.5 mm from the lateral edge of the third ventricle. The STN is usually 4 mm behind the AC-PC midpoint, 12 mm lateral and 4 mm inferior to the AC-PC plane (at the base of the third ventricle).

However, there is significant individual variability in the target localization based on AC-PC coordinates. The advantage of using a high-resolution inversion-recovery sequence MRI is that it allows for anatomical visualization of some borders of the target nuclei, it maximizes gray/white contrast, and it minimizes the inherent distortion present in MRI images. **Fig. 69–2** shows one example of MRI-based target selection for GPi. The lateral (x) and AP (y) coordinates are determined on the axial scan at the level of the AC-PC line, from a point lateral to the midpoint of the AC-PC line and 3 mm medial to the external accessory lamina. The vertical (z) coordinate is determined on the coronal scan closest to the AC-PC line from the superior margin of the lateral edge of the optic tract (OT). Although this targeting algorithm usually places the stereotactic target within a few millimeters in each dimension of the ideal target, physiological localization is important for modification and confirmation of the target location. Direct stereotactic target selection of Vim is difficult because the borders of this small nucleus are not clearly visible. Therefore, the target for the initial microelectrode track is largely based on the standard measurements from the AC-PC line. The STN can be directly visualized on a T2-weighted MRI.

◆ Surgical Technique

Anesthesia

A combination of local anesthesia and intravenous sedation is used for the surgical procedure. The patient is awake during the entire procedure except for the opening and closing, where intravenous sedation is used. Short-acting agents, such as propofol, are used for sedation, and a local anesthetic, 1% lidocaine with 1:100,000 epinephrine, is used for the incision. The use of sedation intraoperatively is limited as much as possible to ensure patient cooperation. Antihypertensive medication may be continuously infused to ensure that the blood pressure remains within acceptable limits.

Positioning

The stereotactic head frame is fastened to the Mayfield head holder and the neck is placed in neutral position. The patient is initially positioned supine for the incision and bony exposure to minimize the risk of air embolism **(Fig. 69–3)**.

◆ Skin Incision and Exposure

The Leksell frame coordinates are set, and the slide on the arc of the Leksell frame is set at 90 degrees, so that the entry is in a parasagittal plane. The arc is rotated about its axis so that it makes an angle of 60 degrees with the AC-PC line. The entry point is marked on the skin. After local anesthetic is infiltrated, a 4 to 5 cm incision (dotted line in **Fig. 69–3**) is made approximately 1 cm posterior to the entry point. The entry point, which is usually 1 cm anterior to the coronal suture, is marked on the bone. A bur hole is then placed at the entry point measuring 1.5 cm in diameter. After adequate hemostasis is obtained, the dura is coagulated and opened widely. Cortical vessels are dissected and mobilized away from the instrument passes. The patient is then placed in a reclining, semi-seated position at about 30 to 45 degrees for the microelectrode recording **(Fig. 69–3)**. Together with the use of fibrin glue to seal the opening, this minimizes cerebrospinal fluid (CSF) loss, adds to patient comfort, and reduces artifact during neuronal recording.

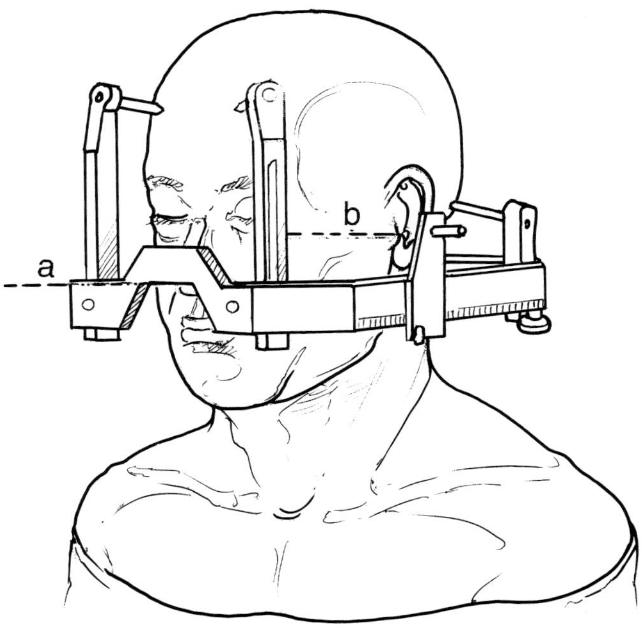

Figure 69–3 Patient position for incision and bony exposure and for microelectrode recording

Microelectrode Mapping

Localization of the Internal Segment of the Globus Pallidus

The authors use the Schaltenbrand and Bailey (SB) human brain atlas as the template for physiological mapping. The initial target point is on the parasagittal lateral 20 mm plane of the SB atlas at the superior border of the optic tract and the inferior border of the GPi. The rationale for selecting this target point is to provide a long trajectory through the GPi, define the position of the optic tract early, and minimize the number of microelectrode passes required for the three-dimensional mapping of GPi.

The microelectrode is advanced, from a frontal approach, in the trajectory based on the stereotactic coordinates of the posterior portion of the GPi. Recording tracts are made in the parasagittal plane from the anterodorsal to the posteroventral direction at an angle of approximately 30 degrees from vertical. The major structures encountered using this approach are the corona radiata, striatum, the external segment of the globus pallidus (GPe) and GPi, the internal and external medullary laminae, the OT, and the internal capsule. The striatum is encountered first, followed by GPe and GPi. **Fig. 69–4** shows the superimposition of the microelectrode tracks on sagittal MRI scans through the basal ganglia. Segments of the track reconstructions are shaded to show striatum (white segment), GPe (stippled segment), and GPi (white triangles, circles, and squares). Movement-related cells are indicated by triangles (leg), circles (arm), and squares (jaw).

The discharge patterns in the above structures are well characterized and are shown in **Fig. 69–5.** The striatal neurons have low spontaneous discharge rates in the range of 1 to 3 Hz. GPe neurons have two distinct patterns of discharge: (1) 80% to 90% of cells have periods of high-frequency discharge (50 ± 21 Hz) separated by pauses; and (2) 10% to 20% of cells discharge at a low frequency (18 ± 12 Hz) with high-frequency short duration bursts. GPi neurons have higher rates of discharge (82 ± 24 Hz) and are more tonic. Border cells may be encountered within the internal and external medullary laminae of the GP and have slower but regular discharge rates (34 ± 19 Hz). The caudolateral portions of the GPi (lateral 18 to 24 in the SB atlas) contain neurons that respond to passive or active movement of the limbs or orofacial structures. Sensorimotor responses are found predominantly in the posterolateral portions of the GPi. The

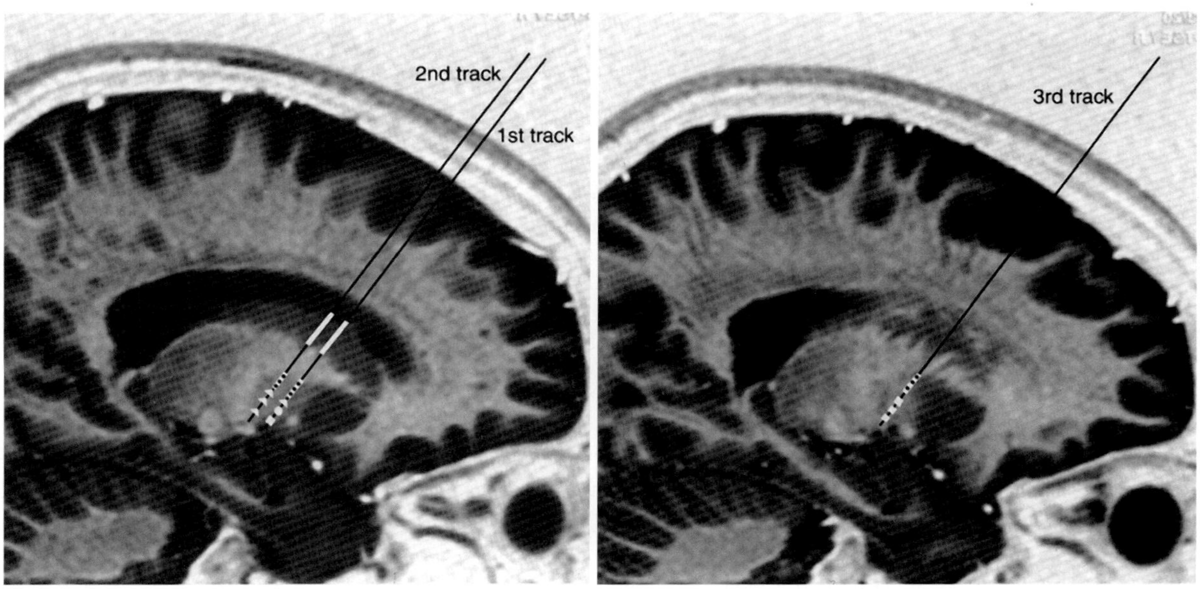

Figure 69–4 Microelectrode tracks on sagittal magnetic resonance imaging scans through the basal ganglia.

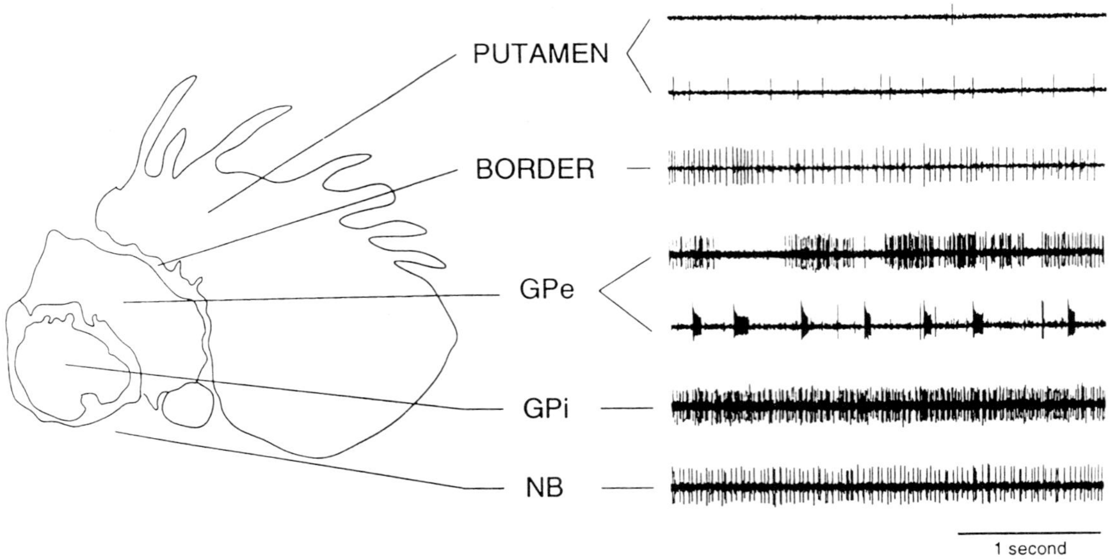

Figure 69–5 Characteristic discharge patterns in structures encountered during microelectrode recording. GPe, globus pallidus externa; GPi, globus pallidus interna; NB,nucleus basalis.

somatotopic organization of the sensorimotor GPi places the leg dorsal and medial to the arm representations. The responses are elicited by moving individual joints on the contralateral limbs. After passing through the GP, the electrode may enter the OT or the corticospinal tract (CST). The CST is identified by stimulation-evoked muscle contractions in the leg, arm, and face. The optic tract is identified by flashing a strobe light in the patient's eyes and listening for high-frequency modulation of the background audio signal. Alternatively, the OT can be identified by microstimulation in which patients report seeing flashes of light in the contralateral visual field.

As the cells, described above, are encountered, their depths are recorded as tick marks on scaled reconstructions of the electrode track. The receptive fields and stimulation thresholds are labeled on the track reconstructions. Subsequent tracks are usually placed anterior or posterior to the initial track to help define the AP dimensions of GPi. After the AP plane is determined, a lateral track is placed to delineate the lateral portion of the GPi. The microelectrode track reconstructions are then superimposed on sagittal sections from a standard human brain atlas, such as the SB atlas, using the surgical team's "best fit." Using this technique, the boundaries of the GPi and surrounding structures are determined relative to the stereotactic coordinate system. This registration is then used to determine the location for placement of the lesion or DBS lead.

Localization of the Nucleus Ventralis Intermedius

Microelectrode localization involves identification and localization of tremor-related cells in the arm area of ventral Vim and identification of the anterior border of nucleus ventrocaudalis (Vc) and the CST. The microelectrode is passed in the parasagittal plane proceeding in the anterodorsal to posteroventral direction. The first target encountered, with advancing of the microelectrode, is the caudate. It has a very slow rate of discharge (0 to 10 Hz). Cells in Vim respond to passive (somatosensory) manipulation, whereas cells in the nucleus Voa and Vop respond more selectively to voluntary movement and less to passive manipulation. The medial-lateral position of the electrode in Vim is based on the somatotopic organization of the cells; from medial to lateral are face/jaw, arm, and leg. The posterior border of Vim is formed by Vc. The anterior border of Vc is characterized by the presence of cells that respond to light touch (tactile cells) and low threshold, microstimulation-induced paresthesias. The lateral border of Vim is adjacent to the CST where microstimulation produces intense short-latency muscle contractions involving more than one limb. As before, the responses to microstimulation, sensory thresholds, and spontaneous activity patterns are recorded.

Localization of the Subthalamic Nucleus

The STN has a high cell density with mean discharge rates of 20 to 30 Hz. The apparent discharge rate is much higher due to the high cell density and simultaneous recording from multiple cells. As the microelectrode passes through the inferior border of STN into substantia Nigra (SNr), the mean discharge rate of individual neurons increases (60 to 80 Hz) and the discharge pattern becomes more tonic. The medial and lateral borders are formed by lemniscal and corticospinal fibers, respectively, and are identified by microstimulation-evoked sensory and motor responses. The track reconstructions are superimposed on standard parasagittal cuts.

Macrostimulation

Macrostimulation involves passing current through the lesioning probe or the DBS electrode. Visual, motor, and cutaneous sensory responses may be evoked by stimulation of OT, CST, and somesthetic pathways, respectively. The response of parkinsonian symptoms to the macrostimulation provides another indication of the accuracy of probe placement. Intraoperative suppression of tremor in the Vim and of rigidity and bradykinesia in STN and GPi are important predictors of a favorable outcome. In the GPi, acute suppression of symptoms of bradykinesia are not always apparent with stimulation, but this does not predict an unfavorable outcome.

Intraoperative testing of the DBS electrode provides the final confirmation for stimulator lead location. For placement of the pallidal lead, proximity of the active contacts to the inferior and posteromedial borders of GPi is indicated by current thresholds for activating the OT and CST, respectively. For placement of the thalamic lead, proximity of active contacts to posterior and lateral borders of Vim is indicated by activation of Vc and CST, respectively. For placement of the STN lead, proximity of active contacts to the medial or inferior borders of STN is indicated by activation of lemniscal fibers, whereas proximity to the lateral border of STN is indicated by activation of the CST.

Fig. 69–6 shows coronal and sagittal MRI of a right pallidal DBS and a left pallidotomy in the same patient. The stimulation electrode contacts are labeled 0 to 3.

Lesioning

Once the target is defined, the recording microelectrode is replaced by the lesioning electrode. Lesion generation is accomplished by using radiofrequency (RF) thermocoagulation. Alternating current at an RF of 500,000 Hz is passed through a monopolar electrode at the lesioning site to a large surface electrode on the patient's skin. The diameter of the coagulum varies from 1 to 4 mm for temperatures from 60° to 90°C for a duration of 60 seconds. Making multiple lesions along a single track or multiple tracks can modify the final lesion size and shape. During lesioning, the size of the lesion is gradually increased by increasing the temperature by 5° or 10° while the patient is examined for any change in strength, speech, or vision.

Closure

Ablative Surgery

After lesioning is completed, the electrode is removed. The fibrin glue is removed and the wound is copiously irrigated with saline. The dural defect is filled with a piece of Gelfoam. The bur hole is covered with methylmethacrylate or a metal plate. The galea is closed with generic interrupted, inverted sutures. The skin is closed with a continuous nylon suture.

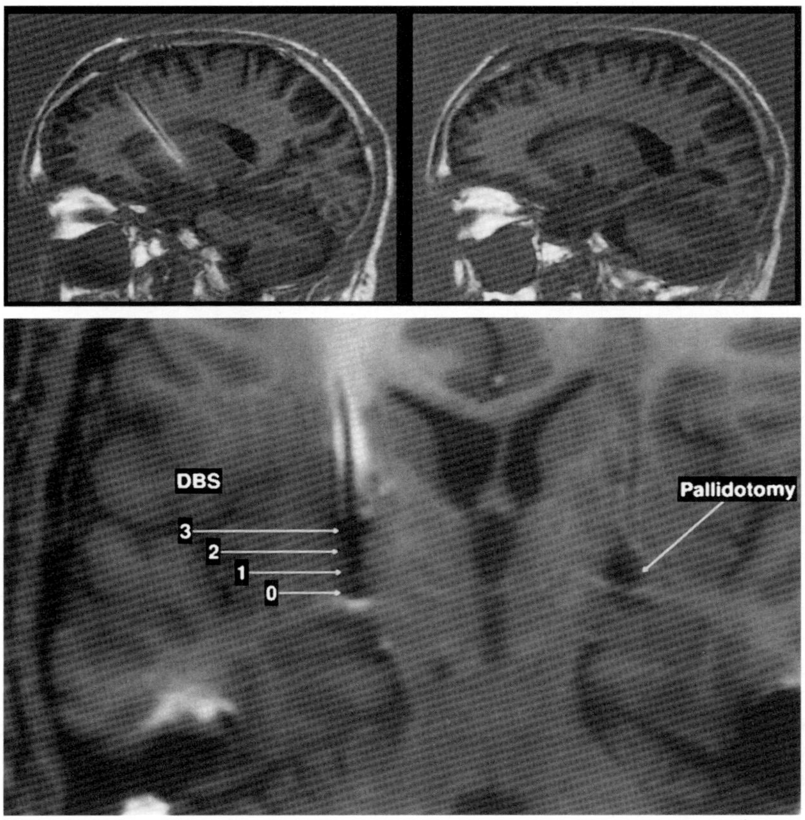

Figure 69–6 Sagittal (top) and coronal (bottom) magnetic resonance imaging of a right pallidal deep brain stimulation (DBS) and a left pallidotomy in the same patient. 0–3, stimulation electrode contacts.

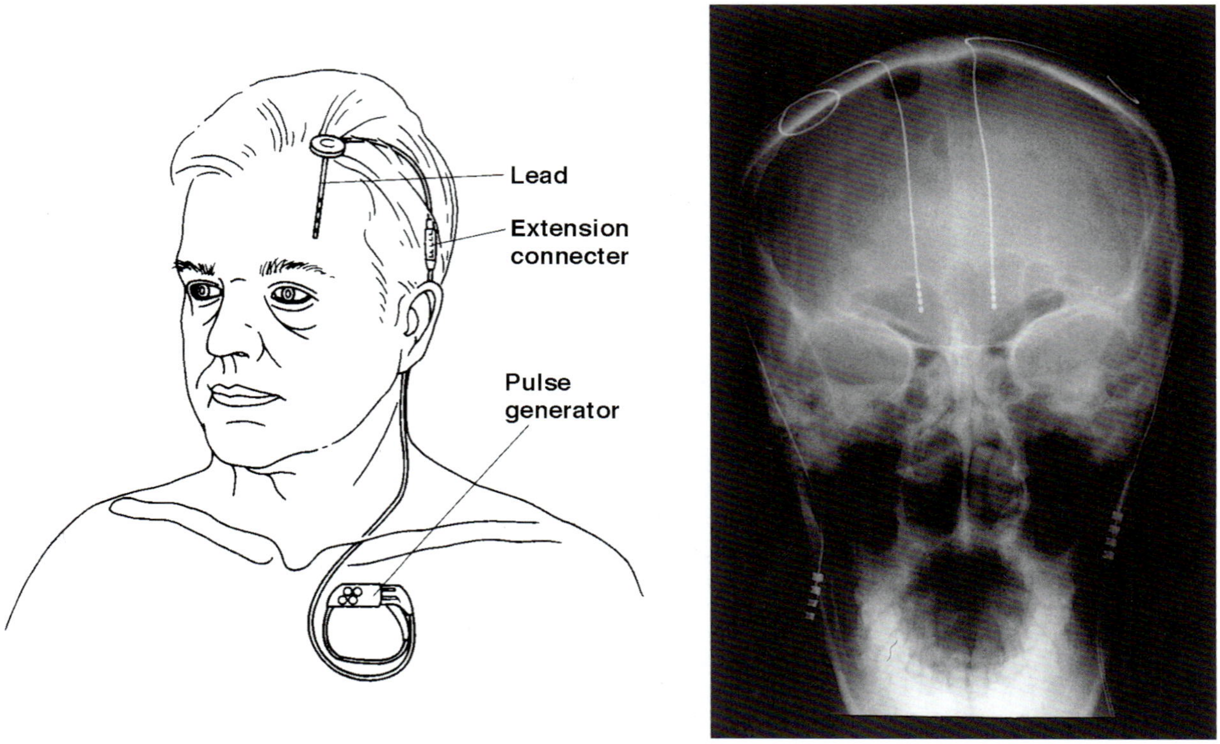

Figure 69–7 (Left) Connections for a complete deep brain stimulation (DBS) system. (Right) Anteroposterior cranial x-ray after placement of a Medtronic quadripolar DBS electrode into the subthalamic nucleus bilaterally. Note the tension release coil on the skull.

Deep Brain Stimulation

The head stage is disassembled and removed carefully, leaving the stimulation electrode in place. The lead is secured to a bur hole cap. The use of a C-arm is highly recommended to prevent and, if necessary, correct any movement of the electrode depth during disassembly or placement of the cap. The distal end of the stimulation electrode is placed in a subcuticular pocket just posterior to the ear. The connector for externalization can be used to help identify the distal lead location in subsequent procedures. The galea and skin are closed as described above. The internalization of the generator can be performed immediately or in a delayed manner. A skin incision is made in the ipsilateral anterior chest a few centimeters inferior to the clavicle. A subcutaneous pocket is created for placement of the generator for stimulation. A skin incision is made just posterior to the ear, and the distal lead of the stimulation electrode is retrieved. The extension cable connecting the electrode to the generator is tunneled under the skin from the posterior auricular incision down to the pocket below the clavicle. The extension cable is connected to the electrode proximally, which rests on the skull surface, and to the generator distally. The generator is placed in the subcutaneous pocket and secured to the pectoralis fascia with silk sutures. The incisions are then irrigated and approximated with inverted, interrupted sutures and closed with subcuticular sutures and Steri-Strips. The connections for a complete DBS system implanted on the left side of the patient are shown in **Fig. 69–7,** which also shows an AP cranial x-ray obtained after the placement of a Medtronic (Jacksonville, FL) quadripolar DBS electrode into the subthalamic nucleus bilaterally. Note the tension release coil on the skull.

◆ Postoperative Care

An MRI or CT scan of the brain is obtained in the postanesthesia unit immediately after the procedure to evaluate for surgical complications. The antiparkinsonian medications are resumed and perioperative antibiotics are continued for 24 hours after surgery. Patients undergoing ablative surgery are usually discharged the following day. Patients undergoing DBS are monitored in the hospital for a few days to adjust the generator parameters for optimal performance. The sutures are usually removed 10 to 14 days after the procedure.

◆ Complications

Ablative Surgery

Internal Segment of the Globus Pallidus

Injuries to the OT or the CST are the two most common complications of lesioning GPi secondary to the close proximity of the inferior border to the OT and the medial border to the CST. Other complications include intracranial hemorrhage, ischemic stroke, and infection. Worsening of speech articulation, verbal fluency, swallowing difficulties, and cognitive deficits (large anterior lesions) have been reported with unilateral pallidotomy, but are two to three times more frequently reported with bilateral pallidotomy.

Nucleus Ventralis Intermedius

Common short-term complications from thalamotomy include lip or hand numbness, dysarthria, hypotonia, confusion, and contralateral weakness. Long-term complications include all the above complications and worsening of preoperative dysarthria or hypophonia, arm dyspraxia, cognitive dysfunction, and occasionally dysmetria.

Deep Brain Stimulation

The complications with DBS have reportedly been minimal. The operative complications in DBS are the same as with lesioning, but the adjustability of stimulation parameters provides the flexibility to minimize side effects while maximizing the beneficial effects. DBS is potentially safer in regions where lesioning might have unacceptable risks such as STN, or contralateral to preexisting Vim or GPi lesions. The same profile of complications is possible but can be minimized or reversed with adjustment of the stimulation parameters. In contrast to bilateral lesioning procedures, bilateral stimulation can be performed without the same increase in complications.

◆ Conclusion

The surgical targets and localization techniques for ablation and DBS have been described. The selection of a target site depends on the patient's symptomatology. Vim stimulation/ablation is efficacious for relief of parkinsonian tremor. DBS procedures offer a potential advantage over ablation in that they are adjustable and reversible. On the other hand, DBS requires considerable postoperative care and periodic battery replacement. In the short-term, Vim DBS has been shown to be just as effective but with fewer side effects than thalamotomy. To determine whether stimulation of the different targets is clinically superior to ablation requires a well-controlled, long-term (5 to 10 years) study with a large number of patients using standardized measures of motor function, patient disability, and quality of life.

Suggested Readings

Alexander GE, Crutcher MD, DeLong MR. Basal ganglia-thalamocortical circuits: parallel substrates for motor, oculomotor, "prefrontal" and "limbic" functions. Prog Brain Res 1990;85:119–146

Bakay RAE, Vitek JL, DeLong MR. Thalamotomy for tremor. In: Rengachary SS, Wilkins RH, eds. Neurosurgical Operative Atlas. Vol 2. Baltimore: Williams & Wilkins; 1992:299–312

Benabid AL, Pollak P, Gao D, et al. Chronic electrical stimulation of the ventralis intermedius nucleus of the thalamus as a treatment of movement disorders. J Neurosurg 1996;84:203–214

Blond S, Siegfried J. Thalamic stimulation for the treatment of tremor and other movement disorders. Acta Neurochir Suppl (Wien) 1991; 52:109–111

Fazzini E, Dogali M, Stereo D, Eidelberg D, Beric A. Stereotactic pallidotomy for Parkinson's disease: a long-term follow-up of unilateral pallidotomy. Neurology 1997;48:1273–1277

Giller CA, Dewey RB, Ginsburg MI, Mendelsohn DB, Berk AM. Stereotactic pallidotomy and thalamotomy using individual variations of anatomic landmarks for localization. Neurosurgery 1998;42:56–62

Guridi J, Lozano AM. A brief history of pallidotomy. Neurosurgery 1997;41:1169–1178

Hutchison WD, Lozano AM, Tasker RR, Lang AE, Dostrovsky JO. Identification and characterization of neurons with tremor-frequency activity in human globus pallidus. Exp Brain Res 1997;113:557–563

Krack P, Pollak P, Limousin P, et al. Subthalamic nucleus or internal pallidal stimulation in young onset Parkinson's disease. Brain 1998;121: 451–457

Laitinen LV, Bergenheim AT, Hariz MI. Leksell's posteroventral pallidotomy in the treatment of Parkinson's disease. J Neurosurg 1992;76: 53–61

Lenz FA, Dostrovsky JO, Kwan HC, Tasker RR, Yamashiro K, Murphy JT. Methods for microstimulation and recording of single neurons and evoked potentials in the human central nervous system. J Neurosurg 1988;68:630–634

Lozano A, Hutchison W, Kiss Z, Tasker R, Davis K, Dostrovsky J. Methods for micro-electrode-guided posteroventral pallidotomy. J Neurosurg 1996;84:194–202

Schuurman PR, Bosch DA, Bossuyt PM, et al. A comparison of continuous thalamic stimulation and thalamotomy for suppression of severe tremor. N Engl J Med 2000;342:461–468

Starr PA, Vitek JL, Bakay RAE. Ablative surgery and deep brain stimulation for Parkinson's disease. Neurosurgery 1998;43:989–1013

Starr PA, Vitek JL, DeLong MR, Mewes K, Bakay RAE. Pallidotomy: theory and technique. In: Techniques in Neurosurgery. Vol 5. Philadelphia: Lippincott Williams & Wilkins; 1999:1–15

Sterio D, Beric A, Dogali M, Fazzini E, Alfaro G, Devinsky O. Neurophysiological properties of pallidal neurons in Parkinson's disease. Ann Neurol 1994;35:586–591

Svennilson E, Torvik A, Lowe R, Leksell L. Treatment of parkinsonism by stereotactic thermolesions in the pallidal region: a clinical evaluation of 81 cases. Acta Psychiatr Scand 1960;35:358–377

Taha JM, Favre J, Baumann TK, Burchief KJ. Tremor control after pallidotomy in patients with Parkinson's disease: correlation with microrecording findings. J Neurosurg 1997;86:642–647

Vitek JL, Bakay RAE, DeLong MR. Microelectrode-guided pallidotomy for medically intractable Parkinson's disease. Adv Neurol 1997;74:183–198

Vitek JL, Bakay RAE, Hashimoto T, et al. Microelectrode-guided pallidotomy: technical approach and its application in medically intractable Parkinson's disease. J Neurosurg 1998;88:1027–1043

70

Spasmodic Torticollis

Ronald R. Tasker

Spasmodic torticollis (ST) is a striking disease whose often dramatic presentation has led to an incorrect diagnosis of psychogenic disease. Today it is considered a focal form of primary dystonia, and the reader is referred to several contemporary reviews.[1–5] The cause is unknown and no underlying responsible pathological change has been identified. ST affects patients of either sex, usually in midlife, often beginning with minor symptoms that progress over 3 to 5 years and then remain fixed in a final postural abnormality that ranges from mild to severe. Only neck muscles are affected and the head usually rotates to either right or left, associated with tilting either toward or away from the side to which the chin turns (**Fig. 70–1**). A small number of patients develop pure antecollis, thrusting the chin on the chest or retrocollis producing the reverse deformity. ST is distinguished from other types of torticollis by the presence of spasmodic contractions in the affected muscles. ST is a postural or action dyskinesia so that unless secondary skeletal changes supervene, the head returns to a normal position when it is no longer being actively supported, as when the patient lies down or sits with the head, neck, and back supported against a firm object. In addition to the postural abnormality, neck pain is often present.

Indications for Surgery

Surgical treatment can be considered when conservative measures have failed and the patient is disabled in the activities of daily living by the abnormal head posture and the associated pain. The posture is particularly aggravated by physical activity such as driving a motor vehicle or crossing a street in traffic, exposing the patient to accidents. A variety of surgical procedures have been suggested for treating ST as outlined in **Table 70–1.** Botulinum toxin injection into the offending muscles is probably the most frequently employed treatment currently.[6] Unfortunately, although the initial results are often very satisfactory, the injections must be repeated about every 3 months; they are expensive, and repeated injections may eventually lose their efficacy. Dorsal column stimulation has seen limited exploitation, and the results appear to be unpredictable,[7,8] though the simplicity and safety of the procedure compared with others have to be kept in mind. Though an early strategy in treating ST, myotomy is seldom used today,[9] and iontophoresis of the labyrinth carries perhaps a 1 in 3 possibility of long-term improvement in symptoms.[10,11] Microvascular decompression of the cranial nerve XI[12,13] is an intriguing option that needs further exploration. Stereotactic procedures with various target sites have been used for many years, but only small series have been reported, again with unpredictable results.[14–20]

The most commonly used operation is a combination of muscle denervation and multiple rhizotomy. The traditional procedure is the so-called Dandy-McKenzie operation.[5,21–25] In McKenzie's hands this consists of selective denervation of the offending sternomastoid muscle in the neck in cases of rotation followed at a second sitting by bilateral anterior

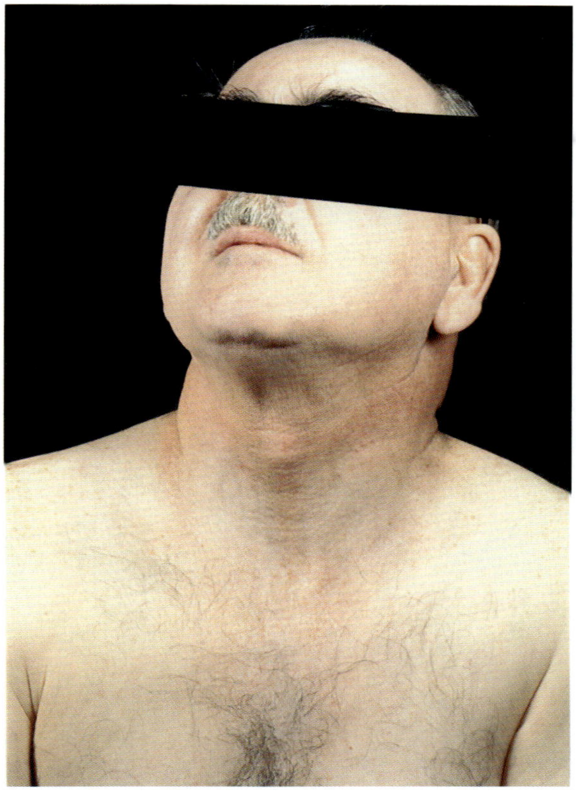

Figure 70–1 Patient with typical rotatory spasmodic torticollis.

rhizotomy from C1 to C3 plus section of the C4 ventral root on the worse affected side. In cases of retrocollis without rotation, only the rhizotomy would be done. However, this procedure has several disadvantages. It is an indiscriminate denervation of the muscles supplied by both anterior and posterior rami throughout the area, all of which may not actually be involved in generating the torticollis. Muscles below C3–C4 often contribute to torticollis, and anterior rhizotomies cannot be done at these lower levels because these roots also supply the upper limbs. Moreover, the operation exposes patients to two rare serious complications: iatrogenic cervical subluxation often with cord compression, presumably the result of interference with facet joints and paralysis of all the local muscles, and myelopathy from inadvertent interruption of a segmental endartery to the cord.[26]

Table 70–1 Treatments Proposed to Treat Spasmodic Torticollis

Botulinum toxin injections
Dorsal column stimulation
Myotomy
Iontophoresis of the labyrinth
Microvascular decompression of cranial nerve XI
Stereotactic
Pallidotomy
Thalamotomy
Other
Multiple neurectomy, muscle denervation
Multiple rhizotomy

In response to these disadvantages Bertrand[3,4,27] has evolved the procedure of multiple posterior ramisectomy accompanied by selective neurectomy of affected muscles wherever possible, the whole procedure being guided by preoperative electromyographic identification of the muscles at fault.

This chapter describes selective denervation of the sternomastoid muscle, the Dandy-McKenzie anterior rhizotomy, and ramisectomy.

◆ Selective Denervation of the Sternomastoid Muscle

Preoperative Studies and Patient Preparation

Although sternomastoid denervation alone is seldom adequate on its own to treat ST, in a small number of cases it may suffice, and so it is usually done first, to be followed, if necessary, by rhizotomy or ramisectomy. It is useful to first carry out diagnostic local anesthetic blockade of the affected sternomastoid muscle to try to predict the result of surgical denervation. The offending muscle is the one that is opposite to the side to which the chin turns, is often hypertrophied, and is the subject of spasmodic contractions. If there is no medical contraindication, 2% lidocaine hydrochloride, 2 to 5 mL, with norepinephrine is injected into the muscle belly about the midpoint of the posterior margin of the sternomastoid in an attempt to block the several sternomastoid branches of cranial nerve XI.

Anesthesia

Selective denervation of the sternomastoid muscle is usually done under general anesthesia without muscle paralysis to facilitate nerve stimulation during the course of the operation.

Positioning

With a pillow under the shoulder on the operative side, the patient's head is rotated to the opposite side.

Operation

A 6 cm incision is made along the posterior margin of the sternocleidomastoid muscle centered on the midpoint between the mastoid process and the sternal manubrium **(Fig. 70–2).** This is deepened until the muscle itself is visualized and the posterior margin cleared, revealing the external jugular vein, great auricular nerve, and anterior cutaneous nerve of the neck **(Fig. 70–3).** Although the accessory nerve lies superficial to the deep fascia of the posterior triangle, it is usually not visible, being covered by connective

Figure 70–2 Incision for selective denervation of the sternomastoid muscle.

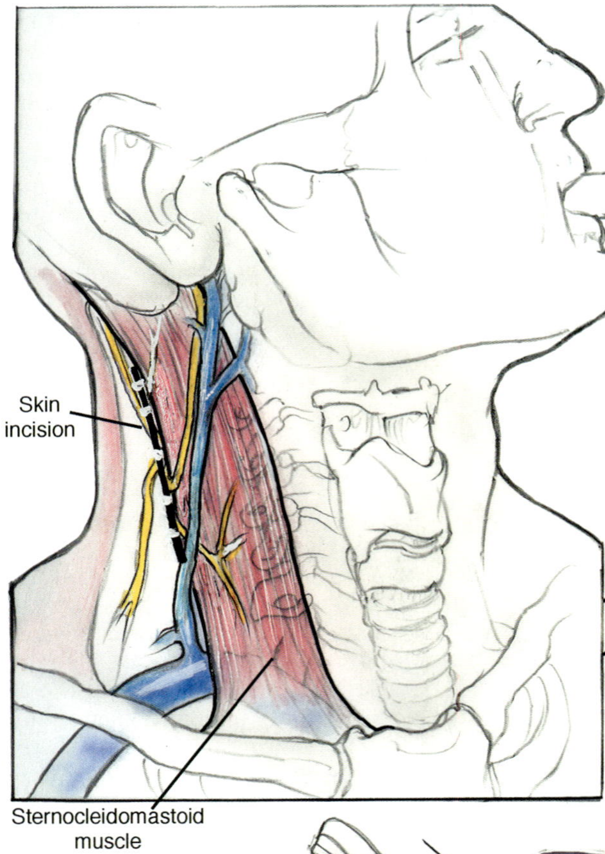

Figure 70–3 Superficial anatomy for sternomastoid denervation.

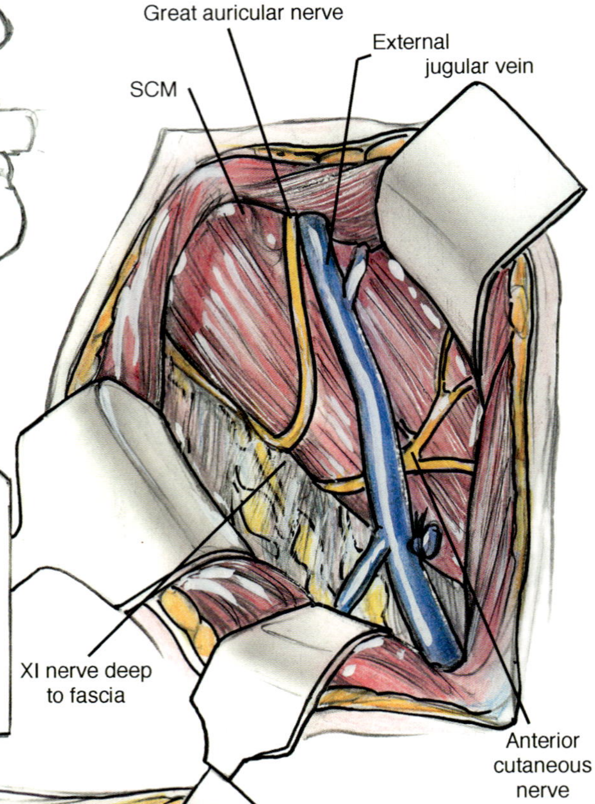

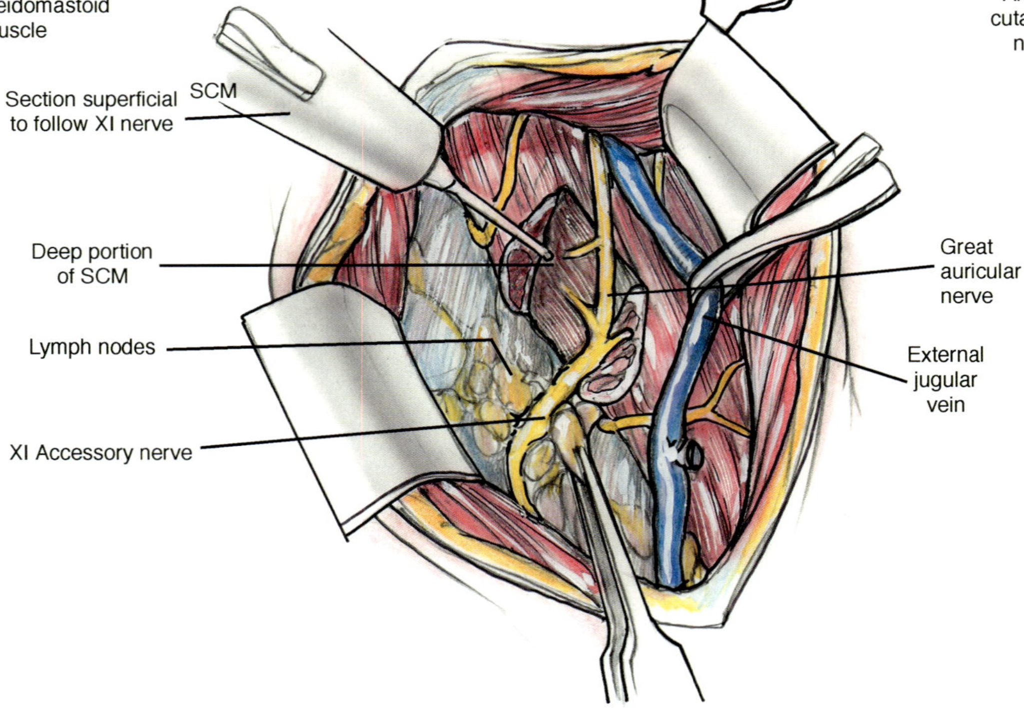

Figure 70–4 Anatomy of cranial nerve XI in the neck during sternocleidomastoid denervation.

tissue and lymph nodes. Its probable location is identified with reference to the great auricular nerve and external jugular vein, often facilitated by electrical stimulation causing contraction in the trapezius muscle. The nerve is identified and cleared and followed rostrally **(Fig. 70–4).** It usually passes through the fibers of the sternocleidomastoid obliquely in an anterosuperior direction toward the jugular foramen; rarely it lies behind the muscle. Fibers of the sternomastoid are divided to lay clear the course of cranial nerve XI through the muscle exposing its three to five sternomastoid branches that pass both superiorly and inferiorly. It is best to divide the muscle completely into the anterior triangle of the neck because the most anterior sternomastoid nerves may lie rostrally. After nerve identity is confirmed by stimulation, the nerves are divided and avulsed distally to discourage regeneration. The main trunk of cranial nerve XI should now be lying free across the sternomastoid, whereupon closure in layers is performed, suturing the aponeurosis of the sternomastoid muscle for cosmetic reasons.

Postoperative Care

No special postoperative care is necessary, and the patient is usually discharged the same day.

Complications

Local hematoma and rarely trapezius weakness from neurapraxia are the only significant complications.

◆ Multiple Anterior Rhizotomy

The second part of the Dandy-McKenzie operation, multiple anterior rhizotomy, is usually performed at a separate sitting after assessment of the results of the sternomastoid denervation in cases of rotatory ST. In a few cases sternomastoid denervation alone may suffice.

Preoperative Studies and Patient Preparation

Plain films of the cervical spine are useful to alert the surgeon to any skeletal problems. Preoperative preparation is the same as for any cervical laminectomy.

Anesthesia, Monitoring, and Patient Positioning

Routine monitoring of sensory evoked potentials and corticospinal function is done. Under general anesthesia the patient is positioned prone with pin fixation of the head, the neck well flexed in such a way that the cervical spine lies horizontal and above the level of the heart to minimize bleeding.

Operation

A midline incision is made from the inion to the spine of C6 and the muscles taken off to reveal the rim of the foramen magnum above and the spines and laminae of C1 to C5 below. A bilateral laminectomy is carried from C1 to C5, and if necessary the occipital rim of the foramen magnum is removed. After a longitudinal midline dural opening and stitching back of the dura to the muscles, the cisterna magna is drained and the attachments of the dentate ligaments to the dura throughout the intended exposure are severed. Under the operating microscope the dorsal roots of C2 to C4 are visualized bilaterally, emerging from the dorsal root line of the spinal cord **(Fig. 70–5A).** By searching in the depths of the exposure the ventral roots of C2, C3 and C4 are identified **(Fig. 70–5A).** The segmental radicular arteries are carefully separated from the ventral roots and the latter then cauterized and divided at C2 and C3 bilaterally and C4 on the worse affected side.

The anatomy at C1 requires special attention **(Fig. 70–5B).** Rostral to the level of the dorsal root at C2, cranial nerve XI is identified with its spinal and, more cephalad, cranial contributions. It lies deep to the level of the C2 dorsal roots with the fibers arising from the branchial cleft of the spinal cord. Because the sternocleidomastoid has been selectively denervated in the neck (if necessary), cranial nerve XI is not disturbed intraspinally. However, deep to it the motor root of C1 is sought coming off the cord in line with the already sectioned motor roots of C2 and below. It is usually small and passes out along the inferior margin of the vertebral artery. It is very carefully separated from any segmental arteries, cauterized, and divided after a careful search for and severing of any anastomoses between it and cranial nerve XI; any apparent infrequently present dorsal root fibers at C1 are also divided (not shown in **Fig. 70–5**). Closure is done in the usual way with careful attention to hemostasis and dural closure.

Postoperative Care

The patient is preferably monitored in an intensive care or step-down unit for the first day postoperatively to avoid any respiratory complications. A soft collar increases the patient's comfort over the first few days, and the usual analgesic procedures for a postoperative laminectomy are used. Patients often report feeling that "my head is going to fall off" for the first few days postoperatively. An early physiotherapy program is organized to help with neck posture and mobility.

Complications

Serial plain films of the cervical spine postoperatively will help guard against the risk of iatrogenic cervical subluxation. Careful microdissection of the radicular arteries greatly reduces the risk of ischemic myelopathy. We have not seen significant dysphagia as a complication of the procedure or any respiratory complications if C4 is preserved unilaterally.

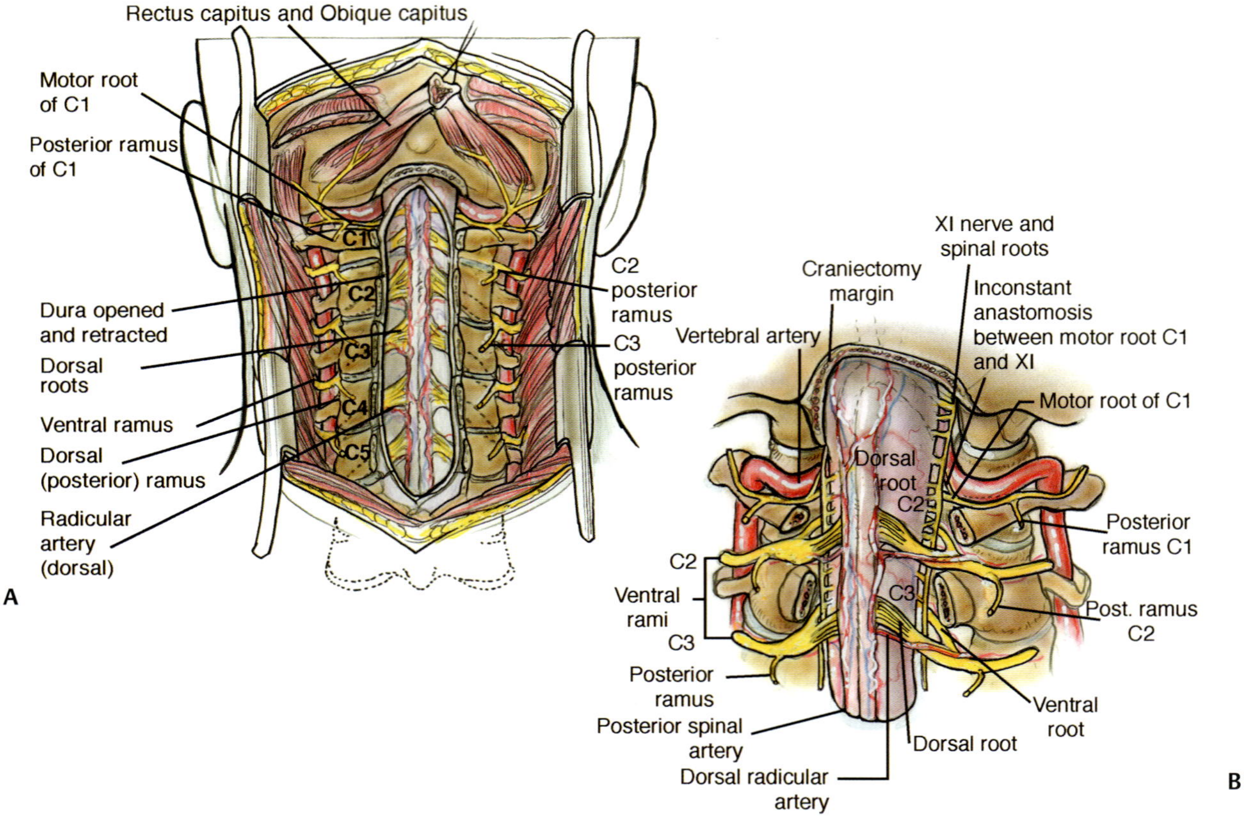

Figure 70–5 Exposure for the anterior rhizotomy portion of the Dandy-McKenzie operation. **(A)** After bilateral laminectomy C1–C5. **(B)** C1 anatomy.

◆ Multiple Posterior Ramisectomy

This procedure, like the Dandy-McKenzie anterior rhizotomy, is preceded by or accompanied by selective sternomastoid denervation in the neck in rotatory cases where electromyography (EMG) studies or local anesthetic blockade show that the sternomastoid makes a significant contribution. This description of the operation is based on publications by Bertrand and his colleagues.

Preoperative Studies

The ramisectomy is aimed at denervating the muscles, which have been shown by EMG analysis to be major contributors to the ST deformity. The operation is based on the premise that the major innervations of the muscles involved in ST are from the posterior rami as listed in **Table 70–2.** According to this analysis, the only muscles involved in ST innervated by anterior rami of the cervical nerves are the levator scapulae, sternocleidomastoid, and trapezius. **Table 70–3** lists several other neck muscles supplied by anterior rami of the upper cervical nerves, but their contribution, if any, to ST is unclear.

Anesthesia

The procedure is performed under general anesthesia with short-acting muscle paralysis to allow intraoperative stimulative studies.

Table 70–2 Innervation of Muscles Involved in Spasmodic Torticollis

Muscle	Nerve Supply
Levator scapulae	VR of C3 and C4
Longissimus capitis	PR of C3 to C8
Obliquus capitis inferior	PR of C1 and C2
Obliquus capitis superior	PR of C1
Rectus capitis posterior major	PR of C1
Rectus capitis posterior minor	PR of C1
Semispinalis capitis	PR of C1 to C6
Semispinalis cervicis	PR of C4 to C8
Splenius capitis	PR of C2 to C6
Splenius cervicis	PR of C4 to C8
Sternocleidomastoideus	Cranial nerve XI, VR of C2 and C3
Trapezius	Cranial nerve XI, VR of C3 and C4

PR, posterior ramus; VR, ventral ramus.

From Bertrand CM, Molina-Negro P, Bouvier G, Benabou R. Surgical treatment of spasmodic torticollis. In: Youmans JR, ed. Neurological Surgery. 4th ed. Philadelphia: Saunders; 1996: 3701–3712.

Table 70–3 Muscles Supplied by Cervical Anterior Rami

Deep Branches—Medial Series	
Communicating branches with	
Hypoglossal	C1, C2
Vagus	C1, C2
Sympathetic	C1, C2, C3, C4
Muscular branches to	
Rectus capitis lateralis	C1
Rectus capitis anterior	C1, C2
Longus capitis	C1, C2, C3
Longus colli	C2, C3, C4
Inferior root of ansa cervicalis	C2, C3
Phrenic	C3, C4, C5
Lateral Series	
Trapezius	C2
Levator scapulae	C3, C4
Scalenus medius	C3, C4

Source: Warwick R, Williams PL, eds. Gray's Anatomy. 35th ed. New York: Longman; 1993:1036.

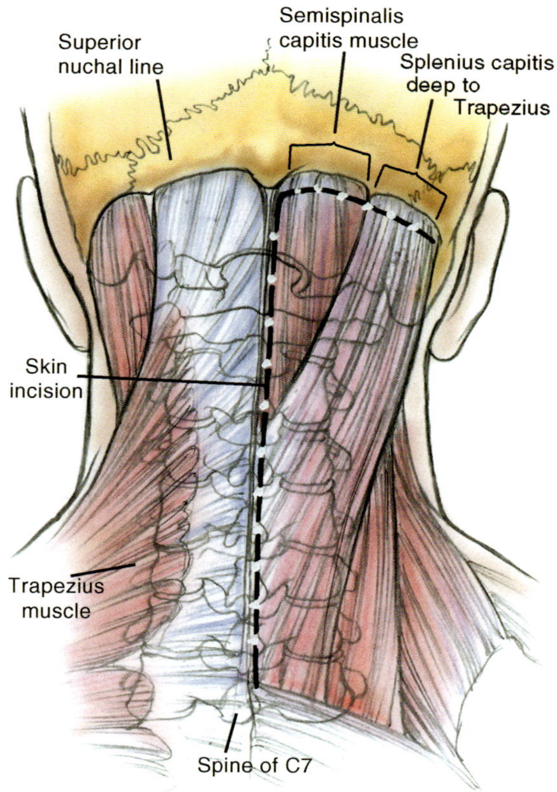

Figure 70–6 The incision and exposure for Bertrand's multiple ramisectomy procedure. (Adapted from Youmans JR, ed. Neurological Surgery. 4th ed. Philadelphia: Saunders; 1996:3708.)

Positioning

As Bertrand et al[3] prefer to do the procedure, the patient is placed in the sitting position, and the usual monitoring techniques are set up, including an esophageal stethoscope, intraarterial pulmonary artery pressure, and central venous pressure monitoring to guard against air embolism. This procedure is usually done on one side with the patient's head fixed in the Gardner headrest, the neck flexed, and the head turned slightly toward the opposite side, although bilateral procedures can be done simultaneously, with the same positioning, except that the head is not turned.

Procedure

An L-shaped incision is made over the attachments of the nuchal muscles to the skull starting at the midline and extending laterally and the longitudinal limb of the incision is carried in the midline to the spine of C7 **(Figs. 70–6** and **70–7).** The trapezius, splenius, and supraspinatus capitis muscles are divided along the horizontal limb of the incision just below their attachments to the skull and their whole muscle mass retracted laterally. The muscles are then carefully dissected in the natural plane of cleavage from the posterior arches of C1 and C2 and the articular facets from C2-C3 to C5-C6. The procedure is then pursued under magnification; Bertrand recommends magnifying glasses and frontal light rather than a microscope. The C1 root is located under the vertebral artery at the level of the notch of the posterior arch of C1 from which it is dissected peripherally. Medial stimulation is performed to avoid denervation of the muscles supplied by the anterior ramus of C1 (omohyoid, stylohyoid, and thyrohyoid) to avoid dysphagia, although the author has not seen this complication after complete anterior rhizotomy at C1 and C2. However, the anterior ramus is not regularly located. When the posterior ramus has been isolated and its identity confirmed by stimulation, it is clipped and divided proximally. The distal portion is avulsed to discourage regeneration (but not the proximal!). Section of the inferior oblique muscle facilitates exposure of the C1 and C2 roots, the latter emerging between the posterior arches of the atlas and axis. Their anterior ramus lies deep and can be identified by stimulation-induced contraction of throat muscles; if it is identified, it is spared. The posterior ramus of C2 is then sectioned distal to any identified anterior ramus, and the peripheral portions avulsed. The posterior rami of C3 to C6 are located with the help of stimulation deep to the semispinatus capitis between the corresponding articular facets, where they rise up from the depths in the notch seen on an anteroposterior (AP) view of these structures **(Fig. 70–7).** They are followed as far as possible toward their corresponding intervertebral foramina below to identify and allow the section of early branches especially prevalent at C3. After proximal clipping and dividing, the distal portions are avulsed and further stimulation is used to search for remaining elements of the posterior rami. If simultaneous bilateral ramisectomy is to be done, Bertrand cautions against carrying out the ramisectomy lower than C5. Closure is performed in the usual way.

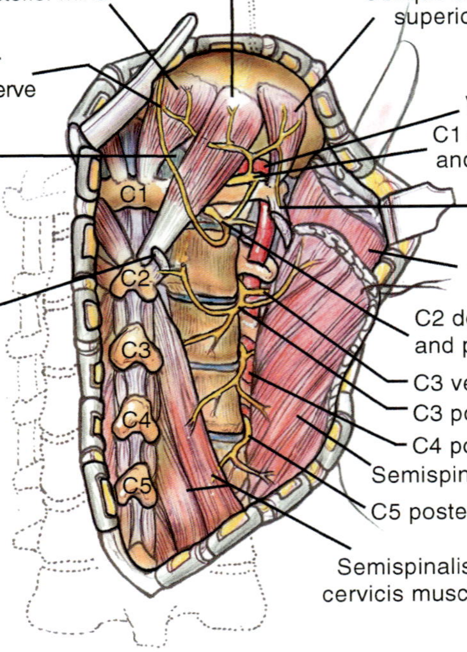

Figure 70–7 Detail of the rostral portion of the exposure in Fig. 70–6 showing the sectioning of the sternomastoid, splenius, and trapezius as well as of the inferior oblique.

Postoperative Care

The patient requires appropriate analgesia postoperatively, and Bertrand recommends nursing in the semisitting position. Within a few days the patient is ready for discharge and is enrolled in an active physiotherapy program for the next 6 to 12 weeks.

In the course of Bertrand's operation it appears that the sensory branch of the posterior ramus of C2, which constitutes the greater occipital nerve, is divided so that occipital numbness is a result of the procedure, with the concomitant small risk of neuropathic pain.

◆ Percutaneous Radiofrequency Division of the Posterior Rami

An alternative strategy is to combine total motor (ventral) rhizotomy at C1 and C2, if indicated by the EMG studies, as in the Dandy-McKenzie procedure, with percutaneous radiofrequency section of the posterior rami at the lower levels, as indicated by the selective EMG studies. It may be simpler to completely denervate the upper cervical muscles at C1 and C2 by intradural section, and this author has never seen dysphagia as a result.

Procedure

The technique is the same as for percutaneous radiofrequency facet denervation. With the patient in the prone position, using general anesthesia and short-acting muscle paralysis to allow intraoperative motor stimulation, the cervical spine is visualized with AP image intensification. The "notches" on the lateral aspects of the articular processes of C3 to C6 are identified (**Fig. 70–7**) and a radiofrequency lesioning electrode for facet denervation, such as that provided by Diros Technology (Toronto, Canada), is introduced to that site. The tip of the needle should reach bone just at the lateral margin of the articular facet as viewed in the AP direction, whereupon stimulation at 2 Hz is performed with a suitable electronic backup such as that produced by Diros. The electrode is repositioned if necessary until 2 Hz contractions are produced segmentally in the paraspinal muscles with voltages at or below 1.0 with the Diros equipment. Suprathreshold stimulation is then applied to ensure that contractions do not occur in muscles supplied by the anterior rami of these nerves below 7 to 10 V. When these criteria have been satisfied, maximum radiofrequency lesions are made, gradually increasing current flow and probe tip temperature until current fall-off occurs. No special preparation or postoperative care is necessary.

Complications

The potential complications of the procedure are damage to anterior rami so as to produce numbness or weakness, particularly in the upper limbs, and damage to radicular arteries, which if they are end arteries to the spinal cord could produce myelopathy, as well as incomplete section of all posterior elements. Damage to ventral rami has never occurred in our hands with use of the stimulation strategy outlined above. The same strategy keeps the electrode tip sufficiently distant from the anterior rami to avoid the radicular arteries. Regeneration of the posterior rami with time is probably no more likely than after the open ramisectomy as performed by Bertrand. The percutaneous procedure can easily be repeated.

◆ Conclusion

The Dandy-McKenzie procedure is the most frequently employed operation for the relief of ST and the one with the longest track record. However, it has its limitations and risks, so that when surgical therapy is indicated, the surgeon should be aware of all options.

References

1. Gildenberg PL, Tasker RR. Spasmodic torticollis. Contemp Neurosurg 1982;4:1–8
2. Tasker RR. Overview of the surgical treatment of spasmodic torticollis. In: Gildenberg PL, Tasker RR, eds. Textbook of Stereotactic and Functional Neurosurgery. New York: McGraw-Hill; 1998:1053–1058
3. Bertrand C, Molina-Negro P, Bouvier G, Benabou R. Surgical treatment of spasmodic torticollis. In: Youmans JR, ed. Neurological Surgery. 4th ed. Philadelphia: Saunders; 1996:3701–3712
4. Bertrand CM. Surgical management of spasmodic torticollis and adult-onset dystonia. In: Schmidek HH, Sweet WH, eds. Operative Neurosurgical Techniques: Indications, Methods, and Results. 3rd ed. Philadelphia: Saunders; 1995:1649–1659
5. Villavicencio AT, Friedman AH. Intradural rhizotomy for the treatment of torticollis. In: Gildenberg PL, Tasker RR, eds. Textbook of Stereotactic and Functional Neurosurgery. New York: McGraw-Hill; 1998:1039–1051
6. Anderson T, Marsden CD. Botulinum toxin for the treatment of spasmodic torticollis and other movement disorders. In: Gildenberg PL, Tasker RR, eds. Textbook of Stereotactic and Functional Neurosurgery. New York: McGraw-Hill; 1998:1059–1069
7. Gildenberg PL. Treatment of spasmodic torticollis by dorsal column stimulation. Appl Neurophysiol 1976;41:113–121
8. Waltz JM. Computerized percutaneous multi-level spinal cord stimulation in motor disorders. Appl Neurophysiol 1982;45:73–92
9. Xinkang C. Selective resection and denervation of cervical muscles in the treatment of spasmodic torticollis: results in 60 cases. Neurosurgery 1981;8:680–688
10. Svien HJ, Cody DTR. Treatment of spasmodic torticollis by suppression of labyrinthine activity: report of a case. Mayo Clin Proc 1969;44: 825–827
11. Davis DH, Duane DD, Swenson MK. Long-term outcome of iontophoresis treatment for torticollis. Stereotact Funct Neurosurg 1996;66:198–201
12. Freckmann N, Hagenah R, Herrmann H-D, Muller D. Bilateral microsurgical lysis of the spinal accessory nerve roots for treatment of spasmodic torticollis: follow-up of 33 cases. Acta Neurochir (Wien) 1986;83:47–53
13. Jho HD, Jannetta PJ. Spasmodic torticollis treated with microvascular decompression of the spinal accessory nerve and the brainstem. J Neurosurg 1989;70:312A
14. Bertrand C, Molina-Negro P, Martinez SN. Combined stereotactic and peripheral surgical approach for spasmodic torticollis. Appl Neurophysiol 1978;41:122–133
15. Essen C, von Augustinsson L, Lindqvist G. VOI thalamotomy in spasmodic torticollis. Appl Neurophysiol 1980;43:159–163
16. Hassler R, Dieckmann G. Stereotactic treatment of different kinds of spasmodic torticollis. Confin Neurol 1970;32:135–143
17. Bertrand C. The treatment of spasmodic torticollis with particular reference to thalamotomy. In: Morley TP, ed. Current Controversies in Neurosurgery. Philadelphia: Saunders; 1976:455–459
18. Cooper IS. Effect of thalamic lesions upon torticollis. N Engl J Med 1964;270:567–572
19. Mundinger F, Riechert T, Dusselhoff J. Long-term results of stereotactic treatment of spasmodic torticollis. Confin Neurol 1972;34: 41–50
20. Sano K, Yoshioka M, Mayanagi Y, Sekino H, Yoshimasu N. Stimulation and destruction of and around the interstitial nucleus of Cajal in man. Confin Neurol 1970;32:118–125
21. McKenzie KG. The surgical treatment of spasmodic torticollis. Clin Neurosurg 1954;2:37–43
22. McKenzie KG. Intrameningeal division of the spinal accessory and roots of the upper cervical nerves for the treatment of spasmodic torticollis. Surg Gynecol Obstet 1924;39:5–10
23. Dandy WE. Operation for treatment of spasmodic torticollis. Arch Surg 1930;20:1021–1032
24. Hamby WB, Schiffer S. Spasmodic torticollis: results after cervical rhizotomy in 50 cases. J Neurosurg 1969;31:323–326
25. Friedman AH, Nashold BS Jr, Sharp R, et al. Treatment of spasmodic torticollis with intradural selective rhizotomies. J Neurosurg 1993; 78:46–53
26. Adams CBT. Vascular catastrophe following the Dandy-McKenzie operation for spasmodic torticollis. J Neurol Neurosurg Psychiatry 1984; 47:990–994
27. Bertrand CM. Surgical management of spasmodic torticollis and adult-onset dystonia with emphasis on selective denervation. In: Schmidek HH, Sweet WH, eds. Operative Neurosurgical Techniques: Indications, Methods, and Results. 2nd ed. New York: Grune & Stratton; 1988: 1261–1269

71

Intraventricular/Subarachnoid Morphine

Amal Abou-Hamden and Ghassan K. Bejjani

Background

The direct application of narcotics within the central nervous system, by the intraventricular or intraspinal routes, allows the use of smaller amounts of the medications by bypassing the hepatic metabolism and the blood–brain barrier, reaching specific receptor sites immediately. Erratic drug absorption and serum protein binding are therefore avoided. Cerebrospinal fluid (CSF) is an ideal drug delivery medium with less enzymatic activity and little protein binding compared with plasma.[1–3] Effective analgesia for severe pain states resistant to oral or parenteral administration of opioids is achieved with minimal systemic toxicity.[1,4–22]

Intraventricular versus Spinal Intrathecal Morphine

Initially used to treat cancer pain,[23–26] spinal intrathecal morphine is being used increasingly in patients with nonmalignant acute and chronic pain.[27–31] Experience with intraventricular morphine, on the other hand, has been almost exclusively limited to intractable cancer pain (**Table 71–1**).

The efficacy of the two sites is comparable, but the distribution of analgesia is limited to the inferior half of the body after lumbar spinal delivery, although it can be as high as the midcervical dermatomes.[10,12,13,22,23,32–34]

Intraventricular Morphine

Intraventricular opioids for cancer pain therapy have been used since the early 1980s.[12–14,32,35–37] Their use has been effective in the treatment of cancer pain at supradiaphragmatic or diffuse sites, particularly for cervical and craniofacial neoplastic pain syndromes, which have had poor results or unacceptable side effects from oral or parenteral morphine (**Table 71–1**).

The intraventricular administration of morphine allows its direct application to the midbrain and brain stem areas for maximal supraspinal analgesia.

At a supraspinal level, there is evidence of a moderate to high density of opiate receptors in the thalamus, amygdala, caudate, putamen, habenular nuclei, interpeduncular nucleus, locus ceruleus, periaqueductal gray, dorsal raphe nucleus, and spinal trigeminal and vagal nuclei.[38–44]

Although it has been established that morphine acts directly on these central opiate receptors, the exact mechanism by which supraspinal analgesia is achieved remains uncertain. It has been proposed that injection of morphine directly into the lateral ventricle, in close proximity to these supraspinal opioid receptors, results in pain modulation by activation of descending antinociceptive pathways that originate in the periaqueductal gray matter and inhibit the transmission of nociceptive impulses at the level of the spinal cord.[38,39,44–48] However, this hypothesis has not been supported by animal research[5] or by a clinical study that showed a facilitation of nociceptive flexion reflexes in patients with head and neck cancer pain relieved by intraventricular morphine.[50]

Patient Selection[1,6,10,51–53]

The main indications for intraventricular morphine administration are the following.[18,12,15,32,37,51]

1. Chronic pain caused by malignant tumors in terminal stages
2. Failure to achieve pain relief by medical treatment, and conventional neuroablative procedures are no longer effective or are not indicated

Table 71–1 Summary of Literature on Intraventricular Morphine

	N	Pain Distribution Diffuse	H&N	Th	A/P	Morphine Dose (mg/24 hours) Min–Max	Drug Delivery Device	Follow-up (days) Range	Average	Analgesia (%)
Leavens, 1982[12]	4	—	—	—	4	0.5–7	V.A.D.	2–90	85	75
Lobato, 1983,1985,1987[15,35,54]	44	12	19	4	9	0.25–16	V.A.D., 1 external pump	6–150	55	97
Roquefeuil, 1984[37]	8	3	1	3	1	0.4–7	V.A.D.	8–210	73	80
Nurchi, 1984[32]	5	3	2	—	—	2–4	V.A.D.	8–48		100
Thiebaut, 1985[22]	32	6	16	2	8	0.1–15	V.A.D.	4–230	50	90
Lenzi, 1985[13,14]	38	5	29	4	—	0.5–2	V.A.D.	4–292	65	95
Obbens, 1987[16]	20	—	—	—	20	3–60	V.A.D.	7–510	98	>55
Weigl, 1987[55]	8	5	3	—	—	1.5–2.7	Pump (Infusaid or Medtronic)	120–660	255	100
Brazenor, 1987[56]	1	1 thalamic infarct				50	First case of implanted pump	444		100
Lazorthes, 1985, 1988, 1995[10,11,57,58]	82	13	23	38	8	0.1–60	V.A.D	12–443	65	80
Blond, 1989[5]	79	19	58	2	—	0.05–3	V.A.D.	3–132	65	94
Dennis, 1990[51]	7	1*	6	—	—	0.1–24.8	Infusaid pump	14–1105	264	83
Reeve, 1990[59]	2	1	1			3–5				
						Diamorphine HCl	V.A.D.	56–588	322	100
Smith, 1991[60]	1	1				1	V.A.D.			
							Stereotaxic placement	140		100
Shoulong, 1991[21]	28					0.05–3	Patient-controlled apparatus (L-224)	5–221	57	96
Schultheiss, 1992[19]	12	6	6	—	—	0.05–6	Manual drug release system	100		100
Lajat, 1992[9]	63					0.5–2.4	V.A.D.	75		75
Cramond, 1993[1]	52	19	16	11	6	0.15–20	V.A.D.	7–525		96
Karavelis, 1996[8]	90	17[67]	27			0.25–4	V.A.D.	1–1362	95	90

H&N, head and neck; Th, thoracic; A/P, abdominopelvic; V.A.D., ventricular access device such as Ommaya or Cordis reservoir.

*Postpolio syndrome.

3. Presence of serious side effects from using oral or systemic opioids
4. Intractable bilateral, midline, or diffuse somatic pain
5. Supradiaphragmatic pain secondary to cervicothoracic cancers
6. Subdiaphragmatic pain after failure of or contraindication to intrathecal spinal administration
7. Absence of risk factors such as coagulopathies, infection, or allergy to morphine

This approach has been shown to be suitable for patients of all ages.[1] Duration of pain before resorting to intraventricular morphine has ranged from 0.5 to 120 months (mean 10 months).[8] A short-term prognosis is not a contraindication, although in some series, patients with less than 1 month life expectancy were excluded.[16]

All factors impacting on the patient's pain must be analyzed and addressed appropriately before and concurrent with the analgesic administration. A family member or a visiting nurse can be trained to administer the medication at home.

Methods of Morphine Delivery

Ventricular Access Devices

The Ommaya reservoir (2 mL) or similar ventricular access devices such as the Cordis (Miami Lakes, FL), 1 mL,[13,14] or a pediatric miniport, 0.2 to 0.5 mL to reduce dead space,[11] have been used as a portal for the administration of intraventricular morphine **(Table 71–1)**.

The daily injections would be expected to increase the risk of infection, dosing errors, and reservoir failure with long-term use. However, the reported incidence of these risks is extremely low.[1,10,13,18,32,37]

It is recommended that bolus injections of morphine through an Ommaya or similar reservoir be used in patients with life expectations of less than 2 months.[19,51]

Morphine Pumps

In 1990 Dennis and De Witty[51] reported their experience with long-term continuous intraventricular infusions of morphine for intractable pain in head and neck cancer by an infusion pump. The advantage of this drug delivery method is a more constant analgesia with steady delivery of morphine reducing peak level side effects.[56] Currently available pumps have versatile programming capabilities so that drug delivery can be individually tailored to the patient's profile; for example, additional boluses can be given to cover pain peaks. However, this is a more expensive option, and its utilization for the delivery of morphine is recommended for patients with a life expectancy of greater than 2 months.[14,51]

Other Methods

Shoulong and his colleagues[21] developed a simple, implanted patient controlled device, celled L224. They reported a long duration of analgesia (average 137 hour) after small doses of morphine.

◆ Preoperative Assessment

The cause and nature of the pain as well as the extent of the disease should be determined. As with any chronic pain management, a multidisciplinary approach is needed.

Computed tomography (CT) of the brain is performed to examine the morphology and dimensions of the cerebral ventricles and to exclude central nervous system (CNS) involvement in the patient's disease.[8]

Some authors have included a requirement for an assessment of the effectiveness and possible risks of subarachnoid morphine prior to administering intraventricular morphine.[15,37]

◆ Surgical Technique

Anesthesia

The procedures are performed under general anesthesia or local anesthesia and sedation if the patient is too ill to tolerate a general anesthetic. A prophylactic antibiotic is given prior to the procedure.

Procedure

Ommaya Reservoir or Other Ventricular Access Device[10,11,14,15,35,52,61]

The patient is placed in a supine position with the neck moderately flexed.

Local anesthesia is used to infiltrate the skin, and an inverted U-shaped incision is made slightly larger than the reservoir. The base of the scalp flap should be directly posterior for maximal denervation of the skin through which the reservoir will be accessed. A bur hole is placed 2 to 3 cm from the midline, 1 cm anterior to the coronal suture (Kocher's point), generally on the right (nondominant) side. The dura is coagulated and incised in a cruciate fashion.

The ventricular catheter is then inserted, aiming for the standard landmarks for the foramen of Monro **(Fig. 71–1)**. The distal catheter tip is ideally located on the floor of the frontal horn of the right lateral ventricle, as close as possible to the foramen of Monro.

The ventricles are often small so confirmation of good catheter position may be achieved by performing a lateral skull x-ray intraoperatively after the injection of 1 to 2 mL of filtered air.

Alternatively, stereotaxic techniques can be used to cannulate small ventricles.[60]

The ventricular catheter (6 to 8 cm) is then connected to a reservoir (Ommaya, Cordis Italia, or pediatric miniport), which is placed beneath the galea and sutured to the pericranium. Patency is ensured by aspirating CSF from the reservoir prior to closure.

Morphine Pump[24,33,51,62]

A right frontal ventricular catheter is inserted as described above. The pump (Infusaid, Norwood, MA; Medtronic, Jacksonville, FL; or Secor) is loaded with morphine and the

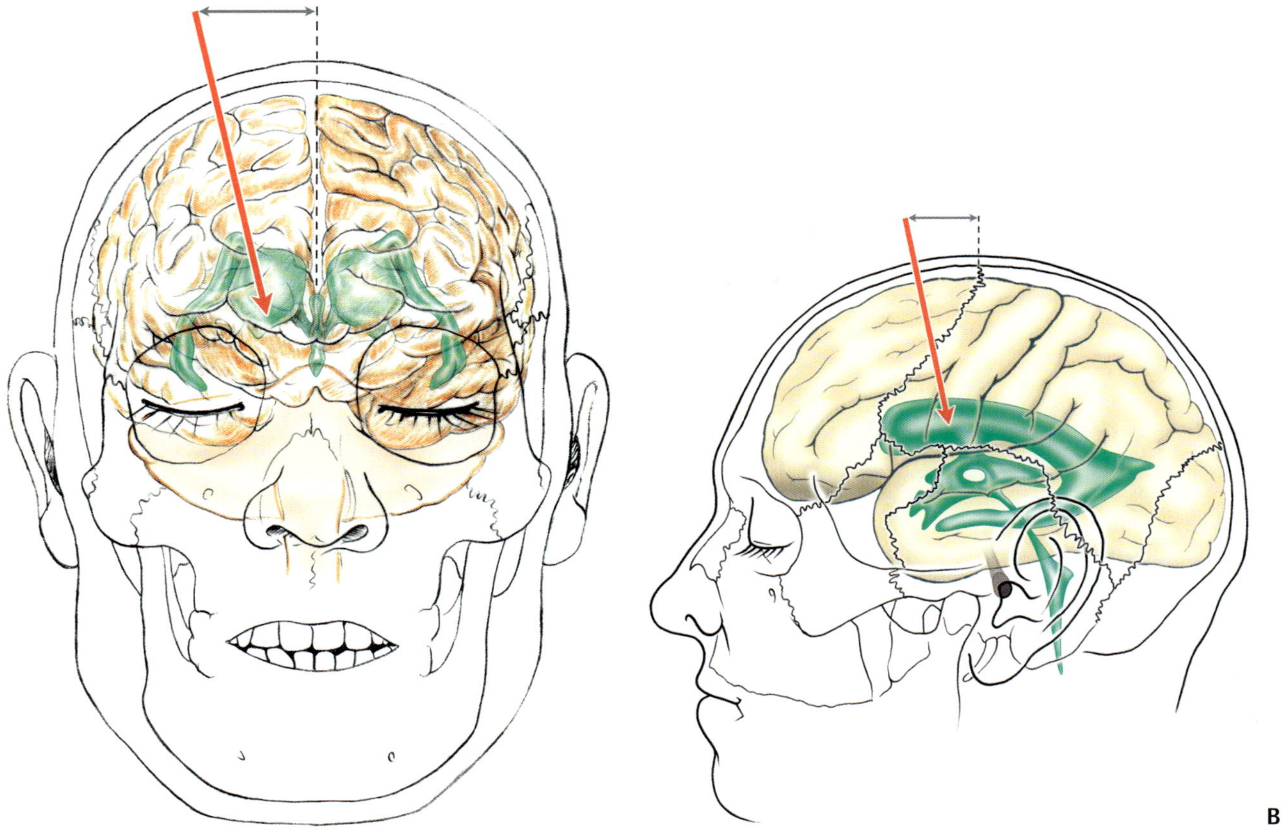

Figure 71–1 **(A)** Aiming from a point 3 cm off the midline and **(B)** 1 cm anterior to the coronal suture toward the medial epicanthus and the external ear canal puts the trajectory along the frontal horn, close to the foramen of Monro.

tubing inside the pump is filled by running it until the medication reaches the outport. The pump is implanted in an infraclavicular or right upper quadrant abdominal subcutaneous pocket, at most 1 cm deep so that the pump reservoir port can be felt. To minimize the risk of wound dehiscence, the incision line must not lie over the pump itself and must be fashioned in such a way as to prevent compromising the vascularity of the flap. Permanent sutures to the fascia are used to hold the pump in place. The tubing should be coiled underneath the pump to prevent its inadvertent puncture when accessing the pump reservoir. Passing the catheter from the pump pocket to the frontal incision is done with a shunt tube passer, and solid connectors are used for connecting the catheters.

Intraventricular Morphine Administration Techniques

For Bolus Injections through a Ventricular Access Device

The relative potency of intraventricular morphine is 10 times that of intrathecal morphine.[19,63] A suitable test dose constitutes 1% of the patient's usual intramuscular (IM) morphine requirement.[16] Initial morphine doses generally range from 0.05 to 1 mg per 24 hours[1,8,11,19] and can be injected soon after the procedure is completed.

Sterile, preservative-free morphine sulfate[12,16,51] or morphine hydrochloride[13,14,37] solution is used. Prior to opiate administration, the skin is disinfected and the reservoir tapped with a 25 gauge needle. A 0.22 mu millipore filter may be placed between the needle and morphine syringe.[11]

Onset of analgesia occurs within 2 to 30 minutes of administration with maximal intensity reached at 15 to 60 minutes.[11,13–15] Most protocols recommend administration every 24 hours.[1,11,14,16,19,37,58] Frequency of injection, once or twice a day, and the dose are determined by the patient's condition and response to treatment. Patients are monitored in the intensive care unit for 24 to 48 hours.[1]

Administration of opioids by other routes may be ceased at the time of ventriculostomy and the dose of intraventricular morphine increased gradually.[1] Usually 5 to 7 days are required to achieve a stable maintenance dose.[1,11,14]

Chronic intraventricular morphine administration has been safely performed on an outpatient basis by either a relative or a visiting nurse.[1,11,14–16,35]

For a Morphine Pump

Dennis and De Witty[51] described connecting the pump-catheter system to an Ommaya reservoir and ventricular catheter. Based on the duration and degree of analgesia achieved by a test dose via the Ommaya reservoir, a dose of morphine for a period of 24 hours was determined and the pump then filled with a concentration of morphine that would provide that daily dose based on the rate at which the pump is emptied. An initial bolus test dose of 0.25 to 0.5 mg is recommended. The dose of infused morphine is adjusted according to the patient's analgesic response. The pump is refilled every 2 to 3 weeks percutaneously.

Weigl et al[55] established the daily morphine requirements by using an external pump before implantation of the pump system.

Intensive respiratory monitoring is required until a safe, effective dose has been determined.

◆ Complications[1,5,8,9,11–13,15,16,19,21,22,32,37,51,55]

The following complications are related to the catheter system, reservoir, or pump:

- Leakage
- Catheter blockage or kinking
- Reservoir malfunction (failure, leak)
- Pump migration, rupture, or failure
- Infection (local sepsis of the implants, transient purulent meningitis)
- Skin breakdown
- Subcutaneous CSF collection or hygromas
- Intracerebral hematoma

The following complications are related to the narcotic drug administration:

- Minor morphine side effects: nausea, vomiting, constipation, urinary retention, pruritus, dizziness, headache, disorientation, euphoria, drowsiness, facial tingling, or diaphoresis. These are almost always transient.
- Major morphine side effects: respiratory depression, visual hallucination, and behavioral disorder. These must be promptly reversed by intravenous naloxone.

Respiratory depression is uncommon, with a reported incidence of 0 to 3.5% of cases and always following the first to third administration.[15] It is managed successfully in all cases with intravenous naloxone, without reversing analgesia. Respiratory depression did not occur during the chronic phase of therapy despite dose escalation. [1,8,12,15,19, 37,69,65]

Seizures have been occasionally observed after systemic, intraspinal, or intraventricular doses (boluses) of morphine in patients suffering from cancer pain.[66,67]

- Tolerance: The use of chronic intrathecal administration of morphine has been shown to lead to the development of opioid tolerance in patients suffering from intractable cancer pain,[18,68] but is much less marked than with parenteral opiates.[69] Only a moderate increase in the daily dose of intrathecal morphine is required (two to three times the initial dose) for satisfactory analgesia without resulting in any central opioid related side effects.

When abrupt increases in opioid requirements occur, possible mechanical complications should be considered and investigated.

◆ Conclusion

Data currently available indicate that intraventricular morphine administration is a feasible, safe, and effective method for the control of otherwise intractable pain of malignant origin.

Clearly, the treatment of chronic pain must be multidisciplinary with support for the patient and family, anticancer treatment, modification of lifestyle, and control of other distressing symptoms.

References

1. Cramond T, Stuart G. Intraventricular morphine for intractable pain of advanced cancer. J Pain Symptom Manage 1993;8:465–473
2. Gustafsson LL, Ackerman S, Adamson H, Garle M, Rane A, Schildt B. Disposition of morphine in cerebrospinal fluid after epidural administration. Lancet 1982;1:796 (letter)
3. Lazorthes Y, Gouarderes C, Verdie JC, et al. Analgesia by intrathecally applied morphine: pharmacokinetics study and application to intractable pain [in French (author's transl).] Neurochirurgie 1980;26: 159–164.
4. Ballantyne J, Carr D, Berkey C, Chalmers T, Mosteller F. Comparative efficacy of epidural, subarachnoid and intracerebroventricular opioids in patients with pain due to cancer. Reg Anesth 1996;21: 542–556
5. Blond S. Morphinothérapie intracérébroventriculaire: a propos de 79 cas. Neurochirurgie 1989;35:52–57
6. Cousins MJ, Mather LE. Intrathecal and epidural administration of opioids. Anesthesiology 1984;61:276–310
7. Follett K, Hitchon P, Piper J. Response of intractable pain to continuous intrathecal morphine: a retrospective study. Pain 1992;49:21–25
8. Karavelis A, Foroglou G, Selviaridis P, Fountzilas G. Intraventricular administration of morphine for control of intractable cancer pain in 90 patients. Neurosurgery 1996;39:57–61 discussion 61–62
9. Lajat Y, Menegalli-Boggelli D, Bensignor Le Henaff M, Resche F. Intracerebral morphine therapy in cancer patients [in French]. Cah Anesthesiol 1992; 40:477–483
10. Lazorthes Y, Verdie JC, Bastide R, Lavados A, Descouens D. Spinal versus intraventricular chronic opiate administration with implantable drug delivery devices for cancer pain. Appl Neurophysiol 1985;48: 234–241
11. Lazorthes YR, Sallerin BA, Verdie JC. Intracerebroventricular administration of morphine for control of irreducible cancer pain. Neurosurgery 1995;37:422–429
12. Leavens ME, Hill CS Jr, Cech DA, Weyland JB, Weston JS. Intrathecal and intraventricular morphine for pain in cancer patients: initial study. J Neurosurg 1982;56:241–245
13. Lenzi A, Galli G, Gandolfini M, Marini G. Intraventricular morphine in paraneoplastic painful syndrome of the cervicofacial region: experience in thirty-eight cases. Neurosurgery 1985;17:6–11
14. Lenzi A, Galli G, Marini G. Intraventricular morphine in the treatment of pain secondary to cancer. In: Schmideck HH, Sweet WH, eds. Operative Neurosurgical Techniques. 3rd ed. Vol 2. New York: Grune & Stratton, 1995:1431–1441
15. Lobato RD, Madrid JL, Fatela LV, Sarabia R, Rivas JJ, Gozalo A. Intraventricular morphine for intractable cancer pain: rationale, methods, clinical results. Acta Anaesthesiol Scand Suppl 1987;85:68–74

16. Obbens EA, Hill CS, Leavens ME, Ruthenbeck SS, Otis F. Intraventricular morphine administration for control of chronic cancer pain. Pain 1987;28:61–68
17. Rawal N, Sjostrand VH, Dahlstrom B, Nydahl PA, Ostelius J. Epidural morphine for postoperative pain relief: a comparative study with intramuscular narcotic and intercostal nerve block. Anesth Analg 1982;61:93–98
18. Sallerin-Caute B, Lazorthes Y, Deguine O, et al. Does intrathecal morphine in the treatment of cancer pain induce the development of tolerance? Clinical study. Neurosurgery 1998;42:44–50
19. Schultheiss R, Schramm J, Neidhardt J. Dose changes in long- and medium-term intrathecal morphine therapy of cancer pain. Neurosurgery 1992;31:664–670
20. Shetter AG, Hadley MN, Wilkinson E. Administration of intraspinal morphine sulfate for the treatment of intractable cancer pain. Neurosurgery 1986;18:740–747
21. Shoulong L, Jianlong W, Rongzeng W, Quan W. Clinical application of a patient-controlled apparatus for ventricular administration of morphine in intractable pain: report of 28 cases. Neurosurgery 1991;29: 73–75
22. Thiebaut JB, Blond S, Farcot MJ, et al. La morphine par voie intraventriculaire dans le traitement des douleurs néoplastiques. Med Hyg (Geneve) 1985;43:636–646
23. Onofrio BM, Yaksh TL, Arnold PG. Continuous low-dose intrathecal morphine administration in the treatment of chronic pain of malignant origin. Mayo Clin Proc 1981;56:516–520
24. Penn RD, Paice JA, Gottschalk W, Ivankovich AD. Cancer pain relief using chronic morphine infusion: early experience with a programmable implanted drug pump. J Neurosurg 1984;61:302–306
25. Tung AS, Tenicela R, Barr G, Winter P. Intrathecal morphine in cancer patients tolerant to systemic opiates. Spinal Opiate Analgesia 1982; 44:138–140
26. Wang K, Nauss L, Thomas J. Pain relief by intrathecally applied morphine in man. Anesthesiology 1979;50:140–151
27. Anderson VC, Burchiel KJ. A prospective study of long term intrathecal morphine in the management of chronic non-malignant pain. Neurosurgery 1999;44:289–300
28. Onofrio BM, Yaksh TL. Long-term pain relief produced by intrathecal morphine infusion in 53 patients. J Neurosurg 1990;72:200–209
29. Paice JA, Penn RD, Shott S. Intraspinal morphine for chronic pain: a retrospective multicenter study. J Pain Symptom Manage 1996; 11:71–80
30. Raphael JH, Sothall JL, Gnanadurai TV, Treharne GJ, Kitas GD. Long-term experience with implanted intrathecal drug administration system systems for failed back syndrome and chronic mechanical low back pain. BMC Musculoskelet Disord 2002;3:17–28
31. Winkelmuller M, Winkelmuller W. Long-term effects of continuous intrathecal opioid treatment in chronic pain of non-malignant etiology. J Neurosurg 1996;85:458–467
32. Nurchi G. Use of intraventricular and intrathecal morphine in intractable pain associated with cancer. Neurosurgery 1984;15: 801–803
33. Penn RD. Drug pumps for treatment of neurologic diseases and pain. Neurol Clin 1985;3:439–451
34. Poletti C, Cohen A, Todd D, Sweet W. Cancer pain relieved by long-term epidural morphine with permanent indwelling system for self-administration. J Neurosurg 1981;55:581–584
35. Lobato RD, Madrid JL, Fatela LV, Rivas JJ, Reig E, Lamas E. Intraventricular morphine for control of pain in terminal cancer patients. J Neurosurg 1983;59:627–633
36. Pawl RP. Intraventricular morphine. Neurosurgery 1986;18:250–251
37. Roquefeuil B, Benezech J, Blanchet P, Batier C, Frerebeau P, Gros C. Intraventricular administration of morphine in patients with neoplastic intractable pain. Surg Neurol 1984;21:155–158
38. Fields HL, Basbaum AI. Brainstem control of spinal pain-transmission neurons. Annu Rev Physiol 1978;40:217–248
39. Gebhart GF. Opiate and opioid peptide effects on brainstem neurons: relevance to nociception and antinociceptive mechanisms. Pain 1982;12:93–140
40. Kuhar MJ, Pert CB, Snyder SH. Regional distribution of opiate receptor binding in monkey and human brain. Nature 1973;245:447–450
41. Martin WR. Pharmacology of opioids. Pharmacol Rev 1983;35: 283–323
42. Pert A, Yaksh T. Sites of morphine induced analgesia in the primate brain: relation to pain pathways. Brain Res 1974;80:135–140
43. Tafani JA, Lazorthes Y, Danet B, et al. Human brain and spinal cord scan after intracerebroventricular administration of iodine-123 morphine. Int J Rad Appl Instrum B 1989;16:505–509
44. Yaksh TL, Rudy TA. Narcotic analgesics: CNS sites and mechanisms of action as revealed by intracerebral injection techniques. Pain 1978; 4:299–359
45. Goudas LC, Langlade A, Serrie A, et al. Acute decreases in cerebrospinal fluid glutathione levels after intracerebroventricular morphine for cancer pain. Anesth Analg 1999;89:1209–1215
46. Le Bars D, Willer JC, De Broucker T. Morphine blocks descending pain inhibitory controls in humans. Pain 1992;48:13–20
47. Meyerson BA. Biochemistry of pain relief with intracerebral stimulation: few facts and many hypotheses. Acta Neurochir Suppl (Wien) 1980;30:229–237
48. Penn RD, Paice JA, Kroin JS. Octreotide: a potent new non-opiate analgesic for intrathecal infusion. Pain 1992;49:13–19. Comment in: Pain 1992;51:261–262; Pain 1993;53:360–361
49. Bouhassira D, Villanueva L, LeBars D. Intracerebroventricular morphine decreases descending inhibitors acting on lumbar dorsal horn neuronal activities related to pain in the rat. J Pharmacol Exp Ther 1988;247:332–342
50. Blond S, Guieu JD, Meynadier J, Le Bars D, Willer JC. Intracerebroventricular morphine, analgesia, and nociceptive spinal reflexes. Lancet 1994;343:857–858
51. Dennis GC, De Witty RL. Long-term intraventricular infusion of morphine for intractable pain in cancer of the head and neck. Neurosurgery 1990;26:404–407
52. Ghajar JB. A guide for ventricular catheter placement: technical note. J Neurosurg 1985;63:985–986
53. Kroin J, Ali A, York M, Penn R. The distribution of medication along the spinal canal after chronic intrathecal administration: clinical study. Neurosurgery 1993;33:226–230
54. Lobato RD, Madrid JL, Fatela LV, Rivas JJ, Sarabia R. Analgesia elicited by low-dose intraventricular morphine in terminal cancer patients. In: Fields HL ed. Advances in Pain Research and Therapy. Vol 9. New York: Raven 1985:673–681
55. Weigl K, Mundinger F, Chrubasik J. Continuous intraventricular morphine- or peptide-infusion for intractable cancer pain. Acta Neurochir Suppl (Wien) 1987;39:163–165
56. Brazenor G. Long-term intrathecal administration of morphine: a comparison of bolus injection via reservoir with continuous infusion by implanted pump. Neurosurgery 1987;21:484–491
57. Lazorthes YR. Intracerebroventricular administration of morphine for control of irreducible cancer pain. Neurosurgery 1995;37:422–429
58. Lazorthes Y, Verdie JC, Caute B, Maranhao R, Tafani M. Intracerebroventricular morphinotherapy for control of chronic cancer pain. Prog Brain Res 1988;77:395–405
59. Reeve WG, Todd JG. Intraventricular diamorphine via Ommaya shunt for intractable cancer pain. Br J Anaesth 1990;65:544–547
60. Smith KA, Frank E. Stereotaxic placement of a ventricular catheter and reservoir for the administration of morphine sulphate. Axone 1991;13:12–15
61. Leavens ME, Aldama-Luebert A. Ommaya reservoir placement: technical note. Neurosurgery 1979;5:264–266
62. Penn RD, Paice JA. Chronic intrathecal morphine for intractable pain. J Neurosurg 1987;67:182–186
63. Leong MS, Calabrese JF, Heit G. Intraventricular administration of morphine and clonidine. Anesthesiology 2001;94:1141–1143
64. Langlade A, Serrie A, Sandouk P, Thurel C, Cunin G. Levels of morphine and metabolites in CSF during respiratory depression after intraventricular morphine injection. Pain 1991;44:175–178
65. Lorenz M, Hussein S, Verner L. Continuous intraventricular clonidine infusion in controlled morphine withdrawal: case report. Pain 2002; 98:335–338
66. Kronenberg MF, Laimer I, Rifici C, et al. Epileptic seizure associated with intracerebroventricular and intrathecal morphine bolus. Pain 1998;75:383–387
67. Parkinson SK, Bailey SL, Little WL, Mueller JB. Myoclonic seizure activity with chronic high-dose spinal opioid administration. Anesthesiology 1990;72:743–745
68. Coombs DW, Saunders RL, Lachance D, Savage S, Ragnarsson TS, Jensen LE. Intrathecal morphine tolerance: use of intrathecal clonidine, DADLE, and intraventricular morphine. Anesthesiology 1985; 62:358–363
69. Dagi TF, Chilton J, Caputy A, Won D. Long-term, intermittent percutaneous administration of epidural and intrathecal morphine for pain of malignant origin. Am Surg 1986;52:155–158

72

Microvascular Decompression for Cranial Nerve Compression Syndromes

Laligam N. Sekhar, Dinko Stimac, and Foad Elahi

This chapter discusses microvascular decompression operations for a variety of cranial nerve syndromes, including trigeminal neuralgia, hemifacial spasm, nervus intermedius neuralgia, disabling positional vertigo, disabling tinnitus, and glossopharyngeal neuralgia. The operative technique for many of these operations is very similar; however, nuances of surgery are very important and make a very big difference between a good outcome and a poor outcome and in the incidence of complications.

◆ Brief Historical Overview

W. James Gardner at the Cleveland Clinic recognized the compression of the trigeminal nerve as being responsible for the facial pain syndrome. Walter Dandy commented on this as well based on the several operations that he performed for trigeminal neuralgia, which involved the section of the trigeminal root from the posterior fossa. However, it remained for Peter Jannetta to perfect this operation for a variety of these syndromes and to popularize them. The validity of the microvascular compression hypothesis has been questioned by C. B. T. Adams. Moller et al have provided the neurophysiological basis of this theory in patients with hemifacial spasm.

◆ Pathogenesis of the Condition

Axons within the central nervous system are covered by myelin, which is generated by oligodendrocytes. This is termed central myelin. In contrast, in the peripheral nerves, the myelin of axons is generated by Schwann cells. When a cranial nerve exits or enters the brain stem, the region of central myelin extends for a variable distance away from the attachment to the brain stem and then transitions into the peripheral myelin. This zone of transition is called the Obersteiner-Redlich zone. It is felt that the area of the nerve that has central myelin is very vulnerable to trauma, especially the trauma that may be caused by repeated pulsations of an artery in contact with the nerve or by compression of a vein in contact with the nerve. This process may then cause demyelination over a focal area and an abnormal conduction or short-circuiting within the axons, which is also called ephaptic transmission. Such abnormality may lead to the production of a variety of hyperactivity syndromes of cranial nerves, which may include trigeminal neuralgia, hemifacial spasm, disabling positional vertigo, tinnitus, glossopharyngeal neuralgia, and nervus intermedius neuralgia. Relief of vascular compression leads to a permanent cure in a high percentage of patients, depending on the clinical syndrome in question, without the production of permanent deficits in the distribution of the cranial nerve.

◆ Indications for Surgery

The indications for microvascular decompression vary with the clinical syndrome. For patients with trigeminal neuralgia, microvascular decompression is indicated for patients who have typical trigeminal neuralgia and have failed or are unable to tolerate medical treatment. Typical trigeminal neuralgia is diagnosed by the history obtained from the patient, which might include the following: sharp, lancinating, and brief episodes of pain with periods of remission in between; the presence of trigger points on the face or the gums; relief with various medications that are used to treat trigeminal neuralgia, such as carbamazepine, diphenylhydantoin, or gabapentin; and the absence of burning or constant pain. Patients with longstanding trigeminal neuralgia may progress to have certain atypical features, such as constant pain or burning pain, which do not contraindicate surgery. Patients with typical trigeminal neuralgia may remember the very first time that they had the pain, and have often been treated by dentists prior to consulting a neurosurgeon. Some patients may mention positional variability of pain and the lack of pain during sleep, especially in the early stages. Patients are considered good candidates for microvascular decompression if they are physiologically able to undergo the operation. Patients who have had previous destructive procedures such as radiofrequency rhizotomy, peripheral nerve sections, or microvascular decompression have a poorer prognosis than patients who have never been operated previously. Patients with atypical facial pain syndromes generally do not respond well to microvascular decompression, although if a blood vessel can be demonstrated to be in contact and is compressive, then the operation is more likely to be successful.

Hemifacial spasm (HFS) is a very typical syndrome that consists of spasm of the facial muscles on one side, particularly around the orbicularis oculi, which spreads to involve the rest of the facial muscles including the platysma. Hemifacial spasm has a typical electromyographic appearance and is very disabling to patients. Nowadays, patients with HFS are frequently treated with botulinum toxin injections initially, and when they seek surgery they are often in an advanced condition. In more advanced stages, patients may exhibit facial weakness and the tonus phenomenon, which creates facial distortion. Hemifacial spasm responds extraordinarily well to microvascular decompression.

Nervus intermedius neuralgia is a condition that involves sharp pain deep in the ear, which may radiate to the temple or to the face. It is thought to be due to hyperactivity of the nervous intermedius, which runs between the facial and vestibulocochlear nerves before joining the facial nerve in the internal auditory canal. Disabling positional vertigo, and disabling tinnitus may have a variety of causes. If the patient is demonstrated to have the vascular compression by magnetic resonance imaging (MRI) scan and has an abnormal auditory brain stem response on the affected side, then the patient may respond well to a microvascular decompression operation.

Glossopharyngeal neuralgia is an intermittently painful syndrome similar to trigeminal neuralgia that involves the throat primarily but may also spread to involve the ear and the upper neck area.

◆ Preoperative Investigations

The preoperative workup of patients with cranial nerve compression symptoms includes an MRI scan with thin sections of the posterior fossa to make sure that the patient does not have an extraaxial tumor, a giant aneurysm, an arteriovenous malformation, multiple sclerosis, or a brain stem tumor. Additionally, thin-section MR angiography with a three-dimensional reconstruction protocol can demonstrate the vascular compression in many cases. Compression of the nerves by large vessels such as the vertebral artery or the basilar artery is readily demonstrated, whereas compression by the smaller vessels such as the superior cerebellar artery (SCA) or posterior inferior cerebellar artery (PICA) or venous compressions are harder to demonstrate. In routine MR scans, the T2-weighted image is more helpful for demonstrating vascular compression.

In addition, physiological tests appropriate to the nerve in question should be obtained. For instance, patients with disabling positional vertigo or tinnitus must undergo an audiogram and auditory brain stem response. If the diagnosis of hemifacial spasm is doubtful, the electromyography and nerve conduction studies of the facial nerves should be obtained. Some of the patients with cranial nerve compression syndromes are elderly, and a careful preoperative medical workup is necessary.

◆ Surgical Technique

Positioning, Neuromonitoring, and Anesthesia

All patients undergoing surgery for cranial nerve decompression syndromes are placed in the lateral decubitus position with the head held in three-point pin fixation and slightly turned toward the surgeon. For patients with trigeminal neuralgia, the operation can be performed with the patient in the supine lateral position with the head turned strongly toward the contralateral side. However, in patients who are obese with a short neck, or patients who have poor mobility of the neck, this position is more risky because the head cannot be turned completely, and there is a greater risk of kinking the vertebral arteries in this position. A standard neuroanesthetic technique, which emphasizes brain relaxation, is used for these operations. However, for hemifacial spasm surgery and for surgery of the eighth nerve, monitoring of facial function is necessary. So these patients cannot be relaxed. For these patients, it is also important to monitor the lateral spread obtained by antidromic stimulation of the facial nerve, which may be the only abnormality under anesthesia in a patient with hemifacial spasm. All patients undergo monitoring of the auditory brain response and somatosensory evoked potentials during the operative procedure. Monitoring of the vocal cord electromyogram (EMG) activity may be considered during operations for glossopharyngeal neuralgia. The senior author commonly employs a lumber drain with slow drainage of ~30 cc of fluid during these operations to relax the brain during craniotomy, which facilitates the early part of the operation.

Retrosigmoid Craniotomy

The important goals of the retrosigmoid (retromastoid) craniotomy/craniectomy are adequate exposure, avoidance

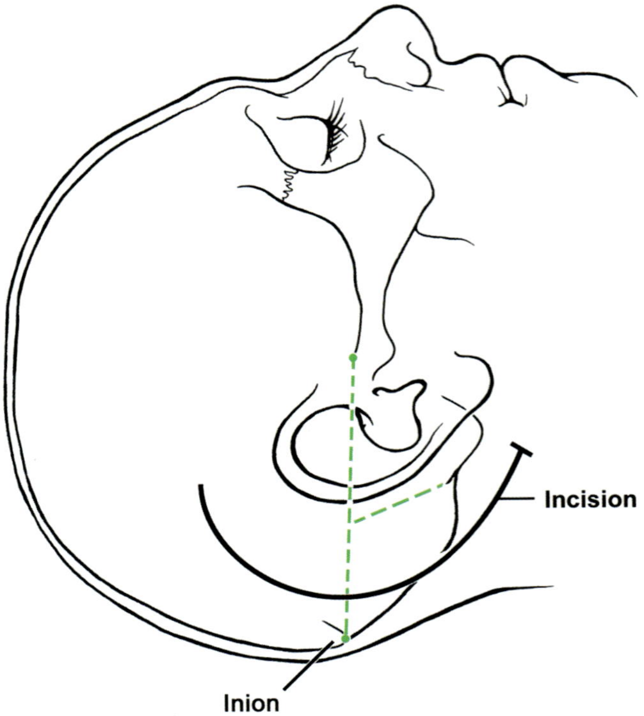

Figure 72–1 Incision and dotted lines indicating the localization of the transverse and sigmoid sinus.

of injury to the dura or the sigmoid sinus, and prevention of the postoperative headache syndrome. Because of the occurrence of postoperative headache in several patients with the older techniques, the senior author has modified the opening and closure considerably. After the patient is positioned, the presumed location of the transverse sinus is marked on the skin. A line drawn parallel to the zygomatic arch and extended posteriorly generally indicates the transverse sinus (**Fig. 72–1**). When frameless stereotaxy is available, the position of the transverse and sigmoid sinuses can be more accurately defined this way. The preoperative MRI scan should be carefully inspected to evaluate the anatomy of the sinus, the cerebellum, and any anomalous veins. The anatomy is very different in patients with a small posterior fossa or Chiari malformations.

A C-shaped posterior temporal and retroauricular incision is then marked out. The upper limb of the C is used for extracting a fascial dural graft, if needed. The posteriormost curve of the C should be at least 4 cm breadth behind the posterior edge of the mastoid process and defines the posterior extent of the craniotomy because it is difficult to retract the skin posteriorly once the incision is made. The inferior limb is curved just to the edge of the hairline. The skin and subcutaneous tissues are elevated along with the sternomastoid fascia and muscle and retracted anteriorly with sutures and rubber bands attached to the bar of a self-retaining retractor. The lesser occipital nerve is frequently divided by this incision; it is tagged with 4–0 neurolon sutures, and reattached at closure with 7–0 Prolene sutures. The periosteum is then divided along the nuchal line, and the superior portion may be elevated for use as a dural graft, or left in situ. The lower portion along with the muscles attaching to the occipital bone is elevated down to the curving portion of the suboccipital bone (the floor of the posterior fossa) and retracted with sutures and rubber bands. A mastoid emissary vein usually will bleed and be closed with bone wax when the muscles are elevated (**Fig. 72–2**).

The location of the bur hole is crucial (**Fig. 72–3**). It is placed just inferior to and posterior to the junction of the transverse and sigmoid sinuses. If in doubt, it is better to place this hole more inferior and more posterior to avoid damaging the sigmoid sinus. The single bur hole is often adequate to separate the dura mater by using a periosteal elevator. It is important to elevate dura cautiously near the sigmoid sinus, which is easy to lacerate because of the curved bony groove, and the thin outer wall of the sinus. If there is difficulty separating the lower portion of the dura, an additional bur hole may be placed inferiorly. A craniotomy is performed, usually about 3 × 4 cm in dimension, or less in cases of trigeminal neuralgia. It is enlarged laterally to the edge of the sigmoid sinus in all patients, superiorly to the transverse sinus in cases of trigeminal neuralgia, and inferiorly to the floor of the posterior fossa for hemifacial spasm and cranial nerve (CN) VIII and IX cases (**Fig. 72–4**).

The mastoid air cells must be thoroughly waxed. A bleeding emissary vein may be bipolar coagulated. However, some bleeding near the sigmoid sinus may require small packs of oxidized cellulose and tack-up sutures.

Dural Opening and Initial Exposure

When a spinal drain is in place and cerebrospinal fluid (CSF) has been withdrawn, the brain will be slack. When no drain is in place, the lateral cerebellomedullary cistern will have to be opened first to relax the cerebellum. The dura mater is opened in a C-shaped fashion inferior to the transverse sinus and medial to the sigmoid sinus. Two T incisions are made laterally as needed and the dura is tacked up, slightly rotating the sigmoid sinus laterally (**Fig. 72–4**). With gentle retraction of the cerebellum, the neuroendoscope is used to visualize the lateral cerebellomedullary cistern. A 0 degree, 2.5 mm endoscope is held in the left hand, and with gentle pressure on the cerebellum with a Rhoton 6 microdissector (V. Mueller, Chicago, IL) in the right hand, the endoscope is advanced inferolaterally to visualize the cistern. Caution must be exercised not to damage a bridging vein that may be present here. The cistern is opened with an arachnoid knife, which results in drainage of CSF and considerable relaxation of the cerebellum (**Fig. 72–5**).

Hemifacial Spasm ***(Fig. 72–6)***

A self-retaining retractor is placed on the cerebellum, never retracting it more than 1 cm medial to the petrous dura. The arachnoid membrane is opened posterior to CNs IX and X and to VII and VIII. The anterior inferior cerebellar artery (AICA) or a branch of the PICA may be visible emerging laterally between CNs IX and VIII. A tapered self-retaining retractor is gently advanced and placed on the flocculus of the cerebellum. The choroid plexus of the lateral recess may be in the way, and may need to be cauterized to shrink it.

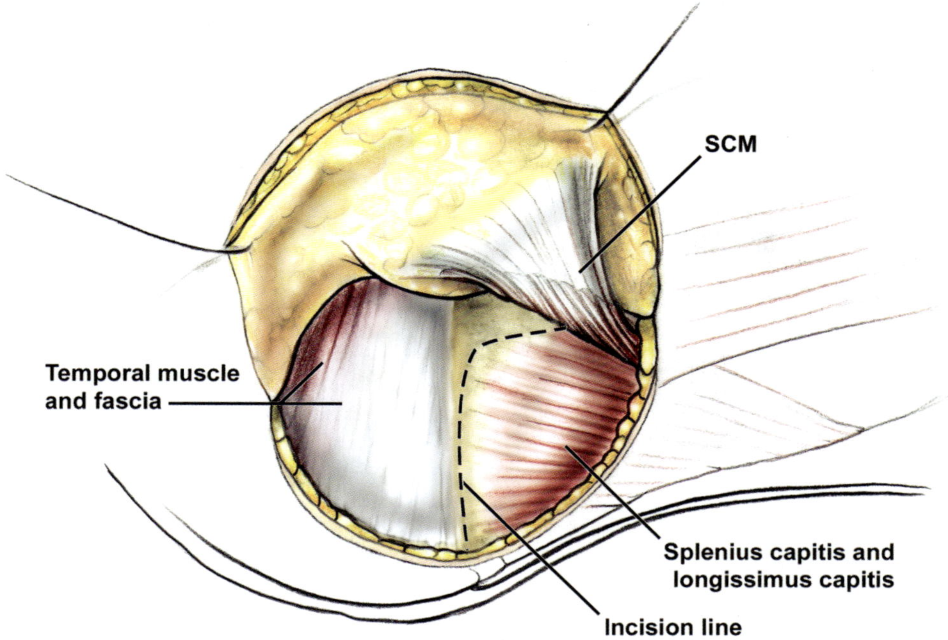

Figure 72–2 The sternocleidomastoid (SCM) muscle and fascia are elevated with the skin opening, revealing the splenius capitis and longissimus capitis muscles. The incision line for muscle detachment is identified from the nuchal line.

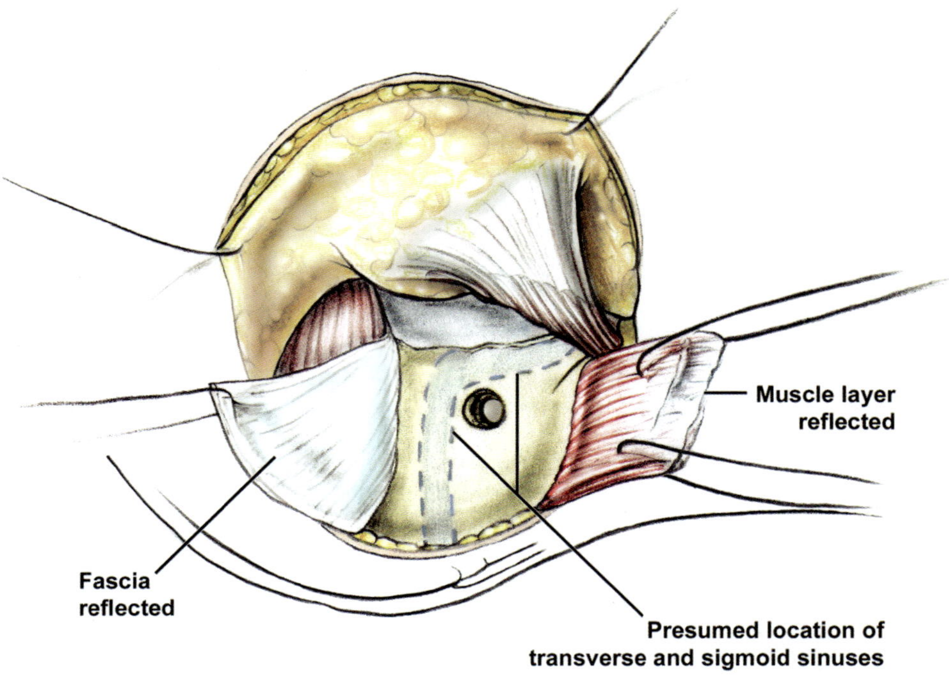

Figure 72–3 The splenius capitis, longissimus capitis, and oblique and rectus muscles are elevated as a single layer. The presumed location of the transverse and sigmoid sinuses is visualized, and a bur hole is made to initiate the craniotomy.

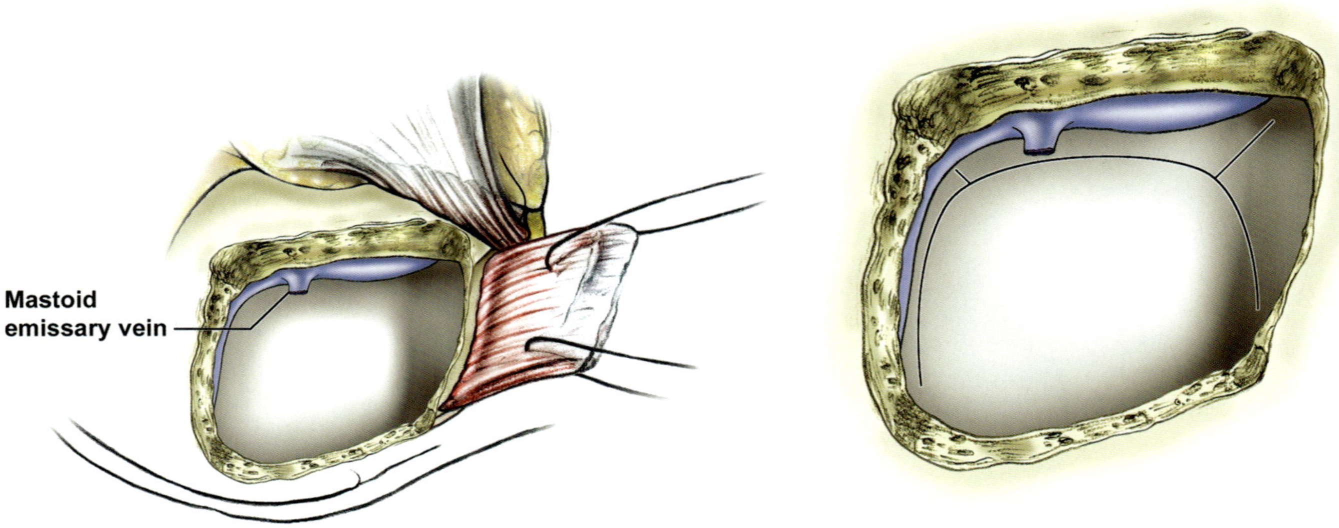

Figure 72–4 The craniotomy and craniectomy have been performed. The edge of the transverse sinus and some of the sigmoid sinus is exposed. (Inset) The mastoid emissary vein is cauterized. The dural incision is shown.

Excessive retraction on the flocculus of the cerebellum will cause deterioration of the brain stem evoked response (BSER), which is an indication to relax the retractor or remove it. The eighth nerve is white in color, posterior, and joins the pons superior to the seventh CN anterior to the lateral recess of the fourth ventricle. The CN VII is grayish in color, anterior to the eighth nerve, and exits the pontomedullary fissure inferior to the eighth nerve. The root-exit zone of the seventh CN lies directly anterior to CN IX and is sometimes hidden from the surgeon's view without excessive brain retraction.

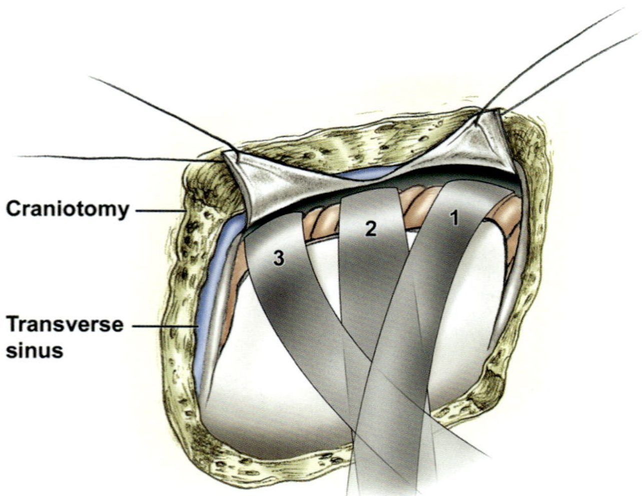

Figure 72–5 In position 1, cerebellar retraction exposes the lateral cerebellomedullary cistern for drainage, and for the exposure of cranial nerves IX and X. In position 2, cerebellar retraction exposes cranial nerves VIII and VII in the cerebellopontine angle cistern. The retractor is placed between positions 1 and 2 to expose the root exit zone of CN VII. The petrosal venous complex is exposed without stretching. In position 3, the retractor initially exposes the petrosal veins (which will be on stretch) and subsequently CN V, just superior to CN VIII.

At this stage, the 0 and 30 degree neuroendoscopes (2.5 mm) are used to visualize the root exit zone of the CN VII. Compressive vascular structures may include the vertebral artery, AICA, PICA, or a small vein. A combination of structures is often present. Any compressive arteries are dissected, mobilized carefully with a Rhoton 6 or 9 microdissector, taking care not to damage any perforating vessels entering the brain stem from those arteries. If the vertebral artery (VA) is compressive, it cannot be decompressed by Teflon felt padding alone. The artery is dissected and mobilized anterior to CNs IX and X and attached to the dura mater anterior to the jugular foramen with an 8–0 nylon stitch passed through the adventitia of the vessel, through the dura, and again through the adventitia, and tied with the artery held away from the nerve. A compressive smaller artery such as the AICA or PICA is mobilized away from the root entry zone of CN VII. If a vein is seen, it is carefully dissected away from the nerve and coagulated with an angled tip bipolar forceps held away from the nerve, using low current, and the vein is cauterized over a distance of 2 mm. It is then divided. Small pieces of shredded Teflon felt rolled in the fashions of cigars are placed between the nerve and AICA or PICA to decompress the nerve.

Any hemifacial spasm in the facial muscles by electromyography often disappears when the arachnoid membrane is opened and the cerebellum falls back, so it cannot be used as a reliable indicator of successful decompression. The disappearance of lateral spread is a reliable indicator of a successful operation and the surgeon must persist until this is accomplished. The use of the neuroendoscope has also improved the success rate of the operation.

At the conclusion of decompression, the neuroendoscope is used once again to view the CN VII and VIII to ensure adequate decompression and to ensure that the arteries are not kinked by the repositioning. Any spasm of the vessels observed may be relieved by coating with 3% papaverine-soaked pledgets of Gelfoam.

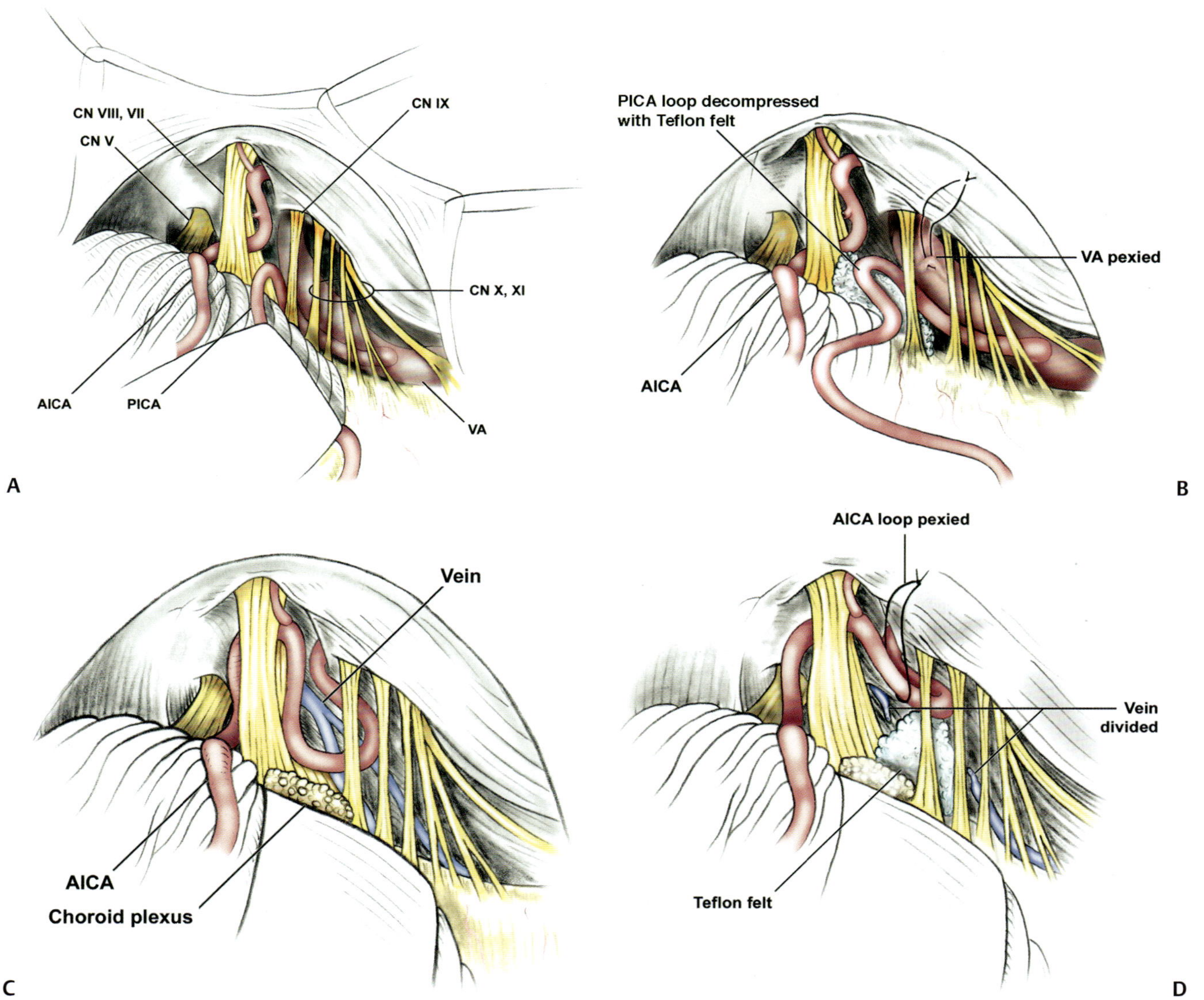

Figure 72–6 Hemifacial spasm. **(A)** Vertebral artery and posterior inferior cerebellar artery (PICA) loop compression of facial nerve. **(B)** The vertebral artery has been pexied, and the PICA loop is decompressed with Teflon felt. **(C)** The anterior inferior cerebellar artery (AICA) and a vein compressing the facial nerve. **(D)** The vein has been cauterized and divided. The AICA loop is lifted up and pexied. Teflon felt provides decompression of the nerve.

◆ Other Cranial Nerve Conditions

Nervus Intermedius Neuralgia

Nervus intermedius neuralgia is characterized by sharp shooting ear pain. Unfortunately, because the ear is also supplied by the trigeminal nerve and the glossopharyngeal nerve, in patients with ear pain syndrome, the trigeminal nerve and the glossopharyngeal nerve also need to be explored for possible vascular compression.

Treatment for nervus intermedius neuralgia consists in sectioning of the nervus intermedius. The nervus intermedius will be visible as one or two fascicles between the seventh and eighth cranial nerves. Gentle retraction of the facial nerve (not the eighth CN) with a Rhoton 6 dissector will reveal the nervus intermedius. It can be mobilized with a Rhoton 9 dissector, and a small segment is excised (simple section may allow regeneration) and submitted for pathology. Although tearing may be affected by the section of the nervus intermedius, patients rarely complain of it. The adequacy of the section of the nerve may be confirmed by the Schirmer's test.

Glossopharyngeal Neuralgia

Glossopharyngeal neuralgia is characterized by the sharp severe and intermittent pain in the throat or in the neck area. Sometimes it may be hard to distinguish between glossopharyngeal and V3 division trigeminal neuralgia, and especially between glossopharyngeal and nervus intermedius neuralgia.

The microsurgical exposure for the glossopharyngeal neuralgia is similar to that for hemifacial spasm. If a vascular compression of the CN IX or upper fascicles of CN X is found (the compressive artery may be PICA or the VA), it is mobilized and held with a stitch to the dura mater near the jugular foramen or with Teflon felt rolls. When the vascular compression is not impressive, then the glossopharyngeal nerve and the upper two fascicles of the vagus nerve are sectioned and a small segment resected. The patient may experience a temporary dysphagia postoperatively and should be warned about this before the operation.

Disabling Positional Vertigo or Tinnitus

Disabling positional vertigo or tinnitus syndrome may occur because of vascular compression of the eighth cranial nerve. Because these disorders can occur from a variety of causes, it is difficult to select the patients preoperatively. The following criteria are helpful in patient selection; however, the success rate even in the best selected patients is around 70%: (1) combination of tinnitus in one ear, disabling positional vertigo, and intermittent ear pain in the same ear; (2) the presence of BSER abnormality in the same side as the ear with tinnitus; (3) duration of disabling tinnitus less than 1 year; and (4) demonstration of arteries on the MRI scans in contact with the seventh and eighth cranial nerves—T2-weighted MRI or the source images of the MR angiograms are most useful for this purpose.

At surgery, compression of the eighth cranial nerve may be present anywhere from the brain stem to the internal auditory canal (IAC), because the root entry zone of the eighth cranial nerve extends into the IAC, the eighth cranial nerve-containing mostly centrally myelinated fibers **(Fig. 72–7)**.

The initial exposure of the eighth cranial nerve is similar to that for hemifacial spasm. However, the eighth cranial nerve has to be displayed completely from the IAC to the brain stem, and in some patients even inside the IAC. The most frequent cause of compression is the AICA, but veins or the PICA may also be responsible. Veins compressing the nerve are cauterized and divided, whereas arteries compressing the nerve are decompressed with small pieces of Teflon felt. Great care must be exercised while mobilizing the AICA to make sure that perforators or the internal auditory artery are not stretched, and that there is no damage to the eighth or seventh cranial nerve. Any change in the auditory brain stem response (ABR) must be corrected by releasing the retractors or by repositioning the Teflon felt. The facial nerve must be stimulated at the brain stem at the end of the procedure to ensure its health. If spasm of the arteries is observed, it can be relieved with papaverine applied with small pieces of Gelfoam soaked in a 3% solution.

If the compression of the nerve is by an AICA loop inside the IAC, it will need to be opened by drilling the petrous bone to allow the adequate mobilization of the AICA loop.

Trigeminal Neuralgia

There are three important considerations in an operation for trigeminal neuralgia: the management of the petrosal vein, the identification of the compressive vessel, and the decompression.

After dural opening, the retractor is placed on the lateral aspect of the cerebellum, posterior to the eighth cranial nerve. This position of the retractor allows the petrosal vein to be visualized without stretching it and causing a tear. If the retractor is placed superolaterally initially, the vein is on stretch and may be torn during coagulation **(Fig. 72–8A,B)**. The arachnoid membrane is opened posterior to CN VIII and the opening is gradually extended upward toward the petrosal vein. The petrosal vein is constituted by two veins that unite in the fashion of an inverted Y, to drain into the superior petrosal sinus. However, in some patients, a cerebellar

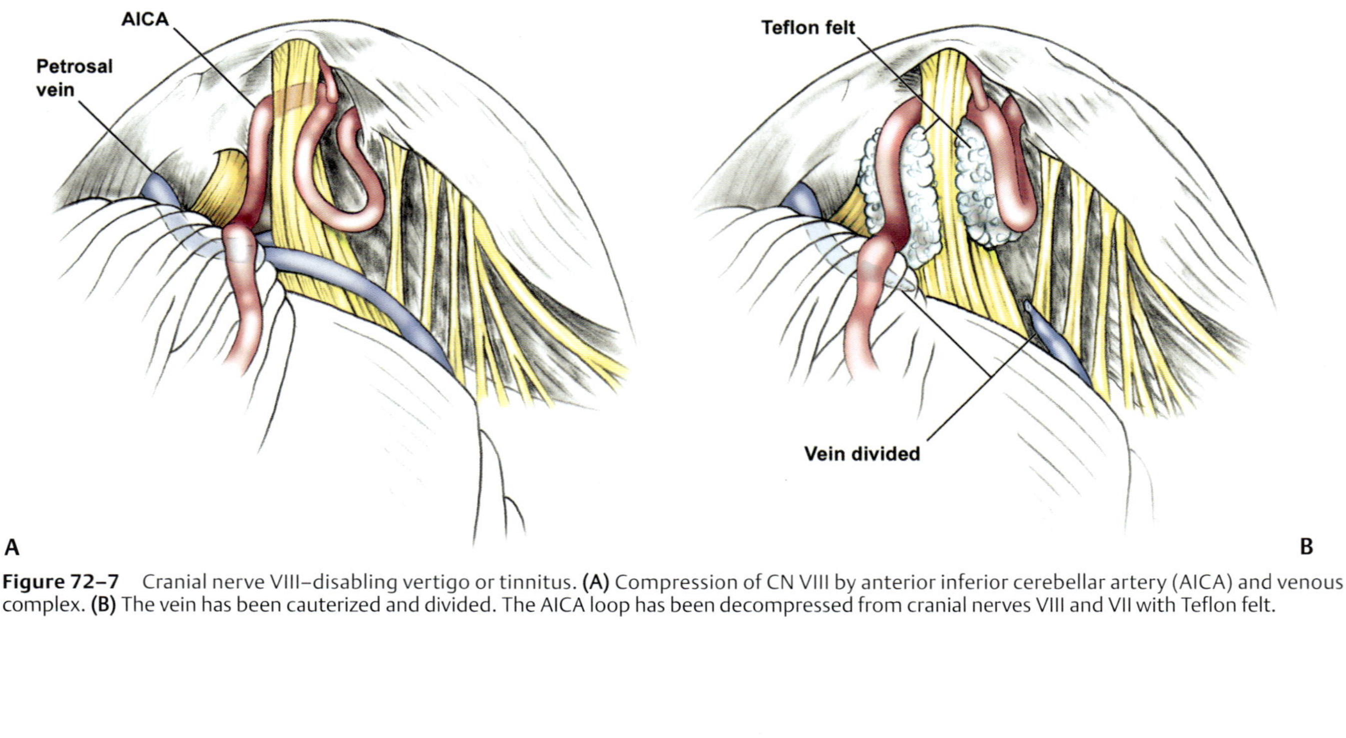

Figure 72–7 Cranial nerve VIII–disabling vertigo or tinnitus. **(A)** Compression of CN VIII by anterior inferior cerebellar artery (AICA) and venous complex. **(B)** The vein has been cauterized and divided. The AICA loop has been decompressed from cranial nerves VIII and VII with Teflon felt.

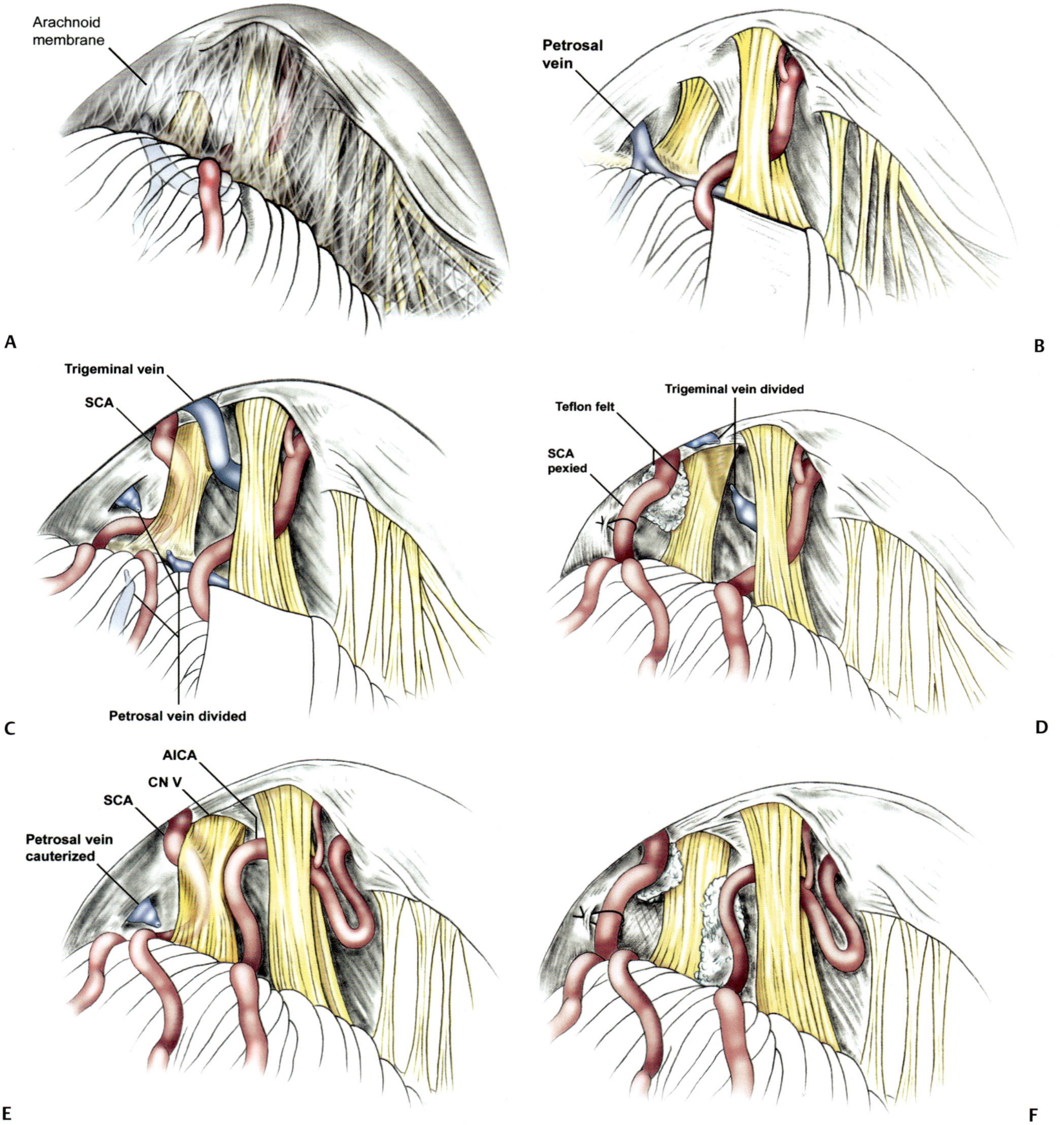

Figure 72–8 Trigeminal neuralgia. **(A)** Initial exposure. **(B)** Initial retraction position puts petrosal venous complex in stretch. **(C)** The petrosal vein has been cauterized and divided. The nerve is compressed by the trigeminal vein and the superior cerebellar artery (SCA). **(D)** The trigeminal vein is cauterized and divided. The SCA is pexied, and two small pieces of Teflon felt are used to decompress the nerve. **(E)** The trigeminal nerve is compressed by the SCA superiorly and anterior inferior cerebellar artery (AICA) inferiorly, causing a scissors-like compression. **(F)** The SCA has been divided and held away with an 8–0 nylon stitch to the tentorium. The AICA has been decompressed with pieces of Teflon felt.

vein may drain into a tentorial venous sinus more superficially, which may result in the vein being torn even with gentle cerebellar retraction. It is wise to look at the anatomy of the vein before the retractor is moved to the superolateral surface of the cerebellum. The arachnoid membrane is opened posterior to the petrosal venous complex. In most patients, the entire petrosal vein may need to be cauterized and divided. In some patients, one of the branches may be preserved. Either the inferior branch of the vein or both branches of the vein are cauterized with bipolar cautery without the vein being under stretch, and then divided. The petrosal vein typically contracts when it is cauterized. If the vein tears during cauterization, it must be divided and then cauterized. Rarely, if the vein is torn near the sinus, it cannot be cauterized. In such a case, the bleeding can be stopped by packing with oxidized cellulose and placing a cotton patty over it.

The initial inspection of the petrosal vein can be made with the 0 or 30 degree neuroendoscope. After the cautery and division of the petrosal vein, the trigeminal nerve is inspected with the endoscope. The retractor is then placed on the superior and lateral aspect of the cerebellum, superior to the eighth nerve. Inspection of the trigeminal nerve reveals the cause of compression, but such inspection must be performed with microvision and with endoscopic vision. The endoscope is particularly useful to look 360 degrees around the nerve roots and to look at the nerve at the entrance to the Meckel's cave; there is a often a vein that compresses the posterior and inferior aspect of the nerve as it drains into the superior petrosal sinus. This vein may be missed if only the microscope is used because of obstruction of vein by a ridge of the petrous bone. The most common cause of vascular compression is the superior cerebellar artery as it comes around the midbrain. The artery frequently has two branches in this location, and one or both may be compressing and grooving the nerve. The arachnoid membrane has to be opened adequately to allow the arteries to be mobilized superiorly from the Meckel's cave all the way to the brain stem. The mobilized artery may be held away from the nerve either by placing a stitch of 8–0 nylon around it and stitching it loosely to the tentorium, avoiding constriction of the artery, or by placing multiple pieces of rolled-up shredded Teflon felt between the nerve and the artery. The Teflon felt pieces are held in place by the tension between the artery and the nerve root and may be aided by a small piece of Gelfoam and fibrin glue **(Fig. 72–8C,D)**.

Other compressive arteries may include the AICA, arterioles, and, rarely, an ectatic basilar artery or a fusiform basilar artery (BA) aneurysm. Compression by the AICA may coexist with the SCA, constricting the nerve on both sides in the form of a pincer. In this case, both vessels must be mobilized and held away from the nerve by Teflon pieces or stitches **(Fig. 72–8E,F)**. Arteriolar constriction may be seen in young patients as the sole cause of trigeminal neuralgia; in such patients the arteriole is simply in the wrong place congenitally. The arteriole can usually be mobilized from the nerve and decompressed. In the senior author's experience, it is not possible to adequately decompress the BA or its aneurysms away from the nerve by a retrosigmoid approach because the artery is fairly fixed in its position. The only solution is to open up Meckel's cave by a transpetrosal approach and then allow the nerve root to be mobilized away from the BA.

Compression of the trigeminal root may also occur by veins. Such venous compression may take the form of a "trigeminal vein" at the entrance to the Meckel's cave, or other unnamed veins close to the brain stem. In the latter case, there are frequently variations of the standard drainage pattern of the petrous vein such that one of the veins forming the petrosal vein is running more anteriorly, compressing the trigeminal root. Most veins compressing the trigeminal root may be cauterized and divided. The only exception to this is anomalous draining veins (venous angiomas) or veins draining a dural arteriovenous malformation (AVM). Anomalous draining veins cannot be occluded. Vein draining dural AVMs must be occluded only after the arterial supply of the dural AVM has been disconnected.

At the conclusion of the decompression procedure, the endoscope must be used again to inspect the nerve root 360 degrees around its circumference to ensure complete decompression. In patients with trigeminal venous compression near Meckel's cave wherein the vein is obstructed by a prominent petrous ridge, the decompression procedure (mobilization of the nerve, cauterization, and division of the vein) may need to be performed mainly under endoscopic vision. In patients with recurrent trigeminal neuralgia, the surgeon may find vessels that were missed during the previous operation, and scar tissue caused by the Teflon felt; most of the Teflon felt must be removed because the original compressive vessel will already be fixed in a new position.

In an occasional patient, no compressive vessel is found despite a typical history of trigeminal neuralgia and adequate inspection by the use of the endoscope. In such patients, section of the anteroinferior half of the nerve may be considered if the pain was in V2 or V3 division (this is not effective if pain is localized to V1). Alternatively, the surgeon may do nothing and treat the patient later with radiosurgery of the nerve root.

Closure

The dura mater is closed under the microscope. Primary closure can usually be accomplished. Small defects may be closed with pieces of muscle or fascia extracted from the wound. Fibrin glue is used for reinforcement. If there is dural shrinkage, a small free graft of pericranium may be employed.

The bone flap is reattached with titanium microplates. Frequently, there are defects in the bone, which are covered with titanium mesh and bone cement. The muscle layers are reattached to the bone or to the titanium plates. The skin is closed as usual.

◆ Postoperative Care

We generally do not administer steroids postoperatively. The patient is observed in the step-down unit or the intensive care unit for a day. Active ambulation is commenced

12 hours after the surgery, and most patients can be discharged 2 to 3 days after the operation. Sutures are removed 1 week after the surgery. Most patients are able to return to work 2 to 4 weeks after discharge depending on their work and recovery. Patients with trigeminal neuralgia who were on many medications preoperatively may need to be tapered over 1 week and stopped.

◆ Complications

Cerebellar contusion and hemorrhage are possible complications. Most of these occur during the opening and initial retraction. A very lateral approach, the use of a lumbar drain, early cisternal drainage, and gentle cerebellar retraction will prevent these complications.

Injury to the sigmoid sinus may occur during the craniotomy or craniectomy. The correct placement of the initial bur hole is important. In older patients, the lateral wall of the sinus becomes adherent to the mastoidal bone and may be damaged if the edge of the sinus is not carefully separated before the craniectomy. Small injuries to the sinus can be managed by placement of oxidized cellulose (Surgicel, Johnson & Johnson Medical Inc., Arlington, TX) or Gelfoam (Upjohn, Kalamazoo, MI) and tack-up sutures. If the tear is large, it is best to apply pressure with cotton patties and expose the sinus further by drilling the bone carefully on the other side. The tear in the sinus is thus repaired with a dural patch, using 6–0 Prolene sutures. This technique is generally preferable to simply packing the sinus closed, especially on the right side; this may result in acute venous obstruction, with serious consequences.

Injury to the CNs, especially to CN VIII, is generally avoided by gentle retraction, careful microtechnique and handling of not only the nerve but also the arteries, and the use of neuromonitoring. If vasospasm of the AICA is observed at surgery, it is relieved by coating the vessel with 3% papaverine solution.

Postoperative CSF leakage through the wound or through the mastoid air cells into the nose is rare. Careful dural closure, fibrin glue application, wax closure of the mastoid air cells, and the trapdoor-like closure of the skin and muscle flaps are steps to use to avoid CSF leaks. CSF leak through the wound may occur more commonly in reoperation cases. In the majority of cases, CSF leakage stops with spinal fluid drainage (30 mL every 8 hours) for 3 days. Very rarely, if leakage through the mastoid air cells continues, reexploration and closure of the fistula may be necessary. Postoperative infection is extremely uncommon. Epidural infection can be manifested by swelling of the wound, fever, and purulent drainage. Reexploration with the removal of the bone flap and all foreign materials, and a 4 to 6 week course of intravenous antibiotics will be curative.

In patients with trigeminal neuralgia, the pain may not abate completely for a few weeks. Patients should be warned about this. Similarly, in patients with hemifacial spasm, the complete subsidence of the spasm initially may be followed by the recurrence of a few spasms. However, if the spasm continues unabated for several weeks, it is a cause for concern and warrants reoperation.

Suggested Readings

Adams CBT. Microvascular compression: an alternative view and hypothesis. J Neurosurg 1989;70:1–12

Adams CBT, Kaye AH, Teddy PJ. The treatment of trigeminal neuralgia by posterior fossa microsurgery. J Neurol Neurosurg Psychiatry 1982;45: 1020–1026

Dandy WE. An operation for the cure of tic douloureux: partial section of the sensory root at the pons. Arch Surg 1929;18:687–734

Dandy WE. The treatment of trigeminal neuralgia by the cerebellar route. Ann Surg 1932;96:787–795

Dandy WE. Concerning the cause of trigeminal neuralgia. Am J Surg 1934; 24:447–455

Dandy WE. Trigeminal neuralgia and trigeminal tic douloureux. In: Davis L, ed. Practice of Surgery. Vol 12. Hagerstown, MD: WF Prior, 1946: 167–187

Jannetta PJ. Arterial compression of the trigeminal nerve at the pons in patients with trigeminal neuralgia. J Neurosurg 1967;26(Suppl 1): 159–192

Jannetta PJ. Microsurgical approach to the trigeminal nerve for tic douloureux. Prog Neurol Surg 1976;7:180–200

Jannetta PJ. Treatment of trigeminal neuralgia by suboccipital and transtentorial cranial operations. Clin Neurosurg 1977;24:538–549

Jannetta PJ. Observations on the etiology of trigeminal neuralgia, hemifacial spasm, acoustic nerve dysfunction and glossopharyngeal neuralgia: definitive microsurgical treatment and results in 117 patients. Neurochirurgia (Stuttgart) 1977;20:145–154

Jannetta PJ. Microsurgery of cranial nerve cross-compression. Clin Neurosurg 1979;26:607–615

Jannetta PJ. Treatment of trigeminal neuralgia by micro-operative decompression. In: Youmans JR, ed. Neurological Surgery. 3rd ed. Philadelphia: Saunders; 1990:3929–3942

Jannetta PJ. Microvascular decompression of the trigeminal nerve root entry zone: theoretical considerations, operative anatomy, surgical techniques, and results. In: Rovit RL, Murali R, Janneta PJ, eds. Trigeminal Neuralgia. Baltimore: Williams & Wilkins; 1990:201–222

Jannetta PJ. Trigeminal disorders: supralateral exposure of the trigeminal nerve in the cerebellopontine angle for microvascular decompression. In: Apuzzo MLJ, ed. Brain Surgery: Complications Avoidance and Management. New York: Churchill Livingstone; 1993: 2085–2096, 2109–2111

Jannetta PJ. Vascular compression is the cause of trigeminal neuralgia. APS J 1993;2:217–227, 237–238

Jannetta PJ, Abbasy M, Maroon JC, Ramos FM, Albin MS. Etiology and definitive microsurgical treatment of hemifacial spasm: operative techniques and results in 47 patients. J Neurosurgery 1977;47:321–328

Moller AR. Vascular compression of cranial nerves, I: History of the microvascular decompression operation. Neurol Res 1998;20:727–731

Nathoo N, Mayberg MR, Barnett GH. W. James Gardner: pioneer neurosurgeon and inventor. J Neurosurg 2004;100:965–973

Rak R, Sekhar LN, Stimac D, Hechl P. Endoscope assisted microvascular decompression Neurosurgery 2004;54:876–882

73

Radiofrequency and Glycerol Rhizotomy for Trigeminal Neuralgia

Rashid M. Janjua and Jamal M. Taha

Trigeminal neuralgia, a condition characterized by unilateral lancinating facial pain, is usually treated effectively by medications (carbamazepine, gabapentin, baclofen, diphenylhydantoin). Patients in whom medical therapy fails, because of either increased pain or adverse effects, require surgical treatment. Treatment options include posterior fossa microvascular decompression, percutaneous ablative procedures (radiofrequency rhizotomy, glycerol rhizotomy, balloon compression), peripheral neurectomy, and radiosurgery. This chapter discusses radiofrequency and glycerol rhizotomy.

Radiofrequency rhizotomy is based on the ability of a graded thermal lesion to produce a relatively selective destruction of pain fibers in the trigeminal root.[1] This procedure was first introduced by Kirshner, modified and popularized by Sweet, and further refined by Tew. Glycerol rhizotomy probably relies on the chemical destruction of medium-size myelinated trigeminal fibers.[2] This procedure, first introduced by Håkanson,[3] rapidly gained popularity due to presumed sparing of facial sensations, an assumption that did not prove correct.

◆ Indications

Percutaneous destructive procedures are recommended for patients with trigeminal neuralgia who are elderly (>60 years) or in poor medical condition, patients with multiple sclerosis associated with trigeminal neuralgia, and patients who develop recurrent pain following microvascular decompression. Microvascular decompression is recommended for young patients in good medical condition, especially if pain involves the ophthalmic division or all three trigeminal divisions, and patients who express concern about postoperative facial numbness.[4]

Among the percutaneous destructive procedures, radiofrequency rhizotomy has the lowest pain recurrence rate (20% in 7 years),[5] whereas glycerol rhizotomy has the highest (50% in 3 years).[6] All destructive procedures produce various degrees of facial numbness. Although glycerol rhizotomy is often claimed to produce minimal dysesthesia, a review of the current literature over the past 10 years does not support this contention.[4] The incidence of dysesthesia and the rate of pain recurrence following mild radiofrequency rhizotomy equal those of glycerol rhizotomy.[4]

Balloon compression selectively destroys large myelinated fibers,[7] making this procedure useful for control of pain in the ophthalmic division without loss of corneal sensation. Mild radiofrequency lesions and glycerol rhizotomy can produce similar results.

◆ Preparation

Preoperatively, a magnetic resonance imaging (MRI) scan is obtained to exclude tumors, cysts, and vascular lesions. Anticoagulant therapy is stopped before surgery, but aspirin may be continued if necessary. Atropine 0.4 mg is administered intramuscularly 30 minutes before surgery to decrease saliva production. A peripheral intravenous access line is secured. Antibiotics are not administered unless indicated (e.g., rheumatoid valvular disease).

◆ Radiofrequency Rhizotomy

Positioning

The procedure is usually performed in the x-ray suite but may be performed in the operating room in medically unstable patients. The patient lies supine with the neck in a neutral position with the arms strapped alongside the body. A grounding pad is attached to the patient. Blood pressure, an electrocardiogram, and pulse oximetry are monitored. The surgeon stands ipsilateral to the patient's affected side.

Needle Placement

Three external landmarks that are marked on the patient's face guide needle placement **(Fig. 73–1A).** Mark 1 is inferior to the pupil, mark 2 is 3 cm anterior to the external auditory meatus along the zygoma, and mark 3 is 2.5 cm lateral to the oral commissure. The skin over mark 3 is prepared with povidone-iodine.

A padded oral airway is placed between the patient's jaws to prevent involuntary biting of the surgeon's finger, which is placed against the lateral pterygoid. Methohexital 40 to 60 mg is administered intravenously. A 100 mm 20 gauge needle (Tew kit, Radionics, Burlington, MA) is inserted through the skin at mark 3 and is directed in the lateral-medial direction toward mark 1, and in the inferior-superior direction toward mark 2 **(Fig. 73–1B).** The needle slides parallel to the surgeon's finger without penetrating the buccal mucosa. Using lateral fluoroscopy, the surgeon directs the cannula toward the intersection of the clivus and the petrous apex, 5 to 10 mm below the sellar floor **(Fig. 73–2A).** Entrance of the cannula into the foramen ovale is signaled by a facial wince, indicating contact with the mandibular nerve. Efflux of cerebrospinal fluid after removal of the stylet indicates, but does not guarantee, cannulation of the trigeminal cistern. Cerebrospinal fluid is obtained from the subtemporal space if the cannula is too deep, or from the gasserian ganglion in cases in which the arachnoid extends distally.

Stimulation and Lesioning

After needle placement, the surgeon changes gloves and replaces the stylet with a Tew curved electrode. The tip of the electrode, which extends up to 5 mm beyond the cannula, is directed caudal within 5 mm proximal to the clival line for third-division pain, straight at the clival line for second-division pain, and cephalad within 5 mm distal to the clival line for first-division pain **(Fig. 73–2B–D).**

The cannula should not be advanced more than 8 mm beyond the clival line to avoid injury of the abducens nerve at Dorello's canal or penetration of the cavernous sinus, the temporal lobe, or the brain stem.

After positioning of the electrode, the patient is allowed to wake up. The correct localization of the electrode tip is confirmed by stimulation using a square-wave pulse of a pulse width of 0.1 msec and a rate of 50 Hz. Stimulation is perceived by the patient as paresthesias or pain in the appropriate division at stimulation amplitudes of 0.3 to 0.6 V. Higher amplitudes may be needed in patients who have had previous destructive surgery. When pain is perceived, it should be differentiated from an attack of trigeminal neuralgia induced by needle placement resulting in nonspecific irritation of the

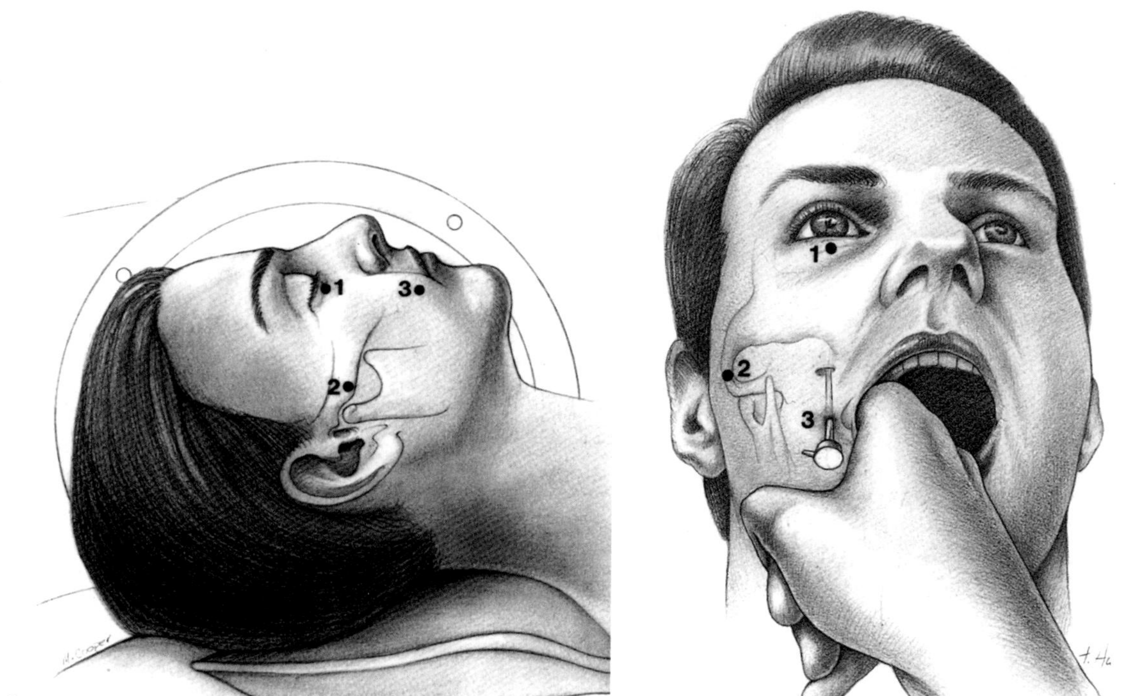

A B

Figure 73–1 **(A)** Patient positioning for radiofrequency rhizotomy. With the head in a neutral position, the following three facial landmarks are marked: 1, inferior to the pupil; 2, 3 cm anterior to the external auditory meatus along the zygoma; and 3, site of needle penetration 2.5 cm lateral to oral commissure. **(B)** Placement of electrode according to Hartel's technique, directing the needle toward the intersection of the planes indicated by points 1 and 2. The surgeon's right-hand index finger prevents the needle from entering the oral cavity. (Reprinted with permission from the Mayfield Clinic.)

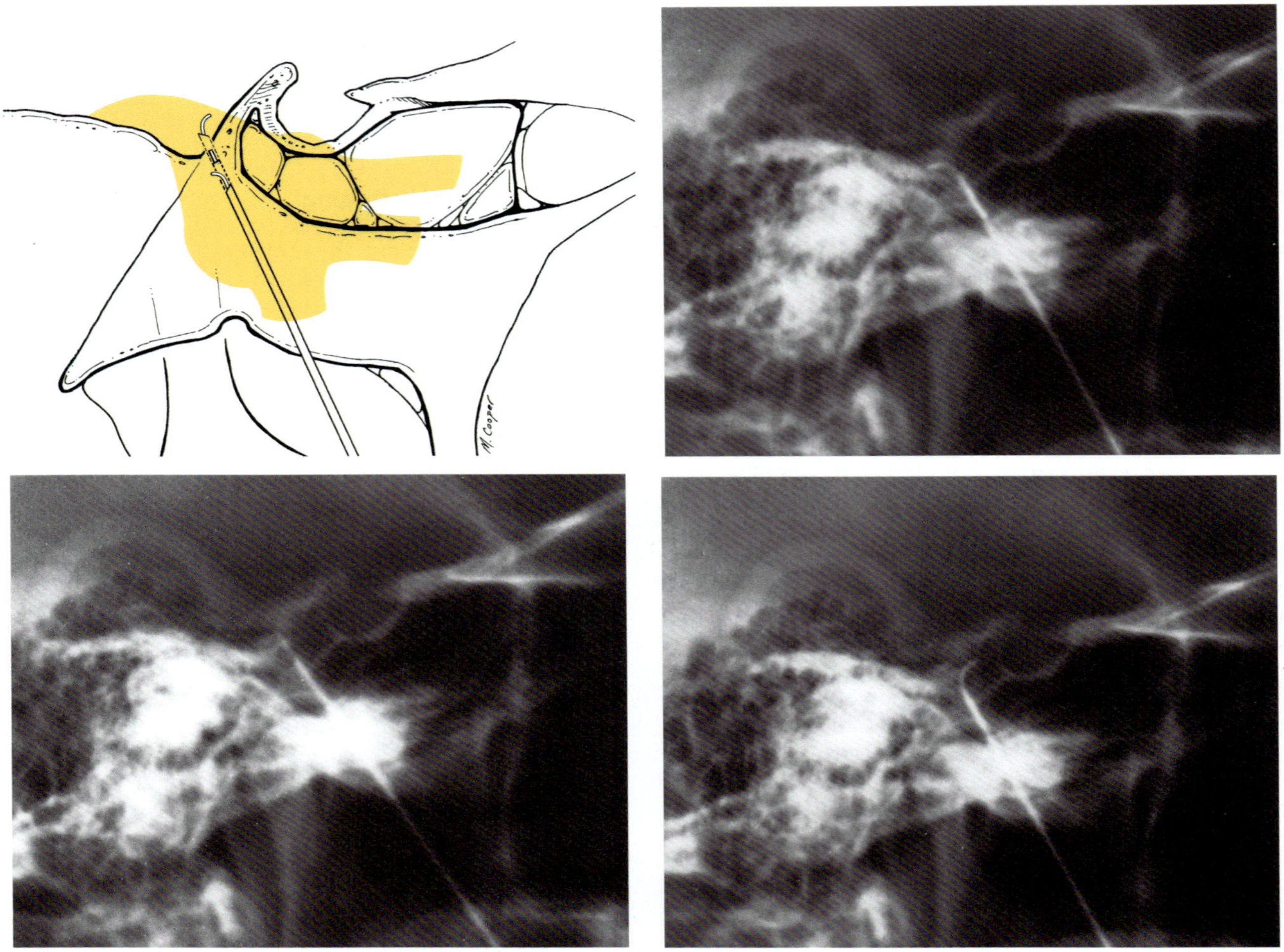

A B C D

Figure 73–2 **(A)** Composite illustration showing the three electrode positions and their relationship to the profile of the clivus, petrous ridge, and trigeminal ganglion for radiofrequency rhizotomy of V1, V2, and V3. The needle is directed toward the intersection of the petrous ridge with the clivus, 5 to 10 mm below the floor of the sella turcica. (Reprinted with permission from the Mayfield Clinic.) **(B)** Lateral fluoroscopic view of needle and electrode position for a V3 lesion. **(C)** Lateral fluoroscopic view of needle and electrode position for a V2 lesion. **(D)** Lateral fluoroscopic view of needle and electrode position for a V1 lesion. (From Fick J, Tew J. Percutaneous radiofrequency rhizolysis for trigeminal neuralgia. In: Neurosurgical Operative Atlas. Vol 1. Park Ridge, IL: American Association of Neurological Surgeons; 1991:405–416, with permission.)

nerve. If stimulation is not achieved in the affected division, the electrode needs to be replaced. This is achieved by one of the following three maneuvers: rotating the electrode lateral (V3) or medial (V1), varying the depth of the electrode in relation to the clival line to move proximal (V3) or distal (V1), or redirecting the needle in a more inferior (V3) or superior (V1) direction. After adequate stimulation has been achieved, the patient is sedated again with 20 to 30 mg of intravenous methohexital. A preliminary lesion is created at 60°C for 60 seconds for V1, 65°C for 65 seconds for V2, and 70°C for 70 seconds for V3. A facial flush may appear in the division being lesioned. During lesioning the corneal reflexes and facial sensations are monitored by using saline drops and reaction to pinprick, respectively.

After lesioning the patient is allowed to wake up again and facial sensations are examined for pinprick both quantitatively and qualitatively. Quantitatively, facial sensations are tested by asking the patient to assess the percentage loss of sensation to pinprick on both sides of the face.

Qualitatively, three modalities are tested: superficial tactile sensation using a wisp of cotton, deep touch sensation (a nongentle stroke by the examiner's finger), and sensation to pinprick. These are tested bilaterally. Deep touch sensation should not be confused with deep pressure sensation.

The ideal lesion produces a loss of sensation to superficial but not deep touch when pressure is applied on the face, and is associated with a 75% or more reduction of sensation to pinprick. A denser thermal lesion can be achieved by increasing the temperature in increments of 5° to 10°C and time in increments of 10 to 15 seconds, to a maximum of 95°C for 90 seconds.

After a lesion is made, the neurological examination is repeated to assess the end result. The needle is then removed, and manual pressure is applied to the entry site for a few minutes. The neurological examination is repeated, emphasizing the extraocular muscles, masseter and pterygoid muscle function, and skin sensations.

Postoperative Care

Ice packs are applied to the face for 4 hours; after that the patient is discharged. Eye drops are administered for 2 weeks, or longer if corneal sensations are lost. The patient is advised to avoid solid food for 1 week. Antiepileptic medications are reduced by half and tapered to discontinue over 2 weeks.

◆ Glycerol Rhizotomy

Positioning

This procedure is preferably performed in the operating room unless the x-ray suite is equipped with a reclining table. The patient lies in the supine position with the head mildly extended (10 degrees) and rotated 15 degrees away from the affected side. The fluoroscope is positioned in anteroposteriorly, and tilted ventrally 30 to 40 degrees **(Fig. 73–3A).** With this method, the foramen ovale can be visualized en face between the mandible laterally and the maxillary sinus medially, just medial and superior to the petrous apex **(Fig. 73–3B).**

Needle Placement

After placement of the mouthpiece and sterilizing the skin, methohexital 30 to 50 mg is administered intravenously and a guiding index finger is placed in the buccal cavity. A 20 gauge spinal needle is inserted 2.5 mm lateral to the oral

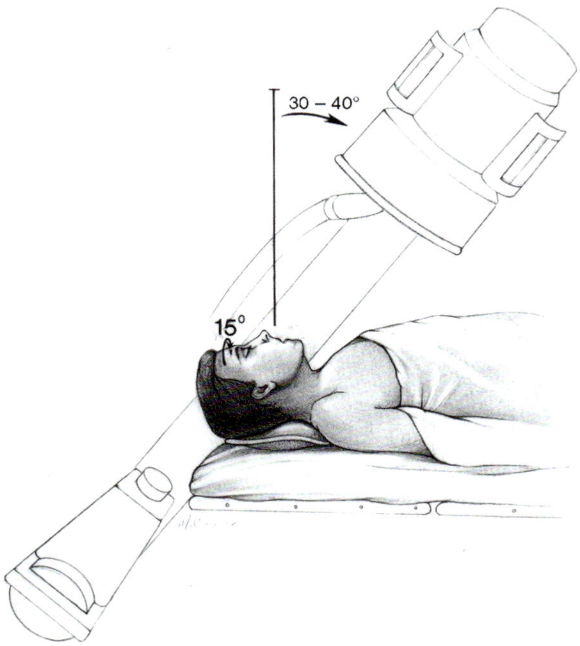

A

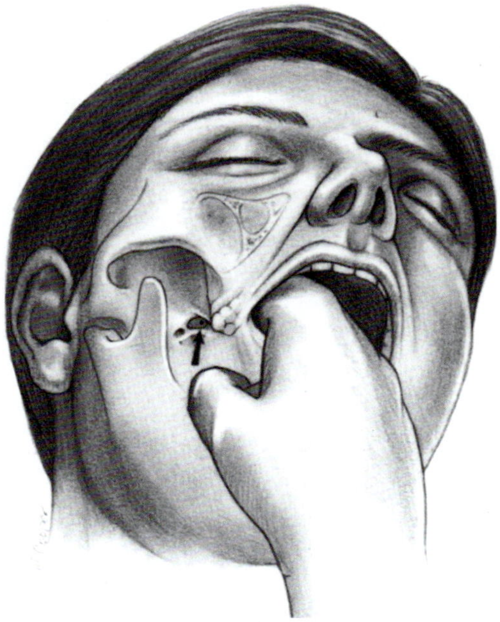

B

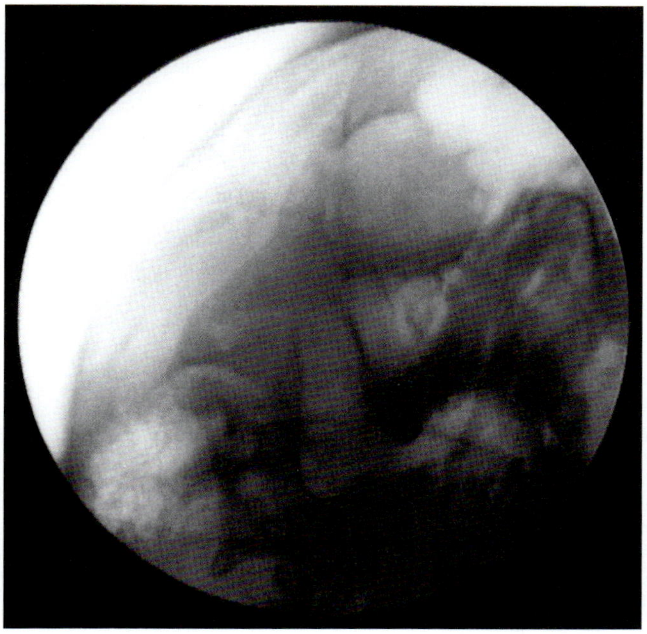

C

Figure 73–3 **(A)** Patient positioning for glycerol rhizotomy. The fluoroscope is positioned anteroposteriorly and tilted ventrally 30 to 40 degrees. The head is extended 10 degrees and rotated ~15 degrees away from the affected side. **(B)** Slight adjustments are made to the fluoroscope position until the foramen ovale is visualized en face between the maxillary sinus and mandible. The needle is guided to the center of the medial half of the foramen ovale (arrow) to enter the trigeminal cistern. Entry into the cistern is confirmed with cerebrospinal fluid efflux after removal of the stylet. (Reprinted with permission from the Mayfield Clinic.) **(C)** Fluoroscopic view showing the foramen ovale en face between the maxillary sinus and the mandible.

commissure, alongside the trajectory of the x-ray beam. Under intermittent fluoroscopic guidance, the needle is directed toward the medial half of the foramen ovale to allow cannulation of the trigeminal cistern. Care should be taken not to penetrate the buccal mucosa. Once the needle engages the foramen ovale, a wince in the face is observed, indicating contact with the mandibular division. A lateral fluorogram is obtained (**Fig. 73–4A**). If cerebrospinal fluid is not obtained, the needle is advanced under lateral fluoroscopy, within 5 mm proximal to the clival line. Efflux of cerebrospinal fluid is necessary for confirmation of needle placement in the cistern. Once this is achieved, the patient is then seated on the reclining table with the head slightly flexed.

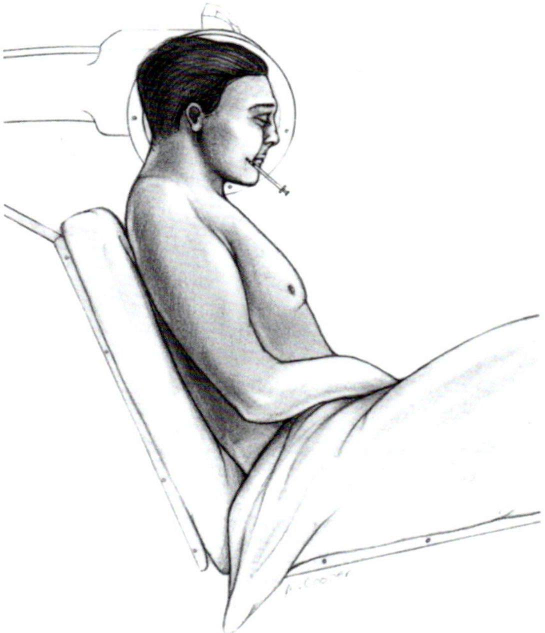

A

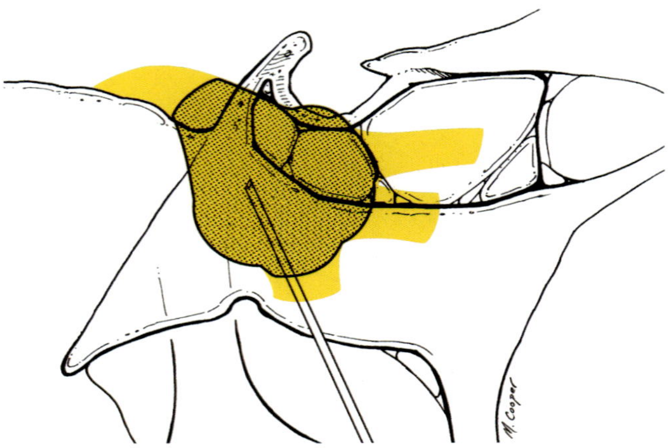

B

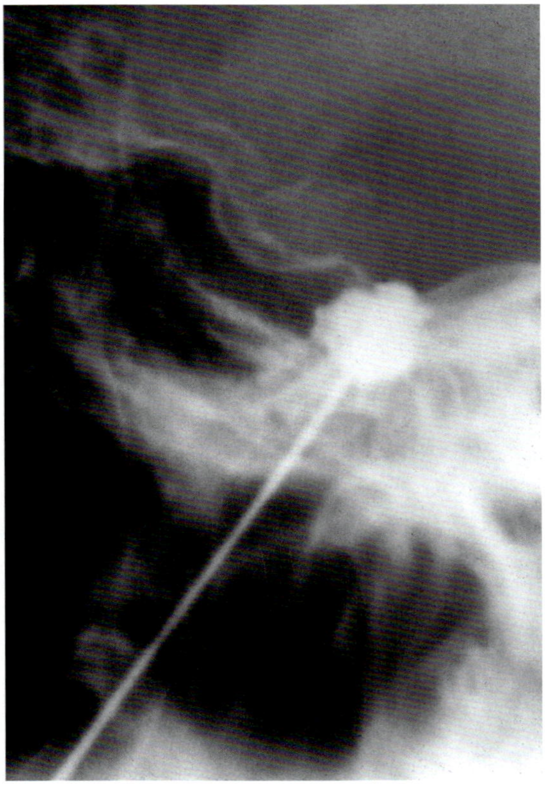

C

Figure 73–4 **(A)** Once correct needle placement is confirmed, the patient is elevated to a semiseated position and the head is slightly flexed. The contrast agent is injected to determine cisternal volume under lateral fluoroscopic view. **(B)** Composite illustration showing the position of the needle in the trigeminal cistern. Stippled area represents the boundaries for the trigeminal cistern. (Reprinted with permission from the Mayfield Clinic.) **(C)** Lateral fluoroscopic view showing the cisternogram, which is used to determine cisternal volume. The cisternogram shows the short extensions of the trigeminal cistern over the three divisions.

Cisternal Imaging and Lesioning

The head is maintained in the neutral position and the patient is seated on the reclining table. A water-soluble contrast agent such as iopamidol is injected to determine cisternal volume, which averages 0.2 to 0.5 mL **(Fig. 73–4B,C)**. The contrast agent is drained through the cannula. If this does not suffice, then the patient is placed in the supine position with the head extended to allow the contrast agent to drain into the posterior fossa. It is drained out completely for V3, 80% for V2, and 60% for V1. The difference between the cisternal volume and the volume of retained contrast agent represents the volume of glycerol that needs to be injected. This method, based on the relative difference between the buoyancy of the contrast agent and that of glycerol, allows relatively selective destruction of the involved division. Glycerol injection is performed with the patient in the sitting position. Patients may experience transient dysesthesia and headache during injection. After the injection is completed, the cannula is removed and the patient is seated for 1 hour with the head flexed.

◆ Complications

Complications that may arise after percutaneous radiofrequency and glycerol rhizotomy can be minimized by strict adherence to details of the procedure, as described above. During needle placement, guidance by fluoroscopy is mandatory to avoid cannulation of the carotid artery, jugular foramen, superior orbital fissure, or other foramina. If the carotid artery is punctured, the needle should be withdrawn, manual pressure applied, and the procedure terminated. Surgery can be repeated 48 hours later.

In radiofrequency rhizotomy, lighter lesions are safer than deeper lesions to avoid complications of sensory deprivation such as dysesthesia, keratitis, and anesthesia dolorosa. With experience, the surgeon learns when to stop. In patients who are unable to communicate, the surgeon can assess the depth of the thermal lesion by evaluating the patient's reaction to pinprick. The surgeon should limit the lesion to the affected dermatome.

In glycerol rhizotomy, we believe that cerebrospinal fluid efflux is essential to ensure direct contact of the nerve fibers with the glycerol, signifying completion of the procedure; however, not all surgeons share this opinion. Thus, we usually do not recommend glycerol rhizotomy for patients who have undergone multiple previous percutaneous ablative procedures.

◆ Conclusion

Both percutaneous radiofrequency and glycerol rhizotomies can effectively treat pain of trigeminal neuralgia with minimal morbidity and mortality. Among the percutaneous ablative procedures, we usually recommend radiofrequency rhizotomy because of its high success rate, low recurrence rate, and minimal morbidity. In our experience, adhering to the technique described, dysesthesia has occurred infrequently. We recommend glycerol rhizotomy to elderly patients who have V1 pain and who cannot tolerate general anesthesia. The finesse required by the procedures can be learned with experience. We strongly encourage inexperienced neurosurgeons to observe experts in the field performing these procedures before attempting one.

References

1. Letcher FS, Goldring S. The effect of radiofrequency current and heat on peripheral nerve action potential in the cat. J Neurosurg 1968;29:42–47
2. Rengachary SS, Watanabe IS, Singer P, Bopp WJ. Effect of glycerol on peripheral nerve: an experimental study. Neurosurgery 1983;13:681–688
3. Håkanson S. Trigeminal neuralgia treated by the injection of glycerol into the trigeminal cistern. Neurosurgery 1981;9:638–646
4. Taha J, Tew JMT Jr. Comparison of surgical treatments for trigeminal neuralgia: reevaluation of radiofrequency rhizotomy. Neurosurgery 1996;38:865–871
5. Taha J, Tew JMT Jr. Therapeutic decisions in facial pain. Clin Neurosurg 1999;45:In press
6. Taha J, Tew JMT Jr. A prospective 15-year follow up of 154 consecutive patients with trigeminal neuralgia treated by percutaneous stereotactic radiofrequency thermal rhizotomy. J Neurosurg 1995;83:989–993
7. Brown JA, Hoeflinger B, Long PB, Axon and ganglion cell injury in rabbits after percutaneous trigeminal balloon compression. Neurosurgery 1996;38:993–1003

74

Percutaneous Balloon Compression for Trigeminal Neuralgia: Technique and Results

Jeffrey A. Brown

Is it better to injure the trigeminal nerve in treating tic pain or to preserve function and decompress it? An appropriate philosophy for treatment would be to relieve each patient's pain using the least invasive approach that causes the lowest morbidity. Numbness is a morbidity of any percutaneous approach to tic douloureux, yet it is frequently more acceptable to patients than the potential morbidity of microvascular decompression: death, ataxia, deafness, facial weakness, or reoperation for spinal fluid leak.[1,2]

Whereas microvascular decompression treats the cause of tic douloureux, percutaneous procedures, such as balloon compression, ignore the cause of the "short circuit" that is the source of pain. Instead they injure either the fibers that transmit the tic pain or the fibers that turn on the switch triggering a painful tic shock. Balloon compression injures the trigeminal nerve by mechanically compressing these myelinated fibers until they are injured.[3]

How do surgeons choose the most appropriate procedure for treatment of tic pain? To an extent they select the procedure for which they are best trained and experienced. Ideally, they tailor the procedure to the symptoms experienced by each patient. A young woman with multidivisional pain and convincing evidence of vascular compression on a magnetic resonance imaging (MRI) scan should be offered a microvascular decompression first. We as neurosurgeons usually agree on this approach. The patient may not. She may not wish to take the risk inherent in a posterior fossa craniectomy. The ability to injure fibers of the first division by thermal rhizotomy, yet preserve the corneal reflex, is based on experience and judgment. Alternatively, a judgment must be made regarding the volume of glycerol to inject to achieve first-division pain relief.

With balloon compression there is no real need for such subtlety. Once the balloon catheter is positioned correctly, balloon pressure is easily measured and the duration of compression is in general unchanged. The position of the balloon correlates with the fiber divisions to be injured. First-division fiber injury does not require more experience, but instead is dependent only on the location of the balloon in the porous and over the ganglion.

Why perform balloon compression instead of other percutaneous procedures?

Compression selectively injures large myelinated fibers, not those small fibers that mediate the corneal reflex. It is thus less likely to injure the corneal reflex.

Compression can injure fibers in multiple divisions in a single compression, reducing the operating time needed to complete the procedure.

The procedure may be performed under general anesthesia. It does not require patient cooperation. The mean age of patients with trigeminal neuralgia who require surgery is 65 years. This elderly population often has trouble communicating, especially when partially sedated, making the selective procedures more difficult to complete.

Indications

Percutaneous balloon compression is indicated for patients who have classical trigeminal neuralgia and have failed medical therapy. This group includes patients who are intolerant of or allergic to anticonvulsants or for whom the medications' other effects are significant. Patients with multiple sclerosis who also have trigeminal neuralgia can be treated by compression. Balloon compression alleviates lancinating pain even when patients have a concurrent trigeminal neuropathy. This trigeminal neuropathy probably represents a later stage of trigeminal neuralgia. The disease progresses from an infrequent, intermittent, unpredictable pain onset to a nearly continuous pain with an underlying, aching residual component over time. What has been described as atypical facial pain does not respond to balloon compression.[4] Atypical pain is usually a dysesthetic or neuropathic pain, the words for which the patient has difficulty identifying. With these patients it may be appropriate to use descriptive pain scales to best identify the nature of the patient's discomfort. Contralateral masseter weakness is a relative contraindication because balloon compression often causes temporary masseter weakness. Bilateral masseter/pterygoid weakness is not incapacitating. Young patients are also candidates for balloon compression if they are willing to accept the associated mild to moderate numbness that occurs after surgery. Elderly patients tolerate the short general anesthetic well, perhaps better than an intravenous anesthetic. Intravenous anesthesia does not protect the airway as well as general anesthetic nor does it control intraoperative pain as consistently.

◆ Preparation

Preoperative imaging of the posterior fossa with MRI is obtained. Only rarely is there an intracranial lesion present. With MRI, using fine axial slices, the vascular loop of the superior cerebellar artery appears as a curvilinear signal-void focus medial to the proximal portion of the trigeminal nerve on T1-weighted axial images. MRI may even show the deformity of the root entry zone. Better images are possible if the operating neurosurgeon monitors the MRI scan acquisitions to ensure that the images cut through the trigeminal nerve at the pontine level.

Skull radiographs of the foramen ovale are done by a modified submental imaging technique. These images predict those patients in whom the foramen cannot be visualized or is too small to allow penetration of the embolectomy catheter. This image is obtained by extending the neck 15 degrees and rotating the head toward the opposite side by 15 degrees, then shooting an image at a submental angle of 25 degrees. The radiologist should review the images obtained to ensure that the foramen is optimally seen.

A general anesthetic is used. Arrhythmias potentially may occur if the pacemaker is triggered by the bradycardia that occurs intraoperatively. An electrocardiogram should therefore be reviewed before surgery. Patients with a history of "cold sores" should receive acyclovir a day or two before surgery. If started after the onset of the sore, the medication is ineffective in halting the viral syndrome's course.

◆ Surgical Technique

Approach

It is easiest if the procedure is done in the angiography suite using multiplanar imaging. A portable C-arm imaging unit with digital enhancement may be used if the procedure is performed in the operating room. The more advanced the radiological adjuncts, the more easily the cannula can be positioned. Three views are used: modified submental, modified anterior-posterior, and lateral.

Anesthesia

Atropine blocks the trigeminal depressor response. The occurrence of the depressor response helps to confirm the degree of nerve compression; therefore, it is best not to use atropine. Instead use an external or esophageal pacemaker. General anesthesia is induced, usually with isoflurane or propofol. After induction with anesthesia, the external pacemaker is positioned on the chest or an esophageal pacer is inserted set to trigger at 40 beats/minute. The anesthesiologist must test the pacemaker to ensure that it will capture when triggered. The depressor response consists of both bradycardia and brief hypotension, often with a reflex hypertension after triggering the pacemaker. It is consistently different from the pressor response (tachycardia and hypertension) seen during radiofrequency rhizotomy. Different fibers are injured in these procedures. The pacemaker responds move quickly than the anesthesiologist can by injecting intravenous atropine. Blocking the depressor response eliminates an excellent monitor of the degree of nerve injury.[5]

Positioning

Position the patient supine with the head in neutral position. This may be done by placing a roll beneath the neck or shoulders. To obtain the modified submental view, the imaging unit is directed at an angle of about 25 to 30 degrees submental, then 15 degrees toward the side of the planned procedure. The foramen ovale is seen just medial to the mandible, lateral to the maxilla, and just above the petrous bone. The foramen should be centered in the video image (**Fig. 74–1**).

After the 14 gauge blunt cannula is positioned at the foramen, an anteroposterior view is imaged. The petrous bone is centered radiographically within the margins of the ipsilateral orbit. There is a dip in the petrous bone medially that corresponds to the porus trigeminus. The guiding stylet and balloon catheter tip are positioned in the lateral side of this dip, at the edge of the petrous bone, and in the center for V2 or V1 pain (**Fig. 74–2**). For an accurate understanding of the location of the stylet position, the petrous bones are aligned and the tip of the balloon stylet is centered in the image intensifier.

A digital balloon pressure monitor is fixed to the fluoroscopy table opposite the surgeon, at the patient's waist level. Imaging monitors are positioned toward the head of the table opposite the side of surgery. The surgeon controls the imaging units with a joystick. The anesthesiologist's equipment is positioned at about the level of the patient's waistline to accommodate the movements of the imaging unit. A long endotracheal connecting tube is needed from the anesthesiologist's machine.

A disposable kit is available that includes all the equipment needed for the procedure except for the radiographic dye. After sterile preparation, the entry point is marked with a pen. The eyes are lubricated and taped shut. Towels drape off the sterile face and a long drape is placed over the neck and chest. The balloon catheter and insufflation syringe are placed on this sterile field.

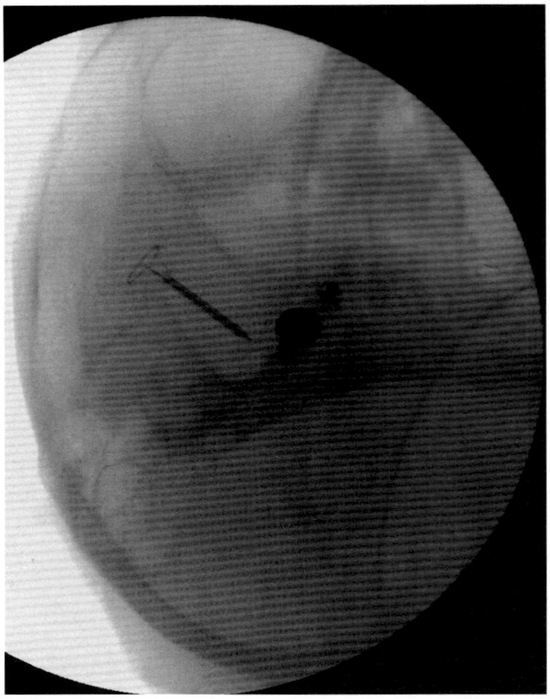

Figure 74–1 Modified submental fluoroscopic image. Needle is positioned in the foramen ovale. Note the medial maxillary sinus, inferior petrous bone, and lateral mandible.

Operative Procedure

A mark is made on the cheek 2 to 3 cm lateral to the angle of the lip, slightly more lateral for first-division pain treatment. The skin is nicked with the no. 11 blade. A sharp obturator is inserted into the 14 gauge blunt cannula and used to penetrate the skin of the cheek. The blunt obturator replaces the sharp one. The cannula is angled parallel to the beam of the image intensifier. The beam is directed toward the center of the foramen ovale. As the foramen is engaged, the depressor response briefly occurs. The tactile feedback and the depressor response will help to prevent penetration beyond the foramen. If a concurrent lateral view is obtainable, this also is beneficial. On the lateral view the cannula can be seen at the level of the middle fossa skull base. The blunt obturator is removed and a straight guiding stylet inserted. Sometimes there is venous bleeding at the skull base. Advancing the cannula slightly until it engages the foramen can prevent this.

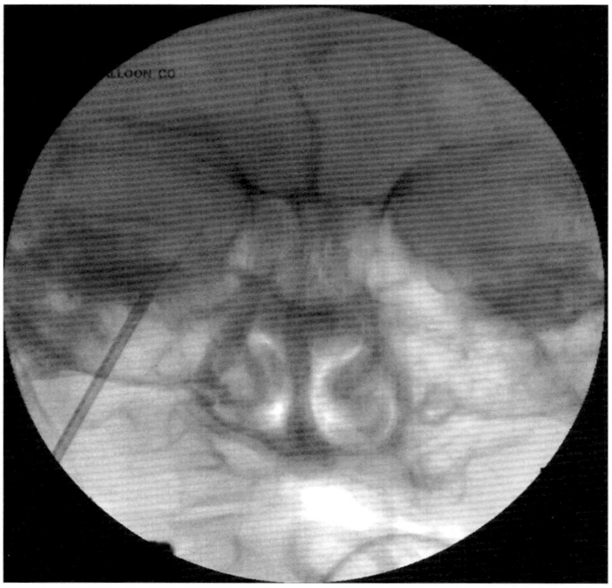

Figure 74–2 Modified anterior posterior image. The catheter stylet is directed to the midportion of the porus trigeminus, its tip at the edge of the petrous ridge. The petrous ridge is positioned radiographically in the midportion of the orbit.

The guiding stylet is directed toward the dip in the petrous bone representing the proximal entrance to Meckel's cave. For third-division pain, the stylet should be directed to the lateral porus, and for second-division pain, to the center. If the patient has first-division pain, the cannula should be directed from a more lateral approach and the guiding stylet directed to the medial porus. The entrance to Meckel's cave is usually 17 mm beyond the foramen ovale. The guiding stylet creates a path through which the catheter easily passes. A curved stylet can be used to reach the medial porus or to redirect the path toward the porus if the cannula entrance angle is lateral. Once the track has been made, the stylet is removed and the catheter advanced to the same position at the edge of the petrous bone. Lateral and modified anteroposterior (AP) views are used to confirm the catheter location. The catheter has an inner thin wire that allows its position to be verified on the image intensifier. The catheter is soft and blunt and should limit the risk of hemorrhage if used alone, but if the catheter does not reach the entrance to Meckel's cave, then the retrogasserian fibers will not be compressed by the balloon. It is here that the highest pressures are obtained. At the entrance to Meckel's cave, the balloon compresses the retrogasserian fibers against the firm edge of the dura and petrous ridge because the dura splits, allowing the nerve to pass into Meckel's cave. This opening is 9 × 2 mm.

When the balloon inflates within the porus, there is a characteristic "pear" shape (**Fig. 74–3**). If the catheter tip is short of the porus, then the numbness created will be less and limited to the third division. No harm has yet to occur from allowing the balloon to slip into the posterior fossa, but the operation will not succeed regardless. For second- or third-division trigeminal pain, the balloon catheter is properly positioned when the catheter stylet hugs the petrous bone, its end just beyond the radiographic clival line. For first-division pain, the balloon catheter is positioned medially in the porus trigeminus as seen on the AP view and more superiorly above the petrous bone on the lateral view (**Fig. 74–4**). The insufflation syringe is filled using the 18 gauge needle with 10 mL of 180 mg% water soluble iodine dye.

The balloon can be inflated with 0.75 to 1 mL of radiographic dye by using an insufflator with an attached pressure transducer. This is available in the disposable kit. When properly inflated, using a 4 French (F) balloon catheter, the intraluminal balloon pressure is 1100 to 1500 mm Hg, or 1.2 to 1.4 atmospheres. Overinflation can cause temporary cranial nerve VI palsy or severe numbness. The balloon is inflated for 1 minute, or up to 1 ½ minutes if there have been multiple recurrences and more significant compression is sought. The insufflator has the slight disadvantage of not providing concurrent sensory

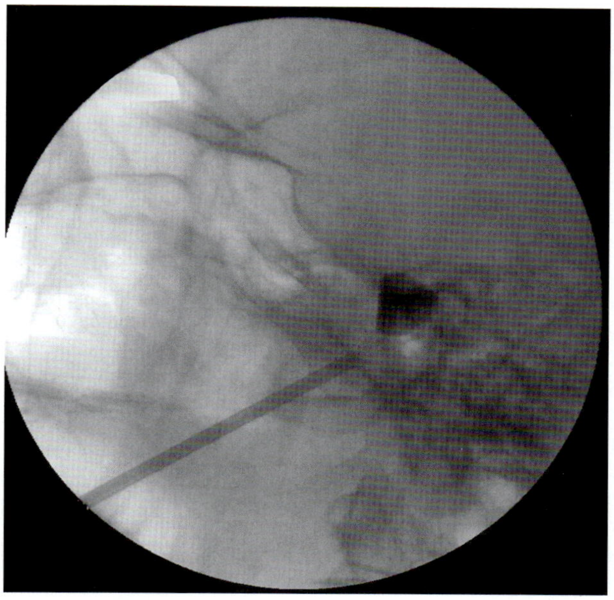

Figure 74–3 Lateral fluoroscopic image showing the inflated balloon during compression.

feedback, but the advantage of precise pressure measurement. It is not necessary to remove air from the catheter. Rupture of the balloon has never led to any morbidity; certainly not leading to any risk from subarachnoid or subdural air release, and should not occur if the blunt cannula is used.

When properly inflated, the pear shape is seen and the depressor response usually occurs. Should the pacemaker be triggered, it is only briefly, and often is followed by a hypertensive response that may be treated with an increase in anesthetic. After deflation, the balloon and catheter are removed concurrently and the cheek is compressed against the maxilla for 5 minutes. Blood-tinged cerebrospinal fluid will drip through the cannula if the catheter is removed separately. The presence of cerebrospinal fluid does not correlate with the success of the procedure.

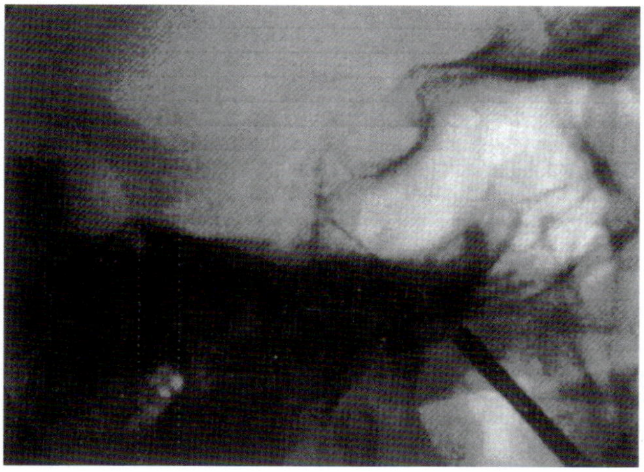

Figure 74–4 Lateral fluoroscopic image showing balloon in position for first division pain. The balloon is directed relatively superior and medially compared to the position for fluid position pain.

◆ Morbidity

Two thirds of patients develop mild to moderate numbness at a mean balloon pressure of 1.2 to 1.3 atmospheres. There is usually jaw weakness. The jaw deviates to the side of the weakness. This will recover over the first month. Presumably because of temporary muscular jaw imbalance, temporomandibular jaw pain can occur. It can be treated until resolution, with antiinflammatory medications. The aching quality of the pain, aggravated by chewing and tenderness palpable at the temporomandibular joint is diagnostic, and the pain should be distinguished from the pain of residual trigeminal neuralgia. The tensor tympani motor branch when weakened will weaken the patient's ability to correct the eustachian tube for air pressure changes. This can be temporarily uncomfortable but will recover. Dysesthesias when present are usually described as intermittent crawling sensations, not burning pain.

Severe headache, fever, and nuchal rigidity have occurred in five patients. This resolves within 48 hours without permanent sequelae and probably represents the effects of subarachnoid blood, too small to detect on computed tomography. Antibiotics are not needed and treatment is symptomatic for the headache. Use of the available disposable cannula system rather than a sharp needle to place the catheter eliminates the risk of this complication.

Temporary diplopia has occurred. This probably was from overinflation of the balloon and compression of nerve in the cavernous sinus. If the intraluminal pressure is measured, rather than using a tuberculin syringe to inflate the balloon, then this is unlikely to occur. The size of Meckel's cave can vary. The corneal reflex has a better chance of being preserved if balloon pressure is measured. The corneal reflex is mediated by unmyelinated fibers that are preserved by balloon compression. If damage does occur, then the patient should be evaluated by an ophthalmologist as a baseline soon after surgery for corneal abrasions. Regular use of eyedrops is recommended, and keratitis has never occurred.

Several cases of external carotid fistula occurred in earlier patients when a beveled needle was used to introduce the catheter and should not occur if a cannula and blunt obturator system are used.[6] Similarly, a case report has been published showing inflation of the balloon in the cavernous sinus creating a fistula.[7] In this instance a beveled needle was introduced beyond the foramen ovale into the sinus inappropriately. Lateral or biplane fluoroscopy to monitor the cannula position will make this complication unlikely. The cannula should not penetrate beyond the foramen. Anesthesia dolorosa has not happened in any series published. By measuring balloon pressure and limiting compression to 1 minute, this is less likely.

◆ Complications

Puncture of the oral mucosa is unlikely if one switches to a blunt obturator after puncturing the skin. If it does occur, another needle system should be used. An inability to visualize the foramen ovale can be predicted preoperatively by obtaining skull radiographs in the position to be used during surgery.

It is safe to estimate the position of the foramen on the modified submental view, especially if a concurrent lateral view is used, because the cannula and obturator are blunt.

The most likely cause of an inability to obtain a pear shape is either that the catheter tip is positioned lateral to the porus trigeminus and is inflating in the middle fossa lateral to the ganglion, or it is short of the porus and inflating over the ganglion. If this occurs, the balloon catheter should then be removed and the guiding stylet repositioned. Its position should be monitored using the modified AP view. If a pear shape and adequate balloon pressure still do not occur, then it is possible that the dura has been perforated by the catheter and it is inflating in the subarachnoid space of the middle fossa. Cadaver studies suggest that the catheter is not likely to do this, however. Often, if the cannula is removed completely, and then repositioned, it is possible to achieve the proper balloon position and inflation shape. If the catheter is introduced so that its equator is beyond the edge of the dura in the porus trigeminus, this will tend to occur during inflation. Once it does happen, it will tend to do so repeatedly with reinflation. The catheter should be held back during inflation to stop this from recurring. One of the available kits provides a lock to hold the catheter in position during inflation.

Balloon rupture occurred more often if a needle was used to introduce the catheter. No complications have been seen when it has happened. If the patient is allergic to iodine and there is concern, preoperative prophylaxis with steroids is an option. However, since the dye is not injected intravenously and is used in low volume, allergic reaction is only a theoretical risk.

◆ Results

One hundred eighty-three patients were treated from 1983 to 1997 at the Medical College of Ohio.[8,9] Their mean age was 64 years with the youngest 27 and the oldest 95 years old. Thirty-seven percent had first-division pain. Thirty-percent had previous destructive operations. Six percent had multiple sclerosis. The mean evaluation period in this series was 5 years, ranging from 2 months to 13 years. There was 93% initial pain relief. Sixty-one percent had numbness. This was mild to moderate in 94%. The incidence of masseter/pterygoid weakness was 19%. Overall, the recurrence rate was 25%. If patients required reoperation, the success rate was 68%. For patients who had first-division pain, the percentage of patients pain free was 69% compared with 62% in patients with second-division, third-division, or second- and third-division pain.

Taha and Tew[10] published a series of 154 consecutive patients treated by thermal rhizotomy in a 15-year prospective evaluation. Their initial pain relief was 91%. When there was mild hypalgesia, as there is in balloon compression, the incidence of dysesthesias is comparable, 7%. Their incidence of absent or depressed corneal reflex was higher, corresponding to the difference in fiber-type injury created by thermal rhizotomy. Thermal rhizotomy does not selectively destroy myelinated versus unmyelinated fibers. The incidence of motor weakness was also comparable overall to that seen in balloon compression, 14%.

When there is mild hypalgesia with thermal rhizotomy, the recurrence rate is higher than with dense hypalgesia, and recurrence tends to occur in less than 4 years. Dense hypalgesia is needed to maintain a recurrence rate of 25%, and this leads to a median pain-free survival of 14 years. If mild hypalgesia is the end point, then recurrence occurs in a mean of 3 years.

◆ Conclusion

One must adapt a philosophy appropriate to the tolerance of each patient. Patients with severe pain who are older may tolerate dense hypalgesia better than a younger patient. The younger patient may require reoperation many times over a lifetime. This should be quite acceptable as long as the numbness is not bothersome. Long-term pain relief concurrent with bothersome dysesthesias may not be worthwhile to the patient, especially given the ease of reoperation and the relatively low risk involved. The goal is the optimal treatment of this cruel and obscure illness, which causes some violent facial motions and some hideous grimaces that are an insurmountable obstacle to the reception of food, which banishes sleep, which makes speech choppy or slurred, which causes motions that are vague and intermittent, and nevertheless so frequent as to be felt several times in a day, in an hour, and sometimes give no respite but are renewed every minute.[11]

References

1. Brisman R. Surgical treatment of trigeminal neuralgia. Semin Neurol 1997;17:367–372
2. Sweet WH. Percutaneous methods for the treatment of trigeminal neuralgia and other faciocephalic pain; comparison with microvascular decompression. Semin Neurol 1988;8:272–279
3. Preul MC, Long PB, Brown JA, Velasco ME, Weaver MT. Autonomic and histopathological effects of percutaneous trigeminal ganglion compression in the rabbit. J Neurosurg 1990;72:933–940
4. Gouda JJ, Brown JA. Atypical facial pain and other pain syndromes: differential diagnosis and treatment. Neurosurg Clin North Am 1997;8:87–100
5. Brown JA, Preul MC. Trigeminal depressor response during percutaneous microcompression of the trigeminal ganglion for trigeminal neuralgia. Neurosurgery 1988;23:745–748
6. Revuelta R, Nathal E, Balderrama J, Tello A, Zenteno M. External carotid artery fistula due to microcompression of the gasserian ganglion for the relief of trigeminal neuralgia. J Neurosurg 1993;78:499–500
7. Kuether TA, O'Neill OR, Nesbit GM, Barnwell SL. Direct carotid cavernous fistula after trigeminal balloon microcompression gangliolysis: case report. Neurosurgery 1996;39:853–855
8. Brown JA, McDaniel MD, Weaver MT. Percutaneous trigeminal nerve compression for treatment of trigeminal neuralgia: results in 50 patients. Neurosurgery 1993;32:570–573
9. Brown JA, Gouda JJ, Sangvai DG. Percutaneous balloon compression for trigeminal neuralgia: results in 183 consecutive patients [abstract]. J Neurosurg 1998;88:417A
10. Taha JM, Tew JM. Treatment of trigeminal neuralgia by percutaneous radiofrequency rhizotomy. Neurosurg Clin N Am 1997;8:31–39
11. Andre N. Observations Practiques sur les maladies de l'urethre et sur plusiers faits convulsif. Paris, 1756.

75

Repair of Cranial Nerve VII

Chris Danner, John Dornhoffer, and Mark Linskey

Facial nerve dysfunction is one of the most disfiguring cranial nerve neuropathies and can be devastating both physically and psychologically. Potential physical handicaps include risks of vision loss secondary to functional loss of the orbicularis oculi, whereas psychological handicaps include loss of self-esteem and well-being from a loss of facial expression and embarrassing events that result from oral incompetence. It is important to restore the integrity of the seventh cranial nerve to regain both form and function to the face. Reestablishing facial symmetry, oral competence, and corneal protection does this. Based on the etiology of the facial verve injury, there are different options to reestablish facial nerve integrity. With the new onset of skull-base techniques virtually any tumor in the infratemporal fossa and cerebellopontine angle is amenable to surgical resection. This leads to an increased likelihood of developing nerve damage from retraction and possible resection of the facial nerve to accomplish adequate tumor removal. This in turn leads to an increased need for facial nerve reconstruction.

◆ General Neurorrhaphy Techniques

The free ends of the facial nerve need to be adequately prepared to minimize connective tissue ingrowth and maximize neuronal transmission between the anastomosed nerve endings. The fibrotic tissue ingrowth that occurs with less than perfect nerve coaptation blocks neural fibers from efficiently crossing the gap between the two nerves and significantly decreases the functional result. Fibrotic ingrowth is minimized by removing the first 5 mm of epineurium from the proximal and distal nerve stump[1] (**Fig. 75–1**). This procedure also enables adequate inspection of the anastomotic ends to ensure proper coaptation of nerve fascicles. It cannot be overemphasized that the nerve graft proximal and distal stumps need to be handled atraumatically. This is achieved by holding only the epineurium with microforceps when manipulating the nerve.

Both the proximal and distal ends should have 3 to 5 mm of extra length to ensure tensionless anastomosis. Tension increases the amount of fibrotic ingrowth and subsequently decreased the number of axons that are able to propagate distally. If there is any tension on the approximated nerve endings, better functional results would be achieved if an interposition nerve graft is placed between the proximal and distal nerve stumps. Donor sites and harvest of the nerve graft are discussed later.

Once the nerve endings have been adequately prepared, placing sutures in the epineurium approximates them. Suturing nerve endings should be minimized and only the absolute minimum used to stabilize the anastomosis. Typically one to two 10–0 epineural sutures are all that are required to stabilize the anastomotic site if it occurs intracranially or within the temporal bone. If the anastomosis occurs in the soft tissues outside the confines of the temporal bone, three to four epineural sutures may be needed.

Primary anastomosis will give the best result and is always initially attempted. Mobilization of the infratemporal portion of the facial nerve is performed when possible to gain additional length. If tensionless coaptation is not achieved after the above measures are performed, then an autologous nerve is harvested for an interposition graft, or a crossover graft is performed if the proximal stump is unavailable or believed to be nonfunctional.[2–4]

The final axon population after anastomosis is only 40% of the original population. Axons can be directed from less to more anatomically critical areas by ligating unwanted peripheral nerve branches. Directing newly developing axons to more anatomically critical areas maximizes the axon count where it is most wanted and increases the strength of innervated mimetic muscles.[5]

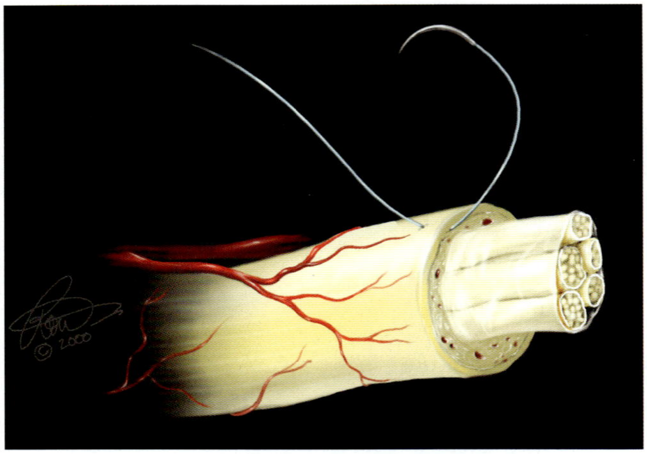

Figure 75–1 Before suturing the nerve, the epineurium should be trimmed. The proper placement of suture through trimmed epineurium is shown.

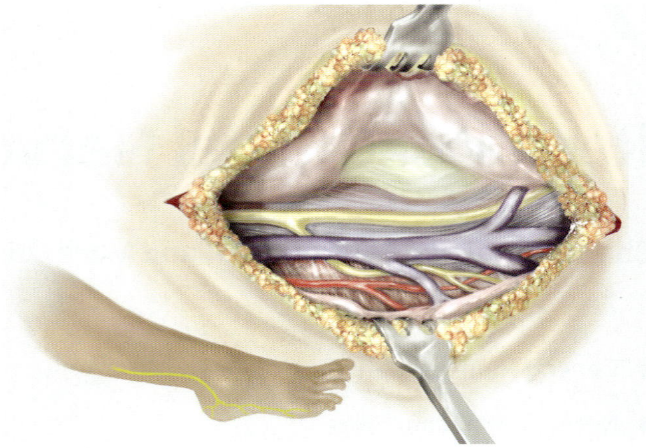

Figure 75–3 Location of the sural nerve, posterior to the lateral malleolus, and it follows the course of the lesser saphenous vein.

◆ Nerve Graft Donor Sites

Great Auricular Nerve

The great auricular nerve is the first choice when less than 10 cm of nerve graft is needed. It usually lies within the surgical field and has a diameter that is similar to that of the facial nerve. It is easily found by bisecting the distance between the angle of the mandible and mastoid tip **(Fig. 75–2)**. A skin incision is made in the skin crease over the upper one third of the sternocleidomastoid muscle. The dissection is taken through the subcutaneous fat to the platysma muscle. The nerve lies immediately under the platysma. Care must be exerted when dividing the platysma fibers so the great auricular nerve is not inadvertently divided. The proximal and distal ends of the recipient nerve need to be adequately cleaned of their epineural sheath prior to harvesting the graft. This minimizes the time the graft is outside the body and thus minimizes Schwann cell degeneration.[6–9]

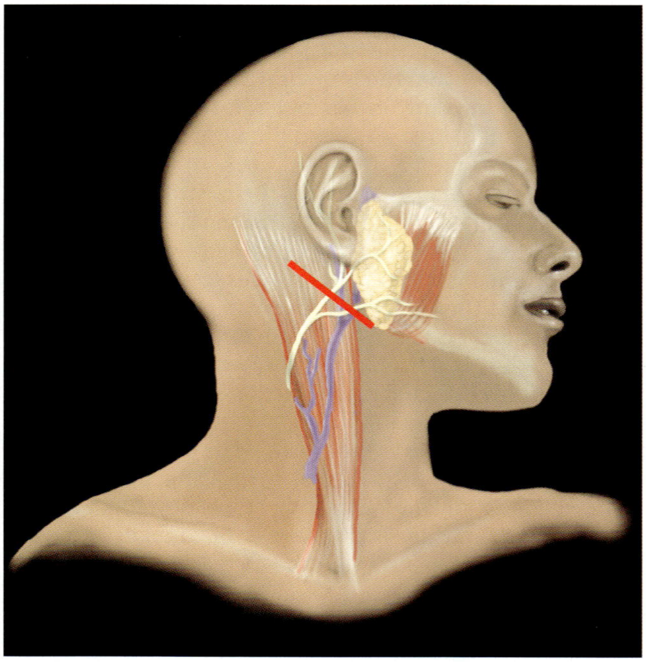

Figure 75–2 The great auricular nerve is located halfway between the mastoid tip and angle of the mandible.

Sural Nerve

Even though the diameter is similar to the facial nerve, the sural nerve is often the second choice for a donor nerve after the great auricular, secondary to its unfavorable branching pattern and inconvenient location. However, the sural nerve is the first choice when greater than 10 cm of graft length is needed. Up to 35 cm of nerve graft may be obtained when dissection is continued to the distal ramifications (n. cutaneus dorsalis lateralis and rami calcanei laterales). Its location is easily identified posterior to the lateral malleolus. There it lies in close approximation to the lesser saphenous vein[7,9] **(Fig. 75–3)**.

◆ Surgical Technique

The technique used to correct a disrupted facial nerve after tumor removal depends on where the discontinuity occurs. Different techniques are employed to correct intracranial, intratemporal, and distal facial nerve discontinuities.

Intracranial Facial Nerve Discontinuity

Intracranial nerves lack a significant perineurium, and if suture techniques are employed, a single 10–0 nylon placed through the center of the nerve is most appropriate. The suture is placed 1 to 2 mm from the cut end. Placing one simple suture through the distal and proximal nerve endings achieves good approximation of the nerve ends while minimizing trauma. Other intracranial anastomotic techniques have been described using collagen splints and tissue glues and are mentioned for completeness. The authors feel the results achieved with a single through-and-through suture are good and do not warrant the extra expense and time needed with the use of collagen splints and tissue glues.

If a splint is used, pulling the proximal nerve stump through the rolled end of a collagen splint and placing the distal end of the splint in the porus acusticus adds stability to the splint.[6] The nerve graft is then laid on the splint for support. Placing the splint in the porus gives additional support in the constant flux of cerebrospinal fluid (CSF). The proximal and distal nerve ends are cut and are stabilized with fibrin glue. Cyanoacrylates are no longer used as tissue glues because of their neurotoxicity.[6,10]

Extracranial Nerve Anastomosis

Intratemporal (Distal End Lies within the Temporal Bone)

Nonserviceable Hearing

A subtotal petrosectomy is completed for nerve exposure when performing facial nerve anastomosis and when the distal nerve stump lies within the temporal bone of a nonhearing ear. The temporal bone will have already been partially drilled to expose and remove the temporal bone tumor. If not already done, a simple mastoidectomy is completed. The sigmoid sinus is skeletonized from the sinodural angle to the digastric ridge. The air cells are cleared from the sinodural angle and the tegmen is then exposed up to the antrum. The horizontal semicircular canal is exposed. The bone between the horizontal canal and the digastric ridge is then slowly painted with the drill until the descending portion of the facial nerve is visualized (**Fig. 75–4**). The nerve is then skeletonized from the horizontal canal to the stylomastoid foramen. Next a labyrinthectomy is performed skeletonizing the internal auditory canal (IAC). Now the entire course of the facial nerve should be visualized from the IAC to the stylomastoid foramen. If the geniculate ganglion is intact, the origin of the greater superficial petrosal nerve is transected. This releases the facial nerve, and the first genu located at the geniculate ganglion can be straightened, adding 1 to 2 cm to the length of the nerve. This may be enough to perform a primary anastomosis between the distal and proximal trunks. If the proximal stump is intracranial, then an intracranial anastomosis is performed as earlier described. A new fallopian canal is cut where there is remaining bone. The canal should be deep enough to accommodate the entire nerve. This can be drilled directly over the jugular bulb from the IAC to the stylomastoid foramen or it can be directed anteriorly over the otic capsule or posteriorly behind the sigmoid. The nerve graft is placed in this canal to help stabilize the anastomosis and also provide blood supply to the nerve. The proximal and distal nerve ends are laid end to end in the new fallopian canal and reinforced with fibrin glue and overlaid with a collagen sheet to prevent fibrotic in growth.[6,11] No sutures are needed for the intratemporal anastomosis.

Serviceable Hearing

Facial nerve anastomosis in a hearing ear is performed by exposing the proximal and distal nerve stumps without disturbing the inner ear or middle ear structures. A mastoidectomy is performed to expose the facial nerve as described earlier. If the proximal nerve stump is located near or proximal to the geniculate ganglion, a middle fossa approach is used to gain access to the IAC and the facial nerve (**Fig. 75–5**). The meatal opening (entrance to the fallopian canal from the IAC) is a fibrous dural band that encompasses the circumference of the facial nerve.[6,9] This is the

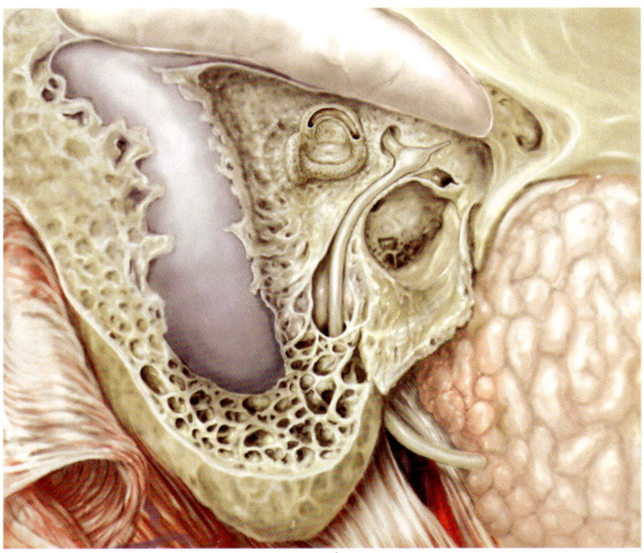

Figure 75–4 Transmastoid exposure of the descending portion of the facial nerve.

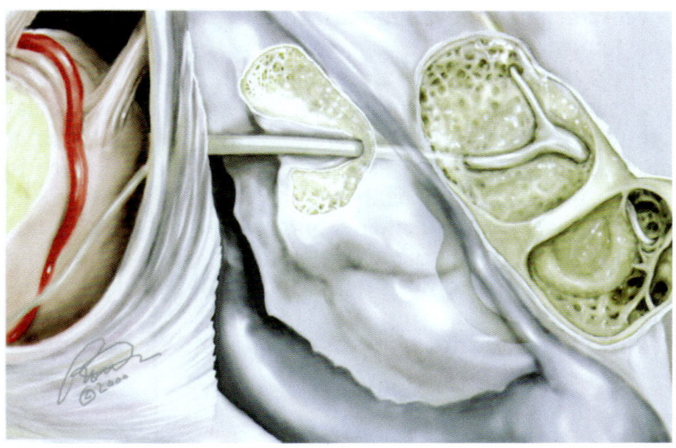

Figure 75–5 The middle fossa exposure of the internal auditory canal (IAC) and tympanic portions of the facial nerve.

narrowest point in the course of the facial nerve. If the labyrinthine portion of the facial nerve is exposed during the dissection of the facial nerve, the dural band at the meatus must be opened to prevent nerve strangulation from edema. However, opening the meatal dural band causes an influx of CSF, making the proximal neural anastomosis unstable. The proximal anastomosis must then be stabilized with a single 10–0 epineural suture. The distal end of the anastomosis is secured by laying the distal and proximal nerve ends in the newly drilled fallopian canal as described earlier. The coapted nerve endings are then reinforced with a collagen sheet and fibrin glue.

Extratemporal Facial Discontinuity

Proximal Stump Present

In performing a facial nerve anastomosis when the distal branch is beyond the confines of the temporal bone, the proximal branch is first isolated by a combined middle fossa transmastoid approach as described above.[11] If the distal stump is unavailable and only the peripheral facial nerve endings are available for anastomosis, the proximal stump may be bipartitioned to allow adequate surface area to anastomose two nerve grafts. These two grafts are then anastomosed to the temporal-facial and cervical-facial divisions of the facial nerve distally.[6] If a suboccipital or retrosigmoid approach is used for tumor extirpation, facial nerve reconstruction may be accomplished using Dott's method.[11,12] The proximal intracranial anastomosis is performed as described above. The nerve graft is then brought out through the cranium and tunneled under the sternocleidomastoid (SCM) to lie in position next to the facial nerve trunk for anastomosis.[12]

Proximal Stump Absent

Crossover nerve grafts are performed only when the proximal nerve stump is unavailable for anastomosis or is thought to be nonfunctional. This can be caused either by nerve resection next to the brain stem or degeneration of axons in an intact nerve that has become evident only after 6 to 12 months of absent facial movement.[13] There are several different options for crossover nerve grafts. The most successful and widely popularized is the hypoglossal facial anastomosis.

The hypoglossal is the preferred nerve in crossover nerve grafts because it is a strong nerve that not only gives facial symmetry at rest but also through training can elicit facial movement **(Fig. 75–6)**. Also, its cortical representation is similar to that of the facial nerve, making mimetic movements easier to perform. The anastomosis may be accomplished by sacrificing the hypoglossal nerve and performing an end to end anastomosis with the facial nerve or performing an end to side anastomosis. There are several variations of the end to side anastomosis (jump graft,[14] distal split,[15] proximal split[16]). The end to end anastomosis sacrifices the hypoglossal nerve, causing tongue atrophy and mild articulation difficulties, but it is associated with stronger facial movements. The end to side anastomosis does preserve some tongue function, although the tongue tends to be weak. This weakness is easily compensated for but may not be desirable if the patient already suffers from multiple cranial nerve palsies.[3,14,16–19]

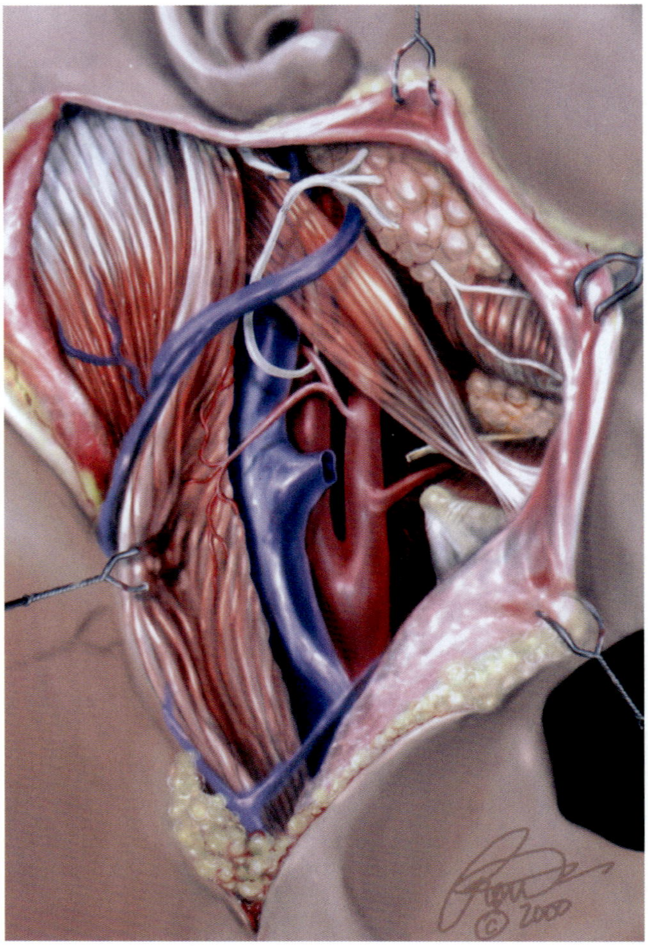

Figure 75–6 Hypoglossal facial nerve anastomosis. The hypoglossal nerve is cut distal along its course to give additional length.

Other cranial nerve facial crossover grafts have been performed with success but are associated with excessive donor site morbidity and are mentioned here only for completeness. They include the accessory nerve, phrenic, and third division of the trigeminal. Also, cross-facial sural nerve anastomosis is an option for facial reanimation. However, because of its prolonged recovery time and weak muscle tone, often requiring adjunctive plastic surgical procedures, this procedure is not used.[12,20]

References

1. Hausamen J, Schmelzeisen R. Current principles in microsurgical nerve repair. Br J Oral Maxillofac Surg 1996;34:143–157
2. Samii M, Matthies C. Management of 1000 vestibular schwannomas (acoustic neuromas): the facial nerve-preservation and restitution of function. Neurosurgery 1997;40:684–694
3. Stephanian E, Sekhar L, Janecka I, Hirsch B. Facial nerve repair by interposition nerve graft: results in 22 Patients. Neurosurgery 1992;31:73–77
4. Spector JG, Lee P, Peterein J, Roufa D. Facial nerve regeneration through autologous nerve grafts: a clinical and experimental study. Laryngoscope 1991;101:537–554
5. Mattox D, Felix H, Fish U, Lyles A. Effect of ligating peripheral branches on facial nerve regeneration. Otolaryngol Head Neck Surg 1988;98:558–563
6. Fisch U, Lanser MJ. Facial nerve grafting. Otolaryngol Clin North Am 1991;24:691–708
7. Janecka I, Sekar L, Stephanian E. Facial nerve management and reconstructive techniques. In: Sekhar L, Janecka I, eds. Surgery of Cranial Base Tumors. New York: Raven; 1993:435–447
8. Jackson CG. Basic surgical principles of neurotologic skull base surgery. Laryngoscope 1993;103:29–44
9. Fisch U. Facial nerve grafting. Otolaryngol Clin North Am 1974;7:517–529
10. Fisch U, Rouleau M. Facial nerve reconstruction. J Otolaryngol 1980;9:487–492
11. Holt J. The stylomastoid area: anatomic-histologic study and surgical approach. Laryngoscope 1996;106:396–400
12. Scaramella LF, Tobias E. Facial nerve anastomosis. Laryngoscope 1973;83:1834–1840
13. Guntinas-Lichius O, Angelov DN, Stennert E, Neiss WF. Delayed hypoglossal-facial nerve suture after predegeneration of peripheral facial nerve stump improves the innervation of mimetic musculature by hypoglossal motoneurons. J Comp Neurol 1997;387:234–242
14. May M, Sobolol S, Mester S. Hypoglossal-facial nerve interpostional-jump graft for facial reanimation without tongue atrophy. Otolaryngol Head Neck Surg 1991;104:818–825
15. Arai H, Sato K, Yanai A. Hemihypoglossal-facial nerve anastomosis in treating unilater facial palsy after acoustic neurinoma resection. J Neurosurg 1995;82:51–54
16. Cusimano M, Sekhar L. Partial hypoglossal to facial nerve anastomosis for reinnervation of the paralyzed face in patients with lower cranial nerve palsies: technical note. Neurosurgery 1994;35:532–534
17. Pitty LF, Tator CH. Hypoglossal-facial nerve anastomosis for facial nerve palsy following surgery for cerebellopontine angle tumors. J Neurosurg 1992;77:724–731
18. Atlas M, Lowinger D. A new technique for hypoglossal-facial nerve repair. Laryngoscope 1997;107:984–991
19. Sawamura Y, Abe H. Hypoglossal-facial nerve side to end anastomosis for preservation of hypoglossal function: results of delayed treatment with a new technique. J Neurosurg 1997;86:203–206
20. Scaramella L. Cross-face facial nerve anastomosis: historical notes. Ear Nose Throat J 1996;75:343–354

76

Occipital Neurectomy and Decompression

Ghassan K. Bejjani and Amal Abou-Hamden

◆ The Greater Occipital Nerve and the Sensory Innervation of the Posterior Scalp

Although the function of the greater occipital nerve per se is not crucial, when it is dysfunctional it may create a significant handicap, causing the condition known as occipital neuralgia. The greater occipital nerve provides the majority of the sensory supply to the posterior scalp. Three other nerves provide a smaller contribution to the posterior scalp (lesser occipital nerve, third occipital nerve, and greater auricular nerves) (**Figs. 76–1** and **76–2**). The innervation of the posterior scalp corresponds to the second and third dermatomes. Procedures used to treat greater occipital neuralgia aim at either the nerve itself or its origin from the cervical roots.

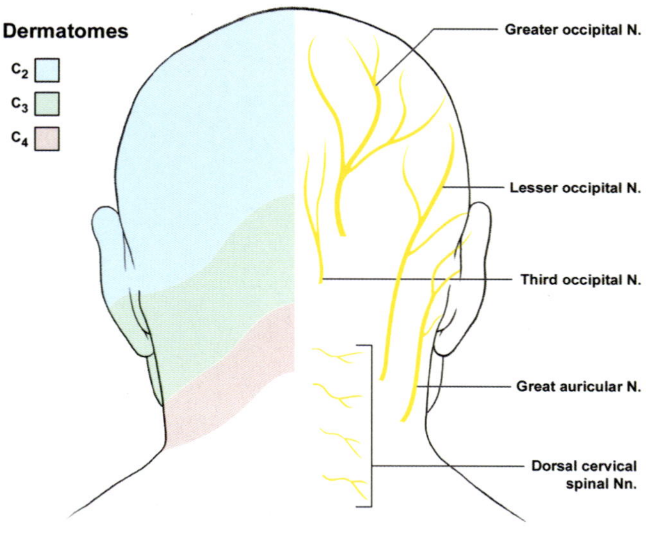

Figure 76–1 Posterior view of the scalp. The innervation is shown by dermatomes (left) and by nerves (right).

◆ Definition and Clinical Presentation

Occipital neuralgia is defined by the Headache Classification Committee of the International Headache Society as a "paroxysmal jabbing pain in the distribution of the greater or lesser occipital nerves, accompanied by diminished sensation or dysaesthesia in the affected area." It is commonly associated with tenderness over the concerned nerve, sometimes with a positive Tinel's sign. Aching pain may persist between the paroxysms. The condition is temporarily relieved by local anesthetic block of the appropriate nerve. Other descriptors of the pain are "shooting, electric, exploding."

◆ Differential Diagnosis

Occipital neuralgia has to be differentiated from nonneuralgic occipital pain. The main common denominator is the location. The lancinating character of occipital neuralgia differentiates it from nonneuralgic occipital pain. Nonneuralgic occipital pain is a much more common occurrence in which the pain lacks the jabbing paroxysms. The pain is described as dull, aching, and pressure-like. It is nonparoxysmal with slower variations in the degree of pain. The pain is more

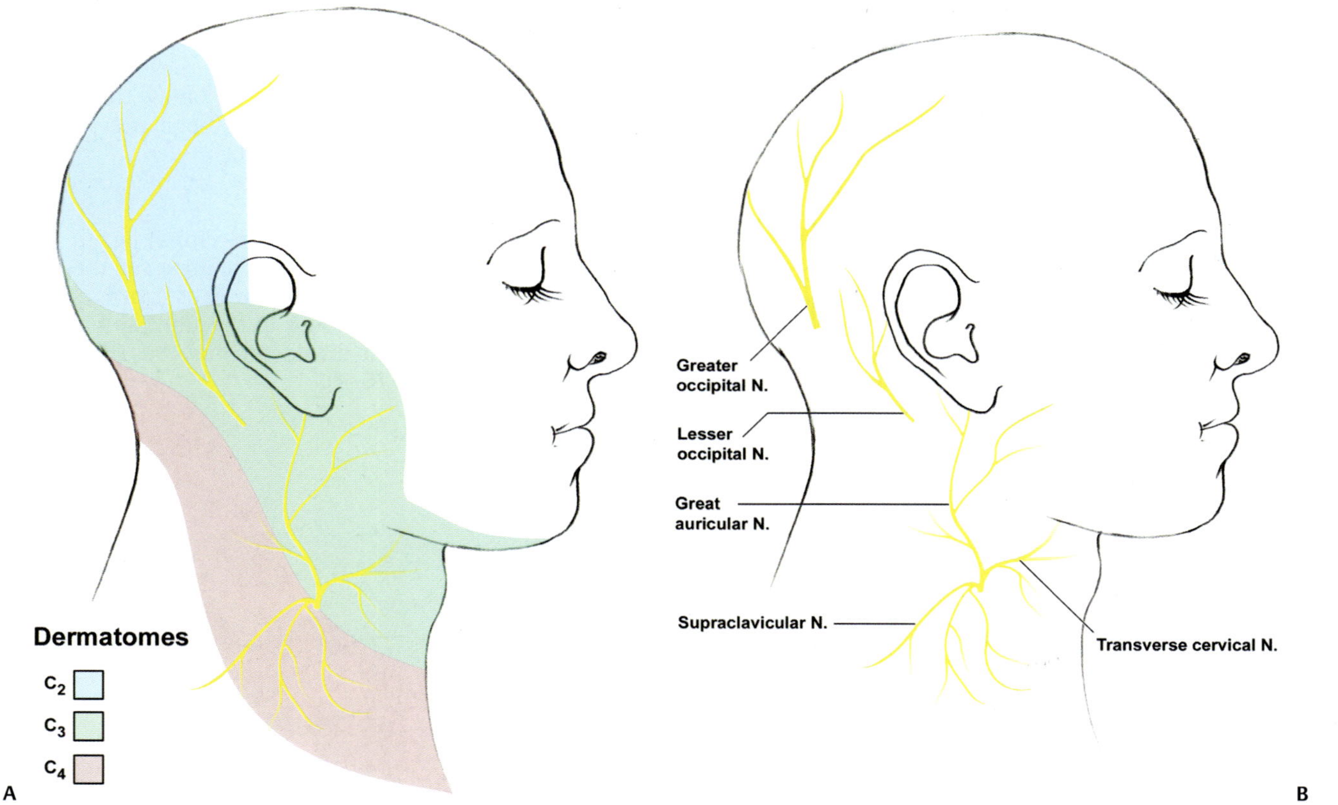

Figure 76–2 Lateral view of the scalp. The innervation is shown **(A)** by dermatomes and **(B)** by nerves.

diffuse, irradiating to adjacent areas: neck, shoulders, forehead, temples, and retro-orbital area.

◆ Etiology

A history of cervical trauma or whiplash injury is elicited in some cases. Other possible etiologies are nerve entrapment in the postsurgical setting by scar or sutures, direct nerve injury (greater occipital, lesser occipital, posterior auricular nerve), myofascial syndrome (posterior cervical myositis or fasciitis), metabolic (diabetes), infectious (syphilis, mastoiditis, pachymeningitis), and cervical nerve root irritation (cervical spine trauma, osteoarthritic spondylosis, neoplasms, vascular anomalies, Chiari malformation, bony anomalies of the occipitocervical junction).

◆ Investigations

The diagnosis of occipital neuralgia is clinical. Investigations should focus on finding an underlying etiology.

If there is a history of trauma, then static and dynamic cervical spine x-rays are indicated to rule out bony injury or spinal instability. Cervical spine magnetic resonance imaging (MRI) is helpful in assessing soft tissue damage or neural compression.

In the absence of a history of trauma, radiological and metabolic investigations should focus on other possible etiologies. Brain and cervical spine MRI will rule out intracranial mass lesions or the presence of Chiari malformation.

◆ Indications

Occipital neuralgia should be managed conservatively with reassurance, observation, heat, gentle massage, and analgesics or nonsteroidal antiinflammatory drugs. Local blocks may be useful, and they may be diagnostic and therapeutic. Acupuncture has been tried also.

◆ Surgical Treatment

Surgical intervention is reserved for disabling cases resistant to conservative management. The site of intervention is along the occipital nerve course: the dorsal nerve roots of the upper cervical nerves, the C2 ganglion, and the greater occipital nerve (usually as it pierces the semispinalis, or at the superior nuchal line). There are a variety of surgical options, mostly decompressive or ablative. Ablative procedures can be percutaneous (occipital nerve, C2 ganglion) or open. We will review the relevant surgical anatomy and then the various surgical procedures used to treat this condition.

◆ Surgical Anatomy

Rootlets of C2 and C2 Ganglion

The dorsal rootlets of C2 join into the dorsal C2 root and C2 ganglion (**Fig. 76–3**). The C2 ganglion is extradural in location. It lies deep to the inferior oblique, posterior to the lateral atlantoaxial joint (against the inferior articular process of C1), under the arch of C1, and lateral to the lateral border of the posterior atlantoaxial membrane. The ventral and dorsal roots of C2 join to form the C2 spinal nerve, which divides shortly afterward into a dorsal and a ventral ramus. A dense venous plexus surrounds the ganglion and nerve roots. In turn, an investing fascia surrounds these structures. This fascia is continuous with the posterior atlantoaxial membrane medially.

The Dorsal Ramus of the C2 Spinal Nerve

The dorsal ramus of C2 emerges between the posterior arch of the atlas and the lamina of the axis, below the inferior oblique muscle and posterior to the vertebral artery. It then divides into a lateral and a medial branch.

The lateral branch supplies twigs to the splenius, longus capitis, and semispinalis capitis.

The medial branch is the greater occipital nerve. It ascends obliquely between the inferior oblique and the semispinalis capitis. It pierces the semispinalis capitis and the trapezius near their attachment to the skull and ascends with the occipital artery to divide into branches that supply the posterior scalp (**Fig. 76–4**).

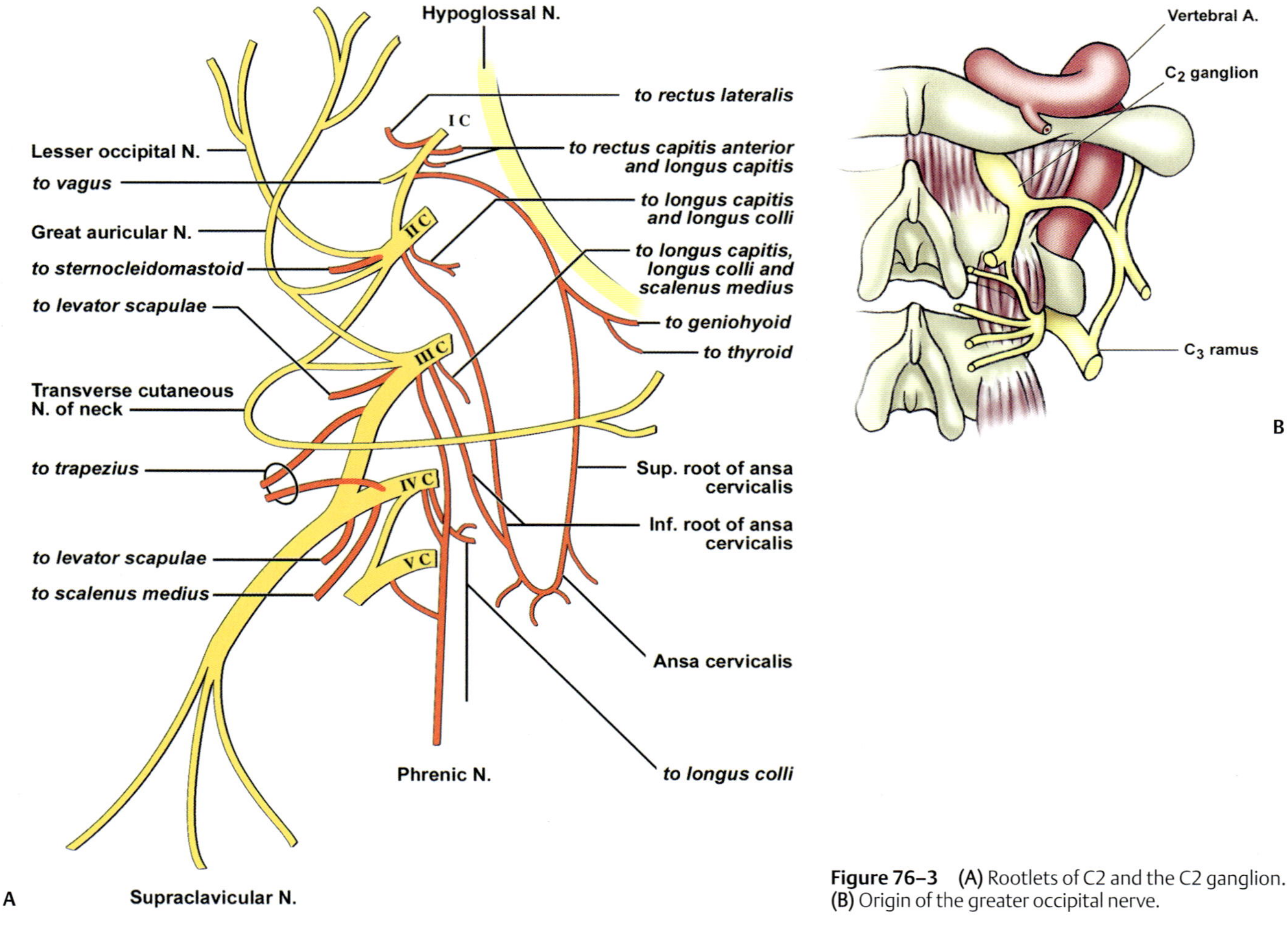

Figure 76–3 **(A)** Rootlets of C2 and the C2 ganglion. **(B)** Origin of the greater occipital nerve.

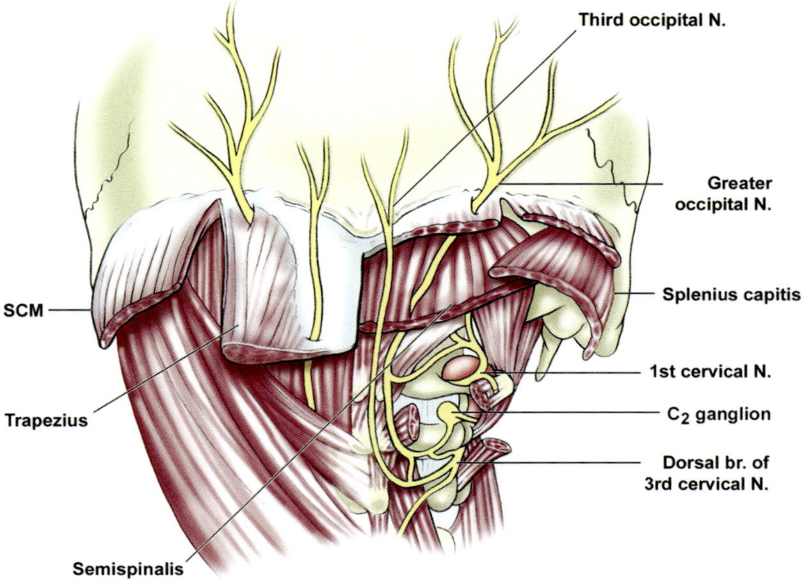

Figure 76–4 Trajectory of the greater occipital nerve. SCM, sternocleidomastoid.

◆ Choice of the Surgical Procedure

There are no studies proving the superiority of one surgical technique over another. The choice is mostly based on the surgeon's preference and level of comfort with a particular intervention. There is a declining success rate on long-term follow-up for most of these procedures.

Occipital neurectomy is the least invasive of the open procedures and is done under local anesthesia. However, a more proximal etiology of pain will lead to failure. It also leads to anesthesia of the posterior scalp. Also, there is the potential for fiber regeneration, neuroma formation, and recurrence.

Rhizotomies address a more proximal etiology of the pain. However, some pain fibers enter through the anterior nerve rootlets, which may explain why the published success rate is not as elevated as would be expected. It is also a more invasive procedure. C2 gangliectomies address the issues of regeneration and incomplete denervation because the neuronal cell bodies are completely destroyed, preventing regeneration.

Percutaneous Injection of the Greater Occipital Nerve

The patient is placed in the sitting position with the head flexed. The external occipital protuberance is felt. Then palpation is carried more laterally on the involved side, to a point just lateral to the insertion of the erector spinae muscles. This point is usually 2.5 cm lateral to the occipital protuberance. After prepping the skin, a 23 gauge needle is inserted gently until the bone is reached. It is then slightly withdrawn, and the injection performed. If block of the lesser occipital nerve is also indicated, the needle is the angled laterally along the skull and the injection performed all the way to the mastoid process.

Surgical Exposure and Decompression/Resection of the Greater Occipital Nerve

The scalp is adequately shaved and prepped along the superior nuchal line ipsilateral to the pathology. Local anesthetic is used. A lazy-S–shaped or linear incision is performed ~2 cm off the midline, along the course of the greater occipital nerve (GON) as it crosses the nuchal line, to expose the cervical fascia (**Fig. 76–5**). The dissection is carried through the latter to expose the nerve (**Fig. 76–6**) that lies adjacent to the occipital artery. The GON is exposed. At this point it may be sectioned (less likely avulsed) or decompressed. Avulsion carries the risk of spinal cord avulsion injury. The first compression point may be the point where the GON emerges from the trapezius fascia. This opening is enlarged and the GON followed proximally for 5 to 7 cm to the point where it emerges from the semispinalis muscle (**Fig. 76–7**). This is another potential compression point that will need to be freed. In decompression cases, the trapezius fascia is left open, and the subcutaneous and cutaneous layers closed.

Surgical Exposure and Selective Dorsal Rhizotomy of the Upper Cervical Nerve Roots

The patient is induced into general anesthesia and placed in the prone position with the head flexed. A midline incision is made from the occiput to the level of C4 approximately. The dissection is carried through the midline raphe, disinserting the cervical muscles to expose unilaterally the arch of C1 and the laminae of C2, C3, and possibly C4, depending on the extent of rhizotomy desired. Unilateral laminectomies are performed. The dura is opened and the dorsal nerve roots exposed. They are located posterior to the dentate ligament. Interconnecting fibers between the rootlets are identified. Dorsal rhizotomies are then performed, with care taken to avoid damage to the spinal accessory nerve fibers.

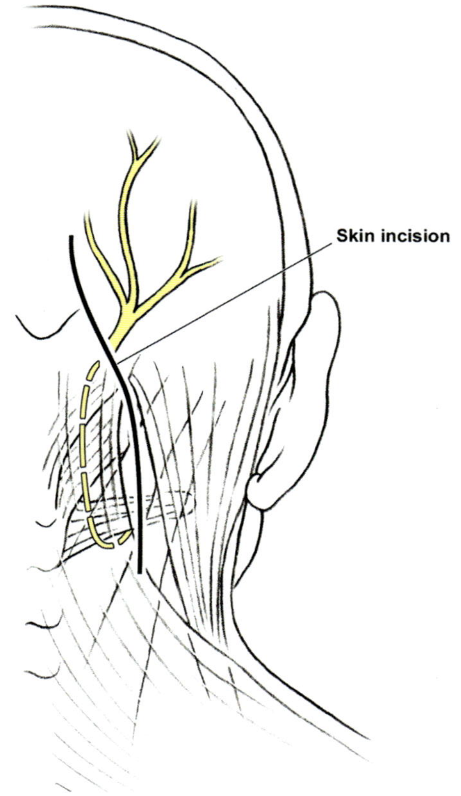

Figure 76–5 Outline of the skin incision.

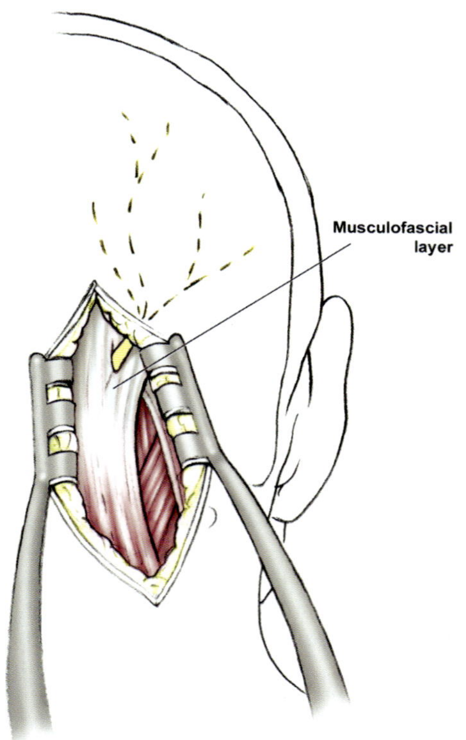

Figure 76–6 Exposure of the emergence of the greater occipital nerve through the musculofascial layer.

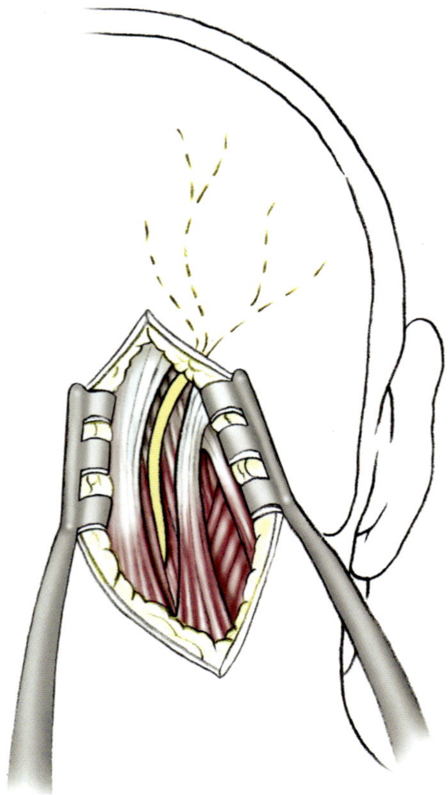

Figure 76–7 Muscular dissection and decompression of the greater occipital nerve.

Surgical Exposure and Resection of the C2 Ganglion

The patient is induced into general anesthesia and placed in the prone position with the head flexed. A midline incision is made from the occiput to the level of C3 approximately. The dissection is carried through the midline raphe, disinserting the cervical muscles to expose the arch of C1 and the laminae of C2. The operating microscope is useful for the remaining dissection. The venous plexus engulfing the C2 ganglion is coagulated and incised. The C2 ganglion is identified as a thickened part of the C2 rami. Occasionally the inferior border of the C1 arch is removed to facilitate exposure. The proximal and distal elements of the C2 ganglion are identified, dissected, cauterized, and incised. The ganglion is then removed and sent for pathological analysis. The dura is usually preserved. Closure is then performed in the usual fashion.

◆ Conclusion

Occipital neuralgia can be a disabling entity. Surgical treatment is reserved for patients with intractable and disabling pain despite conservative medical management. Several different procedures may be performed. The success rate goes down with long-term follow-up with all the various procedures. There is no evidence to support the superiority of one procedure over the others. The choice is still largely a matter of surgeon's preference and level of comfort.

Suggested Readings

Bogduk N. The anatomy of occipital neuralgia. Clin Exp Neurol 1981;17:167–184

Bogduk N. The clinical anatomy of the cervical dorsal rami. Spine 1982;7:319–330

Dubuisson D. Treatment of occipital neuralgia by partial posterior rhizotomy at C1–3. J Neurosurg 1995;82:581–586

Horowitz MB, Yonas H. Occipital neuralgia treated by intradural dorsal nerve root sectioning. Cephalalgia 1993;13:354–360

Lozano A. Microsurgical C-2 gangliectomy for chronic intractable occipital pain. J Neurosurg 1998;89:359–365

Lozano A. Treatment of occipital neuralgia. In: Gildenberg PL, Tasker RR, eds. Textbook of Stereotactic and Functional Neurosurgery. New York: McGraw-Hill; 1998:1729–1733

Maxwell RE. Craniofacial pain syndromes: an overview. In: Wilkins RH, Rengachary SS, eds. Neurosurgery. New York: McGraw-Hill; 1996:3909–3919

Murphy JP. Occipital neurectomy in the treatment of headache. Md State Med J 1969;18:62–66

Stechison M, Mullin BB. Surgical treatment of greater occipital neuralgia: an appraisal of strategies. Acta Neurochir (Wien) 1994;131:236–240

Section X

Craniocerebral Trauma

77

General Principles of Craniocerebral Trauma and Traumatic Hematomas

Jack Jallo and Raj K. Narayan

Trauma continues to be a leading cause of death and disability throughout society. In the United States, injury from trauma is a leading cause of death during the first four decades of life. Head injury contributes significantly to mortality in over half of trauma-related deaths; for each death, at least two survivors suffer some permanent disability usually secondary to head injury. Accurate data regarding the incidence of head injury is lacking because there is no nationwide registry. With this limitation in mind, the average incidence of traumatic brain injury (TBI) in the United States is conservatively estimated to range from 180 to 220 per 100,000 per year. Of the approximate 500,000 new cases per year in a population of 250 million, about 50,000 patients die before reaching the hospital, about 450,000 are admitted, and an indeterminate number do not seek medical attention. Of those seen in a hospital, injuries are classified as mild in 80%, moderate in 10%, and severe in 10%.

Although it was originally believed that most, if not all, of the injury resulting from trauma occurred at the moment of impact, we now know that only part of the injury occurs at impact. This initiating injury sets into motion a series of biochemical processes that have ultrastructural concomitants. Several laboratories have convincingly demonstrated in a variety of animal models that modification of these processes by pharmacological or other means can significantly protect the injured brain and improve the ultimate neurological outcome. Unfortunately, this protection has not yet been successfully demonstrated clinically.

Another concept well documented in recent years has been the deleterious effects of secondary insults on the injured brain. Clearly common posttraumatic events, such as raised intracranial pressure (ICP), hypotension, hypoxia, hyperthermia, hyperglycemia, infection, and others, can markedly affect the outcome. Careful attention to detail in the prevention or prompt treatment of these secondary insults appears to be largely responsible for the improved outcomes after severe TBI during the past several decades.

Classification of Head Injuries

Head injuries may be classified in a number of ways, including by mechanism, severity, and morphology.

Classification by Mechanism

Based on mechanism, head injury may be classified as blunt or penetrating, or as open or closed. Blunt head injuries may be open or closed. Penetrating injuries are by definition open. Open head injuries have an elevated risk of cerebrospinal fluid (CSF) leak and infection. Penetrating injuries are usually due to gunshot or stab wounds, whereas closed injuries are usually due to motor vehicle accidents, falls, or assault.

Penetrating injuries in a civilian environment usually result from handgun use. Missile size and velocity are important because these factors determine the amount of energy that is transmitted to the brain. The energy carried by the bullet is determined by the formula:

$$KE = \frac{1}{2} MV^2$$

where KE is the kinetic energy, M is the mass, and V is the velocity of the missile.

The extent of injury caused by a bullet depends on the velocity and type of bullet. Deformable, hollow-point bullets produce more severe damage by expanding on impact and producing a larger diameter cavity.

Classification by Severity

A number of scales available to measure injury severity include the Abbreviated Injury Scale, Reaction Level Scale, and Injury Severity Scale, to name a few. The most commonly used brain injury severity scale, the Glasgow Coma Scale (GCS), is the sum of three scores (eye opening, *best* motor response, and verbal response). The score should be ascertained after resuscitation because the neurological examination can be markedly altered by hypotension or hypoxia. A maximum score of 15 describes the patient who follows commands, is fully oriented, and has spontaneous eye opening. At the other extreme, a GCS of 3 describes the patient without motor or verbal responses or eye opening to a noxious stimulus.

According to the GCS, coma is generally defined as a score of ≤ 8, representing patients who do not follow commands, speak, or open their eyes. Head injury is further classified using the GCS as mild (score 14–15), moderate (score 9–13), or severe (score 3–8). The patient who is intubated receives a letter score of "T" to replace the verbal score. In a comatose patient, the best motor response is the most important prognostic feature.

Classification by Morphology

Based on morphology, head injuries are broadly divided into skull fractures and intracranial lesions.

Skull Fractures

Skull fractures involve the skull base or cranial vault. Fractures of the cranial vault may be linear or stellate, depressed or nondepressed, and open or closed. In general, fractures that require surgical repair are open with evidence of dural laceration or depressed beyond the inner table of the skull. Patients with a skull fracture also have a much greater likelihood of harboring an intracranial hematoma. Fractures of the skull base are associated with an increased risk for CSF leak and cranial nerve injury.

Intracranial Lesions

Intracranial lesions are broadly categorized as focal or diffuse; both can occur in the same patient. Focal lesions include subdural or epidural hematomas, contusions, and intracerebral hematomas; these frequently represent surgical emergencies. Diffuse lesions are concussions or diffuse axonal injury.

Diffuse axonal injury may be one of the most important factors determining outcome in blunt head injury. It is also the most common cause of coma in the absence of an intracranial mass lesion. Diffuse axonal injury is seen most often in patients injured in vehicular accidents and sometimes in patients after low-velocity injuries (e.g., falls). Diffuse axonal injuries are characterized by distinct microscopic features that include axonal swellings, which are widely distributed in the cerebral white matter, corpus callosum, and upper brain stem; gross hemorrhagic lesions of the corpus callosum; and gross hemorrhagic lesions involving one or both dorsolateral quadrants of the rostral brain stem.

Subdural hematomas, which are the most common focal intracerebral lesions, occur in approximately 30% of patients with severe head injury. When acute, these lesions have the highest morbidity and mortality of all traumatic focal lesions because of underlying parenchymal injury and intracranial hypertension. Subdural hematomas are also frequently associated with cerebral contusions, intracerebral hematomas, and brain lacerations. Subdural hematomas typically arise from torn bridging veins between the cerebral cortex and the major venous sinuses, but may also arise from laceration of cortical vessels with accumulation of blood between the arachnoid and dura mater.

Epidural hematomas, which are less common than subdural hematomas, have a better overall outcome if they are detected and evacuated quickly because parenchymal brain injury is minimal. Outcome after evacuation of an epidural hematoma directly relates to the level of consciousness before surgery. These hematomas classically arise from a laceration of the middle meningeal artery caused by a skull fracture. They may also develop slowly as a result of diploic bleeding from skull fractures. With epidural hematomas, blood accumulation between the skull and dura results in a lens-shaped or biconvex collection.

Contusions and intracerebral hematomas are common traumatic intracerebral lesions that may be found in isolation, or associated with other lesions such as subdural hematomas, epidural hematomas, subarachnoid hemorrhage, or skull fractures. Contusions and intracerebral hematomas represent a continuum. Contusions are bruises of the brain characterized by extravasation of blood from small, lacerated vessels, whereas intracerebral hemorrhages are large blood clots in the brain parenchyma. Contusions are sometimes described as coup or countercoup; they refer to abnormalities seen directly below the site of impact or those located on the diametrically opposite side of the brain. Most contusions are seen in the inferior frontal or temporal lobes and do not require evacuation. However, careful clinical observation and follow-up computed tomographic (CT) scans are very helpful to assess the evolution of these lesions and determine the need for surgery based primarily on the degree of mass effect.

Subarachnoid hemorrhage (bleeding into the subarachnoid space) is the most common form of hemorrhage resulting from head trauma. Although traumatic subarachnoid hemorrhage may be the only manifestation of head injury, it is frequently associated with other lesions such as contusions, hematomas, or fractures. Even when surgical intervention is not indicated in cases of subarachnoid hemorrhage found in isolation, the patient should be monitored for intracranial hypertension, cerebral vasospasm, and subsequent hydrocephalus.

◆ Emergency Room Management

During the past 3 decades, the implementation of emergency medical services and regionalized trauma systems has substantially improved survival rates from head injury and reduced the incidence of preventable deaths. Key factors contributing to better outcomes include the establishment of an airway, adequate oxygenation, fluid resuscitation, spinal stabilization, tamponade of external hemorrhage, and rapid transport to an appropriate trauma facility. Standardization of care for patients with head injuries has been advanced by the evidence-based *Guidelines for the Management of Severe Head Injury* published by the American Association of Neurological Surgeons with the support of the Brain Trauma Foundation.[1] These guidelines are well integrated into the consensus-based Advanced Trauma Life Support (ATLS) course of the American College of Surgeons Committee on Trauma. Care is optimal when there is a designated trauma team, a readily available CT scan and neurosurgeon, and a continuously staffed and available operating room and intensive care unit for treating patients with neurotrauma.

Mild Head Injury

The evaluation of patients with mild head injuries must identify those at risk for developing potentially lethal complications. About 80% of all head injuries are classified as mild. After suffering a mild head injury, 1 to 2% of patients deteriorate, lapsing into coma or requiring neurosurgical intervention. The sequelae that can result from mild brain injury include cognitive dysfunction and problems with attention, problem solving, speech, affect, and personality. Dizziness, headaches, and loss of smell are also common.

Initial management of head injury is the same for patients whether the injury is mild or severe—that is, the identification and treatment of any associated injuries. We generally advocate the routine use of CT scanning even for patients with mild injuries because missing a developing mass may have disastrous consequences. A patient with both a normal exam and a normal CT scan of the head may be sent home under the care of a caregiver. Although magnetic resonance imaging (MRI) is more sensitive than CT scanning in the detection of brain injury, MRI is not routinely performed in the acute setting. Scanning is always performed in patients with a GCS score of <15 or in the presence of focal neurological deficits, altered mental status, open injury, history of significant loss of consciousness, or intoxication.

Much debate has centered on the use of skull x-rays for patients with mild head injury. The use of skull x-rays is important as a diagnostic aid when CT scanning is unavailable; fortunately, CT is available at most institutions in the United States. In the presence of a skull fracture on plain radiographs, the likelihood of finding an intracranial pathology on a CT scan increases 400-fold. Therefore, a CT scan of the head is highly recommended when plain films reveal a significant skull fracture.

Moderate to Severe Head Injury

Along the continuum of head injury, a patient classified with a moderate to severe injury is more likely to have an intracranial hematoma. Subdural and epidural hematomas are grouped together as extraaxial hematomas, and hematomas in the cranium are referred to as intraaxial hematomas. An important early consideration in these patients is to determine when surgery is indicated. Defining the indications for surgical evacuation of intracranial hematomas is not a simple exercise. The brief summary of general principles included here is by no means comprehensive, and many exceptions exist to any rule in this context.

◆ Radiographic Studies

Possible imaging studies available to supplement the initial neurological evaluation include plain skull x-rays, CT scanning, MRI, transcranial Doppler ultrasonography, positron emission tomography (PET) or single photon emission computed tomography (SPECT) imaging, near-infrared spectroscopy, and xenon CT. Despite the variety of imaging modalities available, CT scanning is the cornerstone of the diagnostic imaging for trauma patients. Since its clinical introduction in the 1970s, CT has revolutionized the evaluation and management of patients with brain injuries. The advent of CT scanning markedly diminished the importance of skull x-rays, pneumoencephalograms, and cerebral angiography in the acute radiological evaluation of head trauma. Advantages of CT include its rapid, safe, and noninvasive nature. Its accuracy in the anatomical localization of hematomas, skull fractures, metallic foreign bodies, and hydrocephalus ultimately allows for rapid diagnosis, triage, and surgical evacuation of mass lesions.

Shortcomings of CT imaging include poor visualization of vascular lesions (e.g., arterial dissections, traumatic aneurysms), fractures at the vertex, and somewhat poor visualization of the posterior fossa. Traumatic aneurysms, although uncommon, have a tendency to rupture; these aneurysms are usually pseudoaneurysms, meaning that the vascular adventitia is not intact. These aneurysms also tend to be more peripheral and less likely to occur at vascular branch points. Clinical suspicion of an arterial dissection or aneurysm should be raised, and cerebral angiography should be considered when there is unexpected deterioration after head injury or delayed intracranial hemorrhage.

MRI offers a number of advantages in the evaluation of brain injury, including greater sensitivity when compared with CT in the detection of acute abnormalities and delayed effects of head trauma. The advantages of MRI include visualization of shearing injuries and nonhemorrhagic contusions, improved localization with multiplanar imaging, improved imaging of posterior fossa injury, and the capability to follow the evolution of a hemorrhage. The disadvantages of MRI include longer imaging times in potentially critically ill patients, requirement for MRI-compatible monitoring and ventilator equipment, and poor visualization of bone and subarachnoid hemorrhage.

◆ Indications for Surgery

The management of a condition as diverse as head injury uses a number of guidelines (rather than strict rules) proven to be useful. Some of these practices are based on hard data, some on clinical prejudice, and some on an irresistible desire to simplify a hopelessly complicated problem. In its simplest form, our criterion for considering an acute mass lesion operable is a midline shift of 5 mm or more. A nonsurgical approach is certainly justified in a patient with a small hematoma with minimal shift who is alert and neurologically intact. However, the patient's condition may deteriorate, and close observation is critical. If a significant change develops in mental status, a repeat CT scan should be obtained immediately.

We generally operate on all patients with severe head injuries who have an intracranial mass lesion and ≥ 5 mm midline shift unless they are brain dead. This practice is based on evidence that a few patients with bilaterally nonreactive pupils, impaired oculocephalic responses, and decerebrate posturing can nevertheless make a good recovery. In one series, three of 19 such patients who underwent maximal treatment ended up in the "good" or "moderately disabled" category despite their initially forbidding constellation of signs.

The management of brain contusions is somewhat less clear cut. The only study that provided some guidance in this area was that by Galbraith and Teasdale.[2] In their series of 26 patients with acute traumatic contusions who were initially managed without surgery, all patients with an intracranial pressure exceeding 30 mm Hg eventually deteriorated and required surgery, whereas only one patient with ICP levels < 20 mm Hg deteriorated. Patients in the 20 to 30 mm Hg range were about evenly divided between those who required surgical treatment and those who did not.

In one study, 130 head-injured patients with pure contusions were managed with CT scanning and, as needed, ICP monitoring in a neurosurgical intensive care unit (NICU) setting. We found that patients with brain contusions who could follow commands at admission did not require ICP monitoring and typically did well with monitoring by simple observation. However, those who could not follow commands (in the absence of a focal lesion in the speech area) often had intracranial hypertension and required ICP monitoring. Most patients with a shift of ≥ 5 mm required surgery.

Conclusive evidence demonstrates that patients with large (> 30 mL) temporal lobe hematomas have a much greater risk of developing tentorial herniation than those with frontal or parieto-occipital lesions. One should therefore lean toward early surgery in cases of large hematomas. The same holds true for posterior fossa hematomas.

When CT scanning is unavailable, decisions regarding surgery may be based on air ventriculography and ICP measurements; such tests are rarely performed in centers in the United States. A midline shift of ≥ 5 mm indicates a need for immediate surgical decompression. In cases without midline shift but with the elevation of ICP above 20 mm Hg, angiography should be performed to rule out bilateral balancing lesions.

When angiography is performed in patients with severe head injuries, the following findings are considered as indications for surgical treatment. First, an intra- or extraaxial mass lesion causes a shift of the anterior cerebral vessels across the midline of > 5 mm. Second, an extraaxial mass lesion is > 5 mm from the inner table associated with any degree of anterior or middle cerebral artery displacement. Third, bilateral extraaxial mass lesions lie > 5 mm from the inner table. Except for patients who have marked brain atrophy, such intracranial masses will usually cause major elevations of ICP. Finally, a temporal lobe intraaxial mass lesion causes a major elevation of the middle cerebral artery or any degree of midline shift. These patients are in a precarious position because only slight swelling can cause a tentorial herniation syndrome, which progresses rapidly.

For surgical candidates, mannitol (1 to 2 g/kg body weight) is administered and the patient is promptly transported to the operating room. The patient should be mildly hyperventilated to achieve an arterial $PaCO_2$ of 25 to 30 mm Hg. As in all the maneuvers undertaken thus far, time is of the essence. The sooner the mass lesion is evacuated, the greater the possibility of good recovery. If no surgical lesion is found on CT, the patient is carefully monitored in the NICU, both clinically and with various physiological parameters [i.e., ICP and cerebral perfusion pressure (CPP) recordings, serial CT scans]. Any persistent rise in ICP above 20 mm Hg that cannot be explained readily and reversed, or any deterioration in neurological status warrants prompt repetition of the CT scan followed by the appropriate corrective measures.

◆ Anesthesia

Two particular concerns in the anesthetic management of trauma patients are elevated ICP and aspiration. Because head-injured patients with altered levels of consciousness are at high risk for aspiration, the anesthetic induction requires modification. Rapid sequence induction is performed to minimize this risk. The patient is preoxygenated and denitrogenated by breathing 100% oxygen before being rendered unconscious by the rapid administration of an intravenous induction agent; this is followed by a rapid-acting neuromuscular blocking agent. The patient is intubated while an assistant applies pressure to the cricoid cartilage to occlude the esophagus and prevent regurgitation. Intubation is performed without manual ventilation because this may force anesthetic gases into the stomach, leading to gastric dilatation, regurgitation, and aspiration of gastric contents. If the patient cannot be intubated quickly and begins to desaturate, mask ventilation is begun and another attempt is made after reoxygenation. Cricoid pressure is maintained until proper placement of the endotracheal tube is confirmed.

Patients with severe head injuries are presumed to have elevated ICPs; as such, care is taken to prevent further ICP elevation during intubation. Pretreatment with narcotics or intravenous lidocaine may be useful in this regard. It is incumbent on both the anesthesia and surgical teams to ensure adequate cerebral perfusion throughout the course of surgery.

◆ Surgical Techniques

Basic Trauma Craniotomy

The patient is positioned supine **(Fig. 77–1A)** and the head is turned almost 90 degrees to the appropriate side. A shoulder roll is used to facilitate head turning. A lateral

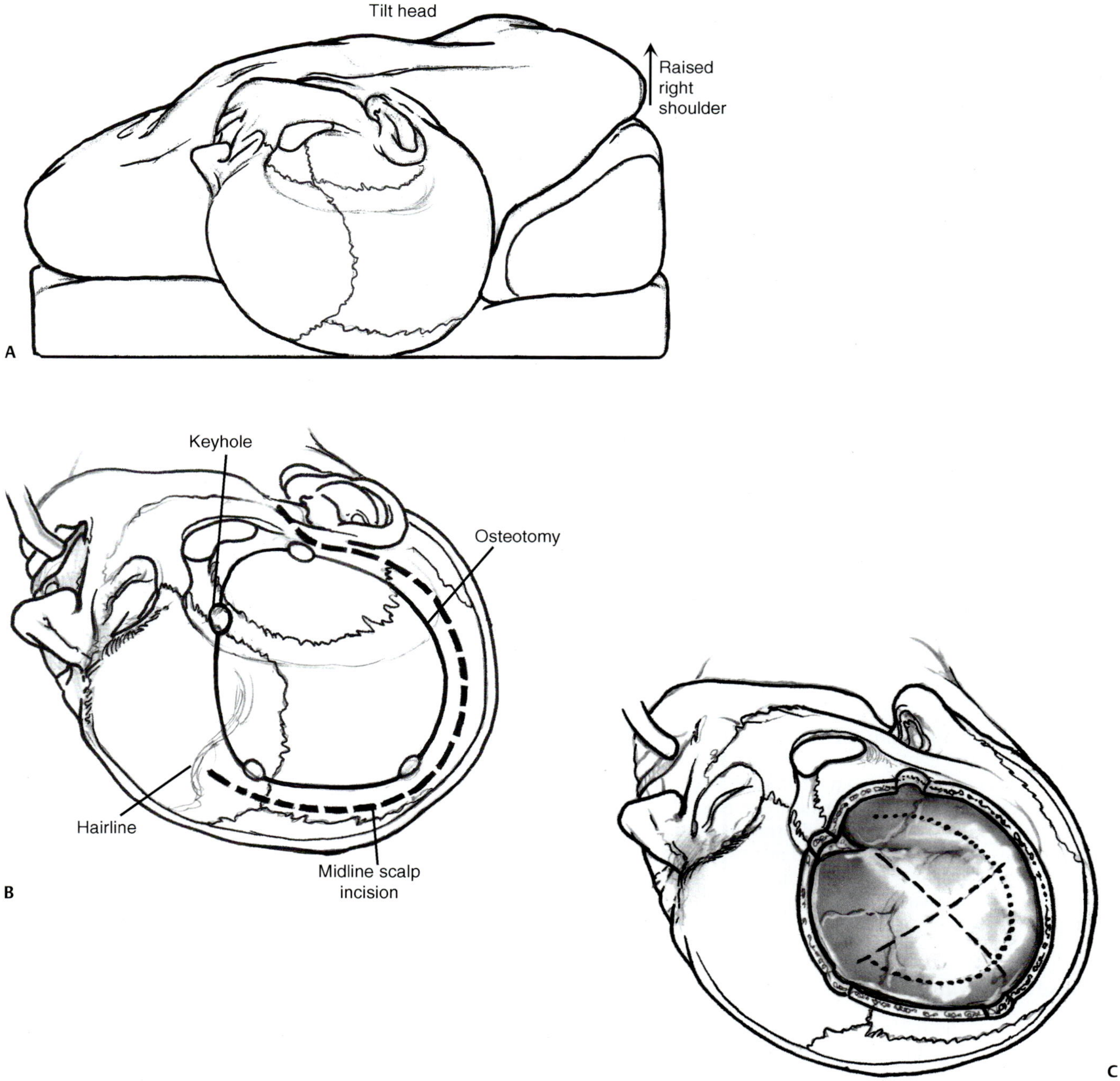

Figure 77–1 Basic craniotomy for a traumatic intracranial hematoma. In general, large craniotomies are recommended for traumatic intracranial hematomas. **(A)** The patient is positioned supine with a roll under one shoulder; the head is turned to the side opposite the lesion. **(B)** A large reverse question-mark skin flap is created that extends along the midline to the forehead and sweeps backward over the parietal region and down to a fingerbreadth in front of the ear. The inferior end of the incision is generally down to the zygomatic arch. **(C)** Depending on the location of the hematoma, a craniotomy flap is elevated. The dura is then opened in a cruciate (or tristar) manner.

position may be used if the cervical spine is not cleared and there is a high suspicion of a cervical spine fracture. The head is elevated above the heart to facilitate venous drainage. A horseshoe, donut, or three-pin headholder is used to facilitate positioning. The scalp is shaved, prepped with alcohol and Betadine, and draped.

An incision is marked that extends from 1 cm anterior to the tragus to just above the helix of the ear where it begins to curve posteriorly over the parietal boss. The incision turns anteriorly to the midline and then forward until just beyond the hairline (**Fig. 77–1B**). Hemostasis and analgesia at the scalp edge are facilitated with the use of a local anesthetic with epinephrine injected along the marked incision line. The incision is made with a no. 10 scalpel. Raney clips are placed at the skin edge to achieve hemostasis.

The scalp and temporalis muscle are reflected as a single unit to reduce the risk of injury to the frontalis branch of the facial nerve branch. A craniotomy is performed, making sure that one bur hole is just above the zygomatic arch and another is made at the keyhole to ensure adequate access to the floor of the temporal and frontal fossa, respectively (**Fig. 77–1C**).

Subdural Hematoma

After the dura is opened, the hematoma and contused brain are removed. With a thin subdural hematoma and a swollen brain, the dura should be opened carefully to avoid cortical laceration (**Fig. 77–2A**). The hematoma and underlying cerebral contusions are then evacuated by careful suction and irrigation (**Fig. 77–2B**). The subdural space is then explored and the origin of the hematoma identified if possible.

Hemostasis is then achieved with the use of bipolar electrocautery, Gelfoam, Surgicel, Nu Knit, Avitene, or other such hemostatic agents. A Valsalva maneuver performed at the end of the decompression is helpful to verify the security of the hemostasis. The dura is closed in a watertight fashion, either primarily or with a graft. Graft options include autologous pericranium or fascia lata, allogeneic grafts (bovine pericardium), and artificial substitutes (e.g., Gore-Tex).

Dural tacking sutures are then placed around the craniotomy margin and centrally to the bone flap to prevent a postoperative epidural hematoma. The bone flap is replaced and secured with nonabsorbable suture or cranial plates. A subgaleal drain may be placed and brought out through a separate incision. The scalp is closed in a two-layer closure with 2-0 Vicryl for the galea and staples for the skin. Patients who were comatose preoperatively undergo placement of a ventriculostomy.

Epidural Hematoma

The craniotomy is based over the hematoma (**Fig. 77–3A**). After removal of the bone flap, the hematoma is removed with suction, irrigation, and cup forceps (**Fig. 77–3B**). The lacerated vessel is identified and bleeding controlled with bipolar electrocautery or tamponade (**Fig. 77–3C**). After removal of the epidural hematoma, a small opening in the dura may be made to rule out the presence of a subdural hematoma. If the dura is opened, it is closed in a watertight fashion.

The dura is then tacked up to the perimeter of the craniotomy, the bone flap is reapplied, and the scalp closed as described earlier.

Intracerebral Hematoma

A standard trauma craniotomy is often needed for these lesions because of their frequent association with other traumatic lesions. After the dura is opened, a limited cortical incision is made through already traumatized or noneloquent brain (**Fig. 77–4**). Intraoperative ultrasound may be helpful to localize lesions that are deep to the cortical surface. The hematoma is then evacuated and hemostasis achieved with bipolar electrocautery and hemostatic agent.

◆ Special Circumstances

Special circumstances in the care of patients with head injuries can include those patients with temporal hematomas, intraoperative brain swelling, injuries to the venous sinus, and air embolism.

Temporal Hematoma

For the comatose patient with evidence of herniation and a temporal mass lesion, the temporal bur hole is placed first and a small craniectomy is performed (**Fig. 77–5**). The craniectomy may allow for aspiration of some of the underlying hematoma and decompress the brain until the rest of the craniotomy can be completed. However, this maneuver is not always effective.

Intraoperative Brain Swelling

Brain edema may be suspected on the preoperative head CT if there is only a thin subdural hematoma associated with significant midline shift. A disconcerting situation may arise after removal of the subdural hematoma with the herniation of brain tissue through the craniotomy site. Causes of the brain swelling include brain edema and hyperemia, or ipsilateral and contralateral intracerebral hematoma. Systemic problems (e.g., hypertension, hypotension, hypoventilation, ventilator malfunction) should be ruled out in conjunction with the anesthesia team. Adequate venous drainage should be verified; the patient's head should be elevated (if not done earlier). Simultaneously, the patient may be further sedated and paralyzed, mannitol should be given rapidly, and a ventriculostomy should be attempted to allow CSF drainage. A search is undertaken to detect any occult hematoma. Ipsilateral and contralateral intracranial hematomas may be identified with intraoperative ultrasound or CT.

Pentobarbital coma and frontal or temporal lobectomy may be used to control refractory brain swelling. In these cases, the dura must be augmented to expand the craniospinal volume. The bone flap may be left out and the scalp separated from the pericranium along the edge of the

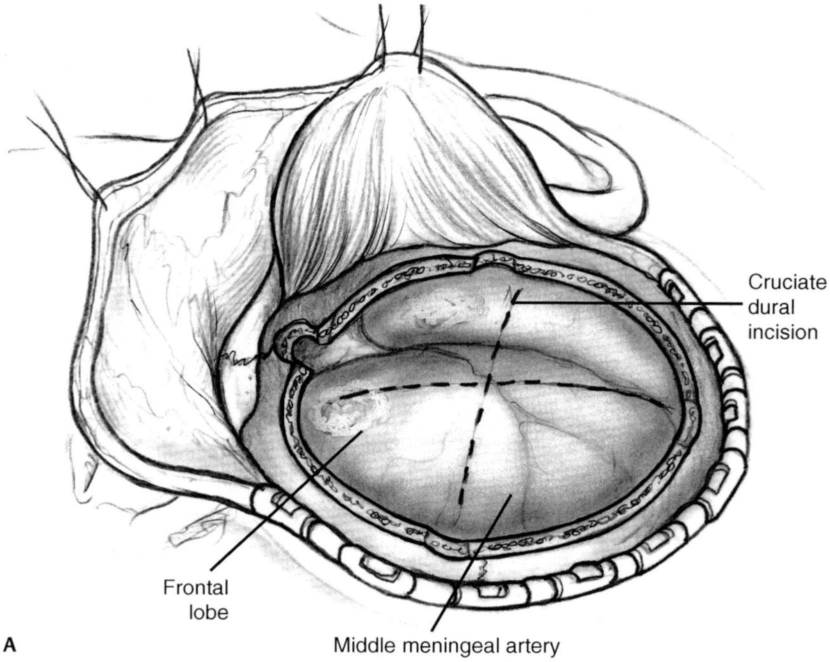

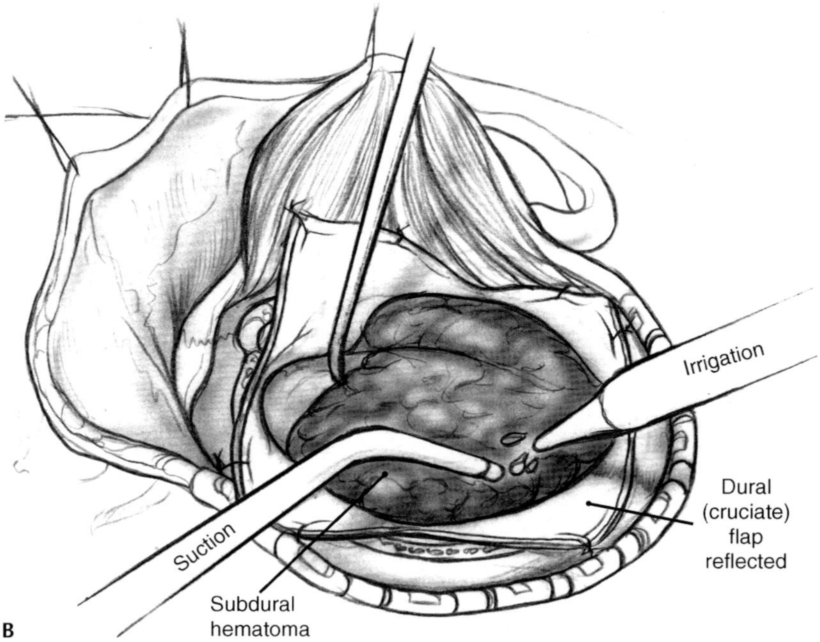

Figure 77–2 Basic craniotomy for a subdural hematoma (shown in Fig. 77–1). **(A)** After the dura covering the temporal lobe is opened, **(B)** the subdural hematoma is removed with suction and irrigation. The source of bleeding is identified and hemostasis is achieved. A dural pouch may be created with various dural substitutes to allow for brain swelling. If substantial brain swelling is anticipated, the bone flap is not replaced but is stored in a freezer or implanted into an abdominal wall pouch on the right side. The margins of the scalp are undermined to allow for maximum expansion of the decompressive craniotomy.

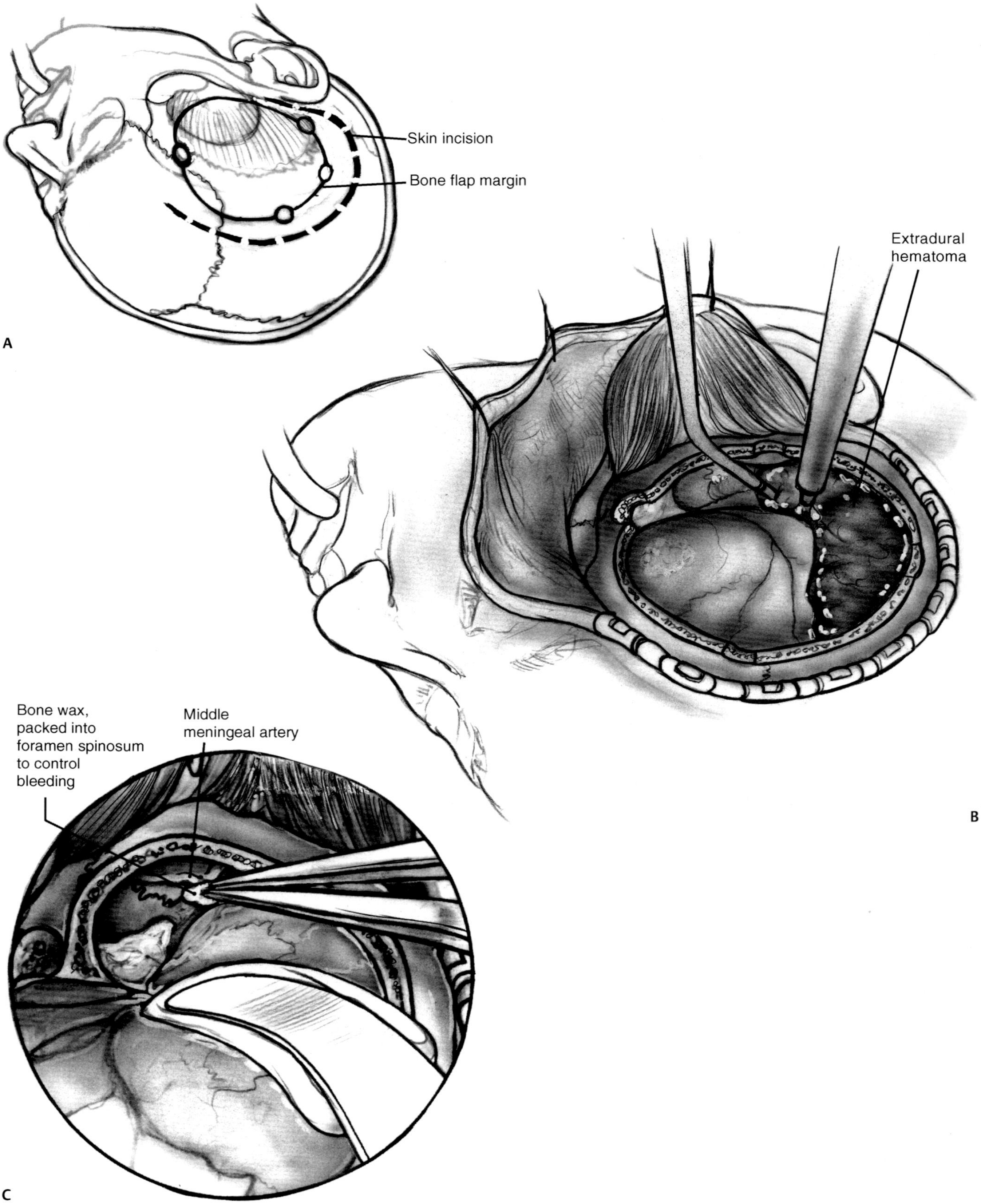

Figure 77–3 Craniotomy for epidural hematoma. **(A)** A small flap is generally created. **(B)** These hematomas usually occur in the temporal region caused by bleeding from the middle meningeal artery and occur in other areas. Although dura does not have to be opened, an opening can be made to look for any subdural bleeding. **(C)** Bone wax is packed into the foramen spinosum to control bleeding.

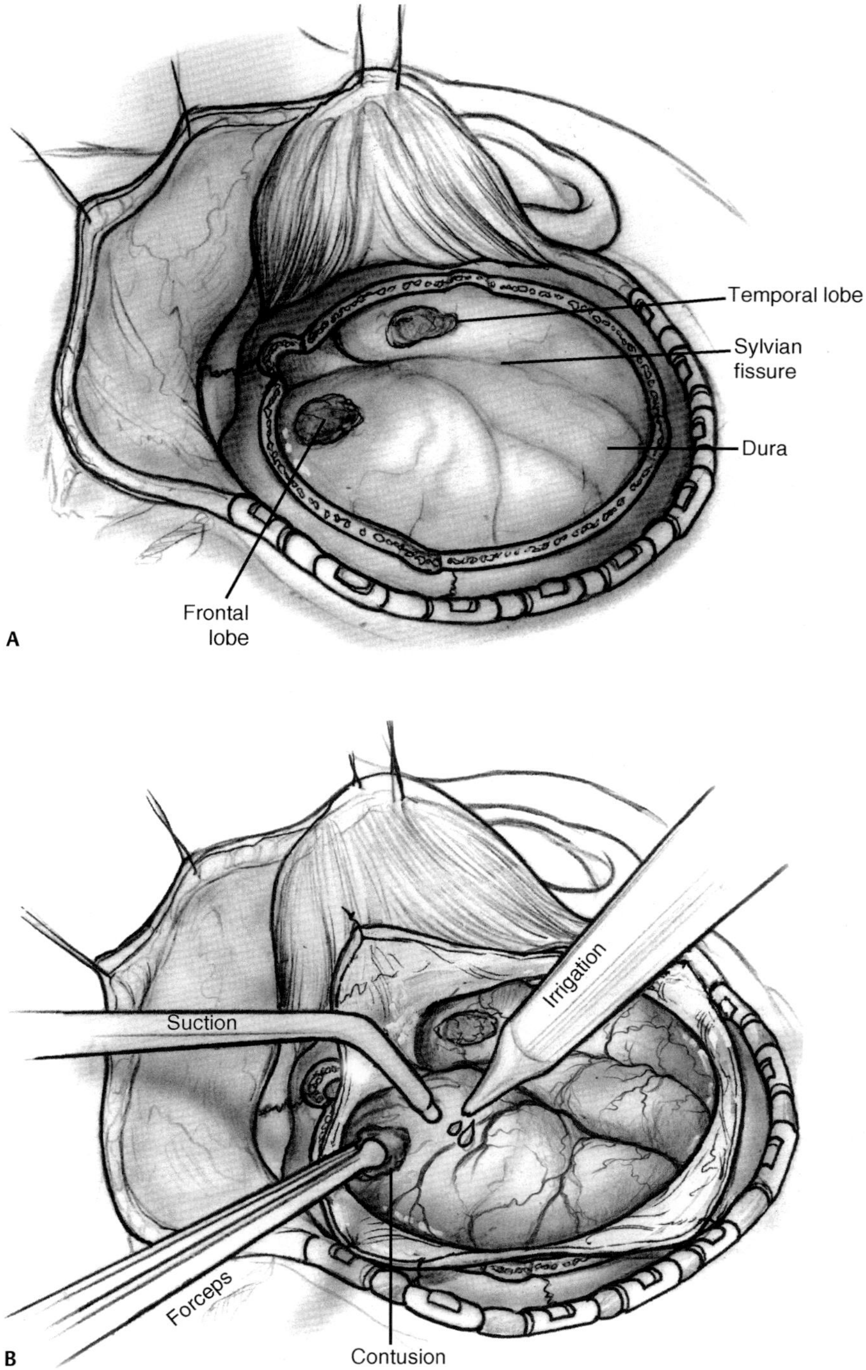

Figure 77–4 Craniotomy for intracerebral hematoma. **(A)** Brain contusions can coalesce into larger hematomas, which are usually seen in the frontal or temporal lobes. **(B)** A craniotomy may be performed for clot evacuation of the intracerebral hematoma causing significant mass effect. In this situation, the surgeon may create a dural expansion pouch and leave the bone flap out.

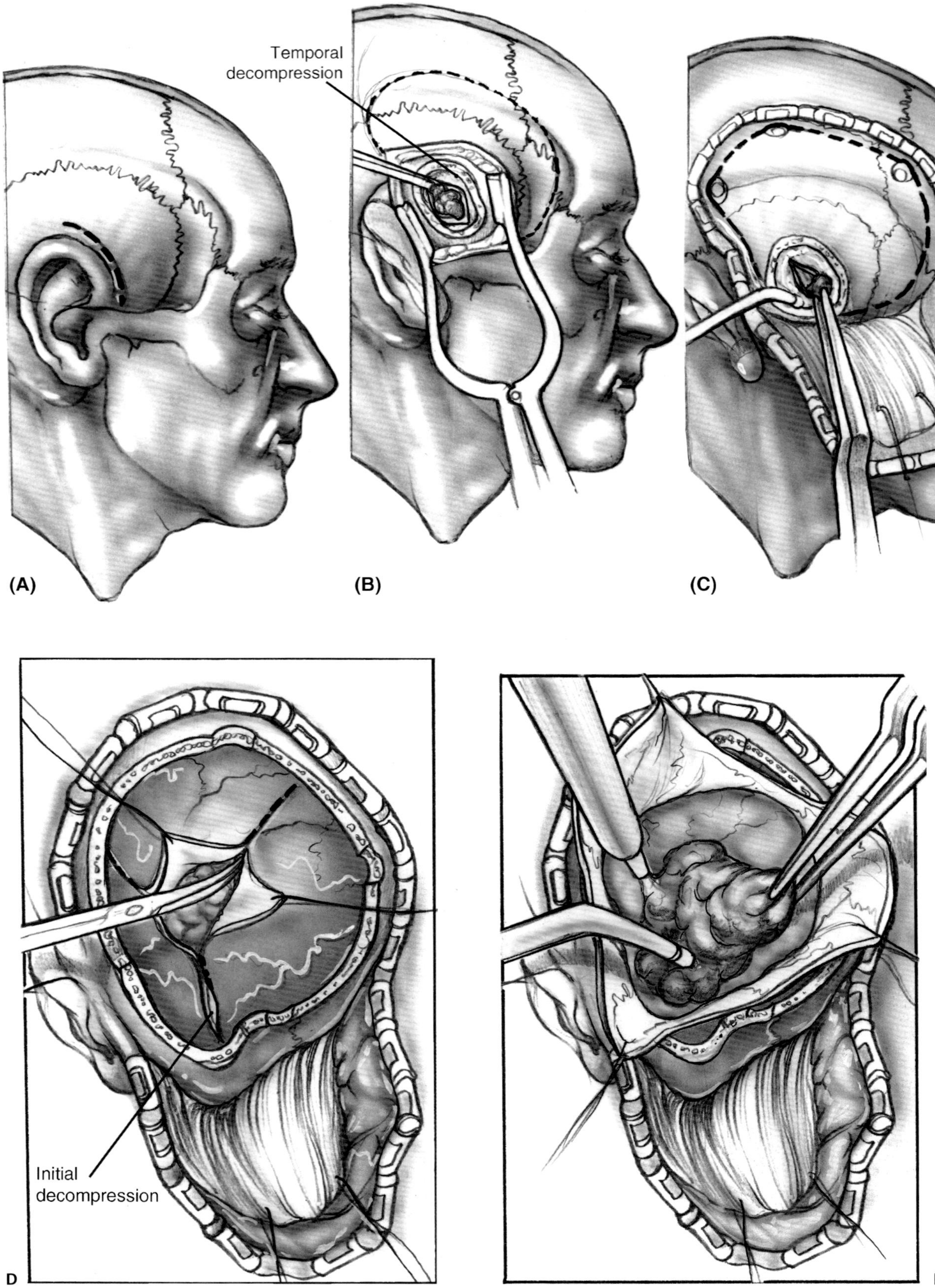

Figure 77–5 Urgent decompression for a hematoma in the temporal lobe. **(A)** A preauricular incision is made though the skin and muscle layers to quickly access the one. **(B)** If a patient presents with a dilated pupil on one side associated with an epidural, subdural, or intracerebral hematoma, an urgent craniotomy can be performed. **(C)** After creation of a temporal bur hole, the hematoma is aspirated. Because this strategy is not always successful, we generally prefer to treat the patient with large doses of mannitol and perform a complete craniotomy. However, if the patient cannot get to the operating room immediately, a limited decompression may be helpful. **(D)** Dural incision. **(E)** Clot evaluation.

craniotomy to facilitate expansion of the scalp flap. In bilateral decompressive craniectomies, the anterior end of the falx may be cut after ligation of the anterior end of the superior sagittal sinus to allow the frontal lobes to expand. A postoperative CT is usually obtained to detect unexpected pathologies, thus assisting in planning further management.

Venous Sinus Injuries

In cases where the injury may involve a major venous sinus, the surgeon needs to be prepared for massive hemorrhage and air embolism. Venous sinus hemorrhage is usually controlled by tamponade with hemostatic agents or small pieces of crushed muscle. Small tears in a sinus may be repaired primarily, whereas larger tears may be patched. Ligation may be the simplest treatment for injuries in noncritical areas (e.g., nondominant transverse sinus or anterior third of the superior sagittal sinus). In rare instances more complex posterior sinus injuries may require placing a shunt in the sagittal sinus prior to reconstruction. However, this procedure is rarely performed.

Air Embolism

Air embolism of clinical significance, which is an uncommon complication during trauma craniotomies, may be diagnosed by a drop in end-tidal CO_2 or a 1 to 2% increase in the expired nitrogen concentration. Precordial Doppler ultrasound is also helpful to detect air emboli in the right atrium. Preoperative placement of a right atrial catheter is helpful for the aspiration of embolized air. Other measures that can prevent air embolus include maintaining adequate blood volume (normovolemia) and avoiding extreme positioning elevation in which the head is above the heart. In the event of an air embolism, the surgical field should be flooded with saline and packed with wet sponges, the head of the bed should be dropped below the level of the patient's heart, and the cut bone surfaces should be waxed. The left lateral decubitus position is helpful in trapping air in the apex of the right atrium, but this position can be difficult to achieve during surgery. The patient is also placed on 100% inspired oxygen.

◆ Conclusion

The outcome of a head injury has improved substantially during the past few decades because of several organizational improvements including better trauma care systems, early CT scanning, surgery for hematomas, and improved neurocritical care. There have been no significant breakthroughs in the pharmacological treatment of traumatic brain injury. Appropriate medical and surgical management can nevertheless make a very substantial impact on the patient's ultimate potential for recovery.

References

1. Bullock R, Chestnut R, Clifton G, et al. Guidelines for the management of severe head injury. J Neurotrauma 1996:13;639–734
2. Galbraith S, Teasdale G. Predicting the need for operation in the patient with an occult traumatic intracranial hematoma. J Neurosurg 1981:55;75–81
3. Kanter MJ, Robertson CS. Measurement of intracranial pressure. Intensive Care World 1990:7;16–19

78

Surgical Management of Cranial Trauma

Karin S. Bierbrauer

The treatment of missile wounds to the brain has changed over the years, whereas the principles guiding the treatment of cranial fractures have remained relatively constant. Improvements in the range and efficacy of antibiotics to treat central nervous system (CNS) infections, for example, may have contributed not only to treatment decisions but also to outcomes. Most changes that have occurred, however, are probably the direct result of the more sophisticated imaging techniques that have evolved over the years. The almost universal availability of computed tomographic (CT) scanning in medical centers that treat patients with head injuries has allowed for very precise preoperative determination of the extent and location of any intracranial injuries that may be associated with an open fracture or penetrating missile. This has, in many instances, alleviated or reduced the need for exploratory surgery as well as the need for exploratory maneuvers during surgery, such as opening the dura in a patient with an open depressed skull fracture to ascertain whether there is an associated underlying subdural or intraparenchymal hemorrhage. The very fact that these are traumatic injuries means that not only do neurosurgeons have to address the cranial injury but also they have to take into account the presence of trauma to other body systems and any associated hemodynamic instability, and they have to be prepared to treat any concomitant elevations in intracranial pressure (ICP).

◆ Indications

The indications for operating on cranial fractures vary depending, in part, on whether or not the skin and galea have been violated overlying the fracture. A simple linear cranial vault fracture, however, can usually be managed nonoperatively, whether open or closed. Any overlying laceration can often be sutured in the emergency department setting after aseptic irrigation, utilizing nonabsorbable suture. Every attempt should be made to incorporate the galeal layer into the closure to minimize scalp bleeding, which can be profuse and even of hemodynamic significance in small children.

The indications for operative intervention for a depressed skull fracture are dependent on several factors. Many closed depressed skull fractures can be corrected nonoperatively with management tempered by the surgeon's judgment. Fractures depressed a depth less than the width of the skull itself, without an underlying mass lesion and not causing significant cosmetic deformity, are among those frequently managed conservatively. Consideration may be given to elevating those fractures that are in a cosmetically important area such as near the orbital rim or low forehead to alleviate any unsightly depression. It seems clear that the incidence of seizures is not affected by whether or not the bone fragments are elevated.[1] Likewise, because an associated neurological deficit may have been caused by cortical injury at the moment of impact rather than any compressive effects of the residual bone fragments, elevating the fracture to alleviate a neurological deficit is usually reserved for those cases where the neurological deficit is worsening. In these cases, an associated expanding hematoma will often be found.

Most open depressed fractures require operative debridement for thorough debridement, irrigation, and cleansing of the bone fragments, repair of any underlying dural lacerations, and evacuation of underlying intra- or extraaxial hematomas as indicated. Those fractures overlying major dural sinuses require special attention. The surgeon must weigh the risk of elevating the bone fragments against the risk of progressive sinus thrombosis. Profuse life-threatening bleeding can occur as the bone fragments are manipulated if there is an underlying tear in the sinus. On the other hand, prolonged compression of a dural venous sinus can lead to intracranial hypertension and other complications of venous sinus thrombosis.

Basilar skull fractures rarely require operative intervention, although these patients must be carefully monitored for associated complications such as cerebrospinal fluid (CSF) rhinorrhea, otorrhea, or cranial nerve VII (or VIII) palsies. These findings can be delayed (up to 2 weeks postinjury for facial nerve palsies) and therefore may not become manifest during the initial hospitalization. The indications for operative intervention to treat a CSF leak associated with a basilar skull fracture are those cases where the leak fails to resolve spontaneously or after conservative measures such as elevation of the head, spinal drainage, or even acetazolamide have failed. Some of these surgical procedures can now be done via extracranial approaches utilizing techniques such as transparanasal sinus endoscopy where appropriate. The surgical treatment of facial nerve palsies or pareses remains controversial, with some authors advocating facial nerve exploration and repair in cases of immediate-onset total paralysis, and a more conservative course that may include short-term oral corticosteroids for those patients with delayed onset paralysis or only paresis.[2]

Most missile injuries to the skull, on the other hand, require surgical debridement. Although some newer literature[3] is available suggesting a nonoperative approach utilizing antibiotics and limited debridement and closure in some select cases, the mainstay of current therapy remains operative. Even tangential wounds, where the patient is often neurologically intact or with just a focal deficit from a cortical contusion, should usually be explored if there is any depression of the skull seen on CT scan images.

Another lingering area of controversy is the management of the patient who arrives with a severe penetrating missile injury that has traversed and consequently irrevocably injured large areas of the brain, whose neurological exam reveals only some minimal brainstem-level function even after resuscitation. When faced with such a patient, whose outlook for functional recovery is virtually nil, the appropriateness of aggressive operative intervention is a matter that needs to be carefully discussed with the family. Poor prognostic signs for patients with civilian (i.e., low-velocity), cerebral gunshot wounds include missile injuries that have traversed the midline and/or entered the ventricular system, low admission Glasgow Coma Scale (GCS) score (all patients with GCS 3 on admission died as a result of their injuries in one published study) and the presence of intracranial hematomas.[4]

However, because prognosticating an outcome can be difficult, it does occasionally happen that a patient who is not expected to live will, in fact, survive. If there has been no or inadequate surgical repair initially in the expectation that the patient will rapidly succumb to the injury (usually by herniation from increased ICP), the consequences of persistent cutaneous CSF fistulas or intracranial content oozing from an open wound can be devastating, not only medically but in terms of nursing care and psychological impact on the family. Therefore, when in doubt as to whether a patient would benefit from surgical debridement and exploration, it is best to err on the side of operating.

◆ Preparation

In this era, CT scanning is the mainstay of imaging for patients with both skull fractures and missile injuries. The role of plain skull x-rays in imaging the neurologically intact patient in the emergency department who has sustained a minor closed head injury to look for a linear skull fracture remains controversial, especially with the ready availability of CT scanning in most medical centers. Plain skull x-rays still have an important role, however, in imaging the patient who has sustained penetrating trauma because they may provide details of bony injury and missile fragments obscured by intra- or extracranial metallic artifact on CT scans. Even when the CT image is viewed on settings appropriate for bone windows, this characteristic artifact produced by metallic fragments can obscure large areas of the image. CT can help with imaging other foreign bodies like wood or glass that may be embedded in a wound, although plain films will also detect glass fragments. Larger wood splinters, such as those in the orbit, may be localized with the help of ultrasound if necessary.

Magnetic resonance imaging (MRI) also has a role in certain select patients. It is particularly helpful in evaluating a dural venous sinus injury such as may be found underlying a depressed skull fracture. If MRI is unavailable, a contrast-enhanced CT can be obtained to look for an "empty delta" sign reflective of sinus occlusion. Magnetic resonance venography (MRV) may be utilized in some of these cases to avoid the need for venous-phase angiography to assess the patency of the underlying sinus. It may also give information about associated findings such as a Chiari I malformation that may affect treatment decisions and not be readily apparent on CT imaging.

Angiography remains the mainstay of imaging in detecting posttraumatic aneurysms that are usually small and peripherally located. Angiography may also be indicated in cases of cranial fracture with an embedded implement, such as a knife, where intracranial vascular injury is suspected. The role of magnetic resonance angiography (MRA) and CT angiography in evaluating these lesions may also expand in the future.

Although imaging the patient with a cranial fracture or missile injury is readily and quickly accomplished in most medical centers in this era, it must never take the place of a thorough general and neurological examination of the patient. The patient must be medically stable prior to the trip to the x-ray department, and interventions must be undertaken as appropriate to prevent, detect, and treat hypoxemia and hypotension, both initially and throughout the management phase of the head-injured patient. Seizures must be recognized and treated appropriately. Unrecognized associated abdominal or chest trauma may lead to hypovolemic shock that also can impair cerebral perfusion pressure.

Establishment of appropriate airway support is necessary in many patients with a depressed level of consciousness, although prophylactic severe hyperventilation therapy is no longer advocated on a routine basis.[5] The indications for the administration of hyperosmolar agents such as mannitol to the patient with a head injury who does not yet have an ICP monitor include signs of transtentorial herniation or progressive neurological deterioration.[6] These agents should certainly be used judiciously, if at all, in the patient with multisystem trauma who may already be hypovolemic. Replacement of the fluid lost by diuresis when these agents are used may help avoid any undesired hypotension. Intermittent boluses of mannitol (0.25 to 1.0 g/kg body weight) may be used to control elevations of ICP once an ICP monitor is in place. This requires careful monitoring of serum osmolarity, serum sodium, and the patient's volume status via a Foley catheter. A central venous access line or even a Swan-Ganz catheter is also often placed for close monitoring of the patient's fluid status.

Routine blood work for the patient with a serious head injury in the emergency department setting will often also include a toxicology screen to look for other agents that may contribute to a depressed level of consciousness. In anticipation of surgical intervention, crossmatching of blood is often a part of the routine serologic evaluation. Patients with penetrating injuries to the head are particularly prone to the development of disseminated intravascular coagulopathy (DIC). A coagulation profile is often indicated, both acutely and later during treatment, especially if unexpected oozing is noted during surgical intervention.

◆ Surgical Technique

Anesthesia

Intraoperative anesthesia for the patient who is undergoing elevation of a depressed skull fracture or treatment of a missile injury is in accordance with standard anesthetic practice for intracranial procedures. The possibility of very rapid blood loss must be anticipated in those patients where injury to an underlying dural venous sinus is suspected. The prevention and detection of an air embolus is also a consideration in these patients. Special venous access lines to aspirate air from the right atrium of the heart as well as precordial Doppler monitoring to listen for the characteristic sound of an air embolus may be necessary. Blood products should be readily available as necessary, including fresh frozen plasma and platelets for those patients developing DIC due to the massive release of tissue thromboplastin that can occur with missiles that injure large areas of brain tissue.

Sophisticated intraoperative monitoring techniques such as motor mapping or cranial nerve electromyograms (EMGs) are rarely necessary in the setting of these acute traumatic brain injuries. Surgical exploration in the head-injured patient is usually limited to areas of the brain that have already been injured by a missile or other perforating or penetrating object, so there is rarely a need for corticotomy through healthy tissue or exploration along intact white matter tracts.

Positioning

Positioning the patient in the operating room setting is done to maximize surgical exposure while minimizing risk to the patient. Therefore, although a slightly elevated position of the head may facilitate the surgeon's view of a vertex injury, it may also increase the risk of air embolus. Air embolism can result from exposed diploic skull veins and not just from large dural venous sinuses. Obstruction of venous outflow from the head or increased airway resistance such as might be caused by overly zealous flexion of the head should be avoided. An adequate wide exposure, as in all neurosurgical trauma cases, is imperative, and in the case of missile injuries should include both entrance and exit sites. The need for postoperative ICP monitoring in many of these patients means that the needed scalp exposure for such a monitor, including any tunneling pathways as might be utilized for a ventriculostomy, must be anticipated. If it is anticipated that a patient with a subfrontal or orbitofrontal missile injury may require a fascia lata graft, the patient's thigh should be included in the prep.

Adequate padding of bony prominences and vulnerable peripheral nerves such as the ulnar and peroneal nerves should prevent iatrogenic nerve injury. Children who are too young for rigid skull pin fixation and who are placed into horseshoe head holders for occipital and suboccipital exposure are at risk for orbital pressure injuries, especially if the head position is changed during the case by overly vigorous manipulation of the bone with rongeurs. The placement of chest rolls for prone cases should allow for adequate chest ventilation and avoid venous congestion.

Initial Exposure

In the rare case of a ping-pong fracture in an infant with intact underlying dura, the fracture may be elevated by making a small incision near the edge of the fracture. A small bur hole is then made with a drill if there is no adjacent open cranial suture. Once the epidural plane has been identified, the fracture can then gently be elevated by sliding an elevator under the fracture. Careful scrutiny of the preoperative CT scan to be sure there is no associated hematoma that needs to be evacuated is important in these patients. Downward levering motion with the elevating instrument needs to be avoided so as not to injure the skull and brain under the fulcrum point.

The incision for the elevation of closed depressed fractures should avoid non–hair-bearing areas of the head because one of the primary indications for this operation is cosmesis. Planning an incision for open depressed fractures is very similar, in principle, to that done for missile wounds to the head. It is often best to incorporate the laceration or jagged missile entry or exit wound into the incision rather than trying to isolate the macerated skin in the middle of a standard horseshoe-shaped incision. A lazy-S–type incision often works very well in this setting, especially if the area of surgical interest is centered in the S. This type of incision often allows greater exposure than a simple linear incision extending out from the fracture or entrance wound. In the case of a small laceration overlying a depressed fracture near the orbital rim, it may be best to plan a modified bicoronal or other elongated incision behind the hairline and close the laceration separately rather than achieving an inadequate exposure through the laceration and thereby being forced to compromise surgery or dramatically enlarge an already unsightly frontal laceration. It is important to preserve blood supply to any surgical flaps. If, for example, the supraorbital artery on one side has been traumatized by the initial injury and one is planning a bicoronal flap, then one should try to preserve the anterior branch of the superficial temporal artery by making the incision posterior to the course of the artery on the involved side.

If the need for a pericranial graft is anticipated for dural closure, extra allowance should be made in planning the incision. Likewise, it is easy to underestimate the peripheral extent of the inner table involvement of a depressed cranial fracture by palpation, and therefore allowance should be made for the need to extend an incision as needed.

Surgical Procedure

Depressed Skull Fractures

One of the main operative goals of elevating an open depressed fracture is thorough debridement. If the skin edges are macerated, contaminated, or severely contused, excision of the involved edges may be indicated. Rotational flaps are rarely necessary but should be anticipated if large areas of the scalp have been denuded at the time of injury. The fact that the fracture will usually be directly under the planned curvilinear incision line is rarely problematic if a good galeal closure is achieved. At the time of opening one can begin to anticipate the need for a pericranial graft and the depth of the incision judged accordingly. In small children needless stripping of the pericranium over intact skull is to be avoided due to the ensuing blood loss as the underlying denuded bone bleeds. Even in older patients it is a good idea to preserve as much pericranium as possible to cover the bone fragments at the time of closure. This helps smooth out the repaired area so the patient is less disturbed by any underlying irregularity, such as can occur from sutures or wires holding the bone fragments in place. Likewise, if the fracture underlies the temporalis muscle, it is ideal to try to reclose that layer over the fragments as well.

Many fractures, be they open or closed, will be comminuted and the bone fragments in-driven under the adjacent inner table to such a degree that a small bur hole placed adjacent to the fracture is necessary to identify the epidural space and begin the gentle piecemeal removal of the bone fragments. If possible, this bur hole should be placed over an area of intact dura to avoid further injuring any underlying contused brain tissue. Removal of the bone fragments should not be rushed but rather done in an orderly fashion as the fragments loosen. A punch or rongeur is often useful here to remove small portions of bone as necessary to allow the fragments to loosen enough to be removed safely without further injuring the underlying dura or cortex.

In some cases where the underlying dura is felt to be intact and there is a central area of depression in a more greenstick or ping-pong type of fracture, one can excise the entire depressed area circumferentially in toto using a high-speed drill once the epidural space is identified with a small bur hole. The entire bone fragment can then be replaced in one piece after reshaping it. Instruments borrowed from the craniofacial trays such as a Tessier rib bender can be very helpful in restoring a natural contour to a depressed, misshapen bone fragment.

Once the depressed fragments have been removed, they are inspected for signs of gross contamination that would preclude their being replaced in the wound even after vigorous irrigation and cleansing. Cultures of the wound and bone and devitalized tissue should be sent for later tailoring of antibiotic coverage should an infection develop. At the time of initial surgery, and for a brief postoperative period, routine antibiotic prophylaxis, especially for soft tissue coverage, usually suffices unless there are extenuating circumstances such as paranasal sinus penetration by the fracture. Unless the wound is very old or unusually contaminated, the bone fragments are replaced at the end of the procedure utilizing suture, wire, or miniplates, depending on the surgeon's preference and the cosmetic needs of the particular patient (wires, for example, tend to be unsightly under a small child's thin scalp). The infection rate, even when the bone fragments are replaced in the setting of an open depressed fracture, if the wound is meticulously debrided and irrigated, should be quite low.[7]

In the event there is an underlying dural laceration, the craniectomy must expose the entire extent of the dural opening. In the case of a growing fracture of childhood (leptomeningeal cyst) exposing this dural laceration usually reveals that it extends beyond the confines of the fracture edges. Repairing this defect in the dura is the most important part of the procedure. Any obvious hematoma and devitalized brain tissue seen may be gently removed, although the removal of partially contused brain tissue that may have some potential for recovery especially in eloquent areas of the brain requires the neurosurgeon's judgment and skill. In an effort to minimize leaving foreign objects in the wound, hemostasis is best achieved with judicious use of bipolar cautery rather than indiscriminate packing with various hemostatic agents. Dural repair should be watertight and may require grafting. If the paranasal sinuses are involved, the mucosa is usually stripped, using a small drill if necessary, and then the residual cavity can be filled with various agents such as temporalis muscle, pericranium, or absorbable gelatin sponge. A pericranial graft can then be reflected over the sinus and sewn to the dura to further isolate it from the intracranial contents.

Prior to replacing the bone fragments such that maximum bone coverage is achieved for areas of non–hair-bearing scalp, epidural tack-up sutures may be prudent to avoid a postoperative epidural hematoma. Special attention should be given to the area of the orbital rim if this is involved with the fracture. This is one area where plating may be quite helpful to reconstruct the brow line if it has been extensively shattered.

Special scenarios involving these types of fractures when they are near the vertex or ear of the patient arise when they overlie a major dural venous sinus. This type of patient may rapidly deteriorate after admission in a relatively good neurological grade—the so-called talk and die syndrome. Not all fractures overlying a dural sinus need to be elevated, especially if there is no overlying laceration and no mass effect on the underlying sinus. (In addition to careful serial clinical examination looking for evidence of early papilledema, MRV may be helpful in making this determination.

Angiography remains the gold-standard study of choice when the status of the sinus remains unclear.)

If a decision is made to remove these fragments overlying a rent in a sinus, then extensive preparation to anticipate any problems is often needed. Anesthesia issues regarding possible blood loss and air embolus should be discussed with the anesthesiologist. The surgical exposure should be such to allow for control of the sinus both proximally and distally prior to lifting out the offending bone fragments. This usually necessitates the placement of several additional bur holes. One should always proceed very cautiously because the jagged fracture edges in fact may have lacerated the sinus but are tamponading it. The laceration in the sinus, once it is exposed, can often be repaired directly or with a muscle or pericranial patch or rotational dural flap sewn over absorbable gelatin sponge or oxidized cellulose. Alternatives in the anterior third of the sagittal sinus include ligation of the sinus to control bleeding. When this is not an option, as in the posterior portion of the superior sagittal sinus, uncontrolled bleeding can sometimes be temporarily controlled with digital pressure and suction long enough to allow for repair. If this is not sufficient to allow visualization of the surgical field due to brisk bleeding, a proximal sinotomy may be needed to allow the placement of an inflatable Fogarty balloon catheter. In cases where an interposed graft is necessary for the permanent repair of a large sinus laceration that cannot be repaired any other way, an autogenous saphenous vein graft may be utilized after temporarily shunting the blood through an interposed shunt to allow time to sew the graft into place.[8]

Missile Wounds

The goals of surgery in treating a patient with a gunshot wound to the head are the debridement of devitalized tissue, removal of in-driven debris, evacuation of any large hematoma, the control of any active bleeding, and the creation of a meticulous dural and galeal closure. Doing this well the first time to prevent the need for reoperation cannot be stressed enough. The scalp incisions have already been discussed earlier in the chapter, but, in short, a linear or curvilinear incision incorporating the entrance or exit wounds usually works best unless there is an unusual associated finding such as a large, hemispheric, subdural hematoma that mandates a more standard trauma flap.

The scalp is opened such that the bony defect created by the missile is centrally incorporated into the planned craniotomy or craniectomy. As much periosteum as possible is preserved during this stage because these patients almost inevitably require dural patch grafting. The bony opening should be large enough to allow for thorough debridement of the bullet tract, as described later, so a small circumferential craniectomy starting at the exposed fracture edges is usually necessary (and sufficient). If there is bleeding from a dural sinus, exposed paranasal air sinuses, or a subfrontal exposure necessary for a skull-base repair, then a craniotomy may be more appropriate. A formal craniotomy bone flap may be replaced at the end of the procedure, but small contaminated bone fragments in general are not replaced. Certainly foreign implants like acrylics should be avoided in the acute setting.

Once an adequate bony removal has been accomplished, the dural defect is exposed and enlarged as needed. (If the dura is intact, as with a tangential wound, it should be opened if preoperative imaging has shown an underlying mass lesion.) Any readily accessible bone or bullet fragments or other contaminated foreign objects can be carefully removed and cultured at this point. The bullet track is then identified and preserved with self-retaining retractors gently held in place until thorough debridement of the track is completed. This debridement is best accomplished by squeezing warm irrigant solution from a large Asepto (Venice, CA) bulb syringe into the surface of the track. This washes most of the debris to the surface and precludes the need for deep suctioning, which in itself can lead to further bleeding. This gentle irrigation also stops most small bleeding points deep in the track if one perseveres with patience.

In the Vietnam War era studies, as many as 50 to 60% of retained bone fragments were found to be contaminated with organisms such as gram-positive cocci, usually *Staphylococcus*, and less frequently, *Streptococcus* and various gram-negative rods.[9] Therefore, any readily accessible bone fragments should be removed. Intraoperative ultrasound can be helpful in locating these fragments, but those fragments in eloquent gray and white matter, in the deep gray nuclei, near a potentially lacerated dural sinus, or those that are at a great distance from the entrance of the track may be best left in place. These are situations where the surgeon's judgment is of paramount importance in weighing the risk of leaving a potentially contaminated object deep in the brain against the real possibility of imparting further neurological injury in an attempt to retrieve such a fragment. The indications for overly vigorous attempts to retrieve the bullet fragment(s) are even less clear because the rate of contamination for these projectiles is even less than for the bone fragments. Bullet fragments within the ventricular system may migrate, however, and for that reason an attempt is often made to retrieve them at the time of surgery.

Any residual bleeding points are then controlled with bipolar cautery after copious irrigation of the track. The dura is then closed in a watertight fashion with synthetic absorbable suture and autologous grafts as necessary. The prevention of CSF cutaneous fistulas and CSF rhinorrhea is a key goal of this operation, and this step should not be neglected. Fibrin glue, now available in commercial preparations, can be used as an adjunct to achieving a watertight closure in difficult skull-base injuries. Exit wounds are treated in a similar fashion to that described earlier for entry wounds.

◆ Closure

The skin is closed in single or double layers depending on the age of the injury, with single-layer nonabsorbable suture used for more contaminated or older wounds. Any undue tension on the wound can compromise the closure and should be avoided, with transposition or other flaps as indicated or relaxing galeal incisions for lesser problematic areas.

◆ Postoperative Care

The principles of postoperative care that apply to any head-injured patient apply to these patients as well. Patients with a GCS score of 8 or less usually have an ICP monitor placed at the time of surgical repair. Ventricular drainage in the patient with a severe missile injury with intraventricular blood has the obvious advantage of allowing an extra modality to treat, not just diagnose, elevations of ICP. Other maneuvers to control intractable elevations of ICP include the prevention and treatment of hyperthermia, maintenance of euvolemia, avoidance of systemic hypotension, provision of adequate sedation and ventilation, attention to maintenance of venous outflow from the head by simple positional maneuvers of the head, prevention and treatment of seizures, and more aggressive maneuvers such as limited hyperventilation (with jugular venous oxygen saturation monitoring if available), osmotic diuretics, induction of relative systemic hypertension to improve cerebral perfusion pressure, and even less proven modalities such as barbiturate coma in cases of severe intractable ICP elevation.

Extensive uncontrollable edema in the white matter adjacent to the track of a missile injury is a common, often terminal, cause of intractable intracranial hypertension with loss of cerebral perfusion pressure. Unfortunately, this often proves fatal even despite the most aggressive maneuvers, both surgical and medical.

Repeat imaging is indicated if there is any possibility of a surgically treatable cause of ICP elevation such as postoperative hematomas or acute obstructive hydrocephalus due to intraventricular blood or migration of a bullet fragment. Sometimes lobectomy of a severely contused nondominant frontal or temporal lobe is done to help lower ICP. Neurological deterioration in some cases may be due to intracranial hypertension from dural venous sinus occlusion and may require elevation of bone fragments overlying a sinus.

Proper attention to electrolyte management in these severely injured patients is very important because abnormalities of electrolytes such as sodium may add to a depressed neurological status. The syndrome of inappropriate antidiuretic hormone secretion not infrequently complicates the postoperative course of these patients. Avoiding excess free water by administering isotonic rather than hypotonic fluids in the acute phase, therefore, may help not only by minimizing brain edema but also by helping prevent iatrogenic hyponatremia.

The use of prophylactic antibiotics remains somewhat controversial in treating these open wounds, especially if they are fresh and "clean." Because the goal of surgery is rapid and thorough wound debridement, one could argue that broad-spectrum antibiotics, particularly for a prolonged period of time postoperatively, may not be necessary, and may in fact select out resistant organisms or even fungi. First-generation cephalosporins in the immediate perioperative period for soft tissue coverage may suffice in many cases, even where debridement has been delayed.[10]

The use of anticonvulsants can be justified, at least in the acute phase,[11] in patients who have sustained a gunshot wound with obvious cortical injury because 30 to 50% of patients with civilian missile wounds have posttraumatic epilepsy. These anticonvulsants are often continued long-term because of concerns about the high incidence of late epilepsy in these patients. The routine use of anticonvulsants in patients with depressed skull fractures is more controversial, and factors sometimes used to help make that decision include the presence of early epilepsy, posttraumatic amnesia of $>$ 24 hours' duration, and the presence of dural and cortical laceration.[12] Seizure prevention can be very important in the acute phase management of patients with high ICPs. The potentially deleterious effects of a seizure on the patient whose ICP is already difficult to control can therefore also be used in the decision-making phase about the use of anticonvulsants.

Those patients who survive with a large or otherwise unsightly cranial defect may require cranioplasty. This should probably be delayed about 6 months in most cases. The choice of materials to use in reconstructing the defects ranges from autologous rib or split skull grafts to acrylic or newer compounds available that are based on the hydroxyapatite molecule or bone matrix. Proper dural closure at the time of the first operation, even in cases where the bone is not replaced for reasons of contamination or severe brain swelling, makes delineation of the planes at the time of reoperation much easier.

Some patients with intraventricular or subarachnoid blood at the time of injury develop posthemorrhagic hydrocephalus that does not resolve after the acute phase. In those rare cases where the hydrocephalus appears to be obstructive, a third ventriculocisternostomy may be tried as an alternative to permanent shunting. Those patients with communicating hydrocephalus who do go on to a shunting procedure will sometimes have a lumboperitoneal shunt placed rather than a ventriculoperitoneal shunt. Reports of scoliosis, nerve root irritation, and acquired Chiari I malformations make lumbar shunting procedures less attractive in children.[13]

◆ Complications

Special surgical situations may arise that can complicate the operative or postoperative management of these patients. Missile wounds that traverse the midline can leave bullet fragments quite remote from the entrance wound. Even though not all bullet fragments must be retrieved if not readily accessible, intraventricular fragments may be washed out or endoscopically retrieved after locating them with ultrasound or ventriculoscope guidance. The problems associated with dural venous sinus injuries have already been addressed earlier in the chapter.

Facio-orbito-frontal wounds can lead to several potential complications, including infections, CSF leaks, bleeding, and cranial nerve injuries. Missile wounds that cause these surgically challenging wounds often enter the skull through the floor of the anterior fossa (as with suicide-type gunshot wounds), the sphenoid wing, or the floor of the temporal fossa. A bifrontal approach is often best to allow for adequate visualization of the floor of the anterior fossa, debridement of injured subfrontal cortex, and repair or patching of dural lacerations overlying the orbits or cribriform plate. Exenteration of involved air sinuses is often necessary.

Attempts to reconstruct the bony floor using acrylics or other foreign substances are not usually necessary and may increase the likelihood of infection. Dural repair, using a vascularized pericranial flap where appropriate for extensive dural lacerations that cannot be primarily repaired, is much more important and may prevent not only CSF rhinorrhea, but also less common delayed complications such as orbital encephaloceles. Fibrin glue may be useful in this setting to reinforce a dural repair. An ophthalmological consultation should be obtained very early on in any patient with an orbital injury. If the patient has sustained disruption of the globe with visual loss, enucleation may be a consideration within the first 10 days to prevent injury to the noninvolved eye by the rare but serious complication of sympathetic ophthalmia.

Temporal fossa wounds caused by missiles are often associated with fractures of the petrous bone that may lead to sensorineural hearing loss as well as facial nerve injury. Of more immediate significance can be the complications arising from associated vascular injuries, not only to the dural sinuses as already discussed, but also to the internal or external carotid arteries. In the latter case, where there is brisk bleeding from the ear at presentation, occlusion of the involved vessels by interventional neuroradiology techniques may be necessary after packing the external ear canal to provide temporary tamponading. If this fails, direct surgical exploration may become necessary to stop bleeding in these cases of severe vascular arterial injury. Conductive hearing loss as well as chronic infections from impacted epidermal elements in the mastoid air cells may complicate these type of injuries in addition to the more commonly and acutely noted CSF otorrhea.

Tangential missile wounds in the civilian setting can be deceptive. Debridement of these wounds is usually advised even without associated parenchymal injury. Complications arising from vertex tangential wounds can lead to a typical picture of proximal arm and distal leg paresis with cortical sensory loss. Although no specific treatment is available for this type of deficit that arises from cortical contusions of frontoparietal paramedian cortex, it is helpful to recognize this syndrome because the injury may be difficult to see on the original imaging study due to bony artifact on these high CT cuts.

The onset of DIC in patients with penetrating wounds can be rapid and is often heralded by uncontrollable oozing in the surgical field. Although it can be seen in the setting of any severe closed head injury, patients with gunshot wounds to the head are especially likely to develop this problem. This complication is characterized by consumption of clotting factors with abnormal intravascular clotting. Despite aggressive treatment with replacement of clotting factors and blood products, it continues to carry a high mortality rate.

With careful attention to operative detail as described above, many CSF leaks can be avoided. Should they still occur postoperatively in the form of rhinorrhea, otorrhea, or cutaneous fistulas, workup should include a search for readily treatable underlying causes of elevated ICP such as hydrocephalus. CSF drainage by ventriculostomy or spinal drainage as dictated by the individual case may then be necessary and adequate to treat the problem. In patients where that is not the case, other treatment measures that can be instituted range from conservative maneuvers such as elevating the head of the bed to the administration of acetazolamide to patients who will not be aversely affected by the accompanying metabolic acidosis and mild dehydration. If the leak persists, then surgical reexploration may be necessary. In select cases, extracranial approaches such as mastoidectomy may be indicated.

Infection is another postoperative complication that can often be avoided by careful attention during the original surgical debridement. If it develops, it may be in the form of meningitis, subdural empyema, or intracranial abscess. The latter two complications usually require reoperation in addition to the administration of broad-spectrum antibiotics. Bur holes placed directly over the subdural collections rather than a large craniotomy flap to drain an empyema may suffice in this age of accurate preoperative localization of any loculations by CT imaging. If a patient develops an unexplained fever about 3 to 5 weeks after a cranial missile injury, an abscess must be suspected and appropriate imaging undertaken to look for it because an untreated abscess may rupture into the ventricular system with an associated high mortality rate. Deep small abscesses may be localized with stereotactic guidance to allow for needle aspiration if there is no implicated foreign object in the abscess cavity that one feels needs to be removed as well.

Postoperative nuchal rigidity, even when associated with fever, should also raise the possibility of subarachnoid hemorrhage due to a traumatic aneurysm in addition to the above concerns about postinjury meningitis after penetrating head trauma. These aneurysms are usually peripherally located with irregular contours and absence of a well-defined neck. This latter feature often makes microsurgical excision, rather than clipping, of the aneurysm the treatment modality that one is forced to choose.

Traumatic carotid cavernous fistulas are another vascular complication seen with complicated penetrating wounds. These patients usually develop bruits, chemosis, and proptosis with or without cranial nerve palsies in the affected eye. Usually the cause is a direct injury to the intracavernous portion of the internal carotid artery, and therefore the fistula is of the high-flow type. Because spontaneous resolution of these types of fistulas is rare and because they may lead to retinal ischemia, obliteration of the fistula by interventional radiological techniques is usually indicated.

◆ Illustrative Cases

The following two cases illustrate some of the difficulties in surgical decision making and the complexities of management that one may encounter when treating the patient with a depressed skull fracture overlying the sagittal sinus (case 1) and the patient with a complex orbitofrontal civilian gunshot wound (case 2).

Case 1

A 9-year-old boy fell off a fence, striking the back of his head on a railroad tie. He presented with an obvious open

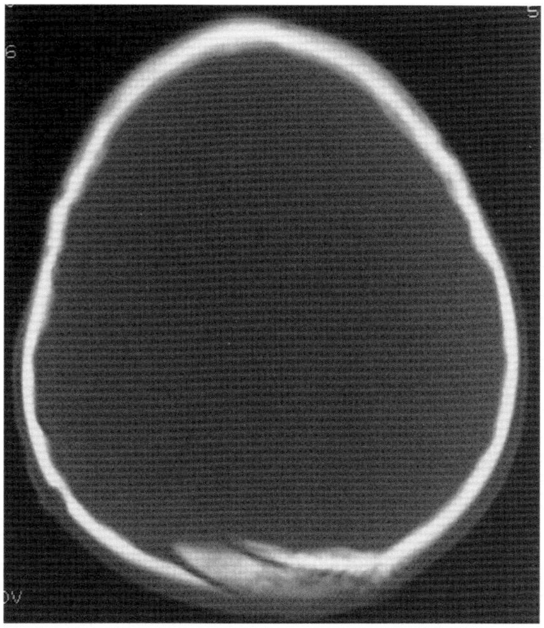

Figure 78–1 Bone setting window of computed tomographic image showing midline depressed skull fragments of occipital bone.

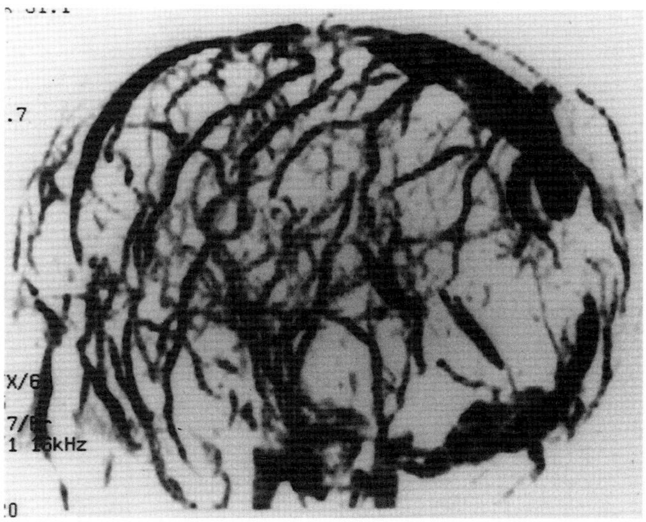

Figure 78–2 Magnetic resonance venography showing lack of flow through the superior sagittal sinus in the area of fracture.

depressed midline skull fracture overlying the posterior (occipital) aspect of the superior sagittal sinus **(Fig. 78–1)**. His GCS score was 15, and because of this good neurological grade, the relative lack of gross contamination of the wound, and the concerns about a possible underlying injury to the sagittal sinus, a decision was made to irrigate and debride the fracture in the operating room but to leave the fragments embedded in/on the sagittal sinus in place to avoid possible catastrophic bleeding from a part of the sinus that could not safely be ligated. Postoperatively, however, he began to complain of neck pain and exhibited slowly progressive signs of elevated ICP with the onset of bilateral cranial nerve VI palsies, relative bradycardia with heart rate in the 60s, and papilledema. MRV showed virtually no flow through the sagittal sinus underlying the fracture **(Fig. 78–2)**, and MRI showed an associated Chiari I malformation with areas of abnormal signal intensity in the deep mesial cerebellar hemispheres and tonsils suggestive of ischemia **(Fig. 78–3)**. He was taken back to the operating room where the remaining fracture fragments over the sinus were elevated without incident, and a suboccipital craniectomy and C1 laminectomy with

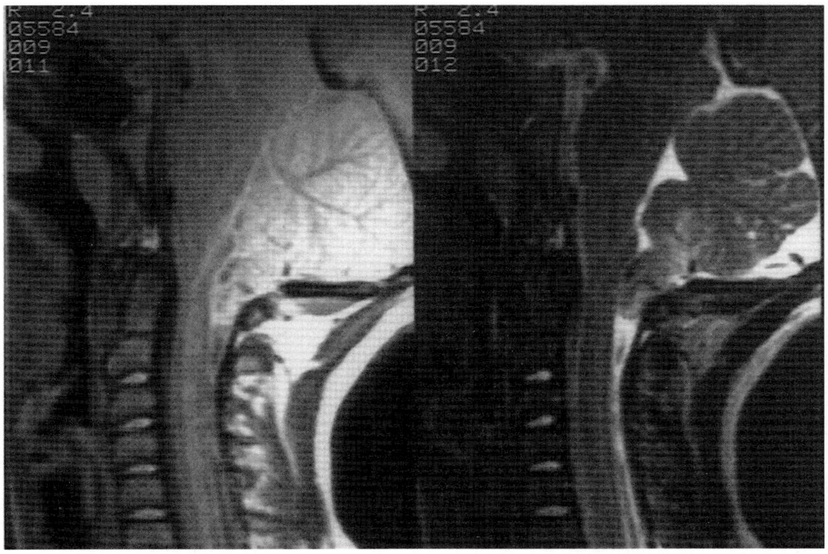

Figure 78–3 Magnetic resonance imaging showing herniated cerebellar tonsils with abnormal signal characteristics suggestive of ischemia.

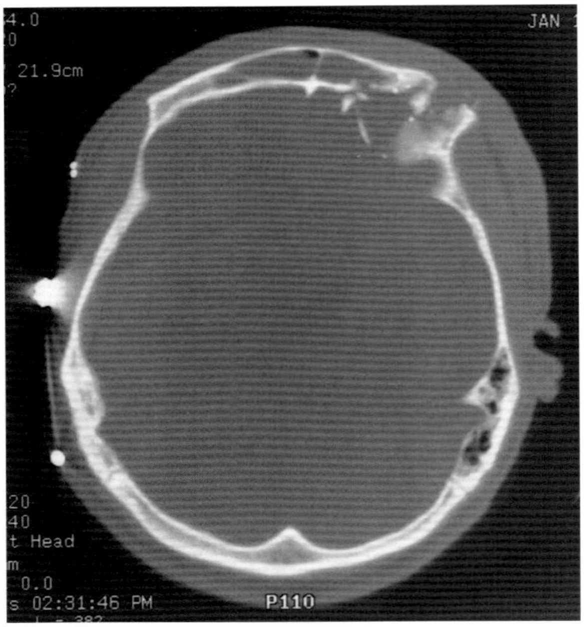

Figure 78–4 Bone setting window of computed tomography showing disruption of the left orbital roof by bullet fragments.

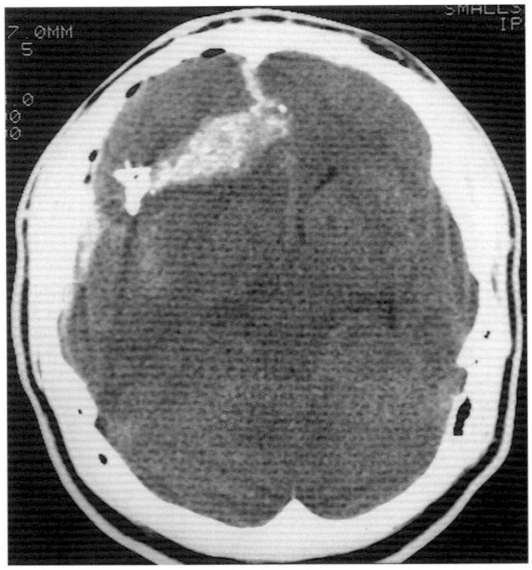

Figure 78–5 Axial computed tomographic image showing the bullet track crossing the midline into the contralateral deep frontal lobe.

dural patch graft was done to treat the Chiari malformation. Small portions of the cerebellar tonsils were found to be necrotic, suggesting that perhaps the Chiari malformation was indeed secondary to the injury rather than congenital, or at least aggravated by the fracture if it was a preexisting condition. Subsequent to this, he made a full and uneventful recovery with full resolution of all his symptoms.

Case 2

A 17-year-old boy sustained a facio-orbito-frontal gunshot wound that entered the left supraorbital region, traversed the frontal lobes as it crossed the midline anterior to the ventricles, and came to rest in the posterior right frontal lobe (**Figs. 78–4** and **78–5**). His initial GCS score was 5, with fixed and dilated pupils. He was taken to the operating room, where only a limited debridement of the facial/forehead entry wound was undertaken. An ICP monitor was also placed and his ensuing hospital course over the next week focused on the successful medical management of his severely elevated ICP. It became apparent, though, as the initial severe periorbital edema subsided that he was developing progressive proptosis of the left eye. He was found to have an orbital encephalocele with protrusion of the inferior portion of the left frontal lobe through a dural and bony defect in the orbital roof created by the pathway of the bullet (**Fig. 78–6**). Reoperation via a large bifrontal exposure was then undertaken using a team approach that included a neurosurgeon, plastic surgeon, and ophthalmologist. A ventriculostomy was placed to aid in brain relaxation. A generous left frontal bone flap incorporating the fracture fragments around the orbital rim was elevated. The fractured left frontal sinus was seen to be filled with brain tissue. Its posterior wall was removed, the mucosa was excised, and the remaining sinus cavity was drilled out and filled with pericranium and muscle. The large dural laceration extending from the orbital rim posteriorly toward the orbital apex was completely identified after gently lifting the frontal lobe. Ventricular drainage and a slightly extended positioning of the head facilitated the necessary frontal lobe retraction. The fractured fragments of the orbital roof were removed to allow debridement of the brain contents within the orbit. The periorbita was opened and there was found to be no direct injury to the globe once the compressive effects of the traumatic encephalocele were alleviated. A free pericranial graft was then used to achieve a watertight dural closure of the subfrontal dural defect using interrupted synthetic absorbable suture. A vascularized pericranial flap, which had been carefully preserved during the initial opening, was then swung posteriorly to reconstruct and reinforce the orbital roof. The orbital rim was reconstructed using split-thickness skull graft from the frontal bone craniotomy flap and titanium miniplates. The patient made a surprisingly good neurological recovery, even to the extent of returning to school. He was maintained on long-term phenytoin therapy for seizure control.

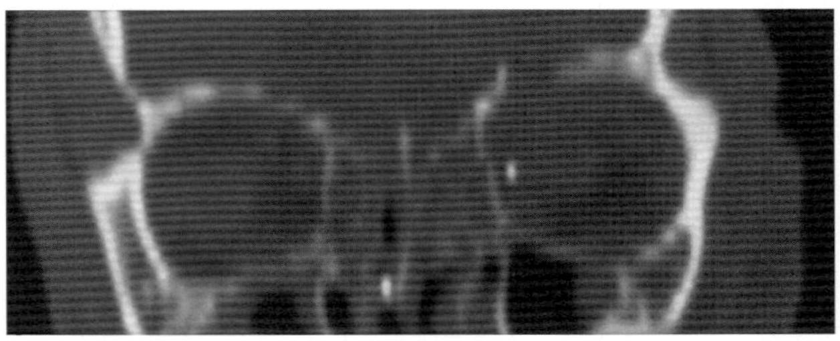

Figure 78–6 Coronal computed tomographic image on bone window setting showing a disrupted orbital roof with abnormal soft tissue density in the orbit displacing the globe laterally.

◆ Conclusion

The management of cranial missile wounds and skull fractures encompasses several diagnostic skills and acumen, the need for thoughtful decision making, and attention to operative detail to help prevent many postoperative dilemmas. Although none of the surgical techniques described in this section of the book are particularly unique to the treatment of these types of injuries, failure to attend to these wounds properly, diligently, thoroughly, and carefully the first time can lead to several potentially preventable problems and prolonged complications.

References

1. Jennett B, Miller JD, Braakman R. Epilepsy after non-missile depressed skull fracture. J Neurosurg 1974;41:208–216
2. Jackler RK. Facial auditory, and vestibular nerve injuries associated with basilar skull fractures. In: Youmans JR, ed. Neurological Surgery, 3rd ed. Philadelphia: WB Saunders; 1990:2305–2316
3. Brandvold B, Levi L, Feinsod M, et al. Penetrating craniocerebral injuries in the Israeli involvement in the Lebanese conflict, 1982–1985: analysis of a less aggressive surgical approach. J Neurosurg 1990;72: 15–21
4. Clark WC, Muhlbauer MS, Watridge CB, et al. Analysis of 76 civilian craniocerebral gunshot wounds. J Neurosurg 1986;65:9–14
5. Bullock R, Chesnut RM, Clifton GC, et al. The use of hyperventilation in the acute management. In: Guidelines for the Management of Severe Head Injury, Section 9. Brain Trauma Foundation; 1995
6. Bullock R, Chesnut RM, Clifton GC, et al. The use of mannitol in severe head injury. In: Guidelines for the Management of Severe Head Injury, Section 10. Brain Trauma Foundation; 1995
7. Miller JD, Jennett WB. Complications of depressed skull fractures. Lancet 1968;2:991–995
8. Becker DP, Gade GF, Young HF, Feuerman TF. Diagnosis and treatment of head injury in adults. In: Youmans JR, ed. Neurological Surgery. 3rd ed. Philadelphia: WB Saunders; 1990:2104–2105
9. Carey M, Young H, Mathis J, Forsythe J. A bacteriological study of craniocerebral missile wounds from Vietnam. J Neurosurg 1971;34:145–154
10. Bierbrauer KS, Tindall SC. Gunshot wounds to the head and spine. Contemp Neurosurg 1987;9:1–5
11. Temkin NR, Dikmen SS, Wilensky AJ, et al. A randomized, double-blind study of phenytoin for the prevention of post-traumatic seizures. N Engl J Med 1990;323:497–502
12. Cooper PR. Depressed skull fracture. In: Apuzzo ML, ed. Brain Surgery: Complication Avoidance and Management. New York: Churchill Livingstone; 1993:1274
13. Kushner J, Alexander E Jr, Davis CH Jr, et al. Kyphoscoliosis following lumbar subarachnoid shunts. J Neurosurg 1971;34:783–791

79

Venous Sinus Repair during the Treatment of Meningiomas

Marc Sindou

The propensity of meningiomas to recur after surgery is linked to the degree of radicality in surgical resection. Total removal of the tumor is more likely to achieve a cure than subtotal removal, regardless of the histological type. Therefore, complete surgical resection is the optimal treatment.

In meningiomas involving the major dural venous sinuses (superior sagittal sinus, transverse sinus, torcular), the treatment is problematic. If total removal is accomplished in these types of meningiomas, and venous sinuses and afferent veins cannot be spared, catastrophic complications may occur.

That is why two main approaches have traditionally been advocated when dealing with these meningiomas. Some authors consider invasion of the sinuses as a deterrent to complete removal; in their opinion the sinuses are to be respected in spite of a higher risk of recurrence. Other authors have adopted a more aggressive approach advocating total removal and venous reconstruction to restore the venous drainage. This chapter endorses the latter view.

◆ Indications

Meningiomas invading the major dural sinuses, especially the ones involving the superior sagittal sinus, can be classified into six types (grades), according to degree of sinus invasion **(Fig. 79–1)**.

An attempt at a total removal is the best warranty of a low rate of recurrences. By following this policy, the recurrence rate in our series was only 2.5% (two cases out of 80 meningiomas involving major sinuses; average follow-up of 8 years).

The possibility or impossibility of resecting the eventual intrasinus fragment can only be ascertained by an exploration of the sinus and its lumen. According to our experience of 80 meningiomas invading the major dural sinuses, we think that venous reconstruction should be performed whenever possible, even if the sinus is occluded by the tumor. In a significant number of cases, the occluded portion of the sinus cannot be resected safely because of the frequent necessity to sacrifice the collateral venous pathways encountered on the surgical approach, as illustrated in **Fig. 79–2.** In our series, the three patients who died after surgery had a complete occlusion of the sinus prior to operation and did not benefit from sinus reconstruction. Patches can be performed using locally harvested dura mater or fascia.

Bypasses must consist of autologous vein (saphenous when a long graft is needed, external jugular vein when only a short graft is necessary) and not of prosthesis. In our series the six patients who had a Gore-Tex bypass thrombosed within the first week.

Immediate patency essentially depends on the driving pressure within the dural venous system. This was apparent in our observations. The absence of long-term patency does not necessarily mean that venous reconstruction was not useful. Progressive occlusion of the venous repair would have given time for compensatory venous pathways to develop. In our series, only the sudden occlusion of a bypass performed with Gore-Tex prosthesis was followed by a neurological aggravation. It was due to acute intracranial pressure, which, although severe, was totally reversible after 2 months of intensive care therapy.

According to our experience (Sindou and Malloy, 1995 and 1998) we recommend the following procedures according to the type of meningioma:

- Type I: excision of outer layer, leaving a clean and glistening dural surface, and coagulation of dural attachment
- Type II: removal of intraluminal fragment through the recess, then repair of the dural defect by resuturing the access or by closing it with a patch, or, provided it is not stenosing, sealing of the opening with aneurysm clip **(Fig. 79–3)**
- Type III: resection of sinus wall and repair with a patch **(Figs. 79–4** and **79–5)**
- Type IV: resection of both invaded walls and reconstruction of the two resected walls by a patch

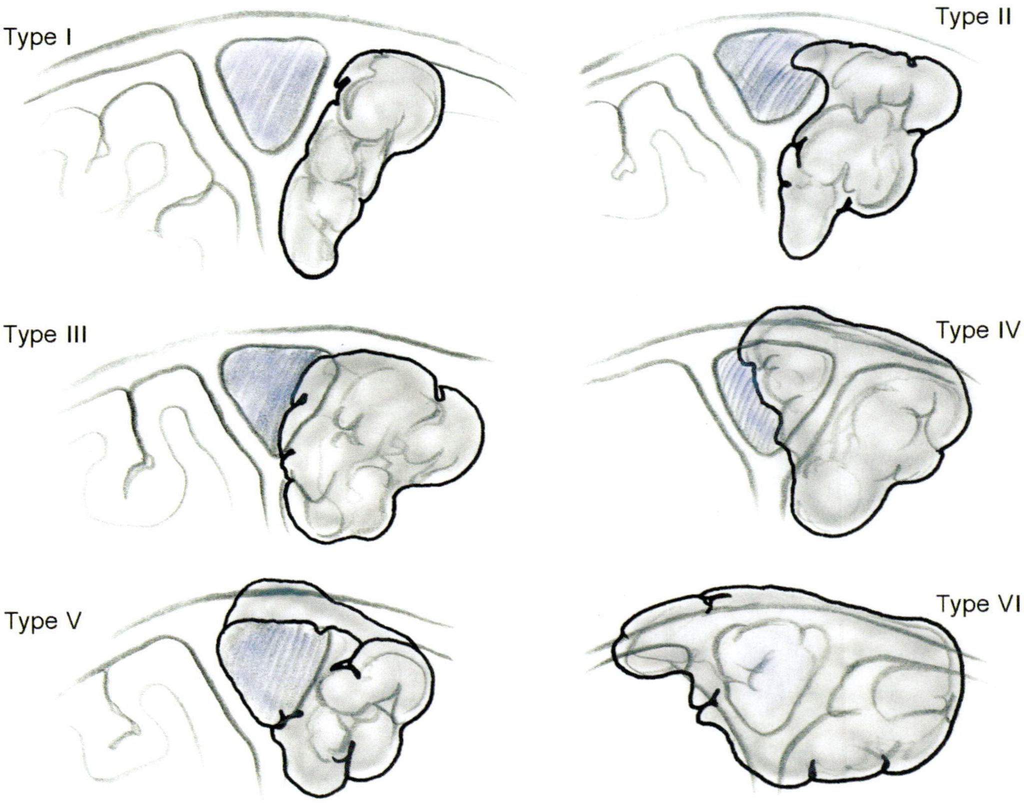

Figure 79–1 Classification of meningiomas according to the degree of dural venous sinus involvement. Type I: meningioma attached to outer surface of the sinus wall. Type II: lateral recess invaded. Type III: lateral wall invaded. Type IV: entire lateral wall and roof of the sinus both invaded. Types V and VI: sinus totally occluded, one wall being free of tumor in type V. This classification is a simplified one from Krause and Merrem, and Bonnal and Brotchi.

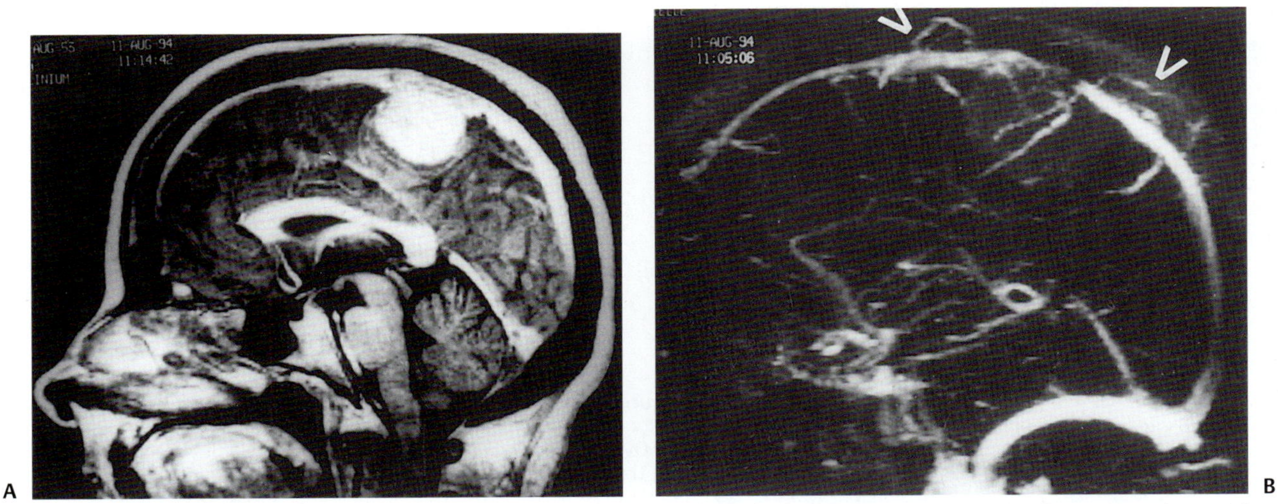

Figure 79–2 Parasagittal Type III meningioma; middle third of superior sagittal sinus. **(A)** Preoperative sagittal magnetic resonance (MR) imaging; T1 sequence after gadolinium. **(B)** Preoperative venous MR, showing subtotal occlusion of the sinus lumen and compensatory drainages through intraosseous emissary veins that communicate with extracranial circulation (white open arrowheads). Exposure can destroy these collateral drainages and lead to brain swelling.

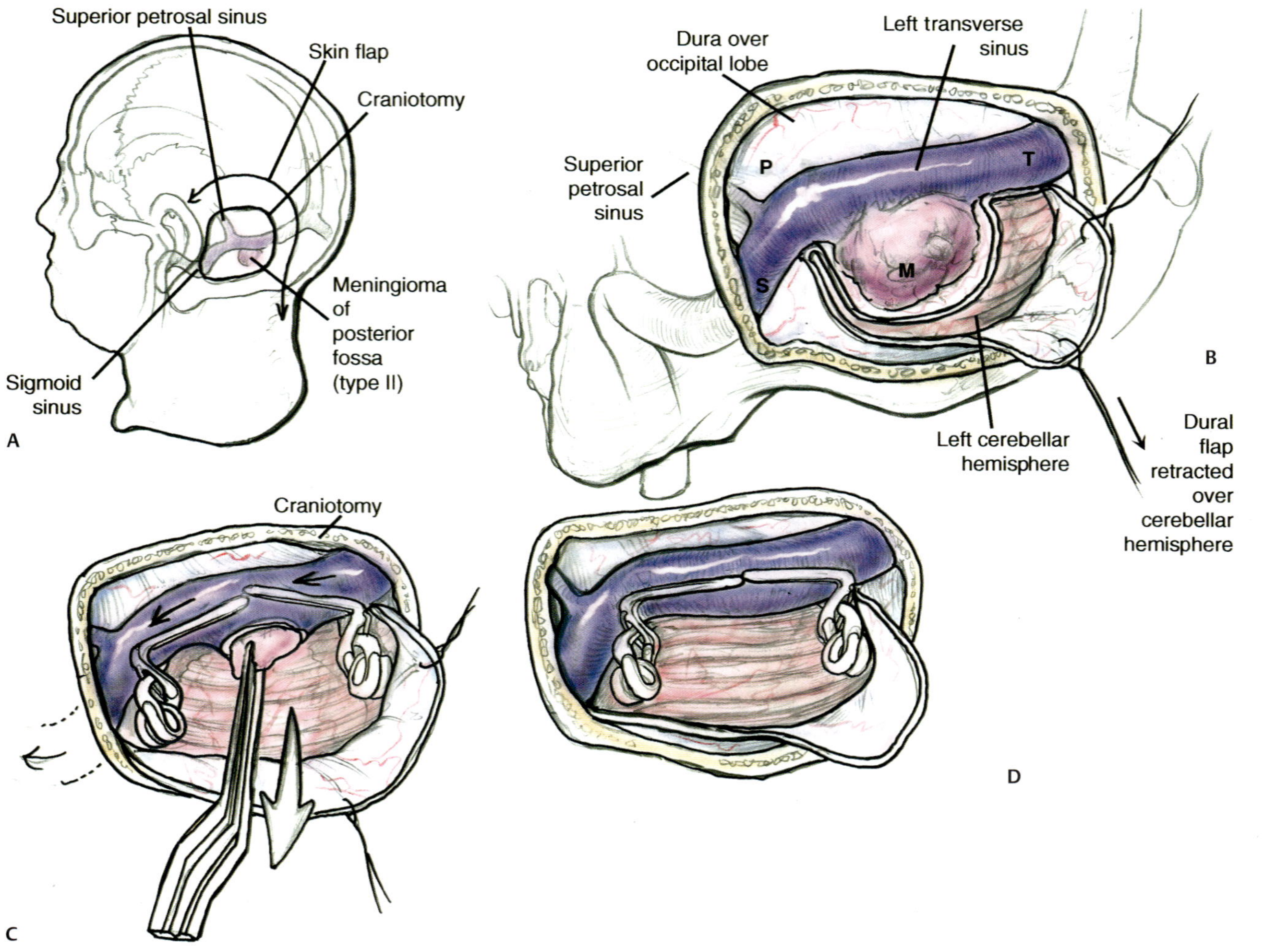

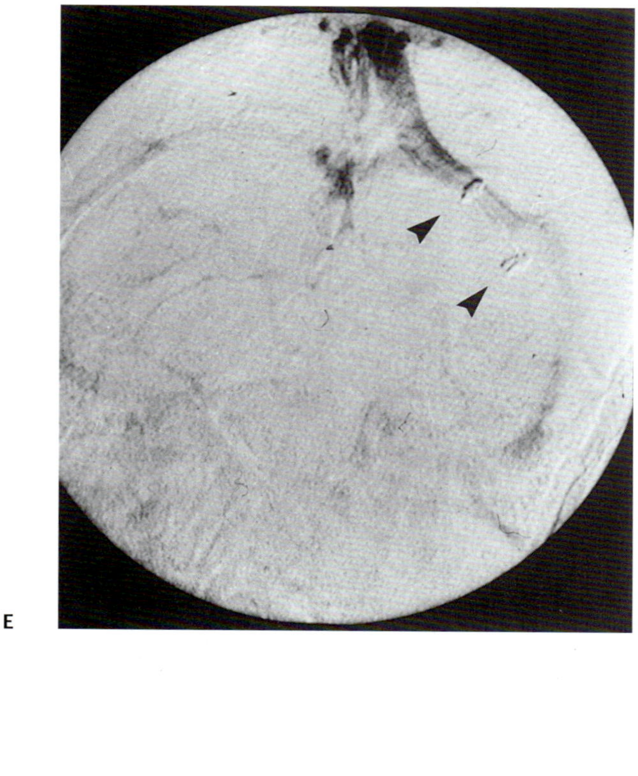

Figure 79–3 Meningioma of posterior fossa convexity, invading the posterior-inferior recess (type II) of left transverse sinus (which is dominant). **(A)** Overview of the surgical steps. **(B)** First step. M, meningioma type II; T, left transverse sinus (dominant); S, sigmoid portion of left lateral sinus; P, superior petrosal sinus. **(C)** Second step. Temporary clamping of transverse sinus to remove intrasinus portion of the meningioma. **(D)** Third step. Closure of the transverse sinus wound after resection of intrasinus fragment, using two angled clips (Sugita type), with lumen patent. **(E)** Venous phase of postoperative digital subtraction angiography, anteroposterior view, showing that the left transverse (unique) sinus is patent after tumor resection and posteroinferior recess repair (two clips designated by arrowheads).

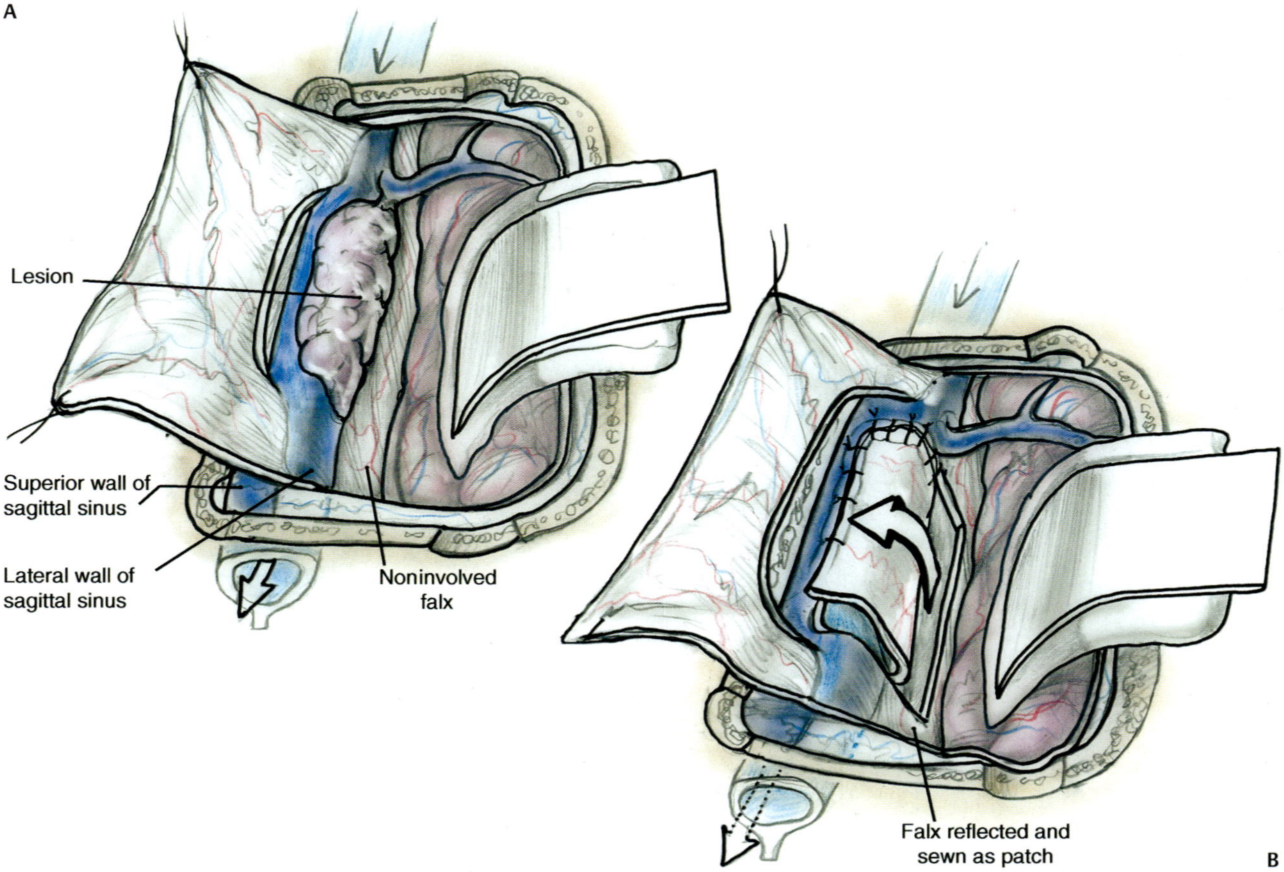

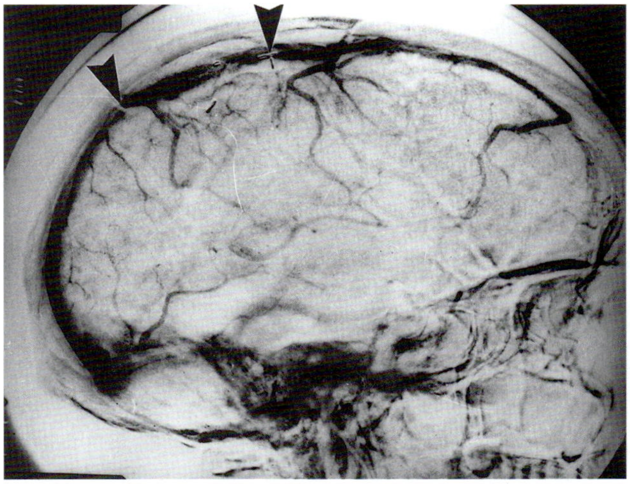

Figure 79–4 Type III parasagittal meningioma; middle third portion of superior sagittal sinus (SSS). **(A)** Before and **(B)** after removal of the extra- and intrasinus portions of the meningioma. The wall is repaired with patching by simple reflection of the falx (which was not invaded in this case). **(C)** Venous phase of postoperative digital subtraction angiography (lateral view) performed on the 21st postoperative day. The patched portion of the sinus (between arrowheads) is patent.

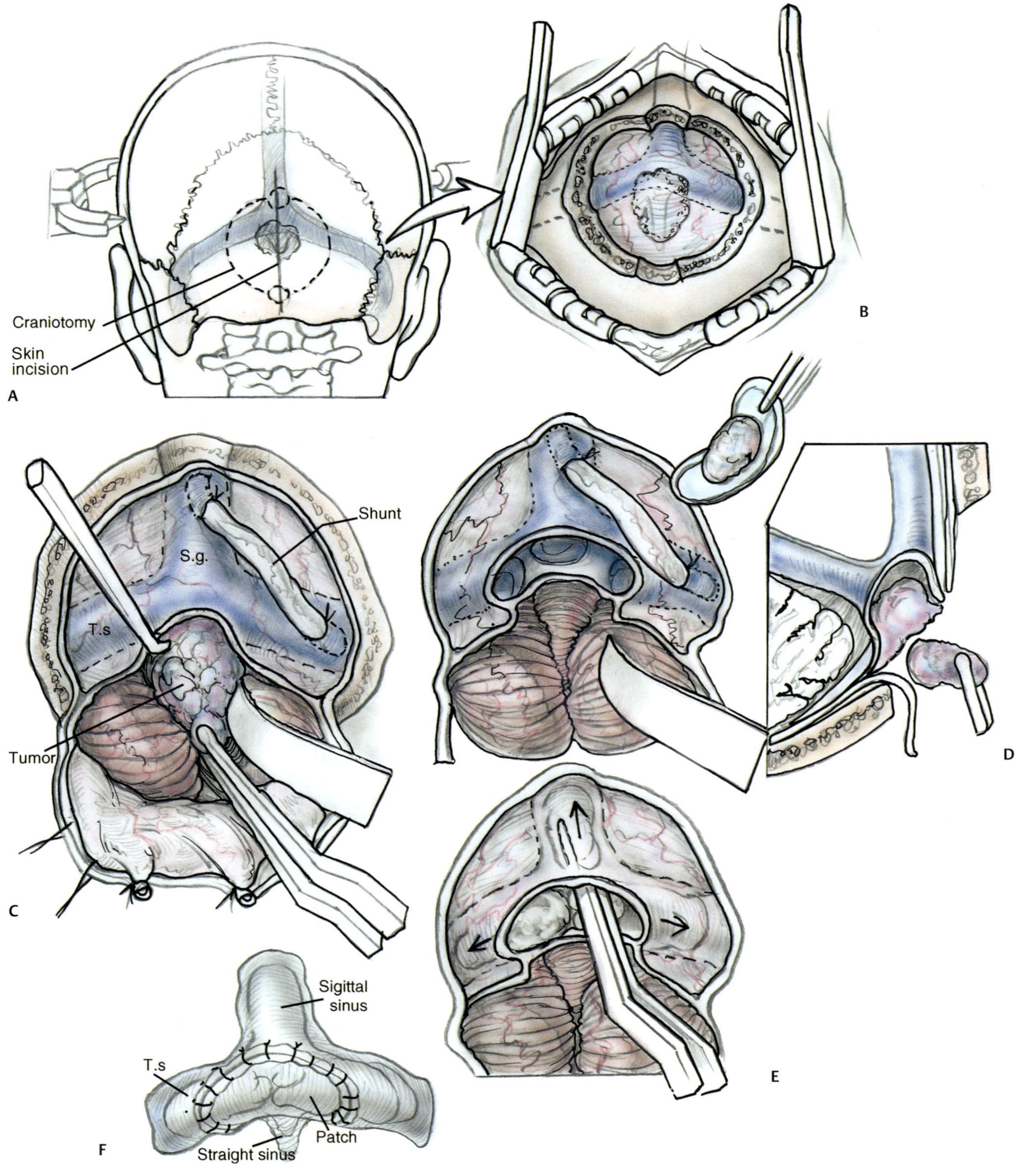

Figure 79–5 Type III torcular meningioma: surgical steps. **(A)** Landmarks. **(B)** Exposure through occipital craniotomy. **(C)** Suboccipital intradural infratentorial approach; resection of the tumor outside the torcular[DK7]; temporary shunting (silicone tube) between sagittal sinus and right transverse sinus. **(D)** Resection of (invaded) inferior wall of the torcular and removal of the intraluminal fragment of the tumor; straight sinus visible. **(E)** Packing of Surgicel pledgets inside the lumen for bleeding control of sagittal, both transverse and straight, sinuses. **(F)** Repair of the inferior wall of the torcular meningioma with a patch. Surgicel pledgets were removed before the last suture. Then the temporary shunt was withdrawn and two sinusotomies, which served for shunt insertion, were closed.

- Type V: the opposite wall to the tumor side is free of tumor. Thus we think that it is preferable to reconstruct with a patch the two invaded walls after their resection (**Figs. 79–6** and **79–7**), rather than to perform a bypass. This type can be distinguished from type VI only by direct surgical exploration of the sinus lumen.
- Type VI: removal of involved portion of sinus and restoration by venous bypass. The site of the bypass is on the sagittal sinus for meningiomas involving the sagittal sinus (SS) (**Fig. 79–8**) between the SS and the external jugular vein for meningiomas totally occluding the posterior third and the torcular (**Fig. 79–9**), between the transverse sinus (TS) and the external jugular vein for meningiomas involving the TS.

Preoperative Studies

Computed tomography (CT) and magnetic resonance imaging (MRI) with and without contrast medium provide the key to diagnosis. MRI (T1-weighted sequences with and without gadolinium injection, and T2 sequences) is more effective in delineating the tumor and differentiating it from surrounding structures; in particular, it can determine the feasibility of dissection. Gadolinium enhancement of the invaded dura allows the site of exposure to be predicted. However, it must be kept in mind that enhancement of the dura adjacent to the main tumor mass may indicate actual tumor invasion or may simply indicate hyperemia. Venous MR offers additional useful information on venous system involvement. But MR angiography does not succeed in providing a reliable exploration of the tumor vascularization and heonodynamics. Therefore, angiography through the transfemoral arterial route is still of value prior to establishing the detailed surgical strategy.

Selective bilateral internal and external carotid substraction angiography as well as vertebral angiography (of the arterial phase) serve to determine the dural and cortical-pial supply ipsilateral or contralateral to the tumor. The arterial phase is useful to predict the difficulty of dissection of the capsule from the cortex when there is a pial vascular supply. When meningeal supply is important, preoperative embolization may be of some value in producing tumor necrosis and reducing the operative risks to the patient by diminishing the blood loss that accompanies resection of these tumors.

The late venous phases with bilateral filling of the sagittal sinus are required for the exact evaluation of sinus patency and collateral venous pathways. Oblique views can depict the superior sagittal sinus (SSS) throughout its entire course. Various degrees of sinus occlusion can be observed, from simple compression with narrowing of the sinus lumen to intraluminal defect to total occlusion. Complete occlusion may be assumed from nonvisualization of segments of the sinus and from collateral venous channel development. The pattern of venous drainage and venous collateral channels must be established preoperatively to determine the surgical approach

Surgical Techniques

Positioning

Placing the patient in the semisitting (lounging) position allows a good venous return without increased intracranial pressure. Air embolism, although possible, is not a frequent risk because of the relatively high level of the intracranial venous pressure in these patients. The problem can be avoided or safely controlled in experienced surgical hands.

Exposure and Initial Steps

1. The operative exposure should be as extensive as possible. The skin flap and craniotomy should extend across the midline to permit visualization of both sides of the sinus and about 3 cm outside the margins of the occluded sinus. However, such a large access should be reconsidered if there are scalp, pericranial, or diploic collateral venous pathways, which may be impaired during the approach.
2. Afferent tumor arteries within the dura should be coagulated or clipped before being cut.
3. The dura is incised in a circumferential manner around the margin of the tumor insertion on the dura of the convexity and along the border of the corresponding portion of the superior sagittal sinus.
4. The microscope is installed.
5. The attachment of the meningioma to the lateral wall of the sinus and to the neighboring falx is disinserted from the structures by using the cutting effect of the bipolar coagulation forceps. This deprives the tumor of its dural-meningeal arterial feeders.
6. Then intracapsular debulking is performed so that the meningioma can be dissected from the underlying cortex. Under the microscope an extraarachnoidal plane of dissection must be carefully searched. If it is absent, the plane of dissection becomes subpial because of pia mater incorporation to the tumor capsula (Sindou and Allayson, 1998).

Sinus Surgery Procedure

- Because there are frequent discrepancies between images and anatomical findings, the sinus should be explored through a short incision to disclose any intrasinus fragment.
- Temporary control of venous bleeding from the sinus and afferent veins is easily obtained by packing small pledgets of hemostatic material (Surgicel, Johnson & Johnson Medical, Viroflay, France) in the lumen and at the ostia of afferent veins. Balloons should not be used because they do not pass easily through the sinus septa and may injure the sinus endothelium. Vascular clamps and aneurysm clips should be avoided as much as possible because they may injure the sinus walls and afferent veins.

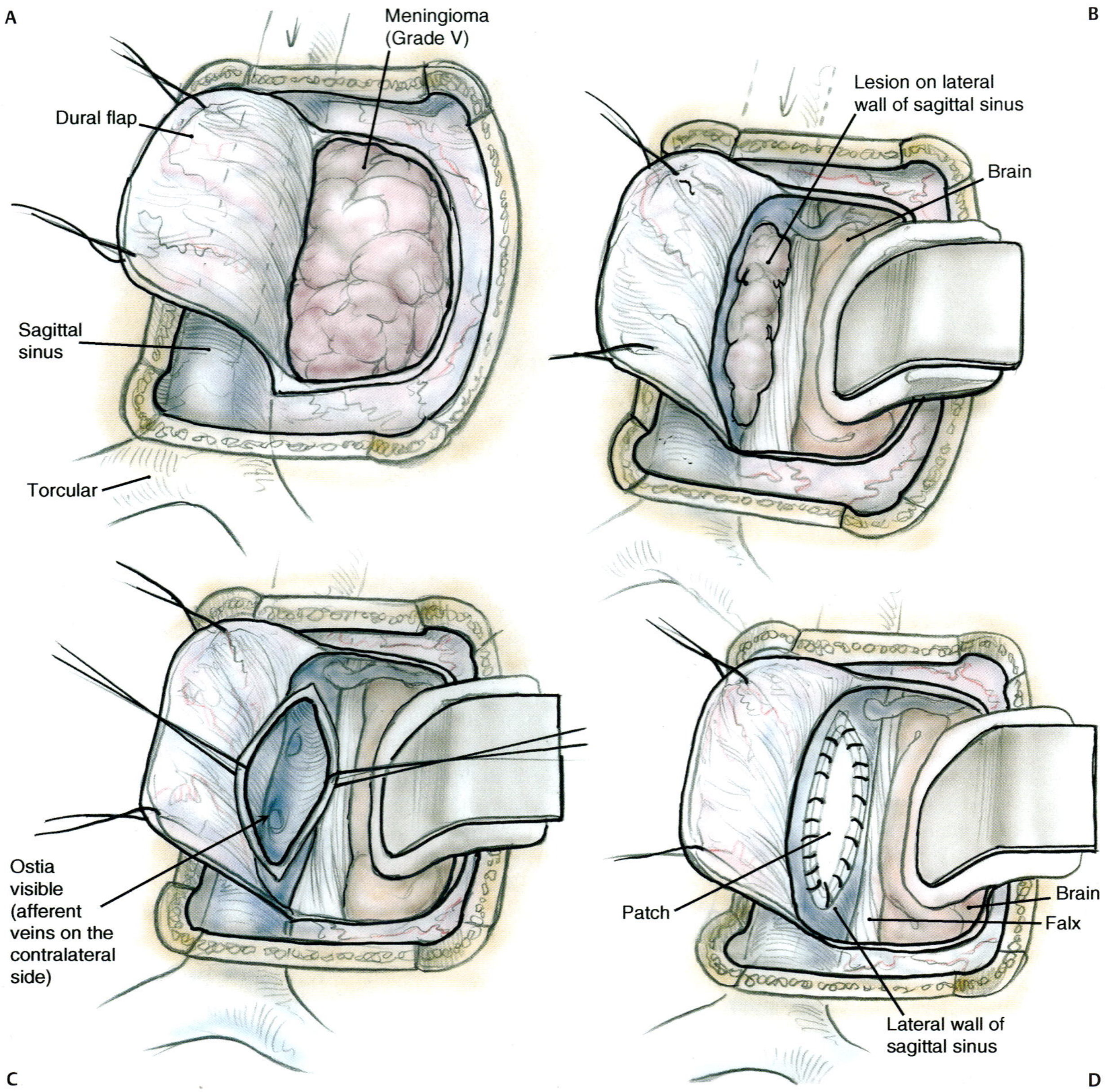

E

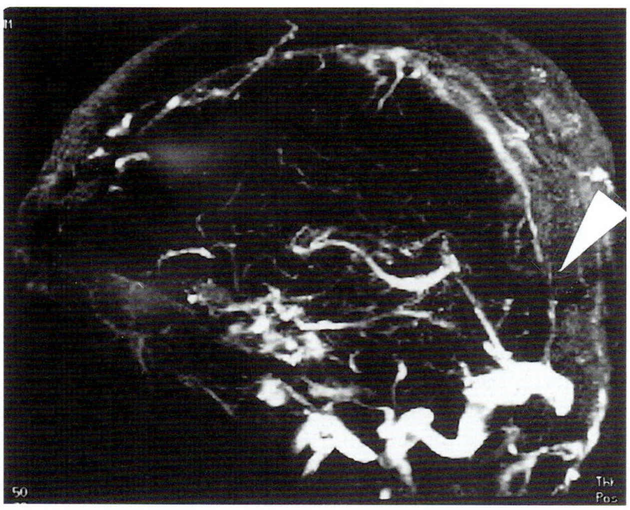

Figure 79–6 Right (Type V) parasagittal meningioma of posterior third: surgical steps. **(A)** First step. Exposure of the meningioma. **(B)** Second step. After removal of the tumor outside the superior sagittal sinus (SSS), one can see that the right wall is invaded. **(C)** Third step. After removal of the intraluminal fragment, the ostia of two afferent veins entering the SSS through the left wall are visible. **(D)** Fourth step. Repair of the resected right wall by means of a patch made of fascia lata and sutured with two running hemisutures. **(E)** Fifth step. Postoperative control by venous magnetic resonance (MR). Venous MR (sagittal view) performed after 2 months of follow-up shows patency of the unobstructed and repaired SSS (posterior third) (white arrowhead).

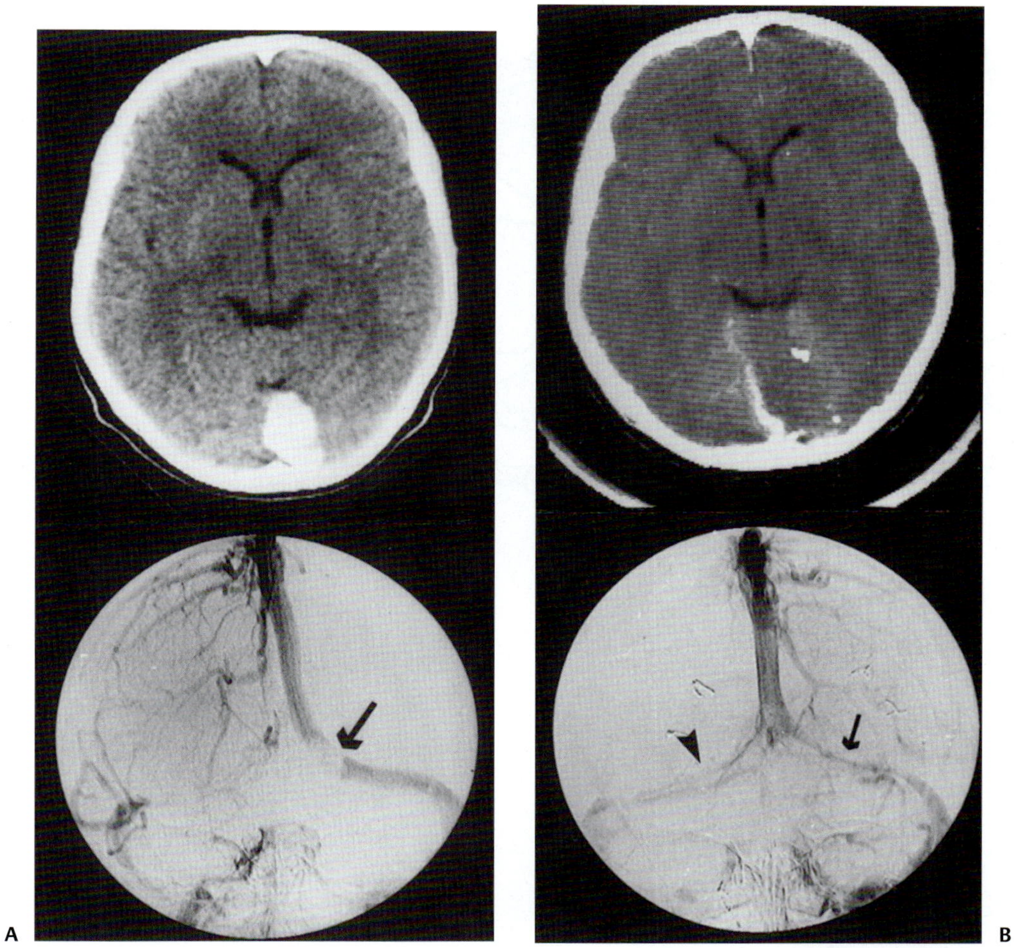

Figure 79–7 Type V torcular meningioma. **(A)** Preoperative axial computed tomograhy (CT) with contrast medium (upper view) and anteroposterior view of venous phase of digital subtraction angiography (DSA) showing the torcular meningioma occluding totally the right transverse sinus and subtotally the left one (arrow) (lower view). **(B)** Postoperative axial CT showing complete removal of the tumor (upper view) and postoperative DSA (after 2 weeks) demonstrating patency of both right (arrowhead) and left (arrow) transverse sinuses (lower view).

- Bridging veins, especially in the rolandic outflow area, should be preserved by dissecting them free from adjacent brain and tumor.
- Venous reconstruction is performed using patches or bypasses, with two hemirunning sutures (Prolene 8.0, Laboratoire ETHNOR, Neuilly/Seine, France). Although the autologous vein would appear as the most suitable material for use as a patch, vein harvesting seems excessive for patching only. The locally situated dura mater, fascia temporalis, and pericranium have a structure rigid enough for blood to flow inside and for use as patche Fascis temporalis seems to be the best material for patching. When a bypass is performed, the graft should not be compressed by increased intracerebral pressure, which reduces flow even further.

Postoperative Care

To facilitate bypass patency after surgery, blood pressure, volume, and viscosity must be carefully monitored. Heparin therapy (two times control valve) is recommended for at least 21 days to avoid clotting the reconstructed sinus and three months' aspirin to allow endothelialization of the sinus walls.

◆ Conclusion

Our surgical experience with meningiomas invading major dural sinuses (80 cases out of a total series of 425 intracranial meningiomas of all sites) leads us to advocate, whenever possible, total removal of the tumor, which results in a low recurrence rate of 2.5% over the last 15 years.

The only way to be certain of the absence of wall invasion or intraluminal tumor fragment is to explore the wall(s) and open the lumen, respectively; this necessitates reconstructing the sinus.

Venous circulation restoration should be performed whenever possible, even if the sinus was occluded preoperatively. Contrary to established opinion, the portion of the venous sinus completely occluded by the tumor cannot be resected safely in most cases because of impairment of collateral venous pathways during surgical approach.

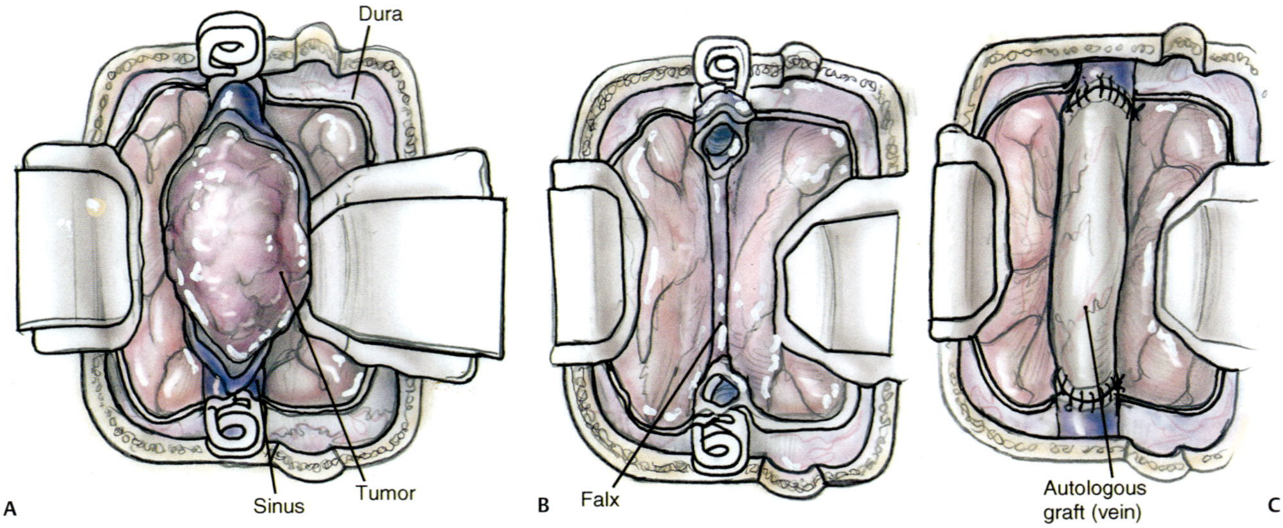

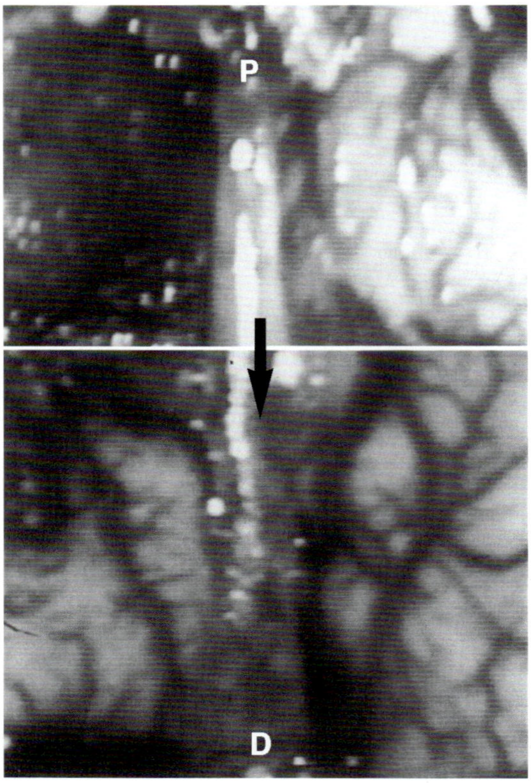

Figure 79–8 Type VI parasagittal meningioma totally invading and occluding the anterior half of the posterior third of superior sagittal sinus. **(A)** Drawing of the tumor. **(B)** Total removal of the meningioma together with the totally invaded portion of the sinus and proximal and distal temporary clamping of the sinus with aneurysm clips (of Sugita type). **(C)** Venous circulation restored with a venous autologous graft harvested from the (external) jugular vein and mounted as a bypass of end to end type at both anastomoses. **(D)** Operative microsurgical view (taken from the intraoperative videotape), after completion of the venous bypass. Proximal (P) and distal (D) end to end anastomoses. Bypass is patent and circulating (arrow flow).

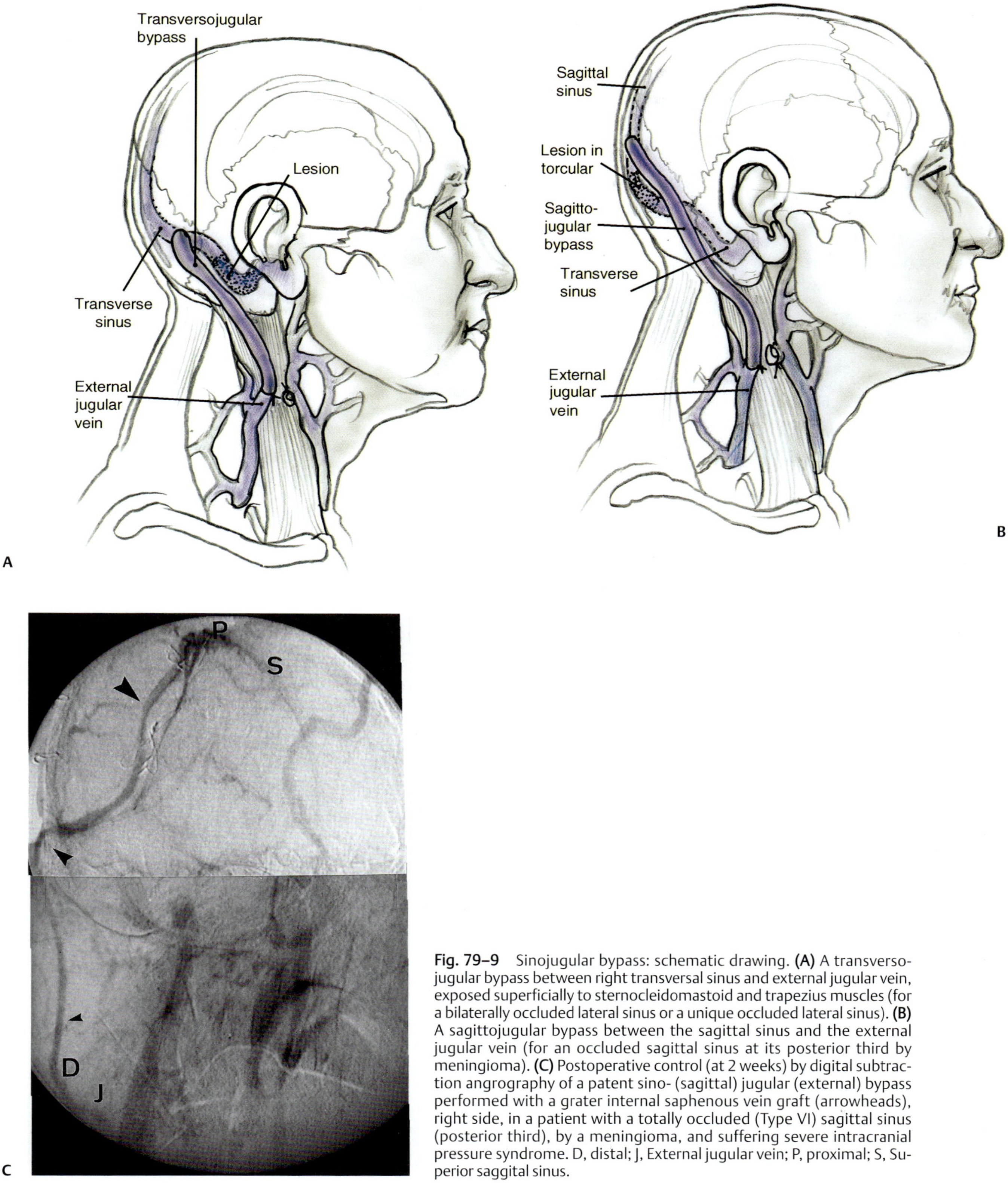

Fig. 79–9 Sinojugular bypass: schematic drawing. **(A)** A transversojugular bypass between right transversal sinus and external jugular vein, exposed superficially to sternocleidomastoid and trapezius muscles (for a bilaterally occluded lateral sinus or a unique occluded lateral sinus). **(B)** A sagittojugular bypass between the sagittal sinus and the external jugular vein (for an occluded sagittal sinus at its posterior third by meningioma). **(C)** Postoperative control (at 2 weeks) by digital subtraction angrography of a patent sino- (sagittal) jugular (external) bypass performed with a grater internal saphenous vein graft (arrowheads), right side, in a patient with a totally occluded (Type VI) sagittal sinus (posterior third), by a meningioma, and suffering severe intracranial pressure syndrome. D, distal; J, External jugular vein; P, proximal; S, Superior saggital sinus.

Patches can be done using dura mater or fascia, and locally harvested. Bypasses must consist of autologous vein (the saphenous or external jugular vein, depending on the desired length). Gore-Tex always causes thrombosis.

Even with autologous material, occlusion of the bypass may occur more or less rapidly (fortunately, most often without apparent clinical deficit). Early thrombosis of graft reconstruction is ascribed to the unique flow characteristics of the system: the driving pressure within the dural venous system is low, the more so as collateral flow has developed.

The absence of patency does not necessarily mean that venous reconstruction was not useful. Progressive occlusion of the venous repair would have given time for compensatory venous pathways to develop. In any case, strategy decisions should be reevaluated during the surgical procedure; one should be ready to stop the operation at any time and to complete it later, especially if brain swelling occurs.

Suggested Readings

Bonnal J. La chirurgie conservatrice et réparatrice du sinus longitudinal supérieur. Neurochirurgie 1982;28:147–172

Bonnal J, Brotchi J. Surgery of the superior sagittal sinus in parasagittal meningiomas. J Neurosurg 1978;48:935–945

Hakuba A. Reconstruction of dural sinus involved in meningioma. In: Al Mefty O, ed. Meningiomas. New York: Raven; 1991:371–382

Hakuba A. Surgery of the Intracranial Venous System. Tokyo: Springer-Verlag; 1996

Hakuba A, Huh Cw, Tsujikawa S, Nishimura S. Total removal of a parasagittal meningioma of the posterior third of the sagittal sinus and its repair by autologous vein graft: case report. J Neurosurg 1979;51:379–382

Merrem G. Die parasagittalen meningeome. Fedor KRAUSE-Gedächtnivorlesung. Acta Neurochir (Wien) 1970;23:203–216

Sindou M, Alaywan M. Most intracranial meningiomas are not cleavable tumors: anatomic-surgical evidence and angiographic predictability. Neurosurgery 1998;42:476–480

Sindou M, Hallacq P. Microsurgery of the venous system in meningiomas invading the major dural sinuses. In: Hakuba A, ed. Surgery of the Intracranial Venous System. Tokyo: Springer-Verlag; 1996:226–236

Sindou M, Hallacq P. Venous reconstruction in surgery of meningiomas invading the sagittal and transverse sinuses. Skull Base Surg 1998;8:57–64

Sindou M, Mazoyer Jf, Fischer G, Pialat J, Fourcade C. Experimental bypass for sagittal sinus repair: preliminary report. J Neurosurg 1976;44:325–330

Sindou M, Mercier P, Bokor J, Brunon J. Bilateral thrombosis of the transverse sinuses: microsurgical revascularization with venous bypass. Surg Neurol 1980;13:215–220

Steiger HJ, Reulin HJ, Huber P, Boll J. Radical resection of superior sagittal sinus meningioma with venous interposition graft and reimplantation of the rolandic veins. Acta Neurochir (Wien) 1989;100:108–111

80

Surgical Management of Cerebrospinal Fluid Leaks

Bizhan Aarabi, Bert W. O'Malley, Jonathan E. Martin, and Howard M. Eisenberg

◆ Historical Background and Overview

The first clinical description of cerebrospinal fluid (CSF) leakage was by Bidloo in the 17th century.[1] In 1884 Chiari[2] documented a pathoanatomical communication between ethmoid sinuses and a pneumatocele in the left frontal lobe in a patient with CSF rhinorrhea. In penetrating brain injury, Cushing suspected ventricular involvement when the clinical course was complicated by CSF leakage. Dandy[3,4] visualized and repaired a dural tear at the base of skull with tensor fascia lata. Cairns[5] in 1937 classified CSF rhinorrhea into acute, delayed, traumatic, operative, and spontaneous. CSF leaks were considered significant harbingers of mortality and morbidity in all the recent military conflicts since the Vietnam War. In a regression model CSF leak was an independent variable contributing to deep central nervous system (CNS) infections in military missile head wounds.[6]

Head trauma is the major cause of mortality and morbidity between the ages of 1 and 44. Each year close to 50,000 Americans die from traumatic brain injury. Approximately 10 to 20% of patients with closed head injury (CHI) have basal skull fracture and 1 to 3% of all head injuries have CSF leakage.[7,8] CSF leakage is more frequent in penetrating brain trauma.[6] Between 20 and 50% of patients with CSF fistulas eventually have infection of the CNS, often with undesirable consequences if treated conservatively.[1,9,10] Over 80% of CSF leaks are cranionasal and 20% cranioaural.[11,12] Discontinuous skull fractures are characteristic of penetrating brain trauma and predispose to significant intracranial infections.[6]

◆ Pathophysiology

The cribriform plate, paranasal air sinuses, and tegmen in closed head trauma and the scalp in penetrating brain trauma are the sites most frequently encountered in CSF leaks[8,13] (**Fig. 80–1**). Although the majority of the CNS infections that are due to CSF leaks in CHI are caused by pneumococci, deep infections following leaks from penetrating head injury are due to highly virulent gram-negative bacteria.[6] One does not have to have a CSF leak to develop meningitis after a skull-base fracture, and trauma could be quite minor.[3,4,9,11,14,15] Once leakage stops spontaneously, there could be resumption of CSF flow at any time.[15]

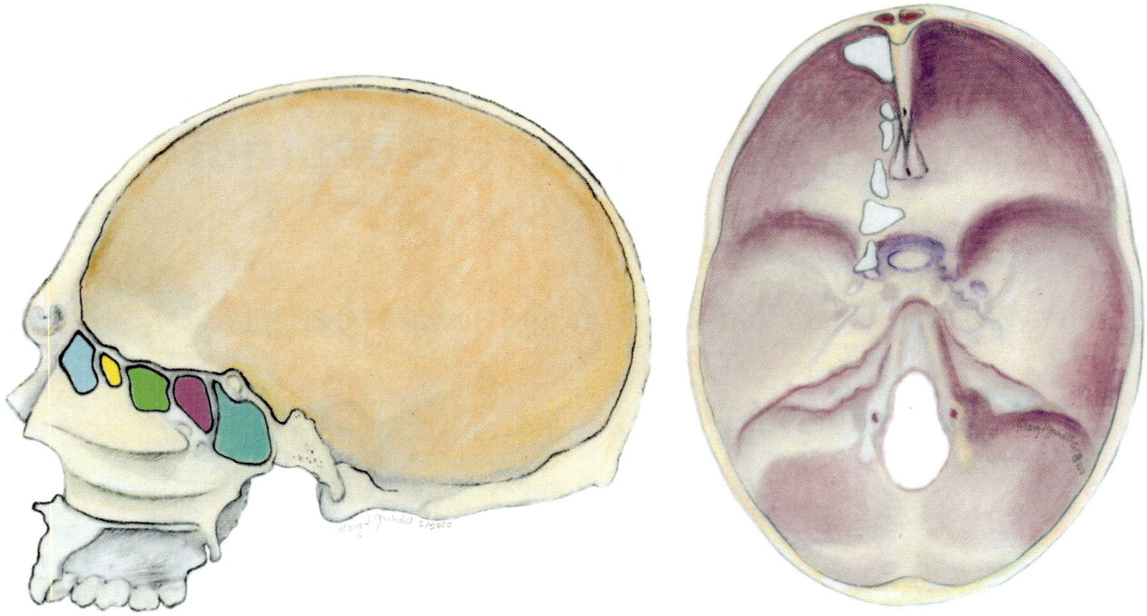

A B

Figure 80–1 **(A)** Lateral and **(B)** basal views of skull showing the paranasal air sinuses.

◆ Diagnostic Studies

Besides plain x-rays and computed tomography (CT) **(Fig. 80–2)**, intrathecal radioimmunosorbent assay (RISA),[16,17] fluorescein, and contrast material can help localize the exact site of leakage prior to surgery or intraoperatively **(Fig. 80–3)**. Metrizamide cisternography as reported first by Drayer and Manelfe in 1977 and magnetic resonance imaging (MRI) of the brain could precisely visualize the site of the dural tear and traumatic meningocele **(Fig. 80–4)**.[18–28]

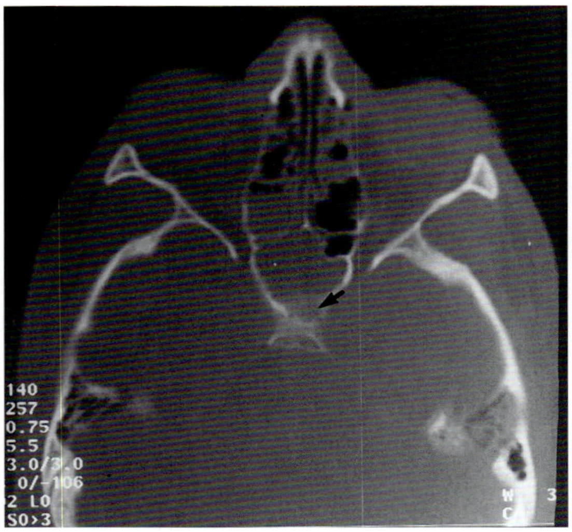

A

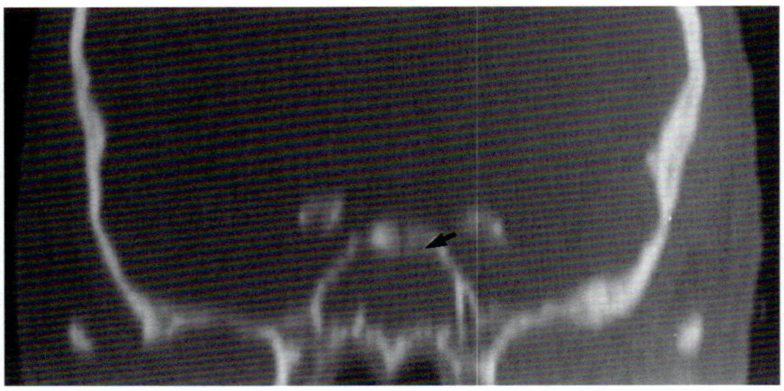

B

Figure 80–2 **(A)** Thin cut coronal and **(B)** basal views of computed tomography showing a fracture through the basisphenoid into the sphenoid sinus.

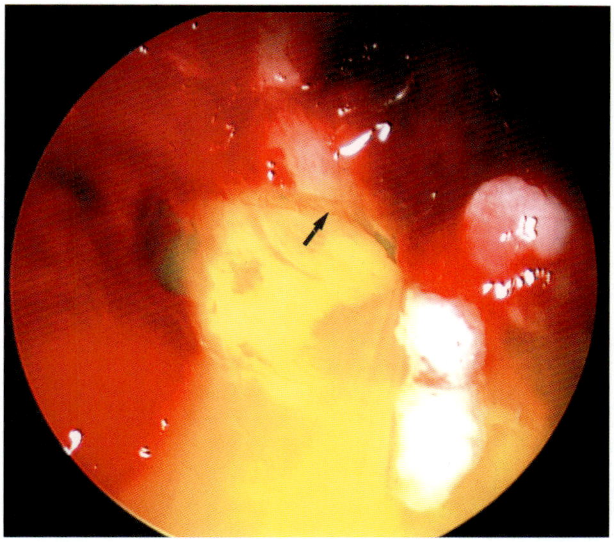

Figure 80–3 Endoscopic visualization of cerebrospinal fluid leak (arrow) mixed with fluorescein through a fracture line inside the sphenoid sinus.

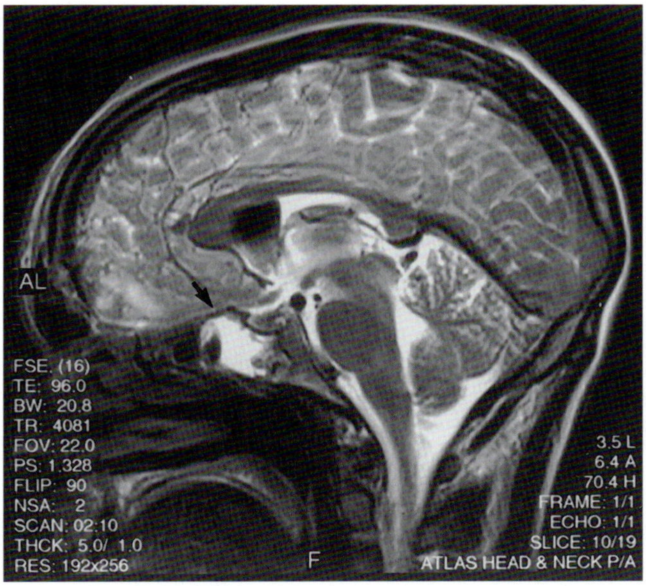

Figure 80–4 Sagittal view of magnetic resonance imaging (T2-weighted images) showing presence of cerebrospinal fluid leak into the sphenoid sinus.

◆ Conservative Management of Cerebrospinal Fluid Leaks

Over 80% of the CSF leaks in CHI are through the anterior fossa and 20% from the ear. The majority of these CSF leaks stop if followed for up to 4 weeks. With long-term follow-up of leaks and conservative management, these leaks could have a 20 to 50% chance of meningitis.[29,30] Coverage of the patients with antibiotics in the face of persistent CSF leakage is controversial.[12,34] To ensure that conservative management is effective, several of the following strategies could be employed: (1) head elevation up to 30 degrees, (2) daily lumbar punctures, (3) continuous lumbar drainage, and (4) fluid restriction with or without acetazolamide. If conservative management is not effective and CSF leaks don't stop, surgical repair is indicated within 1 to 2 weeks. Conservative management of CSF leaks due to the penetrating head injury (PHI) should be pursued with great caution so as not to expose patients to the risks of gram-negative meningitis.[6] CSF fistulas from Penetrating head injury scalp should be repaired at the earliest possible time.

◆ Surgical Technique

Cranial Approach to Cerebrospinal Fluid Leaks

The patient is kept on antibiotics, diphenylhydantoin, and steroids. The approach is either unilateral or bifrontal. The objectives of this approach are (1) to stay close to the base of the skull, (2) to have enough exposure so that the surgeon would be able to repair the dura up to the sphenoid ridge and the tuberculum sella, (3) to save the pericranium to cover the frontal fossa, and (4) to save the frontalis branches of the facial nerve and the supratrochlear and supraorbital nerves.

Positioning

The operating table is flexed and the back is brought up so that the patient's head stays above the chest for better facilitation of the venous drainage.

Skin Incision

The skin incision design could be either curvilinear for a unilateral approach or bicoronal for a bilateral approach. The skin is infiltrated with 0.5% Marcaine with 1/200,000 adrenaline

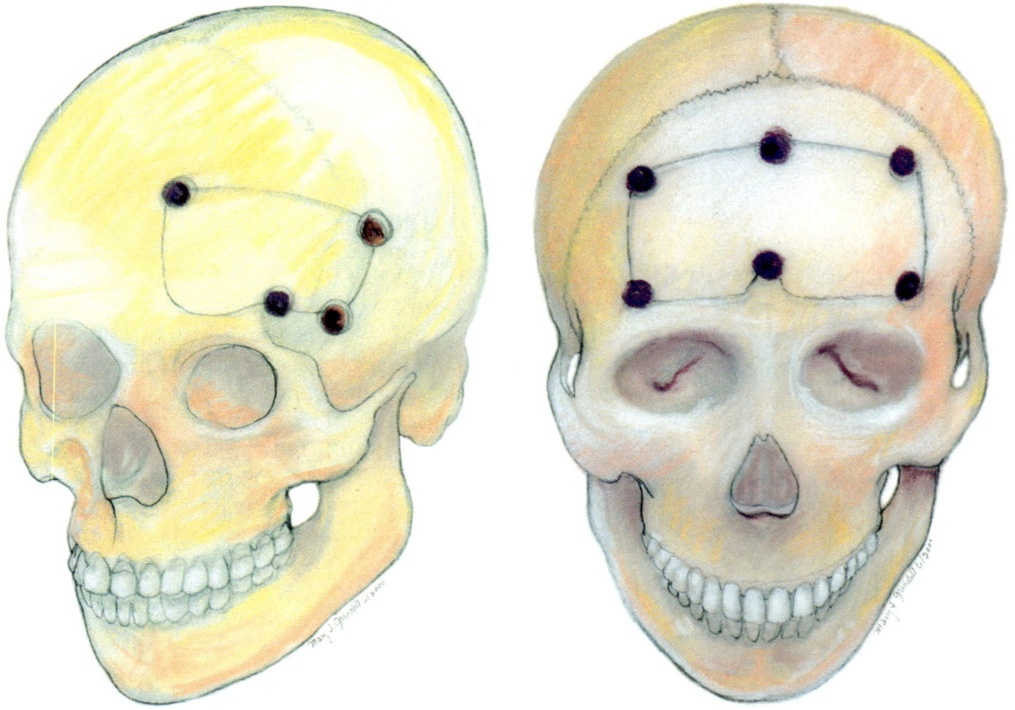

A B

Figure 80–5 **(A)** Unilateral or **(B)** bilateral approach to the base of the anterior fossa.

for better control of bleeding. Upon reflecting the skin, one should try to stay deep to the temporal fat pad so that the frontalis branches of facial nerve are saved. In bicoronal incisions one should stay deep to the galea aponeurotica to save the branches of the supratrochlear and supraorbital nerves. At times the frontal bone has formed a thin canal through which the nerves are passed. In this case the canals should be opened to dislocate the nerves instead of severing them. The pericranium is saved to use it to cover the entire frontal fossa in case there is an extra barrier against CSF leakage.[31]

Craniotomy Design

The craniotomy could be unilateral or bilateral and close to the frontal base and the sphenoid wing **(Fig. 80–5)**. One has to isolate the temporalis muscle close to the superior temporal line. In bilateral frontal craniotomies we need to ligate and cut the most anterior aspect of the sagittal sinus close to the crista galli. In many of the fractures of the anterior fossa close to the anterior ethmoids and cribriform plate it is very difficult to save the olfactory nerves; however, it is possible to dissect free those nerves under the microscope and save them if the chance exists for the patient to have a sense of smell in the future.

Exposure

Exposure of the dural defect could be either extradural or intradural.[1,7] It is advisable to either insert a lumbar drain or evacuate CSF from the prechiasmatic cisterns and to infuse mannitol to prepare ample space so that the frontal lobes can be elevated without contusion. Extradural exposure involves dissecting the dura from the skull base until the defect is reached. Following exposure of the defect, the two arms of a self-retaining retractor are placed on each side and the defect is repaired by dural substitute in a watertight fashion **(Fig. 80–6)**. In older patients, because of the significant adhesion of the dura to the frontal base, it is recommended to have an intradural exposure and repair of dura **(Fig. 80–7)**. Following repair of the dura the stitch line is covered by fibrin glue and the galeal flap is used to cover the floor of the entire frontal fossa.[32,33] To prevent leakage from the line of fracture in the frontal sinus, hydroxyapatite is used as a sealant.[39]

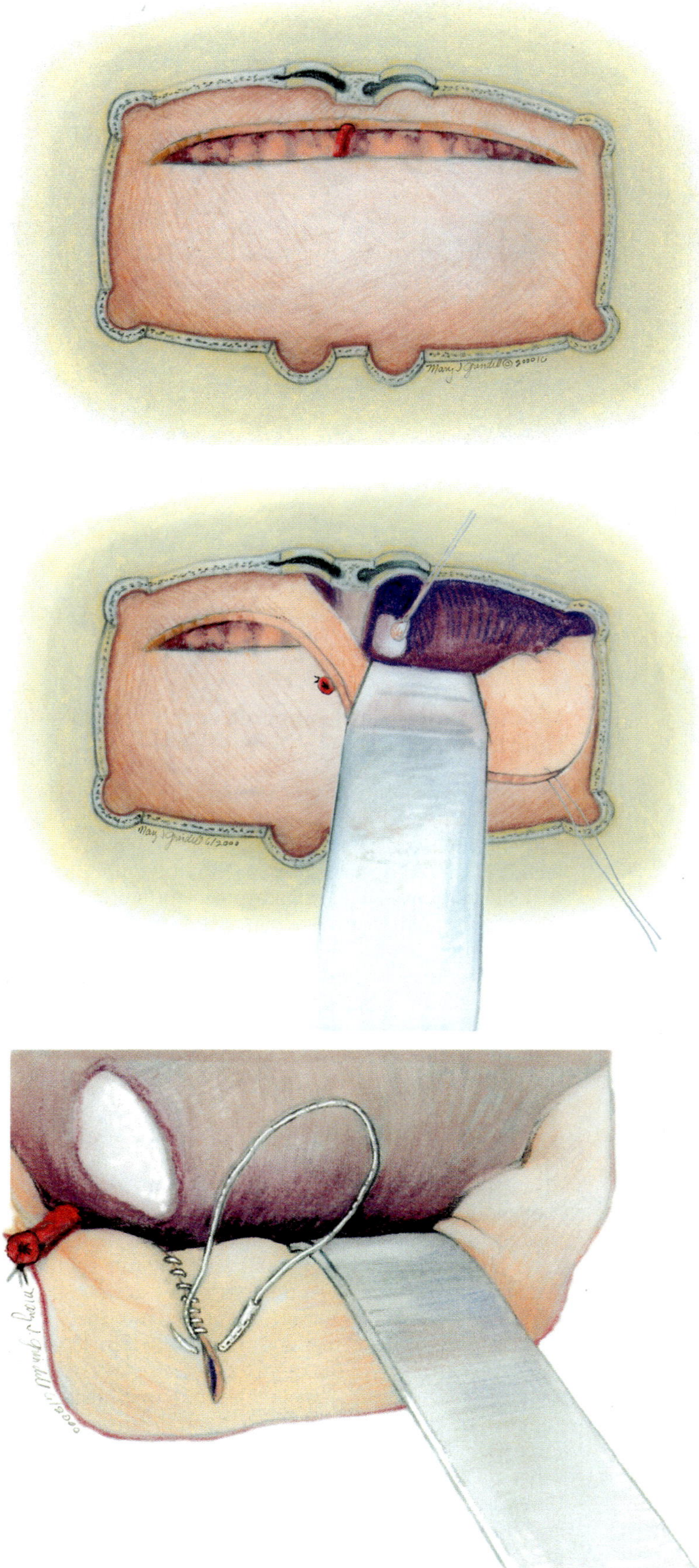

A

B

C

Figure 80–6 Extradural exposure of a cerebrospinal fluid fistula and repair of the defect in a watertight fashion. **(A)** Craniotomy performed and bifrontal dura opened. Bifrontal craniotomy and opening of the dura is perfouned in order to drain the cerebrospinal fluid and relax the exposure. **(B)** Extradural dissection to visualize the leak. Gradually the dura of the right frontal dura is dissected off the floor, exposing a defect on the floor of the fossa. **(C)** Repair of dural defect is closed with neurolon watertight.

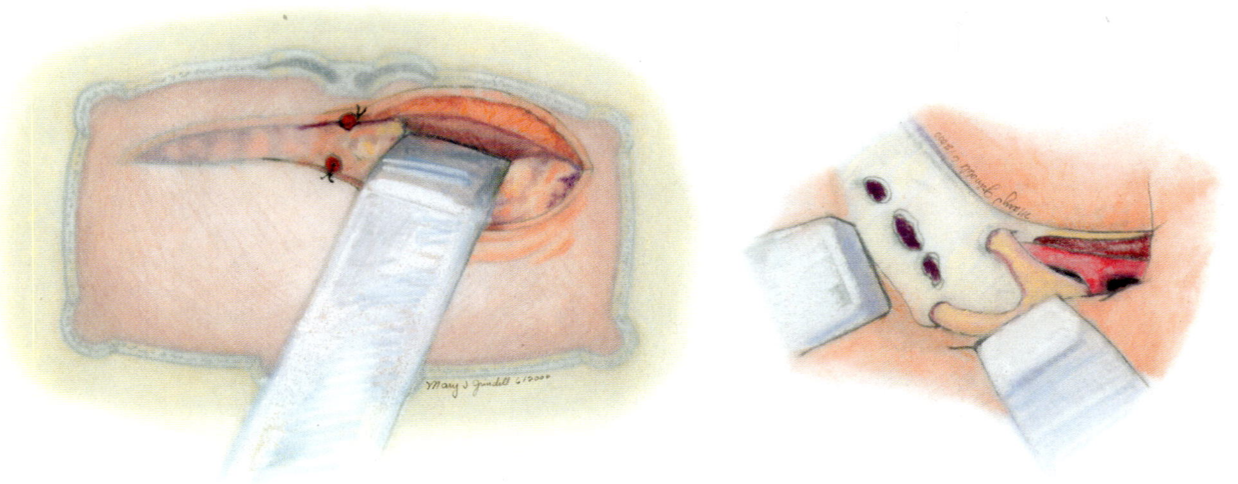

A B

Figure 80–7 Intradural exposure of a crebrospinal fluid. **(A)** Craniotomy, dural opening and brain retraction. Superior sagittal sinus is doubly ligated and cut; then the right frontal lobe is elevated to expose the floor of the fossa **(B)** Site of leak is seen in the ethmoidal area. Exposure of optic nerves and chiasm indicates the defective floor of the frontal fossa.

◆ Postoperative Course

The patient should be kept on antibiotics for 5 to 7 days after the operation. The spinal drain can be used for a few days.

◆ Transnasal Endoscopic Approach to Cerebrospinal Fluid Leak Repair

CSF rhinorrhea from anterior cranial base defects may result from head trauma, tumor surgery, or surgery for inflammatory diseases of the paranasal sinuses. Conservative management of CSF leaks includes head elevation and bed rest, serial lumbar punctures, and lumbar drains. Should profuse drainage occur or drainage persist after conservative therapy, then surgical intervention is warranted. Surgical repair of anterior defects may be performed through a frontal craniotomy as discussed previously, via an external ethmoidectomy, or transnasally using an endoscopic technique.[35–49] Repair of CSF fistulas from posterior or middle cranial fossa and temporal bone defects is discussed later in this chapter. The classic frontal craniotomy approach carries the morbidity of permanent anosmia from mobilization or section of the olfactory bulbs at the cribriform plate as well as risks associated with retraction or elevation of the frontal lobes. Although craniotomy approaches have been considered definitive procedures, the recurrence rate has been reported as high as 27% after the primary surgery and 10% after revision surgery.[43,44] The following section focuses on the endoscopic surgical approach to repair of anterior cranial fossa CSF leaks.

Preoperative Diagnostic Evaluation

As mentioned previously, CT scan with intrathecal nonionic contrast may provide localization of the cranial base defect and site of the CSF leak. Alternatively, intrathecal fluorescein (0.2 to 0.5 mL of 5% diluted into 10 mL of CSF) may be administered upon endoscopic examination to identify the defect intraoperatively **(Fig. 80–3)**.

Endoscopic Repair of Sphenoid Cerebrospinal Fluid Fistulas

Patients are usually placed under general anesthesia and a lumbar drain may be placed if desired or in cases of large fistulas. The nasal cavity and sphenoseptal junction are injected with 1% lidocaine with 1:100,000 epinephrine. Patients usually receive a cephalosporin antibiotic in the perioperative period. Diagnostic nasal endoscopy is performed and the skull-base defect (as seen on CT), or site of active leak or fluorescein drainage is identified. An endoscopic sphenoidotomy is performed with through-cut forceps or microdebriders at the anatomical location of the natural ostia (medial to the middle turbinate and just posterior to the superior turbinate). The ostial opening is enlarged to allow adequate visualization, and the mucosa is dissected and removed from the sinus **(Fig. 80–8)**. Should an encephalocele be the etiology of the CSF leak, the mucosa is dissected free from the mass, and the encephalocele is either reduced through the bony defect into its original position or resected if necrotic or nonviable tissue is evident. Large bony defects may be repaired using free septal cartilage or bone grafts or even turbinate bone grafts. Fat is then harvested from the abdomen and placed into the sphenoid sinus **(Fig. 80–9)**. Fibrin glue is then applied to support the graft and further seal the defect. Gelfoam and possibly antiseptic gauze packing may be placed to provide additional support of the graft and prevent air from entering the intracranial cavity during extubation or in the case of Valsalva episodes in the immediate postoperative period. Patients are usually maintained at bed rest for 4 to 5 days with lumbar drainage to gravity. Antibiotic therapy is typically maintained until all nasal packing has been removed.

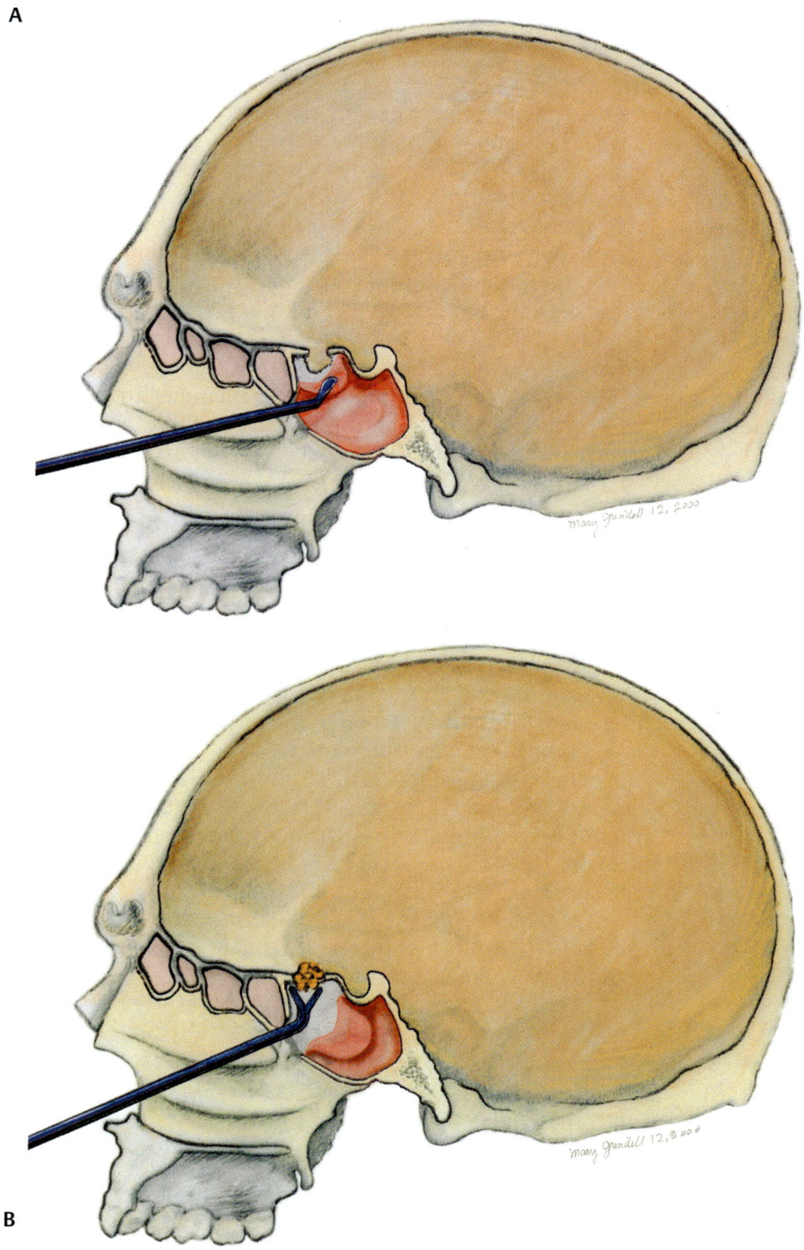

Figure 80–8 Endoscopic sphenoidotomy, and elevation of sphenoid mucosa surrounding the skull-base defect and cerebrospinal fluid fistula. **(A)** Surgeon's attempt to dissect and reduce herniated brain inside the sphenoid sinus. For larger defects, herniated intracranial tissue may be dissected and reduced or resected if it is strangulated and grossly necrotic. **(B)** Surgeon's attempt to resect strangulated and herniated brain inside the sphenoid sinus cerebrospinal fluid.

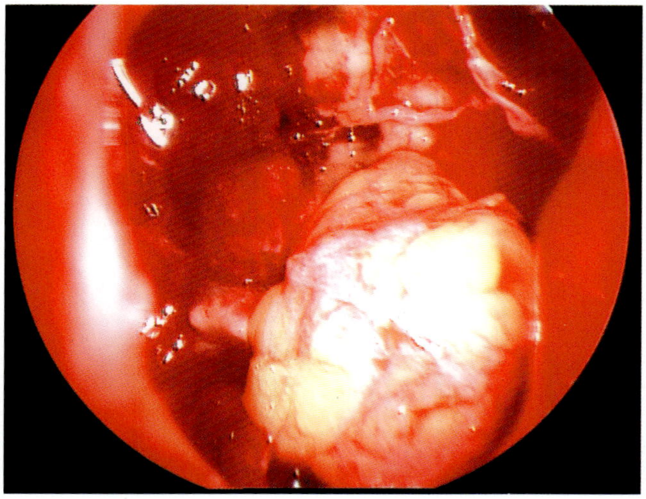

Figure 80–9 Closure of a fistulous tract and bony defect at the roof of the sphenoid sinus and reinforcement with fatty material.

Endoscopic Repair of Ethmoid or Cribriform Plate Fistulas

In general, the repairs of cribriform or ethmoid defects and CSF leaks follow the same pattern of preoperative evaluation, anesthesia, lidocaine with epinephrine injection, perioperative antibiotics, and use of lumbar drains. Nasal sinus endoscopy is performed bilaterally, and ethmoid or cribriform defects with active CSF leakage or fluorescein drainage are identified. A partial or complete ethmoidectomy is performed to provide access to the defect, and the mucosa is carefully dissected from the bony margins and surrounding superior septum and ethmoid sinus cavities. For defects greater than 0.5 cm, free septal cartilage or bone grafts, or turbinate bone and mucosa grafts may be used to close the defect and provide additional support to prevent herniation of intracranial contents. Some authors advocate pedicled superior septal mucosa or middle turbinate mucosa/bone grafts,[46,48] but we have not found this technique to be of any additional benefit. Abdominal fat is harvested and placed over the bony defect or support grafts and then autologous or synthetic fibrin glue is applied to secure the grafts. Gelfoam and adaptic gauze packing is placed and maintained for 3 to 5 days postoperatively.

Success Rates and Complications of Endoscopic Repair of Cerebrospinal Fluid Fistulas

Our success rates parallel those reported in the literature, which range from 90 to 100% after primary or focused revision endoscopic procedures.[35,37,38,41,44] In general, success or failure has not correlated with the size of the skull-base defect. Complications are not common but include nasal obstruction and synechiae, chronic or recurrent sinusitis, and hyposmia or anosmia. More serious and potentially fatal complications such as meningitis or frontal lobe abscess are rare but have been reported.[38]

Repair of Temporal Bone and Middle Cranial Fossa Cerebrospinal Fluid Fistulas

The most common cause of CSF leak in the temporal bone and ear is accidental trauma followed by surgery for chronic inflammatory ear disease or tumors. CSF leak occurs in about 0.5 to 6% of patients with radiographic evidence of temporal bone fractures.[37] Longitudinal temporal bone fractures result in CSF leaks more frequently than transverse fractures. In general, longitudinal fractures extend through the posterior bony external auditory canal and into the tegmen, where they subsequently tear the temporal lobe dura. The tympanic membrane is often ruptured and CSF exits the temporal bone either directly through the external bony canal fracture or through the tympanic membrane defect manifesting as clear otorrhea. Transverse fractures course perpendicular to the long axis of the temporal bone and may course across the internal auditory canal, resulting in facial nerve or auditory nerve injury. The integrity of the tympanic membrane is usually maintained and CSF passes down the eustachian tube into the nasopharynx. Diagnosis of CSF leaks from the temporal bone includes fine-cut axial and coronal temporal bone CT scans and intrathecal nonionic contrast studies as discussed in previous sections.

Surgical Repair of Temporal Bone Cerebrospinal Fluid Leaks

The choice of surgical approach is governed by the location of the actual site of CSF leak. Defects in the tegmen and middle fossa dura are exposed via mastoidectomy or atticotomy and defects in the posterior fossa dura require complete mastoidectomy. Isolated defects in the tegmen tympani of the middle ear space may require only tympanotomy for exposure and repair. For larger middle fossa defects, a small extradural craniotomy through the squamous temporal bone in combination with a mastoidectomy may facilitate fascia, bone, or cartilage graft placement and enhance the success of the repair **(Fig. 80–10)**.

After performing the mastoidectomy, the leak site and possible herniation of intracranial contents are identified and the bony defect surrounding the dural tear is debrided of mucosa and loose bone fragments **(Fig. 80–11)**. The opening may be enlarged as needed to allow adequate exposure and placement of the tissue graft. A small dissector is used to elevate dura intracranially from the surrounding defect margins and a free tissue graft is inserted through the opening so that it covers the dural tear and is supported circumferentially by bone **(Fig. 80–12)**. The choice of graft material includes temporalis fascia, fascia lata, periosteum, perichondrium, and homo- or allograft material. Composite grafts such as conchal cartilage or septal cartilage with attached perichondrium may also be chosen for larger defects. After placement of the graft, additional fat grafting or temporalis muscle graft and fibrin glue are used to reinforce the repair and close the defect. Lumbar drainage of CSF may be done intraoperatively and for 3 to 5 days postoperatively.

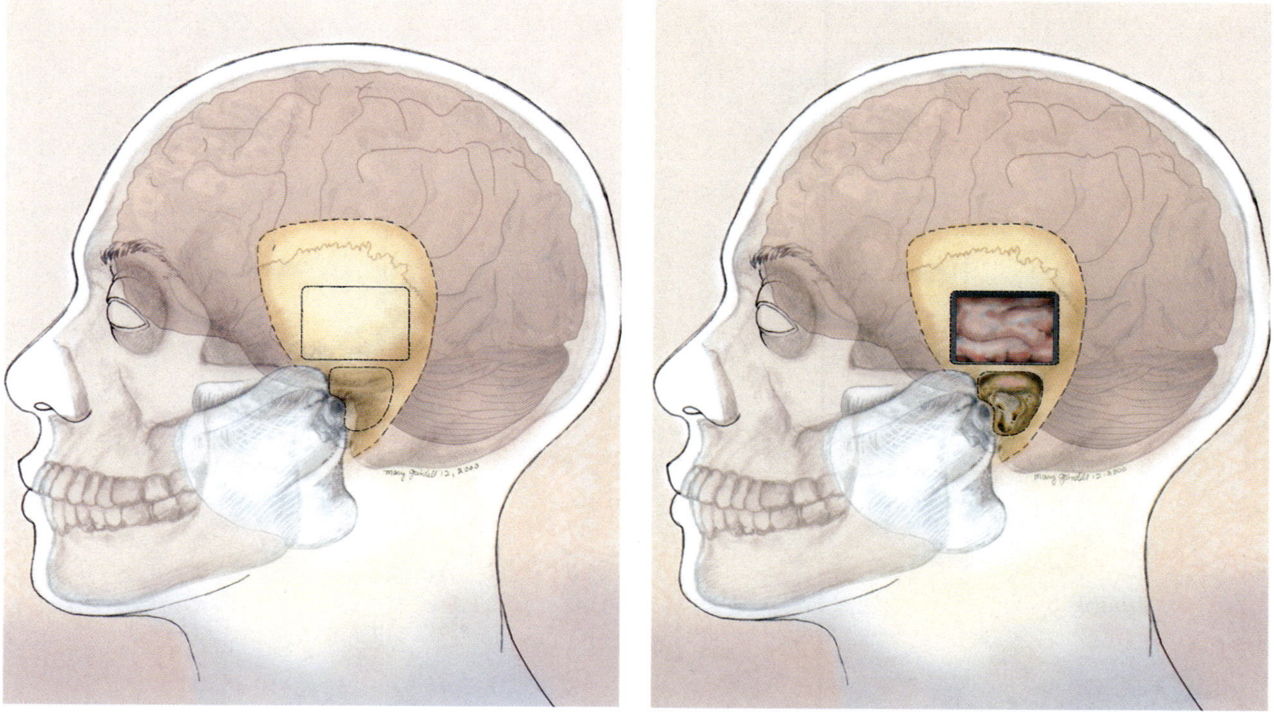

A B

Figure 80–10 (A) Exposure and markings for a combined transmastoid and middle cranial fossa approach to the skull-base defect and crebrospinal fluid fistula. (B) Postcraniotomy and mastoidectomy view.

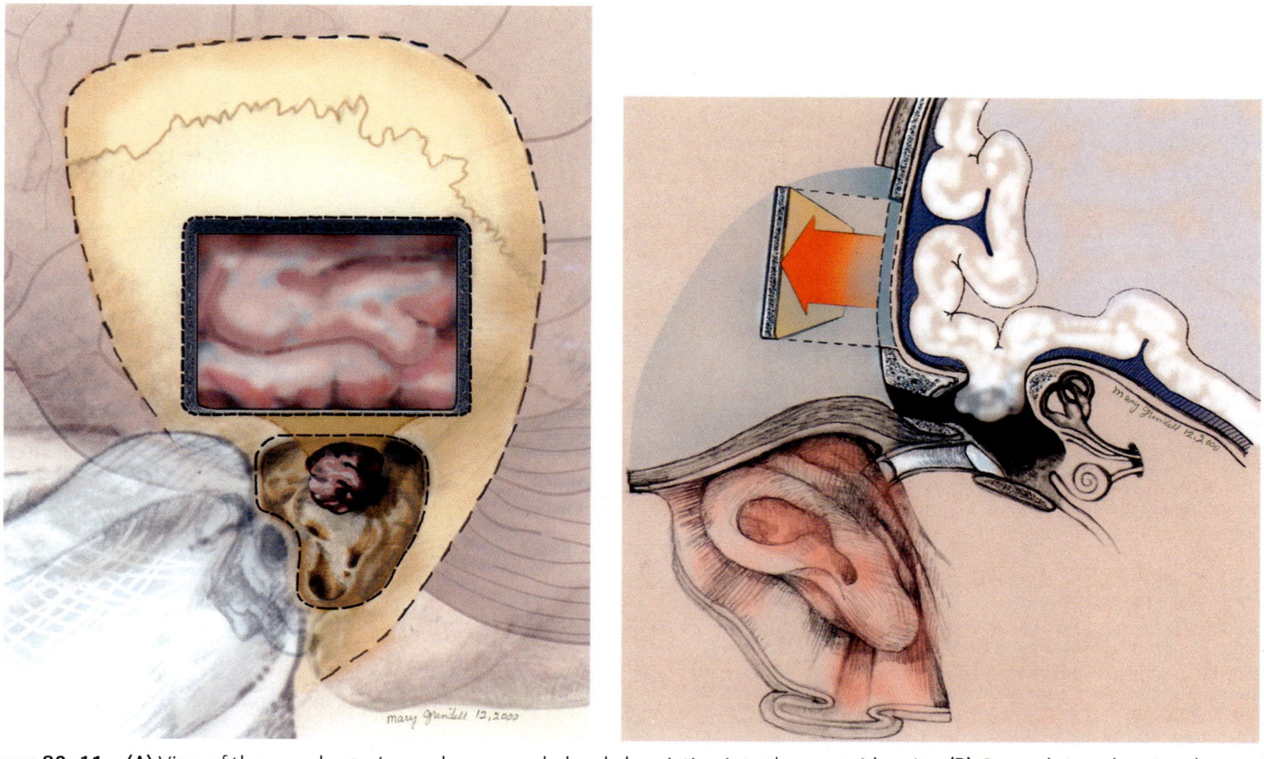

A B

Figure 80–11 (A) View of the pseudomeningocele or encephalocele herniating into the mastoid cavity. (B) Coronal view showing the combined transmastoid and middle cranial fossa approach to the site of the cerebrospinal fluid fistula.

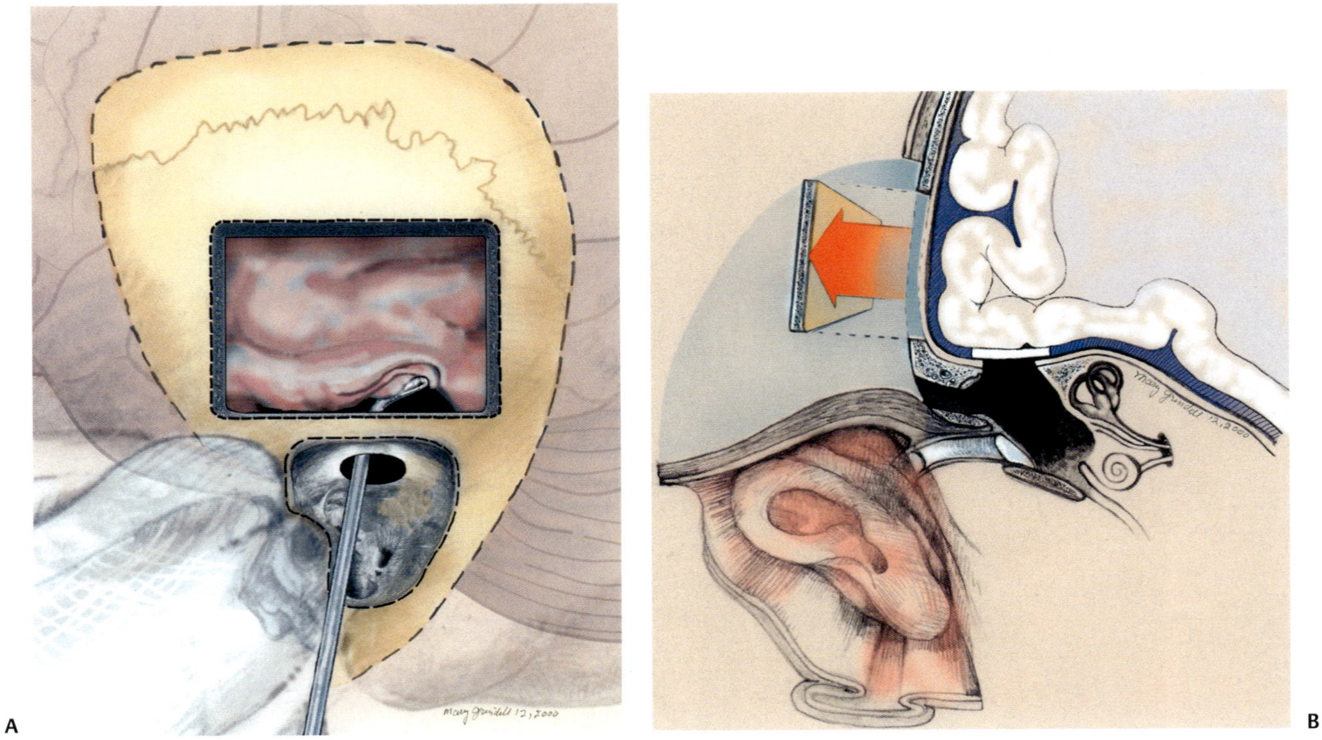

Figure 80–12 (A) Reduction of the pseudomeningocele or encephalocele through the mastoid cavity along with middle cranial fossa exposure. (B) Coronal view demonstrating closure of the skull-base defect with cartilage or bone graft and/or fascia.

References

1. Lewin W. Cerebrospinal fluid rhinorrhea in nonmissile head injuries. Clin Neurosurg 1966;12:237–252
2. Chiari H. Uebereinen Fall, von Luflonsammlong in Der Ventrikeln des Menschlichen Gehoins. Ztsch Heirk 1884;5:383–384
3. Dandy WE. Pneumocephalus (intracranial pneumatocele or aerocedle). Arch Surg 1926;12:949–982
4. Dandy WE. Treatment of rhinorrhea and otorrhea. Arch Surg 1944;49: 75–85
5. Cairns H. Injuries of the frontal and ethmoidal sinuses with special reference to cerebrospinal rhinorrhoea and aerocele. J Laryngol 1937;52:589–623
6. Aarabi B, Taghipour M, Alibaii E, Kamgarpour A. Central nervous system infections after military missile head wounds. Neurosurgery 1998;42:500–507
7. Aarabi B, Leibrock LG. Neurosurgical approaches to cerebrospinal fluid rhinorrhea. Ear Nose Throat J 1992;71:300–305
8. Coleman CC. Fracture of the skull involving the paranasal sinuses and mastoids. JAMA 1947;109:1613–1616
9. Calvert CA, Cairns H. Discussion on injuries of the frontal and ethmoidal sinuses. Proc R Soc Med 1942;35:805–810
10. Lewin W. Cerebrospinal fluid rhinorrhea in closed head injuries. Br J Surg 1954;171:1–18
11. Jamieson KG, Yelland JDN. Surgical repair of the anterior fossa because of rhinorrhea, aerocele, or meningitis. J Neurosurg 1973;39:328–331
12. Leech PJ, Paterson A. Conservative and operative management for cerebrospinal-fluid leakage after closed head injury. Lancet 1973;1: 1013–1016
13. Davis EDD. Discussion on injuries of the frontal and ethmidal sinuses. Laryngology 1942;805:13–18
14. Adson AW, Uihlein A. Repair of defects in ethmoid and frontal sinuses resulting in cerebrospinal rhinorrhea. Arch Surg 1949;58:623–634
15. Russell T, Cummins BH. Cerebrospinal fluid rhinorrhea 34 years after trauma: a case report and review of the literature. Neurosurgery 1984;15:705–706
16. Ashburn WL, Harbert JC, Briner WH, et al. Cerebrospinal fluid rhinorrhea studied with the gamma scintillation camera. J Nucl Med 1968; 9:523–529
17. DiChiro G, Ommaya AK, Ashburn WL, et al. Isotope cisternography in the diagnosis and follow-up of cerebrospinal fluid rhinorrheas. J Neurosurg 1968;28:522–529
18. Ahmadi J, Weiss MH, Segall HD, Schultz DH, Zee CS, Giannotta. Evaluation of cerebrospinal fluid rhinorrhea by metrizamide computed tomography cisternography. Neurosurgery 1985;16:54–60
19. Drayer BP, Wilkins RH, Boehnke M, et al. Cerebrospinal fluid rhinorrhea demonstrated by metrizamide CT cisternography. AJR Am J Roentgenol 1977;129:149–151
20. Eljamel MS, Pidgeon CN, Toland J, Phillips JB, O'Dwyer AAJ. MRI cisternography, and localization of CSF fistulae. Br J Neurosurg 1994;8: 433–437
21. Friedman JA, Ebersold MJ, Quast LM. Persistent posttraumatic cerebrospinal fluid leakage. Neurosurgery Focus 2000;9:1–5
22. Gupta V, Goyal M, Mishra N, Gaikwad S, Sharma A. MR evaluation of CSF fistulae. Acta Radiol 1997;38:603–609
23. Levy LM, Gulya AJ, Davis SW, et al. Flow-sensitive magnetic resonance imaging ion the evaluation of cerebrospinal fluid leaks. Am J Otol 1995;16:591–596
24. Manelfe C, Guiraud B, Tremoulet M. Diagnosis of CSF rhinorrhea by computerized cisternography using metrizamide. Lancet 1977;2:1073
25. Sillers MJ, Morgan CE, Gammal EL. Magnetic resonance cisternography and thin coronal computerized tomography in the evaluation of cerebrospinal fluid rhinorrhea. Am J Rhinol 1997;11:387–392
26. Stafford Johnson DBS, Brennan P, Toland J, O'Dwyer AJ. Magnetic resonance imaging in the evaluation of cerebrospinal fluid fistulae. Clin Radiol 1996;51:837–841
27. Stone JA, Castillo M, Neelon B, Mukherji SK. Evaluation of CSF leaks: high-resolution CT compared with contrast-enhanced CT and radionuclide cisternography. AJNR Am J Neuroradiol 1999;20:706–712
28. Zeng Q, Xiong L, Jinkins JR, et al. Intrathecal gadolinium-enhanced MR myelography and cisternography: a pilot study in human patients. AJR Am J Roentgenol 1999;173:1109–1115
29. Teachenor FR. Intracranial complications of fracture of skull involving frontal sinus. JAMA 1927;88:987–989
30. Thompson St C. The Cerebrospinal Fluid: Its Spontaneous Escape from the Nose. London: Cassell; 1989

31. Costa H, Baptista A, Vaz R, et al. The galea frontalis myofascial flap in anterior fossa CSF leaks. Br J Plast Surg 1993;46:503–507
32. Dunn CJ, Goa KL. Fibrin sealant; a review of its use in surgery and endoscopy. Drugs 1999;58:863–886
33. Gnjidic Z, Tomac D, Negovetic L, et al. Fibrin sealants in the management of cerebrospinal fistulae. Biomed Prog 1994;7:39–42
34. Klastersky J, Sadeghi M, Brihaye J. Antimicrobial prophylaxis in patients with rhinorrhea or otorrhea: a double-blind study. Surg Neurol 1976;6:111–114
35. Amedee RG, Mann WJ, Gilsbach J. Microscopic endonasal surgery for repair of CSF leaks. Am J Rhinol 1993;7:1–4
36. Anand VK, Murali RK, Glasgold MJ. Surgical decisions in the management of cerebrospinal fluid rhinorrhea. Rhinology 1995;33:212–218
37. Applebaum EL, Chow JM. Cerebrospinal fluid leaks. In: Cummings CW, Fredrickson JM, Harker LA, Krause CJ, Richardson MA, Schuller DE, eds. Paranasal Sinuses, Otolaryngology Head and Neck Surgery. Vol 2. 3rd ed. St. Louis: Mosby, 1998:1189–1197
38. Dodson EE, Gross CW, Swerdloff JL, et al. Transnasal endoscopic repair of cerebrospinal fluid rhinorrhea and skull base defects: a review of twenty-nine cases. Otolaryngol Head Neck Surg 1994;111:600–605
39. Friedman M, Venkatesan TK, Caldarelli DD. Composite mucochondral flap for repair of cerebrospinal fluid leaks. Head Neck 1995;17: 414–418
40. Marshall AH, Jones NS, Robertson IJA. An algorithm for the management of CSF rhinorrhea illustrated by 36 cases. Rhinology 1999;37: 182–185
41. Mattox DE, Kennedy DW. Endoscopic management of cerebrospinal fluid leaks and cephaloceles. Laryngoscope 1990;100:857–862
42. Ng Matthew, Maceri DR, Levy MM, Crockett DM. Extracranial repair of pediatric traumatic cerebrospinal fluid rhinorrhea. Arch Otolaryngol Head Neck Surg 1998;124:1125–1130
43. Papay FA, Maggiano H, Dominquez S, et al. Rigid endoscopic repair of paranasal sinus cerebrospinal fluid fistulas. Laryngoscope 1989;99: 1195–1201
44. Park J-I, Strelzow VV, Firedman WH. Current management of cerebrospinal fluid rhinorrhea. Laryngoscope 1983;93:1294–1300
45. Ray BS, Bergland RM. Cerebrospinal fluid fistula: clinical aspects, techniques of localization and methods of closure. J Neurosurg 1967;30:399–405
46. Weisman RA. Septal chondromucosal flap with preservation of septal integrity. Laryngoscope 1989;99:267–271
47. Wetmore RF, Duhaime AC, Klausner RD. Endoscopic repair of traumatic CSF rhinorrhea in a pediatric patient. Int J Pediatr Otorhinolaryngol 1996;36:109–115
48. Yessenow RS, McCabe BF. The osteo-mucoperiosteal flap in repair of cerebrospinal fluid rhinorrhea: a 20-year experience. Otolaryngol Head Neck Surg 1989;101:555–558
49. Yoon JH, Lee JG, Kim SH, Park IY. Microscopical surgical management of cerebrospinal fluid rhinorrhea with free grafts. Rhinology 1995;33: 208–211

81

Motor Cortex Stimulation for Neuropathic Pain

Nikki Maartens, Dawn Carroll, Dipankar Nandi, Sarah L. F. Owen, Ioannis Panourias, and Tipu Z. Aziz

Chronic neuropathic pain conditions, including central post-stroke pain and posttraumatic peripheral neuralgias, represent the cruelest and most difficult conditions that specialist pain centers or neurosurgeons might be called upon to manage. Clinically, pharmacological interventions have marginal effect on these conditions, and most surgical therapies have little effect.

Electrical stimulation with bipolar currents, in or near the internal capsule, and its positive effect on centrally mediated pain was documented more than 20 years ago.[1,2] Interest in motor cortex stimulation (MCS) has since developed in the search for an effective treatment in management of central post-stroke pain, although it has since been shown to be useful for other peripheral neuropathic pain conditions, including trigeminal neuralgia and facial pain. Tsubokawa et al's[3] first reports on the effectiveness of MCS for neuropathic pain was based on experience attained from 25 patients treated over a 10-year period, using intermittent cortical stimulation. The overall response rate first reported by Tsubokawa et al in 1990 was 75%, with long-term benefits for up to 7 months, in a patient group that was known to be resistant to all available pain therapies that had been tried. Tsubokawa et al[4] later went on to publish their findings based on a series of 11 patients with thalamic pain who had undergone implantation of MCS. Eight of the 11 patients tested went on to have internal systems implanted, having reported 73% relief on a visual analog scale (VAS) during initial trial stimulation during surgery. Three of these patients had no response at all. In the eight patients who did respond, pain relief was generally reported within 5 minutes, and these positive effects faded within 10 minutes.

Relief of pain was achieved within ranges of 3 to 8 V, at a level that did not result in muscle spasm. Five of the eight responsive patients continued to achieve the same level of pain relief for a follow-up period of 2 years, receiving intermittent stimulation five to seven times a day. In three patients; however, the relief gradually subsided over a 1-year period. Subsequent to this, there has been growing supportive evidence from published case reports and case series to suggest that stereotactic epidural MCS is an effective treatment for some patients with intractable neuropathic pain. Variable response rates to this procedure have been cited in the literature, in patients with central and peripheral neuropathic pain, and with implantations performed by various techniques.[4–21] The published evidence suggests a positive response in between 44 and 100% of treated patients. Long-term benefits are reported in between 0 and 100% of those patients who responded to initial titration. There is some evidence for a decrease in response over time in some patients. The response rates quoted vary between 0 and 100% with series of larger than five averaging a 50% response. Adverse effects following MCS have been documented in some patients. Effects attributed to surgery include reports of epidural clots.[13] Other effects directly attributed to MCS include epileptic and focal seizures, aphasia and dysphasia, fatigue in the upper limbs, and burning sensations in the area of stimulation.[7,13,16,17,22] Seizures occurred only during titration of MCS, and no seizures or other complications have been reported in the published literature as a result of long-term stimulation at optimum settings.

◆ Indications

Patients with chronic neuropathic pain that has failed to respond to conventional analgesic interventions are considered eligible for surgical implantation of a motor cortex stimulator device (Medtronic Itrel II or III, Jacksonville, FL).

◆ Preoperative Investigations

Predicting those patients who are likely to benefit from stimulation is a major clinical problem. Response does not appear to be condition specific. Barbiturate sensitivity and opioid insensitivity have been suggested as possible predictors of response.[4,21,23,24] Transcranial magnetic stimulation may be another useful predictor of response.[14,23,25–27] However, such preoperative testing is no guarantee of a successful outcome because as not all patients who respond to propofol respond to MCS, and equally morphine insensitive patients have been shown to respond.[23] Preoperative single photon emission computed tomography (SPECT) scans showing parietal hypoperfusion also have not increased the success rate.[23] We have not, therefore, routinely performed any specific investigations other than computed tomographic (CT) and magnetic resonance imaging (MRI) scans of the brain, preoperative chest x-ray, electrocardiogram (ECG), blood count, clotting screen, chemistry, and crossmatch.

◆ Surgical Technique

At the Radcliffe Infirmary, the procedure is performed in two stages. Under general anesthesia the patient is positioned such that the side contralateral to pain lies uppermost with a sandbag under the same shoulder to prevent venous congestion **(Fig. 81–1)**. The central sulcus is positioned using standard anatomical landmarks **(Fig. 81–2)**, but no other image guidance is used. The patient's hair is not shaved but is then cleansed with chlorhexidine shampoo followed by alcoholic chlorhexidine **(Fig. 81–3)**. After draping the operative field, a ∩-shaped incision is marked out 3.0 cm either side of the central sulcus and extending to the midline for the leg, and for faciobrachial pain the exposure ends 2.0 cm lateral to the midline. A free bone flap is raised leaving the dura intact, following which the bone flap is tied down with three Vicryl sutures. The wound is closed in layers over a drain for 24 hours and the patient is wakened.

The following week the patients' scalp and temporalis muscle are infiltrated with 0.25% bupivacaine under intravenous sedation. The scalp is prepared as above with the patient's head in a horseshoe headrest and draped. The scalp is then reopened and retracted laterally and the bone flap removed **(Fig. 81–4)**. The patient is wide awake and cooperative by this time. We then use a four-lead

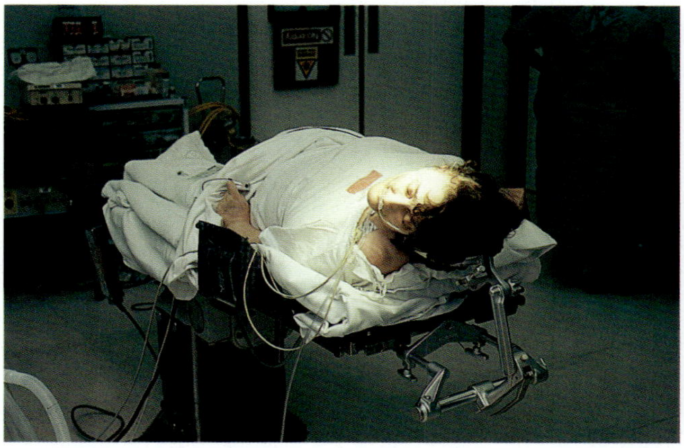

Figure 81–1 The patient is positioned comfortably on the operating table with the craniotomy side uppermost.

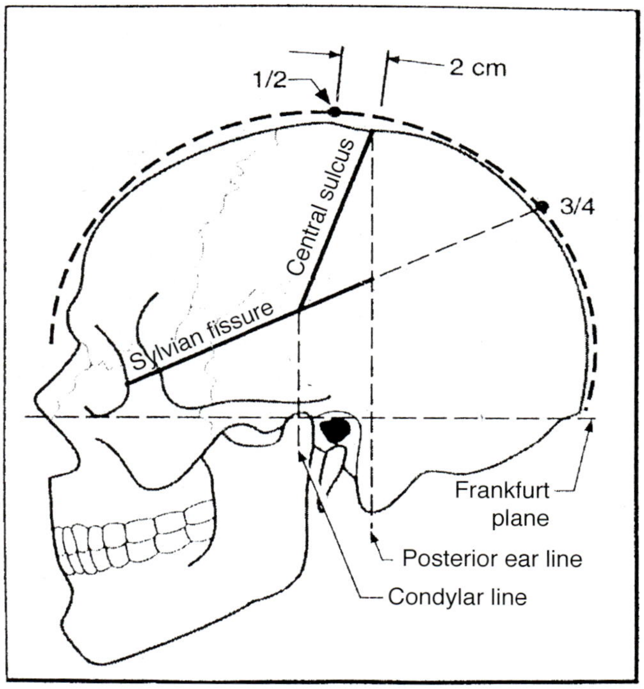

Figure 81–2 We use standard anatomical landmarks as illustrated to make the craniotomy. Face and hand would thus be lateral and the leg medial.

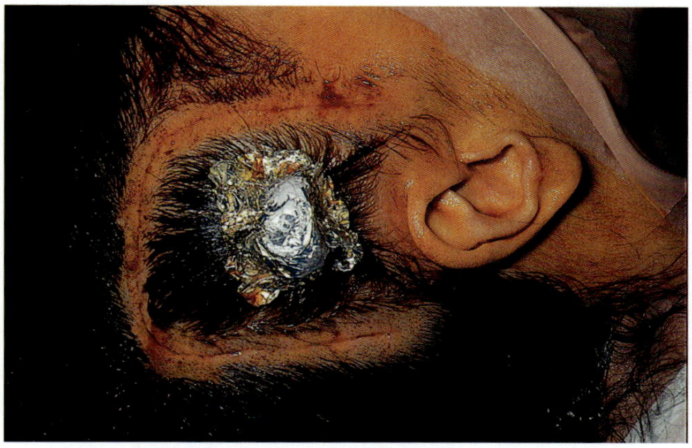

Figure 81–3 We do not shave the patient's head. The scalp and hair are cleansed with aqueous and alcohol chlorhexidine and the hair secured with aluminum foil away from the incision line.

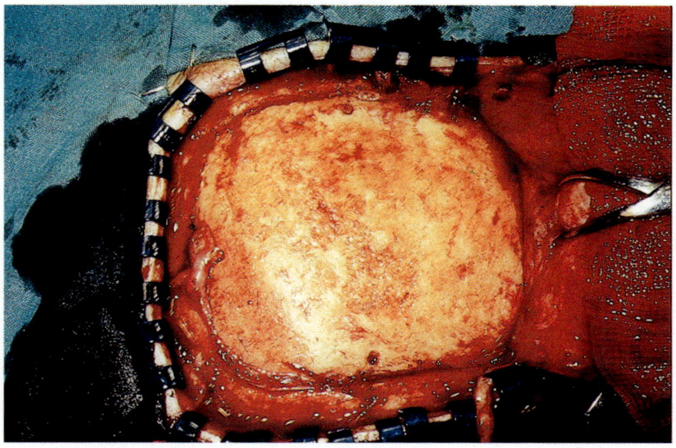

Figure 81–4 The scalp is reopened and retracted to expose the craniotomy flap made the previous week.

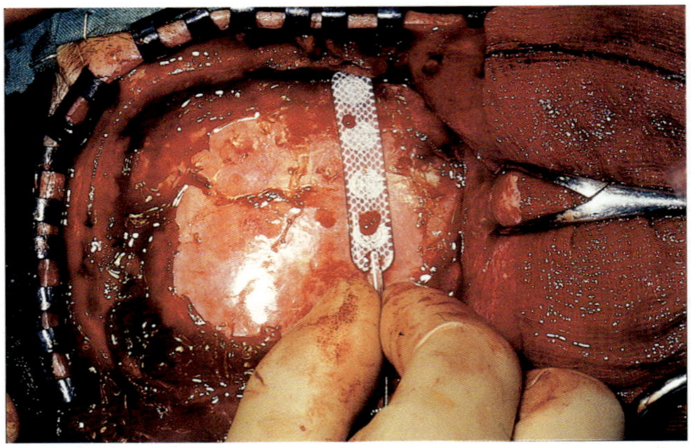

Figure 81–5 The dura is exposed and the Lamitrode (Medtronic) electrode is positioned extradurally over the motor region to elicit motor responses.

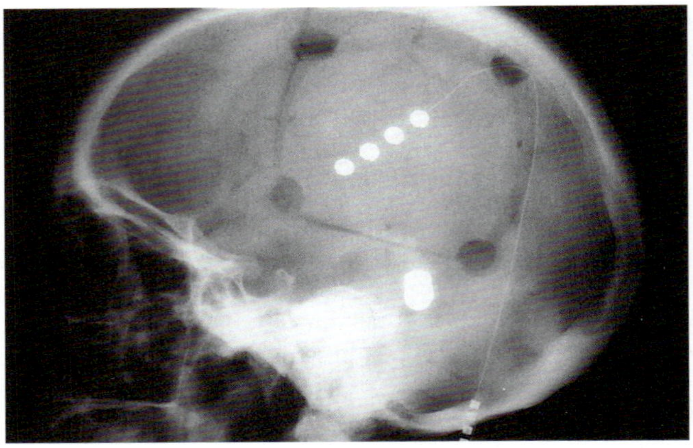

Figure 81–7 Motor cartex electrodes in place.

Resume (Medtronic, Minneapolis, MN,) electrode with the extension lead running out of the operative field to an external stimulator. The electrode is then moved over the dura parallel to the line of the central sulcus while we apply stimuli to elicit motor contractions in the area of pain or, in phantom limb pain, until the patient reports sensations, usually of muscle contractions in the nonexistent limb (**Figs. 81–5** and **81–6**). The stimulus parameters for exploration are 5 to 10 Hz, and 3 to 5.0 V for demarcation of the motor strip. If the patient feels any discomfort from pressure on the dura, a swab soaked in lignocaine is placed over the dura for local anesthesia.

Once the best placement has been identified, the electrode is secured to the dura with silk sutures, the bone flap wired back in place, and most of the wound closed in two layers, except posteroventrally, where the free end of the lead is placed under the skin and interrupted suture placed (**Fig. 81-7**). This allows the drapes to be removed, and the patient is anesthetized and redraped to incorporate the scalp neck and upper chest. The posterior part of the scalp wound is reopened, the free electrode connected to the extension lead, which is then tunneled to a subcutaneous, subclavicular pocket to be connected to an Itrel III (Metronic, Minneapolis, MN) pacemaker (**Fig. 81-8**). All wounds are then closed in two layers and the patient is wakened. Antibiotics are given for up to 3 days. No attempts to program the stimulation parameters are made on this admission. All patients are put on anticonvulsants for the long term.

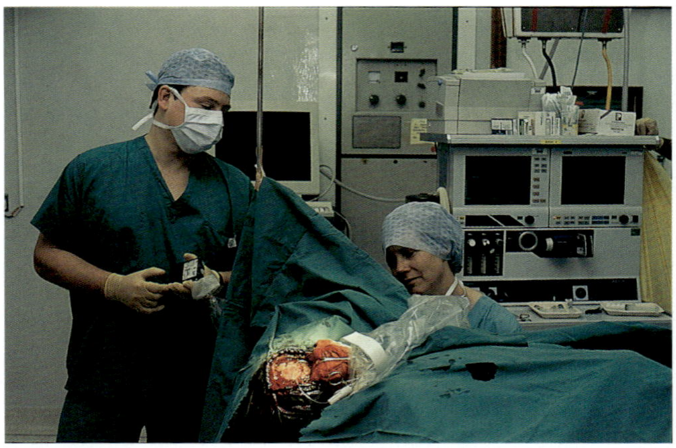

Figure 81–6 The operating room setup. The specialist nurse is speaking to the patient and drapes separate the patient from the assistant, who is controlling the stimulator from the operating field.

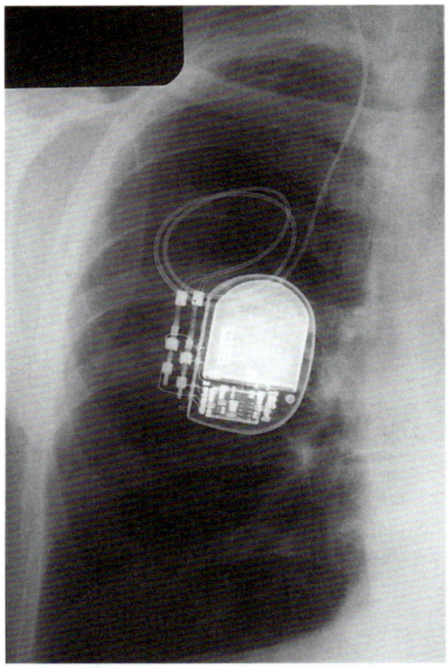

Figure 81–8 The Iatrel III pacemaker has been buried in a subcutaneous pocket.

◆ Postoperative Care

Within 6 weeks postoperatively the patients are routinely admitted to the pain relief unit for a week to optimize the stimulation parameters to achieve the best possible analgesia. All assessments of pain are done independently of the surgeon and the specialist nurse. Patients are then followed up on a regular basis, either by telephone or on an outpatient basis, by the specialist nurse.

◆ Results

Details of the 12 patients treated in Oxford between November 1995 and February 1999 have been previously reported in detail and are shown in **Table 81–1.**[28] A motor response was seen in all 12 patients during intraoperative stimulation, and all 12 patients went on to have full internal implantation of the MCS device. The effects of the procedure on pain relief were then independently assessed in the pain relief unit. The following outcome measures were used:

- Pain intensity: four-point verbal rating scale (3, severe; 2, moderate; 1, mild; 0, none) and 10-point numerical scale (0–10)
- McGill Pain Questionnaire
- Pain relief: 5-point scale (0, none; 1, slight; 2, moderate; 3, good; 4, complete) and percent of pain relief
- Volunteered and observed adverse effects
- Stimulator parameters (amplitude, pulse width, pulse rate, electrode settings)
- Use of other analgesic interventions

Six of the 12 patients treated responded positively (>50% relief) to intermittent motor cortex stimulation (patients 1, 2, 4, 5, 8, and 12). The remaining six patients (3, 6, 7, 9, 10, and 11) failed to achieve any pain relief despite extensive attempts during titration, and their stimulators were eventually switched off. Of those patients who reported pain relief, five (patients 1, 2, 4, 5, and 8) benefited from long-term intermittent stimulation. Only one patient reported complete relief of pain (patient 4). His pain did not return even when the stimulator was switched off. Patients 1 and 12 reported 50% and 70% pain relief, respectively, after the initial titration of the stimulator parameters, but the pain relief gradually diminished in both patients after 2 to 3 weeks. Disappointingly, we failed to reproduce these same positive results, despite multiple attempts at retitration in both patients. Patient 1 had his stimulator explanted and patient 12 eventually had his stimulator switched off.

Patients 2, 5, and 8 took part in a within-patient randomized, double-blind, repeated crossover study in which they were randomly allocated to receive 10 sequential treatment periods of active and no treatment periods in 1999.[28] Each treatment period was for a minimum of 1 hour and lasted for a time period that was sufficient for the patients to make a judgment as to whether the stimulator was currently switched on or off during each treatment because of clinically relevant subjective changes (increases or decreases) in their pain. Patients 5 and 8 were able to judge correctly (because of subjective changes in their pain) when they had received the active and no stimulation treatments on eight of 10 occasions because of clinically relevant changes (decrease/increase) in their pain. Patient 2 could guess correctly which treatment she had received on only four of 10 occasions. She reported that the study treatment periods were not sufficiently long for her to have made a reliable judgment.

Pain relief was achieved with intermittent cortical stimulation, and patients typically received 15 minutes of active stimulation every 3 to 4 hours each day. No epileptic seizures were seen in the patients who gained pain relief from stimulation. A seizure was induced in two patients who did not achieve any reproducible motor response or pain relief during the postoperative test stimulation despite the presence of a positive motor response during intraoperative test stimulation **(Table 81–1).**

Six patients failed to respond to MCS, despite extensive attempts to find optimum stimulation parameters during postoperative titration. Details of these patients are summarized in **Table 81–1.** No clear motor response was ever elicited postoperatively in four of these six patients (patients 3, 6, 7, and 9), neither were there any clinically observable signs of active stimulation after full implantation in these patients. Patient 9 was a clear technical failure because he succeeded in wiping the ID number from his internally implanted programming device when repairing large hi-fi speakers, and he inflicted deliberate damage to the stimulator leads by rotating the pulse generator under his skin repeatedly. Patients 10 and 11 were the only patients in whom there was a clear and reproducible motor response postoperatively. This was demonstrated by muscle spasm and feelings of tightness on the same side of the pain. There was a clear dose response for these motor signs, and epileptic seizures were induced at high voltages in both these patients during titration. These symptoms were quickly reversed once the stimulation was stopped. Such extreme effects were not seen in any other patients, even at high levels of stimulation (10.0 V in patient 9).

◆ Discussion

This chapter has assessed the literature that is available and compared the findings with our own experience prior to recommending it as a technique to other groups. We believe the procedure is effective in 50% of patients with neuropathic pain, although certain subgroups may fare better. Patients with post-stroke pain with a mild hemiparesis probably do better than those with a dense one, and phantom limb pain appears to be one of the best indications.

Until we understand patient selection better and are more able to predict outcome, motor cortex stimulation should be performed within the context of a multidisciplinary pain management team. Continued assessment of successfully implanted patients in *N* of 1 trials will help identify the most suitable candidates.

Table 81–1 Results for Patients Treated with Motor Cortex Stimulation (MCS)

No.	Diagnosis (Year of Onset)	Site of pain/ Characteristics/ Year of Onset	Age/ Sex	Date 1st Stage MCS (2nd Stage)	Summary Adverse Effects/ Complications	Optimum Stimulator Settings	Current Pain Relief / Duration Relief	Comment
1 (DB)	Post-stroke (thalamic infarct) 1991	Hemibody constant severe	62 m	Nov. 95 (Nov. 95)	Subdural hematoma, secondary wound infection; explant Apr. 96	Not documented	>50% 2–3 weeks	Initial pain relief (>50%) lasted 2–3 weeks; patient died of unrelated cause Jun. 96
2 (SB)	Posttraumatic neuralgia (brain stem gunshot injury) 1993	Face, neck, arm, shoulder constantly severe	54 f	Jul. 96 (Jul. 96)	Tender over implant; secondary wound infection; high-amplitude stimulation gave sensation of tightness in area of pain, impaired speech	amp 2.1 volts pw 450 µsec pr 20 Hz	50–60% 36 months	>50% relief overall; titration limited by tightness and other symptoms
3 (TB)	Post-stroke (thalamic infarct) 1985	Facial constantly severe	80 m	Mar. 96 (Mar. 98)	—	None found	None	No relief; no clear postop motor response
4 (RN)	Post-stroke (occipital infarct) 1990	Hemibody constantly severe	70 m	Jul. 96 (Dec. 96)	Itrel 2 affected by exposure to external magnetic field	amp 5.0 volts pw 450 µsec pr 15 Hz	100% 31 months	No pain since Oct. 98; stimulator switched off Feb. 99 with no recurrence of pain; patient died unrelated cause July 99
5 (CW)	Phantom + stump 1992	Leg constantly severe	48 m	Jan. 97 (Jan. 97)	Higher amplitudes gave tightness in area of pain	amp 7.0 volts pw 450 µsec pr 25 Hz	70% phantom 0% stump 30 months	Good relief phantom pain; no relief of stump pain
6 (ME)	Neurofibromatosis 1990	Arm constantly severe	55 f	Jan. 97 (Jan. 97)	No postop motor response	None found	None	No pain relief; no postop motor response; stimulation discontinued
7 (JC)	Post-stroke (thalamic infarct)	Hemibody constantly severe	63 f	Mar. 97 (Mar. 97)		None found	None	No clear reproducible postop motor response; no pain relief; stimulation discontinued
8 (AG)	Phantom limb 1975	Arm and hand constantly severe	56 f	Apr. 97 (Apr. 97)	Secondary wound infection; pain over implant site	amp 2.5 volts pw 450 µsec pr 75 Hz	Arm 75% Hand 5% 27 months	Good long-term relief of phantom pain
9 (MP)	Phantom limb 1979	Arm constantly severe	39 m	Oct. 97 (Oct. 97)	No evidence of any postop motor response; possible contact with external magnetic field	None found	None	Technical failure; stimulation discontinued

Table 81–1 *(Continued)*

10 (DT)	Post-stroke (brain stem) + trigeminal neuralgia 1992	Facial burning constantly; severe episodically	80 f	Feb. 98 (Mar. 98)	Fit induced during postop titration (9.6 V); no pain relief, despite clear motor response during postop titration	None found	None	Clear reproducible postop motor response (8 V); no pain relief; stimulation discontinued
11 (EM)	Brachial plexus avulsion 1976	Hand and arm constantly, but variable intensity	36 f	Nov. 99 (Jan. 2000)	Strong motor response elicited during intraop test stimulation; fit during intraop test stimulation and postop titration	None found	None	Evidence for motor response postop, no pain relief; stimulation discontinued
12 (RD)	Post-stroke 1997	Hemibody constantly moderate to severe	68 m	Mar. 99 (Mar. 99)	Strong motor response elicited during intraop test stimulation	Awaiting retitration	2 weeks relief from initial postoperative titration; awaiting further titration	Complete relief of pain from propofol; initial postop titration produced 70% relief of pain in arm and hand, lasting 2–3 weeks

amp; amplitude; MCS, motor cartex stimulation; pw, pulse width; pr, pulse rate frequency.

References

1. Adams JE, Hosobuchi Y, Fields HL. Stimulation of internal capsule for relief of chronic pain. J Neurosurg 1974;41:740–744
2. Hosobuchi Y, Adams JE, Rutkin B. Chronic thalamic and internal capsule stimulation for the control of central pain. Surg Neurol 1975;4: 91–92
3. Tsubokawa T, et al. Motor cortex stimulation for control of thalamic pain. Abstracts: VIth World Pain Congress, 1990:491
4. Tsubokawa T, Katayama Y, Yamamoto T, Hirayama T, Koyama S. Chronic motor cortex stimulation in patients with thalamic pain. J Neurosurg 1993;78:393–401
5. Canavero S, Bonicalzi V. Therapeutic extradural cortical stimulation for central and neuropathic pain: a review. Clin J Pain 2002; 18: 48–55
6. Canavero S, Bonicalzi V. Motor cortex stimulation. J Neurosurg 2001; 94:688–689
7. Ebel H, Rust D, Tronnier V, Boker D, Kunze S. Chronic precentral stimulation in trigeminal neuropathic pain. Acta Neurochir (Wien) 1996;138:1300–1306
8. Fujii M, Ohmoto Y, Kitahara T, et al. Motor cortex stimulation therapy in patients with thalamic pain [in Japanese]. No Shinkei Geka 1997; 25:315–319
9. Herregodts P, Stadnik T, De Ridder F, D'Haens J. Cortical stimulation for central neuropathic pain: 3-D surface MRI for easy determination of the motor cortex. Acta Neurochir Suppl 1995;64:132–135
10. Hosobuchi Y. Motor cortical stimulation for control of central deafferentation pain. Adv Neurol 1993;63:215–217
11. Katayama Y, Tsubokawa T, Yamamoto T, Hirayama T, Miyazaki S, Koyama S. Characterization and modification of brain activity with deep brain stimulation in patients in a persistent vegetative state: pain-related late positive component of cerebral evoked potential. Pacing Clin Electrophysiol 1991;14:116–121
12. Katayama Y, Tsubokawa T, Yamamoto T. Chronic motor cortex stimulation for central deafferentation pain: experience with bulbar pain secondary to Wallenberg syndrome. Stereotact Funct Neurosurg 1994;62:295–299
13. Meyerson BA, Lindblom U, Linderoth B, Lind G, Herregodts P. Motor cortex stimulation as treatment of trigeminal neuropathic pain. Acta Neurochir Suppl (Wien) 1993;58:150–153
14. Migita K, Uozumi T, Arita K, Monden S. Transcranial magnetic coil stimulation of motor cortex in patients with central pain. Neurosurgery 1995;36:1037–1040
15. Nguyen JP, Lefaucher JP, Le Guerinel C, et al. Motor cortex stimulation in the treatment of central and neuropathic pain. Arch Med Res 2000;31:263–265
16. Peyron R, Garcia-Larrea L, Deiber MP, et al. Electrical stimulation of precentral cortical area in the treatment of central pain: electrophysiological and PET study. Pain 1995;62:275–286
17. Rainov NG. Fels C, Heidecke V, Burkert W. Epidural electrical stimulation of the motor cortex in patients with facial neuralgia. Clin Neurol Neurosurg 1997;99:205–209
18. Saitoh Y, Shibata M, Hirano S, Hirata M, Mashimo T, Yoshimine T. Motor cortex stimulation for central and peripheral deafferentation pain: report of eight cases. J Neurosurg 2000;92:150–155
19. Saitoh Y, Shibata M, Sanada Y, Mashimo T. Motor cortex stimulation for phantom limb pain. Lancet 1999;353:212
20. Tsubokawa T, Katayama Y, Yamamoto T, Hirayama T, Koyama S. Treatment of thalamic pain by chronic motor cortex stimulation. Pacing Clin Electrophysiol 1991;14:131–134
21. Yamamoto T, Katayama Y, Hirayama T, Tsubokawa T. Pharmacological classification of central post-stroke pain: comparison with the results of chronic motor cortex stimulation therapy. Pain 1997;72:5–12
22. Nguyen JP, Keravel Y, Feve A, et al. Treatment of deafferentation pain by chronic stimulation of the motor cortex: report of a series of 20 cases. Acta Neurochir Suppl 1997;68:54–60
23. Canavero S, Bonicalzi V. Cortical stimulation for central pain. J Neurosurg 1995;83:1117
24. Canavero S, Bonicalzi V. The neurochemistry of central pain: evidence from clinical studies, hypothesis and therapeutic implications. Pain 1998;74:109–114
25. Maertens de Noordhout A, Pepin JL, Schoenen J, Delwaide PJ. Percutaneous magnetic stimulation of the motor cortex in migraine. Electroencephalogr Clin Neurophysiol 1992;85:110–115
26. Urban PP, Hopf HC, Fleischer S, Zorowka PG, Muller-Forell W. Impaired cortico-bulbar tract function in dysarthria due to hemispheric stroke: functional testing using transcranial magnetic stimulation. Brain 1997;120(pt 6):1077–1084
27. Rollnik JD, Wustefeld S, Dauper J, et al. Repetitive transcranial magnetic stimulation for the treatment of chronic pain: a pilot study. Eur Neurol 2002;48:6–10
28. Carroll D, Joint C, Maartens N, Shlugman D, Stein J, Aziz TZ. Motor cortex stimulation for chronic neuropathic pain: a preliminary study

82

Soft Tissue Reconstruction of Complex Cranial Defects: A Primer

Michael Olding

- **Indications for Soft Tissue Reconstruction**
- **Coverage of Important Structures**
- **Prevention of Cerebrospinal Fluid Leak and Separation of Cranial Contents**
- **Restoration of Contour**
- **Preoperative Studies**
- **Surgical Technique**
  - Anesthesia
  - Flaps
  - Closure
- **Postoperative Care**
  - Monitoring
- **Complications**

More aggressive surgical treatment of craniofacial tumors, particularly cranial base tumors, has been accompanied by an increased need for more complex reconstructive techniques. Although this need has been addressed primarily by the use of free flaps, a better understanding of the vascular supply to these free flaps has fostered renewed interest in and understanding of the vascular anatomy of local and regional flaps. As a result, improved survival rates of these less complex flaps have made them a more attractive alternative. The reconstructive staff member of the multidisciplinary team must be well versed in all of these available techniques. For the more complicated coverage problems, alternatives are limited and require special microsurgical skills.

More than one reconstructive technique may be available to achieve the desired result; however, the simplest method may not always be the best, particularly if its potential failure rate is higher than a more complex choice. Additional factors that must be considered in choosing the best technique include tumor size and type (malignant versus benign), history of previous surgery, radiation, embolization, and likelihood of additional surgery. Each of these parameters influences the outcome and potential complication rate, and therefore the coverage choice. The "ideal" reconstructive option should be reliable, have limited donor site morbidity, be performed in one stage at the time of tumor resection, and resolve the problem.

The questions regarding the type of reconstruction that must be addressed for each case are essentially the same. What are the goals of the procedure? What flaps are available for coverage? Which flap provides the optimal result and yet does not burn any bridges for reconstructive techniques that might be required in the future? The selection process used to address these questions is euphemistically termed the "reconstructive ladder" **(Table 82–1).** This mental list of the techniques available (in order of increasing complexity) only serves as a general quick reference guide

Table 82–1 Reconstructive Ladder

Skin graft			
	Split- or full-thickness		
Flap			
	Local		
		Scalp flap plus split-thickness skin graft (STSG)	
		Pericranial, galeal-frontalis	
		Temporalis muscle	
	Regional		
		Pectoralis major	
		Trapezius	
		Others	
			Latissimus dorsi
			Sternocleidomastoid
			Omentum
			Deltopectoral
	Distant (free)		
		Latissimus dorsi	
		Rectus abdominis	
		Radial forearm	
		Others	
			Scapular/parascapular
			Omentum

because each coverage problem presents its own unique set of complicating factors.

When is soft tissue coverage needed? This decision-making process is one that requires discussion between the neurosurgeon and the plastic surgeon *prior* to the procedure. Even if it is not ultimately required, the patient is always apprised of the coverage alternatives and their attendant risks and complications in the preoperative consultation. Indications for soft tissue reconstruction are coverage, separation of cranial contents, and restoration of contour.

◆ Indications for Soft Tissue Reconstruction

1. Coverage of important structures (bone, neurovascular)
2. Separation of cranial contents and prevention of cerebrospinal fluid (CSF) leak
3. Restoration of contour (aesthetic considerations)

◆ Coverage of Important Structures

Some of the more commonly encountered reconstructive problems are coverage ones, particularly of exposed bone. Many but not all of these types of problems are best prevented by considering the underlying vasculature of the scalp and previous surgical incisions. Although primary wound closure of exposed cranial bone is usually possible due to its robust blood supply, disregard for the vascular anatomy of the scalp with subsequent scalp necrosis unnecessarily complicates a simple case and causes additional disfigurement.

The scalp has an amazing vascular supply and can be reliably elevated over long distances, even across the midline. Inclusion of a "named" vessel or one of its branches (occipital, posterior auricular, superficial temporal and to a lesser degree supratrochlear and supraorbital) in the elevated scalp only increases the probability of survival **(Fig. 82–1)**. Remember, revascularization of the entire scalp can potentially be accomplished with anastomosis of only one vascular pedicle! Poorly planned incisions and resultant scalp necrosis can usually be avoided.

If primary closure of the scalp is not possible, closure may be obtained with a "flap." A flap, unlike a "graft," carries its own blood supply with it rather than cannibalizing that blood supply from the recipient bed. Thus a flap is moved from one part of the body to another, remaining attached (local or regional flap), or detached and revascularized via microvascular anastomoses (free flap). The flaps can include skin, muscle, or a combination of the two (myocutaneous), as well as fat, fascia, and rarely bone.

When the skull is exposed and devoid of periosteum, local scalp rotation flaps are usually the best alternative. They are simple to design and rapidly executed **(Fig. 82–2)**. A named artery or its branch is included in the flap whenever possible. If the integrity of a vessel within the flap is in question, a Doppler can be utilized to map out its course. When a named artery is not included, the flap is designed with a wide base. The size of the defect dictates the flap size to be elevated, but the flap is always designed slightly larger and longer than necessary to avoid any possible tension on the flap (which only further compromises the blood supply). Scalp flaps tend to be "stiff" and noncompliant (especially if they have been previously elevated or irradiated) and have an obligatory "dog ear" at the pivot point of the flap. Although the donor site can be occasionally closed primarily or with a second smaller flap (especially when the donor site is in a more posterior location), a split-thickness

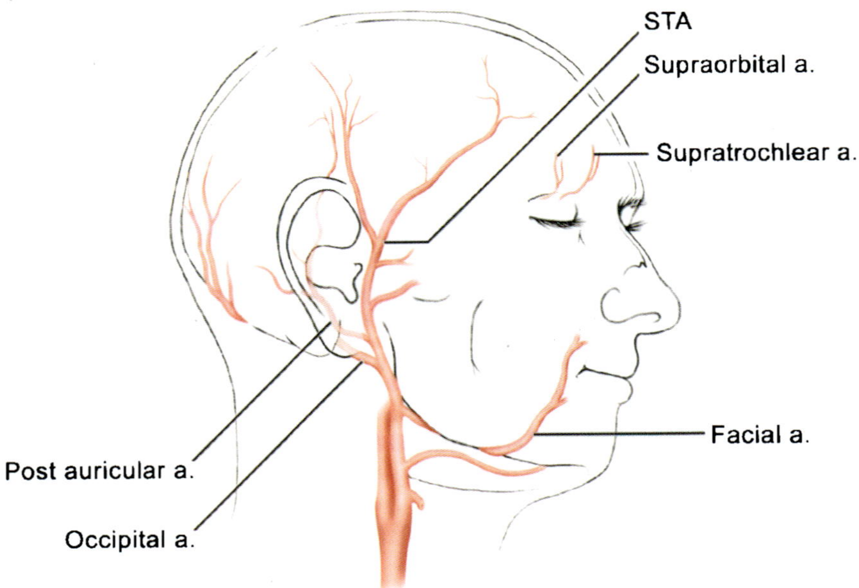

Figure 82–1 Vascular anatomy of the scalp. STA, superficial temporal artery.

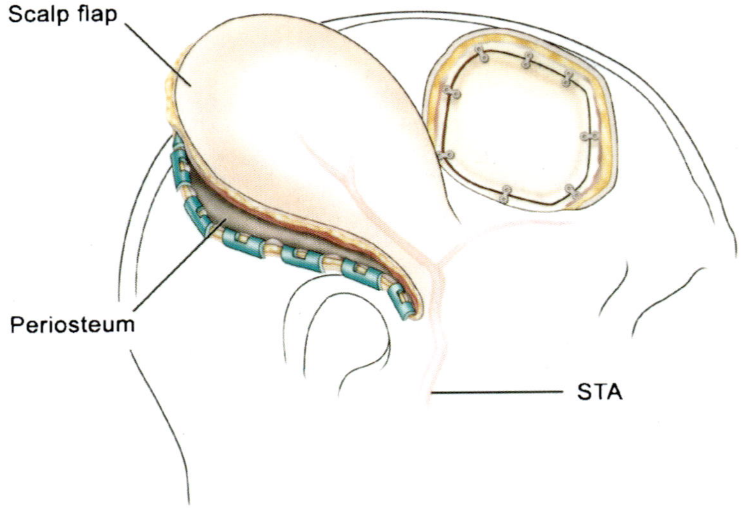

A

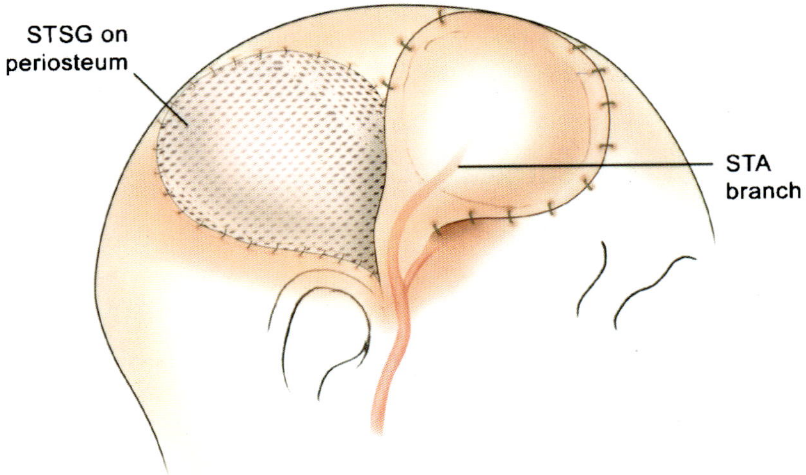

B

Figure 82–2 **(A)** Cranial defect with exposed bone devoid of periosteum. **(B)** Scalp rotation flap and split-thickness skin graft (STSG) covering the donor site. STA, superficial temporal artery.

skin graft placed on intact periosteum prevents tension on the flap and therefore maintains more reliable perfusion **(Table 82–2)**. These flaps are often very unaesthetic, however, because of the non–hair-bearing skin graft placed on the donor site. In some cases, this problem may be addressed later via tissue expansion of the remaining hair-bearing scalp. Intact periosteum must be maintained at the flap donor site because a split-thickness skin graft (STSG) will not take on cortical bone. Larger defects not amenable to local flap coverage and the more complex defects require regional or distant flap coverage.

Table 82–2 Principles of Local Scalp Flap Elevation

1. Know the vascular anatomy, and include a vessel in the flap.
2. Keep the base of the flap wide.
3. Construct the flap slightly larger and longer than anticipated.
4. Never place it under excessive tension.
5. Preserve the donor site periosteum so it can be covered with a skin graft rather than attempt primary closure.

◆ Prevention of Cerebrospinal Fluid Leak and Separation of Cranial Contents

The inability to separate the intradural space from the paranasal sinuses and oronasopharynx can result in CSF leaks and infection including osteomyelitis. Although consideration should be given to reconstruction of all the resected layers, bony reconstruction of the cranial base is rarely warranted. The added risk of nonvascularized bone in a contaminated bed is to be avoided. The goal should be the presence of a well-vascularized tissue (and therefore bacterial barrier) between the cranial contents and the surrounding contaminated paranasal sinuses and oropharynx. Additional vascularized tissue, therefore, is particularly important in anterior and middle cranial base defects.

If a watertight closure of the dura requires a patch (nonvascularized) at the site of a direct connection to the paranasal sinuses, then vascularized tissue should be used to overlie the nonvascularized dural patch. Local flaps (pericranial or galeal) are a simple reliable source, but they have limited reach and volume and may be unavailable due to previous surgery. The reach of regional flaps (pectoralis

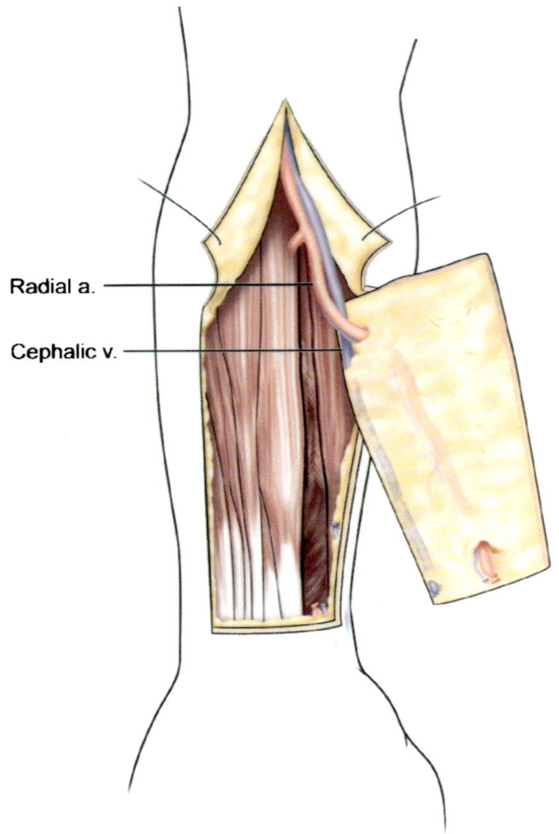

Figure 82–3 Radial forearm flap.

major and trapezius flaps) is limited in the cranial direction by the vascular leash. In the face of previous surgery or radiation or very large defects, distant (i.e., free flap) coverage is needed. Larger volume flaps (latissimus dorsi and rectus abdominis free flaps) are preferred for larger defects to eliminate dead space. Muscle flaps are particularly helpful in abnormally shaped narrow defects where the muscle easily contours to fit an irregularly shaped defect. In addition, the ability to reduce bacterial contamination using well-vascularized muscle is far superior to skin flaps.

For most cranial base defects a thin flap placed intracranially with a relatively large surface area is required for separation of the cranial from surrounding contaminated areas. No flap is more suited for this purpose than the radial forearm free flap **(Fig. 82–3).** It has a long pedicle that can reach from as far away as the neck vessels to the midline base of the anterior fossa. This flap of skin, subcutaneous tissue, and forearm fascia is pliable and can be tailored to cover a large, irregularly shaped surface area defect. Additionally, the large luminal diameter of the radial artery and venae comitantes make it easy to anastomose to a recipient vessel.

◆ Restoration of Contour

Although aesthetic appearance may be compromised because of more pressing functional considerations, it is always considered when choosing the type of tissue reconstruction. Smaller defects like the unwanted hollow that occurs behind the lateral orbital rim with transposition of the temporalis muscle can be addressed later in a secondary reconstructive procedure. If, however, a larger volume defect is created, the replacement tissue is tailored to fill the externally visible defect completely at the time of tissue resection. If the "filler" is primarily muscle, the defect is initially overcorrected to allow for volume loss (25 to 50%), which occurs secondary to denervation and secondary muscle atrophy. Not only is the volume replaced, but if specialized tissue (e.g., hair-bearing scalp) is needed, it is replaced with like tissue if available.

◆ Preoperative Studies

Although an angiogram may be required in particularly difficult cases (especially following multiple operations) and rarely to visualize the recipient artery for a free tissue transfer, the Doppler has largely supplanted the need for any preoperative studies.

◆ Surgical Technique

Anesthesia

These reconstructions are usually done at the time of tumor extirpation and therefore require endotracheal anesthesia. In the case of free tissue transfer, an aspirin suppository (325 mg) is administered just prior to the microvascular anastomosis to decrease platelet adhesion and theoretically reduce the incidence of thrombosis at the anastomotic site.

Flaps

Local Flaps

Pericranium

The combination of periosteum of the skull and its overlying loose connective tissue is collectively termed the pericranium. It provides a thin layer based anteriorly or laterally to cover anterior cranial defects. There are perforators from the galea and the two can be raised together to increase the reliability of the flap. Although it can be elevated as a random flap, the deep divisions of the supratrochlear and supraorbital vessels are included whenever possible. Pericranial flaps are more limited in scope and reliability than galeal-frontalis flaps, but they are excellent for smaller, more focal defects.

Galeal-Frontalis Flap

The galeal-frontalis flap **(Fig. 82–4)** is a dense, well-vascularized structure sandwiched between the frontalis muscle anteriorly and occipitalis muscle posteriorly and extends laterally as the superficial temporal fascia. It can be elevated as the continuation of the frontalis muscle and is particularly useful if placed in the floor of anterior cranial base

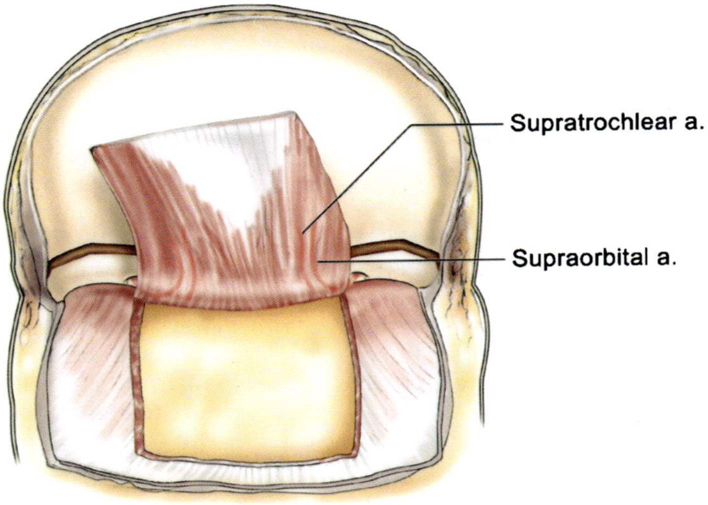

Figure 82–4 Galeal-frontalis flap.

defects to separate cranial from nasopharyngeal cavities. The robust blood supply is based on the supraorbital and supratrochlear vessels anteriorly, and laterally from the superficial temporal and posterior auricular vessels and posteriorly from the occipital vessels. The flap can be based on any of these vessels depending upon the location and size of the defect; however, because the need is greatest in the anterior cranial vault area, most are elevated on the supratrochlear and supraorbital vessels. The flap may have a wide base or if necessary a narrow pedicle so long as that pedicle contains the vessel. It provides a well-vascularized layer that can be easily contoured to cover odd-shaped defects. It provides no bulk, however, and therefore is of little use to fill defects.

Temporalis Muscle

The temporalis muscle is a relatively small muscle and therefore has limited use potential. It originates from the temporal fascia and inserts into the coronoid process. It has its own defined blood supply (deep temporal branch of the internal maxillary artery), which enters near the base of the muscle, and therefore it can be rotated around an arc to cover not only the orbit but some small intracranial defects. Its loss represents no functional deficit. It can be easily contoured to the defect dimensions.

Regional Flaps

When there is inadequate local tissue, regional flaps are considered. They have the advantage of being located away from the head and neck and therefore are often not subject to previous surgical trauma or radiation. The most commonly used flaps have muscle as a component of the flap, and the pectoralis major and trapezius are the workhorses. They rely on their skin extensions to reach the critical area to be covered, and, unfortunately, these areas are often unreliably perfused. In general, the pectoralis major myocutaneous flap (muscle and overlying skin) can be thought of as useful for the anterior and lateral reaches of the head and neck, and the trapezius myocutaneous flap for the posterior and lateral areas. As regional flaps, neither reaches the cranial base.

Pectoralis Major

Prior to the advent of microsurgery, the pectoralis major **(Fig. 82–5)** with its overlying skin extension was the flap used for most complex head and neck reconstructions. Due to the reliable vascular anatomy, it can be elevated rapidly

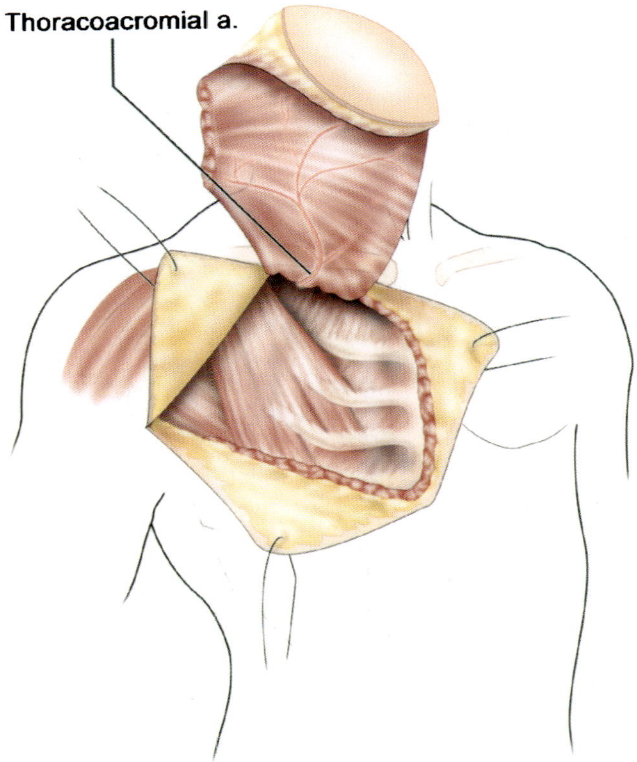

Figure 82–5 Pectoralis major flap.

and safely. The blood supply is based on a branch of the middle third of the axillary artery, the thoracoacromial artery. The vessels are adherent to the undersurface of the pectoralis in the clavipectoral fascia, which separates easily in a plane superficial to the pectoralis minor. The entire muscle can survive on this one vessel, which enables it to be "flipped" cranially over the clavicle. The length of the flap can be prolonged to reach the cranial base by including some of the upper portions of the anterior rectus fascia; however, any skin island extended beyond the muscle has a tenuous blood supply. Other disadvantages include its potential donor site morbidity, especially in women where the breast shape may be altered significantly due to excision of a medial skin paddle. These flaps are less reliable than free flaps, and the coverage distance is limited to the upper third of the lateral cranium. If the flap is brought subcutaneously beneath the neck skin, a large subcutaneous pocket must be created to prevent mechanical constriction of the muscle and death due to venous congestion. If it is not brought through a subcutaneous pocket, the pedicle must be divided at a second stage.

Trapezius Flap

The trapezius myocutaneous flap **(Fig. 82–6)** is used less frequently in part because there are fewer requirements for occipital and posterolateral regional flaps where this flap is especially useful. (There are no sinuses or oropharyngeal cavities posteriorly to be covered.) Although its arc of rotation can reach the skull base, it is a long reach. The muscle has multiple blood supplies and can be raised on the descending or ascending transverse cervical artery. The most commonly used and most reliable is the vertically oriented trapezius flap designed with a vertical axis centered between the cervical spine and the scapula. A surprisingly long flap can be reliably elevated to reach the skull base and upper portions of the posterolateral scalp. The upper fibers of the trapezius muscle must be left undisturbed to prevent a resultant shoulder drop. The donor site defect can be closed primarily. It is not the muscle that performs the needed coverage but the skin paddle overlying it. This thick skin paddle is difficult to shape to the dimensions needed to fill the contours of an irregular space. Other regional flaps are available, but they are farther away and more useful as free flaps (latissimus dorsi), are small (sternocleidomastoid), require entry into the abdominal cavity (omentum), or require a prior "delay" procedure (deltopectoral flap). They are a poor second choice.

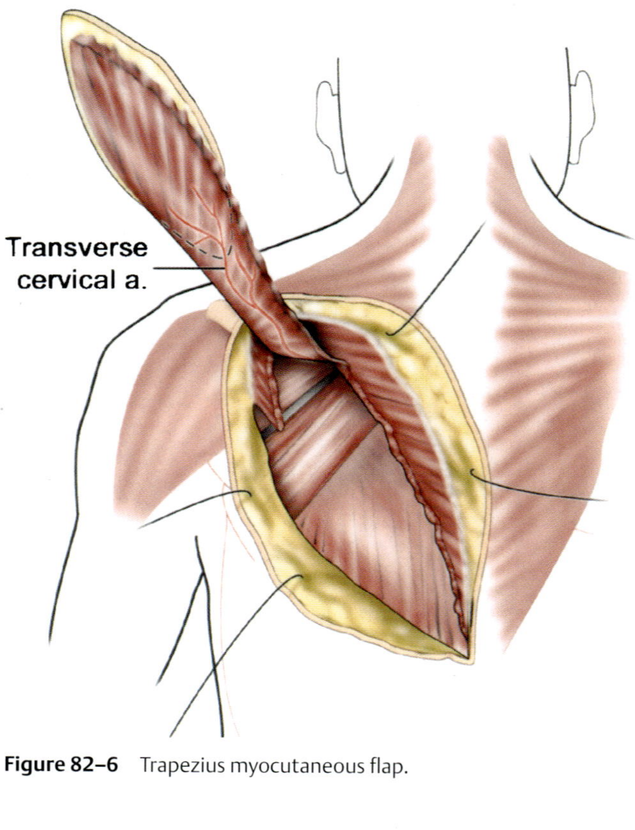

Figure 82–6 Trapezius myocutaneous flap.

Free Flaps

Although more conventional methods of reconstruction are always considered, free flaps have become the preferred method for reconstruction of large complex defects of the cranium, especially central cranial base defects that cross the midline. They are also the first choice for separation of the cranial cavity from the nasopharynx when pericranial or galeal-frontalis flaps do not reach or are no longer available. Occasionally, complex defects may require ingenious combinations of free and local or regional flaps to provide adequate reconstructions. Because their arc of rotation is essentially unlimited (except by the location of a nearby recipient artery and vein) free flaps are far more flexible in design. Large volumes of tissue can be transferred reliably. Success rates for free tissue transfer are greater than 95% at most centers. Free flaps are particularly advantageous because the muscle or fascia can be molded to plug defects of irregular shapes, and it is this portion of the flap rather than the poorly perfused distal skin extension of a regional flap that is used to reconstruct the defect.

Disadvantages of free flaps are prolonged operative time, need for special techniques, and the difficulty monitoring a "buried" flap (in the case of cranial base reconstruction). The choice of free flap may depend on surgeon expertise and preference, but the most commonly used free flaps for cranial defects are the ones that are also the most reliable and have the longest vascular pedicle. They are the rectus abdominis and the latissimus dorsi muscle flaps with or without overlying skin, the radial forearm flap, and the scapular and parascapular flaps to a lesser degree because of their short vascular pedicle and rigid nature of the skin island.

Advantages

1. Reliable
2. Massive volume
3. New well-vascularized tissue

Disadvantages

1. Time consuming
2. Special expertise

3. Donor site morbidity
4. Requires recipient vessels

In general, free flaps are chosen for larger defects and can be used to plug sizable, irregularly shaped holes. If significant amounts of overlying fat are included with the flap, they can be used for very large and deep surface defects to preserve overall contour. Muscle is also the tissue of choice in infected or heavily contaminated wounds and has been shown experimentally to reduce bacterial counts better then corresponding skin flaps. Myocutaneous free flaps, especially the latissimus dorsi and rectus abdominis, have long anatomically consistent vascular pedicles, making them ideal for deeply seated large defects. The most difficult reconstructive problems however, are the deeply placed cranial base defects, especially those near the midline. Here the passageway beneath the brain is narrow and tortuous and does not easily accommodate the bulk of a free myocutaneous flap.

Radial Forearm Flap

The radial forearm flap **(Fig. 82–3)** is ideally suited for the most difficult defects of the cranial base near and crossing the midline, and in previously irradiated patients. Its advantages are a long, vascular pedicle of sizable diameter and thin, pliable tissue that can be used to cover dural patches and separate cranial from nasopharyngeal cavities. It can be harvested in the supine position. Disadvantages are its donor site deformity. It does remove one of the two major vessels supplying the hand, and exposes tendons if the skin graft overlying them does not survive. It has supplanted the rectus abdominis free flap in cranial base reconstruction.

Rectus Abdominis Muscle

The rectus abdominis myocutaneous flap **(Fig. 82–7)** is the second most commonly used free flap for cranial base reconstruction. Because it is located anteriorly, it can be elevated while the extirpation is under way. Because there is no need to turn the patient for harvesting, the operative time is shorter than for the latissimus dorsi, which requires turning the patient to the lateral position. The overlying skin and fat are reliable if the flap is designed near the perforators around the umbilicus. It is ideal for contour defects because a large amount of fat can be included, which tends to plug defects and yet unlike muscle does not atrophy with time. If used to cover surface contour defects, however, significant weight fluctuations can result in over- or undercorrection of the contour abnormality. Its disadvantages are primarily related to the possibility of donor site hernia. In addition, its vascular pedicle is considerably shorter than the radial forearm flap.

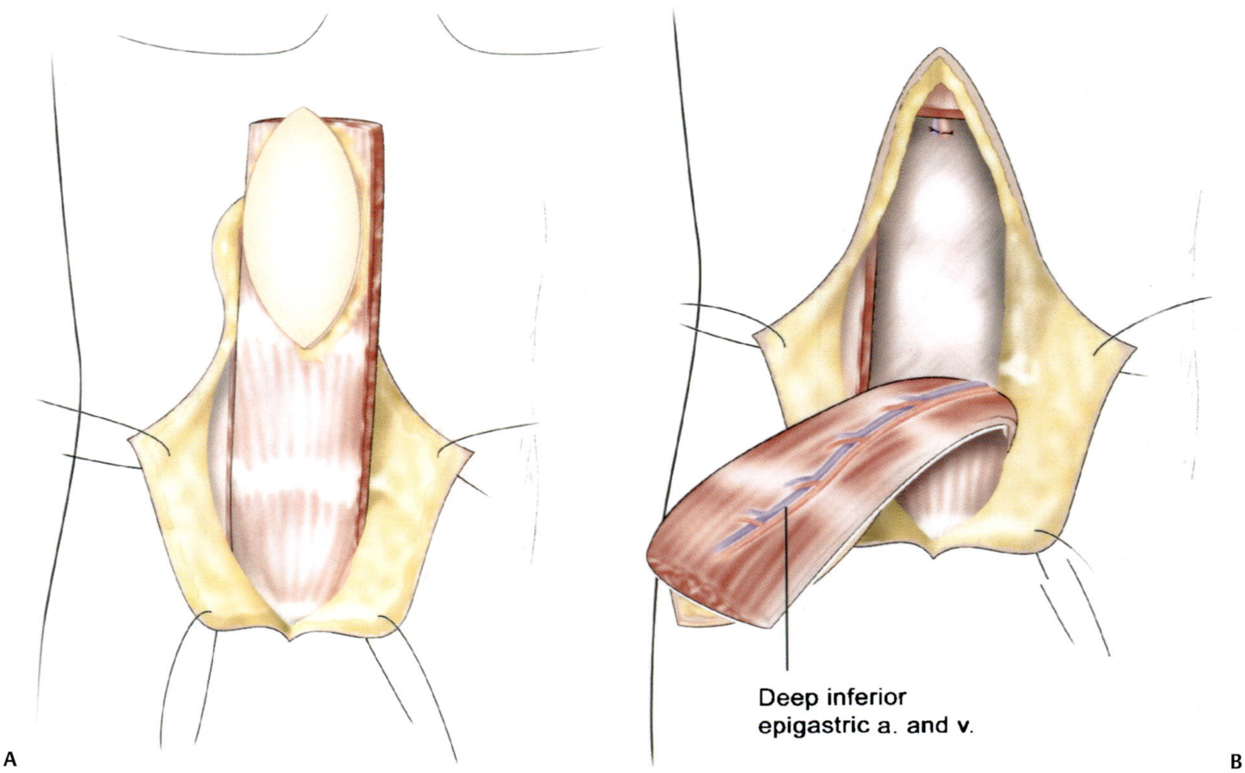

Figure 82–7 **(A)** Rectus abdominis myocutaneous flap. **(B)** The deep inferior epigastric artery on the undersurface of the muscle is the dominant blood supply.

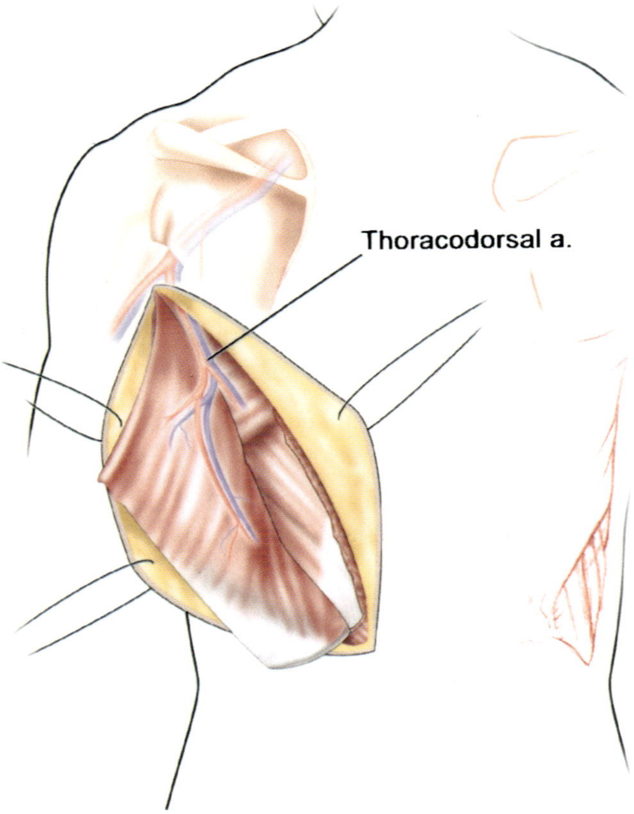

Figure 82–8 Latissimus dorsi flap.

Latissimus Dorsi

The latissimus dorsi **(Fig. 82–8)** is a large, flat muscle (and overlying skin island if necessary) that is particularly useful for large multidimensional defects of the scalp. The vascular pedicle is long and the vessels are of large caliber. There is minimal shoulder weakness when harvested and the donor site can be closed primarily. Because the patients must be positioned laterally for muscle harvest, the length of the procedure is increased. It is the choice for coverage of extremely large scalp defects, which are not amenable to local flap and split graft coverage.

Closure

If the primary indication for a flap is prevention of a CSF leak, then the proper insetting of the flap to fill dead space and separate sterile from contaminated areas is required. Meticulous attention to the closure is necessary and often difficult due to the need to operate in a deep space. Tacking sutures are placed at the margins, and if necessary, holes are drilled in the bone for placement. Mechanical constriction of the vascular pedicle results in venous congestion. Therefore, small amounts of bone are removed if necessary to accommodate the pedicle, and a temporary skin graft is preferred rather than primary closure if there is any concern about too much tension on the pedicle.

◆ Postoperative Care

Monitoring

The most common method of flap monitoring is visual inspection on an hourly basis for the first 24 hours. An assessment of the flap color, capillary refill, turgor, and temperature, and Doppler assessment of the vascular pedicle, are made by the physician or trained medical professional. If the flap is congested because of venous thrombosis or mechanical compression or twisting of the pedicle, the flap will be bluish in color, with a rapid capillary refill, swollen, and ultimately (but as a late sign) cold. The arterial Doppler pulse will still be present.

If the arterial anastomosis has thrombosed or if there is insufficient arterial input, the flap will be white, with little or no capillary refill, not swollen, and cold. The loss of Doppler signal distal to the anastomosis is usually the first sign of arterial obstruction. Once recognized, a return to the operating room for exploration is not only mandatory, it is urgent, to prevent flap necrosis. If the entire flap is buried in the cranial base, Doppler signals are the best way of monitoring the free flap but are less optimal than visual inspection. Although an angiogram may be used to determine patency, it is only needed for confirmation, not assessment.

◆ Complications

The most dreaded postoperative complication following reconstruction of complex cranial defects is flap necrosis. It is best prevented by proper planning, avoidance of any tension on the flap, especially the vascular pedicle, and postoperative monitoring. If it does necrose often, another flap can be harvested and transferred into the area. This second procedure is made more difficult by the postoperative edema. The coverage alternatives are usually fewer, and therefore a movement *up* a “rung” of the reconstructive ladder (i.e., more complicated alternative) is required.

Section XI

Management of Hydrocephalus

83

Using a Programmable Valve with a Hydrostatic Pressure Offset Device

Gary Magram

Programmable valves function as differential valves and are similar to fixed opening pressure valves. The major advantage is that they allow the physician noninvasively to change the valves' opening pressure. The technique of implantation is essentially the same as with conventional valves and only requires attention to a few details.

This chapter reviews the implantation of a programmable valve, the pathophysiological rationale for using a programmable valve with a hydrostatic offset device, and programming strategies.

A shunt is a device that diverts fluid from one body cavity to another. Cerebrospinal fluid (CSF) flows through a shunt from a higher pressure or level to a lower pressure or level. The rate at which CSF flows through a shunt is determined by the resistance of the shunt. A valve regulates both the direction of flow and whether the shunt is open or closed. Without a valve the intracranial pressure (ICP) and fluid level will equilibrate with the absorbing cavity's (peritoneal cavity, pleural cavity, or right atrium) fluid pressure and level. Physiologically the arachnoid villi function as valves with an opening pressure between the subarachnoid space and the intracranial venous sinuses. The normal ICP is approximately the intracranial venous sinus pressure (SP) plus the opening pressure of the arachnoid villi (OP_{av}), plus the CSF outflow resistance (R_o) times the CSF production ($Q_{csf.production}$) or

$$ICP = SP + OP_{av} + (R_o \times Q_{csf.production}).$$

Because the CSF outflow resistance is normally low, the ICP is mostly determined by the intracranial venous pressure and opening pressure of the arachnoid villi. In hydrocephalus the outflow resistance increases, making CSF production a contributing factor to ICP **(Fig. 83–1)**. Similarly, when a shunt is inserted the ICP eventually approaches the absorbing cavity pressure (P_{ac}) plus the shunt valves' opening pressures [the opening pressure of the programmable valve (OP_{pv}) plus the opening pressure of the hydrostatic offset device (OP_{hv})] or $ICP_{shunted} = P_{ac} + OP_{pv} + OP_{hv}$ **(Fig. 83–2)**.

A ventriculoperitoneal (VP) shunt diverts CSF from the ventricle to the peritoneum. When an individual with a VP shunt is supine, CSF layers on the dorsal aspect of the peritoneum.

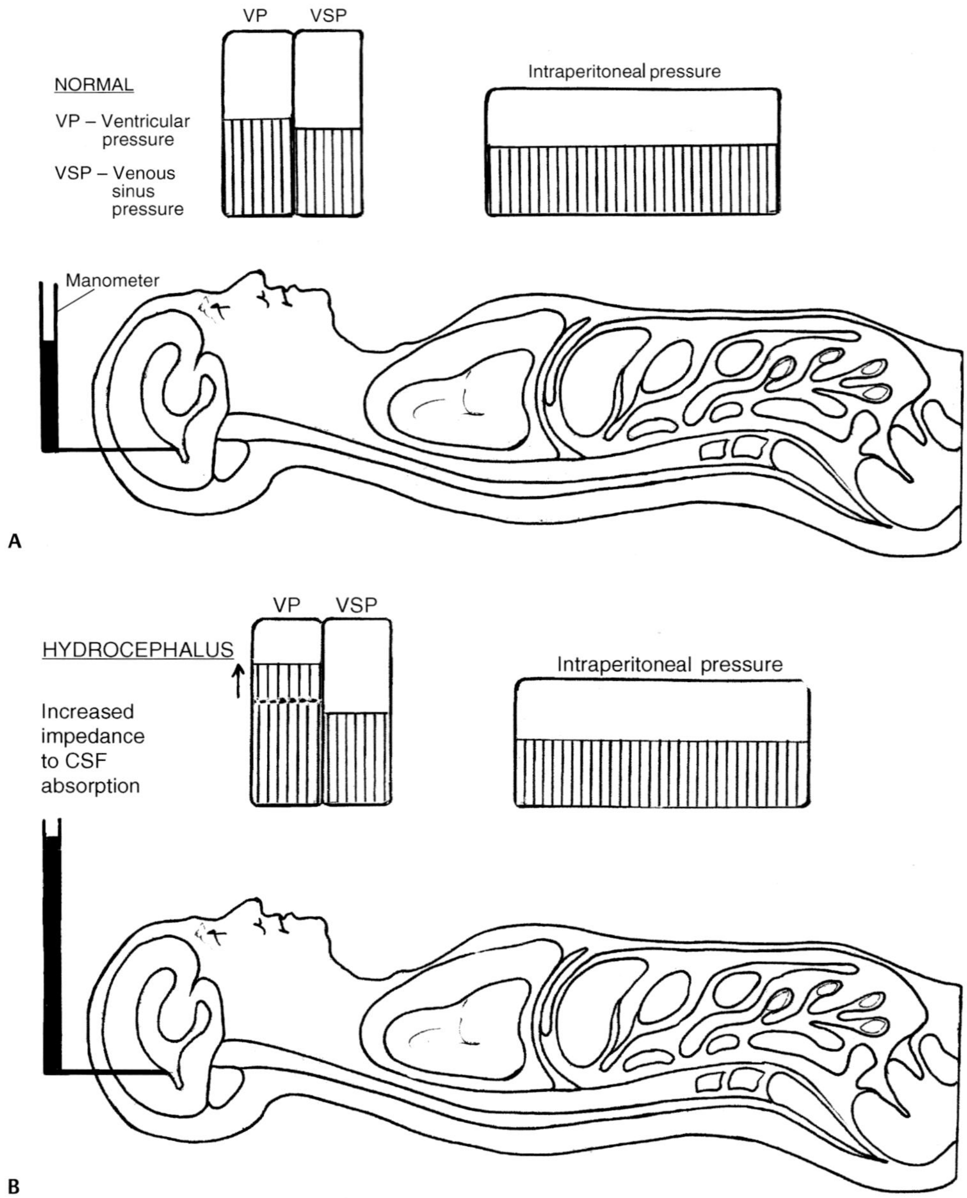

A

B

Figure 83–1 **(A)** Physiological differential pressures. In a healthy individual the ventricular pressure (VP) or intracranial pressure is slightly greater than the venous sinus pressure. In the horizontal position the venous sinus pressure on average exceeds the intraperitoneal pressure. **(B)** Hydrocephalus. Hydrocephalus is associated with an increased impedance to cerebrospinal fluid (CSF) absorption. The increased impedance requires a greater differential pressure between the ventricular pressure and the venous sinus pressure for CSF to be absorbed.

In the vertical position, CSF layers down into the pelvis. If no valve is present, then the intraventricular pressure (fluid level) tends to equilibrate with the peritoneal pressure (fluid level). The programmable valve's opening pressure influences the ICP in both the horizontal and vertical position. The target ICP (the estimated normal ICP after shunt insertion) is proportional (but not equal) to the peritoneal pressure plus the shunt valve's opening pressure.

The problems with selecting a valve's opening pressure are numerous. It is difficult to determine the optimal target ICP, the target ICP in a horizontal position is very different from the target ICP in a vertical position, and it is difficult to measure the intraperitoneal pressure. The vertical target ICP is significantly less than the horizontal target ICP. When vertical both CSF and blood tend to flow downward, lowering the ICP by 150 mm H_2O or more. The vertical target ICP is proportional to the peritoneal pressure plus the hydrostatic pressure difference between the ventricles and the peritoneum, plus the programmable valve's opening pressure plus any hydrostatic valves (gravity assistant, or gravity compensatory accessory [Integra, Plainsboro, NJ]) opening pressure **(Fig. 83–3).** A programmable vertically activated valve is not commercially available, making it necessary to reoperate on some patients to adjust their vertical valve opening pressure. This is especially problematic as a child grows and in a chronically shunted patient who is used to a low vertical ICP.

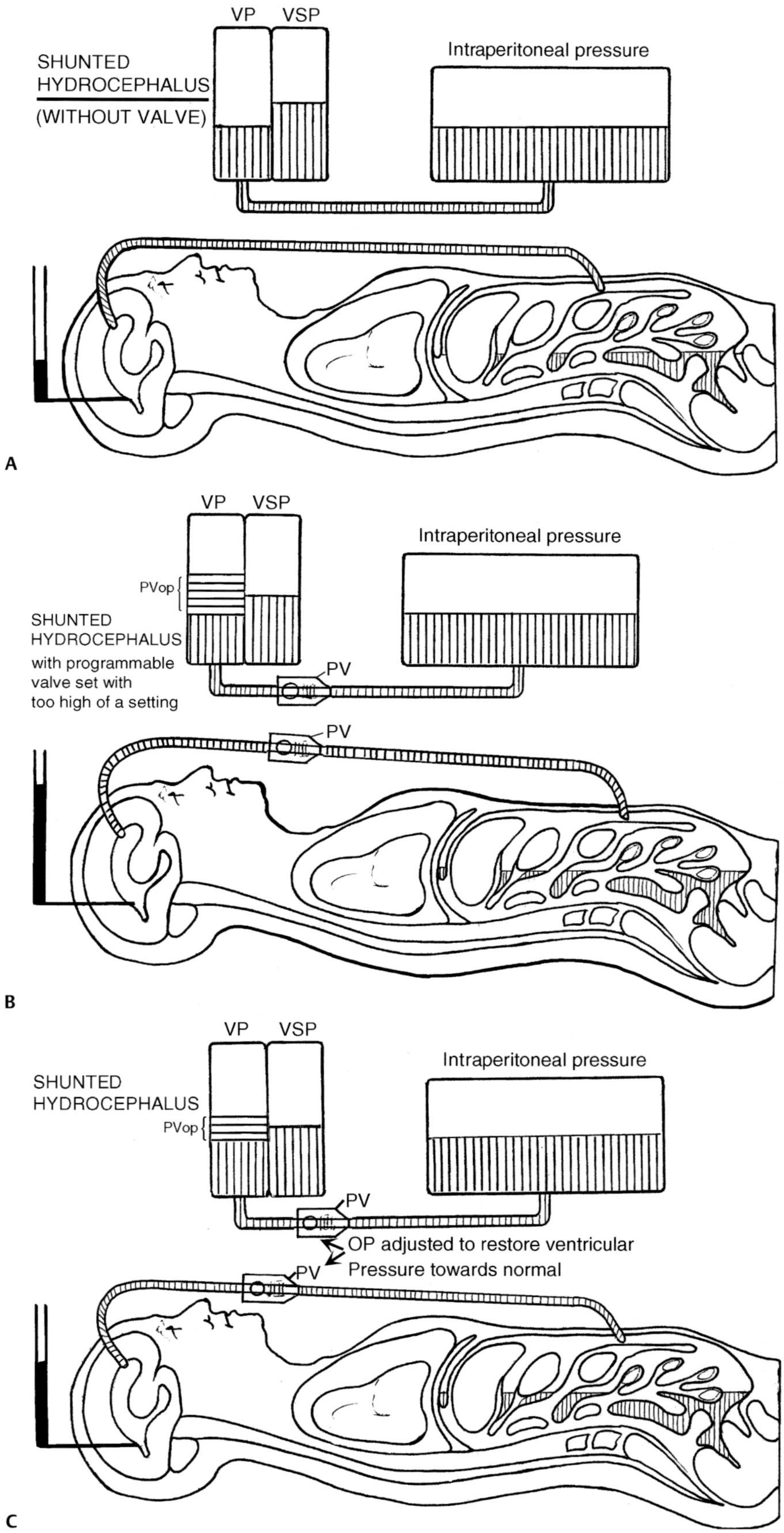

Figure 83–2 **(A)** A ventricular pressure (VP) shunt without a valve. A valveless shunt allows the ventricular pressure to equilibrate with the lower intraperitoneal pressure. Overdrainage can result in the ventricular pressure becoming lower than the venous sinus pressure. **(B)** Shunted hydrocephalus with a programmable valve set at too high of a setting (PV_{op} too high). **(C)** Reprogrammed valve. Decreasing the programmable valve's opening pressure adjusts the shunt, lowering the ventricular pressure toward normal. VSP, Venous sinus pressure.

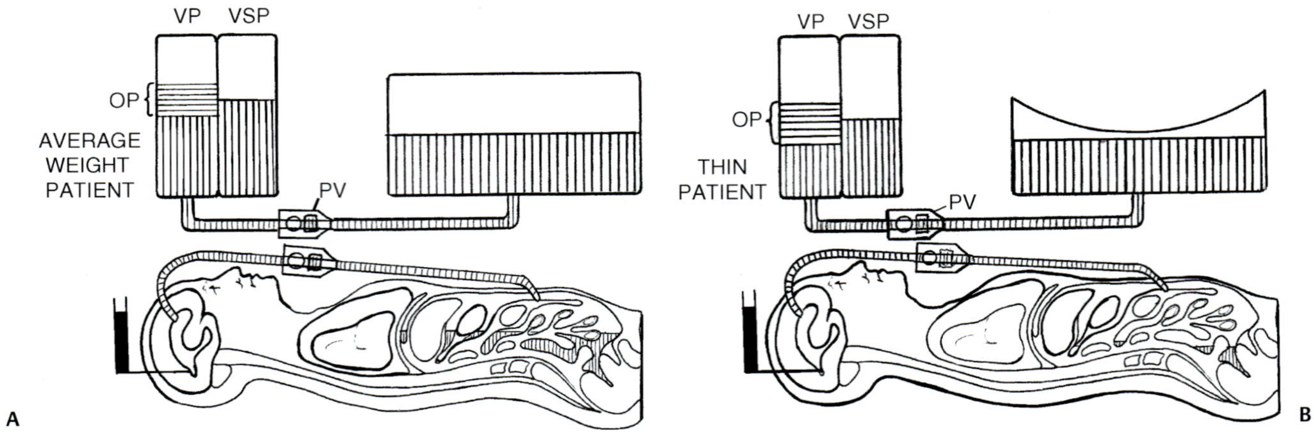

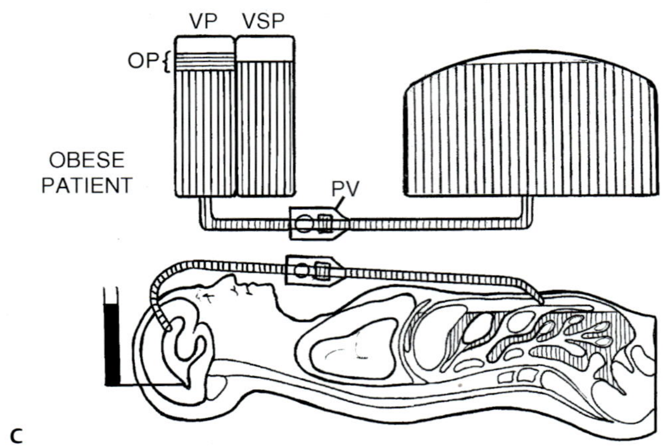

Figure 83–3 Adjusting the programmable valve's opening pressure to compensate for patients with different intraperitoneal pressures. **(A)** A patient of average weight. **(B)** A thin patient has a lower intraperitoneal pressure and may require a slightly higher opening pressure setting than **(C)** an obese patient. OP, opening pressure; PV, programmable valve.

An individual patient's need for CSF diversion can change over time and it is very difficult to predict with accuracy the optimal valve opening pressure for any particular patient. Although many patients tolerate a variety of opening pressures due to healthy compensatory mechanisms or a normal intracranial compliance, some patients have an altered compliance and can be sensitive to small changes in the valve's opening pressure. Because it is not possible to predict which patients are going to require a change in their valve's opening pressure, programmable valves are being used with greater frequency.

For many patients the target ICP is not their ideal ICP (the ICP at which they are least symptomatic and are able to optimally function). Although it might be possible to bring the ICP within a normal range with a conventional nonprogrammable valve, many patients' ICP can be optimized (symptoms minimized) by using a programmable valve.

◆ Implantation

The programmable valve needs to be implanted in a location that will facilitate easy reprogramming and imaging. A strong magnet placed directly over the valve can potentially change the valve's setting. The magnet for a vagal nerve stimulator and for a cochlear implant should be kept away from the valve. Therefore, it is preferable to implant a programmable valve on the side opposite a cochlear implant. Because the valves are differential pressure valves, they potentially can be implanted at any level between the ventricular catheter and the distal cavity insertion site. If a Medtronic Strata valve (Jacksonville, FL) is used, the Delta chamber (Medtronic Neurologic Technologies, Goleta, CA) needs to be positioned at about the level of the proximal openings into the ventricular catheter. Placing a Strata valve above these openings will increase the pressure required to open the Delta chamber. Placing a Strata valve below these openings results in a hydrostatic column of fluid above the valve, making it easier for the Delta chamber to open, negating its effectiveness as a siphon regulatory device.

Placing a programmable valve on the side of the head facilitates both imaging and programming. The Codman Hakim programmable valve (CHPV) (Codman, Raynham, MA) can be used for a lumbar peritoneal shunt as well as placed over the chest if there is a problem with placing it under the scalp. Programmable valves should be placed over a bony surface so that when a programmer is placed over the valve the valve doesn't get pushed inward. The magnetic strength of the programmer falls off dramatically over a slight distance (by the fourth power of the distance). Therefore, if the patient has a lot of adipose tissue between the skin and the valve or if the valve is placed deep in the neck or in the soft tissues over the flank, then the valve can be very difficult to program.

◆ Selecting a Configuration

The configuration of the valve is largely a matter of surgeon preference. A valve with a pumping chamber is designed for use in a ventriculoatrial shunt. The pumping chamber has two one-way valves that allow for flushing out the atrial catheter and preventing aspiration of blood into the catheter when the pumping chamber is released. The pumping chamber allows for sampling of CSF by means of a shunt tap, but the pressure recorded from a shunt tap is the ICP minus the valve's opening pressure. Also it is not possible to inject a medication or contrast into the ventricular catheter by means of the pumping chamber because there are one-way valves on either end of the pumping chamber. Therefore, the valves with a pumping chamber are also available with a prechamber. The prechamber can be used for sampling CSF, measuring the pressure in the ventricular catheter, or injecting a medication or contrast agent into the ventricle. These cylindrical valves can be easily twisted and placed upside down during implantation. There is a black dot on the side that should face out over the distal antireflux valve. During implantation careful attention needs to be given to ensure that this black dot is facing outward.

Valves with in-line reservoirs just proximal to the programmable valve are easy to identify for tapping and programming. Most neurosurgeons are familiar with this configuration. Because valves with in-line reservoirs are shorter in length than the cylindrical valve with a pumping chamber and prechamber, they can be more easily placed posteriorly, if a parietal or occipital approach is used.

Antibiotic-impregnated catheters are now available (Codman's Bactiseal catheters). Because these catheters contain medications, they have expiration dates requiring them to be packaged separately from the valves. Antibiotic-impregnated catheters should be opened immediately prior to implantation and should not be soaked. Soaking the catheters results in the antibiotic being released into the solution. After these catheters are implanted, any fluid that is aspirated from the distal catheter will have a slight orange tinge as the rifampin dissolves into the CSF. The catheters maintain a fairly high concentration of antibiotic immediately adjacent to the plastic for about 4 weeks. This is one of their advantages over IV prophylactic antibiotics.

Valves with integral connectors are designed to be used with these antibiotic-impregnated catheters. Otherwise, if a valve with an integrated distal catheter is used, it is necessary to cut off the distal catheter and interpose a straight connector to attach an antibiotic-impregnated catheter.

◆ Programming the Valve Prior to Implantation

It is a common practice to open the valve and soak it in an antibiotic solution prior to implantation. With programmable valves it is recommended that the valve be programmed in the package prior to implantation. When the operating room (OR) staff is unfamiliar with programmable valves, it helps to mention to the circulating nurse that the valve needs to be programmed in its package prior to the package being opened. It is not necessary to soak the valves nor is it recommended. The valves do not require any testing, and opening the package just prior to implantation might lessen the risk of contamination.

Two types of devices are available to offset the hydrostatic column of CSF that increases the differential pressure across a shunt when a patient is in a vertical position. One is a gravity compensatory accessory and the other is a gravity or shunt assistant. Both need to be oriented in a vertical position and are preferably placed in the subcutaneous shunt tract over the chest. They can be placed anywhere along the distal tubing and are sometimes placed under the scalp. If they are placed in a cranial caudal direction under the scalp behind an ear, the valve might be inappropriately activated or deactivated if the patient looks up or down. If the patient is standing and looks up or down, the valve will be deactivated if the patient looks up or down, and if the patient is supine and flexes the neck, the device will be inappropriately activated. The gravity compensatory accessory requires an additional incision, whereas the gravity assistant can often be fastened into the distal tubing and pulled down the shunt tract. Both devices have arrows, and careful attention needs to be given to make sure that they are inserted in the proper direction. A disadvantage of these devices is that they tether the distal shunt in the subcutaneous tissues. In a growing child this can be problematic and can contribute to a shunt disconnection. The distal tubing proximal to the chest valve can be lengthened when a child outgrows the hydrostatic offset valve and needs to have one of higher opening pressure inserted.

◆ Selection of the Initial Opening Pressure

Programmable valves are used to attempt to adjust the flow rate of CSF through the shunt to match a patient's requirements for CSF diversion. The shunt flow rate required to restore the intracranial fluid dynamics toward normal depends not only on the degree to which the CSF circulation is impaired but also on numerous individual parameters. These parameters include the patient's age, compliance, height, weight, chronicity of hydrocephalus, degree of macrocephaly, ventricular size, and sensitivity to pressure changes.

The flow rate through the valve is related to the differential pressure across the valve and resistance of the tubing. The resistance of the tubing can be decreased by shortening the tubing but once implanted remains constant. The differential pressure across the valve is related to the intraventricular pressure, the valve's opening pressure, and the absorptive receptacle pressure. A patient with a partial CSF circulatory impairment might require a limited quantity of CSF to be diverted through the shunt because some of the CSF can still circulate and be absorbed through natural pathways at a normal ICP. A patient with an almost complete obstruction requires almost all of the CSF that is produced to be diverted through the shunt. In most circumstances it is impossible to determine the extent of CSF circulatory impairment. Therefore, it is not possible to predict prior to implantation the quantity of CSF that needs to be diverted through a shunt. Having a shunt with a fixed flow rate to match the estimated adult CSF production rate results in an excess of CSF being diverted in the majority of cases, and especially in young children.

Even more complicated are the numerous physiological changes [changes in intraabdominal pressure from supine to sitting or standing, intracranial venous pulse pressure changes secondary to respiration, intracranial arterial pressure changes during rapid eye movement (REM) sleep, etc.] that are taking place in individual patients over time and the changes in their pathology (scar formation, absorption of blood products, opening up of alternative CSF absorptive pathways, acquired aqueductal stenosis) that alter their requirements for CSF diversion. For these reasons, having a programmable valve that can have the flow rate increased by lowering the valve's opening pressure or have the flow rate decreased by increasing the opening pressure is beneficial.

It is not possible to accurately predict the ICP that results after inserting a valve with a particular opening pressure. However, the change in the ICP that results from a change in the valve's opening pressure setting directly correlates with the magnitude of the change in the valve's opening pressure setting. An estimate of the ICP in the horizontal position can be made by adding the supine absorbing receptacle pressure (intraperitoneal pressure in the case of a VP shunt) to the valve's opening pressure **(Fig. 83–2)**. An estimate of the ICP in the vertical position (ICP_v) can be made by subtracting the hydrostatic column of fluid that forms in the shunt when vertical (HP) from the valve's programmable valve (PV_{op}) plus hydrostatic offset device (HV_{op}) opening pressures plus the vertical absorbing receptacle or cavity pressure (P_{ac}):

$$ICP_v = PV_{op} + HV_{op} + P_{ac} - HP$$

Initial Intraventricular Pressure

The higher the preshunt intraventricular pressure, the lower the patient's compliance and the greater the drop in intraventricular pressure from a limited flow rate. Programming the valve to a higher setting limits the flow through the shunt and allows a gradual change in the ICP.

Patient's Age

The central nervous system's CSF circulation changes significantly with age and especially during the first several years of life and in old age. The presence of an open fontanel increases the cranial compliance. An infant's brain has a high water content and is more compliant. As the lipid content of the brain increases with maturation, the brain's compliance decreases. The CSF production rate increase as the brain grows, changing the necessary flow rate through a shunt as the brain grows. As a child matures, so do the arachnoid villi, allowing for greater CSF absorption. Therefore, the shunt flow rate that is optimal during infancy is unlikely to be optimal as the child matures. A programmable valve allows adjustments to be made to titrate the shunt's flow rate to the growing child's needs.

An elderly patient with an atrophic brain has a decreased intracranial compliance, and a lower CSF production rate, both requiring a shunt with a lower flow rate.

Height

The greater the height of the patient, the greater the hydrostatic component contributing to CSF flow when the patient is in a vertical position. Infants spend the majority of time in a horizontal position. When a child begins to sit up and later when the child begins to walk, hydrostatic changes begin to increase the differential pressure across the valve during the vertical position. Therefore, as children grow, they not only increase in height but they also spend a greater duration of the day in a vertical position. One alternative is to increase the valve's opening pressure to compensate for the hydrostatic increase in differential pressure. Another alternative is to insert a siphon regulatory device or hydrostatic offset device.

Adding a gravity assistant to a programmable valve minimizes the adjustment needed to compensate for changes in position **(Fig. 83-4)**. As a general guide, a 00/10 gravity accessory is used in newborns, a 00/15 in infants, a 00/20 in children, a 00/25 in shorter adults, a 00/30 in average adults, and a 00/35 in taller adults. A more accurate method is to measure the hydrostatic column that develops when going from a horizontal to a vertical position.

Cerebrospinal Fluid Outflow Resistance

Hydrocephalus results from interference with the circulation of water in the central nervous system (CNS). The degree to which the ventricles enlarge and the pressure increases is determined by the CSF outflow resistance and the CNS compliance. The greater the outflow resistance, the greater the intraventricular pressure. And for a given outflow resistance, the greater the compliance, the larger the ventricles.

The greater the CSF production rate, the greater the force or pressure required for the CSF to flow out or be absorbed. Therefore, if the production rate is lowered (i.e., by acetazolamide) the ICP is also lowered for any given outflow resistance. A shunt "short circuits" the system or provides an alternative pathway for the CSF outflow. As the flow through the shunt is decreased (by increasing the valve's opening pressure) the flow through the natural outflow pathway increases. The pressure that it takes for the CSF to flow through the natural pathways without a shunt is the outflow resistance pressure (B in **Fig 83-1**). This pressure is also the limit to which the ICP will rise if a shunt is turned off. If the outflow resistance pressure is less than the shunt's opening pressure the CSF produced will flow through the natural pathways, and further increases in the valve's opening pressure will not result in any further elevation in the ICP.

For example, the outflow resistance pressure for a patient with normal pressure hydrocephalus (NPH) is only slightly above normal. In NPH if the valve's opening pressure setting is too high, the ICP remains normal and there is little or no flow through the shunt. A patient with a complete obstructive hydrocephalus has a markedly elevated outflow resistance pressure. In this situation, if the valve's opening pressure setting is too high the ICP will be elevated with almost all of the CSF still flowing through the shunt.

Weight

The more obese the patient, the greater the intraperitoneal pressure and therefore the lower the differential pressure across the valve. To achieve a higher flow rate through a shunt in an obese patient, the valve's opening pressure needs to be lowered. If a patient loses a significant amount of weight, then the intraperitoneal pressure can decrease, requiring an increase in the valve's opening pressure setting **(Fig. 83–3).**

Pregnancy

During the third trimester of pregnancy the intraperitoneal pressure can increase, resulting in underdrainage when the patient is horizontal and the development of headaches. Decreasing the valve's opening pressure may help relieve the headaches. Another alternative is to insert a ventriculopleural shunt in women of childbearing age.

Chronicity

Many of the compensatory changes that the CNS can make occur slowly, and cannot occur rapidly after a shunt is inserted. For instance, a sudden decrease in CSF volume may not be able to be compensated for by an expansion of the extracellular fluid compartment (expansion of the brain). Starting out with a high opening pressure setting and gradually decreasing the valve's opening pressure setting might allow for a gradual expansion of the extracellular fluid compartment (brain expansion). Similarly, many patients who have been chronically shunted with fixed opening pressure valves develop compensatory changes for the very low ICP (in some up to −400 mm H_2O pressure) that can occur when they are in a vertical position. Patients used to such low vertical ICPs can become symptomatic if a hydrostatic offset device is inserted. Therefore, the target ICP for a chronically shunted patient can differ significantly from that of a patient undergoing an initial shunt insertion.

Ventriculomegaly and Macrocephaly

Both ventriculomegaly and macrocephaly require a limited and gradual increase in CSF diversion through the shunt. This allows for the gradual compensatory changes to occur,

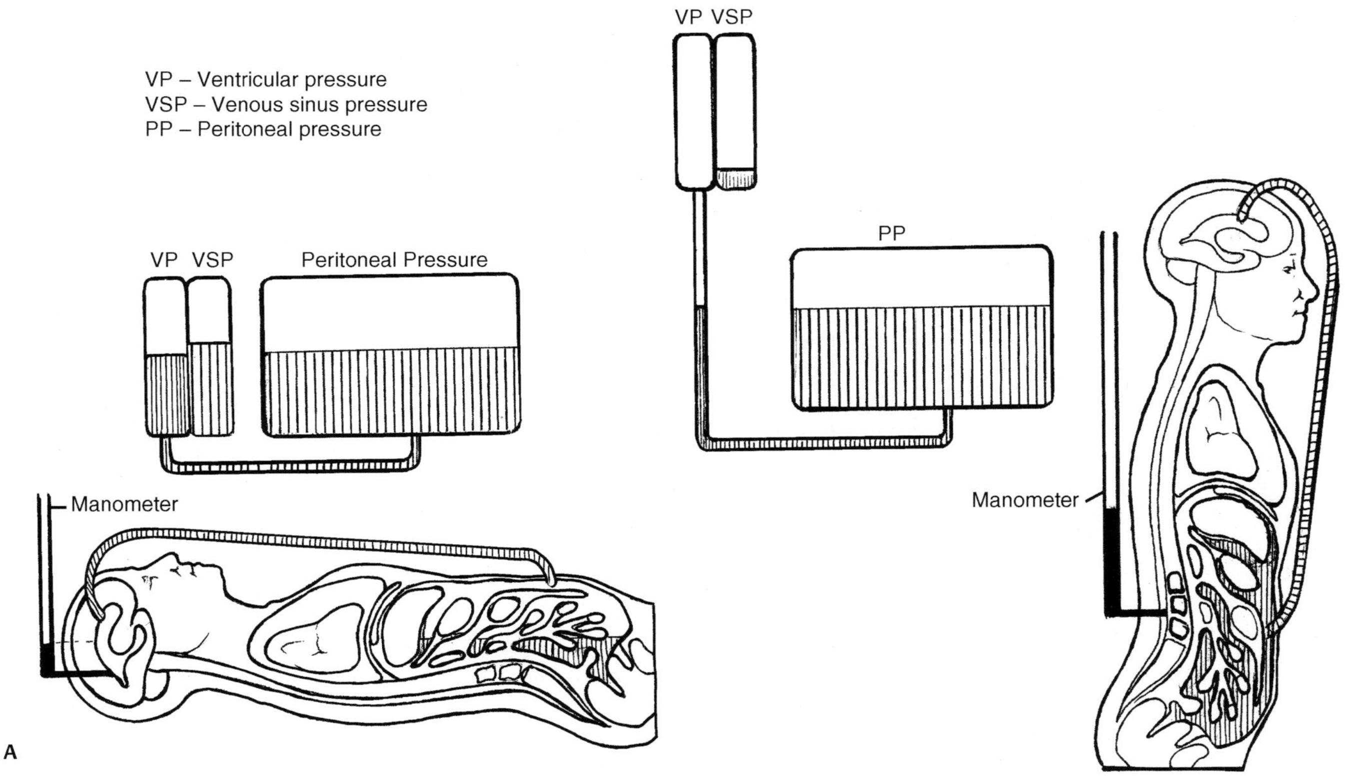

Figure 83–4 Positional changes. **(A)** Going from a horizontal to a vertical position with a valveless shunt results in the ventricular pressure (VP) falling to the lower level of the peritoneum.

(Continued on page 962)

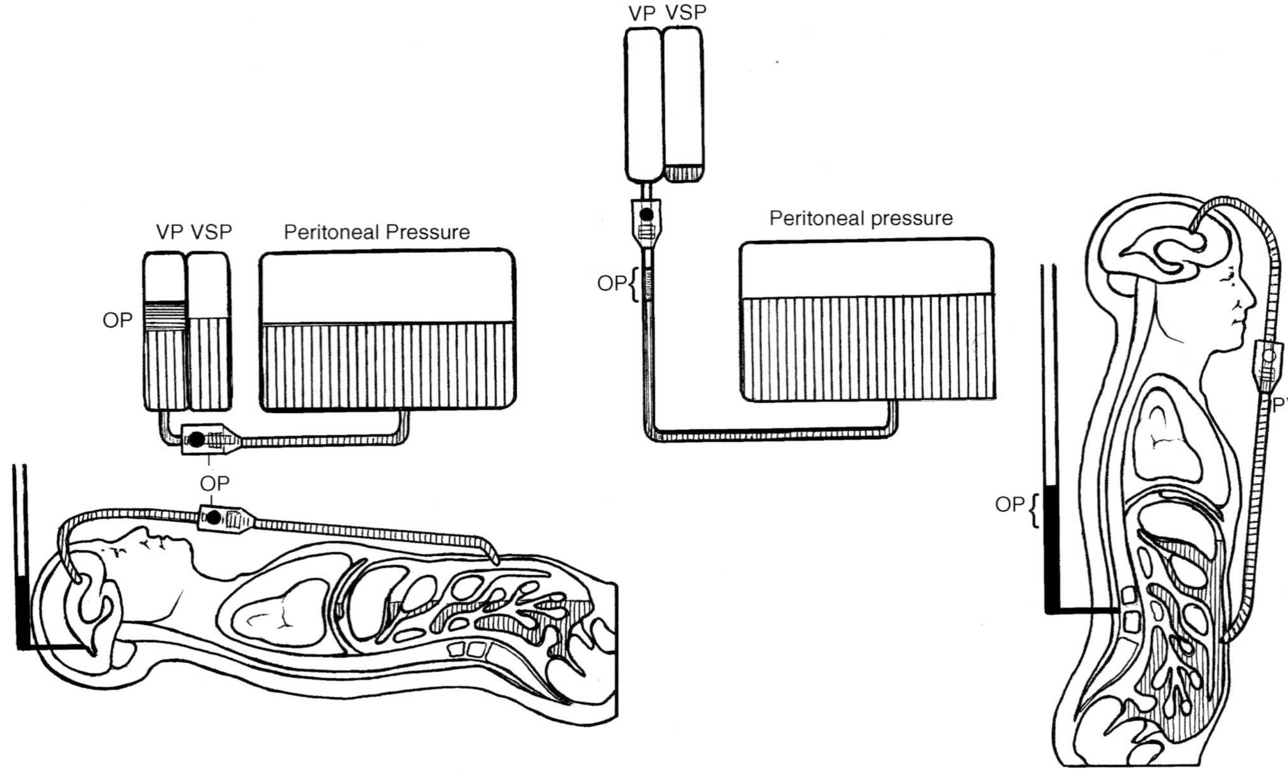

B

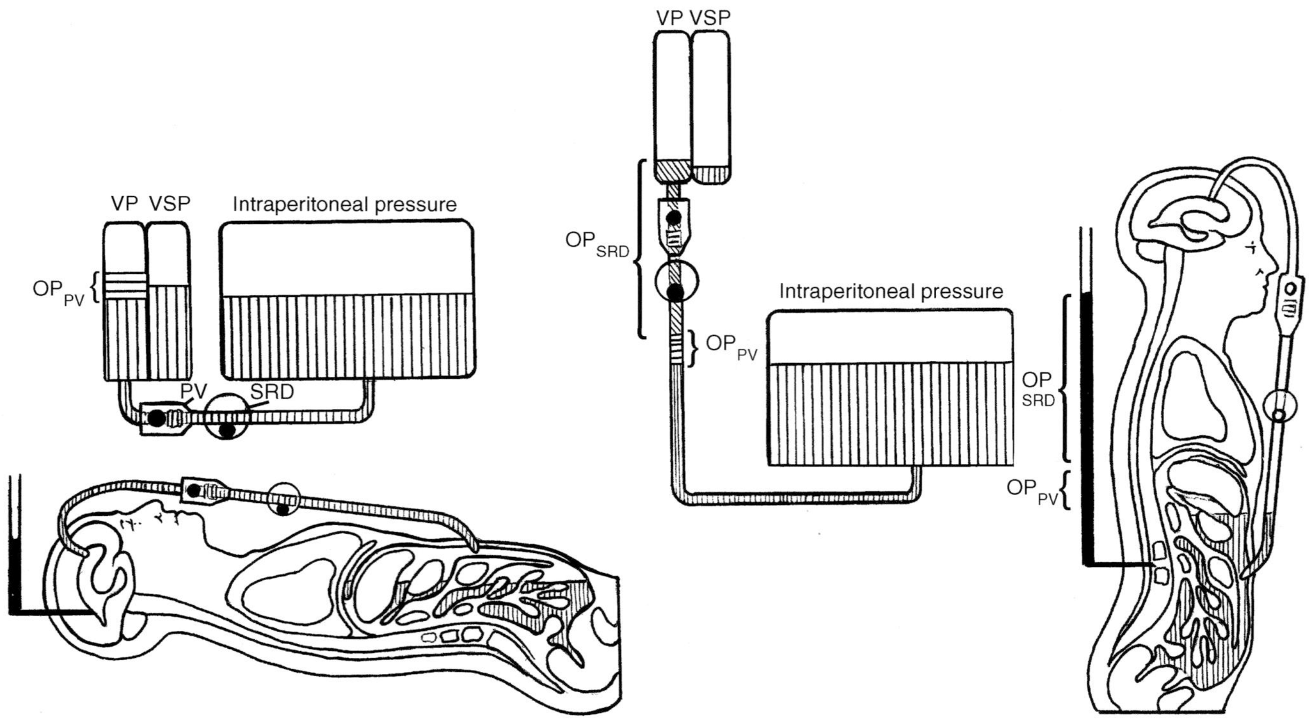

C

(Continued) **Figure 83–4** **(B)** A programmable valve increases the VP by the valve's opening pressure setting in both a horizontal and a vertical position. A setting that normalizes the VP in the horizontal position might be insufficient to compensate for the lower level of the peritoneum in the vertical position. **(C)** A siphon regulatory device increases the opening pressure in the vertical position but not in the horizontal position. VSP, Venous sinus pressure.

such as expansion of the extracellular space, the gradual growth of a child's brain, or a decrease in the cranial volume. The cranial volume can decrease in an infant by the sutures overriding and in an older child or adult by thickening of the calvarium.

Compliance

Compliance is the change in volume that results from a given change in pressure. A highly compliant nervous system readily stores and releases fluid, whereas a nervous system with a limited compliance takes a great deal of force to change its volume. A system with limited compliance has an elevated intracranial pulse pressure. The pulse pressure is elevated because it takes a much greater force to change the intracranial blood volume during systole and promote cerebral perfusion. A greater pulse pressure or lower compliance results in a greater flow rate through a valve when the valve is open.

When a valve is open the flow rate is inversely proportional to the shunt's resistance. Most shunts come with a 1.2 mm internal diameter distal catheter that offers very little resistance to the flow of CSF (especially at low flow rates of less than 20 mL per hour). With a low resistance catheter when the differential pressure across the shunt exceeds the valve's opening pressure, then the flow permitted through the shunt can far exceed the CSF production rate. Increasing the shunt's resistance to flow can significantly decrease the flow through the shunt. Increasing resistance can be accomplished by using a catheter with a smaller internal diameter and greater length or by using a valve with a siphon guard (Codman). A siphon guard essentially increases the resistance by 10-fold whenever the siphon guard is activated. A patient with a siphon guard, therefore, drains 10 times less fluid than a standard programmable shunt when the flow rate through the shunt is sufficient to activate the siphon guard.

Because there are so many parameters that interplay in determining flow through a shunt, it is not possible to precisely select the optimal opening pressure for a particular patient. A strategy of optimizing the valve's setting or programming the valve based on clinical circumstance is outlined below.

◆ Indications for Changing the Opening Pressure

Not only is it necessary to change the valve's opening pressure to optimize the shunt's initial flow rate but as a patient's requirements for CSF diversion change, it is of benefit to be able to noninvasively change the valve's opening pressure. There is no simple universal strategy for changing the opening pressure. The decision of how much and how often to change a valve's setting depends on an integration of three factors: the clinical setting, imaging findings, and ICP. In general changes should not exceed 40 mm H_2O pressure within a 24-hour period unless the patient is under close observation and in a setting where urgent readjustments can readily take place.

Clinical Indications

Headaches, dizziness, fatigue, nausea, and bradyphrenia are some of the common clinical indications for changing the valve's opening pressure. These symptoms can be associated with either over- or underdrainage. Most commonly a severe headache with nausea and vomiting is associated with underdrainage and a need for lowering the opening pressure. Symptoms of fatigue, dizziness, and chronic, less intense headaches with a preference for resting in bed are associated with overdrainage and a need for increasing the opening pressure of the valve. The easiest method to distinguish between over- and underdrainage is to measure the ICP, which generally requires a shunt tap unless the patient has an implanted TeleSensor (Radionics, Dublin, Ireland). The difference between the measured opening intraventricular pressure and the desired intraventricular pressure is then calculated. This difference closely approximates the required change in the valve's setting. For instance, if an obese patient has a shunt tap pressure of 150 mm H_2O in the horizontal position and the programmable valve is set at 120, then the valve might have to be reprogrammed to 80 to bring the intraventricular pressure down to 110.

If a patient has spontaneously restored the normal CSF circulation and no longer needs a shunt, then the shunt can be leading to low pressure symptoms and the ICP will remain abnormally low until the shunt is essentially turned off.

◆ Imaging Studies

If a shunt is overdraining, then either the brain will expand as extracellular fluid is retained, or extracerebral collections will form if the ventricles collapse and the brain is unable to expand sufficiently to compensate for the change in intracranial CSF volume. In an infant or growing child, extracerebral collections can spontaneously resolve as the brain grows, the sutures override, or the skull thickens. If a child with extracerebral collections is asymptomatic and the promotion of cortical expansion is a goal, then the valve might be left at a low setting or have the setting increased only slightly. In an adult, and especially in an elderly individual or a patient who has encephalomalacia, a radiated brain, or atrophy, extracerebral CSF collections are prone to bleed and place the patient at significant risk for developing a symptomatic acute subdural hematoma. Therefore, extracerebral collections in these patients are treated more aggressively by increasing the valve's setting.

◆ Shunt Strategies

Infant with Congenital Hydrocephalus

Infants normally have a lower ICP and a greater compliance due to the presence of open sutures and fontanels. They also spend the majority of the day in a horizontal position. A higher intracranial compliance results in a lower intracranial pulse pressure. The flow through the valve is proportional to the differential pressure across the valve [inflow pressure (intraventricular pressure + hydrostatic pressure) − outflow pressure (opening pressure of the valve + absorbing receptacle pressure)] and inversely proportional to the resistance of the shunt. Therefore, a lower intraventricular pressure requires a lower valve opening pressure setting to obtain the same flow rate. Infants have smaller brains that produce less CSF, and therefore they require lesser flow rates. Furthermore, little hydrostatic pressure is applied across the valve during infancy because of the small length and limited time spent in a vertical or sitting position. As children grow, their length increases and the duration that they spend in a vertical position increases. This increases the differential pressure across the valve. Because most valves have little resistance, a small increase in the differential pressure across the valve can result in a potential flow rate that far exceeds the rate of production. Therefore, as the child grows it may be necessary to increase the valve's opening pressure to prevent overdrainage. The addition of a 0/10 pediatric gravity assistant by Aesculap (Central Valley, PA) will only be active when the child is in a vertical position. The combination of a programmable valve and a 0/10 pediatric gravity assistant can allow the child to grow for a couple of years and maintain a physiological intracranial volume distribution (80% brain, 10% blood, and 10% CSF). This combination of valves can prevent the volume distribution associated with the slit ventricle (close to 90% brain and extracellular fluid and 10% blood with very little CSF secondary to shunt overdrainage). When the child gains sufficient height, it becomes necessary to change the gravity assistant to a higher vertical opening pressure.

When a shunt is inserted into an infant there are two opposing goals: first, to maximize the reconstitution of the cortical mantle, and second, to prevent the overriding of the sutures with the potential for a secondary craniosynostosis. A common strategy is to start off with a valve opening pressure of 70 mm H_2O and then slowly increase the opening pressure as needed to keep the sutures from overlapping. The infant is followed with frequent head ultrasounds, and as soon as the ventricles become less than normal in size, the opening pressure of the valve is increased in order to maintain some CSF in the ventricles. If the patient has a healthy brain that can readily reconstitute its volume, then an increase in the opening pressure reestablishes the physiological distribution of the intracranial contents. If the brain is damaged, then despite a low opening pressure the brain might not expand and large ventricles might persist even with overriding sutures. In this situation, the opening pressure is adjusted (increased slightly despite persistently enlarged ventricles) to keep the fontanel soft to very slightly sunken in a horizontal position. This allows the maintenance of sufficient CSF to prevent overriding sutures and yet allow for as much brain expansion as possible.

Infant with Intraventricular Hemorrhage

An infant with an intraventricular hemorrhage (IVH) and symptomatic hydrocephalus must reach a size and maturity that allows the insertion of a shunt. Usually once the child is over 32 weeks' gestation and/or over 1800 g in weight then the risk of necrotizing enterocolitis (NEC) is low enough to attempt a peritoneal catheter insertion. Prior to this if CSF diversion is required due to symptoms, then a ventriculosubgaleal shunt is recommended. Many children with IVH spontaneously improve over time. This can occur within weeks after the bleed, obviating the need for a shunt, or over a prolonged period. As the child grows, the arachnoid granulations mature, and the fontanels close, changing the intracranial fluid dynamics. With the child spending a greater proportion of the day in a vertical position, the intracranial venous sinus pressure drops, increasing the differential pressure across the arachnoid villi. After a shunt is inserted, the opening pressure should be slowly increased as tolerated. This is done by evaluating the fullness of the anterior fontanel, the ultrasound appearance, and the clinical appearance of the child. In this manner some children can be weaned from their shunt as their normal absorptive pathways mature or existing pathways open up.

◆ Normal Pressure Hydrocephalus: Idiopathic versus Secondary

Normal pressure hydrocephalus (NPH) by definition entails normal ICP. Some patients present with a syndrome of gait disturbance, dementia, or incontinence associated with ventriculomegaly but are found to have elevated CSF pressures. These patients have a chronic active hydrocephalus (and typically benefit from a shunt) and probably should not be included in the category of NPH. Secondary NPH refers to a similar clinical syndrome but with a known etiology (meningitis, traumatic or spontaneous subarachnoid hemorrhage, or postradiation). Secondary hydrocephalus is more likely to improve with CSF diversion than is the idiopathic variety. Patients with idiopathic NPH are at risk for overdrainage, and it is difficult to predict which patients will have a sustained improvement after shunting. A useful screening test is a lumbar puncture. If the patient has a significant improvement after a lumbar puncture, then it is reasonable to consider a shunt. If the patient fails to improve and if the opening pressure is low (less than 90 mm H_2O), then it is very unlikely that the patient will benefit from a shunt. If the patient has an opening pressure above 100 mm H_2O and fails to respond to a lumbar puncture, then a 3-day in-hospital trial of controlled CSF drainage by means of a lumbar catheter can be performed. If the patient improves with this trial, then this improvement serves as a baseline for the expected improvement that might be accomplished by shunting.

There are multiple strategies that can be used for programming a programmable valve in the NPH patient. The first and simplest is to insert the valve with an opening pressure of 200 mm H_2O[DK10] and slowly lower the opening pressure. This is time-consuming for both the patient and the doctor. The second is to insert a valve with an opening pressure of 150 mm H_2O and then make adjustments as needed. The third is to take the patient's central venous pressure (CVP), height, and weight into consideration. The valve setting is increased for a greater height and lowered for a greater weight. With the above approaches it can be difficult to find a valve setting that is adequate for both the horizontal and the vertical position. What typically occurs is that the valve must be set at a high opening pressure to prevent overdrainage when vertical. This high setting impedes drainage at night when the patient is horizontal.

Inserting a shunt assistant plus the addition of a shunt assistant (Aesculap, Inc., Center Valley, PA) can limit the likelihood of overdrainage when the patient is vertical and yet allow for sufficient drainage when the patient is horizontal. The distance between the external auditory meatus and the top of the abdomen is measured. From this distance 15 cm is subtracted and the shunt assistant with a vertical opening pressure closest to but not greater than this value is inserted. Typically the programmable valve is set at 120 mm H_2O and a 00/25 shunt assistant is inserted. Postoperatively the valve's setting is adjusted based on imaging studies, the clinical response, and the intraventricular pressure. If the patient fails to improve to the extent that the patient improved preoperatively after the removal of CSF, then the valve setting is lowered by 20 mm H_2O until an opening pressure of 100 mm H_2O, and after this by 10 mm H_2O until the patient improves. Imaging studies [computed tomographic (CT) scans] are usually taken postoperatively, at 2 weeks, 2 to 6 months, and 1 year to evaluate the ventricular size and to detect any extracerebral collections. Imaging studies are taken more frequently if there is a clinical deterioration or if there has been a significant change in the valve setting.

If on an imaging study an extracerebral collection is detected, then the opening pressure needs to be increased, and the magnitude of the change is determined after measuring the CSF pressure. Similarly, if the patient fails to improve (improved gait, thinking more quickly, less incontinence, etc.) after decreasing the setting by 40 mm H_2O, then the CSF pressure is measured (by means of a Telesensor, shunt tap, or lumbar puncture). The same method should be used to measure the pressure each time a shunt tap is performed. This helps in comparing intrareservoir pressure readings. The patient sits or remains in a vertical position for at least 20 minutes and then assumes a horizontal position. Shortly thereafter the CSF pressure is measured. The CSF pressure should always be slightly greater than the estimated CVP. If the CSF pressure is less than the estimated CVP, then the difference between the measured pressure and the estimated CVP is used as a guide for how much to increase the programmable valve's setting. When a patient is in a horizontal position, an ICP less than the CVP can only occur if the shunt is overdraining CSF. For example, if the estimated CVP is 80 mm H_2O and the horizontal CSF pressure is 40 mm H_2O, then the valve setting should be increased by 40. Leaving a patient with a CSF pressure less than the CVP will increase the risk of subdural formation and symptoms of overdrainage.

If patients complain of dizziness, increasing unsteadiness, or headaches upon assuming a vertical position, then they might be overdraining and the opening pressure is similarly adjusted.

Following the above strategy maximizes the patient's potential for improvement and lessens the risk of symptomatic overdrainage and extracerebral fluid collections.

◆ Pseudotumor Cerebri or Benign Intracranial Hypertension

Patients with pseudotumor cerebri can have markedly elevated ICP, as well as elevated intraperitoneal pressures if the patient is obese. Often these patients benefit from high valve settings in addition to a gravity assistant. The gravity assistant is chosen in a similar fashion by measuring the length of the chest, and the programmable valve is set at ~170 mm H_2O opening pressure. The higher the ICP, the greater the differential pressure across the valve and the greater the flow rate. Increasing the valve setting lessens the shunt flow rate, minimizing the possibility of a proximal obstruction. Depending on the patient's symptoms and follow-up ICP readings, the opening pressure is adjusted accordingly. Often, lumboperitoneal shunts are inserted for pseudotumor cerebri. The complication rate (CSF leak, shunt disconnection, or outward migration of the intrathecal catheter) is just as high, and there is the rare possibility of downward cerebellar herniation. The availability of frameless neuronavigation and endoscopy make insertion of a ventricular catheter into a small frontal horn possible, and therefore VP shunts are now an option for patients with pseudotumor cerebri.

◆ Treating Headaches Related to Overdrainage or Underdrainage

Treating headaches can sometimes be extremely difficult. Patients can have headaches from either overdrainage or underdrainage. Although some patients can distinguish between the two, most patients cannot, and they just complain of a headache. Typically if the headache is increased when vertical and relieved when horizontal, it is thought to be a headache due to loss of CSF. However, when a patient has a hydrostatic offset device, a vertical headache can be due to underdrainage. The best way to distinguish between over- and underdrainage is to take pressure measurements with the patient horizontal and sitting. If magnetic resonance imaging (MRI) with gadolinium demonstrates marked enhancement and thickening of the meninges, then the patient is most likely suffering from overdrainage headaches, and the opening pressure of the programmable valve should be increased. If the ICP is close to the patient's CVP (60 to 90 mm H_2O) when horizontal and drops to about the level of angle of the jaw when vertical, then it can be very problematic to decide which way to change the opening pressure. In this situation changing the opening pressure by lowering it 20 mm H_2O and asking the patient how this affects the headaches might help to identify if the patient is over- or underdraining. If the headaches improve, then the patient was underdraining, and if they remain the same or get worse, then the patient might have been overdraining.

In some patients it can be very difficult to titrate the valve for both the horizontal and vertical position. In these patients the insertion of an ICP monitor can be of help. The programmable valve is adjusted in the morning after the patient assumes a vertical position to minimize symptoms and approach a target ICP of –5 cm H_2O. The valve is readjusted in the evening for the horizontal position to achieve an ICP of close to 10 cm H_2O. The difference between these adjustments is the needed shunt assistant valve adjustment. For example, if a patient required a vertical setting of 140 mm H_2O and a horizontal setting of 90 mm H_2O and had a shunt assistant with a vertical opening pressure of 100 mm H_2O, then the shunt assistant would be changed to a shunt assistant with an opening pressure of 150 mm H_2O.

When a patient has a partial proximal obstruction, then shunt pressures become unreliable. If a patient has a reservoir that is slow to refill and CSF surrounding the ventricular catheter as seen on an MRI or CT, then a proximal revision might be needed because changing the opening pressure by opening the valve often does not provide relief to the headache, and increasing the valve's opening pressure might exacerbate the headache.

It can be very difficult to separate a partial proximal obstruction from a functional overdrainage headache in a patient with slitlike ventricles. If the patient improves with acetazolamide, then the patient might very well have a partial obstruction or an opening pressure that is too high. If the patient improves with increasing the opening pressure, then the patient was overdraining. Often the patient must be given a trial with either changing the opening pressure or with acetazolamide to distinguish between over- and underdrainage because a shunt tap fails to give an answer. In general, if a shunt tap in a patient with CSF in any portion of the ventricle system demonstrates sluggish flow, then there is a partial proximal obstruction.

If there are slitlike ventricles and there is excellent CSF flow on a shunt tap, then the recorded intrareservoir pressure probably is representative of the ICP, and can be used to give an initial guide to changing the opening pressure. Once again the difference between the measured intrashunt pressure and the estimated CVP is used as a guide to the magnitude of the change in the programmable valve. If the estimated CVP is 6 to 8 cm H_2O and the shunt tap in a horizontal position reveals an ICP of 4 cm H_2O, then the setting should be increased by 2 cm H_2O, whereas if the ICP measured 10 cm H_2O, then lowering the valve's opening pressure by 2 cm (or 20 mm) H_2O might help. One of the most rewarding shunt interventions is the alleviation of persistent headaches. This can be done either by simply increasing the valve's opening pressure setting if the patient is found to have a low ICP when horizontal, or by inserting a gravity assistant of a higher opening pressure if the patient has a low ICP when vertical.

◆ Treating Subdural or Extracerebral Fluid Collections

Patients with extracerebral collections need to have the flow rate through their shunts decreased. Depending on the symptoms, a decision can be made about draining the extracerebral collections or simply changing the valve's opening pressure. If the patient is not under distress and does not have a focal impairment due to the extracerebral collection, then surgery might be avoidable, and an attempt should be made to increase the opening pressure of the shunt. To determine the magnitude of this increase, a measurement of the intraventricular pressure in the horizontal and vertical position is helpful. For the horizontal position, if the intraventricular pressure measures less than the CVP, then the opening pressure of the programmable valve is increased until the intraventricular pressure approaches or slightly exceeds the estimated CVP. For the vertical position, the difference between the level of the measured ICP and a point ~10 cm below the external auditory meatus is used as a guide to the magnitude of the opening pressure change recommended for the gravity assistant. The patient is followed by another CT scan in about 10 to 14 days, and further adjustments are made until there is resolution of the extracerebral collections.

If the patient with extracerebral collections is symptomatic with headaches or symptomatic from mass effect or shift, then the collection or collections are drained and the valve's opening pressure setting is increased to 200 mm H_2O. The patient is observed carefully, and as soon as the extracerebral collections resolve on CT, the valve is reopened carefully. Most often adding a gravity assistant to prevent excessive outflow when the patient is in a vertical position decreases the likelihood of a recurrent extracerebral collection.

◆ Promote Shunt Independence

Not infrequently a patient presents with a communicating hydrocephalus that is secondary to an inflammatory process (posthemorrhagic, postoperative, postinfectious), and if the patient fails to improve within a reasonable time period, then a permanent shunt is inserted. It is very difficult to predict when a patient no longer needs a shunt. Any patient can deteriorate unpredictably after removal or ligation of a shunt. Now with a programmable valve the shunt can be almost turned off to test if a patient has become shunt independent. If the patient becomes symptomatic or if an imaging study shows progressive ventricular enlargement, then the shunt can be reopened noninvasively. Typical scenarios include trauma, aneurysmal subarachnoid hemorrhage, or a post-Chiari decompression with a symptomatic pseudomeningocele. Over the course of close to a year, some of these patients can either reestablish their normal circulation and become shunt independent or become symptomatic from excessive CSF drainage. For patients with a programmable valve, the valve setting can be slowly increased weekly until signs or symptoms of hypertensive hydrocephalus develop. If the patient tolerates a setting of 200 for a period of 3 months, then consideration can be given to either ligating the shunt or inserting an on-off valve in the occluded position. Depending on the patient's circumstances, the valve and distal catheter can eventually be removed. If the ventricular catheter is adherent, it is left in place.

◆ Using a Programmable Valve in Combination with a Third Ventriculostomy or a Fenestration of an Arachnoid Cyst

A patient with a newly diagnosed obstructive hydrocephalus secondary to a tectal glioma can undergo a third ventriculostomy without the implantation of any hardware. However, there are numerous shunted patients who present with a proximal obstruction, and the question arises if they are a candidate for a third ventriculostomy. Such patients include those with an initial diagnosis of an obstructive hydrocephalus and those with a resolved communicating hydrocephalus and an acquired aqueductal stenosis. For these patients an attempt at a third ventriculostomy is reasonable, but it is difficult to know with certainty that the subarachnoid pathways are sufficiently open. Performing the third ventriculostomy and placing a programmable valve set at 200 mm H_2O with a shunt assistant allows the patient to safely undergo a third ventriculostomy. Postoperatively the ventricles might enlarge on the imaging study. If the ICP becomes elevated or the patient becomes symptomatic, then the valve's setting can be lowered to alleviate the symptoms. An external ventricular drain cannot be left in place long enough to allow for late deterioration and has the added risk of infection and additional hospital days. A ventricular catheter and reservoir is another alternative that allows for taping of the reservoir and conversion to a shunt should the patient fail the attempt at a third ventriculostomy.

Similarly, there is a controversy concerning the best approach for a patient with an arachnoid cyst. Some of these patients can effectively be treated by endoscopic fenestration of the cyst to the open subarachnoid space. In general, if a patient is found to have a markedly elevated CSF pressure, then a shunt is required. If the intracyst pressure is unremarkable, then a fenestration might be sufficient. Leaving a shunt with a programmable valve set at 200 mm H_2O and providing appropriate shunt assistance allows the patient to undergo a fenestration of the arachnoid cyst and to be followed. Postoperatively, if symptoms persist or the intracyst pressure is elevated as measured by a shunt tap, then the valve's opening pressure is lowered.

◆ Contraindications

The contraindications to using a programmable valve are the same as with any valve (infection or excessively bloody CSF). There are no specific contraindications to the use of a programmable valve. Some patients require numerous shunt revisions, and it is not infrequently that a surgeon will test a programmable valve in such a patient. The programmable valve only helps if the problem was related to a mismatch between the patient's needs and the valve's opening pressure setting. Not uncommonly the patient has a different problem, such as complex hydrocephalus, and therefore the programmable valve does not help. Complex hydrocephalus is when there is more than one obstructed CSF compartment, such as communicating and obstructive hydrocephalus, or a loculated ventricle. In this case all the compartments need to be communicated and the catheters preferentially should be connected to one distal catheter.

Another common problem is the child with a slitlike ventricle who has the openings of the ventricular catheter in the shunt tract or a sleeve. Simply changing the valve's opening pressure does not help this situation. Instead, endoscopically repositioning the ventricular catheter into a free and open portion of the ventricle permits easier CSF outflow. Subsequent to repositioning the catheter, the opening pressure of the valve is increased and a hydrostatic offset device is added to promote the maintenance of some CSF in the ventricle. Sometimes this helps alleviate the symptoms associated with a slit ventricle syndrome. However, often the problem is one of decreased intracranial compliance, and simply changing the opening pressure does not restore the intracranial compliance toward normal. A cranial vault expansion or a subtemporal decompression increases the intracranial compliance and is sometimes helpful in alleviating symptoms of a slit ventricle syndrome. Inserting a programmable valve with a hydrostatic offset device in a newly shunted infant can promote the retention of intraventricular CSF and might lessen the development of a slit ventricle syndrome.

The need for MRI is not a contraindication to the use of a programmable valve. Every patient or guardian needs to be aware that going into an MRI machine can change the valve setting. After an MRI the valve can be reprogrammed back to its original setting, or a lateral skull x-ray can be obtained to see if the valve setting changed.

◆ Conclusion

Programmable valves and hydrostatic offsetting devices make it possible to optimize shunt flow in both a horizontal and a vertical position. These devices are simple to use and can lessen the high complication rate associated with shunts.

84

Endoscopic Third Ventriculostomy

Kerry Crone

During the past 75 years numerous procedures have been developed to bypass the obstructive component in noncommunicating hydrocephalus. The earliest and more frequent procedures required an open craniotomy to communicate the ventricular system with the basal cisterns.[1,2] Less invasive procedures must have been equally attractive because Mixter[3] in 1923 performed the first endoscopic third ventriculostomy by passing a sound from the third ventricle into the interpeduncular cistern.

◆ Indications

There is a general consensus that the best candidates to undergo this procedure are patients with adolescent- or adult-onset nontumoral aqueductal stenosis and those who have never undergone diversionary spinal fluid procedures.[4–6] When these strict criteria are followed, the procedure has a success rate approaching 90%. However, the procedure is appropriate in many additional situations. For example, Hirsch et al[6] reported a success rate of 80% in children older than 2 years and 70% in children younger than 2 years.

Controversial candidates for third ventriculostomy are patients with obstructive hydrocephalus related to myelomeningocele, congenital aqueductal stenosis, tumors, or infection. Although third ventriculostomy may successfully treat obstructive hydrocephalus associated with myelomeningocele or resulting from congenital aqueductal stenosis, the results are poorer and less predictable, approaching 60% and 50%, respectively.[5]

Additional indications include tumors in the posterior third ventricle or periaqueductal region. Biopsy with third ventriculostomy provides a safe, effective, and less invasive approach to deal with many of these lesions.

Contraindications for third ventriculostomy include previous whole-brain irradiation, aberrant variable anatomy of the third ventricle, and tumors that may occupy the floor of the ventricle.[7]

◆ Preparation

Magnetic resonance imaging (MRI) is essential to display the anatomy of the third ventricle, prepontine interpeduncular cistern, and periaqueductal region. Cine-MRI may be useful to access aqueductal flow when the fourth ventricle is moderately enlarged. However, no study can reliably access spinal fluid absorption over the convexities.

◆ Surgical Technique

Anesthesia

Although the procedure is performed typically under general endotracheal anesthesia, local anesthesia can be used in critically ill or elderly patients for whom general anesthesia would be considered a high risk. No specialized intraoperative neurophysiological monitoring is required.

Positioning

The patient is positioned supine in a horseshoe cerebellar headrest with a small roll placed under the shoulders to elevate the chest 10 to 15 degrees **(Fig. 84–1).**

Procedure

Following the induction of general or local anesthesia, a small area of the scalp is shaved clean of hair. The television monitor positioned opposite the surgeon provides an unobstructed view during the endoscopic procedure.

After standard preparation of the scalp and draping of the patient, a 3 cm vertical incision based on the coronal suture is made 2.5 cm from the midline. A 1 cm bur hole is created slightly anterior to the coronal suture. The dura is incised

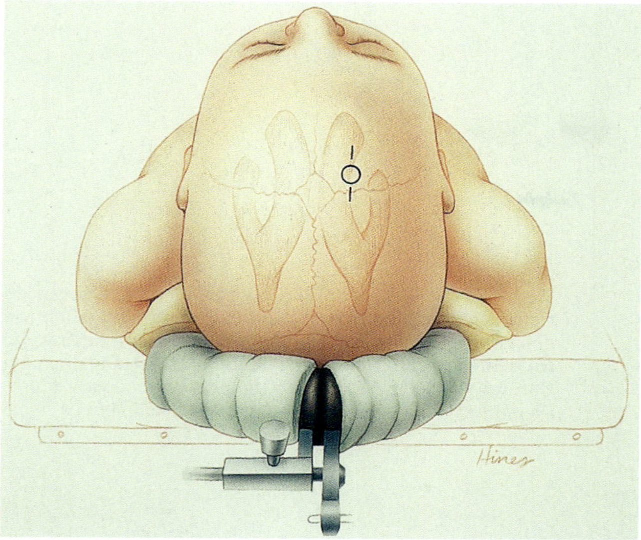

Figure 84–1 The patient is positioned supine in a horseshoe cerebellar headrest with a small roll placed under the shoulders to elevate the chest 10 to 15 degrees. A 3 cm vertical incision based on the coronal suture is made 2.5 cm from the midline. A 1 cm bur hole is created slightly anterior to the coronal suture. (Reprinted with permission from the Mayfield Clinic.)

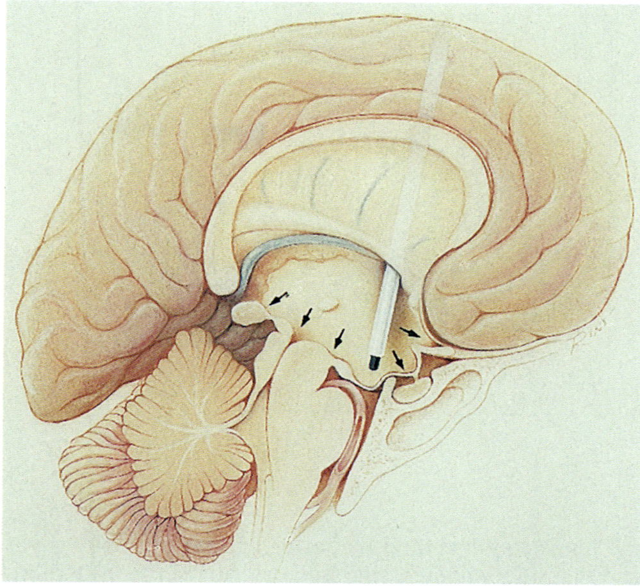

Figure 84–3 The tip of the flexible scope can be moved to visualize the optic recess, infundibular recess, mamillary bodies, aqueduct of Sylvius, suprapineal recess, and in rare instances, the roof of the third ventricle. (Reprinted with permission from the Mayfield Clinic.)

and coagulated to permit entry of the introducer. A 12.5 French peel-away sheath introducer is used to cannulate the lateral ventricle **(Fig. 84–2)**. The central stylet is withdrawn and the endoscope is inserted into the lateral ventricle.

The surgeon should inspect the lateral ventricle and identify the foramen of Monro, choroid plexus, and venous confluens. The endoscope is advanced into the third ventricle, at which time the mamillary bodies, infundibulum, and optic chiasm should come into view **(Fig. 84–3)**. If a flexible scope has been used, the tip of the scope can be moved to visualize the aqueduct, suprapineal recess, and, in rare instances, the roof of the third ventricle. If a rigid scope has been used, the 0 degree lens scope may be exchanged for a 30 or 70 degree scope to view the anatomy of the posterior third ventricle.

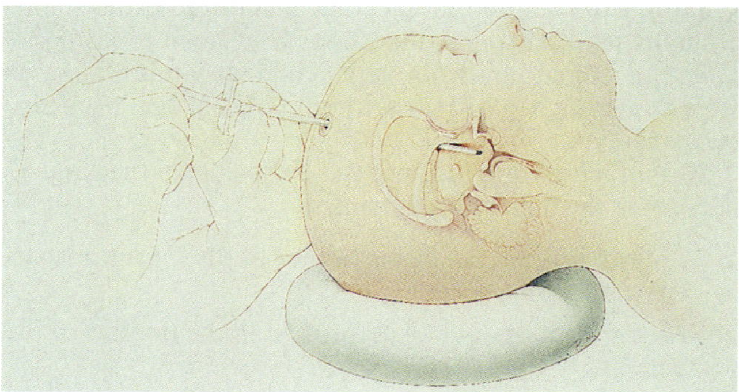

Figure 84–2 The dura is incised and coagulated to permit entry of the introducer. A 12.5 French peel-away sheath introducer is used to cannulate the lateral ventricle. The flexible endoscope is inserted through the cannula and guided through the foramen of Monro to enter the third ventricle. (Reprinted with permission from the Mayfield Clinic.)

The floor of the third ventricle is usually attenuated and pulses freely with each heartbeat. Many of the structures may be visualized beneath the attenuated floor including the clivus, dorsum sellae, and basilar artery **(Fig. 84–4)**. The site for fenestration is selected. If the floor is transparent,

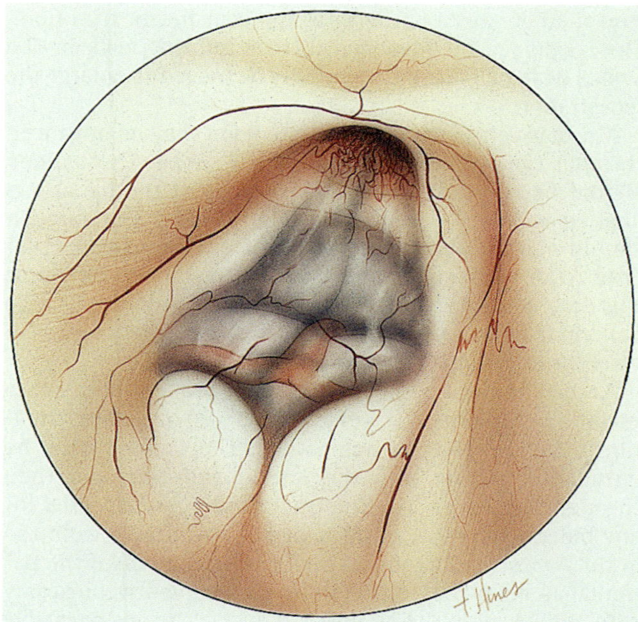

Figure 84–4 The floor of the third ventricle is attenuated between the infundibular recess anteriorly and the mamillary bodies posteriorly. Typically the infundibular recess is stained with a multitude of small blood vessels. Structures that may be visualized beneath the attenuated floor include the clivus, dorsum sellae, pons, and basilar artery. (Reprinted with permission from the Mayfield Clinic.)

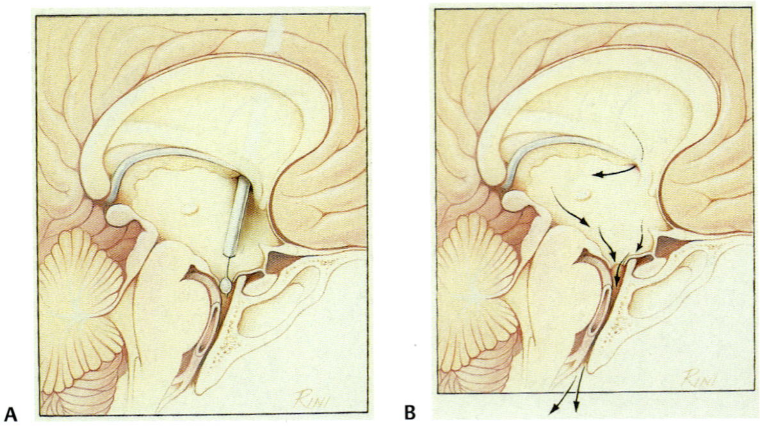

Figure 84–5 **(A)** A small Fogarty balloon may be advanced through the endoscope and should be inflated when the epicenter of the balloon is aligned with the fenestration. **(B)** Hydrocephalus is relieved by cerebrospinal fluid drainage through the fenestration into the interpeduncular cistern. (Reprinted with permission from the Mayfield Clinic.)

the fenestration should be performed between the clivus and mamillary bodies, slightly posterior to the infundibulum. If the floor is translucent or opaque, the inexperienced surgeon should consider abandoning the procedure to avoid inadvertent serious injury to the basilar artery. In such a circumstance, an experienced surgeon will select the stained area of the floor of the third ventricle that is immediately posterior to the infundibular recess.

Various techniques have been described to perform the fenestration.[5,8–10] If the floor is attenuated, it is easiest to bring the scope into direct contact with the floor and gently advance the entire scope through the floor into the interpeduncular cistern. If the floor is not attenuated or translucent, monopolar cautery may be used to create a slight tuft in the floor just posterior to the infundibulum. Rapid irrigation then creates a pathway to the translucent firm floor. The scope can be advanced further into the cistern. The swivel head of a flexible scope may be moved to enlarge the fenestration.

Alternatively, a small Fogarty balloon may be advanced through the working channel of the scope. The balloon should be inflated when the epicenter of the balloon is aligned with the fenestration **(Fig. 84–5A)**. The surgeon should neither inflate the balloon in the interpeduncular cistern nor withdraw the balloon into the third ventricle, as this may inadvertently tear small perforating vessels. The balloon is deflated and then withdrawn to allow egress of cerebrospinal fluid (CSF) **(Fig. 84–5B)**.

A small amount of bleeding is often seen following fenestration of the floor. Observation as well as gentle irrigation usually results in hemostasis. The scope should be withdrawn slowly into the lateral ventricle and then through the entry tract. The tract should be inspected for any bleeding vessels as the scope is withdrawn from the brain. A ventriculostomy catheter is placed only if the patient has been previously shunted. The ventriculostomy catheter is kept in the off position during the postoperative period.

A small circular pledget of Gelfoam is placed into the bur hole, followed by a small titanium bur hole plate. This maneuver provides excellent protection against spinal fluid leakage. The scalp is closed in an anatomical fashion.

◆ Postoperative Care

The patient is observed in a special care unit for the first 24 hours. Frequent neurological checks are made throughout this period to detect any signs of elevated intracranial pressure. If a ventriculostomy was placed at the time of surgery, it may be used to continuously monitor intracranial pressure. The catheter may be removed the following day. Computed tomography is usually performed prior to discharge to detect any evidence of hemorrhage or acute ventricular enlargement. The patient is discharged on the second postoperative day.

◆ Complications

Despite the minimally invasive nature of third ventriculostomy, a variety of complications may occur related to structures in and around the floor of the third ventricle. The most serious and life-threatening risk is injury to the basilar artery or its branches. Hemorrhage, stroke, or false aneurysmal formation may be seen following injury to the basilar artery.[11] Damage to adjacent hypothalamic nuclei in the third ventricle and cranial nerves in the interpeduncular cistern may produce disturbances in endocrine function, mentation, and cranial nerve palsies. Diabetes insipidus, the syndrome of inappropriate section of antidiuretic hormone, amenorrhea, and trance-like states have been reported.[4,12] Subdural hematoma from ventricular decompression, as well as meningitis with or without CSF leakage, have also occurred.[4,5]

Most of these complications can be avoided if the surgeon adheres to the following guidelines:

1. Fenestration should be performed at the most transparent portion of the floor.
2. Fenestration should be performed in the midline of the patient.
3. Blunt perforation is preferable to cautery or the use of sharp instruments.

On the basis of excellent results and low morbidity, third ventriculostomy is rapidly becoming the preferred treatment for acquired aqueductal stenosis.

References

1. Dandy WE. An operative procedure for hydrocephalus. Bull Johns Hopkins Hosp 1922;33:189–190
2. White JC, Michelsen JJ. Treatment of obstructive hydrocephalus in adults. Surg Gynecol Obstet 1942;74:99–109
3. Mixter WJ. Ventriculoscopy and puncture of the floor of the third ventricle. Boston Med Surg J 1923;188:277–278
4. Grant JA. Third ventriculostomy: a review. Surg Neurol 1997;47:210–212
5. Jones RF, Kwok BC, Stening WA, Vonau M. Neuroendoscopic third ventriculostomy: a practical alternative to extracranial shunts in non-communicating hydrocephalus. Acta Neurochir Suppl 1994;61:79–83
6. Hirsch JF, Hirsch E, Sainte-Rose C, et al. Stenosis of the aqueduct of Sylvius: etiology and treatment. J Neurosurg Sci 1986;30:29–39
7. Teo C, Jones R. Management of hydrocephalus by endoscopic third ventriculostomy in patients with myelomeningocele. Pediatr Neurosurg 1996;25:57–63
8. Sainte-Rose C. Third ventriculostomy. In: Manwaring KH, Crone KR, eds. Neuroendoscopy, vol 1. New York: Mary Ann Liebert; 1992: 47–62
9. Drake JM. Ventriculostomy for the treatment of hydrocephalus. Neurosurg Clin N Am 1993;4:657–666
10. Baskin JJ, Manwaring KH, Rekate HL. Ventricular shunt removal: the ultimate treatment for the slit ventricle syndrome. J Neurosurg 1998;88:478–484
11. McLaughlin MR, Wahlig JB, Kaufman AM, Albright AL. Traumatic basilar aneurysm after endoscopic third ventriculostomy: case report. Neurosurgery 1997;41:1400–1403
12. Lowry DW, Lowry DL, Berga SL, Adelson PD, Roberts MM. Secondary amenorrhea due to hydrocephalus treated with endoscopic ventriculocisternostomy: case report. J Neurosurg 1996;85: 1148–1152

Section XII

Central Nervous System Infections

85

Epidural Abscess, Subdural Empyema, and Brain Abscess

Lisa L. Guyot, Colleen B. Duffy, Murali Guthikonda, and Sabareesh Kumar Natarajan

Early in the 19th century, surgeries for pyogenic infections of the brain had an extremely high mortality rate and were often performed by pure chance after cases of trauma. The first documented successful case was performed by the French surgeon S. F. Morand in 1752 in which he drained a temporoethmoidal abscess of otic origin. In 1888, William Macewen delivered an address to the British Medical Association that emphasized two important principles of cerebral surgery: the development of aseptic surgery based on Lister's work and the development of the principles of cerebral localization.[1] In 1893 he published the landmark monograph "Pyogenic Infective Diseases of the Brain and Spinal Cord," discussing the details of surgical anatomy, pathology and symptoms of cerebral abscess and meningitis, thrombosis of intracranial sinuses, treatment, and results. He presented 30 cases of intracranial abscesses: 25 cerebral and cerebellar cases with 19 surgeries and 18 recoveries; five extradural abscesses, all of which recovered following surgery—results comparable to those of modern neurosurgery. The principles of early recognition and drainage of intracranial suppurative disease have been further enhanced with the development of antibiotics and the introduction of computed tomography (CT) and magnetic resonance imaging (MRI).[2]

The intracranial abscesses can be classified based on the anatomical location as epidural, subdural, and intracerebral **(Fig. 85–1)**. Most abscesses are pyogenic and rarely caused by mycobacteria, fungi, or parasites.

◆ Epidural Abscess

Intracranial extradural abscesses (EAs) arise as a result of direct extension from the paranasal sinuses, infections of the orbit, or osteomyelitis of the skull, which can occur postoperatively[3] or after trauma. They tend to be localized infections limited by the dural adherence to the overlying bone. Sinusitis may lead to intracranial extension through two different routes[4]: (1) directly through intervening tissues by sinus wall erosion, via naturally existing foramina (e.g., cribriform plate), or through congenital or traumatic defects and across the meninges; and (2) indirectly through retrograde thrombophlebitis via the valveless diploic veins (of Breschet).[5]

Most patients with EA present with a dull headache and fever with possible tenderness over the affected sinuses or area of trauma. If left untreated, the EA may expand, resulting in increased intracranial pressure. The infection may extend through the dura to cause meningitis, cerebritis, subdural or brain abscess, or thrombosis of the venous sinuses.

Preparation

Preoperative studies include CT of the brain and sinuses, with and without intravenous contrast. The scans may show evidence of dural or cortical enhancement suggestive of early meningoencephalitis or subdural empyema. MRI may show the changes of meningeal and cortical enhancement better and earlier than does CT, but CT may also show evidence of

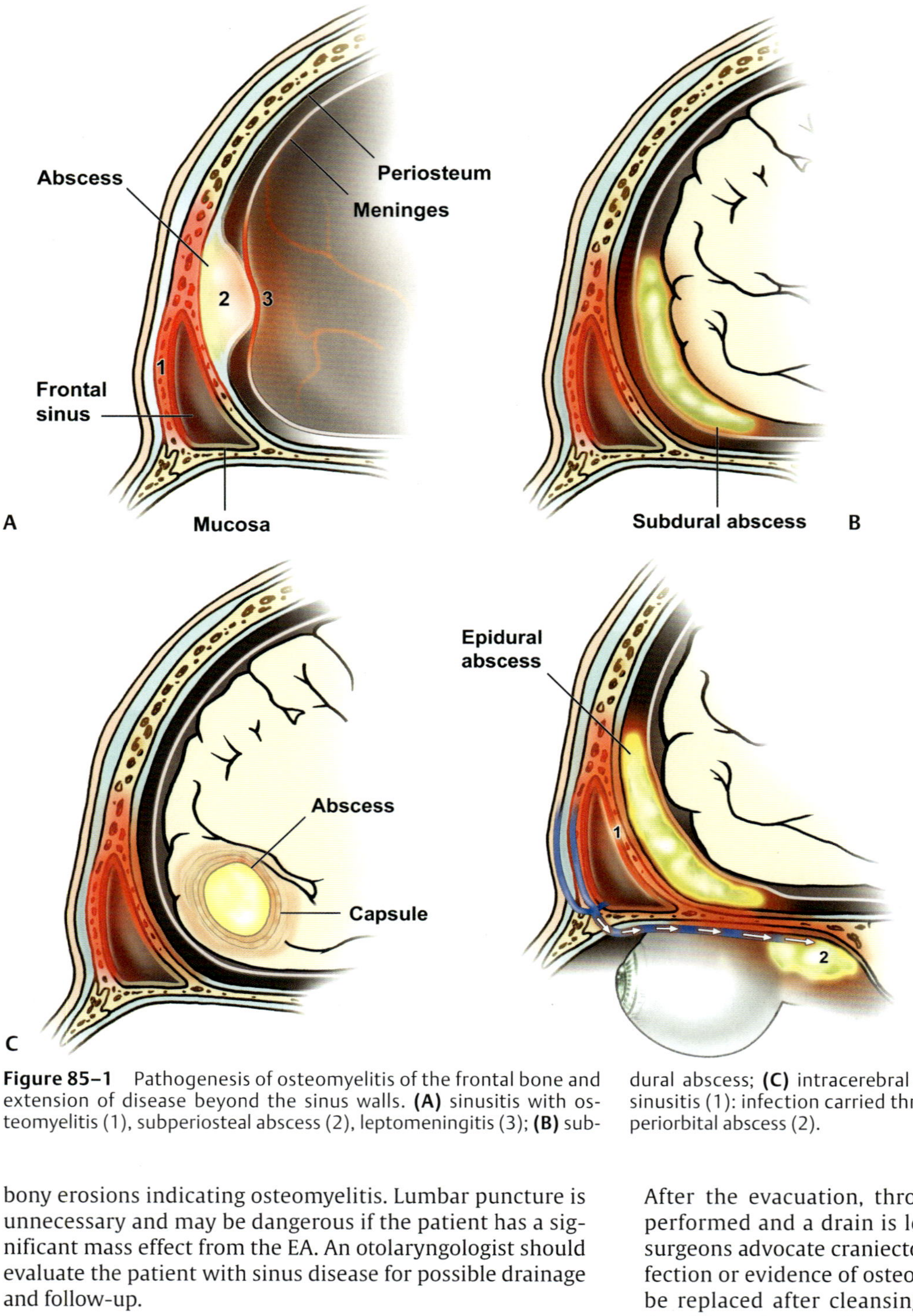

Figure 85–1 Pathogenesis of osteomyelitis of the frontal bone and extension of disease beyond the sinus walls. **(A)** sinusitis with osteomyelitis (1), subperiosteal abscess (2), leptomeningitis (3); **(B)** subdural abscess; **(C)** intracerebral abscess; **(D)** epidural abscess with sinusitis (1): infection carried through communicating veins causing periorbital abscess (2).

bony erosions indicating osteomyelitis. Lumbar puncture is unnecessary and may be dangerous if the patient has a significant mass effect from the EA. An otolaryngologist should evaluate the patient with sinus disease for possible drainage and follow-up.

Surgical Technique

Patients with epidural abscesses require surgical evacuation through bur holes or a craniotomy. If the fluid collection is small, a single bur hole centered over the collection allows the fluid to be drained, thus relieving the mass effect. Bacteriological studies may be obtained at the same time. If the fluid collection spans a wider area, two bur holes are placed. After the evacuation, through and through irrigation is performed and a drain is left in the epidural space. Some surgeons advocate craniectomy. If there is no superficial infection or evidence of osteomyelitis of the bone flap, it may be replaced after cleansing in an antimicrobial solution. Aerobic and anaerobic cultures of the purulent material should be sent for laboratory analysis as well as fungal and acid-fast bacillus (AFB) cultures if indicated.

Management of Overlying Sinus

If the infection seems to arise from a sinus, it is recommended that there be simultaneous treatment of the intracranial component and the sinusitis. Frontal sinusitis followed by mastoiditis is most commonly associated with epidural abscess. In cases involving multiple sinuses, the otolaryngologists may drain the sinuses percutaneously or endoscopically.

Technique for Frontal Epidural Abscess Drainage with Frontal Sinus Involvement

The patient is placed in the supine position. A bicoronal incision is made and the scalp is elevated superficial to the periosteum. An osteoplastic frontal craniotomy is completed depending on the location of the abscess. The dura is elevated from the roof of the orbit and the posterior wall of the frontal sinus. By utilizing a high-speed drill, the posterior wall of the frontal sinus is removed and the mucosa is stripped. The inner surface of the anterior wall of the frontal sinus is decorticated using a large diamond bur and all the mucosal islands are removed. The nasolacrimal duct is obliterated with a small piece of temporalis muscle and covered with a pericranial flap rotated from the scalp. A tissue adhesive (Tisseel; Baxter Healthcare Corp., Glendale, CA) is applied to augment the sinus obliteration. The epidural abscess is evacuated and cultures are obtained. The bone flap is replaced and secured with plates and screws.

In cases where the frontal sinus is large, a Caldwell view of the skull is obtained and the frontal sinus outlined on the film. A template of the frontal sinus is cut and sterilized. The template is used to outline the frontal sinus and the outer table is cut with a high-speed drill and elevated, leaving the periosteum attached to the bone flap. This exposes the inner wall of the frontal sinus, which can then be drilled away, exposing the epidural space. The abscess can then be drained from the epidural space without doing a formal craniotomy.

Mastoid-Related Brain Abscess

If mastoiditis is the source of intracranial abscess, a complete mastoidectomy is performed. The mastoid-related abscesses usually involve the temporal region or the posterior fossa. Depending on the location, a temporal or occipital craniotomy is performed to drain the EA. The dura is inspected carefully for any signs of involvement without violating its integrity. The dura should not be opened unless subdural empyema is strongly suspected on the radiological studies.

Postoperative Care

Antimicrobial therapy should be continued for 4 to 6 weeks with close monitoring of the patient's clinical status. Antimicrobial therapy alone may be used to treat patients with very small fluid collections, and the choice of antibiotic varies with the age of the patient and the site of the infection. Anticonvulsants are not necessary if the infection is localized to the epidural space and has not invaded the dura.

◆ Subdural Empyema

Subdural empyema (SDE) develops primarily as a result of the spread of infection from the paranasal sinuses, after a penetrating trauma or following a craniotomy infection. The frontal and ethmoid sinuses are responsible in over half the cases.[6] SDE can also be the result of a hematogenous spread in cases of meningitis or infection of a preexisting subdural hematoma.

The presenting clinical signs and symptoms may be more dramatic than with EA due to the involvement of the meninges and the underlying cortex. Patients may present with seizures, lethargy, or focal neurological deficits, in addition to generalized symptoms of headache and fever. Septic venous thrombosis may result in cortical venous or dural venous sinus thrombosis, which can lead to venous infarction or hydrocephalus.

Preparation

The preoperative workup is similar to that for EA. MRI is more sensitive in detecting SDE.

Surgical Technique

Surgical options include drainage via bur holes, craniotomy, or craniectomy, if preoperative evaluation detects signs of osteomyelitis. Aggressive debridement of infected granulation tissue could produce significant hemorrhage and should be avoided. The wound is copiously irrigated. The dura should be closed primarily or by using an autograft (pericranium). Synthetic substitutes should not be used.

Postoperative Care

Anticonvulsant therapy should be initiated immediately because of the high risk of seizures. The duration of treatment remains controversial ranging from 6 weeks to 2 years.[7] Antimicrobial therapy should continue for 6 weeks with frequent clinical assessment of the patient and by radiological studies to evaluate resolution of the infection.

◆ Brain Abscess

The etiology of the brain abscess may be predicted by the presence of single or multiple lesions. Single lesions most commonly present as direct extension of infections of the paranasal sinuses, mastoid, or middle ear or as the result of penetrating trauma. Multiple lesions tend to occur as a result of hematogenous spread from skin lesions, endocarditis, pulmonary or periodontal infections, or the presence of cyanotic heart disease.[8] Despite the known association of a given bacterial organism to a specific site, the primary source may not be found in about 20 to 30% of cases.

Patients with brain abscess frequently present with focal symptoms related to the location of the mass lesion, as well as generalized symptoms of increased intracranial pressure (ICP). The symptoms can be out of proportion to the size of the brain abscess, attributed to the significant vasogenic edema associated with the abscess. Mild pyrexia is common and temperature elevations greater than 101.5°F often indicate the presence of a systemic infection. Patients with a brain abscess may experience a sudden worsening of their headache with new onset of meningismus; this could indicate rupture of the abscess into the ventricular system resulting in increased mortality (> 80%).[9]

Preparation

Contrast-enhanced CT of the brain will reveal the presence of an abscess. MRI done with contrast enhancement is very sensitive in detecting early cerebritis, but a CT is sufficient to evaluate the capsule of the lesion and can also detect any associated osteomyelitis of the adjacent bone. Classifications have been proposed that divide the infections into the cerebritis or capsule stage based on varying enhancement patterns seen on CT/MRI **(Fig. 85–2).**

Patients who present with a lesion suspicious for an abscess should be investigated for the presence of any systemic infection. Blood cultures, urinalysis, and a chest x-ray should be completed as initial screening studies. Other laboratory studies include a peripheral leukocyte count, which is elevated in only 60 to 70% of patients, and an erythrocyte sedimentation rate, which is elevated in ~90% of patients. A serum C-reactive protein can be helpful if there is a suspicion of a brain tumor as opposed to an abscess. A study showed that 90% of patients with an abscess had serum C-reactive proteins greater than 28 mg/L.[10] In high-risk (sexually active or intravenous drug abusers) and immune-compromised patients (organ transplant recipients or patients receiving chemotherapy), an HIV test and serum toxoplasma titers should be drawn. A lumbar puncture should not be performed because it might be dangerous in the presence of a large mass lesion and generally yields nonspecific results.

Antimicrobial therapy appropriate to the suspected organism should be started immediately in unstable patients. This might alter the culture results and should be avoided if possible. Antimicrobials can be started after adequate cultures have been obtained, if the patient's neurological status is stable.

The use of corticosteroids in brain abscess remains controversial.[11] Several studies have shown that steroids can delay or inhibit the formation of an abscess capsule, which is felt to be the primary limiting factor in the spread of infection. However, patients with significant mass effect due to the infection may benefit from the reduction in edema afforded by the steroids. The use of steroids must be individualized based on the neurological deficit related to the amount of mass affect and the potential risk of the spread of infection in an immune-compromised patient.

Anticonvulsants should be started immediately due to the high risk of seizures in these patients. They should be continued for 1 to 2 years and tapered if the patient remains seizure free and has no electroencephalograpic (EEG) findings consistent with epileptiform discharges.

Surgical Technique

Treatment strategies of brain abscess depend on the stage at which it presents, its size, and its accessibility. Britt and Enzmann[12] developed a four-stage model of brain abscess evolution based on histopathological data: stage of *early cerebritis* (days 1–3), representing an early inflammatory response; stage of *late cerebritis* (days 4–29), in which pus formation enlarges the necrotic center of the abscess, and fibroblasts lay down a reticulin network that is a precursor to the capsule; stage of *early encapsulation* (days 10–13), representing a well developed capsule with demarcation from the surrounding brain parenchyma; and finally the *late capsule stage* (days 14 and on), in which the capsule matures. Obana and Rosenblum[13] have shown that abscesses

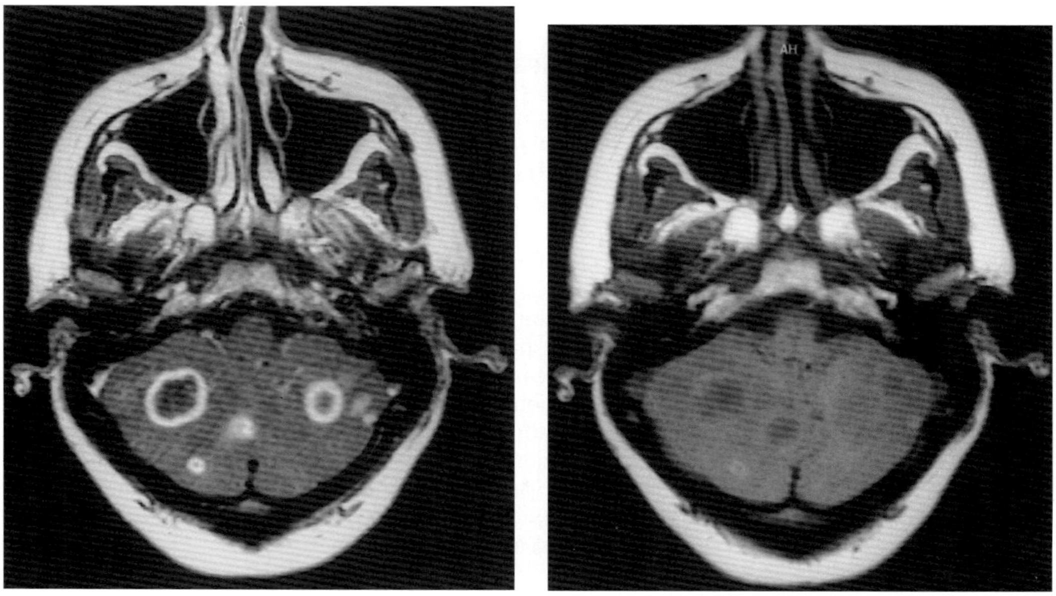

A B

Figure 85–2 A 39-year-old woman with a history of status asthmaticus, on mechanical ventilation and high-dose steroids, presented with right-sided hemiplegia, right sixth cranial nerve palsy, and grand mal seizures. Biopsy showed diagnosis of aspergillosis. Magnetic resonance imaging was done **(A)** with and **(B)** without contrast.

with a diameter less than 1.7 cm can be treated medically and no abscess greater than 2.5 cm in diameter resolved without surgical intervention.

If a patient has a documented bacteremia with positive cultures, one may opt to treat with systemic antibiotics with good central nervous system (CNS) penetration. If the cultures are not definitive or in an immune-compromised patient who may harbor more than one organism, it is best to obtain a biopsy and direct culture of the CNS lesion and to proceed with definitive antibiotic therapy.

Bur Hole Aspiration

A needle biopsy/aspiration can be done under local anesthesia with sedation. The biopsy needle can be guided by stereotactic methods[14] using either a frame-based or frame-less system. A ventricular cannula or any aspiration cannula supplied by the vendor of the stereotactic system can be used. A single bur hole is made at the site of planned needle insertion, and using stereotactic coordinates, the needle is advanced through the meninges. The entry point is chosen that will allow the shortest trajectory to the target or one that avoids any vital parts of the brain including the ventricular system or any major vessels. If more than one abscess is large and loculated, they may require multiple sites of entry and multiple bur holes for aspiration. The dura and the underlying pia-arachnoid are coagulated, and a sharp opening is made before advancing the cannula, otherwise the thickened leptomeninges may push the cortex away from the calvarium resulting in subdural hematoma formation. Following the aspiration, the needles are withdrawn. Instillation of any antibiotic solution is not indicated into the abscess cavity. The aspiration should be done gently to avoid excessive suction that might result in hemorrhage into the cavity. Occasionally a ventricular catheter may be left in the abscess cavity and the contents aspirated in the ensuing 1 or 2 days.

If a stereotactic system is not available, one may perform a small trephine at the expected site of the abscess. Utilizing a 7.5 Hz ultrasonic probe, the abscess can be localized and a needle or a catheter can be advanced into the cavity. The advantages of intraoperative ultrasound-guided drainage is real-time monitoring of the amount of aspirant, gauging the extent of collapse of the capsule and any development of hemorrhagic complications. These techniques can be performed under local anesthesia with intravenous sedation, especially in medically unstable patients who cannot tolerate general anesthetic **(Fig. 85–3).**

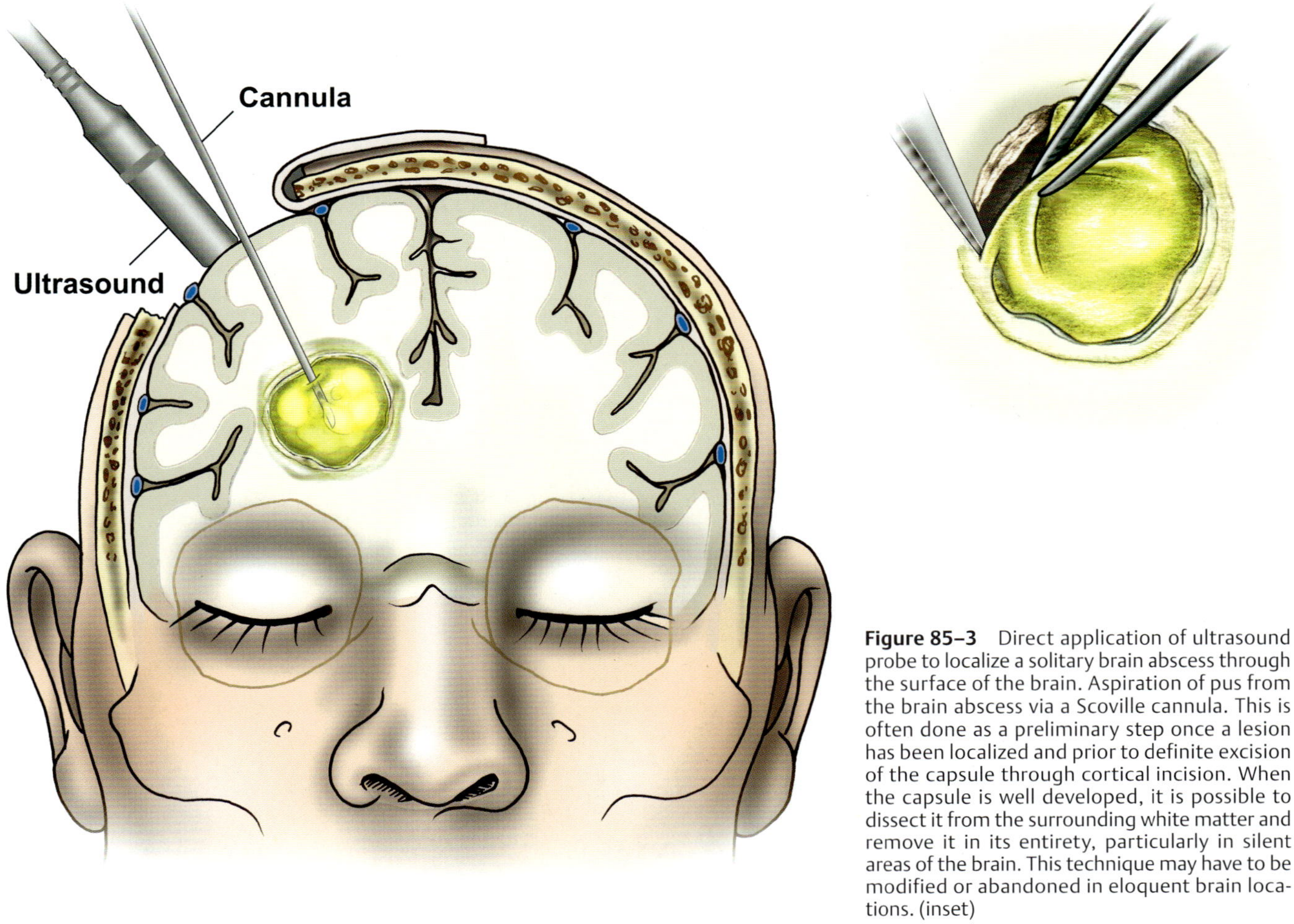

Figure 85–3 Direct application of ultrasound probe to localize a solitary brain abscess through the surface of the brain. Aspiration of pus from the brain abscess via a Scoville cannula. This is often done as a preliminary step once a lesion has been localized and prior to definite excision of the capsule through cortical incision. When the capsule is well developed, it is possible to dissect it from the surrounding white matter and remove it in its entirety, particularly in silent areas of the brain. This technique may have to be modified or abandoned in eloquent brain locations. (inset)

Excision

Consideration should be given for complete excision of the lesion if it is located in an easily accessible and noneloquent area of the brain and if it has a well-defined capsule that will allow complete excision. This technique may be particularly useful in cases of posttraumatic abscesses in which there is foreign material that should be debrided or fungal abscesses, which are often resistant to medical therapy. Stereotactic-guided placement of a craniotomy or trephination site will allow for a small incision. After performing the craniotomy and localizing the abscess, the sulcus overlying the abscess is opened using an operative microscope and magnification. The abscess cavity is usually located at the depth of the sulcus. The capsule can be punctured with a large cannula, and once the contents are aspirated the capsule is dissected away from the adjacent white matter (**Fig. 85–3**).

If there are multiple abscesses, two facts must be considered: the size, and the extent of mass effect from the abscesses and its location. Priority should be given to draining the abscess that is causing the most symptoms from mass effect. In case of multiple small abscesses, the most easily accessible lesion located in the least eloquent area of the brain should be biopsied. Special consideration should be given to abscesses that are located adjacent to a ventricular wall because the capsule at this site is thinner due to the limited blood supply. Studies have shown that intraventricular rupture of an abscess is associated with a high mortality rate approaching 80%.[9] Abscesses in these locations should be aspirated, multiple times if necessary, regardless of the size. In the case of rupture, the patient should be treated with intravenous and intrathecal antibiotics.

Postoperative Care

Postoperatively, patients should be left on antimicrobial therapy for 6 weeks and, in cases of multiple abscesses, up to 3 months. Patients should have frequent contrast-enhanced CT scans in the postoperative period to verify the response to antibiotics. It is not uncommon for the enhancement to persist for months on MR studies in spite of appropriate antibiotic coverage and excellent clinical response. The optimal treatment of intracranial abscesses depends on many factors, and it must be individualized based on the characteristics of both the patient and infectious agent.

◆ Conclusion

Intracerebral brain abscess was a common disease with poor outcome before the advent of antibiotics, which has made the disease curable. Unfortunately, with the emergence of HIV infections and aggressive chemotherapy for cancer, brain abscess secondary to opportunistic organisms has become a common entity. Fortunately, the multiple diagnostic, surgical, and treatment modalities now available have improved neurological outcome from this serious disease.

References

1. Canale D. William Macewen and the treatment of brain abscesses: revisited after one hundred years. J Neurosurg 1996;84:133–142
2. Loftus C, Ostenbach R, Biller J. Diagnosis and management of brain abscesses. In: Wilkins R, Rengachary S, eds. Neurosurgery. 2nd ed. New York: McGraw-Hill; 1996:3285–3298
3. Hlavin M, Kaminski H, Fenstermaker R, White R. Intracranial suppuration: a modern decade of postoperative subdural empyema and epidural abscess. Neurosurgery 1994;34:974–981
4. Dolan R, Chowdhury K. Diagnosis and treatment of intracranial complication complications of paranasal sinus infections. J Oral Maxillofac Surg 1995;53:1080–1087
5. Lerner D, Zalzal G, Choi S, Johnson D. Intracranial complications of sinusitis in childhood. Ann Otol Rhinol Laryngol 1995;104:288–293
6. Giannoni C, Stewart M, Alford E. Intracranial complications of sinusitis. Laryngoscope 1997;107:863–867
7. Haines S, Mampalam T, Rosenblum M, Nagib M. Cranial and intracranial bacterial infections. In: Youmans J, ed. Neurological Surgery. 3rd ed. Philadelphia: WB Saunders; 1990:3707–3735
8. Takeshita M, Kagawa M, Yato S, et al. Current treatment of brain abscess in patients with cyanotic heart disease. Neurosurgery 1997;41:1270–1279
9. Mathisen G, Johnson J. Brain abscess. Clin Infect Dis 1997;25:763–779
10. Hirschberg H, Bosnes V. C-reactive protein levels in the differential diagnosis of brain abscesses. J Neurosurg 1987;67:358–360
11. Quartey GR, Johnston JA, Rozdilsky B. Decadron in the treatment of cerebral abscesses: an experimental study. J Neurosurg 1976;45:301–310
12. Britt R, Enzmann D. Clinical stages of human brain abscesses on serial CT scans after contrast infusion. J Neurosurg 1998;59:972–989
13. Obana WG, Rosenblum ML. Nonoperative treatment of neurosurgical infections. Neurosurg Clin North Am 1992;3:359–373
14. Dyste G, Hitchon P, Menezes A, VanGilder J, Greene G. Stereotaxic surgery in the treatment of multiple brain abscesses. J Neurosurg 1988;69:188–194

Section XIII

Stereotactic Surgery

86

Gamma Knife Radiosurgery for Tumors and Movement Disorders

Douglas Kondziolka and L. Dade Lunsford

Stereotactic radiosurgery has become an important and widely used treatment technique for the management of benign and malignant brain tumors. Ongoing analysis of results has led to refinements in technique and improved understanding of both the target and normal tissue dose response. An evolution in patient selection together with better imaging and computer workstations have led to improved results. Because long-term survival can be expected for most patients with benign disorders of the brain, both short- and long-term outcomes after radiosurgery must be documented. In this report, we present data from the first 18 years of experience at the University of Pittsburgh as part of an overall series of over 7,500 radiosurgery cases.

◆ Meningiomas

Surgical resection of a meningioma and its dural base is the preferred treatment for patients who harbor these tumors. Because these usually benign tumors may be associated closely with critical vascular, cranial nerve, and parenchymal brain structures, such complete resection may not be feasible in some patients.[1] Because recurrence after incomplete resection is quite likely, consideration of alternative or adjuvant strategies is important. Currently, these include stereotactic radiosurgery or the delivery of fractionated external beam radiation.[2–5] To date, hormonal therapies and chemotherapy have played only a limited and investigational role in the management of meningiomas.

Since 1987, over 1,000 patients with meningiomas had stereotactic radiosurgery at the University of Pittsburgh. In an evaluation of the first 380 with longer term follow-up, prior surgical resection was performed in 208 patients (55%) and 27 (7.1%) had undergone what was believed to be a "gross" total resection. Thirty-five patients (9.2%) had failed prior fractionated external beam radiation therapy. At the time of radiosurgery, 277 patients (73%) had evidence of a neurological deficit. The locations of meningiomas are listed in **Table 86–1** and most were at the cranial base.

Technique of Radiosurgery

All patients undergo radiosurgery under local infiltration anesthesia with mild sedation as necessary. Stereotactic magnetic resonance imaging (MRI) is used. We first obtain a contrast-enhanced sagittal scout sequence followed by an axial contrast-enhanced volume acquisition divided into 1 mm contiguous axial slices **(Fig. 86–1)**. This study provides high-resolution imaging of the tumor. Before 1991, patients had radiosurgery using stereotactic computed tomography (CT) guidance.[6] Coronal reformatted images are important in patients with parasagittal or cavernous sinus region tumors.[4] Images are sent via the Ethernet into the GammaPlan(r) computer workstation. Image integrated isodose plans are created to shape the irregular tumor borders. Skull-base and parasagittal meningiomas in particular attain unusual shapes along the dural surfaces and extend

Table 86–1 Brain Locations of 350 Meningiomas for Radiosurgery

Location*	Number of Patients
Cavernous sinus	109
Petrous apex	43
Petroclival	29
Parasagittal	33
Tentorium	29
Torcular herophili	8
Falx	17
Convexity	15
Clivus	6
Tuberculum sellae	7
Sphenoid ridge	20
Planum sphenoidale	6
Clinoid	6
Olfactory groove	7
Foramen magnum	4
Jugular foramen	4
Intraventricular	3
Pineal region	2
Orbit	1
Posterior fossa	1

*Primary location, but may include adjacent locations.

into different intracranial compartments. Multiple isocenter planning is used in most patients. In particular, 4 and 8 mm isocenters are important to tailor the dose toward the corners of tumors and to maintain a steep dose falloff toward structures such as the brain stem or optic chiasm.[2,7]

After dose planning is performed, selection of the dose is completed by the neurosurgeon together with the radiation oncologist and medical physicist. We delivered a mean dose to the tumor margin of 15 Gy and a mean maximum dose of 30 Gy. The mean tumor volume in this series was 4.0 mL (range, 0.12–28.5). A 50% or greater isodose line was used in 352 patients (93%) of this series.

Results of Meningioma Radiosurgery

After radiosurgery, all patients returned to their preoperative activities immediately. We previously completed an analysis of 99 patients with 5- to 10-year follow-up after radiosurgery. Most patients had diminished tumor volumes after 2 years of follow-up. Of 97 patients with serial imaging follow-up, 61 tumors were smaller (63%), 31 remained unchanged in size (32%), and five enlarged (5%). Resection was performed after radiosurgery in six patients.

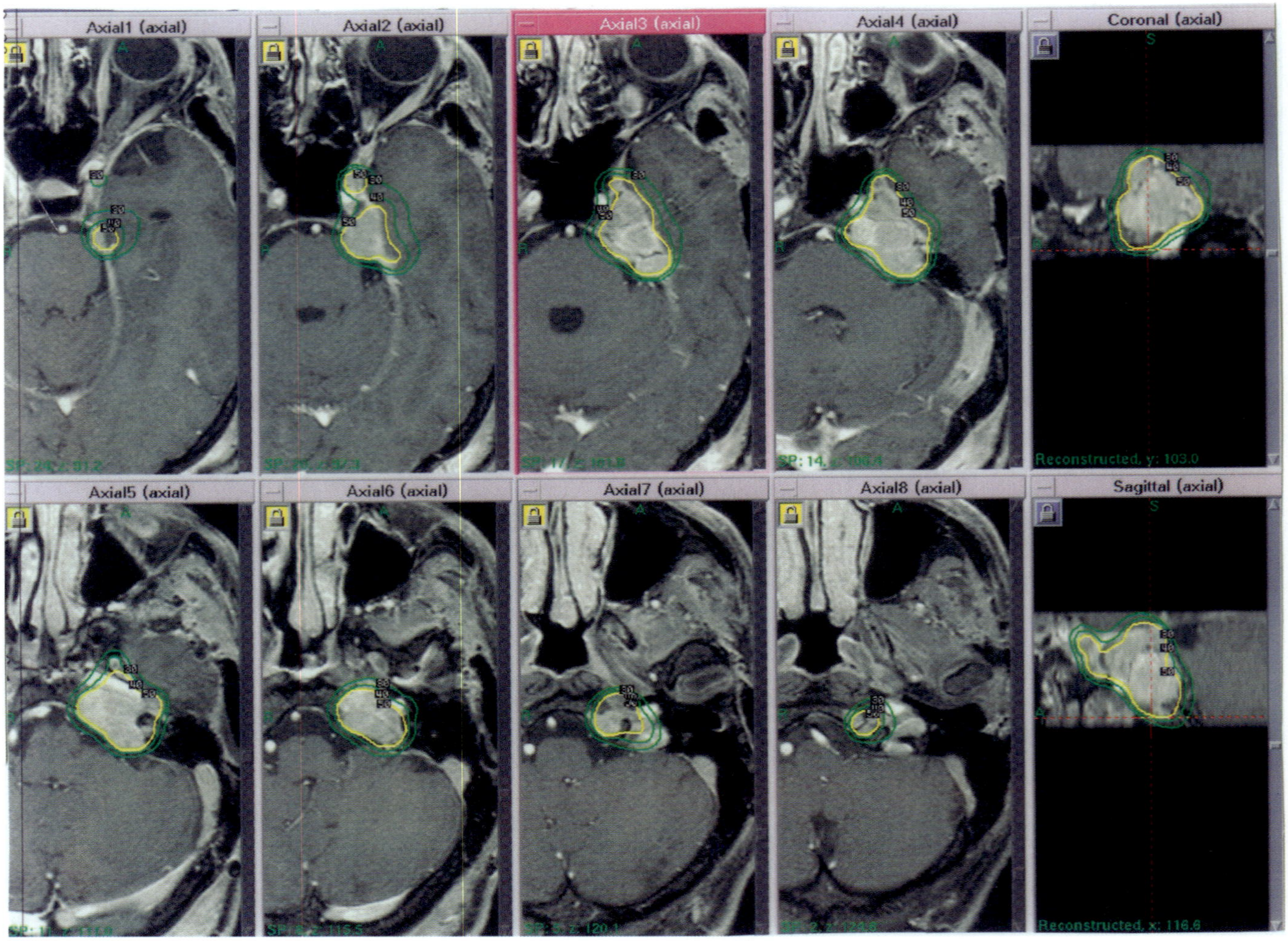

Figure 86–1 Gamma knife radiosurgery dose plan in a 52-year-old man with a petrous apex meningioma. Radiosurgery was performed with five 14 mm and five 8 mm isocenters to deliver 14 Gy to the 50% isodose line targeted to the tumor margin. Coronal and sagittal images are shown on the right. Note the conformal radiosurgery plan that follows the cranial base and tapers into the posterior cavernous sinus.

We characterized the pattern of imaging failure according to growth of the treated tumor or growth of a new separate or adjacent tumor. The failure rate from radiosurgery of the treated tumor mass was 4.9 ± 2.8% at 53–120 months. The total failure rate for *any* subsequent tumor growth in any location was 11.3 ± 4.2% at 63 to 120 months. Local tumor progression after radiosurgery was related to a history of prior resection ($p = .02$) and history of multiple meningiomas ($p < .00001$). Only one patient had resection of a meningioma after radiosurgery (for continued visual symptoms without tumor growth) if no prior resection had been performed ($n = 42$).

Indications for Radiosurgery

Current indications for meningioma radiosurgery include newly diagnosed, recurrent, or residual tumors after prior resection. In many patients, the imaging findings are typical and can be used to make the diagnosis of a meningioma. Patients with atypical imaging findings should undergo histological sampling before treatment. However, for small or medium-sized tumors consistent with meningiomas, radiosurgery may be an option. At this time we do not believe that radiosurgery should be a first-line approach for patients with convexity meningiomas where the likelihood of cure is high after resection. Radiosurgery is not often performed for optic nerve sheath tumors. However, for skull-base tumors or parasagittal tumors, we think that radiosurgery is an excellent management alternative. Although some surgeons believe in resection of as much of the tumor as possible and then follow the residual tumor with serial imaging studies, we believe this subtotal approach is inadequate for most patients. Current radiosurgery systems are not designed to approach spinal meningiomas.

In our initial experience, we advocated that a distance of at least 5 mm be present between the tumor margin and the optic nerve or chiasm.[2] However, with current high-resolution imaging techniques and sophisticated high-speed workstations, radiosurgery dose plans with the B gamma knife can be constructed so that only 1 mm may be necessary between the tumor margin and the chiasm if this proximity occurs only at one point. An extremely steep falloff in dose can be created at this point and the radiation shifted elsewhere (such as into the skull base). This has allowed the use of radiosurgery for tumors more closely related to the optic chiasm.

Advantages over Alternative Approaches

Brain tumor radiosurgery allows minimally invasive tumor management that is highly effective and associated with a low morbidity rate. As primary management for high-risk tumors, or as adjuvant therapy for residual or recurrent tumors, radiosurgery has become the most important new tumor therapy of the last decade.

Movement disorder radiosurgery can provide an effective clinical result in patients for whom more traditional procedures are not considered.

Disadvantages Compared with Alternative Approaches

Radiosurgery should be used for small or medium-sized lesions. When larger volumes are irradiated, the morbidity rate increases. Fractionated radiotherapy provides better treatment for large and diffuse tumors. When prompt improvement in neurological function is required, a resection should be considered. The results of movement disorder radiosurgery are just beginning to be reported. A higher success rate likely is attainable with electrode-based techniques, but with increased risk.

◆ Vestibular Schwannomas

Stereotactic radiosurgery has become a common therapeutic choice for patients with acoustic tumors (vestibular schwannomas). In 1987 we began a prospective assessment of the response of patients with acoustic tumors to gamma knife radiosurgery. Both early and later (5–10 year) outcomes were determined through the use of serial imaging studies, neurophysiological tests, and physician-based evaluations.[8]

Over 1,100 patients underwent stereotactic radiosurgery for an acoustic tumor (vestibular schwannoma) at the University of Pittsburgh over an 18-year period. These included patients with solitary tumors and those with neurofibromatosis type 2 (NF2).

In an evaluation of the first 502 patients, prior resection had been performed in 111 patients (24%). Twenty patients had two resections, five patients had three resections, and two patients had four or more resections. Normal facial function (House-Brackmann grade 1) was present in 382 patients (83%).[9] "Useful" hearing before radiosurgery was noted by 29% of patients.

In patients with NF2, prior resection was performed in 15. Two resections were performed in three patients and four resections in another three patients. Normal facial function before radiosurgery was present in 69%, normal trigeminal function in 80%, and useful hearing (Gardner/Robertson grades 1 + 2) in 31%.

Indications for Radiosurgery

We now believe that all patients with newly diagnosed, residual, or recurrent acoustic tumors (less than 3 cm in extracanalicular diameter) are now suitable radiosurgery candidates **(Fig. 86–2)**.[8] Radiobiology studies showed that the doses used caused tumor regression in a human xenograft model. Patients with larger tumors are not as good candidates because of the dose reduction necessary to reduce the rate of adverse radiation-related effects. In our first 3 years' experience, we accepted elderly patients, those with concomitant medical problems that argued against resection, patients with residual or recurrent tumors after resection, and patients with preserved hearing function. By 1991 we began to offer radiosurgery to all patients with acoustic tumors regardless of age, prior surgical history, or symptoms.[10–12] We continued to observe older patients (over 70 years) with small and minimally symptomatic tumors and recommended management only for imaging-defined tumor growth or progressive symptoms.[3]

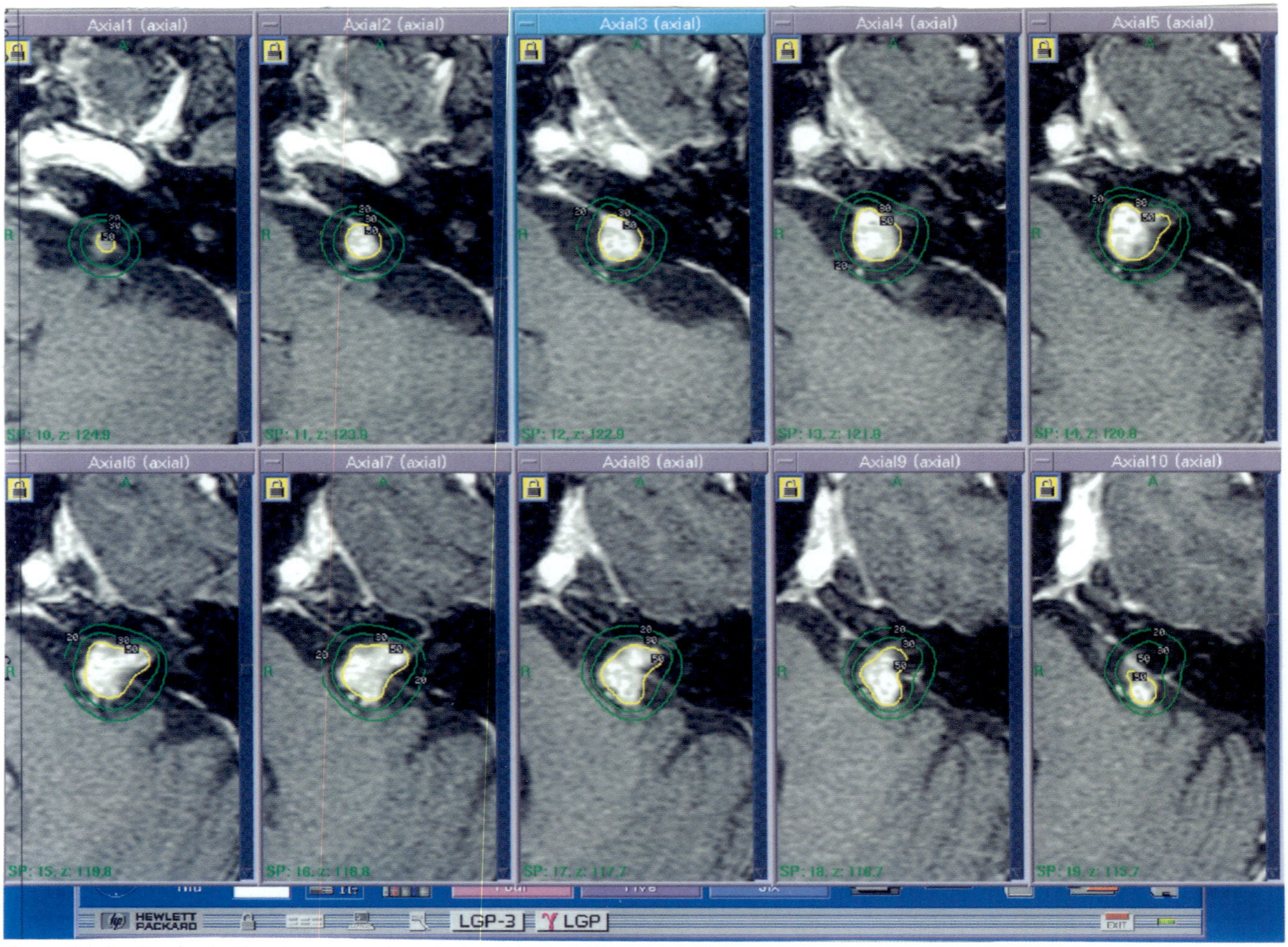

Figure 86–2 Gamma knife radiosurgery dose plan in a 64-year-old woman with an acoustic tumor. The plan was created with one 8 mm and five 4 mm isocenters to deliver 13 Gy to the 50% isodose margin (yellow line). One mm magnetic resonance images are shown.

◆ Evolution of Technique and Effect on Cranial Nerve Outcomes

Refinements in technique followed a continued review of results. When we found an approximate 30% rate of facial or trigeminal nerve morbidity, albeit delayed and usually mild, we reduced the tumor margin dose by an average of 2 Gy. Our initial attempts to preserve useful hearing in NF2 patients with radiosurgery proved unsuccessful. For that reason, we more cautiously used radiosurgery for patients with good hearing, doing so only after tumor growth had been documented and after patients learned lip reading or signing if the tumor was on their only hearing side.

In 1991 we began to use MRI-based stereotactic planning because CT-based planning did not show well the intracanalicular portion of the tumor. With MRI, we could image the tumor and regional neural structures in greater detail. This facilitated the use of multiple small irradiation isocenters for more conformal radiosurgery. With this type of radiosurgery, cranial nerve morbidity dropped precipitously, and by 1995, facial and trigeminal nerve side effects were below 7% for extracanalicular tumors and below 2% for intracanalicular tumors. These rates have dropped even further with improved dose-planning techniques. Similarly, our analysis of hearing preservation in NF2 patients showed significant gains. Whereas no patient maintained hearing at a Gardner-Robertson I or II level before 1992 (0/5), six out of nine patients did so after 1992 with improved radiosurgery techniques. At the same time, the high rate of tumor growth control was maintained.

◆ Pituitary Tumors

The second patient who underwent gamma knife radiosurgery in Sweden had a pituitary adenoma (1968).[14] An even longer experience exists in the use of charged-particle irradiation for pituitary adenomas. Radiosurgery for endocrine-active pituitary tumors was first performed in the late 1950s with charged particles. At the Lawrence Berkeley Laboratory, Lawrence, Tobias and colleagues primarily used the plateau range of protons or helium ions to deliver doses of 50 to

150 Gy in four fractions to adrenocorticotropic hormone (ACTH)- and prolactin-producing tumors and 30 to 50 Gy to patients with acromegaly.[15] Despite the long-term experience in radiosurgery (in a small number of patients), fractionated radiation therapy has been the conventional treatment for unresectable pituitary adenomas. Rates of tumor growth control have been reported to vary from 76 to 97%.[7,9]

Surgical Technique

Over an 18-year interval, 260 patients with pituitary adenomas were treated by stereotactic radiosurgery with the 201 source cobalt-60 Leksell gamma knife. The age of the patients varied from 9 to 88 years (mean = 46 years). In an earlier review, 24 patients (28%) had endocrine-inactive tumors. There were 29 patients (33%) with ACTH-secreting tumors, 20 patients (23%) with growth hormone-secreting tumors, 12 patients (14%) with prolactinomas, and two patients (2%) with tumors producing both growth hormone and prolactin. Ten patients (11%) received stereotactic radiosurgery as the initial treatment modality for their tumors. Of the 77 patients who had been treated by microsurgery prior to radiosurgery, 74 (96%) had a transsphenoidal tumor resection and 17 (22%) had a transcranial approach to the tumor. Eighteen patients (23%) who had residual or recurrent tumor after microsurgery also had fractionated radiotherapy (mean dose 45.6 Gy) prior to radiosurgery. Four of the patients with ACTH-producing adenomas also had bilateral adrenalectomy before radiosurgery.

The dose to the tumor margin was selected to minimize the risk of visual deficit and provide the highest potential for growth control and normalization of hormone production. These doses were chosen based on tumor volume and previous history of radiotherapy.[16] The mean radiation dose to the tumor margin was 19.2 Gy (9.6–30 Gy). When necessary, individual collimators within each helmet were plugged to shift peripheral isodose curves away from the optic nerve, chiasm, or tract to limit the dose to the optic apparatus to less than 9 Gy. Customized beam blocking techniques have improved sellar and parasellar radiosurgery planning by allowing more desirable radiation falloff curves. Presently, much of the falloff can be directed into bone, air sinus, or less critical brain structures **(Fig. 86–3)**.

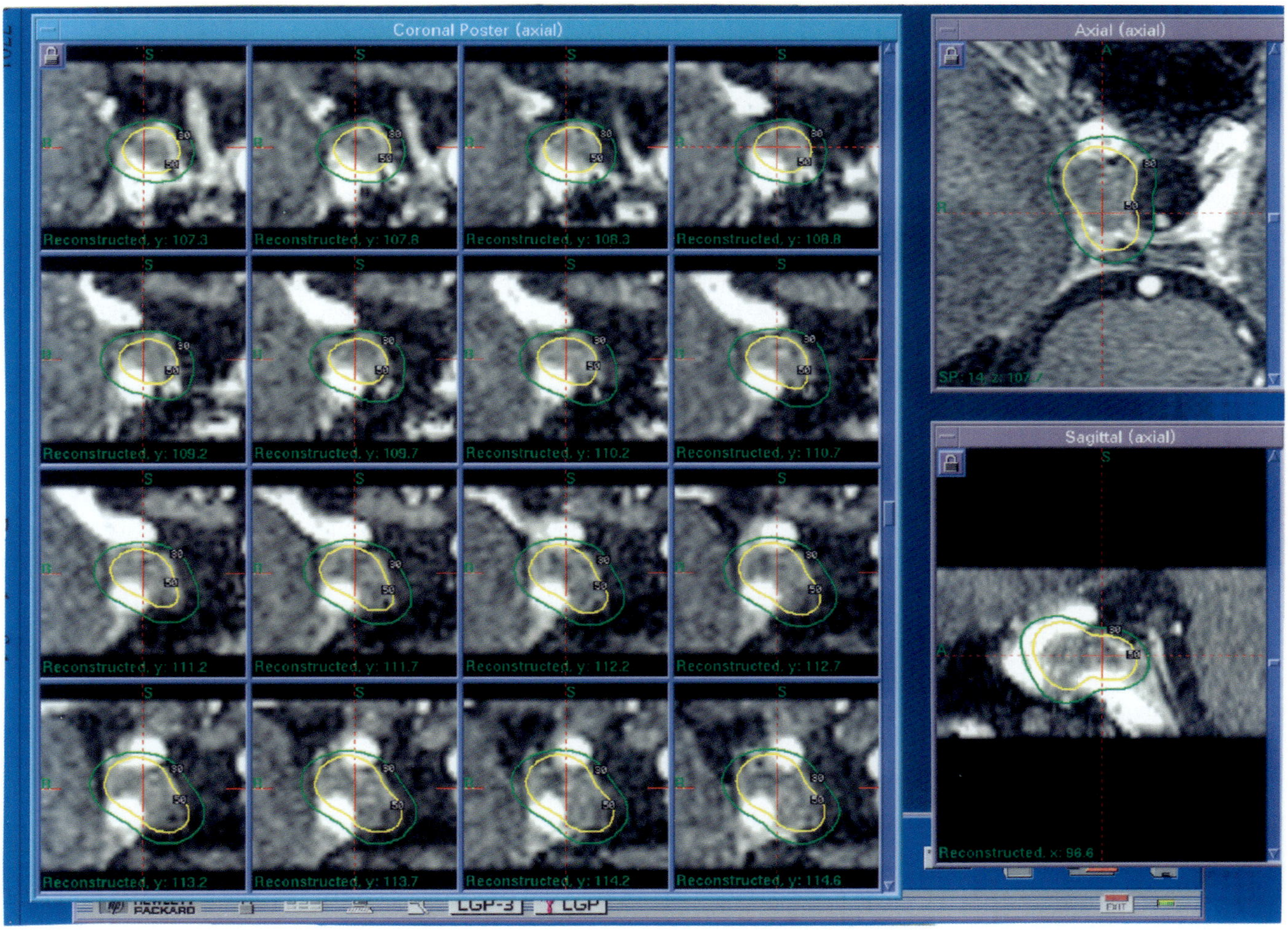

Figure 86–3 Coronal magnetic resonance images at radiosurgery for a pituitary tumor in a 65-year-old man after prior transsphenoidal resection. Gamma knife surgery was performed for a tumor in the cavernous sinus using three 8 mm isocenters to deliver 16 Gy to the 50% isodose margin at the tumor surface. The optic chiasm and nerves are well below the 30% isodose line.

Tumor Growth Control

Follow-up was available in 71 out of 87 patients (82%) over a period of 3 to 103 months (mean = 32 months). Growth control of the tumor enclosed within the prescription isodose line was achieved in 67 patients (94%); tumor volume decreased in 33 patients (46%) and was unchanged in 34 patients (48%). Tumor volume increased in four patients (6%) despite radiosurgery. Three of these four patients had had previous microsurgery (once, twice, and four times) as well as fractionated radiotherapy. Two patients with invasive prolactinomas developed new remote nodules of tumor in the cavernous sinus and along the optic tract and received second radiosurgical procedures. One of these tumors decreased in size and the other one was stable at 3 and 5 months, respectively, after the second gamma knife procedure.

Cushing's Disease

In the group of patients with ACTH-producing tumors, endocrinologic follow-up was available in 21 out of 29 cases (72%). Normalization of pituitary-adrenal function occurred in 11 of these 21 patients (52%) over a period of 4 to 39 months (mean = 16 months).

Acromegaly

Endocrinologic follow-up was available in 16 out of 20 (80%) acromegalic patients treated with the gamma knife. Fourteen of these 16 patients had both growth hormone and somatomedin-C levels tested; two patients only had analysis of somatomedin-C, and one patient was evaluated only by growth hormone levels. Growth hormone levels became normal in 10 of 14 (71%) of patients at a mean follow-up of 29 months (14–52 months). One of these patients continues to take octreotide and one takes bromocriptine. Three out of 14 patients (21%) had a greater than 50% reduction in growth hormone levels by 37 months (13–72 months) following radiosurgery.

◆ Movement Disorders

The origin of stereotactic radiosurgery parallels the developmental history of functional neurosurgery. Leksell[17] initially conceived the idea of closed-skull, single-session irradiation of a precisely defined intracranial target in 1951. He applied this concept immediately to functional neurosurgery. At that time, functional destruction of normal brain required thermal energy, or chemical injection such as phenol. Leksell cross-fired photon or proton radiation beams to achieve a similar goal. The initial radiosurgical concept was to create *small*, precisely defined focal destruction of a functional target, which was defined by image guidance. Whereas the ganglionic portion of the trigeminal nerve could be indirectly located using plain radiographs or cisternograms, deep brain targets required air or positive contrast ventriculography; direct visualization of the target for functional radiosurgery required the later development of computed imaging technology. Leksell first coupled an orthovoltage x-ray tube to his early generation stereotactic frame.[17] Later he worked with physicist Borje Larsson to cross-fire proton beams,[18] and subsequently a modified linear accelerator.

Dose Selection for Parenchymal Functional Radiosurgery

Early animal experiments showed consistent lesion creation at doses at or above 150 Gy.[19,20] Correspondingly, patients treated in initial studies received doses at or above that level, and Steiner recommended doses between 160 and 180 Gy in their cancer pain series. Although information was available on dose effects, little was known regarding the time required for necrosis to occur. Clinical data showed that pain relief occurred usually within 3 weeks after radiosurgery. In rat experiments at 200 Gy using a single 4 mm isocenter, we found a consistent relationship for lesion generation that substantiated observations from that human study.[21] Doses of 200 Gy were delivered to the rat frontal brain and then the brain was studied at 1, 7, 14, 21, 60, and 90 days after irradiation. At 1 and 7 days, the brain continued to appear normal. By 14 days, the parenchyma appeared slightly edematous within the target volume. However, by 21 days, a complete circumscribed volume of necrosis was identified within the radiation volume (4 mm diameter). This remained consistent thereafter. Thus, the clinical observation of pain relief at 21 days noted by Steiner et al was correlated with laboratory findings at the 200 Gy dose.

The ablative radiosurgery lesion appears as a punched-out, circumscribed volume of complete parenchymal necrosis with cavitation. Within a 1 to 3 mm rim that characterizes the steep falloff in radiation dose, normalization of the tissue appearance is found. In this zone, blood vessels appear thickened and hyalinized, and often protein extravasation can be identified. The brain is edematous in this region, either from an increase in extracellular fluid or from the intracellular swelling of gliosis. Acute or chronic inflammatory cells are present. MRI demonstrates all of these features after radiosurgical thalamotomy: a sharply defined, contrast-enhanced rim that defines the low signal lesion (on short TR images) surrounded by a zone of high-signal (on long TR images) brain tissue.[9] Friehs and colleagues[22] collected imaging data from four centers that created functional radiosurgery lesions ($n = 56$). They found that maximum doses in excess of 160 Gy were more likely to produce lesions larger than expected and recommended single 4 mm isocenter lesions at doses below 160 Gy.

The limitation of radiosurgery technology as a lesion generator stems from the inability to reliably control the effects of dose and volume. When a larger brain target may be desirable, the sharp falloff in dose outside the target becomes less steep with increasing volume. The risk of adverse radiation effects outside the target volume becomes problematic.[23] At small volumes (i.e., single 4 mm collimator), the radiosurgery-created lesion appears reliable.

Imaging in Functional Surgery

Because physiological information is excluded from the targeting component of a functional radiosurgery procedure, high-quality stereotactic neuroimaging must be performed. The imaging must be accurate because small volumes are irradiated. In addition, the imaging must be of sufficient resolution to identify the target structure but also show important regional tissues. MRI is the preferred imaging tool for functional radiosurgery.[24,25]

Accurate stereotactic MRI-based localization should be confirmed at each institution.[26] Although some centers fuse MRI data with CT data, many groups believe this unnecessary if the accuracy and precision of MRI is proven. CT poorly shows most functional targets such as the trigeminal nerve, basal ganglia, or thalamus, and should not be used as the sole method of planning unless the patient has a contraindication to MRI. Contrast-enhanced, volume acquisition MRI sequences divided into 1 mm slice thicknesses provide graphic definition of nerve and brain structures. The addition of fast inversion recovery MRI sequences helps to separate gray and white matter structures and has been an important improvement in thalamotomy and pallidotomy targeting for radiofrequency electrode-based surgery or radiosurgery. Despite these imaging improvements, the targeting of physiologically abnormal brain regions such as groups of kinesthetic thalamic tremor cells using imaging alone remains indirect.

Radiosurgical Thalamotomy

Ventrolateral thalamotomy for the management of tremor related to Parkinson's disease remains a proven and time-honored procedure within functional neurosurgery. Traditionally, thalamotomy has involved imaging definition of the thalamic target, placement of an electrode into the thalamus, physiological recording and stimulation at the target site, and creation of a lesion. Radiosurgical thalamotomy by definition avoids placement of the electrode and evaluation of the physiological response. In radiosurgery, imaging definition alone is used to determine lesion placement. Through the use of contrast ventriculography, CT imaging, and more recently stereotactic MRI scan, thalamotomy using the gamma knife has been performed at centers across the world.[24,27,28] We select a target $^{1}/_{4}$ of the anterior-posterior commissure (AC-PC) distance in front of the posterior commissure plus 1 mm, 2 mm superior to the AC-PC line (so the inferior extent of the lesion goes to the AC-PC line), and 12 to 15 mm lateral depending on the third ventricle width. We select this distance as third ventricle width divided by 2 + 11 mm. The target is then checked for its proximity to the internal capsule on fast inversion recovery MRI sequences.

Although radiosurgery can abolish tremor, many surgeons currently believe that better results might be achieved when neurophysiological testing is included in the surgery. Radiosurgical thalamotomy, if performed, should be performed by surgeons experienced in radiofrequency thalamotomy and deep brain stimulator placement. Nevertheless, excellent tremor abolition can be achieved with gamma knife radiosurgery **(Fig. 86–4)**.

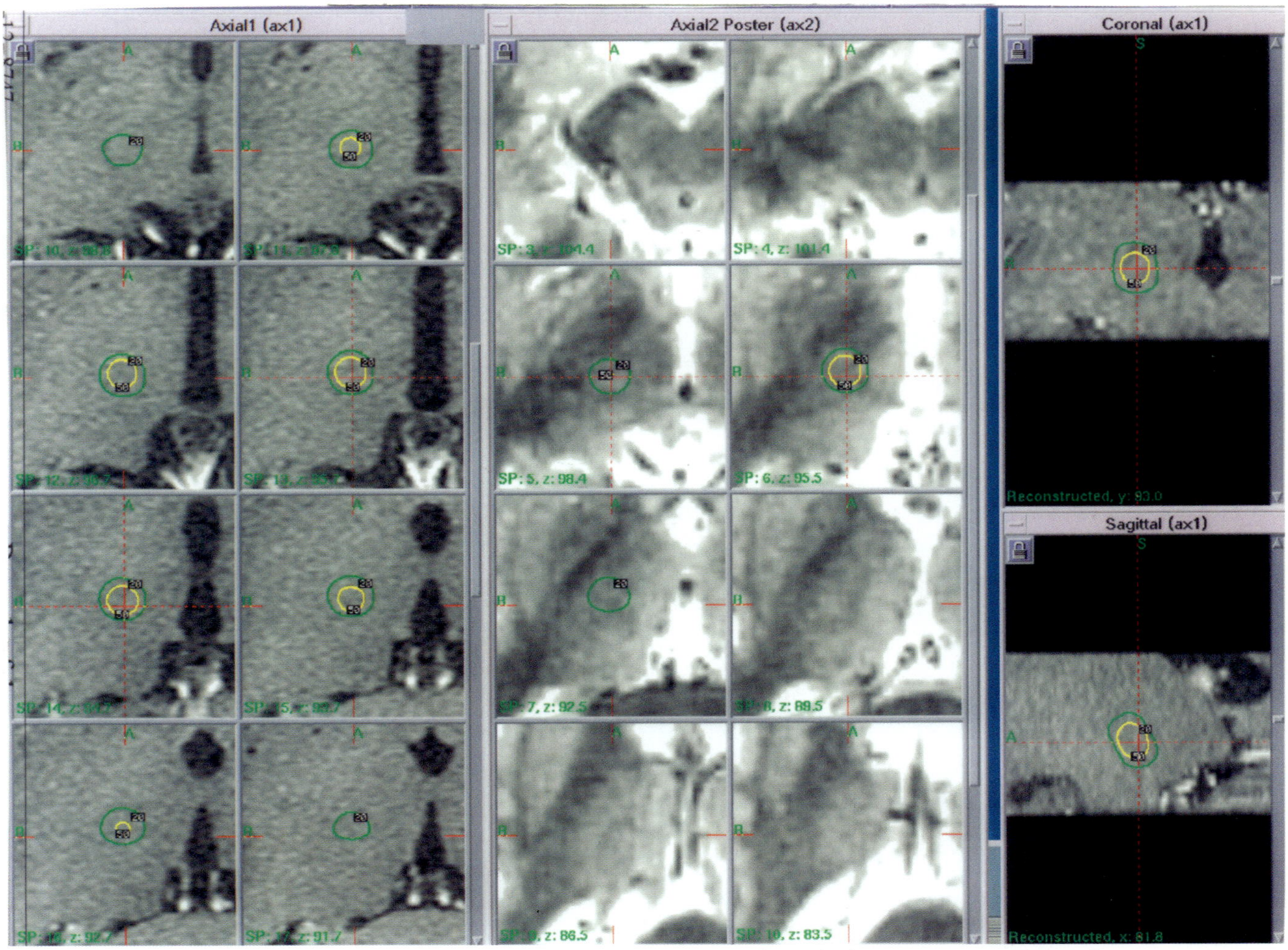

Figure 86–4 Gamma knife radiosurgery plan for left essential tremor. The right thalamotomy was planned with a single 4 mm isocenter targeted to the ventral intermediate nucleus of the thalamus. One mm contrast-enhanced volume acquisition and 3 mm fast inversion recovery sequence images are shown. The patient was 77 years old and had other concomitant medical problems.

References

1. Lunsford LD. Contemporary management of meningiomas: radiation therapy as an adjuvant and radiosurgery as an alternative to surgical removal? J Neurosurg 1994;80:187–190
2. Duma C, Lunsford LD, Kondziolka D, Harsh G, Flickinger JC. Stereotactic radiosurgery of cavernous sinus meningiomas as an addition or alternative to microsurgery. Neurosurgery 1993;32:699–705
3. Goldsmith BJ, Wara WM, Wilson CB, Larson DA. Postoperative irradiation for subtotally resected meningiomas: a retrospective analysis of 140 patients treated from 1967 to 1990. J Neurosurg 1994;80: 195–201
4. Kondziolka D, Flickinger JC, Perez B. Judicious resection and/or radiosurgery for parasagittal meningiomas. Neurosurgery 1998;43:405–414
5. Maire JP, Caudry M, Guerin J, et al. Fractionated radiation therapy in the treatment of intracranial meningiomas: local control, functional efficacy, and tolerance in 91 patients. Int J Radiat Oncol Biol Phys 1995;33:315–321
6. Kondziolka D, Lunsford LD, Coffey RJ, Flickinger J. Stereotactic radiosurgery of meningiomas. J Neurosurg 1991;74:552–559
7. Subach B, Lunsford LD, Kondziolka D, Bissonette D, Flickinger J. Stereotactic radiosurgery for petroclival meningiomas. Neurosurgery 1998;42:437–445
8. Kondziolka D, Lunsford LD, McLaughlin M, et al. Long-term outcomes after acoustic tumor radiosurgery: the physician's and patient's perspective. N Engl J Med 1998;339:1426–1433
9. Leksell L, Herner T, Leksell D, Persson B, Lindquist C. Visualization of stereotactic radiolesions by nuclear magnetic resonance. J Neurol Neurosurg Psychiatry 1985;48:19–20
10. Ogunrinde OK, Lunsford LD, Flickinger JC, Kondziolka D. Cranial nerve preservation after stereotactic radiosurgery of small acoustic tumors. Arch Neurol 1995;52:73–79
11. Ogunrinde OK, Lunsford LD, Flickinger JC, et al. Stereotactic radiosurgery for acoustic tumors in patients with useful preoperative hearing: results at two years. J Neurosurg 1994;80:1011–1017
12. Pollock BE, Lunsford LD, Kondziolka D, et al. Outcome analysis of acoustic neuroma management: a comparison of microsurgery and stereotactic radiosurgery. Neurosurgery 1995;36:215–229
13. Bederson JB, von Ammon K, Wichmann W, et al. Conservative treatment of patients with acoustic tumors. Neurosurgery 1991;28:646–651
14. Backlund EO, Rahn T, Sarby B, de Schryver A, Wennerstrand J. Closed stereotaxic hypophysectomy by means of 60-cobalt gamma radiation. Acta Radiol Ther Phys Biol 1972;11:545–555
15. Levy RP, Fabrikant JI, Frankel KA, et al. Heavy-charged-particle radiosurgery of pituitary gland: clinical results of 840 patients. Stereotact Funct Neurosurg 1991;57:22–35
16. Flickinger JC, Kondziolka D, Lunsford LD, et al. Evolution in technique for vestibular schwannoma radiosurgery and effect on outcome. Int J Radiat Oncol Biol Phys 1996;36:275–280
17. Leksell L. The stereotaxic method and radiosurgery of the brain. Acta Chir Scand 1951;102:316–319
18. Larsson B, Leksell L, Rexed B, Sourander P, Mair W, Andersson B. The high-energy proton beam as a neurosurgical tool. Nature 1958;182:1222–1223
19. Andersson B, Larsson B, Leksell. Histopathology of late local radiolesions in the goat brain. Acta Radiol Ther Phys Biol 1970; 9: 385–394
20. Rexed B, Mair W, Sourander P, Larsson B, Leksell L. Effect of high energy protons on the brain of the rabbit. Acta Radiol 1960;53: 289–299
21. Kondziolka D, Lunsford LD, Claassen D, Maitz A, Flickinger J. Radiobiology of radiosurgery, I: The normal rat brain model. Neurosurgery 1992;31:271–279
22. Friehs G, Noren G, Ohye C, et al. Lesion size following gamma knife treatment for functional disorders. Stereotact Funct Neurosurg 1996;66(Suppl 1):320–328
23. Kihlstrom L, Guo WY, Lindquist C, Mindus P. Radiobiology of radiosurgery for refractory anxiety disorders. Neurosurgery 1995;36:294–302
24. Duma CM, Jacques DB, Kopyov OV, Mark RJ, Copcutt B, Farokhi HK. Gamma knife radiosurgery for thalamotomy in Parkinsonian tremor: a five-year experience. J Neurosurg 1998;88:1044–1049
25. Young RF, Shumway-Cook A, Vermeulen S, Grimm P, Blasko J, Posewitz A. Gamma knife radiosurgery as a lesioning technique in movement disorder surgery. J Neurosurg 1998;89:183–193
26. Kondziolka D, Dempsey PK, Lunsford LD, et al. A comparison between magnetic resonance imaging and computed tomography for stereotactic coordinate determination. Neurosurgery 1992;30:402–407
27. Hirato M, Ohye C, Shibazaki T, Nakamura M, Inoue H, Andou Y. Gamma knife thalamotomy for the treatment of functional disorders. Stereotact Funct Neurosurg 1995;64(Suppl 1):164–171
28. Otsuki T, Jokura H, Takahashi K, et al. Stereotactic gamma-thalamotomy with a computerized brain atlas: technical case report. Neurosurgery 1994;35:764–768

87

Linear Accelerator (LINAC) Radiosurgery

Kelly D. Foote, William A. Friedman, Francis J. Bova, and John M. Buatti

Stereotactic radiosurgery is the application of a single, high dose of radiation to a stereotactically defined target volume. It is a unique hybrid of surgery and radiotherapy that has become an important tool for the treatment of various intracranial lesions. Advantages and disadvantages of radiosurgery compared with conventional neurosurgery and conventional radiation therapy are summarized in **Table 87–1.** Unlike most procedures in neurosurgery, radiosurgery requires

Table 87–1 Radiosurgery versus Conventional Treatments

Advantages	
Compared with Surgical Resection	Compared with Conventional Radiation
Noninvasive, outpatient procedure	Single treatment
No recovery time for the patient	More accurate radiation delivery
Virtually no acute complications	Less radiation of normal brain
Access to deep brain lesions with no trauma to superficial structures	Avoids common radiation-related side effects
Relatively inexpensive	Shorter treatment-to-effect latency
Disadvantages	
Compared with Surgical Resection	Compared with Conventional Radiation
Months to years delay between treatment and effect	Requires head ring placement
Will not immediately eliminate the risk of hemorrhage from an arteriovenous malformation	Does not exploit radiobiological differences in tissue sensitivity
The treated lesion is not removed	
Limited long term follow-up data	

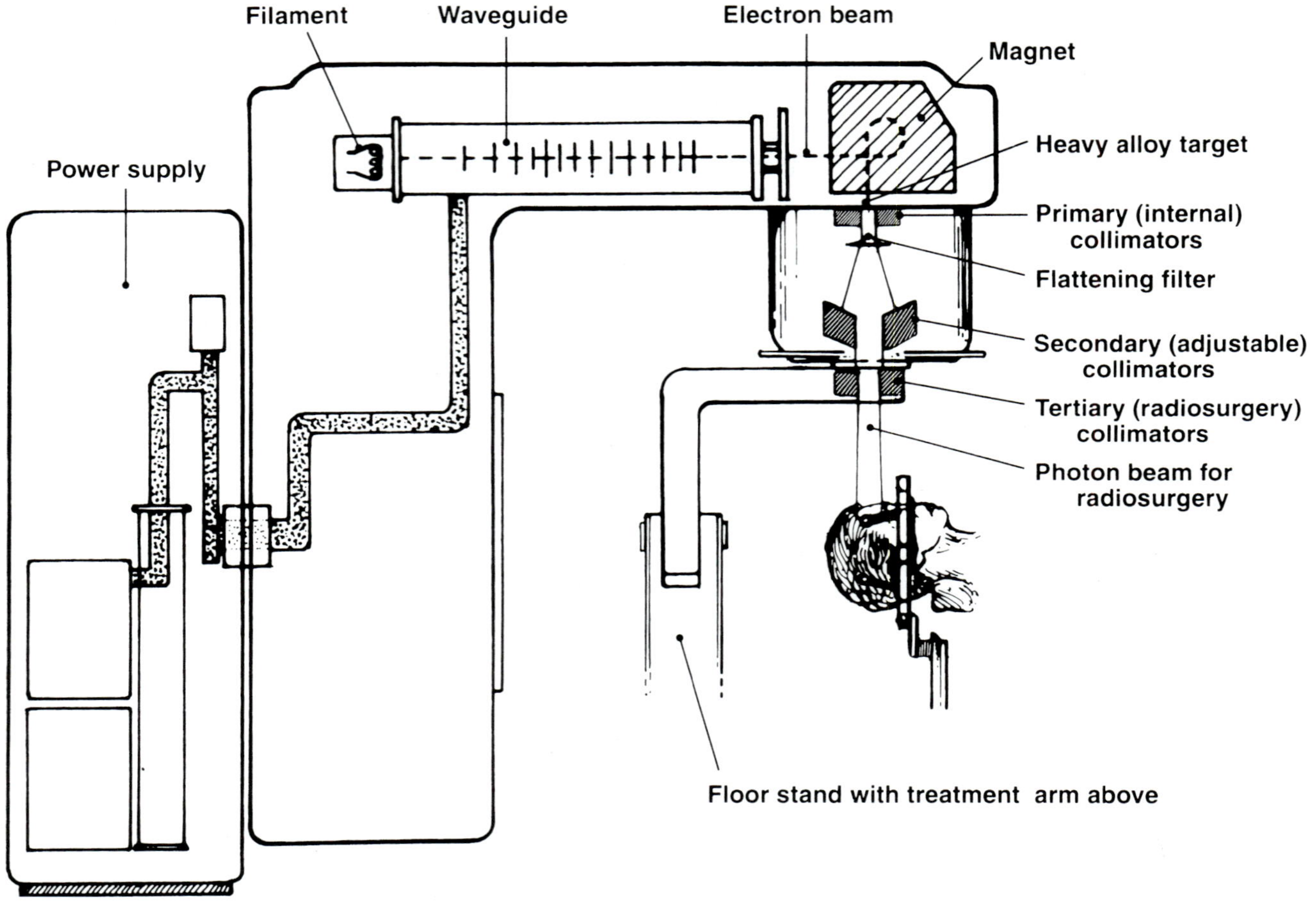

Figure 87–1 The linear accelerator. A linear accelerator is a complex machine capable of producing x-rays for radiation treatments. The power supply generates a large amount of energy that is channeled to the filament shown. This energy causes the filament to emit electrons, which are then accelerated to higher energies using a (microwave) waveguide. Their direction is altered by the magnet so that they impact on a heavy metal alloy target. This results in the production of x-rays, which are then collimated or shaped by both primary and secondary collimators (jaws) within the linear accelerator head. This beam is further collimated for radiosurgery by the tertiary radiosurgery collimator. In the University of Florida system, this tertiary collimator is within the treatment arm of the floor stand.

a multidisciplinary approach that incorporates the unique expertise of three separate medical disciplines (neurosurgery, radiation oncology, and medical physics) to produce an optimal result.

The goal of radiosurgery is to deliver a high dose to the target and a minimal and, it is hoped, harmless dose to normal tissue just a few millimeters away. Unlike the conventional radiation oncologist, the radiosurgeon relies more on extreme accuracy of radiation delivery than on radiobiological differences in tissue sensitivity and repair capacity.

The modified linear accelerator (LINAC) **(Fig. 87–1)** is a popular modality for the delivery of radiosurgical treatment and a description of its use is presented here. This chapter discusses the preparation for, and the delivery of, a typical LINAC radiosurgery treatment. The day of radiosurgery is described, beginning with head ring application, and followed by imaging, treatment planning, dose selection, and, finally, radiosurgery treatment delivery. Because assessment of treatment efficacy and of complications requires prolonged follow-up, we present our recommended schedule of follow-up for commonly treated abnormalities.[1]

◆ Indications for Radiosurgery

Indications for radiosurgery include selected arteriovenous malformations,[2] selected acoustic schwannomas,[3] selected meningiomas,[4] selected metastases,[5] radiation boost for malignant gliomas,[6] and other lesions such as nonacoustic schwannomas, selected pituitary tumors,[7] pineal region tumors, and possibly trigeminal neuralgia. The selection of lesions most suited for treatment with radiosurgery is based on several criteria, both general and specific to the lesion being considered. Factors that commonly enter into patient selection include pathology, lesion size, lesion location/proximity to eloquent or radiosensitive structures, amenability to surgical resection, prior surgery, patient age/medical fitness, and patient preference.

◆ Preoperative Evaluation and Studies

As with any neurosurgical procedure, the history, physical examination, and diagnostic imaging are critical for patient selection and documentation of any preexistent neurological deficits. In addition, a special protocol magnetic resonance imaging (MRI) scan, suited for image fusion with stereotactic head computed tomography (CT), is obtained the day before radiosurgery to facilitate dose planning for lesions that are poorly visualized on CT scan.

◆ The Day of Radiosurgery

Head Ring Application

Current stereotactic radiosurgical methodology requires attachment of a stereotactic head ring. The rigidly attached ring allows us to acquire spatially accurate information from angiography, CT, and MRI. The images obtained with this ring establish fixed relationships between the ring and the target lesion that are later translated during treatment planning so that the treatment target is accurately placed at the precise isocenter of the radiation delivery device. Because the stereotactic head ring is bolted to the treatment delivery device, it also immobilizes the patient during treatment. At the University of Florida, a modified Brown-Roberts-Wells (BRW) head ring **(Fig. 87–2)** is used. Most LINAC radiosurgical centers use some variation of this equipment.

In general, patients are premedicated with 10 mg of oral diazepam given approximately a half hour before ring application. Premedication is optional. No skin shaving or preparation is required. After the ring is assembled, with post drives and posts approximately positioned for application, the surgeon places the ring roughly in position. The post drives are moved in or out until the post tips rest loosely against the patient's skin. As a rule, the front pin holes are positioned about an inch above the supraorbital ridges and in the midpupillary planes. The back pins are positioned just above the external occipital protuberance and ~2 inches from the midline. Having the patient slightly flex the head usually facilitates ring placement. In this position, the pins are usually perpendicular to the skull surface and therefore very unlikely to become dislodged.

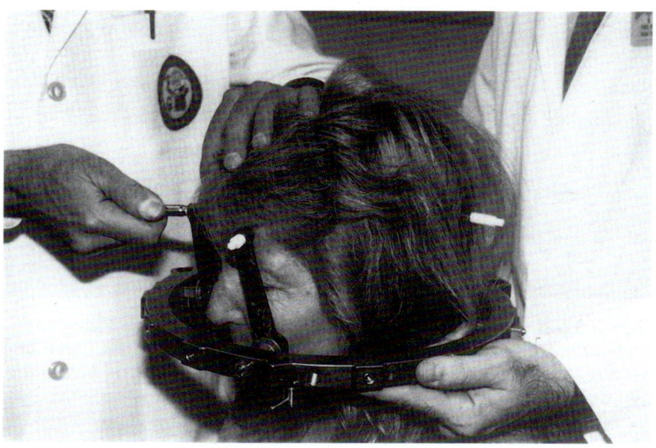

Figure 87–2 Placement of the modified Brown-Roberts-Wells (BRW) head ring.

As soon as the head ring is in final position for attachment, an assistant firmly stabilizes the ring from behind the patient while local anesthetic is injected through each of the post tip holes into the underlying skin. A wheal is raised with a solution containing equal parts of 0.5% lidocaine and 0.25% bupivacaine. This solution provides quick onset of anesthetic action as well as long duration.

Approximately 1 minute after anesthetic injection, the pins are inserted into the post holes and screwed through the skin until they rest against the skull. Using the pin wrench, we tighten the pins until the wrench cannot easily be turned using the thumb and first finger only. Care should be taken to avoid accidentally placing the pins into a bur hole or onto a bone flap from a prior craniotomy. Occasionally it is necessary to obtain skull fixation with three pins as opposed to the normal four because a large bone flap interferes.

At the conclusion of this procedure, the patient is transferred to a wheelchair and transported to the diagnostic radiology department for the next step (imaging) in the radiosurgery process.

Stereotactic Angiography

If the lesion to be treated is an arteriovenous malformation (AVM), stereotactic angiography is frequently the next step after head ring placement. The patient, with stereotactic head ring in place, is transported to the angiography suite. The radiologists prep and drape in the normal manner, as for any angiogram. Typically, a multiple vessel study is performed to fully define the vascular abnormality. In our institution, this "survey" is performed using digital imaging, to increase speed and reduce the amount of angiographic dye required. When the primary vascular distribution of the lesion is identified, the angiographic localizer **(Fig. 87–3)** is attached to the head ring. A set of scout films (or fluoroscopic views) verifies that all eight fiducial markers are seen on the lateral and anteroposterior (AP) views. A cut film angiographic sequence is then performed. Typically, rapid imaging through the arterial phase is performed to optimize AVM nidus visualization.

An AP and a lateral film that best image the AVM nidus are then selected. The nidus is outlined with a film marking pencil. These films are taped to a digitizer board. Using a mouselike device, the fiducial points and nidus outline are transferred to the computer screen. Using geometric methods, the computer determines the AP, lateral, and vertical stereotactic coordinates of the center of the nidus. The demagnified AP and lateral nidus diameters are also computed.

Angiography is the prime imaging modality for diagnosis and anatomical characterization of cerebral AVMs. It is also the time-honored means to judge the result of their treatment. For planning microsurgical or endovascular treatment of an AVM, angiography is clearly the gold standard. Because of its inherent limitations as a two-dimensional database representing a three-dimensional structure, however, stereotactic angiography alone frequently fails to indicate the true size and shape of the AVM, leading to errors in dose planning.[8] For radiosurgery, the two most critical

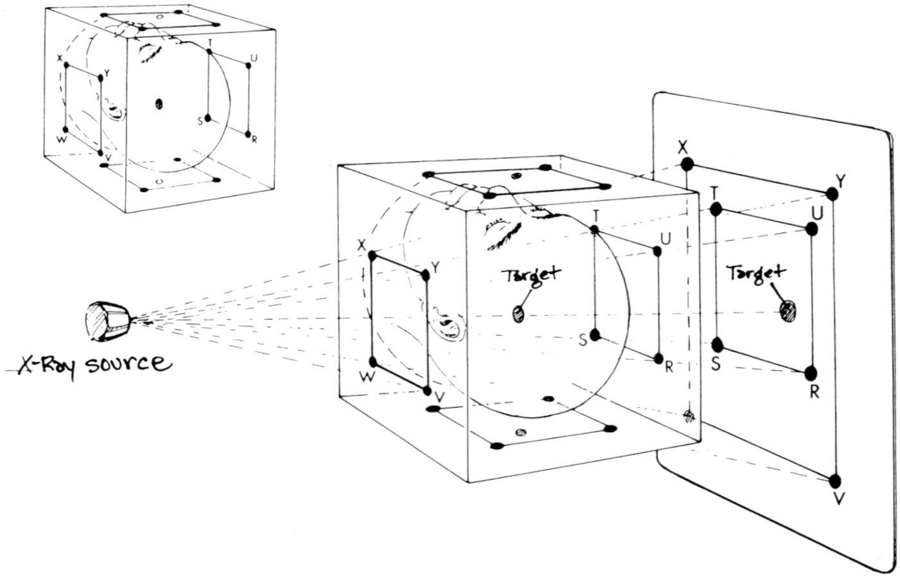

Figure 87–3 Stereotactic angiography. An angiographic localizer box is attached to the Brown-Roberts-Wells head ring. The localizer contains labeled fiducials in the anterior, posterior, right, and left sides of the box (here represented by the unlabeled points on the anterior and posterior of the box and labeled points on the lateral sides connected to make rectangles). Because the true geometry of these fiducial points is known, the location and size of the target in relation to the head ring can be calculated from the measured distances on the semiorthogonal angiographic images. The projection of the target on the semiorthogonal radiograph is shown on the lateral film along with the fiducials. An identical process is used for the anteroposterior angiographic film. In practice, a computer performs these calculations.

features of AVM anatomy are the tridimensional size and shape of the nidus. Underestimation of the target size may result in treatment failure. Overestimation of size results in the inclusion of normal brain within the treatment volume. Misrepresentation of an irregular target shape may lead to radiation damage of normal brain tissue. This, when affecting an eloquent area, may result in a neurological deficit. To avoid these errors, we recommend supplementing the two-dimensional database of a stereotactic angiogram with truly three-dimensional images of the AVM. We usually perform a thin-section CT scan through the area of the AVM nidus. Serial 1 mm cuts are performed while intravenous contrast is infused. This nearly always yields a very clear three-dimensional picture of the nidus.

Stereotactic Magnetic Resonance Imaging and Image Fusion

Stereotactic MRI for use in radiosurgical treatment planning can be obtained in one of two ways: (1) by using a customized, MRI compatible, head ring and localizer coupled to a specially tuned MRI coil to minimize the spatial inaccuracies that result from perturbation of the magnetic field, or (2) through the use of computer-generated image annealing software programs, commonly termed *image fusion*.

Image fusion techniques allow MRI images acquired without the stereotactic head ring to be used for treatment planning. The MRI scan used for image fusion is routinely obtained the day before treatment. Images acquired for image fusion use the standard diagnostic MRI head coil and the scan is not limited to the area of interest but includes the entire head. The scan technique uses volumetric image acquisition with a modified T1-weighted sequence. This technique allows rapid image acquisition so that movement during the MRI is minimized. Image fusion eliminates many of the hardware incompatibility problems involved with using MRI for treatment planning.[9] The volumetric scan technique also allows 1.5 mm slices, similar to the CT technique. Image resolution is identical to that used for diagnostic MRI scanning. **Fig. 87–4** is an example of an image-fusion treatment database being compared with a CT

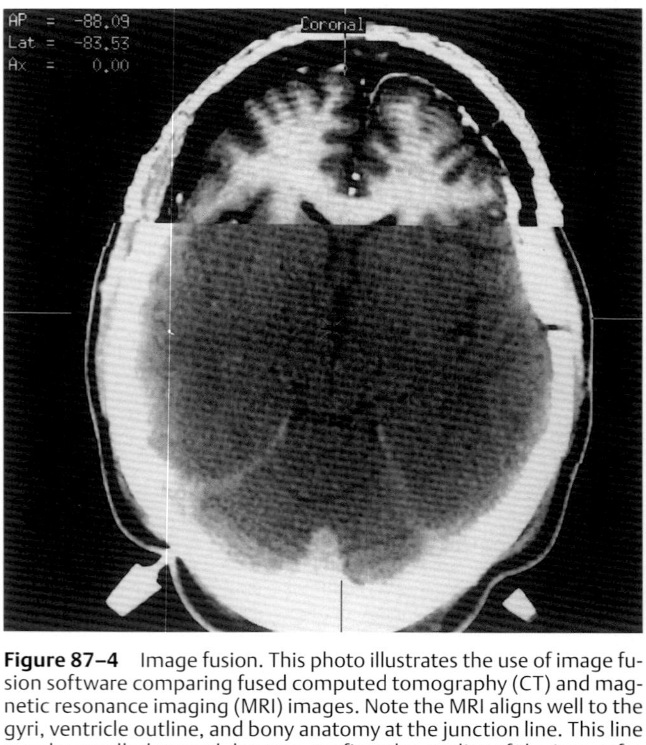

Figure 87–4 Image fusion. This photo illustrates the use of image fusion software comparing fused computed tomography (CT) and magnetic resonance imaging (MRI) images. Note the MRI aligns well to the gyri, ventricle outline, and bony anatomy at the junction line. This line may be scrolled up and down to confirm the quality of the image fusion. Attention to appropriate image annealing is critical to ensure that the nonstereotactically acquired MRI is registered accurately to the stereotactic CT scan.

treatment database before beginning treatment planning. Treatment planning using MRI is likely to increase in the coming years because many radiosurgical lesions are suboptimally imaged on CT scans.

Stereotactic Computed Tomographic Scan

After ring application and, if necessary, stereotactic angiography, the patient is transported to the CT scanner. A special bracket is attached to the head of the CT table, replacing the usual CT head holder. Bolts on the undersurface of the head ring attach it to this bracket, holding the head ring (and the patient's head) stationary and in a fixed, nonrotated position in relation to the CT couch. After securing the head ring to the CT table, the CT localizer is attached to the ring **(Fig. 87–5)**. A CT scanogram is obtained, and the gantry angle is adjusted so that the gantry is exactly parallel to the plane of the head ring, which simplifies calculations but is not a strict requirement of this procedure. The next step is to indicate where to start and stop the series of axial scans and what slice thickness to use.

We always start the scan at the top of the head. A series of sequential, 5 mm thick axial scans is obtained down to the area of the target lesion. At that point, sequential slice thickness is changed to 1 mm. After the lesion is believed to be totally imaged, 5 mm slices are resumed to the base of the skull. This strategy provides maximum resolution through the target region but, by using thicker slices in the nontarget brain regions, reduces the number of scan slices, scanning time, and computer memory requirements. If the CT image is to be fused with a preoperative MRI scan, 1 mm slices are obtained from the top of the head to the base of the localizer to optimize image fusion accuracy.

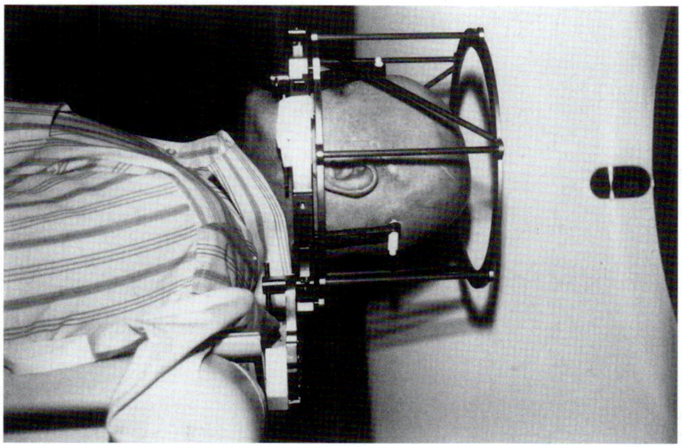

Figure 87–5 A patient ready for computed tomographic image acquisition. After the bracket is attached to the table, the patient is secured to the table bracket by the bolts in the undersurface of the Brown-Roberts-Wells ring shown. Then the localizer is attached, the swivel locks are tightened, and the patient is ready for scanning. Note that the pin wrench is taped to the undersurface of the ring and should remain with the patient at all times in case the frame must be removed in an emergency.

Contrast Injection

Patients should not eat or drink anything after midnight the day of the scan, in case contrast material causes nausea or other adverse reactions. Nonionic contrast material is preferred because it significantly reduces the incidence of side effects. These side effects are especially undesirable in restrained patients (clamped to the table). Typically, in adults, 100 cm^3 of contrast material is used. Scan images are scrutinized during the study to make sure the lesion is well visualized for subsequent dose planning. If not, a repeat scan may be done after more contrast material is injected, or after a further time delay to allow contrast material to infuse into the lesion.

When imaging brain tumors, intravenous contrast material is usually injected just before the scanning begins. For AVMs, a special injection technique is used. No contrast material is injected until the top of the target area is reached. Then 100 cm^3 of contrast material is rapidly infused (1 cm^3 per second) intravenously as the 1 mm target CT slices are acquired. Scanning while infusing the contrast medium results in a superior image of relevant vascular structures (feeding arteries, the nidus, and draining veins) composing the AVM.

Image Processing

CT images (80 to 150 CT slices per patient) are next transferred to the dosimetry planning computer. A program in the dosimetry computer automatically identifies the nine fiducial rods surrounding each axial image. Using geometric equations, the computer determines the AP, lateral, and vertical position of each point (pixel) in each CT slice. This information is then replotted in the computer's memory and all CT images are mathematically referenced to the head ring, which remains fixed to the patient's head. Hence, any point seen on the CT scan image is co-identified as a Cartesian coordinate related to the head ring. Furthermore, because the entire head is scanned and is represented as a conglomeration of unique pixels in the computer, the distance from the scalp to any target point can be mathematically determined from any point along the image. This information is vital for dose calculations, because attenuation of each entering radiation beam is proportional to the target depth for that beam. Rapid calculation of dose distribution for hundreds of beams represented by arcs of radiation requires a defined three-dimensional image within the computer. This image is defined during image processing before treatment planning. Any stereotactic angiography or MRI images are similarly converted to this type of coherent, three-dimensional database.

◆ Radiosurgery Treatment Planning

Once the necessary stereotactic images have been acquired and transferred to the treatment-planning computer, the next step is to plan the precise delivery of radiation. This is accomplished through the use of a computer workstation and specialized treatment planning software tools.

Goals

An ideal radiation treatment plan would deliver 100% of the desired dose to the treatment target and none to the normal brain. This is not possible in reality, but the primary goal of radiosurgery treatment planning is to achieve a plan that conforms to the target as closely as possible, as defined by radiation *isodose shells*. Isodose shells are volumes bounded by surfaces that receive the same radiation dose, expressed as a specified percentage of the maximum radiation dose. Several treatment planning tools are available for adjusting the shape of treatment isodose shells so that they fit even highly irregular target shapes. Regardless of its shape, the entire target must be treated within the prescription isodose shell (most commonly the 70 or 80% line), with as little normal brain included as possible.

Another goal of dose planning is to adjust the dose gradient such that critical brain structures near the target receive the lowest possible dose of radiation. In addition, most LINAC radiosurgeons strive to produce a treatment dose distribution that maximizes uniformity (homogeneity) of dose throughout the entire target volume.

◆ Dose Concentration through the Use of Intersecting Beams

Radiation dose can be concentrated on a given deep target by focusing multiple radiation beams so they intersect at the target. As illustrated in **Fig. 87–6,** the relative dose delivered to the (nontarget) tissue along the entry and exit

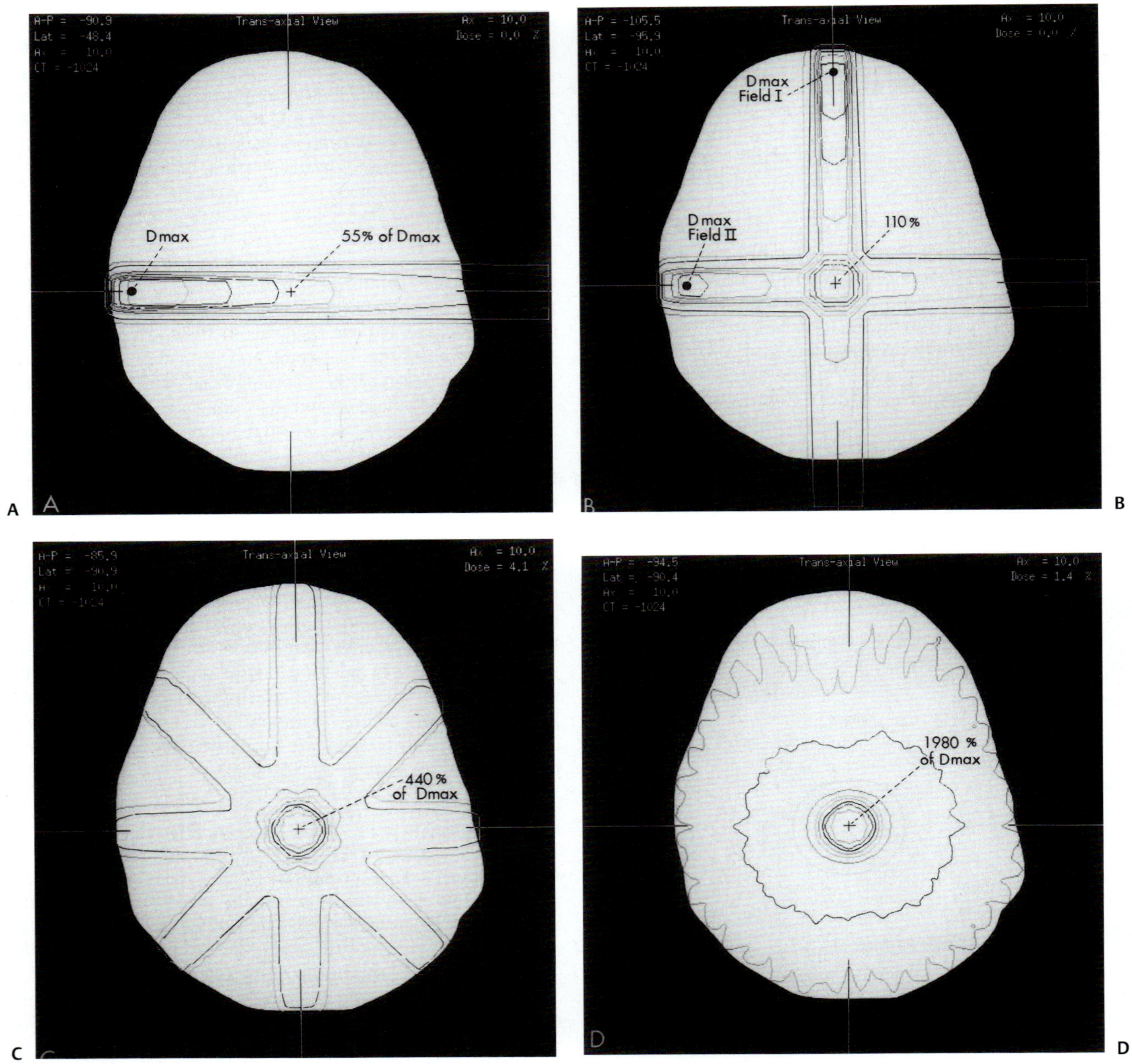

Figure 87–6 Dose concentration by the addition of multiple radiation beams. This example shows **(A)** a single field, **(B)** two fields, **(C)** eight fields, and **(D)** 36 fields of radiation focused on a target. Note that the target (cross-hairs) gets 55% of the maximum (Dmax) of **(A)** one field, **(B)** 110%, **(C)** 440%, and **(D)** 1980% of the dose from any individual field. The radiosurgery paradigm is the equivalent of hundreds of radiation

paths of a given beam is very low compared with the dose at the intersection (target/isocenter) of multiple beams. The concept of using multiple beams is extended by the radiosurgery treatment paradigm used for LINAC and gamma knife systems. Gamma knives use 201 separate cobalt sources, all aimed at one target. LINACs use multiple, noncoplanar arcs of radiation, all focused on one target. In the stereotactic paradigm, the equivalent of hundreds of radiation beams is focused on a selected target.

◆ Treatment Planning Tools

In practice, a set of beam attenuation curves is determined for each size of collimator (beam-shaping device) used in radiosurgery. In this way, the dose contributed by each radiation beam to a target at a given depth is defined. Typically, beam diameters of 5 to 40 mm are available for standard LINAC radiosurgery. The distance each beam will travel through tissue before it reaches the target is readily computed during treatment planning from the reconstructed CT scans. Using the predetermined, collimator-specific attenuation data and the known depths to target, dosimetry software programs can rapidly compute and display the isodose information for any proposed combination of radiation beams and target dose desired.

Arc Elimination

In general, we begin treatment planning by directing nine equally spaced arcs of radiation at the center of the target **(Fig. 87–7)**. Each arc span is 100 degrees, and each arc is spaced 20 degrees from its neighboring arcs. This results in a spherical dose distribution, with the dose falling off equally in all directions.

Many radiosurgical targets are not perfectly spherical; rather, they are shaped more like an elongated sphere (ellipsoidal). It is relatively easy to change the spherical dose

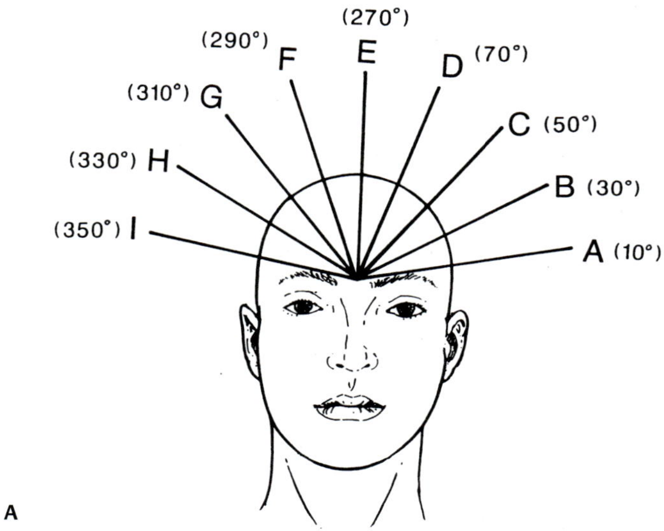

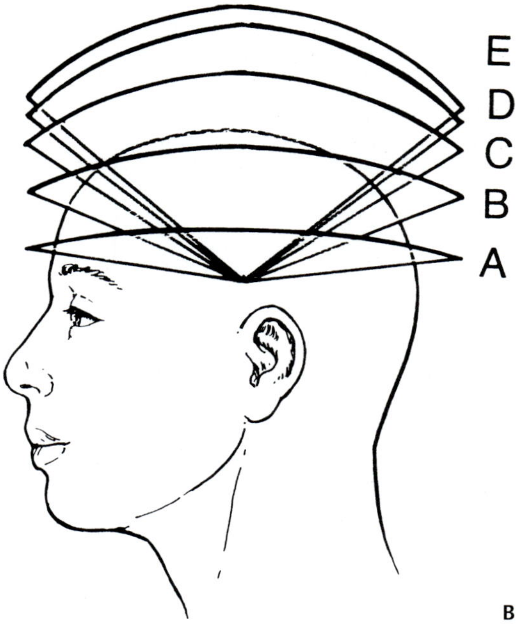

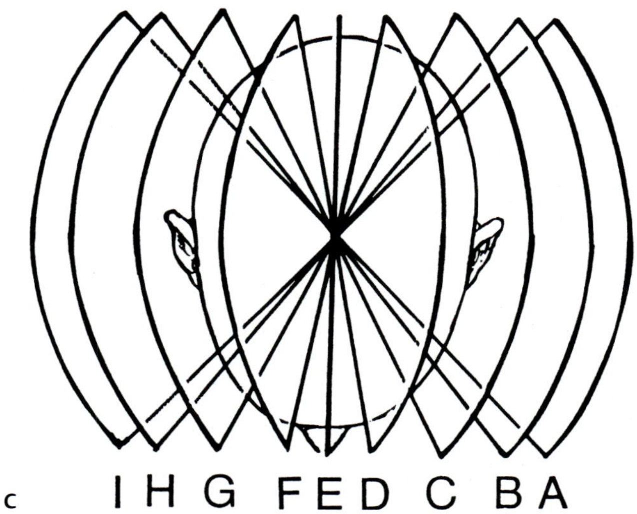

Figure 87–7 A standard nine-arc set. Radiosurgery treatment planning at the University of Florida begins with nine equally spaced arcs of radiation. **(A)** Coronal orientation of the nine arcs. Treatment table angles (in degrees) to deliver each arc are noted in parentheses and each arc is lettered A to I. **(B)** Lateral view showing the arc orientations. **(C)** Superior view of the nine arcs lettered to coincide with each table angle shown in **(A)**.

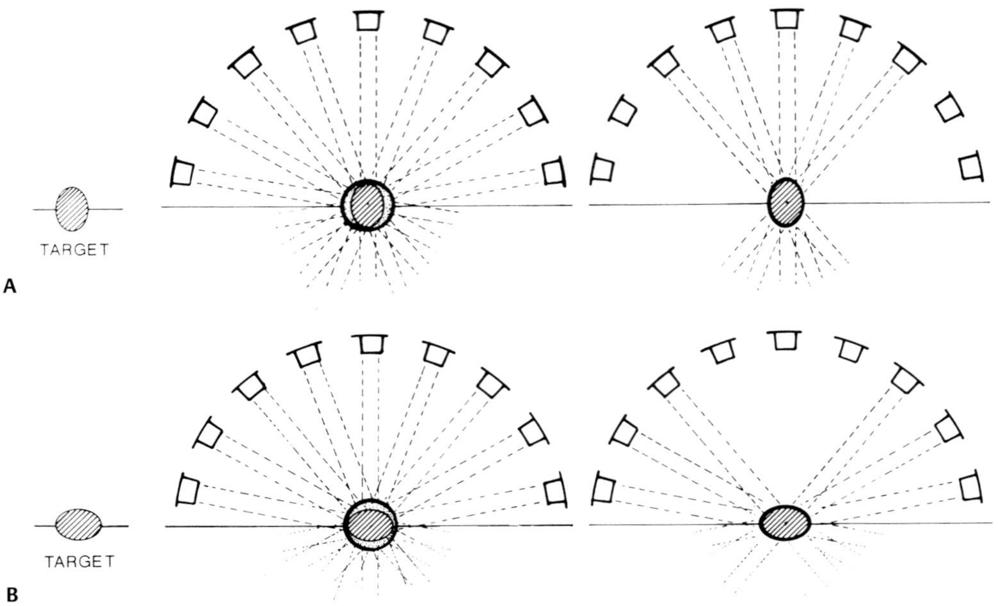

Figure 87–8 Arc elimination. **(A)** An ellipsoidal target in the coronal plane with a principal axis in the superior-inferior direction is represented by the crosshatched region. The spherical dose distribution created by the nine-arc radiosurgery starting point is shown with a bold line. Each arc is represented by a schematic collimator and each entering radiation beam by dotted lines. Note that the isodose line does not conform to the target (see stippled region surrounding the target but within the bold line). By eliminating arcs of radiation perpendicular to the long axis (the more horizontal arcs) of the ellipsoidal target, the dose distribution (bold line) conforms to the target and the stippled area is eliminated. **(B)** An ellipsoidal target in the coronal plane with a principal axis in the medial-lateral direction. Again the target is crosshatched and the dose distribution of the minimum-size nine-arc treatment plan is adjacent. The stippled area illustrates the lack of conformality of the isodose line (bold) to the target. By eliminating arcs of radiation perpendicular to the principal axis of the target (the more vertical arcs), the conformality is significantly better and the stippled area outside the target is eliminated.

distribution into an ellipsoidal distribution with LINAC radiosurgery systems. All that is required is to eliminate the arcs (reduce their weight to zero) that are most perpendicular to the long axis of the ellipsoid. This technique is illustrated in **Fig. 87–8.** A corollary to this method is that elimination of an arc reduces the spread of radiation in the principal direction of the eliminated arc. For example, when treating an acoustic schwannoma, it is desirable to minimize the radiation given to the medially located brain stem. This is effectively accomplished by eliminating the four most horizontal arcs (which would enter or exit through the brain stem). The radiation dose is elongated into the superior-inferior direction, where less critical structures are located, and the spread of radiation over the medially located brain stem is reduced. Alternatively, when treating a pituitary tumor, the adjacent critical structure is the optic chiasm, which is located superior to the tumor. Eliminating the three most vertical arcs reduces the spread of radiation in the superior-inferior direction, but increases the spread in the lateral direction where less sensitive structures (cavernous sinuses) are located. This dose gradient modification might be called the "Jell-O principle" of radiosurgery. If one compresses a spherical Jell-O mold in one direction, it will elongate in another. By using the tool of arc elimination and by understanding the Jell-O principle, both the primary goal of conforming to the target and the secondary goal of sparing critical structures may be approached. In radiosurgery treatment planning designed to avoid critical structures, the elongated portion of the Jell-O mold is in the direction of the least critical structures.

For any target that is approximately ellipsoidal and has its principal axis anywhere in the coronal plane, treatment can be planned by eliminating the arcs that are most perpendicular to its principal axis. In addition, arc elimination maximizes the dose gradient in the direction of the eliminated arc. This strategy is the most frequently used treatment planning method in LINAC radiosurgery and, by itself, results in a conformal treatment plan for many radiosurgical lesions.

Differential Collimator Sizes

The overall weight of an arc can be changed (increased or reduced), rather than completely eliminated, by increasing or reducing the size of the beam (i.e., collimator size) used for the arc. **Fig. 87–9** illustrates the use of this method to fine-tune an elliptical dose distribution. If the most horizontal collimators are reduced in size, the distribution becomes less elongated in the superior-inferior direction because the height is most controlled by the horizontal beams. Conversely, decreasing the size of the more vertically oriented arcs diminishes the lateral spread of the overlapping tubes of radiation and creates a distribution of the same height that is slightly more narrow. Hence, as an alternative to arc elimination, different collimator sizes can be

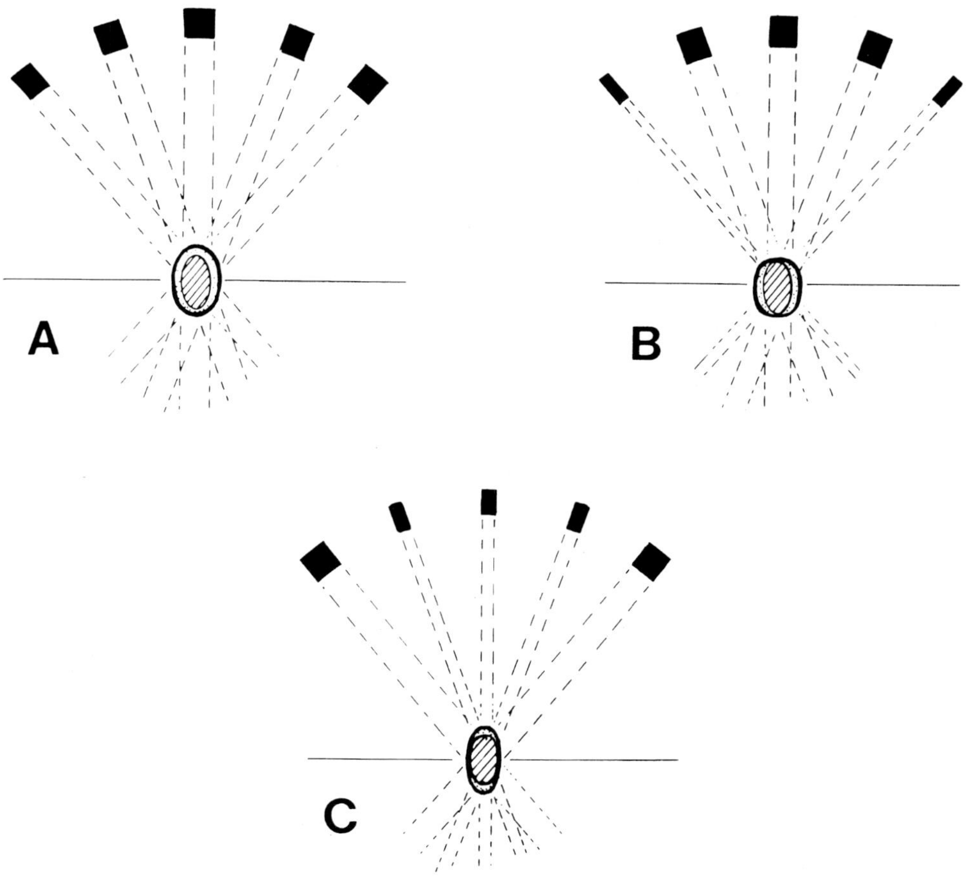

Figure 87–9 Differential collimator sizes. **(A)** A dose distribution elongated in the superior-inferior direction created by eliminating the four most horizontal arcs. **(B)** A reduction in the collimator size on the most horizontal of the remaining arcs reduces the height of the distribution without appreciable change in the width. **(C)** Reduction of the collimator size in the three most vertically oriented arcs makes the dose distribution less wide (thinner) with an elongation (height) that is the same. These changes in differential collimator sizes allow fine-tuning of the ellipsoidal distributions to account for different ratios of the principal to nonprincipal axis. Changes in collimator sizes have relatively little effect on the lower isodose lines in a radiosurgery dose distribution compared with arc elimination.

used on different arcs. This strategy results in slightly more or less severe elongation (i.e., ratio of principal to nonprincipal axis) of the treatment isodose configuration, with much less change in elongation of the lower isodose lines into surrounding tissue.

As a practical matter, differential collimator sizes and arc elimination are often used in combination to fine-tune the shape of the treatment isodose curve. This is especially useful when arc elimination is used primarily to reduce irradiation to surrounding structures.

Altering Arc Start and Stop Angles

Typically, we use arcs spanning 100 degrees, starting 30 degrees off the superior vertical and ending 50 degrees off the inferior vertical **(Fig. 87–10A).** This results in the particular AP orientation (sagittal plane) of the isodose curves shown. Sometimes the target lesion has a significantly different AP orientation. For example, if a lesion is tilted anteriorly or posteriorly compared with the standard isodose orientation, its orientation can be more closely approximated by changing the vertical arc angles. This decreases the total arc span and orients the arc in closer parallel to the long axis of the target.

Another application of this tool emerges because critical structures are sometimes located immediately anterior or posterior to the target lesion. In this case, one would like to maximally reduce the dose gradient in the AP direction. This is readily accomplished by decreasing the arc span **(Fig. 87–10B).** Narrow arcs effectively elongate the lower isodose lines in the superior inferior direction, while narrowing them in the AP direction (another application of the Jell-O principle).

In summary, arc start and stop angles can be adjusted so that the principal AP vector of the arc more closely matches the AP orientation of the target. In addition, reducing the arc span can be used to maximize the AP dose gradient.

Multiple Isocenters

Arc weighting is used in treatment planning for lesions that are ellipsoidal in the coronal plane **(Figs. 87–8** and **87–9).**

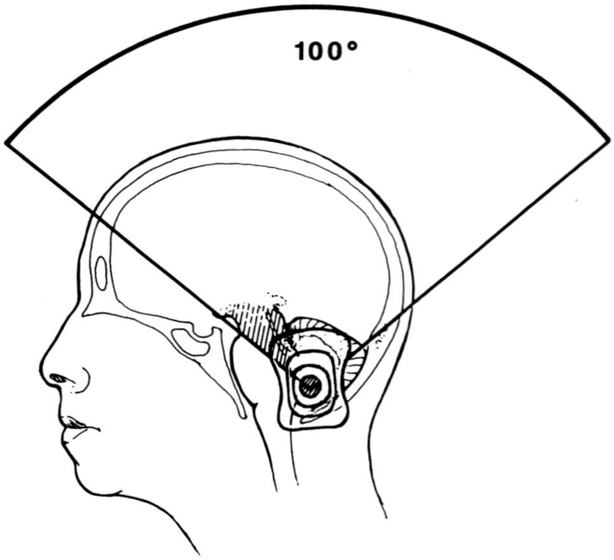

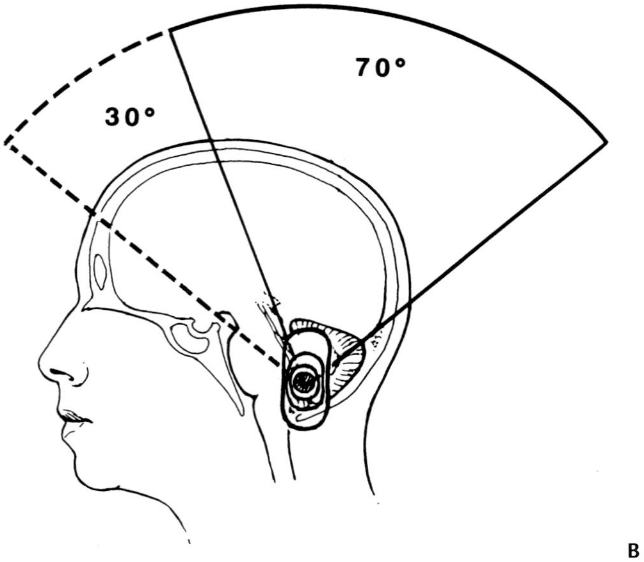

Figure 87–10 Altering arc start and stop angles. Altering the arc start/stop angles can improve conformality and dose gradient by changing the anteroposterior tilt of the field in the sagittal plane. **(A)** Schematic representation of a target immediately posterior to the brain stem. This shows the typical dose distribution obtained with a standard nine-arc plan in the sagittal plane. Note: The anterior portion of this representative arc transgresses the critical neural structure, the brain stem. This area that we want to avoid is crosshatched in the illustration. **(B)** By altering the anterior portion of each arc, the dose gradient is improved. In this case, the anterior 30 degrees of each arc (the segment traversing the brain stem) is removed. The resulting dose distribution (illustrated) has a superior dose gradient (sharper dose falloff) anteriorly near the critical neurological structure, the brain stem.

Changing arc start and stop angles is used to more closely match the AP tilt of lesions that are primarily elongated in a superior-inferior direction **(Fig. 87–10).** If a lesion is ellipsoidal but primarily elongated in the AP direction (axial plane), however, multiple isocenters must usually be used to produce a conformal plan. Likewise, if the lesion is nonspherical and nonellipsoidal, multiple isocenters must be used.

To use multiple isocenters, the three-dimensional (3D) shape of the lesion must be ascertained. This is accomplished by viewing sequential axial CT or MRI images from the top to the bottom of the image, or, optimally, a 3D viewing window more easily accomplishes the same purpose. If the lesion is generally cylindrical, two isocenters are used. If it is generally triangular, three isocenters are used. If it is generally shaped like a rectangular solid, four isocenters are used. Occasionally, more isocenters are necessary to conform to a lesion of very irregular shape.

Once the 3D shape of the lesion and the number of isocenters needed are determined, the isocenters must be positioned. This is accomplished by computer reconstruction of the plane through the lesion that contains its principal axis. The isocenters are roughly positioned, in the appropriate orientation (line, triangle, or rectangle), on this plane. The size of each isocenter is selected. A spacing chart that lists collimator sizes and the optimal spacing for combinations of multiple collimators is consulted. Then, using a computer spacing tool, the isocenter positions are fine-tuned by moving them to the optimal spacing. We typically treat multiple isocenter lesions to the 70% isodose line, maintaining relative dose homogeneity.

With this strategy, multiple isocenter plans can be rapidly constructed. This interactive process is tremendously aided by fast computation times, as many adjustments are often necessary. Multiple isocenter planning requires training, practice, and real expertise to be applied optimally. **Fig. 87–11** illustrates the use of a two-isocenter plan to treat an irregularly shaped acoustic schwannoma.

University of Florida Treatment Planning Algorithm

A strategy is required for selecting and applying the dose-planning tools described above to optimize radiosurgical treatment for a given target lesion. The algorithm generally used at the University of Florida is shown in **Fig. 87–12.**[1]

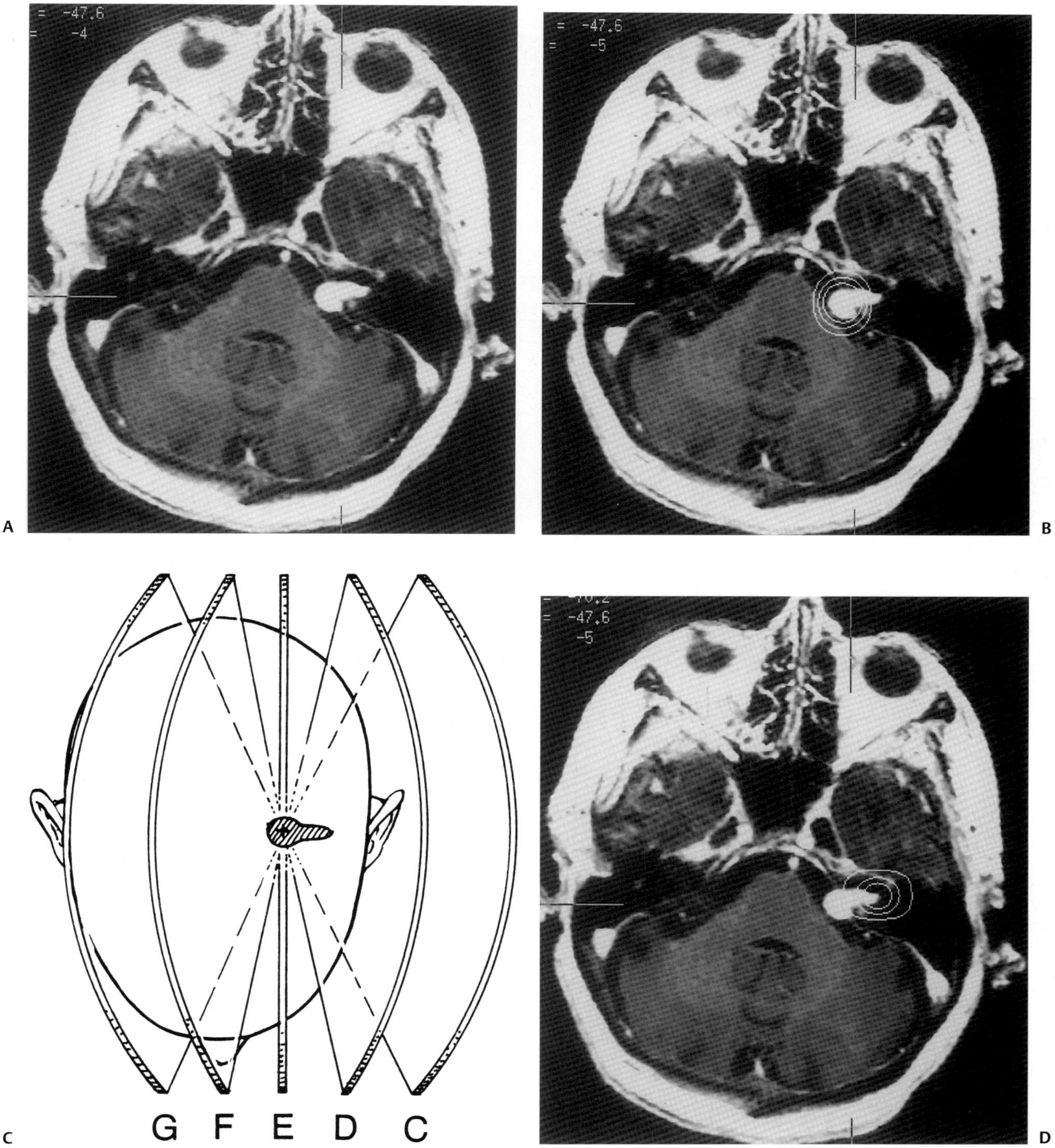

Figure 87–11 Multiple isocenters. This is an illustration of the use of multiple isocenters to treat an irregularly shaped lesion. **(A)** Magnetic resonance imaging (MRI) of an acoustic schwannoma best treated with a two-isocenter plan. Note that the lesion is small but has prominent intracranial and intracanalicular components. Use of MRI as opposed to computed tomographic scans allows adequate visualization of both of these components. Planning begins by identifying this plane and then distributing two isocenters with appropriately small collimators on the intracranial and intracanalicular components (14 mm for the intracranial component and 10 mm for the intracanalicular component in this case). **(B)** The dose distribution for the first (intracranial) isocenter is shown with **(C)** the axial arc set typically used to protect the medial brain stem. Isodose lines 80%, 40%, and 16% are shown. **(D)** The second (intracanalicular) isocenter is then positioned using

(*Continued on page 1002*)

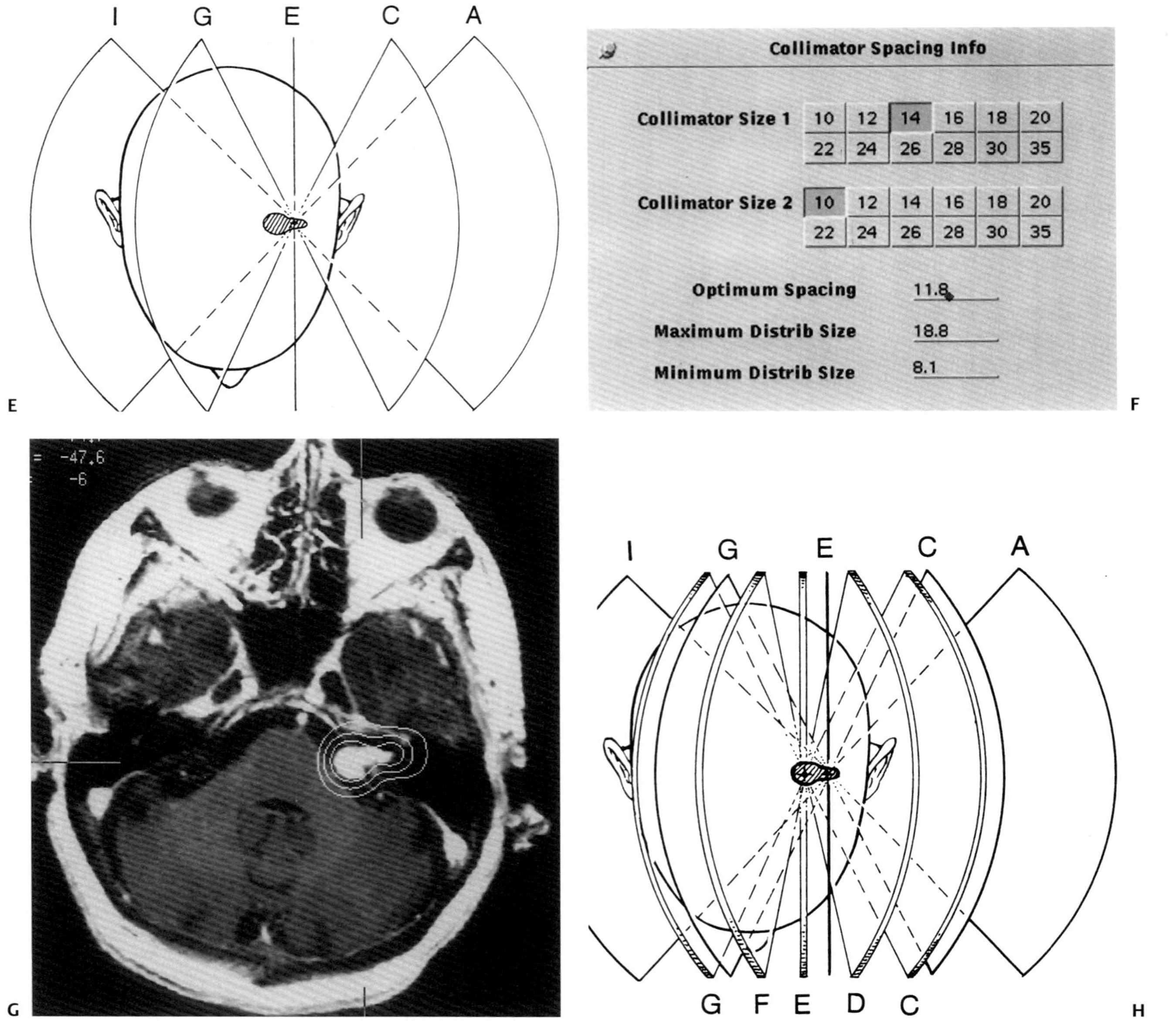

(*Continued*) **Figure 87–11** **(E)** an equally distributed five-arc set. Next, the isodose lines represented are changed to the 70%, 35%, and 14% isodose shells required by multiple isocenter planning. **(F)** The spacing tool is then checked. The isocenters are moved to the ideal spacing, and the composite distribution is reviewed. The ideal spacing is a starting point, but several iterative changes may be needed to achieve optimal spacing for a given case. **(G)** The resulting conformal distribution is shown in the axial view, and **(H)** schematically. Isodose lines 80%, 40%, and 16% are shown. The second (intracanalicular) isocenter is then positioned using an equally distributed five-arc set.

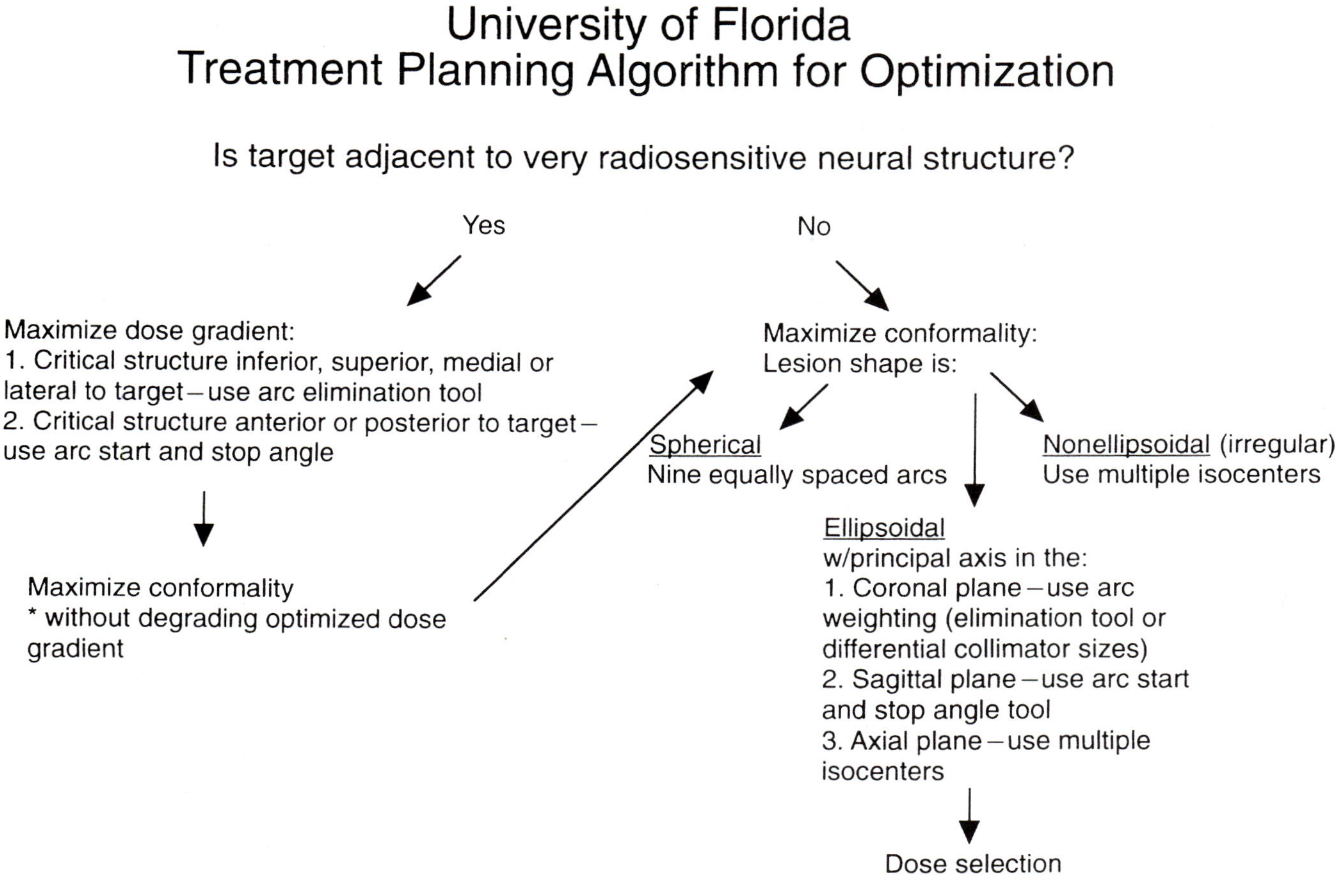

Figure 87–12 The University of Florida stereotactic radiosurgery treatment planning algorithm.

◆ Dose Selection

After a treatment plan is optimized, the radiation dose, expressed in gray (Gy), is selected. In general, the dose is prescribed to the isodose line (or shell, in reality) that conforms to the periphery of the target lesion. For example, a typical dose prescription would be "12.5 Gy to the 80% isodose line." When the 80% isodose line corresponds to the periphery of the lesion, the maximum delivered dose, or 100% of the dose (which lies near the center of the lesion), is 25% higher than the prescribed dose at the 80% isodose line (12.5/0.8 = 15.6 Gy in this example). The lower the isodose line to which the treatment dose is prescribed, the greater the difference between the prescribed treatment dose and the maximum dose; in other words, the greater the dose inhomogeneity across the target.

Dose selection requires a detailed understanding of the radiosurgical literature; many reports provide historical dose guidelines for different radiosurgical situations.[2–7] **Tables 87–2** and **87–3** present some basic principles of dose selection and common doses used for various lesions, respectively. In practice, the selection of a safe and effective radiosurgical dose prescription requires experience and a close interaction between the neurosurgeon, radiation oncologist, and radiation physicist.

Table 87–2 General Principles of Dose Selection

First, do no harm	In general, select the lowest dose that provides the desired therapeutic effect.
Dose–volume relationships	The dose prescribed must be lowered as the treatment volume increases to avoid excessive complications.
Adjacent critical structures	Limit the single-fraction dose to the optic nerves to 7.5 Gy. The brain stem, facial, trigeminal, and cochlear nerves are also relatively radiosensitive, although not as sensitive as the optic nerves.
Lesion location	Lesions in "eloquent" brain areas are often treated with a slightly lower dose of radiation.
Preexisting deficits	Complications are more likely to develop in patients with preexisting neurological deficits, so treat such patients with lower radiation doses.
Previous treatment	If the patient has had any prior radiation treatment, downward adjustments in radiosurgical dose may be required.

Table 87–3 Commonly Used Radiosurgery Doses

Arteriovenous Malformations	Acoustic Schwannomas and Meningiomas	Malignant Gliomas	Metastases
12.5 to 20 Gy	≤ 2 cm, 15 Gy 2 to 3 cm, 12.5 Gy >3 cm, 10 Gy	External beam radiotherapy (e.g., 60 Gy in 40 fractions) Radiosurgical boost ≤ 2 cm, 15 Gy > 2 cm, 10 to 12.5 Gy	12.5 to 20 Gy

◆ Radiation Delivery

Linear accelerators (depicted in **Fig. 87–13** with a radiosurgical subsystem and patient attached) are the most common source of therapeutic radiation. They are mounted on a rotating gantry that arcs vertically over the patient and focuses the x-ray beam on a fixed point in space (the isocenter of the LINAC). The patient table rotates about the same isocenter in a horizontal arc, which allows arcs of radiation to be delivered to the isocenter (target) from variable angles as depicted in the treatment planning discussion above. The inherent mechanical inaccuracy of the average LINAC in defining its isocenter can be up to 4 mm. This degree of accuracy is adequate for conventional radiotherapy but is not acceptable for radiosurgery, which relies on exquisite spatial accuracy in radiation delivery as explained above. An attachable subsystem that converts a standard LINAC into a precision radiosurgical instrument is required. One such system, designed at the University of Florida, employs a series of specialized bearings that virtually eliminate inaccuracy due to imperfections of gantry and table rotation. This system achieves mechanical accuracy within 0.2 ± 0.1 mm for defining the treatment isocenter of beam delivery.[10]

Radiosurgery Treatment Delivery Setup

Before treatment, the standard radiotherapy LINAC must be converted to a radiosurgery treatment device by attachment of the radiosurgery isocentric subsystem. This requires 8 to 12 minutes by our treatment team (generally consisting of two or three people).

◆ Radiosurgery Treatment Target Verification

Once the treatment plan is generated and the room is assembled, the system is ready for treatment. To deliver a treatment, the target lesion must be placed at the isocenter of the machine. Before delivering treatment, a verification system is

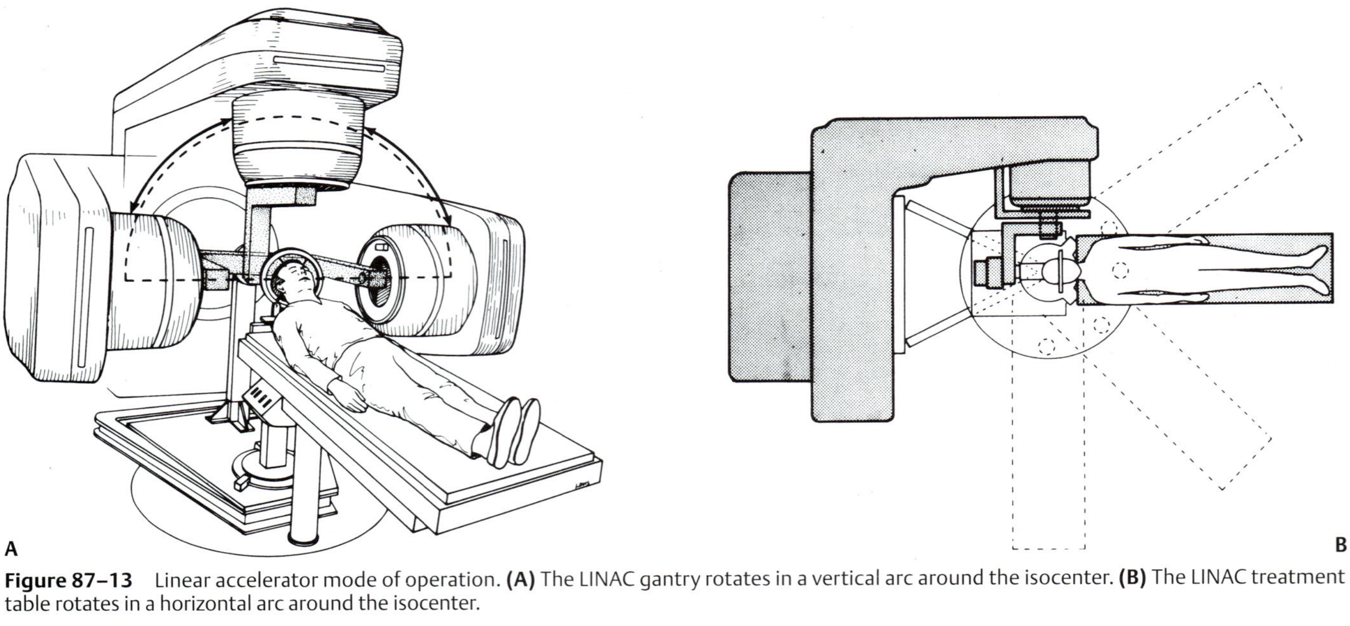

Figure 87–13 Linear accelerator mode of operation. **(A)** The LINAC gantry rotates in a vertical arc around the isocenter. **(B)** The LINAC treatment table rotates in a horizontal arc around the isocenter.

used to ensure that the treatment isocenter defined in the treatment plan is indeed that which is set on the subsystem. This verification also tests to ensure that the subsystem relationship to the isocenter is stable and hence will deliver the treatment to that properly defined target accurately.

The verification system used is a modification of the Lutz-Winston system: The treatment isocenter coordinates are set on the stereotactic radiosurgery subsystem and on a modified BRW phantom base. The phantom and a mock head ring are then used to position a steel ball at the treatment plan isocenter. X-ray film is then attached to the radiosurgery collimator arm and a series of x-rays is taken from various arc and couch positions. This ensures that the phantom target is exactly at the LINAC isocenter and remains so with variation of the gantry and table arcs.

◆ Radiosurgery Treatment Delivery

The treatment collimator is changed to meet the treatment plan specification. The patient is then brought into the treatment room and positioned supine on the treatment couch. The alignment bolts on the undersurface of the head ring are used to firmly attach the patient to the bracket on the radiosurgery ("isocentric") subsystem in a similar manner to that illustrated previously for CT positioning.

At this point, the patient is in position for treatment and the final interlocks are activated. A switch disables the table ram that controls height, and the ram collar lock is tightened as a second method of ensuring that the table height is fixed throughout treatment. The mechanical locks for the lateral and axial table movements are also tightened so that they will not move during the treatment.

The treatment procedure is again explained to the patient and the first table position and gantry rotation are set according to the prescription. Two independent persons on the treatment team verify all positions, and the radiation is then delivered to each specified arc in the sequence.

If a collimator is changed in the middle of a treatment plan, we recommend that the gantry be rotated away from the patient so that the risk of accident during the change is minimized.

If a multiple isocenter plan is used, then the subsequent isocenters are set on the isocentric subsystem without releasing the patient. To move the patient more than a few millimeters, however, the table position and sometimes the table height may need to be changed. Therefore, the interlocks are removed and the patient is adjusted to maintain the body in a comfortable position in relationship to the head, whose position in space is determined by the isocentric subsystem to which it is rigidly fixed. After achieving the correct position for the new isocenter, the interlocks are all reinstituted. After repositioning the patient, the new treatment isocenter is confirmed by independent readings of two members of the treatment team. If all readings agree, the treatment of the new isocenter proceeds as the first.

After treatment of all isocenters is complete, the patient is released from the stereotactic radiosurgery subsystem and allowed to sit up on the treatment couch. The table interlocks are released and the patient is lowered into a comfortable position for the neurosurgeon to remove the head ring. The pins are removed and the ring released. Any slight bleeding that occurs with pin removal is managed with local pressure. The patient is then permitted to leave.

◆ Patient Follow-Up

Radiosurgery is unlike conventional neurosurgery because the effects of treatment are seen only months later. The patients go home the day of treatment exactly as they were prior to the procedure. The efficacy of the procedure and incidence of complications can only be assessed with months or years of careful follow-up. For this reason, physicians delivering radiosurgery treatment must be committed to rigorous follow-up procedures. In general, we see our patients or request information on them regularly, at varying intervals according to the disease treated. Our recommended follow-up schedule for commonly treated lesions is shown in **Table 87–4.**[1]

Table 87–4 Radiosurgery Patient Follow-up Recommendations

Type of Lesion	Follow-Up*	Imaging
AVM (benign)	Every 12 mos for 3 years	MRI/MRA every 12 months until lesion is resolved or 3 years; after resolution or 3 years, an angiogram confirms ablation or is used for retreatment planning
Acoustic schwannoma (benign)	Every 12 mos	12 months for a minimum of 5 years (then as clinically indicated)
Meningioma (benign)	Every 12 mos	12 months for a minimum of 5 years (then as clinically indicated)
Pineocytoma (benign)	Every 12 mos	12 months for a minimum of 5 years (then as clinically indicated)
Pituitary adenoma (benign)	Every 12 mos	12 months for a minimum of 5 years (then as clinically indicated)
Gliomas (malignant)	Every 3 mos	MRI at 3-month intervals for 2 years and then every 6 months
Metastases (malignant)	Every 3 mos	MRI at 3 months and every 6 months thereafter for a minimum of 2 years, then every 12 months

*All patients should have follow-up indefinitely at yearly intervals except as noted.
MRI, magnetic resonance imaging; MRA, magnetic resonance angiography.

◆ Complications

Radiosurgery has few, if any, acute complications. The only acute complication seen in our patients has been a rare increase in seizure activity in the first 48 hours after radiosurgery in patients previously exhibiting seizure activity.

It is important to detect delayed complications early so that appropriate treatment measures can be expeditiously instituted. For example, steroids may produce dramatic improvement in patients with radiation-induced brain edema. As another example, a patient with a transient seventh nerve palsy needs instruction pertaining to eye care, to prevent corneal ulceration while the nerve is recovering. The following general principles should be observed in managing complications:

1. The most important method of managing complications is to prevent complications from occurring through precise dosimetry planning, accurate dose delivery, and selection of the lowest effective radiation dose. *It is critically important to avoid including normal tissue in the radiosurgical treatment field.*
2. If the above principle is diligently pursued, radiation-induced complications are almost always transient. They typically occur after a latent period of 6 to 14 months and run a course to total or near-total resolution in 3 to 6 months. It is important to reassure patients that the problem is usually transient.
3. Steroids are valuable in relieving the symptoms of radiation-induced brain edema. We typically use dexamethasone, starting with 4 mg four times a day and then steadily tapering the dosage to the lowest dose consistent with normal neurological function. Frequent neurological examinations and radiographic procedures are often helpful in guiding therapy.
4. To improve the results of radiosurgery, all complications must be scrupulously documented. This requires a commitment to careful follow-up of all treated patients indefinitely.

◆ Conclusion

Stereotactic radiosurgery is, of necessity, a team endeavor. It requires the expertise of specially trained representatives from the fields of neurosurgery, radiation oncology, and radiation physics. It is a rapidly evolving and improving treatment modality that represents an important weapon in the neurosurgical armamentarium against various intracranial lesions.

References

1. Friedman WA, Buatti JM, Bova FJ, Mendenhall WM. Linac Radiosurgery: a Practical Guide. New York: Springer-Verlag; 1998
2. Friedman WA, Bova FJ, Mendenhall WM. LINAC radiosurgery for arteriovenous malformations: the relationship of outcome to size. J Neurosurg 1995;82:180–189
3. Mendenhall WM, Friedman WA, Buatti JM, Bova FJ. Preliminary results of linear accelerator radiosurgery for acoustic schwannoma. J Neurosurg 1996;85:1013–1019
4. Lunsford LD. Contemporary management of meningiomas: radiation therapy as an adjuvant and radiosurgery as an alternative to surgical removal. J Neurosurg 1994;80:187–190
5. Buatti JM, Friedman WA, Bova FJ, Mendenhall WM. Treatment selection factors for stereotactic radiosurgery of intracranial metastases. Int J Radiat Oncol Biol Phys 1995;32:1161–1166
6. Sarkaria JN, Mehta MP, Loeffler JS, et al. Radiosurgery in the initial management of malignant gliomas: Survival comparison with the RTOG recursive partitioning analysis. Int J Radiat Oncol Biol Phys 1995;32:931–941
7. Witt TC, Kondziolka D, Flickinger JC, et al. Stereotactic radiosurgery for pituitary tumors. In: Kondziolka D, ed. Radiosurgery, 1995. Basel, Switzerland: Karger; 1996:55–65
8. Bova FJ, Friedman WA. Stereotactic angiography: an inadequate database for radiosurgery? Int J Radiat Oncol Biol Phys 1991;20:891–895
9. Alexander E III, Loeffler JS, Holupka EJ, et al. Magnetic resonance image-directed stereotactic neurosurgery: use of image fusion with computerized tomography to enhance spatial accuracy. J Neurosurg 1995;83:271–276
10. Friedman WA, Bova FJ. The University of Florida radiosurgery system. Surg Neurol 1989;32:334–342

Section XIV

Minimally Invasive Surgery

88

Fluid-Filled Neuroendoscopy (Cerebrospinal Fluid Neuroendoscopy)

Gary Magram

◆ Cerebrospinal Fluid Neuroendoscopy

A major distinction in neuroendoscopy is the fluid medium through which the light travels. Cerebrospinal fluid (CSF) neuroendoscopy differs from pneumoneuroendoscopy in several important ways. First, it is much more difficult to keep a liquid medium clear. Second, hemostasis is limited in a liquid medium. Third, access to the fluid cavity is restricted by the size of the scope or sheath.

Pneumoneuroendoscopy is mostly used as an adjunct to microsurgery. The air is at atmospheric pressure and generally replaces the CSF in the subarachnoid space. Clinical applications of pneumoneuroendoscopy include looking around aneurysms, cranial nerves, or the brain stem in an effort to avoid retraction. The scopes are generally rigid rod lens endoscopes with excellent optics and resolution. Angled scopes (15, 30, 45, and even up to 90 degrees) are available. Although instruments can be passed through a sheath, it is also possible to pass instruments alongside of the endoscope and to view the endoscope as it is entering the microsurgical field. Except for smoke, which can be easily aspirated away, the field of view generally remains clear in pneumoneuroendoscopy. Particulate debris or blood falls downward without obscuring the image. Hemostasis is still possible with a bipolar electrode or angled bipolar electrode passed along the endoscope. A binocular microscope allows for depth perception, helping the surgeon estimate the depth of the endoscope. The opening for pneumoneuroendoscopy is typically sufficiently large to allow for adequate irrigation without an excessive buildup of pressure. Furthermore, the larger opening in an air-filled cavity or the subarachnoid space permits a larger endoscope and a greater degree of freedom to change the endoscopes trajectory.

CSF neuroendoscopy is often used as a minimally invasive alternative to microneurosurgery. An advantage is that the procedure can be performed through a bur hole instead of a craniotomy. Therefore, a goal of CSF neuroendoscopy is to keep the diameter of the endoscope or sheath as small as possible. This goal of minimizing the diameter limits the size and number of working channels and irrigation channels. Whereas with pneumoneuroendoscopy the trajectory is similar to that for the open microscope, with CSF neuroendoscopy the trajectory must be planned. Hemostasis is difficult with CSF neuroendoscopy. Small vessels (less than 0.5 mm in diameter) can sometimes be coagulated with a monopolar or bipolar instrument. If a larger vessel or high-pressure artery or arteriole is injured, then the field needs to be irrigated until the bleeding stops. Therefore, it is important to avoid even slight trauma to surrounding structures such as the choroid plexus.

◆ Choice of Endoscope

Both rod lens endoscopes and fiberoptic endoscopes are available for CSF neuroendoscopy. In general the image with a rod lens endoscope is higher in resolution and allows for the recording of a superior image; however, a 10,000-pixel fiber optic endoscope offers sufficient resolution to perform endoscopic procedures. Higher resolution (30,000 pixel) and reusable fiberoptic endoscopes are also available. A major advantage of fiberoptic endoscopes is that they come in various disposable models, which eliminates the need for sterilization. Sterilization can be difficult through the small-diameter irrigating channel of the endoscope. The 1.1 mm fiberoptic endoscopes come with an irrigating channel and are malleable. The rod lens endoscopes are reusable but much more expensive. Rod lens endoscopes require careful handling and are expensive to repair if dropped or bent. Depending on the hospital's sterilization department, it may be more cost-effective to use disposable endoscopes than to pay for repairs of rod lens endoscopes. There are small-diameter rod lens pediatric cystoscopes and ear, nose, and throat (ENT) endoscopes for sinus work; however, when these endoscopes are used without a metal sheath they bend very easily. For a small-diameter endoscope to be used inside a catheter, the disposable ones are preferable. For larger diameter endoscopes with working channels, either rod lens or disposable fiberoptic endoscopes will prove satisfactory.

◆ Irrigation

There are two types of neuroendoscopic irrigation: high pressure/low volume and low pressure/high volume. High-pressure irrigation is performed through a small-diameter irrigating channel with a high resistance and requires forceful inflow. It is used primarily for a focal application, such as displacing a blood clot or moving a membrane. Low-pressure irrigation requires a larger diameter channel and is used to wash out or exchange all the fluid within a compartment. Low-pressure irrigation can be achieved by having an intravenous (IV) bag of either Ringer's lactate or normal saline suspended slightly above the inflow channel and connected to the inflow channel by standard IV fluid tubing. With either type of irrigation it is essential to ensure adequate outflow. This can be accomplished either by having a large-diameter, low-resistance outflow channel, or by frequent removal of any instruments in a working channel to prevent the excessive buildup of irrigation fluid. Complications can arise from either a prolonged elevation in intracranial pressure (ICP) or too rapid distension of a cavity. Brief periods of elevated pressure can be well tolerated provided they do not excessively distend the cavity. Therefore, it is not sufficient to monitor only the intracavity pressure when irrigating because some patients have very compliant cavities. A patient with a very compliant ventricle can suffer from a stretchlike injury from too rapid and excessive distension before a typically elevated intraventricular pressure is recorded.

If a lot of irrigation is going to take place during an endoscopic procedure, then it is helpful to use a peel-away sheath catheter with an inner diameter greater than the outer diameter of the endoscope. This allows for outflow of CSF around the endoscope. Alternatively, a larger endoscope with an extra irrigation outflow channel can be used. Such endoscopes are heavier, more expensive, and often require a larger perforation through the brain. A 9 French peel-away sheath allows the passage of a 1.1 mm endoscope with an irrigating channel as well as an instrument and still provides sufficient room for the outflow of irrigation fluid. Using a working instrument parallel to the endoscope can be challenging, and it is a lot easier to pass an instrument down a working channel. Endoscopes that are less than 3.6 mm in diameter and have a working channel and inflow irrigation channel can easily be passed through a 12 French peel-away sheath catheter. In this situation the 12 French peel-away sheath still provides sufficient room to prevent the excessive buildup of irrigation fluid.

For the placement of a ventricular catheter a peel-away sheath is often not practical. First, it increases the risk of a postoperative leak of CSF around the catheter. Such a leak can lead to a collection of CSF around the valve. Second, for a shunt revision, the old tract is not large enough to atraumatically pass a sheath. If it is necessary to work through a previous shunt tract, then the tract can sometimes be gradually dilated with endoscopic dilators. For the placement of a shunt, if the CSF is clear, then it is often not necessary to irrigate. Sometimes the patient can have a minimally dilated ventricle and after the old shunt is removed the ventricle collapses. Careful irrigation can distend the ventricle to permit navigation and placement of the ventricular catheter in a new position in the ventricle. If irrigation is needed through a ventricular catheter, then after installing a few milliliters of fluid the endoscope should be removed; if the fluid drips out, then a larger volume can be used. The volume of irrigation is gradually increased by a couple of milliliters until the fluid squirts out after removal of the endoscope from the catheter. Exceeding this volume of irrigation can potentially limit the cerebral perfusion.

◆ Endoscopic Ventricular Catheter Placement

The 1.1 mm diameter endoscope is useful for both primary ventricular catheter placement and proximal catheter revision. Although it is not crucial where the openings into the ventricular catheter are placed within the ventricle, it is crucial that the openings be in the proper cavity and not in a shunt tract. The ventricular catheter most commonly obstructs secondary to overdrainage of CSF. Any surrounding tissue, be it choroid plexus or ependymal lining, can obstruct the lumen of the catheter. The advantage of placing the ventricular catheter openings away from the choroid plexus is not that it prevents obstruction, but rather that if the catheter becomes obstructed, the risk of a serious intraventricular bleed is less if the surrounding tissue is avascular. Without the use of an endoscope, the ventricular catheter can take a surprising trajectory and end up in the interhemispheric fissure or the sylvian fissure, or embedded into the medial wall of the ventricle. With the aid of the endoscope, the catheter can be guided to make sure it is within the ventricle and placed if possible away from the choroid plexus.

Prior to the availability of a 1.1 mm endoscope there was a high incidence of recurrent proximal shunt obstruction. Ensuring that the ventricular catheter is in a "clean" region of the ventricle can lessen the incidence of recurrent proximal obstruction. After a shunt is inserted in a dilated ventricle, the ventricle decreases in size, and as it decreases in size the outside wall approximates the inner wall, increasing the cortical mantle thickness and elongating the shunt tract.

As a child's head circumference increases, eventually the proximal catheter openings can reside within the shunt tract, leading to a partial proximal obstruction. In this situation a new longer ventricular catheter needs to be inserted. If the ventricles are small, then blindly trying to insert the longer catheter can result in its penetrating the medial wall of the ventricle. Using an endoscope permits the ventricle to be slightly dilated and the trajectory changed to guide the ventricular catheter into the ventricle. If the trajectory leading to the ventricle is almost perpendicular to the collapsed ventricle, it can be difficult to get the catheter to bend. By bending the disposable endoscope, the ventricular catheter can be placed using a gentle curved trajectory and advanced into the ventricle.

When an obstructed catheter is attached inside the ventricle, the endoscope is very helpful in ensuring that the lumen is free of tethering attachments. If vascular intraventricular tissue is found, then a wire can be inserted to the appropriate depth and the tissue coagulated. After coagulating the tissue, the endoscope can be passed through the tissue, freeing the catheter of any tethering attachments. Simply coagulating the tissue may not be sufficient to prevent tearing of tethering attachments and resultant bleeding with removal of an obstructed catheter. Of course, if a greater amount of coagulation is used, the tissue surrounding the catheter can also be coagulated, lessening the risk of bleeding with removal, but this increases the risk of injuring the surround tissue. Mechanically cleaning the lumen of the ventricular catheter minimizes the use of intracatheter coagulation.

◆ Endoscopic Fenestration of the Septum Pellucidum

Endoscopic fenestration is used to treat a loculated lateral ventricle. This is typically caused by either a third ventricular obstructing lesion (colloid cyst, craniopharyngioma, or giant cell astrocytoma) or scarring at the foramen of Monro (an intraventricular hemorrhage or infection). The alternative to fenestration is the insertion of a catheter into the obstructed ventricle. In selected cases the remainder of the CSF circulation is normal, and fenestration of the septum can eliminate the need for a shunt.

The technique used to fenestrate the septum depends on whether the procedure is an initial procedure or being done at the time of a shunt revision. As an initial procedure, the bur hole is placed a little more lateral and posterior to the standard approach to the frontal horn. A bur hole several centimeters lateral to the sagittal suture and just in front of the coronal suture allows for a trajectory that is more perpendicular to the septum. A medial bur hole results in a trajectory that is more parallel to the septum, making fenestration difficult. A 12 French peel-away sheath catheter is introduced into the lateral aspect of the frontal horn, and an endoscope with a working channel is introduced into the frontal horn. After entering the frontal horn, the foramen of Monro and septal vein are identified. The endoscope is directed cephalad and anterior to the foramen and an avascular region of the septum is selected. An endoscopic bipolar electrode is then passed through the working channel and the septum is fenestrated by gently twisting the bipolar against the septum. After the small perforation is made the endoscope will be looking into the contralateral ventricle. The endoscope can then be gently moved in multiple directions to enlarge the opening, a no. 3 Fogarty balloon can be inflated in the opening to enlarge it, or an instrument can be spread open in the fenestration.

◆ Third Ventriculostomy

Indications

Fenestrating the thinned-out floor of the third ventricle can eliminate the need for a shunt in most patients with an isolated ventricular outlet obstruction. For patients with either a communicating hydrocephalus or more than one site of obstruction, a third ventriculostomy is not sufficient. Although the isolated obstruction is most commonly located in the aqueduct of Sylvius, it can also be at the fourth ventricular outlet.

Some patients who have been shunted for intraventricular hemorrhage develop a secondary aqueductal stenosis with resolution of their communicating hydrocephalus. At the time of a proximal ventricular catheter obstruction, many of these patients might be able to be made shunt free by performing a third ventriculostomy. Shunted patients who are having shunt-related problems can be tested to see if they might be candidates for a third ventriculostomy by performing a computed tomographic (CT) contrast ventricular study. To perform this study, the shunt reservoir is tapped and contrast is injected through the reservoir while occluding the distal tubing. The patient is then placed in a sitting position and asked to tilt the head forward for a minute or two, and then a CT scan is obtained from the upper cervical spine to above the ventricles. If contrast is observed to be in the basilar cisterns and in the upper cervical subarachnoid space, then the patient is not a candidate for a third ventriculostomy. If both the lateral and third ventricles fill or all four ventricles fill without contrast in the subarachnoid space, then the patient may benefit from a third ventriculostomy.

Contraindications

A past medical history of a shunt infection or meningitis is associated with a high third ventriculostomy failure rate. During endoscopy the floor of the third ventricle needs to be inspected for an almost transparent portion. If the floor of the third ventricle has not been thinned out to an almost transparent membrane, then it is probably better to perform a shunt. Fenestrating an almost transparent membrane will not lead to a neurological impairment. Fenestrating a white membrane, even in the midline, can lead to an injury to the hypothalamus (usually reversible over time) and is unlikely to be a successful third ventriculostomy because ventricular outlet obstruction typically does thin out the floor of the third ventricle, the exception being a rare shunted patient with an acquired aqueductal stenosis. It can be difficult to evaluate the floor of the third ventricle on a magnetic resonance imaging (MRI) or CT scan, especially if the patient has a shunt with slitlike ventricles. Slitlike ventricles are not a contraindication to a third ventriculostomy in a shunted patient. Although it may not be possible to use a larger diameter endoscope in a patient with small ventricles, it is possible to atraumatically navigate into the third ventricle with a 1.1 mm disposable endoscope. Once shunted, the third ventricle may go from a spherical shape to a slitlike shape; however, if the floor was thinned out prior to the shunt, it will remain thinned out.

Third Ventriculostomy as an Initial Procedure

The patient is placed on the operating room (OR) table in a supine position with the head very slightly flexed and the head of the bed slightly elevated. This elevates the entrance site, compared with a horizontal position with the head in a neutral position. The advantages of this position are that it allows the ventricles to retain more liquid and minimizes the frontal horn pneumocephalus that results with a more horizontal approach. A right frontal approach is used. The scalp incision is made anterior and medial to the proposed bur hole in case the procedure needs to be converted to a shunt. This avoids having the incision over the shunt valve or tubing. A generous scalp incision away from the bur hole will lessen the risk of CSF leak and allow for the insertion of a shunt should it be needed. The bur hole is placed close to the midline but lateral to the superior sagittal sinus, typically 2 cm from the midline. Placing the bur hole just in front of the coronal suture permits a more anterior trajectory toward the clivus and away from the basilar artery. A generous bur hole allows for adjusting the trajectory of the endoscope. The superficial diameter of the bur hole needs to be larger for a thicker skull. The opening in the dura needs to be greater than for a shunt catheter, and typically is ~4 mm in diameter. The cortex is inspected to make sure there are no large veins. The pia is bipolared and the 12 French peel-away sheath is introduced into the dilated frontal horn. A trajectory of aiming just in front of the ipsilateral ear and toward the ipsilateral inner canthus typically results in entering the right frontal horn by 4 cm. CSF is seen to flow from the inner stylet of the peel-away sheath catheter, and can be collected for routine testing. Holding the peel-away sheath in place, the inner stylet is removed and the 3.5 mm channel endoscope is guided down into the frontal horn. The foramen of Monro is identified. The trajectory from the bur hole to the entrance into the ventricle can be changed to a new trajectory from the bur hole to the foramen of Monro. Movement from this latter trajectory should be kept to a minimum. When the endoscope is in the third ventricle and the foramen is out of visualization, movement of the endoscope can inadvertently traumatize the foramen. If the trajectory is changed to visualize the posterior third ventricle, the choroid plexus or veins on the posterior aspect of the foramen can be injured, and changing the trajectory to visualize the anterior third ventricle can traumatize the ipsilateral fornix. The peel-away sheath can either be held in place or peeled down and fastened in place. If only the endoscope is held, then it is possible for the sheath to slide down along the endoscope and traumatize the choroid plexus at the foramen of Monro. This is particularly likely to occur when the end of the peel-away sheath is out of view while the proximal end of the endoscope is in the third ventricle.

The floor of the third ventricle is examined. The two mamillary bodies are visualized posteriorly. With chronically dilated third ventricles, the mamillary bodies can be displaced posterolaterally, not having the typical rounded appearance. Anteriorly, the vascularized infundibular recess is seen. An avascular, thinned out portion of the floor in the midline, approximately midway between the infundibular recess and the mamillary bodies, is chosen for the fenestration. Sometimes the top of the basilar artery and the posterior cerebral arteries can be visualized through the thinned-out floor. A probe such as the end of the endoscopic bipolar electrode is used to make the perforation. The endoscope is backed up until it just enters the third ventricle through the foramen, so that when an instrument is introduced through the channel, there is a safe distance for it to come into view as it exits from the proximal end of the scope. If the proximal end of the scope is just outside of the foramen, then as the bipolar electrode exits it can possibly injure the foramen. The bipolar electrode comes into view from the side. The tip of the bipolar electrode is bent slightly so that it can be rotated toward the center of the field of view. Once the bipolar electrode is in view, the endoscope and bipolar electrode are advanced toward the targeted site for the fenestration. The view through the endoscope is two-dimensional, so it can be difficult to determine visually the depth of the bipolar electrode. As the bipolar electrode touches and moves the floor of the third ventricle toward the clivus, the bipolar electrode is gently twisted until if perforates the floor of the third ventricle. At this point, either a no. 3 Fogarty balloon is inflated in the perforation to dilate it or an endoscope forceps is spread to gently enlarge the perforation. The problem with the balloon dilatation is that the balloon tends to inflate either above or below the perforation and it is difficult to get the balloon to dilate in the perforation. If the balloon dilates in the third ventricle, then the field of view is obscured. The balloon needs to be frequently inflated and deflated with very minor movements to gradually enlarge the perforation. The inflated balloon should not be pulled through the perforation because it can tear the floor and stretch the surrounding structures. Slowly spreading a forceps in the perforation can enlarge the perforation to ~4 mm or more. Once the perforation is made, the floor of the third ventricle should be seen to pulsate. A nonpulsating floor indicates that there is a lack of free flow of fluid between the third ventricle and the interpeduncular cistern. After enlarging the fenestration, the endoscope can be introduced through the floor to visualize the basilar artery and cranial nerves. If the membrane of Lilliquist is seen below the perforation, then this membrane needs to be perforated as well.

The instruments are withdrawn and the endoscope is pulled back to visualize the fenestration. If there is bleeding from the edges of the fenestration, then continuous irrigation is performed until the bleeding stops and the field is clear. If there is bleeding from the choroids plexus, it can sometimes be controlled by touching the site with the endoscopic bipolar electrode. If bipolar coagulation is used, the debris should be irrigated out.

A piece of Gelfoam is prepared the size of the bur hole. After removing the endoscope and the peel-away sheath, the endoscopic tract is covered with the Gelfoam to prevent any blood from the scalp edges from entering through the tract during closure. The galea is approximated with absorbable sutures and the scalp closed in a watertight fashion.

Inserting an external ventricular drain prior to closure is reserved for cases in which there was a very symptomatic elevation in ICP preoperatively or in cases in which significant bleeding occurred. For a patient with a typical aqueductal stenosis and an uneventful third ventriculostomy, an external drain is not routinely used. If there is some doubt about the success of the third ventriculostomy, then a ventricular catheter attached to a bur hole reservoir can be inserted prior to closure. The ventricular catheter is passed through the peel-away sheath after removal of the endoscope, and then the sheath is peeled away. This ensures that the catheter enters the ventricle and does not take another trajectory through the tract. The bur hole reservoir can be tapped if the patient becomes symptomatic postoperatively. The advantage of the reservoir is that not uncommonly patients become symptomatic in a delayed fashion. The reservoir permits not only a measure of the ICP and withdrawal of CSF but also the insertion of contrast for a CT ventriculogram.

A CT ventriculogram is a useful postoperative test. Patients who are not symptomatic can be followed by an MRI cine-flow study to visualize the pulsatile flow through the fenestration. The advantages of the CT ventriculogram include that it allows for sampling of the fluid and measuring the intraventricular pressure, and it more definitively demonstrates the circulation of the contrast. With a well-functioning third ventriculostomy, the contrast will immediately fill the interpeduncular cistern and be visualized in the upper cervical subarachnoid space. After a delay, the contrast will be seen in the sylvian fissures and then later in the more rostral subarachnoid space. If the patient is symptomatic or if the intraventricular pressure is elevated, then even if contrast is seen to flow through the fenestration, the absorption is not sufficient and shunting will have to be considered. If the contrast study shows that there is neither flow through the aqueduct nor flow through the fenestration, then repeating the third ventriculostomy can be considered.

Performing a Third Ventriculostomy in a Shunted Patient

Some patients with shunts can be made independent of their shunt by having the surgeon perform a third ventriculostomy and eliminate flow through their shunt. If the patient has a functioning shunt, then the pulsatile flow through the third ventriculostomy will be dampened and might not be sufficient to keep the fenestration open. Depending on the patient's clinical status, one of numerous approaches may be selected. If the patient has a distally obstructed or disconnected parietal or occipital shunt, then a frontal approach can be used and the posterior reservoir tapped if needed postoperatively. If the patient has a frontal shunt, then the existing tract is used to create the third ventriculostomy and a new ventricular catheter and reservoir are left in place postoperatively. Either a programmable valve set to the highest setting in combination with a shunt assistant or an on-off valve can be inserted into the shunt to prevent CSF from flowing through the shunt after an attempted third ventriculostomy. If the patient becomes symptomatic, the shunt can then be opened.

If the ventricles are small and the patient does not have a frontal catheter, then a frameless stereotactic neuronavigation system can be used to gain access to the frontal horn and optimize the trajectory through the foramen of Monro to the floor of the third ventricle.

For patients with a frontal ventricular catheter, the existing tract can be used. First, the existing ventricular catheter is endoscopically freed and removed. Then a new ventricular catheter is endoscopically guided into the frontal horn. Careful attention needs to be given to irrigation in this situation so as to not overdistend the ventricle or excessively elevate the intraventricular pressure. After the surgeon identifies the foramen of Monro, the endoscope is passed into the third ventricle and the site for perforation selected. The tip of the 1.1 mm endoscope can be used to make the perforation by gently twisting it against the floor and visualizing the perforation as it is being made. If the prior tract from the frontal bur hole is too anterior, it might not be possible to safely make a perforation. In many cases the bur hole is slightly too far anterior, not permitting visualization of the anterior floor of the third ventricle. In these situations gently bending the 1.1 mm endoscope to give the scope an anteriorly directed curve might permit perforation of the floor. After the floor is perforated, the endoscope is kept in place and the ventricular catheter slowly and gently advanced, helping to dilate the perforation. In some circumstances it is possible to slide a no. 3 Fogarty balloon alongside the endoscope down the tract, and advance the Fogarty through the foramen under visualization and then into the perforation. The perforation is dilated using the balloon.

It is important to inspect below the fenestration to make sure there are no other membranes obstructing flow. If during inspection a lot of arachnoiditis is visualized, then the chances are lessened that the third ventriculostomy will be sufficient to control the hydrocephalus.

◆ Endoscopic Removal of a Colloid Cyst

Colloid cyst can be treated endoscopically with less risk for morbidity than with a standard microsurgical or stereotactic approach. Although the goal is removal of the cyst, sometimes it is better to leave a portion of the cyst attached to the internal cerebral veins than risk injury to these venous structures. An endoscope with at least one working channel and a peel-away sheath catheter are used. The entering bur hole should be a couple of centimeters in front of the coronal suture and at least several centimeters from the midline so that the scope is facing the foramen of Monro. Although a frameless neuronavigation system may be very helpful for optimizing the trajectory in patients without ventriculomegaly, it probably is not necessary for those patients with moderate to marked ventriculomegaly. The peel-away sheath is introduced into the right frontal horn and then endoscopically guided toward the foramen of Monro. Typically, the blue to darkly colored cyst is seen in the foramen, often covered by choroid plexus. The endoscopic bipolar electrode is introduced and the choroids plexus over the cyst is coagulated to shrink it away from the cyst. The cyst itself can also be shrunk. The bipolar electrode is used to coagulate an opening into the cyst, and typically yellowish, greenish, or dark fluid will exude from the perforation. A 3 French pediatric feeding tube can then be inserted into the perforation and the contents aspirated. Following removal of the feeding tube, an endoscopic forceps can be used to gently manipulate the cyst. Sometimes the cyst can be gently pulled out from the foramen and then pulled out along with the endoscope. If resistance is encountered, then the endoscopic bipolar electrode and scissors can be used to remove as much of the cyst as can be safely removed. The remainder of the cyst is coagulated. The endoscope can then be advanced into the third ventricle to make sure there is not obstruction. The ventricles are irrigated until clear. A ventricular drain or a ventricular catheter and a bur hole reservoir can be left in place if there is concern about hydrocephalus. For a patient with an uneventful cyst decompression or removal and a normal preoperative intraventricular pressure, the wound can be closed without a ventricular drain.

◆ Endoscopic Emptying of a Craniopharyngioma

A craniopharyngioma cyst can expand into the third ventricle. If the bulk of the lesion is cystic and not solid, then an endoscopic approach is an option. The approach is similar to that used to remove a colloid cyst, except the bur hole is just in front of the coronal suture. An endoscope with a working channel and a peel-away sheath are used. If the ventricles are not enlarged, then a frameless neuronavigation system is helpful in directing the peel-away sheath into the ventricle. The endoscope is inserted and the cyst should be readily apparent in the foramen of Monro. The cyst pushes up the floor of the third ventricle so there are multiple layers to be fenestrated. Trying to fenestrate the cyst with a blunt-tipped instrument can be difficult because the cyst can be pushed downward. Using a bipolar electrode the cyst and its covering can be coagulated until the cyst wall is perforated. A no. 3 pediatric feeding tube is passed through the working channel and then down through the perforation. The contents of the cyst are aspirated, and then the cyst and the ventricles are irrigated until clear. The endoscope with the working channel is removed and the sheath left in place. A ventricular catheter is then endoscopically guided into the cyst using the 1.1 mm endoscope. The catheter is guided down to the bottom of the cyst and a bur hole reservoir attached to the catheter. The wound is closed in the usual manner. After about 2 weeks the patient is reimaged by MRI. The cyst can then be percutaneously aspirated and this procedure repeated until the cyst shrinks down to a size that can be treated by either conventional radiation or radiosurgery.

◆ Endoscopic Biopsy of an Intraventricular Lesion

Frameless stereotactic neuronavigation is used to plan the trajectory and optimal entrance site for a biopsy of an intraventricular lesion (unless the patient has hydrocephalus with a lesion in or near the foramen of Monro). For a posterior third ventricular lesion a bur hole just behind the hairline and close to the midline is used. The probe for the frameless neuronavigation is used to make a tract along the desired trajectory, and then the peel-away sheath is passed down this tract into the ventricle. The endoscope is advanced toward the lesion. If the lesion is found to be highly vascular, then it might be better to approach the lesion microsurgically. Otherwise, the bleeding from a biopsy of most other lesions usually stops spontaneously with irrigation. The peel-away sheath should allow for sufficient outflow to prevent pressure buildup associated with plentiful irrigation. After inserting an endoscopic biopsy forceps into the lesion and obtaining a biopsy, it is sometimes possible to coagulate the site with the endoscopic bipolar electrode. The ventricles are irrigated until clear. If the lesion was associated with an intraventricular obstruction, then either a septal fenestration or third ventriculostomy can be performed at the same time. A ventricular catheter and bur hole reservoir can be left in place, if there is concern over possible postoperative hydrocephalus or a need for future CSF sampling or injection of chemotherapy.

◆ Endoscopic Aqueductal Fenestration for a Trapped Fourth Ventricle

For patients with an isolated fourth ventricular outlet obstruction and an open aqueduct it might be possible to perform a third ventriculostomy. If the patient has aqueductal stenosis and a trapped fourth ventricle, then consideration can be given to endoscopically opening the aqueduct. Thin sagittal MRI images through the aqueduct are helpful in selecting candidates for this procedure. If the aqueduct has an elongated stenosis, then it might not be possible to safely open the aqueduct endoscopically. However, if the aqueduct has a funnel-like dilatation extending from the posterior third ventricle, and a focal short region of stenosis, then it is often possible to fenestrate this septum or stenotic region using the 1.1 mm endoscope. To visualize the posterior third ventricle, the entering bur hole is placed several centimeters from the midline and just behind the hairline. The anterior horn of the lateral ventricle is entered and a ventricular catheter is endoscopically guided down through the foramen of Monro. If the patient already has a ventricular shunt in place and has a small decompressed frontal horn, then frameless neuronavigation can be used to guide the endoscope.

Using the MRI the distance from the caudal fourth ventricle to the midportion of the third ventricle is measured and the distance between the midportion of the anterior horn and the third ventricle is measured. Side openings are made in the ventricular catheter at these distances, so that after placement the ventricular catheter will function as a stent between the ventricles. Typically a side hole is made 4 and 6 cm from the proximal tip of the catheter. After entering the third ventricle, the posterior commissure is identified and the funnel-shaped entrance into the aqueduct is followed until the obstruction is identified. Following this same trajectory, the thinned-out membrane is perforated and the endoscope and catheter advanced into the fourth ventricle. The catheter is secured at the entering bur hole site and the endoscope is withdrawn. Either the ventricular catheter is connected to a shunt or, if a functioning posterior shunt is already in place, the catheter is connected to a bur hole reservoir.

89

Endoscope-Assisted Microsurgery of Aneurysms and Tumors

Dinko Stimac, Laligam N. Sekhar, and Ramin Rak

The neuroendoscope is an excellent tool to complement microneurosurgery because the views it provides are different from those provided by the microscope. Each modality has its own advantages, which can be very useful to the neurosurgeon when operating on basal lesions such as aneurysms or tumors.

Advantages and Disadvantages of Endoscope and Microscope

The operating microscope is a well-established tool for neurosurgery. Microscope technology has steadily improved, but development has plateaued in recent years. The surgical microscope is similar to a telescope, viewing structures from a distance. It provides a wide field of view that is not easily obscured by various structures and instruments in the field or by blood. Instruments can be easily moved in and out of the operative space. Both hands of the surgeon and frequently those of the assistant can be used for instruments and for operating or assisting. On the other hand, the view of structures is from a distance, is a straight line, and is limited by the extent of the exposure and the maneuverability of the microscope. The surgeon may not be able to look around corners without displacing a structure (e.g., aneurysm, tumor) during the operation. However, the surgeon has a three-dimensional view, with a good sense of depth perception.

The endoscope is more like a periscope. The view is from close to the structure. It can be introduced through a small space, and it can look around corners and inside "caves." Its disadvantages are that the view is two-dimensional, the judgment of distance is difficult except by movement of the scope closer to or farther from the lesion, and the view can be easily obstructed by blood in the field, by other operative debris, or by fogging of the lens.

The surgeon has to hold the endoscope or use a holder. When it is held by the holder, there is the danger of damaging neurovascular structures if there is accidental bumping of the holder. When held with the hand, the surgeon loses the availability of a hand for manipulation of the structures. Instruments for use with the endoscope are not well developed, and traditional microsurgical tools, such as the bipolar cautery, may not be useful because they are not used for working through a very small opening. So the surgeon can often "look but cannot touch" with the endoscope.

Bleeding instantly obscures the view through the endoscope. It is a problem for the microscope also, but because of the wide field of view, suction can be readily employed to clean the field and stop the bleeding. Fogging is also a problem with the endoscope, and the endoscope may need to be taken out and cleaned when it occurs. A scrubbing or irrigating device can be useful for cleaning blood and fog from the endoscope but adds to the diameter of the device and to its weight.

Endoscopic Surgery versus Endoscope-Assisted Microsurgery

Endoscopic cranial surgery is performed through the paranasal sinuses or the ventricular system; for example, endoscopic pituitary surgery, ventriculoperitoneal shunt

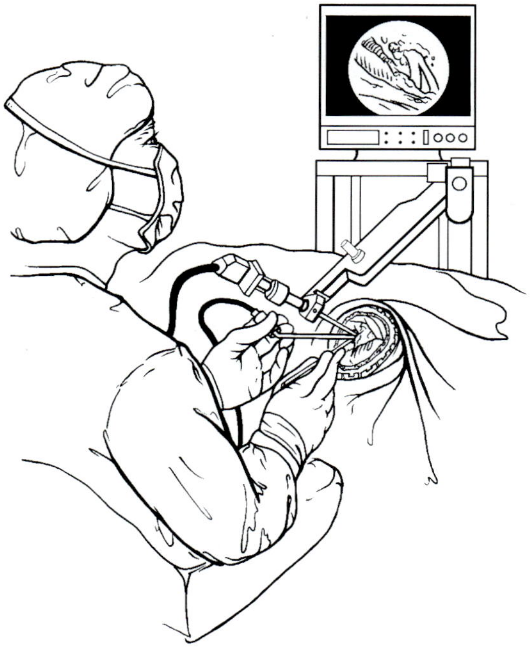

A

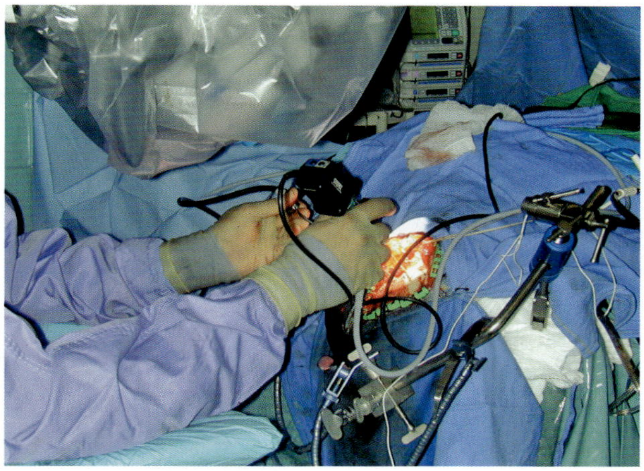

B

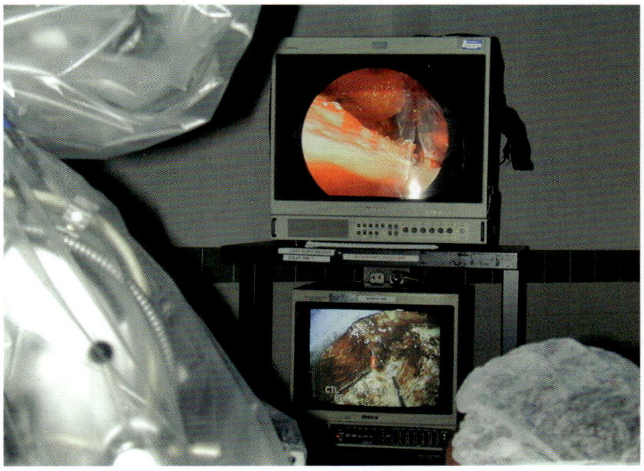

C

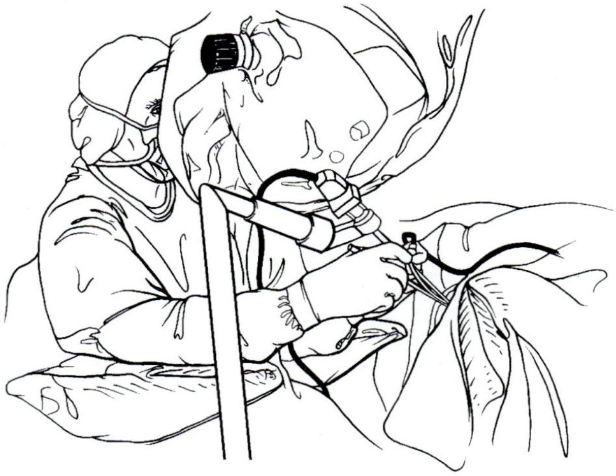

D

Figure 89–1 (A) Endoscopic cranial surgery is done only with an endoscope, and the operative microscope is not in use. **(B,C)** Endoscope-assisted microsurgery uses the endoscope as an adjunctive instrument to make surgery easier and safer. **(D)** A firm, stable endoscope holder is useful for some endoscope-assisted cranial microsurgery.

insertion, third ventriculostomy (**Fig. 89–1A**). *Endoscope-assisted microsurgery* (EAM) can be performed wherever the surgical microscope is used. It is most useful for intracranial aneurysms, microvascular decompression, and basal tumors, such as acoustic neuroma (**Fig. 89–1B,C**). This chapter discusses endoscope-assisted microneurosurgery.

◆ Equipment and Instruments

The equipment consists of an endoscope, Endoscrub device (Medtronic-Xomed, Jacksonville, FL), endoscope connection to the microscope or the monitor, recorder and printer, and specialized instruments for EAM.

Endoscopes can be flexible or rigid. Because of the need to have high resolution, rigid endoscopes are generally used for EAM (**Fig. 89–2**). Hopkins rod lens endoscopes of diameter 4.0 mm or 2.7 mm, with the angle of view 0, 30,

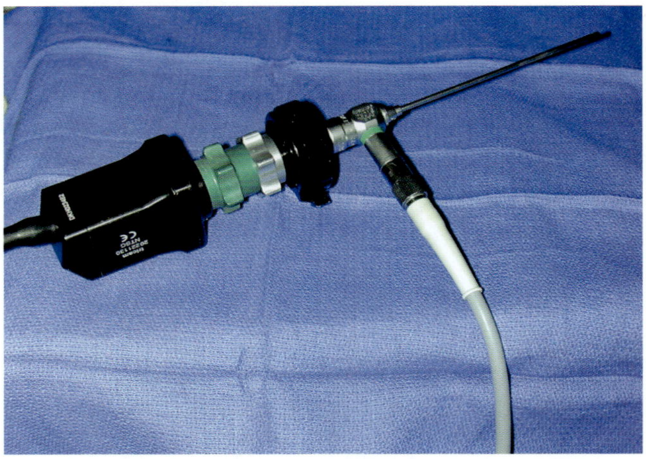

Figure 89–2 Rigid rod-lens endoscope with camera. This endoscope is easy to use, well balanced, and specially adapted for endoscope-assisted microsurgery.

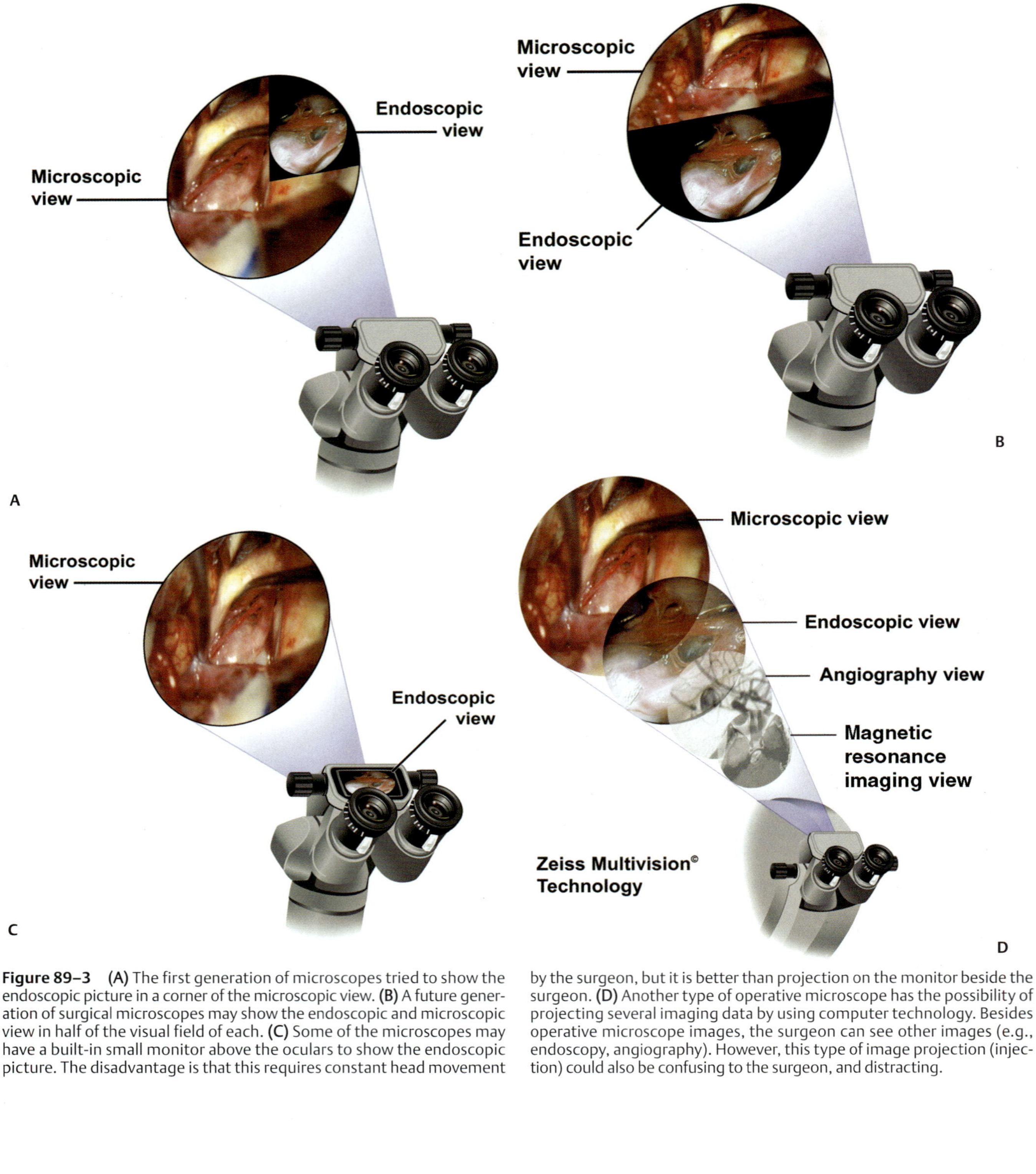

Figure 89–3 **(A)** The first generation of microscopes tried to show the endoscopic picture in a corner of the microscopic view. **(B)** A future generation of surgical microscopes may show the endoscopic and microscopic view in half of the visual field of each. **(C)** Some of the microscopes may have a built-in small monitor above the oculars to show the endoscopic picture. The disadvantage is that this requires constant head movement by the surgeon, but it is better than projection on the monitor beside the surgeon. **(D)** Another type of operative microscope has the possibility of projecting several imaging data by using computer technology. Besides operative microscope images, the surgeon can see other images (e.g., endoscopy, angiography). However, this type of image projection (injection) could also be confusing to the surgeon, and distracting.

45, and 70 degrees are used. The Endoscrub is a device to wash the endoscope free of blood during surgery. Endoscope holders available may be too bulky for use, such as the Mitaka holder (Mitaka Kohki, Tokyo, Japan), and the Aesculap (Central Valley, PA) holder. The surgeon has to be careful with the endoscope when it is fixed to a holder because of the potential to damage neighboring structures.

The endoscope is connected to a camera that produces an image projected on a videoscreen **(Fig. 89–1C)**. The image may be projected into the microscope (Zeiss Multivision Technology, Zeiss Co., Thornwood, NJ) **(Fig. 89–3)** or as a picture on the video screen **(Fig. 89–4)**. An alternative is to place the endoscope screen between the oculars of the microscope **(Fig. 89–3)**.

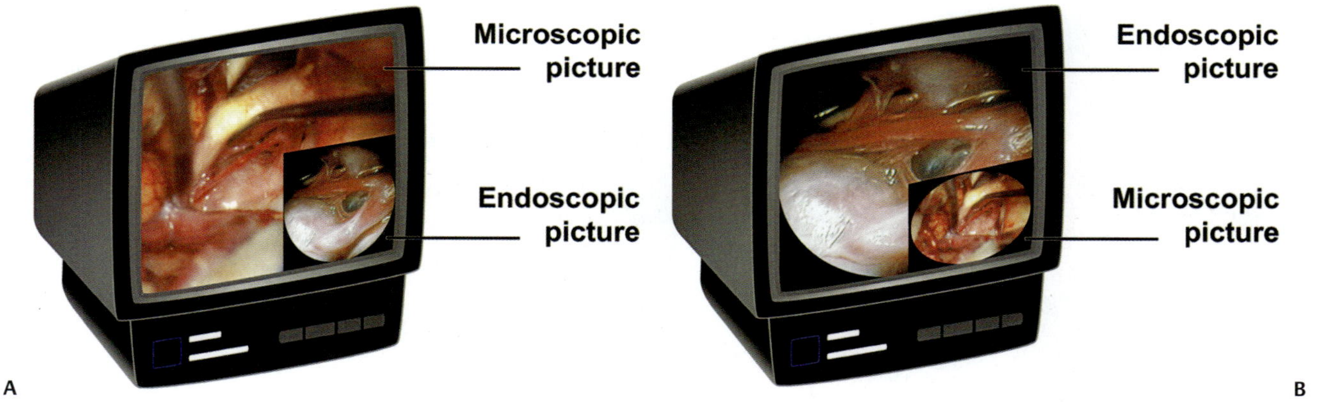

Figure 89–4 Endoscope-assisted microsurgery. **(A)** After positioning the endoscope in the surgical field by means of an operative microscope, surgeons can switch their view to the monitor, simultaneously checking the microscopic and endoscopic views. **(B)** If the endoscopic view is of great importance, the system can be switched to show the endoscopic view as the main view.

◆ Use of the Endoscope in Aneurysm Surgery: Operative Technique

After aneurysm exposure is obtained, the endoscope can be used to look around the aneurysm. However, if the endoscope is close to the aneurysm, a temporary clip must be placed on the feeding vessel to reduce the danger of rupture. The endoscope is frequently used to look behind aneurysms for perforators or for other vessels. The endoscope is more important after aneurysm clipping to judge if the clip has completely occluded the aneurysm neck and to see if any branches are within the blades of the clip. The endoscope may be fixed with a holder such that one can watch the posterior aspect of an aneurysm as clipping of the aneurysm under microscopic vision is in progress (**Fig. 89–5**).[4,11,12,14–16]

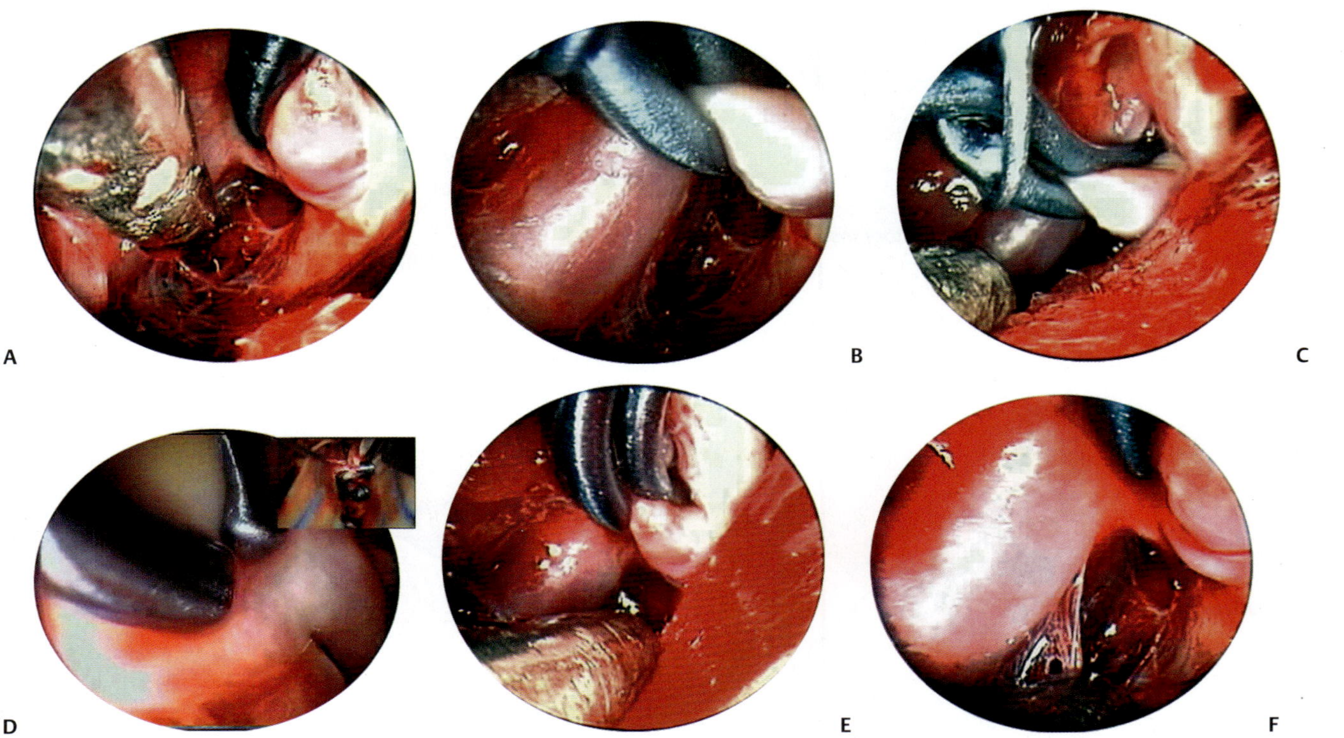

Figure 89–5 **(A)** Endoscopic view of a clipped aneurysm. **(B)** Endoscopic view of a clipped aneurysm **(C)** Endoscopic view of a clipped aneurysm **(D–E)** Aneurysm successfully clipped with two curved clips. **(F)** Unsuccessfully clipped aneurysm neck—needed clip replacement and readjustment.

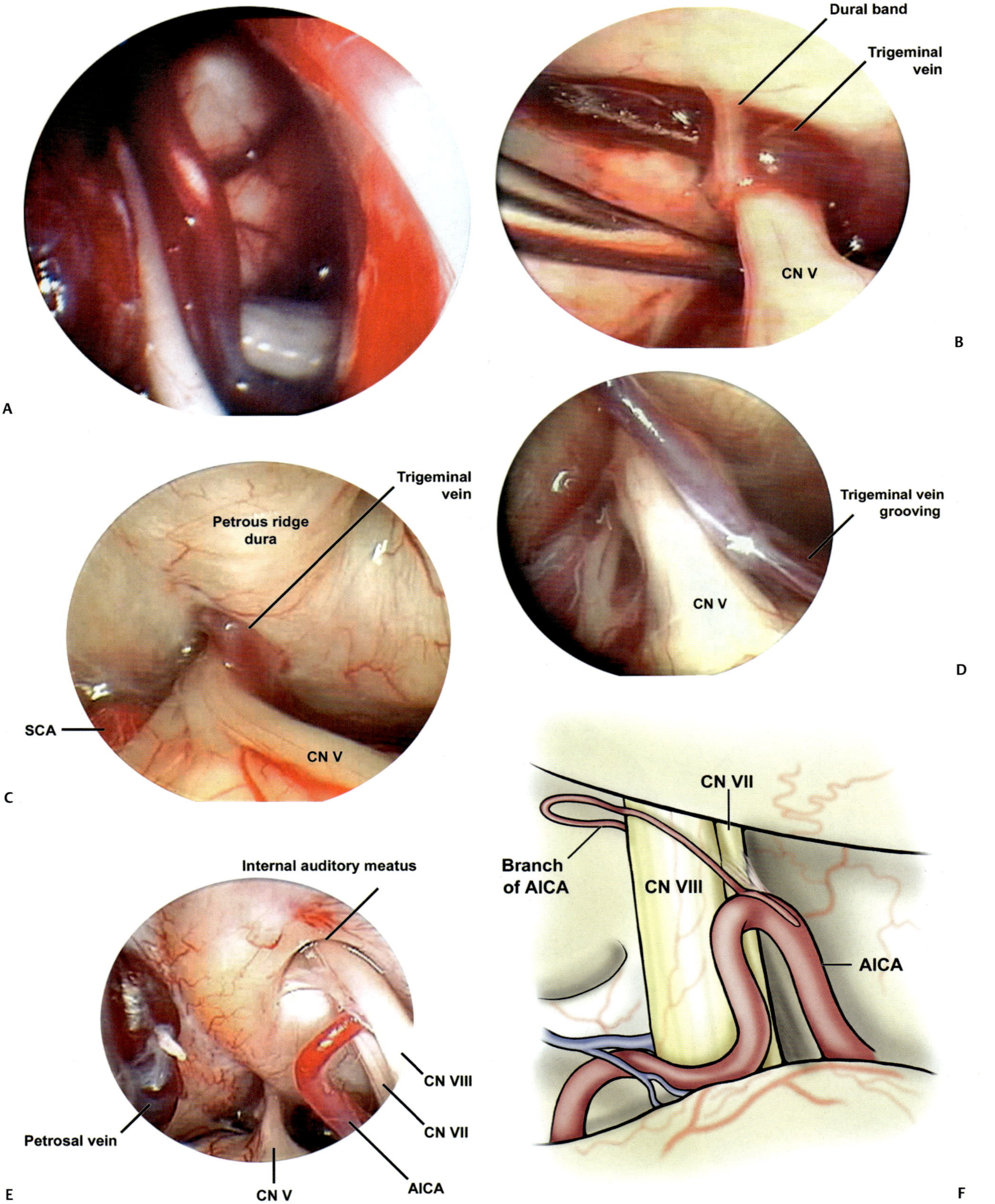

Figure 89–6 **(A)** Endoscopic view of a case of hemifacial spasm. **(B–D)** The trigeminal vein frequently compresses the nerve in a patient with trigeminal neuralgia. **(E)** The anterior inferior cerebellar artery (AICA) passes between cranial nerves (CNs) VII and VIII, causing tinnitus and disabling positional vertigo. **(F)** Drawing of the AICA and vein compressing CN VIII.

◆ Endoscope-Assisted Microvascular Decompression

The endoscope is very useful for microvascular decompression (MVD) of cranial nerves (CNs) V and VII. After retromastoid craniotomy and craniectomy, and dural opening, the endoscope may be used to open the cerebellomedullary cistern and to look for bridging veins, which may be torn during cerebellar retraction. Once CN V or VII is exposed, the endoscope is then used to look for compressive vessels, especially in areas poorly visible to the microscope. During and after the decompression, the endoscope may be used to verify decompression.[1–3,8,13]

During MVD of CN V, the endoscope is especially useful for looking at the inferior and medial aspect of the nerve and the lateral aspect of the nerve at the entrance to Meckel's cave. A trigeminal vein, entering Meckel's cave and compressing the inferior aspect of the nerve, may be hidden by a ridge of petrous bone under microscopic view. It may be the only compressive vessel in some patients. In certain cases, dissection, coagulation, and division of the vein may have to be done under endovision **(Fig. 89–6B–D).**

During hemifacial spasm operations, it is often difficult to see the root exit zone of CN VII completely under microvision without excessive cerebellar retraction. When a 30 or 45 degree endoscope is used, small arteries or frequently a vein may be found to be a compressive element. The endoscope may also be useful to look for compression inside the internal auditory canal in cases of tinnitus or disabling positional vertigo **(Fig. 89–6E,F).**

◆ Endoscope-Assisted Surgery of Cranial Base Tumors

The endoscope can be very useful for cranial base tumor surgery. Pituitary tumors can be resected with endovision alone. In general, with the exception of small tumors confined to the sella, the senior author (DS) nowadays prefers endoscope-assisted (DS) microneurosurgery. After a routine transsphenoidal opening, the endoscope is used to confirm the anatomy such as the carotid and optic nerve prominences, sella, and tuberculum sellae region. After the

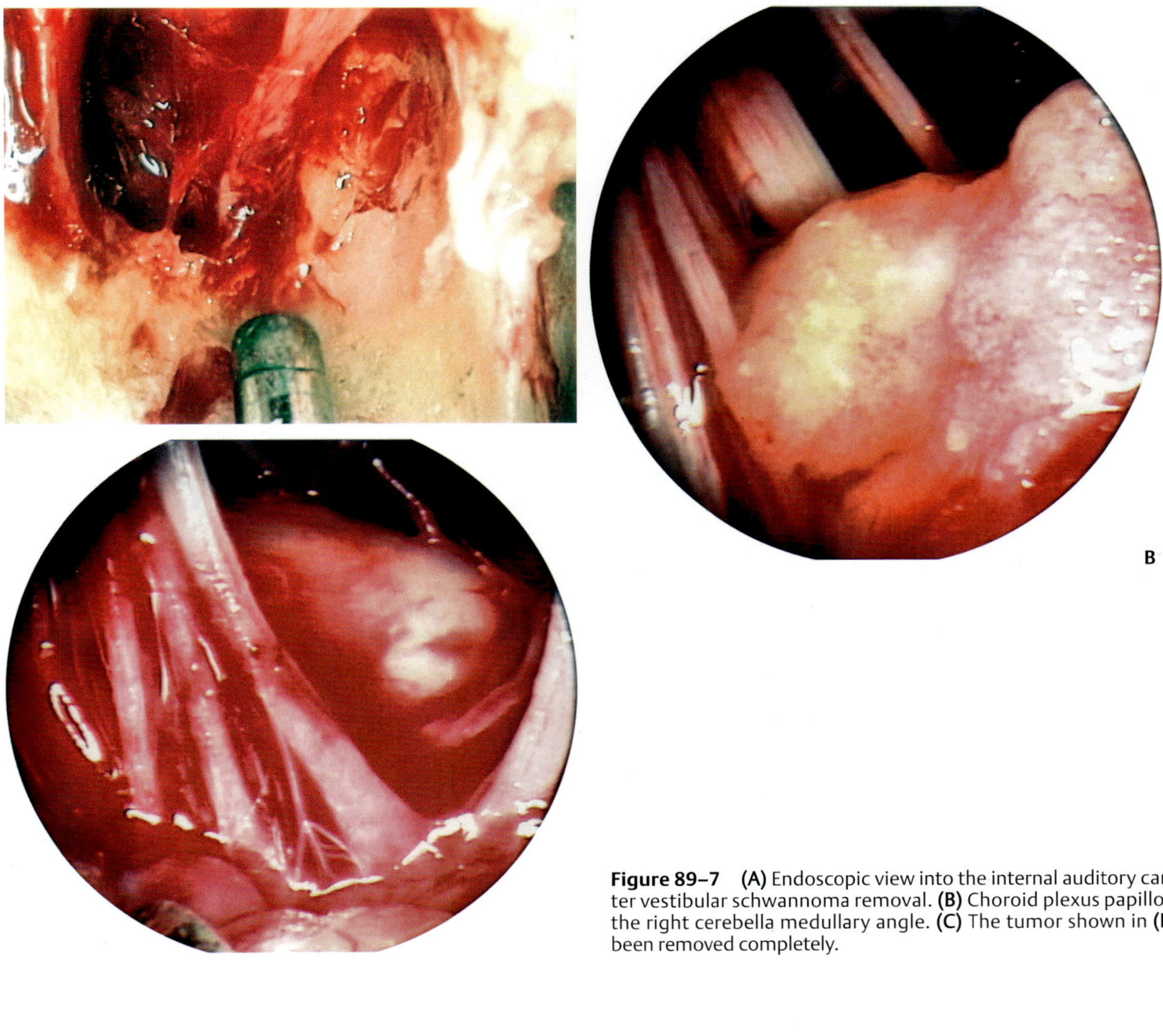

A B C

Figure 89–7 **(A)** Endoscopic view into the internal auditory canal after vestibular schwannoma removal. **(B)** Choroid plexus papilloma in the right cerebella medullary angle. **(C)** The tumor shown in **(B)** has been removed completely.

sellar dura is opened and the tumor is removed, the endoscope is useful to visualize the cavernous sinus region, including the cavernous internal carotid artery (ICA), intracavernous tumor, diaphragma sellae, and suprasellar tumor. The Endoscrub device is very useful for this surgery, and tumor removal can be performed under endovision.

Transsphenoidal and transethmoidal CSF leaks can often be repaired with purely endoscopic surgery. Repair of the leak area is performed with fascia lata or abdominal fascia and fat graft. A septal mucosal flap may also be used for repair of the leak.

During basal meningioma surgery, the endoscope is useful to look around corners and to view neurovascular structures such as the ICA, the optic nerve, the abducens nerve, the basilar artery, or the anterior inferior cerebellar artery (AICA). At the end of tumor resection, it is useful to look around corners to ensure complete resection of tumor. Small pieces of residual tumor may be resected under the endoscopic view. In such situations, the endoscope is held with the left hand, and bipolar cautery and scissors are held with the right hand. A third hand is necessary for the suction device. It may be held by a holder or an assistant, or a Spetzler-Shaw (NMT Co., Phoenix, AZ) microsuction device (malleable microsuction) is placed inside the surgical space (**Figs. 89–1D** and **89–7**).[5–7,9,10,17]

During acoustic neuroma surgery, the endoscope is useful to visualize tumors inside the internal auditory canal (IAC). A 30 or 45 degree endoscope may be used for this purpose. The endoscope allows the lateral extent of drilling to be limited to 1 cm, avoiding injury to the posterior semicircular canal. The lateral portion of the tumor near the fundus is removed under endovision, using a Rhoton 16 or 17 dissector (Codman Co., Boston, MA) or a Shea-Robertson (V. Mueller, Chicago, IL) excavator (**Fig. 89–7A**). The endoscope is also used to look for air cells that may have been opened by the drilling. In cases where the tumor is confined to the medial aspect of the IAC, the endoscope may be used to resect the tumor without opening the IAC.

◆ Pitfalls and Complications

Training with the use of the endoscope in the cadaver laboratory is helpful to the surgeon. Endoscope equipment is in great demand in hospitals, and the neurosurgical nursing team must be experienced in its usage and have the refined technical support for maintaining the equipment.

The main problems with endoscope usage are obscuration of the field by blood or fogging, the absence of any side vision, the problems with holders, and the current non-availability of equipment and technology that allow the surgeon to work entirely with endovision in most operative situations. Current-generation endoscopes also do not provide binocular vision. For all these reasons, endoscope-assisted neurosurgery is much easier than endoscopic surgery for most neurosurgeons.

◆ Conclusion

We expect significant progress in this field based on improvements in equipment and on the coordination of the endoscope and microscope.

References

1. Abdeen K, Kato Y, Kiya N, Yoshida K, Kanno T. Neuroendoscopy in microvascular decompression for trigeminal neuralgia and hemifacial spasm: technical note. Neurol Res 2000;22:522–526
2. Badr-El-Dine M, El-Garem HF, Talaat AM, Magnan J. Endoscopically assisted minimally invasive microvascular decompression of hemifacial spasm. Otol Neurotol 2002;23:122–128
3. El-Garem HF, Badr-El-Dine M, Talaat AM, Magnan J. Endoscopy as a tool in minimally invasive trigeminal neuralgia surgery. Otol Neurotol 2002;23:132–135
4. Fischer J, Mustafa H. Endoscopic-guided clipping of cerebral aneurysms. Br J Neurosurg 1994;8:559–565
5. Gangemi M, Maiuri F, Colella G, Sardo L. Endoscopic surgery for large posterior fossa arachnoid cysts. Minim Invasive Neurosurg 2001;44:21–24
6. Hayashi N, Cohen AR. Endoscope-assisted far-lateral transcondylar approach to the skull base. Minim Invasive Neurosurg 2002;45:132–135
7. Hopf NJ, Perneczky A. Endoscopic neurosurgery and endoscope-assisted microneurosurgery for the treatment of intracranial cysts. Neurosurgery 1998;43:1330–1337
8. Jarrahy R, Berci G, Shahinian HK. Endoscope-assisted microvascular decompression of the trigeminal nerve. Otolaryngol Head Neck Surg 2000;123:218–223
9. Jho HD. Endoscopic pituitary surgery. Pituitary 1999;2:139–154
10. Jho HD, Carrau RL. Endoscopic endonasal transsphenoidal surgery: experience with 50 patients. J Neurosurg 1997;87:44–51
11. Kalavakonda C, Sekhar LN, Ramachandran P, Hechl P. Endoscope-assisted microsurgery for intracranial aneurysms. Neurosurgery 2002; 51:1119–1127
12. Kato Y, Sano H, Nagahisa S, et al. Endoscope-assisted microsurgery for cerebral aneurysms. Minim Invasive Neurosurg 2000; 43:91–97
13. King WA, Wackym PA, Sen C, Meyer GA, Shiau J, Deutsch H. Adjunctive use of endoscopy during posterior fossa surgery to treat cranial neuropathies. Neurosurgery 2001;49:108–116
14. Perneczky A, Boecher-Schwarz HG. Endoscope-assisted microsurgery for cerebral aneurysms. Neurol Med Chir (Tokyo) 1998;38(suppl):33–34
15. Takaishi Y, Yamashita H, Tamaki N. Cadaveric and clinical study of endoscope-assisted microneurosurgery for cerebral aneurysms using angle-type rigid endoscope. Kobe J Med Sci 2002;48:1–11
16. Taniguchi M, Takimoto H, Yoshimine T, et al. Application of a rigid endoscope to the microsurgical management of 54 cerebral aneurysms: results in 48 patients. J Neurosurg 1999;91:231–237
17. Tatagiba M, Matthies C, Samii M. Microendoscopy of the internal auditory canal in vestibular schwannoma surgery. Neurosurgery 1996;38:737–740

90

Endoscope-Assisted Microvascular Decompression

Jacques Magnan and Hani E. L. Garem

In 1934, Dandy[1] suggested that idiopathic cases of trigeminal neuralgia are due to artery–nerve compressions in the cerebellopontine angle (CPA). Jannetta defended this theory, which also explained the etiology of other conditions such as hemifacial spasm,[2] idiopathic unilateral disabling tinnitus,[3] and disabling positional vertigo.[4] Accordingly, the concept of microvascular decompression as a causal treatment for these conditions was born.

In 1959, Gardner performed microvascular decompression for a case of trigeminal neuralgia, but it was Jannetta[5] who codified and popularized it in the 1970s. He performed it under the operating microscope through a suboccipital approach using a cerebellar retractor. Later, Zini et al[6] used the modified enlarged middle cranial fossa approach to decompress the facial nerve in cases of hemifacial spasm.

In the 1990s Magnan et al[7,8] renewed interest in microvascular decompression and modified it by introducing the endoscope as a complementary tool. CPA endoscopy had already been described by the French surgeon Doyen[9] in 1917, and described again by Oppel and Mulch[10] in 1979 when they performed it through a retrolabyrinthine approach, but this technique had very few disciples at that time.

The minimally invasive keyhole retrosigmoid approach is preferred in endoscopic microvascular decompression because it provides a direct and excellent approach to the CPA. Endoscopy is used in combination with the operating microscope. It has the advantage of offering an unobstructed panoramic view of all components of the CPA, unlike the monoaxial one offered by the operating microscope. It "displaces" the surgeon's eye inside the CPA and allows "looking around corners" without the need for excessive cerebrospinal fluid (CSF) drainage because the view is as clear inside the CPA as it is outside it. Unlike the previously mentioned approaches, this endoscopic retrosigmoid approach does not require cerebellar retraction, and the anatomical relations between vascular and neural elements remain undisturbed. This allows the precise identification of conflicts in all cases, and it can identify the grayish indentation caused by the offending vessel, which corresponds precisely to the conflict's site. This makes endoscopy superior to using the operating microscope alone in this field. Thus, it offers an atraumatic, less invasive, and precise guide to the site of pathology in the CPA (**Fig. 90–1**).

However, endoscopy might have a few disadvantages. It does not offer binocular vision, and the heat produced at its tip can damage the nervous elements if it is kept in contact with the cranial nerves for a long time.

Endoscopic-assisted microvascular decompression is the best and most logical functional surgical treatment for cases resulting from a neurovascular conflict in the CPA. It gives excellent long-term results with a low rate of morbidity. The retrosigmoid approach provides direct and easy access to the CPA.

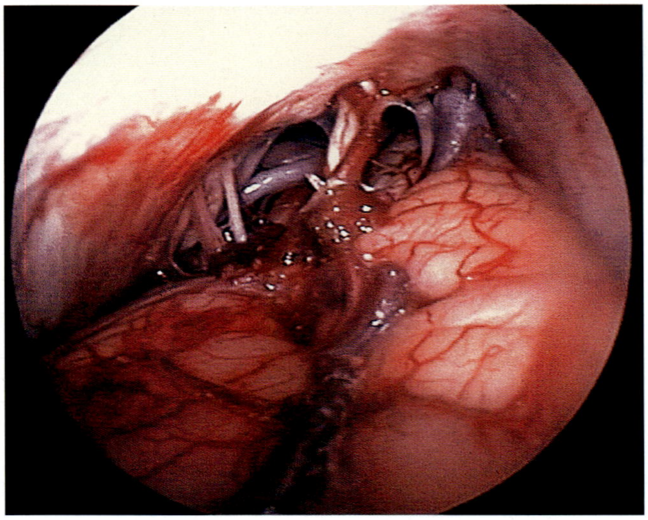

Figure 90–1 Endoscopic view of the left cerebellopontine angle showing, from right to left, the trigeminal nerve and Dandy's vein, the acousticofacial nerve bundle, and the lower cranial nerves (endoscope 4 mm diameter, 0 degree). Advantages of endoscopy are its panoramic view, there is no retraction or dislocation of neural structures, and the precise guidance to the site of the neurovascular conflict.

◆ Indications

- Trigeminal neuralgia
- Hemifacial spasm
- Unilateral disabling tinnitus
- Disabling positional vertigo
- Glossopharyngeal neuralgia
- Microvascular decompression in cases of idiopathic blood hypertension is still very controversial.

◆ Alternative Treatments

Medical Treatment

Drugs such as carbamazepine (Tegretol) are used as an initial treatment in cases of trigeminal neuralgia[11] and hemifacial spasm,[12] but they are either inefficient or of limited efficiency.

Vestibular suppressants have only a temporary effect in cases of disabling positional vertigo.

Injections

Botulin toxin injections are used in cases of hemifacial spasm, but their action is through the production of facial paralysis, which is not tolerated by all patients.[13] Their efficiency is of limited duration.

Percutaneous retrogasserian glycerol injection into the cistern of Meckel's cave through a needle guided by fluoroscopy can be used in the treatment of trigeminal neuralgia. It can produce lasting pain relief, but, because it is technically difficult and has many side effects, especially sensory ones, it is not the treatment of choice.[14]

Injection treatments can be reserved for patients with repeated failure after surgery, for those who are refusing surgery, and for those who have a contraindication for surgery.

Nonsurgical Treatment

Puncturing the trunk or extracranial branches of the facial nerve and the retrogasserian portion of the trigeminal nerve with a needle heated by electrocoagulation or radiofrequency is a treatment modality of hemifacial spasm[12] and trigeminal neuralgia,[14] respectively. Intolerance to the pain induced by this technique, its side effects (such as severe facial paralysis), and the high rate of recurrence made this treatment unpopular.

Balloon compression of the trigeminal nerve for the treatment of trigeminal neuralgia has been attempted. This method consists of introducing a Fogarty catheter percutaneously through a trocar until it reaches Meckel's cave, where it is inflated for a period of 1 to 10 minutes. This technique produced facial sensory troubles in 18% of cases, and its efficiency still needs further evaluation.[15] These modalities of treatment are suggested as an alternative for patients refusing surgery or having a contraindication for surgery.

Surgical Treatment

Surgical interventions other than microvascular decompression in cases of hemifacial spasm or trigeminal neuralgia are all palliative and falling into disuse. Partial resection or longitudinal incision of the facial nerve[16,17] had been suggested in cases of hemifacial spasm. However, these procedures have limited efficiency, recurrence is frequent, and they invariably induce facial nerve paralysis or facial sensory troubles according to the operated cranial nerve.

Retrogasserian rhizotomy for trigeminal neuralgia[14] is reserved for failed cases of microvascular decompression. It has the disadvantage of producing the loss of facial sensation. In cases of disabling positional vertigo, vestibular neurotomy usually controls any episodic vertigo, but it does not alter the constant unsteadiness seen in these patients.[18]

◆ Preoperative Studies

Magnetic Resonance Imaging

For all cases, three-dimensional Fourier transform (3DFT) Magnetic Resonance Imaging (MRI) with special T2 sequences [constructive interference in study state (CISS)], postcontrast special Tl sequences (TurboFLASH), and magnetic resonance angiography (MRA) are performed to show the presence of a conflict and its location. It also excludes the presence of other pathologies that can induce the operated condition (acoustic neuroma, meningioma, cholesteatoma) and cause hemifacial spasm, trigeminal neuralgia, tinnitus, or vertigo.

Electromyography

In cases of hemifacial spasm, electromyography (EMG) shows an abnormal synkinetic response, which will disappear after facial nerve decompression.

Auditory Brain Stem Response (ABR)

Abnormal brain stem auditory evoked potential latencies associated with an MRI showing eighth-nerve compression is considered a sufficient argument for surgical options in the treatment of vertigo, tinnitus, or hearing loss.[19,20]

◆ Surgical Technique

Anesthesia

General endotracheal anesthesia is administered, profound and balanced, with the complementary use of analgesics, hypnotics, or neuroleptics (Diprivan, Sulphentanyl). Before opening the dura mater, the patient is hyperventilated to obtain hypocapnia to diminish the intracranial pressure, which helps spontaneous cerebellar retraction. This step allows an easy penetration in the CPA without the use of a cerebellar retractor. Progress in this type of anesthesia has made it unnecessary to use lumbar puncture, and mannitol 206 mg infusion helps spontaneous cerebellar retraction.

Neurophysiological Monitoring

Facial Nerve Monitoring

Facial nerve monitoring is used during microvascular decompression for hemifacial spasm, tinnitus, or positional vertigo. It helps the surgeon to avoid or stop any maneuver that can threaten the facial nerve. In addition, it can be used as an indicator of the success of the decompression procedure, as the spontaneous firing activity of the facial nerve detected by the monitoring at the beginning of the intervention stops after a successful decompression of the nerve.

Cochlear Nerve Monitoring

Intraoperative ABR monitoring of the cochlear nerve is used during microvascular decompression for tinnitus or positional vertigo. It can help to prevent cochlear nerve injury. The return of the ABR to normal intraoperatively is a sign of good prognosis. Unfortunately, the return to normal is not always constant.

Positioning

The patient is placed in the dorsal decubitus position, with the head flexed and turned to the contralateral side.

Cutaneous Landmarks for the Craniotomy

Two lines should be identified. The first one is horizontal and corresponds to the superior occipital line. It is the posterior prolongation of a line joining the outer catheter of the eye to the superior border of the external auditory canal (Frankfurt line). This line demarcates the tentorial level and separates the middle cranial fossa from the posterior fossa. It passes along the zygomatic arch.

The second line is oblique, passing along the posterior border of the mastoid. It demarcates the sigmoid sinus. Usually, the sinus is slightly anterior to this line. The craniotomy is to be done in the posteroinferior quadrant drawn by the intersection of those two lines, overriding the inferior occipital line (**Fig. 90–2**).

Skin Incision and Craniotomy

The skin incision is curvilinear, 6 to 8 cm long, passing over the posterior part of the craniotomy area, about one fingerbreadth behind the oblique line. The cutaneous flap is anteriorly based, whereas the underlying musculoperiosteal flap is fashioned so it is posteriorly based.

The mastoid emissary vein is identified. Burring for the craniotomy is done in the previously mentioned site, centered on this vein using a cutting bur head. Bone dust is collected to make a bone pâté used during closure. The craniotomy is usually 20 mm in diameter. In cases of hemifacial spasm, because the flocculus might hide the root entry zone (REZ) of the facial nerve, where it is the most common site for the conflict, or compression the craniotomy is slightly extended inferiorly toward the mastoid tip, which gives it an elliptical form.

When the sigmoid sinus (blue in color) and the posterior fossa dura (white in color) are reached, the surgeon uses the operating microscope. A diamond bur head is used to saucerize the craniotomy edges to get a maximal view of the CPA and facilitate the passage of the instruments afterward. The craniotomy must reach the posterior border of the sigmoid sinus anteriorly, but it is not necessary to skeletonize it.

All opened mastoid air cells should be obliterated using bone pâté and Horsley bone wax to avoid CSF leakage through these cells to the middle ear, and eventually through the eustachian tube. Hemostasis must be done before opening the dura.

Opening of the Dura Mater and Penetration in the Cerebellopontine Angle

The best moment to open the dura is when transmitted CSF pulsations are clearly seen—a sign of spontaneous cerebellar retraction. If these pulsations are not clear, the anesthetist is asked to increase the hyperventilation.

Two transfixing punctures of ~2 mm are made in the superior and inferior parts of the dura to allow some CSF to escape. This helps the spontaneous cerebellar retraction. The opening of the dura is completed by making a U-shaped incision so as to form an anteriorly based dural flap. This flap is suspended anteriorly using a stitch or fibrin glue.

A fine neurosurgical cottonoid to protect the cerebellum is introduced following the posterior surface of the temporal bone in an anteroinferior direction to reach the lower cranial nerve area, and then up to the acousticofacial bundle. The arachnoid wrapping is dissected to expose the neurovascular structures under the operating microscope (**Fig. 90–3**).

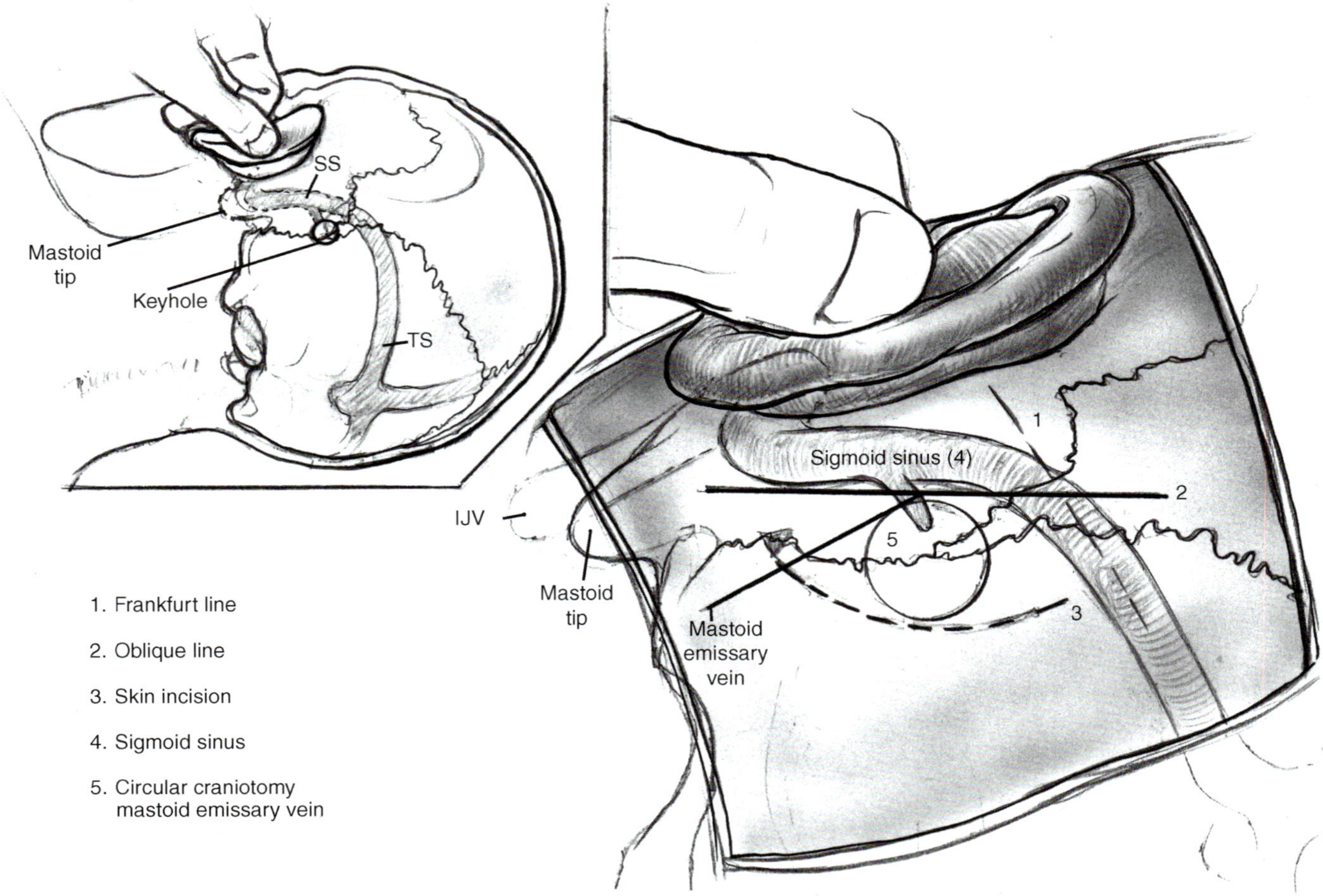

Figure 90–2 Cutaneous landmarks. 1, The Frankfurt line; 2, the oblique line along the posterior margin of the mastoid process; 3, the curvilinear skin incision about one fingerbreadth behind the oblique line; 4, the sigmoid sinus; 5, circular craniotomy and mastoid emissary veins. IJV, internal jugular vein; SS, Sigmoid sinus; TS, Transverse sinus.

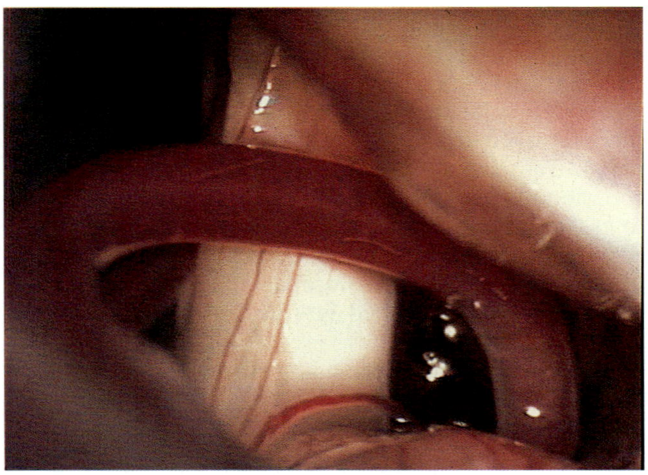

Figure 90–3 Microscopic view of the cerebellopontine angle (CPA) through a keyhole retrosigmoid approach in a case of right hemifacial spasm toward the acousticofacial nerve bundle.

Cerebellopontine Angle Endoscopy

Now an initial CPA exploration is performed with the endoscope to identify its different elements and explore the suspected sites of a neurovascular conflict.[21–23] The CPA is endoscopically divided into two zones separated by the acousticofacial bundle **(Fig. 90–4)**.

The superior zone (above the acousticofacial bundle) is the trigeminal zone where the trigeminal nerve and Meckel's cave are meticulously inspected **(Fig. 90–5).** The most common compressing vessel of the trigeminal nerve is the superior cerebellar artery (SCA).

The inferior zone (below the acousticofacial bundle) is the lower cranial nerves zone, inspected in cases of hemifacial spasm, tinnitus, or positional vertigo. In cases of hemifacial spasm, a vertebral artery in high position and a posterior inferior cerebellar artery (PICA) are the most common offending vessels at the REZ of the facial nerve **(Fig. 90–6).** In cases of tinnitus or positional vertigo, the AICA is the

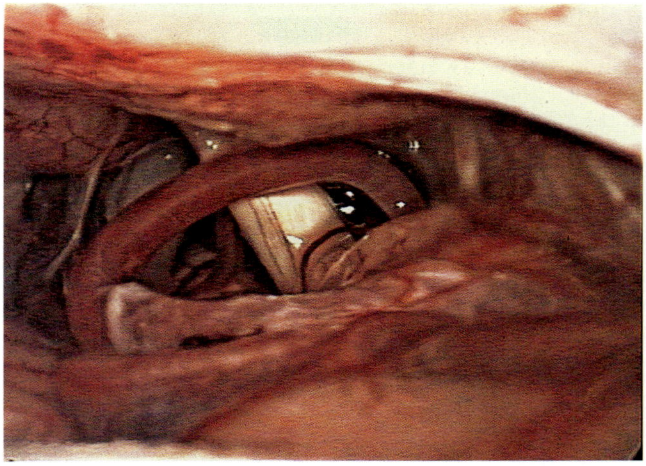

Figure 90–4 Endoscopic view of the same case showing an overview of the whole CPA. The site of the offending vessel and the root entry zone of the facial nerve still hidden by the flocculus will be discovered because of the assisted endoscopic procedure (endoscope 4 mm diameter, degree).

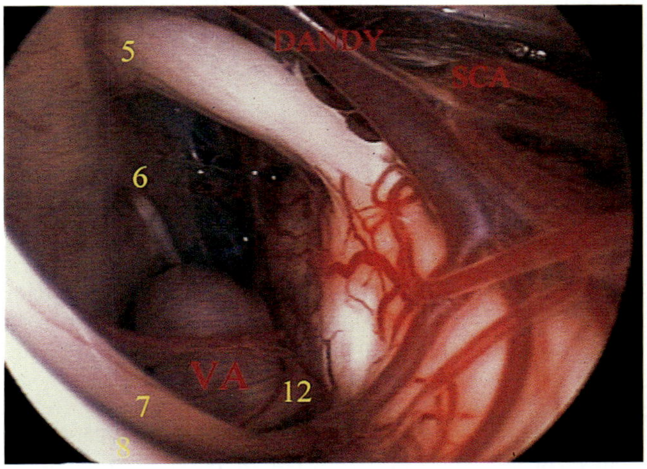

Figure 90–5 Endoscopic view of a left trigeminal zone showing the trigeminal nerve (5) from Meckel's cave to the pons, Dandy's vein, and the caudal and cranial branches of the superior cerebellar artery (SCA). In this case of hemifacial spasm, the vertebral artery (VA), which is seen from above, is in high position (endoscope 4 mm diameter, degree).

most common offending vessel to the eighth nerve especially at the porus of the IAC.

The useful endoscopes include a 4 mm outside diameter, 6 cm long, zero degree; a 4 mm outside diameter, 11 cm long, 30 degrees; and a 2.7 mm outside diameter, 12 cm long, 30 degrees. They are sterilized by autoclaving. To maintain asepsis, a camera is attached to the endoscope and the endoscopic examination is followed on a monitor rather than directly.

Microvascular Decompression Procedure

Whatever the site of the neurovascular compression, microvascular decompression aims to change the offending vessel axis and to keep it away from the offended cranial nerve.

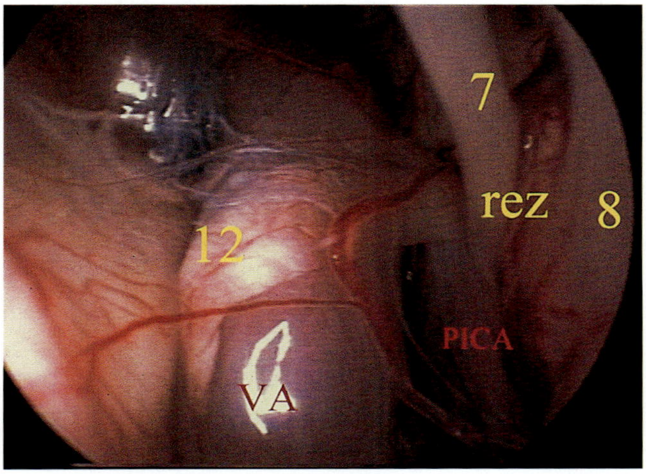

Figure 90–6 Endoscopic view of the lower cranial nerve zone of the same patient. The tip of the endoscope is below the acousticofacial bundle. The root exit zone (REZ) is under control. The vertebral artery (VA) and posterior inferior cerebellar artery (PICA) are both compressing the facial nerve and distorting the hypoglossal nerve (12) (endoscope 4 mm diameter, zero degree).

This surgical procedure is done under the operating microscope. First, the offending artery is carefully mobilized using a microelevator or a microhook. Further meticulous and careful dissection allows the artery's axis of direction to change. The decompression is completed by inserting one or more small Teflon pads between the artery and the nerve and adjusting it with a microinstrument. Teflon is an inert material very well tolerated in the CPA and other parts of the body. If a vein is involved in the conflict and cannot be mobilized safely, it is coagulated using bipolar coagulation after verifying by means of a preoperative MRI assessment that it is not a predominant one.

The operation ends with another CPA endoscopy to assess the quality of the surgery and the correct positioning of the Teflon pad, and to verify the absence of contact between the decompressed nerve and all adjacent vascular structures. The endoscope allows the surgeon to perform this assessment without disturbing the Teflon pad's correct position H.

Closure

Before closure, the small cottonoids in the CPA are removed. The operating field is usually bloodless. If, however, small bleeding areas on the cerebellum are found, they are stopped by using bipolar coagulation or by covering them with a piece of Surgicel, which is further covered by a fibrin glue layer.

The dura mater is sutured meticulously using 5–0 silk sutures. Gaps between sutures are covered by pieces of muscle and then covered by a fibrin glue layer to get a tightly sealed closure. Before closing the dura completely, the CPA is filled with physiological saline at body temperature to extrude air, which can cause postoperative headache. The dura is covered by a piece of Surgicel and a fibrin glue layer. The craniotomy is then filled with a mixture of bone pâté and fibrin glue. An additional layer of adipose tissue can be used. The musculoaponeurotic flap is sutured in place, and finally the subcutaneous layer is sutured followed by skin closure. The duration of the intervention is usually between 1½ and 2½ hours.

◆ Postoperative Care

The patient stays in the recovery room for 2 hours and is then transferred to a hospital room without the necessity of additional care in the intensive care unit (ICU).

Antibiotic therapy begins during the intervention and continues intravenously for 5 days.

The patient leaves the hospital on the eighth postoperative day, and the cutaneous sutures are removed on the 15th postoperative day. The return to normal daily activity is determined during the regular follow-up.

◆ Complications

Endoscopic-assisted microvascular decompression is a functional operation and should be a minimally invasive one, so caution must be taken to avoid any serious complications.The first problem that can be encountered in microvascular decompression is identifying the precise site of the conflict and the offending vessels in it. The nerve can be offended by one or more vessels in hidden areas that can only be explored by the endoscope without cerebellar retraction.

A second problem can be met during the decompression procedure itself. Perforating or labyrinthine arteries originating at the AICA can anchor it, and render its decompression difficult or insufficient, as injury to these branches can affect the inner ear. The AICA itself can compress the facial nerve by passing between it and the eighth nerve, or it can even compress the eighth nerve inside the internal auditory canal (IAC), which renders the procedure of decompression impossible and dangerous in both conditions. In cases of hemifacial spasm, the offending vessel may become embedded in the lateral part of the brain stem and be very difficult to decompress.

It is also important for the surgeon to verify that the decompression procedure was successfully performed, which, again, can only be done by the endoscopic assessment.

Trauma

Trauma to the vascular or nervous system can occur due to clumsy manipulation of the endoscope or other instruments in the CPA. Careful manipulation is mandatory. The endoscope should be kept in contact with the nerves for a short time only (less than 1 minute) to avoid injury produced by its hot tip. Nerve trauma can result in facial paralysis or paresis, or hearing troubles. Here, the surgeon's experience plays a major role in the avoidance of such complications.

Cerebrospinal Fluid Leak

Meticulous dura closure, careful obliteration of opened mastoid air cells, fashioning the skin and musculoaponeurotic flaps so as to be oppositely based (anterior and posterior, respectively), and allowing tight closure are all precautions that contribute to decreasing the incidence of a CSF leak. If a CSF leak occurs, conservative measures are taken first. A tight bandage (if the leak occurs through the wound), repeated lumbar puncture, and administration of diuretics usually stop the leak. If the leak does not respond to these measures, surgical reintervention is done through the previous skin incision.

Delayed Facial Nerve Paresis

Immediate postoperative facial nerve paralysis has never been reported, but rarely delayed paresis occurs around the second postoperative week. It is treated as a case of Bell's palsy using corticoids. A viral origin is suspected. It might be due to a quiescent virus that flourishes in the postoperative period and profits from the "infraclinically fragile" facial nerve. This was realized after the observation of recurrent herpes labialis infection, which flourished after some CPA interventions. A systematic intravenous administration of antiviral drugs (Zovirax) has been done as a prophylaxis in the immediate postoperative period without a significant efficiency. The facial nerve recovers completely within 1 month.

References

1. Dandy W. Concerning the cause of trigeminal neuralgia. Am J Surg 1934;24:447–455
2. Jannetta P. Neurovascular compression in cranial nerve and systemic disease. Ann Surg 1980;192:518–525
3. Jannetta P, Resnick D. Cranial rhinopathies. In: Youmans J, ed. Neurological Surgery. Philadelphia: WB Saunders; 1996:3563–3574
4. Jannetta P. Neurovascular cross compression in patients with hyperactive dysfunction of the eighth cranial nerve. Surg Forum 1975;26: 467–469
5. Jannetta P. Microvascular decompression. In: Rovit R, Murali R, Jannetta P, eds. Trigeminal Neuralgia. Baltimore: Williams & Wilkins; 1990:201–222
6. Zini C, Gandolfi A, Piazza F. Les voies suspetreuses élargies et retrosigmoides: indications et détails techniques. Rev Laryngol Otol Rhinol (Bord) 1988;109(Suppl):173
7. Magnan J, Chays A, Lepetre C, et al. Surgical perspectives of the endoscopy of the cerebellopontine angle. Am J Otol 1994;15:366–370
8. Magnan J, Caces F, Locatelli P, et al. Hemifacial spasm: endoscopie vascular decompression. Otolaryngol Head Neck Surg 1997;117: 308–314
9. Doyen F. Historical perspective. In: Rovit R, Murali R, Jannetta P, eds. Trigeminal Neuralgia. Baltimore: Williams & Wilkins; 1990:17
10. Oppel F, Mulch G. Selective trigeminal root section via an endoscopic transpyramidal retrolabyrinthine approach. Acta Neurochir Suppl (Wien) 1979;28:565–571
11. Jacob R, Rhoton A Jr. Diagnosis and non-operative management of trigeminal neuralgia. In: Youmans J, ed. Neurological Surgery. Philadelphia: WB Saunders; 1996:3376–3385
12. Digre K, Carbett J. Hemifacial spasm: differential diagnosis, mechanisms, treatment. In: Jankovic J, Tolosa E, eds. Advances in Neurology. New York: Raven; 1988:151–173
13. Yoshimura D, Aminoff M, Tansi T, et al. Treatment of hemifacial spasm with botulinum toxin. Muscle Nerve 1992;15:1045–1049
14. Burchiel K. Alternative treatment for trigeminal neuralgia and other cranial neuralgias. In: Youmans J, ed. Neurological Surgery. Philadelphia: WB Saunders; 1996:3416–3427
15. Fraioli B, Ferrante L, Santoro A, et al. Recent progress in the treatment of trigeminal neuralgia: glycerol into the trigeminal cistern and percutaneous gasserian compression by means of Fogarty's catheter. Acta Neurochir (Wien) 1984;33(Suppl):507–510

16. Fisch U. Selective neurectomy for facial hyperkinesia. In: Portmann M, ed. The Facial Nerve. New York: Masson; 1985:49–53
17. Fan Z. Intracranial longitudinal splitting of facial nerve: a new approach for hemifacial spasm. Ann Otol Rhinol Laryngol 1993;102: 108–109
18. Schwaber M, Hall J. Cochleovestibular nerve compression syndrome, I: Clinical features and audiovestibular test findings. Laryngoscope 1992;102):1020–1029
19. Bergsneider M, Becker D. Vascular compression syndrome of the vestibular nerve: a critical analysis. Otolaryngol Head Neck Surg 1995;112:118–123
20. Möller M, Möller A, Janenetta P, et al. Vascular decompression surgery for severe tinnitus: selection criteria and results. Laryngoscope 1993; 103:421–427
21. Jarrahy R, Berci G, Shahinian H. Endoscope assisted microvascular decompression of the trigeminal nerve. Otolaryngol Head Neck Surg 2000;123:218–223
22. Badr-El-Dine M, El Garem H, Talaat A, et al. Endoscopically assisted minimally invasive microvascular decompression of hemifacial spasm. Otol Neurotol 2002;23:122–128
23. El Garem H, Badr-El-Dine M, Talaat A, et al. Endoscopy as a tool in minimally invasive trigeminal neuralgia surgery. Otol Neurotol 2002;23:132–138

91

Endoscope-Assisted Transsphenoidal Surgery

Hae-Dong Jho and Sun-Ho Lee

- Indications for Endoscopic Transsphenoidal Surgery
- Preparation
- Equipment for Endoscopic Transsphenoidal Surgery
- Endoscopic Endonasal Approaches to the Midline Skull Base
- Patient Positioning and Preparation
- Surgical Technique for Endoscopic Pituitary Surgery
- Surgical Technique for Anterior Fossa Skull-Base Surgery
- Surgical Technique for Cavernous Sinus and Optic Nerve Surgery
- Surgical Technique for Clival and Posterior Fossa Surgery
- Postoperative Management
- Complications
- Conclusion

Transsphenoidal pituitary surgery has evolved over the past century to the current microscopic transseptal approach, which has been the standard surgical treatment for pituitary adenomas for many years.[1] Different routes to gain access to the sella through the sphenoidal sinuses have been tried, among which the sublabial transseptal approach has been the most popular. To avoid orodental complications and discomfort induced by a sublabial incision, a transnasal transseptal approach was introduced and has been widely used. As an alternative to the sublabial or transnasal transseptal approach, an endonasal approach has been revived.[2,3] When the senior author (HDJ) developed transsphenoidal endoscopy, an endonasal route was used.[4]

Interest in the neurosurgical implementation of endoscopy has been sporadic for many years since ventriculoscopy was adopted for a choroid plexus operation in the early 1900s. The use of an endoscope during sublabial transseptal transsphenoidal surgery was reported in 1963 by Guiot et al.[5] However, the use of endoscopes in transsphenoidal pituitary surgery had not been practical until functional endoscopy for sinonasal disorders was developed with improved rod-lens optics in Europe 2 decades ago.[6–9] The rapid development of endoscopic sinus surgery has improved surgical techniques as well as the equipment. Subsequently, over the past 10 years, the once conventional surgical treatment of paranasal sinuses has been replaced completely with functional endoscopic sinus surgery. Naturally, sinus endoscopy has been utilized for the repair of cerebrospinal fluid (CSF) leakage. The first successful endoscopic transsphenoidal pituitary surgery was reported by Jankowski et al[10] in 1992. They reported three patients who had undergone transsphenoidal pituitary surgery through a middle turbinectomy approach. However, they later changed to a transseptal technique. This endonasal approach to the sella was not new. In 1909, Hirsch performed his first successful transsphenoidal surgery through multiple-staged operations with an endonasal approach.[1] Despite his successful transsphenoidal surgery via an endonasal route, he subsequently changed his surgical technique to a sublabial transseptal approach. The endonasal route was revived for microscopic pituitary surgery by Griffith and Veerapen[3] in 1987. Cooke and Jones[2] in 1994 reported excellent outcome when an endonasal route was adopted for microscopic pituitary surgery, demonstrating a lack of sinonasal and dental complications.

The senior author has used a sinonasal endoscope in transsphenoidal pituitary surgery for several years.[4,11–15] Initially, an endoscope was adopted as a supplementary tool during the standard conventional sublabial transseptal approach. As the senior author became more confident in employing the endoscope alone as the visualizing tool, he developed an endonasal endoscopic transsphenoidal technique, which has been used with satisfactory outcome in more than 150 operations between 1993 and 1998. Meanwhile, there has been rapid evolution of surgical technique and development of surgical instrumentation in transsphenoidal endoscopy. The authors believe in the very promising future of endonasal endoscopy for pituitary surgery. Neurosurgeons who wish to acquire experience with the endoscope in pituitary tumor surgery should start by using the endoscope during conventional microscopic transsphenoidal surgery. Currently, many pituitary surgeons have already adopted the endoscope as a supplementary visualizing tool during their microscopic transsphenoidal pituitary surgeries.[17–19] Sole use of the endoscope at first may be cumbersome, but it is something that in time surgeons can get used to. Once familiar with the use of surgical instruments under endoscopic visualization, the neurosurgeon may replace the operating microscope with the endoscope as the sole visualizing tool. Endonasal endoscopy for pituitary surgery carries a steep learning curve approximately for the first 30 operations. Frustration associated with early experience is common. Since endonasal endoscopy was first used for transsphenoidal surgery by the senior author in 1993, he has expanded its use to anterior skull-base surgery, cavernous sinus surgery, and clival posterior fossa surgery.[15] The surgical access gained by endonasal endoscopy ranges from the crista galli to the foramen magnum. The midline skull base, within a width of ~2 cm, can be approached with this technique. Although further instrumental improvement is required for dural and bony skull-base reconstruction, this endonasal endoscopic approach to the midline skull base proves to be promising.

There are many advantages with using this endoscopic endonasal technique.[20] In conjunction with an endonasal route that does not require sublabial or nasal incisions, this endoscopic technique preserves physiological sinonasal anatomy, does not require the use of a transsphenoidal retractor, and does not require any sort of postoperative nasal packing. Subsequently, postoperative pain and discomfort is very minimal and patients can be discharged quickly. The main advantage of this endoscopic technique is that the angled lens endoscope can directly visualize hidden anatomical corners as well as the diaphragma sella and the suprasellar region. By rotating the angled lens endoscope, the corners of the sella and sphenoidal sinus can also be directly visualized. A close endoscopic view of the juncture of tumor and pituitary gland tissue seems to enhance the chance of complete resection of the tumor. The disadvantages of transsphenoidal endoscopy are the flat two-dimensional monitor-generated images, and the reduced clarity and sharpness of the images. In time, stereoscopic endoscopes and improved videocamera systems will overcome these shortcomings. Having an endoscopic shaft located at the center of the surgical corridor could be a hindrance for some surgeons and difficult to get used to. Another disadvantage is the steep learning curve for neurosurgeons who are not familiar with sinus endoscopy. One of the major concerns often imparted by microscopic pituitary surgeons has been the possibility of uncontrollable bleeding within such a limited exposure. However, controlling bleeding has not been a problem in the authors' experiences. Although the actual operation time for a transsphenoidal endoscopic procedure may be initially longer than a microscopic operation for a surgeon during his first few attempts, the time will become comparable or decrease once the surgeon becomes accustomed to this technique. This chapter describes an endoscopic endonasal approach to the sella as well as to the midline skull base, such as the anterior cranial fossa, optic nerve, cavernous sinuses, and clival posterior fossa.

◆ Indications for Endoscopic Transsphenoidal Surgery

Indications for endoscopic transsphenoidal pituitary surgery are very similar to those for conventional microscopic transsphenoidal surgery. Patients with hormonally inactive pituitary adenomas are operated on when the tumors cause symptomatic compression of the optic pathway, hypopituitarism, pituitary apoplexy, or severe intolerable headaches. Patients with hormonally active pituitary adenomas causing acromegaly, hyperthyroidism, and Cushing's disease are operated on as the first choice of treatment. Patients with prolactinomas are operated on when they are not responsive to dopaminergic medications or develop intolerable side effects with the medication. Other mass lesions at the pituitary fossa have also been operated on for a simple biopsy or for total resection. Because this technique can directly visualize the suprasellar portion of the tumor with an angled-lens endoscope or by further anterior fossa exposure, the need to use a transcranial approach for pituitary adenomas has been rare even if the tumors are predominantly suprasellar.

After experience accumulated, portions of tumor invading the patient's cavernous sinus have also been operated on using this endoscopic technique. Intracranial tumors at the anterior fossa skull base have been operated on when the tumors are located within a 2 cm width of the midline skull base. The most common tumors that have been treated have been meningiomas at the olfactory groove, planum sphenoidale, and tuberculum sella. Clival and posterior fossa tumors have also been operated on with this endoscopic technique. Although this technique has been used primarily in patients with pituitary lesions, the authors have also employed it in treatment for various other skull-base lesions such as craniopharyngiomas, meningiomas at the olfactory groove, planum sphenoidale and tuberculum sella, germinomas, epidermoid, posterior fossa clival chordomas, CSF leakage, and clival meningiomas.

Patients with Cushing's disease often have a very narrow nasal airway due to swollen hypertrophic mucosa. Among the more than 150 patients who have undergone endoscopic transsphenoidal surgery by the senior author, only two patients with Cushing's disease required a two-nostril technique. An endoscope was inserted through one nostril and the surgical instruments were inserted through the other. Reoperation by this endoscopic technique for patients who have undergone previous transsphenoidal surgery is relatively easy because an anterior sphenoidotomy has already been done as part of the previous surgery, and submucosal dissection is not required.

◆ Preparation

Magnetic resonance imaging (MRI) scans of the brain with and without contrast enhancement are done in all patients. Thinly sliced coronal and sagittal views of MRI scans are integral for pituitary adenomas. Computed tomography (CT) scans of the skull base are selectively obtained when review of detailed bony anatomy is necessary. Endocrine evaluations are performed in all patients with pituitary adenomas and other lesions located in the vicinity of the pituitary gland. A formal neuro-ophthalmological evaluation is performed in patients with macroadenomas and other tumors located near the optic system. Hypopituitarism is treated preoperatively. Although stress doses of a steroid were used perioperatively in our earliest patients, steroids are no longer used when the patient's pituitary-adrenal function is normal preoperatively. Instead, an a.m. cortisol level is measured the day following surgery to confirm that it is higher than 18 g/dL. If the a.m. cortisol level is below 18 g/dL, postoperative treatment is instituted with oral hydrocortisone 20 mg q a.m. and 10 mg q p.m. until the pituitary-adrenal axis is proven to be normal. For patients with hypocortisolism, perioperative stress doses of steroids are used. For patients with Cushing's disease, dexamethasone is administered postoperatively with an oral 1 mg b.i.d. regimen. When dexamethasone is used instead of hydrocortisone, serum cortisol and urinary free cortisol levels can be measured early postoperatively to judge the postoperative outcome of Cushing's disease.

◆ Equipment for Endoscopic Transsphenoidal Surgery

Appropriate surgical equipment is absolutely necessary to perform successful endoscopic pituitary surgery. This endoscopic surgical technique differs from microscopic surgery. It is essential that this technique be learned and practiced before application. The required surgical instruments are endoscopes with 0, 30, and 70 degree lenses and their accessories include a video imaging system and a light source, an endoscope lens cleansing device, a rigid endoscope holder, and various surgical instruments specifically designed for endoscopic surgery. The endoscopes we use are rod-lens rigid endoscopes. The diameter of the endoscope must be 4 to 5 mm because the quality of the video image markedly drops when the diameter is reduced to 3 mm or less. The length has to be at least 18 cm or longer. Endoscopic optics and the relative video images continue to improve. Digital enhancing mechanisms for endoscopic video images have recently improved the clarity of monitored endoscopic images. Although a high-definition camera is available, it has not been widely used yet. When this high-definition video camera is used in conjunction with endoscopy, the quality of the endoscopic images improves drastically.

An endoscope holder is an essential and required piece of equipment. To perform this operation successfully, the endoscope holder has to be able to hold the endoscope firmly. It should be compact and slender so as to sacrifice as little operating space as possible. The endoscopic holder now available commercially is not yet adequate. There are two types that are currently available. One is a simple manual holder with multiple joints that can be tightened by hand. The other is a holder with joints that are tightened or released by a nitrogen gas powered mechanism. The latter, though more expensive, should prove to be a promising and convenient device once fully developed. The endoscope holder must also be able to be mounted to an operating table as well as to various neurosurgical head-holding devices. Endoscope holders not only provide stable video images but also allow a surgeon to freely use both hands. The holder currently used by the authors is a custom-made manual type that is incorporated with a Greenberg retractor system.

An endoscopic lens-cleansing device is another useful tool and is required to cleanse the lens so the operation can be performed without interruption. The device consists of a battery-powered motor, disposable irrigation tubing, and an endoscope-cleansing sheath. The irrigation tubing is connected to a saline bag hung on a pole. The tubing is threaded through a battery-powered motor that controls the intensity of irrigation including forward and reverse. This irrigation device, controlled by a foot pedal, pushes saline forward to clean the lens. When the foot pedal is released, the motor reverses its rotary direction and draws the saline back for a second or two. This action clears water drops from the end of the endoscope. It facilitates maintenance of a clean endoscopic lens throughout surgery. The two main flaws with this device are the short duration of reverse flow interval and the inadequate seal at the proximal end of the endoscope sheath, which is easily broken. Inserting the endoscope through the cleansing sheath, even with lubrication, may damage the small rubber ring seal. The damaged seal results in the leakage of water bubbles, which obscures the video image. A more dependable endoscope lens-cleansing device needs to be developed in the future.

Inclusive among the various essential surgical instruments are a monopolar Bovie-suction 8 or 9 French (F) cannula, bipolar suction cannulas sized 8 or 9F, and a single blade bipolar coagulator, which are very useful tools for hemostasis. They are all disposable and inexpensive. A monopolar Bovie-suction cannula is malleable and insulated. A bipolar suction cannula or a single blade bipolar coagulator that has two cables, one at the core and the other at the shell, to produce bipolar functioning are used for dural or intradural hemostasis. The suction cannulas we use are 5, 7, 9 and 11F. The 9 and 11F suction cannulas are used for the nasal portion of the operation. The 5 and 7F suction cannulas are used for tumor resection in the sella. The tips of the suction cannulas are shaped to be straight as well as curved upward and downward with various lengths. These curved instruments are helpful for accessing remote anatomical corners.

Titanium microclips have been used as a dural suturing device, but further improvement in the currently available clips is required. They have proven to be difficult to apply and are easily dislodged due to their nonpenetrating clip mechanism. In addition, the device was not designed for and is too short for skull-base surgery through a nostril. Other instruments used are a micropituitary rongeur, pituitary rongeur, ethmoid rongeurs, high-speed drill, micro-Kerrison rongeurs, pituitary ring curets, Jannetta 45 degree microdissector, single blade Kurze scissors, and a specially designed septal breaker that was developed to expedite anterior sphenoidotomy. A septal breaker functions by opening the alligator-toothed mouth at the tip and then fracturing the nasal septum and vomer at the sphenoidal rostrum. Its use facilitates fracturing the thick bone at the vomer. A high-speed drill is very useful when the sphenoidal sinuses are small and not well pneumatized. The endoscope has to be mounted to the endoscope holder for the use of a drill. A high-speed drill and a suction cannula can be inserted next to the endoscope shaft without difficulty. A suction cannula has to be placed next to the drill bit to prevent clouding of the endoscope lens by bone dust.

◆ Endoscopic Endonasal Approaches to the Midline Skull Base

Endoscopic endonasal approaches to the midline skull base can be made through three different surgical routes. The first is a paraseptal approach that is made between the nasal septum and middle turbinate **(Fig. 91–1A).** The middle turbinate is pushed laterally and the nasal septum is fractured toward the contralateral side. For an anterior skull-base approach, an ethmoidectomy is required. This paraseptal approach has been adopted for surgery involving the pituitary, cavernous sinus, optic nerve, anterior fossa, and clivus. Most of the authors' endoscopic endonasal surgery has been performed with the paraseptal approach. The second route is a middle turbinectomy approach **(Fig. 91–1B).** When a wider surgical corridor is required, a middle turbinectomy is performed in addition to the septal fracture made toward the contralateral side. This middle turbinectomy approach can be used for surgery at the anterior fossa, optic nerve, cavernous sinus, pituitary, and clival posterior fossa. Although this middle turbinectomy approach provides substantial space for maneuvering of surgical equipment, the reconstruction of the skull base can be problematic when solid intranasal structures are required for support. The third route is a middle meatal approach that is made between the middle turbinate and the lateral wall of the middle meatus **(Fig. 91–1C).** This middle meatal approach can be used for a limited anterior fossa skull-base approach and an approach to the optic nerve and cavernous sinus. An ethmoidectomy is required for anterior fossa access through the middle meatal approach.

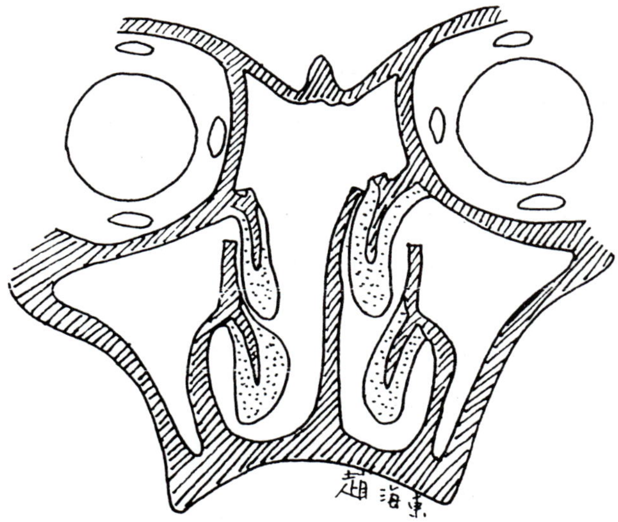

A

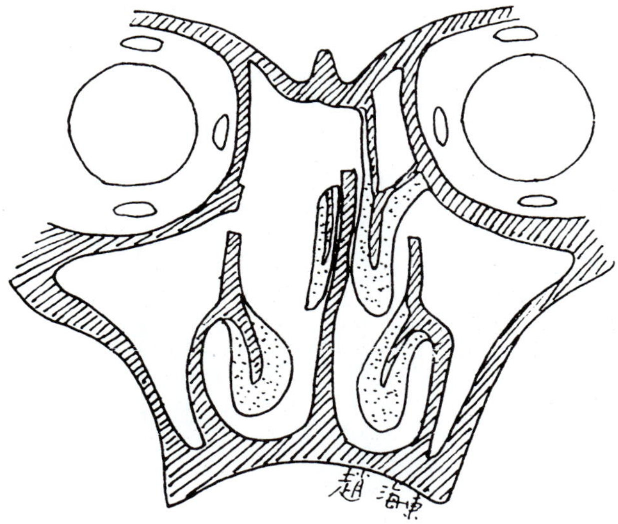

B

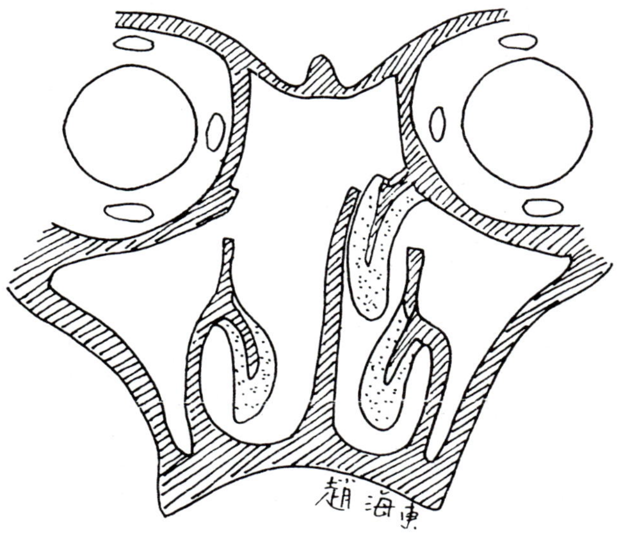

C

Figure 91–1 Schematic drawings of three different endoscopic endonasal surgical approaches to the skull base. **(A)** The paraseptal approach, the most commonly used approach by the authors, is made between the nasal septum and middle turbinate. The middle turbinate is pushed laterally and the nasal septum is fractured at its basal attachment and displaced contralaterally. It can be used for surgery at the anterior cranial base, optic nerves, cavernous sinus, pituitary and clivus. **(B)** The middle meatal approach is made through the middle meatus. The middle turbinate is pushed medially and an ethmoidectomy is performed to access the skull base. This approach can be used for surgery at the anterior cranial fossa, optic nerve, and cavernous sinus. **(C)** The middle turbinectomy approach is performed with resection of the middle turbinate. It provides a much wider surgical corridor for the surgeon facilitating maneuvering of surgical instruments.

◆ Patient Positioning and Preparation

The patient is positioned supine. General anesthesia is induced and maintained with orotracheal intubation. To prevent kinking of the endotracheal tube, an endotracheal tube incorporating an inner wire is used. A Doppler cardiac monitor is used, although no instance of air embolism has been encountered with this operation. The oropharynx is packed with a 2 inch gauze roll to prevent blood accumulation. Ophthalmic ointment is placed on the cornea and conjunctiva. The eyelids are closed and sealed with soft vinyl adhesives. A three-pin head clamp was utilized for head fixation in our earlier patients. The endoscopic holding device was usually mounted to the head clamp when draping was completed. Now, a head clamp fixation device is not used, and the endoscopic holder is mounted to the operating table after completion of the sterile draping. The patient's torso is elevated ~20 degrees to reduce venous bleeding at the time of surgery. The patient's hips and knees are gently flexed with padding for comfort. The patient's head is rotated toward the surgeon as needed, usually ~20 degrees **(Fig. 91–2).** This head rotation does not disturb the surgeon's anatomical orientation because the endoscopic camera can be rotated accordingly. For this pituitary operation, the head is positioned horizontally with the forehead–chin line parallel to the operating room floor. This head positioning will naturally render 25 degree cephalad angulation of the endoscope shaft when it is inserted while aiming toward the sella between the middle turbinate and nasal septum. This 25 degree cephalad angulation of the endoscope shaft renders comfort to the surgeon who operates under the video images. With the patient's head positioned horizontally, insertion of the endoscope into the nasal cavity will naturally expose the middle turbinate.

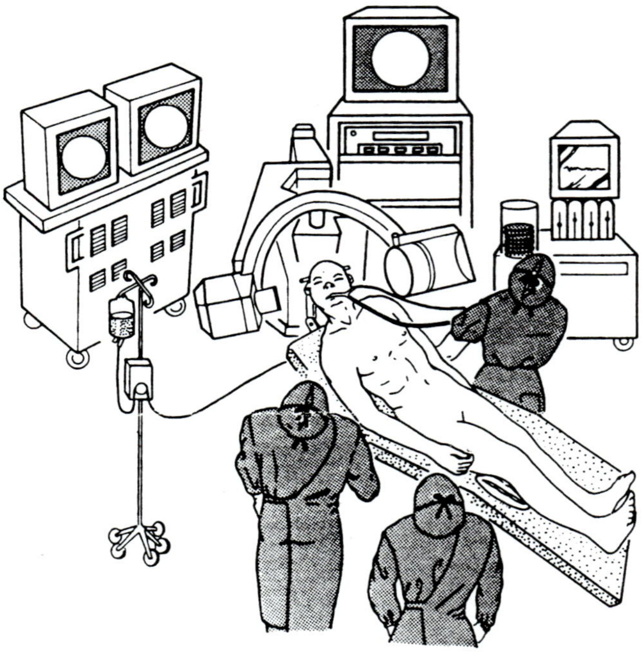

Figure 91–2 Schematic drawing of the arrangement of the operating room and patient's positioning that the authors utilize. A fluoroscopic C-arm is used selectively with patients undergoing surgery at the anterior fossa or clival posterior fossa, or for pituitary patients with complex sinonasal anatomy. The video monitor is placed a few feet in front of the surgeon, and the endoscopic cleansing system is placed to the left of the video monitor or fluoroscopic C-arm. The patient's torso is elevated 20 degrees with the hips and knees flexed for comfort. The head is rotated toward the surgeon at about 10 to 20 degrees. The head is laid horizontally for pituitary surgery, in 15 degree extension for anterior fossa surgery and at 15 degree flexion for clival surgery. This specific head positioning will render ~25 degree cephalad angulation of the endoscope shaft when the endoscope is inserted and aimed at the surgical target. This 25 degree cephalad angulation of the endoscope shaft facilitates surgeon comfort when the surgeon operates under the video monitor.

When the anterior fossa is to be explored, the head is extended ~15 degrees. When the clival or posterior fossa region is explored, 15 degree flexion is applied. This specific modification of head positioning allows the surgeon to maintain the cephalad incline of the endoscope shaft similar to that in pituitary surgery. Although it was used in our earlier patients, a fluoroscopic C-arm is now only used selectively in patients with anterior fossa or posterior fossa tumors or with patients with complex sinonasal anatomy. The lens-cleansing motor is placed next to the video monitor. When a fluoroscopic C-arm is used, the video monitor is placed at the right side of the C-arm and the lens-cleansing motor at the left. Foley catheterization has been used selectively only in patients who are expected to require longer operating hours or have high risk of developing diabetes insipidus.

A single dose of cephazolin 1 g is given intravenously as a prophylactic antibiotic. Clindamycin 900 mg is mixed in a bag of 250 mL of normal saline, which is used as the irrigation fluid for the endoscope-cleansing device. The nasal cavity, entire face, and abdominal wall is prepared with iodoform. The abdominal wall is prepared because fat graft placement is often required and is harvested from the abdominal wall though a small infraumbilical incision. Although we used vasoconstrictors early in our series, the topical use of a vasoconstrictor and the local infiltration of a vasoconstrictor have been completely eliminated. When vasoconstrictors are not used, the hemostasis achieved intraoperatively is maintained postoperatively, resulting in minimal dripping of nasal blood. It has been our experience that patients have much less nasal bleeding postoperatively when vasoconstrictors are not used. The use of vasoconstrictors may render a surgical field bloodless intraoperatively; however, it seems to be followed by a rebound effect postoperatively. When the aseptic draping has been completed, the endoscopic holder is mounted and a 0 degree endoscope is connected to the camera system, light source, and lens-cleansing device. The intensity of the endoscope light is increased to 100% and the white balance of the video images is established. The surgical equipment including the drill and endoscope cleansing system is then tested for proper functioning.

◆ Surgical Technique for Endoscopic Pituitary Surgery

The nasal cavity is inspected and the middle turbinate is identified **(Fig. 91–3A).** Three to four cotton patties, $^{1}/_{2} \times 3$ inches, are inserted to widen the space between the middle

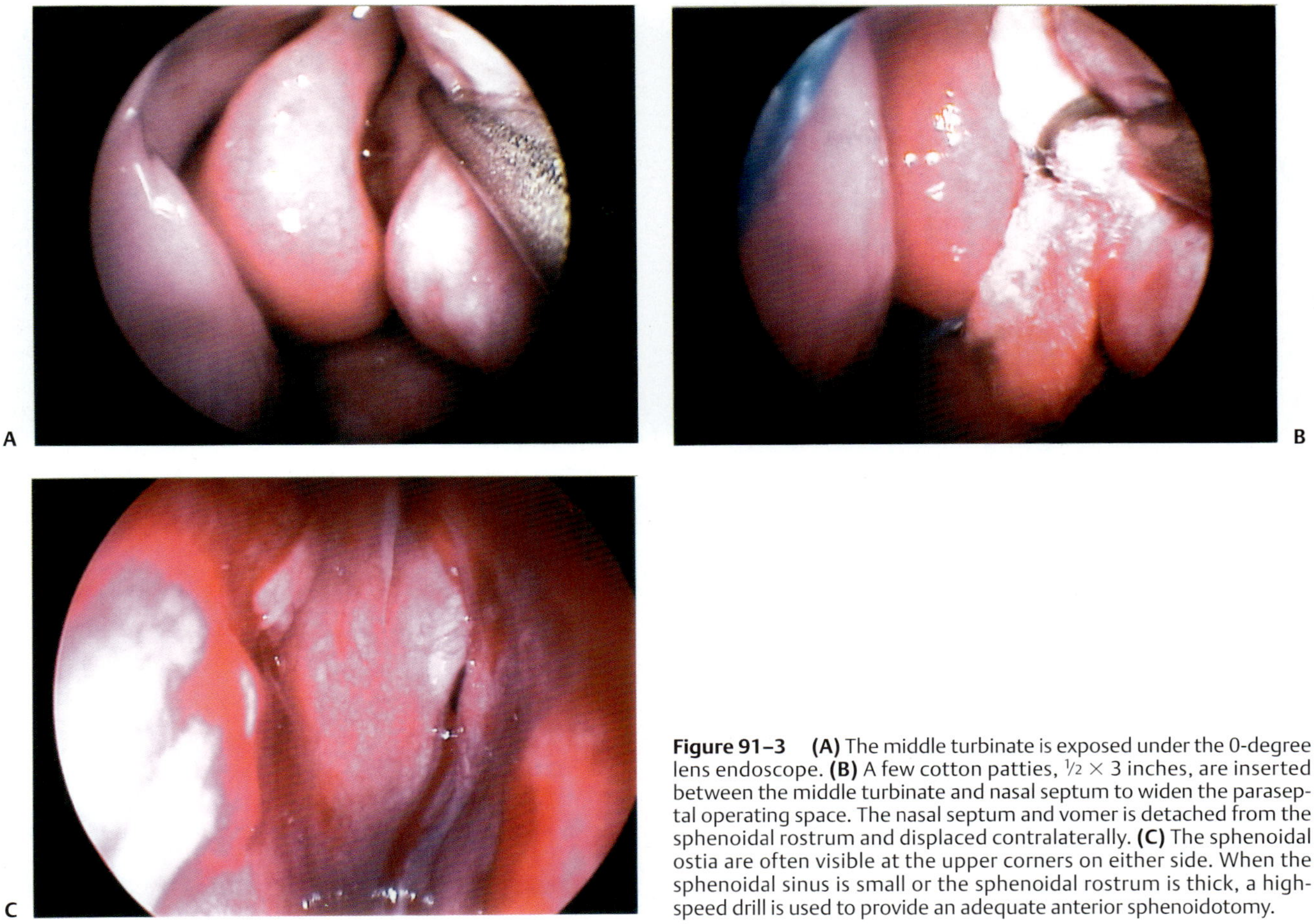

Figure 91–3 **(A)** The middle turbinate is exposed under the 0-degree lens endoscope. **(B)** A few cotton patties, ½ × 3 inches, are inserted between the middle turbinate and nasal septum to widen the paraseptal operating space. The nasal septum and vomer is detached from the sphenoidal rostrum and displaced contralaterally. **(C)** The sphenoidal ostia are often visible at the upper corners on either side. When the sphenoidal sinus is small or the sphenoidal rostrum is thick, a high-speed drill is used to provide an adequate anterior sphenoidotomy.

turbinate and nasal septum **(Fig. 91–3B)**. When the cotton patties are removed, bleeding occurs from the mucosa at the rostrum of the sphenoidal sinus. The mucosa over the rostrum of the sphenoidal sinus is coagulated and divided with an 8F suction-monopolar coagulator. The sphenoidal ostium is often visible at the lateral corner of the sphenoidal rostrum ~1 cm rostral to the inferior margin of the middle turbinate **(Fig. 91–3C)**. However, a consistent landmark is the inferior margin of the middle turbinate, which leads to the clivus ~1 cm below the floor of the sella **(Fig. 91–4)**. The septal breaker is used to fracture the nasal septum and vomer at the rostrum of the sphenoidal sinus. Submucosal dissection is performed along the contralateral side of the sphenoidal rostrum. The contralateral sphenoidal ostium can then be seen. The sphenoidal sinuses are laterally penetrated along either side with a suction cannula. This penetration is easiest near the sphenoidal ostium. Starting from this lateral penetration site into the sphenoidal sinuses, a series of penetrations are made along the lateral gutter of the anterior wall of the sphenoidal sinus. The anterior wall of the sphenoidal sinus is removed with ethmoidal and Kerrison rongeurs. Each blade of the mouth of an ethmoidal rongeur is inserted into the lateral penetration site at the sphenoidal rostrum and the bone is fractured and removed. Attention is paid so as not to strip the sphenoidal sinus mucosa. When the sinus mucosa is stripped inadvertently, the subsequent bleeding from the bony wall can be cumbersome. Removal of the sphenoidal mucosa is limited to the anterior sphenoidotomy hole. The mucosa located behind the anterior wall of the sphenoidal sinuses is removed with Kurze scissors. When the bone is thick, a high-speed drill is used with a ball-type 5 mm cutting bit **(Fig. 91–3C)**. An anterior sphenoidotomy is performed of about 1.5 to 2 cm in width. The sphenoidal septum is removed as needed for full exposure of the sella. Further rostral extension of the anterior sphenoidotomy is adjusted accordingly when the floor of the sella is identified. Meticulous control of bleeding is made with electrocoagulation. When the endoscope is inserted into the sphenoidal sinuses, a panoramic view of the posterior wall of the sphenoidal sinuses comes under direct visualization. With the sella being at the center, the view of the anatomy that is demonstrated is as follows: the clival indentation is at the bottom, the petrous carotid bony protuberances are at the 5 and 7 o'clock points, the tuberculum sella is superior to the sella, the optic protuberances are at the 2 and 10 o'clock positions and the cavernous sinuses are at the 3 and 9 o'clock positions **(Fig. 91–5)**. Once the anterior sphenoidotomy is completed, an endoscope is mounted to the endoscope holder. The endoscope tip is advanced to a point in front of the sella for a close-up view. The mucosa on the anterior wall of the sella is coagulated and removed.

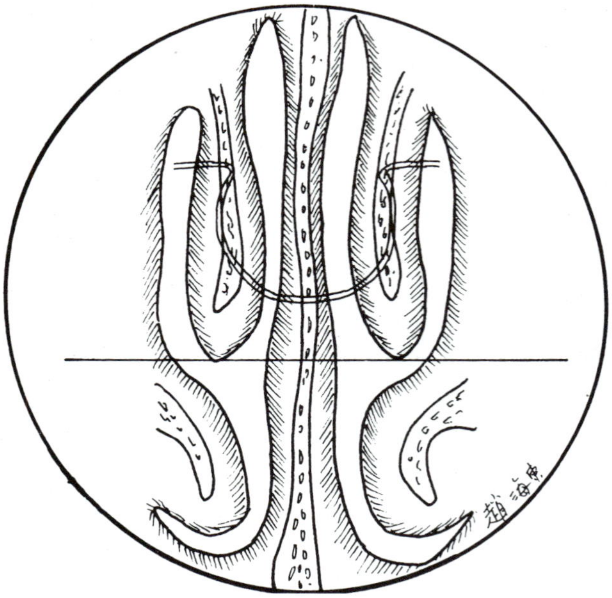

A

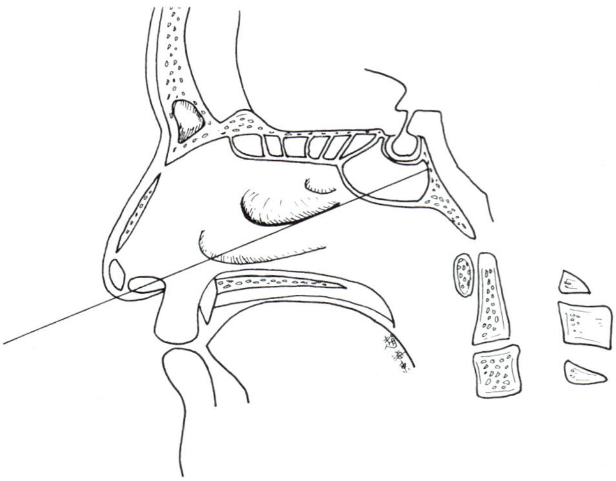

B

Figure 91–4 Schematic drawings of the **(A)** coronal and **(B)** sagittal views of the nasal cavity demonstrate the anatomical landmark leading to the sella. The line drawn along the inferior margin of the middle turbinate leads to the clivus at approximately 1 cm inferior to the floor of the sella. The lower extent of the anterior sphenoidotomy is made at this line. Once the floor of the sella is identified, the rostral extent of the anterior sphenoidotomy is adjusted accordingly.

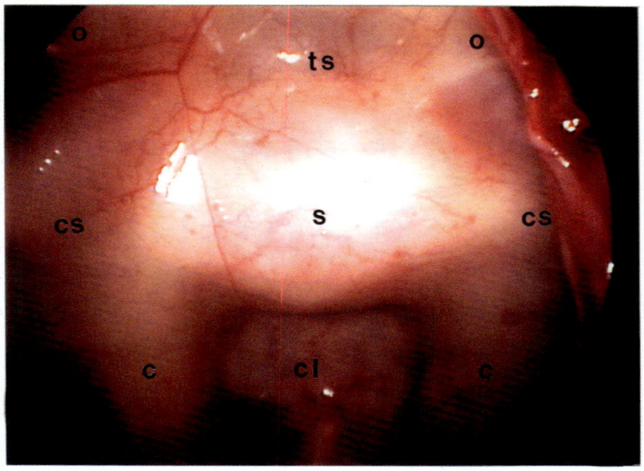

A

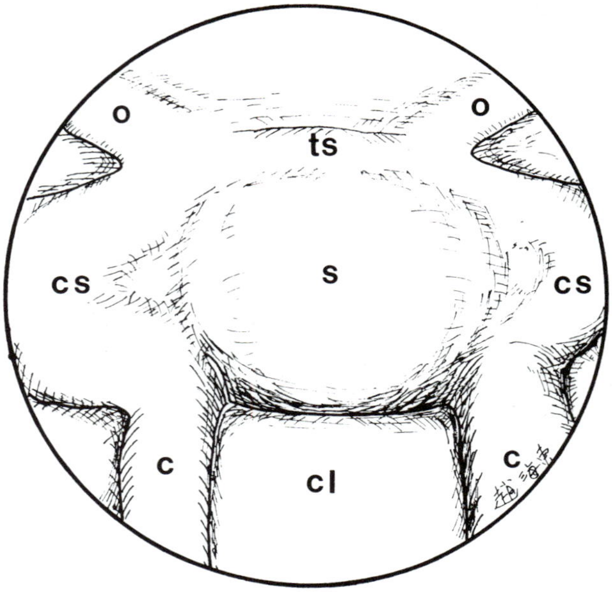

B

Figure 91–5 An endoscopic view under **(A)** a 0 degree lens and **(B)** a schematic drawing of the sphenoidal sinuses. When the anterior sphenoidotomy has been completed, the endoscopic view of the sphenoidal sinuses is panoramic. The clival indentation (cl) is at the bottom, the bony protuberances covering the petrous carotid artery (c) are at the 5 and 7 o'clock positions, the sella (s) is at the center, the cavernous sinuses (cs) are seen laterally, the tuberculum sella (ts) is superiorly, and the optic protuberances (o) are at the 10 and 2 o'clock positions.

The bony anterior wall of the sella is penetrated with a small bone curet. Through this small hole, the anterior wall of the sella is opened from cavernous sinus to cavernous sinus laterally, and from the tuberculum sella to the sellar floor vertically. If further rostral exposure is required, the bony wall at the tuberculum sella and planum sphenoidale can be also removed. The dura mater is coagulated along the periphery with a single-blade bipolar coagulator. The dura is incised horizontally along the inferior margin of the sella with a Jannetta 45 degree microdissector. The dura mater is incised in circular fashion with curved Kurze microscissors and removed for biopsy. In cases of microadenomas the tumor is removed with a small ring curet from the suspected location as suggested by the MRI scan. Attention is paid so as not to lose the tumor specimen by suctioning. The tumor specimen is sampled and sent to a neuropathologist.

When tumor tissue is curetted out, the thin shell of the normal pituitary tissue is shaved along the tumor cavity to enhance the chance of cure when dealing with a hormonally active microadenoma. For macroadenomas, the tumor is removed at the floor of the sella first with downward-angled curets and suction cannulas. When the inferior portion of the tumor has been completely removed, the dura mater or intercavernous sinus at the floor of the sella can be visualized directly. The lateral portion of the tumor is removed with upward-angled curets and straight or upward-angled suction cannulas. The tumor is dissected and removed along the medial wall of the cavernous sinus. The thin venous wall of the cavernous sinus is visualized when the lateral portion of the tumor is completely removed. Then, the superior portion of the tumor is removed with both upward-angled ring curets and suction cannulas. The tumor is removed at the periphery along the diaphragma sella first. When the diaphragma sella is defined at the periphery, the tumor is progressively removed by moving toward the center. When the tumor is soft in consistency, the tumor tissue descends after progressive tumor removal. When the tumor removal has advanced from the periphery of the diaphragma sella toward the center, the medial edge of the diaphragma sella is often definable with the remaining suprasellar portion of the tumor at the center. This portion of the tumor is removed further with two upward-angled suction cannulas or one upward-angled ring curet in one hand and one upward-angled suction cannula in the other. A fibrotic tumor requires more aggressive curetting as well as the use of pituitary microrongeurs. When the suprasellar portion of the tumor is removed, the thinned pituitary tissue, as well as the arachnoid membrane behind it, bulges down displaying a dimple at the center. The shape of this bulging resembles a lily. The central dimple is where the pituitary stalk is attached **(Fig. 91–6A).** The tumor resection cavity is thoroughly inspected with a 30 degree angled lens endoscope. By rotating the 30 degree lens endoscope, the surgeon can directly inspect the suprasellar area, the medial walls of the cavernous sinuses, and the floor of the sella. Any suspicious tumor remnants are removed during this inspection. Attention is paid so as not to rupture the arachnoidal membrane to prevent CSF leakage.

During the removal of tumor tissue, surgical instruments should be used gently without any force that would apply traction to the pituitary stalk. Traction injury to the pituitary stalk renders the risk of postoperative diabetes insipidus. When the tumor resection cavity is large or if a CSF leak occurs intraoperatively, an abdominal fat graft is placed at the tumor resection cavity. The abdominal fat graft is harvested through an infraumbilical transverse skin incision about 1 to 2 cm in length. The abdominal incision is closed in subcuticular fashion. The anterior wall of the sella is reconstructed with autogenous bone or titanium mesh **(Fig. 91–6B).** The sphenoidal sinus is kept aerated. No foreign material is laid in the sphenoidal sinuses. In case of a fibrotic suprasellar tumor that does not descend by tumor removal at the sella, further rostral exposure becomes necessary at the tuberculum sella and planum sphenoidale as mentioned earlier. In that case, the fibrotic tumor is dissected from the surrounding structures with a microdissection technique. When a fibrotic suprasellar tumor is removed by further rostral exposure, the optic nerves, chiasm, pituitary stalk and anterior cerebral arteries then come under direct endoscopic view. When the anterior cranial fossa is opened for tumor removal, the dural defect is reconstructed with a cadaveric dural graft that is sutured with microclips. The bony skull base is reconstructed with autogenous bone or titanium mesh. In this case the sphenoidal sinus is stripped of its mucosa and packed with an abdominal fat graft to secure a watertight seal. The middle turbinate, which had been displaced laterally, is placed back to its normal position and the operation is finished.

A

B

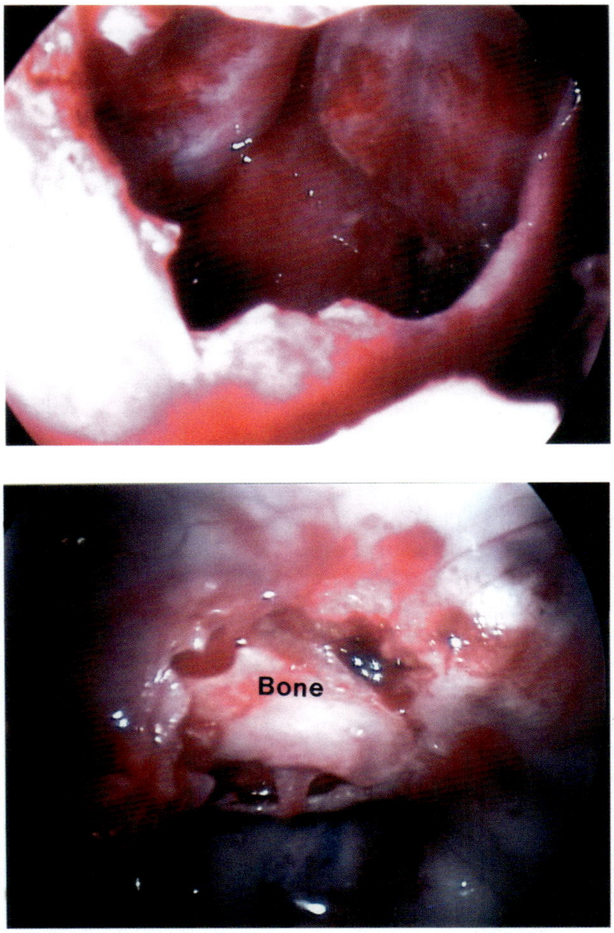

Figure 91–6 The suprasellar portion of the tumor is removed from the periphery of the tumor along the diaphragm sella. Tumor removal is advanced centripetally. The thinned pituitary tissue and arachnoidal membrane behind it will descend with brain pulsation. **(A)** Once the tumor is removed, a central dimple can be noted, which indicates the attachment point of the pituitary stalk. When the tumor resection cavity is large or intraoperative cerebrospinal fluid leak is encountered, an abdominal fat graft is placed in the sella. **(B)** The anterior wall of the sella is reconstructed with a piece of bone.

◆ Surgical Technique for Anterior Fossa Skull-Base Surgery

As mentioned earlier, the patient's head is extended ~15 degrees to maintain 25 degree cephalad angulation of the endoscope shaft when the endoscope is inserted into the nasal cavity and aimed at the floor of the anterior cranial fossa. A fluoroscopic C-arm is used to provide guidance to the vertical dimension of the anterior fossa. The aforementioned middle meatal approach is used for repair of CSF leakage or removal of small tumors located eccentrically at the unilateral midline. The paraseptal approach is utilized in most other circumstances. The middle turbinectomy approach is avoided, if possible, to utilize the middle turbinate as a supportive structure for skull-base reconstruction. The following surgical procedure is based on the paraseptal approach. The details of the surgical technique of the middle meatal approach do not vary much from that of the paraseptal approach. For the removal of anteriorly located olfactory groove meningiomas, the surgical trajectory is primarily determined by fluoroscopic guidance. The middle turbinate is displaced laterally and the perpendicular plate of the nasal septum is fractured and displaced contralaterally. Ethmoidectomy is performed with ethmoidal rongeurs. Hemostasis is obtained with a suction-coagulator. Anterior and posterior ethmoidal arteries are coagulated and divided. The anterior skull base is opened with a high-speed drill or Kerrison rongeurs. The dura mater is opened with Kurze scissors. The tumor is debulked at its center first followed by further removal at the periphery with fine dissection. Often, tumor removal becomes bloodless because the main blood supply to the tumor, which was derived from the ethmoidal arteries, had already been taken care of by the surgical approach itself. Small cotton patties are placed behind the tumor when the tumor is progressively dissected from the surrounding brain tissue. For removal of tumors at the planum sphenoidale or tuberculum sella, the surgical approach is made in similar fashion to that of the previously described pituitary surgery. Once an anterior sphenoidotomy is established, further rostral exposure is made under fluoroscopic guidance. When the tumor is excised, a roll of a cadaveric dura is inserted and laid intradurally. The dura graft is sutured with titanium microclips. The skull base is covered with titanium mesh for bone reconstruction. In addition, the ethmoidectomy site is filled with an abdominal fat graft **(Fig. 91–7).** When the nasal septum and middle turbinate is placed back to normal position, the abdominal fat graft tissue is well supported. Nasal packing is not necessary and is not used. Postoperative pain or discomfort is minimal. The patients are often discharged the day following surgery.

A

B

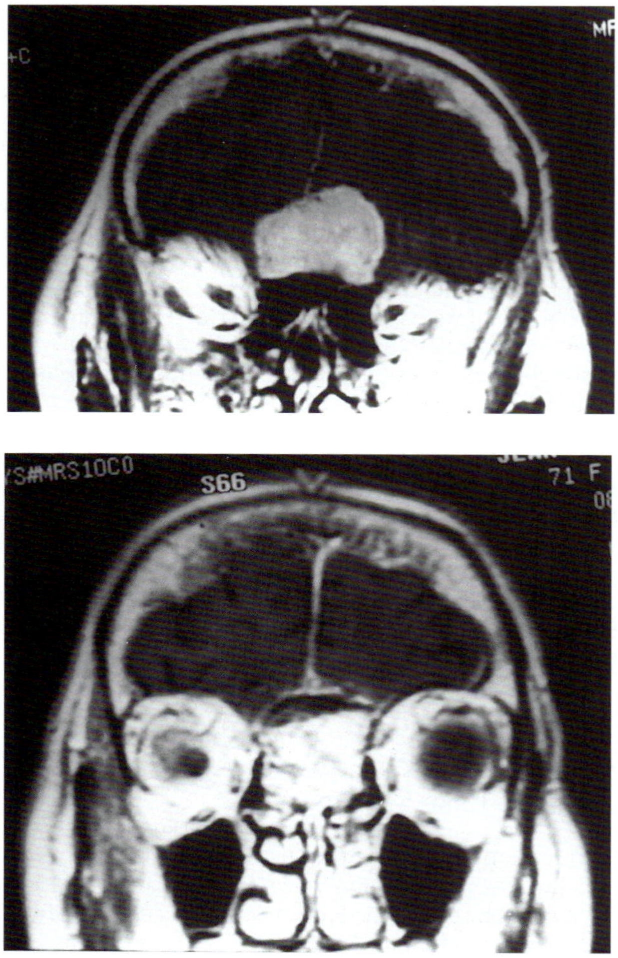

Figure 91–7 **(A)** A preoperative magnetic resonance imaging (MRI) scan, coronal view, reveals a contrast-enhancing meningioma in a 72-year-old woman. The tumor was totally removed through a paraseptal approach. The cranial base was reconstructed with dural graft suturing, titanium mesh placement for bone, and fat graft placement at the ethmoidectomy site. **(B)** A postoperative MRI scan, coronal view, demonstrates removal of the tumor, dural reconstruction, and fat graft placement.

◆ Surgical Technique for Cavernous Sinus and Optic Nerve Surgery

Although surgical access can be made via one of three aforementioned approaches, the paraseptal approach is most frequently used. The surgical technique is again similar to the pituitary surgery described earlier. Once an anterior sphenoidotomy is made, the anterior sphenoidotomy is adjusted to adequately expose the cavernous sinus or the optic nerve. The bone wall of the cavernous sinus or optic nerve is opened with a 1-mm Kerrison rongeur. For a pituitary adenoma invading the cavernous sinus, the sellar and suprasellar portion of the tumor is removed prior to removal of the tumor from the cavernous sinus. The cavernous sinus is entered from the medial wall behind the carotid artery syphon. Inside the C-shaped carotid artery syphon, the tumor is excised with no. 5 or 7 upward-curved suction cannulas. Once the tumor is excised, the inner surface of the lateral wall of the cavernous sinus can be viewed directly. Care has to be exercised so as not to traumatize the lateral wall of the cavernous sinus because of the cranial nerves that are embedded there. The carotid artery is wrapped with abdominal fat graft material to prevent its bare exposure into the sphenoidal sinus. The sphenoidal sinus is also packed with abdominal fat graft material to protect the carotid artery. The procedure is concluded as described in the pituitary surgery discussion.

◆ Surgical Technique for Clival and Posterior Fossa Surgery

Fluoroscopic guidance is used for vertical orientation at the lower clivus. Surgical access is made with the paraseptal approach. An anterior sphenoidotomy is made as described for pituitary tumor surgery. Further caudal clival exposure is made with a high-speed drill. The lateral landmarks are the carotid protuberances. The midline width of the clivus between the carotid arteries is a little less than 2 cm. The tumors that most commonly have been operated on with this technique are chordomas. The tumor is excised with pituitary rongeurs and suction cannulas. The dura is opened for removal of clival meningiomas or other intradural tumors. The dural reconstruction is performed with abdominal fat graft placement. Titanium microclips have not worked for dural graft repair because the clip applier has proved to be too short to reach the clival dura. This procedure again concludes in similar fashion to that of our pituitary operation.

◆ Postoperative Management

Patients are hospitalized overnight and are most often discharged the following day. Postoperatively, patients may experience a few drops of nasal bleeding when they raise their head from a lying position. This does not require a nasal sling or any particular treatment. It stops once the accumulated blood in the sphenoidal sinuses has drained. Patients are encouraged to perform positional drainage of this accumulated blood from the sphenoidal sinus cavity. This small amount of bloody drainage dwindles and abates over a few days. Postoperative discomfort is minimal and often does not require strong analgesics.

Oral antibiotics (clarithromycin 500 mg b.i.d. for 5 days) have been used routinely postoperatively. A formal endocrine evaluation, visual examination, nasal examination, and postoperative MRI scans are all obtained within 6 weeks postoperatively.

◆ Complications

Postoperative CSF leakage is a major potential complication. Among the first 100 patients of the authors' series, three patients developed postoperative CSF leakage. All were repaired immediately with endoscopic reexploration and the placement of abdominal fat graft. Once a CSF leak is confirmed, the authors believe that it is advantageous to repair the leak immediately surgically rather than exert CSF diversion. Immediate repair of CSF leakage enhances rapid recovery, lessens the chance of meningitis, and shortens the patient's hospital stay compared with less aggressive treatments such as lumbar spinal drainage. Although the possibility of an insecure CSF seal has always been our major concern, especially in anterior fossa or transclival posterior fossa surgery, we do not use a postoperative lumbar drain. As mentioned earlier, early detection and prompt surgical repair have been the strategy utilized for postoperative CSF leakage. Further instrumental improvement is also required for providing secure dural graft placement by direct watertight closure.

In our earlier patients postoperative diuresis was an annoying problem that often prolonged the patients' hospital stays. Its clinical presentation had often mimicked that of diabetes insipidus. Because the amount of intraoperative fluid administration has been adjusted judiciously, postoperative diuresis from fluid overload has not occurred. Pitressin is used immediately when diabetes insipidus is confirmed by exhibition of the classic symptoms of polyuria and polydipsia, clear diluted urine with low urinary specific gravity, and increased serum osmolarity and sodium concentration. Postoperative hyponatremia occurs in such a delayed fashion that extended hospitalization for that reason alone would not make any difference in its management unless the patients are kept in the hospital for 1 to 2 weeks. Synechia between the middle turbinate and nasal septum has occurred in two of our earlier patients, and one patient developed delayed sphenoidal sinusitis. The patients with synechia were asymptomatic and did not require treatment. The sinusitis was treated with oral antibiotics. Synechia can be avoided with increased endoscopic surgical experience.

◆ Conclusion

This chapter described an endoscopic endonasal approach to the sella as well as to the midline skull base from the crista galli to the foramen magnum.

References

1. Landolt AM. History of transsphenoidal pituitary surgery. In: Landolt AM, Vance ML, Reilly PL, eds. Pituitary Adenomas. New York: Churchill Livingstone; 1996:307–314
2. Cooke RS, Jones RAC. Experience with the direct transnasal transsphenoidal approach to the pituitary fossa. Br J Neurosurg 1994; 8:193–196
3. Griffith HB, Veerapen R. A direct transnasal approach to the sphenoid sinus. Technical note. J Neurosurg 1987;66:140–142
4. Jho HD, Carrau RL, Ko Y. Endoscopic pituitary surgery. In: Wilkins RH, Rengachary SS, eds. Neurosurgical Operative Atlas. Vol 5. Baltimore: Williams & Wilkins; 1996:1–12
5. Guiot J, Rougerie J, Fourestier A, et al. Intracranial endoscopic explorations [in French]. Presse Med 1963;71:1225–1228
6. Rodziewicz GS, Kelly RT, Kellman RM, Smith MV. Transnasal endoscopic surgery of the pituitary gland: technical note. Neurosurgery 1996;39:189–193
7. Sethi DS, Pillay PK. Endoscopic management of lesions of the sella turcica. J Laryngol Otol 1995;109:956–962
8. Shikani AH, Kelly JH. Endoscopic debulking of a pituitary tumor. Am J Otolaryngol 1993;14:254–256
9. Stammberger H. Endoscopic endonasal surgery: concepts in treatment of recurring rhinosinusitis, II: Surgical technique. Otolaryngol Head Neck Surg 1986;94:147–156
10. Jankowski R, Auque J, Simon C, Marchal JC, Hepner H, Wayoff M. Endoscopic pituitary tumor surgery. Laryngoscope 1992;102: 198–202
11. Carrau RL, Jho HD, Ko Y. Transnasal-transsphenoidal endoscopic surgery of the pituitary gland. Laryngoscope 1996;106:914–918
12. Jho HD. Endoscopic endonasal pituitary surgery: technical aspects. Contemporary Neurosurgery 1997;19:1–7
13. Jho HD, Carrau RL. Endoscopy assisted transsphenoidal surgery for pituitary adenoma. Technical note. Acta Neurochir (Wien) 1996; 138: 1416–1425

14. Jho HD, Carrau RL. Endoscopic endonasal transsphenoidal surgery: experience with 50 patients. J Neurosurg 1997;87:44–51

15. Jho HD, Carrau RL, Mclaughlin ML, Somaza SC. Endoscopic transsphenoidal resection of a large chordoma in the posterior fossa Acta Neurochir (Wien) 1997;139:343–348

16. Jho HD, Carrau RL, Ko Y, Daly M. Endoscopic pituitary surgery: an early experience. Surg Neurol 1997;47:213–223

17. Gamea A, Fathi M, El-Guindy A. The use of the rigid endoscope in trans-sphenoidal pituitary surgery. J Laryngol Otol 1994;108:19–22

18. Heilman CB, Shucart WA, Rebeiz EE. Endoscopic sphenoidotomy approach to the sella. Neurosurgery 1997;41:602–607

19. Helal MZ. Combined micro-endo trans-sphenoid excisions of pituitary macroadenomas. Eur Arch Otorhinolaryngol 1995;252: 186–189

20. Cappabianca P, Alfieri A, de Divitiis E. Endoscopic endonasal transsphenoidal approach to the sella: towards functional endoscopic pituitary surgery (FEPS). Minim Invasive Neurosurg 1998;41:66–73

Index

Page numbers followed by an f or t refer to figures and tables respectively.

B

D

E

F

G

N

O

S

T

U

V

W

X

Y

Z